Comprehensive
Clinical Nephrology

3rd Edition

John Feehally MA DM FRCP
Consultant Nephrologist
University Hospitals of Leicester
Professor of Renal Medicine
University of Leicester
Leicester, United Kingdom

Jürgen Floege MD
Professor of Medicine
Director, Division of Nephrology and Clinical Immunology
University Hospital
Aachen, Germany

Richard J Johnson MD
J. Robert Cade Professor of Nephrology
Chief of Nephrology, Hypertension, and Transplantation
University of Florida
Gainesville, Florida, USA

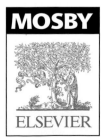

MOSBY

ELSEVIER

1600 John F. Kennedy Blvd.
Ste 1800
Philadelphia, PA 19103-2899

COMPREHENSIVE CLINICAL NEPHROLOGY

ISBN-13: 978-0-323-04602-2
ISBN-10: 0-323-04602-9

Previous editions copyrighted 2003, 2000

ISBN-13: 978-0-323-04602-2
ISBN-10: 0-323-04602-9

Acquisitions Editor: Susan Pioli
Developmental Editor: Arlene Chappelle

**Cover: Three-dimensional rendering of a rat glomerulus showing podocytes double-labeled
with anti-vimentin (blue) and anti-WT1 (brown) antibodies. Optical sections were collected at
the Indiana Center for Biological Microscopy using a two-photon fluorescence microscope and
Voxx software, and provided by Carrie Phillips.**

Printed in China.

Last digit is the print number: 9 8 7 6 5 4 3 2

We dedicate this book to

Our mentors in nephrology—especially Bill Couser, Stewart Cameron, and Karl M. Koch

Our colleagues and collaborators, as well as others whose research continues to light the way

Our wives and families who have once again endured the preparation of this third edition with unfailing patience and support

Our patients with renal disease for whom it is a privilege to care

Contributors

Horacio J Adrogué MD
Baylor College of Medicine
Houston, TX
USA
14: Respiratory Acidosis, Respiratory Alkalosis, and
Mixed Disorders

Venkatesh Aiyagari MBBS DM
University of Illinois at Chicago
Chicago, IL
USA
38: Neurogenic Hypertension, Including Hypertension
Associated with Stroke or Spinal Cord Injury

Robert J Alpern MD
Yale University
School of Medicine
New Haven, CT
USA
11: Normal Acid-Base Balance
12: Metabolic Acidosis

Charles E Alpers MD
University of Washington Medical Center
Seattle, WA
USA
20: Membranoproliferative Glomerulonephritis and
Cryoglobulinemic Glomerulonephritis

Kerstin Amann MD
University of Erlangen–Nürnberg
Erlangen
GERMANY
71: Cardiovascular Disease in Chronic Kidney Disease

Thomas E Andreoli MD MACP
University of Arkansas College of Medicine
Little Rock, AR
USA
7: Disorders of Extracellular Volume

Gerald B Appel MD
Columbia University College of Physicians and
   Surgeons
New York, NY
USA
18: Focal and Segmental Glomerulosclerosis: Genetic
and Spontaneous Causes
24: Lupus Nephritis

Stephen R Ash MD FACP
HemoCleanse, Inc.
Ash Access Technologies
Lafayette, IN
USA
82: Diagnostic and Interventional Nephrology

Arif Asif MD
University of Miami
Miller School of Medicine
Miami, FL
USA
82: Diagnostic and Interventional Nephrology

Pierre Aucouturier PhD
Pierre and Marie Curie University
Paris
FRANCE
26: Renal Amyloidosis and Glomerular Diseases with
Monoclonal Immunoglobulin Deposition

George L Bakris MD FACP
Rush University Medical Center
Chicago, IL
USA
32: Essential Hypertension
34: Pharmacologic Treatment of Hypertension

Rashad S Barsoum MD FRCP FRCPE
Cairo University
Cairo
EGYPT
25: Glomerular Diseases Associated with Infection
53: The Kidney in Schistosomiasis

Chris Baylis PhD
University of Florida
Gainesville, FL
USA
40: Renal Physiology in Normal Pregnancy

William M Bennett MD
Legacy Good Samaritan Hospital
Portland, OR
USA
101: Principles of Drug Dosing and Prescribing in Renal
Failure

Tomas Berl MD
University of Colorado
Denver, CO
USA
8: Disorders of Water Metabolism

Suresh Bhat MBBS MS MCh
Medical College
Kerala
INDIA
51: Tuberculosis of the Urinary Tract

Gemma Bircher BSc (Hons) SRD MSc
Leicester General Hospital
Leicester
UNITED KINGDOM
77: Gastroenterology and Nutrition in Chronic Kidney
Disease

Nicholas R Brook BSc MSc BM MD MRCS
University of Leicester
Leicester
UNITED KINGDOM
92: Kidney Transplantation Surgery

Christopher Brown MD
Ohio State University Medical Center
Columbus, OH
USA
69: Retarding Progression of Kidney Disease

Emmanuel A Burdmann MD PhD
São José do Rio Preto Medical School
São José do Rio Preto
BRAZIL
25: Glomerular Diseases Associated with Infection

David A Bushinsky MD
University of Rochester
Rochester, NY
USA
54: Nephrolithiasis and Nephrocalcinosis

J Stewart Cameron CBE MD FRCP
Melmerby
Cumbria
UNITED KINGDOM
24: Lupus Nephritis

Giovambattista Capasso MD
Second University of Naples
Naples
ITALY
2: Renal Physiology

Michele Ceruti MD
Mario Negri Institute for Pharmacological Research
Bergamo
ITALY
28: Thrombotic Microangiopathies, Including Hemolytic
Uremic Syndrome

Steven J Chadban BMed (Hons) PhD FRACP
Royal Prince Alfred Hospital
Camperdown, NSW
AUSTRALIA
96: Recurrent Disease in Kidney Transplantation

Karen E Charlton PhD MPhil MSc
Medical Research Council of South Africa
Cape Town
SOUTH AFRICA
33: Nonpharmacologic Prevention and Treatment of
Hypertension

Ignatius KP Cheng MBBS PhD FRACP FRCP
   FHKCP FHKAM
University of Hong Kong
HONG KONG
67: Hepatorenal Syndrome

Glenn M Chertow MD MPH
University of California–San Francisco
San Francisco, CA
USA
97: Outcomes of Renal Transplantation

John O Connolly PhD MRCP
Royal Free Hospital
London
UNITED KINGDOM
49: Congenital Abnormalities of the Renal Tract

William G Couser MD
University of Washington School of Medicine
Seattle, WA
USA
19: Membranous Nephropathy

Vivette D'Agati MD
New York–Presbyterian Hospital
Columbia University Medical Center
New York, NY
USA
18: Focal and Segmental Glomerulosclerosis: Genetic and Spontaneous Causes

Gabriel M Danovitch MD
David Geffen School of Medicine at UCLA
Los Angeles, CA
USA
94: Medical Management of the Kidney Transplant Recipient

Simon J Davies BSc MD FRCP
Keele University
Keele
UNITED KINGDOM
86: Complications of Peritoneal Dialysis

Connie L Davis MD
University of Washington School of Medicine
Seattle, WA
USA
91: Evaluation and Preoperative Management of Kidney Transplant Recipient and Donor

John M Davison MD
University of Newcastle upon Tyne
Newcastle upon Tyne
UNITED KINGDOM
40: Renal Physiology in Normal Pregnancy

Paul E de Jong MD PhD
University Medical Center Groningen
Groningen
THE NETHERLANDS
48: Sickle Cell Disease

Sevag Demirjian MD
Cleveland Clinic Foundation
Cleveland, OH
USA
66: Intensive Care Unit Nephrology

Wayne Derman MBChB PhD FACSM
University of Cape Town
Cape Town
SOUTH AFRICA
33: Nonpharmacologic Prevention and Treatment of Hypertension

Gerald F DiBona MD
University of Iowa College of Medicine
Iowa City, IA
USA
31: Normal Blood Pressure Control and the Evaluation of Hypertension

Haresh Dodeja MD DNB (Nepho) MNAMS
Wockhardt Hospitals Ltd.
Mumbai
INDIA
100: Poisoning and Drug Overdose

Ciaran C Doherty MD FRCP FRCPI
Belfast City Hospital
Belfast
UNITED KINGDOM
77: Gastroenterology and Nutrition in Chronic Kidney Disease

Tilman B. Drüeke MD
Necker Hospital
Paris
FRANCE
10: Disorders of Calcium, Phosphate, and Magnesium Metabolism

Kai-Uwe Eckardt MD
University of Erlangen–Nürnberg
Erlangen
GERMANY
72: Anemia in Chronic Kidney Disease

Gunilla Einecke MD
University of Alberta
Edmonton, Alberta
CANADA
89: Immunologic Principles of Kidney Transplantation
90: Immunosuppressive Agents Used in Transplantation

Frank Eitner MD
RWTI I University of Aachen
Aachen
GERMANY
79: Acquired Cystic Kidney Disease and Malignancies in Chronic Kidney Disease

A Ahsan Ejaz MD
University of Florida
Gainesville, FL
USA
65: Nondialytic Management of Acute Renal Failure

Marlies Elger PhD
University of Heidelberg
Heidelberg
GERMANY
1: Renal Anatomy

Mohsen El Kossi MD MRCP
University of Sheffield
Sheffield
UNITED KINGDOM
68: Epidemiology and Pathophysiology of Chronic Kidney Disease: Natural History, Risk Factors, and Management

Meguid El Nahas PhD FRCP
University of Sheffield
Sheffield
UNITED KINGDOM
68: Epidemiology and Pathophysiology of Chronic Kidney Disease: Natural History, Risk Factors, and Management

Franklin H Epstein MD
Beth Israel Deaconess Medical Center
Boston, MA
USA
41: Renal Complications in Pregnancy

Pieter Evenepoel MD PhD
University Hospital Leuven
Leuven
BELGIUM
78: Dermatologic Manifestations of Chronic Kidney Disease

Ronald J Falk MD
University of North Carolina
Chapel Hill, NC
USA
23: Renal and Systemic Vasculitis

John Feehally MA DM FRCP
University of Leicester
Leicester
UNITED KINGDOM
15: Introduction to Glomerular Disease: Pathogenesis and Classification
16: Introduction to Glomerular Disease: Clinical Presentations
21: IgA Nephropathy and Henoch-Schönlein Nephritis
100: Poisoning and Drug Overdose

Leon Ferder MD
Ponce School of Medicine
Ponce, Puerto Rico
USA
62: Geriatric Nephrology

Evelyne A Fischer MD PhD
Pasteur Institute
Paris
FRANCE
57: Acute Interstitial Nephritis

Jonathan S Fisher MD FACS
Scripps Clinic and Green Hospital
La Jolla, CA
USA
98: Pancreas and Islet Transplantation

John M Flack MD MPH
Wayne State University
Detroit, MI
USA
39: Hypertension in African Americans

Jürgen Floege MD
RWTH University of Aachen
Aachen
GERMANY
15: Introduction to Glomerular Disease: Pathogenesis and Classification
16: Introduction to Glomerular Disease: Clinical Presentations
21: IgA Nephropathy and Henoch-Schönlein Nephritis
75: B$_2$-Microglobulin–derived Amyloid
79: Acquired Cystic Kidney Disease and Malignancies in Chronic Kidney Disease

Giovanni B Fogazzi MD
Ospedale Maggiore Policlinico
Milano
ITALY
4: Urinalysis

John W Foreman MD
Duke University Medical Center
Durham, NC
USA
47: Fanconi Syndrome and Other Proximal Tubule Disorders

Toshiro Fujita MD
University of Tokyo School of Medicine
Tokyo
JAPAN
59: Chronic Interstitial Nephritis

Rijk OB Gans MD PhD
University Medical Center Groningen
Groningen
THE NETHERLANDS
48: Sickle Cell Disease

F John Gennari MD
University of Vermont
Burlington, VT
USA
13: Metabolic Alkalosis

Michael Gersch MD
University of Florida
Gainesville, FL
USA
81: Vascular Access for Hemodialysis

Scott J Gilbert MD
Tufts–New England Medical Center
Boston, MA
USA
3: Assessment of Renal Function

Richard J Glassock MD
David Geffen School of Medicine at UCLA
Los Angeles, CA
USA
*27: Other Glomerular Disorders, Including Congenital
   Nephrotic Syndrome*

Esther A González MD FACP
St. Louis University
St. Louis, MO
USA
*74: Bone and Mineral Metabolism in Chronic Kidney
   Disease*

Philip B Gorelick MD MPH FACP
University of Illinois at Chicago
Chicago, IL
USA
*38: Neurogenic Hypertension, Including Hypertension
   Associated with Stroke or Spinal Cord Injury*

Barbara Greco MD
Western New England Renal and Transplant
   Associates
Springfield, MA
USA
*61: Atheromatous and Thromboembolic Renovascular
   Disease*

Peter Gross MD
Universitätsklinikum Carl Gustav Carus
Dresden
GERMANY
46: Inherited Disorders of Sodium and Water Handling

Lisa Guay-Woodford MD
University of Alabama at Birmingham
Birmingham, AL
USA
44: Other Cystic Kidney Diseases

Ambreen Gul MD
Tufts–New England Medical Center
Boston, MA
USA
3: Assessment of Renal Function

Nabil Haddad MD
Ohio State University Medical Center
Columbus, OH
USA
69: Retarding Progression of Kidney Disease

Philip F Halloran MD PhD FRCPC
University of Alberta
Edmonton, Alberta
CANADA
89: Immunologic Principles of Kidney Transplantation
*90: Immunosuppressive Agents Used in
   Transplantation*

Kevin PG Harris MA MBBS MD FRCP
Leicester General Hospital
Leicester
UNITED KINGDOM
55: Urinary Tract Obstruction

Lee A Hebert MD
Ohio State University Medical Center
Columbus, OH
USA
69: Retarding Progression of Kidney Disease

Peter Heduschka MD
Universitätsklinikum Carl Gustav Carus
Dresden
GERMANY
*46: Inherited Disorders of Sodium and Water
   Handling*

Luis G Hidalgo BSc
University of Alberta
Edmonton, Alberta
CANADA
89: Immunologic Principles of Kidney Transplantation

Walter Hörl MD PhD FRCP
Medical University of Vienna
Vienna
AUSTRIA
*73: Other Blood and Immune Disorders in Chronic
   Kidney Disease*

Thomas Hooton MD
University of Washington
Seattle, WA
USA
50: Urinary Tract Infections in Adults

Ashley B Irish MBBS FRACP
Royal Perth Hospital
Perth, WA
AUSTRALIA
60: Myeloma and the Kidney

Bertrand L Jaber MD FASN
Tufts University School of Medicine
Boston, MA
USA
84: Acute Complications of Hemodialysis

Sunjay Jain MD FRCS (Urol)
St. James's University Hospital
Leeds
UNITED KINGDOM
56: Urologic Issues for the Nephrologist

J Ashley Jefferson MD MRCP
University of Washington
Seattle, WA
USA
63: Pathophysiology and Etiology of Acute Renal Failure

J Charles Jennette MD
University of North Carolina
Chapel Hill, NC
USA
23: Renal and Systemic Vasculitis

Richard J Johnson MD
University of Florida
Gainesville, FL
USA
*15: Introduction to Glomerular Disease: Pathogenesis
   and Classification*
32: Essential Hypertension
62: Geriatric Nephrology

Bruce Kaplan MD
University of Illinois at Chicago
Chicago, IL
USA
*93: Prophylaxis and Treatment of Kidney Transplant
   Rejection*

S Ananth Karumanchi MD
Beth Israel Deaconess Medical Center
Boston, MA
USA
41: Renal Complications in Pregnancy

Clifford E Kashtan MD
University of Minnesota
Minneapolis, MN
USA
45: Alport's and Other Familial Glomerular Syndromes

Bertram L Kasiske MD
Hennepin County Medical Center
Minneapolis, MN
USA
95: Chronic Allograft Nephropathy

Markus Ketteler MD
RWTH University of Aachen
Aachen
GERMANY
71: Cardiovascular Disease in Chronic Kidney Disease

Nitin Khosla MD
Rush University Medical Center
Chicago, IL
USA
34: Pharmacologic Treatment of Hypertension

Klaus Konner MD
University of Cologne
Cologne
GERMANY
81: Vascular Access for Hemodialysis

Peter Kotanko MD
Renal Research Institute
New York, NY
USA
83: Hemodialysis: Technology, Adequacy, and Outcomes

Wilhelm Kriz MD
University of Heidelberg
Heidelberg
GERMANY
1: Renal Anatomy

Martin K Kuhlmann MD
Renal Research Institute
New York, NY
USA
83: Hemodialysis: Technology, Adequacy, and Outcomes

Dirk R Kuypers MD PhD
University Hospital Leuven
Leuven
BELGIUM
78: Dermatologic Manifestations of Chronic Kidney Disease

Bernard Lacour PhD
Necker Hospital
Paris
FRANCE
10: Disorders of Calcium, Phosphate, and Magnesium Metabolism

Jonathan RT Lakey PhD MSM
University of Alberta
Edmonton, Alberta
CANADA
98: Pancreas and Islet Transplantation

Estelle V Lambert BS MS PhD
University of Cape Town
Cape Town
SOUTH AFRICA
33: Nonpharmacologic Prevention and Treatment of Hypertension

Norbert Lameire MD
University Hospital Gent
Gent
BELGIUM
64: Epidemiology, Clinical Evaluation, and Prevention of Acute Renal Failure

William J Lawton MD
University of Iowa
Iowa City, IA
USA
31: Normal Blood Pressure Control and the Evaluation of Hypertension

Edgar V Lerma MD FACP FASN
University of Illinois at Chicago
Chicago, IL
USA
62: Geriatric Nephrology

Andrew S Levey MD
Tufts–New England Medical Center
Boston, MA
USA
3: Assessment of Renal Function

Nathan W Levin MD
Renal Research Institute
New York, NY
USA
83: Hemodialysis: Technology, Adequacy, and Outcomes

Jeremy Levy MA PhD ILTM FRCP
Charing Cross Hospital
London
UNITED KINGDOM
88: Plasma Exchange

Julia Lewis MD
Vanderbilt University
Nashville, TN
USA
61: Atheromatous and Thromboembolic Renovascular Disease

Felix FK Li MBBS MRCP FRCP FHKCP FHKAM
University of Hong Kong
HONG KONG
67: Hepatorenal Syndrome

Stuart L Linas MD
University of Colorado
Denver, CO
USA
9: Disorders of Potassium Metabolism

Friedrich C Luft MD FACP FRCP (Edin)
Franz Volhard Clinic
Helios Klinikum–Berlin
Berlin
GERMANY
31: Normal Blood Pressure Control and the Evaluation of Hypertension

Kelvin Lynn MB ChB FRACP
Christchurch Hospital
Christchurch
NEW ZEALAND
58: Vesicoureteral Reflux and Reflux Nephropathy

Iain C Macdougall BSc MD FRCP
King's College Hospital
London
UNITED KINGDOM
72: Anemia in Chronic Kidney Disease

Nicolaos E Madias MD
Tufts University School of Medicine
Boston, MA
USA
14: Respiratory Acidosis, Respiratory Alkalosis, and Mixed Disorders

Colm C Magee MD MPH
Brigham and Women's Hospital
Boston, MA
USA
97: Outcomes of Renal Transplantation

Christopher L Marsh MD FACS
Scripps Clinic and Green Hospital
La Jolla, CA
USA
98: Pancreas and Islet Transplantation

Mark R Marshall MD
University of Auckland
Auckland
NEW ZEALAND
87: Acute Renal Replacement Therapy in the Intensive Care Unit

Kevin J Martin MB BCh BAO FACP
St. Louis University
St. Louis, MO
USA
74: Bone and Mineral Metabolism in Chronic Kidney Disease

Philip D Mason BSc PhD MBBS FRCP
The Churchill Hospital
Oxford
UNITED KINGDOM
17: Minimal Change Disease

Anette Melk MD PhD
University of Heidelberg
Heidelberg
GERMANY
90: Immunosuppressive Agents Used in Transplantation

J Kilian Mellon MD FRCS
University of Leicester
Leicester
UNITED KINGDOM
56: Urologic Issues for the Nephrologist

Edgar L Milford MD
Brigham and Women's Hospital
Boston, MA
USA
97: Outcomes of Renal Transplantation

Mohammadreza Mirbolooki MD
University of Alberta
Edmonton, Alberta
CANADA
98: Pancreas and Islet Transplantation

Rebeca D Monk MD
University of Rochester
Rochester, NY
USA
54: Nephrolithiasis and Nephrocalcinosis

Bruno Moulin MD
Louis Pasteur University
Strasbourg
FRANCE
26: Renal Amyloidosis and Glomerular Diseases with Monoclonal Immunoglobulin Deposition

Masaomi Nangaku MD PhD
University of Tokyo School of Medicine
Tokyo
JAPAN
59: Chronic Interstitial Nephritis

Samar A Nasser PA-C MPH
Wayne State University
Detroit, MI
USA
39: Hypertension in African Americans

Guy H Neild MD FRCP FRCPath
Middlesex Hospital
London
UNITED KINGDOM
49: Congenital Abnormalities of the Renal Tract

Charles G Newstead MBBS MRCP (UK) MD
FRCP
St. James's University Teaching Hospital
Leeds
UNITED KINGDOM
*91: Evaluation and Preoperative Management of Kidney
Transplant Recipient and Donor*

M Gary Nicholls MB ChB MD FRACP FRCP (Glas,
Edin, Lond) FACC FAHA
UAE University
Al-Ain
UNITED ARAB EMIRATES
36: Endocrine Causes of Hypertension

Michael L Nicholson MD FRCS
Leicester General Hospital
Leicester
UNITED KINGDOM
92: Kidney Transplantation Surgery

Shannon M O'Connor BS
Wayne State University
Detroit, MI
USA
39: Hypertension in African Americans

Akinlolu O Ojo MD PhD
University of Michigan Medical School
Ann Arbor, MI
USA
*99: Kidney Disease in Liver, Cardiac, Lung, and
Hematopoietic Cell Transplantation*

Ali J Olyaei PharmD
Oregon Health and Science University
Portland, OR
USA
*101: Principles of Drug Dosing and Prescribing in Renal
Failure*

W Charles O'Neill MD
Emory University
Atlanta, GA
USA
82: Diagnostic and Interventional Nephrology

Vuddhidej Ophascharoensuk MD
Chiang Mai University
Chiang Mai
THAILAND
25: Glomerular Diseases Associated with Infection

Deirdre A O'Sullivan MD
Mayo Clinic
Rochester, MN
USA
43: Autosomal Dominant Polycystic Kidney Disease

Emil P Paganini MD
The Cleveland Clinic
Cleveland, OH
USA
65: Nondialytic Management of Acute Renal Failure
66: Intensive Care Unit Nephrology
*87: Acute Renal Replacement Therapy in the Intensive
Care Unit*

Biff F Palmer MD
University of Texas Southwestern Medical School
Dallas, TX
USA
11: Normal Acid-Base Balance
12: Metabolic Acidosis

Chirag Parikh MD PhD FACP
Yale University
New Haven, CT
USA
8: Disorders of Water Metabolism

Rosaleen B Parsons MD
Fox Chase Cancer Center
Philadelphia, PA
USA
5: Imaging

Brian JG Pereira MD
Tufts University School of Medicine
Boston, MA
USA
84: Acute Complications of Hemodialysis

Phuong-Chi T Pham MD
David Geffen School of Medicine at UCLA
Los Angeles, CA
USA
*94: Medical Management of the Kidney Transplant
Recipient*

Phuong-Thu T Pham MD
David Geffen School of Medicine at UCLA
Los Angeles, CA
USA
*94: Medical Management of the Kidney Transplant
Recipient*

Richard G Phelps MB BChir PhD MRCP
University of Edinburgh
Edinburgh
UNITED KINGDOM
*22: Antiglomerular Basement Membrane Disease and
Goodpasture's Disease*

Barbara Pirovano ScD
Azienda Ospedaliera Treviglio–Caravaggio
Treviglio
ITALY
4: Urinalysis

Marc A Pohl MD
The Cleveland Clinic
Cleveland, OH
USA
35: Renovascular Hypertension

Martin R Pollak MD
Brigham and Women's Hospital
Boston, MA
USA
*18: Focal and Segmental Glomerulosclerosis: Genetic
and Spontaneous Causes*

Didier Portilla MD
University of Arkansas College of Medicine
Little Rock, AR
USA
7: Disorders of Extracellular Volume

Charles D Pusey DSc FRCP FRCPath FMedSci
Imperial College School of Medicine
London
UNITED KINGDOM
88: Plasma Exchange

Brian Rayner MB ChB MMed FCP (SA)
University of Cape Town
Cape Town
SOUTH AFRICA
*33: Nonpharmacologic Prevention and Treatment of
Hypertension*

Hugh C Rayner MA MB MD FRCP DipMedEd
Birmingham Heartlands Hospital
Birmingham
UNITED KINGDOM
80: Approach to Renal Replacement Therapy

Giuseppe Remuzzi MD FRCP
Mario Negri Institute for Pharmacological Research
Bergamo
ITALY
*28: Thrombotic Microangiopathies, Including Hemolytic
Uremic Syndrome*

Helmut G Rennke MD
Brigham and Women's Hospital
Boston, MA
USA
*15: Introduction to Glomerular Disease: Pathogenesis
and Classification*

A Mark Richards MB ChB MD PhD DSc FRACP
FAHA FRSNZ
Christchurch School of Medicine and Health
Sciences
Christchurch
NEW ZEALAND
36: Endocrine Causes of Hypertension

Bengt Rippe MD PhD
University of Lund
Lund
SWEDEN
*85: Peritoneal Dialysis: Principles, Techniques, and
Adequacy*

Eberhard Ritz MD
University of Heidelberg
Heidelberg
GERMANY
*29: Pathogenesis, Clinnical Manifestations, and Natural
History of Diabetic Nephropathy*
*30: Prevention and Treatment of Diabetic
Nephropathy*

R Paul Robertson MD
University of Washington
Seattle, WA
USA
98: Pancreas and Islet Transplantation

Bernardo Rodríguez-Iturbe MD
Hospital Universitario and Universidad del Zulia
Maracaibo, Zulia
VENEZUELA
25: Glomerular Diseases Associated with Infection
32: Essential Hypertension

Pierre M Ronco MD PhD
Université Curie
Paris
FRANCE
26: Renal Amyloidosis and Glomerular Diseases with
   Monoclonal Immunoglobulin Deposition

Jérôme A Rossert MD PhD
Paris–Descartes University School of Medicine
Paris
FRANCE
57: Acute Interstitial Nephritis

Piero Ruggenenti MD
Mario Negri Institute for Pharmacological Research
Bergamo
ITALY
28: Thrombotic Microangiopathies, Including Hemolytic
   Uremic Syndrome

Sean Ruland DO
University of Illinois–Chicago
Chicago, IL
USA
38: Neurogenic Hypertension, Including Hypertension
   Associated with Stroke or Spinal Cord Injury

F Paolo Schena MD
University of Bari
Bari
ITALY
20: Membranoproliferative Glomerulonephritis and
   Cryoglobulinemic Glomerulonephritis

Robert W Schrier MD
University of Colorado
Denver, CO
USA
63: Pathophysiology and Etiology of Acute Renal Failure

Julian Lawrence Seifter MD
Brigham and Women's Hospital
Boston, MA
USA
76: Neurologic Complications of Chronic Kidney Disease

David G Shirley BSc PhD
Royal Free and University College Medical School
London
UNITED KINGDOM
2: Renal Physiology

William L Simpson Jr MD
Mount Sinai Medical Center
New York, NY
USA
5: Imaging

Jack D Sobel MD
Wayne State University School of Medicine
Detroit, MI
USA
52: Fungal Infection of the Urinary Tract

Peter Stenvinkel MD PhD
Karolinska University Hospital at Huddinge
Stockholm
SWEDEN
71: Cardiovascular Disease in Chronic Kidney Disease

Jan C ter Maaten MD PhD
University Medical Center Groningen
Groningen
THE NETHERLANDS
48: Sickle Cell Disease

Stephen C Textor MD
Mayo Clinic
Rochester, MN
USA
35: Renovascular Hypertension

Peter S Topham MB ChB MD FRCP
Leicester General Hospital
Leicester
UNITED KINGDOM
6: Renal Biopsy

Vicente E Torres MD
Mayo Clinic
Rochester, MN
USA
43: Autosomal Dominant Polycystic Kidney Disease

A Neil Turner PhD FRCP
Royal Infirmary
Edinburgh
UNITED KINGDOM
22: Antiglomerular Basement Membrane Disease and
   Goodpasture's Disease

Robert J Unwin BM PhD FRCP
Royal Free and University College of Medicine
London
UNITED KINGDOM
2: Renal Physiology

Ashish Upadhyay MD
Tufts University School of Medicine
Boston, MA
USA
84: Acute Complications of Hemodialysis

Wim Van Biesen MD PhD
University Hospital Gent
Gent
BELGIUM
64: Epidemiology, Clinical Evaluation, and Prevention of
   Acute Renal Failure

Raymond Vanholder MD PhD
University Hospital Gent
Gent
BELGIUM
64: Epidemiology, Clinical Evaluation, and Prevention of
   Acute Renal Failure

R Kasi Visweswaran MBBS MD DM MNAMS
Ananthapuri Hospitals and Research Institute
Kerala
INDIA
51: Tuberculosis of the Urinary Tract

Haimanot Wasse MD MPH
Emory University
Atlanta, GA
USA
82: Diagnostic and Interventional Nephrology

I David Weiner MD
University of Florida
Gainesville, FL
USA
9: Disorders of Potassium Metabolism
37: Endocrine Causes of Hypertension: Aldosterone

David C Wheeler MD FRCP
Royal Free and University College Medical School
London
UNITED KINGDOM
70: Clinical Evaluation and Management of Chronic
   Kidney Disease

David Williams MBBS PhD FRCP
University College Hospital
London
UNITED KINGDOM
42: Pregnancy with Pre-existing Kidney Disease

John D Williams MD FRCP
Cardiff University School of Medicine
Cardiff
UNITED KINGDOM
86: Complications of Peritoneal Dialysis

Christopher G Winearls MB ChB D Phil FRCP
Oxford Radcliffe Hospitals
Oxford
UNITED KINGDOM
70: Clinical Evaluation and Management of Chronic
   Kidney Disease

Charles S Wingo MD
University of Florida
Gainesville, FL
USA
9: Disorders of Potassium Metabolism
37: Endocrine Causes of Hypertension: Aldosterone

Karl L Womer MD
University of Florida
Gainesville, FL
USA
93: Prophylaxis and Treatment of Kidney Transplant
   Rejection

Preface

For this third edition of *Comprehensive Clinical Nephrology*, the two established editors, John Feehally and Richard J. Johnson, have been joined by Jürgen Floege, whose expertise and energy have contributed enormously to this new edition that we are confident will build on the popular success of the book.

We continue to offer a text for fellows, practicing nephrologists, and internists that covers all aspects of the clinical work of the nephrologist including fluid and electrolytes, hypertension, diabetes, dialysis, and transplantation. We recognize that this single volume does not compete with multivolume, highly referenced texts, and it remains our goal to provide "comprehensive" coverage of clinical nephrology yet also ensure that enquiring nephrologists can find the scientific issues and pathophysiology that underlie their clinical work.

For this edition all chapters have again been extensively revised and updated in response to the advice and comments that we have received from many readers and colleagues. The number of references for each chapter has been further increased to improve access to additional in-depth reading. A new chapter has been added on Intensive Care Unit Nephrology and the section on Chronic Kidney Disease and the Uremic Syndrome has been reworked with new chapters on dermatologic and neurologic complications.

By popular demand we continue to offer readers a CD-ROM of the images from the book that we are pleased to see used in lectures and seminars in many parts of the world.

John Feehally

Jürgen Floege

Richard J. Johnson

Contents

Contents

Section 17: Drugs and the Kidney

CHAPTER

1 Renal Anatomy

Wilhelm Kriz and Marlies Elger

INTRODUCTION

The complex structure of the mammalian kidney is best understood in the unipapillary form that is common to all small species. Figure 1.1 is a schematic coronal section through such a kidney with a cortex enclosing a pyramid-shaped medulla the tip of which protrudes into the renal pelvis. The medulla is divided into an outer and an inner medulla; the outer medulla is further subdivided into an outer and an inner stripe.

STRUCTURE OF THE KIDNEY

The specific components of the kidney are the nephrons, the collecting ducts, and a unique microvasculature.[1] The multipapillary kidney of humans contains roughly one million nephrons; however, the number is quite variable. This number is already established during prenatal development; after birth, new nephrons cannot be developed, and a lost nephron cannot be replaced.

Nephrons

A nephron consists of a renal corpuscle (glomerulus) connected to a complicated and twisted tubule that finally drains into a collecting duct (Figs. 1.2 and 1.3). Based on the location of renal corpuscles within the cortex, three types of nephron can be distinguished: superficial, midcortical, and juxtamedullary nephrons. The tubular part of the nephron consists of a proximal tubule and a distal tubule connected by Henle's loop[2] (see later discussion).

There are two types of nephron, those with long Henle's loops and those with short loops. Short loops turn back in the outer medulla or even in the cortex (cortical loops). Long loops turn back at successive levels of the inner medulla.

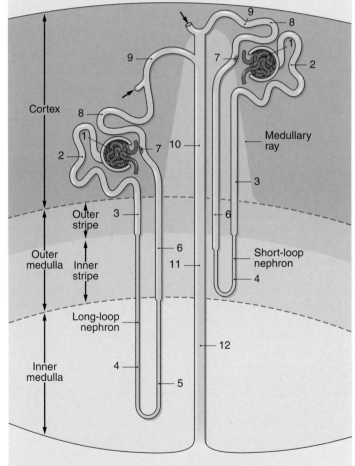

Nephrons and the collecting duct system

1. Renal corpuscle
2. Proximal convoluted tubule
3. Proximal straight tubule
4. Descending thin limb
5. Ascending thin limb
6. Distal straight tubule (thick ascending limb)
7. Macula densa
8. Distal convoluted tubule
9. Connecting tubule
10. Cortical collecting duct
11. Outer medullary collecting duct
12. Inner medullary collecting duct

Figure 1.2 Nephrons and the collecting duct system. Shown are short-looped and long-looped nephrons, together with a collecting duct (not drawn to scale). *Arrows* denote confluence of further nephrons.

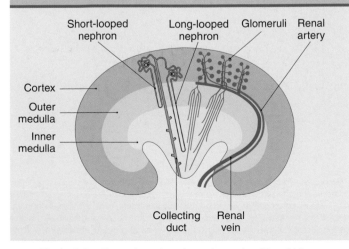

Coronal section through a unipapillary kidney

Figure 1.1   Coronal section through a unipapillary kidney.

Subdivisions of the nephron and collecting duct system

Section	Subsections
Nephron	
Renal corpuscle	Glomerulus: the term used most frequently to refer to the entire renal corpuscle
	Bowman's capsule
Proximal tubule	Convoluted part
	Straight part (pars recta) or thick descending limb of Henle's loop
Intermediate tubule	Descending part or thin descending limb of Henle's loop
	Ascending part or thin ascending limb of Henle's loop
Distal tubule	Straight part or thick ascending limb of Henle's loop: subdivided into a medullary and a cortical part; the latter contains in its terminal portion the macula densa
	Convoluted part
Collecting duct system	
Connecting tubule	Includes the arcades in most species
Collecting duct	Cortical collecting duct
	Outer medullary collecting duct subdivided into an outer and an inner stripe portion
	Inner medullary collecting duct subdivided into basal, middle, and papillary portions

Figure 1.3   Subdivisions of the nephron and collecting duct system.

Collecting Ducts

A collecting duct is formed in the renal cortex when several nephrons join. A connecting tubule (CNT) is interposed between a nephron and a cortical collecting duct. Cortical collecting ducts descend within the medullary rays of the cortex. They traverse the outer medulla as unbranched tubes. On entering the inner medulla, they fuse successively and open finally as papillary ducts into the renal pelvis (see Figs. 1.2 and 1.3).

Microvasculature

The microvascular pattern of the kidney (see Figs 1.1 and 1.4) is also similarly organized in mammalian species.[1,3] The renal artery after entering the renal sinus finally divides into the interlobar arteries, which extend toward the cortex in the space between the wall of the pelvis (or calyx) and the adjacent cortical tissue. At the junction between cortex and medulla, they divide and pass over into the arcuate arteries, which also branch. They give rise to the cortical radial arteries (interlobular arteries) that ascend radially through the cortex. No arteries penetrate the medulla.

Afferent arterioles generally arise from cortical radial arteries; they supply the glomerular tufts. Aglomerular tributaries to the capillary plexus are rarely found. As a result, the blood supply of the peritubular capillaries of the cortex and the medulla is exclusively postglomerular. Glomeruli are drained by efferent arterioles. Two basic types can be distinguished: cortical and juxtamedullary efferent arterioles. Cortical efferent arterioles, which derive from superficial and midcortical glomeruli, supply the capillary plexus of the cortex.

The efferent arterioles of juxtamedullary glomeruli represent the supplying vessels of the renal medulla. Within the outer stripe of the medulla, they divide into the descending vasa recta and then penetrate the inner stripe in cone-shaped vascular

bundles. At intervals, individual vessels leave the bundles to supply the capillary plexus at the adjacent medullary level.

Ascending vasa recta drain the renal medulla. In the inner medulla, they arise at every level, ascending as unbranched vessels. They traverse the inner stripe within the vascular bundles. The ascending vasa recta that drain the inner stripe may either join the vascular bundles or may ascend directly to the outer stripe between the bundles. All the ascending vasa recta traverse the outer stripe as individual wavy vessels with wide lumina interspersed among the tubules. Since true capillaries derived from direct branches of efferent arterioles are

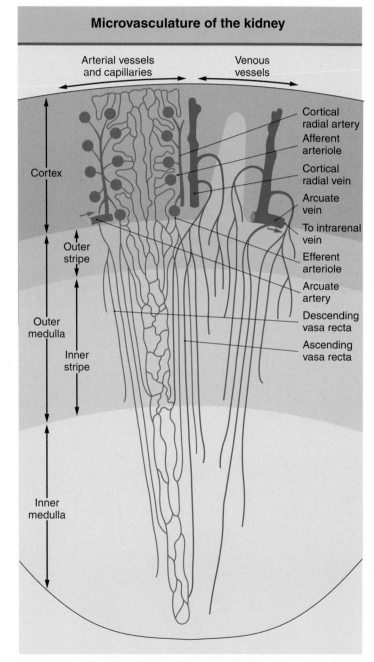

Microvasculature of the kidney

Arterial vessels and capillaries   Venous vessels

Cortex

Outer stripe

Outer medulla

Inner stripe

Inner medulla

Cortical radial artery
Afferent arteriole
Cortical radial vein
Arcuate vein
To intrarenal vein
Efferent arteriole
Arcuate artery
Descending vasa recta
Ascending vasa recta

Figure 1.4   Microvasculature of the kidney. Afferent arterioles supply the glomeruli and efferent arterioles leave the glomeruli and divide into the descending vasa recta, which, together with the ascending vasa recta, form the vascular bundles of the renal medulla. The vasa recta ascending from the inner medulla all traverse the inner stripe within the vascular bundles, whereas most of the vasa recta from the inner stripe of the outer medulla ascend outside the bundles. Both types traverse the outer stripe as wide, tortuous channels.

relatively scarce, it is the ascending vasa recta that form the capillary plexus of the outer stripe. Finally, the ascending vasa recta empty into arcuate veins.

The vascular bundles represent a countercurrent exchanger between the blood entering and that leaving the medulla. In addition, the organization of the vascular bundles results in a separation of the blood flow to the inner stripe from that to the inner medulla. Descending vasa recta supplying the inner medulla traverse the inner stripe within the vascular bundles. Therefore, blood flowing to the inner medulla has not been exposed previously to tubules of the inner or outer stripe. All ascending vasa recta originating from the inner medulla traverse the inner stripe within the vascular bundles; thus, blood that has perfused tubules of the inner medulla does not subsequently perfuse tubules of the inner stripe. However, the blood returning from either the inner medulla or the inner stripe afterward does perfuse the tubules of the outer stripe. It has been suggested that this arrangement in the outer stripe functions as the ultimate trap to prevent solute loss from the medulla.

The intrarenal veins accompany the arteries. Central to the renal drainage of the kidney are the arcuate veins, which, in contrast to arcuate arteries, do form real anastomosing arches at the corticomedullary border. They accept the veins from the cortex and the renal medulla. The arcuate veins join to form interlobar veins, which run alongside the corresponding arteries.

The intrarenal arteries and the afferent and efferent arterioles are accompanied by sympathetic nerve fibers and terminal axons representing the efferent nerves of the kidney.[1] Tubules have direct contact to terminal axons only when they are located around the arteries or the arterioles. As stated by Barajas,[4] "the tubular innervation consists of occasional fibers adjacent to perivascular tubules." The density of nerve contacts to convoluted proximal tubules is low; contacts to straight proximal tubules, thick ascending loops of the limbs of Henle, and collecting ducts (located in the medullary rays and the outer medulla) have never been encountered. The vast majority of tubular portions have no direct relationships to nerve terminals. Afferent nerves of the kidney are commonly believed to be sparse.[5]

NEPHRON

Renal Glomerulus (Renal Corpuscle)

The glomerulus comprises a tuft of specialized capillaries attached to the mesangium, both of which are enclosed in a pouch-like extension of the tubule, that is, Bowman's capsule (Figs 1.5 and 1.6). The capillaries together with the mesangium are covered by epithelial cells (podocytes), forming the visceral epithelium of Bowman's capsule. At the vascular pole, this is reflected to become the parietal epithelium of Bowman's capsule. At the interface between the glomerular capillaries and the mesangium on one side and the podocyte layer on the other side, the glomerular basement membrane (GBM) is developed. The space between both layers of Bowman's capsule represents the urinary space, which at the urinary pole continues as the tubule lumen.

When entering the tuft, the afferent arteriole immediately divides into several (two to five) primary capillary branches,

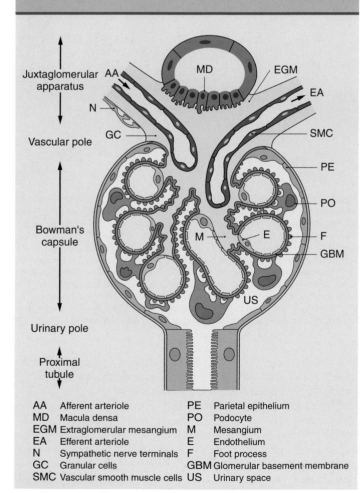

Renal corpuscle and juxtaglomerular apparatus

AA	Afferent arteriole	PE	Parietal epithelium
MD	Macula densa	PO	Podocyte
EGM	Extraglomerular mesangium	M	Mesangium
EA	Efferent arteriole	E	Endothelium
N	Sympathetic nerve terminals	F	Foot process
GC	Granular cells	GBM	Glomerular basement membrane
SMC	Vascular smooth muscle cells	US	Urinary space

Figure 1.5 Renal corpuscle and juxtaglomerular apparatus (JGA). (Adapted with permission from Kriz W, Kaissling B: Structural organization of the mammalian kidney. In Seldin D, Giebisch G [eds]: The Kidney. Philadelphia, Lippincott Williams & Wilkins, 2000, pp 587–654.)

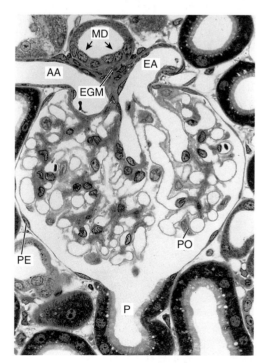

Figure 1.6 Longitudinal section through a glomerulus (rat). At the vascular pole, the afferent arteriole (AA), the efferent arteriole (EA), the extraglomerular mesangium (EGM), and the macula densa (MD) are seen. At the urinary pole, the parietal epithelium (PE) transforms into the proximal tubule (P). PO, podocyte (light microscopy: ×390).

each of which gives rise to an anastomosing capillary network representing a glomerular lobule. In contrast to the afferent arteriole, the efferent arteriole is already established inside the tuft by confluence of capillaries from each lobule.[6] Thus, the efferent arteriole has a significant intraglomerular segment located within the glomerular stalk.

Glomerular capillaries are a unique type of blood vessel made up of nothing but an endothelial tube (Figs 1.7 and 1.8). A small stripe of the outer aspect of this tube directly abuts the mesangium; a major part bulges toward the urinary space and is covered by the GBM and the podocyte layer. This peripheral portion of the capillary wall represents the filtration area. The glomerular mesangium represents the axis of a glomerular lobule to which the glomerular capillaries are attached.

Glomerular Basement Membrane

The GBM serves as the skeleton of the glomerular tuft. It represents a complexly folded sack with an opening at the glomerular hilum (see Fig. 1.5). The outer aspect of this GBM sack is completely covered with podocytes. The interior of the sack is filled with the capillaries and the mesangium. As a result, on its inner aspect, the GBM is in touch either with capillaries or with the mesangium. At any transition between these two locations, the GBM changes from a convex pericapillary into a concave perimesangial course; the turning points are called mesangial angles.

In electron micrographs of traditionally fixed tissue, the GBM appears as a trilaminar structure made up of a lamina densa bounded by two less dense layers: the lamina rara interna

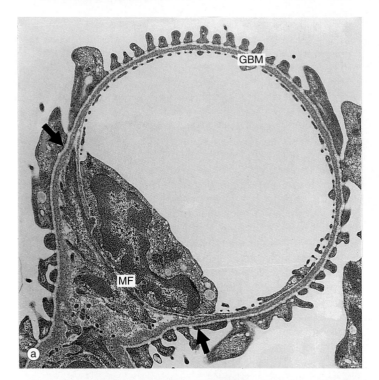

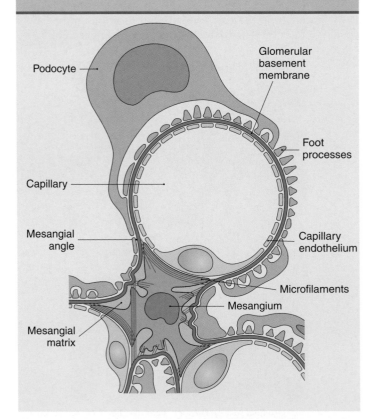

Figure 1.7 Peripheral portion of a glomerular lobule. This shows a capillary, the axial position of the mesangium, and the visceral epithelium (podocytes). At the capillary–mesangial interface, the capillary endothelium directly abuts the mesangium.

Peripheral portion of a glomerular lobule

- Podocyte
- Glomerular basement membrane
- Foot processes
- Capillary
- Capillary endothelium
- Mesangial angle
- Microfilaments
- Mesangium
- Mesangial matrix

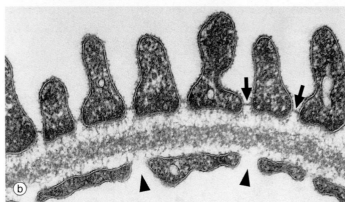

Figure 1.8 Glomerular capillary. *a*, The layer of interdigitating podocyte processes and the glomerular basement membrane (GBM) do not completely encircle the capillary. At the mesangial angles (*arrows*), both deviate from a pericapillary course and cover the mesangium. Mesangial cell processes, containing dense bundles of microfilaments (MF), interconnect the GBM and bridge the distance between the two mesangial angles. *b*, Filtration barrier. The peripheral part of the glomerular capillary wall comprises the endothelium with open pores (*arrowheads*), the GBM, and the interdigitating foot processes. The GBM shows a lamina densa bounded by the lamina rara interna and externa. The foot processes are separated by filtration slits bridged by thin diaphragms (*arrows*) (transmission electron microscopy: *a*, ×8770; *b*, ×50,440).

and externa (see Fig. 1.8). Recent studies using freeze techniques reveal only one thick dense layer directly attached to the bases of the epithelium and endothelium.[7]

The major components of the GBM include type IV collagen and laminin, heparan sulfate proteoglycans, as in basement membranes at other sites. Type V and VI collagen and nidogen have also been demonstrated. However, the GBM has several unique properties, notably a distinct spectrum of type IV collagen and laminin isoforms. The mature GBM is made up of type IV collagen consisting of α_3, α_4, and α_5 chains (instead of α_1 and α_2 chains of most other basement membranes) and of laminin-11 consisting of α_5, β_2, and γ_1 chains.[8] Type IV collagen is the antigenic target in Goodpasture's disease (see Chapter 22), and mutations in the genes of the α_3, α_4, and α_5 chains of type IV collagen are responsible for Alport's syndrome (see Chapter 45).

Current models depict the basic structure of the basement membrane as a three-dimensional network of type IV collagen.[7] The type IV collagen monomer consists of a triple helix of length 400 nm that has a large noncollagenous globular domain at its C-terminal end called NC1. At the N terminus, the helix possesses a triple helical rod of length 60 nm: the 7S domain. Interactions between the 7S domains of two triple helices or the NC1 domains of four triple helices allow type IV collagen monomers to form dimers and tetramers. In addition, triple helical strands interconnect by lateral associations via binding of NC1 domains to sites along the collagenous region. This network is complemented by an interconnected network of laminin 11 resulting in a flexible, nonfibrillar polygonal assembly that is considered to provide mechanical strength to the basement membrane and to serve as a scaffold for alignment of other matrix components.

The electronegative charge of the GBM mainly results from the presence of polyanionic proteoglycans. The major proteoglycans of the GBM are heparan sulfate proteoglycans, among them perlecan and agrin. Proteoglycan molecules aggregate to form a meshwork that is kept highly hydrated by water molecules trapped in the interstices of the matrix.

Mesangium

Three major cell types occur within the glomerular tuft, all of which are in close contact with the GBM: mesangial cells, endothelial cells, and podocytes. In the rat, the numerical ratio has been calculated to be 2:3:1. The mesangial cells, together with the mesangial matrix, establish the glomerular mesangium. In addition, some studies suggest that macrophages bearing HLA-DR/Ia–like antigens may also rarely be found in the normal mesangium.

Mesangial Cells Mesangial cells are quite irregular in shape with many processes extending from the cell body towards the GBM (see Figs 1.7 and 1.8). In these processes, dense assemblies of microfilaments are found that contain actin, myosin, and α-actinin.[9] The processes are attached to the GBM either directly or through the interposition of microfibrils (see later discussion). The GBM represents the effector structure of mesangial contractility. Mesangial cell–GBM connections are especially prominent alongside the capillaries, interconnecting the two opposing mesangial angles of the GBM.

Mesangial Matrix The mesangial matrix fills the highly irregular spaces between the mesangial cells and the perimesangial GBM, anchoring the mesangial cells to the GBM.[6] The ultrastructural organization of this matrix is incompletely understood. In specimens prepared by a technique that avoids osmium tetroxide and uses tannic acid for staining, a dense network of elastic microfibrils is seen. A large number of common extracellular matrix proteins have been demonstrated within the mesangial matrix, including several types of collagens (IV, V, and VI) and several components of microfibrillar proteins (fibrillin and the 31-kd microfibril-associated glycoprotein). The matrix also contains several glycoproteins (fibronectin is most abundant) as well as several types of proteoglycans.

Endothelium

Glomerular endothelial cells consist of cell bodies and peripherally located, attenuated, and highly fenestrated cytoplasmic sheets (see Figs 1.7 and 1.8). Glomerular endothelial pores lack

diaphragms, which are only encountered in the endothelium of the final tributaries to the efferent arteriole.[6] The round-to-oval pores have a diameter of 50 to 100 nm. The luminal membrane of endothelial cells is negatively charged because of its cell coat of several polyanionic glycoproteins, including podocalyxin. In addition, the endothelial pores are filled with sieve plugs mainly made up of sialoglycoproteins.[10]

Visceral Epithelium (Podocytes)

The visceral epithelium of Bowman's capsule comprises highly differentiated cells, the podocytes (see Figs 1.7 and 1.9). In the developing glomerulus, podocytes have a simple polygonal shape. In rats, mitotic activity of these cells is completed soon after birth together with the cessation of the formation of new nephron anlagen. In humans, this point is already reached during prenatal life. The differentiation of the adult podocyte phenotype with the characteristic cell process pattern (see later discussion) is associated with the appearance of several podocyte-specific proteins, including podocalyxin, nephrin, podocin, synaptopodin, and GLEPP-1.[11,12] Differentiated podocytes are unable to replicate; therefore, in the adult, degenerated podocytes cannot be replaced. In response to an extreme mitogenic stimulation (e.g., by basic fibroblast growth factor 2), these cells may undergo mitotic nuclear division; however, the cells are unable to complete cell division, resulting in bi- or multinucleated cells.[12]

Podocytes have a voluminous cell body that floats within the urinary space. The cell bodies give rise to long primary processes that extend toward the capillaries, to which they affix by their most distal portions and by an extensive array of foot processes. The foot processes of neighboring podocytes regularly interdigitate with each other, leaving between them meandering slits (filtration slits) that are bridged by an extracellular structure, the slit diaphragm (see Figs 1.7 through 1.10). Podocytes are polarized epithelial cells with a luminal and a basal cell membrane domain; the latter corresponds to the sole plates of the foot processes that are embedded into the GBM. The border

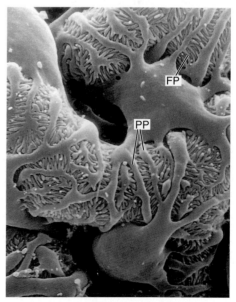

Figure 1.9 Glomerular capillaries in the rat. The urinary side of the capillary is covered by the highly branched podocytes. The interdigitating system of primary processes (PP) and foot processes (FP) lines the entire surface of the tuft extending also beneath the cell bodies. The foot processes of neighboring cells interdigitate but spare the filtration slits in between (scanning electron microscopy: ×2200).

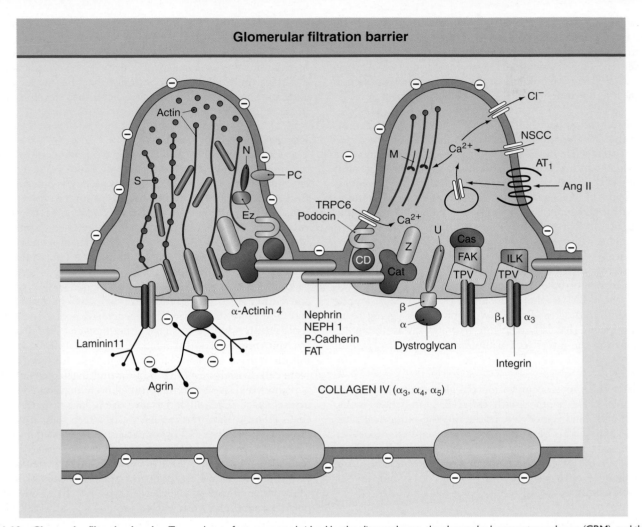

Glomerular filtration barrier

Figure 1.10 Glomerular filtration barrier. Two podocyte foot processes bridged by the slit membrane, the glomerular basement membrane (GBM), and the porous capillary endothelium are shown. The surfaces of podocytes and of the endothelium are covered by a negatively charged glycocalix containing the sialoprotein podocalyxin (PC). The GBM is mainly composed of type IV collagen (α_3, α_4, and α_5) of laminin 11 (α_5, β_2, and γ_1 chains) and the heparan sulfate proteoglycan agrin. The slit membrane represents a porous proteinaceous membrane composed of (as far as known) nephrin; NEPH1, 2, and 3; P-cadherin; and FAT1. The actin-based cytoskeleton of the foot processes connects to both the GBM and the slit membrane. Regarding the connections to the GBM, β_1/α_3 integrin dimers specifically interconnect the TVP complex (talin, paxillin, vinculin) to laminin 11; the β and dystroglycans interconnect utrophin to agrin. The slit membrane proteins are joined to the cytoskeleton via various adaptor proteins, including podocin, zonula occludens protein 1 (ZO-1; Z), CD2-associated protein (CD), and catenins (Cat). Among the nonselective cation channels (NSCC), TRPC6 associates with podocin (and nephrin; not shown) at the slit membrane. Only the angiotensin II (Ang II) type 1 receptor (AT1) is shown as an example of the many surface receptors. Additional abbreviations: Cas, p130Cas; Ez, ezrin; FAK, focal adhesion kinase; ILK, integrin-linked kinase; M, myosin; N, NHERF2 (Na^+-H^+ exchanger regulatory factor); S, synaptopodin. (Modified from Endlich K, Kriz W, Witzgall R: Update in podocyte biology. Curr Opin Nephrol Hypertens 2001;10:331–340.)

between basal and luminal membrane is represented by the slit diaphragm.[13]

The luminal membrane and the slit diaphragm are covered by a thick surface coat that is rich in sialoglycoproteins (including podocalyxin and podoendin) and is responsible for the high negative surface charge of the podocytes. By comparison, the abluminal membrane (i.e., the soles of podocyte processes) contains specific transmembrane proteins that connect the cytoskeleton to the GBM. Two systems are known; first, $\alpha_3\beta_1$ integrin dimers that interconnect the cytoplasmic focal adhesion proteins vinculin, paxillin, and talin with the α_3, α_4, and α_5 chains of type IV collagen and, second, β-α-dystroglycans that interconnect the cytoplasmic adapter protein utrophin with agrin and laminin α_5 chains in the GBM.[11] In addition, a sub-podocyte space has also been recently recognized that can be altered by changes in ultrafiltration pressure and might theoretically be involved in the regulation of glomerular filtration.[12] Other membrane proteins, such as the C3b receptor and gp330/megalin, are present over the entire surface of podocytes.[13]

In contrast to the cell body (harboring a prominent Golgi system), the cell processes contain only a few organelles. A well-developed cytoskeleton accounts for the complex shape of the cells. In the cell body and the primary processes, microtubules and intermediate filaments (vimentin, desmin) dominate. Microfilaments form prominent U-shaped bundles arranged in the longitudinal axis of two successive foot processes in an overlapping pattern. Centrally, these bundles are linked to the microtubules of the primary processes, and peripherally, they are linked to the GBM by integrins and dystroglycans (see previous discussion). α-Actinin 4 and synaptopodin establish the podocyte-specific bundling of the microfilaments.

The filtration slits (see Figs. 1.8 and 1.10) are the sites of convective fluid flow through the visceral epithelium. They have a constant width of about 30 to 40 nm. They are bridged by the slit diaphragm. This is a proteinaceous membrane whose molecular composition is presently not fully understood. Chemically fixed and tannic acid–treated tissue reveals a zipper-like structure with a row of pores approximately 14 nm^2 on either side of a central bar. At present, the following proteins are known to establish this membrane and/or to mediate its connection to the actin cytoskeleton of the foot processes: nephrin, p-cadherin, FAT1, NEPH1-3, and podocin.[14] However, how these molecules interact with each other to establish a size-selective porous membrane is unknown.

Parietal Epithelium

The parietal epithelium of Bowman's capsule consists of squamous epithelial cells resting on a basement membrane (see Figs 1.5 and 1.6). The flat cells are filled with bundles of actin filaments running in all directions. The parietal basement membrane differs from the GBM in that it comprises several dense layers that, in addition to type IV, contain type XIV collagen. The predominant proteoglycan of the parietal basement membrane is a chondroitin sulfate proteoglycan.[1]

Filtration Barrier

Filtration through the glomerular capillary wall occurs along an extracellular pathway including the endothelial pores, the GBM, and the slit diaphragm (see Figs. 1.8 and 1.10). All these components are quite permeable for water; the high permeability for water, small solutes, and ions results from the fact that no cell membranes are interposed. The hydraulic conductance of the individual layers of the filtration barrier is difficult to study. In a mathematical model of glomerular filtration, the hydraulic resistance of the endothelium was predicted to be small, whereas the GBM and filtration slits contribute roughly one half each to the total hydraulic resistance of the capillary wall.[15]

The barrier function of the glomerular capillary wall for macromolecules is selective for size, shape, and charge.[13] The charge selectivity of the barrier results from the dense accumulation of negatively charged molecules throughout the entire depth of the filtration barrier, including the surface coat of endothelial cells, and the high content of negatively charged heparan sulfate proteoglycans in the GBM. Polyanionic macromolecules, such as plasma proteins, are repelled by the electronegative shield originating from these dense assemblies of negative charges.

The crucial structure accounting for the size selectivity of the filtration barrier appears to be the slit diaphragm.[13] Uncharged macromolecules up to an effective radius of 1.8 nm pass freely through the filter. Larger components are more and more restricted (indicated by their fractional clearances, which progressively decrease) and are totally restricted at effective radii >4 nm. Plasma albumin has an effective radius of 3.6 nm; without the repulsion from the negative charge, plasma albumin would pass through the filter in considerable amounts.

Stability of the Glomerular Tuft

The main challenge for the glomerular capillaries is to combine selective leakiness with stability. The walls of capillaries do not appear to be capable of resisting high transmural pressure gradients. Several structures/mechanisms are involved in counteracting the distending forces to which the capillary wall is constantly exposed. The locus of action of all these forces is the GBM.

Two systems appear to be responsible for the development of stabilizing forces. A basic system consists of the GBM and the mesangium. Cylinders of the GBM, in fact, largely define the shape of glomerular capillaries. These cylinders, however, do not completely encircle the capillary tube; they are open toward the mesangium. Mechanically, they are completed by contractile mesangial cell processes that bridge the gaps of the GBM

between two opposing mesangial angles, permitting the development of wall tension.[16]

Podocytes act as a second structure-stabilizing system. Two mechanisms appear to be involved. First, in addition to mesangial cells, podocytes stabilize the folding pattern of glomerular capillaries by fixing the turning points of the GBM between neighboring capillaries (mesangial cells from inside, podocytes from outside).[16] Second, podocytes may contribute to structural stability of glomerular capillaries by a mechanism similar to that of pericytes elsewhere in the body. Podocytes are attached to the GBM by foot processes that cover almost entirely the outer aspect of the GBM. The foot processes possess a well-developed contractile system connected to the GBM. Since the foot processes are attached at various angles on the GBM, they may function as numerous small, stabilizing patches on the GBM, counteracting locally the elastic distention of the GBM.[9]

Renal Tubule

The renal tubule is subdivided into several distinct segments: a proximal tubule, an intermediate tubule, a distal tubule, a CNT, and the collecting duct (see Figs. 1.1 and 1.3).[1,2] Henle's loop comprises the straight part of the proximal tubule (representing the thick descending limb), the thin descending and the thin ascending limbs (both thin limbs together represent the intermediate tubule), and the thick ascending limb (representing the straight portion of the distal tubule), which includes the macula densa. The CNT and the various collecting duct segments form the collecting duct system.

The renal tubules are outlined by a single-layer epithelium anchored to a basement membrane. The epithelium is a transporting epithelium consisting of flat or cuboidal epithelial cells connected apically by a junctional complex consisting of a tight junction (zonula occludens), an adherens junction, and, rarely, a desmosome. As a result of this organization, two different pathways through the epithelium exist (Fig. 1.11): a transcellular pathway, including the transport across the luminal and the basolateral cell membrane and through the cytoplasm, and a paracellular pathway through the junctional complex and the lateral intercellular spaces. The functional characteristics of the paracellular transport are determined by the tight junction,

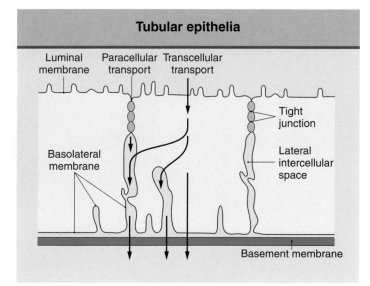

Figure 1.11 Tubular epithelia. Transport across the epithelium may follow two routes: transcellular across luminal and basolateral membranes and paracellular through the tight junction and intercellular spaces.

7

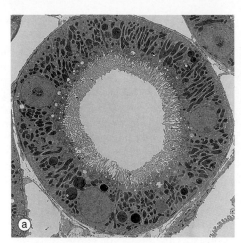
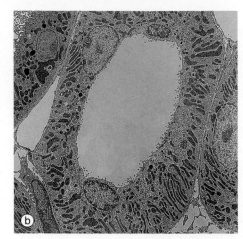

Figure 1.12   Tubules of the renal cortex. *a,* Proximal convoluted tubule is equipped with a brush border and a prominent vacuolar apparatus in the apical cytoplasm. The rest of the cytoplasm is occupied by a basal labyrinth consisting of large mitochondria associated with basolateral cell membranes (transmission electron microscopy: ×1530). *b,* Distal convoluted tubule also has interdigitated basolateral cell membranes intimately associated with large mitochondria; in contrast to the proximal tubule, the apical surface is amplified only by some stubby microvilli (transmission electron microscopy: ×1830).

which differs markedly in its elaboration in the various tubular segments. The transcellular transport is determined by the specific channels, carriers, and transporters included in the apical and basolateral cell membranes. The various nephron segments differ markedly in function, distribution of transport proteins, and responsiveness to hormones and drugs such as diuretics.

Proximal Tubule

The proximal tubule reabsorbs the bulk of filtered water and solutes (Fig. 1.12). The epithelium shows numerous structural adaptations to this role. The proximal tubule has a prominent brush border (increasing the luminal cell surface area) and extensive interdigitation by basolateral cell processes (increasing the basolateral cell surface area). This lateral cell interdigitation extends up to the leaky tight junction, thus increasing the tight junctional belt in length and providing a greatly increased passage for the passive transport of ions. Proximal tubules have large prominent mitochondria intimately associated with the

basolateral cell membranes where the Na$^+$-K$^+$-adenosine triphosphatase (ATPase) is located; this machinery dominates the transcellular transport. The luminal transporter for Na$^+$ entry specific for the proximal tubule is the Na$^+$-H$^+$ exchanger. The high hydraulic permeability for water is rooted in abundant occurrence of the water channel protein aquaporin-1. A prominent lysosomal system is known as the apical vacuolar endo-cytotic apparatus and is responsible for the reabsorption of macromolecules (polypeptides and proteins such as albumin) that have passed through the glomerular filter. The proximal tubule is generally subdivided into three segments (known as S$_1$, S$_2$, S$_3$, or P$_1$, P$_2$, P$_3$) that differ considerably in cellular organization and, consequently, also in function.[17]

Henle's Loop

Henle's loop consists of the straight portion of the proximal tubule, thin descending and (in long loops) thin ascending limbs, and the thick ascending limb (see Figs 1.2 and 1.13). The thin

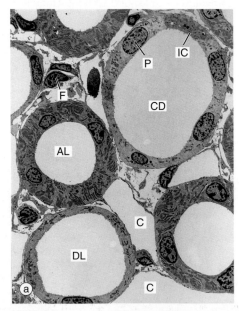
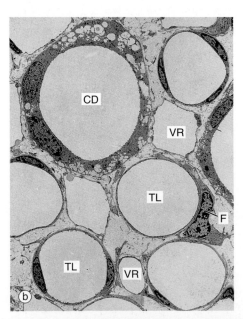

Figure 1.13   Tubules in the medulla. *a,* Cross section through the inner stripe of the outer medulla. A descending thin limb of a long loop (DL), medullary thick ascending limbs (AL), and a collecting duct (CD) with principal cells (P) and intercalated cells (IC) are shown. C, peritubular capillaries; F, fibroblast. *b,* In the inner medulla cross section, thin descending and ascending limbs (TL), a collecting duct (CD), and vasa recta (VR) are seen (transmission electron microscopy: *a,* ×990; *b,* ×1120).

descending limb, like the proximal tubule, is highly permeable for water (the channels are of aquaporin-1), whereas, beginning exactly at the turning point, the thin ascending limb is impermeable for water. The specific transport functions of the thin limbs contributing to the generation of the osmotic medullary gradient are under debate.

The thick ascending limb is often called the diluting segment. It is water impermeable but reabsorbs considerable amounts of salt, resulting in the separation of salt from water. The salt is trapped in the medulla, whereas the water is carried away into the cortex where it may return into the systemic circulation. The specific transporter for Na^+ entry in this segment is the luminal Na^+-K^+-$2Cl^-$ cotransporter, which is the target of diuretics such as furosemide. The tight junctions of the thick ascending limb have a comparatively low permeability. The cells heavily interdigitate by basolateral cell processes, associated with large mitochondria supplying the energy for the transepithelial transport. The cells synthesize a specific protein, the Tamm-Horsfall protein, and release it into the tubular lumen. This protein is thought to be important later for preventing the formation of kidney stones. In contrast to the proximal tubule, the luminal membrane is only sparsely amplified by microvilli. Just before the transition to the distal convoluted tubule, the thick ascending limb contains the macula densa, which adheres to the parent glomerulus (see juxtaglomerular apparatus).

Distal Convoluted Tubule

The epithelium is fairly highly differentiated, exhibiting the most extensive basolateral interdigitation of the cells and the greatest density of mitochondria in all nephron portions (see Fig. 1.12). Apically, the cells are equipped with numerous microvilli. The specific Na^+ transporter of the distal convoluted tubule is the luminal Na^+-Cl^- cotransporter, which is the target of thiazide diuretics.

COLLECTING DUCT SYSTEM

The collecting duct system (see Fig. 1.2) includes the CNT and the cortical and medullary collecting ducts. Two nephrons may join at the level of the CNT, forming an arcade that, cytologically, is a CNT. Two types of cell line the CNT: the CNT cell, which is specific to the CNTs, and the intercalated cell, which also occurs

later in the collecting duct. The CNT cells are similar in cellular organization to the collecting duct cells (CD cells). Both cell types share sensitivity to vasopressin (antidiuretic hormone [ADH]; see later discussion); the CNT cell, however, lacks sensitivity to mineralocorticoids.

Collecting Ducts

The CDs (see Fig. 1.13) may be subdivided into cortical and medullary ducts, the latter into outer and inner medullary ducts; the transitions are gradual. Like the CNT, the CDs are lined by two types of cell: CD cells (principal cells) and intercalate cells (IC cells). The latter decrease in number as the CD descends into the medulla and are absent from the papillary collecting ducts.

The CD cells (Fig. 1.14a) are simple, polygonal cells increasing in size toward the tip of the papilla. The basal surface of these cells is characterized by invaginations of the basal cell membrane (basal infoldings). The tight junctions have a large apicobasal depth, and the apical cell surface has a prominent glycocalyx. Along the entire collecting duct, these cells contain a luminal shuttle system for aquaporin-2 under the control of vasopressin, providing the potential to switch the water permeability of the collecting ducts from zero (or at least from low) to permeable.[18] A luminal amiloride-sensitive Na^+ channel is involved in the responsiveness of cortical collecting ducts to aldosterone. The terminal portions of the collecting duct in the inner medulla express the urea transporter UTB1, which, in an ADH-dependent fashion, accounts for the recycling of urea, a process that is crucial in the urine-concentrating mechanism.[19]

The second cell type, the IC cell (Fig. 1.14b), is present in both the CNT and the collecting duct. There are at least two types of IC cells, designated A and B cells, distinguished based on structural, immunocytochemical, and functional characteristics. Type A cells have been defined as expressing H^+-ATPase at their luminal membrane; they secrete protons. Type B cells express the H^+-ATPase at their basolateral membrane; they secrete bicarbonate ions and reabsorb protons.[20]

With these different cell types, the collecting ducts are the final regulators of fluid and electrolyte balance, playing important roles in the handling of Na^+, Cl^-, and K^+ as well as acid and base. The responsiveness of the collecting ducts to vasopressin enables an organism to live in arid conditions, allowing it to produce a concentrated urine, and, if necessary, a dilute urine.

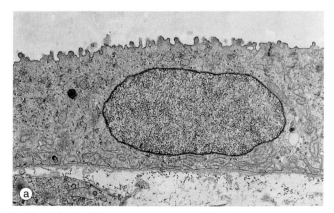
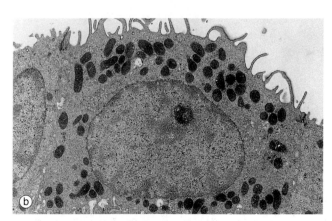

Figure 1.14 Collecting duct cells. *a,* Principal cell (CD cell) of a medullary collecting duct. The apical cell membrane bears some stubby microvilli covered by a prominent glycocalyx; the basal cell membrane forms invaginations. Note the deep tight junction. *b,* Intercalated cells, type A. Note the dark cytoplasm (*dark cells*) with many mitochondria and apical microfolds; the basal membrane forms invaginations (transmission electron microscopy: *a,* ×8720; *b,* ×6970).

JUXTAGLOMERULAR APPARATUS

The juxtaglomerular apparatus (JGA; see Fig. 1.5) comprises the macula densa, the extraglomerular mesangium, the terminal portion of the afferent arteriole with its renin-producing granular cells (nowadays also often termed juxtaglomerular cells), and the beginning portions of the efferent arteriole.

The macula densa (see Figs. 1.6 and 1.15a) is a plaque of specialized cells in the wall of the thick ascending limb at the site where the limb attaches to the extraglomerular mesangium of the parent glomerulus. The most obvious structural feature is the narrowly packed cells with large nuclei, which account for the name macula densa. The cells are anchored to a basement membrane, which blends with the matrix of the extraglomerular mesangium.[1] The cells are joined by tight junctions with very low permeability and have prominent lateral intercellular spaces. The width of these spaces varies under different functional conditions.[1] The most conspicuous immunocytochemical difference between macula densa cells and any other epithelial cell of the nephron is the high content of neuronal nitric oxide synthase-1[21] and of cyclooxygenase-2.[22]

The basal aspect of the macula densa is firmly attached to the extraglomerular mesangium, which represents a solid complex of cells and matrix that is penetrated neither by blood vessels nor lymphatic capillaries (see Figs 1.5 and 1.15a). Like the mesangial cells proper, extraglomerular mesangial cells are heavily branched. Their processes, interconnected among each other by gap junctions, contain prominent bundles of microfilaments and are connected to the basement membrane of Bowman's capsule as well as to the walls of both glomerular arterioles. As a whole, the extraglomerular mesangium interconnects all structures of the glomerular entrance.[6]

The granular cells are assembled in clusters within the terminal portion of the afferent arteriole (see Fig. 1.15b), replacing ordinary smooth muscle cells. Their name refers to the specific cytoplasmic granules in which renin, the major secretion product of these cells, is stored. They are the main site of the body where renin is secreted. Renin release occurs by exocytosis into the surrounding interstitium. Granular cells are connected to the extraglomerular mesangial cells, to adjacent smooth muscle cells, and to endothelial cells by gap junctions. They are densely innervated by sympathetic nerve terminals. Granular cells are modified smooth muscle cells; under conditions requiring enhanced renin synthesis (e.g., volume depletion or stenosis of the renal artery), additional smooth muscle cells located upstream in the wall of the afferent arteriole may transform into granular cells.

The structural organization of the JGA suggests a regulatory function. There is agreement that some component of the distal urine (probably Cl^-) is sensed by the macula densa and this information is used first to adjust the tone of the glomerular arterioles, thereby producing a change in glomerular blood flow and filtration rate. Even if many details of this mechanism are still subject to debate, the essence of this system has been verified by many studies, and it is known as the tubular glomerular feedback mechanism.[23]

Second, this system determines the amount of renin that is released, via the interstitium, into the circulation, thereby acquiring great systemic relevance.

RENAL INTERSTITIUM

The interstitium of the kidney is comparatively sparse. Its fractional volume in the cortex ranges from 5% to 7% (with a tendency to increase with age). It increases across the medulla from cortex to papilla: in the outer stripe, it is 3% to 4% (the lowest value of all kidney zones; this is interpreted as forming a barrier to prevent loss of solutes from a hyperosmolar medulla into the cortex); in the inner stripe, it is 10%; and in the inner medulla, it is up to ~30%. The cellular constituents of the interstitium are resident fibroblasts, which establish the scaffold frame for renal corpuscles, tubules, and blood vessels. In addition, there are varying numbers of migrating cells of the immune system, especially dendritic cells. The space between the cells is filled with extracellular matrix, namely, ground substance (proteoglycans, glycoproteins), fibrils, and interstitial fluid.[24]

From a morphologic point of view, fibroblasts are the central cells in the renal interstitium. They are interconnected by

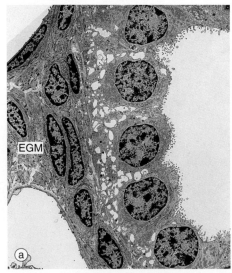
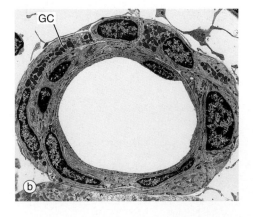

Figure 1.15 Juxtaglomerular apparatus. *a,* Macula densa of a thick ascending limb. The cells have prominent nuclei and lateral intercellular spaces. Basally they attach to the extraglomerular mesangium (EGM). *b,* Afferent arteriole near the vascular pole. Several smooth muscle cells are replaced by granular cells (GC) containing accumulations of renin granules (transmission electron microscopy: *a,* ×1730; *b,* ×1310).

specialized contacts and adhere by specific attachments to the basement membranes surrounding the tubules, the renal corpuscles, the capillaries, and the lymphatics.

Renal fibroblasts are difficult to distinguish from interstitial dendritic cells on a morphologic basis because both may show a stellate cellular shape and both display substantial amounts of mitochondria and endoplasmic reticulum. They may, however, easily be distinguished by immunocytochemical techniques. Dendritic cells constitutively express the major histocompatibility complex class II antigen and may express antigens such as CD11c, whereas fibroblasts in the renal cortex (not in the medulla) contain the enzyme ecto-5'-nucleotidase (5'-NT).[25] A subset of 5'-NT–positive fibroblasts of the renal cortex synthesize epoetin.[25] Under normal conditions, these fibroblasts are exclusively found within the juxtamedullary portions of the cortical labyrinth. When there is an increasing demand for epoetin, the synthesizing cells extend to more superficial portions of the cortical labyrinth and, to a lesser degree, to the medullary rays.[26]

Fibroblasts within the medulla, especially within the inner medulla, have a particular phenotype known as lipid-laden interstitial cells. The cells are oriented strictly perpendicularly toward the longitudinal axis of the tubules and vessels (running all in parallel) and contain conspicuous lipid droplets. These fibroblasts of the inner medulla produce large amounts of glycosaminoglycans and, possibly related to the lipid droplets, produce vasoactive lipids, in particular prostaglandin E_2.[24]

The intrarenal arteries are accompanied by a prominent sheath of loose interstitial tissue (Fig. 1.16); the renal veins are in apposition to this sheath but not included in it. Intrarenal

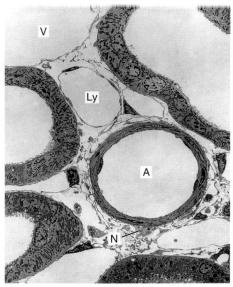

Figure 1.16 Intrarenal arteries in a periarterial connective tissue sheath. Cross section through a cortical radial artery surrounded by the sheath containing the renal nerves (N) and lymphatics (LY). A vein lies outside the sheath (transmission electron microscopy: ×830).

nerve fibers and lymphatics run within this periarterial tissue. Lymphatics start in the vicinity of the afferent arteriole and leave the kidney running within the periarterial tissue sheath toward the hilum. Together with the lymphatics, the periarterial tissue constitutes a pathway for interstitial fluid drainage of the renal cortex; the renal medulla has no lymphatic drainage.

REFERENCES

1. Kriz W, Kaissling B: Structural organization of the mammalian kidney. In Seldin D, Giebisch G (eds): The Kidney. Philadelphia, Lippincott Williams & Wilkins, 2000, pp 587–654.
2. Kriz W, Bankir L: A standard nomenclature for structure of the kidney. The Renal Commission of the International Union of Physiological Sciences (IUPS). Pflugers Arch 1988;411:113–120.
3. Rollhäuser H, Heinke W: Das Gefässsystem der Rattenniere. Z Zellforsch Mikrosk Anat 1964;64:381–403.
4. Barajas L: Innervation of the renal cortex. Fed Proc 1978;37: 1192–1201.
5. DiBona G, Kopp U: Neural control of renal function. Physiol Rev 1997;77:75–197.
6. Elger M, Sakai T, Kriz W: The vascular pole of the renal glomerulus of rat. Adv Anat Embryol Cell Biol 1998;139:1–98.
7. Inoue S: Ultrastructural architecture of basement membranes. Contrib Nephrol 1994;107:21–28.
8. Miner J: Renal basement membrane components. Kidney Int 1999; 56:2016–2024.
9. Kriz W, Elger M, Mundel P, Lemley K: Structure-stabilizing forces in the glomerular tuft. J Am Soc Nephrol 1995;5:1731–1739.
10. Rostgaard J, Qvortrup K: Electron microscopic demonstrations of filamentous molecular sieve plugs in capillary fenestrae. Microvasc Res 1997;53:1–13.
11. Endlich K, Kriz W, Witzgall R: Update in podocyte biology. Curr Opin Nephrol Hypertens 2001;10:331–340.
12. Neal CR, Crook H, Bell E, et al: Three-dimensional reconstruction of glomeruli by electron microscopy reveals a distinctive restrictive urinary subpodocyte space. J Am Soc Nephrol 2005;16:1223–1235.
13. Pavenstadt H, Kriz W, Kretzler M: Cell biology of the glomerular podocyte. Physiol Rev 2003;83:253–307.
14. Mundel P, Kriz W: Structure and function of podocytes: An update. Anat Embryol 1995;192:385–397.
15. Drumond M, Deen W: Structural determinants of glomerular hydraulic permeability. Am J Physiol 1994;266:F1–F12.
16. Kriz W, Endlich K: Hypertrophy of podocytes: A mechanism to cope with increased glomerular capillary pressures? Kidney Int 2005;607: 373–374.
17. Maunsbach A: Functional ultrastructure of the proximal tubule. In Windhager E (ed): Handbook of Physiology: Section on Renal Physiology. New York: Oxford University Press, 1992, pp 41–108.
18. Sabolic I, Brown D: Water channels in renal and nonrenal tissues. News Physiol Sci 1995;10:12–17.
19. Bankir L, Trinh-Trang-Tan M: Urea and the kidney. In Brenner B (ed): The Kidney. Philadelphia, WB Saunders, 2000, pp 637–679.
20. Madsen K, Verlander J, Kim J, Tisher C: Morphological adaptation of the collecting duct to acid-base disturbances. Kidney Int 1991;40(Suppl 33):S57–S63.
21. Mundel P, Bachmann S, Bader M, et al: Expression of nitric oxide synthase in kidney macula densa cells. Kidney Int 1992;42:1017–1019.
22. Harris R, McKanna J, Akai Y, et al: Cyclooxygenase-2 is associated with the macula densa of rat kidney and increases with salt restriction. J Clin Invest 1994;94:2504–2510.
23. Klamt B, Koziell A, Poulat F, et al: Frasier syndrome is caused by defective alternative splicing of WT1 leading to an altered ratio of WT1 +/– KTS splice isoforms. Hum Mol Genet 1998;7:709–714.
24. Kaissling B, Hegyi I, Loffing J, Le Hir M: Morphology of interstitial cells in the healthy kidney. Anat Embryol 1996;193:303–318.
25. Bachmann S, Le Hir M, Eckardt K: Co-localization of erythropoietin mRNA and ecto-5'-nucleotidase immunoreactivity in peritubular cells of rat renal cortex indicates that fibroblasts produce erythropoietin. J Histochem Cytochem 1993;41:335–341.
26. Kaissling B, Spiess S, Rinne B, Le Hir M: Effects of anemia on the morphology of the renal cortex of rats. Am J Physiol 1993;264: F608–F617.

CHAPTER 2

Renal Physiology

David G. Shirley, Giovambattista Capasso, and Robert J. Unwin

INTRODUCTION

The prime function of the kidney is to maintain a stable *milieu intérieur* by the selective retention or elimination of water, electrolytes, and other solutes. This is achieved by three processes: (1) filtration of circulating blood from the glomerulus to form an ultrafiltrate of plasma in Bowman's space; (2) selective reabsorption (from tubular fluid to blood) across the cells lining the renal tubule; and (3) selective secretion (from peritubular capillary blood to tubular fluid).

GLOMERULAR STRUCTURE AND ULTRASTRUCTURE

The process of urine formation begins by the production of an ultrafiltrate of plasma. Chapter 1 provides a detailed description of glomerular anatomy and ultrastructure; therefore, only brief essentials to an understanding of how the ultrafiltrate is formed are given here. The glomerulus is a tuft of capillaries supplied and drained by afferent and efferent arterioles, respectively. The pathway for ultrafiltration of plasma from the glomerulus to Bowman's space consists of the capillary endothelium, the capillary basement membrane, and the visceral epithelial cell layer (podocytes) of Bowman's capsule; the podocytes have large cell bodies that float in Bowman's space and make contact with the basement membrane only by foot processes. Mesangial cells, which fill the spaces between capillaries, have contractile properties and are capable of altering the capillary surface area available for filtration.

What is filtered is determined principally by size and to a much lesser extent by charge. The size cutoff is not absolute; resistance to filtration begins at an effective molecular radius of slightly less than 2 nm, while substances with an effective radius exceeding ~4 nm are not filtered at all. The capillary endothelial cells have relatively large gaps (50- to 100-nm diameter) between them and the podocytes' foot processes have slitlike pores (30- to 40-nm diameter) between them, but the latter are partially occluded by zipper-like structures (the slit diaphragms), so the real gap is much smaller. It is believed that these slitlike pores constitute the main filtration barrier, although both the endothelium (by preventing the passage of blood cells) and the basement membrane contribute. The podocytes and the endothelial cells carry fixed negative charges from glycoproteins on their surface, and the basement membrane is rich in heparan sulfate proteoglycans. These fixed negative charges further restrict the filtration of large negatively charged ions, mainly proteins (Fig. 2.1). This explains why albumin, despite an effective radius (3.6 nm) that would allow significant filtration based on size alone, is normally virtually excluded. If these fixed negative charges are lost, as in some forms of early or mild glomerular disease (e.g., minimal

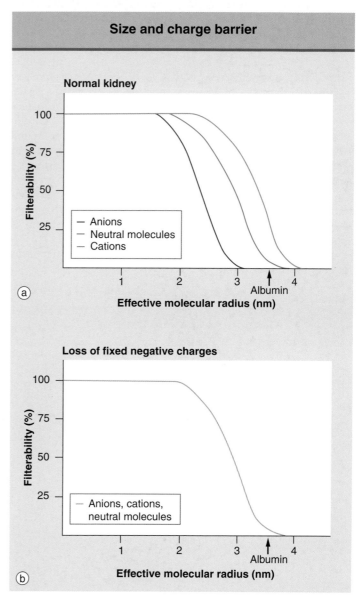

Size and charge barrier

Normal kidney

(a) Effective molecular radius (nm)

Loss of fixed negative charges

(b) Effective molecular radius (nm)

Figure 2.1   Size and charge barrier: effects of size and electrical charge on filterability. *a,* Normal kidney. *b,* Loss of fixed negative charge. One hundred percent filterability indicates that the substance is freely filtered, that is, its concentration in Bowman's space equals that in glomerular capillary plasma. For molecules and small ions (e.g., Na^+, Cl^-), charge has no effect on filterability, but for ions whose effective molecular radius exceeds ~1.6 nm, anions are filtered less easily than neutral molecules or cations. Thus, insignificant amounts of albumin (anion) are normally filtered. If the fixed negative charges of the glomerular basement membranes are lost, as in early minimal change nephropathy, charge no longer influences filterability; consequently, significant albumin filtration occurs.

change nephropathy), albumin filterability increases and protein-uria results.

GLOMERULAR FILTRATION RATE AND RENAL BLOOD FLOW

At the level of the single glomerulus, the driving force for glomerular filtration (the *net ultrafiltration pressure*) is determined by the net hydrostatic and oncotic (colloid osmotic) pressure gradients between glomerular plasma and the filtrate in Bowman's space. The rate of filtration (single-nephron glomerular filtration rate) is determined by the product of the net ultrafiltration pressure and the *ultrafiltration coefficient*, the latter being a composite of the surface area available for filtration and the hydraulic conductivity of the glomerular membranes. Therefore, the single-nephron glomerular filtration rate is

$$K_f\,[(P_{gc} - P_{bs}) - (\pi_{gc} - \pi_{bs})],$$

where K_f is the ultrafiltration coefficient, P_{gc} is glomerular capillary hydrostatic pressure ($\sim$45 mm Hg), π_{bs} is Bowman's space hydrostatic pressure ($\sim$10 mm Hg), π_{gc} is glomerular capillary oncotic pressure ($\sim$25 mm Hg), and p_{bs} is Bowman's space oncotic pressure (0 mm Hg). Thus, net ultrafiltration pressure is around 10 mm Hg at the afferent end of the capillary tuft. As filtration of protein-free fluid proceeds along the glomerular capillaries, π_{gc} increases, and, at a certain point toward the efferent end, π_{gc} may equal the net hydrostatic pressure gradient, that is, the net ultrafiltration pressure may fall to zero: so-called *filtration equilibrium* (Fig. 2.2). In humans, complete filtration equilibrium is approached, but rarely (if ever) achieved.

The total rate at which fluid is filtered into all the nephrons (glomerular filtration rate [GFR]) is typically 120 ml/min per 1.73 m^2 surface area, but the normal range is wide. In the population as a whole, GFR declines with age (see Chapter 62), but this is not inevitable in every individual: longitudinal studies have shown that, in up to 30% of elderly subjects, GFR is stable and that a fall in GFR depends on blood pressure, protein intake, and associated renal or cardiovascular disease.[1]

GFR can be measured using renal clearance techniques. The renal clearance of any substance not metabolized by the kidneys is the volume of plasma required to provide that amount of the substance excreted in the urine per unit time; this virtual volume can be expressed mathematically as

$$C_y = U_y \times V/P_y,$$

where C_y is the renal clearance of y, U_y is the urine concentration of y, V is the urine flow rate, and P_y is the plasma concentration of y. If a substance is freely filtered by the glomerulus and is not reabsorbed or secreted by the tubule, then its renal clearance equals GFR, that is, it measures the volume of plasma filtered through the glomeruli per unit time. Measurement of GFR and its pitfalls is described in detail in Chapter 3 and is considered only briefly here. The substance that best fits the criteria for a marker of GFR is the polysaccharide inulin. However, partly because it has to be infused intravenously, measurement of inulin clearance is cumbersome and inappropriate for routine clinical investigation. In contrast, the clearance of endogenous creatinine is convenient and easy to measure and provides a reasonable approximation of GFR in normal subjects. Unfortunately, because some creatinine is secreted into proximal tubules and the proportion secreted increases in renal failure, creatinine clearance overestimates true GFR in this situation. As an alternative to creatinine clearance, the plasma disappearance of endogenous cystatin C, the radiocontrast agent iohexol, or a marker radiolabeled with a gamma emitter (e.g., ^{51}Cr-ethylenediamine tetraacetic acid, ^{99m}TC-diethylenetriamine pentaacetic acid), following a single intravenous injection, is often used (see Chapter 3).

MEASUREMENT OF RENAL PLASMA FLOW

The use of the clearance technique and the availability of substances that undergo both glomerular filtration and tubular secretion have made it possible to measure renal plasma flow (RPF). Para-amino hippurate (PAH) is an organic acid that is filtered by the glomerulus and actively secreted by the proximal tubule. The amount that is found in the final urine is the sum of the PAH filtered plus the component that is secreted. When the plasma concentration of PAH is lower than 10 mg/dl, most of the PAH reaching the peritubular capillaries is cleared by tubular secretion and little PAH appears in renal venous plasma. Under these circumstances, the amount of PAH transferred from the plasma to the tubular lumen via filtration and secretion (i.e., the amount found in the final urine) approximates the amount of PAH delivered to the kidneys in the plasma. Therefore,

$$RPF \times P_{PAH} = U_{PAH} \times V$$
$$\text{or } RPF = (U_{PAH} \times V)/P_{PAH} = \text{PAH clearance},$$

where U_{PAH} and P_{PAH} are the concentrations of PAH in the urine and plasma, respectively, and V is the urine flow rate. Renal blood flow (RBF) can be calculated as

$$RBF = [RPF/(100 - \text{hematocrit})] \times 100.$$

The most important limitation of this method is the renal extraction of PAH. The latter is always less than 100%. At high

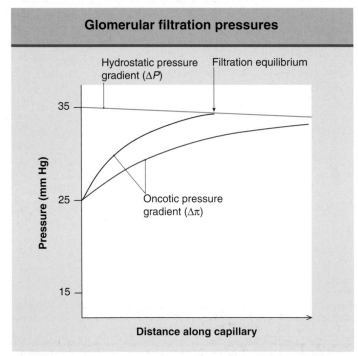

Glomerular filtration pressures

Figure 2.2 Glomerular filtration pressures along a glomerular capillary. The hydrostatic pressure gradient ($\Delta P = P_{gc} - P_{bs}$) is relatively constant along the length of a capillary, whereas the opposing oncotic pressure gradient ($\Delta\pi = \pi_{gc}$) increases as protein-free fluid is filtered, thereby reducing net ultrafiltration pressure. Two curves are shown, one where filtration equilibrium is reached and one where it is merely approached.

plasma concentrations (>10 to 15 mg/dl), fractional tubular secretion of PAH declines and significant amounts appear in the renal veins; under these circumstances, PAH clearance seriously underestimates RPF. There are also diseases that can produce either toxins or weak organic acids (e.g., liver and renal failure) that interfere with PAH secretion or cause tubular damage leading to inhibition of PAH transport. Finally, certain drugs, like probenecid, are organic acids and therefore compete with PAH for tubular secretion and reduce PAH clearance.

AUTOREGULATION OF RENAL BLOOD FLOW AND GLOMERULAR FILTRATION RATE

Although acute variations in arterial blood pressure inevitably cause corresponding changes in RBF and GFR, the latter are short lived, and, provided the blood pressure remains within the normal range, compensatory mechanisms come into play after a few seconds to return both RBF and GFR to near normal.[2] This is the phenomenon of *autoregulation* (Fig. 2.3). Autoregulation is brought about predominantly by changes in the caliber of the afferent arterioles and is believed to result from a combination of two mechanisms:

1. A *myogenic reflex*, whereby the afferent arteriolar smooth muscle wall constricts automatically when renal perfusion pressure rises.
2. *Tubuloglomerular feedback* (*TG feedback*), whereby an increased delivery of NaCl to the *macula densa* region of the nephron (a specialized plaque of cells situated near the end of the loop of Henle), resulting from increases in blood pressure, RBF, and GFR, causes vasoconstriction of the afferent arteriole supplying that nephron's glomerulus.

Because these mechanisms restore both RBF and P_{gc} toward normal, the initial change in GFR is also reversed. The TG

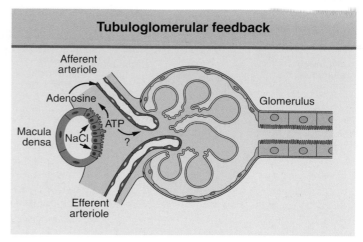

Figure 2.4 Tubuloglomerular feedback. Changes in the delivery of NaCl to the macula densa region of the thick ascending limb of the loop of Henle cause changes in the afferent arteriolar caliber. The response is mediated by adenosine and/or adenosine triphosphate (ATP) and modulated by other locally produced agents such as angiotensin II and nitric oxide. Increased macula densa NaCl delivery results in afferent arteriolar constriction, thereby reducing GFR.

feedback system is possible because of the anatomic arrangement in the kidney such that the macula densa region of each nephron is in close contact with its own glomerulus and afferent and efferent arterioles (Fig. 2.4). This structural complex is known as the *juxtaglomerular apparatus*.

There is evidence that the major mediator of TG feedback is adenosine, acting on adenosine A_1 receptors in the afferent arteriole.[3] Increased NaCl delivery to the macula densa leads to increased NaCl uptake by these cells, which in turn triggers adenosine triphosphate (ATP) release into the surrounding extracellular space.[4] Nucleotidases present in this region are then thought to degrade the ATP to adenosine, although there is also some evidence that ATP itself might have a direct vasoconstrictor effect (acting on afferent arteriolar $P2X_1$ purinoceptors). The sensitivity of TG feedback is modulated by locally produced angiotensin II (Ang II), nitric oxide, and certain eicosanoids (see later discussion).

Despite the underlying influence of autoregulation, which usually maintains RBF and GFR relatively constant in the mean arterial pressure range ~80 to 180 mm Hg, a number of extrinsic factors (nervous and humoral) can alter renal hemodynamics. Independent or unequal changes in the resistance of afferent and efferent arterioles, together with alterations in K_f (the latter thought to result largely from mesangial cell contraction/relaxation, although some evidence also implicates contractile elements in the podocytes that line Bowman's capsule), can result in disproportionate, or even contrasting, changes in RBF and GFR. In addition, within the kidney, changes in vascular resistance in different regions of the renal cortex can alter the distribution of blood flow, for example, diversion of blood from outer to inner cortex in hemorrhagic shock.[5] Figure 2.5 indicates how, in principle, changes in afferent and efferent arteriolar resistance will affect net ultrafiltration. Some of the better known vasoactive factors that alter renal hemodynamics are listed in Figure 2.6 and are discussed in the final section of the chapter. In addition, recent studies suggest that disease of the renal afferent arteriole, such as occurs in hypertension and progressive kidney disease, may also interfere with renal autoregulatory mechanisms, leading to either inadequate or excessive renal vasoconstriction in response to stimuli.

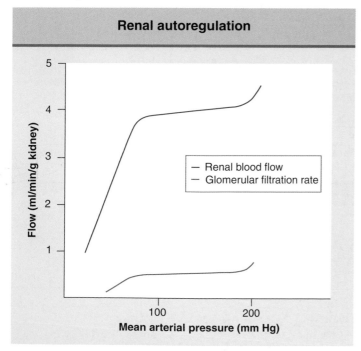

Figure 2.3 Renal autoregulation of renal blood flow and glomerular filtration rate. If mean arterial blood pressure is in the range ~80 to 180 mm Hg, fluctuations in blood pressure have only marginal effects on renal blood flow and glomerular filtration rate. This is an intrinsic mechanism and can be modulated or overridden by extrinsic factors.

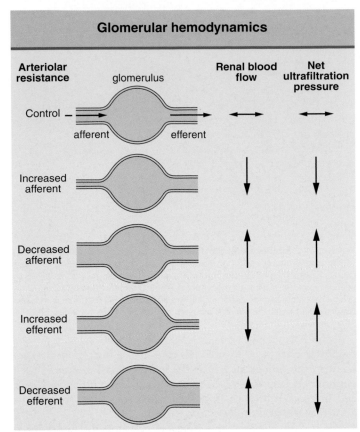

Glomerular hemodynamics

| Arteriolar resistance | glomerulus | Renal blood flow | Net ultrafiltration pressure |

Figure 2.5 Glomerular hemodynamics. Changes in afferent or efferent arteriolar resistance will alter renal blood flow and (usually) net ultrafiltration pressure. However, the effect on ultrafiltration pressure depends on the *relative* changes in afferent/efferent arteriolar resistance. The overall effect on glomerular filtration rate will depend not only on renal blood flow and net ultrafiltration pressure but also on the ultrafiltration coefficient (K_f; see Fig. 2.6).

TUBULAR TRANSPORT MECHANISMS: BASIC PRINCIPLES

Vectorial transport, that is, net movement of substances from tubular fluid to blood (reabsorption) or vice versa (secretion), requires that the cell membrane facing the tubular fluid (luminal or apical) must have different properties from the membrane facing the blood (peritubular or basolateral). In this *polarized* epithelium, certain transport proteins are located in one membrane (apical or basolateral), while others are located in the other, thus allowing the net movement of substances across the cell (transcellular route). The *tight junction*, which is a contact point found close to the apical side of adjacent cells, limits water and solute movement between cells (paracellular route).

Solute transport across cell membranes uses either passive or active mechanisms.

Passive Transport

1. *Simple diffusion* always occurs down an electrochemical gradient, which is a composite of the concentration gradient and the electrical gradient. In the case of an undissociated molecule, only the concentration gradient is relevant, whereas in the case of a charged ion, the electrical gradient must also be considered. Simple diffusion does not require a direct energy source, although an active transport process (see later discussion) is usually necessary to establish the initial concentration and/or electrical gradients.

2. *Facilitated diffusion* (or carrier-mediated diffusion) depends on an interaction of the molecule or ion with a specific membrane carrier protein that eases, or facilitates, its passage across the cell membrane's lipid bilayer. In almost all instances of carrier-mediated transport in the kidney, two or more ions or molecules share the carrier, one moiety moving

Physiologic and pharmacologic factors with effects on glomerular hemodynamics

	Afferent Arteriolar Resistance	Efferent Arteriolar Resistance	Renal Blood Flow	Net Ultrafiltration Pressure	K_f	GFR
Renal sympathetic nerves	↑↑	↑	↓	↓	↓	↓
Epinephrine	↑	↑	↓	→	?	↓
Adenosine	↑	→	↓	↓	?	↓
Cyclosporine	↑	→	↓	↓	?	↓
NSAIDs	↑↑	↑	↓	↓	?	↓
Angiotensin II	↑	↑↑	↓	↑	↓	↓→
Endothelin-1	↑	↑↑	↓	↑	↓	↓
High protein diet	↓	→	↑	↑	→	↑
Nitric oxide	↓	↓	↑	?	↑	↑ (?)
Atrial natriuretic peptide (high dose)	↓	→	↑	↑	↑	↑
Prostaglandins E_2/I_2	↓	↓	↑	↑	?	↑
Calcium channel blockers	↓	→	↑	↑	?	↑
ACE inhibitors/angiotensin receptor blockers	↓	↓↓	↑	↓	↑	?*

Figure 2.6 Physiologic and pharmacologic influences on glomerular hemodynamics. The overall effect on glomerular filtration rate (GFR) will depend on renal blood flow, net ultrafiltration pressure, and the ultrafiltration coefficient (K_f), the latter being controlled by mesangial cell contraction/relaxation. The effects shown are those seen when the agents are applied (or inhibited) in isolation; the actual changes that occur are dose dependent and are modulated by other agents. *In clinical practice, GFR is usually either decreased or unaffected. ACE, angiotensin converting enzyme; NSAIDs, nonsteroidal anti-inflammatory drugs.

down its electrochemical gradient, the other(s) against (see later discussion).

3. *Diffusion through a membrane channel* (or pore) formed by specific integral membrane proteins is also a form of facilitated diffusion because it enables charged and lipophobic molecules to pass through the membrane at a high rate.

Active Transport

When an ion is moved directly against an electrochemical gradient ("uphill"), a source of energy is required, and this is known as *active* transport. In cells, this energy is derived from metabolism: ATP production and its hydrolysis. The most important active cell transport mechanism is the sodium pump, which extrudes Na^+ from inside the cell in exchange for K^+ from outside the cell.[6] In the kidney, it is located only in the basolateral membrane. It derives energy from the enzymatic hydrolysis of ATP; hence, its more precise description as Na^+,K^+-ATPase. It exchanges $3Na^+$ ions for $2K^+$ ions, which makes it electrogenic since it extrudes a net positive charge from the cell. It is an example of a *primary* active transport mechanism. Other well-defined primary active transport mechanisms in the kidney are the proton-secreting H^+-ATPase, important in H^+ secretion in the distal nephron, and Ca^{2+}-ATPase, partly responsible for calcium reabsorption.

Activity of the basolateral Na^+, K^+-ATPase is key to the operation of all the passive transport processes outlined earlier. It ensures that the intracellular Na^+ concentration is kept low (10 to 20 mmol/l) and the K^+ concentration high ($\sim$150 mmol/l), compared with their extracellular concentrations ($\sim$140 and $\sim$4 mmol/l, respectively). Sodium entry into tubular cells down the electrochemical gradient maintained by the sodium pump is either through Na^+ channels (in the distal nephron) or linked (coupled) via specific membrane carrier proteins to the influx (*symport* or *cotransport*) or efflux (*antiport* or *countertransport*) of other molecules or ions: in various parts of the nephron, glucose, phosphate, amino acids, K^+, and Cl^- can all be cotransported with Na^+ entry, while H^+ and Ca^{2+} can be countertransported against Na^+ entry. In each case, the nonsodium molecule or ion is transported against its electrochemical gradient, using energy derived from the "downhill" movement of sodium. Their ultimate dependence on the *primary* active sodium pump makes them *secondary* active transport mechanisms.

TRANSPORT IN SPECIFIC NEPHRON SEGMENTS

Given a typical GFR, approximately 180 l of (largely protein-free) plasma are filtered each day, necessitating massive reabsorption by the nephron as a whole. Figure 2.7 shows the major transport mechanisms operating along the nephron (with the exception of the loop of Henle, which is dealt with separately).

Proximal Tubule

As indicated in Chapter 1, the first part of the nephron, the proximal tubule, is well adapted for bulk reabsorption. The epithelial cells have microvilli (brush border) on their apical surface, providing a large absorptive area, while the basolateral membrane is thrown into folds that similarly enhance surface area. The cells are rich in mitochondria (concentrated near the basolateral membrane) and lysosomal vacuoles, and the tight junctions between adjacent cells are in fact relatively leaky. The *proximal convoluted tubule* ([PCT] pars convoluta) makes up the first two thirds of the proximal tubule; the final third is the *proximal straight tubule* (pars recta).

Based on subtle structural and functional differences, the proximal tubule epithelium is subdivided into three types: S1 makes up the initial short segment of the PCT; S2, the remainder of the PCT and the cortical segment of the pars recta; and S3, the medullary segment of the pars recta. The proximal tubule as a whole is responsible for the bulk of Na^+, K^+, Cl^-, and HCO_3^- reabsorption, and the nearly complete reabsorption of glucose, amino acids, and low molecular weight proteins (e.g., retinol binding protein, α- and β-microglobulins) that have penetrated the filtration barrier. Most other filtered solutes are also reabsorbed to some extent in the proximal tubule (e.g., $\sim$60% of calcium, $\sim$80% of phosphate, $\sim$50% of urea). The wall of the proximal tubule is highly permeable to water, so no quantitatively significant osmotic gradient can be established; thus, most filtered water ($\sim$65%) is also reabsorbed at this site. In the final section of the proximal tubule (late S2 and S3), there is some *secretion* of weak organic acids and bases, including most diuretics and *p*-aminohippurate.

Loop of Henle

The loop of Henle is defined anatomically as comprising the pars recta of the proximal tubule (thick descending limb), the thin descending and ascending limbs, the thick ascending limb (TAL), and the macula densa. In addition to its role in the continuing reabsorption of solutes (Na^+, Cl^-, K^+, Ca^{2+}, Mg^{2+}), this part of the nephron is responsible for the kidney's ability to generate a concentrated or dilute urine and is discussed in more detail later.

Distal Nephron

The distal tubule is made up of three segments: the *distal convoluted tubule* (DCT), where thiazide-sensitive NaCl reabsorption (via an apical cotransporter) occurs (see Fig. 2.7); the *connecting tubule* (CNT), whose function is essentially intermediate between that of the DCT and that of the next segment; and the *initial collecting duct*, which is of the same epithelial type as the cortical collecting duct. Two cell types make up the cortical collecting duct. The predominant type, the *principal cell* (see Fig. 2.7), is responsible for Na^+ reabsorption and K^+ secretion (as well as for water reabsorption; see later discussion). Sodium ions enter principal cells from the lumen via apical Na^+ channels (ENaC) and are extruded by the basolateral Na^+, K^+-ATPase. This process is electrogenic and sets up a lumen-negative potential difference. Potassium ions enter principal cells via the same basolateral Na^+, K^+-ATPase and leave via K^+ channels in both membranes; however, the smaller potential difference across the apical membrane (owing to Na^+ entry) favors K^+ secretion into the lumen. The other cells in the late distal tubule and cortical collecting duct, the *intercalated cells*, are responsible for secretion of H^+ (by α-intercalated cells) or HCO_3^- (by β-intercalated cells) into the final urine (see Fig. 2.7). The medullary collecting duct consists largely of modified principal cells that reabsorb Na^+ but do not secrete K^+.

Figures 2.8 and 2.9 show schematically the sites of Na^+ and K^+ reabsorption/secretion along the nephron. Figure 2.10 shows the pathophysiologic consequences of known genetic defects in some of the major transporters in the nephron (see Chapter 46).

GLOMERULOTUBULAR BALANCE

Because the proportion of filtered sodium that is excreted in the urine is so small (normally <1%), it follows that, in the absence of any compensatory changes in reabsorption, even small changes in the filtered load would cause major changes in the amount excreted. For example, if GFR were to increase by 10% and the

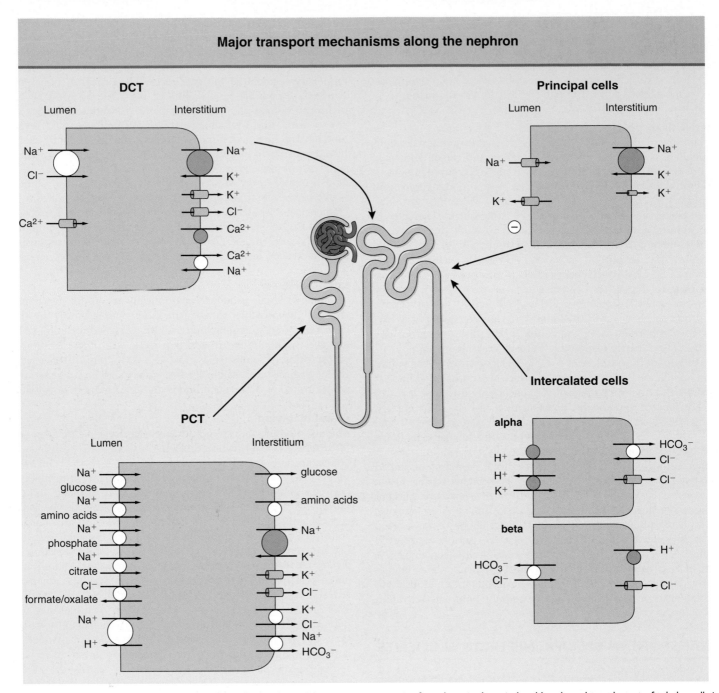

Figure 2.7   Major transport mechanisms along the nephron. Major transport proteins for solutes in the apical and basolateral membranes of tubular cells in specific regions of the nephron. Stoichiometry is not indicated; it is not 1:1 in all cases. *Pink circles* represent primary active transport; *white circles* represent carrier-mediated transport (secondary active); *cylinders* represent ion channels. In the PCT, Na^+ enters the cell via a Na^+-H^+ exchanger and a series of cotransporters; in the DCT, Na^+ enters the cell via the thiazide-sensitive Na^+-Cl^- cotransporter; and in the principal cells of the cortical collecting duct (CCD), Na^+ enters via a channel (ENaC). In all cases, Na^+ is extruded from the cells via the basolateral Na^+,K^+-ATPase. Transporters in the thick ascending limb of Henle are dealt with separately (see Fig. 2.12). DCT, distal convoluted tubule; PCT, proximal convoluted tubule.

rate of reabsorption were to remain unchanged, sodium excretion would increase more than 10-fold. However, an intrinsic feature of tubular function is that the extent of sodium reabsorption in a given nephron segment is roughly proportional to the sodium delivery to that segment. This is the phenomenon of *glomerulotubular balance*. Perfect glomerulotubular balance would mean that both sodium reabsorption and sodium excretion changed in exactly the same proportion as the change in GFR, but in fact glomerulotubular balance is usually somewhat less than perfect. Thus, if GFR *were* to increase by 10%, overall reabsorption in the

nephron would increase, not by 10%, but by slightly less. Most studies of glomerulotubular balance have focused on the proximal tubule. However, succeeding nephron segments exhibit the same property, so if the load to the loop of Henle and/or to the distal tubule is increased, some of the excess is mopped up. This is part of the reason why diuretics acting on the proximal tubule are relatively ineffective compared with those acting further downstream: with the latter, there is less scope for buffering their effects. It is also the reason why combining two diuretics that act on different nephron segments is a particularly effective strategy.

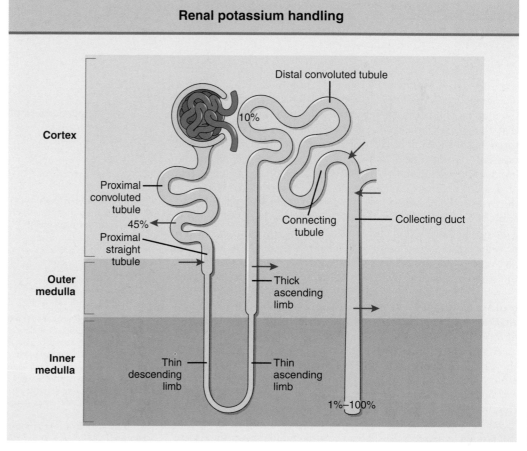

Renal sodium handling

Figure 2.8 Renal sodium handling along the nephron. Figures outside the nephron represent the approximate percentage of the filtered load reabsorbed in each region. Figures within the nephron represent the percentages remaining. Most filtered sodium is reabsorbed in the proximal tubule and loop of Henle; normal day-to-day control of sodium excretion is exerted in the distal nephron.

Renal potassium handling

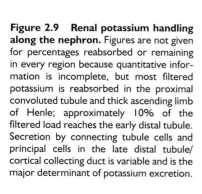

Figure 2.9 Renal potassium handling along the nephron. Figures are not given for percentages reabsorbed or remaining in every region because quantitative information is incomplete, but most filtered potassium is reabsorbed in the proximal convoluted tubule and thick ascending limb of Henle; approximately 10% of the filtered load reaches the early distal tubule. Secretion by connecting tubule cells and principal cells in the late distal tubule/cortical collecting duct is variable and is the major determinant of potassium excretion.

Defects in transport proteins resulting in renal disease	
Transporter	Consequence of Mutation
Proximal Tubule	
Apical Na$^+$-cystine cotransporter	Cystinuria
Apical Na$^+$-glucose cotransporter (SGLT2)	Renal glycosuria
Basolateral Na$^+$-HCO$_3^-$ cotransporter	Proximal renal tubular acidosis
Intracellular Cl$^-$ channel (ClC5)	Dent's disease
Thick Ascending Limb	
Apical Na$^+$-K$^+$-2Cl$^-$ cotransporter	Bartter syndrome type 1
Apical K$^+$ channel	Bartter syndrome type 2
Basolateral Cl$^-$ channel	Bartter syndrome type 3
Basolateral Cl$^-$ channel accessory protein	Bartter syndrome type 4
Ca^{2+}-sensing receptor (activating mutation)	Bartter syndrome type 5
Distal Convoluted Tubule	
Apical Na$^+$-Cl$^-$ cotransporter	Gitelman's syndrome
Collecting Duct	
Apical Na$^+$ channel (principal cells)	*Overexpression*: Liddle disease *Underexpression*: pseudohypoaldosteronism type 1
Basolateral Cl$^-$/HCO$_3^-$ exchanger (intercalated cells)	Distal renal tubular acidosis
Apical H$^+$-ATPase (intercalated cells)	Distal renal tubular acidosis (with or without deafness)

Figure 2.10   Defects in transport proteins resulting in renal disease.

The mechanism of glomerulotubular balance is not fully understood. As far as the proximal tubule is concerned, physical factors operating across peritubular capillary walls may be involved. Glomerular filtration of (essentially protein-free) fluid means that the plasma leaving the glomeruli in efferent arterioles and supplying the peritubular capillaries has a relatively high oncotic pressure, which favors uptake of fluid reabsorbed from the proximal tubules. Similarly, the passage of blood through two sets of resistance vessels (afferent and efferent arterioles) means that the hydrostatic pressure in peritubular capillaries is particularly low, again favoring fluid uptake. If GFR were reduced in the absence of a change in RPF, peritubular capillary oncotic pressure would also be reduced, and the tendency to take up fluid reabsorbed from the proximal tubule would be diminished. It is thought that some of this fluid might leak back through the (leaky) tight junctions, thereby reducing net reabsorption (Fig. 2.11). This mechanism could only work if GFR changed in the absence of a corresponding change in RPF: if the two change in parallel (i.e., unchanged *filtration fraction*), there will be no change in oncotic pressure.

A second contributory factor to glomerulotubular balance in the proximal tubule might be the filtered loads of glucose and amino acids. If these loads increase (due to increased GFR), the rates of sodium-coupled glucose and amino acid reabsorption in the proximal tubule will also increase.

Although the renal sympathetic nerves and certain hormones can influence reabsorption in the proximal tubule (e.g., Ang II) and

loop of Henle (e.g., vasopressin), under normal circumstances, the combined effects of autoregulation (see previous discussion) and glomerulotubular balance ensure that a relatively constant load of glomerular filtrate is delivered to the distal tubule. It is in the final segments of the nephron that normal day-to-day control of sodium excretion is exerted. In this regard, recent evidence points toward important roles for the late DCT and the CNT, as well as for the collecting duct.[7] The hormone *aldosterone*, secreted from the adrenal cortex, stimulates the basolateral sodium pump in principal cells and CNT cells, and also increases the number of sodium channels in the apical membrane (see Fig. 2.7). This not only stimulates sodium reabsorption but, by further depolarizing the apical membrane, also facilitates potassium secretion in the late distal tubule/cortical collecting duct. The actions of aldosterone are mediated by mineralocorticoid receptors within principal cells (and CNT cells). These receptors have equal affinity in vitro for aldosterone and adrenal *glucocorticoids*. Circulating concentrations of the latter vastly exceed those of aldosterone, but, in vivo, the mineralocorticoid receptors show specificity for aldosterone due to the presence along the distal nephron of the enzyme *11β-hydroxysteroid dehydrogenase 2*, which inactivates glucocorticoids in the vicinity of the receptor.[8]

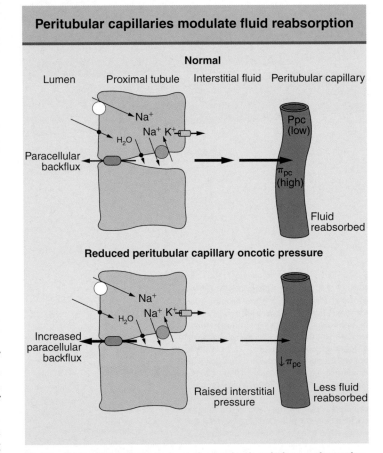

Figure 2.11   Physical factors and proximal tubular reabsorption. Influence of peritubular capillary oncotic pressure on net reabsorption in proximal tubules. Uptake of reabsorbate into peritubular capillaries is determined by the balance of hydrostatic and oncotic pressures across the capillary wall. Compared with those in systemic capillaries, the peritubular capillary hydrostatic (P_{pc}) and oncotic (π_{pc}) pressures are low and high, respectively, so that uptake of proximal tubular reabsorbate into the capillaries is favored. If peritubular capillary oncotic pressure decreases (and/or hydrostatic pressure increases), less fluid is taken up, interstitial pressure increases, and more fluid may leak back into the lumen paracellularly; net reabsorption in proximal tubules would therefore be reduced.

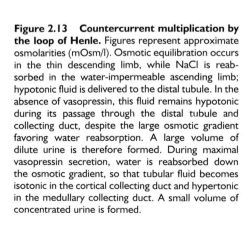

Transport mechanisms in the thick ascending limb

Figure 2.12   Transport mechanisms in the thick ascending limb of Henle. The major cellular entry mechanism is the Na^+-K^+-$2Cl^-$ cotransporter. The transepithelial potential difference drives paracellular transport of Na^+, K^+, Ca^{2+}, and Mg^{2+}.

COUNTERCURRENT SYSTEM

A major function of the loop of Henle is the generation and maintenance of the interstitial osmotic gradient that increases from the renal cortex ($\sim$290 mOsm/kg) to the tip of the medulla ($\sim$1200 mOsm/kg). The anatomic loop of Henle reabsorbs approximately 40% of filtered Na^+, mostly in the TAL, and approximately 25% of filtered water in the pars recta and thin descending limb. The thin descending limb is permeable to water but relatively impermeable to Na^+, whereas both the thin ascending limb and the TAL are essentially impermeable to water; in the thin ascending limb, Na^+ is reabsorbed passively, but in the TAL, it is reabsorbed actively. Active Na^+ reabsorption in the TAL is again driven by the basolateral sodium pump, which maintains a low intracellular Na^+ concentration, allowing Na^+ entry from the lumen via the Na^+-$2Cl^-$-K^+ cotransporter and, to a much lesser extent, the Na^+-H^+ exchanger (Fig. 2.12). The apical Na^+-$2Cl^-$-K^+ cotransporter is unique to this nephron segment and is the site of action of loop diuretics such as furosemide and bumetanide. Na^+ exits the cell via the sodium pump, and Cl^- and K^+ exit via basolateral ion channels and a K^+-Cl^- cotransporter. K^+ also re-enters the lumen (recycles) through apical membrane potassium channels. Re-entry of K^+ into the tubular lumen is necessary for normal operation of the Na^+-$2Cl^-$-K^+ cotransporter, presumably because the availability of K^+ is a limiting factor for the transporter (the K^+ concentration in tubular fluid being much lower than those of Na^+ and Cl^-). K^+ entry is also partly responsible for generating the lumen-positive potential difference found in this segment. This potential difference drives additional Na^+ reabsorption through the paracellular pathway: for each Na^+ reabsorbed transcellularly, another one is reabsorbed paracellularly (see Fig. 2.12).[9] Other cations (K^+, Ca^{2+}, Mg^{2+}) are also reabsorbed by this route. The reabsorption of NaCl along the TAL in the absence of significant water reabsorption means that the tubular fluid leaving this segment is *hypotonic*; hence, its other name of the *diluting segment*.

The U-shaped, countercurrent arrangement of the loop of Henle, the differences in permeability of the descending and ascending limbs to Na^+ and water, and active Na^+ reabsorption in the TAL are the basis of *countercurrent multiplication* and generation of the medullary osmotic gradient (Fig. 2.13). Fluid

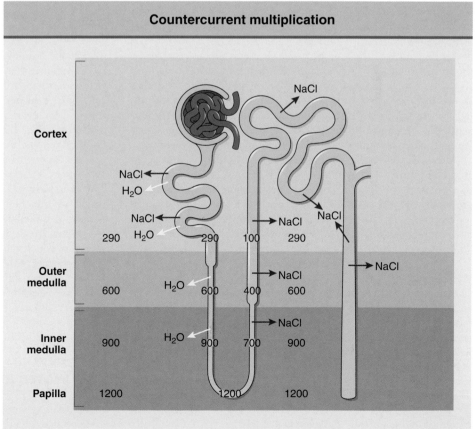

Countercurrent multiplication

Figure 2.13   Countercurrent multiplication by the loop of Henle. Figures represent approximate osmolarities (mOsm/l). Osmotic equilibration occurs in the thin descending limb, while NaCl is reabsorbed in the water-impermeable ascending limb; hypotonic fluid is delivered to the distal tubule. In the absence of vasopressin, this fluid remains hypotonic during its passage through the distal tubule and collecting duct, despite the large osmotic gradient favoring water reabsorption. A large volume of dilute urine is therefore formed. During maximal vasopressin secretion, water is reabsorbed down the osmotic gradient, so that tubular fluid becomes isotonic in the cortical collecting duct and hypertonic in the medullary collecting duct. A small volume of concentrated urine is formed.

entering the descending limb from the proximal tubule is isotonic (~290 mOsm/kg). However, the increased medullary osmolarity resulting from NaCl reabsorption in the water-impermeable ascending limb induces water reabsorption from the thin descending limb, thereby increasing the osmolarity and NaCl concentration of the fluid delivered to the ascending limb. These events, combined with continuing NaCl reabsorption in the ascending limb, result in a progressive increase in medullary osmolarity from corticomedullary junction to papillary tip. A similar osmotic gradient exists in the thin descending limb, while at any level in the ascending limb, the osmolarity is less than in the surrounding tissue. Thus, hypotonic (~100 mOsm/kg) fluid is delivered to the distal tubule. Ultimately, the energy source for countercurrent multiplication is active Na^+ reabsorption in the TAL. As already indicated, Na^+ reabsorption in the thin ascending limb is passive; this is thought to be made possible by a mechanism involving urea.

Role of Urea

The thin limbs of the loop of Henle are relatively permeable to urea (ascending > descending), but more distal nephron segments (TAL and beyond) are urea impermeable up to the final part of the inner medullary collecting duct. By this stage, vasopressin-dependent water reabsorption in the collecting ducts (see later discussion) has led to a high urea concentration within the lumen, which in turn leads to reabsorption of urea into the interstitium by vasopressin-sensitive urea transporters along the terminal portion of the inner medullary collecting duct.[10] The interstitial urea exchanges with vasa recta capillaries (see later discussion), in which uptake is facilitated by a specific urea carrier mechanism, and some urea enters the S3 segment of the pars recta and the descending and ascending thin limbs of the loop of Henle; it is then returned to the inner medullary collecting ducts to be reabsorbed. The net result of this recycling process is to add urea to the inner medullary interstitium, thereby increasing interstitial osmolality, which in turn increases water abstraction from the thin descending limb of the loop of Henle. It is this process that raises the intraluminal Na^+ concentration in the thin descending limb and sets the scene for passive Na^+ diffusion from the thin ascending limb into the surrounding inner medullary interstitium. It is worth emphasizing, however, that in the final analysis, it is *active* Na^+ reabsorption in the TAL, diluting the tubular fluid that enters the distal nephron, which makes such a system possible.

Although this model for passive Na^+ reabsorption in the thin ascending limb is an attractive one, it is only fair to point out that not all experimental evidence concerning the permeability properties of the thin limbs is consistent with the model's requirements.[11] Thus, the details of the mechanisms operating in the inner medulla are still far from settled.

Vasa Recta

The capillaries that supply the medulla also have a special anatomic arrangement. If they passed through the medulla as a more usual capillary network, they would soon dissipate the medullary osmotic gradient due to equilibration of the latter with the isotonic capillary blood. This does not happen to any appreciable extent, because the U-shaped arrangement of the *vasa recta* ensures that solute entry and water loss in the *descending* vasa recta are offset by solute loss and water entry in the *ascending* vasa recta. This is the process of *countercurrent exchange* and is entirely passive (Fig. 2.14).

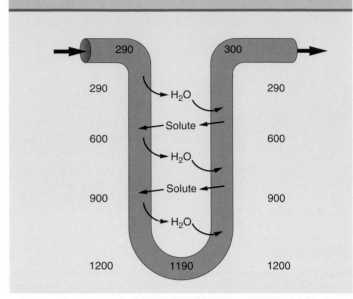

Figure 2.14 Countercurrent exchange by the vasa recta. Figures represent approximate osmolarities (mOsm/l). The vasa recta capillary walls are highly permeable, but the U-shaped arrangement of the vessels minimizes the dissipation of the medullary osmotic gradient. Nevertheless, because equilibration across the capillary walls is not instantaneous, a certain amount of solute is removed from the interstitium.

Renal Medullary Hypoxia

Countercurrent exchange by the medullary capillaries applies also to oxygen, which diffuses from descending to ascending vasa recta, bypassing the deeper regions. This phenomenon, combined with ongoing energy-dependent salt transport in the (outer medullary) TAL, has the consequence that medullary tissue is relatively hypoxic. Thus, the partial pressure of oxygen normally decreases from ~50 mm Hg in the cortex to ~10 mm Hg in the inner medulla.[12] Administration of furosemide, by inhibiting oxygen consumption in the TAL, increases medullary oxygenation. As part of the adaptation to this relatively hypoxic environment, medullary cells have a higher capacity for glycolysis than do cells in the cortex. Moreover, a number of *heat shock proteins* are expressed in the medulla; these assist cell survival by restoring damaged proteins and inhibiting apoptosis.[12]

The degree of medullary hypoxia depends on the balance between medullary blood flow and oxygen consumption in the TAL. The former is controlled by contractile cells, called *pericytes*, which are attached to the descending vasa recta. In health, this balance is modulated by a variety of autocrine/paracrine agents (e.g., nitric oxide, eicosanoids, adenosine; see later discussion), several of which can increase medullary oxygenation by simultaneously reducing both pericyte contraction and TAL transport. There is evidence that some cases of radiocontrast-induced nephropathy result from disturbance of this balance between oxygen supply and demand, with consequent hypoxic medullary injury in which the normal cellular adaptations are overwhelmed, with subsequent apoptotic and necrotic cell death.

VASOPRESSIN (ANTIDIURETIC HORMONE) AND WATER REABSORPTION

Vasopressin, or antidiuretic hormone, is a nonapeptide synthesized in specialized neurons of the supraoptic and paraventricular nuclei. It is transported from these nuclei to the posterior pituitary and released in response to increases in plasma osmolality and decreases in blood pressure. Osmoreceptors are found in the hypothalamus, and there is also input to this region from arterial baroreceptors and atrial stretch receptors. The actions of vasopressin are mediated by three receptor subtypes: V_{1a}, V_{1b}, and V_2 receptors. V_{1a} receptors are found in vascular smooth muscle and are coupled to the phosphoinositol pathway; they cause an increase in intracellular Ca^{2+}, resulting in contraction. (V_{1a} receptors have also been identified in the apical membrane of several nephron segments, although their role is not clear.) V_{1b} receptors are found in the anterior pituitary, where vasopressin modulates adrenocorticotropic hormone release. V_2 receptors are found in the basolateral membrane of principal cells in the late distal tubule and the whole length of the collecting duct; they are coupled to a G_s protein and thereby to cyclic adenosine monophosphate generation, which ultimately leads to the insertion of water channels (*aquaporins*) into the apical membrane of this otherwise water-impermeable segment (Fig. 2.15). In the X-linked form of nephrogenic diabetes insipidus (the most common hereditary cause), the V_2 receptor is defective.[13]

Several aquaporins have been identified in the kidney.[14] Aquaporin-1 is found in apical and basolateral membranes of the proximal tubule and thin descending limb of Henle and is responsible for the permanently high water permeability of these segments. Aquaporins-3 and -4 are constitutively expressed in the basolateral membrane of principal cells in collecting duct epithelium. It is aquaporin-2 that is responsible for the variable water permeability of the collecting duct. Acute vasopressin release causes shuttling of aquaporin-2 from intracellular vesicles to the apical membrane, while chronically raised vasopressin levels increase aquaporin-2 expression. The apical insertion of aquaporin-2 allows reabsorption of water, driven by the high interstitial osmolality achieved and maintained by the countercurrent system. Vasopressin also contributes to the effectiveness of this system by increasing Na^+ reabsorption in the TAL and urea reabsorption in the inner medullary collecting duct. In the (rare) autosomal recessive and (even rarer) autosomal dominant forms of nephrogenic diabetes insipidus, aquaporin-2 is abnormal and/or fails to translocate to the apical membrane.[14]

Interestingly, aquaporin-2 dysfunction also appears to underlie the well-known urinary concentrating defect associated with hypercalcemia. Increased intraluminal Ca^{2+} concentrations, acting via an apically located calcium-sensing receptor, interfere with the insertion of aquaporin-2 channels in the apical membrane of the medullary collecting duct. In addition, stimulation of a calcium receptor in the basolateral membrane of the TAL inhibits solute transport in this nephron segment, thereby reducing the medullary osmotic gradient.[15]

INTEGRATED CONTROL OF RENAL FUNCTION

Lack of space precludes an account of the mechanisms regulating plasma levels of individual ions such as potassium, calcium, phosphate, and bicarbonate (see Chapters 9 through 11). Instead, we focus on those mechanisms directed toward the control of *effective circulating volume*, a poorly defined and unmeasurable volume that reflects the degree of fullness of the vasculature. Effective circulating volume normally varies in direct proportion to the extracellular fluid volume (ECFV). However, this relationship breaks down in heart failure, cirrhosis, and nephrotic syndrome, when effective circulating volume is reduced even though ECFV is not, triggering inappropriate renal fluid retention and contributing to the edema characteristic of these conditions. Renal control of effective circulating volume is achieved by regulating the *sodium* content of the body. Osmoreceptor-mediated control of vasopressin secretion and thirst ensures that extracellular fluid osmolarity and therefore sodium concentration are closely regulated. Thus, by controlling the extracellular sodium *content*, extracellular *volume* is also controlled. Effective circulating volume is monitored largely by intravascular receptors located in the aorta and carotid sinuses (baroreceptors), the renal afferent arterioles, and the atria of the heart. The effector mechanisms usually work in concert to influence both glomerular filtration and tubular reabsorption, but in the interests of clarity they are described individually.

Renal Interstitial Hydrostatic Pressure

Acute increases in arterial blood pressure lead to natriuresis (*pressure natriuresis*). Since autoregulation is not perfect, part of this response is mediated by increases in RBF and GFR (see Fig. 2.3), but the main cause is reduced tubular reabsorption, which appears to result largely from an increase in renal interstitial hydrostatic pressure (RIHP). An elevated RIHP could reduce net reabsorption in the proximal tubule by increasing paracellular backflux through the tight junctions in the tubular wall (see Fig. 2.11). There is good evidence that the increase in RIHP is dependent on intrarenally produced *nitric oxide*.[16] Moreover, increased nitric oxide production in macula densa cells (which contain the neuronal [type I] isoform of nitric oxide synthase [nNOS]) blunts the sensitivity of TG feedback (see later discussion), thereby allowing increased NaCl delivery to the distal nephron without incurring a TG feedback–mediated decrease in GFR.[17]

A further renal action of nitric oxide results from the presence of inducible (type II) nitric oxide synthase in glomerular mesangial cells. Local production of nitric oxide counteracts the mesangial

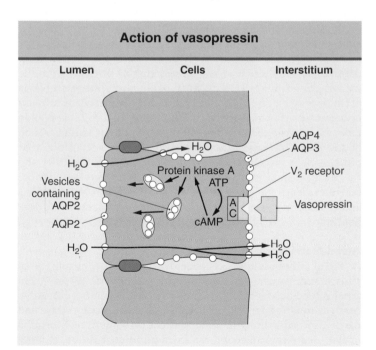

Figure 2.15 Mechanism of action of vasopressin (antidiuretic hormone). The hormone binds to V_2 receptors on the basolateral membrane of collecting duct principal cells and increases intracellular cyclic adenosine monophosphate (cAMP) production, causing, via intermediate reactions involving protein kinase A, insertion of preformed water channels (aquaporin-2 [AQP-2]) into the apical membrane. The water permeability of the basolateral membrane, which contains aquaporins-3 and -4, is permanently high. Therefore, vasopressin secretion allows transcellular movement of water from lumen to interstitium. AC, adenylate cyclase.

23

contractile response to agonists such as Ang II and endothelin (see later discussion). Finally, nitric oxide may have a role in the regulation of medullary blood flow. Locally synthesized nitric oxide offsets the vasoconstrictor effects of other agents on the pericytes of the descending vasa recta and additionally reduces Na^+ reabsorption in the TAL; both actions will help protect the renal medulla from hypoxia (see previous discussion).

Renal Sympathetic Nerves

Reductions in arterial pressure and/or central venous pressure result in reduced afferent signaling from arterial baroreceptors and/or atrial volume receptors, which elicits a reflex increase in renal sympathetic nervous discharge. This reduces urinary sodium excretion in at least three ways:

1. Constriction of afferent and efferent arterioles (predominantly afferent), thereby directly reducing RBF and GFR and indirectly reducing RIHP
2. Direct stimulation of sodium reabsorption in the proximal tubule and the TAL of the loop of Henle
3. Stimulation of *renin* secretion by afferent arteriolar cells (see later discussion)

Renin Angiotensin Aldosterone System

The renin angiotensin aldosterone system is central to the control of ECFV and blood pressure. The enzyme renin is synthesized and stored in specialized afferent arteriolar cells that form part of the juxtaglomerular apparatus (see Fig. 2.4) and is released into the circulation in response to

- Increased renal sympathetic nervous discharge
- Reduced stretch of the afferent arteriole following a reduction in renal perfusion pressure (reduced arterial pressure)
- Reduced delivery of NaCl to the macula densa region of the nephron

Renin catalyzes the production of the decapeptide angiotensin I from circulating angiotensinogen (synthesized in the liver); angiotensin I is in turn converted to the octapeptide *Ang II* by the ubiquitous angiotensin-converting enzyme. Ang II has a number of actions pertinent to the control of ECFV and blood pressure:

- It causes general arteriolar vasoconstriction, including renal afferent and (particularly) efferent arterioles, thereby increasing arterial pressure but reducing RBF. The tendency of P_{gc} to increase is offset by Ang II–induced mesangial cell contraction and reduced K_f; thus, the overall effect on GFR is unpredictable.
- It directly stimulates sodium reabsorption in the proximal tubule.
- It stimulates *aldosterone* secretion from the zona glomerulosa of the adrenal cortex. As described earlier, aldosterone stimulates sodium reabsorption in the distal tubule and collecting duct.

Eicosanoids

Eicosanoids are a family of metabolites of arachidonic acid, produced enzymatically by three systems: cyclooxygenase (of which two isoforms exist: COX-1 and COX-2, both constitutively expressed in the kidney), cytochrome P-450, and lipoxygenase. The major renal eicosanoids produced by the COX system are *prostaglandin E_2* and *prostaglandin I_2*, both of which are renal vasodilators and act to buffer the effects of renal vasoconstrictor agents such as Ang II and norepinephrine; and *thromboxane A_2*, a vasoconstrictor. Prostaglandin E_2 is also believed to have tubular effects, inhibiting sodium reabsorption in the TAL of the loop of Henle and in the collecting duct. Its action in the TAL, together

with a dilator effect on vasa recta pericytes, is another paracrine regulatory mechanism that helps to protect the renal medulla from hypoxia.

The metabolism of arachidonic acid by renal cytochrome P-450 enzymes yields *epoxyeicosatrienoic acids* (EETs), *20-hydroxyeicosatetraenoic acid* (20-HETE), and *dihydroxyeicosatrienoic acids* (DHETs). These compounds appear to have a multiplicity of autocrine/paracrine/second messenger effects on the renal vasculature and tubules that have yet to be fully unraveled.[18] Like prostaglandins, EETs are vasodilator agents, whereas 20-HETE is a potent renal arteriolar constrictor and may be involved in the vasoconstrictor effect of Ang II as well as the TG feedback mechanism. 20-HETE also constricts vasa recta pericytes and may be involved in the control of medullary blood flow. Recent work suggests that locally produced 20-HETE and EETs can inhibit sodium reabsorption in the proximal tubule and TAL.[19] Indeed, there is evidence that cytochrome P-450 metabolites of arachidonic acid contribute to the reduced proximal tubular reabsorption seen in pressure natriuresis.

The third enzyme system that metabolizes arachidonic acid, the lipoxygenase system, is activated (in leukocytes, mast cells, and macrophages) during inflammation and injury and is not considered here.

COX-2 is present in macula densa cells, and there is good evidence that it occupies a critical role in the stimulation of renin release in response to reduced NaCl delivery to the macula densa.[20] A low-sodium diet increases COX-2 expression in the macula densa and simultaneously increases renin secretion; the renin response is absent in COX-2 knockout mice. Furthermore, in the rabbit isolated juxtaglomerular apparatus, selective inhibition of COX-2 virtually abolishes renin release in response to reduced luminal NaCl at the macula densa. It is likely, therefore, that the hyporeninemia observed during administration of non-steroidal anti-inflammatory drugs is largely a consequence of COX-2 inhibition. The principal COX-2 product responsible for enhancing renin secretion is thought to be prostaglandin E_2.

As already indicated, nNOS (type I) is also present in macula densa cells, and there is clear evidence that nitric oxide from the macula densa blunts TGF.[21] Nitric oxide also appears to play a permissive role in renin secretion, although the mechanism is not understood. The increase in macula densa COX-2 expression induced by a low-sodium diet is attenuated during administration of selective nNOS inhibitors, which has led to speculation that nitric oxide is responsible for the increase in COX-2 activity and the resulting increase in juxtaglomerular renin secretion.[22] More recent evidence, however, is less conclusive. The roles of COX-2 and nNOS, both established and putative, are shown diagrammatically in Figure 2.16.

Atrial Natriuretic Peptide

If blood volume increases significantly, the resulting atrial stretch stimulates the release of *atrial natriuretic peptide* from atrial myocytes. This hormone increases sodium excretion, partly through suppression of renin and aldosterone release and partly through a direct inhibitory effect on sodium reabsorption in the medullary collecting duct. An additional action of atrial natriuretic peptide may be to increase GFR, since high doses cause afferent arteriolar vasodilatation and mesangial cell relaxation (thus increasing K_f; see Fig. 2.6).

Endothelins

Endothelin-1 (ET-1) through -3 are a family of peptides with potent vasoconstrictor action, to which the renal vasculature is exquisitely

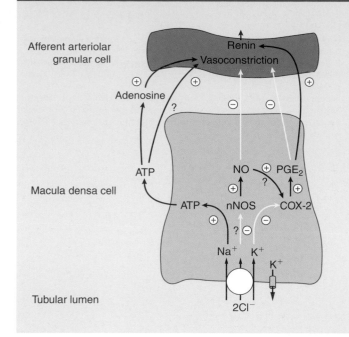

Interactions between macula densa and afferent arteriole

Figure 2.16 Interactions between macula densa and afferent arteriole: proposed mediators of renin secretion and tubuloglomerular feedback. Both cyclooxygenase-2 (COX-2) and neuronal nitric oxide synthase (nNOS) enzyme systems are present in macula densa cells. Increased NaCl delivery to the macula densa stimulates NaCl entry into the cells via the $Na^+-K^+-2Cl^-$ cotransporter. This causes afferent arteriolar constriction, through adenosine and/or adenosine triphosphate (ATP), and also inhibits COX-2 activity; the latter effect might be mediated partly through inhibition of (nNOS-mediated) nitric oxide (NO) production. Generation of prostaglandin E_2 by COX-2 stimulates renin release. Prostaglandin E_2 (PGE_2) also modulates vasoconstriction, as does nitric oxide.

sensitive.[23] Endothelins function primarily as autocrine or paracrine agents. The kidney is a rich source of endothelins, the predominant isoform being ET-1. ET-1 is generated throughout the renal vasculature, including afferent and efferent arterioles (where it causes vasoconstriction, possibly mediated by 20-HETE) and mesangial cells (where it causes contraction, i.e., decreases K_f). Consequently, renal ET-1 causes profound reductions in RBF and GFR (see Fig. 2.6). The effects, if any, of endothelins on tubular function are not clear; tubular endothelin receptors are found mainly in the collecting duct, and their activation inhibits sodium and water reabsorption. There is evidence that ET-1 may be involved in disturbed renal function in pathologic conditions such as congestive heart failure and radiocontrast-induced acute renal failure; however, its role in normal renal physiology remains to be clarified.

Purines

It is likely that in the future an increasing number of autocrine or paracrine agents will need to be added to the list of controlling factors. Prime candidates for such a role are the purines (ATP, adenosine diphosphate [ADP], adenosine, and uric acid). Purinoceptors are subdivided into P1 and P2 receptors. The former are responsive to adenosine and are more usually known as adenosine receptors (A_1, A_{2a}, A_{2b}, and A_3), while the latter, responsive to nucleotides (ATP and/or ADP), are further subdivided into P2X (ligand-gated ion channels) and P2Y (metabotropic) receptors, each category having a number of subtypes. As indicated earlier, A_1 and $P2X_1$ receptors are found in afferent arterioles and mediate vasoconstriction. All three categories of purinoceptor are also found along the nephron, sometimes on the basolateral membrane, sometimes on the apical membrane, and sometimes both.[24] Locally produced adenosine enhances proximal tubular reabsorption, while luminal ADP inhibits it.[25] In the collecting duct, basolateral ATP inhibits vasopressin-sensitive water reabsorption, and basolateral or luminal ATP inhibits sodium reabsorption.[24] Finally, a recent investigation suggests that the end product of purine metabolism, uric acid, may cause renal vasoconstriction, possibly by inhibiting endothelial release of nitric oxide, an action that may be mediated by entry into vascular cells via an organic anion transporter.[26] Further studies will be necessary before the physiologic roles of endogenous purines in normal tubular physiology are clarified.

CONCLUSION

The balance between glomerular filtration and tubular reabsorption allows precise control of overall sodium excretion and consequently of ECFV, the key to long-term blood pressure regulation. It is notable that, with the exception of aldosterone (the factor largely responsible for day-to-day fluctuations in sodium excretion), those agents prominent in the control of sodium excretion also have direct vascular effects, both within the kidney and systemically. Thus, there are elements in place for an integrated regulatory system that not only controls blood *volume* but contributes also to the circulatory *capacity*. Such a system, if its complexities can be unraveled, might conceivably provide a target for future antihypertensive therapeutic strategies.

REFERENCES

1. Fliser D, Ritz E, Franek E: Renal reserve in the elderly. Semin Nephrol 1995;15:463–467.
2. Persson PB: Renal blood flow autoregulation in blood pressure control. Curr Opin Nephrol Hypertens 2002;11:67–72.
3. Thomson SC: Adenosine and purinergic mediators of tubuloglomerular feedback. Curr Opin Nephrol Hypertens 2002;11:81–86.
4. Komlosi P, Fintha A, Bell PD: Renal cell-to-cell communication via extracellular ATP. Physiology 2005;20:86–90.
5. Shirley DG, Walter SJ: A micropuncture study of the renal response to haemorrhage in rats: Assessment of the role of vasopressin. Exp Physiol 1995;80:619–630.
6. Skou JC: The influence of some cations on an adenosine triphosphatase from peripheral nerves. Biochem Biophys Acta 1957;23:394–401.
7. Meneton P, Loffing J, Warnock DG: Sodium and potassium handling by the aldosterone-sensitive distal nephron: The pivotal role of the distal and connecting tubule. Am J Physiol Renal Physiol 2004;287:F593–F601.
8. Bailey MA, Unwin RJ, Shirley DG: In vivo inhibition of renal 11β-hydroxysteroid dehydrogenase in the rat stimulates collecting duct sodium reabsorption. Clin Sci 2001;101:195–198.
9. Greger R: Ion transport mechanisms in thick ascending limb of Henle's loop of mammalian nephron. Physiol Rev 1985;65:760–795.
10. Sands JM: Renal urea transporters. Curr Opin Nephrol Hypertens 2004;13:525–532.
11. Chou C-L, Knepper MA, Layton HE: Urinary concentrating mechanism: The role of the inner medulla. Semin Nephrol 1993;13:168–181.
12. Neuhofer W, Beck F-X: Cell survival in the hostile environment of the renal medulla. Annu Rev Physiol 2005;67:531–555.
13. Rosenthal W, Seibold A, Antaramian A, et al: Molecular identification of the gene responsible for congenital nephrogenic diabetes insipidus. Nature 1992;359:233–235.
14. Nielsen S, Frøkiær J, Marples D, et al: Aquaporins in the kidney: From molecules to medicine. Physiol Rev 2002;82:205–244.

15. Ward DT, Riccardi D: Renal physiology of the extracellular calcium-sensing receptor. Pflugers Arch 2002;445:169–176.
16. Nakamura T, Alberola AM, Salazar FJ, et al: Effects of renal perfusion pressure on renal interstitial hydrostatic pressure and Na^+ excretion: Role of endothelium-derived nitric oxide. Nephron 1998;78:104–111.
17. Thorup C, Persson AEG: Macula densa derived nitric oxide in regulation of glomerular capillary pressure. Kidney Int 1996;49:430–436.
18. Maier KG, Roman RJ: Cytochrome P450 metabolites of arachidonic acid in the control of renal function. Curr Opin Nephrol Hypertens 2001;10:81–87.
19. Sarkis A, Lopez B, Roman RJ: Role of 20-hydroxyeicosatetraenoic acid and epoxyeicosatrienoic acids in hypertension. Curr Opin Nephrol Hypertens 2004;13:205–214.
20. Breyer MD, Harris RC: Cyclooxygenase 2 and the kidney. Curr Opin Nephrol Hypertens 2001;10:89–98.
21. Vallon V: Tubuloglomerular feedback in the kidney: Insights from gene-targeted mice. Pflugers Arch 2003;445:470–476.
22. Welch WJ, Wilcox CS: What is brain nitric oxide doing in the kidney? Curr Opin Nephrol Hypertens 2002;11:109–115.
23. Kohan DE: Endothelins in the normal and diseased kidney. Am J Kidney Dis 1997;29:2–26.
24. Unwin RJ, Bailey MA, Burnstock G: Purinergic signaling along the renal tubule: The current state of play. News Physiol Sci 2003;18:237–241.
25. Bailey MA: Inhibition of bicarbonate reabsorption in the rat proximal tubule by activation of luminal $P2Y_1$ receptors. Am J Physiol Renal Physiol 2004;287:F789–F796.
26. Sanchez-Lozada LG, Tapia E, Santamaria J, et al: Mild hyperuricemia induces severe cortical vasoconstriction and perpetuates glomerular hypertension in normal rats and in experimental chronic renal failure. Kidney Int 2005;67:237–247.

CHAPTER

3 Assessment of Renal Function

Ambreen Gul, Scott J. Gilbert, and Andrew S. Levey

INTRODUCTION

The kidney has excretory and endocrine functions. The level of the glomerular filtration rate (GFR) is accepted as an overall index of excretory function, although in some circumstances it is advisable to assess tubular function in addition to GFR. Currently, the serum level of creatinine, an endogenous filtration marker, is most commonly used as an index of kidney function. In our opinion, GFR estimates should replace the serum creatinine level as the standard method for the clinical assessment of excretory kidney function.

PHYSIOLOGIC VARIABILITY OF THE GLOMERULAR FILTRATION RATE AND THE NORMAL VALUE

GFR is a product of the average filtration rate of each single nephron, the filtering unit of the kidneys, multiplied by the number of nephrons in both kidneys.[1] The normal level of GFR varies according to age, sex, body size, physical activity, diet, pharmacologic therapy, and physiologic states such as pregnancy. The normal level for GFR is approximately 130 ml/min/1.73 m² for men and 120 ml/min/1.73 m² for women, with considerable variation among individuals.[2,3] GFR is conventionally adjusted for body surface area, which can be computed from height and weight, and is expressed per 1.73 m² surface area, the mean surface area of young men and women. GFR is approximately 8% higher in young men than in women of the same age and declines with age; the mean rate of decline is approximately 0.75 mL/min per year after the age of 40.[4] During pregnancy, GFR increases by about 50% in the first trimester and returns to normal immediately after delivery. GFR has a diurnal variation and is 10% lower at midnight as compared to the afternoon.[5] Within an individual, GFR is relatively constant over time,[2] but varies considerably among people, even after adjustment for the known variables.[3]

Reductions in GFR can be due either to a decline in the nephron number (as in chronic kidney disease [CKD]) or a decline in the single nephron GFR (SNGFR) from physiologic or hemodynamic alterations. An increase in SNGFR due to increased glomerular capillary pressure or glomerular hypertrophy can compensate for a decrease in nephron number, and therefore the level of GFR may not reflect the loss of nephrons. As a result, there may be substantial kidney damage before GFR decreases.[6]

MEASUREMENT OF THE GLOMERULAR FILTRATION RATE

GFR cannot be measured directly. Instead, it is measured as the urinary clearance of an ideal filtration marker.

Concept of Clearance

Clearance of a substance is defined as the volume of plasma cleared of a marker by excretion per unit of time. The clearance of substance "x" (C_x) can be calculated as $C_x = A_x / P_x$, where A_x is the amount of x eliminated from the plasma, P_x is the average plasma concentration, and C_x is expressed in units of volume per time. Clearance does not represent an actual volume, but rather a virtual volume of plasma that is completely cleared of the substance per unit of time. The value for clearance is related to the efficiency of elimination: the greater the rate of elimination, the higher the clearance. Clearance of substance x is the sum of the urinary and extrarenal clearance; for substances that are eliminated by renal and extrarenal routes, plasma clearance exceeds urinary clearance.

Urinary Clearance

The amount of substance x excreted in the urine can be calculated as the product of the urinary flow rate (V) and the urinary concentration (U_x). Therefore, urinary clearance is defined as follows:

$$C_{(x)} = (U_x \times V)/P_x.$$

Urinary excretion of a substance depends on filtration, tubular secretion, and tubular reabsorption. Thus, the magnitude of urinary clearance reflects the mechanism of excretion. For substances that are filtered but neither secreted nor reabsorbed, the urinary excretion equals the filtered load, and urinary clearance equals GFR.

Such substances are ideal filtration markers because their urinary clearance can be used as a measure of GFR. For substances that are filtered and secreted, urinary clearance exceeds GFR, and for substances that are filtered and reabsorbed, urinary clearance is less than GFR.

Exogenous Filtration Markers

Inulin, a 5200-d uncharged polymer of fructose, was the first substance described as an ideal filtration marker and remains the gold standard against which other markers are evaluated. It is freely filtered at the glomerulus and neither secreted nor reabsorbed by the renal tubule. It is nontoxic and physiologically inert; thus, it can be infused for measurement of GFR. The ideal protocol for inulin clearance requires a continuous intravenous infusion to achieve a steady state and bladder catheterization with multiple timed urine collections.[7] Because this technique is cumbersome, and inulin measurement requires a difficult chemical assay, this method has not been used widely in clinical practice and remains largely a research tool.[1] Other exogenous substances including iohexol, ^{51}Cr-ethylenediamine tetraacetic acid, ^{99m}Tc-diethylenetriamine pentaacetic acid, and ^{125}I-iothalamate also fulfill the criteria for ideal filtration markers (Fig. 3.1). Alternative

Exogenous filtration markers for estimation of GFR		
Marker	Method of Administration	Comments
Inulin	Continuous IV	Gold standard
^{125}I-iothalamate	Bolus IV or SC	Potential problem of thyroid uptake of ^{125}I, tubular secretion of iothalamate leading to overestimation of GFR
^{99m}Tc-DTPA	Bolus IV	Dissociation of ^{99m}Tc leads to plasma protein binding and underestimation of GFR
^{51}Cr-EDTA	Bolus IV	10% lower clearance than inulin
Iohexol	Bolus IV	Low incidence of adverse effects; comparable to inulin

Figure 3.1   Exogenous filtration markers for estimation of glomerular filtration rate. ^{51}Cr-EDTA, ethylenediamine tetraacetic acid; GFR, glomerular filtration rate; ^{99m}Tc-DTPA, ^{99m}Tc-diethylenetriamine.

protocols to assess clearance have also been validated, including bolus subcutaneous injection, spontaneous bladder emptying, and plasma disappearance rather than urinary clearance. These measurement protocols are too complicated for routine clinical practice in most centers; thus, GFR is usually measured or estimated using endogenous filtration markers.

Endogenous Filtration Markers

The most commonly used endogenous filtration markers in clinical practice include creatinine and urea. More recently, cystatin C has shown great promise. A comparison of these markers is outlined in Figure 3.2.

Measurement of Urinary Clearance

Urinary clearance requires a timed urine collection for measurement of urine volume and concentration and measurement of serum concentrations. Calculations of clearance are done according to the equation

$$C_{(x)} = (U_x \times V)/P_x.$$

Special care must be taken to avoid incomplete urine collections, which will limit the accuracy of the clearance calculation. In a complete urine collection, creatinine excretion should be 20 to 25 and 15 to 20 mg/kg/day in healthy young men and women, respectively. If the serum level is not constant during the urine

Comparison of creatinine, urea, and cystatin C as filtration markers			
Variable	Creatinine	Urea	Cystatin C
Molecular Properties			
Weight	113 d	60 d	13,000 d
Structure	Amino acid derivative	Organic molecular product of protein metabolism	Nonglycosylated basic protein
Physiologic Determinants of Serum Level			
Generation	Varies, according to muscle mass and dietary protein; lower in elderly persons, women, and Caucasians	Varies, according to dietary protein intake and catabolism	Thought to be constant by all nucleated cells
Handling by the kidney	Filtered, secreted, and excreted in the urine	Filtered, reabsorbed, and excreted in the urine	Filtered, reabsorbed, and catabolized
Extrarenal elimination	Yes; increases at reduced GFR	Yes; increases at reduced GFR	Preliminary evidence of increases at reduced GFR
Use in Estimating Equations for GFR			
Demographic and clinical variables as surrogates for physiologic determinants	Age, sex, and race; related to muscle mass	Not applicable	Unknown
Accuracy	Accurate for GFR <60 ml/min/ 1.73 m^2	Fairly accurate	Unknown
Assay			
Method	Colorimetric or enzymatic	Direct measurement, enzymatic calorimetric, and electrochemical	PENIA
Assay precision	Very good except at low range	Precise with standard deviation on repetitive measurement of 0.47%–1.72%	Precise throughout range
Clinical laboratory practice	Multiple assays; widely used nonstandard calibration	Multiple assays; enzymatic and calorimetric more commonly used	Single dominant method; not on most auto-analyzers; not standardized
Reference standard	IDMS	IDMS	None at present

Figure 3.2 Comparison of creatinine, urea, and cystatin C as filtration markers. GFR, glomerular filtration rate; IDMS, isotope dilution gas chromatography–mass spectrometry; PENIA, particle-enhanced nephelometric immunoassay. (Adapted from Stevens LA, Levey AS: Chronic kidney disease in the elderly—how to assess risk. N Engl J Med 2005;352:2122–2124. Copyright © 2005 Massachusetts Medical Society. All rights reserved.)

collection as in acute renal failure or when assessing residual renal function in dialysis patients, it is also necessary to obtain additional blood samples during the urine collection to estimate the average serum concentration.

Estimation of the Glomerular Filtration Rate from Steady-State Serum Levels and Formulas

During steady state, a constant plasma level of a substance is maintained since generation, the sum of exogenous and endogenous production is equal to urinary excretion and extrarenal elimination. In steady state, the plasma level is related to the reciprocal of the level of GFR, but is also influenced by extrarenal elimination, tubular secretion and reabsorption, and generation.

Estimating equations incorporate demographic and clinical variables as surrogates of these physiologic determinants of the plasma concentration other than GFR and provide a more accurate estimate of GFR than the reciprocal of the serum level alone.

CREATININE

Creatinine, a 113-d end product of muscle catabolism, is the most commonly used endogenous filtration marker. Advantages of creatinine include its ease of measurement and the low cost and widespread availability of the assay.

Creatinine is derived by the metabolism of phosphocreatine in muscle as well as from dietary meat intake. Creatinine generation is proportional to muscle mass, which can be estimated from age, gender, race, and body size. Figure 3.3 lists factors that can affect creatinine generation.

Creatinine is released into the circulation at a constant rate. It is not protein bound and freely filtered across the glomerulus.

It is also secreted by the tubules[8]; hence, creatinine clearance exceeds GFR. Several commonly used medications, including cimetidine and trimethoprim, competitively inhibit creatinine secretion and reduce creatinine clearance. These medications thus lead to a rise in the serum creatinine concentration without effect on GFR (see Fig. 3.3).

In addition, creatinine is contained in intestinal secretions and can be degraded by bacteria. If serum levels are increased (when GFR is reduced), the amount of creatinine eliminated via this extrarenal route is increased. Antibiotics can raise the serum level of creatinine by destroying intestinal flora, thereby interfering with extrarenal elimination as well as by reduction of the GFR. The rise in serum creatinine following inhibition of tubular secretion and extrarenal elimination is greater in patients with a reduced GFR. Clinically, it can be difficult to distinguish a rise in serum creatinine due to inhibition of creatinine secretion or extrarenal elimination from a decline in GFR, but processes other than a true decline in GFR should be suspected if urea levels remain unchanged despite a significant change in serum creatinine in a patient with an initially reduced GFR.

Figure 3.4 demonstrates the wide range of GFR for a given serum creatinine level. For example, a serum creatinine level of 1.5 mg/dl (132 μmol/l) may correspond to a GFR from approximately 20 to 90 ml/min/1.73 m^2.

Creatinine clearance is usually computed from the creatinine excretion in a 24-hour urine collection and single measurement of serum creatinine in the steady state. This method has several drawbacks. First, creatinine clearance systematically overestimates GFR due to tubular creatinine secretion. This overestimation is magnified at lower levels of kidney function. Second, the challenges of achieving a complete urine collection limit the accuracy.

Factors affecting serum creatinine concentration		
	Effect on Serum Creatinine	Mechanism/Comment
Age	Decrease	Reduction in creatinine generation due to age-related decline in muscle mass
Female Sex	Decrease	Reduction in creatinine generation due to reduced muscle mass
Race		
African American	Increase	Higher creatinine generation rate to higher average muscle mass in African Americans; not known how muscle mass in other races compares to that of African Americans or Caucasians
Diet		
Vegetarian diet	Decrease	Decrease in creatinine generation
Ingestion of cooked meats and creatinine supplements	Increased	Transient increase in creatinine generation; however, may be blunted by transient increase in GFR
Body Habitus		
Muscular	Increase	Increased muscle generation due to increased muscle mass ± increased protein intake
Malnutrition/muscle wasting/amputation	Decrease	Reduced creatinine generation due to reduced muscle mass ± reduced protein intake
Obesity	No change	Excess mass is fat, not muscle mass, and does not contribute to increased creatinine generation
Medications		
Trimethoprim, cimetidine, fibric acid derivatives other than gemfibrizol	Increase	Reduced tubular secretion of creatinine
Keto acids, some cephalosporins	Increase	Interference with alkaline picrate assay for creatinine

Figure 3.3 Factors affecting serum creatinine concentration. (From Stevens LA, Levey AS: Measurement of kidney function. Med Clin North Am 2005;89: 457–473, with permission.)

Measured glomerular filtration rate (GFR) versus serum creatinine

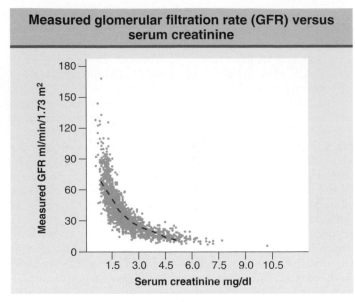

Figure 3.4 Measured glomerular filtration rate (GFR) versus serum creatinine. Each point represents the baseline measurement of Modification of Diet in Renal Disease Study participants (N = 1628). *Dashed line* represents the fitted line plotted from the 2.5 to 97.5 percentile of GFR estimates. Note the wide range of creatinine values for a given GFR. Serum creatinine 1.5 mg/dl (132 μmol/l) is near the upper limit of the reference range in many clinical laboratories and could reflect a GFR from approximately 15 to 90 ml/min/1.73 m² depending on the age, sex, and race of an individual.

Formulae for Estimating the Glomerular Filtration Rate from Serum Creatinine

GFR can be estimated from serum creatinine using equations that use age, sex, race, and body size as surrogates for creatinine generation. The two most commonly used equations are the Cockcroft-Gault formula and Modification of Diet in Renal Disease (MDRD) Study equation.

Cockcroft-Gault Formula

The Cockcroft-Gault formula (Fig. 3.5) includes age, sex, and body weight in addition to serum creatinine.[9] There is an adjustment factor for women that is based on a theoretical assumption of 15% reduction in creatinine generation due to lower muscle

mass. This formula systematically overestimates creatinine clearance in patients who are edematous or overweight, while most likely underestimating it in people of African origin. Furthermore, since the formula predicts creatinine clearance, it is an overestimate of GFR. Comparison to normal values for creatinine clearance requires computation of body surface area and adjustment to 1.73m².

Modification of Diet in Renal Disease Study Equation

The MDRD Study equation was originally expressed as a six-variable equation using serum creatinine, urea, and albumin concentrations in addition to demographic variables to predict GFR. A revised four-variable equation (see Fig. 3.5) has minimal bias and precision and accuracy close to those of the six-variable equation. From here on, we refer to the four-variable MDRD Study equation as the MDRD Study equation. This equation has now been validated in African Americans, people with diabetic kidney disease, and kidney transplant recipients, three groups not included in large numbers in the original MDRD Study. Its validity is independent of the etiology of kidney disease.[10] The equation appears to underestimate GFR in populations with higher levels of GFR, such as patients with type 1 diabetes without microalbuminuria and people undergoing kidney transplant donor evaluation. It has not been validated in children, pregnant women, the elderly (age >70 years), or other racial or ethnic subgroups. Figure 3.6 shows the measured GFR (with iothalamate) compared to the estimated GFR using the MDRD Study equation, estimated creatinine clearance using the Cockcroft-Gault formula, and measured creatinine clearance in the MDRD Study cohort population.[11] In this study and others, the MDRD Study equation had greater precision and greater overall accuracy than that of measured creatinine clearance and of the Cockcroft-Gault formula, even when the latter was adjusted for body surface area and corrected for systematic bias.[10] Neither equation is expected to work as well in patients with extreme levels for creatinine generation, such as amputees, large or small individuals, patients with muscle-wasting conditions, or people with high or low levels of dietary meat intake (see Fig. 3.3). In addition, estimating equations depend critically on the assumption of a steady state since the serum creatinine level lags behind the change in GFR. Thus, in a patient with a rapidly declining GFR (rising serum creatinine), GFR estimate will exceed the

Formulae for estimating GFR		
Cockcroft-Gault Formula		
Male	$C_{cr} = \dfrac{(140 - age) \times weight}{72 \times P_{cr}(mg/dl)}$ *or*	$C_{cr} = \dfrac{(140 - age) \times weight}{0.814 \times P_{cr}(\mu mol/l)}$
Female	$C_{cr} = \dfrac{(140 - age) \times weight \times 0.85}{72 \times P_{cr}(mg/dl)}$ *or*	$C_{cr} = \dfrac{(140 - age) \times weight \times 0.85}{0.814 \times P_{cr}(\mu mol/l)}$
MDRD Study Equation (Four-Variable Equation)		
GFR (ml/min/1.73 m²) = $186 \times P_{cr}(mg/dl)^{-1.154} \times Age^{-0.203} \times 0.742$ (if female) $\times 1.210$ (if black) *or* GFR (ml/min/1.73 m²) = $186 \times \left[\dfrac{P_{cr}(\mu mol/l)}{88.4}\right]^{-1.154} \times Age^{-0.203} \times 0.742$ (if female) $\times 1.210$ (if black)		
MDRD Study Equation with Standardized Serum Creatinine (Four-Variable Equation)		
GFR (ml/min/1.73 m²) = $175 \times$ Standardized $P_{cr}(mg/dl)^{-1.154} \times Age^{-0.203} \times 0.742$ (if female) $\times 1.210$ (if black) *or* GFR (ml/min/1.73 m²) = $179 \times \left[\dfrac{Standardized\ P_{cr}(\mu mol/l)}{88.4}\right]^{-1.154} \times Age^{-0.203} \times 0.742$ (if female) $\times 1.210$ (if black)		

Figure 3.5 Formulae for estimating glomerular filtration rate. Age in years, weight in kilograms. The Modification of Diet in Renal Disease (MDRD) Study equation calculator can also be found online (*http://www.nephron.com/mdrd/default.html*).

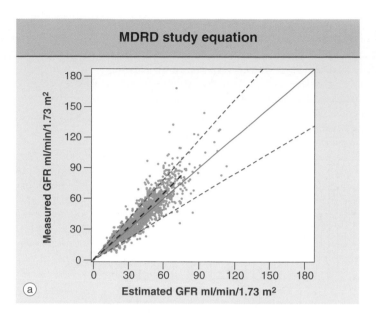

MDRD study equation

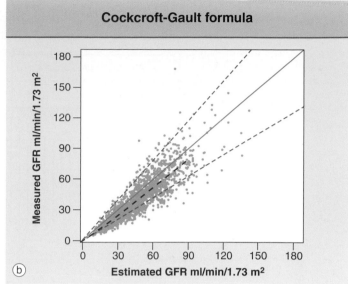

Cockcroft-Gault formula

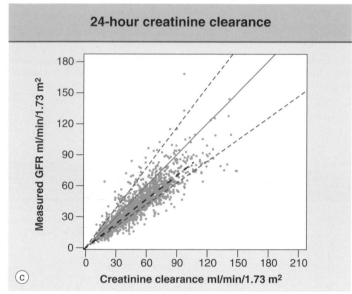

24-hour creatinine clearance

Figure 3.6 Measurements and estimates of glomerular filtration rate (GFR). GFR using urinary clearance of ^{125}I-iothalamate versus GFR estimated by the Modification of Diet in Renal Disease Study participants (N = 1628). *Green diagonal line* represents the line of identity. *Red dashed line* represents the fitted line plotted from the 21.5 to 97.5 percentile of GFR estimates. *Blue dashed lines* represent the difference between estimated and measured GFR of ±30%.[11] *a,* Modification of Diet in Renal Disease Study equation; *b,* Cockcroft-Gault formula; *c,* 24-hour creatinine clearance. (From Stevens LA, Coresh J, Greene T, Levey AS: Assessing kidney function—measured and estimated glomerular filtration. N Engl J Med 2006;354:2473–2483. Copyright © Massachusetts Medical Society. All rights reserved.)

true GFR, and, conversely, in a patient with a rising GFR (declining serum creatinine), GFR estimate will be lower than the true GFR.

Creatinine Assay

Accurate, standardized, and reproducible creatinine measurements are critical to the estimation of GFR. The most commonly used assay for measuring serum creatinine, the alkaline picrate (Jaffe) assay, detects and quantifies the color reaction. Chromogens other than creatinine are known to interfere with the assay, giving rise to errors. In normal subjects, up to 20% of the color reaction in creatinine assays is due to substances other than creatinine (noncreatinine chromogens).[12] Enzymatic assays do not detect noncreatinine chromogens and yield lower serum levels than the alkaline picrate assays. Calibration of assays to adjust for this interference is not standardized across laboratories, as highlighted in Figure 3.7.

In one study, the average coefficient of variation (reproducibility) of serum creatinine measured in laboratories was 8%; however, there was a 13% average overestimation of serum creatinine compared to the reference standard.[13] Differences in calibration of serum creatinine assays to the reference standard accounted for 85% of the difference between laboratories rather than imprecision of measurement. Noncreatinine chromogens are not retained as GFR declines; thus, the variability among laboratories is relatively higher at lower serum creatinine levels (higher GFR).

In the United States, in an effort to address the heterogeneity in creatinine assays, the College of American Pathologists has prepared fresh-frozen serum pools with known creatinine levels that are traceable to a primary reference at the U.S. National Institute of Standards and Technology. This enables standardization of creatinine measurements and calibration of equipment.[14]

The four-variable MDRD equation has now been re-expressed for use with standardized serum creatinine, which is approximately 5% lower than the serum levels using the original MDRD Study assay[11,15] (see Fig. 3.5). As of 2006 in the United Kingdom, it is a national requirement that all hospital laboratories provide routine reporting of the estimated GFR using the MDRD Study equation with standardized creatinine measurement.

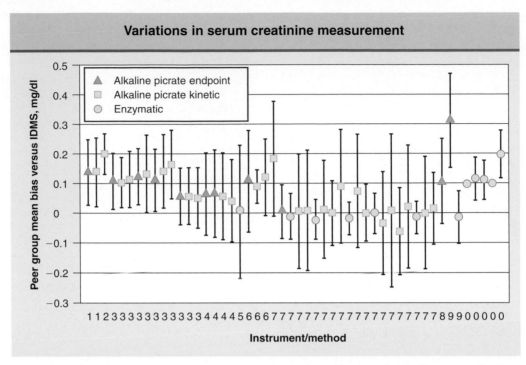

Figure 3.7   Variations in serum creatinine measurement. Bias of serum creatinine measurements using three different chemical methods compared to isotope dilution gas chromatography–mass spectrometry (IDMS), the reference method. The numbers on the horizontal axis identify equipment from 10 different manufacturers used for the analyses. Error bars indicate 1.96 × standard deviation for distribution of participant results. The error bars that appear missing are smaller than the plot symbol. (From Miller WG, Myers GL, Ashwood ER, et al: Creatinine measurement: State of the art in accuracy and interlaboratory harmonization. Arch Pathol Lab Med 2005;129:297–304, with permission. Copyright © 2005 College of American Pathologists.)

Until standardization is complete, the variability in the calibration of creatinine assays will remain an important limitation of the use of GFR estimating equations, especially at higher levels of estimated GFR (Fig. 3.8). This has important consequences for clinicians trying to compare the level of kidney function based on serum creatinine reported by different laboratories, especially when the estimated GFR is more than 60 ml/min/1.73 m². Standardization will reduce but not completely eliminate the error at higher levels of GFR. For this reason, we recommend reporting GFR estimates as a numeric value only if GFR estimate is less than 60 ml/min/1.73 m² and is more than 60 ml/min/1.73 m² for higher values.

UREA

The serum urea level has limited value as an index of GFR, in view of widely variable urea generation and tubular reabsorption.

Urea is a 60-d end product of protein catabolism by the liver. Factors associated with the increased generation of urea include protein loading from hyperalimentation or absorption of blood after a gastrointestinal hemorrhage. Catabolic states due to infection, corticosteroid administration, or chemotherapy also increase urea generation. Decreased urea generation is seen in severe malnutrition and liver disease.

Urea is freely filtered by the glomerulus and then passively reabsorbed in both the proximal and distal nephrons.[8] Owing to the tubular reabsorption, urinary clearance of urea underestimates kidney function. Reduced kidney perfusion in the setting of volume depletion and states of antidiuresis is associated with increased urea reabsorption. This leads to a greater decrease in

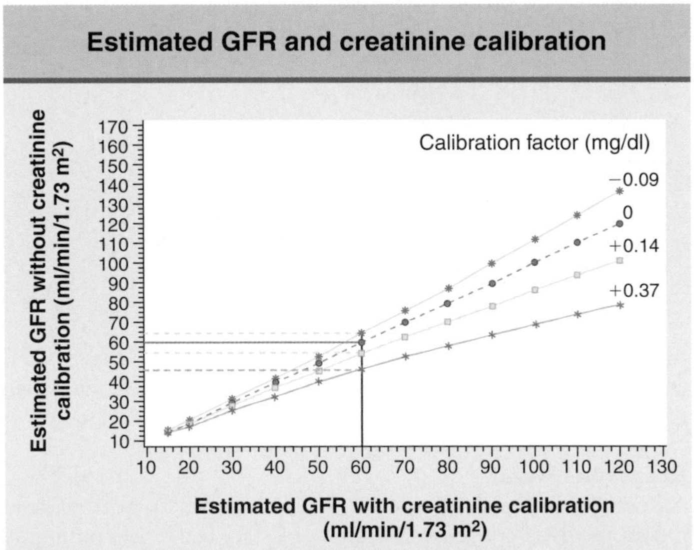

Estimated GFR and creatinine calibration

Figure 3.8   Estimated glomerular filtration rate (GFR) with and without creatinine calibration for a 60-year-old black male. Lines represent estimated GFR values with and without calibration of serum creatinine assay over the 95% confidence interval for calibration differences (factors) observed from the survey of the College of American Pathologists for a 60-year-old black male. A calibration factor of zero indicates no difference between laboratories in serum creatinine assay. For an estimated GFR less than 60 ml/min/1.73 m², a mean calibration difference of 0.14 mg/dl is associated with an error in GFR estimates of –9.1%. The upper and lower limits of the 95% confidence intervals are –0.09 mg/dl and +0.37 mg/dl, respectively. The error in GFR estimates over this range is from +7.6% to –21.9%. (From Murthy K, Stevens LA, Stark PC, Levey AS: Variation in the serum creatinine assay calibration: A practical application to glomerular filtration rate estimation. Kidney Int 2005;68:1884–1887, with permission.)

urea clearance than the concomitant decrease in GFR. At levels of GFR less than approximately 20 ml/min/1.73 m^2, the overestimation of GFR by creatinine clearance due to creatinine secretion is approximately equal to the underestimation of GFR by urea clearance due to urea reabsorption.

CYSTATIN C

Low molecular weight proteins have long been proposed as good markers of GFR as they are freely filtered. Cystatin C (see Fig. 3.2) is a 130-d protein that is unique in that it appears to be produced at a constant rate by all nucleated human cells. Its low molecular mass and its high isoelectric point allow it to be freely filtered by the glomerular membrane. After filtration, cystatin C is reabsorbed and catabolized by the tubular epithelial cells, with only small amounts excreted in the urine.[16] Thus, cystatin C generation cannot be quantitated by urinary excretion, nor can its urinary clearance be measured. Cystatin C is very stable in serum but readily degraded in urine. Cystatin C levels in surveys of normal adults range from 0.54 to 1.55 mg/l, with slight variability depending on the assay used.[17] The serum concentration of cystatin C remains constant from approximately 1 to 50 years of age and appears to be largely independent of height, gender, and muscle mass. There is some suggestion that liver disease, thyroid disease, and large doses of corticosteroids may increase production of cystatin C. Higher levels of cystatin C are observed from birth to 4 months of age and in the elderly.[17] It is thought that the elevation after the age of approximately 70 years is related to the age-associated decline in GFR. However, a population-based study showed that even after adjusting for creatinine clearance, age, male sex, higher body mass index, and higher C-reactive protein levels were significantly related to cystatin C level,[18] suggesting the presence of determinants of cystatin C level in addition to GFR.

With an acute decline in GFR, one study demonstrated that the cystatin C level increases before that of serum creatinine.[19] The presence of cystatin C in the urine of patients with kidney disease indicates that the ability of the kidney to reabsorb and degrade cystatin C may be affected at low levels of GFR. However, it is not clear whether this effect interferes with the direct relationship between cystatin C and GFR in patients with CKD.

In studies that have compared serum cystatin C and creatinine, cystatin C appears to be a better filtration marker. When compared to creatinine-based estimating equations, such as the MDRD Study equation or the Cockcroft-Gault formula, there is no clear advantage of cystatin C.[8] These studies also showed the superiority of serum cystatin C as a GFR marker compared to other low molecular mass proteins, such as ß$_2$-microglobulin, retinol-binding protein, and complement factor D. Some studies show that elevations in cystatin C level are a better predictor of the risk of cardiovascular disease and total mortality than an estimated GFR based on serum creatinine. Whether this is due to its superiority as a filtration marker or to confounding by determinants of cystatin C and creatinine other than GFR remains to be determined.[8] Cystatin C is measured using the Dade particle-enhanced nephelometry immunoassay.[20] Little is known about the comparability of assays across laboratories. Widespread adoption of serum cystatin C for the estimation of GFR is not recommended until more research and laboratory standardization are in place.

CLINICAL APPLICATION OF ESTIMATED GLOMERULAR FILTRATION RATE IN CHRONIC KIDNEY DISEASE

Estimation of GFR is necessary for the detection, evaluation, and management of CKD. Current guidelines recommend testing patients at increased risk of CKD for albuminuria or a reduced estimated GFR, and staging the severity of CKD by the level of the estimated GFR.[21] Using serum creatinine alone as an index of GFR is unsatisfactory and can lead to delays in detection of CKD and misclassification of the severity of CKD. Use of estimating equations allows for direct reporting of GFR estimates by clinical laboratories whenever serum creatinine is measured. Many organizations now recommend GFR estimates as the primary method of clinical assessment of kidney function.[21,22] All current estimating equations are less accurate at higher levels of the estimated GFR (>60 ml/min/1.73 m^2) in patients with factors affecting serum creatinine other than GFR (see Fig. 3.3) and in the nonsteady state. In these situations, more accurate GFR estimates require a clearance measurement, using either an exogenous filtration marker or a timed urine collection for creatinine clearance. In the future, improved estimating equations using creatinine and possibly cystatin C will allow more accurate GFR estimates.

MARKERS OF TUBULAR DAMAGE

Low Molecular Weight Proteins

Low molecular weight proteins in plasma are readily filtered by the glomerulus and are subsequently reabsorbed by the proximal tubule in normal subjects, with the result that only small amounts of the filtered proteins appear in the urine. The urinary excretion of these proteins rises when proximal tubular reabsorption is impaired. Since there is no distal tubular reabsorption, measurement of urinary low molecular weight proteins has been widely accepted as a marker of proximal tubular damage. β$_2$-Microglobulin (11,800 d), the light chain of the class I major histocompatibility antigens, α$_1$-macroglobulin (33,000 d), a glycosylated protein synthesized in the liver, and retinol-binding protein are measured in clinical practice. β$_2$-Microglobulin is unstable in acidic urine (pH <6), leading to underestimation; α$_1$-macroglobulin is stable and not readily affected by urine pH.

N-Acetyl-β-glucosaminidase

N-Acetyl-β-glucosaminidase (NAG) is a hydrolytic enzyme distributed throughout the nephron, but its activity is two to four times higher in the proximal tubule than in other nephron segments. The molecular weight of 130,000 to 140,000 d is too large for filtration by the glomerulus, so most urinary NAG originates from tubular cells. Urinary NAG excretion rises in tubular cell injury from a variety of insults including drug nephrotoxicity, kidney transplant rejection, and tubulointerstitial nephritis. In glomerular disease, a part of urinary NAG may have originated from the plasma and been filtered; since sustained glomerular proteinuria will damage the proximal tubule, this may cause a further rise in urinary NAG. Urinary NAG is therefore useful for the early diagnosis of tubular damage in the absence of glomerular injury. It has been used in the early diagnosis of transplant rejection with some success, but its main value in clinical practice now lies in the early detection of drug nephrotoxicity. For example, an increase in urinary NAG excretion appears early in the course of aminoglycoside toxicity before any increase in plasma creatinine level or the appearance of ß$_2$-microglobulin in urine.[23] Other urinary markers of tubular damage under investigation are shown in Figure 64.13.

MEASUREMENT OF TUBULAR FUNCTION

Techniques for assessing proximal and distal tubular function are discussed in the chapters listed:

- Sodium handling (Chapter 7: "Disorders of Extracellular Volume").
- Concentrating and diluting capacity (Chapter 8: "Disorders of Water Metabolism").
- Potassium handling (Chapter 9: "Disorders of Potassium Metabolism").
- Urinary acidification (Chapter 11: "Normal Acid-Base Balance" and Chapter 12: "Metabolic Acidosis").

REFERENCES

1. Perrone RD, Madias NE, Levey AS: Serum creatinine as an index of renal function: New insights into old concepts. Clin Chem 1992;38: 1933–1953.
2. Smith H: The Kidney: Structure and Function in Health and Disease. New York: Oxford University Press, 1951, p 1072.
3. Wesson LG: Physiology of the Human Kidney. New York: Grune & Stratton, 1969, p 712.
4. Lindeman RD, Tobin JD, Shock NW: Association between blood pressure and the rate of decline in renal function with age. Kidney Int 1984;26:861–868.
5. Wesson LG Jr: Electrolyte excretion in relation to diurnal cycles of renal function. Medicine (Baltimore) 1964;43:547–592.
6. Stevens LA, Levey AS: Measurement of kidney function. Med Clin North Am 2005;89:457–473.
7. Smith HW, Chasis H, Goldring W, Ranges HA: Glomerular dynamics in the normal human kidney. J Clin Invest 1940;19:751–764.
8. Stevens LA, Levey AS: Chronic kidney disease in the elderly—how to assess risk. N Engl J Med 2005;352:2122–2124.
9. Cockcroft DW, Gault MH: Prediction of creatinine clearance from serum creatinine. Nephron 1976;16:31–41.
10. Coresh J, Stevens L: Kidney function estimating equations: Where do we stand? Curr Opin Nephrol Hypertens 2006;15:276–284.
11. Stevens LA, Coresh J, Greene T, Levey AS: Assessing kidney function—measured and estimated glomerular filtration. N Engl J Med 2006;354: 2473–2483.
12. Doolan PD, Alpen EL, Theil GB: A clinical appraisal of the plasma concentration and endogenous clearance of creatinine. Am J Med 1962;32:65–79.
13. Ross JW, Miller WG, Myers GL, Praestgaard J: The accuracy of laboratory measurements in clinical chemistry: A study of 11 routine chemistry analytes in the College of American Pathologists Chemistry Survey with fresh frozen serum, definitive methods, and reference methods. Arch Pathol Lab Med 1998;122:587–608.
14. Miller WG, Myers GL, Ashwood ER, et al: Creatinine measurement: State of the art in accuracy and interlaboratory harmonization. Arch Pathol Lab Med 2005;129:297–304.
15. Levey AS, Eckardt KU, Tsukamoto Y, et al: Definition and classification of chronic kidney disease: A position statement from Kidney Disease: Improving Global Outcomes (KDIGO). Kidney Int 2005;67: 2089–2100.
16. Filler G, Bokenkamp A, Hofmann W, et al: Cystatin C as a marker of GFR—history, indications, and future research. Clin Biochem 2005;38: 1–8.
17. Randers E, Erlandsen EJ: Serum cystatin C as an endogenous marker of the renal function—a review. Clin Chem Lab Med 1999;37:389–395.
18. Knight EL, Verhave JC, Spiegelman D, et al: Factors influencing serum cystatin C levels other than renal function and the impact on renal function measurement. Kidney Int 2004;65:1416–1421.
19. Herget-Rosenthal S, Marggraf G, Husing J, et al: Early detection of acute renal failure by serum cystatin C. Kidney Int 2004;66:1115–1122.
20. Stowe H, Lawrence D, Newman DJ, Lamb EJ: Analytical performance of a particle-enhanced nephelometric immunoassay for serum cystatin C using rate analysis. Clin Chem 2001;47:1482–1485.
21. K/DOQI clinical practice guidelines for chronic kidney disease: Evaluation, classification, and stratification. Am J Kidney Dis 2002;39: S1–266.
22. Levey AS, Coresh J, Balk E, et al: National Kidney Foundation practice guidelines for chronic kidney disease: Evaluation, classification, and stratification. Ann Intern Med 2003;139:137–147.
23. Gibey R, Dupond JL, Alber D, et al: Predictive value of urinary N-acetyl-beta-D-glucosaminidase (NAG), alanine-aminopeptidase (AAP) and beta-2-microglobulin (beta 2M) in evaluating nephrotoxicity of gentamicin. Clin Chim Acta 1981;116:25–34.
24. Murthy K, Stevens LA, Stark PC, Levey AS: Variation in the serum creatinine assay calibration: A practical application to glomerular filtration rate estimation. Kidney Int 2005;68:1884–1887.

Urinalysis

Giovanni B. Fogazzi and Barbara Pirovano

INTRODUCTION

Urinalysis is one of the basic tests to evaluate the presence and severity of kidney and urinary tract disease. When a patient is first seen by a nephrologist, urinalysis including microscopy should always be performed. Urinalysis is informative in all renal disease; both positive and negative urinary findings help in the correct evaluation of the patient. Dipsticks are the most widely used method for urinalysis, but the nephrologist should be aware of their limitations, especially in detecting urine proteins other than albumin. Urine microscopy should ideally be performed by trained nephrologists rather than clinical laboratory personnel, who are usually unaware of the clinical correlates of the findings. This chapter describes the physicochemical features of the urine as well as urine microscopy and then describes the main urinary profiles seen in common renal diseases.

COLLECTION OF SPECIMENS

The way urine is collected and handled in the laboratory is of the highest importance since this can greatly influence the results. Recent European urinalysis guidelines[1] suggest that written instructions are given to the patient about urine collection. Strenuous physical exercise (e.g., running or a soccer match) must be avoided in the 72 hours preceding the collection to avoid exercise-induced proteinuria and/or hematuria or cylindruria. In females, urinalysis should also be avoided during menstruation since blood contamination can easily occur. The first or second morning urine specimen is recommended.[1]

After the washing of hands, females should spread the labia, and males withdraw the foreskin of the glans. The external genitalia are then washed and wiped dry with a paper towel, and the urine is collected after discarding the first portion.[1] The same procedures can also be used for children, while for small infants, bags for urine are often used, even though these carry a high probability of contamination. A suprapubic bladder puncture may occasionally be necessary. Urine can also be collected through a bladder catheter. However, this may cause hematuria in itself, while permanent indwelling catheters are almost invariably associated with bacteriuria, leukocyturia, hematuria, and candiduria.

The container for urine should be provided by the laboratory or bought in a pharmacy. It should be clean and have a capacity of at least 50 to 100 ml, with a diameter opening of at least 5 cm to allow easy collection of urine by both female and male. It should also have a wide base to avoid accidental spillage and should be capped.[1]

Several elements (but especially leukocytes) can lyse rapidly after collection, and the best means to preserve the specimens

to minimize this is uncertain. Refrigeration of specimens at +2°C to +8°C assists preservation, but may allow precipitation of phosphates or uric acids, which can hamper examination of the sample. Formaldehyde, glutaraldehyde, "cellFIX," a formaldehyde-based fixative,[2] and tubes containing a lyophilized borate-formate sorbitol powder[3] are good particle preservatives for the formed elements of urine.

PHYSICAL PARAMETERS

Color

In normal conditions, the color of urine ranges from pale to dark yellow and amber, depending on the concentration of the urochrome. Abnormal changes in color can be due to pathologic conditions, drugs, or foods.

The main *pathologic conditions* that can cause color changes of the urine are gross hematuria, hemoglobinuria, myoglobinuria (pink, red, brown, or black urine); jaundice (dark yellow to brown urine); chyluria (white milky urine); massive uric acid crystalluria (pink urine); and porphyrinuria and alkaptonuria (red urine turning black on standing).

The main *drugs* that can be responsible for abnormal urine color are rifampin (rifampicin) (yellow-orange to red urine); phenytoin (red urine); chloroquine and nitrofurantoin (brown urine); triamterene and blue dyes of enteral feeds (green urine); methylene blue (blue urine); and metronidazole, methyldopa, and imipenem-cilastatin (darkening on standing).

Among *foods*, it is worth remembering the following: beetroot (red urine), senna and rhubarb (yellow to brown or red urine), and carotene (brown urine).

Turbidity

Normal urine is usually transparent. Urine can be turbid due to an increased concentration of any urine particle. The most frequent causes of turbidity are urinary tract infections, heavy hematuria, and contamination from genital secretions. The absence of turbidity is not a reliable criterion to judge a urine sample since pathologic samples can be perfectly clear.

Odor

Some rare pathologic conditions confer a characteristic odor to the urine. These are maple-syrup urine disease (maple syrup odor), phenylketonuria (musty or mousy odor), isovaleric acidemia (sweaty feet odor), and hypermethioninemia (rancid butter or fishy odor). Ketones may confer a sweet or fruity odor to urine, while bacterial urinary tract infection is often associated with a pungent odor, which is due to the production of ammonia.

Relative Density

Relative density can be measured by a number of methods:

Specific gravity (SG) is a function of the number and weight of the dissolved particles and is influenced by urine temperature, proteins, glucose, and radiocontrast media. It can be measured by a urinometer, which is a weighted float marked with a scale from 1.000 to 1.060. The urinometer is simple and quick to use, but needs at least 25 ml of urine.

SG of 1.000 to 1.003 is consistent with marked urinary dilution such as observed with diabetes insipidus or water intoxication. SG of 1.010 is often called "isosthenuric" urine since it is of similar SG (and osmolality) as plasma, so is often observed in conditions in which urinary concentration is impaired (such as acute tubular necrosis [ATN] or chronic kidney disease). If SG is >1.032, glycosuria should be considered, whereas SG >1.040 almost always indicates the presence of some extrinsic osmotic agent (such as contrast).

Osmolality depends on the number of particles present and is measured by an osmometer. It is not influenced by urine temperature and protein concentrations. However, high glucose concentrations significantly increase osmolality (10 g/l of glucose = 55.5 mOsm/l).

Refractometry is based on measurement of the refractive index, which depends on the weight and the size of solutes per unit volume, and correlates well with osmolality.[4] Refractometers are simple to use and have the major advantage of requiring only one drop of urine. For these reasons, we suggest the use of refractometry rather than SG, even though the factors that can interfere with SG can also interfere with refractometry.

Dry chemistry is incorporated into dipsticks. In the presence of cations, protons are released by a complexing agent and produce a color change in the indicator bromthymol blue from blue via blue-green to yellow. Due to its simplicity, this method is the most widely used. However, underestimation occurs with urine pH >6.5, while overestimation is found with urine protein concentration >7.0 g/l. In addition, nonionized molecules, such as glucose and urea, are not detected. Not surprisingly, this method does not strictly correlate with the results obtained by osmolality[4] and refractometry.[5]

CHEMICAL PARAMETERS

pH

pH is generally evaluated by a dipstick in which a mixed pH indicator covers the pH range 5.0 to 8.5 to 9.0. Using dipsticks, significant deviations from true pH are observed for values <5.5 and >7.5. Therefore, a pH meter with a glass electrode is mandatory when an accurate measurement is necessary.[1]

The pH of the urine reflects the presence of hydrogen ions due to secretion of acid in the collecting duct, but this does not necessarily reflect the overall acid load in the urine as most of the acid is excreted as ammonia. A low pH is often observed with metabolic acidosis (in which acid is secreted), with high protein meals (which generate more acid and ammonia), and with volume depletion (in which aldosterone is stimulated resulting in an acid urine). Indeed, low urinary pH may help to distinguish prerenal acute renal impairment from ATN (which is typically associated with a higher pH). High pH is often observed with renal tubular acidosis (especially distal, type 1, see Chapter 12), with vegetarian diets (due to minimal nitrogen and acid generation), and with infection with urease-positive organisms (such as *Proteus*) that generate ammonia from urea.

Measurement of urine pH is also needed for the interpretation of urinalysis (see "Leukocyte Esterase" and "Microscopy" sections).

Hemoglobin

Hemoglobin is usually detected by a dipstick based on the pseudoperoxidase activity of the heme moiety of hemoglobin, which catalyzes the reaction of a peroxide and a chromogen to produce a colored product. The presence of hemoglobin is shown as green spots, which are due to intact erythrocytes, or as a homogeneous diffuse green pattern. The latter is common with marked hematuria, due to the high number of erythrocytes that cover the whole pad surface. It may also be observed if lysis of erythrocytes has occurred on standing or as a consequence of alkaline urine pH and/or a low relative density (especially <1.010).

The most important false-positive results occur from the presence of hemoglobinuria deriving from intravascular hemolysis, myoglobinuria deriving from rhabdomyolysis, and high concentration of bacteria with pseudoperoxidase activity (Enterobacteriaceae, staphylococci, and streptococci).[6]

False-negative results are mainly due to ascorbic acid, a strong reducing agent, which can result in low-grade microscopic hematuria being completely missed.[7]

Detection of hemoglobin by dipstick has a high specificity and a low sensitivity.[8,9]

Glucose

Glucose is also commonly detected by dipstick. Glucose, with glucose oxidase as catalyst, is first oxidized to gluconic acid and hydrogen peroxide. Then, through the catalyzing activity of a peroxidase, hydrogen peroxide reacts with a reduced colorless chromogen to form a colored product. This test is sensitive to concentrations of 0.5 to 20 g/l. When more precise quantification of urine glucose is needed, enzymatic methods such as hexokinase must be used.

False-negative results occur in the presence of ascorbic acid and bacteria, while false-positive findings may be observed in the presence of oxidizing detergents and hydrochloric acid.

Protein

Physiologic proteinuria does not exceed 150 mg/24 hours for adults and 140 mg/m² for children.

Proteinuria is usually detected by dipstick, which relies on proteins in a buffer causing a change of pH proportional to their concentration. Thus, the dipstick changes color from pale green to green and blue according to the pH changes induced by proteins. This method is highly sensitive to albumin (detection limit, about 0.20 g/l), which has 16 binding sites for the chromogen contained in the pad, while it has little sensitivity to other proteins such as immunoglobulin light chains, which have only 1.5 to 2 binding sites for the chromogen. Dipsticks allow only a rough quantification of urine albumin, which is expressed on a scale from 0 to +++ or ++++ according to the manufacturer. For a reliable quantification of total protein, other methods are necessary, such as turbidimetric or dye-binding techniques. The latter are based on the interaction between copper ions and the carbamide group of proteins and have the same sensitivity for all proteins and minimal interference from drugs, radiographic contrast media, and colored metabolites.

Protein quantification is expressed as g/l or g/24 h. The latter method is still widely used; however, the 24-hour urine collection is time-consuming, subject to error due to overcollection or undercollection, and impractical for many patients. The recommended alternative to 24-hour urine collection is the measurement of the protein:creatinine ratio, which can be calculated in random urine samples, but preferably in first urine specimens, which correlate better with 24-hour urine excretion.[10] Since protein excretion follows a circadian rhythm (highest during the day and lowest overnight) and creatinine excretion is fairly constant over 24 hours, the time of collection may influence the results of the protein:creatinine ratio. Therefore, in the follow-up, the spot sample for the protein:creatinine ratio should always be collected at the same time of the day.[11]

The *qualitative analysis* of proteinuria is currently performed by electrophoresis on cellulose acetate or agarose after protein concentration or using very sensitive stains such as silver or gold. Sodium dodecyl sulfate–polyacrylamide gel electrophoresis (SDS-PAGE) can be used to identify the different urine proteins based on molecular weight and to characterize the proteinuria pattern.[12]

A newer approach is to measure single urinary proteins as markers in the diagnosis, prognosis, and treatment of glomerular and tubular disease. For instance, in idiopathic membranous nephropathy, the urinary excretion of β_2-microglobulin has been reported as a good predictor of poor prognosis,[13] while the combination of IgG and α_1-microglobulin excretion predicts the renal outcome and the response to therapy.[14]

For the identification of *Bence Jones proteinuria* (free immunoglobulin light chains in the urine), immunofixation is the recommended method.[15]

Selectivity of proteinuria in nephrotic syndrome is still today assessed by the ratio of the clearance of IgG (molecular weight 160,000) to the clearance of transferrin (molecular weight 88,000).[16] Highly selective proteinuria, ratio <0.1, in nephrotic children suggests the diagnosis of minimal change disease (MCD) and predicts steroid responsiveness. A recent study suggests that the selectivity of proteinuria combined with SDS-PAGE and the excretion of α_1-microglobulin predicts the outcome and response to therapy in conditions such as MCD, focal segmental glomerulosclerosis, and membranous nephropathy.[17]

Leukocyte Esterase

This dipstick evaluates the presence of leukocytes on the basis of an indoxyl esterase activity released from *lysed* neutrophil granulocytes and macrophages. This feature explains why, especially in urine with an alkaline pH and/or a low relative density, there frequently is a positive dipstick with negative microscopy. The detection limit of the dipstick is 20×10^6 white blood cells per liter.

False-positive results are very rare, for example, when formaldehyde is used as urine preservative. False-negative results occur in the presence of high glucose or protein concentrations (20 g/l and 5 g/l, respectively) or in the presence of cephalothin and tetracycline (strong inhibition), cephalexin (moderate inhibition), or tobramycin (mild inhibition). It should also be remembered that the sensitivity of dipstick for leukocyte esterase is reduced by high SG values since these prevent leukocyte lysis. Sensitivity varies from 76% to 94% and specificity from 68% to 81%,[18,19] which can also depend on different experimental conditions used during leukocyte esterase investigation.

Nitrites

This dipstick test reveals the presence of bacteria that have the capability of reducing nitrates to nitrites due to nitrate reductase activity, which is present in most gram-negative uropathogenic bacteria, but low or absent in *Pseudomonas* spp, *Staphylococcus albus*, and *Enterococcus* spp. Test positivity also requires a diet rich in nitrates (vegetables), which form the substrate for nitrite production, and sufficient bladder incubation time. Thus, it is not surprising that the sensitivity of this test is low, with specificity >90%.[20]

Bile Pigments

Measurements of urinary urobilinogen and bilirubin concentrations have lost their clinical value in the detection of liver disease following the introduction of liver enzyme examination from plasma.

Ketones

This dipstick reveals the presence of acetoacetate and acetone (but not β-hydroxybutyrate), which are excreted into urine during diabetic acidosis, or during fasting, vomiting, or strenuous exercise. It is based on the reaction of the ketones with nitroprusside. Figure 4.1 summarizes the main false-negative and false-positive results that can occur with urine dipstick testing.

Urine dipstick testing		
Parameter	False-Negative Results	False-Positive Results
Specific gravity	Reduced values in the presence of glucose, urine pH >6.5	Increased values in the presence of protein >7 g/l, keto acids
pH	Reduced values in the presence of formaldehyde	—
Hemoglobin	Ascorbic acid, delayed examination, high density of urine, formaldehyde (>0.5 g/l)	Myoglobin, microbial peroxidases, oxidizing agents, hydrochloric acid
Glucose	Ascorbic acid, bacteria	Oxidizing detergents, hydrochloric acid
Albumin	Immunoglobulin light chains, tubular proteins, globulins, abnormally colored urine, hydrochloric acid	Urine pH ≥9, quaternary ammonium detergents, chlorhexidine, polyvinylpyrrolidone
Leukocyte esterase	High density of urine, high vitamin C intake, protein >5 g/l, glucose >20 g/l, cephalosporins, nitrofurantoin	Oxidizing detergents, formaldehyde (>0.4 g/l), sodium azide, abnormally colored urine due to beet
Nitrites	No vegetables in diet, short bladder incubation time, vitamin C, bacteria that do not reduce nitrates to nitrites	Abnormally colored urine
Ketones	Improper storage	Free sulfhydryl groups (e.g., captopril), L-dopa, abnormally colored urine

Figure 4.1 **Urine dipstick testing.** Main false-negative and false-positive results of urine dipsticks.

URINE MICROSCOPY

Urine microscopy is an integral part of urinalysis and adds valuable information to the physicochemical investigation, especially when performed by a trained nephrologist.[21] However, reliable results can be achieved only with standardized methodology.[1] The urine sediment can contain cells, lipids, casts, crystals, organisms, and contaminants.

Methods

The first or second urine of the morning should be collected, following the procedures described previously (see "Urine Collection"). Then, as soon as possible to avoid the lysis of elements, an aliquot of urine is centrifuged and concentrated, after which a standardized volume of resuspended urine should be transferred to the slide and covered with a coverslip of defined size. The use of noncentrifuged samples, advocated by some authors, greatly reduces the sensitivity of the sample, especially for rare but important particles such as erythrocyte casts.

International guidelines suggest the use of a phase contrast microscope in order to improve the identification of the particles. Filters to polarize light are also mandatory for the correct identification of lipids and crystals[1] (Fig. 4.2).

At least 10 microscopic fields, in different areas of the sample, should be examined at both low and high magnification.[1] More extensive examination may be required in certain clinical settings. For instance, for patients with isolated microscopic hematuria of unknown origin, we always examine 50 low power ($\times$160) fields to evaluate the presence of erythrocyte casts.

For a correct examination, both pH and relative density of the sample should be known. Both alkaline pH and low relative density (especially <1.010) favor the lysis of erythrocytes and leukocytes, which can cause discrepancies between dipstick readings and the microscopic examination (see "Hemoglobin" and "Leukocyte Esterase" sections). Alkaline pH also impairs the formation of casts and favors the precipitation of phosphates.

When slides and coverslips are used, the elements observed are quantified as number per microscopic field, while when counting chambers are used the elements are quantified as number per milliliter. Counting chambers allow a precise quantitation of particles, but are rarely used in everyday practice.

Cells

The cells of the urine sediment derive from the circulation (i.e., erythrocytes, leukocytes, and macrophages) and from the epithelia lining the urinary tract (i.e., renal tubular cells, uroepithelial cells, and squamous cells).

Erythrocytes

Erythrocytes have a diameter of 4 to 7 μm. There are two main types of urinary erythrocytes: isomorphic, with regular shapes and contours, derived from the urinary excretory system, and dysmorphic, with irregular shapes and contours, which are of glomerular origin[22] (Fig. 4.3a and b). Some authors define hematuria as nonglomerular when isomorphic erythrocytes predominate (>80% of total erythrocytes) and as glomerular when dysmorphic erythrocytes prevail (>80% of total erythrocytes).[23] Other investigators, including ourselves, recommend that a diagnosis of glomerular hematuria can also be made when the two types of cells are in the same proportion (so-called mixed hematuria)[24] or when at least 5% of erythrocytes examined are acanthocytes,[25] a subtype of dysmorphic erythrocytes with a characteristic appearance that is due to the presence of one or more blebs protruding from a ring-shaped body (see Fig. 4.3b, inset).

The distinction between glomerular and nonglomerular hematuria is of particular importance for the management of patients with isolated microscopic hematuria, allowing an early separation of patients with hematuria caused by a glomerular disease from those with a urologic disorder.[26] However, the evaluation of erythrocyte morphology is subjective and requires experience, which has limited its widespread introduction into clinical practice.

Erythrocyte dysmorphism is thought to be the result of a dual injury: deformation of the erythrocyte while passing through gaps of the glomerular basement membrane followed by physico-chemical insults occurring while the erythrocyte passes through the tubular system.[27]

In patients with a glomerular disease, the *number* of urinary erythrocytes may also be of clinical significance. In proliferative glomerular diseases, the number of erythrocytes is significantly higher than in patients with nonproliferative forms.[28]

Procedures for preparation and examination of the urine sediment used in the authors' clinic and laboratory
Written instructions to the patients for urine collection
Collection in disposable containers of the second urine of the morning after discarding the first few milliliters of urine
Sample handling and analysis within 2 hours after collection
Centrifugation of a 10-ml aliquot of urine at 400g for 10 minutes
Removal by suction of 9.5 ml of supernatant urine
Gentle but thorough resuspension with a pipette of the sediment in the remaining 0.5 ml of urine
Transfer by a pipette of 50 μl of resuspended urine to a slide
Covering of sample with a 24- $\times$ 32-mm coverslip
Examination of the urine sediment by a phase contrast microscope at $\times$160 and $\times$400
Use of polarized light to identify doubtful lipids and crystals
Match the microscopic findings with dipstick for pH, density, hemoglobin, and leukocyte esterase
Cells expressed as lowest to highest number seen per high-power field, casts as number per low-power field, all the other elements on a scale from 0 to ++++

Figure 4.2 Procedures for preparation and examination of the urine sediment.

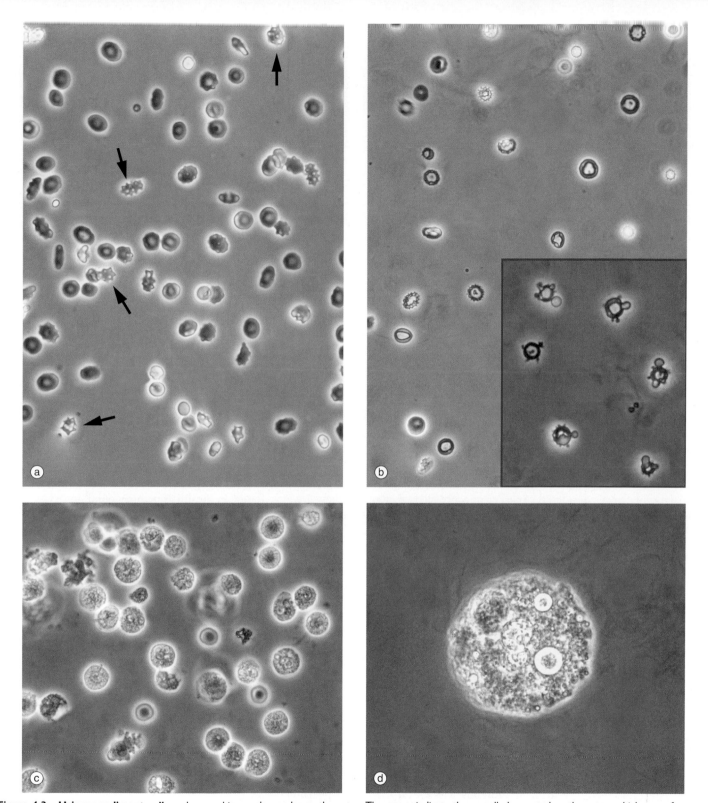

Figure 4.3 Urinary sediment cells. *a*, Isomorphic nonglomerular erythrocytes. The *arrows* indicate the so-called crenated erythrocytes, which are a frequent finding in nonglomerular hematuria. *b*, Dysmorphic glomerular erythrocytes. The dysmorphism consists mainly in irregularities of the cell membrane. *Inset*, Acanthocytes with their typical ring-formed cell bodies with one or more blebs of different sizes and shapes. *c*, Neutrophils. Note their typical lobulated nucleus and granular cytoplasm. *d*, A granular phagocytic macrophage (diameter about 60 μm). *Figure continues on following page.*

Leukocytes

Neutrophils (diameter 7 to 13 μm) are the leukocytes most frequently found in the urine. They are easily identified due to their granular cytoplasm and lobulated nucleus (see Fig. 4.3c). Neutrophils are a marker of lower and upper urinary tract infections. However, especially in young women, they are frequently found due to urine contamination from genital secretions. They can also be found in glomerulonephritis (GN), especially the proliferative forms,[28] and interstitial nephritis, either acute or chronic.

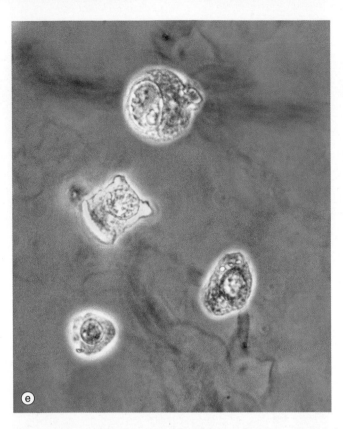

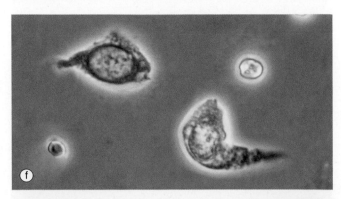

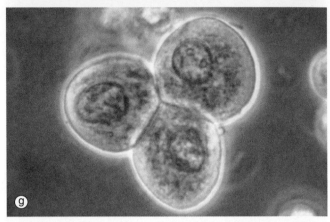

Figure 4.3, cont'd e, Different types of renal tubular cells. f, Two cells from the deep layers of the uroepithelium. g, Three cells from the superficial layers of the uroepithelium. Note the difference in shape and nucleus:cytoplasm ratio existing between the two types of uroepithelial cells. (All images by phase contrast microscopy: original magnification ×400.)

Eosinophils, once considered a marker of acute allergic interstitial nephritis, are now regarded as nonspecific elements, found in various types of GN, prostatitis, chronic pyelonephritis, urinary schistosomiasis, cholesterol embolism, and so on.[29] Eosinophiluria in the evaluation of acute interstitial nephritis is discussed further in Chapter 57.

Lymphocytes are an early marker of acute cellular rejection in renal allograft recipients, but their identification requires staining, and this technique is not widely used in clinical practice.

Macrophages
Macrophages have only recently been identified in urinary sediments. They are of variable size (diameter 15 to >100 μm) and variable appearance: granular, phagocytic, and vacuolar (see Fig. 4.3d). In addition, in patients with the nephrotic syndrome, they can be engorged with lipid droplets, thus appearing as the so-called "oval fat bodies."[30] Using monoclonal antibodies with cytofluorimetry, immunostaining, or immunofluorescence techniques, they have been found in the urine of patients with active GN, nonselective proteinuria,[30] or IgA nephropathy.[31] In our experience, based on phase contrast microscopy alone, they are frequent and abundant in the urine of patients with polyomavirus BK infection (see later discussion). However, the diagnostic value of urinary macrophages is not yet fully defined, and further studies are needed.

Renal Tubular Cells
These cells derive from the exfoliation of the tubular epithelium. Tubular cells in the urine differ in size (diameter ~11 to 15 μm) and shape (from roundish to rectangular or columnar; see Fig 4.3e). Tubular cells are a marker of tubular damage. Therefore,

they are not found in health, but are found in ATN, acute interstitial nephritis, and acute cellular rejection of a renal allograft. In smaller numbers, they are also found in glomerular diseases.[28]

In ATN, tubular cells are usually damaged and necrotic while in other conditions, such as glomerular diseases, they usually have a normal appearance. Tubular cells are very often associated with tubular cell casts (also known as epithelial casts), although the two are not always seen together.[28]

Uroepithelial Cells
These cells derive from the exfoliation of the uroepithelium, which lines the urinary tract from calyces to the bladder in women and to the proximal urethra in men. It is a multilayered epithelium, with small cells in the deep layers and much larger cells in the superficial layers.

The cells of the deep layers (diameter ~13 to 20 μm; see Fig. 4.3f), when in large amounts, are a marker of urologic diseases, such as neoplasia or stones.[32] The cells of the superficial layers (diameter ~20 to 40 μm; see Fig. 4.3g) are a common finding, especially in urinary tract infections.

Squamous Cells
These cells (diameter 45 to 65 μm) derive from the urethra or from the external genitalia. When in large amounts, they indicate urine contamination from genital secretions.

Lipids
Lipids in the urine have the appearance of spherical, translucent, yellow drops of different size. They can be free in the urine (isolated or in clusters; Fig. 4.4a) or fill the cytoplasm of tubular

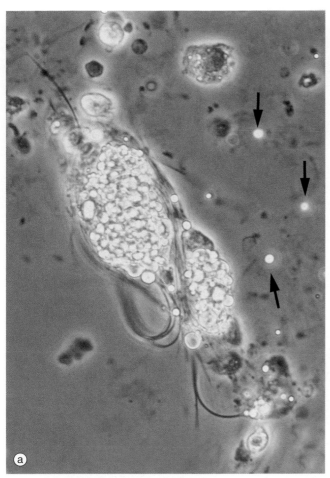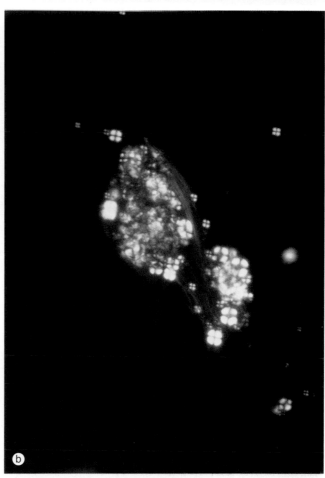

Figure 4.4 Two large aggregates of lipid droplets. Scattered in the specimen there also are isolated fatty droplets (*arrows*). *a*, As seen by phase contrast microscopy. *b*, Under polarized light, which shows the typical Maltese crosses with their symmetric arms (original magnification ×400). (For full morphologic details about these particles, see Fogazzi and colleagues.[32])

epithelial cells or macrophages.[30] When entrapped within casts, lipids form fatty casts. Finally, they can also appear as cholesterol crystals (see "Crystals" section). Lipid drops under polarized light have the appearance of Maltese crosses (see Fig. 4.4b).

Lipids in the urine are typical of glomerular diseases associated with marked proteinuria, usually but not invariably in the nephrotic range. They can also be found in sphingolipidoses such as Fabry's disease. In this condition, they appear as fat particles with an irregular membrane protrusion, which form Maltese crosses under polarized light and show typical myelin bodies with electron microscopy.[33]

Casts

Casts are elements with a cylindrical shape that form in the lumen of distal renal tubules and collecting ducts. Their matrix is Tamm-Horsfall glycoprotein (also called uromodulin), which is secreted by the cells of the thick ascending limb of the loop of Henle. Trapping of particles within the cast matrix results in casts with different appearances and clinical significance (Fig. 4.5). For instance, the trapping within the matrix of cells (erythrocytes, leukocytes, or tubular cells) causes the appearance of erythrocytic, leukocytic, or epithelial casts. Degradation processes occurring within the casts can transform leukocyte or tubular cell casts into coarse granular casts. Finely granular casts, instead, are mostly due to the trapping within the matrix of the casts of lysosomes containing serum ultrafiltered proteins.

- *Hyaline casts* are colorless elements, with a low refractive index (Fig. 4.6a). Therefore, they are easily seen with phase contrast microscopy, but can be overlooked when bright-field microscopy is used. Hyaline casts can be seen in normal urine. When seen in patients with renal disease, they are usually associated with other types of casts.
- *Hyaline-granular casts* contain granules within the hyaline matrix (see Fig 4.6b). Rare but possible in normal individuals, they are common in patients with GN of whatever type.[28]
- *Granular casts* can be either finely granular (see Fig. 4.6c) or coarsely granular. Both types are typical of patients with a renal disease.
- *Waxy casts* derive their name from their appearance, which is similar to that of melted wax (see Fig. 4.6d). The nature of waxy casts is still unknown. They are typical of patients with renal failure, and, in our experience, they are also frequent in patients with rapidly progressive GN.
- *Fatty casts* contain variable amounts of lipid droplets, either isolated, in clumps, or packed. They are typical of glomerular diseases associated with marked proteinuria or the nephrotic syndrome.
- *Erythrocyte casts* may contain a few erythrocytes (see Fig. 4.6e) or so many that the matrix of the cast cannot be identified. In patients with hematuria, the finding of erythrocyte casts clearly indicates that hematuria is of glomerular origin. Therefore, their search is of particular importance in

Clinical significance of urinary casts

Cast	Main Clinical Associations
Hyaline	Normal subject and renal disease
Hyaline-granular	Normal subject and renal disease
Granular	Renal disease
Waxy	Renal insufficiency, rapidly progressive renal disease
Fatty	Marked proteinuria, nephrotic syndrome
Erythrocytic	Glomerular bleeding, proliferative/necrotizing glomerulonephritis
Hemoglobin	The same as the erythrocytic cast + hemoglobinuria
Leukocytic	Acute interstitial nephritis, acute pyelonephritis, proliferative glomerulonephritis
Epithelial	Acute tubular necrosis, acute interstitial nephritis, glomerulonephritis
Myoglobin	Rhabdomyolysis
Bacterial/fungal	Bacterial/fungal infection in the kidney

Figure 4.5   Main clinical significance of urinary casts.

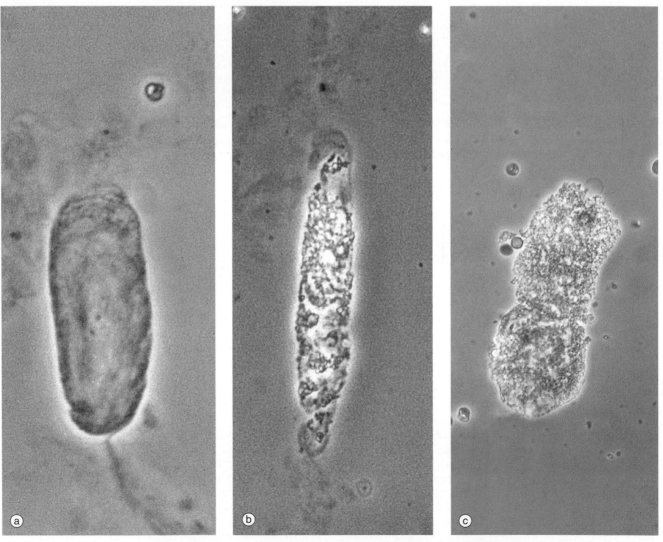

Figure 4.6   Casts. *a*, Hyaline cast. *b*, Hyaline-granular cast. *c*, Finely granular cast.

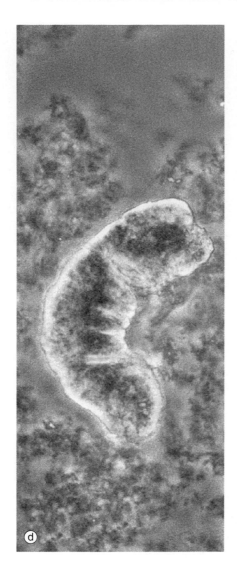

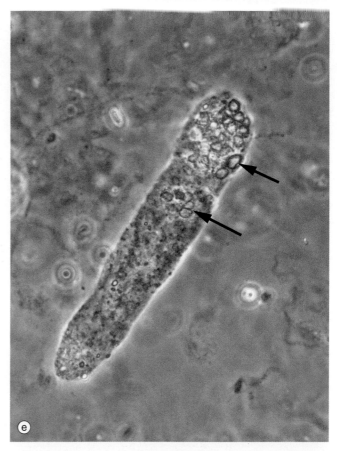

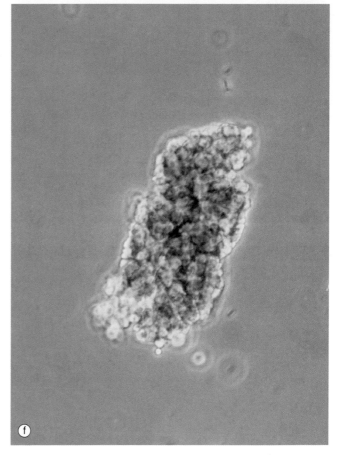

Figure 4.6, cont'd *d*, Waxy cast. *e*, Erythrocyte cast. The *arrows* indicate the erythrocytes embedded in the matrix of the cast. *f*, Hemoglobin cast with its typical brownish hue.   *Figure continues on following page.*

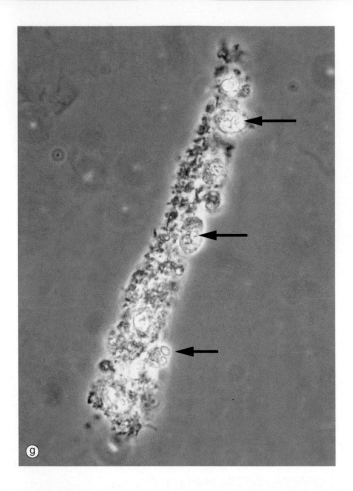

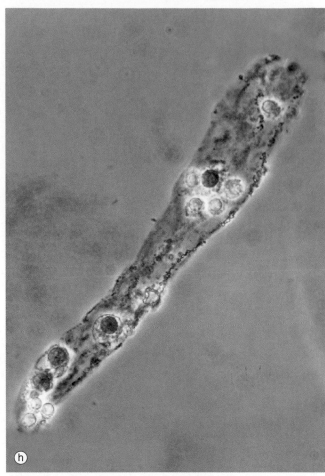

Figure 4.6, cont'd *g*, Leukocyte cast. The polymorphonuclear leukocytes are identifiable due to their lobulated nucleus (*arrows*). *h*, Epithelial cast. Renal tubular cells are identifiable thanks to their large nucleus. (All images by phase contrast microscopy: original magnification ×400.) (For full morphologic details about these particles, see Fogazzi and associates.[32])

patients with isolated microscopic hematuria of unknown origin.

- *Hemoglobin casts* have a brownish hue and often a granular appearance deriving from the degradation of erythrocytes entrapped within the casts (see Fig. 4.6f). Therefore, hemoglobin casts have the same clinical meaning as erythrocyte casts. However, they may also derive from free hemoglobinuria in patients with intravascular hemolysis.
- *Leukocyte casts* contain variable amounts of polymorphonuclear leukocytes (see Fig. 4.6g). They are found in acute pyelonephritis and acute interstitial nephritis. In GN, they are the rarest type of casts.[28]
- *Epithelial casts* contain variable numbers of tubular cells, which can be identified based on their prominent nucleus (see Fig. 4.6h). Epithelial casts are a typical finding in ATN and acute interstitial nephritis of whatever cause. However, they are also frequent in glomerular disorders[28] and in the nephrotic syndrome.
- *Myoglobin casts* contain myoglobin and may be similar to hemoglobin casts (see Fig. 4.6f), from which they can be distinguished through knowledge of the clinical setting. They are observed in the urine of patients with acute renal failure (ARF) associated with rhabdomyolysis.
- *Casts containing microorganisms* (bacteria and yeasts) clearly indicate that the infection is located in the kidneys.
- *Casts containing crystals* indicate that crystals derive from the renal tubules.

- *Mixed casts*, such as the granular-waxy and granular-cellular, have the same significance as their separate components.

Crystals

There are several types of urine crystals. Their correct identification requires combined knowledge of crystal morphologies, urine pH, and appearance under polarizing light.[32] Examination of the urine for crystals is informative in the assessment of patients with stone disease, with some rare inherited metabolic disorders, and with suspected drug nephrotoxicity. The following are the main crystals of the urine.

Uric Acid Crystals and Amorphous Uric Acids

Uric acid crystals have a typical amber color and a wide spectrum of appearances, which ranges from rhomboids to barrels to less defined shapes (Fig. 4.7a). These crystals are found only in acid urine (pH 5.8 or lower), and under polarizing light show a beautiful polychromatic appearance.

Amorphous uric acids are tiny granules of irregular shape, which also precipitate in acid urine. They are identical to amorphous phosphates, which, however, precipitate in alkaline pH. In addition, while uric acids polarize light, phosphates do not.[32]

Calcium Oxalate Crystals

There are two types of calcium oxalate crystals. Bihydrated (or Wedellite) crystals most often have a bipyramidal appearance

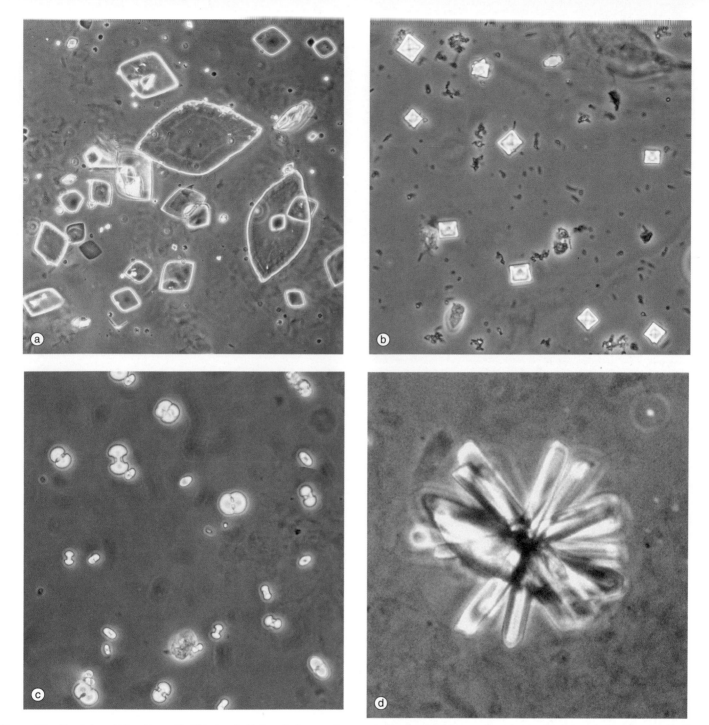

Figure 4.7 **Crystals.** *a*, Uric acid crystals. This rhomboid shape is the most frequent. *b*, Bihydrated calcium oxalate crystals with their typical appearance of a "letter envelope." *c*, Different types of monohydrated calcium oxalate crystals. *d*, A starlike calcium phosphate crystal. *Figure continues on following page.*

(see Fig. 4.7b), while monohydrated (or Whewellite) crystals are ovoid, dumbbell-shaped, or biconcave disks (see Fig. 4.7c). Both types of calcium oxalate crystals precipitate at pH 5.4 to 6.7. Bihydrated crystals do not polarize light while monohydrated crystals do.

Calcium Phosphate Crystals and Amorphous Phosphates

Calcium phosphate crystals are pleomorphic crystals, appearing as prisms, starlike particles, or needles of various sizes and shapes (see Fig. 4.7d). They can also appear as plates with a granular surface. These crystals precipitate in alkaline urine

(pH about 7.0) and, with the exception of plates, they polarize light intensely.

Amorphous phosphates are tiny particles identical to amorphous uric acids. However, they precipitate at a pH of about 7.0 and do not polarize light.

Triple Phosphate Crystals

These crystals contain magnesium ammonium phosphate and in most instances have the appearance of "coffin lids" (see Fig. 4.7e). They are found only in alkaline urine (pH about 7.0) and polarize light strongly.

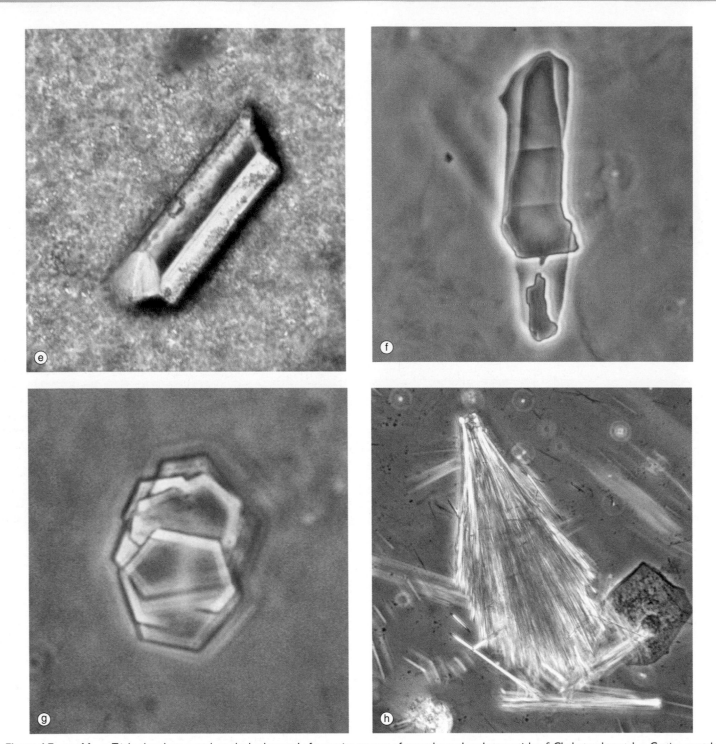

Figure 4.7, cont'd *e,* Triple phosphate crystal, on the background of a massive amount of amorphous phosphate particles. *f,* Cholesterol crystal. *g,* Cystine crystals heaped one on the other. *h,* Amoxicillin crystal resembling a branch of a broom bush.

Cholesterol Crystals
They are transparent and thin plates, often clumped together, with sharp edges (see Fig. 4.7f).

Cystine Crystals
These crystals are hexagonal plates with irregular sides, which are often heaped one upon the other (see Fig. 4.7g). They precipitate only in acid urine, especially after the addition of acetic acid and after overnight storage at 4°C. Evaluation of their size can be used to predict the recurrence of cystine stones.[34]

2,8-Dihydroxyadenine Crystals
These are spherical, brownish crystals with radial striations from the center and polarize light strongly.[35]

Crystals Due to Drugs
Many drugs (especially in a setting of drug overdose, dehydration, or hypoalbuminemia in the presence of a urinary pH favoring drug crystallization) can cause transient crystalluria: common examples are the sulfonamide sulfadiazine, the antibiotics amoxicillin (see Fig 4.7h) and ciprofloxacin, the antiviral agents acyclovir and indinavir (see Fig. 4.7i), the vasodilator pyridoxylate,

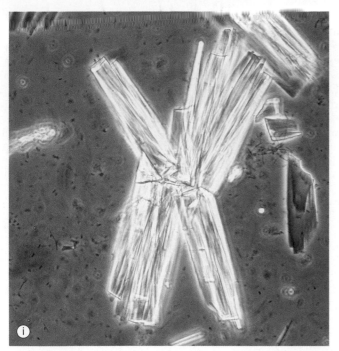

Figure 4.7, cont'd *i*, A large crystal of indinavir. (All images by phase contrast microscopy: original magnification ×400.)

the barbiturate primidone, the vasodilator naftidrofuryl oxalate, and vitamin C.[32]

Drugs should always be considered as a likely cause of atypical crystals.

Clinical Significance of Crystals

The finding in the urine of a few uric acid, calcium oxalate, or calcium phosphate crystals is rather common. In most instances, it is a finding without clinical importance since it reflects a transient supersaturation of the urine due to ingestion of some foods (e.g., meat for uric acid, spinach or chocolate for calcium oxalate, milk or cheese for calcium phosphate) or mild dehydration. However, the persistence of a calcium oxalate or uric acid crystalluria in repeated samples of the same subject may reflect persistent hypercalciuria, hyperoxaluria, or hyperuricosuria. Therefore, in calcium stone formers, the accurate study of crystalluria may be used to evaluate the calcium stone disease activity.[36]

Large numbers of uric acid crystals may be associated with ARF due to acute uric acid nephropathy, while large numbers of monohydrated calcium oxalate crystals, especially with a spindle shape, may be associated with ARF from ethylene glycol intoxication.

Some crystals are always pathologic. This is the case with cholesterol, which is found in patients with marked proteinuria; cystine, which is a marker of cystinuria; and 2,8-dihydroxyadenine, which is a marker of homozygotic deficiency of the enzyme adenine phosphoribosyltransferase. This rare condition causes crystalluria in about 96% of untreated patients who frequently also suffer from radiolucent urinary stone formation, ARF, or even chronic renal failure.[35]

When crystalluria is due to drugs, this may be the only urinary abnormality or it may be associated with hematuria, obstructive uropathy, or ATN due to the precipitation of crystals within the renal tubules. This last possibility has been described with crystals due to sulfadiazine, indinavir,[37] naftidrofuryl oxalate, vitamin C, and amoxicillin.

Organisms

Bacteria are a frequent finding since urine is usually collected and handled under nonsterile conditions and examination is often delayed. Urinary infection can be suspected only if bacteria are found in noncontaminated, freshly voided midstream urine, especially if numerous leukocytes are also present.[38]

Candida, Trichomonas vaginalis, and *Enterobius vermicularis* are mostly common contaminants deriving from genital secretions.

Schistosoma hematobium is a parasite responsible for urinary schistosomiasis. In endemic areas, the examination of the urinary sediment is the most widely used method to diagnose this condition, which causes recurrent bouts of macroscopic hematuria and obstructive uropathy. The diagnosis is based on the finding of the parasite eggs, with their typical terminal spike (see Chapter 53, Fig. 53.4). The eggs are especially found between 10 AM and 2 PM and after strenuous exercise, such as a run.

INTERPRETATION OF THE MAIN URINE SEDIMENT FINDINGS

The examination of the urine sediment, coupled with the quantity of proteinuria and integrated with other urine and blood findings, leads to urine sediment profiles that contribute to the diagnosis of diseases of the urinary tract (Fig. 4.8)

Main urinary sediment profiles		
Renal Disease	Hallmark	Associated Findings
Nephrotic syndrome	Lipiduria Marked cylindruria	Tubular cells Epithelial casts Microscopic hematuria: absent/mild to moderate
Nephritic syndrome	Moderate to severe hematuria Erythrocyte/hemoglobin casts	Mild leukocyturia Tubular cells Epithelial casts Waxy casts
Acute tubular necrosis	Necrotic/damaged renal tubular cells Epithelial and muddy brown granular casts	Variable according to the cause of ATN (e.g., pigmented myoglobin casts in crush syndrome; uric acid crystals in acute uric acid nephropathy)
Urinary tract infection	Leukocytes Bacteria	Superficial epithelial cells Triple phosphate crystals (for infections due to urease-producing bacteria) Leukocyte casts (in renal infection)
Polyomavirus BK infection	Decoy cells	Macrophages

Figure 4.8 Main urinary sediment profiles.

Nephrotic Sediment

The typical nephrotic sediment contains lipids, casts, and tubular cells. Hyaline, hyaline-granular, granular, and fatty casts are seen, while erythrocyte/hemoglobin casts, leukocyte casts, and waxy casts are very rare or absent. Erythrocytes may be totally absent, especially in MCD, or may be in moderate numbers, which occurs in membranous nephropathy and focal segmental glomerulosclerosis. Leukocytes are usually not found.

Nephritic Sediment

Hematuria is the hallmark of the nephritic sediment. Moderate to marked hematuria is present in virtually all cases. More than 100 erythrocytes per high-power field is not uncommon, especially in cases with extracapillary and/or necrotizing glomerular lesions. Leukocyturia is also frequent. Erythrocyte/hemoglobin casts are frequent. Leukocyte and waxy casts can also be observed.

The nephritic sediment may clear with treatment, while its reappearance indicates a relapse of the disease. Therefore, the study of the urine sediment is of special value in recurring proliferative glomerular diseases such as lupus nephritis[39] or systemic vasculitis.[40] However, in rare cases, there may be an active proliferative glomerular disease without the nephritic sediment.

In our experience, it is possible to distinguish proliferative from nonproliferative glomerular diseases by the examination of the urine sediment with 80% sensitivity and 79% specificity. We found that proliferative disorders are associated with significantly higher numbers of erythrocytes, leukocytes, and tubular epithelial cells as well as erythrocyte and epithelial cell casts.[28]

Sediment of Acute Tubular Necrosis

In ATN, the urine sediment contains variable numbers of necrotic/damaged tubular cells and a marked granular and epithelial cylindruria. Epithelial cell casts may predominate at first if there is massive tubular cell injury, but as ATN progresses, the tubular cells become degraded during transit and granular casts are more characteristic, the so-called muddy brown casts of ATN. In addition, depending on the cause of the tubular damage, other elements can be seen. For instance, in rhabdomyolysis, myoglobin pigmented casts can also be found, while in ATN due to intratubular precipitation of crystals (e.g., acute uric acid nephropathy, ethylene glycol poisoning, drugs), there may be massive crystalluria.

Sediment of Urinary Tract Infection

Bacteriuria and leukocyturia are the hallmarks of this condition. Superficial uroepithelial cells are common. Triple phosphate crystals are also present when the infection is caused by urease-producing bacteria such as *Ureaplasma urealyticum* or *Corynebacterium urealyticum*.

The correlation between the urine sediment findings and the urine culture is usually good. False-positive results may occur as a consequence of urine contamination from genital secretions or bacterial overgrowth upon standing. False-negative results may be due to misinterpretation of bacteria (especially with cocci) or the lysis of leukocytes.

Sediment of Infection Due to Polyomavirus BK

In this condition (see Chapter 94), the urinary sediment contains variable numbers of the so-called decoy cells (as a general rule, the higher the number, the more severe the infection). These are mostly renal tubular cells with nuclear changes due to the cytopathic effect of the polyomavirus BK. The main nuclear changes consist of nuclear enlargement ("ground glass appearance"), chromatin margination, abnormal chromatin patterns, and viral inclusion bodies of various sizes and shapes with or without a perinuclear halo. In our experience, these cells can easily be seen by phase contrast microscopy without staining[41] (Fig. 4.9a), while most investigators use Papanicolaou stain[42] (see Fig. 4.9b). Electron microscopy shows the presence of variable amounts of virus particles whose mean diameter is about 45 Å (see Fig. 4.9c). In our experience, in addition to decoy cells, macrophages are also frequent and abundant. The finding of decoy cells in the urine is a sign of reactivation of the viral infection, while for the diagnosis of polyomavirus BK nephropathy, a renal biopsy is mandatory.

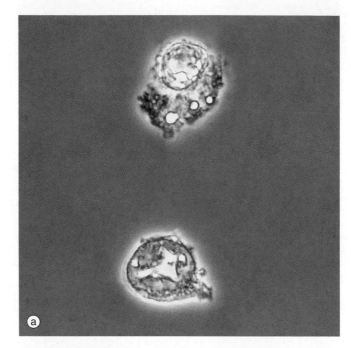

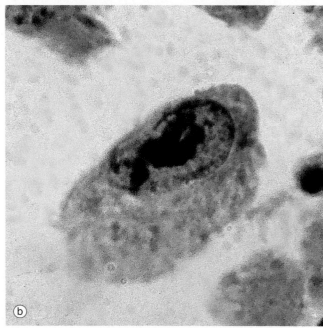

Figure 4.9 **Decoy cells due to polyomavirus BK infection.** *a*, Decoy cells as seen by phase contrast microscopy. Note the enlarged nucleus of the lower cell that contains a large inclusion body (original magnification ×400). *b*, A decoy cell as seen by Papanicolaou stain. Again, note the large nuclear inclusion body (original magnification ×1000).

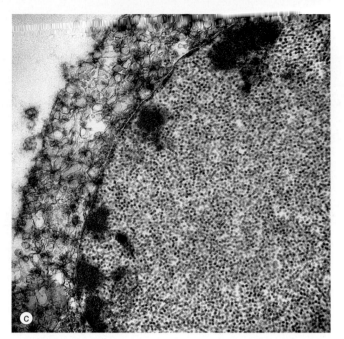

Figure 4.9, cont'd *c*, A decoy cell as seen by transmission electron microscopy (original magnification ×30,000), whose nucleus is engorged with virus particles. Also note various chromatin granules close to nuclear membrane (= chromatin margination).

Nonspecific Urinary Abnormalities

In addition to the urine patterns previously described, urine sediments can demonstrate less defined changes, such as variable casts with or without mild erythrocyturia or leukocyturia, mild crystalluria, and small numbers of superficial transitional cells. In such cases, the correct interpretation of the urinary findings requires adequate clinical information and the results of other diagnostic tests.

AUTOMATED ANALYSIS OF THE URINE SEDIMENT

In the past 10 years, flow cytometry has been applied to the analysis of urinary sediments using stains for nucleic acid and cell membranes in uncentrifuged urine samples. The results appear on a screen as both scattergrams and numeric data.[43]

Flow cytometry allows the identification and quantification of many particles of urine sediments, but does not identify lipids and some types of crystals or casts and cannot distinguish between uroepithelial cells and renal tubular cells. Accuracy is excellent for leukocytes, while erythrocytes are overestimated due to the interference from bacteria, crystals, and yeasts.[44]

Today, flow cytometry is used especially in large laboratories to screen large numbers of samples in a short time. This approach greatly reduces the number of samples that require manual microscopy, which mostly derive from renal patients.

A new technology based on digital imaging software has recently been incorporated in an automated urine analyzer; preliminary evaluations show good precision and accuracy for erythrocytes and leukocytes.[45,46] Evaluation for lipids, crystals, casts, and epithelial cells is in progress.

REFERENCES

1. Kouri T, Fogazzi G, Gant V, et al: European urinalysis guidelines. Scand J Clin Lab Med 2000;60(Suppl 231):1–96.
2. Van der Snoek BE, Koene RAP: Fixation of urinary sediment. Lancet 1997;350:933–934.
3. Kouri T, Vuotari L, Pohjavaara S, et al: Preservation of urine flow cytometric and visual microscopic testing. Clin Chem 2002;48:900–905.
4. Pradella M, Dorizzi RM, Rigolin F: Relative density of urine: Methods and clinical significance. Crit Rev Clin Lab Sci 1988;26:195–242.
5. Dorizzi RM, Caputo M: Measurement of urine relative density using refractometer and reagent strips. Clin Chem Lab Med 1998;36:925–928.
6. Lam MO: False hematuria due to bacteriuria. Arch Pathol 1995;119:717–721.
7. Bridgen ML, Edgell D, McPherson M, et al: High incidence of significant urinary ascorbic acid concentration in a West Coast population—implication for routine analysis. Clin Chem 1992;38:426–431.
8. Grienstead GF, Scott RE, Stevens BS, et al: The Ames Clinitek 200/Multistix P urinalysis method compared with manual and microscopic method. Clin Chem 1987;33:1660–1662.
9. Bank CM, Codrington JF, Van Dieijen-Visser MP, Brombacher PJ: Screening urine specimen populations for normality using different dipsticks: Evaluation of parameters influencing sensitivity and specificity. J Clin Chem Clin Biochem 1987;25:299–307.
10. K/DOQI clinical practice guidelines for chronic kidney disease: Evaluation, classification, and stratification. Am J Kidney Dis 2002;39(Suppl 1):S93–S102.
11. Koopman MG, Krediet RT, Koomen GCM, et al: Circadian rhythm of proteinuria: Consequences of the use of urinary protein:creatinine ratios. Nephrol Dial Transplant 1989;4:9–14.
12. Bazzi C, Petrini C, Rizza V, et al: Characterization of proteinuria in primary glomerulonephritides. SDS-PAGE patterns: Clinical significance and prognostic value of low molecular weight ("tubular") proteins. Am J Kidney Dis 1997;29:27–35.
13. Reichert LJM, Koene RAP, Wetzels FM: Urinary excretion of β_2-microglobulin predicts renal outcome in patients with idiopathic membranous nephropathy. J Am Soc Nephrol 1995;6:1666–1669.
14. D'Amico G, Bazzi C: Urinary protein and enzyme excretion as markers of tubular damage. Curr Opin Nephrol Hypertens 2003;12:639–643.
15. Graziani M, Merlini GP, Petrini C: IFCC Committee on Plasma Protein. Guidelines for the analysis of Bence Jones protein. Clin Chem Lab Med 2003;41:338–346.
16. Cameron JS, Blandford G: The simple assessment of selectivity in heavy proteinuria. Lancet 1966;ii:242–247.
17. Bazzi C, Petrini C, Rizza V, et al: A modern approach to selectivity of proteinuria and tubulointerstitial damage in nephrotic syndrome. Kidney Int 2001;58:1732–1741.
18. Kutter D, Figueiredo G, Klemmer L: Chemical detection of leukocytes in urine by means of a new multiple test strip. J Clin Chem Clin Biochem 1987;25:91–94.
19. Skjold AC, Stover LR, Pendergrass JH, et al: New DiP-and-read test for determining leukocytes in urine. Clin Chem 1987;33:1242–1245.
20. Lundberg JO, Carlsson S, Engstrand L, et al: Urinary nitrite: More than a marker of infection. Urology 1997;50:189–191.
21. Tsai JJ, Yeun JY, Kumar VA, Don BR: Comparison and interpretation of urinalysis performed by a nephrologist versus a hospital-based clinical laboratory. Am J Kidney Dis 2005;46:820–829.
22. Fairley K, Birch DF. Hematuria: A simple method for identifying glomerular bleeding. Kidney Int 1982;21:105–108.
23. Fasset RG, Horgan BA, Mathew TH: Detection of glomerular bleeding by phase contrast microscopy. Lancet 1982;i:1432–1434.
24. Rizzoni G, Braggion F, Zacchello G: Evaluation of glomerular and nonglomerular hematuria by phase-contrast microscopy. J Pediatr 1983;103:370–374.
25. Dinda AK, Saxena S, Guleria S, et al: Diagnosis of glomerular hematuria: Role of dysmorphic red cells, G1 cells and bright field microscopy. Scand J Clin Lab Invest 1997;57:203–208.

26. Schramek P, Gergopoulos M, Schuster FX, et al: Value of urinary erythrocytes morphology in assessment of symptomless microhematuria. Lancet 1989;ii:1316–1319.

27. Rath B, Turner C, Hartley B, Chantler C: What makes red cells dysmorphic in glomerular hematuria? Paediatr Nephrol 1992;6:424–427.

28. Fogazzi GB, Saglimbeni L, Banfi G, et al: Urinary sediment features in proliferative and nonproliferative glomerular diseases. J Nephrol 2005;18:703–710.

29. Nolan CR, Kelleher SP: Eosinophiluria. Clin Lab Med 1988;8:555–565.

30. Hotta O, Yusa N, Kitamura H, Taguma Y: Urinary macrophages as activity markers of renal injury. Clin Chim Acta 2000;297:123–133.

31. Maruhashi Y, Nakajima M, Akazawa H, et al: Analysis of macrophages in urine sediments in children with IgA nephropathy. Clin Nephrol 2004;62:336–343.

32. Fogazzi GB, Ponticelli C, Ritz E: The Urinary Sediment. An Integrated View, 2nd ed. Oxford: Oxford University Press, 1999.

33. Sessa A, Meroni M, Battini G, et al: Renal transplantation in patients with Fabry disease. Nephron 2002;91:348–351.

34. Daudon M, Cohen-Solal F, Barbey F, et al: Cystine crystal volume determination: A useful tool in the management of cystinuric patients. Urol Res 2003;31:207–211.

35. Edvarsson V, Palsson R, Olafsson I, et al: Clinical features and genotype of adenine phosphoribosyltransferase deficiency in Iceland. Am J Kidney Dis 2001;38:473–480.

36. Daudon M, Jungers P: Clinical value of crystalluria and quantitative morphoconstitutional analysis of urinary calculi. Nephron Physiol 2004;98:31–36.

37. Kopp JB: Renal dysfunction in HIV-1 infected patients. Curr Infect Dis Rep 2002;4:449–460.

38. Vickers D, Ahmad T, Coulthard MG: Diagnosis of urinary tract infection in children: Fresh urine microscopy or culture? Lancet 1991;338:767–770.

39. Hebert LA, Dillon JJ, Middendorf DF, et al: Relationship between appearance of urinary red blood cell/white blood cell casts and the onset of renal relapse in systemic lupus erythematosus. Am J Kidney Dis 1995;26:432–438.

40. Fujita T, Ohi H, Endo M, et al: Levels of red blood cells in the urinary sediment reflect the degree of renal activity in Wegener's granulomatosis. Clin Nephrol 1998;50:284–288.

41. Fogazzi GB, Cantù M, Saglimbeni L: "Decoy cells" in the urine due to polyomavirus BK infection: Easily seen by phase-contrast microscopy. Nephrol Dial Transplant 2001;16:1496–1498.

42. Drachemberg RC, Drachenberg CB, Papadimitriou JC, et al: Morphological spectrum of polyomavirus disease in renal allografts: Diagnostic accuracy of urine cytology. Am J Transplant 2001;1:373–381.

43. Delanghe JR, Kouri TT, Huber AR, et al: The role of automated urine particles flow cytometry in clinical practice. Clin Chim Acta 2000;301:1–18.

44. Fenili D, Pirovano B: The automation of sediment urinalysis using a new urine flow cytometer (UF-100(TM)). Clin Chem Lab Med 1998;36:909–917.

45. Alves L, Ballester F, Camps J, Joven J: Preliminary evaluation of the Iris IQ 200 automated urine analyzer. Clin Chem Lab Med 2005;43:967–970.

46. Wah DT, Wises PK, Butch AW: Analytic performance of the iQ200 automated urine microscopy analyzer and comparison with manual counts using Fuchs-Rosenthal cell chambers. Am J Clin Pathol 2005;123:290–296.

Imaging

Rosaleen B. Parsons and William L. Simpson, Jr.

IMAGING STRATEGY

This chapter discusses the range of available imaging methods and their role in the diagnosis and management of renal disease. The correct choice of imaging will minimize the time and cost of effective evaluation. In the past 5 years, there has been a major shift in the imaging approach for kidney disease. For example, the patient who presented in the past with painless hematuria would undergo plain radiography followed perhaps by ultrasound and intravenous contrast urography (IVU), but computed tomography (CT) is often the first study now ordered in this scenario. The use of three-dimensional (3-D) ultrasound and ultrasound contrast agents has expanded the role of ultrasound from a static process to a dynamic imaging tool that can be used to provide detailed information regarding perfusion. The role of magnetic resonance imaging (MRI) is also expanding as faster pulse sequences and kidney-specific contrast agents are developed. The choice of imaging technique may also be influenced by the comorbid state of the patient. For example, a technique avoiding radiographic contrast may be preferred for those at high risk for contrast nephrotoxicity (discussed at the end of this chapter). The first-choice imaging techniques in common clinical situations are shown in Figure 5.1.

ULTRASOUND

Ultrasound examination of the kidneys is relatively inexpensive and provides a rapid way to assess renal location, contour, and size. Nephrologists are increasingly undertaking straightforward ultrasound examination: the practical techniques, as well as the appropriate interpretative skills, are discussed in Chapter 82. Portable ultrasound is available and is essential in the pediatric or emergency setting. Obstructing renal calculi can be readily detected, and renal masses can be identified as cystic or solid. In cases of suspected obstruction, the progression or regression of hydronephrosis is easily evaluated. Color Doppler imaging permits assessment of renal vascularity and perfusion. Unlike the other imaging modalities, ultrasound is highly dependent on the operator's skills.

Kidney Size

The kidney is imaged in transverse and sagittal planes and is normally 9 to 12 cm in length in adults. Abnormal renal size is the most common sign identified on renal imaging. Differences in renal size can be detected with all imaging modalities. The common causes of enlarged and shrunken kidneys are shown in Figure 5.2.

First-choice imaging techniques in renal disease	
Renal Failure, Unknown Cause	Ultrasound
Hematuria	CT
Proteinuria/nephrotic syndrome	CT urography
Hypertension	
With normal renal function	CT angiography including imaging of the adrenal glands
With impaired renal function	MR angiography
Renal artery stenosis	
With normal or impaired renal function	MR angiography
Renal infection	CT
Hydronephrosis detected by ultrasound	IVU (if renal function is preserved) or ^{99}Tc-DTPA renography
Retroperitoneal fibrosis	Contrast-enhanced CT
Papillary necrosis	Contrast-enhanced CT
Cortical necrosis	Contrast-enhanced CT
Renal vein thrombosis	Contrast-enhanced CT
Renal infarction	Contrast-enhanced CT
Nephrocalcinosis	CT

Figure 5.1   First-choice imaging techniques in common clinical situations. CT, computed tomography; IVU, intravenous urography; MR, magnetic resonance.

Renal Echo Pattern

The normal cortex is hypoechoic compared with the fat-containing echogenic renal sinus (Fig. 5.3). The cortical echotexture may be isoechoic or hypoechoic compared with the liver or spleen.[1] In children, the renal pyramids are hypoechoic, and the cortex is characteristically hyperechoic compared with the liver and the spleen.[2] In adults, an increase in cortical echogenicity is a sensitive marker for parenchymal renal disease but is nonspecific (Fig. 5.4). Decreased cortical echogenicity can be found in acute pyelonephritis and acute renal vein thrombosis.

The normal renal contour is smooth, and the cortical mantle should be uniform and slightly thicker toward the poles. Two benign masses that can be seen with ultrasound are the dromedary hump and the column of Bertin. The column of Bertin results from bulging of cortical tissue into the medullary portion of the kidney. On ultrasound, it is seen as a mass with similar echotexture to the cortex but found within the central renal sinus (Fig. 5.5). The renal pelvis and proximal ureter are anechoic. An extrarenal pelvis refers

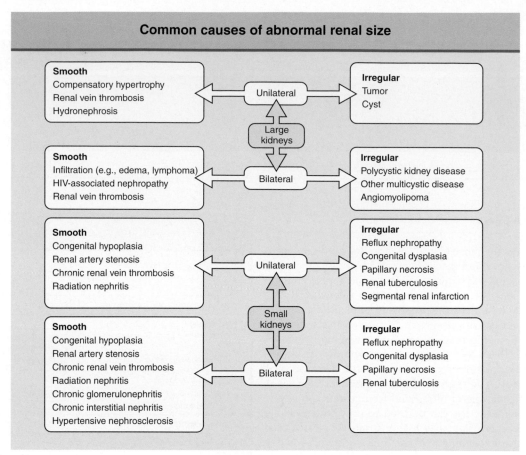

Common causes of abnormal renal size

Smooth
Compensatory hypertrophy
Renal vein thrombosis
Hydronephrosis

Irregular
Tumor
Cyst

Unilateral

Large kidneys

Smooth
Infiltration (e.g., edema, lymphoma)
HIV-associated nephropathy
Renal vein thrombosis

Irregular
Polycystic kidney disease
Other multicystic disease
Angiomyolipoma

Bilateral

Smooth
Congenital hypoplasia
Renal artery stenosis
Chronic renal vein thrombosis
Radiation nephritis

Irregular
Reflux nephropathy
Congenital dysplasia
Papillary necrosis
Renal tuberculosis
Segmental renal infarction

Unilateral

Small kidneys

Smooth
Congenital hypoplasia
Renal artery stenosis
Chronic renal vein thrombosis
Radiation nephritis
Chronic glomerulonephritis
Chronic interstitial nephritis
Hypertensive nephrosclerosis

Irregular
Reflux nephropathy
Congenital dysplasia
Papillary necrosis
Renal tuberculosis

Bilateral

Figure 5.2 Common causes of abnormal renal size.

to the renal pelvis location outside the renal hilum. The ureter is not identified beyond the pelvis in nonobstructed patients.

Obstruction can be identified by the presence of hydronephrosis (Fig. 5.6) Obstructing renal calculi can be readily detected (Fig. 5.7). The upper ureter will also be dilated if obstruction is distal to the pelviureteral junction (see Fig. 5.6c). False-negative ultrasound examination with no hydronephrosis occasionally occurs in early obstruction.

Renal Cysts
Cysts can be identified as anechoic lesions and are a frequent coincidental finding during renal imaging. Ultrasound readily

identifies renal masses as cystic or solid (Figs. 5.8 and 5.9). Differentiation of cysts as simple or complex is required to plan intervention. The classification developed by Bosniak for the CT characterization of renal cysts can be applied to the ultrasound features and is widely used[3,4] (Fig. 5.10).

Simple Cysts
A simple cyst on ultrasound is anechoic, has a thin or imperceptible wall, and demonstrates through-transmission because of the relatively rapid progression of the sound wave through fluid compared with adjacent soft tissue.

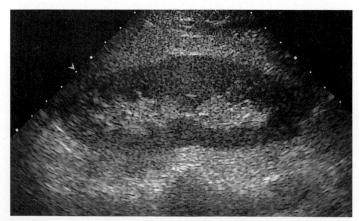

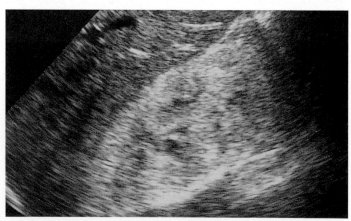

Figure 5.3 Normal sagittal renal ultrasound. The cortex is hypoechoic compared with the echogenic fat containing the renal sinus.

Figure 5.4 HIV-associated nephropathy. Enlarged echogenic kidney with lack of corticomedullary distinction. Bipolar length of kidney is 14.2 cm.

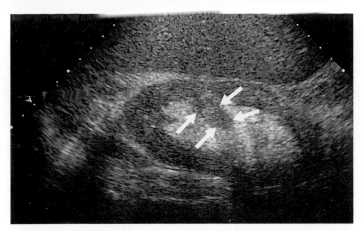

Figure 5.5 Sagittal renal ultrasound. Column of Bertin is present *(arrows)* and is easily identified because of the similar echo texture to the cortex.

Complex Cysts

Complex cysts contain calcifications, septations, and mural nodules. Instead of being anechoic, they may contain internal echoes representing hemorrhage, pus, or protein. Complex cysts may be benign or malignant, the latter strongly suggested by cyst wall nodularity, septations, and vascularity. Complex cysts identified by ultrasound require further evaluation by contrast CT (or MRI) to identify abnormal contrast enhancement of the cyst wall, mural nodule, or septum. See also Chapter 56.

Bladder

Color-flow Doppler evaluation of the bladder in well-hydrated patients can be used to identify a ureteral jet. The jet is produced when peristalsis propels urine into the bladder, the incoming urine having a specific gravity higher relative to the urine already in the bladder (Fig. 5.11). Absence of the ureteral jet can indicate total ureteral obstruction.

Renal Vasculature

Color Doppler investigation of the kidneys provides a detailed evaluation of the renal vascular anatomy, particularly in renal transplants. The main renal arteries can be identified in most patients (Fig. 5.12). Power Doppler is an alternative method of evaluating the renal vasculature, which is a more sensitive indicator of flow than is color Doppler. Unlike color Doppler, it does not provide any information about flow direction, and it cannot be used to assess vascular waveforms. It is, however, exquisitely sensitive for detection of renal parenchymal flow and has been used to identify cortical infarction.

Renal Artery Duplex Scanning

Renal artery stenosis is an uncommon cause of hypertension but is potentially curable with angioplasty or surgery. The role of gray scale and color Doppler sonography in screening for renal artery stenosis is controversial.

The underlying principle is that a narrowing in the artery will cause a velocity change commensurate with the degree of stenosis as well as a change in the normal renal arterial waveform downstream from the lesion. Long-standing renal artery stenosis often results in a decrease in renal size.

The entire length of the renal artery should be examined for the highest-velocity signal. The origins of the renal arteries are important to identify because this is a common area affected by atherosclerosis. Within the kidney, medullary branches and cortical branches in the upper, middle, and lower thirds should be included in the Doppler examination in order to attempt to detect stenosis in accessory renal arteries.

There are proximal and distal criteria for diagnosing renal artery stenosis of more than 60%. The proximal criteria detect changes in the Doppler signal at the site of stenosis. These include

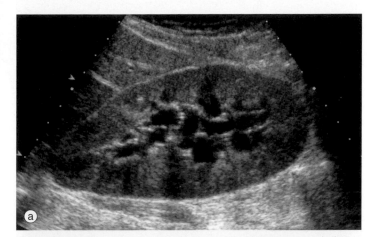

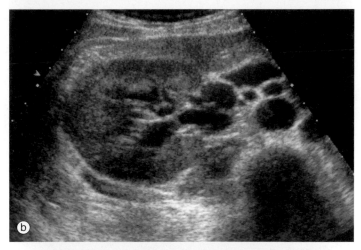

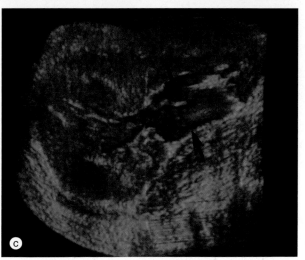

Figure 5.6 Renal ultrasound demonstrating hydronephrosis. *a,* Sagittal image. *b,* Transverse image. *c,* Transverse three-dimensional surface-rendered image with *arrows* indicating the dilated proximal ureter.

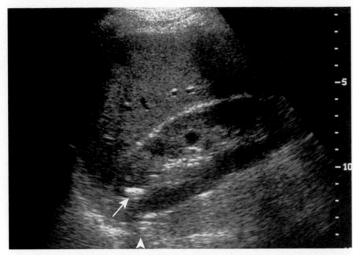

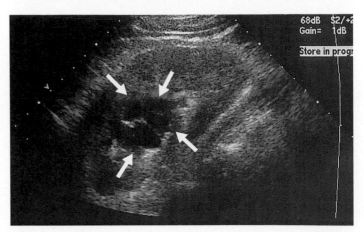

Figure 5.9   Sagittal renal ultrasound showing a complex cyst (arrows).

Figure 5.7   Sagittal ultrasound showing an upper pole renal calculus (arrow). Note the acoustic shadowing *(arrowhead)*.

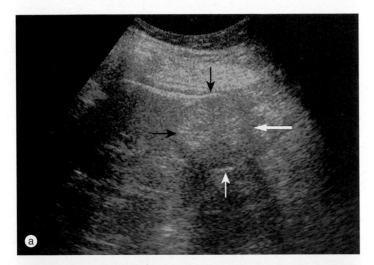

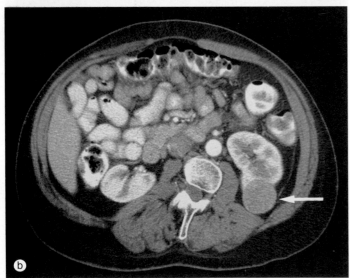

Figure 5.8   Evaluation of a renal mass. *a*, Sagittal ultrasound showing a large hyperechoic mass arising from the lower pole *(arrows)*. *b*, Corresponding contrast computed tomography scan showing a renal cell carcinoma *(arrow)*.

high systolic velocity and turbulence. The distal criteria detect a change in the arterial waveform downstream from a stenosis. The change in waveform can be expressed mathematically using the resistive index, which is a ratio defined as the end-diastolic velocity (EDV) subtracted from the peak systolic velocity (PSV) divided by the peak systolic velocity [(PSV − EDV)/PSV]. The arterial resistive index in the normal kidney is 0.70 to 0.72.

There are four proximal criteria:
1. Peak systolic velocity of 200 cm/second or greater
2. Ratio of peak systolic velocity in the renal artery to the aorta of greater than 3.5
3. Turbulent flow in the poststenotic region
4. Lack of detectable Doppler signal in a visualized renal artery, which denotes occlusion of the artery

Using these criteria, sensitivities and specificities ranging from 0% to 98% and 37% to 98%, respectively, have been reported.[5,6] Lack of sensitivity and specificity are attributable in part to a large number of technical failures.

The distal criteria are related to detection of a tardus parvus waveform distal to a stenosis. The normal renal arterial waveform demonstrates a rapid systolic upstroke and an early systolic peak (Fig. 5.13a). The waveform becomes dampened downstream from a stenosis. This consists of a slow systolic acceleration (tardus) and a decreased and rounded systolic peak (parvus; see Fig. 5.13b). It also results in a decrease in the resistive index.

There are four distal criteria:
1. Loss of the early systolic peak
2. Slope of the systolic upstroke (acceleration) reduced to less than 300 cm/second
3. Acceleration time of greater than 0.07 second
4. Resistive index change of greater than 5% between the left and right kidneys

Using these distal criteria, sensitivities and specificities of 66% to 100% and 67% to 94%, respectively, have been reported.[7,8]

Combining the proximal and distal criteria improves the detection of stenoses. Sensitivity of 96.7% and specificity of 98% can be achieved when both the extrarenal and intrarenal arteries are examined.[9] However, reliable results require a skilled and experienced sonographer and a long examination time. Other limitations include inability to identify the entire course of the renal artery in some patients owing to the patient body habitus or bowel gas. Patients must also hold their breath to stop respiratory motion in order to obtain a good, reliable Doppler spectral tracing. The

Classification and evaluation of simple and complex renal cysts			
Classification	Ultrasound Characteristics	Intervention	CT Characteristics
Type I: simple cyst	Anechoic, thin walled	None	Water density Thin, imperceptible wall No septa, calcifications, solid components No enhancement
Type II: minimally complicated	Mural calcification, thin septation (s)	Contrast CT to assess complicated vascularity: if enhancement >12 HU use surgical intervention	Few hairline thin septations Fine calcification in wall or septa No enhancement Uniformly high attenuation lesions < 3 cm that do not enhance
Type IIF: complicated	Course calcification, thick septation(s), mural nodules	Contrast CT to assess complicated vascularity: if enhancement >12 HU, use surgical intervention	Increased number of hairline thin septations Minimal thickening of the wall or septation Minimal enhancement of the thin septation (s) or wall May contain thick or nodular calcification but no enhancement Totally intrarenal nonenhancing high-attenuation lesions ≥3 cm
Type III: indeterminate	Calcification, septations, mural nodules	Contrast CT to assess complicated vascularity: if enhancement >12 HU, use surgical intervention	Thickened irregular walls or septations Enhancement of the irregular walls or septations
Type IV: malignancy	Mural nodules, vascularization	Surgery	Thickened irregular walls or septations Enhancement of the irregular walls or septations Enhancing soft-tissue components in addition to the wall or septation

Figure 5.10   The Bosniak classification and evaluation of simple and complex renal cysts. CT, computed tomography; HU, Hounsfield units.

Doppler angle should be kept at 60 degrees or less; the tortuosity of some renal arteries often makes this difficult. Finally, 10% to 20% of patients have accessory renal arteries that are small and often missed on Doppler studies.[5]

These factors add to the controversy over duplex scanning and have led to the advocacy of CT angiography or magnetic resonance angiography (MRA) as a faster and more reliable screening tool. At present, the choice between this technique and MRA will depend on local expertise and preference. For further discussion of the diagnosis and management of renovascular disease, see Chapter 61.

Contrast and Three-Dimensional Ultrasound

Ultrasound contrast agents have been studied in Europe for some time. Initially introduced to assess cardiac perfusion, they are being used to evaluate hepatic and renal perfusion. The first agents were albumin-coated, air-filled spheres that were quite unstable. Advances in microsphere technology and experimentation with other gases such as octafluoropropane have resulted in prolonged intravascular viability. The agents are injected intravenously, and the kidney is interrogated with phase inversion ultrasound. Once exposed to the ultrasound beam, the spheres burst, resulting in a reflective interface that enhances the image.

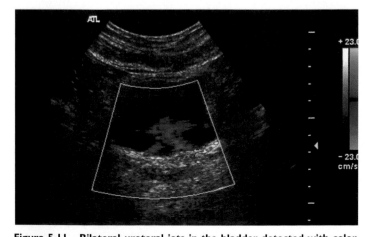

Figure 5.11   Bilateral ureteral jets in the bladder detected with color Doppler ultrasound. This is a normal appearance.

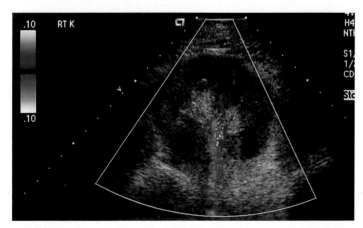

Figure 5.12   Transverse color Doppler ultrasound of the kidney. The artery is shown as *red*, and the vein as *blue*.

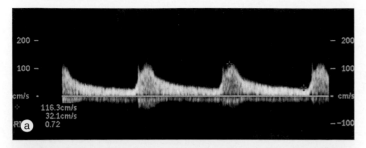

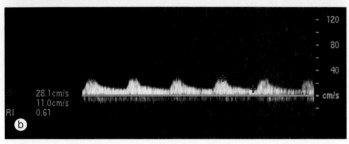

Figure 5.13 **Renal artery color Doppler and spectral tracing.** *a,* Normal renal arterial tracing showing the rapid systolic upstroke and early systolic peak velocity (~100 cm/s). *b,* Tardus parvus waveform demonstrating the slow systolic upstroke (acceleration) and decreased peak systolic velocity (~20 cm/s) associated with renal artery stenosis. Note different scales on vertical axis.

Preliminary studies evaluating renal perfusion in dysfunctional kidneys show reduced flow compared with normal kidneys (Fig. 5.14).

Two-dimensional (2-D) ultrasound images can be reconstructed into a 3-D volume image using a process similar to 3-D reconstructions for MRI and CT. Limitations of ultrasound include lack of an acoustic window, patient body habitus, and poor patient cooperation. With 3-D technology, images need only be acquired in one imaging plane, and are then reconstructed and viewed in any axis. Although the current techniques are time-consuming, technical improvements should decrease reconstruction time. Potential applications include vascular imaging and fusion with MRI or positron emission tomography (PET) scanning.

PLAIN RADIOGRAPHY AND INTRAVENOUS UROGRAPHY

The use of IVU has receded as cross-sectional imaging by CT or MRI has become more widely applied to the renal tracts. Contrast urography now has few primary indications in many centers, but may still be a key investigation in parts of the world where economic limitations mean cross-sectional imaging is not available. However, plain radiography (often called a KUB—kidneys, ureter, bladder), traditionally a preliminary part of contrast urography, still has an important role in the identification of soft-tissue masses, bowel gas pattern, calcifications, and renal location.

Renal Calcification

Most renal calculi are radiodense and visible on plain films. Calculi that are radiolucent on plain films are usually detected as filling defects on IVU. CT demonstrates nonopaque stones, which include uric acid, xanthine, and struvite stones. However, both CT and plain films may not detect calculi associated with protease inhibitor therapy.[10] Oblique films are sometimes obtained when a suspicious upper quadrant calcification is detected. Rotating the patient can aid in determining whether such a calcification is renal in origin.

Nephrocalcinosis may be medullary (Fig. 5.15a and b) or cortical (see Fig. 5.15c) and is localized or diffuse. The common causes of nephrocalcinosis are shown in Figure 5.16 (see also Chapter 54).

Intravenous Contrast Urography

Before administering contrast, an abdominal compression device may be placed. Its purpose is to maintain the excreted contrast in the upper tract and to distend the renal pelvis and calyces. A series of films is obtained following the contrast injection. The first film is usually performed at 30 seconds, when the renal parenchyma is at peak enhancement. Subtle renal masses are often detected only on these early films. Additional films of the entire abdomen are obtained at 5 minutes when there is renal excretion of contrast; on these films, the ureters are best evaluated. Prone films may be required to visualize the entirety of the ureter. A filled bladder film is obtained, and a postvoid film of the bladder assesses bladder emptying and is useful for

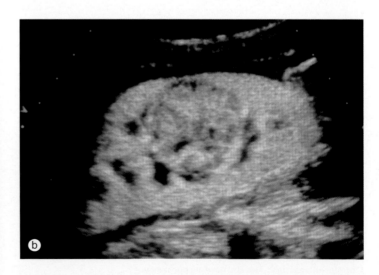

Figure 5.14 **Contrast ultrasound.** *a,* Sagittal renal ultrasound with a large central renal cell cancer (*arrows*). *b,* Central cancer better seen following contrast injection. (Courtesy of Dr. Christoph F. Dietrich.)

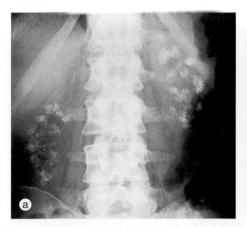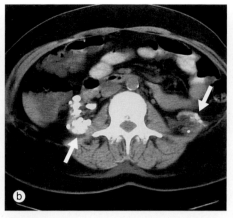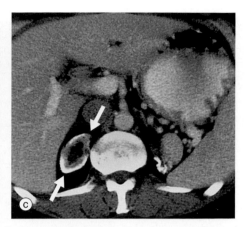

Figure 5.15 Nephrocalcinosis. *a*, Plain film showing bilateral medullary nephrocalcinosis in a patient with distal renal tubular acidosis. *b*, Noncontrast computed tomography (CT) scan in a patient with hereditary oxalosis and dense bilateral renal calcification *(arrows)*. The left kidney is atrophic. *c*, CT scan showing cortical nephrocalcinosis in the right kidney *(arrows)* following cortical necrosis.

evaluation of the distal ureters, which may be obscured by a distended contrast-filled bladder.[2]

Kidneys

Evaluation of the kidneys on IVU (and also on CT or MRI) should include their number, location, axis, size, contour, and degree of enhancement. In the normal patient, the kidneys are located in the superior portion of the retroperitoneum with the upper poles directed medially and the lower poles directed laterally. Renal size is variable, but a normal kidney should be about three to four lumbar vertebral bodies in length. The renal outline should be smooth and sharply demarcated from the retroperitoneal fat. Renal enhancement begins about 30 seconds after contrast administration and should be symmetric. Enhancement progresses centrally from the cortex, with excretion evident in the ureters by

5 minutes. Asymmetry of renal enhancement can be indicative of renal arterial disease.

Pelvicalyceal System

The pelvicalyceal system is best evaluated on the early abdominal films. Normally, there are about 10 to 12 calyces per kidney. The calyces drain into the infundibula, which in turn empty into the renal pelvis (Fig. 5.17). The infundibulum and renal pelvis should have smooth contours without filling defects. When more than one calyx drains into an infundibulum, it is considered a compound calyx; this anatomic variation is frequently seen in the polar regions. The normal calyx is gently cupped. Calyceal distortion occurs with papillary necrosis and reflux nephropathy.

Ureters

The ureters should be seen segmentally, owing to incomplete visualization of the ureter related to active peristalsis, on the abdomen films after 5 minutes. The ureters should be free of filling defects and smooth. In the abdomen, the ureters lie in the retroperitoneum, passing anterior to the transverse processes of

Patterns and causes of nephrocalcinosis	
Area Affected	**Causes**
Medullary	
Disturbed calcium metabolism	Hyperparathyroidism Sarcoidosis Idiopathic hypercalciuria Milk-alkali syndrome Hypervitaminosis D
Other systemic metabolic disease	Oxalosis
Other tubular disease	Distal renal tubular acidosis Dent disease Hyperoxaluria Bartter syndrome Medullary sponge kidney
Other	Papillary necrosis
Cortical	
	Cortical necrosis
	Chronic glomerulonephritis
	Trauma

Figure 5.16 Nephrocalcinosis. Patterns and common causes of nephrocalcinosis.

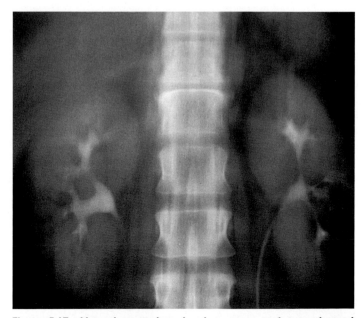

Figure 5.17 Normal parenchymal enhancement and normal renal excretion. Early postcontrast tomogram in intravenous urography.

57

the vertebral bodies. In the pelvis, the ureters course laterally and posteriorly, eventually draining into the posteriorly located vesicoureteral junction. At the vesicoureteral junction, the ureters gently taper. Medial bowing or displacement of the ureter is often abnormal and should be further evaluated.

Bladder

The midline urinary bladder lies posterior to the symphysis pubis. Its cephalad extent varies in relation to bladder distention. The bladder should be rounded in configuration and smooth walled. Benign indentations on the bladder include the uterus, prostate gland, and bowel.

RETROGRADE PYELOGRAPHY

Retrograde pyelography is performed when the ureters are poorly visualized on other imaging studies or when samples of urine need to be obtained from the kidney for cytology or culture. Patients who have severe contrast allergies can be evaluated with retrograde pyelography. The examination is performed by placing a catheter through the ureteral orifice under cystoscopic guidance and advancing it into the renal pelvis. Using fluoroscopy, the catheter is slowly withdrawn while radiographic contrast material is injected. This technique provides excellent visualization of the renal pelvis and ureter and can be used for cytologic sampling from suspect areas.

ANTEGRADE PYELOGRAPHY

Antegrade pyelography is performed through a percutaneous renal puncture and is resorted to when a retrograde pyelogram is not possible. Ureteral pressures can be measured, hydronephrosis evaluated, and ureteral lesions identified. The examination is often performed as a prelude to nephrostomy placement. Both antegrade and retrograde pyelography are invasive and should only be performed when other studies are inadequate.

ILEAL CONDUITS

Following cystectomy, or bladder failure, there are numerous types of urinary diversion that can be surgically created. There are continent or incontinent diversions; they are placed percutaneously or surgically by single- or multistaged procedures. One of the most common diversions is the ileal conduit: an ileal loop is isolated from the small bowel, and the ureters are implanted into the loop. This end of the loop is closed, whereas the other end exits through the anterior abdominal wall. This type of conduit can be evaluated by an excretory study or a retrograde study. The excretory or antegrade study is performed and monitored in the same way as an IVU. A retrograde examination, also referred to as a "loop-o-gram," is obtained when the ureters and conduit are suboptimally evaluated on the excretory study. A Foley catheter is placed into the stoma, and contrast is then slowly instilled. The ureters should fill by reflux because the ureteral anastomoses are not of the antireflux variety (Fig. 5.18).

CYSTOGRAPHY

A cystogram is obtained when more detailed radiographic evaluation of the bladder is required. A voiding cystogram is performed to identify ureteral reflux and to assess bladder function and urethral anatomy. In the trauma setting, adequate distention of the bladder is essential for evaluation of suspected bladder

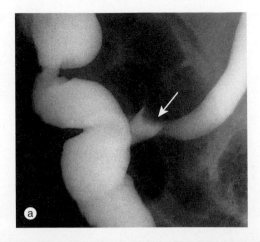

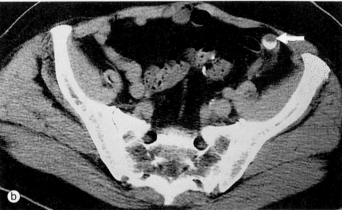

Figure 5.18   Ileal conduit. *a,* "Loop-o-gram." A recurrent transitional carcinoma is present in the reimplanted left ureter *(arrow). b,* Computed tomography scan clearly showing the tumor as a filling defect in the anterior aspect of the opacified ureter *(arrow).*

perforations. Incomplete bladder filling can result in missed perforations on IVU or CT. A Foley catheter is placed into the bladder and the urine drained. Contrast is then placed through the catheter, and the bladder is filled under fluoroscopic guidance. Early supine frontal and oblique films are obtained while the bladder is filling. Ureteroceles are best identified on early films. When the bladder is full, multiple films are obtained with varying degrees of obliquity. Reflux may be seen on these films. To obtain a voiding cystogram, the catheter is removed, and the patient voids. The contrast is followed into the urethra, and spot films are obtained. Occasionally, bladder diverticula are seen only on the voiding films. When the patient has completely voided, a final film of the bladder is obtained that can be used to assess the amount of residual urine as well as the mucosal pattern. Radionuclide cystography is an alternative often used in children to avoid passing a urethral catheter. It is useful in the diagnosis of reflux, but does not provide the detailed anatomy that is seen with contrast cystography.

COMPUTED TOMOGRAPHY

CT examination of the kidneys is performed to evaluate suspect renal masses, to locate ectopic kidneys (Figs. 5.19 and 5.20), to investigate calculi, to assess retroperitoneal masses, and for evaluating the extent of parenchymal involvement in patients with pyelonephritis. The major improvement in CT technology in the

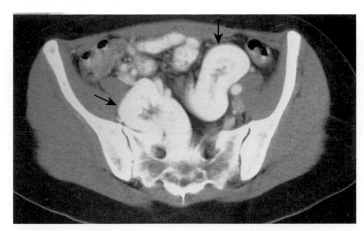

Figure 5.19 Computed tomography scan showing bilateral pelvic kidneys (*arrows*).

early 1990s was the introduction of helical scanners, which allow a large volume of the body to be scanned in a fraction of the time required with the earlier machines. The abdomen and pelvis can be scanned at 3-mm intervals with one to two breath-held acquisitions. This eliminates motion artifact, which was previously a significant problem. In the late 1990s, multidetector row CT was introduced. This results in multiple slices of information (currently 64-slice machines are commercially available) being acquired simultaneously, allowing the entire abdomen and pelvis to be covered in one breath-hold using submillimeter intervals.

The kidneys lie in the retroperitoneum. This space can be seen with MRI but is better detected with CT. It consists of three compartments: the anterior pararenal space, the perinephric space, and the posterior pararenal space. The anatomy of the spaces influences the spread of infectious and inflammatory processes (Figs. 5.21 through 5.23). The perinephric space is open anteriorly across the midline and encompasses the aorta and inferior vena cava. Thus, the right and left perinephric spaces are in potential communication across the midline. The perinephric space is bordered by the anterior and posterior perirenal fascia, also known as Gerota's fascia. The posterior pararenal space contains only fat and is not typically involved with inflammatory processes. The anterior pararenal space is open across the midline and contains the duodenum, pancreas, and ascending and descending colon (see Fig. 5.21).

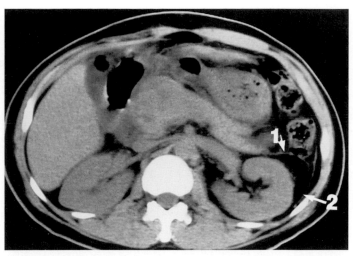

Figure 5.21 Noncontrast computed tomography scan through the mid-abdomen showing the retroperitoneal spaces. The kidney is situated in the perirenal space. The fascia surrounding the kidney is known as Gerota's fascia and comprises anterior (1) and posterior (2) fascial planes.

Tissue Density

The Hounsfield unit (HU) is a measurement of relative tissue densities determined with CT. Simple benign renal cysts have water density ranging from –20 to +20 HU. Soft-tissue measurements range between 30 and 80 HU. Bone density is high (400–1000 HU), whereas air is low (–1000 HU). Fat density ranges from –80 to –100 HU. The values vary somewhat among different machines and can vary depending on the imaging parameters selected. Fat, water, and some soft-tissue densities can look identical to the eye, so such measurement is essential.

Contrast and Noncontrast Computed Tomography

CT examination of the kidneys can be performed with or without intravenous contrast. Noncontrast imaging allows the kidneys to be evaluated for the presence of calcium deposition and hemorrhage, which are obscured following contrast administration (see Fig. 5.15b). Noncontrast CT is the examination of choice in patients with renal colic and suspected nephrolithiasis.[11,12]

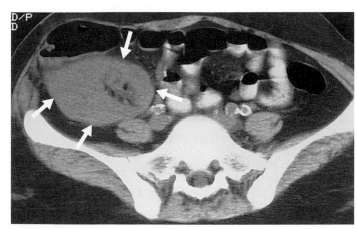

Figure 5.20 Computed tomography scan showing normal renal transplant (*arrows*).

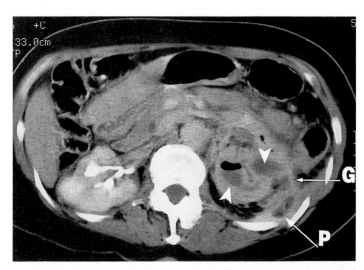

Figure 5.22 Emphysematous pyelonephritis. Contrast-enhanced computed tomography scan showing gas (*arrowheads*) within an enlarged left kidney and marked enhancement of Gerota's fascia (G) and the posterior perirenal space (P) indicative of inflammatory involvement.

59

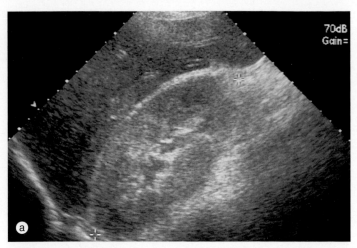

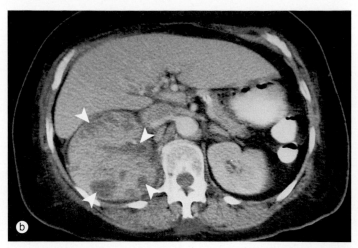

Figure 5.23 **Acute pyelonephritis.** *a,* Ultrasound demonstrates an enlarged echogenic kidney. Bipolar length of kidney is 12.9 cm. *b,* Computed tomography scan with contrast obtained 24 hours later demonstrates multiple nonenhancing abscesses *(arrowheads).*

Typically, the kidneys are imaged after contrast administration. With helical scans, the kidneys can be imaged initially during the cortical medullary phase and then later during the excretory phase. The kidneys should be similar in size and show equivalent enhancement and excretion. During the cortical medullary phase, there is brisk enhancement of the cortex. The cortical mantle should be intact. Any disruption of the cortical enhancement requires further evaluation: it may be caused by acute pyelonephritis (see Fig. 5.23) or infarction (Fig. 5.24). During the excretory phase, the entire kidney and renal pelvis enhance. Delayed excretion can be a finding in obstruction (Fig. 5.25) but also in renal parenchymal disease such as acute tubular necrosis.

CT urography has almost completely replaced IVU (Fig. 5.26). It can be helpful in the evaluation of renal infection, masses, and collecting system or ureteral abnormalities. It can identify a possible obstructing calculus as well as the extent of parenchymal and perinephric involvement. The degree of enhancement can be assessed in both solid masses and complex cysts (Bosniak category IIF–IV; see Fig. 5.10). The study consists of unenhanced images from the kidneys through the bladder for detection of calculi. Contrast is then administered, and the kidneys are imaged in the corticomedullary phase for evaluation of the renal vasculature as well as in the nephrographic phase for evaluation of the renal parenchyma. A compression device can be used as in IVU. Delayed images through the kidneys and bladder are performed for evaluation of the opacified and distended collecting system, ureters, and bladder.[13,14] Once the axial images have been obtained, they can be reformatted into coronal or sagittal planes to optimize visualization of the entire collecting system. The study can be tailored to the individual clinical scenario. For example, the corticomedullary phase can be eliminated to decrease the radiation dose if there is no concern about a vascular abnormality or no need for presurgical planning. A diuretic or saline bolus can be administered after the contrast to better distend the collecting system and ureters during the excretory phase. Various protocols for CT urography are recommended, with variations in the number of phases, the number of contrast injections, and different methods of hydration.

Computed Tomography Angiography
Helical scanning facilitates CT angiography, which can produce images that are similar to conventional angiography but are less invasive. A bolus of contrast is administered, and the images are obtained at 0.5- to 3-mm consecutive intervals. The contrast bolus

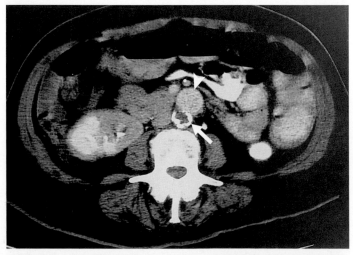

Figure 5.24 **Renal infarction involving the medial half of the right kidney following aortic bypass surgery.** CT scan shows densely calcified wall of the native aorta *(arrow).* The aortic graft is anterior to the native aorta *(arrowhead).*

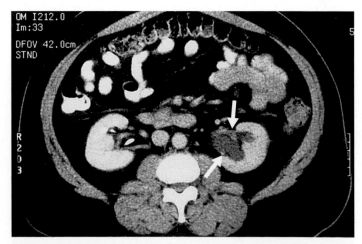

Figure 5.25 **Delayed excretion in the left kidney secondary to a distal calculus.** Contrast CT scan showing dilated left renal pelvis *(arrows).*

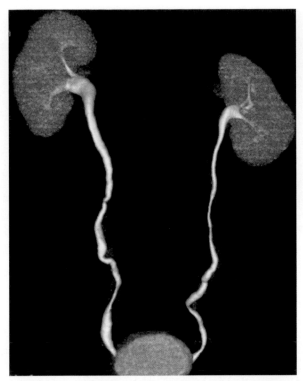

Figure 5.26 Computer-reformatted, volume-rendered CT urogram obtained from axial CT acquisition.

is timed for optimal enhancement of the aorta. The images are then reconstructed at a workstation. The aorta and branch vessels are well demonstrated (Fig. 5.27). This technique has been used with success for assessment of the renal vascular supply in patients undergoing renal donor transplant evaluation (see Chapter 92). It can be used to screen for renal artery stenosis as well, with sensitivity of 96% and specificity of 99% for the detection of hemodynamically significant stenosis compared with digital subtraction angiography.[15] Other advantages of CT angiography include the depiction of accessory renal arteries as well as nonrenal causes of hypertension such as adrenal masses.

Limitations of Computed Tomography

There are some limitations of CT. The cradle that the patient lies on has a weight limit, which varies by manufacturer: 200 kg (~450 lb) is the upper extreme. Obese patients often have suboptimal scans because of poor intravenous access and extensive artifact caused by the excess weight. This can be a particular

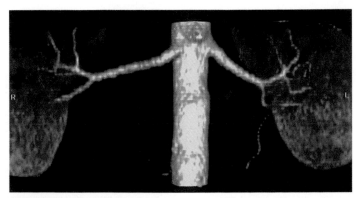

Figure 5.27 Three-dimensional reformatted CT angiogram of the normal renal arteries.

problem in the abdomen and retroperitoneum. Finally, CT is very sensitive to metal and patient motion. Retroperitoneal clips and intramedullary rods will cause extensive streak artifact, which severely degrades the images. Uncooperative patients who are unable to remain motionless due to pain or neurologic impairment will also have suboptimal studies. Intensive care unit and critically ill patients can be scanned by CT as long as they are stable enough to be transported to the CT suite because the scanners are not portable. Ultrasound can be an alternative to CT in these situations.

MAGNETIC RESONANCE IMAGING

MRI should only rarely be the first examination used to evaluate the kidneys, but typically it is an adjunct to another imaging technique. The major advantage of MRI over the other imaging modalities is direct multiplanar imaging, whereas CT is limited to slice acquisition in the axial plane of the abdomen, and coronal and sagittal planes are acquired only by reconstruction of the axial data, which can lead to loss of information.

Tissues contain an abundance of hydrogen, the nuclei of which are positively charged protons. These protons spin on their axis, producing a magnetic field (magnetic moment). When a patient is placed in a strong magnetic field in an MRI scanner, the protons align along the direction of, or in the opposite direction to, the field. When the radiofrequency pulse is applied, some of the protons aligned with the field will absorb energy and reverse their direction. This absorbed energy is given off as a radiofrequency pulse as the protons relax (return to their original alignment), producing a voltage in the receiver coil. The coil is the hardware that covers the region of interest. For renal imaging, a body coil or torso coil is used. Relaxation is a 3-D event giving rise to two parameters: T1 relaxation results in the recovery of magnetization in the longitudinal (spin–lattice) plane, whereas T2 results from the loss of transverse (spin–spin) magnetization. A rapid-sequence variant of T2 in common use is fast spin echo (FSE). Hydrogen ions move at slightly different rates in the different tissues. This difference is used to select imaging parameters that can suppress or aid in the detection of fat and water. Fluid, such as urine, is dark or low in signal on T1-weighted sequences and bright or high in signal on FSE sequences. Fat is bright on T1 and not as bright on FSE sequences (Fig. 5.28). When MRI is performed, the sequences and imaging planes selected must be tailored to the individual case.

Standard imaging usually includes T1 and FSE sequences. The imaging plane varies depending on the clinical concerns. Usually, one sequence is performed in the axial plane. Sagittal images cover the entire length of the kidney and can make some subtle renal parenchymal abnormalities more conspicuous (Fig. 5.29).

On T1-weighted sequences, the normal renal cortex is higher in signal than the medulla, producing a distinct corticomedullary differentiation, which becomes indistinct in parenchymal renal disease. It is analogous to the echogenic kidney seen on ultrasound. On FSE sequences, the corticomedullary distinction is not as sharp but should still be present.

Contrast Magnetic Resonance Imaging

As with CT, intravenous contrast can be administered to allow further characterization of the lesions. Gadolinium is a paramagnetic contrast agent that is frequently used in MRI and is much less nephrotoxic than iodinated contrast.[16] Gadolinium can be used in patients with moderate to severe renal dysfunction.[17,18] Paramagnetic contrast agents are currently being evaluated for measurement of glomerular function.

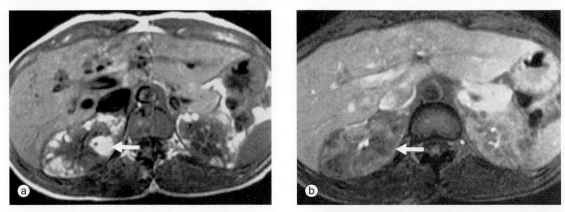

Figure 5.28   **Magnetic resonance imaging of tuberous sclerosis.** There are multiple renal angiomyolipomas. *a,* T1-weighted image. The tumors are high in signal on T1 because of their fat; the *arrow* shows the largest. *b,* T1-weighted image with fat suppression. The fat within the tumors is now low in signal (*arrow*).

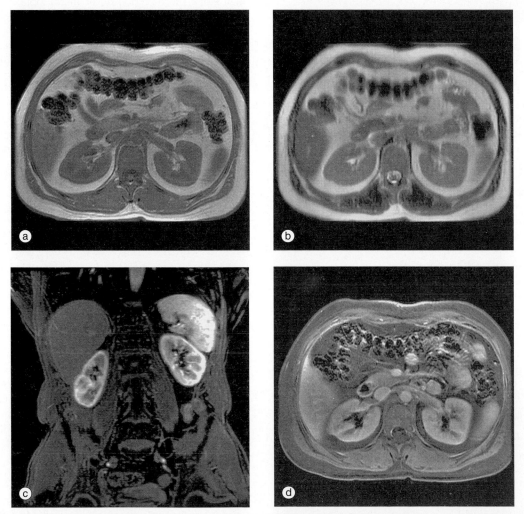

Figure 5.29   Normal magnetic resonance images through the kidneys. *a,* T1-weighted image. Note the distinct corticomedullary differentiation. *b,* Fast spin-echo image. The urine within the collecting tubules causes the high signal within the renal pelvis on this sequence. *c,* Coronal T1-weighted, fat-suppressed image following contrast administration. *d,* Axial T1-weighted, fat-suppressed image following contrast administration.

After injection of gadolinium, the vessels appear high in signal, or white, on T1-weighted sequences. For renal imaging, a bolus administration of gadolinium is administered followed by a rapid type of T1 sequence called gradient-echo imaging. Multiple images can be obtained in a single breath-held acquisition. This technique is useful for lesion characterization in patients who cannot obtain iodinated contrast. As with contrast-enhanced CT, the kidneys initially show symmetric cortical enhancement, which progresses to excretion. A delay in enhancement can be seen with renal artery stenosis.

Magnetic Resonance Urography

There are two techniques for performing magnetic resonance urography (MRU).[19,20] The first technique is sometimes called *static MRU*. Because urine contains abundant water, it will demonstrate high signal on a T2-weighted image, so a heavily T2-weighted sequence accentuates the static fluid in the collecting system and ureters, which stands out against the background soft tissues. Static MRU can be performed rapidly, which is a benefit when imaging children. It does have disadvantages. Any fluid in the abdomen or pelvis, such as fluid collections or fluid in small bowel, will demonstrate similar bright signal that can obscure superimposed structures. Also, the collecting system and ureters need to be distended to get good images.

The second technique is often referred to as *excretory MRU*. It is similar to CT urography. Gadolinium injection intravenously is followed by T1-weighted imaging. This technique allows some assessment of renal function because the contrast is filtered by the kidney and excreted into the urine. The opacified collecting system and ureters are depicted well, even when negative, and a diuretic can be administered to dilate the renal pelvis and ureters if necessary. A limitation of MRU is in the detection of calculi because it does not depict calcification well.

CT and MRU are comparable examinations, and the choice of modality is a matter of local preference. CT urography is the better choice in the evaluation of urinary tract calculi. MRU is better suited in cases with iodinated contrast allergy or impaired renal function. In addition, MRU can be used to reduce radiation exposure in children.

Magnetic Resonance Angiography

MRA can be performed with or without intravenous contrast, although contrast is preferable. The aorta and branch vessels are beautifully demonstrated (Fig.5.30). This technique is performed to evaluate the renal arteries for stenosis and is less invasive than angiography (Fig. 5.31). Technical advances, including faster sequences, have greatly improved the current state of MRA. It has a sensitivity of 97% and a specificity of 93% when compared with digital subtraction angiography for the detection of renal artery stenosis.[21] It has become the primary screening modality in patients with hypertension, declining renal function, or iodinated contrast allergy.[22] Where MRA is unavailable, Doppler ultrasound is used.

Disadvantages of Magnetic Resonance Imaging

MRI, like CT, has some disadvantages. The table and gantry are confining, so claustrophobic patients may be unable to cooperate. Patients with some types of internal metallic hardware such as pacemakers cannot undergo MRI. With the new, fast, breath-hold imaging techniques, patients need to be able to cooperate with breath-holding instructions to minimize motion-related artifacts.

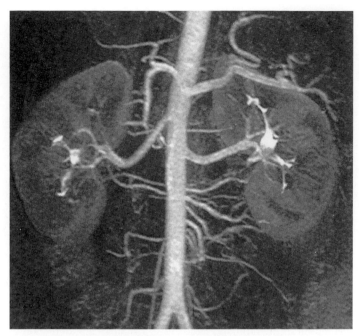

Figure 5.30 Magnetic resonance angiography. Coronal three-dimensional image following contrast administration showing normal renal arteries.

MRI can be used in intensive care unit and critically ill patients if they are stable enough to be transported to the MRI suite and have no implanted metallic devices. Ventilated patients can undergo MRI; however, specific MRI-compatible, nonferromagnetic ventilators and other life support devices must be used.

Measurement of Glomerular Filtration Rate with Computed Tomography and Magnetic Resonance Imaging

Methods for quantifying renal blood flow and split renal function by CT and MRI have recently been described.[23–25] The attenuation of the accumulated contrast within the kidney is directly proportional to the GFR, so the difference between the attenuation of

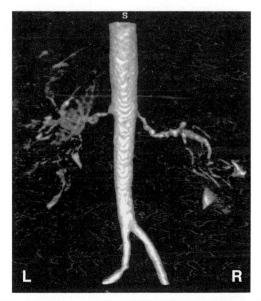

Figure 5.31 Magnetic resonance angiography. Coronal three-dimensional image showing fibromuscular dysplasia of the proximal right renal artery.

the kidney before and after contrast administration can be calculated as an indicator of GFR. Taking into account the renal volume, the function of each kidney can be determined. Both modalities yield similar information; however, MRI is used more in pediatric patients and in those with renal impairment or contrast allergy. This technique has not yet gained widespread acceptance, and renal scintigraphy remains the standard method for determination of renal function (discussed later).

ANGIOGRAPHY

In the past, angiography was frequently performed for diagnosis, a role that has gradually been replaced by cross-sectional imaging. Angiography is now most often performed for therapeutic intervention such as embolotherapy or angioplasty and stenting, preceded by diagnostic angiography to evaluate the renal arteries for possible stenosis (Figs. 5.32 and 5.33). Although CT and MRA techniques are improving, they remain inferior to conventional angiography for detection of accessory renal arteries, which are often small and bilateral and not infrequently a cause of hypertension. There is also a role for diagnostic angiography in the evaluation of medium and large vessel vasculitis and detection of renal infarction.

The conventional angiogram is performed through arterial puncture followed by catheter placement in the aorta. An abdominal aortogram is obtained to identify the renal arteries. Selective renal artery catheterization can be performed as necessary. Contrast is administered intra-arterially, and the images are obtained with conventional film or digital subtraction angiography. Conventional angiography is superior to digital angiography but requires higher doses of contrast material. Digital subtraction angiography uses computer reconstruction and manipulation to generate the images, with the advantage that previously administered and excreted contrast material and bones can be digitally removed to better visualize the renal vasculature.

RENAL VENOGRAPHY

Venography is not routinely performed. Previously, it was obtained for evaluation of renal vein thrombosis and gonadal vein thrombosis, but it has largely been replaced with Doppler ultrasound, followed by contrast-enhanced CT or MRI in equivocal cases.

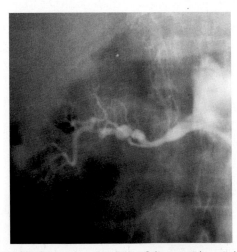

Figure 5.32 Fibromuscular dysplasia. Selective right renal arteriogram demonstrating typical beaded appearance. (Courtesy of Dr. Harold Mitty.)

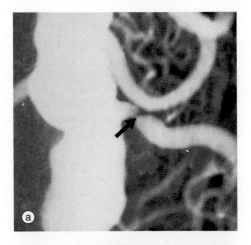

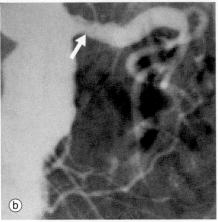

Figure 5.33 Left renal artery stenosis and angioplasty. a, Aortogram demonstrating a tight left renal artery stenosis (arrow). b, Postangioplasty image with marked improvement of the stenosis (arrow). (Courtesy of Dr. Harold Mitty.)

RADIONUCLIDE SCINTIGRAPHY

Unlike the other imaging modalities, scintigraphy provides a noninvasive means to obtain both qualitative and quantitative information about the kidneys. The gamma ray camera captures the photons from a radiotracer within the patient and generates an image. Images can be obtained over the entire body or portions of the body. Single-photon emission computed tomography (SPECT) is a specialized type of imaging whereby the emitted photons are measured at multiple angles similar to CT. There are three categories of radiotracers used in renal imaging, which differ in their mode of renal clearance: glomerular filtration, tubular secretion, and tubular retention agents (Fig. 5.34).

Scintigraphy remains superior to the other imaging modalities in the evaluation of renal flow and function. It is the study of choice for the evaluation of functional obstruction and in the evaluation of renal transplants, and is particularly valuable when ultrasound evidence of obstruction is equivocal.

It also provides an accurate assessment of renal function, which assists, for example, in estimating the reduction in renal function to be expected following nephron-sparing surgery in the management of patients with multifocal renal cancers. Both CT angiography and MRA have replaced nuclear medicine in the evaluation of renal artery stenosis. Suspected benign renal masses, such as a column of Bertin, can be easily diagnosed with either contrast-enhanced CT or MRI replacing DMSA scintigraphy. Although there has been some investigation of CT, MRI, and contrast-enhanced ultrasound

Choice of radionuclide in renal imaging	
Glomerular filtration rate	99mTc-DTPA
Glomerular filtration rate with renal impairment	99mTc-MAG3, 131I-OIH
Effective renal plasma flow	99mTc-MAG3, 131I-OIH
Renal scarring	99mTc-DMSA, 99Tc-GH
Renal pseudotumor	99mTc-DMSA
Upper renal tract obstruction	99mTc-DTPA
Upper renal tract obstruction with renal impairment	99mTc-MAG3

Figure 5.34   Choice of radionuclide in renal imaging.

for the evaluation of renal function, scintigraphy remains the preferred modality.

Glomerular Filtration Agents
Glomerular filtration agents are cleared by the glomerulus and can be used to measure the glomerular filtration rate (GFR). Technetium-99 (99mTc)-labeled diethylenetriamine pentaacetic acid (DTPA), is the most common glomerular agent used for imaging and can also be used for GFR calculation. In patients with poor renal function, mercaptoacetyl triglycine (99mTc-labeled MAG3) and o-iodohippurate ([131I]OIH) are superior to DTPA.[26,27]

Tubular Secretion Agents
Agents handled primarily by tubular secretion are used to estimate effective renal plasma flow because of their higher renal extraction and clearance. Both [131I]OIH and 99mTc-MAG3 are secreted from the proximal tubule. The clearance rate for [131I]OIH in normal patients is 500 to 600 ml/min and for 99mTc-MAG3 is 340 ml/min.[28]

Tubular Retention Agents
Tubular retention agents include 99mTc-labeled dimercaptosuccinate (DMSA) and 99mTc-labeled glucoheptonate (GH). These agents provide excellent cortical imaging and can be used in suspected renal scarring or infarction, and for clarification of renal pseudotumors.

Renogram
A renogram is generated by scintigraphy and provides information about blood flow, renal uptake, and excretion. Time–activity graphs are produced that plot flow of the radiotracer into each kidney relative to the aorta. Peak enhancement and clearance of the tracer are also plotted. DTPA, MAG3, and OIH can be used to generate the renogram. The relative radiotracer uptake can be measured and can provide split or differential information about renal function (Fig. 5.35).

The blood pool or flow images are obtained following injection of the radiotracers. Images are obtained with the gamma ray camera every few seconds for the first minute. The second component of the renogram evaluates renal function by measuring radiotracer uptake and excretion by the kidney. In normal patients, the peak concentration occurs between 3 and 5 minutes after injection tracer. Delayed transit of the isotope will alter the curve of the renogram.

In cases of suspected obstructive uropathy, a diuretic renogram can be obtained. A loop diuretic is injected intravenously when radiotracer activity is present in the renal pelvis; a computer-generated washout curve is obtained. In patients with true obstruction, activity will remain in the renal pelvis, whereas it will quickly decrease in patients without an obstruction (Fig. 5.36).

Captopril Renogram
Captopril renography was developed to detect renal artery stenosis. It relies on changes in scintigraphic findings that are exaggerated by administration of an angiotensin-converting enzyme inhibitor, usually captopril. A baseline renogram is performed using 99mTc-DTPA or 99mTc-MAG3. After captopril, findings indicative of renal artery stenosis include delayed time to maximum radioactivity, cortical retention of the isotope, and a decrease in the GFR of the ipsilateral kidney. The limitations of captopril renography include poor sensitivity in renal insufficiency and with bilateral renal artery stenosis. It has now been almost completely replaced by CT or MRA.

Cortical Imaging
Renal cortical imaging is performed with 99mTc-GH or 99mTc-DMSA. Information about renal size, location, and contour can be obtained (Fig. 5.37). The study is most commonly used for

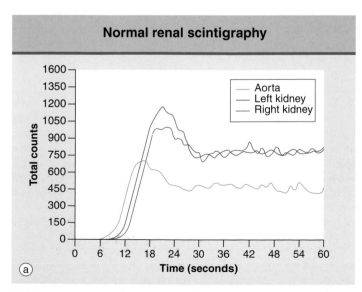

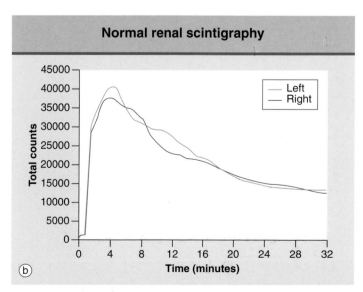

Figure 5.35   Normal 99mTc-labeled DTPA study: time–activity curves. *a*, Early (0–1 min), showing renal blood flow. *b*, Later (0–30 min), showing renal uptake and excretion of tracer. (Courtesy of Dr. Chun Kim.)

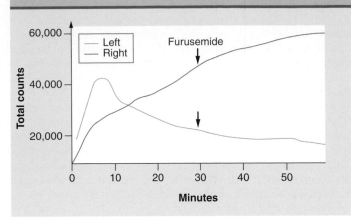

Diuresis renogram showing obstructed right kidney

Figure 5.36   Diuresis renogram showing obstructed right kidney. Isotope continues to accumulate in the right kidney despite intravenous furosemide (given at ↓). Isotope excretion in left kidney is normal.

evaluation of renal scarring, particularly in children (see Chapter 58), and for clarification of renal pseudotumors, such as a suspected column of Bertin in which an apparent mass on ultrasound will produce no abnormality on radionuclide scanning. Split renal function can also be determined from cortical imaging. Pinhole imaging (using a pinhole collimator, which magnifies the kidney to provide more anatomic detail than with planar imaging) and, more recently, SPECT imaging have been found useful for detection of cortical defects caused by inflammation or scarring. Cortical imaging may be better than ultrasound in the evaluation of the young patient with urinary tract infection.[29]

Vesicoureteral Reflux

In children with suspected vesicoureteral reflux, a standard cystogram is obtained. If reflux is shown, the child is subsequently followed up with radioisotope cystography, which exposes the child to a lower radiation dose and can be used to quantitate the bladder capacity when reflux occurs. The study is performed following placement of technetium pertechnetate into the bladder. Images are obtained during voiding.

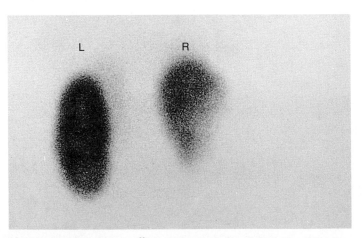

Figure 5.37   Renal infarct. ^{99m}Tc-DMSA scan in a newborn with a right lower pole infarct secondary to an embolus from an umbilical catheter. (Courtesy of Dr. Chun Kim.)

Renal Transplants

Renal transplants are easily evaluated with scintigraphy. As with the normal kidneys, information about blood flow and function can be determined. Postoperative complications are also well delineated. Ultrasound is often a complementary investigation, and choice of imaging modality in part depends on local expertise and preference.

RADIOLOGIC CONTRAST AGENTS

Contrast agents continue to have a role in many imaging techniques. A tri-iodinated benzene ring forms the chemical basis for all intravascular contrast agents. Conventional contrast agents have high osmolality, about five times greater than plasma osmolality. This feature makes them excellent for renal opacification but also contributes to their toxicity. Modifications to the benzene ring have led to newer contrast agents, including low osmolar and more recently iso-osmolar nonionic agents, which are less nephrotoxic.

Intravascular contrast material rapidly passes through the capillary pores into the interstitial, extracellular space and into the renal tubules through glomerular filtration.[30] In patients with normal renal function, the kidneys eliminate almost all the contrast agent. Extrarenal routes of excretion include the liver and bowel wall and account for less than 1% of elimination but can increase when renal function is compromised. The half-time for elimination in patients with normal renal function is 1 to 2 hours, compared with 2 to 4 hours in dialysis patients.[31,32]

The overall incidence of contrast reactions for all agents is 3.1% to 4.7%.[33,34] Twenty percent of patients who have a contrast reaction will experience a reaction upon re-exposure that may be similar or worse. Contrast reactions can be anaphylactoid or chemotoxic reactions. The former mimic an allergic response, whereas the latter are believed to be mediated by direct toxic effects of the contrast. The exact mechanism of contrast reaction is not known but is likely multifactorial. Formation of antigen–antibody complexes, complement activation, protein binding, and histamine release have all been cited as possible mechanisms.

Reactions may be minor, intermediate, or severe. Minor reactions include heat sensation, nausea, and mild urticaria. Intermediate reactions include vasovagal reaction, bronchospasm, and generalized urticaria. Severe reactions include profound hypotension, pulmonary edema, and cardiac arrest. The use of low osmolar or iso-osmolar contrast reduces the incidence of minor and intermediate contrast reactions. The incidence of death related to high osmolar contrast is reported to be 1 in 40,000. Immediate treatment of reactions should be directed toward the symptoms.

Contrast Nephrotoxicity

Renal failure associated with contrast administration has been reported as the third most common cause of in-hospital renal failure.[35] Patients with normal renal function rarely develop contrast-induced renal failure. In patients with serum creatinine levels higher than 1.5 mg/dl (132 μmol/l), iodinated contrast should be used with caution because the risk for contrast-induced renal failure is increased. Nephrotoxicity ranges in severity from a nonoliguric transient fall in GFR to severe renal failure requiring dialysis. The major risk factor for developing acute renal failure is the combination of pre-existing renal insufficiency and diabetes. Other risk factors include cardiovascular disease, the use of diuretics, advanced age (>75 years), multiple myeloma in dehydrated patients, hypertension, uricosuria, and high dose of contrast. Both ionic and nonionic contrast media can induce nephrotoxicity, although nonionic contrast is significantly less nephrotoxic. In end stage renal disease, fluid overload may follow the use of contrast because of thirst provoked by the osmotic load.

The two major theories for the pathogenesis of contrast-induced acute renal failure include renal vasoconstriction, perhaps mediated by alterations in nitric oxide, and direct nephrotoxicity of the contrast agent. There is some evidence that people with diabetes and heart failure have altered nitric oxide metabolism, which may account for their increased risk for contrast-induced nephrotoxicity. Tubular injury produces oxygen free radicals possibly as a result of the vasoconstriction. In animal studies, reduction in antioxidant enzymes associated with hypovolemia contributes to the injury.[36] Hydration is the mainstay of prevention; acetylcysteine, a thiol-containing antioxidant given in conjunction with hydration, has not proved consistently to be protective.[37] In most patients, the renal failure is transient, and the patients recover without incident.

Low or iso-osmolar contrast agents should be used and the doses reduced. Repetitive, closely performed contrast studies should be avoided. In high-risk patients, alternative imaging studies, ultrasound, MRI, or noncontrast CT should always be considered. The prevention and management of contrast nephrotoxicity are discussed further in Chapter 64.

REFERENCES

1. Katzberg RW: Urography into the 21st century: New contrast media, renal handling, imaging characteristics and nephrotoxicity. Radiology 1997;204:297–312.
2. O'Neill WC: Perianal anatomy. In O'Neill WC (ed): Atlas of Renal Ultrasonography. Philadelphia, Saunders, 2001, pp 3–10.
3. Bosniak MA: Difficulties in classifying cystic lesions of the kidney. Urol Radiol 1991;13:91–93.
4. Bosniak MA: Problems in the radiologic diagnosis of renal parenchymal tumors. In Olsson CA, Sawczuk IS (eds): Urologic Clinics of North America. Philadelphia, WB Saunders, 1993, pp 217–230.
5. Berland LL, Koslin DB, Routh WD, Keller FS: Renal artery stenosis: Prospective evaluation of diagnosis with color duplex US compared with angiography. Radiology 1990;174:421–423.
6. Olin JW, Piedmonte MR, Young JR, et al: The utility of ultrasound duplex scanning of the renal arteries for diagnosing significant renal artery stenosis. Ann Intern Med. 1995;122:833–838.
7. Kliewer MA, Tupler RH, Carroll BA, et al: Renal artery stenosis: Analysis of Doppler waveform parameters and tardus-parvus pattern. Radiology 1993;189:779–787.
8. Schwerk WB, Restrepo IK, Stellwaag M, et al: Renal artery stenosis: Grading with image-directed Doppler US evaluation of renal resistive index. Radiology 1994;190:785–790.
9. Radermacher J, Chavan A, Schaffer J, et al: Detection of significant renal artery stenosis with color Doppler sonography: Combining extrarenal and intrarenal approaches to minimize technical failure. Clin Nephrol 2000; 53:333–343.
10. Blake SP, McNicholas MM, Raptopoulos V: Nonopaque crystal deposition causing ureteric obstruction in patients with HIV undergoing Indinavir therapy. Am J Radiol 1998;171:717–720.
11. Sommer FG, Jeffrey RB Jr, Rubin GD, et al: Detection of ureteral calculi in patients with suspected renal colic. Value of reformatted non-contrast helical CT. Am J Radiol 1995;165:509–513.
12. Lanoue MZ, Mindell HJ: The use of unenhanced helical CT to evaluate suspected renal colic. Am J Radiol 1997;169:1579–1584.
13. Joffe SA, Servaes S, Okon S, Horowitz M: Multi-detector row CT urography in the evaluation of hematuria. Radiographics 2003;23:1441–1455.
14. Caoili EM, Cohan RH, Korobkin M, et al: Urinary tract abnormalities: Initial experience with CT urography. Radiology 2002;222:353–360.
15. Wittenberg G, Kenn W, Tschammler A, et al: Spiral CT angiography of renal arteries: Comparison with angiography. Eur Radiol 1999;9:546–551.
16. Prince MR, Arnoldus C, Frisoli JK: Nephrotoxicity of high dose gadolinium compared with iodinated contrast. J Magn Reson Imaging 1996;6: 162–166.
17. Tombach B, Bremer C, Reimer P, et al: Renal tolerance of a neutral gadolinium chelate (gabobutrol) in patients with chronic renal failure: results of a randomized study. Radiology 2001;218:651–657.
18. Townsend RR, Cohen DL, Katholi R, et al: Safety of intravenous gadolinium (Gd-BOPTA) infusion in patients with renal insufficiency. Am J Kidney Dis 2000;36:1207–1212.
19. Kawashima A, Glockner JF, King BF: CT urography and MR urography. Radiol Clin North Am 2003;41:945–961.
20. Nolte-Ernsting CC, Staatz G, Tacke J, Gunther RW: MR urography today. Abdom Imaging 2003;28:191–209.
21. Tan KT, van Beek EJR, Brown PWG, et al: Magnetic resonance angiography for the diagnosis of renal artery stenosis: A meta-analysis. Clin Radiol 2002;51:617–624.
22. Marcos HB, Choyke PL: Magnetic resonance angiography of the kidney. Semin Nephrol 2000;20:450–455.
23. Krier JD, Ritman EL, Bajzer Z, et al: Noninvasive measurement of concurrent single-kidney perfusion, glomerular filtration and tubular function. Am J Physiol Renal Physiol 2001;281:F630–F638.
24. Nilsson H, Wadstrom J, Andersson LG, et al: Measuring split renal function in renal donors: Can computed tomography replace renography? Acta Radiol 2004;45:474–480.
25. Lee VS, Rusinek H, Noz ME, et al: Dynamic three-dimensional MR renography for the measurement of single kidney function: Initial experience. Radiology 2003;227:289–294.
26. Taylor A, Nally JV: Clinical applications of renal scintigraphy. Am J Radiol 1995;64:31–41.
27. Taylor A Jr, Ziffer JA, Echima D: Comparison of Tc-99m MAG3 and Tc-99m DTPA in renal transplant patients with impaired renal function. Clin Nucl Med 1990;15:371–378.
28. Taylor A, Eshima D, Christian PE, et al: A technetium-99m MAG3 kit formulation: Preliminary results in normal volunteers and patients with renal failure. J Nucl Med 1988;29:616–662.
29. Mastin ST, Drane WE, Iravani A: Tc 99m DMSA SPECT imaging in patients with acute symptoms or history of UTI: Comparison with ultrasonography. Clin Nucl Med 1995;20:407–412.
30. Morris TW, Fischer HW: The pharmacology of intravascular radiocontrast media. Annu Rev Pharmacol Toxicol 1986;26:143–160.
31. Norby A, Tvedt KE, Halgunset J, Haugen OA: Intracellular penetration and accumulation of radiographic contrast media in the rat kidney. Scanning Microsc 1990;4:651–666.
32. Bahlmann J, Kruskemper HL: Elimination of iodine containing contrast media by hemodialysis. Nephron 1973;19:25–55.
33. Shehadi WH: Adverse reactions to intravascularly administered contrast media. Am J Radiol 1975;124:145–152.
34. Katayama H, Yamaguchi K, Kozuka T, et al: Adverse reactions to ionic and nonionic contrast media: A report from the Japanese committee on the safety of contrast media. Radiology 1990;175:616–618.
35. Cohan RH, Dunnick NR: Intravascular contrast media: adverse reactions. Am J Radiol 1987;149:665–670.
36. Yoshioka T, Fogo A, Beckman JK: Reduced activity of antioxidant enzymes underlies contrast media-induced renal injury in volume depletion. Kidney Int 1992;41:1008.
37. Barrett BJ, Parfrey PS: Preventing nephropathy induced by contrast medium. N Engl J Med 2006;354:379–386.

INTRODUCTION

Percutaneous renal biopsy was first described in the early 1950s by Iversen and Brun[1] and Alwall.[2] In these reports, the biopsies were performed with the patients in the sitting position using a suction needle and intravenous urography (IVU) for guidance. An adequate tissue diagnosis was achieved in less than 40% of these early cases. In 1954, Kark and Muehrcke[3] reported a modified technique that used the Franklin-modified Vim-Silverman needle and the patient in the prone position. In addition, although IVU was still used for guidance, an exploring needle was used to localize the kidney before insertion of the biopsy needle. With these modifications, a tissue diagnosis was made in 96% of cases and no major complications were reported. Since then, the approach to the renal biopsy procedure has remained largely unchanged, although the advent of ultrasonography and the refinement of biopsy needle design have offered significant improvements. Renal biopsy is now able to provide a tissue diagnosis in more than 95% of cases with a life-threatening complication rate of less than 0.1%.

INDICATIONS FOR RENAL BIOPSY

The indications for renal biopsy are listed in Figure 6.1. Ideally the information obtained from a renal biopsy should identify a specific diagnosis, reflect the level of disease activity, and allow informed decisions about treatment to be given. Although the renal biopsy is not always able to fulfill these criteria, it remains a valuable clinical tool and is of particular benefit in the following clinical situations.

Nephrotic Syndrome

Routine clinical and serologic examination of patients with nephrotic syndrome usually allows the clinician to determine whether a systemic disorder is present. In adults and older children without systemic disease, there is no reliable way to predict the glomerular pathology with confidence by noninvasive criteria alone; therefore, a renal biopsy should be performed. In children aged between 1 year and puberty, a presumptive diagnosis of minimal change disease (MCD) can be made. Renal biopsy is reserved for nephrotic children with atypical features (microscopic hematuria, reduced complement levels, renal impairment, failure to respond to steroids).

Acute Renal Failure

In most patients with acute renal failure (ARF), the cause can be determined without a renal biopsy. Obstruction, reduced renal perfusion, and acute tubular necrosis are usually evident from other lines of investigation. In a minority of patients, however, a confident diagnosis cannot be made, and in these circumstances, a renal biopsy should be performed as a matter of urgency so that appropriate treatment can be started before irreversible renal injury develops. This is particularly the case if ARF is accompanied by an active urine sediment.

Systemic Disease Associated with Renal Dysfunction

Patients with diabetes mellitus and renal dysfunction do not usually require a biopsy if the clinical setting is compatible with diabetic nephropathy (isolated proteinuria, diabetes of long duration, evidence of other microvascular complications). However, if the presentation is atypical (proteinuria associated with microscopic hematuria, absence of retinopathy or neuropathy [in patients with type 1 diabetes], onset of proteinuria less than 5 years from documented onset of diabetes, uncharacteristic change in renal function or renal disease of acute onset, the presence of immunologic abnormalities), a renal biopsy should be performed.

Indications for renal biopsy
Nephrotic Syndrome
Routinely indicated in adults; in prepubertal children only if clinical features atypical of minimal change disease
Acute Renal Failure
Indicated if obstruction, reduced renal perfusion, and acute tubular necrosis have been ruled out.
Systematic Disease with Renal Dysfunction
Indicated in patients with small vessel vasculitis, anti–glomerular basement membrane disease, and systemic lupus erythematosus; those with diabetes only if atypical features present
Non-nephrotic Proteinuria
May be indicated if proteinuria > 1g/24 h
Isolated Microscopic Hematuria
Indicated only in unusual circumstances
Unexplained Chronic Renal Failure
May be diagnostic, e.g., identify IgA nephropathy even in "end-stage kidney"
Familial Renal Disease
Biopsy of one affected member may give diagnosis and minimize further investigation of family members
Renal Transplant Dysfunction
Indicated if ureteral obstruction, urinary sepsis, renal artery stenosis, and toxic calcineurin inhibitor levels are not present

Figure 6.1   Indications for renal biopsy. See text for further discussion.

The advent of serologic testing for antineutrophil cytoplasmic antibodies with antimyeloperoxidase or antiproteinase-3 specificity and for antiglomerular basement membrane antibodies has made it possible to make a confident diagnosis of renal small vessel vasculitis or Goodpasture's disease without invasive measures in most patients. Nonetheless, a renal biopsy should still be performed in order to confirm the diagnosis and to clarify the extent of active inflammation versus chronic fibrosis and hence the potential for recovery. This information may be important in helping to determine the value of commencing or continuing immunosuppressive therapy, particularly in patients who may tolerate immunosuppression poorly.

The diagnosis of lupus nephritis can initially be based on noninvasive criteria including urine protein excretion, renal function, and urine sediment abnormalities. In addition, some would argue that this information can be used to gauge the severity of renal involvement and inform decisions about initial immunosuppressive treatment. However, a renal biopsy will clarify the underlying pathologic lesion, the level of acute activity, and the extent of chronic fibrosis, thereby providing robust guidance for evidence-based therapy.

Other systemic diseases such as amyloidosis, sarcoidosis, allergic drug reactions, and myeloma can be diagnosed with a renal biopsy. However, since these diagnoses can usually be made using other investigative approaches, a renal biopsy is indicated only if the diagnosis remains uncertain or if knowledge of renal involvement would change management.

Renal Transplant Dysfunction

Renal allograft dysfunction in the absence of ureteral obstruction, urinary sepsis, renal artery stenosis, or toxic levels of calcineurin inhibitors requires a renal biopsy to determine the cause. In the early post-transplantation period, this is most useful in differentiating acute rejection from acute tubular necrosis and the increasingly prevalent BK virus nephropathy. Later, renal biopsy can differentiate late acute rejection from chronic allograft nephropathy, recurrent or *de novo* glomerulonephritis, and calcineurin-inhibitor toxicity. The location of the renal transplant just below the anterior abdominal wall facilitates biopsy of the allograft and allows repeated biopsies when indicated. This has encouraged many units to adopt a policy of routine protocol biopsy to detect subclinical acute rejection and renal scarring that would require therapeutic alterations (see Chapter 93).

Non-nephrotic Proteinuria

The value of renal biopsy in this setting is not clear. All conditions that result in nephrotic syndrome can cause non-nephrotic proteinuria with the exception of MCD. However, the benefit of specific treatment with steroids and other immunosuppressive agents in this clinical setting probably does not justify the risk of significant drug-related side effects. In patients with protein excretion rates of more than 1 g/day, there is convincing evidence that generic treatment with strict blood pressure control, and angiotensin-converting enzyme inhibitors and angiotensin receptor blockers alone or in combination reduces proteinuria and reduces the risk of developing progressive renal dysfunction.[4] Nonetheless, although the renal biopsy may not lead to an immediate change in management, it can be justified in these circumstances since it will provide prognostic information, may identify a disease for which a different therapeutic approach is indicated, and may provide clinically important information about the future risk of disease recurrence following renal transplantation.

Isolated Microscopic Hematuria

Patients with microscopic hematuria should initially be evaluated to identify structural lesions such as renal stones or tumors and urothelial malignancy if older than the age of 40 years. The absence of a structural lesion suggests that the hematuria may have a glomerular source. Biopsy studies have identified glomerular lesions in between 50% and 75% of biopsies.[5,6] In all series, IgA nephropathy has been the most common lesion followed by thin basement membrane nephropathy. In the absence of proteinuria and hypertension, the prognosis for these conditions is excellent and since specific therapies are not available, renal biopsy in this setting is not necessary. Biopsy should be performed only if the result would provide reassurance to the patient, avoid repeated urologic investigations, or provide specific information (e.g., in the evaluation of potential living kidney donors), or for life insurance and employment purposes.

Unexplained Chronic Renal Failure

Renal biopsy can be informative in the patient with unexplained chronic renal failure with normal-sized kidneys since, in contrast to ARF, it is often difficult to determine the underlying cause based on clinical criteria alone. Studies have suggested that in this setting, the biopsy demonstrated pathology that was not predicted in almost half of cases.[7] It should be pointed out, however, that if both kidneys are small (<9 cm on ultrasonography), the risks of the biopsy are increased and the diagnostic information available from the biopsy may be limited by extensive glomerular and tubulointerstitial fibrosis. Even in this setting, however, immunofluorescence studies may be informative. For example, glomerular IgA deposition may be identifiable even in the presence of advanced structural damage.

Familial Renal Disease

A renal biopsy can be helpful in the investigation of patients with a family history of renal disease; a biopsy performed on one affected family member may secure the diagnosis for the whole family and avoid the need for repeated investigation. Conversely, a renal biopsy may unexpectedly identify disease that has an inherited basis, thereby stimulating evaluation of other family members.

VALUE OF THE RENAL BIOPSY

Biopsy Adequacy

In the assessment of a renal biopsy, the number of glomeruli in the sample is the major determinant of whether the biopsy will be diagnostically informative.[8]

The first issue to be considered is how good the renal biopsy is at identifying focal diseases. For a focal disease such as focal segmental glomerulosclerosis [FSGS], the diagnosis can potentially be made on a biopsy containing a single glomerulus that contains a typical sclerosing lesion. However, the probability that FSGS is *not* present in a patient with nephrotic syndrome and minimal changes on the biopsy is dependent on the actual proportion of abnormal glomeruli in the kidney and the number of glomeruli obtained in the biopsy specimen. For example, if 20% of glomeruli in the kidney have sclerosing lesions and five glomeruli are sampled, there is a 35% chance that all the glomeruli in the biopsy will be normal and that the biopsy will miss the diagnosis. By contrast, in the same kidney, if 10 or 20 glomeruli are sampled, the chance of missing all normal glomeruli is reduced to 10% and <1%, respectively, and the biopsy is more discriminating. This argument assumes that if segmental lesions are present in the biopsy, they are identified, and this chance is increased if the biopsy specimen is sectioned at multiple levels.

A further issue is how the number of glomeruli in the biopsy sample reflects the true extent of glomerular involvement in the kidney. Unless all glomeruli are affected equally, the probability that the observed involvement in the biopsy accurately reflects true involvement in the kidney depends on the number of glomeruli sampled and the proportion of affected glomeruli in the kidney. For example, in a biopsy containing 10 glomeruli of which three are abnormal (30%), there is a 95% probability that the actual glomerular involvement is between 7% and 65%. In the same kidney, if the biopsy contained 30 glomeruli with 30% being abnormal, the 95% confidence intervals are narrowed to 15% and 50%.

Therefore, the interpretation of the biopsy needs to take into account the number of glomeruli obtained. A typical biopsy sample will contain 10 to 15 glomeruli and will be diagnostically useful. Nonetheless, it must be appreciated that because of the sampling issue, a biopsy sample of this size will occasionally be unable to diagnose focal diseases and at best will provide imprecise guidance on the extent of glomerular involvement.

An adequate biopsy should also provide samples for immunofluorescence and electron microscopy. It is helpful for the biopsy cores to be viewed under an operating microscope after being taken to ensure that they contain cortex and that when the cores are divided, the immunofluorescence and electron microscopy samples contain glomeruli as well.

If insufficient material for a complete pathologic evaluation is obtained, discuss how to proceed with the pathologist before placing the tissue in fixative so that the material can be processed in a way that will provide maximum information for the specific clinical situation. For example, if the patient has heavy proteinuria, most information will be gained from electron microscopy since it can demonstrate podocyte foot process effacement, focal sclerosis, electron-dense deposits of immune complexes, and the organized deposits of amyloid and therefore potentially provide a diagnosis.

Is the Renal Biopsy a Necessary Investigation?

The role of the renal biopsy has been much debated. As stated previously, a renal biopsy should be able to identify a specific diagnosis, reflect the level of disease activity, and guide treatment decisions. Early studies suggested that renal biopsies provided diagnostic clarity in the majority of cases but that this information did not alter the management of most patients with the exception of those with heavy proteinuria or systemic disease.[9] More recent prospective studies have suggested that the pathologic diagnosis is different from that predicted on clinical grounds in 50% to 60% of patients, resulting in an altered therapeutic approach in 20% to 50% of cases.[10] This is particularly apparent in patients with heavy proteinuria or ARF in whom the biopsy findings altered management in more than 80% of cases.[11]

PREBIOPSY EVALUATION

This evaluation identifies issues that may compromise the safety and success of the procedure (Fig. 6.2). It should determine whether the patient has two normal-sized unobstructed kidneys, sterile urine, controlled blood pressure, and no bleeding

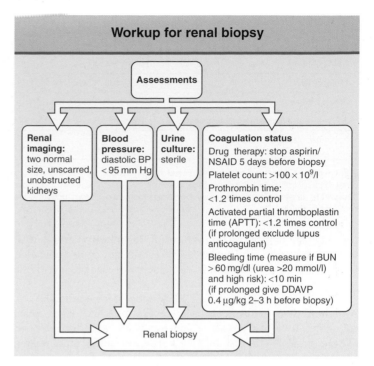

Figure 6.2 Workup for renal biopsy.

diathesis. A thorough history should be taken to identify evidence of a bleeding diathesis such as previous prolonged surgical bleeding, spontaneous bleeding, family history of bleeding, and the ingestion of medication that increases bleeding risk (including antiplatelet agents and warfarin).

An ultrasound scan should be performed to assess kidney size and to identify significant anatomic abnormalities such as solitary kidney, polycystic or simple cystic kidneys, malpositioned kidneys, horseshoe kidneys, small kidneys, or hydronephrosis.

The value of the bleeding time in patients undergoing renal biopsy is controversial. The predictive value of the bleeding time for postrenal biopsy bleeding has never been prospectively tested. Retrospective studies, however, demonstrated a three- to fivefold increase in bleeding complications after renal biopsy in patients with prolonged bleeding times.[12,13] Prospective studies of percutaneous liver biopsy patients showed a fivefold increase in bleeding complications in those with uncorrected bleeding times.[14] A consensus document concluded that the bleeding time is a poor predictor of postsurgical bleeding but that it does correlate with clinical bleeding episodes in uremic patients.[15] Since many patients undergoing renal biopsy have renal dysfunction, many centers measure the prebiopsy bleeding time and administer 1-desamino-8-D-arginine vasopressin (desmopressin or DDAVP) if it is prolonged beyond 10 minutes. In our center, we no longer measure the bleeding time but routinely administer DDAVP to those patients with significant renal impairment (BUN >55 mg/dl [urea >20 mmol/l] or serum creatinine >3 mg/dl [250 μmol/l]). Either of these two approaches is acceptable practice.

Contraindications to Renal Biopsy

The contraindications to renal biopsy are listed in Figure 6.3. The major contraindication to percutaneous renal biopsy is a bleeding diathesis. If the disorder cannot be corrected and the biopsy is deemed indispensable, alternative approaches such as open biopsy, laparoscopic biopsy, or transvenous (usually

Contraindications to renal biopsy	
Kidney Status	Patient Status
Multiple cysts	Uncontrolled bleeding diathesis
Solitary kidney	Uncontrolled blood pressure
Acute pyelonephritis/perinephric abscess	Uremia
Renal neoplasm	Obesity Uncooperative patient

Figure 6.3   Contraindications to renal biopsy. Most contraindications to renal biopsy are relative rather than absolute; when clinical circumstances necessitate urgent biopsy, they may be overridden, apart from uncontrolled bleeding diathesis.

transjugular) biopsy can be performed. Inability to comply with instructions during the biopsy is a further major contraindication to renal biopsy. Sedation or, in extreme cases, general anesthesia may be necessary.

Hypertension (>160/95), hypotension, perinephric abscess, pyelonephritis, hydronephrosis, severe anemia, large renal tumors, and cysts are relative contraindications to renal biopsy. Where possible, they should be corrected before undertaking the biopsy.

The presence of a solitary functioning kidney is considered to be a contraindication to percutaneous biopsy. If a biopsy is indicated, it has been argued that direct visualization is required at the time of biopsy. However, the postbiopsy nephrectomy rate of 1/2000 to 1/5000 is comparable to the mortality rate associated with the general anesthetic required for an open procedure. Therefore, in the absence of risk factors for bleeding, percutaneous biopsy of a solitary functioning kidney can be justified.

RENAL BIOPSY TECHNIQUE

Percutaneous Renal Biopsy
Native Renal Biopsy
In our center, the kidney biopsy is performed by nephrologists using continuous (real-time) ultrasound guidance and disposable automated biopsy needles. We use 16-gauge needles as a compromise between the greater tissue yield of larger needles and the trend to fewer bleeding complications of smaller needles.[16,17] For most patients, premedication or sedation is not required. The patient is laid prone and a pillow is placed under the abdomen at the level of the umbilicus to straighten the lumbar spine and splint the kidneys. Figure 6.4 demonstrates the anatomic relationships of the left kidney. Ultrasonography is used to localize the lower pole of the kidney where the biopsy will be performed (usually the left kidney). An indelible pen mark is used to indicate the point of entry of the biopsy needle. The skin is sterilized with either Betadine or chlorhexidine solution. A sterile fenestrated sheet is placed over the area to maintain a sterile field. Local anesthetic (2% lidocaine [lignocaine]) is infiltrated into the skin at the point previously marked. While the anesthetic takes effect, the ultrasound probe is covered in a sterile sheath. Sterile ultrasound jelly is applied to the skin, and under ultrasound guidance, a 10-cm, 21-gauge needle is guided to the renal capsule and further local anesthetic infiltrated into the perirenal tissues and then along the track of the needle on withdrawal. A stab incision is made through the dermis to ease passage of the biopsy needle. This is passed under ultrasound guidance to the kidney capsule (Fig. 6.5). As the needle approaches the capsule, the

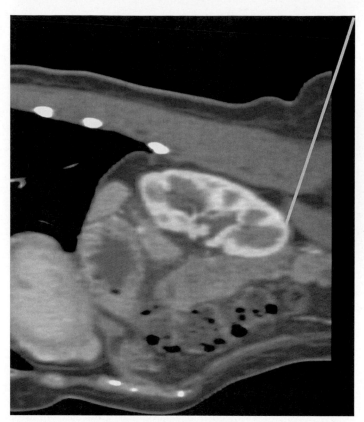

Figure 6.4   Computed tomography through the left kidney. The angle of approach of the needle is demonstrated. Note the relative adjacency of the lower pole of the kidney to other structures, particularly the large bowel.

patient is instructed to take a breath until the kidney is moved to a position such that the lower pole rests just under the biopsy needle and then to stop breathing. The biopsy needle tip is advanced to the renal capsule, and the trigger mechanism is released, firing the needle into the kidney (Fig. 6.6). The needle is immediately withdrawn, the patient asked to resume

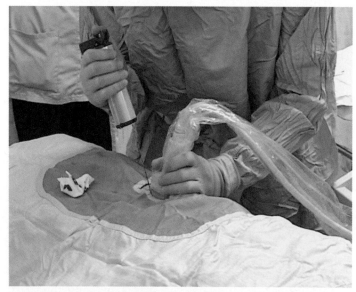

Figure 6.5   Renal biopsy procedure. The biopsy needle is introduced at an angle of approximately 70 degrees to the skin and is guided by continuous ultrasonography. The operator is shown wearing a surgical gown. This is not strictly necessary; sterile gloves and maintenance of a sterile field are sufficient.

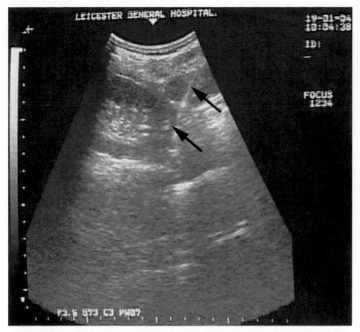

Figure 6.6   Renal biopsy. Ultrasound scan demonstrating the needle entering the lower pole of the left kidney. The *arrows* indicates the needle track that appears as a fuzzy white line.

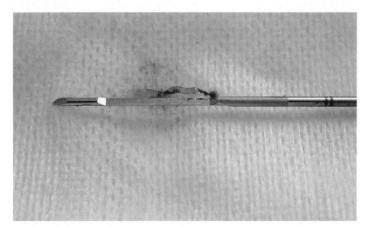

Figure 6.7   Renal biopsy. A core of renal tissue is demonstrated in the sampling notch of the biopsy needle.

breathing, and the contents of the needle examined (Fig. 6.7). We examine the tissue core under an operating microscope to ensure that renal cortex has been obtained (Fig. 6.8). A second pass of the needle may be necessary to obtain additional tissue for immunofluorescence and electron microscopy. If insufficient tissue is obtained, further passes of the needle are made. However, in our experience, if the needle is passed more than four times, a modest increase in the postbiopsy complication rate is observed.

Once sufficient renal tissue has been obtained, the skin incision is dressed and the patient is rolled directly into bed for observation.

No single fixative has been developed that allows good-quality light microscopy, immunofluorescence, and electron microscopy to be performed on the same sample. In our center, therefore, the renal tissue is divided into three samples and placed in formalin for conventional light microscopy, normal saline for subsequent snap-freezing in liquid nitrogen for immunofluorescence, and gluteraldehyde for electron microscopy.

There are a number of variations of the percutaneous renal biopsy technique. While the majority of biopsies are guided by ultrasound, some operators choose to use it only to localize the kidney and determine the depth and angle of approach of the needle, then performing the biopsy without further ultrasound guidance. The success and complication rates appear to be no different from those seen with continuous ultrasound guidance. For technically challenging biopsies, computed tomography can be used to guide the biopsy needle.

Renal Transplant Biopsy

The overall approach to the biopsy of the transplant kidney is similar to that of the native kidney. However, it is facilitated by the proximity of the kidney to the anterior abdominal wall and the lack of movement on respiration. The biopsy of the kidney is performed under real-time ultrasound guidance using an automated biopsy needle. In most cases, the renal transplant biopsy is performed to identify the cause of acute allograft dysfunction. In these circumstances, the aim is to identify acute rejection and therefore the diagnosis can be made on a formalin-fixed sample alone. If vascular rejection is suspected, a snap-frozen sample for C4d immunostaining should also be obtained.

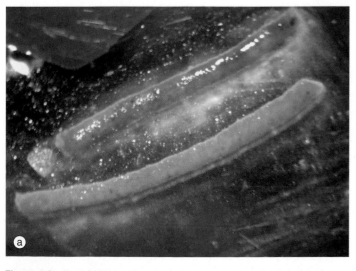

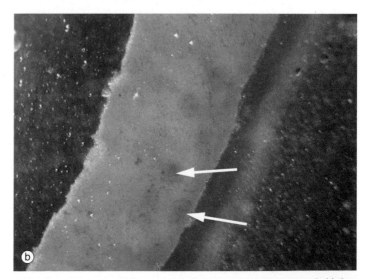

Figure 6.8   Renal biopsy. The appearance of renal biopsy material under the operating microscope. *a*, Low-power view showing two good-sized cores. *b*, Higher magnification view showing the typical appearance of glomeruli (*arrows*).

If recurrent or *de novo* glomerulonephritis is suspected in patients with chronic allograft dysfunction, additional samples for electron microscopy and immunofluorescence microscopy should be collected.

Postbiopsy Monitoring

Following the biopsy, the patient is placed supine and subjected to strict bed rest for 6 to 8 hours. The blood pressure is monitored frequently, the urine is examined for macroscopic hematuria, and the skin puncture site examined for excessive bleeding. If there is no evidence of bleeding following biopsy, the patient is sat up in bed initially and subsequently allowed to mobilize. If macroscopic hematuria develops, bed rest is continued until the bleeding settles. Conventionally, patients have been kept in hospital for 24 hours after a biopsy to be observed for complications. Recently, however, day case renal biopsy with same-day discharge after 6 to 8 hours of observation has become increasingly popular for both native and renal transplant biopsies. This has been largely driven by the financial and resource implications of overnight hospital admission and has been justified by the perception that the significant complications of renal biopsy will become apparent during this shortened period of observation. This view has been challenged recently by a study of 750 native renal biopsies that showed that only 67% of major complications (i.e., those that either required blood transfusion or an invasive procedure or resulted in urinary tract obstruction, septicemia, or death) were apparent by 8 hours after biopsy.[18] The authors concluded that the widespread application of an early discharge policy after renal biopsy was not in the patient's best interest and that a 24-hour period of observation was preferable. In our center, approximately half of our renal biopsies are performed as day cases. The patient population is selected to avoid those with the highest risk of complications, for example, impaired renal function (creatinine >3 mg/dl [250 µmol/l]), small kidneys, and uncontrolled hypertension. In addition, we require that the patient is not allowed to be alone at home for at least one night after the biopsy. This selection policy has proved to be safe. Of the last 287 day case biopsies performed in our unit, 7% developed a self-limiting postbiopsy complication within 8 hours that required a short hospital admission. Two patients returned after same-day discharge with biopsy-related complications: one with macroscopic hematuria 24 hours after the biopsy and one with loin pain due to a perirenal hematoma 4 days after biopsy. Both settled with conservative management. In this author's opinion, day-case renal biopsy is acceptably safe when a low-risk patient group is selected.

Alternatives to the Percutaneous Approach

When the percutaneous approach is contraindicated, other approaches to renal biopsy have been described. The choice of technique depends on the safety, morbidity, recovery period, and adequacy of the technique but probably above all on the local expertise that is available.

Transvenous (Transjugular or Transfemoral) Renal Biopsy

This technique, which was developed by accident, was described in 1990 by Mal and colleagues.[19] While performing a transjugular liver biopsy, the renal vein was inadvertently entered, a biopsy sample was taken, and renal tissue was identified on pathologic examination. The patient had no postprocedure complications. Transvenous sampling of the kidney is theoretically safer than the percutaneous approach because the needle passes from the venous system into the renal parenchyma and is directed away from large blood vessels. In addition, it is suggested that any bleeding that occurs should be directed back into the venous system and if capsular perforation develops, significant bleeding points can be immediately identified and controlled by coil embolization. Others argue that coil embolization of the punctured vein is unhelpful since significant bleeding either into a perirenal hematoma or the urine indicates an arterial breach that requires selective angiography and arterial embolization.

The transjugular route for renal biopsy cannot be regarded as routine since it requires specialist skill and additional time and is significantly more expensive than the percutaneous approach. The main indication for this approach is an uncontrollable bleeding diathesis. It has also been advocated for use in a variety of other situations: patients receiving artificial ventilation in the intensive therapy unit; the need to obtain tissue from more than one organ including the kidney, liver, or heart; large-volume ascites that precludes the prone position; uncontrolled hypertension; morbid obesity; severe respiratory insufficiency; solitary right kidney; failed percutaneous approach; and coma.

The patient lies supine and the right internal jugular vein is cannulated. A guidewire is passed into the inferior vena cava and a catheter is passed over the guidewire and selectively into the right renal vein. The right kidney is preferred because the right renal vein is shorter and enters the vena cava at a more favorable angle than the left. A sheath is passed over the catheter into the renal vein and located in a suitable peripheral location with the aid of contrast enhancement. Finally, the biopsy device is passed through the sheath and samples taken. Two sampling techniques have been described. Early studies used a modified Colapinto aspiration biopsy needle; recent studies used a side-cut biopsy needle system. Compared to the Colapinto system, the side-cut needle avoids the tissue distortion produced by the aspiration needle, yields larger samples thereby reducing the number of needle passes, and has a smaller diameter that facilitates a more peripheral location of the needle that theoretically reduces the risk of renal pelvis injury. It does, however, have a higher incidence of capsular perforation.

Once samples have been taken, contrast is injected into the biopsy track to identify capsular perforation and embolization coils are inserted if brisk bleeding is identified.

The quality of renal tissue obtained by transjugular biopsy is variable, with studies reporting diagnostic yields of between 73% and 98.2%.[20,21] The complication rate appears to be comparable to that seen with percutaneous renal biopsy, which is reassuring given that these are high-risk patients.

Open Renal Biopsy

This has been established as a safe alternative to percutaneous biopsy when uncorrectable contraindications exist. The largest study reported a series of 934 patients in which tissue adequacy was 100% with no major complications.[22] Nonetheless, although this is an effective approach with minimal postprocedure complications, the risk of general anesthesia and the delayed recovery time have prevented its widespread adoption. It may still, however, be performed when a renal biopsy is required in patients who are otherwise undergoing an abdominal surgical procedure.

Laparoscopic Renal Biopsy

This procedure requires general anesthesia and two laparoscopic ports in the posterior and anterior axillary lines to gain access to the retroperitoneal space. Laparoscopic biopsy forceps are used to obtain cortical biopsy samples, and the biopsy sites are coagulated with laser and packed to prevent hemorrhage. In the most recent and largest study, adequate tissue was obtained in 96% of the 74 patients included.[23] Significant bleeding occurred in three patients, the colon was injured in one, and a biopsy was performed inadvertently on the spleen and liver in two others. This latter complication was subsequently averted by the use of intraoperative ultrasound to define the anatomy in difficult cases.

Transurethral Renal Biopsy

This novel approach has been described in a single patient.[24] The procedure was performed with an 18-gauge needle via cystoscopy. Twenty-eight glomeruli were obtained and a small subcapsular hematoma was identified on routine postbiopsy computed tomography. The benefit of this approach is yet to be determined.

COMPLICATIONS OF RENAL BIOPSY

The complication rates compiled from large series of renal biopsies are shown in Figure 6.9. Hemorrhagic complications have persisted despite apparent improvements in technique and equipment, but serious complications have become less common. It should be noted, however, that more recent series included fewer higher risk patients with severe renal impairment.

Pain

A dull ache around the needle entry site is inevitable when the local anesthetic wears off, and patients should be warned about this. This ache often requires no treatment or just simple analgesia with paracetamol or paracetamol/codeine combinations. More severe pain should raise the possibility of a significant perirenal hemorrhage. Opiates may be necessary for pain relief, and appropriate investigations to clarify the severity of the bleed should be performed. Patients with macroscopic hematuria may develop clot colic and describe the typical severe pain associated with ureteral obstruction.

Hemorrhage

A degree of perirenal bleeding accompanies every renal biopsy. The mean decrease in hemoglobin after a biopsy is approximately 1 g/dl.[25] Significant perirenal hematomas are almost invariably associated with severe loin pain. Both macroscopic hematuria and painful hematoma are seen in 3% of patients after biopsy. The initial management is strict bed rest and maintenance of normal coagulation indices. If bleeding is brisk and associated with hypotension or prolonged and fails to settle with bed rest,

Complications of renal biopsy		
	1952–1977 (%)	1990 to Present (%)
Number	14,492	3884
Hematoma	1	3
Gross hematuria	3	3
Arteriovenous fistula	0.1	0.2
Surgery	0.3	1 case
Death	0.12	1 case

Figure 6.9 Complications of renal biopsy. The data for 1952 to 1977 are taken from 20 series including 14,492 patients.[27] The 1990 to present data are from eight series including 3884 patients.[18,25,28–33]

renal angiography should be performed to identify the source of bleeding. Coil embolization can be performed during the same procedure, and this has largely eliminated the need for open surgical intervention and nephrectomy.

Arteriovenous Fistula

Most postbiopsy arteriovenous fistulas are detected by Doppler ultrasonography or contrast-enhanced computed tomography and when looked for specifically can be found in as many as 18% of patients. Since most are clinically silent and more than 95% resolve spontaneously within 2 years,[26] they should not be routinely sought. In a small minority, they can lead to macroscopic hematuria, hypertension, and renal impairment, in which case, embolization is appropriate.

Other Complications

A variety of other rare complications have been reported including biopsy performed on other organs (liver, spleen, pancreas, bowel, and gallbladder), pneumothorax, hemothorax, calyceal-peritoneal fistula, dispersion of carcinoma, and the Page kidney. This latter complication results from compression of the kidney by a perirenal hematoma leading to renin-mediated hypertension.

Death

Death resulting directly from the renal biopsy has become much less common according to recent biopsy series when compared to earlier reports. The vast majority of deaths are the result of uncontrolled hemorrhage in high-risk patients, particularly those with ARF.

REFERENCES

1. Iversen P, Brun C: Aspiration biopsy of the kidney. 1951. J Am Soc Nephrol 1997;8:1778–1787.
2. Alwall N: Aspiration biopsy of the kidney, including a report of a case of amyloidosis diagnosed through aspiration biopsy of the kidney in 1944 and investigated at an autopsy in 1950. Acta Med Scand 1952;143: 430–435.
3. Kark RM, Muehrcke RC: Biopsy of kidney in prone position. Lancet 1954;266:1047–1049.
4. Wolf G, Ritz E: Combination therapy with ACE inhibitors and angiotensin II receptor blockers to halt progression of chronic renal disease: pathophysiology and indications. Kidney Int 2005;67:799–812.
5. Copley JB, Hasbargen JA: "Idiopathic" hematuria. A prospective evaluation. Arch Intern Med 1987;147:434–437.
6. Topham PS, Harper SJ, Furness PN, et al: Glomerular disease as a cause of isolated microscopic hematuria. Q J Med 1994;87:329–335.
7. Kropp KA, Shapiro RS, Jhunjhunwala JS: Role of renal biopsy in end stage renal failure. Urology 1978;12:631–634.
8. Corwin HL, Schwartz MM, Lewis EJ: The importance of sample size in the interpretation of the renal biopsy. Am J Nephrol 1988;8:85–89.
9. Paone DB, Meyer LE: The effect of biopsy on therapy in renal disease. Arch Intern Med 1981;141:1039–1041.
10. Turner MW, Hutchinson TA, Barre PE, et al: A prospective study on the impact of the renal biopsy in clinical management. Clin Nephrol 1986; 26:217–221.
11. Richards NT, Darby S, Howie AJ, et al: Knowledge of renal histology alters patient management in over 40% of cases. Nephrol Dial Transplant 1994;9:1255–1259.
12. Diaz-Buxo JA, Donadio JV Jr: Complications of percutaneous renal biopsy: An analysis of 1,000 consecutive biopsies. Clin Nephrol 1975;4:223–227.
13. Nass K, O'Neill WC: Bedside renal biopsy: Ultrasound guidance by the nephrologist. Am J Kidney Dis 1999;34:955–959.
14. Boberg KM, Brosstad F, Egeland T, et al: Is a prolonged bleeding time associated with an increased risk of hemorrhage after liver biopsy? Thromb Haemost 1999;81:378–381.

15. Peterson P, Hayes TE, Arkin CF, et al: The preoperative bleeding time test lacks clinical benefit: College of American Pathologists' and American Society of Clinical Pathologists' position article. Arch Surg 1998;133:134–139.

16. Riehl J, Maigatter S, Kierdorf H, et al: Percutaneous renal biopsy: Comparison of manual and automated puncture techniques with native and transplanted kidneys. Nephrol Dial Transplant 1994;9:1568–1574.

17. Doyle AJ, Gregory MC, Terreros DA: Percutaneous native renal biopsy: Comparison of a 1.2-mm spring-driven system with a traditional 2-mm hand-driven system. Am J Kidney Dis 1994;23:498–503.

18. Whittier WL, Korbet SM: Timing of complications in percutaneous renal biopsy. J Am Soc Nephrol 2004;15:142–147.

19. Mal F, Meyrier A, Callard P, et al: Transjugular renal biopsy. Lancet 1990;335:1512–1513.

20. Cluzel P, Martinez F, Bellin MF, et al: Transjugular versus percutaneous renal biopsy for the diagnosis of parenchymal disease: Comparison of sampling effectiveness and complications. Radiology 2000;215:689–693.

21. Jouet P, Meyrier A, Mal F, et al: Transjugular renal biopsy in the treatment of patients with cirrhosis and renal abnormalities. Hepatology 1996;24:1143–1147.

22. Nomoto Y, Tomino Y, Endoh M, et al: Modified open renal biopsy: Results in 934 patients. Nephron 1987;45:224–228.

23. Shetye KR, Kavoussi LR, Ramakumar S, et al: Laparoscopic renal biopsy: A 9-year experience. BJU Int 2003;91:817–820.

24. Leal JJ: A new technique for renal biopsy: The transurethral approach. J Urol 1993;149:1061–1063.

25. Burstein DM, Korbet SM, Schwartz MM: The use of the automatic core biopsy system in percutaneous renal biopsies: A comparative study. Am J Kidney Dis 1993;22:545–552.

26. Bennett AR, Wiener SN: Intrarenal arteriovenous fistula and aneurysm. A complication of percutaneous renal biopsy. Am J Roentgenol Radium Ther Nucl Med 1965;95:372–382.

27. Parrish AE: Complications of percutaneous renal biopsy: A review of 37 years' experience. Clin Nephrol 1992;38:135–141.

28. Eiro M, Katoh T, Watanabe T: Risk factors for bleeding complications in percutaneous renal biopsy. Clin Exp Nephrol 2005;9:40–45.

29. Fraser IR, Fairley KF: Renal biopsy as an outpatient procedure. Am J Kidney Dis 1995;25:876–878.

30. Hergesell O, Felten H, Andrassy K, et al: Safety of ultrasound-guided percutaneous renal biopsy—retrospective analysis of 1090 consecutive cases. Nephrol Dial Transplant 1998;13:975–977.

31. Manno C, Strippoli GF, Arnesano L, et al: Predictors of bleeding complications in percutaneous ultrasound-guided renal biopsy. Kidney Int 2004;66:1570–1577.

32. Marwah DS, Korbet SM: Timing of complications in percutaneous renal biopsy: What is the optimal period of observation? Am J Kidney Dis 1996;28:47–52.

33. Stiles KP, Hill C, LeBrun CJ, et al: The impact of bleeding times on major complication rates after percutaneous real-time ultrasound-guided renal biopsies. J Nephrol 2001;14:275–279.

CHAPTER

7 Disorders of Extracellular Volume

Didier Portilla and Thomas E. Andreoli

EXTRACELLULAR FLUID COMPARTMENT

In healthy adults, body water constitutes approximately 60% of the total body weight. It exists in two compartments: the intracellular fluid (ICF) compartment containing two thirds of total body water and the extracellular fluid (ECF) compartment containing the remaining one third. The capillary endothelial membrane further divides the ECF into two compartments. The intravascular or plasma fluid compartment makes up one fourth of the ECF and the extravascular compartment makes up the remaining three fourths of the ECF volume.[1] The extravascular compartment is composed of two fractions: interstitial volume and transcellular water (25% and 4% of total body water, respectively). Transcellular fluid includes cerebrospinal fluid, gastrointestinal fluids, and the fluids in the eye and serous surfaces (Fig. 7.1).

The composition of the ECF is quite similar to that of the intravascular compartment, with some difference as a result of disparity in the protein concentration between the plasma and interstitial space. The difference in the electrolyte concentration between these two compartments is determined by the effect of the Donnan equilibrium, and, therefore, the concentration of diffusible cations is about 4% greater in plasma water and the concentration of diffusible anions is lower by the same percentage[2] (Fig. 7.2).

Concentrations of ions in plasma, plasma water, and interstitial fluid

	Plasma (mmol/l)	Plasma Water (mmol/l)	Interstitial Fluid (mmol/l)
Sodium	140	151	148
Potassium	4.5	5.0	5.0
Calcium	2.5	2.8	2.0
Magnesium	0.85	0.9	0.75
Chloride	104	112	115
Bicarbonate	24	26	27
Phosphate	1.0	1.05	1.15

Figure 7.2 Concentrations of ions in plasma, plasma water, and interstitial fluid.

The ICF and ECF compartments are in osmotic equilibrium because virtually all cell membranes in the body are freely permeable to water. The ECF volume is determined primarily by the total amount of osmotically active solutes in the compartment. Sodium salts, by virtue of being the most abundant solutes in the ECF, are the most important determinants of ECF volume. The amount of sodium in the ECF is, therefore, regulated tightly. ECF sodium deficiency results in renal sodium retention and excess ECF sodium promotes increased urinary excretion of sodium.

The most fundamental characteristic of fluid and electrolyte homeostasis is the maintenance of ECF volume and circulatory stability. In normal humans, despite significant day-to-day variations in the intake of salt and water, the ECF volume is maintained within a normal range, varying by only 1% to 2%.[3] Maintaining the appropriate ECF volume is critical because it determines the mean arterial pressure and left ventricular filling volume. Furthermore, ECF bathes all cells and is therefore responsible for the delivery of oxygen and nutrients and the removal of metabolic products.

Effective Arterial Blood Volume
The blood volume that is detected by volume sensors (see later discussion) can be referred to as the effective arterial blood volume (EABV).[4] In other words, EABV is the amount of arterial blood required to adequately "fill" the capacity of the arterial circulation. ECF volume and EABV can be independent of each other (Fig. 7.3). In addition, the concept of volume/capacitance ratio is even more important than the absolute EABV in disease states such as sepsis.

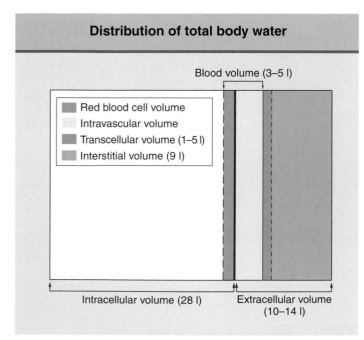

Distribution of total body water

- Red blood cell volume
- Intravascular volume
- Transcellular volume (1–5 l)
- Interstitial volume (9 l)

Blood volume (3–5 l)

Intracellular volume (28 l)

Extracellular volume (10–14 l)

Figure 7.1 Distribution of total body water into different compartments. The volumes are for an average 70-kg adult.

Relationship of effective arterial blood volume and total extracellular fluid in various disease states					
Compartment	Volume Depletion	Nephrosis	Congestive Heart Failure	Arteriovenous Fistula with Congestive State	Renal Artery Stenosis
Total extracellular fluid volume	↓	↑	↑	↑	↑
Total blood volume	↓	Variable	↑	↑	↑
Arterial blood volume	↓	Variable	↓	↑	↓
Effective arterial blood volume	↓	Variable	↓	↓	↑
Renal blood flow	↓	Variable	↓	↓	↓

Figure 7.3 Relationship of effective arterial blood volume and total extracellular fluid in various disease states.

FACTORS REGULATING EXTRACELLULAR FLUID HOMEOSTASIS

The characteristic feature of the body fluid homeostatic mechanism is that the composition of the body fluid compartments remains remarkably constant despite wide daily variations in solute and water intake.[5] The homeostatic mechanism also invariably protects the ECF volume in circumstances when multiple physiologic variables are threatened simultaneously; this can sometimes occur at the expense of aggravating another electrolyte disorder.[6,7] For example, a patient with volume depletion who is replenished with water, and not sodium, will retain water and become hyponatremic, thereby preventing circulatory collapse. Here, fluid balance is maintained at the expense of electrolyte imbalance, specifically, hypotonicity of body fluids.

The integrated homeostatic response involves two key components (Fig. 7.4): an afferent limb that contains sensors that detect changes in effective circulating volume and an efferent limb that regulates the rate of sodium excretion by the kidney.[8,9]

Afferent Limb: Volume Sensors
Volume detectors reside at several sites in the vasculature (Fig. 7.5) and serve as the most sensitive volume receptors that monitor changes in circulatory function within that compartment.[10] They can be broadly classified as low-pressure baroreceptors, high-pressure baroreceptors, intrarenal sensors, and hepatic and central nervous system sensors.

Low-Pressure Baroreceptors
Low-pressure baroreceptors are located on the venous side of the central circulation and assess the filling of the central venous circulation. They are very sensitive and monitor changes in the intrathoracic volume and are designed to defend against ECF volume expansion and its deleterious pulmonary consequences. The low-pressure baroreceptors include the cardiac atria and the cardiopulmonary receptors.

Cardiac Atrial Receptors   Receptors in the cardiac atria transduce atrial wall stretch. Increased venous return increases the discharge rate of these receptors, and stretch and tension impulses travel along cranial nerves IX and X to the hypothalamic and medullary centers in the brain. This, in turn, decreases the renal sympathetic nerve activity, leading to natriuresis. The resultant hemodynamic changes counteract the original stimuli from volume expansion.

Humoral alterations that assist in counteracting the increase in central blood volume also occur as a response to atrial stretch. The hypothalamus responds to an increase in atrial stretch by inhibiting the release of arginine vasopressin (vasopressin or antidiuretic hormone [ADH]) and adrenocorticotropic hormone.

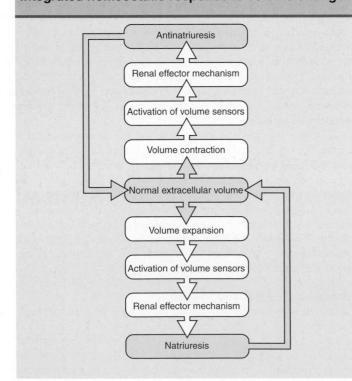

Integrated homeostatic response to volume changes

- Antinatriuresis
- Renal effector mechanism
- Activation of volume sensors
- Volume contraction
- Normal extracellular volume
- Volume expansion
- Activation of volume sensors
- Renal effector mechanism
- Natriuresis

Figure 7.4 A general overview of the integrated homeostatic response system regulating extracellular fluid volume during volume contraction and expansion.

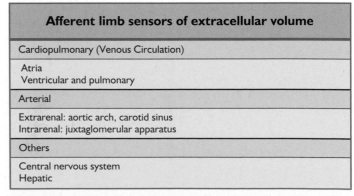

Afferent limb sensors of extracellular volume
Cardiopulmonary (Venous Circulation)
Atria Ventricular and pulmonary
Arterial
Extrarenal: aortic arch, carotid sinus Intrarenal: juxtaglomerular apparatus
Others
Central nervous system Hepatic

Figure 7.5 Afferent limb (volume) sensors of the integrated homeostatic response system for extracellular volume.

Vasopressin induces free water retention and adrenocorticotropic hormone stimulates mineralocorticoid release from the adrenal gland. The inhibition of these hormones in response to atrial stretch leads to salt and water diuresis. Furthermore, decreased renal sympathetic activity, specifically β-adrenergic activity, lowers renal renin production, which in turn decreases levels of angiotensin II (Ang II).[10] This facilitates natriuresis and contributes to the lowering of blood pressure. Distention of the cardiac atria also results in release of atrial natriuretic peptide (ANP) (atriopeptin) from the myocytes. ANP induces renal excretion of sodium and water and may also increase the capacitance of the central circulatory bed, thus lowering central venous pressure (CVP). ANP does not seem to play an important role in daily salt and water balance, and its most important role is in pathophysiologic states that affect ECF volume homeostasis. Volume contraction leads to a decrease in CVP, which in turn decreases the discharge rate of these atrial receptors, leading to renal salt and water conservation.

Cardiopulmonary Sensors   The central circulation contains low-pressure receptors in the left ventricle and the pulmonary vascular bed. When CVP decreases, the rate of discharge from these cardiopulmonary receptors is low, which leads to a decrease in the inhibition of the vasomotor center in the brain and subsequent increase in sympathetic outflow. The net result is an increase in heart rate, peripheral vascular resistance, antinatriuresis, and antidiuresis, all of which lead to increases in blood pressure and cardiac output and to volume conservation. Conversely, an increase in CVP increases the rate of discharge from these receptors, which eventually leads to natriuresis and sympathetic withdrawal.

High-Pressure Baroreceptors

High-pressure baroreceptors, located at the bifurcation of the carotid artery (carotid sinus body) and the aortic arch (aortic body), work independently from the low-pressure sensors. They assess the pressure of the arterial circulation and are designed to maintain mean arterial pressure at a constant level and protect the brain from wide fluctuations in perfusion pressure.

Underfilling of the arterial tree leads to activation of these receptors. Signals from these receptors travel to the vasomotor center in the brain, which in turn signals the kidney to retain sodium. The latter is accompanied by increases in sympathetic nerve activity and plasma norepinephrine levels and by increases in vasopressin and endothelin levels.[9,10] The catecholamine response increases blood pressure by increasing the heart rate and arteriolar resistance. The increase in arteriolar resistance promotes transfer of fluid from the interstitium to the vascular compartment.

Overfilling of the arterial tree elicits the opposite response. It decreases the discharge rate from these baroreceptors, which finally results in natriuresis and decreased catecholamine response. In addition, left ventricular distention will also release brain natriuretic peptide (nesiritide) that has similar actions as ANP to increase renal blood flow (RBF) and induce natriuresis.

Intrarenal Sensors: Juxtaglomerular Apparatus

The kidney plays an important role in the afferent limb of volume homeostasis. The intrarenal sensors are formed by the renal juxtaglomerular apparatus (JGA). Renin, an acid protease, is released from the JGA into the plasma when intrarenal sensors detect volume contraction. Renin catalyzes the release of angiotensin I from angiotensinogen. This is the rate-limiting step in the formation of Ang II. Subsequently, angiotensin-converting

enzyme (ACE) catalyzes the cleavage of angiotensin I to Ang II, which is the cardinal stimulus to aldosterone production and, by itself, is a potent vasoconstrictor.

Renin production is regulated by three major mechanisms[7]:
1. *Change in renal perfusion pressure*. A decrease in perfusion pressure can lead to increased renin release by the specialized cells of the macula densa, which can directly sense the reduced perfusion pressure.
2. *Solute delivery to the macula densa cells*. An increase in the concentration of sodium chloride near the macula densa cells results in inhibition of renin release; conversely, there is increased release when sodium delivery is decreased.
3. *Influence of renal sympathetic nerves*. Activation of the β-adrenoceptors in the juxtaglomerular cells results in renin release from the macula densa cells.

It appears that the reductions in renal perfusion pressure and solute delivery to macula densa cells involve a complex interplay between the cyclooxygenase (COX) enzyme system and the nitric oxide synthase (NOS) system. More specifically, the enzyme NOS-1 in macula densa cells is activated by reductions and solute delivery to the macula densa. In turn, NOS-1 activates expression of the COX-2 enzyme, which enhances renal prostaglandin E_2 (PGE_2) synthesis and consequently afferent renal arteriolar dilatation. COX-2 stimulation of PGE_2 also stimulates renin secretion and subsequent Ang II production that acts to stimulate efferent arteriolar constriction. These processes act in concert to help maintain the glomerular filtration rate (GFR) under conditions of renal hypoperfusion.

Hepatic and Central Nervous System Sensors

Several other volume sensors contribute to the afferent limb of the volume homeostasis loop. They are located in various organs in the body, for example, the central nervous system and the portohepatic circulation. The physiologic significance and the exact mechanism of action of these sensors remain to be defined.

Efferent Limb: Effector Elements

The stimulation of the afferent volume sensing system leads to activation of the efferent limb, where the kidney is the major effector organ in the body fluid volume homeostasis loop. The ECF volume is mainly regulated by alteration in renal sodium excretion.[11] Several factors that influence renal sodium handling are listed in Figure 7.6.

Major renal efferent mechanisms regulating extracellular fluid volume
Glomerular filtration rate

Physical factors
    At the level of the proximal tubule
    Beyond the proximal tubule

Humoral effector mechanisms
    Renin angiotensin aldosterone system
    Vasopressin
    Catecholamines
    Prostaglandins
    Kinin-kallikrein system
    Atrial natriuretic peptide
    Endothelium-derived factors

Renal sympathetic nerves

Figure 7.6   Major renal efferent mechanisms regulating excretion of sodium and controlling extracellular fluid volume.

Glomerular Filtration

The amount of sodium excreted by the kidney is dependent on the filtered load of sodium. The determinants of the filtered load of sodium include GFR and the serum sodium concentration. In the human kidney, >1000 mmol (23 mg) of sodium are filtered each hour. Of this, about 990 mmol (22.8 mg) are reabsorbed from the renal tubules. Consequently, any fluctuation in GFR can, in principle, affect the renal handling of sodium.

The transfer of fluid across a capillary wall is governed by the hydrostatic pressure gradients and plasma oncotic pressure gradients, expressed by the Starling equation[12]: $J_v = K_f (\Delta P - \sigma \Delta \pi)$, where J_v is the rate of fluid transfer between the capillary and interstitial compartments, K_f is the water permeability of the capillary bed (also termed the glomerular capillary ultrafiltration coefficient), ΔP is the hydrostatic pressure difference between capillary and interstitial fluids, σ is the permeability of the solute to the membrane, in case of glucose $\sigma = 1$, while urea and sodium have a 0 refraction coefficient, and $\Delta \pi$ is the oncotic pressure difference between capillary and interstitial fluids.

Determinants of Glomerular Filtration

There are four major determinants of glomerular filtration[9]:
1. The balance of Starling forces acting across the capillary wall; the glomerular capillary hydraulic pressure and the oncotic pressure of Bowman's space favor filtration, whereas the hydraulic pressure of Bowman's space and glomerular oncotic pressure tend to retard it.
2. The ultrafiltration coefficient K_f, which reflects the glomerular permeability and the total filtration area of the glomerular capillaries.
3. Changes in plasma protein composition that affect the rate of filtrate formation.
4. The rate at which plasma flows through the glomeruli.

Renal Autoregulation

Renal autoregulation is a phenomenon by which GFR is maintained fairly constant in the presence of perturbations that otherwise would result in its variation. For example, constricting the renal artery can lead to modest alteration in renal perfusion pressure without altering either GFR or RBF.

The afferent arteriolar resistance is an important determinant of the net glomerular filtration pressure. The RBF and GFR are maintained under tight control by two intrarenal mechanisms that contribute to adjustments in arteriolar resistance during changes in arterial pressure. The first, known as the myogenic mechanism, is a pressure-sensitive mechanism that is an inherent property of smooth muscle cells. An increase in renal arterial pressure causes stretching of the afferent arteriolar smooth muscle cells. This in turn triggers afferent arteriolar constriction, preventing transmission of the high arterial pressure to the glomerular capillaries. A decrease in renal arterial pressure results in the opposite effect.

The second mechanism, tubuloglomerular feedback, is a phenomenon whereby increased sodium delivery to the macula densa controls afferent arteriolar tone.[13] Here, an increase in intravascular pressure leads to an increase in GFR and increased delivery of sodium chloride to the macula densa. This causes an increase in afferent arteriolar resistance and subsequently decreases GFR back to normal.[14] These changes in afferent arteriolar tone are mediated principally by the interplay between vasodilatory factors, principally the prostaglandins, ANP, and nitric oxide, and vasoconstrictive agents, primarily adenosine, adenosine triphosphate, vasopressin, Ang II, endothelins, and the adrenergic effectors epinephrine and norepinephrine. In addition, it has been proposed that mild levels of hyperuricemia can increase renin production in the afferent arteriole.[15] Finally, both the myogenic mechanism and tubuloglomerular feedback are impaired in circumstances that result in consistent renal hypoperfusion, such as renal artery stenosis.

Glomerulotubular Balance

Glomerulotubular balance is a fundamental property of the kidney whereby changes in GFR automatically induce a proportional change in the rate of proximal tubular sodium reabsorption. Thus, the fractional reabsorption of sodium in the proximal tubule is maintained constant in the setting of increases or decreases in GFR. However, in the event that there is volume contraction, glomerulotubular balance is set upward (resulting in a higher fractional reabsorption), whereas with volume expansion glomerulotubular balance is set downward (resulting in a decrease in fractional reabsorption).

Tubular Reabsorption of Sodium

The control of tubular sodium reabsorption is more important than GFR in the regulation of urinary sodium excretion. The net urinary sodium excretion is the balance between the filtered load of sodium and the amount of sodium reabsorbed from the nephron. As mentioned previously, about 99% of the total filtered sodium is reclaimed from the renal tubules. This occurs via four major cell types located along the length of the nephron, as illustrated in Figure 7.7. The proximal nephron reclaims about 70% and the loop of Henle accounts for about 20% of the glomerular filtrate. In the distal nephron, about 5% of the filtered sodium is reabsorbed in the distal convoluted tubule, and the final 2% to 4% is reabsorbed in the collecting duct.

Physical Factors

Physical factors act through peritubular capillary Starling forces to influence the renal handling of sodium at the level of the proximal tubule as well as beyond this nephron segment. This effect is independent of GFR, hormones, and renal sympathetic nerves.

In the proximal nephron, the peritubular capillary network is closely linked to the glomerular capillary bed through the efferent arteriole. Consequently, changes in the physical determinants of GFR influence the hydrostatic and oncotic pressures in the peritubular capillaries.[9] The hydrostatic pressure is significantly lower in the peritubular capillaries than in the glomerular capillaries. Also, because the peritubular capillaries receive blood from the glomerulus, the plasma oncotic pressure is high at the outset as a result of previous filtration of protein-free fluid. The renal interstitial hydrostatic pressure and the peritubular oncotic pressure are important regulators of the absolute rate of reabsorption of proximal tubule absorbate.[16]

Beyond the proximal tubule, there is substantial evidence that the natriuresis induced by volume expansion is also determined in part by physical factors. Increased distal delivery of fluid from the proximal tubule is associated with an increase in fractional sodium reabsorption along the loop of Henle. Furthermore, the loop of Henle has the capacity to increase fractional sodium reabsorption in response to changes in the delivered load of sodium from the proximal tubule. However, there also occurs, with an absolute increase in distal sodium delivery, an absolute increase in net sodium excretion.

One important mechanism to increase net sodium excretion is pressure natriuresis. This is a phenomenon in which an increase

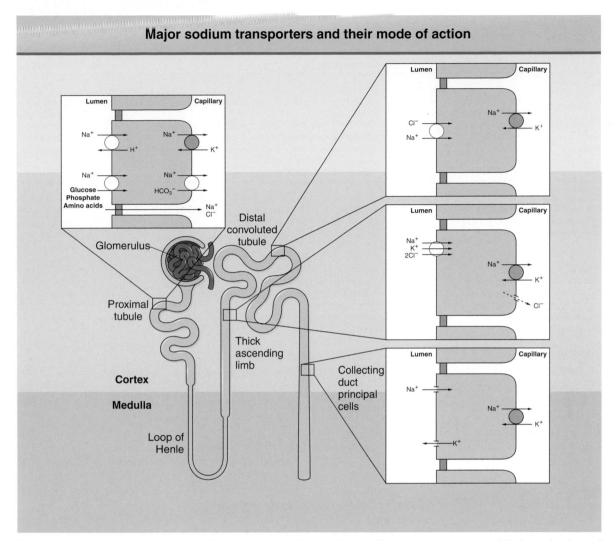

Major sodium transporters and their mode of action

Figure 7.7 Structure of the nephron showing the four major cell types where sodium transport occurs and their mechanisms of action.

in renal perfusion pressure (such as from a sudden increase in systemic pressure) results in a marked increased excretion of sodium and vice versa. The mechanism may at first seem puzzling since the response of the renal cortex to increases in perfusion pressure, which receives >95% of RBF, is to increase afferent resistance, thereby maintaining GFR and RBF (renal autoregulation, see previous discussion). However, there is evidence that changes in perfusion pressure in the medulla are transmitted into the capillary network, where it is thought to increase interstitial pressure and facilitate a natriuretic response that involves both nitric oxide and activation of the angiotensin receptor type 2.

Humoral Mechanisms
Renin Angiotensin Aldosterone System
Volume contraction of the ECF leads to renal hypoperfusion, which enhances renin release by the JGA. Renal renin release into the plasma accelerates the formation of Ang II, the direct actions of which on the kidneys tend to be antinatriuretic.[17] These effects occur at relatively low concentrations of Ang II. The first effect of Ang II is a direct vasoconstrictor action, predominantly on the efferent arteriole, with a subsequent increase in intraglomerular pressure and modulation of peritubular Starling forces; this results in enhanced proximal sodium and water reabsorption. Ang II also directly stimulates the proximal tubular reabsorption of sodium independently of changes in renal

or systemic hemodynamics. It stimulates catecholamine release from the renal nerves and enhances production of vasodilatory prostaglandins. Furthermore, it stimulates the adrenal gland to produce aldosterone, which increases the reabsorption of sodium in the distal parts of the nephron.

Vasopressin
Changes in blood osmolality of 1% can lead to vasopressin release from the posterior pituitary gland. In addition, vasopressin is also released in response to a 7% to 10% decrease in EABV (nonosmotic volume stimulus). This hormone, when bound by the vasopressin V_2 receptors on basolateral membranes of medullary thick ascending limbs and collecting ducts, enhances water permeability and absorption from the collecting duct and also stimulates sodium chloride reabsorption from the thick ascending limb of the loop of Henle and from the cortical collecting duct. The systemic vasoconstrictor action of vasopressin, mediated by vasopressin binding to V_1 receptors in vascular smooth muscle, also helps in the defense against perceived ECF volume contraction.

Catecholamines
Epinephrine and norepinephrine induce sodium retention by directly stimulating sodium reabsorption at the proximal tubule and the loop of Henle. They also activate the renin angiotensin

Characteristics of hormones regulating renal sodium excretion			
Mediators	Site of Production	Site of Action	Tubular Actions
Vasoconstrictors			
Angiotensin II	Circulating/local generation	Glomerular arterioles, proximal tubule	Sodium retention
Aldosterone	Adrenal glands	Distal tubule	Sodium retention
Vasopressin	Hypothalamus	Thick ascending limb (TAL) of loop of Henle, distal tubule	Water retention
Catecholamines	Adrenal glands	Glomerular arterioles, proximal tubule	Sodium retention
Renal sympathetics	Kidneys	Glomerular arterioles, proximal tubule	Sodium retention
Endothelin I	Endothelium	Glomerular arterioles, IMCD	Natriuresis
Na^+-K^+-ATPase inhibitors	Adrenal glands	Tubular Na^+-K^+-ATPase	Natriuresis
Vasodilators			
Atrial natriuretic peptide	Cardiac atria	CCD/IMCD	Natriuresis
Brain natriuretic peptide	Brain	CCD/IMCD	Natriuresis
C-type natriuretic peptide	Endothelium	CCD/IMCD	Natriuresis
Urodilatin	Renal tubules	CCD/IMCD	Natriuresis
Nitric oxide	Endothelium	Glomerular arterioles, distal nephron	Natriuresis
Prostaglandins E and I	Kidneys	Glomerular tubules, TAL, IMCD, CCD	Natriuresis
Bradykinin-kallikrein	Distal nephron	Glomerular tubules, IMCD	Natriuresis
Dopamine	Proximal tubular cells	Afferent arterioles, proximal nephron	Natriuresis

Figure 7.8 Characteristics of hormones regulating renal sodium excretion. ATP, adenosine triphosphatase; CCD, cortical collecting duct; IMCD, inner medullary collecting duct.

aldosterone system and induce a preferential vasoconstriction at the level of the efferent arteriole to maintain the intraglomerular pressure in response to volume contraction. Dopamine, when administered in low concentrations, causes renal vasodilation and enhances glomerular filtration; dopamine may also have a direct role in augmenting renal sodium excretion by decreasing tubular sodium absorption.

Prostaglandins

Prostaglandins are autacoids derived from the metabolism of arachidonic acid. The important renal prostaglandins include PGE_2, PGI_2, and thromboxane. PGE_2 and PGI_2 have natriuretic properties and influence renal sodium handling in the collecting ducts and the loop of Henle. They also play an active role in regulating renal hemodynamics. PGE_2 also antagonizes the action of ADH on sodium absorption in the thick ascending limb and on water absorption in collecting ducts.

Two COX enzymes are principally involved in modulating prostaglandin production. COX-1, which is constitutively expressed, augments PGE_2 production in collecting ducts and thus leads to reductions in the rates of sodium and water absorption in collecting ducts. Second, COX-2 is expressed both in the renal interstitium and, as noted previously, by macula densa cells under the influence of NOS-1. Thus, prostaglandin production catalyzed by COX-2 participates in modulating tubuloglomerular feedback (see previous discussion) and in antagonizing the effects of vasopressin on sodium absorption in medullary thick ascending limbs and on sodium and water absorption in collecting ducts.

Atrial Natriuretic Peptide

ANP is a polypeptide synthesized by the cardiac myocytes that has natriuretic properties. In the kidney, ANP exerts hemodynamic and tubular actions that eventually lead to increased urinary excretion of sodium and water.[18] At the level of the glomerulus, ANP induces vasodilatation of the afferent arteriole, thereby leading to increases in GFR and in the filtered load of sodium. ANP also inhibits sodium reabsorption in the inner medullary collecting duct by activating production of cGMP, a

known intracellular messenger of nitric oxide. ANP inhibits the action of several hormones; it inhibits renin release, reduces aldosterone secretion by the adrenal cortex, and blocks some of the vasoconstrictive effect of Ang II.

Other Hormones

Several other hormones influence renal sodium excretion (Fig. 7.8). Whereas the renal sodium-regulating properties of some of these hormones have been elucidated, the exact roles of others in volume homeostasis have yet to be determined.

Renal Nerves

The sympathetic nervous system is present in all segments of the renal vasculature and tubules. It innervates the afferent and efferent arterioles of the glomerulus and regulates urinary sodium and water excretion by changing hemodynamics.[19] It also exerts a direct effect on innervated tubules to regulate the renal reabsorption of sodium from the proximal nephron. ECF volume contraction increases the activity of the renal sympathetic nerves.

Sympathetic nerves, specifically β-adrenergic fibers, enhance the release of renin from the JGA, thereby increasing the level of Ang II and aldosterone. They also interact with other hormonal systems including vasopressin and ANP.

EXTRACELLULAR FLUID VOLUME CONTRACTION

Since the ECF represents one third of total body water and one fifth of total body weight, volume contraction occurs when the functional ECF volume is <20% of the total body weight or <15 liters in a 70-kg adult. The reduction in ECF volume usually occurs simultaneously from both the interstitial and intravascular compartments and is determined by whether the volume loss is primarily solute-free water or a combination of salt and water.[20] Since only one twelfth of the total body water resides in the vascular space, the loss of solute-free water has a lesser effect on intravascular volume.[21] However, most of the sodium is confined to the ECF space and a combined loss of sodium and water results in significant intravascular volume depletion.

Etiology and Pathogenesis

Volume contraction is a result of increased salt and water loss from renal and extrarenal sources that exceeds total intake. Renal losses of salt and water (Fig. 7.9) can be secondary to either a loss of effector mechanisms for salt and water conservation or intrinsic renal diseases that cause alterations in the output mechanism.[7] Extrarenal fluid losses (Fig. 7.10), when inadequately replaced, can also lead to volume depletion.

Renal Losses of Salt and Water
Genetic Mechanisms

A major advance in the study of inherited disorders of salt-wasting syndromes has been the demonstration that Bartter and Gitelman's syndromes result from mutation of specific ion transport proteins expressed by cells of the distal nephron.[22,23] The dysfunction of the thiazide-sensitive sodium-chloride cotransporter (NCC1) in Gitelman's syndrome and the bumetanide-sensitive sodium-potassium-chloride cotransporter (NKCC2) in Bartter syndrome cause salt wasting, ECF volume depletion, secondary hyperaldosteronism, and hypokalemia (see Chapter 46 for details).

Chronic Diuretic Abuse

Chronic diuretic abuse is a frequent cause of ECF volume contraction seen in clinical practice and usually leads to renal salt wasting, volume contraction, and metabolic acid-base abnormalities. Acetazolamide and other proximal tubule diuretics inhibit proximal renal absorption of sodium bicarbonate, resulting in volume contraction and hyperchloremic, hypokalemic metabolic acidosis. Loop diuretics such as furosemide inhibit sodium chloride absorption in the thick ascending limb of the loop of Henle, thus causing renal salt and water loss and hypokalemic metabolic alkalosis. Competitive inhibitors of aldosterone, such as spironolactone, or nonaldosterone inhibitors of collecting duct sodium absorption, such as triamterene and amiloride, can cause renal salt wasting, volume depletion, and hyperkalemic, hyperchloremic metabolic acidosis. Diuretics are discussed in more detail at the end of the chapter.

Osmotic and Other Diureses

Osmotic diuresis results in obligatory renal loss of salt and water. This can occur in uncontrolled diabetes secondary to the failure to reabsorb glucose from the tubular fluid; in mannitol diuresis; and in urea diuresis, which can occur in burn patients

Conditions associated with renal loss of salt and water

Salt and Water
Diuretic abuse
Osmotic diuresis
Postobstructive diuresis
Salt-losing tubular nephropathies: medullary cystic disease, Bartter syndrome, chronic interstitial renal diseases
Aldosterone insufficiency: Addison's disease, hyporeninemic hypoaldosteronism
Water
Diabetes insipidus: pituitary, nephrogenic

Figure 7.9   Conditions associated with renal loss of salt and water.

Conditions associated with extrarenal loss of salt and water

Dermal losses Sweat Burns Insensible loss
Hemorrhage
Gastrointestinal losses Upper: vomiting, nasogastric suction Lower: diarrheal disorder, tube drainage, fistula Sequestrational losses: intestinal obstruction, pancreatitis, muscle injury, rhabdomyolysis

Figure 7.10   Conditions associated with extracellular loss of salt and water.

with abnormally high rates of urea production. Other common conditions associated with diuresis include postobstructive diuresis after relief of complete or partial urinary tract obstruction and the diuretic phase of acute tubular necrosis, in which loss of sodium and water usually accompanies recovery from acute tubular necrosis.

Aldosterone Deficiency

Aldosterone deficiency frequently leads to renal sodium wasting. It can occur from destruction of the adrenal gland, as seen in Addison's disease, or secondary to hyporeninemic hypoaldosteronism, which may occur in disease states like diabetes and other chronic renal interstitial disease.

Other Causes

Less common conditions associated with excessive renal salt and water losses include renal tubular acidosis, Bartter syndrome, and some chronic tubular and interstitial renal diseases. Medullary cystic kidney disease (and the related juvenile nephronophthisis) are genetically transmitted types of chronic interstitial disease with medullary cysts that are classically associated with salt wasting (see Chapter 44).

Renal Water Loss

Diabetes insipidus, either pituitary (impaired secretion of vasopressin) or nephrogenic (impaired renal response to vasopressin), can result in profound volume depletion from obligatory loss of marked amounts of free water; which can sometimes exceed 10 to 15 liters daily (see Chapter 8). This scenario is particularly manifest in patients with diabetes insipidus who are denied free access to water.

Extrarenal Losses
Dermal Fluid Losses

Dermal fluid losses can result from excessive sweating caused by prolonged exercise or by high ambient temperature or fever. Professional athletes can lose as much as 5 liters of sweat within one game. This is especially important when losses are not replaced by appropriate salt and water intake. Burns can lead to large amounts of fluid losses through the affected areas, with resultant profound ECF volume contraction.

"Sequestrational" Losses

"Sequestrational" losses occur when ECF is lost into body compartments. In intestinal obstruction, the fluid collects within the bowel lumen; in pancreatitis, the fluid is sequestered in the retroperitoneal space; and in cirrhosis, within the peritoneal cavity as ascites. Severe trauma and muscle injuries can cause significant sequestration of fluid, sufficient to cause volume depletion.

Hemorrhage
Hemorrhage, both internal and external, can lead to significant loss of intravascular volume and cause volume contraction.

Gastrointestinal Losses
Gastrointestinal losses are commonly associated with volume contraction as a result of loss of significant amounts of digestive secretions. Upper gastrointestinal losses can occur from vomiting and from nasogastric suctioning; these are usually accompanied by metabolic alkalosis. Lower gastrointestinal alkaline fluid losses from diarrhea and fistulas lead to metabolic acidosis.

Clinical Manifestations
The clinical findings in states of volume contraction result from the underfilling of the arterial tree and the renal and hemodynamic responses to this underfilling. Signs and symptoms of volume depletion depend on the interplay of four major factors: the magnitude of fluid loss, the rate of volume loss, the nature of the losses, and, finally, the responsiveness of the vasculature to volume reduction. An accurate history and a careful physical examination are extremely important in the clinical assessment of ECF volume contraction. A rapid reduction in body weight is a reliable indicator of ECF volume loss. The symptoms of ECF volume contraction are nonspecific and can range from minimal symptoms to severe circulatory collapse. In mild or partially compensated volume contraction, particularly when it is gradual, the patient may exhibit symptoms of mild postural dizziness, thirst, and weakness. In more advanced stages of volume depletion, particularly those occurring more acutely, the symptoms include recumbent hypotension, tachycardia, and reduced urinary output. Finally, with severe volume contraction, the combination of profound fluid loss and sympathetic hyperactivity results in circulatory collapse characterized by confusion, oliguria, very low blood pressure (detectable by Doppler studies only), cold clammy extremities, and recumbent tachycardia. The lack of physical findings does not exclude the presence of mild to moderate ECF volume contraction. In postoperative patients, blood volume losses of 7% to 10% are frequently associated with normal blood pressure and only minimally reduced CVP. Orthostatic hypotension (a decrease in systolic blood pressure of >20 mm Hg or a decrease in diastolic blood pressure of >10 mm Hg with change from recumbency to standing) may be one of the early manifestations of moderate volume depletion if accompanied by an increase in pulse rate (typically an increase in heart rate >20 beats per minute on standing). A low jugular venous pressure noted with the patient lying at ≤45 degrees is also useful, particularly in patients with thin necks. Skin turgor and the moistness of the mucous membranes are valuable indicators of volume depletion in infants but are unreliable in adults. In young adults, reduction of skin turgor is usually associated with profound volume contraction; the normal loss of skin elasticity makes skin turgor difficult to assess in older patients. Furthermore, dry mucous membranes are a common occurrence in mouth breathers independent of external volume status and, therefore, may be unreliable.

Diagnosis
The blood pressure, pulse, loss of body weight, and clinical features provide an initial assessment of circulatory dynamics.

Nevertheless, evaluation of hemodynamic parameters, serum, and urinary indices are helpful in characterizing the cause and severity of volume contraction.[24]

Hemodynamic Monitoring
Clinical findings may be unreliable or inconclusive in moderate degrees of volume contraction, and invasive hemodynamic monitoring may be required in critically ill patients who are hemodynamically unstable. The hemodynamic parameters frequently measured include CVP, pulmonary capillary wedge pressure (PCWP), cardiac output, arterial pressures, and systemic vascular resistance. However, most of these parameters may be within normal limits when blood volume has been reduced by 5% to 10%. Consequently, a fluid challenge may be necessary in the evaluation of patients in whom volume deficit is thought to be a contributing factor to a reduced cardiac output.

The exact volume of such a "fluid challenge" is determined by the clinical circumstance. In individuals with no underlying cardiovascular disease, 500 ml of normal saline administered over 90 minutes is reasonable. However, in elderly patients, those with documented cardiovascular disease, or starved individuals, it is prudent to reduce the volume administered to 300 ml of normal saline over a 3-hour interval and then evaluate the patients' hemodynamic status before proceeding with more aggressive hydration.

Serum Indices of Volume Contraction
Measurement of serum blood urea nitrogen (BUN) and creatinine concentration may assist in the diagnosis of volume contraction. Volume contraction causes increased tubular reabsorption of urea, leading to an increased serum BUN:creatinine ratio. This prerenal azotemia is characterized by a serum BUN:creatinine ratio (mg/dl)/(mg/dl) of >20 compared to the normal ratio of 10. Plasma volume contraction may also result in hemoconcentration (increased hematocrit) and a relative increase in serum albumin.

Urinary Indices
The initial renal response to a decrease in EABV is a decrease in urine volume and a reduction in sodium excretion (see Chapter 64). The urinary sodium concentration and fractional excretion of sodium are indices of renal sodium avidity. Fractional excretion of sodium (%) is calculated according to the following equation:

$$FE_{Na} = [U_{Na} \times P_{creat}/P_{Na} \times U_{creat}] \times 100,$$

where U_{Na} and U_{creat} are urinary sodium and creatinine concentrations, respectively, and P_{Na} and P_{creat} are serum sodium and creatinine concentrations, respectively. In a volume-contracted state, the urinary sodium concentration is generally <10 to 15 mmol/l and the fractional excretion of sodium is usually <1%.

The urinary sodium indices are not reliable determinants of volume contraction in some situations. The urinary sodium may be elevated in states of upper gastrointestinal fluid losses associated with vomiting and gastric drainage. Here, the metabolic alkalosis causes obligatory renal sodium wasting as a consequence of bicarbonaturia, which requires cations for electroneutrality. Therefore, in this situation, the urinary chloride concentration is a more reliable index of renal salt avidity. Volume-contracted states associated with obligatory renal sodium wasting, such as with diuretic use, will also make the urinary sodium indices unreliable. Finally, patients with preexisting renal impairment and elderly patients may have higher than expected urinary sodium concentrations and fractional sodium excretion for the degree of volume contraction.

Other important urine parameters in volume-contracted states include urine osmolality and specific gravity. A urine/plasma creatinine ratio of >40:1 and a specific gravity of ≥1.020 also are suggestive of a prerenal state.

Treatment

The most important goal in the treatment of volume contraction is the expansion of the ECF volume by replacing the fluid deficits. In general, the composition of the replacement fluid should resemble the lost fluid and the rate, amount, and route of administration will vary with the particular circumstance. Increasing oral intake of salt and water may be sufficient with mild volume contraction. Absorption of sodium is also facilitated in the gut if glucose is coadministered. Excessive intake of hypotonic fluids in marathon runners can result in fatal hyponatremia. Immediate administration of intravenous fluids is required in more severe states of ECF volume contraction. The amount of replacement fluid should be adjusted not only to correct the established volume contraction, but also to replace the ongoing fluid losses. However, in elderly patients and patients with congestive heart failure (CHF), one must be very careful to avoid volume overload and pulmonary congestion.

Solutions containing sodium as the principal solute preferentially expand the ECF volume. Infusion of 1 liter of normal (isotonic) saline can result in an increase in plasma volume by about 250 ml; the remaining portion is distributed in the interstitial compartment. Isotonic saline remains the fluid of choice in patients with hypernatremia and volume contraction, not only because restoration of volume status takes preference over the correction of hypernatremia and hyperosmolality but also because the administration of isotonic saline solution to hypernatremic patients is still hypo-osmolar when compared to their serum osmolality. In subjects with marked hypernatremia (serum sodium >160 mmol/l), it is reasonable to administer either half normal saline or normal saline, but one must be careful not to correct the serum sodium too rapidly due to the risk of cerebral edema; in subjects with severe hypernatremia, a correction of 6 to 8 mmol/24 hours is recommended (see Chapter 8).

Colloid-containing solutions such as albumin and plasma preferentially expand the intravascular compartment and should be limited to situations in which patients are hemodynamically unstable and rapid correction of intravascular volume is critical. This is because the half-life of albumin is usually short, and the cost of albumin administration is very high. Furthermore, a meta-analysis found an association between albumin infusion and mortality risk in critically ill patients[25]; however, it remains controversial as to whether this represents cause and effect or whether it simply reflects the fact that the more seriously ill patients were given greater amounts of colloid. In a recent study, the use of either 4% albumin or normal saline for fluid resuscitation in critically ill patients resulted in similar mortality rates.

A physical examination should be performed frequently and laboratory parameters followed closely during the process of volume repletion. Monitoring of CVP and PCWP may be beneficial in patients who are critically ill with severe volume depletion. Hemodynamic monitoring may also be beneficial in patients with poor tolerance to volume expansion. It is important to remember that because volume contraction is accompanied by vasoconstriction, transient changes in PCWP may not accurately reflect the volume status of the patient. The initial elevation in PCWP is usually the result of fluid infusion onto a vasoconstricted, low-capacity vascular bed. This should not be misinterpreted to indicate adequacy of volume repletion.

EXTRACELLULAR FLUID EXPANSION

ECF volume expansion states are characterized by an increase in total body water, usually accompanied by an increase in total body sodium. They are associated with edema formation, which refers to the accumulation of excessive amounts of salt and water in the interstitial space.

Etiology and Pathogenesis

Volume expansion develops when the intake of salt and water exceeds the total renal and extrarenal volume losses. These disorders are usually associated with avid renal sodium and water retention that persists despite the ECF volume expansion. Three general kinds of physiologic derangement account for most edematous states (Fig. 7.11).

Disturbance in Starling Forces

Derangement in the Starling forces leads to expansion of the interstitial compartment at the expense of the ECF volume. Volume excess disorders are associated with a decrease in capillary oncotic pressure and/or an increase in capillary hydrostatic pressure. In other words, edema is a result of either an increase in movement of fluid to the interstitial space or a decrease in uptake of interstitial fluid into the intravascular compartment. Last, inadequacy in lymphatic drainage of the interstitial compartment can contribute to edema formation.

Cardiac disorders such as right heart failure or constrictive pericarditis are frequently associated with high systemic venous pressure.[26] Local elevations in pulmonary or venous pressures may also occur in conditions such as left heart failure, portal vein obstruction, or venacaval obstruction. In nephrotic syndrome, the reduction in plasma oncotic pressure may lead to a decrease in removal of interstitial fluid and a tendency for fluid to transude from the capillaries to the interstitium. In hepatic cirrhosis, there is a combination of increased venous pressures (portal hypertension) and decreased plasma oncotic pressure (hypoalbuminemia) that contributes to the development of ascites and edema.[26,27]

Disorders associated with extracellular fluid volume excess
Disturbed Starling Forces: Reduced Effective Circulating Volume, Edema Formation
Systematic venous pressure increases: right heart failure, constrictive pericarditis Local venous pressure increases: left heart failure, vena cava obstruction, portal vein obstruction Reduced oncotic pressure, nephrotic syndrome Combined disorders: cirrhosis
Primary Hormone Excess: Increased Effective Circulating Volume
Primary aldosteronism Cushing's syndrome Syndrome of inappropriate secretion of vasopressin
Primary Renal Sodium Retention: Increased Effective Circulating Volume
Acute glomerulonephritis

Figure 7.11 Classification of disorders associated with extracellular fluid volume excess based on the type of physiologic derangement. (Adapted from Andreoli TE: Disorders of fluid volume, electrolytes and acid-base balance. In Wyngaarden JB, Smith LH Jr, Bennett JC [eds]: Cecil Textbook of Medicine, 18th ed. Philadelphia: WB Saunders, 1992, pp 499–527.)

Alterations in Starling forces across the capillary bed are responsible for the initiation of edema formation. However, the maintenance of edema occurs because the baroreceptors perceive a reduced effective circulating volume and this stimulates renal sodium and water retention.[26] This arterial "underfilling" is, therefore, a result of the disease process limiting the ability of the heart to transfer blood from the venous to the arterial circuit. The combination of renal sodium and water retention coupled with continued salt and water intake leads to worsening of the edematous state.

Primary Hormonal Excesses

Disorders giving rise to primary hormonal excesses are characterized by increased circulating volume as a result of unregulated overproduction of mineralocorticoids or vasopressin. Mineralocorticoid excess states such as primary hyperaldosteronism lead to avid renal sodium retention and ECF volume expansion and hypertension. The syndrome of inappropriate vasopressin (ADH) production (SIADH) is a condition associated with water retention and subsequent volume expansion that involves both the ECF and the ICF. This leads to dilutional hyponatremia, which is a hallmark of this condition.

Edema is usually absent in both of these disorders. Instead, patients with primary hyperaldosteronism or SIADH reach a volume-expanded steady state in which output usually equals intake. This phenomenon, seen both in SIADH and in hyperaldosteronism, occurs in part because volume expansion resets glomerulotubular balance (see previous discussion) downward, that is, in the direction of reducing fractional proximal sodium absorption.

Primary Renal Sodium Retention

Abnormal renal sodium retention may sometimes occur when the effective circulating volume is normal. An example of such abnormal sodium retention is acute glomerulonephritis, in which unidentified renal mechanisms are primarily responsible for salt retention and edema formation. This occurs without alteration in GFR or EABV, indicating that this disease clearly represents "overfilling."

Pathophysiology of Renal Salt Retention
Congestive Heart Failure

CHF is associated with a reduction in the EABV along with increased filling pressures in the atrium and venous circuit "behind" the failed ventricle. The "backward" theory[12] suggests that the elevation of CVPs secondary to cardiac pump failure leads to increased peripheral venous pressure and subsequent alteration of the Starling forces at the capillary level, resulting in edema. The "backward failure" theory certainly is adequate to explain the symptoms of CHF. However, the "backward failure" theory does not account for fluid retention. Thus, the most pure example of "backward failure" is the sudden pulmonary edema, so-called flash pulmonary edema, that occurs in patients with diastolic dysfunction.

The "forward failure" theory argues that reduced filling of the arterial tree and, consequently, inadequate renal perfusion, result in sodium retention. In turn, if cardiac pump failure is present, much of this fluid will be accumulated on the venous side of the circulation. To summarize, "backward failure" explains the accumulation of fluid on the venous side of the circulation, but "forward failure" accounts for sodium retention by inadequate renal perfusion. In modern terms, the purest form of "backward failure" is, as noted previously, the sudden pulmonary edema of

Renal sodium retention in congestive heart failure

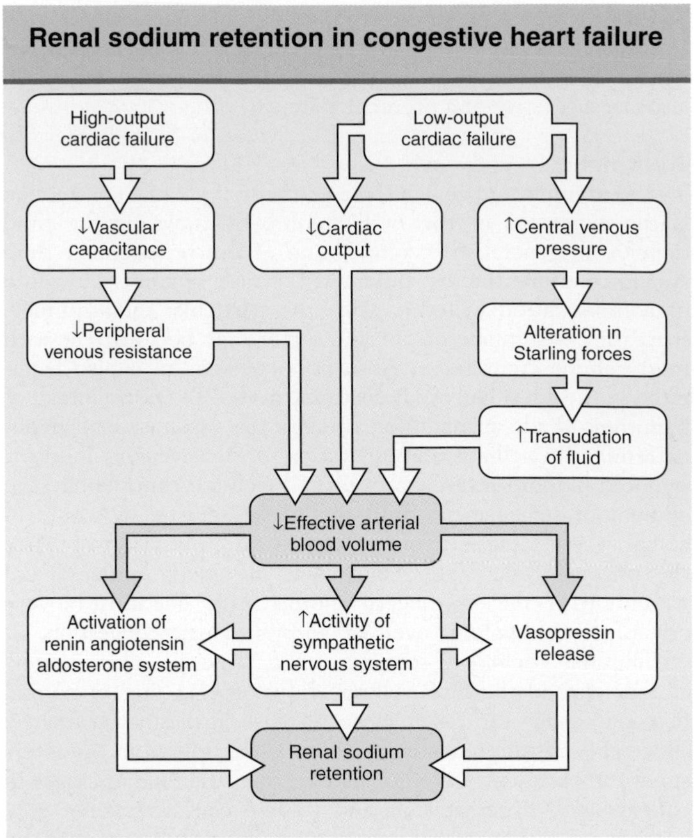

Figure 7.12 **Pathophysiology of renal sodium retention in congestive heart failure.**

diastolic dysfunction, while "forward failure" is accounted for best by systolic pump failure and the attendant accumulation of fluid in the venous side of the circulation (Fig. 7.12).

Put differently, an inability to transfer fluid either from the interstitium to veins, or from the veins to arteries, results in what has picturesquely been referred to as "inadequate filling of the arterial tree." The latter, whether in CHF, cirrhosis, or the nephrotic syndrome, is perceived by the kidneys as a volume-contracted state.[26,27] Moreover, as a perceived reduction in effective blood volume becomes increasingly severe, there occurs not only sodium retention but water retention due to nonosmotic vasopressin release. As a consequence, hyponatremia in edematous states, particularly cirrhosis and CHF, is a particularly ominous condition. For example, several studies have indicated that, in cirrhosis, serum sodium concentrations <125 mmol/l are commonly associated with a survival time of <1 year.

There are significant alterations in the afferent limb of volume homeostasis in CHF.[28] There is blunting of the afferent signaling mechanisms emanating from the venous sensing sites. The reduction in cardiac output diminishes the blood flow to the critical sensors in the arterial circuit that detect an underperfused state. Abnormalities in the effector mechanisms are a consequence of primary disturbance in the afferent-sensing mechanism. Alterations in glomerular hemodynamics in CHF include reduced GFR and a disproportionate increase in efferent arteriolar constriction, resulting in increased filtration fraction. As a direct consequence of the glomerular hemodynamics, there is an increase in proximal tubular absorption of filtered sodium load. Elevated Ang II, catecholamines, and vasopressin levels along with resistance to the action of ANP also contribute to the sodium retention in patients with CHF.

Cirrhosis

Cirrhosis results in disarray of hepatic architecture: regenerating nodules compress sinusoids and increase intrasinusoidal hydrostatic pressure with excessive loss of fluid from the hepatic surface into the peritoneal cavity, resulting in ascites. Furthermore, portal hypertension, portosystemic shunting, splanchnic pooling, and hypoalbuminemia characterize cirrhosis. The "underfill" theory suggests that all these factors, along with peripheral vasodilation, leads to decreased EABV (Fig. 7.13). Some investigators[29] have found evidence of increased total plasma volume in cirrhotic patients and therefore proposed the "overfill" theory. However, it is quite likely that what has been termed "overfilling" is the consequence of splanchnic vasodilatation.[27] The latter results, obviously, in a reduction in the volume/capacitance ratio in the systemic venous bed, a decrease in systemic venous return, and an attendant "underfilling" of the arterial tree.

As in CHF, the abnormalities in the effector mechanism are multifactorial. Sodium retention occurs independently of a decrease in GFR and peritubular physical factors may enhance proximal tubular sodium reabsorption. Furthermore, there is activation of the renin angiotensin aldosterone axis, ANP resistance, and sympathetic overactivity, all of which lead to renal tubular sodium retention.

The issue of ANP resistance warrants particular mention.[26] The inner medullary collecting duct is responsible for the net absorption of about 5% of GFR, or approximately 1200 to 1500 mmol/day. The rate of excretion of Na[+] by the inner medullary collecting duct is modulated by the potent cardiac peptide ANP. ANP, working through cyclic guanosine monophosphate (cGMP), blocks apical entry by inhibiting the activity of Na[+] channels.[30] In the present context, it is relevant to note that there are three types of receptors for ANP[31]:

1. ANP_A. This receptor has guanylate cyclase activity, is biologically active, and is present both in glomeruli and in papillary receptors.
2. ANP_B. This receptor also is present in glomeruli and papillae, has guanylate cyclase activity, and is biologically active.
3. ANP_C. This is a clearance receptor that has no guanylate cyclase activity.

There is now a considerable body of evidence indicating that ANP resistance is, in a sense, the last locus of action for producing renal retention of Na[+]. Specifically, in experimental CHF, ANP resistance seems to be the result of a decrease in the density of ANP_A receptor, while in experimental cirrhosis and experimental nephrotic syndrome, ANP resistance is the consequence of an increase in cGMP-phosphodiesterase activity.[32]

Nephrotic Syndrome

Nephrotic syndrome differs from CHF and cirrhosis because it is characterized by intrinsic renal disease and altered renal

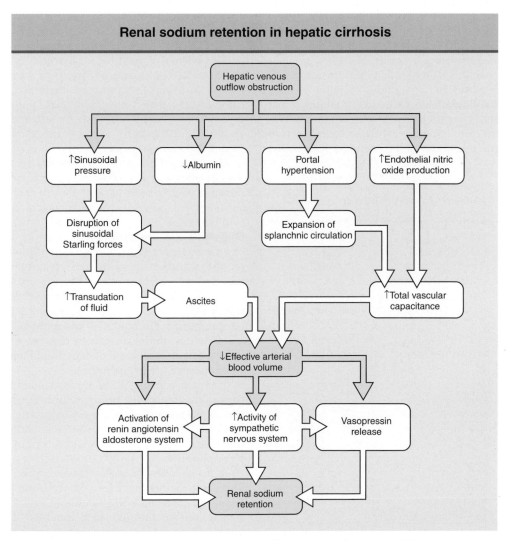

Figure 7.13 **Pathophysiology of renal sodium retention in hepatic cirrhosis.**

function in most patients. Consequently, this syndrome is associated with elevated mean arterial pressures and relatively less impairment of renal sodium excretion.

The pathogenesis of edema in nephrotic syndrome involves two different mechanisms (Fig. 7.14). According to the classic "underfill" hypothesis, nephrotic syndrome results in increased urinary loss of albumin, which subsequently leads to hypoalbuminemia and decreased plasma oncotic pressure. Consequently, the alteration in Starling forces leads to the net efflux of fluid from the intravascular space to the interstitial compartment, which in turn decreases plasma volume and EABV. The reduction in EABV activates the effector mechanism that culminates in renal salt and water retention.

The "underfill" hypothesis has been challenged by some investigators who have proposed the "overfill" hypothesis.[33,34] According to this theory, renal salt and water retention is a primary phenomenon that leads to plasma volume expansion and subsequent exudation of fluid to the interstitium. The hypoalbuminemia and reduced plasma oncotic pressure further worsen the edema. Evidence supporting the "overfill" hypothesis comes from studies that have shown elevated plasma volumes and blood pressure as well as decreased plasma renin and aldosterone levels. Furthermore, hypoalbuminemia and familial analbuminemia do not always lead to edema formation.[33] In evaluating the relative merits of these mechanisms, one should note that the nephrotic syndrome is a heterogeneous disease from a variety of renal lesions. It is therefore possible that both "underfilling" and "overfilling" may have a role in the formation of edema, depending on the nature of the underlying nephropathy.

In general, noninflammatory glomerular diseases, such as minimal change disease, result in nephrotic syndrome associated with low blood volumes and an "underfilling" type of picture, while glomerular diseases associated with interstitial inflammation, such as membranous nephropathy or membranoproliferative glomerulonephritis, are associated with a clinical picture consistent with volume expansion and systemic hypertension

and an "overfilling" picture. It has been postulated that the presence of the interstitial inflammatory cells may facilitate an increase in salt reabsorption and systemic hypertension by releasing mediators that cause renal vasoconstriction.[35]

The effector mechanisms for sodium retention in the nephrotic syndrome are complex and may vary depending on the underlying renal lesion as well as the stage of edema formation. Whereas some animal studies have shown that the collecting duct may be the predominant site for avid renal sodium retention, other studies suggest that increased proximal tubular sodium absorption may also be important. A decrease in GFR and activation of the peritubular physical factors and the renin angiotensin aldosterone system also seem to be operative. Finally, as noted previously, ANP resistance in the inner medullary collecting duct may be a final determinant of sodium acquisitiveness in nephrotic edema.

Clinical Manifestations

Edema is the classic sign of ECF excess but may not be evident until there are 3 or 4 liters of excess. Patients with CHF usually present with a history of dyspnea on exertion, weakness, decreased exercise tolerance, orthopnea, paroxysmal nocturnal dyspnea, and sometimes nocturia. Physical examination reveals increased weight gain, distention of the jugular veins, pulmonary rales, tachycardia, a third heart sound, and peripheral edema. Edema in cardiac disease is usually dependent and presents symmetrically in both lower extremities. Pretibial and ankle edema is frequently seen in the evening in ambulatory patients, and presacral edema is a feature of individuals at bed rest.

The edema of nephrotic syndrome is usually diffuse and manifests itself as anasarca. Periorbital edema is a characteristic feature of nephrotic syndrome. Periorbital edema develops as patients can sleep comfortably flat, unlike in CHF (due to pulmonary edema) or cirrhosis (in which the ascites pushes up against the diaphragm). Some patients may also present with pleural effusions or ascites.

Hepatic cirrhosis presents clinically as ascites and lower extremity edema as a result of portal hypertension and hypoalbuminemia. Other signs of liver disease include jaundice, spider angiomas, palmar erythema, and gynecomastia.

Diagnosis and Treatment

The management of ECF volume-expanded states is dependent on the accurate diagnosis and treatment of the underlying disorder. The cornerstone of therapy in these patients is salt restriction and diuretics. For patients with mild volume expansion, a 3-g/day (130-mmol/d) sodium diet (or 7-g salt diet) may be appropriate. For moderate to severe ECF volume expansion, a 2-g/day (86-mmol/d) sodium diet (or 4.6-g salt diet) should be advocated. Restriction of daily fluid intake should occur only when patients are hyponatremic.

The management of volume-expanded states should aim to correct the underlying primary disorder. Drugs that predispose to salt retention or alter the effect of diuretics need to be discontinued. For example, nonsteroidal anti-inflammatory agents promote renal salt retention and interfere with the efficacy of some diuretics.

ACE inhibitors or angiotensin receptor blockers (ARBs) are important in the treatment of nephrotic syndrome and heart failure. In the nephrotic syndrome, both ACE inhibitors and angiotensin receptor blockers minimize proteinuria. In heart failure, these agents reduce cardiac remodeling and hence protect against diastolic dysfunction and reduce afterload.

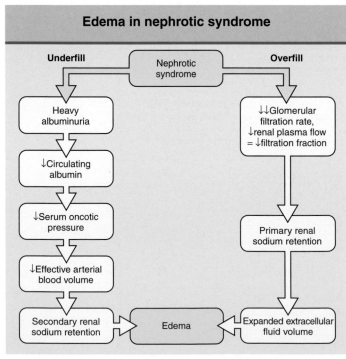

Figure 7.14 Pathophysiology of edema in nephrotic syndrome.

However, because blockade of the renin angiotensin aldosterone axis produces primarily efferent arteriolar relaxation, these agents should be used with caution in patients whose serum creatinine exceeds 2.5 to 3 mg/dl (220 to 265 µmol/l) and not at all in cirrhotic patients, in whom efferent arteriolar dilatation can produce a sharp decline in GFR.

Diuretics

Diuretics are the mainstay of therapy in volume-expanded states and should be used only if symptomatic edema persists despite salt restriction. The characteristics of commonly used diuretics are provided in Figure 7.15. It should be recognized that diuretics such as acetazolamide, furosemide, bumetanide, and torsemide, as well as thiazide diuretics, are all derived from a common parent, sulfanilamide. Thus, the question about being allergic to sulfa drugs must always be asked of a patient prior to instituting therapy with these agents.

A second factor relating to diuretics is the coadministration of agents intended to increase colloid osmotic pressure. For example, albumin infusions have been used in the hope of improving the efficacy of diuretics for many years.[36] However, as noted previously, there is no benefit to diuresis efficacy using an albumin/furosemide combination compared to furosemide alone.[37] Finally, in subjects with chronic renal failure, the excretion of the diuretic agent is impaired and therefore using the intravenous route and/or increasing the dose of the diuretic may be necessary.

Diuretics Acting at the Proximal Tubule

Acetazolamide is the prototype of a proximal tubular diuretic. It is a carbonic anhydrase inhibitor and acts by blocking the proximal tubular reabsorption of sodium bicarbonate.[36,37] The proximal diuretics are relatively mild in their potency because the distal parts of the nephron compensate for the decrease in proximal sodium reabsorption. Prolonged use of acetazolamide can lead to increased urinary excretion of Na^+, K^+, and HCO_3^- and subsequent hyperchloremic metabolic acidosis. This modest alkaline diuresis may be beneficial in some patients with metabolic alkalosis and ECF volume expansion, where isotonic saline cannot be administered. These weak diuretics are rarely used in clinical practice as primary diuretic therapy. Acetazolamide is commonly used to treat open-angle glaucoma and to prevent acute mountain sickness.

Metolazone belongs to the thiazide class of diuretics and acts by a different mechanism from that of the carbonic anhydrase inhibitors. It blocks sodium chloride reabsorption in the proximal and early distal nephron sites by unknown mechanisms. Since the major tubular site for phosphate absorption is the proximal tubule, the phosphaturia accompanying metolazone administration exceeds that with other thiazide diuretics. Metolazone is more commonly used in conjunction with other classes of diuretic, most commonly loop diuretics, where the latter are ineffective when used alone.

Diuretics Acting at the Loop of Henle

Furosemide, bumetanide, and torsemide are loop diuretics that act by inhibiting the coupled entry of sodium, potassium, and chloride across apical plasma membranes in the thick ascending limb of the loop of Henle.[36-38] Approximately 25% of the filtered load of sodium chloride is reabsorbed along the loop of Henle. These diuretics are anions that are bound to protein; as a result, very little of the diuretic reaches the tubules via glomerular filtration. Loop diuretics are secreted into the lumen of the proximal tubule by the organic anion transport system and act on the luminal side of the thick ascending limb of Henle.

Loop diuretics are commonly referred to as "high-ceiling" diuretics mainly because of their potency and because the natriuretic dose-response characteristics of these diuretics are considered more linear than those of all other currently used diuretics. They inhibit potassium reabsorption along the thick ascending limb of the loop of Henle and increase potassium secretion along the distal nephron, which results in significant hypokalemia and metabolic alkalosis. These diuretics impair tubular reabsorption and increase the urinary excretion of calcium and magnesium.

Finally, with respect to the loop diuretics, some workers have proposed the use of continuous infusions of loop diuretics rather than oral pulses or intravenous boluses as a potential means of enhancing diuretic efficiency. Thus far, there are no controlled, paired clinical trials to support this contention. Moreover, it should be recalled that the dose response curve for loop diuretics is nearly linear. Thus, increasing the dose of a single pulse of a loop diuretic, up to the equivalent of 200 mg furosemide intravenously to avoid risk of ototoxicity, remains the most rational approach to diuresis in difficult patients, together with the

Characteristics of the commonly used diuretics based on predominant site of action

Type of Diuretic	Site of Action	Potency	Primary Effect	Secondary Effect	Dose (mg/day)	Complications
Carbonic anhydrase inhibitor	Proximal tubule		↓ Na^+/H^+ exchange	↑ K^+ loss ↑ HCO_3^- loss		Hypokalemia Hyperchloremic acidosis
Acetazolamide		+			250–500	
Loop	Loop of Henle		↓ $Na^+/K^+/2Cl^+$ absorption	↑ K^+ loss ↑ K^+ secretion		Hypokalemic alkalosis
Furosemide		+++			40–500	
Ethacrynic acid		+++			50–400	
Thiazide	Distal tubule		↓ Na^+ absorption	↑ K^+ loss ↑ K^+ secretion		Hypokalemic alkalosis Glucose intolerance Hyperuricemia
Chlorothiazide		++			500–1000	
Hydrochlorothiazide		++			50–100	
Metolazone		++			2.5–10	
Potassium sparing	Collecting duct		↓ Na^+ absorption	↑ K^+ loss ↑ K^+ secretion		Hypokalemic acidosis
Triamterene		+			100–300	
Amiloride		+			5–10	
Spironolactone					100–400	

Figure 7.15   Characteristics of the commonly used diuretics based on predominant site of action.

simultaneous use of other diuretics, notably metolazone and spironolactone.

Diuretics Acting at the Distal Convoluted Tubule

Thiazides are the prototype for this class of diuretic. The distal convoluted tubule reabsorbs about 5% to 10% of the filtered sodium and chloride ions. These diuretics act on the distal convoluted tubule and interfere primarily with sodium and chloride reabsorption. They block sodium entry from the tubular fluid across apical plasma membranes into distal tubular cells.[36-38] Consequently, they limit the diluting ability of the distal nephron but have no effect on the concentration gradient generated by the loop of Henle. Distal convoluted tubule diuretics are anions, similar to the loop diuretics, and are secreted into the proximal nephron by the organic acid anion transport system. The effectiveness of this class of diuretic decreases when GFR drops below 40 ml/min. In some cases, metolazone (2.5 to 5 mg) can be given orally in addition to intravenous furosemide to increase diuresis in patients with GFR less than 40 ml/min.

Distal convoluted tubule diuretics, like loop diuretics, lead to hypokalemic metabolic alkalosis. Thiazides promote urinary magnesium losses, however, and in contrast to the loop diuretics, they increase luminal calcium absorption and decrease urinary calcium losses. Accordingly, these drugs are useful in the treatment of hypercalciuric states, especially calcium nephrolithiasis.

Hyponatremia occurs frequently and results from impaired distal tubular diluting mechanisms.

Diuretics Acting at the Collecting Duct

Triamterene and amiloride are sodium channel blockers that predominantly inhibit sodium reabsorption from the luminal side of the collecting duct. Consequently, there is a decrease in the transepithelial voltage in this segment with secondary inhibition of potassium and hydrogen ion secretion. This effect accounts for their potassium-sparing action. They are secreted into the tubular fluid by the organic cation pathway.

Spironolactone and epleronone are competitive antagonists of aldosterone and cause mild natriuresis and potassium retention.[36-39] They are weak diuretics and their use is limited to conditions of aldosterone excess. Spironolactone has been particularly used in treating disorders characterized by secondary hyperaldosteronism, such as cirrhosis with ascites.

These diuretics are relatively modest in their potency because they act on only a small part (about 3%) of the filtered sodium load. The most common use of collecting duct diuretics is in combination with other classes of diuretic to prevent potassium wasting. The predominant side effect of these agents is hyperkalemia. Spironolactone can cause painful gynecomastia in men and amenorrhea in women. Triamterene can sometimes crystallize in urine.

REFERENCES

1. Share L, Claybaugh JR: Regulation of body fluids. Annu Rev Physiol 1972;34:235–260.
2. Oh MS, Carroll HJ: Regulation of intracellular and extracellular volume. In Arieff AI, DeFronzo RA (eds): Fluid, Electrolyte, and Acid-Base Disorders, 2nd ed. New York: Churchill Livingstone, 1995, pp 1–28.
3. Simpson FO: Sodium intake, body sodium, and sodium excretion. Lancet 1988;2:25–29.
4. Bichet DG, Schrier RW: Cardiac failure, liver disease, and nephrotic syndrome. In Schrier RW, Gottschalk CW (eds): Diseases of the Kidney, 5th ed. Boston: Little, Brown, 1993, pp 2453–2491.
5. Gauer OH, Henry JP, Behn C: The regulation of extracellular fluid volume. Annu Rev Physiol 1970;32:547–595.
6. Briggs JP, Singh I, Sawaya BE, Schnermann J: Disorders of salt balance. In Kokko JP, Tannen RL (eds): Fluid and Electrolytes, 3rd ed. Philadelphia: WB Saunders, 1996, pp 3–62.
7. Andreoli TE: Disorders of fluid volume, electrolytes and acid-base balance. In Wyngaarden JB, Smith LH Jr, Bennett JC (eds): Cecil Textbook of Medicine, 18th ed. Philadelphia: WB Saunders, 1992, pp 499–527.
8. Schrier RW: Body fluid volume regulation in health and disease: A unifying hypothesis. Ann Intern Med 1990;113:155–159.
9. Miller JA, Tobe SW, Skorecki KL: Control of extracellular fluid volume and the pathophysiology of edema formation. In Brenner BW (ed): The Kidney, 5th ed. Philadelphia: WB Saunders, 1996, pp 817–862.
10. Gonzalez-Campoy JM, Knox FG: Integrated responses of the kidney to alterations in extracellular fluid volume. In Seldin DW, Giebisch G (eds): The Kidney: Physiology and Pathophysiology, 2nd ed. New York: Raven Press, 1992, pp 2041–2097.
11. deWardener HE: The control of sodium excretion. Am J Physiol 1978;235:F163–F173.
12. Starling EH: On the absorption of fluid from the connective tissue spaces. J Physiol (Lond) 1896;19:312–326.
13. Briggs JP, Schnermann J: The tubuloglomerular feedback mechanism. Functional and biochemical aspects. Annu Rev Physiol 1989;49:251–273.
14. Thompson SC, Blantz RC: Homeostatic efficiency of tubuloglomerular feedback in hydropenia, euvolemia, and acute volume expansion. Am J Physiol 1993;264:F930–F936.
15. Mazzali M, Hughes J, Kim Y-G, et al: Elevated urine acid increases blood pressure in the rat by a novel crystal-independent mechanism. Hypertension 2001;38:1101–1106.
16. Brenner BM, Falchuh KH, Keinmowitz RI, Berliner RW: The relationship between peritubular capillary protein concentration and fluid reabsorption by the renal proximal tubule. J Clin Invest 1969;48:1519–1531.
17. Hall JE: Control of sodium excretion by angiotensin II: Intrarenal mechanisms and blood pressure regulation. Am J Physiol 1986;250:R960–R972.
18. Zeidel ML, Brenner BM: Actions of atrial natriuretic peptides on the kidney. Semin Nephrol 1987;7:91–97.
19. DiBona GF: Neural control of renal tubular sodium reabsorption and renin secretion: Integrative aspects. Clin Exp Theor Pract 1987;A9(Suppl 1):151–165.
20. Rose BD: Hypovolemic states. In Rose BD (ed): Clinical Physiology of Acid-Base and Electrolyte Disorders, 2nd ed. New York: McGraw-Hill, 1989, pp 279–309.
21. DuBose TD Jr: Salt wastage and salt depletion. In Seldin DW, Giebisch G (eds): The Regulation of Sodium and Chloride Balance. New York: Raven Press, 1990, pp 419–432.
22. Ellison DH: Divalent cation transport by the distal nephron: Insights from Bartter's and Gitelman's syndromes. Am J Physiol Renal Physiol 2000;279:F616–F625.
23. Naesens M, Steels P, Verberckmoes R, et al: Bartter's and Gitelman's syndromes. Nephron Physiol 2004;96:65–78.
24. Gougoux A, Bichet DG: Extracellular fluid volume contraction. In Jacobson HR, Striker GE, Klahr S (eds): The Principles and Practice of Nephrology, 2nd ed. St. Louis, MO: Mosby, 1995, pp 876–879.
25. Cochrane Injuries Group Albumin Reviewers. Human albumin administration in critically ill patients: Systematic review of randomised controlled trials. BMJ 1998;317:235–240.
26. Andreoli TE: Edematous states: An overview. Kidney Int 1997;51(Suppl 59):S2–S10.
27. Schrier RW, Ecder T: Unifying hypothesis of body fluid volume regulation: Implications for cardiac failure and cirrhosis. Mt Sinai J Med 2001;68:350–361.
28. Palmer BF, Alpern RJ, Seldin DW: Pathophysiology of edema formation. In Seldin DW, Giebisch G (eds): The Kidney: Physiology and Pathophysiology, 2nd ed. New York: Raven Press, 1992, pp 2099–2141.
29. Lieberman FL, Denison EK, Reynolds TF: The relationship of plasma volume, portal hypertension, ascites and renal sodium retention in cirrhosis: The overflow theory of ascites formation. Ann NY Acad Sci 1970;170:202–210.
30. Zeidel ML, Silva P, Brenner BM, Seifter JL: cGMP mediates effects of atrial peptides on medullary collecting duct cells. Am J Physiol 1987;252:F551–F559.

31. Vafhieh H, Kahana L, Haramati A, et al: Regulation of renal glomerular and papillary ANP receptors in rats with experimental heart failure. Am J Physiol 1993;265:F119–F125.

32. Lee EYW, Humphreys MH: Phosphodiesterase activity as a mediator of renal resistance to ANP in pathological salt retention. Am J Physiol 1996;271:F3–F6.

33. Seldin DW: Sodium balance and fluid volume in normal and edematous states. In Seldin DW, Giebisch G (eds): The Regulation of Sodium and Chloride Balance. New York: Raven Press, 1990, pp 261–292.

34. Koomans HA, Geers AB, Meiracker AH, et al: Effects of plasma volume expansion on renal salt handling in patients with nephrotic syndrome. Am J Nephrol 1984;4:227.

35. Rodriguez-Iturbe B, Herrera-Acosta J, Johnson RJ: Interstitial inflammation, sodium retention, and the pathogenesis of nephritic edema. Kidney Int 2002;62:1379–1384.

36. Dillingham MA, Schrier RW, Gregor R: Mechanism of diuretic action. In Schrier RW, Gottschalk CW (eds): Diseases of the Kidney, 5th ed. Boston: Little, Brown, 1993, pp 2435–2452.

37. Ghalasani N, Gorski JC, Horlander JC Sr, et al: Effect of albumin/furosemide mixtures on responses to furosemide in hypoalbuminemic patients. J Am Soc Nephrol 2001;12:1010–1016.

38. Brater DC: Drug-induced electrolyte disorders and use of diuretics. In Kokko JP, Tannen RL (eds): Fluid and Electrolytes, 3rd ed. Philadelphia: WB Saunders, 1996, pp 693–728.

39. Brater C: The use of diuretics in congestive heart failure. Semin Nephrol 1994;14:479–484.

Disorders of Water Metabolism

Chirag Parikh and Tomas Berl

PHYSIOLOGY OF WATER BALANCE

The maintenance of the tonicity of body fluids within a narrow physiologic range is made possible by homeostatic mechanisms that control the intake and excretion of water. Vasopressin (antidiuretic hormone [ADH]) governs the excretion of water by its end-organ effect on the renal collecting system. Osmoreceptors located in the hypothalamus control the secretion of vasopressin in response to changes in tonicity.

In steady-state situations, water intake matches water losses. Water intake is regulated by the individual's need to maintain a physiologic serum osmolality of 285 to 290 mOsm/kg. Despite major fluctuations of solute and water intake, the total solute concentration (i.e., the tonicity) of body fluids is maintained virtually constant. The ability both to dilute and to concentrate the urine allows for a wide flexibility in urine flow (see Chapter 2). During water loading, the diluting mechanisms permit excretion of 20 to 25 liters of urine per day and during water deprivation, the urine volume may be as low as 0.5 liter per day.[1–3]

VASOPRESSIN

Vasopressin (also known as arginine vasopressin [AVP] or antidiuretic hormone [ADH]) plays a critical role in determining the concentration of urine. It is a cyclic octapeptide (1099 d) with a three-amino-acid tail and is synthesized and secreted by the specialized supraoptic and paraventricular magnocellular nuclei in the hypothalamus. Vasopressin has a short half-life of about 15 to 20 minutes and is rapidly metabolized in the liver and the kidney.

Osmotic Stimuli for Vasopressin Release
Vasopressin is secreted in response to osmotic and nonosmotic stimuli. Substances that are restricted to the extracellular fluid (ECF), such as hypertonic saline or mannitol, decrease cell volume by acting as effective osmoles and enhancing osmotic water movement from the cell. This stimulates vasopressin release. Urea and glucose cross cell membranes and do not cause any change in cell volume. The "osmoreceptor" cells, located close to the supraoptic nuclei in the anterior hypothalamus, are sensitive to changes in plasma osmolality as small as 1%. In humans, the osmotic threshold for vasopressin release is 280 to 290 mOsm/kg (Fig. 8.1). This system is so efficient that plasma osmolality usually does not vary by more than 1% to 2% despite wide fluctuations in water intake.

Nonosmotic Stimuli for Vasopressin Release
There are several other nonosmotic stimuli for vasopressin secretion. In settings with decreased effective circulating volume (e.g.,

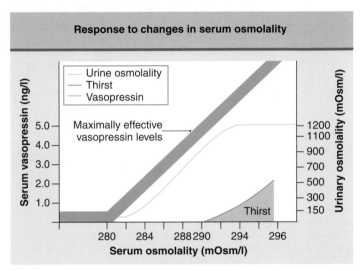

Response to changes in serum osmolality

Figure 8.1   Mechanisms maintaining plasma osmolality. The response of thirst, vasopressin levels, and urinary osmolality to changes in serum osmolality. (Adapted from Narins RG, Krishna GC: Disorders of water balance. In Stein JH [ed]: Internal Medicine. Boston: Little, Brown, 1987, p 794.)

heart failure, cirrhosis, vomiting), discharge from parasympathetic afferent nerves in the carotid sinus baroreceptors increases vasopressin secretion. Other nonosmotic stimuli include nausea, which can lead to a marked increase in circulating vasopressin levels, postoperative pain, and pregnancy. Much higher vasopressin levels can be achieved with hypovolemia than with hyperosmolality, although a large (7%) decrease in blood volume is required before this response is initiated.

Mechanism of Vasopressin Action
Vasopressin binds three types of receptors coupled to G proteins: the V_{1a} (vascular and hepatic), V_{1b} (anterior pituitary), and V_2 receptors. The V_2 receptor is primarily localized in the collecting duct and leads to an increase in water permeability (Fig. 8.2) via aquaporin-2 (AQP-2), which is a member of a family of cellular water transporters.[4,5] The first member, AQP-1, is localized in the apical and basolateral region of the proximal tubule epithelial cells and the descending limb of Henle and accounts for the high water permeability of these nephron segments. Because AQP-1 is constitutively expressed, it is not subject to regulation by vasopressin. In contrast, AQP-2 is found exclusively in apical plasma membrane and intracellular vesicles in the collecting duct principal cells. Vasopressin affects both the short- and long-term regulation of AQP-2. The short-term regulation, also described as the "shuttle hypothesis," explains the rapid and reversible increase (within minutes) in collecting duct water permeability following vasopressin administration. This involves the insertion

Cellular mechanism of vasopressin action

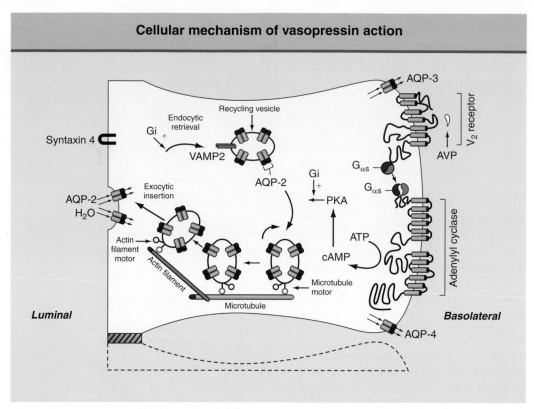

Figure 8.2 Cellular mechanism of vasopressin action. Vasopressin binds to V_2 receptors on the basolateral membrane and activates G proteins that initiate a cascade resulting in aquaporin-2 (AQP-2) insertion in the luminal membrane. This then allows water uptake into the cell. ATP, adenosine triphosphate; AVP, arginine vasopressin; cAMP, cyclic adenosine monophosphate; PKA, protein kinase A; VAMP2, vesicle-associated membrane protein 2. (Adapted from Bichet D: Nephrogenic and central diabetes insipidus. In Schrier R [ed]: Diseases of the Kidney and Urinary Tract, Vol. 3, 8th ed. Philadelphia: Lippincott Williams & Wilkins, 2006.)

of water channels from subapical vesicles into the luminal membrane. Long-term regulation involves vasopressin-mediated increased transcription of genes involved in AQP-2 production and occurs if circulating vasopressin levels are elevated for 24 hours or more. The maximal water permeability of the collecting duct epithelium is increased as a consequence of an increase in the total number of AQP-2 channels per cell. This process is not readily reversible.

AQP-3 and AQP-4 are located on the basolateral membranes of the collecting duct (see Fig. 8.2) and are probably involved in water exit from the cell. AQP-3 is also urea permeable and under the stimulus of vasopressin increases the permeability of the collecting duct to urea, resulting in its movement into the interstitium. AQP-4 is also in the hypothalamus and is a candidate osmoreceptor for the control of vasopressin release. Analysis of the molecular biology of AQP channels and the receptors responsible for vasopressin action have contributed to an understanding of genetically transmitted as well as acquired forms of vasopressin resistance.

THIRST AND WATER BALANCE

The thirst mechanism plays an important role in water balance. Hypertonicity is the most potent stimulus for thirst, with a change of only 2% to 3% in plasma osmolality producing a strong desire to drink water. The osmotic threshold for thirst usually occurs at approximately 290 to 295 mOsm/kg H_2O and is above the threshold for vasopressin release (see Fig. 8.1). It closely approximates the level at which maximal concentration of urine is achieved. Hypovolemia, hypotension, and angiotensin II are also stimuli for thirst. Between the limits imposed by the osmotic

thresholds for thirst and vasopressin release, plasma osmolality may be regulated more precisely by small, osmoregulated adjustments in urine flow and water intake. The exact level at which balance occurs depends on various factors, for example, insensible losses through skin and lungs, the gains incurred from drinking water and eating, and water generated from metabolism. In general, overall intake and output come into balance at a plasma osmolality of 288 mOsm/kg, roughly halfway between the thresholds for vasopressin release and thirst.

QUANTITATION OF RENAL WATER EXCRETION

Urine volume can be considered as having two components. The osmolar clearance (C_{osm}) is the volume needed to excrete solutes at the concentration of solutes in plasma. The free water clearance (C_{water}) is the volume of water that has been added to (positive C_{water}) or subtracted (negative C_{water}) from isotonic urine (C_{osm}) to create either hypotonic or hypertonic urine.

Urine volume flow (V) comprises the isotonic portion of urine (C_{osm}) plus the free water clearance (C_{water}):

$$V = C_{osm} + C_{water}$$

and, therefore,

$$C_{water} = V - C_{osm}.$$

The term C_{osm} relates urine osmolality to plasma osmolality P_{osm} by

$$C_{osm} = \left(\frac{U_{osm} \times V}{P_{osm}} \right)$$

Therefore,

$$C_{water} = V - \left(\frac{U_{osm} \times V}{P_{osm}} \right)$$

$$= V \left(1 - \frac{U_{osm}}{P_{osm}} \right)$$

This relationship describes three key points:
1. hypotonic urine: $U_{osm} < P_{osm}$ and C_{water} is positive
2. isotonic urine: $U_{osm} = P_{osm}$ and there is no C_{water}
3. hypertonic urine: $U_{osm} > P_{osm}$ and C_{water} is negative (water retained)

If excretion of free water in a polyuric patient is unaccompanied by water intake, the patient will become hypernatremic. Conversely, failure to excrete free water in settings of increased water intake can cause hyponatremia. The second equation fails to predict clinically important alterations in plasma tonicity and serum Na^+ concentration because it factors in urea. Urea is an important component of urinary osmolality; however, because it crosses cell membranes readily, it does not establish a transcellular osmotic gradient and does not cause water movement between fluid compartments. Therefore, it does not influence serum Na^+ concentration or the release of vasopressin. As a result, changes in serum Na^+ concentration are predicted by electrolyte free water clearance [$C_{water}(e)$]. The equation can be modified, replacing P_{osm} by plasma Na^+ concentration (P_{Na}) and the urine osmolality by urinary sodium and potassium concentrations ($U_{Na} + U_K$):

$$C_{water}(e) = V \left(1 - \frac{U_{Na} \times U_K}{P_{Na}} \right)$$

If the patient's $U_{Na} + U_K$ is less than the P_{Na}, then $C_{water}(e)$ is positive and the serum Na^+ concentration increases. If $U_{Na} + U_K$ is greater than P_{Na}, then $C_{water}(e)$ is negative and serum Na^+ concentration decreases. In the clinical setting, since the previous equation reflects water clearance with respect to total body osmolality, it is more appropriate to use the modified equation. For example, in a patient with high urea excretion, the original equation would predict negative water excretion and a decrease in serum Na^+ concentration. In actuality, the serum Na^+ concentration increases, a fact that would be accurately predicted if the modified equation were employed. Thus, assessing whether a patient's Na^+ will increase or decrease in the face of the prevailing water excretion as determined in the latter equation is clinically extremely useful.

SERUM SODIUM, OSMOLALITY, AND TONICITY

The countercurrent mechanism of the kidneys, which allows for urinary concentration and dilution, acts in concert with the hypothalamic osmoreceptors via vasopressin secretion to keep serum Na^+ and tonicity within a very narrow range (Fig. 8.3). A defect in the urine-diluting capacity when coupled with excess water intake leads to hyponatremia. A defect in urinary concentrating ability with inadequate water intake leads to hypernatremia.

Serum $Na,^+$ along with its accompanying anions, accounts for nearly all the osmotic activity of the plasma. Calculated serum osmolality is given by $2[Na^+] + BUN$ (mg/dl)/2.8 + glucose (mg/dl)/18, where BUN is blood urea nitrogen. The addition of other solutes to ECF results in an increase in measured osmolality (Fig. 8.4). Solutes that are permeable across cell membranes, such as urea, methanol, ethanol, and ethylene glycol, do not cause water movement and cause hypertonicity without causing cellular

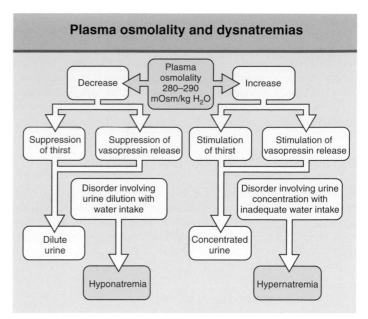

Figure 8.3 Maintenance of plasma osmolality and pathogenesis of dysnatremias. (Adapted with permission from Halterman R, Berl T: Therapy of dysnatremic disorders. In Brady H, Wilcox C [eds]: Therapy in Nephrology and Hypertension. Philadelphia: WB Saunders, 1999, pp 257–269.)

dehydration. Examples of patients with increases in these solutes are those with uremia and ethanol intoxication. By comparison, a patient with diabetic ketoacidosis has an increase in plasma glucose, which cannot move freely across cell membranes in the absence of insulin. Glucose in the ECF causes water to move from the cells to the ECF, thereby leading to cellular dehydration and concomitantly lowering serum [Na^+]. This can be viewed as "translocational" at the cellular level, as the serum [Na^+] does not reflect change in total body water but rather reflects a movement of water from intracellular to extracellular space. A decrease in serum [Na^+] of 1.6 mmol/l occurs for every 100-mg/dl (5.6-mmol/l) increase in plasma glucose. However, this calculation may underestimate the impact of glucose to a decreased concentration of serum sodium and may be closer to 2.5 mmol/l.[7] Other substances known to cause translocational hyponatremia are mannitol, maltose, and glycine (see Fig. 8.4).

Pseudohyponatremia occurs when the solid phase of plasma (usually 6% to 8%) is greatly increased by large increments in either lipids or proteins (e.g., in hypertriglyceridemia and

Effects of osmotically active substances on serum sodium levels	
Substances That Increase Osmolality Without Changing Serum Na^+	Substances That Increase Osmolality and Decrease Serum Na^+ (Translocational Hyponatremia)
Urea	Glucose
Ethanol	Mannitol
Ethylene glycol	Glycine
Isopropyl alcohol	Maltose
Methanol	

Figure 8.4 Effects of osmotically active substances on serum sodium levels.

paraproteinemias). This false result occurs because the method that measures the concentration of Na^+ uses whole plasma and not just the liquid phase. The alternative method involves ion selective potentiometry—direct and indirect. However, only the direct (undiluted) potentiometry measurements, to which most laboratories are now moving, will give the true aqueous sodium activity. Serum osmolality is normal in these settings of pseudo-hyponatremia.

ESTIMATION OF TOTAL BODY WATER

In the normal individual, total body water is approximately 60% of body weight (50% in women and obese individuals). In patients with hyponatremia or hypernatremia, the change in total body water can be calculated from the serum Na^+ concentration, using the following formula:

$$\text{Water excess} = 0.6W \times \left(1 - \frac{[Na^+]_{obs}}{140}\right)$$

$$\text{Water deficit} = 0.6W \times \left(\frac{[Na^+]_{obs}}{140} - 1\right)$$

where $[Na^+]_{obs}$ is observed sodium concentration in mmol/l and W is body weight in kilograms. In general, a change of

10 mmol/l in the serum $[Na^+]$ in a 70-kg individual is equivalent to a change of 3 liters in free water.

HYPONATREMIC DISORDERS

Hyponatremia is defined as serum $[Na^+]$ <135 mmol/l and equates with a low serum osmolarity once translocational hyponatremia and pseudohyponatremia are ruled out (see previous discussion). True hyponatremia develops when normal urinary dilution mechanisms (Fig. 8.5) are disturbed. This may occur via three mechanisms. First, hyponatremia may result from intrarenal factors such as a diminished glomerular filtration rate (GFR) and/or an increase in proximal tubular fluid and Na^+ reabsorption, which decrease distal delivery to the diluting segments of the nephron. Hyponatremia may also result from a defect in Na^+/Cl^- transport out of the water-impermeable segments of the nephrons (the thick ascending limb of Henle [TALH] or distal convoluted tubule). Most commonly, hyponatremia results from continued stimulation of vasopressin secretion by nonosmotic mechanisms despite the presence of serum hypo-osmolality.

Etiology and Classification of Hyponatremia

Once pseudohyponatremia and translocational hyponatremia are ruled out and the patient is established as truly hypo-osmolar, the next step is to classify the patient as hypovolemic, euvolemic, or hypervolemic (Fig. 8.6).[6]

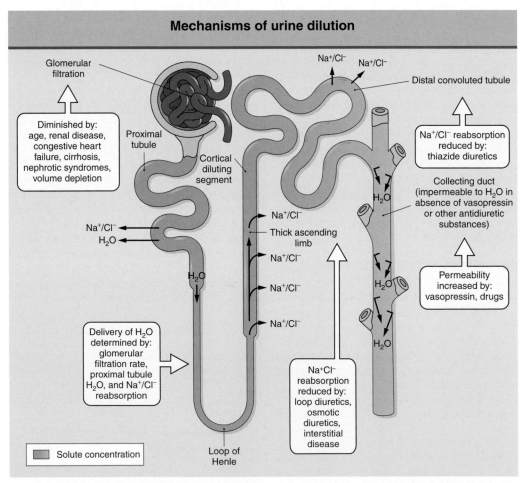

Figure 8.5   Urinary dilution mechanisms. Normal determinants of urinary dilution and disorders causing hyponatremia. (Adapted from Cogan M: Normal water homeostasis. In Cogan M [ed]: Fluid and Electrolytes. Norwalk, CT: Lange, 1991, pp 98–106.)

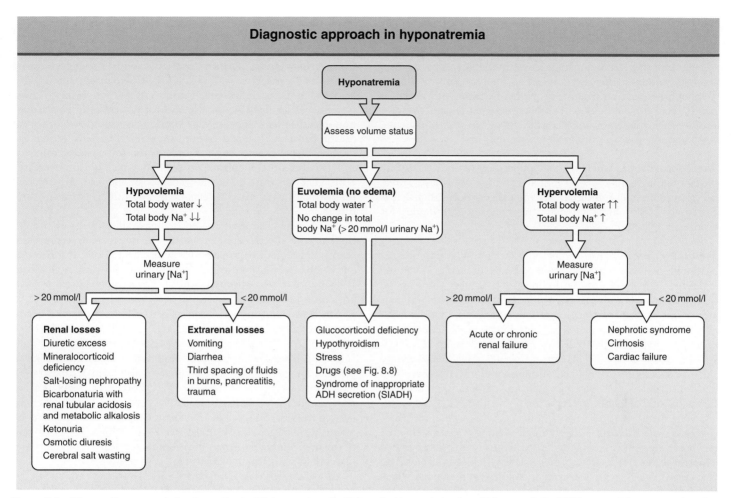

Figure 8.6 Diagnostic approach for the patient with hyponatremia. (Adapted with permission from Halterman R, Berl T: Therapy of dysnatremic disorders. In Brady H, Wilcox C [eds]: Therapy in Nephrology and Hypertension. Philadelphia: WB Saunders, 1999, pp 257–269.)

Hypovolemia: Hyponatremia Associated with Decreased Total Body Sodium

A patient with hypovolemic hyponatremia has both a total body Na^+ and a water deficit, with the Na^+ deficit exceeding the water deficit. This occurs in patients with high gastrointestinal and renal losses of water and solute accompanied by free water or hypotonic fluid intake. The underlying mechanism is the nonosmotic release of vasopressin stimulated by volume contraction, which maintains the secretion of the hormone despite the hypotonic state. Baroreceptors in the aortic arch and carotid sinus and vagal receptors located in the left atrium contribute to the release of vasopressin in response to volume contraction. Measurement of urinary Na^+ concentration is a useful tool in helping to diagnose these conditions (see Fig. 8.6).

Gastrointestinal and Third-Space Sequestered Losses In the setting of diarrhea or vomiting, the kidney responds to volume contraction by conserving Na^+ and Cl^-. A similar pattern is observed in burn patients and in patients with sequestration of fluids in third spaces, as in the peritoneal cavity with peritonitis or pancreatitis, or in the bowel lumen with ileus. In all these situations, the urinary Na^+ concentration is usually <10 mmol/l and the urine is hyperosmolar. An exception to this is in patients with vomiting and metabolic alkalosis. Here the increased HCO_3^- excretion requires simultaneous cation excretion such that urinary Na may be >20 mmol/l despite severe

volume depletion and a urinary Cl^- of <10 mmol/l. Likewise, in chronic renal insufficiency, renal salt conservation is impaired and urine Na may be high.

Diuretics Diuretic use is one of the most common causes of hypovolemic hyponatremia associated with a high urine Na^+ concentration. Loop diuretics inhibit Na^+/Cl^- reabsorption in the TALH. This interferes with the generation of a hypertonic medullary interstitium. Therefore, even though volume contraction leads to increased vasopressin secretion, responsiveness to vasopressin is diminished and free water is excreted. In contrast, thiazide diuretics act in the distal tubule by interfering with urinary dilution rather than urinary concentration, limiting free water excretion. Hyponatremia usually occurs within 14 days of initiation of therapy, although one third of cases present within 5 days. Underweight women and elderly patients appear to be most susceptible. Several mechanisms for diuretic-induced hyponatremia have been postulated, including

- Hypovolemia-stimulated vasopressin release and decreased fluid delivery to the diluting segment
- Impaired water excretion through interference with maximal urinary dilution in the cortical diluting segment
- K^+ depletion, directly stimulating water intake by alterations in osmoreceptor sensitivity and increasing thirst

Water retention can mask the physical findings of hypovolemia, thereby making the patients with diuretic-induced hyponatremia appear euvolemic.

Salt-Losing Nephropathy A salt-losing state sometimes occurs in patients with advanced chronic renal insufficiency (GFR <15 ml/min) and is characterized by hyponatremia and hypovolemia. This may occur in patients with medullary cystic disease, polycystic kidney disease, analgesic nephropathy, chronic pyelonephritis, and obstructive uropathy. Patients with proximal type II renal tubular acidosis exhibit renal Na^+ and K^+ wastage despite only moderate renal insufficiency. In these patients, bicarbonaturia obligates urine Na^+ excretion.

Mineralocorticoid Deficiency Hyponatremia with ECF volume contraction, urine [Na^+] >20 mmol/l, and high serum K^+, urea, and creatinine are indicative of mineralocorticoid deficiency. Decreased ECF volume provides the nonosmotic stimulus for vasopressin release.

Osmotic Diuresis An osmotically active, nonreabsorbable solute obligates the renal excretion of Na^+ and results in volume depletion. In the face of continuing water intake, the diabetic patient with severe glycosuria, the patient with a urea diuresis after relief of urinary tract obstruction, and the patient with mannitol diuresis all undergo urinary losses of Na^+ and water leading to hypovolemia and hyponatremia. Urinary [Na^+] is typically >20 mmol/l. The ketone bodies β-hydroxybutyrate and acetoacetate also obligate urinary electrolyte losses and aggravate renal Na^+ wasting seen in diabetic ketoacidosis, starvation, and alcoholic ketoacidosis.

Cerebral Salt Wasting Cerebral salt wasting is a syndrome that has been described primarily in patients with subarachnoid hemorrhage. In this condition, the primary defect is salt wasting from the kidneys with subsequent volume contraction, which stimulates vasopressin release. The exact mechanism is not understood, but it is postulated that brain natriuretic peptide is related to the increase in urine volume and Na^+ excretion. Differentiation from syndrome of inappropriate ADH release (SIADH) is challenging but important.[9]

Hypervolemia: Hyponatremia Associated with Increased Total Body Sodium

In conditions causing hypervolemia, the total body Na^+ and total body water are increased, the water more than the Na^+, thus causing hyponatremia. These syndromes include congestive heart failure, nephrotic syndrome, and cirrhosis. They are all associated with impaired water excretion (see Fig. 8.6).

Congestive Heart Failure Patients with congestive heart failure have a defect in water excretion. Edematous patients with heart failure have intravascular volume contraction owing to lower systemic mean arterial pressure and cardiac output. This reduction in the "effective circulating volume" is sensed by aortic and carotid baroreceptors and vasopressin is released. In addition, the relative "hypovolemic" state stimulates the renin angiotensin axis and increases norepinephrine production, which in turn decreases GFR. The decrease in GFR leads to an increase in proximal tubular reabsorption and a decrease in water delivery to the distal tubule.

The neurohumoral-mediated decrease in delivery of tubular fluid to the distal nephron and/or an increase in vasopressin secretion mediate hyponatremia by limiting Na^+/Cl^- and water excretion. In addition, low cardiac output and high angiotensin II levels are potent stimuli of thirst. These mechanisms tend to normalize perfusion pressure.

Studies in a rat model of congestive heart failure have demonstrated a marked upregulation of AQP-2 expression in the renal collecting duct cells, resulting in excessive free water absorption[4] (Fig. 8.7). Excessive intracellular targeting of AQP-2 to the apical cell membrane of the collecting duct has also been demonstrated, indicating a hyperactivation of the short-term regulation of AQP-2. These effects are most likely a consequence of high circulating levels of vasopressin. Nonosmotic pathways may also be operative in patients with congestive heart failure. The activation of the nonosmotic pathways of vasopressin release is linked to the increase in sympathetic activity noted in these patients.

As cardiac function improves with afterload reduction, the plasma vasopressin levels decrease along with concomitant improvement in water excretion. The degree of hyponatremia has also been correlated with the severity of cardiac disease and with patient survival, which is significantly reduced when the serum Na^+ decreases to <137 mmol/l. In fact, a serum Na^+ of 125 mmol/l reflects severe heart failure.

Hepatic Failure Patients with cirrhosis and hepatic insufficiency also have increased extracellular volume (i.e., ascites and edema). Because of marked splanchnic venous dilatation, they have an increased plasma volume. Unlike patients with

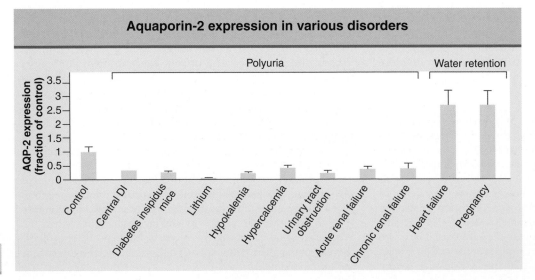

Aquaporin-2 expression in various disorders

Figure 8.7 Changes in aquaporin-2 (AQP-2) expression seen in association with different water balance disorders. Levels are expressed as a percentage of control levels (*leftmost bar*). AQP-2 expression is reduced, sometimes dramatically, in a wide range of hereditary and acquired forms of diabetes insipidus characterized by different degrees of polyuria. Conversely, congestive heart failure and pregnancy are conditions associated with increased expression of AQP-2 levels and excessive water retention. (From Neilsen S, Schrier R [eds]: Diseases of the Kidney and Urinary Tract, Vol. 3, 7th ed. Philadelphia: Lippincott Williams & Wilkins, 2001.)

congestive heart failure, cirrhotic patients have an increased cardiac output because of multiple arteriovenous fistulae in their alimentary tract and skin. In patients with advanced chronic liver disease, splanchnic arterial vasodilatation by nitric oxide is prominent.[10]

Vasodilatation and arteriovenous fistulas lead to a decrease in mean arterial blood pressure and effective cardiac output. As the severity of cirrhosis increases (no ascites to ascites and ascites to hepatorenal syndrome), a progressive increase in plasma renin, norepinephrine, vasopressin, and endothelin is noted. There is also an associated decline in mean arterial pressure and serum Na^+ levels.

The nonosmotic secretion of vasopressin is central to water retention and is related to increased hypothalamic vasopressin mRNA content in cirrhotic rats. Cirrhotic rats that lack vasopressin do not develop hyponatremia. Cirrhotic rats also show increased expression of vasopressin-regulated AQP-2 in their collecting ducts.[4] Unlike the heart failure model, an increase in intracellular trafficking of AQP-2 has not yet been demonstrated.

Nephrotic Syndrome In some patients with nephrotic syndrome, especially children with minimal change disease, hypoalbuminemia and lowered plasma oncotic pressure alter Starling forces leading to intravascular volume contraction. Most patients with nephrotic syndrome appear to have a renal defect in sodium excretion resulting in increased effective circulatory volume. In contrast to the water-retaining disorders discussed previously, in which increased AQP-2 expression is found, in rat models of nephrotic syndrome (i.e., treated with aminonucleoside or Adriamycin [doxorubicin]), expression of AQP-2 and AQP-3 in the renal collecting ducts is downregulated[4] (see Fig. 8.7).

Advanced Chronic Renal Insufficiency Patients with advanced renal insufficiency, either acute or chronic, have a profound increase in fractional excretion of Na^+ to maintain normal salt balance given the overall decreased number of functioning nephrons. Edema usually develops in patients when the Na^+ ingested exceeds the kidneys' capacity to excrete this load. Likewise, if water intake exceeds threshold, a positive water balance ensues and hyponatremia results. At a GFR of 5 ml/min, only 7.2 liters of filtrate is formed daily. Approximately 30%, or 2.2 liters, of this filtered fluid will reach the diluting segment of the nephron. Thus, because of the smaller volumes of fluid that are filtered by the diseased kidney, even with total suppression of vasopressin, a maximum of only 2.2 liters of solute-free water can be excreted daily.

Euvolemia: Hyponatremia Associated with Normal Total Body Sodium

Euvolemic hyponatremia is the most commonly encountered dysnatremia in hospitalized patients.[11] In these patients, no physical signs of increased total body Na^+ are detected. They may have slight excess of volume but are not edematous.

Glucocorticoid Deficiency Glucocorticoid deficiency causes impaired water excretion in patients with primary and secondary adrenal insufficiency. Elevation of vasopressin levels accompanies the water-excretory defect resulting from anterior pituitary deficiency and adrenocorticotropic hormone deficiency. This can be corrected by physiologic doses of glucocorticoids. In addition,

vasopressin-independent factors, such as impaired renal hemodynamics and decreased distal fluid delivery to the diluting segments of the nephron, are also implicated in the defective water handling in glucocorticoid deficiency.

Hypothyroidism Hyponatremia occurs in patients with hypothyroidism, who usually meet the criteria for myxedema coma. The cardiac output and GFR in severe hypothyroidism are often reduced. The decrease in cardiac output lead to nonosmotic release of vasopressin and a reduction in the GFR, which lead to diminished free water excretion through decreased delivery to the distal fluid. The exact mechanism, however, is less clear. In support of a vasopressin-independent mechanism, investigators have found normal suppression of vasopressin after water loading in patients with untreated myxedema.[12] In contrast, in advanced hypothyroidism, elevated levels of vasopressin in the basal state and after a water load have been demonstrated. Although both vasopressin-dependent and vasopressin-independent factors may be operating, hyponatremia is readily reversed by treatment with levothyroxine (thyroxine).

Psychosis Patients with acute psychosis have a propensity to develop hyponatremia. Although psychogenic drugs are commonly associated with hyponatremia, psychosis can cause hyponatremia independently. The pathophysiology involves increased thirst perception, a mild defect in osmoregulation that causes vasopressin to be secreted at lower osmolality, and an enhanced renal response to vasopressin.

Postoperative Hyponatremia Most hospitalized hyponatremic patients are asymptomatic and euvolemic and have measurable vasopressin levels.[13] Postoperative hyponatremia mainly occurs as a result of excessive infusion of electrolyte-free water (hypotonic saline or 5% dextrose in water) and the presence of vasopressin, which prevents its excretion. Hyponatremia can also occur in the postoperative setting despite near-isotonic saline infusion within 24 hours of induction of anesthesia. This occurs mostly through the generation of electrolyte-free water by the kidneys in the presence of vasopressin.[14] In a small subgroup of young females, hyponatremia is accompanied by cerebral edema, leading to seizures and hypoxia with catastrophic neurologic events, particularly after gynecologic surgery. The mechanism has not been fully elucidated, and the patients at highest risk cannot be prospectively identified.

Exercise-Induced Hyponatremia Since long distance running has gained in popularity, the number of reports of hyponatremia in this setting has increased. A recent report conducted during the Boston Marathon revealed that runners with a body mass index (BMI) <20 kg/m^2, whose running time exceeded 4 hours and had the greatest weight gain, had an increased risk of this complication.[15]

Drugs Causing Hyponatremia Drug-induced hyponatremia is mediated by vasopressin analogues such as desmopressin (brand name DDAVP [1-desamino-D-arginine vasopressin]), drugs that enhance vasopressin release, and agents potentiating the action of vasopressin.[16] In other instances, the mechanism is unknown (Fig. 8.8).

Drugs associated with hyponatremia*

Vasopressin Analogs	Drugs That Potentiate Renal Action of Vasopressin
Desmopressin (DDAVP)	Chlorpropamide
Oxytocin	Cyclophosphamide
	Nonsteroidal anti-inflammatory drugs
	Acetaminophen
Drugs That Enhance Vasopressin Release	**Drugs That Cause Hyponatremia by Unknown Mechanisms**
Chlorpropamide	*Haloperidol*
Clofibrate	Fluphenazine
Carbamazepine-oxycarbazepine	Amitriptyline
Vincristine	Thioridazine
Nicotine	Fluoxetine
Narcotics	*Methamphetamine (MDMA or Ecstasy)*
Antipsychotics/antidepressants	Sertraline
Ifosfamide	

Figure 8.8 Drugs associated with hyponatremia. Terms in *italics* are the most common causes. *Not including diuretics. (From Berl T, Schrier R: Disorders of water metabolism. In Schrier R [ed]: Renal and Electrolyte Disorders, 6th ed. Philadelphia: Lippincott Williams & Wilkins, 2003.)

Syndrome of Inappropriate ADH Secretion Despite being the most common cause of hyponatremia in hospitalized patients, SIADH is a diagnosis of exclusion. A defect in osmoregulation causes vasopressin to be inappropriately stimulated, leading to urinary concentration. The common causes of this syndrome are listed in Figure 8.9.

A few causes deserve special mention. Central nervous system (CNS) disturbances such as hemorrhage, tumors, infections, and trauma cause SIADH by excess vasopressin secretion. Small cell lung cancers, cancer of the duodenum and pancreas, and olfactory neuroblastoma cause ectopic production of vasopressin. The cells of these tissues increase vasopressin secretion in response to osmotic stimulation *in vitro*. *Pneumocystis carinii* pneumonia, CNS infections, and malignancies play a role in the development of SIADH in patients with human immunodeficiency virus. Idiopathic cases of SIADH are unusual except in the elderly, in whom as many as 10% of patients have been found to have abnormal vasopressin secretion without known cause.[17]

Several patterns of abnormal vasopressin release have emerged from studies of patients with clinical SIADH.[1] In a third of patients, vasopressin release varied appropriately with the serum Na^+ concentration but began at a lower threshold of serum osmolality, implying a "resetting of the osmostat." In this setting, when serum osmolality is above the new threshold, ingestion of free water leads to water retention in order to maintain the serum Na^+ concentration at the new low level, usually 125 to 130 mmol/l. In the remaining patients, vasopressin release did not correlate with serum Na^+ concentration. Such patients are unable to excrete a solute-free urine. Therefore, ingested water is retained, giving rise to moderate nonedematous volume expansion

Causes of the syndrome of inappropriate ADH release (SIADH)

Carcinomas	Pulmonary Disorders	Nervous System Disorders	Other
Bronchogenic carcinoma	*Viral pneumonia*	*Encephalitis (viral or bacterial)*	AIDS–HIV
Carcinoma of the duodenum	*Bacterial pneumonia*	*Meningitis (viral, bacterial, tuberculous, and fungal)*	*Idiopathic (elderly)*
Carcinoma of the pancreas	*Pulmonary abscess*	*Head trauma*	Prolonged exercise
Thymoma	*Tuberculosis*	*Brain abscess*	
Carcinoma of the stomach	Aspergillosis	*Brain tumors*	
Lymphoma	Positive pressure ventilation	Guillain-Barré syndrome	
Ewing's sarcoma	Asthma	Acute intermittent porphyria	
Carcinoma of the bladder	Pneumothorax	Subarachnoid hemorrhage or subdural hematoma	
Prostatic carcinoma	Mesothelioma	Cerebellar and cerebral atrophy	
Oropharyngeal tumor	Cystic fibrosis	Carvernous sinus thrombosis	
Carcinoma of the ureter		Neonatal hypoxia Hydrocephalus Shy–Drager syndrome Rocky Mountain spotted fever Delirium tremens Cerebrovascular accident (cerebral thrombosis or hemorrhage) Acute psychosis Peripheral neuropathy Multiple sclerosis	

Figure 8.9 Causes of the syndrome of inappropriate ADH release (SIADH). Terms in *italics* are the common causes. AIDS, acquired immunodeficiency syndrome; HIV, human immunodeficiency virus. (From Berl T, Schrier R: Disorders of water metabolism. In Schrier R [ed]: Renal and Electrolyte Disorders, 6th ed. Philadelphia: Lippincott Williams & Wilkins, 2003.)

Diagnostic criteria for the syndrome of inappropriate ADH release
Essential Diagnostic Criteria
Decreased extracellular fluid effective osmolality (<270 mOsm/kg H$_2$O)
Inappropriate urinary concentration (>100 mOsm/kg H$_2$O)
Clinical euvolemia
Elevated urinary Na$^+$ concentration under conditions of normal salt and water intake
Absence of adrenal, thyroid, pituitary, or renal insufficiency or diuretic use
Supplemental Criteria
Abnormal water-load test (inability to excrete at least 90% of a 20-ml/kg water load in 4 hours and/or failure to dilute urine osmolality to <100 mOsm/kg)
Plasma vasopressin level inappropriately elevated relative to the plasma osmolality
No significant correction of plasma Na$^+$ level with volume expansion, but improvement after fluid restriction

Figure 8.10 **Diagnostic criteria for the syndrome of inappropriate ADH release (SIADH).** (From Verbalis J: The syndrome of inappropriate antidiuretic hormone secretion and other hypo-osmolar disorders. In Schrier R [ed]: Diseases of the Kidney and Urinary Tract, 8th ed. Philadelphia: Lippincott Williams & Wilkins, 2006.)

and dilutional hyponatremia. The degree of volume expansion and hyponatremia is limited by the phenomenon of "vasopressin escape." It has been shown that escape from antidiuresis is caused by a decrease in the expression of AQP-2, without a concomitant decrease in the expression of the basolateral AQP-3 and AQP-4.[18] This downregulation appears to depend on the maintenance of volume expansion and is independent of changes in plasma or interstitial osmolality.

The diagnostic criteria for SIADH are summarized in Figure 8.10. When measured, plasma vasopressin levels may be in the "normal" range (up to 10 ng/l). However, these levels are always abnormal given the hypo-osmolar state. In clinical practice, the measurement of AVP levels is rarely needed, as the urinary osmolality provides an excellent surrogate bioassay. Thus, the presence of a less than maximally dilute urine is usually associated with measurable AVP levels.

Clinical Manifestations of Hyponatermia

Most patients with a serum Na$^+$ concentration >125 mmol/l are asymptomatic. Once the serum Na$^+$ concentration decreases to <125 mmol/l, headache, lethargy, nausea, reversible ataxia, psychosis, seizures, and coma may occur as a result of cerebral edema. Rarely, hypotonicity leads to cerebral edema so severe that patients experience increased intracerebral pressure, tentorial herniation, respiratory depression, and death. Hyponatremia-induced cerebral edema primarily occurs with rapid development of hyponatremia, typically in hospitalized patients receiving diuretics or hypotonic fluids in the postoperative setting. Mortality can be as high as 50% in patients with severe hyponatremia if left untreated. Neurologic symptoms in a hyponatremic patient call for prompt and immediate attention and treatment.

The development of cerebral edema largely depends on the cerebral adaptation to hypotonicity. Decreases in extracellular osmolality cause movement of water into cells, increasing intracellular

volume and causing tissue edema.[19] Cellular edema within the fixed confines of the cranium causes an increase in intracranial pressure, leading to the neurologic syndromes described previously. In the vast majority of patients with hyponatremia, mechanisms geared toward volume regulation prevent cerebral edema from developing.

Early in the course of hyponatremia (within 1 to 3 hours), a decrease in cerebral extracellular volume occurs by movement of fluid into the cerebrospinal fluid, which is then shunted back into the systemic circulation. This happens promptly and is evident by the loss of extracellular solutes Na$^+$ and Cl$^-$ as early as 30 minutes after the onset of hyponatremia (Fig. 8.11). If hyponatremia persists for longer than 3 hours, the brain adapts by losing cellular osmolytes, including K$^+$ and organic solutes, which tends to lower the osmolality of the brain without substantial gain of water. Thereafter, if hyponatremia persists, other organic

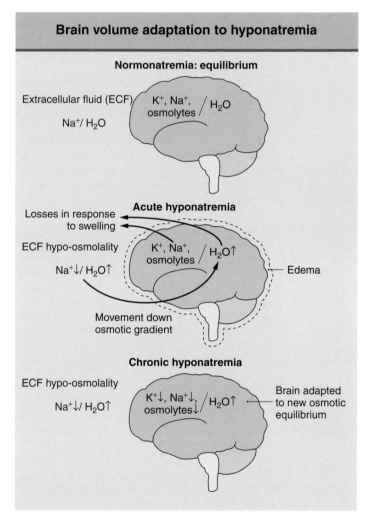

Brain volume adaptation to hyponatremia

Figure 8.11 **Brain volume adaptation to hyponatremia.** Under normal conditions, brain osmolality and extracellular fluid (ECF) osmolality are in equilibrium. Following the induction of ECF hypo-osmolality, water moves into the brain down osmotic gradients, producing brain edema. In response, the brain loses both extracellular and intracellular solutes (see text for details). As water losses accompany the losses of brain solute, the expanded brain volume then decreases back to normal. In chronic hyponatremia, the brain volume eventually normalizes completely, and the brain becomes fully adapted to the ECF hyponatremia. (Adapted from Verbalis J: The syndrome of inappropriate antidiuretic hormone secretion and other hypoosmolar disorders. In Schrier R [ed]: Diseases of the Kidney and Urinary Tract, 8th ed. Philadelphia: Lippincott Williams & Wilkins, 2006.)

osmolytes such as phosphocreatine, myoinositol, and amino acids (e.g., glutamine and taurine) are lost. The loss of these solutes markedly decreases cerebral swelling. It is because of these adaptations that some subjects, particularly the elderly, may have minimal symptoms despite profound ($[Na^+]$ <120 mmol/l) hyponatremia.

Certain patients are at increased risk of developing acute cerebral edema in the course of hyponatremia (Fig. 8.12). For example, hospitalized menstruating females with hyponatremia are more symptomatic and more likely to develop complications of therapy than postmenopausal females or men. This increased risk is independent of the rate of development or the magnitude of hyponatremia. The best approach to management of these patients is to avoid the administration of hypotonic fluids in the postoperative setting. Hyponatremia may occur in the postoperative state even if isotonic fluid is being used if the concentration of $Na^+ + K^+$ in the urine exceeds that in the serum. However, the hyponatremia is mild and has not been reported to be associated with cerebral dysfunction.[14] Children are particularly vulnerable to the development of acute cerebral edema because of physical factors, such as the relatively high ratio of brain to skull volume.

Another neurologic syndrome can occur in hyponatremic patients and is observed as a complication of correction of hyponatremia. The syndrome, termed osmotic demyelination, most commonly affects the central pons of the brainstem and occurs in all ages but appears to be common after orthotopic liver transplantation, with a reported incidence of 13% to 29% at autopsy. Figure 8.12 lists the patients at most risk of osmotic demyelination. The risk of development of central pontine myelinolysis is related to the severity and chronicity of the hyponatremia. It rarely occurs if the serum Na^+ levels are >120 mmol/l and if the hyponatremia is acute in onset (<48 hours). The symptom complex follows a biphasic course. Initially, a generalized encephalopathy associated with a rapid increase in serum Na^+ occurs. Two to 3 days after correction, the classic symptoms of behavioral changes, cranial nerve palsies, and progressive weakness culminating in quadriplegia ("locked-in" syndrome) occur. On T2-weighted magnetic resonance imaging, the lesions are nonenhancing and hyperintense. As these lesions may not appear until 2 weeks after development, a diagnosis of myelinolysis should not be excluded if the imaging is initially negative. The pathogenesis of this syndrome continues to

be investigated. While central pontine myelinolysis was originally considered to be uniformly fatal, it is now evident that some neurologic recovery can occur and that milder forms of the disorder occur as well. As discussed previously, the brain undergoes a multistep adaptation to hyponatremia. Once this adaptation occurs, the brain has no protection from the osmotic stress that accompanies the correction of hyponatremia. Although serum Na^+ and K^+ concentrations return to normal in a few hours, it takes several days for osmotically active solutes in the brain to reach normal levels. This temporary imbalance causes cerebral dehydration and can lead to a potential breakdown of the blood-brain barrier.

Treatment of Hyponatremia

Symptomatology and duration of hyponatremia determine treatment. Acutely hyponatremic patients (hyponatremia developing within 48 hours) are at great risk of developing permanent neurologic sequelae from cerebral edema if the hyponatremia remains uncorrected. Patients with chronic hyponatremia are at risk of osmotic demyelination if the hyponatremia is corrected too rapidly.

Acute Symptomatic Hyponatremia

Acute symptomatic hyponatremia, especially associated with seizures or other neurologic manifestations, almost always develops in hospitalized patients receiving hypotonic fluids (Fig. 8.13).

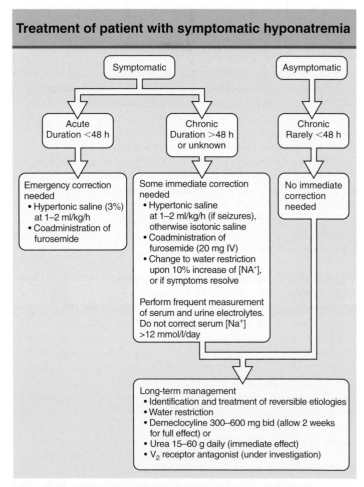

Figure 8.13   Treatment of the patient with symptomatic hyponatremia. (Adapted from Thurman J, Halterman R, Berl T: Therapy of dysnatremic disorders. In Brady H, Wilcox C [eds]: Therapy in Nephrology and Hypertension, 2nd ed. Philadelphia: Saunders, 2003, pp 335–348.)

Hyponatremic patients at risk of neurologic complications	
Acute Cerebral Edema	**Osmotic Demyelination Syndrome (Central Pontine Myelinolysis)**
Postoperative menstruating females	Liver transplant recipients
Elderly women taking thiazides	Alcoholics
Children	Malnourished patients
Polydipsia secondary to psychiatric disorders	Hypokalemic patients
Hypoxemic patients	Burn victims
	Elderly women taking thiazide diuretics
	Hypoxemia

Figure 8.12   Hyponatremic patients at risk of neurologic complications. (From Thurman J, Halterman R, Berl T: Therapy of dysnatremic disorders. In Brady H, Wilcox C [eds]: Therapy in Nephrology and Hypertension, 2nd ed. Philadelphia: Saunders, 2003, pp 335–348.)

Treatment of these patients should be prompt as the risk of acute cerebral edema far exceeds the risk of osmotic demyelination. Serum Na^+ concentration should be ideally corrected by 2 mmol/l per hour until symptoms resolve. It is not necessary to correct the serum Na^+ completely, although it does not appear to be unsafe to do so. Correction may be achieved by administration of hypertonic saline (3% Na/Cl) at the rate of 1 to 2 ml/h/kg body weight.[20,21] The administration of a loop diuretic like furosemide enhances free water excretion and hastens the process of normalization of serum Na^+ concentration. If the patient presents with severe neurologic symptoms, such as seizures, obtundation, or coma, 3% Na/Cl may be infused at higher rates (4 to 6 ml/h/kg body weight). During treatment with hypertonic saline, the patient should be monitored carefully and serum electrolytes should be checked frequently.

Various formulas have been suggested to estimate the rise in serum Na^+ concentration after administration of intravenous fluids.[22] These formulas operate well in static conditions but fail to account for ongoing water and solute losses. A comprehensive formula incorporating the solute and water balance has been suggested.[23] Although the formula is precise, it cannot be used routinely in clinical practice due to its complexity. Frequent monitoring of water and electrolyte intake and output is necessary in such acutely ill patients.

Chronic Symptomatic Hyponatremia

If it is known that hyponatremia has taken more than 48 hours to evolve or if the duration is not known, then therapy for correction of hyponatremia should be prescribed with caution (see Fig. 8.13). Controversy exists as to whether it is the rate of correction or the magnitude of correction of hyponatremia that predisposes to neurologic complications. In clinical practice, it is difficult to dissociate these two variables since a rapid correction rate is usually accompanied by a greater absolute magnitude of correction over a given period of time. Therefore, each of these variables should be considered when designing a treatment regimen. The following guidelines are fundamental to successful therapy[21]:

- Because cerebral water is increased only by approximately 10% in severe chronic hyponatremia, promptly increase the serum Na^+ level by 10% or by approximately 10 mmol/l.

- Do not exceed a correction rate of 1.0 to 1.5 mmol/l in any given hour.
- Do not increase the serum Na^+ by more than 12 mmol/l per 24 hours.

It is important to take into account the rate and electrolyte content of infused fluids and the rate of production and electrolyte content of urine. Once the desired increment in serum Na^+ concentration is obtained, treatment should consist of water restriction.

If correction has proceeded more rapidly than desired (usually because of excretion of hypotonic urine), the risk of osmotic demyelination may be decreased by relowering serum Na^+ with desmopressin and/or administration of 5% dextrose. While these therapies have been demonstrated in experimental animals, there are only case reports of its potential benefit in humans.[24] However, they should be considered in patients who have corrected too rapidly and are at a high risk of developing neurologic symptoms.

Chronic Asymptomatic Hyponatremia

The approach to the chronic asymptomatic patient with hyponatremia is different. Initial evaluation includes looking for an underlying disorder such as hypothyroidism, adrenal insufficiency, and SIADH. In addition, patients' medications should be reviewed and necessary adjustments made.

Patients with idiopathic SIADH should be managed conservatively, because rapid changes in serum tonicity lead to a greater degree of cerebral water loss and possible demyelination. Treatment options are summarized in Figure 8.14.

Fluid Restriction   Fluid restriction is the first-line therapy in patients with chronic asymptomatic hyponatremia. This approach is easy and usually successful if patients are compliant. It involves a calculation of the fluid restriction that will maintain a specific serum Na^+ concentration. The daily osmolar load (OL) and the minimal urinary osmolality $(U_{osm})_{min}$ determine a patient's maximal urine volume (V_{max}).

$$V_{max} = \frac{OL}{(U_{osm})_{min}}$$

Treatment of chronic asymptomatic hyponatremia				
Treatment	Mechanism of Action	Dose	Advantages	Limitations
Fluid restriction	Decreases availability of free water	Variable	Effective and inexpensive; not complicated	Noncompliance
Pharmacologic inhibition of vasopressin action				
Lithium	Inhibits the kidney's response to vasopressin	900–1200 mg/day	Unrestricted water intake	Polyuria, narrow therapeutic range, neurotoxicity
Demeclocyline	Inhibits the kidney's response to vasopressin	300–600 mg twice daily	Effective; unrestricted water intake	Neurotoxicity, polyuria, photosensitivity, nephrotoxicity
V_2 receptor antagonist	Antagonizes vasopressin action		Ongoing trials	
Increased solute (salt) intake				
With furosemide	Increases free water clearance	Titrate to optimal dose; coadministration of 2–3g NaCl	Effective	Ototoxicity, K^+ depletion
With urea	Osmotic diuresis	30–60g/day	Effective; unrestricted water intake	Polyuria, unpalatable, gastrointestinal symptoms

Figure 8.14   Treatment of patients with chronic asymptomatic hyponatremia.

The value of $(U_{osm})_{min}$ is a function of the severity of the diluting disorder. In the absence of circulating vasopressin, it can be as low as 50 mOsm. In a normal North American diet, the daily osmolar load is approximately 10 mOsm/kg (700 mOsm for a 70-kg person). Assuming that a patient with SIADH has a U_{osm} that cannot be lowered to <500 mOsm, the same osmolar load of 700 mOsm allows for only 1.4 liters of urine to be excreted per day. Therefore, if the patient drinks more than 1.4 liters per day, the serum Na^+ concentration will decrease. Measurement of urine Na and K can indicate the degree of water restriction required in a given patient.[25] If the diluting defect is so severe that fluid restriction to <1 liter is necessary or if the patient's serum Na^+ remains low (<130 mmol/l), an alternative approach to treatment such as increasing solute excretion or pharmacologic inhibition of vasopressin should be considered.

Maneuvers That Increase Solute Excretion   If the patient remains unresponsive to fluid restriction, solute intake can be increased to facilitate an obligatory increase in excretion of solute and free water. This can be achieved by increasing oral salt and protein intake in the diet in order to increase the C_{osm} of the urine. Loop diuretics combined with high Na^+ intake (2 to 3 g of additional salt) are effective in the management of hyponatremia. A single diuretic dose (40 mg furosemide) is usually sufficient but should be doubled if the diuresis induced in the first 8 hours is <60% of the total daily urine output.

The administration of urea increases urine flow by causing an osmotic diuresis. This permits a more liberal water intake without worsening the hyponatremia and without altering urinary concentration. The dose for urea is usually 30 to 60 g/day. The major limitations are gastrointestinal distress and unpalatability. Quantitation of electrolyte C_{water} both before and after urea permits demonstration of the effect of the increased solute load.[21]

Pharmacologic Inhibition of Vasopressin   In patients who cannot comply with water restriction, pharmacologic agents can be used. Lithium was the first pharmacologic agent used to antagonize vasopressin action and to be used in the treatment of SIADH. However, because lithium causes neurotoxicity and is unreliable, demeclocycline is now the agent of choice. The drug inhibits the formation and action of cyclic adenosine monophosphate (cAMP) in the renal collecting duct. The onset of action is usually 3 to 6 days after beginning treatment. Its action can be monitored by a decline in urine osmolality. The dose needs to be decreased to the lowest level that keeps the serum Na^+ concentration within the desired range with unrestricted water intake (usually a dose of 600 to 1200 mg/day). The drug is indicated in patients in whom water restriction is ineffective because of high urine:plasma electrolyte ratio or poor compliance. The drug should be given 1 to 2 hours after meals and calcium-, aluminum-, and magnesium-containing antacids should be avoided. Skin photosensitivity may occur and tooth or bone abnormalities may result in the pediatric population. Polyuria leads to noncompliance, and nephrotoxicity also limits its use. The latter commonly occurs in patients with underlying liver disease in whom hepatic metabolism of the drug may be impaired.

The previously described approaches to the treatment of hyponatremia are suboptimal and may soon be superseded by novel oral V_2 receptor antagonists that block vasopressin binding to the collecting duct tubular epithelial cells.[26] OPC-31260 is a selective nonpeptide V_2 receptor antagonist that induces a water diuresis without affecting urine electrolyte or solute excretion. Recent clinical trials have produced the expected effects of enhanced water excretion and correction of hyponatremia in cirrhosis, heart failure, and SIADH.[26] Maximum doses of OPC-31260 increase plasma vasopressin concentrations, suggesting a role of the V_2 receptor in either the clearance or negative-feedback regulation of AVP. No effects on hemodynamic variables or potassium concentrations have been observed. V_2 receptor antagonists should not be used for treatment of hyponatremia due to hypovolemia (where saline is the treatment of choice) or for hyponatremia associated with advanced renal insufficiency (in which the hyponatremia is not mediated by vasopressin).

Hypovolemic Hyponatremia
Neurologic syndromes directly related to hyponatremia are unusual in hypovolemic hyponatremia as both Na^+ and water loss limits any osmotic shifts in the brain. Restoration of ECF volume with crystalloids or colloids interrupts the nonosmotic release of vasopressin. The administration of thiazides in general and to elderly women in particular requires monitoring of Na^+ and advice to restrict water intake. If hyponatremia develops, the drug needs to be discontinued.

Hypervolemic Hyponatremia
The treatment of hyponatremia in hypervolemic states is more difficult as it requires reversing the underlying disorder, be it heart failure or chronic liver disease, responsible for hyponatremia. In patients with congestive heart failure, Na^+ and water restriction is critical. Refractory patients may be treated with a combination of angiotensin-converting enzyme inhibitors and diuretics. The increase in cardiac output that follows decreases the neurohumoral mediated processes that limit water excretion. Loop diuretics diminish the action of vasopressin on the collecting tubules, thereby decreasing water reabsorption. Thiazides should be avoided as they impair urinary dilution and may worsen hyponatremia. The use of V_2 antagonists in congestive heart failure is under active investigation.[27] In patients with cirrhosis, water and sodium restriction is the mainstay of therapy. Loop diuretics increase C_{water} once a negative Na^+ balance has been achieved. In both of these disorders, the V_2 receptor antagonists, which are currently under active investigation, may be useful.[26]

HYPERNATREMIC DISORDERS

Hypernatremia is defined as a serum $[Na^+]$ >145 mmol/l and reflects serum hyperosmolarity. The renal concentrating mechanism represents the first defense mechanism against water depletion and hyperosmolarity. The components of the normal concentrating mechanism are depicted in Figure 8.15. Disorders of urinary concentration reflect perturbations of these determinants and may result from decreased delivery of solute (with decreasing GFR) or the inability to generate interstitial hypertonicity as a consequence of decreased Na^+/Cl^- reabsorption in the ascending limb of the loop (loop diuretics), decreased medullary urea accumulation (poor dietary intake), or alterations in medullary blood flow. Finally, hypernatremia may result from failure to release or respond to AVP. Thirst is the first and most important defense mechanism in preventing hypernatremia.

Etiology and Classification of Hypernatremia
As with hyponatremic patients, patients with hypernatremia fall into three broad categories based on volume status.[28,29] A diagnostic algorithm is helpful in the evaluation of these patients (Fig. 8.16).

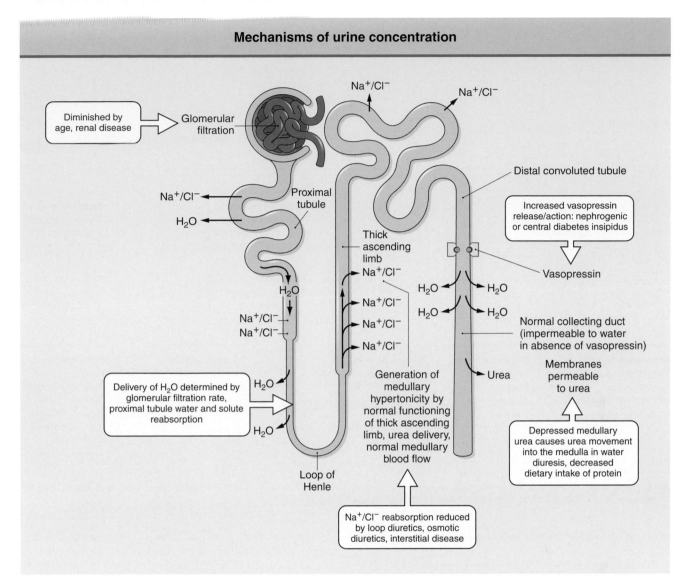

Mechanisms of urine concentration

Diminished by age, renal disease → Glomerular filtration

Na^+/Cl^-

Na^+/Cl^-

Proximal tubule

$Na^+/Cl^- ←$

$H_2O ←$

Distal convoluted tubule

Increased vasopressin release/action: nephrogenic or central diabetes insipidus

Thick ascending limb

Na^+/Cl^-

Vasopressin

H_2O

Na^+/Cl^-

$H_2O ← H_2O$

H_2O

Na^+/Cl^-

$H_2O ← H_2O$

Na^+/Cl^-

Na^+/Cl^-

Normal collecting duct (impermeable to water in absence of vasopressin)

Na^+/Cl^-

Delivery of H_2O determined by glomerular filtration rate, proximal tubule water and solute reabsorption

H_2O

Generation of medullary hypertonicity by normal functioning of thick ascending limb, urea delivery, normal medullary blood flow

Urea

Membranes permeable to urea

H_2O

Depressed medullary urea causes urea movement into the medulla in water diuresis, decreased dietary intake of protein

Loop of Henle

Na^+/Cl^- reabsorption reduced by loop diuretics, osmotic diuretics, interstitial disease

Figure 8.15 Urinary concentrating mechanisms. Determinants of normal urinary concentrating mechanism and disorders causing hypernatremia. (Adapted from Cogan M: Normal water homeostasis. In Cogan M [ed]: Fluid and Electrolytes. Norwalk, CT: Lange, 1991, pp 98–106.)

Hypovolemia: Hypernatremia Associated with Low Total Body Sodium

Patients with hypovolemic hypernatremia sustain losses of both Na^+ and water, but with a relatively greater loss of water. On physical examination, they manifest signs of hypovolemia such as orthostatic hypotension, tachycardia, flat neck veins, poor skin turgor, and sometimes altered mental status. Patients will generally have hypotonic water losses from the kidneys and/or the gastrointestinal tract. In the latter, the urinary Na^+ concentration will be low.

Hypervolemia: Hypernatremia Associated with Increased Total Body Sodium

Hypernatremia with increased total body Na^+ is the least common form of hypernatremia. It results from the administration of hypertonic solutions such as 3% NaCl given as intra-amniotic instillation for therapeutic abortion and $NaHCO_3$ for the treatment of metabolic acidosis, hyperkalemia, and cardiorespiratory arrest. It may also result from inadvertent dialysis against a dialysate with a high Na^+ concentration or from consumption of salt tablets. Hypernatremia is increasingly recognized in hypoalbuminemic azotemic hospitalized patients who are edematous and unable to concentrate their urine.[28]

Euvolemia: Hypernatremia Associated with Normal Body Sodium

Most patients with hypernatremia secondary to water loss appear euvolemic with normal total body Na^+ since loss of water without Na^+ does not lead to overt volume contraction. Water loss per se need not result in hypernatremia unless it is unaccompanied by water intake. Since hypodipsia is uncommon, hypernatremia usually supervenes in those who have no access to water and the very young and old, in whom there may be an altered perception of thirst. Extrarenal water loss occurs from the skin and respiratory tract in febrile or other hypermetabolic states and is associated with a high urine osmolality since the osmoreceptor-vasopressin-renal response is intact. The urine Na^+ concentration varies with the intake. Renal water loss leading to euvolemic hypernatremia results from either a defect in vasopressin production and/or release (central DI) or a failure of the collecting duct to respond to the hormone (nephrogenic DI). Defense against the development of hyperosmolality requires the

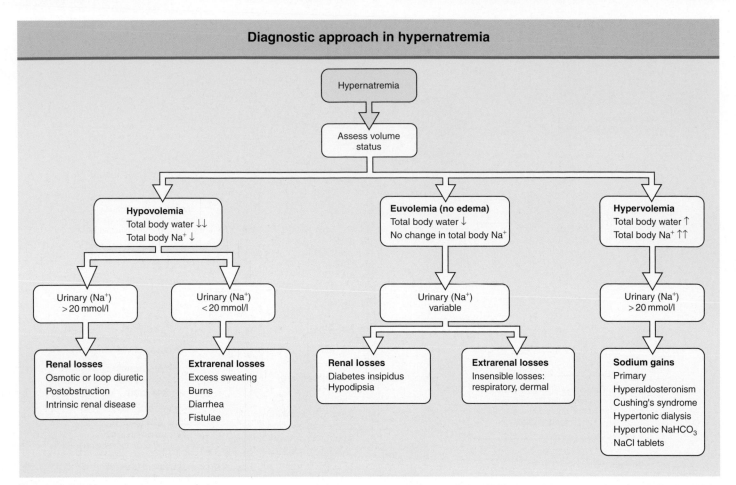

Figure 8.16 **Diagnostic approach in hypernatremia.** (Adapted with permission from Halterman R, Berl T: Therapy of dysnatremic disorders. In Brady H, Wilcox C [eds]: Therapy in Nephrology and Hypertension. Philadelphia: WB Saunders, 1999, pp 257–269.)

appropriate stimulation of thirst and the ability to respond by drinking water.

Polyuric disorders can result from either an increase in C_{osm} or an increase in C_{water} (see the first equation in chapter). An increase in C_{osm} occurs in several settings, notably diuretic use, renal salt wasting, excess salt ingestion, vomiting (bicarbonaturia), alkali administration, and the administration of mannitol as a diuretic, for bladder lavage or for the treatment of cerebral edema. An increase in C_{water} occurs with excess ingestion water (psychogenic polydipsia) or in abnormalities of the renal-concentrating mechanism (diabetes insipidus [DI]).

Diabetes Insipidus DI is a disease characterized by polyuria and polydipsia and is caused by defects in vasopressin action.

Central Diabetes Insipidus
Clinical Features Patients with central and nephrogenic DI and primary polydipsia present with polyuria and polydipsia. The differentiation between these entities can be accomplished by measurements of vasopressin levels and the response to a water deprivation test followed by vasopressin administration (Fig. 8.17). Other clinical features can distinguish compulsive water drinkers (primary polydipsia) from patients with central DI. Central DI usually has an abrupt onset. Patients have a constant need to drink, have a predilection for cold water, and commonly have nocturia. The compulsive water drinker may give a vague history of the onset and has large variations in water intake and urine output. Nocturia is unusual. A plasma osmolality of >295 mOsm/kg suggests central DI and <270 mOsm/kg suggests compulsive water drinking.

Measurements of circulating vasopressin by radioimmunoassay can be used as an alternative to the tedious water deprivation test. Under basal conditions, the measurements of vasopressin levels have not been of practical value since there is a significant overlap among the polyuric disorders. Its measurement following a water deprivation test is more useful (see Fig. 8.17). Measurement of urinary excretion of AQP-2 may also differentiate between primary polydipsia and central DI.[30]

Causes The causes of central DI are listed in Figure 8.18. In 50% of patients, no cause is identified (idiopathic). Central DI in the other 50% is caused by infection, tumors, granuloma, and trauma affecting the CNS. In a survey of 79 children and young adults, the disease was idiopathic in 52%. A significant number of the remaining patients had tumors and Langerhans' cell histiocytosis. These patients had an 80% chance of developing anterior pituitary hormone deficiency compared to 50% in patients with idiopathic disease.[31]

An inherited autosomal dominant form of the disease is caused by point mutations in a precursor gene for vasopressin that causes "misfolding" of the provasopressin peptide preventing its release from the hypothalamic and posterior pituitary neurons.[32] Patients present with a mild polyuria and polydipsia in the first year of life. These children have normal physical and mental development. Rarely, an autosomal recessive central DI associated with diabetes mellitus, optic atrophy, and deafness (Wolfram syndrome) occurs.[33] This is linked to chromosome 4 and involves abnormalities in mitochondrial DNA. In patients

Water deprivation test			
Condition	Urinary Osmolality with Water Deprivation (mOsm/kg H_2O)	Plasma Vasopressin after Dehydration (pg/ml)	Increase in Urinary Osmolality with Exogenous Vasopressin
Normal	>800	>2	Little or no increase
Complete central diabetes insipidus	<300	Undetectable	Substantially increased
Partial central diabetes insipidus	300–800	<1.5	Increase of >10% of urinary osmolality after water deprivation
Nephrogenic diabetes insipidus	<300–500	>5	Little or no increase
Primary polydipsia	>500	<5	Little or no increase

Figure 8.17   Water deprivation test. Test procedure: Water intake is restricted until the patient loses 3% to 5% of his or her body weight or until three consecutive hourly determinations of urinary osmolality are within 10% of each other. (Caution must be exercised to ensure that the patient does not become excessively dehydrated.) Aqueous vasopressin (5 U subcutaneously) is given and urinary osmolality is measured after 60 minutes. The expected responses are given in the table. (From Lanese D, Teitelbaum I: Hypernatremia. In Jacobson HR, Striker GE, Klahr S [eds]: The Principles and Practice of Nephrology, 2nd ed. St Louis, MO: Mosby, 1995, pp 893–898.)

with the Wolfram syndrome, DI is usually partial and gradual in onset.

Treatment   Central DI may be treated with hormone replacement or pharmacologic agents (Fig. 8.19). In acute settings, where renal water losses are extensive, aqueous vasopressin (Pitressin) is useful. It has a short duration of action, allows for careful monitoring, and avoids complications such as water intoxication. This drug should be used with caution in patients with underlying coronary artery disease and peripheral vascular disease as it may cause vascular spasm and prolonged vasoconstriction. For chronic central DI, desmopressin acetate is the agent of choice. It has a long half-life and does not have the significant vasoconstrictive effects of aqueous vasopressin. It is administered at the dose of 10 to 20 µg intranasally every 12 to 24 hours. It is tolerated well, safe to use in pregnancy, and resistant to degradation by circulating vasopressinase. Oral desmopressin (dose 0.1 to 0.4 mg every 12 hours) is available and is second-line therapy. In patients with partial DI, in addition to desmopressin itself, agents that potentiate the release of vasopressin may be used. These agents include chlorpropamide, clofibrate, and carbamazepine.

Congenital Nephrogenic Diabetes Insipidus   One form of congenital nephrogenic DI is due to mutations in the V_2 receptor gene on the X chromosome and clinically manifests only in males, although it can be detected subclinically in females.[3] A rarer autosomal recessive form of nephrogenic DI has also been described and is caused by mutations in the gene for AQP-2.[3] The disease may have variable penetrance. Finally, an autosomal dominant form of nephrogenic DI has been reported in three Japanese families and is due to mutations of the carboxy terminal of AQP-2.[34] Defects in water concentrating ability have also been described with other AQPs such as AQP-1[35] in mice and humans and AQP-3 and AQP-4 in mice only.[4]

Clinical Features   Diagnosis of congenital nephrogenic DI is made when an infant presents with hypo-osmolar urine together with severe dehydration, hypernatremia, vomiting, and fever. In the X-linked variety, unlike females with variable penetrance of the disease, male patients do not concentrate their urine despite severe dehydration and vasopressin administration. Affected patients suffer from repeated episodes of dehydration, hypernatremia, and hyperthermia early in infancy and may suffer from impaired growth and mental retardation. Hydronephrosis is not unusual in these patients as a consequence of the large urine output and some voluntary retention.

Treatment   Neither pharmacologic nor hormonal maneuvers are effective in patients with congenital nephrogenic DI: an intact thirst mechanism is indispensable to life. Since the excretion of solute requires further water losses, rehydration therapy should include hypotonic (2.5%) rather than isotonic (5%) glucose solutions. Solute intake should be kept low (low Na^+ and protein diet). The use of thiazide diuretics has met with some success. They decrease urine output by causing ECF volume contraction, thereby enhancing proximal tubular Na^+ and water reabsorption. The addition of amiloride to hydrochlorothiazide has also been useful. Nonsteroidal anti-inflammatory drugs have been especially well tolerated in children. It should be realized that a change in urine osmolality from 50 to 200 mOsm/kg H_2O is very important, as it translates into substantial reduction in urine output from 10 to 12 to 3 to 4 liters/day. Recently, novel approaches to

Causes of central diabetes insipidus
Congenital
Autosomal dominant
Autosomal recessive
Acquired
Post-traumatic
Iatrogenic (postsurgical)
Tumors (metastatic from breast, craniopharyngioma, pinealoma)
Histiocytosis
Granuloma (tuberculosis, sarcoid)
Aneurysm
Meningitis
Encephalitis
Guillain-Barré syndrome
Idiopathic

Figure 8.18   Causes of central diabetes insipidus. Entries in *italics* are the common causes.

Treatment of central diabetes insipidus			
Disease	Drug	Dose	Interval
Complete central diabetes insipidus	Desmopressin (DDAVP) Desmopressin (DDAVP)	10–20 µg intranasally 0.1–0.4 mg orally	12–24 h Every 12 h
Partial central diabetes insipidus	Desmopressin (DDAVP) Aqueous vasopressin Chlorpropamide Clofibrate Carbamazepine	10–20 µg intranasally 5–10U subcutaneously 250–500mg 500mg 400–600mg	12–24 h 4–6 h 24 h 6 or 8 h 24 h

Figure 8.19   Treatment of central diabetes insipidus.

the treatment of these disorders are emerging. These involve the use of pharmacologic chaperones or phosphodiesterase inhibitors that enhance cyclic guanosine monophosphate production and the insertion of AQP-2 into the membrane to improve urinary concentration.[36,37]

Acquired Nephrogenic Diabetes Insipidus   Acquired nephrogenic DI is more common and rarely as severe as congenital nephrogenic DI. In these patients, the ability to elaborate a maximal concentration of urine is impaired, but urinary concentrating mechanisms are partially preserved. For this reason, urinary volumes are <3 to 4 l/day, which contrasts with the higher values seen in patients with congenital or central DI or compulsive water drinking. The causes and mechanisms of acquired nephrogenic DI are listed in Figure 8.20.

Chronic Renal Failure   Patients with advancing chronic renal failure of any etiology may develop a defect in urinary concentrating ability, but this defect is most prominent in polycystic and medullary cystic diseases. Disruption of inner medullary structures in tubulointerstitial diseases and diminished medullary concentration are thought to play a role, and in experimental models there is also selective downregulation of the V_2 receptor in the inner medulla. AQP-2 expression also decreases in both obstruction and acute and chronic renal failure. It is important to recognize that, in order to achieve daily osmolar clearance, an amount of fluid commensurate with the severity of the concentrating defect is necessary in patients who still make urine.

Electrolyte Disorders   Hypokalemia causes a reversible abnormality in urinary concentrating ability. Hypokalemia stimulates water intake and reduces interstitial tonicity, which relates to the decreased Na^+/Cl^- reabsorption in the TALH. Hypokalemia resulting from diarrhea, chronic diuretic use, and primary aldosteronism also decreases intracellular cAMP accumulation and causes a reduction in vasopressin-sensitive AQP-2 expression (see Fig. 8.7).

Hypercalcemia also impairs urinary concentrating ability, resulting in mild polydipsia. The pathophysiology is multifactorial and includes a reduction in medullary interstitial tonicity caused by decreased vasopressin-stimulated adenylate cyclase in the TALH and a defect in adenylate cyclase activity with decreased AQP-2 expression in the collecting duct.

Pharmacologic Agents   Certain drugs impair urinary concentrating ability. Amphotericin and foscarnet cause a concentrating defect due to their renal toxicity. Demeclocycline reduces renal medullary adenylate cyclase activity, thereby decreasing vasopressin's effect on the collecting ducts. Lithium may cause nephrogenic DI in as many as 50% of patients by causing downregulation of AQP-2 in the collecting duct. Lithium also increases cyclooxygenase-2 expression and urinary prostaglandins in mice, which may contribute to the polyuria.[38] The concentrating defect of lithium may persist even when the drug is discontinued.

Sickle Cell Anemia   Patients with sickle cell disease and trait often have a urinary concentrating defect. In the hypertonic medullary interstitium, the "sickled" red cells cause occlusion of

Acquired nephrogenic diabetes insipidus: causes and mechanisms				
Disease State	Defect in Generation of Medullary Interstitial Tonicity	Defect in cAMP Generation	Downregulation of Aquaporin-2	Other
Chronic renal insufficiency	Yes	Yes	Yes	Downregulation of V_2 receptor message
Hypokalemia	Yes	Yes	Yes	—
Hypercalcemia	Yes	Yes	—	—
Sickle cell disease	Yes	—	—	—
Protein malnutrition	Yes	—	Yes	—
Demeclocycline therapy	—	Yes	—	—
Lithium therapy	—	Yes	Yes	—
Pregnancy	—	—	—	Placental secretion of vasopressinase

Figure 8.20   Acquired nephrogenic diabetes insipidus: causes and mechanisms. cAMP, cyclic adenosine monophosphate.

respond to desmopressin, as desmopressin does not undergo degradation by this enzyme.

Patient groups at risk of development of severe hypernatremia
Elderly patients or infants
Hospitalized patients receiving hypertonic infusions, tube feedings, osmotic diuretics, lactulose, mechanical ventilation
Altered mental status
Uncontrolled diabetes mellitus
Underlying polyuric disorders

Figure 8.21   Patient groups at risk of development of severe hypernatremia. (From Thurman J, Halterman R, Berl T: Therapy of dysnatremic disorders. In Brady H, Wilcox C [eds]: Therapy in Nephrology and Hypertension, 2nd ed. Philadelphia: Saunders, 2003, pp 335–348.)

the vasa recta and papillary damage. The resultant medullary ischemia may impair Na^+/Cl^- transport in the ascending limb and thus diminish medullary tonicity. Although initially reversible, medullary infarcts occur with long-standing sickle cell disease and the concentrating defects become irreversible.

Dietary Abnormalities   Extensive water intake or a marked decrease in salt and protein intake leads to impairment of maximal urinary concentrating ability through a reduction in medullary interstitial tonicity. In low-protein diets and excessive water intake, there is a decrease in vasopressin-stimulated osmotic water permeability. This appears to be promptly reversed with feeding.

Gestational Diabetes Insipidus   In gestational DI, there is an increase in circulating vasopressinase, which is produced by the placenta. Patients are typically unresponsive to vasopressin but

Clinical Manifestations of Hyprenatremia

Certain groups of patients are at increased risk of developing hypernatremia (Fig. 8.21). Signs and symptoms mostly relate to the CNS and include altered mental status, lethargy, irritability, restlessness, seizures (usually in children), muscle twitching, hyperreflexia, and spasticity. Fever, nausea or vomiting, labored breathing, and intense thirst can also occur. In children, the mortality of acute hypernatremia ranges between 10% and 70%. As many as two thirds of survivors have neurologic sequelae. In contrast, mortality in chronic hypernatremia is 10%. In adults, serum Na^+ concentrations >160 mmol/l are associated with a 75% mortality. Hypernatremia in adults occurs in the setting of serious disease, and the mortality figures may reflect the mortality of the underlying diseases rather than hypernatremia per se.

Treatment of Hyprenatremia

Hypernatremia occurs in predictable clinical settings. Thus, preventing its development may be the best therapy. Elderly and hospitalized patients are at very high risk due to impaired thirst mechanisms and their inability to access free water independently and to have it prescribed as needed.[39] Certain clinical situations such as recovery from acute renal failure, catabolic states, therapy with hypertonic solutions, uncontrolled diabetes, and burns should prompt close attention to serum sodium and increased administration of free water.

Hypernatremia always reflects a hyperosmolar state. The primary goal in the treatment of these patients is the restoration of serum tonicity. The treatment regimen depends on the volume status. Specific management options are outlined in Figure 8.22.[21]

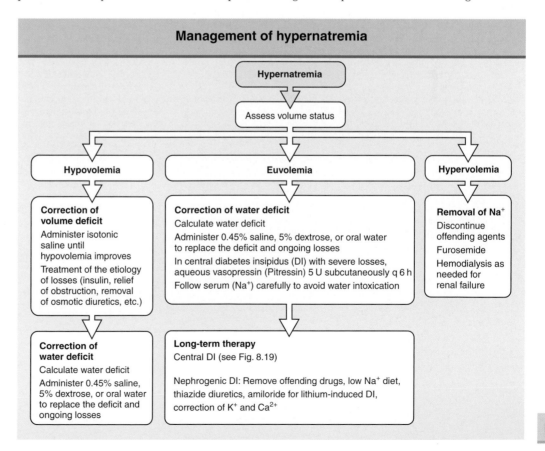

Figure 8.22   Management of hypernatremia. (From Thurman J, Halterman R, Berl T: Therapy of dysnatremic disorders. In Brady H, Wilcox C [eds]: Therapy in Nephrology and Hypertension, 2nd ed. Philadelphia: Saunders, 2003, pp 335–348.)

The rapidity with which hypernatremia should be corrected is a matter of controversy. Some animal studies and case series in pediatric patients suggest that a correction rate of >0.5 mmol/l per hour can cause seizures. Cerebral edema also can be caused by rapid correction of hypernatremia due to the net movement of water into the brain. Most clinicians believe that even in adults correction should be achieved over 48 hours at a rate no greater than 2 mmol/h.

REFERENCES

1. Berl T, Verbalis J: Pathophysiology of water metabolism. In Brenner BM (ed): The Kidney, 7th ed. Philadelphia: WB Saunders, 2004, pp 857–919.
2. Narins RG, Krishna GC: Disorders of water balance. In Stein JH (ed): Internal Medicine. Boston: Little, Brown, 1987, p 794.
3. Bichet D: Nephrogenic and central diabetes insipidus. In Schrier R (ed): Diseases of the Kidney and Urinary Tract, Vol. 3, 8th ed. Philadelphia: Lippincott Williams & Wilkins, 2006.
4. Nielsen S, Frokler J, Marples D, et al: Aquaporins in the kidney: From molecules to medicine. Physiol Rev 2002;82:205–244.
5. Agre P: Aquaporin water channels. Nobel Lecture. Biosci Rep 2004;24:127–148.
6. Halterman R, Berl T: Therapy of dysnatremic disorders. In Brady H, Wilcox C (eds): Therapy in Nephrology and Hypertension. Philadelphia: WB Saunders, 1999, pp 257–269.
7. Hiller TA, Abott RD, Barrett EJ: Hyponatremia: Evaluating the correction factor for hypoglycemia. Am J Med 1999;106:399–403.
8. Cogan M: Normal water homeostasis. In Cogan M (ed): Fluid and Electrolytes. Norwalk, CT: Lange, 1991, pp 98–106.
9. Palmer B: Hyponatremia in patients with central nervous system disease: SIADH versus CSW. Endocrinol Metab Rev 2003;4:182–187.
10. Martin PY, Gines P, Schrier RW: Nitric oxide as mediator of hemodynamic abnormalities and sodium and water retention in cirrhosis. N Engl J Med 1998;339:533–541.
11. Anderson RJ, Chung HM, Kluge R, Schrier RW: Hyponatremia: A prospective analysis of its epidemiology and the pathogenetic role of vasopressin. Ann Intern Med 1985;102:164–168.
12. Iwasaki Y, Oiso Y, Yamauchi K, et al: Osmoregulation of plasma vasopressin in myxedema. J Clin Endocrinol Metab 1990;70:534–539.
13. Anderson RJ: Hospital-associated hyponatremia (clinical conference). Kidney Int 1986;29:1237–1247.
14. Steele A, Gowrishankar M, Abrahamson S, et al: Postoperative hyponatremia despite near-isotonic saline infusion: A phenomenon of desalination. Ann Intern Med 1997;126:20–25.
15. Almond CS, Shin AY, Fortescue EB, et al: Hyponatremia among runners in the Boston Marathon. N Engl J Med 2005;352:1550–1556.
16. Berl T, Schrier R: Disorders of water metabolism. In Schrier R (ed): Renal and Electrolyte Disorders, 6th ed. Philadelphia: Lippincott Williams & Wilkins, 2003.
17. Miller M: Hyponatremia: Age related risk factors and therapy decisions. Geriatrics 1998;53:32–33, 37–38, 41–42.
18. Ecelbarger CA, Nielsen S, Olson BR, et al: Role of renal aquaporins in escape from vasopressin-induced antidiuresis in rat. J Clin Invest 1997;99:1852–1863.
19. Verbalis J: The syndrome of inappropriate antidiuretic hormone secretion and other hypoosmolar disorders. In Schrier R (ed): Diseases of the Kidney and Urinary Tract, 8th ed. Philadelphia: Lippincott Williams & Wilkins, 2006.
20. Soupart A, Decaux G: Therapeutic recommendations for management of severe hyponatremia: Current concepts on pathogenesis and prevention of neurologic complications. Clin Nephrol 1996;46:149–169.
21. Thurman J, Halterman R, Berl T: Therapy of dysnatremic disorders. In Brady H, Wilcox C (eds): Therapy in Nephrology and Hypertension, 2nd ed. Philadelphia: Saunders, 2003, pp 335–348.
22. Adrogue HJ, Madias NE: Hyponatremia. N Engl J Med 2000;342:1581–1589.
23. Barsoum N, Levine B: Current prescriptions for corrections of hypo- and hypernatremia: Are they too simple? Nephrol Dial Transplant 2002;17:1176–1180.
24. Goldszmidt MA, Iliescu EA: DDAVP to prevent rapid correction in hyponatremia. Clin Nephrol 2000;53:226–229.
25. Furst H, Hallows KR, Post J, et al: The urine/plasma electrolyte ratio: A predictive guide to water restriction. Am J Med Sci 2000;319:240–244.
26. Verbalis JG: Vasopressin V2 receptor antagonists. J Mol Endocrinol 2002;29:1–9.
27. Francis GS, Tang WH: Vasopressin receptor antagonists: Will the "vaptans" fulfill their promise? JAMA 2004;291:2017–2018.
28. Kahn T: Hypernatremia with edema. Arch Intern Med 1999;159:93–98.
29. Lanese D, Teitelbaum I: Hypernatremia. In Jacobson HR, Striker GE, Klahr S (eds): The Principles and Practice of Nephrology, 2nd ed. St Louis, MO: Mosby, 1995, pp 893–898.
30. Saito T, Ishikawa S, Ito T, et al: Urinary excretion of aquaporin-2 water channel differentiates psychogenic polydipsia from central diabetes insipidus. J Clin Endocrinol Metab 1999;84:2235–2237.
31. Maghnie M: Diabetes insipidus. Horm Res 2003;59:42–54.
32. Phillips JA: Dominant-negative diabetes insipidus and other endocrinopathies. J Clin Invest 2003;112:1641–1643.
33. Smith CJ, Crock PA, King BR, et al: Phenotype-genotype correlations in a series of Wolfram syndrome families. Diabetes Care 2004;27:2003–2009.
34. Kuwahara M, Iwai K, Ooeda T, et al: Three families with autosomal dominant nephrogenic diabetes insipidus caused by aquaporin-2 mutation in the C-terminus. Am J Hum Genet 2001;69:738–748.
35. King LS, Choi M, Fernandez PC, et al: Defective urinary concentrating ability due to a complete deficiency of aquaporin-1. N Engl J Med 2001;345:175–179.
36. Bernier V, Morello JP, Zarruk A, et al: Pharmacologic chaperones as a potential treatment for X-linked nephrogenic diabetes insipidus. J Am Soc Nephrol 2006;17:232–243.
37. Bouley R, Pastor-Soler N, Cohen O, et al: Stimulation of AQP2 membrane insertion in renal epithelial cells in vitro and in vivo by the cGMP phosphodiesterase inhibitor sildenafil citrate (Viagra). Am J Physiol Renal Physiol 2005;288:F1103–F1112.
38. Rao R, Zhang MZ, Zhao M, et al: Lithium treatment inhibits renal GSK-3 activity and promotes cyclooxygenase 2 dependent polyuria. Am J Physiol Renal Physiol 2005;288:F642–F649.
39. Polderman KH, Schreuder WO, van Schijndel RJ, et al: Hypernatremia in the intensive care unit: An indicator of quality of care? Crit Care Med 1999;27:1105–1108.

CHAPTER 9

Disorders of Potassium Metabolism

I. David Weiner, Stuart L. Linas, and Charles S. Wingo

INTRODUCTION

Potassium disorders are some of the most commonly encountered fluid and electrolyte abnormalities in clinical medicine. They can be asymptomatic or they can be associated with symptoms that range from mild weakness to sudden death. When an abnormal serum potassium level is verified, correction is essential, but inappropriate treatment can worsen symptoms and even lead to death.

NORMAL PHYSIOLOGY OF POTASSIUM METABOLISM

Potassium Intake

Potassium is essential for many cellular functions, present in most foods, and excreted primarily by the kidney. The typical Western diet contains ~70 to 150 mmol of potassium per day. The gastrointestinal tract, particularly the jejunum, ileum, and colon, efficiently absorbs potassium. Dietary potassium intake varies greatly with the composition of the diet. Figure 9.1 summarizes the potassium content of several foods high in potassium.

Potassium content of selected high-potassium foods		
Food	Portion Size	mmol K+
Artichoke, boiled	1, medium	27
Avocado	1, medium	38
Sirloin steak	8 oz	23
Hamburger, lean	8 oz	18
Cantaloupe, cut up	1 cup	13
Grapefruit juice	8 oz	10
Milk	8 oz	10
Orange juice	8 oz	12
Potato, baked	7 oz	22
Prunes	10	16
Raisins	2/3 cup	19
Squash	1 cup	15–20
Tomato paste	1/2 cup	31
Tomato juice	6 oz	10
Banana	Medium size	12

Figure 9.1 Potassium content of selected high potassium foods. (Data adapted from Na-K-Phos Counter, published by the American Association of Kidney Patients, Inc. 1999.)

Potassium Distribution

After gastrointestinal tract absorption, potassium distributes primarily into the intracellular fluid compartment. Potassium is the major intracellular cation, with values from ~100 to 120 mmol/l in the cytoplasm. Total intracellular potassium content is 3000 to 3500 mmol in healthy adults and primarily distributed in muscle (70%), with smaller amounts present in bone, red blood cells, liver, and skin (Fig. 9.2). Only 1% to 2% total body potassium is present in the extracellular fluids. The electrogenic Na^+-K^+-ATPase is present in virtually all cells and transports two K^+ ions into cells in exchange for extrusion of three Na^+, resulting in high intracellular potassium and low sodium concentrations. The ratio of intracellular to extracellular K^+ concentration is a major determinant of cell membrane potential. Normal maintenance of this ratio and membrane potential is critical for normal nerve conduction and muscular contraction.

Addition of potassium to the extracellular fluid compartment results in a shift of potassium from the extracellular to the intracellular fluid compartment. Conversely, extracellular potassium losses result in cellular potassium release into the extracellular fluid, particularly from skeletal muscle. This thereby minimizes changes in the transmembrane potassium ratio and the membrane potential. Accordingly, small changes in extracellular potassium concentration are associated frequently with substantial changes in total body potassium.

Several factors shift potassium from the extracellular to the intracellular pool or, conversely, block the shift and result in increases in the extracellular potassium concentration (Fig. 9.3). Acidosis associated with inorganic anions, such as NH_4Cl or HCl, is associated with hyperkalemia, but the mechanism is not fully understood. In contrast, with organic acidosis (such as lactic acidosis), there is minimal cellular shift of potassium.

Distribution of total body potassium in organs and body compartments			
Organs and Compartments		Body Compartment Concentrations	
Muscle	2650 mmol	Intracellular concentration	150 mmol/l
Liver	250 mmol	Extracellular concentration	4 mmol/l
Interstitial fluid	35 mmol		
Red blood cells	35 mmol		
Plasma	15 mmol		

Figure 9.2 Distribution of total body potassium in organs and body compartments.

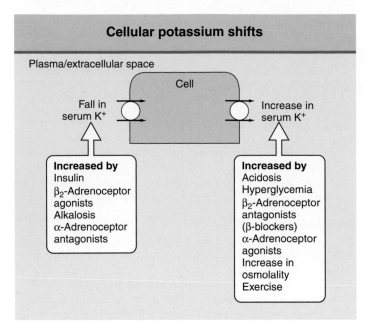

Figure 9.3 Regulation of extracellular/intracellular potassium shifts.

Insulin and β_2-adrenergic receptor activation stimulate Na$^+$-K$^+$-ATPase and, as a result, increase cellular potassium uptake. Insulin directly stimulates the Na$^+$-K$^+$-ATPase pump; this effect is independent of its stimulation of glucose entry. β_2-Adrenergic

receptor activation stimulates Na$^+$-K$^+$-ATPase–mediated potassium uptake. α-Adrenergic activation opposes the effect of β_2-adrenergic receptor stimulation. The effects of insulin and β_2-adrenergic receptor activation are synergistic, as expected, given the differing cellular mechanisms.

Aldosterone lowers serum potassium by two complementary mechanisms. First, aldosterone stimulates cellular potassium uptake due to increased Na$^+$-K$^+$-ATPase activity. Second, aldosterone potentiates potassium excretion by the kidneys and, to a lesser extent, by the gastrointestinal tract.

Changes in plasma osmolality, particularly if acute, can cause cellular potassium shifts. Hyperosmolality results in water movement out of the cells together with a mass movement of potassium; this results in hyperkalemia. In patients with diabetes mellitus, increased plasma glucose levels can increase plasma potassium due to the glucose-induced increase in extracellular osmolality.

Exercise may result in hyperkalemia due to α-adrenergic receptor activation that inhibits Na$^+$-K$^+$-ATPase and results in potassium shifts out of the skeletal muscle cells. The increased serum potassium induces arterial dilation, which increases skeletal muscle blood flow and acts as an adaptive mechanism during exercise. Simultaneous β_2-adrenergic receptor activation stimulates skeletal muscle cellular potassium uptake and minimizes the severity of exercise-induced hyperkalemia, but this can lead to hypokalemia after the cessation of exercise.[1] In patients with pre-existent potassium depletion, postexercise hypokalemia may be severe and rhabdomyolysis may occur.[2]

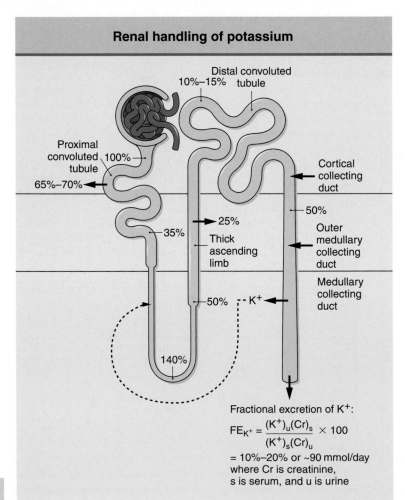

Figure 9.4 Renal handling of potassium.

Renal Potassium Handling with Normal Renal Function

Long-term potassium homeostasis is accomplished predominantly by renal potassium excretion. Potassium is nearly completely filtered by the glomerulus (Fig. 9.4). The majority of filtered potassium is reabsorbed in the proximal tubule, but the rate of reabsorption is not substantially regulated by changes in potassium intake. Potassium is secreted into the luminal fluid of the descending loop of Henle, at least in deep nephrons, and is reabsorbed in the thick ascending loop of Henle by the apical Na^+-K^+-$2Cl^-$ cotransporter (Fig. 9.5a). Because the apical membrane of the thick ascending loop of Henle also secretes potassium via potassium channels, notably Kir 1.1 (ROM potassium channel), modest net potassium reabsorption occurs under normal conditions. However, this can change to net secretion by administration of a loop diuretic or in response to potassium loading. Nevertheless, physiologic conditions do not substantially change loop of Henle net potassium transport. Instead, changes in net potassium secretion and reabsorption in the distal nephron and the collecting duct are the major sites by which the kidney regulates urinary potassium excretion.

Net potassium transport in the collecting duct occurs through distinct cell types that allow fine control of renal potassium excretion. The principal cell of the cortical collecting duct secretes potassium and the intercalated cell reabsorbs potassium (see Fig. 9.5b).

In the principal cell, potassium secretion is coupled to sodium reabsorption. Sodium reabsorption through an apical sodium

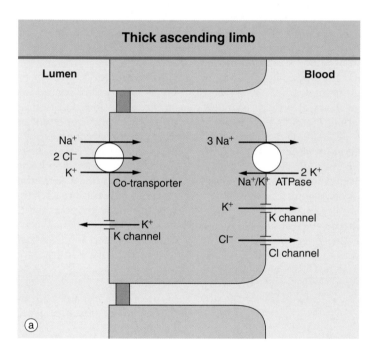

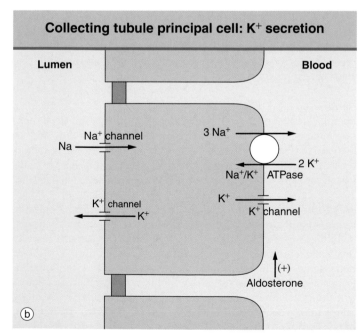

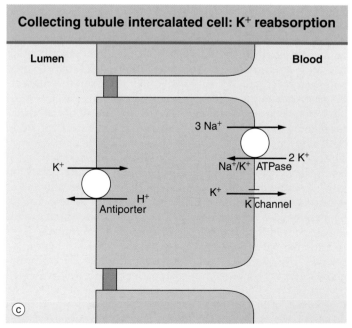

Figure 9.5   A–C, Mechanisms of potassium reabsorption and secretion in the thick ascending limb and the collecting tubule principal and intercalated cells.

channel stimulates basolateral Na^+-K^+-ATPase, and the active turnover of this pump maintains high intracellular potassium concentrations. Potassium is then secreted through apical potassium channels and an apical KCl cotransporter.

Several factors regulate potassium secretion by principal cells. These are, in relative order of importance, luminal flow rate and distal sodium delivery, aldosterone, and extracellular potassium and extracellular pH. An increase in the luminal flow rate reduces luminal potassium concentration, thereby increasing the concentration gradient across the apical membrane, which stimulates potassium secretion. In addition, flow rate directly influences cellular potassium secretion, possibly by modulating the activity of potassium channels through activation of an apical cilia present on principal cells.[3] Conversely, reduced luminal flow, as may occur in prerenal azotemia and obstruction, decreases potassium secretion, and promotes hyperkalemia. Similarly, decreased apical sodium reabsorption from reduced luminal sodium delivery decreases potassium secretion. Potassium-sparing diuretics inhibit sodium reabsorption by blocking apical sodium channels, and thereby inhibit potassium secretion. Conversely, aldosterone increases Na^+-K^+-ATPase expression and stimulates insertion of apical sodium channels, thereby stimulating potassium secretion. Increasing extracellular potassium directly stimulates Na^+-K^+-ATPase activity, which leads to increased potassium secretion. Metabolic acidosis decreases potassium secretion, both through direct effects on potassium channels and through changes in interstitial ammonia concentration, which then decreases potassium secretion.[4]

Collecting duct potassium reabsorption occurs via intercalated cells (see Fig. 9.5c). Intercalated cells reabsorb potassium via an apical H^+-K^+-ATPase that actively secretes H^+ into the luminal fluid in exchange for potassium reabsorption.[5] This active potassium reabsorption by H^+-K^+-ATPase enables urinary potassium excretion to decrease to as little as 15 mmol/day. Metabolic acidosis can also increase H^+-K^+-ATPase, thereby contributing to hyperkalemia.[6]

Renal Potassium Handling in the Face of Chronic Renal Failure

Potassium homeostasis is relatively well preserved, and serum potassium usually remains normal until the glomerular filtration rate is severely reduced. This adaptation is due to increased potassium excretion per nephron, which occurs in the connecting segment and the collecting duct. Increases in gastrointestinal tract potassium excretion also occur and contribute to maintenance of a relatively normal serum potassium concentration. Both aldosterone and subclinical serum potassium increases may contribute to this adaptation. However, patients with renal insufficiency have more difficulty handling an acute potassium load. In patients with baseline hyperkalemia, the amount of potassium that can be distributed into cells in response to hyperkalemia is limited, and such individuals also often exhibit impairment in the maximal rate of potassium excretion.

Patients with chronic kidney disease (CKD) appear to tolerate hyperkalemia with fewer cardiac and electrocardiographic (ECG) abnormalities than patients with well-preserved or normal renal function who experience acute renal failure. The mechanism of this adaptation is incompletely understood. Nevertheless, severe hyperkalemia (serum K^+ >6 mmol/l and/or ECG changes) can have lethal effects and should be aggressively treated.

HYPOKALEMIA

Epidemiology
The incidence of potassium disorders is strongly dependent on the patient population. Less than 1% of normal adults not receiving medicines develop hypokalemia or hyperkalemia; however, a diet with a high sodium and a low potassium content can cause potassium depletion. Thus, hypokalemia generally suggests either an underlying renal or endocrine disorder or effects related to medications.

Clinical Manifestations
Potassium deficiency alters the function of several organs, most prominently, the heart and blood vessels, nerves, muscles, and kidneys. Overall, children and young adults tolerate hypokalemia better than the elderly. Prompt correction is warranted in the presence of ischemic heart disease or in patients receiving digoxin.

Cardiovascular
Hypokalemia is associated with multiple aspects of cardiovascular disease. A low-potassium diet is associated with an increased prevalence of hypertension. Experimentally, hypokalemia increases blood pressure by 5 to 10 mm Hg, and potassium supplementation lowers blood pressure.[7] Potassium deficiency probably increases blood pressure both by stimulating sodium retention, leading to intravascular volume expansion, and by increasing vascular reactivity and can lead to renal injury, salt-sensitive hypertension, and activation of the renin angiotensin system.[7,8] Hypokalemia also increases the risk of ventricular arrhythmias and can lead to an increased risk of sudden cardiac death, particularly in patients who are receiving digoxin.[9]

Hormonal
Hypokalemia impairs both insulin release and tissue sensitivity to insulin, resulting in worsened glucose control in diabetic patients.[10]

Muscular
Hypokalemia hyperpolarizes skeletal muscle cells, thereby impairing muscle contraction. Hypokalemia also reduces skeletal muscle blood flow, possibly by impairing local nitric oxide release, which can predispose patients to rhabdomyolysis during vigorous exercise.[11]

Renal
Hypokalemia leads to several important disturbances of renal function. These include a reduction in medullary blood flow and an increase in renal vascular resistance that may predispose to hypertension, tubulointerstitial and cystic changes, alterations in acid-base balance, and impairment of renal concentrating mechanisms.

Tubulointerstitial and Cystic Changes Potassium depletion causes tubulointerstitial fibrosis through multiple mechanisms, including angiotensin II and endothelin.[12,13] Although usually reversible, chronic hypokalemia can cause renal failure. Potassium depletion also stimulates intrarenal vasoconstrictors (endothelin, local angiotensin II formation) and inhibits intrarenal vasodilators (including kallikrein, nitric oxide, and prostaglandins); these alterations may account for the renal structural changes.[8] In addition, hypokalemia predisposes to renal cyst formation. This finding is accentuated with concomitant hyperaldosteronism and may signal impaired renal function.[14]

Acid Base Metabolic alkalosis is a common consequence of potassium depletion and is due to increased renal net acid excretion. Conversely, metabolic alkalosis may increase renal potassium excretion, resulting in potassium depletion. Severe hypokalemia can lead to respiratory muscle weakness and the development of respiratory acidosis.

Polyuria Severe hypokalemia impairs renal concentrating ability and causes mild polyuria, ~2 to 3 liters/day. Both increased thirst and mild nephrogenic diabetes insipidus contribute to the polyuria.[15] The nephrogenic diabetes insipidus may be due to decreased expression of the collecting duct water channel aquaporin-2.[16]

Hepatic Encephalopathy

Hypokalemia increases renal ammonia production, approximately half of which returns to the systemic circulation via the renal veins. The resulting increase in serum ammonia may worsen hepatic encephalopathy.[17]

Etiology

There are four causes of hypokalemia: pseudohypokalemia, redistribution, extrarenal potassium loss, and renal potassium loss.

Pseudohypokalemia

Large numbers of abnormal white blood cells, such as with acute myeloblastic leukemia, can take up extracellular potassium if blood is stored for prolonged periods at room temperature before the potassium concentration is assayed. This may result in an artificially reduced potassium concentration or pseudohypokalemia. Either rapid separation of the plasma or storing the sample at 4°C can confirm this diagnosis and can enable the clinician to avoid inappropriate treatment.

Redistribution

More than 98% total body potassium is present in the intracellular fluid; movement of relatively small amounts of potassium from the extracellular to the intracellular fluid compartment can alter the extracellular concentration markedly. As discussed previously, many hormones, particularly insulin, aldosterone, and β_2-adrenergic agonists, stimulate transcellular potassium uptake.

Rarely, hypokalemia is due to hypokalemic periodic paralysis.[18] Attacks frequently occur during the night or the early morning or after a carbohydrate-rich meal and are characterized by flaccid paralysis. Genetic abnormalities in a dihydropyridine-sensitive calcium channel underlie some cases.[19]

Nonrenal Potassium Loss

Both the skin and the gastrointestinal tract excrete potassium. Under normal conditions, fluid loss from these organs is small, limiting net potassium loss. Occasionally, excessive sweating or chronic diarrhea can cause substantial potassium loss.[20] Vomiting or nasogastric suction may also result in potassium losses, usually about 5 to 8 mmol/l of gastric contents. These conditions also can lead to increased urinary potassium loss resulting from metabolic alkalosis and secondary hyperaldosteronism.[20]

Renal Potassium Loss

The most common cause of hypokalemia is renal potassium loss. This can occur either because of drugs, endogenous hormone production, or, in rare conditions, intrinsic renal defects.

Drugs Both thiazide and loop diuretics increase urinary potassium excretion, and the incidence of diuretic-induced hypokalemia is both dose and treatment duration related. When adjusted for their natriuretic effect, thiazide diuretics cause more urinary potassium loss than loop diuretics. Certain antibiotics increase urinary potassium excretion. Some penicillin analogues, such as carbenicillin, increase distal tubular delivery of a nonreabsorbable anion, which obligates the presence of a cation such as potassium, thereby increasing urinary potassium excretion.[21] Amphotericin B increases collecting duct potassium secretion; this may occur either with or without simultaneous nephrotoxicity.[22] Cisplatin is a commonly used medication that can induce hypokalemia.[23] Toluene exposure, from sniffing certain glues, can also cause renal tubular acidosis with renal potassium wasting leading to hypokalemia.[24]

Endogenous Hormones Endogenous hormones are important and common causes of hypokalemia. Aldosterone is the most important hormone regulating total body potassium homeostasis and causes hypokalemia both by stimulating potassium uptake into cells and by stimulating renal potassium excretion. Rarely, genetic defects lead to excessive aldosterone production. These include glucocorticoid-remediable aldosteronism, congenital adrenal hyperplasia, and conditions in which glucocorticoid hormones activate the mineralocorticoid receptor (see Chapter 46).

Magnesium Depletion Magnesium deficiency inhibits the kidney's ability to retain potassium and should be suspected if potassium replacement does not correct hypokalemia.[25] This most commonly occurs with diuretic-, aminoglycoside-, and cisplatin-induced hypokalemia.

Intrinsic Renal Defect Intrinsic renal potassium transport defects leading to hypokalemia with alkalosis are rare and include Bartter, Gitelman's, and Liddle syndromes (see Chapter 46).

Bicarbonaturia Bicarbonaturia can result from metabolic alkalosis, distal renal tubular acidosis, or treatment of proximal renal tubular acidosis. In each case, the increased distal tubular bicarbonate delivery increases potassium secretion.

Diagnosis

The evaluation of hypokalemia is summarized in Figure 9.6. One should first rule out pseudohypokalemia or redistribution of potassium from the extracellular to the intracellular space. Insulin, aldosterone or its synthetic analogue fludrocortisone, and sympathomimetic agents, such as theophylline or β_2-adrenergic receptor agonists, are common causes of potassium redistribution.

If neither of these possibilities is present, then the hypokalemia probably represents total body potassium depletion due to renal, gastrointestinal, or skin loss. Renal potassium loss is most frequently due to diuretics, in which secondary hyperaldosteronism is a common contributing cause. High dietary NaCl ingestion worsens renal potassium wasting. Hypomagnesemia frequently complicates diuretic usage and can cause renal potassium wasting. Rarer causes include renal tubular acidosis, diabetic ketoacidosis, and ureterosigmoidostomy. Primary aldosteronism should be considered in the hypertensive patient. Surreptitious diuretic use, vomiting, and Bartter or Gitelman's syndrome should be considered when the cause of the hypokalemia is not obvious and the patient is either normotensive or hypotensive. Finally, excessive potassium loss may result via the skin (excessive sweating) or from diarrhea, vomiting, nasogastric

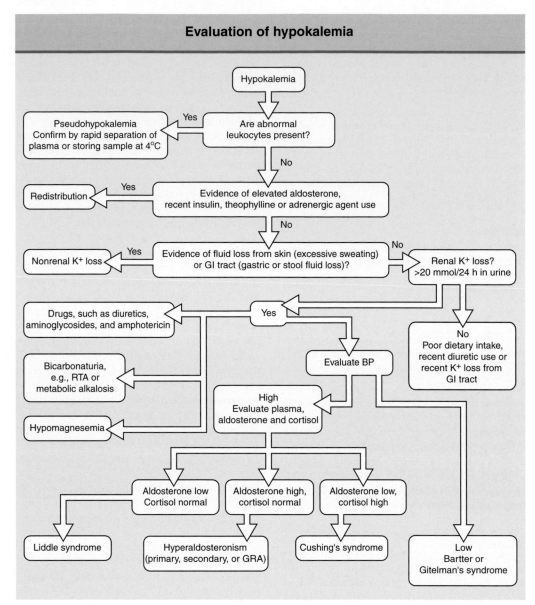

Figure 9.6 **Diagnostic evaluation of hypokalemia.** BP, blood pressure; GI, gastrointestinal; GRA, glucose remediable aldosteronism; RTA, renal tubular acidosis.

suction, or a gastrointestinal fistula. Occasionally, patients are reluctant to admit to self-induced diarrhea, and the diagnosis may need to be confirmed by sigmoidoscopy or direct testing of the stool for cathartic agents.

Treatment

The risks associated with hypokalemia must be balanced against the risks of therapy. Usually, the primary short-term risks are cardiovascular and neuromuscular. In contrast, the primary risk of overaggressive replacement is acute hyperkalemia, with resultant ventricular fibrillation.

Conditions in which hypokalemia requires emergency therapy are rare. The clearest indications are hypokalemic periodic paralysis, severe hypokalemia in a patient requiring emergent surgery, and the patient with an acute myocardial infarction and life-threatening ventricular ectopy. In such cases, administration of 5 to 10 mmol of KCl intravenously over 15 to 20 minutes may be used and can be repeated every 30 minutes until the paralysis or arrhythmias resolve or until the serum potassium is greater

than 3.5 mmol/l. Close monitoring of the serum potassium and ECG changes are necessary to avoid hyperkalemia.

The body responds to chronic hypokalemia due to potassium losses by shifting potassium from the intracellular to the extracellular space. This minimizes the change in the serum potassium. Figure 9.7 summarizes the expected total body potassium depletion that occurs in chronic hypokalemia and illustrates that the total amount of potassium needed to correct hypokalemia may be quite large.

In most conditions, the choice of parenteral versus oral therapy depends on the ability of the patient to take oral medication and the functional integrity of the gastrointestinal tract. If the patient is unable to take oral potassium safely or if gastrointestinal tract absorption is impaired, then intravenous potassium should be administered. Intravenous potassium can be given safely at a rate of 10 mmol/h. Although significant variations can occur between patients, 20 mmol of KCl typically increases the serum potassium by ~0.25 mmol/l.[26] If more rapid replacement is necessary, 20 to 40 mmol/h can be administered through a central venous

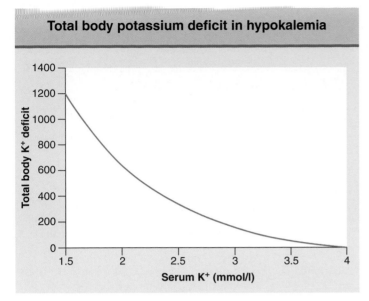

Figure 9.7 Total body potassium deficit in hypokalemia. Because of shift of potassium from the intracellular to the extracellular fluid compartment during chronic potassium depletion, the magnitude of deficiency can be masked and is generally much larger than would be calculated solely from the change in plasma potassium and the extracellular fluid volume.

catheter; simultaneous continuous ECG monitoring should be used to enable early recognition of cardiac effects of potassium.

The parenteral fluids used for potassium administration can affect the response. In patients without diabetes mellitus, dextrose administration increases serum insulin, which stimulates cellular potassium uptake. As a result, if KCl is administered in dextrose-containing solutions, the resulting increase in cellular potassium uptake may exceed the KCl replacement rate and may worsen the hypokalemia.[27]

The risk of hyperkalemia due to potassium replacement is lower with oral potassium. This probably reflects several factors, most prominently hepatic potassium uptake, which minimizes changes in serum potassium levels.

The underlying condition should be treated whenever possible. Patients with diuretic-induced hypokalemia should be re-evaluated to reconsider the need for diuretics. If their use is required, concomitant use of potassium-sparing diuretics may be helpful. Dietary NaCl restriction minimizes diuretic-induced hypokalemia. If indicated for other reasons, β-blockers, angiotensin-converting enzyme inhibitors, and angiotensin receptor blockers can assist in maintaining potassium levels.

Hypomagnesemia can lead to refractoriness to potassium replacement.[25] Correction of the hypokalemia may not occur until the hypomagnesemia is corrected. Patients with unexplained hypokalemia or with diuretic-induced hypokalemia should have their serum magnesium checked and replacement therapy (such as 1 g intramuscularly daily for 3 days) begun, if indicated.

HYPERKALEMIA

Epidemiology
Less than 1% of healthy adults develop hyperkalemia. This low frequency is a testament to the potent mechanisms that can increase renal potassium excretion. Accordingly, chronic hyperkalemia suggests impaired renal potassium excretion. Rarely, pseudohyperkalemia or conditions that shift potassium from the intracellular space to the extracellular space are present.

Clinical Manifestations
Manifestations of hyperkalemia range from asymptomatic to life threatening. The most prominent effect is on the cardiac conduction system. This is demonstrable on electrocardiography (Fig. 9.8, and see Fig. 65.5). The initial effect is a generalized, symmetric increase in T-wave height, known as tenting. More severe hyperkalemia is associated with delayed electrical conduction, resulting in increased PR and QRS intervals. This is followed by progressive flattening and eventual absence of the P waves. Under extreme conditions, the QRS complex widens sufficiently that it merges with the T wave, resulting in a sine-wave pattern. Finally, ventricular asystole or fibrillation can develop. Although a general correlation between the ECG findings and the degree of hyperkalemia is often observed, the ECG progression can be unpredictable.

Hyperkalemia also affects cellular muscular contraction. Skeletal muscle cells are particularly sensitive to hyperkalemia; accordingly, hyperkalemia may cause weakness. With severe hyperkalemia, respiratory failure may occur from paralysis of the diaphragm. Patients with end-stage renal disease may experience perioral paresthesias or "rubbery legs."

Etiology
Hyperkalemia can be due to pseudohyperkalemia, redistribution of potassium from the intracellular to the extracellular space, or imbalances between potassium intake and renal potassium excretion. A diagnostic approach is shown in Figure 9.9.

Pseudohyperkalemia
Serum potassium concentration may be artificially increased due to potassium release from erythrocytes due to hemolysis during the collection process or from release during the clotting process.

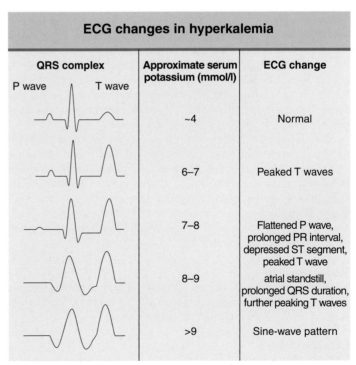

ECG changes in hyperkalemia

QRS complex	Approximate serum potassium (mmol/l)	ECG change
P wave / T wave	~4	Normal
	6–7	Peaked T waves
	7–8	Flattened P wave, prolonged PR interval, depressed ST segment, peaked T wave
	8–9	atrial standstill, prolonged QRS duration, further peaking T waves
	>9	Sine-wave pattern

Figure 9.8 Electrocardiographic (ECG) changes in hyperkalemia. Progressive hyperkalemia results in identifiable ECG changes. These include peaking of the T wave, flattening of the P wave, prolongation of the PR interval, ST segment depression, prolongation of the QRS complex, and, eventually, progression to a sine-wave pattern. Ventricular fibrillation may occur at any time during this progression.

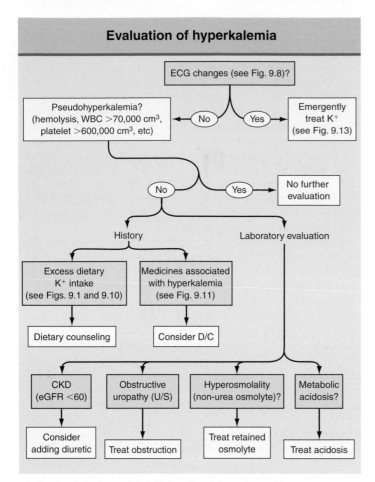

Figure 9.9   Evaluation of hyperkalemia.

Potassium content of common enteral products

	Calories/ml	Potassium (mmol/l)	Sodium (mmol/l)	Osmolality (mOsm/kg)
Ensure	1.06	40	37	470
Ensure Plus	1.50	54	49	690
Glucerna	1.00	40	40	375
Osmolyte	1.06	26	27	300
Pulmocare	1.50	49	57	490
Suplena	2.00	29	34	615
Ultracal	1.06	41	41	310
Vivonex TEN	1.00	20	20	630

Figure 9.10   Potassium content of common enteral products.

Common sources of dietary potassium excess include potassium supplements, salt substitutes, enteral nutrition products, and common foods. As many as 4% of patients receiving potassium supplements develop hyperkalemia. Typical salt substitutes contain 10 to 13 mmol potassium per gram or 283 mmol per tablespoon.[29] Many enteral nutrition products contain 40 mmol/l KCl or more; administration of 100 ml/h provides ~100 mmol/day of KCl (Fig. 9.10). Finally, many food products are particularly high in potassium, and many pharmacies routinely label diuretic medicine bottles with suggestions for the patient to increase potassium intake from dietary sources, such as fresh fruits, particularly bananas. Figure 9.1 summarizes the potassium content of common foods with high potassium.

Impaired Renal Potassium Secretion

The normal kidney possesses a remarkable ability to excrete potassium, so chronic hyperkalemia almost always involves impaired renal potassium excretion. This is particularly important to consider in the elderly because the decreased muscle mass may cause the serum creatinine level to be normal or only slightly elevated despite advanced renal insufficiency. Many commonly used medications impair renal potassium excretion and are discussed in more detail. Obstructive uropathy can lead to hyperkalemia; the hyperkalemia may occur either with or without associated metabolic acidosis. Mineralocorticoid resistance frequently is present; whether this is a receptor deficiency or is related to the interstitial nephritis that occurs is unclear. In many cases, the hyperkalemia may persist for weeks following relief of the obstruction.

Specific Drugs   The renin angiotensin aldosterone system (RAAS) is the primary hormonal system regulating renal potassium excretion. Accordingly, drugs that interfere with this system or that inhibit the cellular mechanisms of renal potassium excretion are frequent causes of hyperkalemia. Classes of medications that inhibit the RAAS are summarized in Figure 9.11.

Prostaglandins increase renal potassium secretion by stimulating renin release and are necessary for collecting duct potassium secretion. Both nonsteroidal anti-inflammatory drugs and cyclooxygenase-2 inhibitors block prostaglandin formation and can cause hyperkalemia. Potassium-sparing diuretics, such as amiloride and triamterene, block the epithelial sodium channel and lead to hyperkalemia by decreasing urinary potassium excretion. The antibiotics trimethoprim and pentamidine have identical effects and can cause hyperkalemia, particularly in the elderly or when used at high doses, such as for *Pneumocystis carinii* pneumonia.[30,31]

This is termed pseudohyperkalemia. Severe leukocytosis (>70,000/cm³) or thrombocytosis (>500,000/cm³) can cause pseudohyperkalemia. Ischemia, from prolonged tourniquet time or limb exercise in the presence of a tourniquet, can lead to pseudohyperkalemia. Rarely, pseudohyperkalemia may occur as a result of rheumatoid arthritis or infectious mononucleosis, and some families have abnormal red blood cell membrane potassium permeability.

Pseudohyperkalemia is diagnosed either when the hyperkalemia is corrected when phlebotomy is performed without a tourniquet and without limb exercise or by showing that the potassium concentration in a serum sample is more than 0.3 mmol/l greater than in a plasma sample obtained simultaneously. Pseudohyperkalemia does not require treatment other than identifying the condition and avoiding inappropriate use of potassium-lowering treatments.

Redistribution

Hyperkalemia may occur as a result of severe hyperglycemia (due to effects of osmolarity), with severe acidosis due to nonorganic acids or with the use of β-blockers.

Excessive Intake

Excessive potassium ingestion rarely causes hyperkalemia if renal function is normal. Under normal conditions, the kidney can excrete hundreds of millimoles of potassium daily.[28] However, if renal potassium excretion is impaired, whether by medications, renal insufficiency, or other causes, excessive potassium intake can contribute to hyperkalemia.

Medications associated with hyperkalemia		
Class	Mechanism	Example
Potassium-containing drug	Increased potassium intake	KCl, penicillin G, potassium citrate
β-adrenergic receptor blocker	Inhibit renin release	Propranolol, metoprolol, atenolol
ACE-I	Inhibit conversion of angiotensin I to angiotensin II	Captopril, lisinopril, etc.
Angiotensin receptor blocker	Inhibit activation of angiotensin I receptor by angiotensin II	Losartan, irbesartan, etc.
Heparin	Inhibit aldosterone synthase, rate–limiting enzyme for aldosterone synthesis	Heparin sodium
Aldosterone receptor antagonist	Block aldosterone receptor activation	Spironolactone, eplerenone
Potassium-sparing diuretic	Block collecting duct apical sodium channel, decreasing gradient for potassium secretion	Amiloride, triamterene, certain antibiotics, specifically trimethoprim and pentamidine
NSAID and COX-2 inhibitor	Inhibit prostaglandin stimulation of collecting duct potassium secretion, inhibits renin release	Ibuprofen
Digitalis glycoside	Inhibit Na^+-K^+-ATPase necessary for collecting duct potassium secretion	Digoxin
Calcineurin inhibitor	Inhibit Na^+-K^+-ATPase necessary for collecting duct potassium secretion	Cyclosporine, tacrolimus

Figure 9.11 Medications associated with hyperkalemia. ACE-I, angiotensin-converting enzyme inhibitor; COX-2, cyclooxygenase-2; NSAID, nonsteroidal anti-inflammatory drug.

Digoxin inhibits the principal cell basolateral Na^+-K^+-ATPase, thereby inhibiting cellular potassium uptake. Hyperkalemia may occur in predisposed patients, such as those with renal failure, even in the absence of toxic levels.[32]

The immunosuppressive drugs cyclosporine and tacrolimus can cause hyperkalemia by inhibiting distal nephron potassium secretion.[33]

Heparin can cause hyperkalemia in susceptible individuals, particularly those with CKD. The primary mechanism appears to be inhibition of aldosterone production. This can occur with both unfractionated (conventional) and fractionated (low molecular weight) heparin and is dose dependent and reversible if the heparin is discontinued.[34] Heparin-associated hyperkalemia is typically moderate and rarely life threatening.

Certain agents that can depolarize skeletal muscle, such as succinylcholine, or that activate potassium-dependent amino acid exchangers, such as lysine or arginine, also can lead to hyperkalemia.

Distinguishing Renal and Nonrenal Mechanisms of Hyperkalemia

In most circumstances, a 24-hour urine K^+ excretion rate will distinguish renal (K^+ <20 mmol/l) from extrarenal (K^+ >40 mmol/l) causes of hyperkalemia. Furthermore, in patients with a low urinary K^+ excretion, administration of fludrocortisone may be used to distinguish aldosterone deficiency (urine K^+ increases to >40 mmol/l) from aldosterone resistance (K^+ remains <20 mmol/l). However, urinary K^+ measurements may be difficult to interpret since K^+ excretion depends on multiple factors, including glomerular filtration rate, tubular lumen flow, diuretic use, and water reabsorption in the distal tubule. As a result, calculation of the transtubular K^+ gradient may be helpful (Fig. 9.12). The transtubular K^+ gradient corrects the urinary K^+ for changes in osmolality that occur with water reabsorption in the collecting duct and provides indirect measurement of net K^+ secretion in the distal nephron. A value less than 5 to 7 in the setting of hyperkalemia implies either

Transtubular potassium gradient	
TTKG is a measurement of net K^+ secretion by the distal nephron after correcting for changes in urinary osmolality and is often used to determine whether hyperkalemia is caused by aldosterone deficiency/resistance or whether the hyperkalemia is secondary to nonrenal causes. TTKG = $(K_u/K_s) \times (S_{osm}/U_{osm})$, where K_u and K_s are the concentration of K^+ in urine and serum, respectively, and U_{osm} and S_{osm} are the osmolalities of urine and serum, respectively.	
TTKG Value	Indication
6–12	Normal
>10	Suggests normal aldosterone action and an extrarenal cause of hyperkalemia
<5–7	Suggests aldosterone deficiency or resistance
After 0.05 mg 9α-fludrocortisone	
>10	Hypoaldosteronism is likely
No change	Suggests a renal tubule defect from either K^+-sparing diuretics (amiloride, triamterene, spironolactone), aldosterone resistance (interstitial renal disease, sickle cell disease, urinary tract obstruction, pseudohypoaldosteronism type I), or increased distal K^+ reabsorption (pseudohypoaldosteronism type II, urinary tract obstruction)

Figure 9.12 Transtubular potassium gradient (TTKG).

Treatment of hyperkalemia				
Mechanism	Therapy	Dose	Onset	Duration
Antagonize membrane effects	Calcium	Calcium gluconate, 10% solution, 10 ml IV over 10 min	1–3 min	30–60 min
Stimulate cellular potassium uptake	Insulin	Regular insulin, 10 U IV, with dextrose, 50%, 50 ml if plasma glucose <250 mg/dl	30 min	4–6 h
	β_2-adrenergic agonist	Nebulized albuterol, 10 mg	30 min	2–4 h
Potassium removal	Sodium polystyrene sulfonate	Kayexalate, 60 g PO, in 20% sorbitol, or 60 g in 250 ml water, per retention enema	1–2 h	4–6 h
	Hemodialysis	—	Immediate	Until dialysis completed

Figure 9.13   Treatment of hyperkalemia.

aldosterone deficiency or resistance, whereas a value greater than 10 suggests excessive K^+ intake and normal distal nephron K^+ handling. In all cases, an accurate estimate of potassium intake is necessary to properly interpret the clinical situation.

Treatment

Therapies for hyperkalemia can be divided into those that block the cardiac effects of hyperkalemia, those that induce cellular potassium uptake, and those that remove potassium from the body. Figure 9.13 summarizes the available treatments and their mechanisms of action, times of onset of action, and durations of action.

Treatment of hyperkalemia should not include $NaHCO_3$ unless the patient is frankly acidotic (pH <7.2) or unless substantial endogenous renal function is present. $NaHCO_3$ therapy can cause volume overload related to the sodium load and has little benefit in patients without endogenous renal function[35]; hypertonic ampules of $NaHCO_3$ can also lead to acute hypernatremia.

Blocking Cardiac Effects

Intravenous calcium administration specifically antagonizes the effects of hyperkalemia on the myocardial conduction system and on myocardial repolarization. Calcium is the most rapid way to treat hyperkalemia and should be given intravenously if unambiguous ECG changes of hyperkalemia are present. Patients with prolonged PR intervals, widened QRS complexes, or absence of P waves should receive intravenous calcium without delay. Effects occur within 1 to 3 minutes and last for 30 to 60 minutes. The dose may be repeated within 5 to 10 minutes if ECG changes persist. If a delay in the institution of dialysis is anticipated, a continuous calcium infusion should be considered.

There are several precautions to observe with intravenous calcium. First, $NaHCO_3$-containing solutions should not be used, because $CaCO_3$ precipitation can occur. Second, hypercalcemia, which occurs during rapid calcium infusion, may potentiate digoxin-related myocardial toxicity. Hyperkalemic patients taking digoxin should be given calcium as a slow infusion over 20 to 30 minutes.

Cellular Potassium Uptake

The second most rapid way to treat hyperkalemia is to stimulate cellular potassium uptake, with either insulin or β_2-adrenergic agonist administration. Insulin rapidly stimulates cellular potassium uptake and should be administered intravenously to ensure predictable bioavailability. Effects on serum potassium are seen generally within 10 to 20 minutes and last for 4 to 6 hours. Glucose is generally coadministered to avoid hypoglycemia, but may not be needed if hyperglycemia coexists. Hyperglycemia in patients with diabetes mellitus can increase serum potassium. If a

delay in instituting dialysis is anticipated, it may be wise to administer a continuous infusion of insulin (4 to 10 U/h) with 10% dextrose and periodically monitor serum glucose and potassium.

β_2-Adrenergic receptor agonists directly stimulate cellular potassium uptake. Intravenous albuterol, 0.5 mg, rapidly increases potassium uptake and can decrease serum potassium by ~1 mmol/l,[36] but is not approved for intravenous use in the United States. Nebulized albuterol, at a dose of 10 or 20 mg, decreases serum potassium by ~0.6 or ~1 mmol/l, respectively, with a rapid onset of action and maximal effect at 90 to 120 minutes.[37] However, β_2-agonist therapy is limited frequently by tachycardia, and as many as 25% of patients do not respond when β_2-agonists are given by nebulizer.[37] A frequent mistake when administering nebulized albuterol is underdosing; the dose for treating hyperkalemia is two to eight times greater than the bronchodilator dose given by nebulizers and is 50 to 100 times greater than that administered by metered-dose inhalers. In severe hyperkalemia, combined therapy with insulin and albuterol may be more effective than either alone.[38]

Potassium Removal

Most cases of severe hyperkalemia are associated with increased total body potassium content. Definitive treatment requires potassium removal.

In selected cases, increasing renal potassium elimination may be adequate. With chronic or mild hyperkalemia, loop or thiazide diuretics increase renal potassium excretion and may be sufficient for therapy. In particular, loop or thiazide diuretics may be the therapy of choice for hyperkalemic renal tubular acidosis.[39] While synthetic mineralocorticoids, such as fludrocortisone, stimulate renal potassium excretion, the accompanying sodium retention and intravascular volume expansion limit their usefulness. Also, mineralocorticoids may contribute to the progression of CKD. Acute hyperkalemia with ECG changes should generally not be treated solely with diuretics because the rate of potassium excretion may not be adequate. Also, most patients with hyperkalemia have underlying renal insufficiency, which limits the acute effectiveness of diuretic therapy. If a rapidly reversible cause of renal failure is identified, such as obstructive uropathy and prerenal azotemia, then treatment of the underlying condition with close observation may be adequate.

A second mode of potassium elimination is with potassium-exchange resins, such as sodium polystyrene sulfonate and calcium resonium. In general, 30 to 60 g should be given, depending on the severity of the hyperkalemia; 1 g removes ~0.5 to 1 mmol of potassium and 60 g reduces serum potassium by ~0.5 mmol/l. It can be administered either orally or rectally as a retention enema. The rate of potassium removal is relatively slow, requiring ~4 hours for full effect, although administering it as a retention enema results in more rapid onset of action. When given orally, it is generally administered with 20% sorbitol or lactulose to avoid constipation. If given as an enema, sorbitol should be avoided because rectal administration of 20% sorbitol may lead to colonic perforation.[40]

Acute hemodialysis is the primary method of potassium removal when renal function is absent and hyperkalemia is persistent or severe. In general, the more severe the hyperkalemia is, the more rapid should be the reduction in plasma potassium. However, care should be exercised in patients with ischemic heart disease and in those predisposed to arrhythmias. If a very low potassium (0 or 1 mmol/l K$^+$) dialysate is used, then the serum potassium should be rechecked after 2 hours. In most cases, the dialysate should contain 2 mmol/l potassium. Continuous dialysis modalities, such as peritoneal dialysis and continuous venovenous hemodialysis, do not remove potassium sufficiently quickly to be used for life-threatening hyperkalemia.

Whereas dialysis is the most rapid method to treat most cases of hyperkalemia, other modes of treatment should not be delayed while waiting to institute dialysis. If dialysis is required at times other than a dialysis unit's regular hours or when hemodialysis vascular access is not already present, then there is frequently a substantial delay before beginning hemodialysis. In these conditions, other therapies should be instituted and continued until hemodialysis can be started.

Specific therapies may be quite valuable in certain causes of hyperkalemia. For example, digoxin-specific Fab fragments are beneficial for severe digitalis toxicity.[41] Patients with acute urinary tract obstruction and subsequent hyperkalemia may be effectively treated with relief of the urinary tract obstruction. Since the rate of potassium excretion in the latter condition may be variable, frequent measurement of plasma potassium is necessary.

REFERENCES

1. Williams ME, Gervino EV, RM Rosa, et al: Catecholamine modulation of rapid potassium shifts during exercise. N Engl J Med 1985;312: 823–827.
2. Aizawa H, Morita K, Minami H, et al: Exertional rhabdomyolysis as a result of strenuous military training. J Neurol Sci 1995;132:239–240.
3. Praetorius HA, Spring KR: The renal cell primary cilium functions as a flow sensor. Curr Opin Nephrol Hypertens 2003;12:517–520.
4. Hamm LL, Gillespie C, Klahr S: NH4Cl inhibition of transport in the rabbit cortical collecting tubule. Am J Physiol 1985;248:F631–F637.
5. Wingo CS, Cain BD: The renal H-K-ATPase: Physiological significance and role in potassium homeostasis. Annu Rev Physiol 1993;55:323–347.
6. Garg LC, Komatsu Y: In vitro and in vivo effects of ammonium chloride on H-K-ATPase activity in the outer medullary collecting duct. Contrib Nephrol 1994;110:67–74.
7. Barri YM, Wingo CS: The effects of potassium depletion and supplementation on blood pressure: A clinical review. Am J Med Sci 1997; 314:37–40.
8. Ray PE, Suga S, Liu XH, et al: Chronic potassium depletion induces renal injury, salt sensitivity, and hypertension in young rats. Kidney Int 2001;59:1850–1858.
9. Siscovick DS, Raghunathan TE, Psaty BM, et al: Diuretic therapy for hypertension and the risk of primary cardiac arrest. N Engl J Med 1994; 330:1852–1857.
10. Knochel JP: Diuretic-induced hypokalemia. Am J Med 1984;77:18–27.
11. Singhal PC, Abramovici M, Venkatesan J, Mattana J: Hypokalemia and rhabdomyolysis. Miner Electrolyte Metab 1991;17:335–339.
12. Suga S, Yasui N, Yoshihara F, et al: Endothelin a receptor blockade and endothelin B receptor blockade improve hypokalemic nephropathy by different mechanisms. J Am Soc Nephrol 2003;14:397–406.
13. Suga S, Mazzali M, Ray PE, et al: Angiotensin II type 1 receptor blockade ameliorates tubulointerstitial injury induced by chronic potassium deficiency. Kidney Int 2002;61:951–958.
14. Ogasawara M, Nomura K, Toraya S, et al: Clinical implications of renal cyst in primary aldosteronism. Endocr J 1996;43:261–268.
15. Berl T, Linas SL, Alisenbrye GA, Anderson RJ: On the mechanism of polyuria in potassium depletion. The role of polydipsia. J Clin Invest 1977;60:620.
16. Marples D, Frokiaer J, Dorup J, et al: Hypokalemia-induced downregulation of aquaporin-2 water channel expression in rat kidney medulla and cortex. J Clin Invest 1996;97:1960–1968.
17. Gabuzda GJ, Hall II: Relation of potassium depletion to renal ammonium metabolism and hepatic coma. Medicine (Baltimore) 1966;45: 481–489.
18. Ahlawat SK, Sachdev A: Hypokalemic paralysis. Postgrad Med J 1999; 75:193–197.
19. Antes LM, Kujubu DA, Fernandez PC: Hypokalemia and the pathology of ion transport molecules. Semin Nephrol 1998;18:31–45.
20. Knochel JP, Dotin LN, Hamburger RJ: Pathophysiology of intense physical conditioning in a hot climate. I. Mechanisms of potassium depletion. J Clin Invest 1972;51:242–255.
21. Gill MA, DuBe JE, Young WW: Hypokalemic, metabolic alkalosis induced by high-dose ampicillin sodium. Am J Hosp Pharm 1977;34: 528–531.
22. O'Regan S, Carson S, Chesney RW, Drummond KN: Electrolyte and acid-base disturbances in the management of leukemia. Blood 1977;49: 345–353.
23. Kintzel PE: Anticancer drug-induced kidney disorders. Drug Saf 2001; 24:19–38.
24. Taher SM, Anderson RJ, McCartney R, et al: Renal tubular acidosis associated with toluene "sniffing." N Engl J Med 1974;290:765–768.
25. Whang R: Magnesium deficiency: Pathogenesis, prevalence, and clinical implications. Am J Med 1987;82:24–29.
26. Kruse JA, Carlson RW: Rapid correction of hypokalemia using concentrated intravenous potassium chloride infusions. Arch Intern Med 1990; 150:613–617.
27. Kunin AS, Surawicz B, Sims EA: Decrease in serum potassium concentration and appearance of cardiac arrhythmias during infusion of potassium with glucose in potassium depleted patients. N Engl J Med 1962;66:288.
28. Rabelink TJ, Koomans HA, Hene RJ, et al: Early and late adjustment to potassium loading in humans. Kidney Int 1990;38:942–947.
29. Sopko JA, Freeman RM: Salt substitutes as a source of potassium. JAMA 1977;238:608–610.
30. Velazquez H, Perazella MA, Wright FS, Ellison DH: Renal mechanism of trimethoprim-induced hyperkalemia. Ann Intern Med 1993;119: 296–301.
31. Kleyman TR, Roberts C, Ling BN: A mechanism for pentamidine-induced hyperkalemia: Inhibition of distal nephron sodium transport. Ann Intern Med 1995;122:103–106.
32. Papadakis MA, Wexman MP, Fraser C, Sedlacek SM: Hyperkalemia complicating digoxin toxicity in a patient with renal failure. Am J Kidney Dis 1985;5:64–66.
33. Tumlin JA, Sands JM: Nephron segment-specific inhibition of Na+/(K+)(ATPase) activity by cyclosporin A. Kidney Int 1993;43:246–251.
34. Oster JR, Singer I, Fishman LM: Heparin-induced aldosterone suppression and hyperkalemia. Am J Med 1995;98:575–586.
35. Allon M: Hyperkalemia in end-stage renal disease: Mechanisms and management. J Am Soc Nephrol 1995;6:1134–1142.
36. Montoliu J, Lens XM, Revert L: Potassium-lowering effect of albuterol for hyperkalemia in renal failure. Arch Intern Med 1987;147:713–717.
37. Allon M, Dunlay R, Copkney C: Nebulized albuterol for acute hyperkalemia in patients on hemodialysis. Ann Intern Med 1989;110: 426–429.
38. Allon M, Copkney C: Albuterol and insulin for treatment of hyperkalemia in hemodialysis patients. Kidney Int 1990;38:869–872.
39. Sebastian A, Schambelan M, Sutton JM: Amelioration of hyperchloremic acidosis with furosemide therapy in patients with chronic renal insufficiency and type 4 renal tubular acidosis. Am J Nephrol 1984;4:287–300.
40. Gerstman BB, Kirkman R, Platt R: Intestinal necrosis associated with postoperative orally administered sodium polystyrene sulfonate in sorbitol. Am J Kidney Dis 1992;20:159–161.
41. Smith TW, Butler VP Jr, Haber E, et al: Treatment of life-threatening digitalis intoxication with digoxin-specific Fab antibody fragments: Experience in 26 cases. N Engl J Med 1982;307:1357–1362.

Disorders of Calcium, Phosphate, and Magnesium Metabolism

Tilman B. Drüeke and Bernard Lacour

HOMEOSTASIS OF CALCIUM AND DISORDERS OF CALCIUM METABOLISM

Distribution of Calcium in the Organism and Calcium Homeostasis

Most calcium is bound and associated with bony structures (99%). Most free calcium, either in diffusible (ultrafilterable) nonionized form or in ionized form (Ca^{2+}), is found in the intra- and extracellular fluid spaces. There is a steep concentration gradient between Ca^{2+} in the intra- and extracellular milieu. Figure 10.1 shows the distribution of calcium in the extracellular and intracellular fluid compartments.

The plasma concentration of Ca^{2+} is tightly regulated. The principal regulatory hormones are parathyroid hormone (PTH) and calcitriol (1,25-dihydroxycholecalciferol). The physiologic role of other calcium regulatory hormones such as calcitonin, estrogens, and prolactin is less clear. Figures 10.2 and 10.3 shows the physiologic defense mechanisms used by the organism to counter changes of serum Ca^{2+} levels. Levels of Ca^{2+} are also influenced by acid-base status, with alkalosis causing a decrease in Ca^{2+} and acidosis having the opposite effect.

Long-term maintenance of calcium homeostasis depends on the adaptation of intestinal Ca^{2+} absorption to the needs of the organism, on the balance between bone accretion and resorption, and on urinary excretion of calcium (see Fig. 10.3).

Intestinal, Skeletal, and Renal Handling of Calcium

Transport of Ca^{2+} across the intestinal wall occurs in two directions: absorption and secretion. Absorption can be subdivided into transcellular and paracellular flow (Fig. 10.4).[1] Many factors play a role in intestinal Ca^{2+} transport. Schematically, those that enhance absorption can be distinguished from those that reduce absorption. Among the former, the daily amount of calcium ingested plays a major role (Fig. 10.5), and its bioavailability is modified by a number of factors. Vitamin D synthesized in the skin from 7-dehydrocholesterol under the influence of sunlight or absorbed from the intestinal tract is hydroxylated in the liver to 25-hydroxyvitamin D and then further hydroxylated to calcitriol in the kidney. Calcitriol is the most important hormonal regulatory factor.[2] After binding to and activating its receptor (vitamin D receptor [VDR]), it increases active transport by inducing the expression of the calcium channel TRPV6, calbindin-D_{9k}, and Ca^{2+}-ATPase (PMCA1b) (see Fig. 10.4).[3] Other hormones, including estrogens, prolactin, growth hormone, and PTH, also stimulate Ca^{2+} absorption, either directly or indirectly.

Increased calcium absorption is required in some physiologic states, such as puberty, pregnancy, and lactation. In all these states, calcitriol synthesis is increased. Intestinal Ca^{2+} absorption is increased in at least two other pathologic conditions: vitamin D excess and acromegaly. Other conditions are associated with a decrease in intestinal Ca^{2+} transport, including a low Ca^{2+} phosphate ratio in the food, a high vegetable fiber and fat content of the diet, corticosteroid treatment, estrogen deficiency, advanced age, gastrectomy, intestinal malabsorption syndromes, diabetes mellitus, and renal failure. The decrease in Ca^{2+} absorption in the elderly probably results from multiple factors in addition to lower serum calcitriol and intestinal VDR levels.[4]

The net balance between Ca^{2+} entry and exit fluxes is positive during skeletal growth in children, zero in young adults, and negative in the elderly. Exchangeable skeletal Ca^{2+} contributes to maintaining extracellular Ca^{2+} homeostasis. Several growth factors, hormones, and genetic factors participate in the differentiation from the mesenchymal precursor cell to the osteoblast and the maturation of the osteoclast from its granulocyte/macrophage precursor cell (Fig. 10.6). The regulation of bone formation and resorption involves a large number of hormones, growth factors, and mechanical factors (Fig. 10.7).[5]

Distribution of calcium in extra- and intracellular spaces

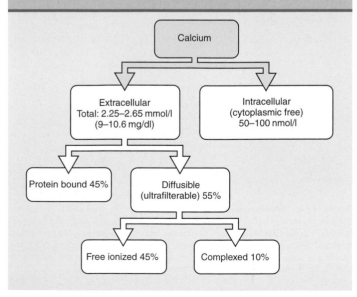

Calcium

Extracellular
Total: 2.25–2.65 mmol/l
(9–10.6 mg/dl)

Intracellular
(cytoplasmic free)
50–100 nmol/l

Protein bound 45%

Diffusible
(ultrafilterable) 55%

Free ionized 45%

Complexed 10%

Figure 10.1   Distribution of calcium in extra- and intracellular spaces.

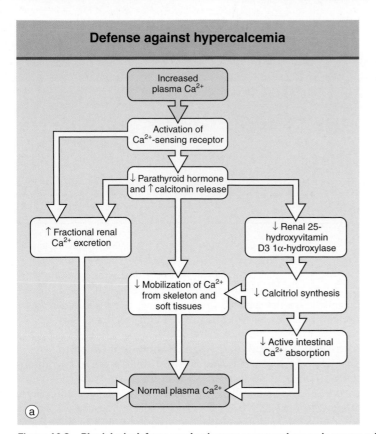

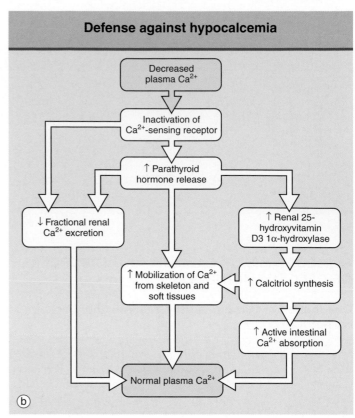

Figure 10.2 Physiologic defense mechanisms to counter changes in serum calcium. *a*, Hypercalcemia. *b*, Hypocalcemia. (Adapted from Kumar R: Vitamin D and calcium transport. Kidney Int 1991;40:1177–1189.)

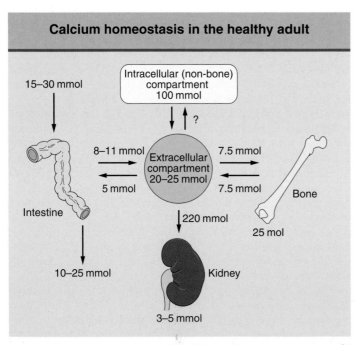

Figure 10.3 Calcium homeostasis in the healthy adult. Net zero Ca^{2+} balance is the result of net intestinal absorption (absorption minus secretion) and urinary excretion, which, by definition, are the same. After its passage into the extracellular fluid, Ca^{2+} enters the extracellular space, is deposited in bone, or is eliminated via the kidneys. Entry and exit fluxes between the extra- and intracellular spaces (skeletal and nonskeletal compartments) are also of identical magnitude under steady-state conditions.

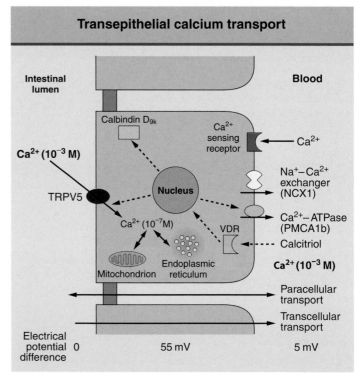

Figure 10.4 Transepithelial calcium transport in the small intestine. Calcium penetrates into the enterocyte via a recently discovered calcium channel (TRPV5) via the brush border membrane along a favorable electrochemical gradient. Under physiologic conditions, the cation is pumped out of the cell at the basolateral side against a steep electrochemical gradient by the adenosine triphosphate–consuming pump Ca^{2+}-ATPase. When there is a major elevation of intracytoplasmic Ca^{2+}, the cation leaves the cell using the Na^+-Ca^{2+} exchanger. Passive Ca^{2+} influx as well as efflux are sensitive to calcitrol, which binds the vitamin D receptor (VDR).

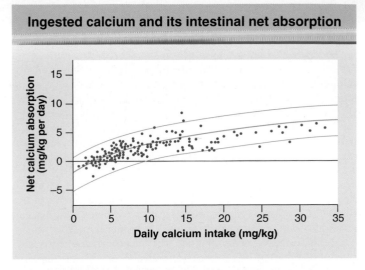

Ingested calcium and its intestinal net absorption

Figure 10.5 Relationship between ingested calcium and its absorption in the intestinal tract (net) in healthy young adults. (From Wilkinson R: Absorption of calcium, phosphorus, and magnesium. In Nordin BEC [ed]: Calcium and Magnesium Metabolism. Edinburgh: Churchill Livingstone, 1976, pp 36–112.)

Mechanisms of osteoblast differentiation

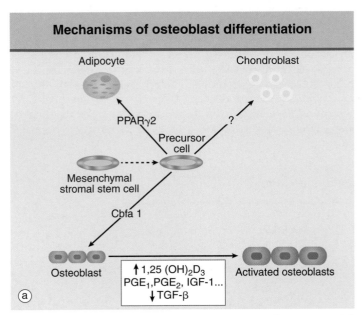

Mechanisms of osteoclast differentiation

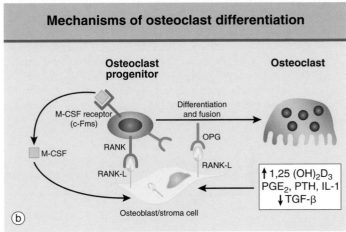

Figure 10.6 Mechanisms of osteoblast differentiation. *a*, The major growth factors and hormones controlling in the differentiation from the mesenchymal precursor cell to the osteoblast. *b*, The major growth factors, cytokines, and hormones controlling osteoblast and osteoclast activity. IL, interleukin; M-CSF, macrophage colony-stimulating factor; OPG, osteoprotegerin; PGE₂, prostaglandin E₂; PTH, parathyroid hormone; RANK-L, receptor activator of nuclear factor–kappaβ ligand; TGF-β, transforming growth factor β.

Determinants of skeletal homeostasis and bone mass

Figure 10.7 Determinants of skeletal homeostasis and bone mass. Physiologic (*black*) and pharmocologic (*red*) stimulators and inhibitors of bone formation and resorption are listed with the relative impact represented by the thickness of the arrows. BMP, bone morphogenetic protein; LRP5, low-density lipoprotein receptor–related protein 5; PTH, parathyroid protein; SERM, selective estrogen-receptor modulator; SOST, sclerostin. (From Harada S, Rodan GA: Control of osteoblast function and regulation of bone mass. Nature 2003;423:349–355.)

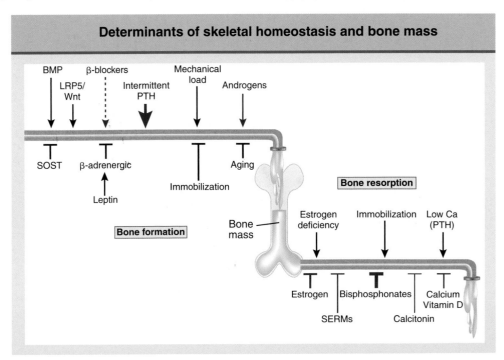

The kidneys play a major role in the short-term, minute-by-minute regulation, while the intestine and the skeleton ensure homeostasis in the mid and long term. To perform its task, the kidney uses a complex system of filtration and reabsorption (Fig. 10.8). The adjustment of blood Ca^{2+} is mainly achieved by modulation of tubular Ca^{2+} reabsorption in response to the body's needs, perfectly compensating minor increases or decreases in the filtered load of calcium at the glomerular level, which is normally about 220 mmol (8800 mg) in 24 hours (see Fig. 10.3). In the proximal tubule, most of the Ca^{2+} is reabsorbed by convective flow (as for Na^+ and water), whereas in the distal segments of the tubule, the transport mechanisms are more complex. In the thick ascending loop, the transport of Ca^{2+} is primarily passive via the paracellular route, depending on the electrical gradient, with the tubular lumen being positive, and also on the presence of claudin-16 in the tight junction. At this step, Ca^{2+} transport is enhanced by PTH, probably via an increase in paracellular permeability, but is reduced by an increase in extracellular Ca^{2+} involving the Ca^{2+}-sensing receptor (CaR_G). In the distal tubule, Ca^{2+} transport is primarily active via the transcellular route, through a recently identified calcium channel (TRPV5) located in the apical membrane and coupled with a specific basolateral calcium-ATPase (PMCa1b) and a Na^+-Ca^{2+} exchanger (NCX1). Both PTH and calcitriol regulate distal tubular transport.

The factors that control the glomerular filtration and tubular reabsorption of Ca^{2+} are numerous.[3,6,7] Elevated renal blood flow and glomerular filtration pressure (during extracellular fluid volume expansion) lead to an increase in filtered load, as do changes in the ultrafiltration coefficient K_f and an increase in glomerular surface. True hypercalcemia also increases ultrafilterable calcium; whereas true hypocalcemia decreases it. PTH decreases glomerular K_f and thus reduces the ultrafiltered calcium load; it also increases Ca^{2+} reabsorption in the distal nephron. However, PTH and PTHrp (PTH-related peptide) also induce hypercalcemia, and, because of the increase in serum calcium, the excretion of filtered calcium is elevated overall. Both extracellular Ca^{2+} and intracellular Ca^{2+} per se reduce tubular calcium reabsorption by activating CaR_G, and the effect of extracellular Ca^{2+} is enhanced by calcimimetics. Metabolic and respiratory acidoses lead to hypercalciuria, the latter via an increase in plasma Ca^{2+} and the former via an inhibitory effect on tubular Ca^{2+} reabsorption. Conversely, alkali ingestion reduces renal excretion of calcium. The enhancing effect of phosphate depletion on urinary calcium elimination can partly occur through changes in PTH and calcitriol secretion. Dietary factors modify urinary excretion of calcium mostly via their effects on intestinal Ca^{2+} absorption. Several classes of diuretics act directly on the tubules: loop diuretics and mannitol favor hypercalciuria, with a major

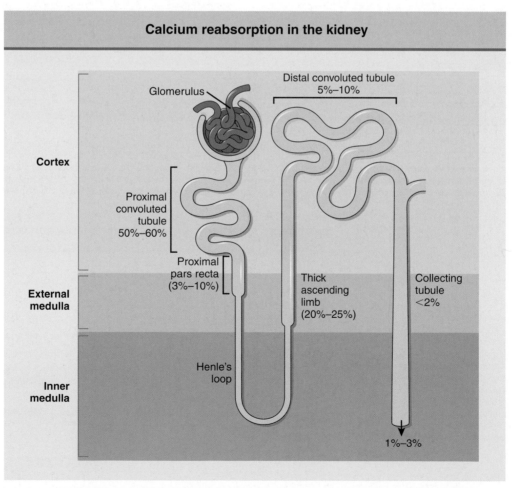

Figure 10.8 Sites of calcium reabsorption in various segments of the renal tubule. The percentage of Ca^{2+} absorbed in various segments following glomerular ultrafiltration is shown. (Redrawn from Puschett JB: Renal handling of calcium. In Massry SG, Glassock RJ [eds]: Textbook of Nephrology. Baltimore: Williams & Wilkins, 1989, pp 293–299.)

impact on the thick ascending limb, whereas the thiazide diuretics and amiloride induce hypocalciuria.

HYPERCALCEMIA

Increased plasma total calcium concentration can result from an increase in plasma proteins (false hypercalcemia) or from an increase in plasma ionized Ca^{2+} (true hypercalcemia). Only the latter leads to clinically relevant hypercalcemia. When only the value for the total plasma calcium is available rather than the free level ions, as is generally the case in clinical practice, plasma Ca^{2+} can be estimated by taking into account plasma albumin: an increase in albumin of 1.0 g/dl reflects a concomitant increase of 0.20 to 0.25 mmol/l (0.8 to 1.0 mg/dl) plasma calcium.

The recently cloned CaR_G has been identified in numerous tissues and its function well defined.[8] Mutations of the gene for CaR_G result in various clinical syndromes characterized either by hypercalcemia or by hypocalcemia (see later discussion). Several other Ca^{2+} receptors have been cloned subsequently. The precise functional properties of one of them, GPRC6A, which is expressed in osteoblasts and clearly distinct from CaR_G, have been recently characterized.[9] Its role in the regulation of osteoblast function and in human disease is still unknown.

Causes of Hypercalcemia

True hypercalcemia results from an increase in intestinal Ca^{2+} absorption, a stimulation of bone resorption, or a decrease in urinary Ca^{2+} excretion. Enhanced bone resorption is the predominant mechanism in most cases of hypercalcemia. The main causes of hypercalcemia are shown in Figure 10.9.

Malignant Neoplasias

The main cause of hypercalcemia is excessive bone resorption induced by neoplastic processes, usually solid tumors. Tumors of the breast, lung, and kidney are the most common, followed by hematopoietic neoplasias, particularly myeloma; other types of lymphoma and leukemia rarely cause hypercalcemia.

Most hypercalcemic tumors act on the skeleton either by direct invasion (metastases) or by producing factors that stimulate osteoclastic activity such as osteoclast-activating factor. A large number of such factors have been described, including most commonly PTHrp, as well as factors activating osteoclasts, transforming growth factors, prostaglandin E, and rarely calcitriol and tumor necrosis factor α, and very rarely PTH. Parathyroid cancer is an extremely infrequent cause of hypercalcemia. Its precise diagnosis is not always easy. Allelic loss in the retinoblastoma tumor-suppressor gene and mutations of the *HRPT2* gene may be involved.

Only eight of the 13 first amino acids of PTHrp are identical with those of the N-terminal fragment of PTH, but the effects of both hormones on target cells are mostly the same. In addition to their common receptor, the PTH/PTHrp receptor, there is at least one other receptor, the PTH_2 receptor. The latter recognizes solely PTH, with similar or identical signal transduction systems. In pathologic conditions, most of the PTHrp in the body is synthesized by solid tumors. Among its numerous actions, it stimulates osteoclastic activity and thus liberates excess quantities of calcium from the skeleton.

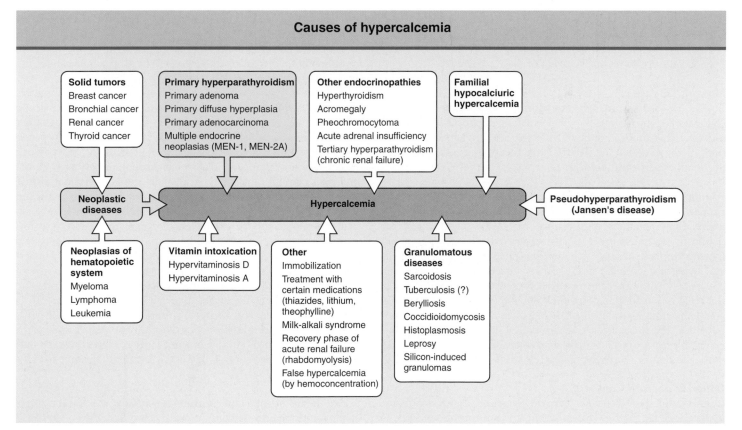

Figure 10.9   Causes of hypercalcemia. *Green boxes* indicate common causes of hypercalcemia. MEN, multiple endocrine neoplasia. (From Puschett JB: Renal handling of calcium. In Massry SG, Glassock RJ [eds]: Textbook of Nephrology. Baltimore: Williams & Wilkins, 1989, pp 293–299.)

Osteoclast-activating factor is secreted by myeloma plasmocytes and the lymphoblasts of malignant lymphomas. They include several members of the cytokine family, interleukins (ILs) such as IL-1α, IL-1β, IL-6, and also tumor necrosis factor α, which all stimulate osteoclast activity.

Prostaglandins of the E series (PGE$_1$ and PGE$_2$) can be secreted in large amounts by some tumors (especially renal tumors) and also stimulate osteoclastic resorption.

Some lymphoid tumors synthesize excess quantities of calcitriol. This capacity has been described in Hodgkin's disease, T cell lymphoma, and leiomyoblastoma.

Primary Hyperparathyroidism

The second most common cause of hypercalcemia is primary hyperparathyroidism. Early diagnosis is achieved through the widespread use of routine plasma calcium determination. In more than 80% of cases, the disease is caused by adenoma of a single parathyroid gland; in 10% to 15%, there is diffuse hyperplasia of all glands and in less than 5%, a parathyroid cancer. Primary hyperparathyroidism can be inherited either as diffuse hyperplasia of the parathyroid glands alone or as a component in multiple glandular hereditary endocrine disorders. Patients with multiple endocrine neoplasia type 1 (MEN1) have various combinations of parathyroid, anterior pituitary, enteropancreatic, and other endocrine tumors, resulting in hypersecretion of prolactin and gastrin, in addition to PTH. This disease is caused by inactivating germ-line mutations of a tumor-suppressor gene (the *MEN1* gene) that is inherited as an autosomal dominant trait. In MEN2A, the thyroid medulla and the adrenal medulla are involved with the parathyroid, resulting in hypersecretion of calcitonin and catecholamines. This disease is caused by activating mutations of the *RET* proto-oncogene. It is also inherited as an autosomal dominant trait. Not all patients with mildly elevated plasma PTH levels develop hypercalcemia. The development of the latter may depend on a concomitant elevation of plasma calcitriol.

Jansen's Disease

Jansen's disease is a rare hereditary form of short-limbed dwarfism characterized by severe hypercalcemia, hypophosphatemia, and metaphyseal chondrodysplasia.[10] It is the result of activating mutations of the gene for the PTH/PTHrp receptor, a particular form of pseudohyperparathyroidism.

Familial Hypocalciuric Hypercalcemia

Familial hypocalciuric hypercalcemia is a hereditary disease due to inactivating mutations in the gene for CaR$_G$[11] with autosomal dominant transmission. It is characterized by moderate chronic hypercalcemia associated with hypophosphatemia, hyperchloremia, and hypermagnesemia. Plasma PTH concentration is normal or moderately elevated. The fractional excretion of calcium is lower than that observed in hyperparathyroidism, and the urine calcium/creatinine ratio is usually <0.01. In patients with this syndrome, hypercalcemia never leads to severe clinical signs (except during the neonatal period, in which malignant hypercalcemia can be observed in the context of severe hyperparathyroidism).

Other Endocrine Causes

Other endocrine disorders can be associated with moderate hypercalcemia, such as hyperthyroidism, acromegaly, and pheochromocytoma. In addition, acute adrenal insufficiency should also be considered in the differential diagnosis, although here hypercalcemia is usually false and results from hemoconcentration. Hypercalcemia also occurs in severe forms of the secondary hyperparathyroidism of chronic renal failure (tertiary hyperparathyroidism). It has been shown that the latter is often the result of monoclonal growth of the parathyroid tissue.[12]

Various Pathologic States

Several other disorders sometimes induce hypercalcemia. Among the granulomatoses, sarcoidosis results in increased plasma Ca^{2+}, particularly in patients exposed to sunlight. The cause is uncontrolled production of calcitriol by macrophages (owing to the presence of the 1α-hydroxylase in the macrophages within the granulomas). Tuberculosis, leprosy, berylliosis, and many other granulomatous diseases are sometimes (but much more rarely than sarcoidosis) the origin of hypercalcemia, probably through the same mechanism.

Other Causes

Hypercalcemia may also result from prolonged bed rest (especially in patients with pre-existing high bone turnover rates, such as children, adolescents, and patients with Paget's disease). Recovery from acute renal failure secondary to rhabdomyolysis-induced renal failure has been associated with hypercalcemia in 25% of cases and is thought to occur as a consequence of mobilization of soft-tissue calcium deposits and through increases in PTH and calcitriol levels. Other causes include intoxication by vitamin D or one of its derivatives, vitamin A overload, and treatment by thiazide diuretics. Large doses of calcium (5 to 10 g/day), especially when ingested with alkali (antacids), can also lead to hypercalcemia and nephrocalcinosis (milk-alkali syndrome).

Clinical Manifestations

The severity of clinical symptoms and signs caused by hypercalcemia depends not only on the degree but also on the velocity of its development. Severe hypercalcemia can be accompanied by few manifestations in some patients because of its slow, progressive development, whereas much less severe hypercalcemia can lead to major disorders if it develops rapidly.

Generally, the first symptoms are increasing fatigue, muscle weakness, inability to concentrate, nervousness, increased sleepiness, and depression. Subsequently, gastrointestinal signs may occur, such as constipation, nausea and vomiting, and, rarely, peptic ulcer disease or pancreatitis. Renal-related signs include polyuria (secondary to nephrogenic diabetes insipidus), urinary tract stones and their complications, and occasionally tubulointerstitial disease with medullary and to a lesser extent cortical deposition of calcium (nephrocalcinosis). Neuropsychiatric manifestations include headache, loss of memory, somnolence, stupor, and, rarely, coma. Ocular symptoms include conjunctivitis from crystal deposition and, rarely, band keratopathy. Osteoarticular pain in primary hyperparathyroidism has become rare in Western countries because of the generally early diagnosis of hypercalcemia. High blood pressure can be induced by hypercalcemia, but it is more frequently a chance association. Soft-tissue calcifications can occur with long-standing hypercalcemia. Electrocardiography may show shortening of the QT interval and coving of the ST wave. Hypercalcemia may also increase cardiac contractility and can amplify digitalis toxicity.

Diagnosis

When the history and clinical examination are not helpful, primary hyperparathyroidism should be investigated first. Although this is only the second most frequent cause, its laboratory diagnosis is at present easier than that of tumoral involvement. In addition to total plasma calcium and ionized Ca^{2+} plasma albumin (or total protein), phosphate, creatinine, total alkaline phosphatases, PTH, and urinary calcium, phosphate and creatinine should be determined. From these results, the tubular phosphate reabsorption and the maximum amount reabsorbed factored for the glomerular filtration rate (GFR), T_mP (see later discussion), can be calculated. Note that prolonged hypercalcemia is often associated with (reversible) increased serum creatinine. Measurement of so-called intact PTH (which also measures N-terminal PTH fragments) may be replaced in the future by that of whole or biointact PTH recognizing the entire peptide only. When plasma PTH is high or abnormally normal with respect to the degree of hypercalcemia, the diagnosis is generally confirmed. Cervical ultrasonography and SESTAMIBI isotope scanning may be performed to locate a parathyroid adenoma, but, in general, experienced surgeons consider these examinations unnecessary before a first neck exploration. However, they are indispensable in case of recurrent hyperparathyroidism. If the plasma PTH level is low-normal or low, the possibility of a neoplastic disorder should be seriously considered. A low serum anion gap may be a clue to multiple myeloma (because occasionally the monoclonal IgG is positively charged). In addition to the usual examinations such as serum protein electrophoresis, measurement of the plasma PTHrp level can now be done in specialized laboratories. Exogenous vitamin D overload is associated with increased serum 25-hydroxyvitamin D levels, and granulomatous diseases such as sarcoidosis are associated with elevated calcitriol levels and with increased serum angiotensin-converting enzyme activity.

Treatment

Treatment is aimed at the underlying cause. However, severe and symptomatic hypercalcemia requires rapid, effective treatment, whatever the cause. Initially, the patient must be rapidly rehydrated with isotonic saline to correct the often marked dehydration. Then loop diuretics can be used, for example, intravenous furosemide at 100 to 200 mg every other hour, in order to facilitate urinary excretion of calcium. Oral intake and intravenous administration of fluids and electrolytes should be carefully monitored, and urinary, fecal, and gastric excretions measured if excessive, especially those of potassium, magnesium, and phosphate. Acid-basic balance should also be carefully monitored. Severe cardiac failure and/or renal insufficiency are contraindications to massive extracellular fluid volume expansion in conjunction with diuretics.

Bisphosphonates have progressively become the treatment of first choice, especially in hypercalcemia associated with cancer.[13] They inhibit bone resorption as well as calcitriol synthesis. They can be administered orally in less severe disease or intravenously in severe hypercalcemia. Frequently used bisphosphonates are clodronate (1600 to 3200 mg/day orally), pamidronate (15 to 90 mg intravenously over 1 to 3 days, once per month), and alendronate (10 mg/day orally). In intravenous administration, doses should be infused in 500 ml of isotonic saline or dextrose over at least 2 hours and up to 24 hours.

Calcitonin is theoretically an ideal drug for the treatment of hypercalcemia. Its effect is rapid (within hours), in particular after intravenous administration. Human, porcine, or salmon calcitonin can be given. Doses vary depending on the type of calcitonin used, for instance, subcutaneous or intramuscular porcine calcitonin 4 IU/kg/day in two to four injections or intravenous salmon calcitonin 4 to 8 IU/kg/day in 500 ml of isotonic saline over 6 hours. In clinical practice, however, calcitonin often has no effect or only a short-term effect because of the rapid development of tachyphylaxis.

Plicamycin (formerly mithramycin) is a cytostatic drug having a remarkable power to inhibit bone resorption. Administration of a single intravenous dose is generally followed by a rapid decline in plasma calcium within a few hours, and this effect lasts several days. However, its use is reserved for malignant hypercalcemia, and its cytotoxic effect and side effects (thrombocytopenia and liver function abnormalities) preclude prolonged administration. The maximal daily dose is 25 µg/kg.

Corticosteroids (0.5 to 1.0 mg/kg predniso(lo)ne daily) are mainly indicated in hypervitaminosis D of endogenous origin, such as sarcoidosis and tuberculosis, and of exogenous origin, such as vitamin D intoxication. The use of ketoconazole, an antifungal agent that can inhibit renal and extrarenal calcitriol synthesis and thus lower plasma calcitriol levels, has also been proposed in hypervitaminosis D. Corticosteroids can also be tried in the treatment of hypercalcemia associated with some hematopoietic tumors such as myeloma and lymphoma and even for some solid tumors such as breast cancer. Of course, prolonged treatment with corticosteroids exposes patients to the classic risks of such therapy.

In rare cases of malignant hypercalcemia, treatment with prostaglandin antagonists, for example, indomethacin or aspirin, can be successful. Hyperkalemia and renal insufficiency may occur with indomethacin. Hypercalcemia caused by thyrotoxicosis can rapidly resolve with intravenous administration of propranolol or less rapidly with oral administration.

In moderate and nonsymptomatic hypercalcemia of primary hyperparathyroidism, treatment with estrogens has been tried, at least in females. The clinical evaluation of the new therapeutic class of CaR_G agonists (calcimimetics) is ongoing for the medical treatment of parathyroid overfunction. In patients with primary hyperparathyroidism, prolonged experience with the calcimimetic drug cinacalcet is presently available, allowing normalization of serum Ca^{2+} in most instances together with a reduction of serum PTH.[14] In long-term dialysis patients with secondary and many cases of so-called tertiary uremic hyperparathyroidism, long-term administration of cinacalcet has been shown to be superior to standard therapy in controlling serum PTH, calcium, phosphorus, and the calcium × phosphorus product.[15] Cinacalcet is also efficacious in patients with parathyroid carcinoma.

HYPOCALCEMIA

As with hypercalcemia, hypocalcemia can be secondary either to a change (reduction in this case) in plasma albumin (false hypocalcemia) or to a change in ionized Ca^{2+} (true hypocalcemia). False hypocalcemia can be excluded by directly measuring plasma Ca^{2+} by determining plasma total protein or albumin levels, by the clinical context, or by other laboratory results. Acute hypocalcemia is often observed during acute hyperventilation and the respiratory alkalosis that follows, regardless of the cause of hyperventilation. Hyperventilation can occur secondary to cardiopulmonary or cerebral diseases.

Causes of Chronic Hypocalcemia
After excluding false hypocalcemia linked to hypoalbuminemia, hypocalcemia can be divided into that associated with elevated and that associated with low plasma phosphate concentration.

Hypocalcemia Associated with Hyperphosphatemia
This form of hypocalcemia is caused by hypoparathyroid states that are idiopathic or acquired (following surgery or radiotherapy or secondary to amyloidosis). Sporadic cases of hypoparathyroidism can occasionally be seen in patients with pernicious anemia

or adrenal insufficiency. Pseudohypoparathyroidism (Albright's hereditary osteodystrophy) is characterized by a particular phenotype including short neck, round face, and short metacarpals, with end-organ resistance to PTH. Chronic renal insufficiency, acute renal failure in its oligoanuric phase (e.g., secondary to rhabdomyolysis), and massive phosphate administration can also lead to hypocalcemia with hyperphosphatemia. At least one form of inherited, familial hypocalcemia is linked to particular activating mutations of the CaR_G.[16]

Hypocalcemia Associated with Hypophosphatemia

Hypocalcemia with hypophosphatemia may occur from vitamin D–deficient states. This may result from insufficient sunlight exposure, dietary deficiency of vitamin D, decreased absorption following gastrointestinal surgery, intestinal malabsorption syndromes (steatorrhea), or hepatobiliary disease (primary biliary cirrhosis). Magnesium deficiency may also result in hypocalcemia, often in conjunction with hypokalemia. The low serum Ca^{2+} appears to result from decreased PTH release and end-organ resistance. Acute renal failure in the polyuric phase may also be associated with hypocalcemia and hypophosphatemia. The main causes of hypercalcemia are shown in Figure 10.10.

Clinical Manifestations

As with hypercalcemia, the symptoms of hypocalcemia depend on the rate of its occurrence and its degree. The most common manifestations, in addition to fatigue and muscular weakness, are increased irritability, loss of memory, a state of confusion, hallucination, paranoia, and depression. The best known clinical signs are Chvostek's sign (tapping of facial nerve branches leading to twitching of facial muscle) and Trousseau's sign (carpal spasm in response to forearm ischemia caused by sphygmomanometer cuff). In acute hypocalcemia, there may be paresthesias of the lips and the extremities, muscle cramps, and sometimes frank tetany, laryngeal stridor, or convulsions. Chronic hypocalcemia can be associated with cataracts, brittle nails with transverse grooves, dry skin, and decreased or even absent axillary and pubic hair, especially in idiopathic hypoparathyroidism, which is often of autoimmune origin.

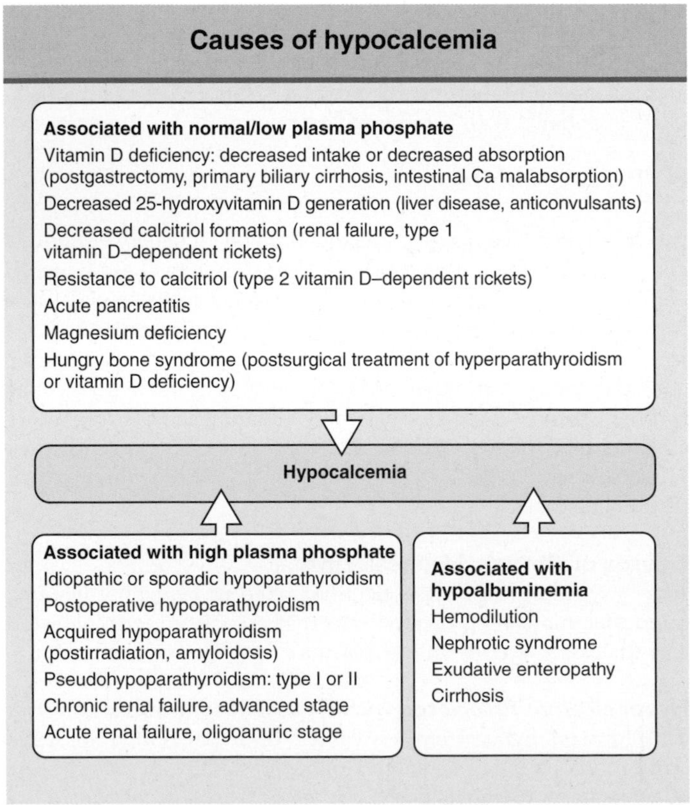

Laboratory and Radiographic Signs

Plasma phosphate is elevated in hypoparathyroidism, pseudohypoparathyroidism, and advanced renal failure, whereas it is decreased in steatorrhea, vitamin D deficiency, acute pancreatitis, and the polyuric phase during recovery from acute renal failure. Plasma PTH is reduced in hypoparathyroidism and also during chronic magnesium deficiency, whereas it is normal or increased in pseudohypoparathyroidism and in chronic renal failure. Urinary calcium excretion is increased only in the treatment of hypoparathyroidism with calcium and/or vitamin D derivatives; it is low in all other cases of hypocalcemia. Fractional urinary calcium excretion is, however, high in hypoparathyroidism, in the polyuric phase during recovery from acute renal failure, and in severe chronic renal failure; it is low in all other cases of hypocalcemia. Urinary phosphate excretion is low in hypoparathyroidism, pseudohypoparathyroidism, and magnesium deficiency; it is high in vitamin D deficiency, steatorrhea, chronic renal failure, and during phosphate administration. Determination of serum 25-hydroxyvitamin D and calcitriol levels may also be useful.

Intracranial calcifications, notably of the basal ganglia, are observed radiographically in 20% of patients with idiopathic hypoparathyroidism, but much less frequently in patients with postsurgical hypoparathyroidism or pseudohypoparathyroidism.

On electrocardiography, the corrected QT interval is frequently prolonged, and there are sometimes arrhythmias. Electroencephalography shows nonspecific signs such as an increase in slow, high-voltage waves.

Treatment

The basic treatment is that of the underlying cause. Severe and symptomatic (tetany) hypocalcemia requires rapid and appropriate treatment. Acute respiratory alkalosis, if present, should be corrected, if possible. When the cause is functional, the simple retention of carbon dioxide, for example, by breathing into a paper bag, may suffice. In other cases and to obtain a prolonged effect, intravenous infusion of calcium salts is most often required. In the setting of seizures or tetany, calcium gluconate should be administered as a bolus (for instance, 90 mg calcium ions in 10 ml) followed by 12 to 24 g over 24 hours in 5% dextrose or isotonic saline. Calcium gluconate is preferred to calcium chloride because of its better clinical tolerability. Intravenously administered calcium chloride can lead to extensive skin necrosis in accidental extravasation.

Treatment of chronic hypocalcemia includes oral administration of calcium salts, thiazide diuretics, or vitamin D. Several oral presentations of calcium are available, each with their advantages and disadvantages. It should be remembered that the amount of elemental calcium of the various salts differs greatly. For example, the calcium content is 40% in carbonate, 36% in chloride, 12% in lactate, and only 8% in gluconate salts. The daily amount prescribed can be 2 to 4 g elemental Ca. Concurrent magnesium deficiency (serum Mg^{2+} <0.75 mmol/l) should be treated either with oral magnesium oxide (250 to 500 mg every 6 days) or with magnesium sulfate: intramuscular (4 to 8 mmol/day) or intravenous (e.g., 12 ml 50% magnesium sulfate in 1000 ml 5% dextrose over 3 to 4 hours).

Causes of hypocalcemia

Associated with normal/low plasma phosphate

Vitamin D deficiency: decreased intake or decreased absorption (postgastrectomy, primary biliary cirrhosis, intestinal Ca malabsorption)

Decreased 25-hydroxyvitamin D generation (liver disease, anticonvulsants)

Decreased calcitriol formation (renal failure, type 1 vitamin D–dependent rickets)

Resistance to calcitriol (type 2 vitamin D–dependent rickets)

Acute pancreatitis

Magnesium deficiency

Hungry bone syndrome (postsurgical treatment of hyperparathyroidism or vitamin D deficiency)

Hypocalcemia

Associated with high plasma phosphate

Idiopathic or sporadic hypoparathyroidism

Postoperative hypoparathyroidism

Acquired hypoparathyroidism (postirradiation, amyloidosis)

Pseudohypoparathyroidism: type I or II

Chronic renal failure, advanced stage

Acute renal failure, oligoanuric stage

Associated with hypoalbuminemia

Hemodilution

Nephrotic syndrome

Exudative enteropathy

Cirrhosis

Figure 10.10 Causes of hypocalcemia.

Treatment of hypocalcemia secondary to hypoparathyroidism is difficult as urinary calcium excretion increases markedly with calcium supplementation and can lead to nephrocalcinosis and loss of renal function. To reduce urinary calcium concentrations, one can treat the patient with thiazide diuretics in association with restricted sodium chloride intake and have the patient drink large amounts of water.

Last, treatment with vitamin D, or rather its most active metabolite calcitriol or its analogue 1α-hydroxycholecalciferol 0.25 to 1.0 μg/day, is the treatment of choice at present for idiopathic or acquired hypoparathyroidism because these compounds are more easily taken by the patients than massive doses of calcium salts. Administration of vitamin D derivatives generally leads to hypercalciuria and, rarely, to nephrocalcinosis. It requires regular monitoring to avoid induction of hypercalcemia and renal disease.

HOMEOSTASIS OF PHOSPHATE

Distribution of Phosphate in the Organism and Phosphate Homeostasis

Apart from its abundance in the skeleton, phosphate is also one of the main components of soft tissues and an integral part of the various cell structures. It participates, directly or indirectly, in most metabolic processes. Phosphorus is found in the organism both as mineral phosphate and organic phosphate (phosphoric esters). The phosphate contained in laboratory samples (food, plasma, urine, feces, tissues) is generally expressed in terms of elemental phosphorus. Phosphorus is, however, transported across cell membranes in the form of phosphate (31 mg/l elemental phosphorus = 1 mmol/l phosphorus in the form of phosphate). Figure 10.11 shows the distribution of phosphate in the extra- and intracellular fluid compartments.

Short-term variations in plasma phosphate are controlled by PTH and calcitriol. Recently fibroblast growth factor (FGF)-23 has been identified as one of the elusive phosphate regulatory hormones, if not the most important one.[17] Several other phosphatonins have been identified subsequently, including secreted frizzled related protein 4 (sFRP-4), matrix extracellular phosphoglycoprotein, and FGF-7.[17] Very recently, the *klotho* gene has also been shown to regulate phosphate homeostasis. Deletion of *klotho* in the mouse induces a hyperphosphatemic phenotype, and *klotho* activates the calcium channel TRPV5.[18]

There are wide daily variations in blood phosphate levels, depending on food intake but also on dietary carbohydrates (negatively) and blood pH. Long-term maintenance of phosphate homeostasis depends mainly on the adaptability of renal tubular reabsorption of phosphate to the needs of the organism. Chronic deficiency in phosphate intake first leads to hypophosphatemia and then to intracellular depletion of phosphate. By comparison, hyperphosphatemia occurs in advanced renal failure even when dietary intake remains within normal limits.

Figure 10.12 shows the balance of ingestion, body distribution, and excretion of phosphate in a healthy human. A young adult requires approximately 0.5 mmol/kg phosphate daily. These needs are much higher in the child during growth. Phosphates are widely found in milk products, meat, eggs, and cereals.

Phosphate entrance into transport epithelia involves a secondary active Na^+/phosphate (Na/Pi) cotransport. Three different Na/Pi cotransporters have been identified and characterized.[19] The type 1 Na/Pi family is present in the renal tubule and may also have anion channel function. It is represented by three members: NPT1, NPT3, and NPT4. Type 2 Na/Pi cotransporters are the key players in phosphate homeostasis and include three members: NPT2a, NPT2b, and NPT2c. Two of them serve specific epithelial transport functions, respectively, in the brush border of the proximal tubule (NPT2a) and of the small intestine (NPT2b), determining Na^+-dependent phosphate (re)absorption. Type 3 Na/Pi cotransporters are ubiquitous. They are composed of Pit1 and Pit2 and may serve housekeeping functions. Type 2 cotransporters are regulated by altered phosphate intake, PTH, calcitriol, and pH. The exit of phosphate at the basolateral side of the intestinal and renal tubular epithelium probably occurs by anionic exchange.

The transcellular transport of phosphate is also controlled by several other metabolic, hormonal, and autocrine/paracrine factors, including growth hormone, insulin-like growth factor-1, insulin,

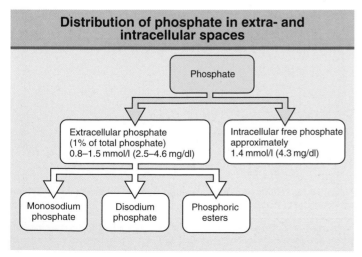

Distribution of phosphate in extra- and intracellular spaces

Phosphate

→ Extracellular phosphate (1% of total phosphate) 0.8–1.5 mmol/l (2.5–4.6 mg/dl)

→ Intracellular free phosphate approximately 1.4 mmol/l (4.3 mg/dl)

→ Monosodium phosphate

→ Disodium phosphate

→ Phosphoric esters

Figure 10.11 Distribution of phosphate in extra- and intracellular spaces.

Phosphate homeostasis in the healthy adult

25–65 mmol

Intracellular (nonbone) compartment 3–5 mmol

Intestine

15–50 mmol

Extracellular compartment 15 mmol

?

40 mmol

40 mmol

Bone

15–25 mol

120–200 mmol

100–170 mmol

15–20 mmol

Kidney

20–50 mmol

Figure 10.12 Phosphate homeostasis in healthy young adults. At net zero balance, identical net intestinal uptake (absorption minus secretion) and urinary loss occur. After its passage into the extracellular fluid, phosphate enters the intracellular space, is deposited in bone or soft tissue, or is eliminated via the kidneys. Entry and exit fluxes between the extra- and intracellular spaces (skeletal and nonskeletal compartments) are also the same under steady-state conditions.

and thyroid hormone. Most importantly, the new family of phosphatonins appears to play a major role in the control of renal tubular phosphate handling. The central role of FGF-23 is based on a number of recent observations both in experimental animals and in humans. Like PTH, it decreases the serum phosphorus concentration by reducing NPT2a, b, and c expression, but, in contrast to PTH, it impairs renal calcitriol synthesis as well.[19]

Intestinal, Skeletal, and Renal Handling of Phosphate

Phosphate transport across the intestinal wall occurs by both the transepithelial and the paracellular route (Fig. 10.13), most of it via Na/Pi cotransport. Absorption is a linear, nonsaturable function of phosphate intake (Fig. 10.14) and amounts to 60% to 75% of intake (15 to 50 mmol/day). Many factors affect phosphate uptake. Calcitriol stimulates Na/Pi cotransport, whereas high Ca^{2+} concentrations decrease phosphate absorption.

Bone permanently exchanges phosphate with the surrounding milieu. Entry and exit of phosphate amount to approximately 100 mmol/day (slowly exchangeable phosphate), for a total skeleton content of approximately 20,000 mmol. The net balance is positive during growth, zero in the young adult, and negative in the elderly.

The kidneys play a major role in controlling extracellular phosphate homeostasis.[20,21] Normally, the daily amount of phosphate excreted in urine equals that absorbed in the intestine. It usually comprises 5% to 20% of ultrafiltered phosphate. The amount of phosphate reabsorbed can be expressed in relation to the amount filtered as tubular reabsorption of phosphate (TRP), which is calculated as

$$[1 - (C_{PO4}/GFR)] \times 100,$$

where C_{PO4} is phosphate clearance. TRP also equals

$$1 - (U_{PO4}S_{creat}/SPO_4 U_{creat}),$$

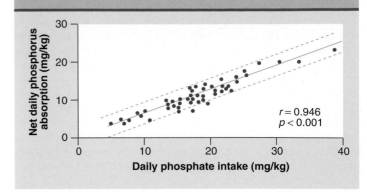

Figure 10.14 Relationship between ingested phosphate and that absorbed in the digestive tract (net absorption) in healthy young adults. (From Wilkinson R: Absorption of calcium, phosphorus, and magnesium. In Nordin BEC [ed]: Calcium and Magnesium Metabolism. Edinburgh: Churchill Livingstone, 1976, pp 36–112.)

where U_{PO4}, S_{PO4}, U_{creat}, and S_{creat} are urinary and serum phosphate and creatinine concentrations, respectively. The maximal TRP factored for GFR (TmP/GFR: Bijvoet index) represents the concentration above which most phosphate is excreted and below which most is reabsorbed. This can be calculated from the plasma phosphate and TRP (Fig. 10.15).

After its passage through the glomerular filter, part of the ultrafiltered phosphate is recovered by the tubule depending on the body's needs. The major part of phosphate is reabsorbed in

Transepithelial phosphate transport

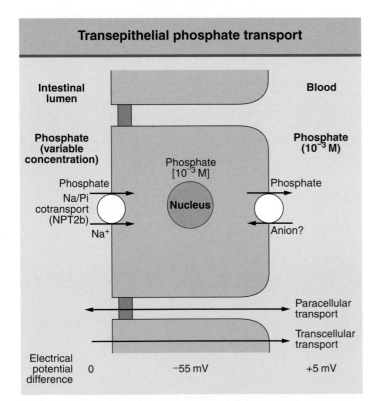

Figure 10.13 Transepithelial phosphate transport in the small intestine. Phosphate enters the enterocyte (influx) via the brush border membrane using the Na^+/Pi cotransport system, with a stoichiometry of 2:1, operating against an electrochemical gradient. Phosphate exit at the basolateral side possibly occurs by passive diffusion or (more probably) by anion exchange.

Nomogram for estimation of the renal threshold phosphate concentration

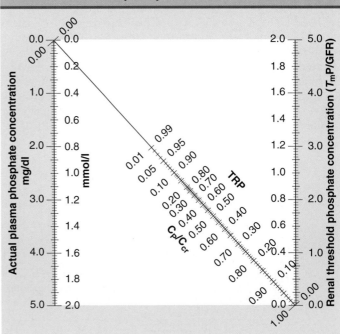

Figure 10.15 Nomogram for estimation of the renal threshold phosphate concentration (T_mP/GFR) without any calculation. A straight line through the appropriate values of phosphate concentration and TRP (amount of phosphate reabsorbed or C_P/C_{cr}, where C is clearance for phosphate [P] or creatinine [cr]) passes through the corresponding value of T_mP/GFR. (From Bijvoet OL: Relation of plasma phosphate concentration to renal tubular reabsorption of phosphate. Clin Sci 1969;37:23–36.)

the proximal convoluted tubule. A large number of endocrine and metabolic factors modulate urinary excretion of phosphate.[21] Factors increasing renal excretion of phosphate include PTH, FGF-23, dietary phosphate, and extracellular volume expansion, whereas calcitriol increases phosphate reabsorption. Adaptation of tubular reabsorption to dietary intake can occur independently of PTH and vitamin D, probably via regulation by the phosphatonins.

HYPERPHOSPHATEMIA

Causes of Hyperphosphatemia
Increased levels of plasma phosphate can be observed in many clinical situations. The most common cause is reduced urinary excretion in renal failure.[22] Although hyperphosphatemia is seen particularly in conditions in which urinary phosphate excretion is perturbed, it can also be caused by increased exogenous or endogenous phosphate supply (Fig. 10.16).

Chronic Kidney Disease
In advanced renal failure, hyperphosphatemia is a practically constant finding owing to phosphate retention. This leads to an increase in ultrafiltered phosphate by the remaining nephrons. At the same time, tubular reabsorption of phosphates progressively decreases under the influence of both PTH and FGF-23. Thus, fractional urinary excretion of phosphates can reach values as high as 60% to 90%. This progressive adaptation of tubular reabsorption maintains plasma phosphate within normal limits until GFR falls to <25 ml/min. In patients with anuric end-stage renal disease, the increase in plasma phosphate results not only from decreased excretion but also from increased PTH, which may further increase plasma phosphate through its action to release calcium and phosphate from bone. The concomitant stimulation of renal calcitriol synthesis by PTH is offset by FGF-23 and decreased functional renal tissue mass.[23] During acute renal failure, plasma phosphate is also high, sometimes even higher than in chronic renal failure, especially in association with infection or rhabdomyolysis.

Hypoparathyroidism
In states of reduced PTH secretion (idiopathic or postsurgical hypoparathyroidism) or resistance to its peripheral action (pseudohypoparathyroidism), tubular reabsorption of phosphate is increased and consequently urinary excretion is diminished. The resulting increase in plasma phosphate leads to an increase in the ultrafiltered load. This results in the regulation of plasma phosphate at a new level.

Chronic Hypocalcemia
Hyperphosphatemia is sometimes observed in association with chronic hypocalcemia with normal or high plasma PTH levels. In the absence of characteristic abnormalities of pseudohypoparathyroidism, the existence of an abnormal form of plasma PTH has been suggested. The latter could result from an abnormal conversion of the prohormone to its secreted form.

Acromegaly
In this condition, hyperphosphatemia results from an increase in tubular reabsorption of phosphate due to stimulation by growth hormone.

Pseudotumoral Calcinosis
This syndrome is seen primarily in black people with hyperphosphatemia, an increase in serum calcium × phosphate product (>65 mg^2/dl^2) and calcitriol, an exaggerated tubular reabsorption of phosphate, and metastatic soft-tissue calcifications. Circulating PTH is not decreased. Recently, mutations in two genes have been identified as candidates: inactivating mutations in GALNT3 and in FGF-23. As a hypothetical explanation for the involvement of two different genes for the same phenotype, it is possible that the glycosyl transferase encoded by GALNT3 is necessary for FGF-23 activity.[19]

Treatment-Induced Hyperphosphatemia
Treatment by bisphosphonates, in particular by etidronate in Paget's disease, can lead to hyperphosphatemia, possibly through an increased liberation of tissue phosphate and/or an increase in renal tubular reabsorption.

Hypercatabolism
Exaggerated phosphate loss by soft tissues can be observed in some states of increased cell lysis, as during the crush syndrome, or in

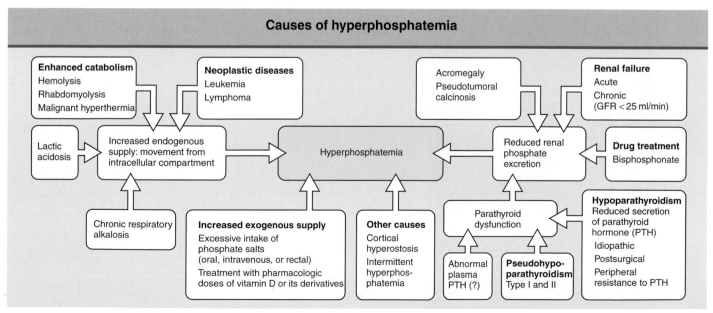

Figure 10.16 Causes of hyperphosphatemia.

some malignancies and their treatment (especially lymphomas and leukemias). Severe hypercatabolic states during severe infection or in diabetic ketoacidosis can also cause hyperphosphatemia by increased cellular release of phosphate (which is usually accompanied with an acute reduction in GFR).

Phosphate Salts and Vitamin D

Massive supply of phosphate, as may occur by laxative or enema use, can sometimes lead to hyperphosphatemia. Similarly, administration of pharmacologic doses of vitamin D can lead to hyperphosphatemia. In this latter case, there is usually hypercalcemia as well.

Respiratory Alkalosis by Prolonged Hyperventilation

Respiratory alkalosis resulting from prolonged hyperventilation is characterized by resistance to the renal action of PTH, hyperphosphatemia, and hypocalcemia. Functional pseudohypoparathyroidism may be present as well since renal phosphate clearance is diminished, whereas plasma PTH is normal, despite hypocalcemia. There is no decrease in urinary calcium excretion.

Clinical Manifestations

Severe hyperphosphatemia can induce hypocalcemia, which stimulates PTH secretion. In addition, it can inhibit renal synthesis of calcitriol, which tends to aggravate hypocalcemia further. The occurrence of severe hypocalcemia with tetany and ectopic calcifications is the most severe manifestation of hyperphosphatemia. Calcification may occur in joints and soft tissues, as well as in the lung, kidney, and conjunctiva. This syndrome is observed in several clinical situations, such as renal failure, hypoparathyroidism, pseudohypoparathyroidism, and pseudotumoral calcinosis. Tumor-like extraskeletal calcifications, however, are more frequently observed in hyperphosphatemia associated with normal or increased plasma Ca^{2+} levels, either as a familial syndrome (very rare) or in uremic patients (rare). Figure 10.17 shows the radiographic appearance of a tumor-like, massive periarticular calcium phosphate deposit in a uremic patient with an extremely high serum calcium × phosphate product. In addition to soft-tissue calcifications, some uremic subjects with

elevated calcium phosphate products may also develop a severe skin condition termed calciphylaxis (see Chapters 74 and 78).

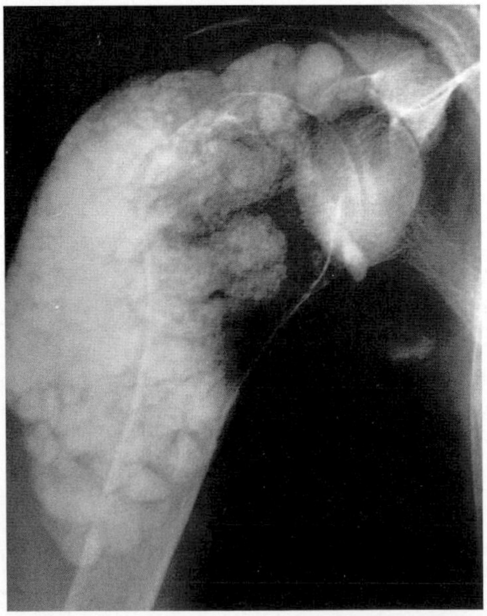

The stimulation of PTH secretion by high phosphate levels is both indirect, secondary to a decrease of plasma Ca^{2+} and calcitriol synthesis, and direct, secondary to a stimulatory effect on the parathyroid gland.

Treatment

Treatment of the underlying cause of hyperphosphatemia should be attempted whenever possible. There are, however, situations, as for example chronic renal failure, in which treatment must remain symptomatic. To this end, oral phosphate binders can be given (see Chapter 74).

HYPOPHOSPHATEMIA

Decreased plasma phosphate levels may reflect phosphate deficiency. They can, theoretically, be observed during a prolonged decrease in phosphate intake. However, as shown in Figure 10.18, several defense mechanisms counter a decrease in plasma phosphate resulting from low intake. Moderately reduced plasma phosphate levels may also be observed in conditions not linked to overall deficiency, for example, in maldistribution between the intra- and extracellular compartments during acute respiratory alkalosis.

When plasma phosphate is 0.8 to 0.3 mmol/l (2.5 to 1.0 mg/dl), the condition is termed moderate hypophosphatemia. When it is less than 0.3 mmol/l (1.0 mg/dl), it is considered to be severe hypophosphatemia.

Causes of Hypophosphatemia

Moderate hypophosphatemia can be caused by genetic diseases or by acquired conditions (Fig. 10.19). The main acquired condition is malnutrition owing to low food intake or anorexia during severe disease or alcoholism; its incidence varies greatly among countries. Another cause is a shift of phosphate into cells, which can occur

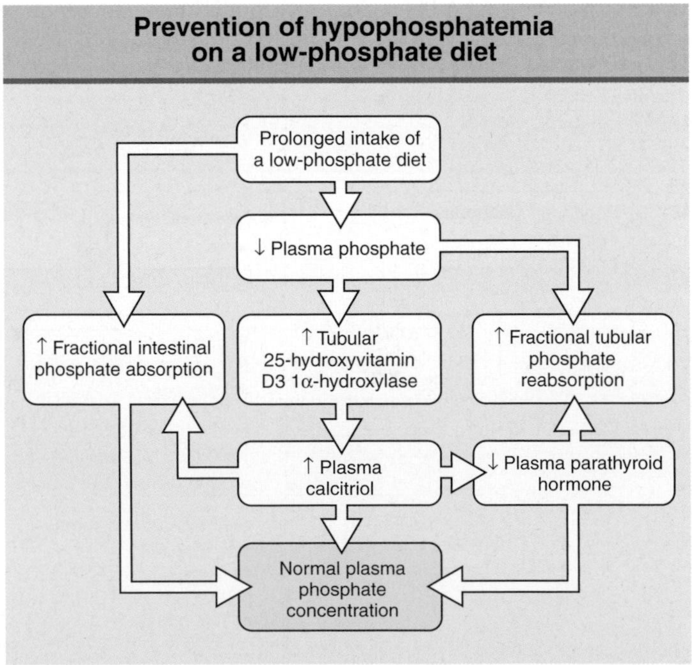

Figure 10.17 Tumor-like extraskeletal calcification in the shoulder.

Prevention of hypophosphatemia on a low-phosphate diet

Prolonged intake of a low-phosphate diet

↓ Plasma phosphate

↑ Fractional intestinal phosphate absorption

↑ Tubular 25-hydroxyvitamin D3 1α-hydroxylase

↑ Fractional tubular phosphate reabsorption

↑ Plasma calcitriol

↓ Plasma parathyroid hormone

Normal plasma phosphate concentration

Figure 10.18 Compensatory mechanisms to prevent hypophosphatemia during a prolonged intake of a phosphate-poor diet.

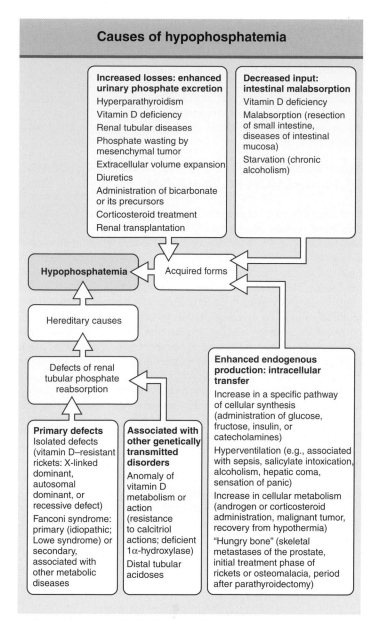

Figure 10.19 Causes of hypophosphatemia.

PHEX, which has significant homology to a family of endopeptidase genes.[24] FGF-23, which is elevated in at least some patients with X-linked hypophosphatemia, may be a substrate for *PHEX*, but this hypothesis has been challenged recently. *PHEX* is mainly expressed in bone. The urinary leak of phosphate is secondary to a decrease in proximal tubular Na/Pi cotransport. Clinical signs are rickets in the child and sometimes osteomalacia and bone deformation in the adult. Hypophosphatemia is associated with normal plasma Ca^{2+}, calcitriol, and PTH and with elevated serum alkaline phosphatases. The TRP is greatly lowered. Isolated inherited hypophosphatemia may also occur rarely in an autosomal dominant (see later discussion) or autosomal recessive pattern.

Autosomal-Dominant Hypophosphatemic Rickets Autosomal-dominant hypophosphatemic rickets is a phosphate wasting disorder characterized by short stature, bone pain, fracture, and lower extremity deformity. It is caused by mutations in the FGF-23 gene that prevent the degradation of the intact peptide.[25]

Fanconi Syndrome Fanconi syndrome (see Chapter 47) is characterized by a complex transport defect of the proximal tubule that results in decreased reabsorption of glucose, amino acids, and bicarbonate in addition to phosphate. It is either primary (idiopathic, Lowe syndrome, Dent disease) or associated with other metabolic diseases (cystinosis, Wilson's disease, and others). In Dent disease and Lowe syndrome, a defective recycling of megalin to the apical cell surface of the proximal tubule has been found, implicating a role in abnormal tubular endocytic function.[26]

In addition to a tubular defect causing phosphate wasting, the activity of renal 1α-hydroxylase may be insufficient, resulting in decreased circulating calcitriol levels and bone disease such as rickets and osteomalacia. Functional disorders associated with the syndrome, such as polyuria and extracellular volume contraction, lead to hyperaldosteronism with hypokalemia and eventually to renal failure.

Hypophosphatemia Linked to Other Inherited Diseases Several rare inherited diseases can be associated with hypophosphatemia, including vitamin D–dependent rickets type 1, caused by a defect of renal 1α-hydroxylase, and type 2, caused by peripheral resistance to the action of calcitriol. Clinical signs are similar to those of vitamin D–deficient rickets, but alopecia also occurs in 50% of cases. In type 1, calcitriol levels are low, whereas in type 2, there is normal circulating 25-hydroxyvitamin D and high calcitriol. Treatment with low doses of calcitriol is sufficient to treat type 1, whereas extremely high doses of calcitriol or alfacalcidol are required for type 2.

Distal Renal Tubular Acidosis (Type I) Distal renal tubular acidosis (type I; see Chapter 12) is associated with hypercalciuria and sometimes nephrocalcinosis. Hypophosphatemia is inconstant. It is possible that the latter only results when there is concomitant vitamin D deficiency.

Acquired Forms of Hypophosphatemia
The number of acquired diseases that can be associated with hypophosphatemia is even greater than inherited diseases and includes hyperparathyroidism and vitamin D deficiency (see Fig. 10.19). True phosphate deficiency associated with total body depletion must be distinguished from enhanced influx of phosphate from the extracellular to the intracellular space or increased skeletal mineralization.

through various mechanisms but especially with the administration of insulin. Although there are a large number of genetic diseases and syndromes, overall, these are rare. Severe forms of hypophosphatemia are all acquired.

Inherited Forms of Hypophosphatemia
Many inherited diseases are associated with chronic hypophosphatemia. These are generally diagnosed in childhood. Permanent low plasma phosphate usually leads to rickets or osteomalacia. The molecular genetic defect has not yet been identified in most cases.

Inherited hypophosphatemia can be subdivided into two groups: primary defects, which are either isolated or associated with tubular disorders (Fanconi syndrome), and defects that are secondary to another genetically transmitted disease, mainly metabolic disorders or disturbances in the action of vitamin D.

X-Linked Hypophosphatemia X-linked hypophosphatemia is a rare, dominantly transmitted disease characterized by hypophosphatemia and isolated phosphate wasting. The mutant gene is

Alcoholism Alcoholism is the most common cause of severe hypophosphatemia in Western countries. The causes are multiple, including insufficient food intake, the use of phosphate binders for intestinal disorders, and excessive phosphate loss in urine secondary to hypomagnesemia, as well as phosphate transfer from the extra- to the intracellular compartment secondary to hyperventilation or glucose infusion in subjects with postalcoholic cirrhosis or in acute abstinence.

Acute Respiratory Alkalosis In intense and short-term hyperventilation, plasma phosphate can sometimes decrease considerably to values as low as 0.1 mmol/l (0.3 mg/dl). Such a decrease is never observed in acute metabolic alkalosis. Hypophosphatemia following acute and intense hyperventilation is probably the result of muscle sequestration of extracellular phosphate. However, it must be remembered that prolonged chronic hyperventilation leads to hyperphosphatemia (see previous discussion).

Diabetic Ketoacidosis During decompensated diabetes associated with acidosis provoked by accumulation of ketone bodies, glycosuria, and polyuria, plasma phosphate can be normal or high, even in the presence of hyperphosphaturia. Correction of this complication by insulin and refilling of the extracellular compartment leads to massive transfer of phosphate into the intracellular compartment, hypophosphatemia, and subsequently less urinary loss of phosphate. Generally, plasma phosphate does not decrease to less than 0.3 mmol/l (0.9 mg/dl), except when there is pre-existing phosphate deficiency.

Oncogenic Hypophosphatemic Osteomalacia Hypophosphatemia associated with tumor-induced osteomalacia results from renal phosphate wasting in patients with mesenchymal tumors (hemangiopericytomas, fibromas, angiosarcomas). The humoral factor secreted by these tumors is FGF-23.[27] This condition can be healed by tumor resection.

Total Parenteral Nutrition Hyperalimentation can also be associated with severe hypophosphatemia through the insulin-mediated shift of phosphate into the cell, particularly if phosphate is omitted from the parenteral nutrition solution. Severe hypophosphatemia can also occur with acute feeding after starvation (as occurred in World War II).

Clinical Manifestations

Clinical manifestations depend more on how rapidly hypophosphatemia has been developing than on its severity and the degree of phosphate deficiency. In practice, they are rarely seen above a serum phosphorus level of 0.65 mmol/l (2.0 mg/dl). They include metabolic encephalopathy, red and white blood cell dysfunction, sometimes hemolysis, and thrombocytopenia. Reduced muscle strength and decreased myocardial contractility (with occasional rhabdomyolysis and cardiomyopathy, respectively) may occur.

Treatment

Generally, phosphate deficiency is not an emergency. First, the mechanism involved should be defined to determine the most appropriate treatment. Diabetic ketoacidosis and acute respiratory alkalosis are typical examples.

When phosphate deficiency is diagnosed, oral treatment by milk products or phosphate salts should always be tried first whenever possible, except in the presence of nephrocalcinosis or

nephrolithiasis with urinary phosphate wasting. In severe symptomatic deficiency, phosphate can also be infused intravenously, in divided doses over 24 hours. In patients undergoing parenteral nutrition, 10 to 25 mmol potassium phosphate should be given for each 1000 kcal. Induction of hyperphosphatemia should be avoided because of the risk of inducing soft-tissue calcifications. The administration of dipyridamole (300 mg divided into four doses per day) has been shown to reduce the urinary excretion of phosphate in patients with a low renal phosphate threshold.[28]

MAGNESIUM HOMEOSTASIS AND DISORDERS OF MAGNESIUM METABOLISM

Distribution of Magnesium in the Organism and Magnesium Homeostasis

Magnesium (Mg) is, after potassium, the second most abundant cation in the intracellular fluid in living organisms. Mg^{2+} is involved in the majority of metabolic processes. In addition, it plays a part in DNA and protein synthesis. It is involved in the regulation of mitochondrial function, in inflammatory processes and immune defense, allergy, growth, and stress, and the control of neuronal activity, cardiac excitability, neuromuscular transmission, vasomotor tone, and blood pressure. The distribution of Mg^{2+} within the intra- and extracellular spaces is shown in Figure 10.20.

Figure 10.21 shows the balance of ingestion, body distribution, and excretion of Mg^{2+} in healthy humans. Mg^{2+} influx into and efflux out of cells are linked to carbohydrate-dependent active transport systems. The stimulation of β-adrenoceptors favors Mg^{2+} outflux, whereas insulin, calcitriol, and vitamin B_6 favor Mg^{2+} entry into cells.

Intestinal and Renal Handling of Magnesium

The intestinal absorption of dietary Mg^{2+} occurs by both a saturable and a passive transport process, the major part being absorbed in the small intestine. The entry step in enterocyte brush border membrane is controlled by the magnesium channel TRPM6, which has been cloned recently and whose functional

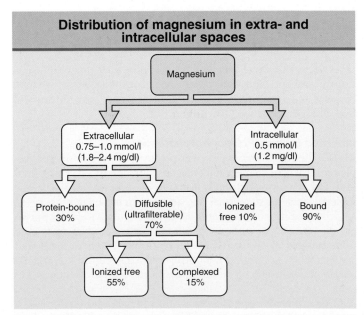

Figure 10.20 Distribution of magnesium in extra- and intracellular spaces.

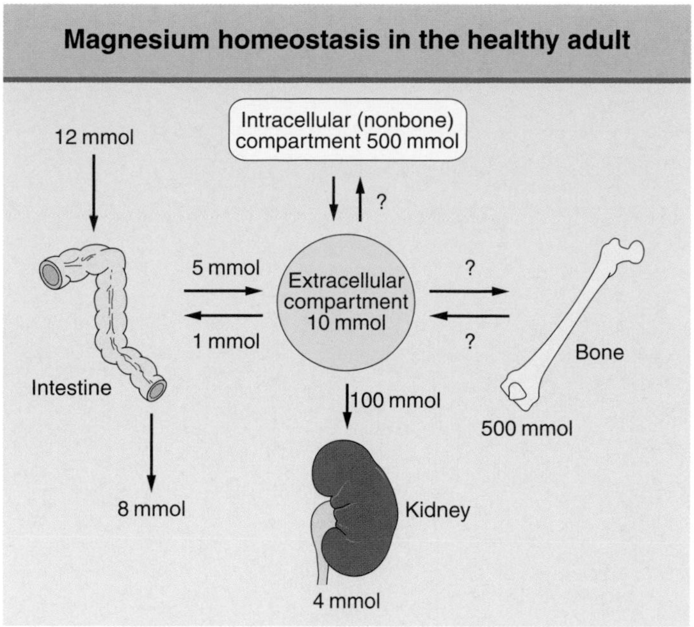

Magnesium homeostasis in the healthy adult

Figure 10.21 Magnesium homeostasis in the healthy young adult. Net zero balance results from net intestinal uptake (absorption minus secretion) equaling urinary loss. After its passage into the extracellular fluid, Mg^{2+} enters the intracellular space, is deposited in bone or soft tissue, or is eliminated via the kidneys. Entry and exit fluxes between the extra- and intracellular spaces (skeletal and nonskeletal compartments) are also of identical magnitude; however, precise values of exchange are still debated.

characterization is in progress.[3] Mg^{2+} absorption can vary by as much as 25% to 60%, with a mean absorption of approximately 30%. There appears to be no adaptation of its intestinal transport in response to chronic changes of dietary magnesium content. However, TRPM6 appears to be downregulated by an increase in intracellular Mg^{2+}.

Various factors modify intestinal Mg^{2+} absorption. High dietary phosphate intake is inhibitory, as is high phytate consumption. The effect of dietary calcium is complex, and vitamin D probably has an enhancing effect. Growth hormone slightly increases Mg^{2+} absorption, whereas aldosterone and calcitonin appear to reduce it. Vitamin B_6 has been reported to enhance it.

Several conditions are associated with anomalies of intestinal Mg^{2+} absorption. A prolonged and severe reduction of dietary magnesium may lead to hypomagnesemia, for example, in chronic alcoholism. The fractional absorption of Mg^{2+} may be reduced in several malabsorption syndromes, intestinal bypass surgery, or fistulas. Malabsorption also occurs with steatorrhea of various causes and in many diarrheal disorders. Severe diarrhea can cause magnesium deficiency quite rapidly. In alcoholism, diarrhea may contribute to reducing intestinal Mg^{2+} absorption.

The long-reported inborn error of intestinal Mg^{2+} absorption has recently been attributed to mutations in the TRPM6 gene.[29] It is associated with profound hypomagnesemia, renal Mg^{2+} wasting, and secondary hypocalcemia. Reduction of intestinal Mg^{2+} absorption has also been observed in patients with hypercalciuria and nephrolithiasis.

Intake of large amounts of magnesium-containing laxatives or antacids can cause a marked increase in Mg^{2+} absorption. However, clinical problems with hypermagnesemia caused by increased magnesium intake arise only when the capacity to excrete Mg^{2+} is reduced.

Mg^{2+} is eliminated by the kidney. Losses via intestinal secretion and sweat are negligible under normal conditions. With an ultrafilterable plasma magnesium concentration of 0.5 to 0.7 mmol/l (80% of total plasma magnesium), the filtered load of magnesium amounts to approximately 104 mmol (or 2500 mg) per day. As the normal urinary magnesium excretion rate is approximately 4 to 5 mmol (or 100 mg) per day, the urinary output represents approximately 5% of the filtered load. The major portion of filtered magnesium is reabsorbed by the renal tubules (25% in the proximal tubule, 65% in the thick ascending loop of Henle, and 5% in the distal convoluted tubule). Figure 10.22 shows a schematic view of the tubular reabsorption of Mg^{2+}.

Mg^{2+} transport in the thick ascending limb is primarily passive via the paracellular route. However, two conditions are necessary for normal Mg^{2+} reabsorption: first, the generation of an electrical, lumen-positive gradient induced by NaCl reabsorption that creates the driving force required for the reabsorption of divalent cations and, second, the expression of claudin-16 in the tight junction, which is responsible for the selectivity of the reabsorption of divalent cations. Different anomalies associated with either NaCl reabsorption or with claudin-16 (formerly called paracellin) expression result in hypermagnesuria (see also later discussion).[30]

In the distal nephron, that is, the distal convoluted tubule and the connecting tubule, Mg^{2+} is reabsorbed via the transcellular route against an uphill electrochemical gradient. The molecular identity of the gatekeeper channel that controls Mg^{2+} entry into the tubular epithelium across the brush border membrane has been discovered recently as TRPM6.[3] It is identical to that of the intestine.

Tubular Mg^{2+} transport is modulated by serum Mg^{2+} and Ca^{2+} and extracellular fluid volume. An increase of plasma Mg^{2+} or Ca^{2+} concentration results in a depression of Mg transport. Extracellular volume expansion produces a decrease in proximal tubular Mg^{2+} reabsorption, in parallel with that of Na^+ and Ca^{2+}. Dietary phosphate restriction results in marked hypercalciuria and hypermagnesuria and can thereby lead to overt hypomagnesemia. PTH, vasopressin, calcitonin, and glucagon increase tubular Mg^{2+} reabsorption, whereas acetylcholine, bradykinin, and atrial natriuretic peptide stimulate urinary Mg^{2+} excretion.

Finally, a number of drugs have been shown to increase renal Mg^{2+} excretion, including the loop diuretics such as furosemide, ethacrynic acid, distal diuretics such as thiazides, and osmotic diuretics such as mannitol and urea. Furthermore, renal Mg^{2+} wasting syndromes have been observed in patients treated with antibiotics such as gentamicin, and antineoplastic agents such as cisplatin and cyclosporine. The precise mechanisms of action(s) of these agents are not all well understood.

HYPERMAGNESEMIA

Elevated plasma Mg^{2+} is seen in patients with acute or chronic renal failure, during the administration of pharmacologic doses of magnesium, in some infants born to mothers who received magnesium for eclampsia, and with the use of oral laxatives or rectal enemas containing magnesium (Fig. 10.23).

Mild hypermagnesemia may also be present in patients with adrenal insufficiency, acromegaly, or familial hypocalciuric hypercalcemia.

Clinical Manifestations

Symptoms and signs are the result of the pharmacologic effects of increased Mg^{2+} concentrations on the nervous and cardiovascular systems. At Mg^{2+} concentrations up to 1.5 mmol/l (3.6 mg/dl), hypermagnesemia is asymptomatic. Deep tendon reflexes are usually lost when plasma magnesium concentration

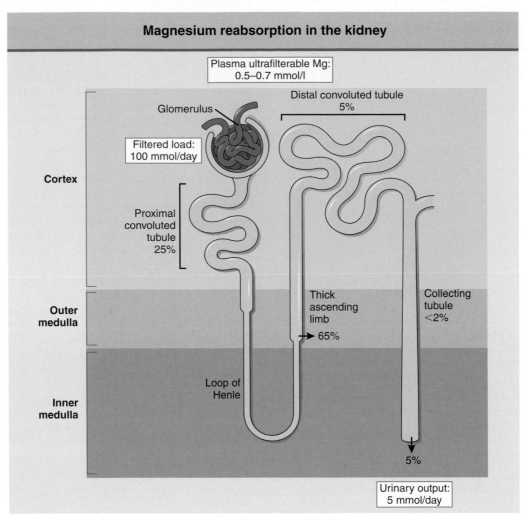

Magnesium reabsorption in the kidney

Figure 10.22 Sites of magnesium reabsorption in various segments of the renal tubule. The percentage absorbed in various segments from the glomerular ultrafiltrate is shown. (Redrawn from Quamme GA: Control of magnesium transport in the thick ascending limb. Am J Physiol 1989;256:F197–F210.)

is greater than 3 mmol/l (7.2 mg/dl). Respiratory paralysis, hypotension, abnormal cardiac conduction, and loss of consciousness may occur as plasma levels of magnesium approach 5 mmol/l (12 mg/dl).

Treatment

Treatment consists of cessation of magnesium administration and the intravenous infusion of calcium salts (calcium gluconate, approximately 90 mg elemental calcium in 10 ml over 5 to 10

minutes intravenously) as initial steps for the management of symptomatic hypermagnesemia.

HYPOMAGNESEMIA AND MAGNESIUM DEFICIENCY

Magnesium deficiency is defined as a decrease in total body magnesium content. Poor dietary intake of magnesium is usually not associated with a marked magnesium deficiency because of the remarkable ability of the normal kidney to conserve Mg^{2+}. However, prolonged and severe dietary magnesium restriction of <0.5 mmol/day can produce symptomatic magnesium deficiency in humans. Severe hypomagnesemia is usually associated with magnesium deficiency. Approximately 10% of patients admitted to a large city hospital in the United States were hypomagnesemic. The incidence may be as high as 65% in medical intensive care units.

Underlying causes are usually diseases of the gastrointestinal tract, in particular malabsorption syndromes including nontropical sprue, and massive resection of the small intestine. Hypomagnesemia can also be induced by prolonged tube feeding without magnesium supplements and by the excessive use of laxatives (Fig. 10.24).

Hypomagnesemia is encountered in about 25% to 35% of patients with acute pancreatitis, is frequently observed in patients

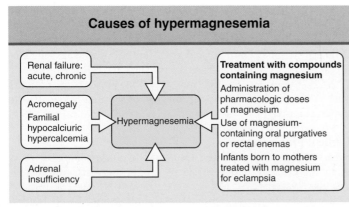

Causes of hypermagnesemia

Renal failure: acute, chronic

Acromegaly Familial hypocalciuric hypercalcemia

Adrenal insufficiency

Hypermagnesemia

Treatment with compounds containing magnesium

Administration of pharmacologic doses of magnesium

Use of magnesium-containing oral purgatives or rectal enemas

Infants born to mothers treated with magnesium for eclampsia

Figure 10.23 Causes of hypermagnesemia.

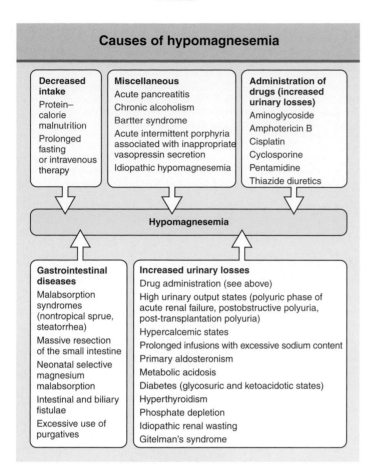

Figure 10.24 Causes of hypomagnesemia.

mutations of the genes of the Na,K,2Cl cotransporter, the rectifying K^+ channel (ROM-K), or the basolateral Cl^- channel in Bartter syndrome are responsible for the abolition of the driving force for Mg^{2+} reabsorption. This results in hypermagnesuria, which, however, is not always associated with hypomagnesemia. Inactivating mutations of the CaR_G gene, whose protein product is a key regulator of NaCl reabsorption in the thick ascending limb via extracellular Ca^{2+} concentration, lead to hypermagnesuria and hypomagnesemia. A mutation of the claudin-16 (previously paracellin-1) gene has been reported to induce a recessive disease characterized by hypomagnesemia, hypermagnesuria, hypercalciuria, and nephrocalcinosis. Mutations in the *TRPM6* gene induce profound hypomagnesemia due to impaired intestinal Mg^{2+} absorption and renal Mg^{2+} wasting, with secondary hypocalcemia.[29]

In the distal convoluted tubule, inactivating mutations of the thiazide-sensitive, electroneutral Na-Cl cotransporter gene (*NCCT*) in Gitelman's syndrome are also responsible for selective renal magnesium wasting and hypomagnesemia.

Recently, hypomagnesemia associated with inappropriate magnesuria has been reported in an autosomal-dominant, isolated familial hypomagnesemia syndrome mapped to chromosome 11q23, which appears to be due to misrouting of the Na^+-K^+-ATPase γ-subunit.[31]

Clinical Manifestations

The main clinical manifestations of moderate to severe magnesium depletion include general weakness and neuromuscular hyperexcitability with hyperreflexia, carpopedal spasm, tremor, and, rarely, tetany. Cardiac findings include a prolonged QT interval and ST depression. There is a predisposition to ventricular arrhythmias and potentiation of digitalis toxicity. Magnesium deficiency can also be associated with hypocalcemia (decreased PTH release and end-organ responsiveness) and hypokalemia (urinary loss). In addition, intracellular K^+ is frequently decreased. Magnesium deficit constitutes a cardiovascular risk factor and also a risk factor in pregnancy for the mother and the fetus.

The diagnosis of moderate degrees of magnesium deficiency is not easy since clinical manifestations may be absent and blood Mg^{2+} levels may not reflect the state of body magnesium. In contrast, a severe magnesium deficit generally goes along with a decrease in blood Mg^{2+} level.

Treatment

Magnesium deficiency is managed with the administration of magnesium salts. Magnesium sulfate is generally used for parenteral therapy (1500 to 3000 mg magnesium sulfate [150 to 300 mg elemental Mg] per day). A variety of magnesium salts are available for oral administration, including oxide, hydroxide, sulfate, lactate, chloride, carbonate, and pidolate. Oral magnesium salts often are not well tolerated. All of them may induce gastrointestinal intolerance, in particular diarrhea.

with chronic alcoholism, and can also be present in patients with poorly controlled diabetes mellitus. Hypomagnesemia can also be observed in patients with hypercalcemic disorders and in primary aldosteronism.

Excessive urinary loss of magnesium occurs in a variety of clinical conditions, leading to hypomagnesemia and magnesium deficiency, even in the face of normal dietary intake. It may result from the overzealous use of diuretics and, therefore, it is important to monitor plasma Mg^{2+} levels in patients with congestive heart failure who are treated with digitalis derivatives and diuretic agents. The administration of other drugs (e.g., gentamicin, cisplatin, and cyclosporine) can also be responsible for hypomagnesemia.

Several familial diseases are associated with hypermagnesuria, with or without hypomagnesemia. They can be associated with inactivating mutations of genes whose abnormal products are responsible for disturbed Mg^{2+} reabsorption in the thick ascending limb of Henle or in the distal nephron. Inactivating

REFERENCES

1. Wasserman RH, Chandler JS, Meyer SA, et al: Intestinal calcium transport and calcium extrusion process at the basolateral membrane. J Nutr 1992; 122:662–671.
2. Wasserman RH, Fullmer CS: Vitamin D and intestinal calcium transport: Facts, speculations and hypotheses. J Nutr 1995;125:1971S–1979S.
3. Hoenderop JG, Bindels RJ: Epithelial Ca2+ and Mg2+ channels in health and disease. J Am Soc Nephrol 2005;16:15–26.
4. Kinyamu HK, Gallagher C, Prahl JM, et al: Association between intestinal vitamin D receptor, calcium absorption, and serum 1,25 dihydroxyvitamin D in normal young and elderly women. J Bone Miner Res 1997;12: 922–928.
5. Mundy GR, Chen D, Zhao M, et al: Growth regulatory factors and bone. Rev Endocr Metab Disord 2001;2:105–115.
6. Bindels RJ: Molecular pathophysiology of renal calcium handling. Kidney Blood Press Res 2000;23:183–184.
7. Hoenderop JG, Nilius B, Bindels RJ: Molecular mechanism of active Ca2+ reabsorption in the distal nephron. Annu Rev Physiol 2002;64: 529–549.

8. Tfelt-Hansen J, Brown EM: The calcium-sensing receptor in normal physiology and pathophysiology: A review. Crit Rev Clin Lab Sci 2005; 42:35–70.

9. Pi M, Faber P, Ekema G, et al: Identification of a novel extracellular cation-sensing G-protein-coupled receptor. J Biol Chem 2005;280:40201–40209.

10. Schipani E, Langman CB, Parfitt AM, et al: Constitutively activated receptors for parathyroid hormone and parathyroid hormone-related peptide in Jansen's metaphyseal chondrodysplasia. N Engl J Med 1996;335:708–714.

11. Thakker RV: Diseases associated with the extracellular calcium-sensing receptor. Cell Calcium 2004;35:275–282.

12. Arnold A, Brown MF, Ureña P, et al: Monoclonality of parathyroid tumors in chronic renal failure and in primary parathyroid hyperplasia. J Clin Invest 1995;95:2047–2054.

13. Stewart AF: Clinical practice. Hypercalcemia associated with cancer. N Engl J Med 2005;352:373–379.

14. Peacock M, Bilezikian JP, Klassen PS, et al: Cinacalcet hydrochloride maintains long-term normocalcemia in patients with primary hyperparathyroidism. J Clin Endocrinol Metab 2005;90:135–141.

15. Block GA, Martin KJ, de Francisco AL, et al: Cinacalcet for secondary hyperparathyroidism in patients receiving hemodialysis. N Engl J Med 2004;350:1516–1525.

16. Pollak MP, Seidman CE, Brown EM: Three inherited disorders in calcium sensing. Medicine 1996;75:115–123.

17. Berndt TJ, Schiavi S, Kumar R: "Phosphatonins" and the regulation of phosphorus homeostasis. Am J Physiol Renal Physiol 2005;289: F1170–F1182.

18. Chang Q, Hoefs S, van der Kemp AW, et al: The beta-glucuronidase klotho hydrolyzes and activates the TRPV5 channel. Science 2005;310:490–493.

19. Prie D, Beck L, Urena P, Friedlander G: Recent findings in phosphate homeostasis. Curr Opin Nephrol Hypertens 2005;14:318–324.

20. Murer H, Hernando N, Forster L, Biber J: Molecular mechanisms in proximal tubular and small intestinal phosphate reabsorption (plenary lecture). Mol Membr Biol 2001;18:3–11.

21. Friedlander G: Autocrine/paracrine control of renal phosphate transport. Kidney Int Suppl 1998;65:S18–S23.

22. Delmez JA, Slatopolsky E: Hyperphosphatemia: Its consequences and treatment in patients with chronic renal disease. Am J Kidney Dis 1992; 19:303–317.

23. Shigematsu T, Kazama JJ, Yamashita T, et al: Possible involvement of circulating fibroblast growth factor 23 in the development of secondary hyperparathyroidism associated with renal insufficiency. Am J Kidney Dis 2004;44:250–256.

24. Brame LA, White KE, Econs MJ: Renal phosphate wasting disorders: Clinical features and pathogenesis. Semin Nephrol 2004;24:39–47.

25. Shimada T, Muto T, Urakawa I, et al: Mutant FGF-23 responsible for autosomal dominant hypophosphatemic rickets is resistant to proteolytic cleavage and causes hypophosphatemia in vivo. Endocrinology 2002;143: 3179–3182.

26. Norden AG, Lapsley M, Igarashi T, et al: Urinary megalin deficiency implicates abnormal tubular endocytic function in Fanconi syndrome. J Am Soc Nephrol 2002;13:125–133.

27. Shimada T, Mizutani S, Muto T, et al: Cloning and characterization of FGF23 as a causative factor of tumor-induced osteomalacia. Proc Natl Acad Sci U S A 2001;98:6500–6505.

28. Prie D, Blanchet FB, Essig M, et al: Dipyridamole decreases renal phosphate leak and augments serum phosphorus in patients with low renal phosphate threshold. J Am Soc Nephrol 1998;9:1264–1269.

29. Schlingmann KP, Sassen MC, Weber S, et al: Novel TRPM6 mutations in 21 families with primary hypomagnesemia and secondary hypocalcemia. J Am Soc Nephrol 2005;16:3061–3069.

30. Unwin RJ, Capasso G, Shirley DG: An overview of divalent cation and citrate handling by the kidney. Nephron Physiol 2004;98:15–20.

31. Meij IC, Koenderink JB, De Jong JC, et al: Dominant isolated renal magnesium loss is caused by misrouting of the Na+,K+-ATPase gamma-subunit. Ann N Y Acad Sci 2003;986:437–443.

Normal Acid-Base Balance

Biff F. Palmer and Robert J. Alpern

INTRODUCTION

The acid-base status of the body is carefully regulated to maintain the arterial pH between 7.35 and 7.45 and the intracellular pH between 7.0 and 7.3. This regulation occurs in the setting of continuous production of acidic metabolites and is accomplished by intracellular and extracellular buffering processes in conjunction with respiratory and renal regulatory mechanisms. The chapter reviews the normal physiology of acid-base homeostasis.

NET ACID PRODUCTION

Both acid and alkali are generated from the diet. Lipid and carbohydrate metabolism result in production of CO_2, a volatile acid, at the rate of approximately 15,000 mmol/day. Protein metabolism yields amino acids, which can be metabolized to form nonvolatile acid and alkali. Amino acids such as lysine and arginine yield acid upon metabolism, while the amino acids glutamate and aspartate and organic anions such as acetate and citrate generate alkali. Sulfur-containing amino acids (methionine and cysteine) are metabolized to sulfuric acid (H_2SO_4), and organophosphates are metabolized to phosphoric acid (H_3PO_4), both strong acids. In general, animal foods are high in proteins and organophosphates, thereby providing a net acid diet, while plant foods are higher in organic anions and provide a net alkaline load. In addition to acid/alkali generated from the diet, there is a small daily production of organic acids including acetic acid, lactic acid, and pyruvic acid. Last, a small amount of acid is generated by the excretion of alkali into the stool. Under normal circumstances, daily net nonvolatile acid production is approximately 1 mmol hydrogen ions (H^+) per kilogram of body weight.

BUFFER SYSTEMS IN REGULATION OF pH

Intracellular and extracellular buffer systems minimize the change in pH during the addition of acid or base equivalents but do not remove acid/alkali from the body. The most important buffer system is that of the bicarbonate ion and carbon dioxide (HCO_3^-/ CO_2). In this system, the $[CO_2]$ concentration is maintained at a constant level set by respiratory control. Addition of acid (HA) leads to conversion of HCO_3^- to CO_2 according to the reaction $HA + NaHCO_3 \rightarrow NaA + H_2O + CO_2$.

HCO_3^- is consumed, but $[CO_2]$ concentration does not change because this is maintained by respiration. The net result is that the acid load has been buffered and pH changes are minimal.

While the HCO_3^-/CO_2 buffer system is the most important of the buffers in extracellular fluid (ECF), other buffers such as plasma proteins and phosphate ions also participate in the maintenance of a stable pH. During metabolic acidosis, the skeleton becomes a major buffer source as acid-induced dissolution of bone

apatite releases alkaline Ca^+ salts and HCO_3^- into the ECF. With chronic metabolic acidosis, this can result in osteomalacia and osteoporosis. The calcium released can result in hypercalciuria and an increased likelihood of renal stones. Within the intracellular compartment, pH is maintained by intracellular buffers such as hemoglobin, cellular proteins, organophosphate complexes, and HCO_3^- as well as by the H^+/HCO_3^- transport mechanisms that serve to transport acid and alkali in and out of the cell.

RESPIRATORY SYSTEM IN REGULATION OF pH

While buffers minimize the changes in pH upon acid/alkali addition, they do not remove acid or alkali from the body. This is accomplished by the lungs and kidneys. The lungs regulate the CO_2 tension, while the kidneys regulate the serum HCO_3^- concentration. While the HCO_3^-/CO_2 buffer system is not the only buffer system, all extracellular buffer systems are in equilibrium. Because the serum HCO_3^- concentration is far greater than that of other buffers, changes in the HCO_3^-/CO_2 buffer pair can easily titrate other buffer systems and, thus, set pH. To understand how the lungs and kidneys function in concert, it is useful to look at the Henderson-Hasselbalch equation:

$$pH = 6.1 + \log \left[\frac{HCO_3^-}{(0.03 \times PaCO_2)}\right]$$

if $PaCO_2$ is measured in mm Hg and

$$pH = 6.1 + \log \left[\frac{HCO_3^-}{(0.225 \times PaCO_2)}\right]$$

if $PaCO_2$ is measured in kPa.

As can be seen, pH is determined by the ratio of HCO_3^- to CO_2. Conditions associated with similar fractional changes in the concentrations of $[HCO_3^-]$ and $[CO_2]$, such as when both are halved, will not change blood pH.

The lungs defend pH by altering alveolar ventilation, which alters the CO_2 excretion rate, and thereby controls the $PaCO_2$ of body fluids. Systemic acidosis stimulates the respiratory center, resulting in increased respiratory drive that lowers the $PaCO_2$. As a result, the fall in blood pH is less than would have occurred in the absence of respiratory compensation. If the fractional change in CO_2 tension were similar to that in serum HCO_3^- concentration, blood pH would not change. However, respiratory compensation rarely normalizes blood pH, and, thus, the fractional change in CO_2 tension is less than the change in the serum HCO_3^- concentration. Quantitatively, the normal respiratory response in metabolic acidosis is a 1.2-mm Hg decrease in $PaCO_2$ for every 1-mmol/l decrease in HCO_3^-, while the increase in $PaCO_2$ in response to metabolic alkalosis averages 0.6 mm Hg for every 1-mmol/L increase in HCO_3^- above baseline.

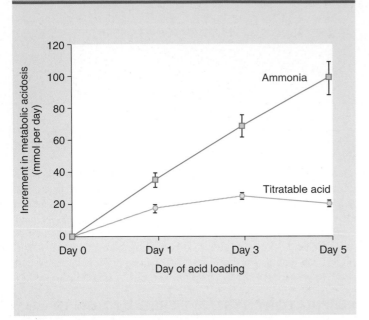

Figure 11.1 Changes in net acid excretion in response to chronic metabolic acidosis. Chronic metabolic acidosis increases net acid excretion dramatically over several days. This figure shows quantitatively the increases in the two major components of net acid excretion: titratable acids and ammonia. Titratable acid excretion increases slightly and predominantly in the first 24 to 48 hours. In contrast, urinary ammonia excretion progressively increases over a period of 7 days, and is responsible for the majority of the increase in net acid excretion in chronic metabolic acidosis. (Data plotted are redrawn from original data of Elkinton JR, Huth EJ, Webster GD Jr, McCance RA: The renal excretion of hydrogen ion in renal tubular acidosis. I. Quantitative assessment of the response to ammonium chloride as an acid load. Am J Medicine 1960;36:554–575.)

RENAL REGULATION OF pH

While buffer systems and respiratory excretion of CO_2 have important roles in maintaining normal acid-base balance, the kidneys provide a critical role in acid-base homeostasis. Under normal conditions, the kidneys generate sufficient net acid excretion to balance the nonvolatile acid produced from normal metabolism. Net acid excretion (NAE) has three primary components, titratable acids, ammonium, and bicarbonate, and is calculated using the following formula:

$$NAE = U_{Am}V + U_{TA}V - U_{HCO_3}V,$$

where $U_{Am}V$ is the rate of NH_4^+ excretion, $U_{TA}V$ is the rate of titratable acid excretion, and $U_{HCO_3}V$ is the rate of HCO_3^- excretion. Under basal conditions, approximately 40% of net acid excretion is in the form of titratable acids and 60% is in the form of ammonia; urinary bicarbonate concentrations and excretion are essentially zero under normal conditions. When acid production increases, the increase in acid excretion is almost entirely due to an increase in excretion of NH_4^+ (Fig. 11.1).

RENAL TRANSPORT MECHANISMS OF HYDROGEN AND BICARBONATE IONS

Glomerulus

The glomerulus is not normally considered to participate in acid-base regulation. However, the glomerulus filters an amount of HCO_3^- equivalent to the serum HCO_3^- concentration multiplied

by the glomerular filtration rate (GFR). Under normal circumstances, the filtered load of HCO_3^- averages approximately 4000 mmol/day. Normal acid-base homeostasis requires both the reabsorption of this filtered bicarbonate and the generation of "new" bicarbonate; the latter replenishes bicarbonate and other alkaline buffers consumed in the process of titrating endogenous acid production. From the standpoint of prevention of or correction of acidosis, GFR is not regulated by alterations in acid or base, and therefore does not contribute to acid-base homeostasis.

Proximal Tubule

The proximal tubule reabsorbs approximately 80% of the filtered load of HCO_3^-. In addition, by titrating luminal pH from 7.4 down to approximately 6.7, the majority of phosphate, the major form of titratable acid, is titrated to its acid form. Last, ammonia synthesis occurs in the proximal tubule.

Figure 11.2 shows a model of the acid-base transport mechanisms of the proximal tubule cell. HCO_3^- absorption from the tubular lumen is mediated by H^+ secretion across the membrane.[1,2] This H^+ secretion is active in that the electrochemical gradient favors H^+ movement from lumen to cell. Two mechanisms have been identified that mediate active apical H^+ secretion. Approximately two thirds occurs via the apical membrane Na^+-H^+ antiporter NHE-3. This protein uses the inward Na^+ gradient to drive H^+ secretion. The Na^+-H^+ exchanger has a 1:1 stoichiometry and is electroneutral. In parallel with the Na^+-H^+ antiporter, there is an apical membrane H^+-ATPase that mediates approximately one third of basal proximal tubular HCO_3^- absorption.

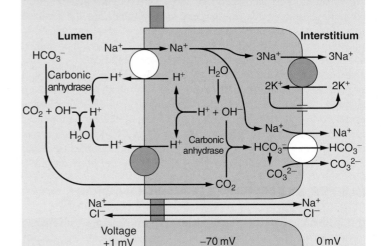

Figure 11.2 Proximal tubule NaHCO₃ reabsorption. The secretion of H^+ into the proximal tubule lumen involves an Na^+-H^+ antiporter and an H^+-ATPase. Apical membrane H^+ secretion generates OH^-, which reacts with CO_2 to form HCO_3^- and CO_3^{2-}, and these exit with an Na^+ on the basolateral membrane Na^+-HCO_3^--CO_3^{2-} cotransporter. The Na^+ absorbed by the Na^+-H^+ antiporter exits the cell on the basolateral membrane Na^+-K^+-ATPase and the Na^+-HCO_3^--CO_3^{2-} cotransporter. The K^+ that enters the cell on the Na^+-K^+-ATPase exits on a basolateral membrane K^+ channel. Carbonic anhydrase catalyzes the conversion of HCO_3^- to CO_2 and OH^- in the lumen and the reverse reaction in the cell. Electrogenic H^+ secretion generates a small lumen-positive voltage that generates a current flow across the paracellular pathway.

Both of these H$^+$ transporters generate base in the cell, which must exit across the basolateral membrane in order to affect transepithelial transport. The primary mechanism by which this occurs is a basolateral Na$^+$-HCO$_3^-$-CO$_3^{2-}$ cotransporter. Because this protein transports the equivalent of two net negative charges, intracellular electronegativity, generated by the basolateral Na$^+$-K$^+$-ATPase, drives net outward movement. The Na$^+$-3HCO$_3^-$ cotransporter NBC1, encoded by the gene *SLC4A4*, mediates the majority of proximal tubule basolateral base exit.[3]

Carbonic anhydrase is present in the proximal tubule cytoplasm and on the apical and basolateral membranes. Carbonic anhydrase subserves a number of functions in the proximal tubule. Apical membrane carbonic anhydrase allows secreted H$^+$ ions, which react with luminal HCO$_3^-$ forming H$_2$CO$_3$ to rapidly dissociate to CO$_2$ + H$_2$O. This CO$_2$ can then diffuse across the apical plasma membrane into the cell. There the process is reversed, using cytoplasmic carbonic anhydrase, generating intracellular H$^+$ and HCO$_3^-$. This H$^+$ "replenishes" the H$^+$ secreted across the apical membrane, resulting in net movement of the HCO$_3^-$ from the luminal solution to the cell cytoplasm. The intracellular HCO$_3^-$ is then secreted across the basolateral plasma membrane as described previously.

Thick Ascending Limb of the Loop of Henle

Tubular fluid arriving at the early distal tubule has a pH and serum HCO$_3^-$ concentration similar to that of the late proximal tubule. Because there is significant water extraction in the loop of Henle, maintenance of a constant serum HCO$_3^-$ concentration requires reabsorption of HCO$_3^-$. The majority of this HCO$_3^-$ absorption appears to be accomplished in the thick ascending limb through mechanisms that appear to be very similar to those present in the proximal tubule. The majority of apical membrane H$^+$ secretion is mediated by the Na$^+$-H$^+$ antiporter NHE-3. In addition, the cells possess a basolateral membrane Na$^+$-HCO$_3^-$-CO$_3^{2-}$ cotransporter, which likely mediates the majority of base efflux. These cells also possess an H$^+$-ATPase, but it is not clear what role it plays in acidification.

Distal Nephron

Approximately 80% of the filtered HCO$_3^-$ is reabsorbed in the proximal tubule, with most, but not all, of the remainder absorbed in the thick ascending limb. One of the functions of the distal nephron is to reabsorb the remaining 5% of filtered HCO$_3^-$. In addition, the distal nephron must secrete a quantity of H$^+$ equal to that generated systemically by metabolism in order to maintain acid-base balance.

The distal nephron is subdivided into several distinct portions that differ in their anatomy and acid secretory properties. Most of these segments transport H$^+$ and HCO$_3^-$ into the luminal fluid, but the main segments appear to be in the collecting duct.[4] The segments of the collecting duct include the cortical collecting duct, the outer medullary collecting duct, and the inner medullary collecting duct. There are two distinct cell types in the cortical collecting duct that can be distinguished histologically: the principal cell and the intercalated cell. The principal cell reabsorbs Na$^+$ and secretes K$^+$ and is discussed further. Depending on chronic acid-base status, the cortical collecting duct is capable of either H$^+$ or HCO$_3^-$ secretion. These functions are mediated by one of two types of intercalated cells: the acid secreting α-intercalated cell and the base secreting β-intercalated cell. Both types of intercalated cells are rich in carbonic anhydrase.

Reabsorption of HCO$_3^-$ in the distal nephron is mediated by apical H$^+$ secretion mediated by the α-intercalated cell. This

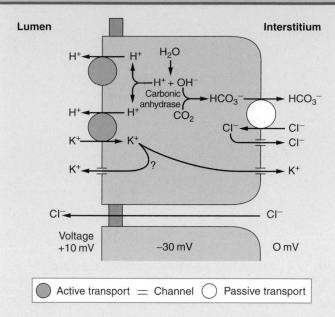

Secretion of H$^+$ in the α-intercalated cell of the cortical collecting duct

Figure 11.3   Secretion of H$^+$ in the α-intercalated cell. Secretion of H$^+$ into the lumen by an H$^+$-ATPase and an H$^+$-K$^+$-ATPase. Apical membrane H$^+$ secretion generates OH$^-$, which reacts with CO$_2$ to form HCO$_3^-$; this exits across the basolateral membrane on a Cl$^-$-HCO$_3^-$ exchanger. The Cl$^-$ that enters the cell on the exchanger recycles across a basolateral membrane Cl channel. The K$^+$ that enters the cell on the H$^+$-K$^+$-ATPase appears to be able to either recycle across the apical membrane or exit across the basolateral membrane, depending on the potassium balance of the individual. Carbonic anhydrase catalyzes the conversion of CO$_2$ and OH$^-$ to HCO$_3^-$ in the cell. Electrogenic H$^+$ secretion generates a lumen-positive voltage, which generates a current flow across the paracellular pathway.

process is mediated by one of two transporters: a vacuolar H$^+$-ATPase and an H$^+$-K$^+$-ATPase (Fig. 11.3). The vacuolar H$^+$-ATPase is an electrogenic pump and similar to, but distinct from, the H$^+$ pump present within many intracellular compartments, such as lysosomes, the Golgi apparatus, and endosomes. At least two H$^+$-ATPase isoforms are present in the kidney, one similar to that present in the stomach and one similar to that present in the colon. H$^+$-ATPase uses the energy derived from adenosine triphosphate hydrolysis to secrete H$^+$ into the lumen and reabsorb K$^+$ in an electroneutral fashion. The activity of the H$^+$-K$^+$-ATPase increases in K$^+$ depletion and thus provides a mechanism by which K$^+$ depletion enhances both collecting duct H$^+$ secretion and K$^+$ absorption.

Active H$^+$ secretion by the apical membrane generates intracellular base that must exit the basolateral membrane. A basolateral Cl$^-$-HCO$_3^-$ exchanger is the mechanism by which this base exit occurs. The Cl$^-$ that enters the cell in exchange for HCO$_3^-$ exits the cell through a basolateral membrane Cl$^-$ conductance channel (see Fig. 11.3).

The HCO$_3^-$ secreting β-intercalated cell is in many respects a mirror image of the α-intercalated cell (Fig. 11.4). It possesses an H$^+$-ATPase on the basolateral membrane, which mediates active H$^+$ extrusion. Alkali that is generated within the cell then exits on an apical membrane Cl$^-$-HCO$_3^-$ exchanger. Importantly, this Cl$^-$-HCO$_3^-$ exchanger appears to be distinct from the basolateral Cl$^-$-HCO$_3^-$ exchanger present in the α-intercalated cell.

The other cortical collecting tubule cell type is the principal cell, and it, too, regulates acid-base transport, albeit indirectly.

Secretion of HCO₃⁻ in the β-intercalated cell of the cortical collecting duct

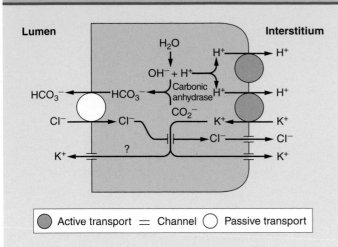

Figure 11.4 Bicarbonate secretion by the β-intercalated cell. Here H⁺ is secreted into the interstitium by an H⁺-ATPase. The OH⁻ generated by basolateral membrane H⁺ secretion reacts with CO_2 to form HCO_3^-, which exits across the apical membrane on a Cl^--HCO_3^- exchanger. The Cl^- that enters the cell on the exchanger exits across a basolateral membrane Cl^- channel. Carbonic anhydrase catalyzes the conversion of CO_2 and OH^- to HCO_3^- in the cell.

Transport of Na⁺ in the principal cell of the cortical collecting duct

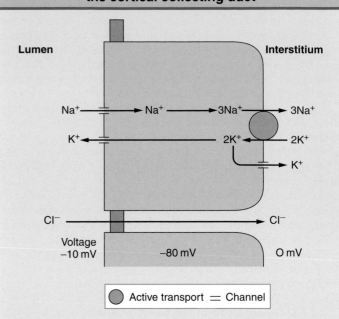

Figure 11.5 The transport of Na⁺ in the principal cell of the cortical collecting duct. Electrogenic Na^+ absorption is mediated by an Na^+ channel. The Na^+ enters the cell across the apical membrane channel and exits the cell on the basolateral membrane Na^+-K^+-ATPase. The K^+ that enters the cell on the basolateral Na^+-K^+-ATPase can be secreted into the luminal fluid by an apical membrane K^+ channel. Electrogenic Na^+ absorption establishes a lumen-negative voltage that drives a paracellular current.

Principal cells mediate electrogenic Na^+ reabsorption that results in a net negative luminal charge (Fig. 11.5). The greater this negative charge is, the lesser the electrochemical gradient for electrogenic proton secretion, and therefore the greater the rate of net proton secretion. Thus, factors that stimulate Na^+ reabsorption indirectly regulate the H^+ secretory rate.

The medullary collecting duct appears to only possess mechanisms for H^+ secretion. This H^+ secretion is mediated by α-intercalated cells, but also is mediated by cells that morphologically appear distinct from intercalated cells yet functionally appear similar.

Net Acid Excretion

For the kidney to generate net acid excretion, it must both reabsorb filtered HCO_3^- and excrete titratable acids and ammonia. Several weak acids, such as phosphate, creatinine, and uric acid, are filtered at the glomerulus and can buffer secreted protons. Of these, phosphate is the most important because of its favorable pKa of 6.80 and its relatively high rate of urinary excretion (~25 to 30 mmol/day). However, the capacity of phosphate to buffer protons is maximized at a urine pH of 5.8, and acid-base disturbances do not, in general, induce substantial changes in urinary phosphate excretion. Other titratable acids, such as creatinine and uric acid, are limited by their lower excretion rates that are not dramatically changed in response to acid-base disturbances. As shown in Figure 11.1, titratable acid excretion is a minor component of the increase in net acid excretion in response to metabolic acidosis.

Ammonia Metabolism

Quantitatively, the most important component of net acid excretion is the NH_3/NH_4^+ system.[5] Unlike titratable acids, the rate of ammonia production and excretion is varied according to physiologic needs. Under normal circumstances, ammonia excretion

accounts for approximately 60% of total net acid excretion, and in response to chronic metabolic acidosis, almost the entire increase in net acid excretion is due to increased ammonia metabolism. Ammonia metabolism involves an interplay between the proximal tubule, thick ascending limb of the loop of Henle, and the collecting duct.

The proximal tubule is responsible for both ammonia production and luminal secretion. Ammonia is synthesized in the proximal tubule predominantly from glutamine metabolism through enzymatic processes in which phosphoenolpyruvate carboxykinase and phosphate-dependent glutaminase are the rate-limiting steps. This results in production of two NH_4^+ and two HCO_3^- ions from each glutamine ion. Ammonia is then preferentially secreted into the lumen. The primary mechanism for this luminal secretion appears to be NH_4^+ transport by the apical Na^+-H^+ antiporter NHE-3.

Most of the ammonia that leaves the proximal tubule does not return to the distal tubule. Thus, there is transport of ammonia out of the loop of Henle. This transport appears to occur predominantly in the thick ascending limb of the loop of Henle and is mediated by at least three mechanisms. First, the lumen-positive voltage provides a driving force for passive paracellular NH_4^+ transport out of the thick ascending limb. Second, NH_4^+ can be transported out of the lumen by the furosemide-sensitive Na^+-K^+-$2Cl^-$ transporter. Last, NH_4^+ can leave the lumen across the apical membrane K^+ channel of the thick ascending limb cell. There is little information as to how NH_4^+ would then leave the cell across the basolateral membrane.

Finally, ammonia is secreted by the collecting duct. Although the traditional thought was that NH_3/NH_4^+ then enters the collecting duct by nonionic diffusion driven by the acid luminal pH, increasing evidence suggests that the nonerythroid glyco-proteins Rhbg and Rhcg may be involved in collecting duct ammonia secretion.[6]

Based on the preceding discussion, ammonia excretion can be regulated by three mechanisms. First, ammonia synthesis in the proximal tubule can be regulated. Chronic acidosis and hypokalemia increase ammonia synthesis, whereas hyperkalemia suppresses ammonia synthesis. Second, ammonia delivery from the proximal tubule to the medullary interstitium can be regulated. In particular, chronic metabolic acidosis increases expression of both NHE-3 and the loop of Henle Na^+-K^+-$2Cl^-$ cotransporter. Hyper-kalemia can inhibit NH_4^+ reabsorption from the thick ascending limb. This may explain the low urinary $[NH_4^+]$ concentrations found in hyperkalemic distal renal tubular acidosis (RTA) in addition to decreased synthesis of ammonia by hyperkalemia. In addition, any interstitial renal disease that destroys renal medullary anatomy may decrease medullary interstitial $[NH_3/NH_4^+]$ concentration. Last, mechanisms that regulate collecting duct H^+ secretion or ammonia transporter expression can regulate ammonia entry into the collecting duct and excretion. However, it is important to recognize that the majority of the mechanisms described involve synthesis of new proteins in order to increase both ammonia production and transport. Accordingly, changes in ammonia excretion may be delayed, and the maximal renal response to chronic metabolic acidosis requires 4 to 7 days.

REGULATION OF RENAL ACIDIFICATION

The precise regulation of acid-base balance requires an integrated system that precisely regulates proximal tubular H^+-HCO_3^- transport, distal nephron H^+-HCO_3^- transport, and ammonia synthesis and transport. Some key determinants of this regulation are reviewed.

Blood pH
The regulation of acid-base balance requires that in states of acidosis net H^+ excretion increase, and in states of alkalosis, net H^+ excretion decrease. This form of regulation involves both acute and chronic mechanisms. In the proximal tubule, acute decreases in blood pH increase the rate of HCO_3^- absorption, and acute increases in blood pH inhibit HCO_3^- absorption. These alterations in the rate of HCO_3^- absorption occur whether the change in pH is the result of changes in $PaCO_2$ or serum HCO_3^- concentration. Similarly, in the collecting duct, acute changes in peritubular serum HCO_3^- concentration and pH regulate the rate of H^+ secretion.

In addition to acute regulation, mechanisms exist for chronic regulation. Chronic acidosis or alkalosis leads to parallel changes in the activities of the proximal tubule apical membrane Na^+-H^+ antiporter and basolateral membrane Na^+-HCO_3^--CO_3^{2-} cotransporter. Metabolic acidosis acutely increases the kinetic activity of NHE-3 through direct pH effects and by phosphory-lation while chronic acidosis increases the number of NHE-3 transporters.[7,8] In addition, chronic acidosis increases proximal tubular ammonia synthesis by increasing the activities of the enzymes involved in ammonia metabolism.

The cortical collecting duct is also modified by chronic acid-base changes. As previously noted, the cortical collecting duct is able to secrete either H^+ ion or HCO_3^-. If animals are fed an acid-rich diet, cells responsible for H^+ secretion increase their activity, whereas cells responsible for HCO_3^- secretion decrease their activity.[9] Conversely, in animals fed an alkali-rich diet, HCO_3^--secreting cells increase their activity and H^+-secreting cells decrease their activity.

Mineralocorticoids, Distal Sodium Delivery, and Extracellular Fluid Volume
Mineralocorticoid hormones are key regulators of distal nephron and collecting duct H^+ secretion. Two mechanisms appear to be involved. First, mineralocorticoid hormone stimulates Na^+ absorption in principal cells of the cortical collecting duct (see Fig. 11.5). This leads to a more lumen-negative voltage that then stimulates H^+ secretion. This mechanism is indirect in that it requires the presence of Na^+ and of Na^+ transport.

A second mechanism is the direct activation of H^+ secretion by mineralocorticoid hormones. The effect of mineralocorticoids is chronic, requiring long exposure, and appears to involve increases in apical membrane H^+-ATPase and basolateral membrane Cl^--HCO_3^- exchanger activity in parallel.[10] This effect is most likely transcriptional, as with other steroid hormones.

Plasma Volume
Changes in plasma volume have important effects on acid-base homeostasis. This effect appears to be related to a number of factors. First, volume contraction is associated with a decreased GFR that lowers the filtered load of HCO_3^- and decreases the load placed on the tubules to maintain net acid excretion. Volume contraction also acutely decreases the paracellular permeability of the proximal tubule. This will tend to decrease HCO_3^- backleak around cells, thereby increasing net bicarbonate reabsorption by the proximal tubule. Third, chronic volume contraction is associated with an adaptive increase in the activity of the proximal tubule apical membrane Na^+-H^+ antiporter NHE-3. Because this transporter contributes to both $NaHCO_3$ and $NaCl$ absorption, both of these capacities will be increased with chronic volume contraction. Last, volume contraction limits distal delivery of chloride. In the presence of chronic metabolic alkalosis, the cortical collecting duct is poised for HCO_3^- secretion. However, collecting duct HCO_3^- secretion requires luminal Cl^- and is inhibited by Cl^- deficiency.

Potassium
Potassium deficiency is associated with an increase in renal net acid excretion. This effect is multifactorial. First, chronic K^+ deficiency increases the proximal tubule apical membrane Na^+-H^+ antiporter and basolateral membrane Na^+-HCO_3^--CO_3^{2-} cotransporter activities. This effect is similar to that seen with chronic acidosis and may be due to intracellular acidosis. Chronic K^+ deficiency also increases proximal tubular ammonia produc-tion. Last, chronic K^+ deficiency leads to an increase in collecting duct H^+ secretion. This appears to be related to increased activity of the apical membrane H^+-K^+-ATPase. Such an effect increases the rate of H^+ secretion and the rate of K^+ reabsorption in the collecting duct. Finally, ammonia, whose production is stimulated by hypokalemia, has direct effects to stimulate collecting duct H^+ secretion. Counterbalancing these effects is that K^+ deficiency decreases aldosterone secretion, which can inhibit distal acidification. Thus, in normal individuals, the net effect of K^+ deficiency is typically a minor change in acid-base balance. However, in those in whom mineralocorticoid secretion

is nonsuppressible (e.g., hyperaldosteronism, Cushing's syndrome), K^+ deficiency can markedly stimulate renal acidification and cause profound metabolic alkalosis.

It should be noted that hyperkalemia appears to have opposite effects on renal acidification. The most notable effect of hyperkalemia is inhibition of ammonia synthesis in the proximal tubule and ammonia absorption in the loop of Henle, thereby resulting in inappropriately low levels of urinary ammonia excretion. This contributes to the metabolic acidosis seen in patients with hyperkalemic distal renal tubular acidosis or type IV RTA.

REFERENCES

1. Alpern RJ: Cell mechanisms of proximal tubule acidification. Physiol Rev 1990;70:79–114.
2. Bobulescu A, Di Sole F, Moe OW: Na/H exchangers: Physiology and link to hypertension and organ ischemia. Curr Opin Nephrol Hypertens 2005;14:485–494.
3. Romero M: Molecular pathophysiology of SLC4 bicarbonate transporters. Curr Opin Nephrol Hypertens 2005;14:495–501.
4. Alpern RJ: Renal acidification mechanisms. In Brenner BM (ed): The Kidney, 5th ed. Philadelphia: Saunders, 1996, pp 455–519.
5. Knepper MA, Packer R, Good DW: Ammonium transport in the kidney. Physiol Rev 1989;69:179–249.
6. Weiner ID: The Rh gene family and renal ammonium transport. Curr Opin Nephrol Hypertens 2004;13:533–540.
7. Moe OW: Acute regulation of proximal tubule apical membrane Na/H exchanger NHE-3: Role of phosphorylation, protein trafficking, and regulatory factors. J Am Soc Nephrol 1999;10:2412–2425.
8. Ambuhl P, Amemiya M, Danczkay M, et al: Chronic metabolic acidosis increases NHE3 protein abundance in rat kidney. Am J Physiol 1996;271:F917–F925.
9. McKinney TD, Burg MB: Bicarbonate transport by rabbit cortical collecting tubules: Effect of acid and alkaline loads in vivo on transport in vitro. J Clin Invest 1977;60:766–768.

12 Metabolic Acidosis

Biff F. Palmer and Robert J. Alpern

Metabolic acidosis is diagnosed by a low arterial blood pH in conjunction with a reduced serum HCO_3^- concentration. Respiratory compensation resulting in a decrease in the $PaCO_2$ is almost always present. It is important to note that a low serum HCO_3^- concentration alone is not diagnostic of metabolic acidosis since it also results from the renal compensation to chronic respiratory alkalosis. Measurement of the arterial pH differentiates between these two possibilities. A recommended approach to a patient with metabolic acidosis is shown in Figure 12.1.

After confirming the presence of metabolic acidosis, the first step in the examination of metabolic acidosis is to calculate the serum anion gap. The anion gap is equal to the difference between the plasma concentrations of the major cation (Na^+) and the major measured anions (Cl^- + HCO_3^-) and is given by the following formula:

$$\text{anion gap} = [Na^+] - ([Cl^-] + [HCO_3^-]).$$

Assessment of low serum HCO_3^- concentration

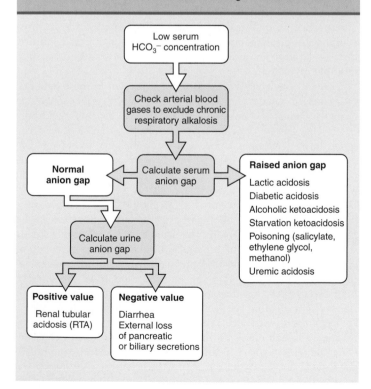

Figure 12.1 Approach to the patient with a low serum HCO_3^- concentration.

Classification of metabolic acidosis

Hyperchloremic normal gap acidosis
  Renal origin
    Proximal renal tubular acidosis (type II RTA)
    Hypokalemic distal renal tubular acidosis (type I RTA)
    Hyperkalemic distal renal tubular acidosis (type IV RTA)
    Renal tubular acidosis of renal insufficiency (GFR usually >15–20 ml/min)
  Extrarenal origin
    Diarrhea
    Gastrointestinal ureteral connections
    External loss pancreatic or biliary secretions

Anion gap metabolic acidosis
  Renal origin
    Uremic acidosis (GFR usually <15–20 ml/min)
  Extrarenal origin
    Lactic acidosis
    Diabetic ketoacidosis
    Starvation ketoacidosis
    Alcoholic ketoacidosis
    Poisoning (ethylene glycol, methanol, salicylate)
    Pyroglutamic acidosis

Figure 12.2 Classification of metabolic acidosis. GFR, glomerular filtration rate; RTA, renal tubular acidosis.

The normal value of the anion gap is approximately 12 ± 2 mmol/l. Because much of the unmeasured anions consist of albumin, the normal anion gap may be decreased by approximately 4 mmol/l for each 1-g/dl decrease in the serum albumin below normal. Because the total number of cations must equal the total number of anions, a decrease in the serum HCO_3^- concentration must be offset by an increase in the concentration of other anions. If the anion accompanying excess H^+ is Cl^-, then the decrease in the serum HCO_3^- concentration is matched by an equal increase in the serum Cl^- concentration. The acidosis is classified as a normal gap or a nonanion gap or a hyperchloremic metabolic acidosis. By contrast, if excess H^+ is accompanied by an anion other than Cl^-, then the decreased HCO_3^- is balanced by an increase in the concentration of the unmeasured anion. The Cl^- concentration remains the same. In this setting, the acidosis is said to be a "high anion gap" or "anion gap" metabolic acidosis. Figure 12.2 lists common causes of metabolic acidosis according to the anion gap.

NONANION (NORMAL ANION) GAP METABOLIC ACIDOSIS

A nonanion gap metabolic acidosis can result from either renal or extrarenal causes. Renal causes of metabolic acidosis occur when renal bicarbonate generation, which results from net acid excretion, does not balance the loss of bicarbonate and other alkali buffers consumed in the buffering of normal endogenous acid production. This failure of net acid excretion is termed renal tubular acidosis (RTA). Extrarenal causes occur when exogenous acid loads, endogenous acid production, or endogenous bicarbonate losses are elevated and exceed renal net acid excretion. The most common extrarenal cause of nonanion gap metabolic acidosis is chronic diarrhea.

A useful method to distinguish renal and extrarenal causes of metabolic acidosis is to measure urinary ammonia excretion.[1] As discussed in Chapter 11, the primary mechanism by which the kidneys generate new bicarbonate to both buffer normal endogenous acid production and respond to metabolic acidosis is through urinary ammonia excretion. Each millimole of urinary ammonia excreted results in the generation of 1 mmol of "new" bicarbonate. Thus, renal causes of metabolic acidosis are characterized by low urinary ammonia excretion rates. In contrast, in extrarenal metabolic acidosis, urinary ammonia excretion is elevated. Unfortunately, most clinical laboratories will not measure urinary ammonia. Instead, one can indirectly assess urinary ammonia concentration using the urinary anion gap (UAG), which is calculated using the following formula:

$$UAG = (U_{Na+} + U_{K+}) - U_{Cl^-}.$$

Under normal circumstances, the UAG is positive, with values ranging from $+30$ to $+50$ mmol/l. A negative value for the UAG suggests increased renal excretion of an unmeasured cation (i.e., a cation other than Na^+ or K^+). One such cation is NH_4^+. With chronic metabolic acidosis due to extrarenal causes, urinary ammonia concentrations, in the form of NH_4Cl, can reach 200 to 300 mmol/l. As a result, the measured cation concentration will be less than the measured anion concentration, which includes the increased urinary Cl^-, and the UAG will be less than zero, and frequently less than -20 mmol/l.

It is important to recognize that the UAG only indirectly reflects the urinary ammonia concentration and, if other unmeasured ions are excreted, can give misleading results. One such example is diabetic ketoacidosis when there is substantial urinary excretion of sodium keto acid salts. Another example, discussed later in more detail, is toluene exposure in which there is increased urinary excretion of sodium hippurate and sodium benzoate. In most cases, these conditions are associated with an elevated anion gap metabolic acidosis, not a nonanion gap metabolic acidosis, and thus are easily distinguishable from diarrhea-induced metabolic acidosis.

It is also important to recognize that urine pH, in contrast to the UAG, does not reliably differentiate acidosis of renal origin from that of extrarenal origin. For example, an acid urine pH does not necessarily indicate an appropriate increase in net acid excretion. If renal ammonia metabolism is inhibited, as occurs with chronic hyperkalemia, there is decreased ammonia available in the distal nephron to serve as a buffer, and small amounts of distal H^+ secretion can lead to a significant urine acidification. In this setting, the urine pH is acid, but net acid excretion is low because of the low ammonia excretion. Similarly, alkaline urine does not necessarily imply a renal acidification defect. In conditions in which ammonia metabolism is stimulated, distal H^+ secretion can be massive and yet the urine remains relatively alkaline because of the buffering effects of ammonia.

METABOLIC ACIDOSIS OF RENAL ORIGIN

Proximal Renal Tubular Acidosis (Type II)

Under normal circumstances, approximately 80% to 90% of the filtered load of HCO_3^- is reabsorbed in the proximal tubule. In proximal RTA, the proximal tubule has a decreased capacity to reabsorb filtered bicarbonate. When serum bicarbonate is normal or near normal, the amount of bicarbonate filtered by the glomerulus exceeds proximal tubule bicarbonate reabsorptive capacity. When this happens, there is increased bicarbonate delivery to the loop of Henle and distal nephron that exceeds their capacity to reabsorb bicarbonate. As a result, a component of filtered bicarbonate appears in the urine. The net effect is that the serum HCO_3^- concentration decreases. Eventually, the filtered bicarbonate load decreases to the point where the proximal tubule is able to reabsorb sufficient filtered bicarbonate that the bicarbonate load to the loop of Henle and the distal nephron is within their reabsorptive capacity. When this process occurs no further bicarbonate is lost in the urine, net acid excretion normalizes, and a new steady-state serum bicarbonate concentration develops, albeit at a lower than normal level.

Hypokalemia is characteristically present in proximal RTA. During the generation of proximal RTA, renal $NaHCO_3$ losses lead to intravascular volume depletion, which in turn activates the renin angiotensin aldosterone system. Distal Na^+ delivery is increased as a result of the impaired proximal reabsorption of $NaHCO_3$. Because of the associated hyperaldosteronism and increased distal nephron Na^+ reabsorption, there is increased K^+ secretion. The net result is renal potassium wasting and the development of hypokalemia. In the steady state, when virtually all the filtered HCO_3^- is reabsorbed in the proximal and distal nephron, renal K^+ wasting is less and the degree of hypokalemia tends to be mild.

Proximal RTA may occur as an isolated defect in acidification, but typically occurs in the setting of widespread proximal tubule dysfunction (Fanconi syndrome)[2] (see Chapter 47). In addition to decreased HCO_3^- reabsorption, patients with the Fanconi syndrome have impaired reabsorption of glucose, phosphate, uric acid, amino acids, and low molecular weight proteins. Various inherited and acquired disorders have been associated with the development of Fanconi syndrome and proximal RTA (Fig. 12.3). The most common inherited cause in children is cystinosis. Most adults with the Fanconi syndrome have an acquired condition that is related to an underlying dysproteinemic condition such as multiple myeloma.

Skeletal abnormalities are commonly present in these patients. Osteomalacia can develop as a result of chronic hypophosphatemia owing to renal phosphate wasting if the Fanconi syndrome is present. These patients may also have a deficiency in the active form of vitamin D because of an inability to convert 25-hydroxyvitamin D_3 to 1,25-dihydroxyvitamin D in the proximal tubule. In contrast to distal RTA, proximal RTA is not associated with nephrolithiasis or nephrocalcinosis.

The diagnosis of proximal RTA should be suspected in a patient with a normal anion gap acidosis and hypokalemia who has an intact ability to acidify the urine to <5.5 while in a steady state.[3] Other findings of proximal tubular dysfunction, such as glycosuria in the setting of a normal serum glucose concentration, hypophosphatemia, hypouricemia, and mild proteinuria, help to support this diagnosis. The UAG is generally greater than zero, indicating the lack of increase in net acid excretion.

Treating patients with proximal RTA can be difficult. Administration of alkali increases the serum bicarbonate concentration, which increases urinary bicarbonate losses, and thereby minimizes subsequent increases in the serum bicarbonate. Moreover, the increased distal sodium load, in combination with increased circulating plasma aldosterone, results in increased renal potassium wasting and worsening hypokalemia. As a result, substantial amounts of the alkali may be needed to be provided as the potassium salt in order to prevent substantial hypokalemia from developing. The most widely available potassium alkali is potassium citrate. Citra-K and Polycitra K are commercially available potassium citrate products. Polycitra is a commercially available product that consists of equimolar amounts of sodium citrate and potassium citrate.

Children with proximal RTA need to be aggressively treated in an attempt to normalize their serum bicarbonate concentration. Doing so can help to minimize the growth retardation that results in children from metabolic acidosis. These children may require large amounts of alkali therapy, typically 5 to 15 mmol/kg/day.

Adults with proximal RTA are frequently not treated as aggressively as children because of the lack of significant metabolic abnormalities or bone disease. Many clinicians will treat these patients with alkali therapy if the serum bicarbonate is <18 mmol/l to prevent the development of more severe acidosis. Whether more aggressive therapy directed toward normalizing the serum bicarbonate is beneficial is unknown. However, the large amounts of alkali required, approximately 700 to 1000 mmol/day for a 70-kg individual, makes this therapeutic approach problematic.

Causes of proximal (type II) renal tubular acidosis

Not associated with Fanconi syndrome
  Sporadic
  Familial
  Disorder of carbonic anhydrase
    Drugs: acetazolamide, sulfanilamide, topiramate[2]
    Carbonic anhydrase II deficiency

Associated with Fanconi syndrome
  Selective (no systemic disease present)
    Sporadic
    Familial
      Autosomal recessive proximal RTA with ocular
        abnormalities: Na^+-HCO_3^- cotransporter (NBC-1) defect
      Autosomal recessive proximal RTA with osteopetrosis and
        cerebral calcification: carbonic anhydrase II defect
      Generalized (systemic disorder present)
  Genetic disorders
    Cystinosis
    Wilson's disease
    Hereditary fructose intolerance
    Lowe syndrome
    Metachromatic leukodystrophy
  Dysproteinemic states
    Myeloma kidney
    Light chain deposition disease
  Primary and secondary hyperparathyroidism
  Drugs and toxins
    Outdated tetracycline
    Ifosfamide
    Gentamicin
    Streptozocin
    Lead
    Cadmium
    Mercury
  Tubulointerstitial disease
    Post-transplantation rejection
    Balkan nephropathy
    Medullary cystic disease
  Others
    Bone fibroma
    Osteopetrosis
    Paroxysmal nocturnal hemoglobinuria

Figure 12.3   Causes of proximal (type II) renal tubular acidosis (RTA).

Hypokalemic Distal Renal Tubular Acidosis (Type I)

In contrast to proximal RTA, patients with distal RTA are unable to acidify their urine, either under basal conditions or in response to metabolic acidosis.[4] This disorder results from a reduction in net H^+ secretion in the distal nephron, which results in continued urinary bicarbonate losses and prevents urinary acidification, thereby minimizing titratable acid excretion and urinary ammonia excretion. As a result, these patients are unable to match net acid excretion to endogenous acid production and acid accumulation ensues. The subsequent metabolic acidosis stimulates reabsorption of bone matrix in order to release the calcium alkali salts present in bone. Over prolonged periods, this can result in progressive osteopenia in adults and in osteomalacia in children.

The pathophysiologic basis for distal RTA can be either impaired H^+ secretion (secretory defect) or an abnormally permeable distal tubule, resulting in increased backleak of normally secreted H^+ (gradient defect). Defects, either genetic or acquired, of all the major proteins involved in collecting duct proton secretion have been shown to cause distal RTA. Certain medications, particularly amphotericin B, result in increased backleak of protons across the apical plasma membrane, thereby leading to a gradient defect form of distal RTA.

For patients with a secretory defect, the inability to acidify the urine below pH 5.5 results from abnormalities in any of the proteins involved in collecting duct H^+ secretion.[5] Some patients may have an isolated defect in the H^+-K^+-ATPase that impairs H^+ secretion and K^+ reabsorption. A defect confined to the vacuolar H^+-ATPase could also lead to renal K^+ wasting but would do so in a more indirect fashion. The development of systemic acidosis tends to diminish net proximal fluid reabsorption with an increase in distal delivery, resulting in volume contraction and activation of the renin aldosterone system. Increased distal Na^+ delivery coupled to increased circulating levels of aldosterone then leads to increased renal K^+ secretion. Defects in the basolateral anion exchanger (AE1) can also cause distal RTA. In this case, the lack of basolateral HCO_3^- exit leads to intracellular alkalinization, which inhibits apical proton secretion.

Patients with distal RTA exhibit low ammonia secretion rates. In part, the decreased secretion is caused by the failure to trap ammonia in the tubular lumen of the collecting duct as a result of the inability to lower the pH of the fluid. In addition, there is likely to be impaired medullary transfer of ammonia because of interstitial disease. Interstitial disease is frequently present in such patients through an associated underlying disease or as a result of nephrocalcinosis or hypokalemia-induced interstitial fibrosis.

In contrast to proximal RTA, patients frequently manifest nephrolithiasis and nephrocalcinosis. This predisposition to renal calcification results from a number of factors. Urinary Ca^{2+} excretion is high secondary to acidosis-induced bone mineral dissolution. Second, luminal alkalinization inhibits calcium reabsorption, resulting in further increases in urinary calcium excretion. Third, calcium phosphate solubility is markedly lowered at alkaline pH. As a result, calcium phosphate nidus formation and calcium phosphate stone formation are accelerated. Stone formation is further enhanced as a result of low urinary citrate excretion. Citrate is metabolized to HCO_3^-, and its renal reabsorption is stimulated by metabolic acidosis, thereby tending to minimize the severity of metabolic acidosis. Urinary citrate also chelates urinary calcium, thereby decreasing ionized calcium concentrations. Accordingly, the decreased citrate excretion that occurs in chronic metabolic acidosis due to distal RTA further contributes to both nephrolithiasis and nephrocalcinosis.

Causes of hypokalemic distal (type I) renal tubular acidosis

Primary
  Idiopathic
  Familial

Secondary
  Autoimmune disorders
    Hypergammaglobulinemia
    Sjögren's syndrome
    Primary biliary cirrhosis
    Systemic lupus erythematosus
  Genetic diseases
    Autosomal dominant RTA: anion exchanger I defect
    Autosomal recessive: H^+-ATPase A4 subunit
    Autosomal recessive with progressive nerve deafness:
      H^+-TPase BI subunit
  Drugs and toxins
    Amphotericin B
    Toluene
  Disorders with nephrocalcinosis
    Hyperparathyroidism
    Vitamin D intoxication
    Idiopathic hypercalciuria
  Tubulointerstitial disease
    Obstructive uropathy
    Renal transplantation

Figure 12.4 Causes of hypokalemic distal (type I) renal tubular acidosis (RTA).

Distal RTA may be a primary disorder, either idiopathic or inherited, but most commonly occurs in association with a systemic disease, of which one of the most common causes is Sjögren's syndrome (Fig. 12.4). There is also a particularly striking association with hypergammaglobulinemic states. Several drugs and toxins have also been linked with the development of this disorder.

A common cause of acquired distal RTA is glue sniffing. Inhalation of toluene from the fumes of model glue, spray paint, and paint thinners can give rise to hypokalemic normal gap acidosis through multiple mechanisms. First, toluene can inhibit collecting duct proton secretion. Second, metabolism of toluene produces the organic acids, hippuric and benzoic acid. These are buffered by sodium bicarbonate, resulting in metabolic acidosis and the production of sodium hippurate and sodium benzoate. If plasma volume is normal, these salts are rapidly excreted in the urine, and a nonanion gap metabolic acidosis develops. If plasma volume is decreased, urinary excretion is limited, they accumulate, and an anion gap metabolic acidosis develops.

The diagnosis of distal RTA should be considered in all patients with a nonanion gap metabolic acidosis and hypokalemia who have an inability to lower the urine pH maximally.[6] A urine pH >5.5 in the setting of systemic acidosis is suggestive of distal RTA, and the finding of a UAG greater than zero is confirmatory. Depending on the duration of the distal RTA, the metabolic acidosis can either be mild or very severe, with a serum bicarbonate as low as 10 mEq/l. Urinary potassium losses lead to the development of hypokalemia. In some cases, the hypokalemia can be quite severe (<2.5 mmol/l), resulting in musculoskeletal weakness and nephrogenic diabetes insipidus. The latter occurs because hypokalemia decreases aquaporin-2 expression in the collecting duct, thereby minimizing the ability to concentrate urine. An abdominal ultrasound scan may reveal nephrocalcinosis.

Correcting the metabolic acidosis in distal RTA can be achieved by administration of alkali in an amount only slightly greater than daily acid production (usually 1 to 2 mmol/kg/day). In patients with severe K^+ deficits, correcting the acidosis with HCO_3^-, particularly if done with sodium alkali salts such as sodium bicarbonate, can lower serum potassium concentration to dangerous levels. In this setting, potassium replacement should begin prior to correcting the acidosis. In general, a combination of sodium alkali and potassium alkali is required for long-term treatment of distal RTA. For the patient with recurrent renal stone disease due to distal RTA, treatment of the acidosis increases urinary citrate excretion, which slows the rate of further stone formation and may even lead to stone dissolution.

Type III Renal Tubular Acidosis

Type III RTA refers to combined proximal and distal RTA that was observed as a transient phenomenon in children and in infants during the 1960s and 1970s. Interestingly, it is almost never seen any more. This has led to the speculation that this condition may have been related to some exogenous factor, possibly high salt intake, and does not reflect a specific renal disorder.

Hyperkalemic Distal Renal Tubular Acidosis (Type IV)

Type IV RTA is a disorder characterized by a disturbance in distal nephron function, resulting in impaired renal excretion of both H^+ and K^+ and giving a hyperchloremic normal gap acidosis and hyperkalemia.[7] The syndrome occurs most often in association with mild to moderate renal insufficiency; however, the magnitude of hyperkalemia and acidosis are disproportionately severe for the observed degree of renal insufficiency. While hypokalemic distal (type I) RTA is also a disorder of distal nephron acidification, type IV RTA is easily distinguished from type I RTA on the basis of several important characteristics that are summarized in Figure 12.5. It should be remembered that type IV RTA is a much more common form of RTA, particularly in adults.

The pathophysiologic basis for this disorder can either be a deficiency in circulating aldosterone or abnormal cortical collecting duct function, or it can be related to hyperkalemia. In either case, a defect in distal H^+ secretion develops. Impaired Na^+ reabsorption by the principal cell leads to a decrease in the luminal electronegativity of the cortical collecting duct, which impairs distal acidification as a result of the decrease in driving force for H^+ secretion into the tubular lumen. The H^+ secretion is further impaired in this segment as well as in the medullary collecting duct, as a result either of the loss of the direct stimulatory effect of aldosterone on H^+ secretion or of an abnormality in the H^+ secreting cell.

Factors differentiating type I and type IV distal RTA

	Type I RTA	Type IV RTA
Serum K^+	Low	High-normal or high
Renal function	Normal or near normal	Stage 3, 4, or 5 chronic kidney disease
Urine pH during acidosis	6.0–6.5	5.5
Serum HCO_3^- (mmol/l)	10–20	16–22

Figure 12.5 Factors differentiating types I and IV distal renal tubular acidosis (RTA).

Another consequence of the decrease in luminal electronegativity in the cortical collecting duct is impaired renal K^+ excretion. In addition, a primary abnormality in the cortical collecting duct transport can also impair K^+ secretion. The development of hyperkalemia adds to the defect in distal acidification by decreasing the amount of ammonia available to act as a urinary buffer.[8] Some evidence suggests that hyperkalemia itself, through its effects on ammonia metabolism, is the primary mechanism by which the metabolic acidosis develops in type IV RTA.

The differential diagnosis of type IV RTA can be divided into those conditions associated with decreased circulating levels of aldosterone and conditions associated with impaired function of the cortical collecting duct. Perhaps the most common disease associated with type IV RTA in adults is diabetes mellitus. In these patients, primary NaCl retention leads to volume expansion and suppression and atrophy of the renin-secreting juxtaglomerular apparatus. Several commonly used drugs such as nonsteroidal anti-inflammatory agents, angiotensin-converting enzyme (ACE) inhibitors, and high doses of heparin, as used for systemic anticoagulation, can lead to decreased mineralocorticoid synthesis. Impaired function of the cortical collecting duct can be a feature of structural damage to the kidney, as in interstitial renal diseases such as sickle cell nephropathy, urinary tract obstruction, or lupus; it may also result from use of certain drugs.[9]

Type IV RTA should be suspected in a patient with a normal gap metabolic acidosis associated with hyperkalemia. The typical patient is in the fifth to seventh decade of life with a long-standing history of diabetes mellitus with a moderate reduction in the glomerular filtration rate (GFR). The plasma HCO_3^- concentration is usually in the range of 18 to 22 mmol/l and the serum K^+ is in the range of 5.5 to 6.5 mmol/l. Most patients are asymptomatic; however, occasionally the hyperkalemia may be severe enough to cause muscle weakness or cardiac arrhythmias. The UAG is slightly positive, indicating minimal ammonia excretion in the urine. Patients in whom the disorder is caused by a defect in mineralocorticoid activity typically have a urine pH <5.5, reflecting a more severe defect in ammonia availability than in H^+ secretion (Fig. 12.6). In patients with structural damage to the collecting duct, the urine pH may be alkaline, reflecting both impaired H^+ secretion and decreased urinary ammonia excretion.

Treatment of type IV RTA is directed at treating both the hyperkalemia and the metabolic acidosis. In many instances, lowering the serum K^+ will simultaneously correct the acidosis.[10] Correction of the hyperkalemia allows for renal ammonia production to increase, thereby increasing the buffer supply for distal acidification. The first consideration in the treatment of patients is to discontinue any nonessential medication that might interfere in either the synthesis or activity of aldosterone or the ability of the kidneys to excrete potassium (Fig. 12.7). ACE inhibitors and angiotensin receptor blockers, however, in general should be continued because of the beneficial effects on cardiovascular disease and their renoprotective benefits in patients with chronic kidney disease (CKD). In patients with aldosterone deficiency who are neither hypertensive nor fluid overloaded, administration of a synthetic mineralocorticoid such as fludrocortisone (0.1 mg/day) can be effective. In patients with hypertension or volume overload, particularly when associated with CKD, administration of either a thiazide or a loop diuretic is frequently effective. Loop diuretics are required in patients with an estimated GFR <30 ml/minute. Loop and thiazide diuretics increase distal Na^+ delivery and, as a result, stimulate K^+ and H^+ secretion in the collecting duct. Alkali therapy (e.g., $NaHCO_3$) can also be used to treat the acidosis and hyperkalemia, but one must

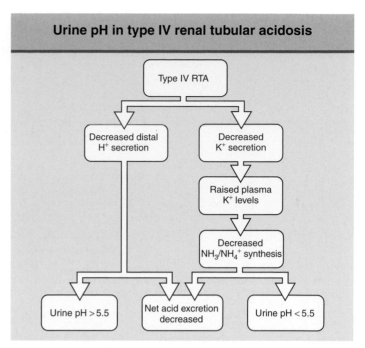

Figure 12.6 Urine pH in type IV renal tubular acidosis (RTA). Net acid excretion is always decreased; however, the urine pH can be variable. In structural disease of the kidney, the predominant defect is usually decreased distal H^+ secretion and the urine pH is >5.5. In disorders associated with decreased mineralocorticoid activity, urine pH is usually <5.5.

closely monitor the patient to avoid volume overload and worsening hypertension.

Renal Tubular Acidosis in Chronic Kidney Disease
Metabolic acidosis in advanced CKD is caused by failure of the tubular acidification process to excrete the normal daily acid load. As functional renal mass is reduced by disease, there is an

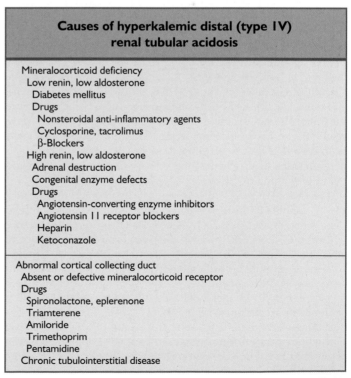

Figure 12.7 Causes of hyperkalemic distal (type IV) renal tubular acidosis.

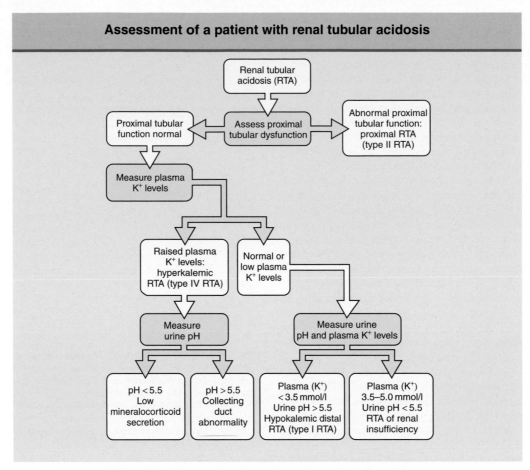

Figure 12.8   Approach to the patient with renal tubular acidosis.

adaptive increase in ammonia production and H+ secretion by the remaining nephrons. Despite increased production of ammonia from each remaining nephron, overall production may be decreased secondary to the decrease in total renal mass. In addition, there is less delivery of ammonia to the medullary interstitium secondary to a disrupted medullary anatomy.[11] The ability to lower the urinary pH remains intact, reflecting the fact that the impairment in distal nephron H+ secretion is less than that in ammonia secretion. Quantitatively, however, the total amount of H+ secretion is small and the acidic urine pH is the consequence of very little buffer in the urine. The lack of ammonia in the urine is reflected by a positive value for the UAG. Differentiating RTA from renal insufficiency from type IV RTA can be difficult, as it is based on the clinician's determination as to whether the severity of metabolic acidosis is out of proportion to the degree of renal insufficiency.

Patients with CKD may develop a hyperchloremic normal gap metabolic acidosis associated with normokalemia or mild hyperkalemia as GFR decreases to <30 ml/min. With more advanced CKD (GFR <15 ml/min), the acidosis may change to an anion gap metabolic acidosis, reflecting a progressive inability to excrete phosphate, sulfate, and various organic acids. At this stage, the acidosis is commonly referred to as uremic acidosis.

Correction of the metabolic acidosis in patients with CKD is achieved by treatment with $NaHCO_3$, 0.5 to 1.5 mmol/kg/day, beginning when the HCO_3^- level is <22 mmol/l. In some cases, nonsodium citrate formulations can be used. Loop diuretics are often used in conjunction with alkali therapy to prevent volume overload. If the acidosis becomes refractory to medical therapy, dialysis needs to be initiated. Recent evidence suggests that

metabolic acidosis in the setting of CKD needs to be aggressively treated, as chronic acidosis is associated with metabolic bone disease and may lead to an accelerated catabolic state in patients with chronic renal failure.[12,13] An overall approach for work-up of metabolic acidosis of renal origin is shown in Figure 12.8.

EXTRARENAL ORIGIN

Diarrhea

Intestinal secretions beyond the stomach, including those of the pancreas and biliary tract, are rich in HCO_3^-. Accelerated loss of this HCO_3^--rich solution can lead to the development of metabolic acidosis. The resultant volume loss signals the kidney to increase NaCl reabsorption; this combined with the intestinal $NaHCO_3$ losses generates a normal anion gap metabolic acidosis. The renal response to the systemic acidosis is to increase net acid excretion markedly. This is primarily accomplished by increasing the urinary excretion of ammonia.[14] Hypokalemia, as a result of gastrointestinal losses, and the low serum pH both stimulate the synthesis of ammonia in the proximal tubule. The increase in availability of ammonia to act as a urinary buffer allows for a maximal increase in H+ secretion by the distal nephron.

Confirming the diagnosis of an extrarenal etiology of the normal anion gap metabolic acidosis is based on demonstrating elevated urinary net acid excretion, thereby differentiating the condition from RTA. Determining the UAG is the best way to distinguish between them. In extrarenal conditions, urinary ammonia excretion is elevated, leading to a negative UAG. In RTA, urinary ammonia excretion is low and the UAG is positive. Examining the urine pH in the patient with normal anion gap metabolic acidosis can be misleading. Urine pH in chronic diarrhea may be >6.0 because of substantial increases in renal ammonia metabolism that result in increased urine pH because of the buffering ability of the ammonia. Although the clinical history should be an easy way to distinguish between these two possibilities, in a patient with surreptitious laxative abuse, this may not be helpful. Finally, confirmation of diarrhea may require colonoscopy to demonstrate characteristic findings of laxative abuse, if this diagnosis is being considered.

Treatment of diarrhea-associated metabolic acidosis is based on treating the underlying diarrhea. If this is not possible, alkali treatment, possibly including potassium alkali to treat simultaneously hypokalemia and metabolic acidosis, is indicated.

Ileal Conduits

Surgical diversion of the ureter into an ileal pouch is sometimes used in the treatment of patients with a neurogenic bladder or after cystectomy. The procedure may rarely be associated with the development of a hyperchloremic normal anion gap metabolic acidosis. Acidosis may occur in part due to reabsorption of urinary NH_4Cl by the intestine. The ammonia is transported through the portal circulation to the liver or is metabolized to urea in order to prevent hyperammonemic encephalopathy. This metabolic process consumes equimolar amounts of bicarbonate and therefore can result in the development of metabolic acidosis. Metabolic acidosis may also develop because urinary Cl^- can be exchanged for HCO_3^- through activation of a Cl^-/HCO_3^- exchanger on the intestinal lumen. In some patients, a renal defect in acidification can develop and exacerbate the degree of acidosis. Such a defect may result from tubular damage caused by pyelonephritis or high colonic pressures, secondarily causing urinary obstruction.

The main factors that influence the development and severity of acidosis are the length of time the urine is in contact with the bowel and the total surface area of bowel exposed to urine. In patients with an ureterosigmoid anastomosis, these factors are increased and the acidosis tends to be more common and more severe than in those patients with an ileal conduit. The latter procedure was designed to minimize the time and area of contact between urine and intestinal surface. Patients with surgical diversion of the ureter who develop a metabolic acidosis should be examined for an ileal loop obstruction since this would lead to an increase in contact time between the urine and the intestinal surface.

ANION GAP METABOLIC ACIDOSIS

Lactic Acidosis

One of the most common causes of anion gap metabolic acidosis is lactic acidosis.[15] Lactic acid is the end product in the anaerobic metabolism of glucose and is generated by the reversible reduction of pyruvic acid by lactic acid dehydrogenase and NADH (reduced nicotinamide adenine dinucleotide), as shown in the following formula:

$$\text{pyruvate} + \text{NADH} + \text{H}^+ \leftrightarrow \text{lactate} + \text{NAD}^+.$$

Under normal conditions, the reaction is shifted toward the right and the normal lactate to pyruvate ratio is approximately 10:1. The reactants in this pathway are interrelated as shown in the following equation:

$$\text{lactate} = K[(\text{pyruvate})(\text{NADH})(\text{H}^+)]/(\text{NAD}^+),$$

where K is the equilibrium constant.

On the basis of this relationship, it is evident that lactate can increase for three reasons. First, lactate can increase as a consequence of increased pyruvate production alone. In this situation, the normal 10:1 lactate-to-pyruvate ratio will be maintained. An isolated increase in pyruvate production can be seen in the setting of intravenous glucose infusions, intravenous administration of epinephrine, and respiratory alkalosis. Lactate levels in these conditions tend to be only minimally elevated, rarely exceeding 5 mmol/l. Second, lactate can increase as a result of an increased $NADH/NAD^+$ ratio. Under these conditions, the lactate-to-pyruvate ratio can increase to very high values. Finally, lactate can increase when there is a combination of increased pyruvate production with an increased $NADH/NAD^+$ ratio. This is usually the case in severe lactic acidosis.

Lactic acidosis is generated whenever there is an imbalance between the production and utilization of lactic acid. The net result is an accumulation of serum lactate and the development of metabolic acidosis. The accumulation of the nonchloride anion lactate accounts for the increase in anion gap. Severe exercise and grand mal seizures are examples of when lactic acidosis can develop as a result of increased production. The short-lived nature of the acidosis in these conditions suggests that a concomitant defect in lactic acid utilization is present in most conditions of sustained and severe lactic acidosis.

A partial list of the disorders associated with the development of lactic acidosis is given in Figure 12.9. Type A lactic acidosis is characterized by disorders in which there is underperfusion of tissue or acute hypoxia. Such disorders include patients with hypotension, sepsis, and acute tissue hypoperfusion as may occur in thrombotic mesenteric ischemia, cardiopulmonary failure, severe anemia, hemorrhage, and carbon monoxide poisoning. Type B lactic acidosis occurs in patients with a variety of disorders that have in common the absence of overt hypoperfusion or hypoxia. These conditions include congenital defects in glucose or lactate metabolism, diabetes mellitus, liver disease, effects of drugs and toxins, and neoplastic diseases.[16–19] It should be pointed out that in clinical practice, many patients will often exhibit features of type A and type B lactic acidosis simultaneously.

The primary goal in the therapy of lactic acidosis is correction of the underlying disorder. Every attempt should be made to restore tissue perfusion and oxygenation if they are compromised.

Causes of lactic acidosis

Type A (tissue underperfusion or hypoxia)
   Cardiogenic shock
   Septic shock
   Hemorrhagic shock
   Acute hypoxia
   Carbon monoxide poisoning
   Anemia

Type B (absence of hypotension and hypoxia)
   Hereditary enzyme deficiency (glucose 6-phosphatase)
   Drugs or toxins
     Phenformin, metformin
     Cyanide
     Salicylate, ethylene glycol, methanol
     Propylene glycol[19]
     Linezolid[17]
     Propofol[16]
     Nucleoside reverse transcriptase inhibitors: stavudine, didanosine[18]
   Systemic disease
     Liver failure
     Malignancy

Figure 12.9   Causes of lactic acidosis.

The role of alkali in the treatment of lactic acidosis is controversial. The controversy has centered on experimental models and clinical observations that indicate administration of HCO_3^- may depress cardiac function and exacerbate the acidemia. In addition, such therapy may be complicated by volume overload, hypernatremia, and rebound alkalosis after the acidosis has resolved. In general, HCO_3^- should be given when the systemic pH decreases to <7.1, as hemodynamic instability becomes much more likely with severe acidemia. In such cases, alkali therapy should be directed at increasing the pH above 7.1; attempts to normalize the pH or $[HCO_3^-]$ concentration should be avoided. Acute hemodialysis is rarely beneficial for lactic acidosis induced by tissue hypoperfusion. The hemodynamic instability that can occur with hemodialysis in these often critically ill patients may worsen the underlying difficulty in tissue oxygenation.

Diabetic Ketoacidosis

Diabetic ketoacidosis is a metabolic condition characterized by the accumulation of acetoacetic acid and β-hydroxybutyric acid. The development of ketoacidosis is the result of insulin deficiency and a relative or absolute increase in glucagon concentration.[20] These hormonal changes lead to increased fatty acid mobilization from adipose tissue and, at the same time, alter the oxidative machinery of the liver such that delivered fatty acids are primarily metabolized into keto acids. In addition, peripheral glucose utilization is impaired and the gluconeogenic pathway in the liver is maximally stimulated. The resultant hyperglycemia results in an osmotic diuresis and volume depletion.

Ketoacidosis results when the rate of hepatic keto acid generation exceeds renal excretion, resulting in increased blood keto acid concentrations. The H^+ accumulation in the extracellular fluid decreases HCO_3^-, whereas the keto acid anion concentration increases. While an anion gap metabolic acidosis is the more common finding in diabetic ketoacidosis, a normal gap metabolic acidosis can also be seen. In early stages of ketoacidosis, when the extracellular volume is near normal, keto acid anions that are produced are rapidly excreted by the kidney as Na^+ and K^+ salts. Excretion of these salts is equivalent to the loss of potential HCO_3^-. This loss of potential HCO_3^- in the urine at the same time that the kidney is retaining NaCl results in a normal gap metabolic acidosis. As volume depletion develops, renal keto acid excretion cannot match production rates, and keto acid anions are retained within the body, thus increasing the anion gap. During treatment, the anion gap metabolic acidosis transforms once again into a normal gap acidosis. Treatment leads to a termination in keto acid production. As the extracellular fluid volume is restored, there is increased renal excretion of the Na^+ salts of the keto acid anions. The loss of this potential HCO_3^- combined with the retention of administered NaCl accounts for the redevelopment of the hyperchloremic normal gap acidosis. In addition, K^+ and Na^+ administered in solutions containing NaCl and KCl enter cells in exchange for H^+. The net effect is infusion of HCl into the extracellular fluid. The reversal of the hyperchloremic acidosis is accomplished over a period of several days as the HCO_3^- deficit is corrected by the kidney.

Diabetic ketoacidosis can lead to very severe metabolic acidosis, with serum bicarbonate levels sometimes <5 mEq/l. This diagnosis should be considered in patients who present with simultaneous metabolic acidosis and hyperglycemia. The diagnosis can be confirmed by demonstrating the presence of retained keto acids. This can be performed either with use of nitroprusside tablets or reagent strips or by serologic assays performed in a routine clinical laboratory. However, the nitroprusside tablets and reagent strips can be misleading in assessing the severity of ketoacidosis as they only detect acetone and acetoacetate and not β-hydroxybutyrate. Acetoacetic acid and β-hydroxybutyric acid are interconvertible, with the $NADH/NAD^+$ ratio being the primary determinant as to which moiety predominates. In the setting of a high ratio, formation of β-hydroxybutyric acid is favored and the nitroprusside test will become less positive or even negative despite significant ketoacidosis. This situation can occur when ketoacidosis is accompanied by lactic acidosis or in the setting of alcoholic ketoacidosis. During treatment, the $NADH/NAD^+$ ratio tends to decline, favoring the formation of acetoacetic acid. As a result, it is common for the nitroprusside test to register more strongly positive during the treatment of diabetic ketoacidosis. Specific assay of β-hydroxybutyurate avoids these limitations.

Treatment of diabetic ketoacidosis involves the use of insulin and intravenous fluids to correct volume depletion. Deficiencies in K^+, Mg^{2+}, and phosphate are common, and, therefore, these electrolytes are typically added to intravenous solutions. However, diabetic ketoacidosis typically presents with hyperkalemia due to the insulin deficiency. Potassium should only be administered after confirmation that hypokalemia is present. It is also important to recognize that insulin administration during treatment of diabetic ketoacidosis will decrease serum potassium levels. If significant hypokalemia is present at the patient's presentation, then potassium supplementation may need to be administered prior to insulin administration in order to avoid possibly life-threatening worsening of the hypokalemia. Alkali therapy is generally not required since administration of insulin leads to the metabolic conversion of keto acid anions to HCO_3^- and allows partial correction of the acidosis. However, HCO_3^- therapy may be indicated in those patients who present with severe acidemia (pH <7.1).

D-Lactic Acidosis

D-Lactic acidosis is a unique form of metabolic acidosis that can occur in the setting of small bowel resections or in patients with a jejunoileal bypass. Such short bowel syndromes create a situation in which carbohydrates that are normally extensively reabsorbed in the small intestine are delivered in large amounts to the colon. In the presence of colonic bacterial overgrowth, these substrates are metabolized into D-lactate and absorbed into the systemic circulation. Accumulation of D-lactate produces an anion gap metabolic acidosis in which the serum lactate is normal since the standard test for lactate is specific for L-lactate. These patients typically present after ingestion of a large carbohydrate meal with neurologic abnormalities consisting of confusion, slurred speech, and ataxia. Ingestion of low carbohydrate meals and antimicrobial agents to decrease the degree of bacterial overgrowth are the principal treatments.

Starvation Ketosis

Abstinence from food can lead to a mild anion gap metabolic acidosis secondary to increased production of keto acids. The pathogenesis of this disorder is similar to that of diabetic ketoacidosis in that starvation leads to relative insulin deficiency and glucagon excess. As a result, there is increased mobilization of fatty acids while the liver is set to oxidize fatty acids to keto acids. With prolonged starvation, the blood keto acid level can reach 5 to 6 mmol/l. The serum $[HCO_3^-]$ concentration rarely decreases to values <18 mmol/l. More fulminant ketoacidosis is aborted by the fact that ketone bodies stimulate the pancreatic islets to release insulin and lipolysis is held in check. This break in the ketogenic process is notably absent in those with insulin-dependent diabetes. There is no specific therapy indicated in this disorder.

Alcoholic Ketoacidosis

Ketoacidosis develops in patients with a history of chronic ethanol abuse, decreased food intake, and often a history of nausea and vomiting. As with starvation ketosis, a decrease in the insulin to glucagon ratio leads to accelerated fatty acid mobilization and alters the enzymatic machinery of the liver to favor keto acid production. However, there are features unique to this disorder that differentiate it from simple starvation ketosis. First, the presence of alcohol withdrawal combined with volume depletion and starvation markedly increases the levels of circulating catecholamines. As a result, the peripheral mobilization of fatty acids is much greater than that typically found with starvation alone. This sometimes massive mobilization of fatty acids can lead to marked keto acid production and severe metabolic acidosis. Second, the metabolism of alcohol leads to accumulation of NADH. The increase in the $NADH/NAD^+$ ratio is reflected by a higher β-hydroxybutyrate-to-acetoacetate ratio. As mentioned previously, the nitroprusside reaction may be diminished by this redox shift despite the presence of severe ketoacidosis. Treatment of this disorder is focused on the administration of glucose. Glucose administration leads to the rapid resolution of the acidosis since stimulation of insulin release leads to diminished fatty acid mobilization from adipose tissue as well as decreased hepatic output of keto acids.

Ethylene Glycol and Methanol Intoxication

Ethylene glycol and methanol intoxication is characteristically associated with the development of a severe anion gap metabolic acidosis. Metabolism of ethylene glycol by alcohol dehydrogenase generates various acids, including glycolic, oxalic, and formic acids. Ethylene glycol is a component of antifreeze and solvents and is ingested by accident or as a suicide attempt. The initial effects of intoxication are neurologic and begin with drunkenness but can quickly progress to seizures and coma. If left untreated, cardiopulmonary symptoms such as tachypnea, noncardiogenic pulmonary edema, and cardiovascular collapse may appear. Twenty-four to 48 hours after ingestion, patients may develop flank pain and renal failure often accompanied by abundant calcium oxalate crystals in the urine (Fig. 12.10). A fatal dose is approximately 100 ml.

Methanol is also metabolized by alcohol dehydrogenase and forms formaldehyde, which is then converted to formic acid. Methanol is found in a variety of commercial preparations such as shellac, varnish, and de-icing solutions and is also known as wood alcohol. As with ethylene glycol ingestion, methanol can be ingested either by accident or as a suicide attempt. Clinically, methanol ingestion is associated with an acute inebriation followed by an asymptomatic period lasting 24 to 36 hours. At this point, abdominal pain caused by pancreatitis, seizures, blindness, and coma may develop. The blindness is due to direct toxicity of formic acid on the retina. Methanol intoxication is also associated with hemorrhage in the white matter and putamen, which can lead to the delayed onset of a Parkinson's disease–like syndrome (see Fig. 12.10). The lethal dose is between 60 and 250 ml. Lactic acidosis is also a feature of methanol and ethylene glycol poisoning and contributes to the elevated anion gap.

Together with the appearance of the anion gap, an osmolar gap is an important clue to the diagnosis of ethylene glycol and methanol poisoning. The osmolar gap is the difference between the measured and calculated osmolality. The formula for the calculated osmolality is as follows:

$$\text{calculated osmolality} = \frac{2 \times Na^+ + BUN}{2.8} + \frac{\text{glucose}}{18} + \frac{\text{EtOH}}{4.6},$$

Ethylene glycol and methanol poisoning
Time course of clinical symptoms and signs after ingestion Ethylene glycol 0–12 hours: inebriation progressing to coma 12–24 hours: tachypnea, noncardiogenic pulmonary edema 24–36 hours: flank pain, renal failure, urinary calcium oxalate crystals Methanol 0–12 hours: inebriation followed by asymptomatic period 24–36 hours: pancreatitis, retinal edema progressing to blindness, seizures >48 hours: putamen and white matter hemorrhage leading to Parkinson's disease–like state
Increased anion gap metabolic acidosis
Increased osmolar gap
Treatment Supportive care Fomepizole (4-methylpyrazole) is agent of choice (competitor of alcohol dehydrogenase): 15 mg/kg IV loading dose, then 10 mg/kg every 12 hours for 48 hours; after 48 hours, increase dose to 15 mg/kg every 12 hours; increase frequency of dosing to 4 hours during hemodialysis Intravenous ethanol (5% or 10% solution) if fomepizole unavailable: loading dose of 0.6 g/kg followed by hourly maintenance dose of 66 mg/kg; increase maintenance dose when there is a history of chronic alcohol use and during hemodialysis Institute hemodialysis to accelerate removal of parent compound and metabolites Bicarbonate therapy to treat acidosis

Figure 12.10 Ethylene glycol and methanol poisoning.

where the blood urea nitrogen (BUN), glucose, and ethanol concentrations are in milligram per deciliter. Including the ethanol concentration in this calculation is important, as many patients who ingest either ethylene glycol or ethanol do so while inebriated from ethanol ingestion. The normal value for the osmolar gap is <10 mOsm/kg. Each 100 mg/dl (161 mmol/l) of ethylene glycol will increase the osmolar gap by 16 mOsm/kg, while methanol contributes 32 mOsm/kg for each 100 mg/dl (312 mmol/l).

In addition to supportive measures, the therapy for ethylene glycol and methanol poisoning is centered on reducing the metabolism of the parent compound and accelerating the removal of the alcohol from the body (see Fig. 12.10). Decreasing metabolism of the parent compound is important since the metabolites rather than the parent compound are primarily responsible for the toxic effects. Fomepizole (4-methylpyrazole) is now the agent of choice to inhibit the enzyme alcohol dehydrogenase and prevent formation of toxic metabolites.[21] If fomepizole is unavailable, then intravenous ethanol can be used to prevent the formation of toxic metabolites. Ethanol has more than a 10-fold greater affinity for alcohol dehydrogenase than other alcohols. Ethanol has its greatest efficacy when levels of 100 to 200 mg/dl are obtained. With both fomepizole and ethanol therapy, hemodialysis therapy should be employed to remove both the parent compound and its metabolites. One final aspect of management is correction of the acidosis. This can be accomplished with use of an HCO_3^- containing dialysate or by intravenous infusion of $NaHCO_3$.

Salicylate

Aspirin (acetylsalicylic acid) is one of the most widely available therapeutic agents and is associated with a large number of accidental or intentional poisonings. At toxic concentrations, salicylate uncouples oxidative phosphorylation and, as a result, leads to increased lactic acid production. In children, keto acid production may also be increased. The accumulation of lactic, salicylic, keto, and other organic acids leads to the development of an anion gap metabolic acidosis. At the same time, salicylate has a direct stimulatory effect on the respiratory center. Increased ventilation lowers the PCO_2, contributing to the development of a respiratory alkalosis. Children primarily manifest an anion gap metabolic acidosis with toxic salicylate levels, while a respiratory alkalosis is most evident in adults.

In addition to conservative management, the initial goals of therapy are to correct systemic acidemia and to increase the urine pH. By increasing systemic pH, the ionized fraction of salicylic acid will increase, and, as a result, there will be less accumulation of the drug in the central nervous system. Similarly, an alkaline urine pH will favor increased urinary excretion since the ionized fraction of the drug is poorly reabsorbed by the tubule. At serum concentrations of >80 mg/dl or in the setting of severe clinical toxicity, hemodialysis can be used to accelerate the removal of the drug from the body.

Pyroglutamic Acidosis

Pyroglutamic acid, also known as 5-oxoproline, is an intermediate in the γ-glutamyl cycle that is important in the synthesis and metabolism of glutathione, the transport of glutathione out of the cell, and uptake of amino acids into the cell. Pyroglutamic acidemia (5-oxoprolinemia) was originally recognized in a patient with a rare congenital deficiency in glutathione synthetase (Fig. 12.11). Subsequently patients with an acquired form of pyroglutamic acidemia have been reported. Affected patients present with severe anion gap metabolic acidosis accompanied by alterations in mental status ranging from confusion to coma. High concentrations of pyroglutamic acid are found in the blood and urine, and plasma concentrations parallel the increase in the anion gap. Many of the reported cases have occurred in critically ill patients receiving therapeutic doses of acetaminophen.[22] In this setting, glutathione levels are reduced due to the oxidative stress associated with critical illness. In addition, the metabolism of acetaminophen depletes glutathione. The reduction in glutathione secondarily leads to increased production of pyroglutamic acid. The diagnosis of pyroglutamic acidosis should be considered in patients with unexplained anion gap metabolic acidosis and recent acetaminophen ingestion.

ALKALI TREATMENT OF METABOLIC ACIDOSIS

A number of treatment options are available for treatment of metabolic acidosis. In general, these can be subdivided into treatments that involve sodium bicarbonate and those that involve citrate. Figure 12.12 summarizes some of the treatment options and modalities available.

Sodium bicarbonate can be administered as oral tablets, as a powder, as a hypertonic sodium bicarbonate bolus, or as isotonic sodium bicarbonate. The latter can be created by adding three ampules ("amps") of sodium bicarbonate (50 mmol/amp) to a liter of 5% dextrose in water (D_5W) solution. This results in an intravenous fluid that is very similar to 5% dextrose in isotonic saline (D_5NS), but has bicarbonate as the anion instead of chloride. It is very useful in the treatment of the volume-depleted patient who requires both volume expansion and alkali administration.

Citrate is available in the liquid preparation, either as sodium citrate, potassium citrate, and citric acid or as a combination of

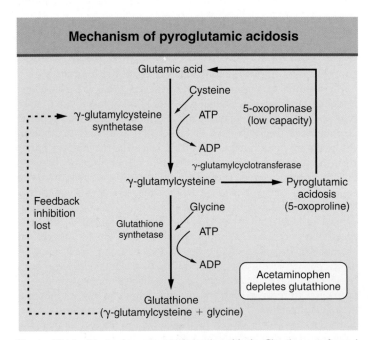

Figure 12.11 Mechanism of pyroglutamic acidosis. Glutathione is formed from γ-glutamylcysteine and glycine in the presence of glutathione synthetase. Glutathione normally regulates the activity of γ-glutamylcysteine synthetase through feedback inhibition. Depletion of glutathione results in increased formation of γ-glutamylcysteine, which in turn is metabolized to pyroglutamic acid (5-oxoproline) and cystine via γ-glutamylcyclotransferase. Pyroglutamic acid accumulates since the enzyme responsible for its metabolism (5-oxoprolinase) is low capacity. ADP, adenosine diphosphate; ATP, adenosine triphosphate.

Alkali treatment options			
	Route	Dose Per Unit	Comments
Sodium bicarbonate tablet	PO	650 mg = 8 mmol	May cause gastric gas
Sodium bicarbonate "amp"	IV	50 mmol in 50 ml	Hypertonic, may cause hypernatremia
D_5W with 3 "amps" of NaHCO₃ per liter	IV	150 mmol/1.15 l or 130 mmol/l	Useful for simultaneous intravascular volume expansion and alkali administration
Sodium citrate/ citric acid (liquid, Bicitra, Cytra-2)	PO	1 mmol of Na⁺ and citrate per milliliter	1 mmol citrate equivalent to 1 mmol HCO₃⁻. Avoid concomitant aluminum-containing medications such as antacids and sucralfate.
Potassium citrate (tablet, Urocit-K)	PO	5 and 10 mmol per tablet	Useful for simultaneous K⁺ and alkali therapy
Citric acid/potassium citrate/sodium citrate (liquid, Cytra-3 Syrup, Polycitra Syrup)	PO	1 mmol of Na⁺ and K⁺ and 2 mmol of citrate per milliliter	Avoid concomitant aluminum-containing medications
Potassium citrate (liquid, Polycitra K)	PO	2 mmol of K⁺ and 2 mmol of citrate per milliliter	Avoid concomitant aluminum-containing medications

Figure 12.12 Alkali treatment options.

these compounds. Many patients find citrate-containing solutions to be a more palatable source of oral alkali therapy than oral sodium bicarbonate. It is important to recognize, however, that oral citrate therapy should not be combined with medications that include aluminum. Citrate, which has a −3 charge under normal conditions, can complex with aluminum (Al^{3+}) in the intestinal tract, resulting in an uncharged moiety that is rapidly absorbed across the intestinal tract and then can dissociate to release free aluminum. This can increase the rate of aluminum absorption dramatically, and in some cases, particularly in patients with severe CKD, has resulted in acute aluminum encephalopathy.

The dose of alkali therapy that is administered is based on both the total body bicarbonate deficit and on the desired rapidity of treatment. Under normal circumstances, the volume of distribution (V_D) for bicarbonate is approximately 0.5 l per kilogram of total body weight. Thus, the bicarbonate deficit, in millimoles, can be estimated from the following formula:

$$\text{bicarbonate deficit} = (0.5 \times LBW_{kg}) \times (24 - HCO_3^-),$$

where LBW_{kg} is the lean body weight in kilograms and 24 is the desired resultant bicarbonate concentration.

Several caveats regarding this equation should be understood. First, edema fluid contributes to the volume of distribution of bicarbonate. Accordingly, an estimation of the amount of edema fluid should be included in this calculation. Second, the volume of distribution for bicarbonate increases as the severity of the metabolic acidosis worsens. When the serum bicarbonate is ≤5 mmol/l, the volume of distribution may increase to ≥1 l/kg.

When acute treatment is desired, it is reasonable to replace approximately 50% of the bicarbonate deficit over the first 24 hours. If "amps" of sodium bicarbonate are used, then it is important to recognize that this is a hypertonic solution and that the increase in the serum sodium concentration will parallel the increase in the serum bicarbonate concentration. Following the initial 24 hours of therapy, the response to therapy and the patient's current clinical condition are reevaluated before making determinations as to future therapy. Acute hemodialysis solely for the treatment of metabolic acidosis is rarely beneficial.

REFERENCES

1. Halperin ML, Richardson RM, Bear R, et al: Urine ammonium: The key to the diagnosis of distal renal tubular acidosis. Nephron 1988;50:1–4.
2. Groeper K, McCann M: Topiramate and metabolic acidosis: A case series and review of the literature. Pediatr Anesth 2005;15:167–170.
3. Rodriguez S: Renal tubular acidosis: The clinical entity. J Am Soc Nephrol 2002;13:2160–2170.
4. Kim S, Lee J, Park J, et al: The urine-blood PCO_2 gradient as a diagnostic index of (H+ATPase) defect distal renal tubular acidosis. Kidney Int 2004;66:761–767.
5. Nicoletta J, Schwartz G: Distal renal tubular acidosis. Curr Opin Pediatr 2004;16:194–198.
6. McSherry E, Sebastian A, Morris RC: Renal tubular acidosis in infants: The several kinds, including bicarbonate-wasting, classic renal tubular acidosis. J Clin Invest 1972;51:499–514.
7. DuBose TD: Hyperkalemic hyperchloremic metabolic acidosis: Pathophysiologic insights. Kidney Int 1997;51:591–602.
8. Hulter HN, Ilnicki L, Harbottle J, Sebastian A: Impaired renal H+ secretion and NH3 production in mineralocorticoid-deficient glucocorticoid-replete dogs. Am J Physiol 1977;232:F136–F146.
9. Palmer BF: Managing hyperkalemia caused by inhibitors of the renin-angiotensin-aldosterone system. N Engl J Med 2004;351:585–592.
10. Sebastian A, Schambelan M, Lindenfeld S, Morris RC: Amelioration of metabolic acidosis with fludrocortisone therapy in hyporeninemic hypoaldosteronism. N Engl J Med 1977;297:576–583.
11. Buerkert J, Martin D, Trigg D, Simon E: Effect of reduced renal mass on ammonium handling and net acid formation by the superficial and juxtamedullary nephron of the rat. J Clin Invest 1983;71:1661–1675.
12. Krieger N, Frick K, Bushinsky D: Mechanism of acid-induced bone resorption. Curr Opin Nephrol Hypertens 2004;13:423–436.
13. Alpern RJ, Sakhaee K: The clinical spectrum of chronic metabolic acidosis: Homeostatic mechanisms produce significant morbidity. Am J Kidney Dis 1997;29:291–302.
14. Garibotto G, Sofia A, Robaudo C, et al: Kidney protein dynamics and ammoniagenesis in humans with chronic metabolic acidosis. J Am Soc Nephrol 2004;15:1606–1615.
15. Madias N: Lactic acidosis. Kidney Int 1986;29:752–774.
16. Casserly B, O'Mahony E, Timm E, et al: Propofol infusion syndrome: An unusual cause of renal failure. Am J Kidney Dis 2004;44:e98–e101.
17. Palenzuela L, Hahn N, Nelson R, et al: Does linezolid cause lactic acidosis by inhibiting mitochondrial protein synthesis? Clin Infect Dis 2005;40: e113–e116.
18. Day L, Shikuma C, Gerschenson M: Mitochondrial injury in the pathogenesis of antiretroviral-induced hepatic steatosis and lactic academia. Mitochondrion 2004;4:95–109.
19. Arroliga A, Shehab N, McCarthy K, Gonzales J: Relationship of continuous infusion lorazepam to serum propylene glycol concentration in critically ill adults. Crit Care Med 2004;32:1709–1714.
20. Foster DW, McGarry JD: The metabolic derangements and treatment of diabetic ketoacidosis. N Engl J Med 1983;309:159–169.
21. Brent J, McMartin K, Phillips S, et al: Fomepizole for the treatment of ethylene glycol poisoning. Methylpyrazole for toxic alcohols study group. N Engl J Med 1999;340:832–838.
22. Tailor P, Raman T, Garganta C, et al: Recurrent high anion gap metabolic acidosis secondary to 5-oxoproline (pyroglutamic acid). Am J Kidney Dis 2005;46:E4–E10.

DEFINITION

Metabolic alkalosis is caused by retention of excess alkali and is manifested by an increase in serum bicarbonate concentration, [HCO_3^-], to >28 mmol/l (or serum [total CO_2] >30 mmol/l).[1,2] The increase in pH that results from retained HCO_3^- induces hypoventilation, producing a secondary increase in arterial P_{CO_2}. Thus, the disorder is characterized by coexisting elevations in serum [HCO_3^-], arterial pH, and P_{CO_2}. Because the kidney normally responds to an increase in [HCO_3^-] by rapidly excreting the excess alkali, sustained metabolic alkalosis only occurs when some additional factor disrupts renal regulation of body alkali stores.

RENAL REGULATION OF BICARBONATE STORES

Bicarbonate ions are freely filtered by the glomerulus and must be completely recaptured from the tubular urine to conserve body alkali stores. Throughout the nephron, H^+ is secreted into the renal tubules, combining with filtered HCO_3^- to produce CO_2 and water. This process removes HCO_3^- from the tubular urine and generates new HCO_3^- in the peritubular blood.[1] Figure 13.1 illustrates the major epithelial transporters and channels that participate in the regulation of renal HCO_3^- reabsorption. In the proximal tubule and ascending limb of the loop of Henle, H^+ is secreted via an Na^+-linked transporter (the Na^+-H^+ exchanger NHE-3). An H^+-ATPase is also present in the proximal tubule (not shown in the figure). In the collecting duct, NHE-3 is not present and H^+ secretion is accomplished primarily by an epithelial H^+-ATPase. The activity of this H^+-ATPase is regulated by aldosterone and by the rate of Na^+ delivery to and reabsorption in the collecting duct. When body K^+ stores are low, a K^+-linked H^+ secretory transporter, H^+-ATPase, is activated, further promoting H^+ secretion in the distal nephron. If excess alkali is ingested, HCO_3^- can re-enter the tubular fluid in the distal nephron via an apical membrane Cl^--HCO_3^- exchanger.[3] This transporter is activated by alkalemia and requires sufficient Cl^- delivery to the distal tubule for Cl^- to be reabsorbed in exchange for secreted HCO_3^-. Because H^+ secretion in the collecting duct will recapture secreted HCO_3^-, excretion of excess alkali requires both stimulation of the Cl^--HCO_3^- exchanger and suppression of the normally active H^+-ATPase. Abnormal stimulation of H^+-secreting transporters or changes in the activity of Na^+-linked Cl^- transporters in the loop of Henle and early distal tubule (see Fig. 13.1) can disrupt the renal regulation of body alkali stores and produce sustained metabolic alkalosis.

PATHOPHYSIOLOGY OF METABOLIC ALKALOSIS

Metabolic alkalosis can be produced by administering HCO_3^- (or a HCO_3^- precursor) or by inducing K^+ or Cl^- depletion.

Potassium and Cl^- depletion are closely linked events in causing sustained metabolic alkalosis, and it is often difficult to determine which ion is the primary culprit. The most common clinical presentation of metabolic alkalosis is associated with Cl^- depletion. Although the term *contraction alkalosis* is often used as a synonym for Cl^- depletion alkalosis, this phrase is confusing because it implies incorrectly that volume contraction causes metabolic alkalosis. The term refers specifically to the increase in

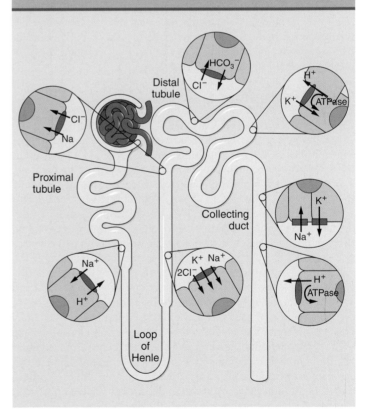

Key ion transport proteins in the nephron

Figure 13.1 Key ion transport proteins and their linkages. Bicarbonate reabsorption is accomplished by H^+ secretion throughout the nephron. This process is directly linked to Na^+ reabsorption via the Na^+-H^+ exchanger and indirectly coupled to Na^+ uptake via a Na^+ channel and parallel H^+-ATPase. Chloride-linked Na^+ reabsorption in the loop of Henle and early distal tubule affects H^+ secretion by determining Na^+ delivery to the collecting duct. Bicarbonate secretion only occurs under conditions of alkalemia via a Cl^--linked exchanger. Potassium reabsorption in states of K^+ depletion is linked to H^+ secretion via an H^+-K^+-ATPase. (From Gennari FJ: Metabolic alkalosis. In Jacobson HR, Striker GE, Klahr S [eds]: The Principles and Practice of Nephrology, 2nd ed. St. Louis: Mosby, 1995, pp 932–941.)

serum [HCO_3^-] that follows only one type of extracellular fluid volume contraction, that caused by selective Cl^- losses. Moreover, a sustained change in renal HCO_3^- reabsorption and acid excretion must occur for this increase to be maintained, and it remains unclear whether volume contraction is necessary or instrumental in inducing this change in renal function.[4,5] More rarely, sustained metabolic alkalosis is the result of primary abnormalities in the regulation of specific ion transporters in the loop of Henle, distal tubule, or collecting ducts. The specific role of each of these factors in the pathogenesis of metabolic alkalosis is discussed.

Exogenous Alkali

The kidney responds rapidly to excess alkali by increasing HCO_3^- excretion, and thus metabolic alkalosis can only be induced transiently by alkali administration when renal function is normal. Even when supplemental $NaHCO_3$ is ingested daily, serum [HCO_3^-] does not increase. When dietary Cl^- intake is severely restricted, however, alkali ingestion produces a significant metabolic alkalosis.[6] If renal HCO_3^- excretion is impaired as a result of renal failure, alkali administration can cause a sustained metabolic alkalosis independent of Cl^- intake.

Potassium Depletion

Induction of K^+ losses by severely restricting dietary K^+ intake produces a small but significant increase in serum [HCO_3^-].[7] When dietary Cl^- intake is concomitantly restricted, however, the resultant alkalosis is four times as great, illustrating the coupled roles of Cl^- and K^+ in regulating renal HCO_3^- reabsorption. Depletion of body K^+ stores is probably the most important factor in producing and sustaining the rarer Cl^--resistant forms of metabolic alkalosis (see later discussion).

Chloride Depletion

Selective Cl^- depletion, induced by vomiting or nasogastric suction, increases serum [HCO_3^-] (Fig. 13.2).[8] The degree of alkalosis generated is greater when H^+ loss also occurs, as in the example shown in Figure 13.2, but it can occur even when H^+ loss is minimized by administering a proton pump inhibitor. In either setting, maintenance of the metabolic alkalosis is dependent on sustaining the depletion of body Cl^- stores. Serum [HCO_3^-] returns to normal when sufficient Cl^- is given to replenish losses. Chloride-depletion metabolic alkalosis causes concomitant K^+ depletion through renal K^+ losses, but Cl^- administration corrects the alkalosis even if the K^+ deficit is deliberately maintained.[9] The role of Cl^- depletion, as opposed to extracellular fluid (ECF) volume depletion, and the contribution of K^+ depletion in sustaining this form of metabolic alkalosis, remains controversial.[4,5,7–9] Dissection of the contribution of each factor is of little importance in the clinic, however, as treatment is dictated by the particular clinical setting, with some patients needing NaCl to replenish extracellular volume, and most needing KCl to treat K^+ depletion. One can generate a metabolic alkalosis, although milder, when a proton pump inhibitor is given, and the Cl^--dependent alkalosis produced by diuretics occurs without evident H^+ loss.

Interplay of K^+, Cl^-, and HCO_3^- Transport by the Kidney

When metabolic alkalosis is induced by Cl^- depletion and dietary Cl^- intake is restricted, a characteristic sequence of changes in renal electrolyte excretion occurs.[8] Sodium and HCO_3^- excretion increase transiently, then decrease rapidly to low levels and K^+ excretion increases. The increase in K^+ excretion is also transient but nonetheless induces significant K^+ depletion (see Fig. 13.2). In the new steady state, urinary K^+ excretion matches intake despite

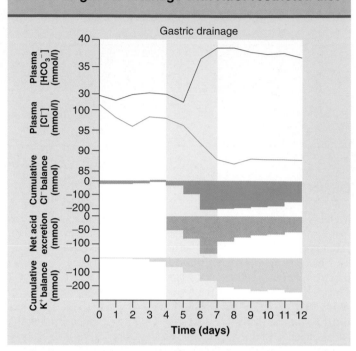

Effects of gastric drainage with NaCl-restricted diet

Figure 13.2 Effect of gastric drainage on plasma [HCO_3^-] and [Cl^-], on Cl^- and K^+ balance, and on net acid excretion in a normal individual ingesting a NaCl-restricted diet. In this subject ingesting a low sodium chloride diet, gastric drainage for 3 days increased plasma [HCO_3^-] by 9 mmol/l, a change that persisted even after gastric drainage was stopped. Potassium depletion occurs as a result of renal K^+ losses during the period of gastric drainage and is not corrected in the postdrainage period despite the daily ingestion of 70 mmol K^+ in the diet. Net acid excretion decreases transiently during the period of gastric drainage, but then returns to control levels in the postdrainage period despite sustained metabolic alkalosis. Chloride depletion is maintained by the low dietary intake of this ion. (From Kassirer JP, Schwartz WB: The response of normal man to selective depletion of hydrochloric acid. Am J Med 1966;40:10–18.)

persistent K^+ depletion. As a result, hypokalemia is a cardinal feature of metabolic alkalosis. Chloride depletion promotes K^+ secretion in the distal nephron through effects on several transport processes and may also impede K^+ reabsorption in the ascending limb of the loop of Henle.[10] Potassium depletion stimulates both H^+ secretion (via the H^+-K^+-ATPase; see Fig. 13.1) and renal NH_4^+ production, facilitating the acid excretion needed to sustain metabolic alkalosis (Fig. 13.3). Chloride depletion also impedes HCO_3^- secretion via the Cl^--HCO_3^- exchanger.[3,10] Continued secretion of aldosterone coupled with impaired distal HCO_3^- secretion also facilitates acid excretion. As a result, acid excretion matches net acid production in the steady state despite systemic alkalemia. When K^+ depletion is unusually severe, renal Cl^- reabsorption is also impaired, possibly due to a limitation in Cl^- transport via the Na^+-K^+-$2Cl^-$ cotransporter (see Fig. 13.1), resulting in persistent Cl^- depletion despite intake or administration of this anion.[10,11]

Primary Abnormalities in Renal Ion Transport

Acquired or inherited abnormalities in ion transport in the loop and distal tubule can cause metabolic alkalosis (Fig. 13.4). These Cl^--resistant forms of metabolic alkalosis account for <1% of all causes, and by far the most common of these is primary hyperaldosteronism.[12] In this disorder, persistently high and unregulated aldosterone secretion promotes Na^+ reabsorption and H^+ and K^+

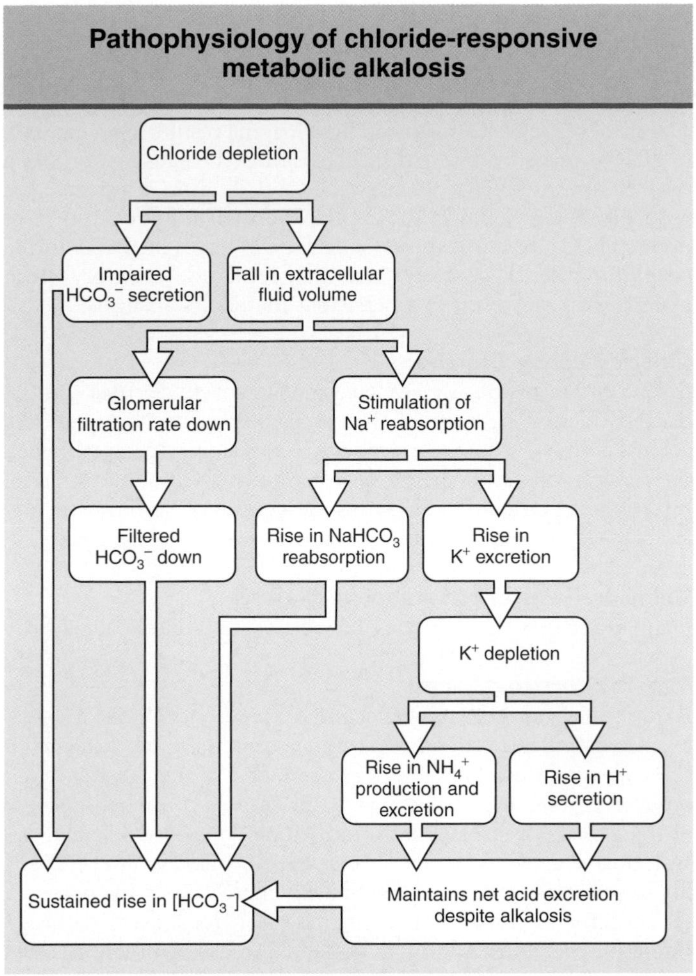

Pathophysiology of chloride-responsive metabolic alkalosis

Figure 13.3 Pathophysiology of chloride-responsive metabolic alkalosis. Chloride depletion decreases extracellular volume and glomerular filtration rate, increases HCO_3^- reabsorption, increases K^+ excretion, and impairs HCO_3^- secretion in the distal nephron. The resultant K^+ depletion further stimulates H^+ secretion and facilitates ammonium (NH_4^+) excretion. These events all contribute to a sustained increase in serum $[HCO_3^-]$. (From Gennari FJ: Metabolic alkalosis. In Jacobson HR, Striker GE, Klahr S [eds]: The Principles and Practice of Nephrology, 2nd ed. St. Louis: Mosby, 1995, pp 932–941.)

Renal ion transport derangements and metabolic alkalosis

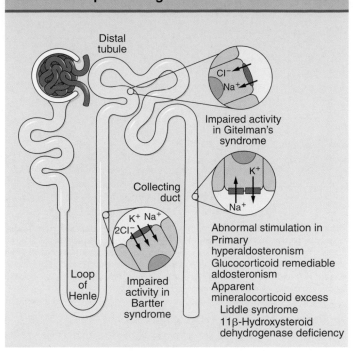

Figure 13.4 Primary derangements in renal ion transport that lead to sustained metabolic alkalosis. The epithelial Na^+ channel in the collecting duct is stimulated abnormally in primary hyperaldosteronism and in three defined genetic abnormalities. One of these causes aldosterone secretion to respond to adrenocorticotropic hormone rather than angiotensin II (glucocorticoid-remediable aldosteronism); one blocks downregulation of the channel (Liddle syndrome), and one allows cortisol to act as a mineralocorticoid (11β-hydroxysteroid dehydrogenase deficiency). Bartter and Gitelman's syndromes are caused by genetic abnormalities that impede the activity of or inactivate Cl^--linked Na^+ reabsorption in two separate transporters in the nephron.

secretion in the collecting duct by stimulating both the epithelial Na^+ channel and H^+-ATPase (see Figs. 13.1 and 13.4). The resultant K^+ depletion promotes NH_4^+ production and stimulates H^+-ATPase activity, facilitating acid excretion and producing metabolic alkalosis despite normal Cl^- intake. Not surprisingly, the degree of alkalosis induced in primary hyperaldosteronism is modulated by both Cl^- and K^+ intake. Other forms of Cl^--resistant alkalosis are caused by genetic mutations in the regulation and function of specific transporters in the loop of Henle and distal nephron (see Fig. 13.4 and Chapter 46).

Secondary Response to an Increase in Serum [HCO₃⁻]
Regardless of the cause, blood pH increases in metabolic alkalosis and elicits characteristic secondary hypoventilation, increasing arterial P_{CO_2}. The response is a potent one, occurring despite the concomitant development of hypoxemia and, in uncomplicated metabolic alkalosis, virtually always prevents blood pH from exceeding 7.60. On average, P_{CO_2} increases by 0.7 mm Hg (0.1 kP) for each 1 mmol/l increase in serum $[HCO_3^-]$. Assuming a normal $[HCO_3^-]$ and P_{CO_2} of 24 mmol/l and 40 mm Hg, respectively, the

predicted P_{CO_2} for any given serum $[HCO_3^-]$ in metabolic alkalosis can be calculated as follows:

$$P_{CO_2}\ (mm\ Hg) = 40 + 0.7 \times ([HCO_3^-]\ (mmol/l) - 24).$$

Although this formula is helpful in determining whether the ventilatory response to metabolic alkalosis is appropriate, it implies a precision that does not exist in nature. Variations of up to 5 to 7 mm Hg between the observed and calculated P_{CO_2} may normally occur. Even in severe metabolic alkalosis (serum $[HCO_3^-]$ >50 mmol/l), however, the P_{CO_2} (in mm Hg) virtually always exceeds the value for the serum $[HCO_3^-]$ (in mmol/l). Figure 13.5 illustrates the ameliorating effect of increasing P_{CO_2} on pH in metabolic alkalosis. While it mitigates the alkalemia, the increase in P_{CO_2} also stimulates renal HCO_3^- reabsorption, increasing serum $[HCO_3^-]$ further.[13] In the clinical setting, this latter effect is small and unimportant.

ETIOLOGIES

For ease of classification, the causes of metabolic alkalosis are subdivided into Cl^--responsive and Cl^--resistant forms. Metabolic alkalosis can also occur in certain settings as a result of alkali ingestion.

Chloride-Responsive Metabolic Alkalosis
Figure 13.6 lists the main causes of Cl^--responsive metabolic alkalosis.

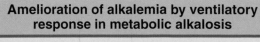

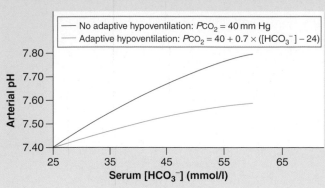

Figure 13.5 Amelioration of alkalemia by the normal ventilatory response to the increase in serum [HCO$_3^-$] in metabolic alkalosis. The red (*upper*) line in the graph illustrates the relationship between arterial pH and serum [HCO$_3^-$] in the absence of adaptive hypoventilation (PCO$_2$ maintained at 40 mm Hg) and the green (*lower*) line, the relationship when PCO$_2$ is increased by the expected level of hypoventilation.

Vomiting or Nasogastric Drainage

Loss of chloride from the upper gastrointestinal tract, often accompanied by concomitant H$^+$ losses, produces a metabolic alkalosis that is sustained until body Cl$^-$ stores are replenished (see Fig. 13.2). With continued emesis or nasogastric suction and without replacement of Cl$^-$ losses, serum [HCO$_3^-$] may rise to very high levels (>45 mmol/l). The use of gastric tissue to augment bladder size (gastrocystoplasty) can occasionally lead to metabolic alkalosis as a result of gastrin-induced Cl$^-$ secretion into the urine.[14]

Diuretic Administration

Diuretics that inhibit specific Cl$^-$ transport proteins in the kidney are the most common cause of metabolic alkalosis (see Fig. 13.6). The thiazides and metolazone inhibit the Na$^+$-Cl$^-$ cotransporter in the early distal tubule, and the loop diuretics inhibit the Na$^+$-K$^+$-2Cl$^-$ cotransporter in the ascending limb of the loop of Henle (see Fig. 13.1). These agents all impair Cl$^-$ reabsorption, causing selective Cl$^-$ depletion, and stimulate K$^+$ excretion by increasing Na$^+$ delivery to the collecting duct. The alkalosis produced is typically mild (serum [HCO$_3^-$] <36 mmol/l), except in patients who continue to ingest excess salt and have extreme renal Na$^+$ avidity. Hypokalemia due to K$^+$ depletion is more prominent and is the major management problem.[15]

Recovery from Chronic Hypercapnia

The renal response to sustained hypercapnia results in an increase in HCO$_3^-$ reabsorption and a decrease in Cl$^-$ reabsorption. As a result, serum [HCO$_3^-$] increases and body Cl$^-$ stores are reduced. When PCO$_2$ is restored to normal, renal excretion of excess HCO$_3^-$ requires repletion of the Cl$^-$ losses incurred during adaptation. If these losses are not replaced, recovery from hypercapnia can result in a persistent metabolic alkalosis.

Chloride-Losing Diarrhea

In two rare forms of diarrhea, congenital chloride diarrhea and the diarrhea caused by some Cl$^-$-secreting villous adenomas of the colon, Cl$^-$ losses in stool can produce metabolic alkalosis.[5] Although the alkalosis could, in theory, be corrected by Cl$^-$ administration, repletion of Cl$^-$ is difficult because of continued stool losses, and the alkalosis is often persistent despite adequate dietary intake.

Chloride-Resistant Metabolic Alkalosis

Figure 13.7 lists the causes of Cl$^-$-resistant metabolic alkalosis.

Mineralocorticoid Excess

Aldosterone and other mineralocorticoids cause metabolic alkalosis by stimulating both the H$^+$-ATPase and epithelial Na$^+$ channel in the collecting duct (see Figs. 13.1 and 13.4). The resultant Na$^+$ retention causes hypertension and also ensures continued delivery of Na$^+$ to the distal nephron, facilitating continued H$^+$ and K$^+$ secretion. The metabolic alkalosis is typically mild (serum [HCO$_3^-$] 30–35 mmol/l) and is associated with more severe hypokalemia (K$^+$ often <3 mmol/l) than in most Cl$^-$-responsive causes.[12] Primary hyperaldosteronism is by far the most common cause of this form of metabolic alkalosis (see Chapter 37), but it can also occur with rarer hereditary defects in cortisol synthesis or in the regulation of aldosterone secretion (see Fig. 13.7). Glucocorticoid-remediable aldosteronism is caused by a mutation that results in aldosterone secretion being stimulated by adrenocorticotropic

Causes of chloride-responsive metabolic alkalosis

Acid loss from the stomach (common)
    Vomiting
    Nasogastric suction

Diuretic administration (common)
    Thiazides
    Metolazone
    Loop diuretics: furosemide, bumetanide, torsemide, ethacrynic acid

Recovery from chronic hypercapnia (rarer)
Gastrocystoplasty (rarer)

Chloride-depleting diarrhea (much rarer)
    Congenital chloride diarrhea
    Villous adenoma of the colon

Figure 13.6 Causes of chloride-responsive metabolic alkalosis.

Causes of chloride-resistant metabolic alkalosis	
Cause	Examples
Mineralocorticoid excess	Primary hyperaldosteronism: adenoma, hyperplasia Cushing's syndrome Adrenocorticotropic hormone–secreting tumor Renin-secreting tumor Glucocorticoid-remediable aldosteronism Adrenogenital syndromes Fludrocortisone treatment α-fluoroprednisolone (inhaled)
Apparent mineralocorticoid excess	Licorice Carbenoxolone Liddle syndrome II-β-Hydroxysteroid dehydrogenase deficiency
Glucocorticoids (high dose)	Methylprednisolone
Impairment of Cl$^-$- linked Na$^+$ reabsorption	Bartter syndrome Gitelman's syndrome
Severe K$^+$ deficiency	Diarrhea

Figure 13.7 Causes of chloride-resistant metabolic alkalosis.

hormone rather than by angiotensin.[16] Fludrocortisone, an oral mineralocorticoid drug, can induce metabolic alkalosis if used inappropriately. Although no longer available in the U.S., habitual use of inhaled 9 α-fluoroprednisolone (still available in a nasal spray in other countries) can cause metabolic alkalosis. Glucocorticoids, when administered in very high doses, increase renal K^+ excretion nonspecifically and produce a mild increase in serum $[HCO_3^-]$.

Apparent Mineralocorticoid Excess Syndromes

Several inherited abnormalities produce a Cl^--resistant metabolic alkalosis that is clinically indistinguishable from hyperaldosteronism, but without measurable aldosterone (see Chapter 46). Liddle syndrome results from a genetic mutation that prevents the removal of epithelial Na^+ channels from the urinary membrane of collecting duct epithelial cells (see Fig. 13.4).[17] As a result, Na^+ reabsorption cannot be downregulated, causing the same cascade of events seen in hyperaldosteronism. Because continuous stimulation of Na^+ reabsorption expands ECF volume, however, aldosterone levels are vanishingly low. In another rare familial disorder, termed the syndrome of apparent mineralocorticoid excess, a mutation inactivates 11β-hydroxysteroid dehydrogenase, an enzyme adjacent to the mineralocorticoid receptor that rapidly converts cortisol to cortisone, minimizing cortisol binding to this receptor.[18] When the enzyme is inactivated, cortisol activates the receptor, stimulating Na^+ reabsorption and K^+ secretion and producing Cl^--resistant metabolic alkalosis and hypertension with low aldosterone levels. Glycyrrhizic acid (a component of natural licorice), carbenoxolone, and gossypol (an agent that inhibits spermatogenesis) all inhibit the activity of 11β-hydroxysteroid dehydrogenase and can cause the same clinical picture.

Impairment of Chloride-Linked Na+ Transport

Bartter and Gitelman's syndromes are two hereditary disorders manifested by Cl^--resistant metabolic alkalosis and hypokalemia, but without hypertension (see Chapter 46). Bartter syndrome is caused by several mutations, all of which have the effect of impeding Cl^--associated Na^+ reabsorption in the ascending limb of the loop of Henle (via the Na^+-K^+-$2Cl^-$ cotransporter; see Fig. 13.4).[19,20] Patients with this syndrome usually present early in life with metabolic alkalosis and volume depletion, features similar to those seen in individuals abusing loop diuretic agents. Gitelman's syndrome is caused by genetic mutations that inactivate the thiazide-sensitive Na^+-Cl^- cotransporter in the early distal tubule (see Fig. 13.4), leading to hypokalemia and metabolic alkalosis similar to that caused by thiazide diuretics.[20] Gitelman's syndrome becomes clinically apparent later in life and differs from Bartter syndrome in that hypomagnesemia and hypocalciuria are prominent features.[19] Although, in theory, Cl^- repletion could correct these disorders, they are Cl^- resistant because any administered Cl^- is rapidly excreted due to the defective transporters.

Severe K+ Deficiency

In patients with severe K^+ depletion (serum K^+ <2 mmol/l), metabolic alkalosis can be sustained despite Cl^- administration.[11] Chloride resistance in this setting is due to impairment of renal Cl^- reabsorption (see earlier discussion). Even partial repletion of K^+ stores rapidly reverses this problem and makes the alkalosis Cl^- responsive.

Alkali Administration

Exogenous alkali produces metabolic alkalosis in individuals with deficient body K^+ or Cl^- stores, due to impaired renal HCO_3^- excretion (Fig. 13.8; see earlier discussion).[6] When acute or

Causes of metabolic alkalosis associated with alkali administration	
Renal Status	Causes
Normal renal function (only in association with K^+ depletion or low NaCl intake)	Alkali intake: $NaHCO_3$, citrate, lactate, acetate, amino acid anions
Renal failure	Milk–alkali syndrome Alkali intake Aluminum hydroxide with K^+ exchange resin

Figure 13.8 Causes of metabolic alkalosis associated with alkali administration.

chronic renal failure is present, alkali administration or ingestion produces metabolic alkalosis independent of K^+ and Cl^- stores because the excess alkali cannot be excreted.[21] Milk-alkali syndrome is characterized by the concomitant presence of metabolic alkalosis and renal insufficiency, brought on by the ingestion of $NaHCO_3$ in combination with excess calcium (either in milk or as $CaCO_3$).[22,23] In this disorder, renal damage is caused by calcium deposition (facilitated by an alkaline urine). The renal damage in turn facilitates the development of metabolic alkalosis if alkali ingestion continues. Metabolic alkalosis is usually mild in these patients unless they develop concomitant vomiting. In hospitalized patients with renal failure, a wide variety of alkali sources or alkali precursors can cause metabolic alkalosis (Fig. 13.9). Although only rarely used now, administration of aluminum hydroxide in combination with sodium polystyrene sulfonate (Kayexalate) can cause metabolic alkalosis because aluminum binds to the resin in exchange for Na^+.[8] As a result, the HCO_3^- normally secreted into the duodenum is neither titrated by H^+ (which was neutralized by the aluminum hydroxide) nor does it form an insoluble salt with aluminum. Instead, it is completely reabsorbed from the gut, increasing serum $[HCO_3^-]$.[21]

Other Causes

Refeeding after starvation causes an abrupt increase in serum $[HCO_3^-]$ from the low levels characteristic of the fasting state.

Potential sources of alkali	
Alkali/Alkali Precursor	Source
Bicarbonate	$NaHCO_3$: pills, intravenous solutions Proprietary brands, e.g., Alka–Seltzer Baking soda $KHCO_3$: pills, oral solutions
Lactate	Ringer's solution, peritoneal dialysis solutions
Acetate Glutamate Propionate	Parenteral nutrition
Citrate	Blood products, plasma exchange, K^+ supplements, alkalinizing agents
Calcium compounds (alkalinizing effect minimal when given orally) Acetate Citrate Carbonate	Calcium supplements, phosphate binders

Figure 13.9 Potential sources of alkali.

In some instances, serum $[HCO_3^-]$ increases transiently above normal, causing a mild metabolic alkalosis. The causes are multiple, including HCO_3^- generation from metabolism of accumulated organic anions and K^+ and Cl^- depletion. Administration of vitamin D causes a small but significant increase in serum $[HCO_3^-]$.[24,25] Hyperparathyroidism in the clinic, however, is not associated with metabolic alkalosis. Hypercalcemia and vitamin D intoxication have been associated with metabolic alkalosis, but in most instances, the alkalosis can be explained by the vomiting that characteristically accompanies these disorders. High aldosterone levels induced by hyperreninemia in renovascular or malignant hypertension are associated with hypokalemia and, occasionally, with very minor increases in serum $[HCO_3^-]$.[21]

CLINICAL MANIFESTATIONS

Mild to moderate metabolic alkalosis is well tolerated, with few clinically important adverse effects. Patients with serum $[HCO_3^-]$ levels as high as 40 mmol/l are usually asymptomatic. The adverse effect of most concern is hypokalemia, which increases the likelihood of cardiac arrhythmias in patients with ischemic heart disease.[26] With more severe metabolic alkalosis (serum $[HCO_3^-]$ >45 mmol/l), arterial PO_2 often decreases to <50 mm Hg ([<6.65 kP] secondary to hypoventilation), and ionized calcium decreases (due to alkalemia). Patients with serum $[HCO_3^-]$ >50 mmol/l may develop seizures, tetany, delirium, or stupor. These changes in mental status are probably multifactorial in origin, due to alkalemia, hypokalemia, hypocalcemia, and hypoxemia.

DIAGNOSIS

Diagnosis of metabolic alkalosis involves three steps (Fig. 13.10). The first is to detect the disorder. The second is to assure oneself that the secondary response (hypoventilation) is appropriate, excluding the possibility that a respiratory acid-base abnormality is also present. The third is to uncover the cause. Detection of metabolic alkalosis is straightforward. The finding of a serum [total CO_2] >30 mmol/l in association with hypokalemia is virtually pathognomonic. The only other cause of an elevated serum $[HCO_3^-]$ is chronic respiratory acidosis, and hypokalemia is not a feature of this disorder (see Chapter 14). Because the diagnosis is usually evident and the disorder is almost always uncomplicated, one need not measure arterial pH and PCO_2 in most patients.

If the alkalosis is severe (serum $[HCO_3^-]$ >40 mmol/l), if the cause of the elevated $[HCO_3^-]$ is unclear, or if a mixed acid-base disorder is suspected, however, one should always measure arterial pH and PCO_2 to fully characterize the disorder (see Fig. 13.10). Measurement of pH and PCO_2 confirms the presence of alkalosis and allows one to estimate whether the degree of hypoventilation is appropriate for the serum $[HCO_3^-]$ (see earlier equation on p. 161). A major deviation in PCO_2 from the expected value indicates the presence of a complicating respiratory acid-base disorder (either respiratory acidosis or alkalosis, see Chapter 14). The anion gap, defined as $[Na^+]$ − $([Cl^-] + [HCO_3^-])$, is not increased in mild to moderate metabolic alkalosis, but can be increased by as much as 3 to 5 mmol/l when alkalosis is severe.[21] If the anion gap is >20 mmol/L, the disorder is most likely complicated by a superimposed metabolic acidosis (see Chapter 12).

In most instances, the third step, elucidating the cause, is also straightforward. More than 95% of metabolic alkalosis is caused either by diuretic use or by Cl^- losses from the upper gastrointestinal tract. This historical information is usually easily obtainable, and attention can be directed toward the appropriate treatment. If the cause is unclear from the history, measurement of urine $[Cl^-]$ can help. Unless the patient has recently taken a diuretic agent, urine $[Cl^-]$ should be <10 mmol/l if the metabolic alkalosis is due to Cl^- depletion. Surreptitious use of diuretics or self-induced vomiting (bulimia) can be a confounding problem. The former behavior presents the greater diagnostic dilemma

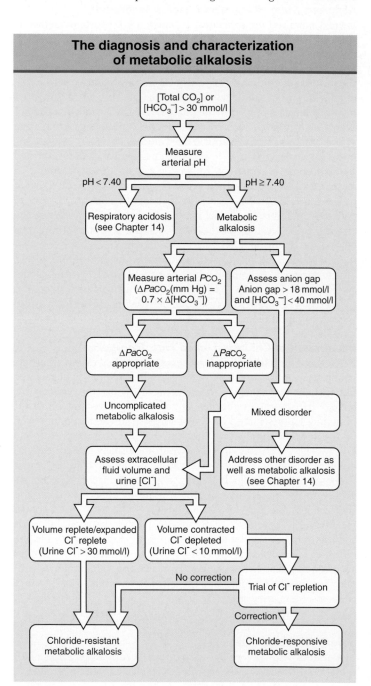

Figure 13.10 Approach to diagnosis and characterization of metabolic alkalosis. To determine with certainty whether an increase in serum $[HCO_3^-]$ signifies the presence of metabolic alkalosis, arterial pH and PCO_2 measurements are necessary. These measurements, along with a calculation of the anion gap, allow one to determine as well whether metabolic alkalosis is the only acid-base disturbance present. Once the acid-base disturbance has been characterized, one can assess extracellular fluid volume and/or measure urine Cl^- concentration to determine whether the disorder is Cl^- responsive or Cl^- resistant. (From Gennari FJ: Metabolic alkalosis. In Jacobson HR, Striker GE, Klahr S [eds]: The Principles and Practice of Nephrology, 2nd ed. St. Louis: Mosby, 1995, pp 932–941.)

because continued diuretic-induced Cl⁻ excretion may lead one to undertake an extensive work-up for rarer forms of metabolic alkalosis. Urinary screens for specific diuretic compounds may be necessary to establish the correct diagnosis. In bulimic patients, urine Cl⁻ excretion should be low (spot urine [Cl⁻] <10 mmol/l). If the cause is not apparent from this analysis, one should consider the Cl⁻-resistant forms of metabolic alkalosis. In these forms of metabolic alkalosis, urine [Cl⁻] is typically >30 mmol/l.

In the patient with hypertension and metabolic alkalosis who is not taking any diuretic agents, the most common cause of Cl⁻-resistant metabolic alkalosis is primary hyperaldosteronism. Measurement of serum renin and serum or urine aldosterone levels can distinguish mineralocorticoid excess syndromes from the rarer syndromes of apparent mineralocorticoid excess (see Fig. 13.7). The details of such a work-up are presented in Chapter 46. In the normotensive or hypotensive patient with Cl⁻-resistant metabolic alkalosis, the diagnoses of either Bartter or Gitelman's syndrome should be entertained. Aldosterone and/or renin levels are not helpful in making these diagnoses because the levels can be low or high, depending on the patient's ECF volume at the time of measurement. Familial genetic studies can establish these diagnoses with high specificity.

TREATMENT

Chloride-Responsive Alkalosis
In the patient with metabolic alkalosis due to nasogastric drainage or vomiting, ECF volume depletion is always a concomitant feature and treatment is straightforward. Administration of intravenous NaCl will correct both the alkalosis and the volume depletion. Potassium losses should also be replaced by oral or intravenous KCl. Typically, the K⁺ deficit is 200 to 400 mmol in patients with mild to moderate metabolic alkalosis induced by upper gastrointestinal Cl⁻ losses. When nasogastric drainage must be continued, H⁺ and Cl⁻ losses can be reduced by administration of drugs that inhibit gastric acid secretion, such as famotidine or omeprazole. In contrast to patients with upper gastrointestinal losses, NaCl administration is not usually required in patients with metabolic alkalosis caused by diuretics unless clinical signs of volume depletion are present. Potassium chloride supplements should be given to minimize K⁺ depletion as well as the metabolic alkalosis. The addition of a K⁺-sparing diuretic such as amiloride, triamterene, spironolactone, and eplerenone can assist in minimizing these abnormalities. Complete repair of diuretic-induced metabolic alkalosis is often difficult because of continued Cl⁻ and K⁺ losses. Fortunately, such a therapeutic goal is not necessary in most instances. A mild metabolic alkalosis is well tolerated, with no clinically significant adverse effects. One should always weigh the medical necessity of the diuretic agent. If the drug can be discontinued, the disorder will resolve so long as the diet contains adequate K⁺ and Cl⁻.

Chloride-Resistant Alkalosis
Management of Cl⁻-resistant alkalosis depends on the underlying cause. If the alkalosis is caused by an adrenal adenoma, the disorder is corrected by surgical removal of the tumor (see Chapter 37). In other forms of primary hyperaldosteronism, the alkalosis can be minimized by dietary NaCl restriction and by aggressive replacement of body K⁺ stores, using supplemental KCl. Spironolactone or eplerenone, competitive inhibitors of

aldosterone, can also correct the disorder. In glucocorticoid-remediable aldosteronism, the disorder is corrected by dexamethasone administration, suppressing ACTH secretion and thereby reducing aldosterone secretion. In the hereditary forms of apparent mineralocorticoid excess (Liddle syndrome and 11β-hydroxysteroid dehydrogenase deficiency), amiloride is the most effective treatment. The metabolic alkalosis (and hypokalemia) seen in Bartter and Gitelman's syndromes is the most difficult to correct. In addition to oral KCl supplements (and magnesium supplements in Gitelman's syndrome), nonsteroidal anti-inflammatory drugs have been used with moderate success. These drugs minimize renal Cl⁻ losses.

Alkali Ingestion
Treatment here is directed at identifying and discontinuing the offending alkali (see Fig. 13.9). One should be diligent in the intensive care unit to look for sources of exogenous alkali. A common offender is the use of acetate as a replacement for Cl⁻ in parenteral nutritional solutions.

SPECIAL PROBLEMS IN MANAGEMENT

Management of metabolic alkalosis is a more difficult undertaking in patients with severe congestive heart failure or renal failure. In patients with heart failure and fluid overload who still have renal function, acetazolamide can be used to reduce serum [HCO₃⁻]. This carbonic anhydrase inhibitor blocks H⁺-linked Na⁺ reabsorption, leading to excretion of both Na⁺ and [HCO₃⁻]. Acetazolamide decreases extracellular volume and lowers serum [HCO₃⁻], but it stimulates K⁺ excretion, exacerbating hypokalemia. When used, it should be accompanied by aggressive K⁺ replacement therapy.

In patients with renal failure, serum [HCO₃⁻] can be reduced in a timely fashion using the appropriate form of renal replacement therapy. Continuous venovenous hemofiltration can remove as much as 20 to 30 l/day of an ultrafiltrate of plasma, and the replacement solution can be modified to control electrolyte composition. Serum [HCO₃⁻] can also be lowered rapidly by continuous slow low-efficiency dialysis, with the dialysate [HCO₃⁻] adjusted to 23 mmol/l. Standard hemodialysis or peritoneal dialysis is less useful because these treatments are designed to add alkali to the blood and the alkali concentration in the dialysate is set at 35 to 40 mmol/l.

If renal replacement therapy cannot be instituted, titration with HCl is an alternative therapy. This approach is limited by the concentration of HCl that can be administered without producing hemolysis or venous coagulation. Although some investigators have used higher concentrations, the recommended safe level of H⁺ is 100 mmol/l (0.1 N HCl). Even at this concentration, HCl must be administered via a central vein. Because the apparent space of distribution of HCO₃⁻ is approximately 50% of body weight, 350 mmol of H⁺ is required to reduce serum [HCO₃⁻] by 10 mmol/l in a 70-kg patient. The volume of fluid required for this titration using HCl, unfortunately, is 3.5 liters. Ammonium chloride (NH₄Cl) or arginine monohydrochloride has also been used to provide H⁺ in a more concentrated solution. These solutions are no longer recommended because they both cause life-threatening problems.[21] The former can cause NH₃ intoxication and the latter can cause severe hyperkalemia.

REFERENCES

1. Gennari FJ, Maddox DM: Renal regulation of acid-base homeostasis. Integrated response. In Seldin DW, Giebisch G (eds): The Kidney. Physiology and Pathophysiology, 3rd ed. Philadelphia: Lippincott Williams & Wilkins, 2000, pp 2015–2053.
2. Gennari FJ: Metabolic alkalosis. In Jacobson HR, Striker, GE, Klahr S (eds): The Principles and Practice of Nephrology, 2nd ed. St. Louis: Mosby, 1995, pp 932–941.
3. Starr RA, Burg MB, Knepper MA: Bicarbonate secretion and chloride absorption in the rabbit cortical collecting ducts. Role of chloride/bicarbonate exchange. J Clin Invest 1985;76:1123–1130.
4. Jacobson HR, Seldin DW: On the generation, maintenance, and correction of metabolic alkalosis. Am J Physiol 1983;245:F425–F432.
5. Galla J: Metabolic alkalosis. J Am Soc Nephrol 2000;11:369–375.
6. Cogan MG, Carneiro MW, Tatsumo J, et al: Normal diet NaCl variation can affect the set point for plasma pH–HCO_3^- maintenance. J Am Soc Nephrol 1990;1:193–199.
7. Hernandez RE, Schambelan M, Cogan MG, et al: Dietary NaCl determines the severity of potassium depletion-induced metabolic alkalosis. Kidney Int 1987;31:1356–1367.
8. Kassirer JP, Schwartz WB: The response of normal man to selective depletion of hydrochloric acid. Am J Med 1966;40:10–18.
9. Kassirer JP, Schwartz WB: Correction of metabolic alkalosis in man without repair of potassium deficiency. Am J Med 1966;40:19–26.
10. Gennari FJ: Hypokalemia in metabolic alkalosis. A new look at an old controversy. In Hatano M (ed): Nephrology. Tokyo: Springer Verlag, 1991, pp 262–269.
11. Garella S, Chazan JA, Cohen JJ: Saline resistant metabolic alkalosis or "chloride-wasting nephropathy." Ann Intern Med 1970;73:31–38.
12. Holland OB: Primary hyperaldosteronism. Semin Nephrol 1995;15:116–125.
13. Madias NE, Adrogue HJ, Cohen JJ: Maladaptive renal response to chronic metabolic alkalosis. Am J Physiol 1980;238:F283–F289.
14. DeFoor W, Minevich E, Reeves D, et al: Gastrocystoplasty: Long-term follow-up. J Urol 2003;170:1647–1650.
15. Gennari FJ: Hypokalemia. N Engl J Med 1998;339:451–458.
16. Lifton RP, Dluhy RG, Powers M, et al: A chimaeric 11β-hydroxylase/aldosterone synthase gene causes glucocorticoid-remediable aldosteronism and human hypertension. Nature 1992;355:262–265.
17. Tamura H, Schild L, Enomoto N, et al: Liddle disease caused by a missense mutation of β subunit of the epithelial sodium channel gene. J Clin Invest 1996;97:1780–1784.
18. Whorwood CB, Stewart PM: Human hypertension caused by mutations in the 11β-hydroxysteroid dehydrogenase gene: A molecular analysis of apparent mineralocorticoid excess. J Hypertens 1996;14(Suppl 5):S19–S24.
19. Guay-Woodford LM: Bartter syndrome: Unraveling the pathophysiologic enigma. Am J Med 1998;105:151–161.
20. Simon DB, Lifton RJ: The molecular basis of inherited hypokalemic alkalosis: Bartter and Gitelman syndromes. Am J Physiol 1996;271:F961–F966.
21. Rimmer JM, Gennari FJ: Metabolic alkalosis. J Intensive Care Med 1987;2:137–150.
22. Orwoll ES: The milk-alkali syndrome: Current concepts. Ann Intern Med 1982;97:242–248.
23. Beall DP, Scofield RH: Milk-alkali syndrome associated with calcium carbonate consumption. Medicine 1995;74:89–96.
24. Hulter HN, Sebastian A, Toto RD, et al: Renal and systemic effects of the chronic administration of hypercalcemia-producing agents: Calcitriol, PTH and intravenous calcium. Kidney Int 1982;21:445–458.
25. Hulter HN, Peterson JC: Acid-base homeostasis during chronic PTH excess in humans. Kidney Int 1985;28:187–192.
26. Schulman M, Narins RG: Hypokalemia and cardiovascular disease. Am J Cardiol 1990;65:4E–9E.

Respiratory Acidosis, Respiratory Alkalosis, and Mixed Disorders

Horacio J. Adrogué and Nicolaos E. Madias

INTRODUCTION

Deviations of systemic acidity in either direction can have adverse consequences and, when severe, can be life threatening. Therefore, it is essential for the clinician to be able to recognize and properly diagnose acid-base disorders, understand their impact on organ function, and be familiar with their treatment and the potential complications of treatment.[1,2]

RESPIRATORY ACIDOSIS (PRIMARY HYPERCAPNIA)

Definition

Respiratory acidosis is the acid-base disturbance initiated by an increase in CO_2 tension of body fluids. The secondary increment in plasma bicarbonate $[HCO_3^-]$ observed in acute and chronic hypercapnia should be viewed as an integral part of the respiratory acidosis.[3] Whole-body CO_2 stores are increased and the level of arterial CO_2 tension ($PaCO_2$) is >45 mm Hg (5.3 kP) in patients with simple respiratory acidosis (measured at rest and

at sea level). An element of respiratory acidosis may still occur with lower levels of $PaCO_2$ in patients residing at high altitude (e.g., 4000 m or 13,000 ft) or with metabolic acidosis in whom a normal $PaCO_2$ is inappropriately high for this condition.[4] Another special case of respiratory acidosis is the presence of arterial eucapnia, or even hypocapnia, occurring together with severe venous hypercapnia, in patients having an acute, profound decrease in cardiac output but relative preservation of respiratory function.[5,6] This disorder is known as pseudorespiratory alkalosis and is discussed under respiratory alkalosis.

Etiology and Pathogenesis

The ventilatory system is responsible for maintaining $PaCO_2$ within normal limits by adjusting alveolar minute ventilation ($\dot{V}A$) to match the rate of CO_2 production. The main elements of ventilation are the respiratory pump, which generates a pressure gradient responsible for air flow, and the loads that oppose such action.

The determinants of CO_2 retention can be viewed as factors imposing an imbalance between the strength of the respiratory pump and the weight of the respiratory loads (Fig. 14.1). When

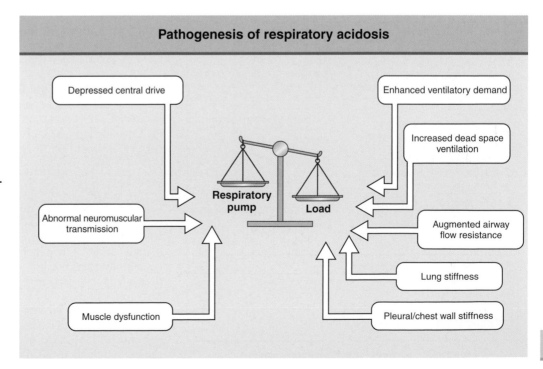

Figure 14.1 Pathogenesis of respiratory acidosis.

Pathogenesis of respiratory acidosis

Depressed central drive

Enhanced ventilatory demand

Increased dead space ventilation

Abnormal neuromuscular transmission

Respiratory pump

Load

Augmented airway flow resistance

Lung stiffness

Muscle dysfunction

Pleural/chest wall stiffness

the respiratory pump is unable to balance the opposing load, respiratory acidosis develops. Respiratory acidosis is divided into acute and chronic forms, taking into consideration the usual mode of onset and duration of the various causes (Figs. 14.2 and 14.3). Life-threatening acidemia of respiratory origin can occur during severe, acute respiratory acidosis or during respiratory decompensation in patients with chronic hypercapnia.

The following equation presents the simplified form of the alveolar gas equation at sea level and when breathing room air (FiO_2, 21%):

$$P_{A}O_2 = 150 - 1.25\ PaCO_2,$$

where $P_{A}O_2$ is alveolar O_2 tension in millimeters of mercury (mm Hg) (to convert values from mm Hg to kP, multiply by 0.1333). The constraints of the alveolar gas equation establish that

Causes of acute respiratory acidosis	
Increased Load	Depressed Pump
Enhanced Ventilatory Demand	Depressed Central Drive

High carbohydrate diet
 High carbohydrate dialysate
  (peritoneal dialysis)
 Sorbent-regenerative
  hemodialysis
	General anesthesia
	 Sedative overdose
	 Head trauma
	 Cerebrovascular accident
	 Obesity hypoventilation syndrome
	 Cerebral edema
	 Brain tumor
	 Encephalitis
	 Brainstem lesion

Increased Dead Space Ventilation	Abnormal Neuromuscular Transmission

Acute lung injury
 Multilobar pneumonia
 Cardiogenic pulmonary edema
 Pulmonary embolism
 Positive pressure ventilation
 Supplemental oxygen
	High spinal cord injury
	 Guillain–Barré syndrome
	 Status epilepticus
	 Botulism, tetanus
	 Crisis in myasthenia gravis
	 Familial periodic paralysis
	 Drugs or toxic agents (e.g., curare,
	  succinylcholine, aminoglycosides,
	  organophosphate poisoning)

Augmented Airway Flow Resistance	Muscle Dysfunction

Upper airway obstruction
  Coma-induced hypopharyngeal
   obstruction
  Aspiration of foreign body or vomitus
  Laryngospasm
  Angioedema
  Inadequate laryngeal intubation
  Laryngeal obstruction postintubation
 Lower airway obstruction
  Status asthmaticus
  Exacerbation of chronic obstructive
   pulmonary disease
	Fatigue
	 Hyperkalemia
	 Hypokalemia

Lung Stiffness	
Atelectasis	
Pleural/Chest Wall Stiffness	
Pneumothorax Hemothorax Flail chest Abdominal distension Peritoneal dialysis	

Figure 14.2 Causes of acute respiratory acidosis.

Causes of chronic respiratory acidosis	
Increased Load	Depressed Pump
Increased Dead Space Ventilation	Depressed Central Drive
Emphysema Pulmonary fibrosis Pulmonary vascular disease	Central sleep apnea Obesity hypoventilation syndrome Methadone/heroin addiction Brain tumor Bulbar poliomyelitis Hypothyroidism
Augmented Airway Flow Resistance	Abnormal Neuromuscular Transmission

Upper airway obstruction
  Tonsillar and peritonsillar
   hypertrophy
  Paralysis of vocal cords
  Tumor of the cords or larynx
  Airways stenosis after prolonged
   intubation
  Thymoma, aortic aneurysm
 Lower airway obstruction
  Chronic obstructive pulmonary
   disease
	High spinal cord injury
	 Poliomyelitis
	 Multiple sclerosis
	 Muscular dystrophy
	 Amyotrophic lateral sclerosis
	 Diaphragmatic paralysis

Lung Stiffness	Muscle Dysfunction
Severe chronic interstitial lung disease	Myopathic disease (e.g., polymyositis)
Pleural/Chest Wall Stiffness	
Kyphoscoliosis Thoracic cage disease Thoracoplasty Obesity	

Figure 14.3 Causes of chronic respiratory acidosis.

patients breathing room air cannot reach $PaCO_2$ levels much greater than 80 mm Hg (10.6 kP) because the degree of hypoxemia that would occur at greater values is incompatible with life. Therefore, extreme hypercapnia occurs only during O_2 therapy, and severe CO_2 retention is often the result of uncontrolled O_2 administration.

Secondary Physiologic Response

Adaptation to acute hypercapnia elicits an immediate increment in plasma HCO_3^- concentration that is explained by titration of non-HCO_3^- body buffers; such buffers generate HCO_3^- by combining with H^+ derived from the dissociation of carbonic acid:

$$CO_2 + H_2O \rightleftharpoons H_2CO_3 \rightleftharpoons HCO_3^- \\ + H^+ + H^+ + B^- \rightleftharpoons HB$$

where B^- refers to the base component and HB refers to the acid component of non-HCO_3^- buffers. This adaptation is completed within 5 to 10 minutes from the increase in $PaCO_2$, and, assuming a stable level of hypercapnia, no further change in acid-base equilibrium is detectable for a few hours.[7] Moderate hypoxemia does not alter the adaptive response to acute respiratory acidosis. However, pre-existing hypobicarbonatemia (whether caused by metabolic acidosis or chronic respiratory alkalosis) enhances the magnitude of the HCO_3^- response to acute hypercapnia; this response is diminished in hyperbicarbonatemic states (whether caused by metabolic alkalosis or chronic respiratory acidosis).[8,9]

The adaptive increase in plasma HCO_3^- concentration observed in the acute phase of hypercapnia is amplified greatly during chronic hypercapnia as a result of HCO_3^- generation by the kidney. In addition, the renal response to chronic hypercapnia includes a reduction in the rate of Cl^- reabsorption, resulting in depletion of the body's Cl^- stores. Completion of the adaptation to chronic hypercapnia requires 3 to 5 days.[7] Quantitative aspects of the secondary physiologic responses to acute and chronic hypercapnia are depicted in Figure 14.4. The renal response to chronic hypercapnia is not altered appreciably by dietary Na^+ or Cl^- restriction, moderate K^+ depletion, alkali loading, or moderate hypoxemia. However, recovery from chronic hypercapnia is crippled by a diet deficient in Cl^-; in this circumstance, despite correction of the level of $PaCO_2$, plasma $[HCO_3^-]$ concentration remains elevated so long as the state of Cl^- deprivation persists, thus creating the entity of posthypercapnic metabolic alkalosis.

Clinical Manifestations

Because clinical hypercapnia almost always occurs with some degree of hypoxemia, it is often difficult to determine whether a specific manifestation is the consequence of the elevated $PaCO_2$ or the reduced PaO_2. Nevertheless, one should bear in mind several characteristic manifestations of neurologic or cardiovascular dysfunction to diagnose the condition accurately and to treat it effectively.[4,7]

Neurologic Symptoms

Acute hypercapnia is often associated with marked anxiety, severe breathlessness, disorientation, confusion, incoherence, and combativeness. A narcotic-like effect is not uncommon in patients with chronic hypercapnia, and drowsiness, decreased alertness, inattention, forgetfulness, loss of memory, irritability, confusion, and somnolence can be observed. Motor disturbances, including tremor, myoclonic jerks, and asterixis, are frequent accompaniments of both acute and chronic hypercapnia. Sustained myoclonus and seizure activity can also develop. Signs and symptoms of increased intracranial pressure (pseudotumor cerebri) are occasionally evident in patients with either acute or chronic hypercapnia, and they appear to be related to the vasodilating effects of CO_2 on cerebral blood vessels. Headache is a frequent complaint. Blurring of the optic discs and frank papilledema can be found when hypercapnia is severe. Hypercapnic coma characteristically occurs in patients with acute exacerbations of chronic respiratory insufficiency, who are treated injudiciously with high-flow O_2.

Cardiovascular Symptoms

Acute hypercapnia of mild to moderate degree is usually characterized by warm, flushed skin, a bounding pulse, sweating, increased cardiac output, and normal or increased blood pressure. By comparison, severe hypercapnia might be attended by decreases in both cardiac output and blood pressure. Cardiac arrhythmias occur frequently in patients with either acute or chronic hypercapnia, especially those receiving digoxin or digitoxin.

Renal Symptoms

Mild to moderate hypercapnia results in renal vasodilation, but acute increments in $PaCO_2$ to levels >70 mm Hg (9.3 kP) induce renal vasoconstriction and hypoperfusion. Salt and water retention commonly attend sustained hypercapnia, especially in the presence of cor pulmonale. In addition to the effects of heart failure on the kidney, multiple other factors might be at play, including the prevailing stimulation of the sympathetic nervous system and the renin angiotensin aldosterone axis, the increased renal vascular resistance, and the elevated levels of antidiuretic hormone and cortisol.

Diagnosis

Whenever CO_2 retention is suspected, blood gas determinations should be obtained.[10] Indeed, accurate laboratory data are a prerequisite for establishing the diagnosis of respiratory acidosis. If the patient's acid-base profile reveals hypercapnia in association with acidemia, at least an element of respiratory acidosis must be present. However, hypercapnia can be associated with a normal or even an alkaline pH if certain additional acid-base disorders are also present. Information from the patient's history, a physical examination, and ancillary laboratory data should be used to assess whether part or all of the increase in $PaCO_2$ reflects an adaptive response to metabolic alkalosis rather than being primary in origin.

Treatment

As previously noted, CO_2 retention, whether acute or chronic, is always associated with hypoxemia in patients breathing room air. Consequently, O_2 administration represents a critical element in the management of respiratory acidosis.[1,11] However, supplemental O_2 may lead to worsening hypercapnia, especially in patients with chronic obstructive pulmonary disease. Although a depressed respiratory drive in CO_2 retention seems to play a role, other factors might largely account for the worsening hypercapnia in response to supplemental O_2 therapy. These include an increase in dead space ventilation and ventilation/perfusion $[\dot{V}/\dot{Q}]$ mismatch due to the loss of hypoxic pulmonary vasoconstriction, and the Haldane effect (the decreased hemoglobin affinity for

Secondary response to alterations in acid-base status			
Condition	Initiating Mechanism	Expected Response: Change in $[HCO_3^-]$ or $PaCO_2$	Maximal Level of Response
Respiratory acidosis	Increase in $PaCO_2$		
Acute		Increase in $[HCO_3^-] \approx 0.1\ PaCO_2$	30 mmol/l
Chronic		Increase in $[HCO_3^-] \approx 0.3\ PaCO_2$	45 mmol/l
Respiratory alkalosis	Decrease in $PaCO_2$		
Acute		Decrease in $[HCO_3^-] \approx 0.2\ PaCO_2$	16–18 mmol/l
Chronic		Decrease in $[HCO_3^-] \approx 0.4\ PaCO_2$	12–15 mmol/l
Metabolic acidosis	Decrease in $[HCO_3^-]_p$	Decrease in $PaCO_2 \approx 1.2\ [HCO_3^-]$	10 mm Hg (1.3 kP)
Metabolic alkalosis	Increase in $[HCO_3^-]_p$	Increase in $PaCO_2 \approx 0.7\ [HCO_3^-]$	65 mm Hg (8.7 kP)

Figure 14.4 Secondary response to alterations in acid-base status.

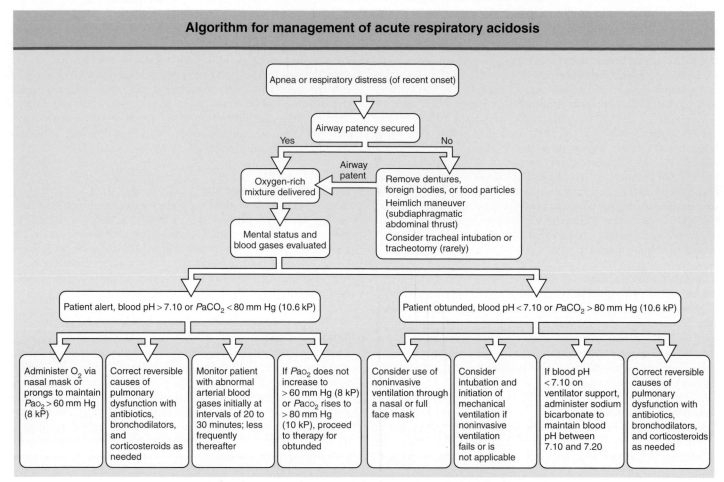

Figure 14.5 Algorithm for the management of acute respiratory acidosis.

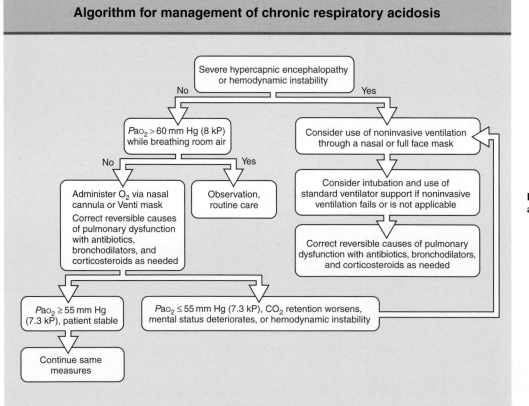

Figure 14.6 Algorithm for the management of chronic respiratory acidosis.

CO_2 in the presence of increased O_2 saturation), which mandates an increase in ventilation to eliminate the excess CO_2.[7]

A synopsis of the management of acute respiratory acidosis and chronic respiratory acidosis is presented in Figures 14.5 and 14.6. Whenever possible, treatment must be directed at removing or ameliorating the underlying cause. Immediate therapeutic efforts should focus on securing a patent airway and restoring adequate oxygenation by delivering an O_2-rich inspired mixture. Mechanical ventilation must be initiated in the presence of apnea, severe hypoxemia unresponsive to conservative measures, or progressive respiratory acidosis ($PaCO_2$ >80 mm Hg [10.6 kP]).[7] Vigorous treatment of pulmonary infections, bronchodilator therapy, and removal of secretions can offer considerable benefit. Naloxone will reverse the suppressive effect of narcotic agents on ventilation. Avoidance of tranquilizers and sedatives, gradual reduction of supplemental oxygen (aiming at a PaO_2 of about 60 mm Hg [8 kP]), and treatment of a superimposed element of metabolic alkalosis will optimize the ventilatory drive.

Noninvasive mechanical ventilation delivered through a nasal or full facial mask is being used with increasing frequency to avert possible complications of endotracheal intubation. However, if the patient is unstable or noninvasive ventilation fails, intubation should be carried out to allow invasive ventilatory support. Minute ventilation should be raised so that the $PaCO_2$ gradually returns to near its long-term baseline and excretion of excess HCO_3^- by the kidneys is accomplished (assuming that Cl^- is provided).

By contrast, overly rapid reduction in the $PaCO_2$ risks the development of posthypercapnic alkalosis, with potentially serious consequences. Should posthypercapnic alkalosis develop, it can be ameliorated by providing Cl^-, usually as the potassium salt, and administering the HCO_3^- wasting diuretic acetazolamide at doses of 250 to 375 mg once or twice daily.

Traditionally, the goal of treatment with mechanical ventilation had been to restore $PaCO_2$ and arterial blood pH to the normal values of 40 mm Hg and 7.40, respectively. This strategy led to the widespread use of tidal volumes of 10 to 15 ml/kg body weight. However, large tidal volumes often lead to alveolar overdistention and volutrauma. Therefore, an alternative approach that uses a lung-protective ventilatory strategy and allows $PaCO_2$ to increase, called permissive hypercapnia (or controlled mechanical hypoventilation), has been successfully applied to prevent barotrauma and cardiovascular collapse.[4,12] In this form of treatment, lower tidal volumes of <6 ml/kg body weight and lower peak inspiratory pressures are used. Further, $PaCO_2$ is allowed to increase but rarely exceeds 80 mm Hg, and blood pH can decrease to as low as 7.00 to 7.10, while maintaining adequate oxygenation. The increased respiratory drive associated with permissive hypercapnia causes extreme discomfort, making sedation necessary. Because the patients commonly require neuromuscular blockade as well, accidental disconnection from the ventilator can cause sudden death. There are several contraindications to the use of permissive hypercapnia, including cerebrovascular disease, brain edema, increased intracranial pressure, and convulsions and depressed cardiac function, arrhythmias, and severe pulmonary hypertension. Notably, most of these entities may occur secondary to permissive hypercapnia itself, especially when hypercapnia is associated with substantial acidemia. In fact, some experimental evidence indicates that correction of acidemia attenuates the adverse hemodynamic effects of permissive hypercapnia.[13] It appears prudent, although still controversial, to keep the blood pH at approximately 7.30 by administering intravenous alkali when controlled hypoventilation is prescribed.[1,14]

RESPIRATORY ALKALOSIS (PRIMARY HYPOCAPNIA)

Definition

Respiratory alkalosis is the acid-base disturbance initiated by a reduction in CO_2 tension of body fluids. The secondary decrease in plasma HCO_3^- concentration observed in acute and chronic hypocapnia should be viewed as an integral part of the respiratory alkalosis. Whole-body CO_2 stores are decreased and the level of $PaCO_2$ is <35 mm Hg (4.7 kP) in patients with simple respiratory alkalosis who are at rest and at sea level. An element of respiratory alkalosis may still occur with higher levels of $PaCO_2$ in patients with metabolic alkalosis, in whom a normal $PaCO_2$ is inappropriately low for this primary metabolic disorder.

Etiology and Pathogenesis

Respiratory alkalosis is the most frequent acid-base disorder encountered since it occurs in normal pregnancy and with high-altitude residence.[2,15] It is also the most common acid-base abnormality in critically ill patients, occurring either as the simple disorder or as a component of mixed disturbances; indeed, in such patients, its presence may constitute a grave prognostic sign, especially if $PaCO_2$ levels are <20 to 25 mm Hg (2.7 to 3.3 kP). The presence of hypocapnia signifies transient or persistent alveolar hyperventilation relative to the prevailing CO_2 production, thus leading to negative CO_2 balance; primary hypocapnia might also originate from the extrapulmonary elimination of CO_2 by a dialysis device or extracorporeal circulation (e.g., heart-lung machine).

Figure 14.7 gives the major causes of respiratory alkalosis.[6] In the vast majority of patients, primary hypocapnia reflects alveolar hyperventilation owing to increased ventilatory drive. The latter might represent signals arising from the lung, the peripheral chemoreceptors (carotid and aortic), or the brainstem chemoreceptors or influences originating in other centers of the brain. The response of the brainstem chemoreceptors to CO_2 can be augmented by systemic diseases (e.g., liver disease, sepsis), pharmacologic agents, volition, and other influences. Hypoxemia is a major stimulus of alveolar ventilation, but PaO_2 values <60 mm Hg (8 kP) are required to elicit this effect consistently. Not uncommonly, alveolar hyperventilation is the result of maladjusted mechanical ventilators, psychogenic hyperventilation, some psychiatric conditions, and lesions involving the central nervous system.

In states of severe circulatory failure, arterial hypocapnia may coexist with venous and, therefore, tissue hypercapnia; under these conditions, the body CO_2 stores have been enriched so that respiratory acidosis rather than respiratory alkalosis is present. This entity, which we have termed pseudorespiratory alkalosis, develops in patients with profound depression of cardiac function and pulmonary perfusion but relative preservation of alveolar ventilation, including patients with advanced circulatory failure and those undergoing cardiopulmonary resuscitation. The severely reduced pulmonary blood flow limits the CO_2 delivered to the lungs for excretion, thereby increasing the venous PCO_2. However, the increased ventilation-to-perfusion ratio causes a larger than normal removal of CO_2 per unit of blood traversing the pulmonary circulation, thereby giving rise to arterial eucapnia or frank hypocapnia. A progressive widening of the arteriovenous difference in pH and PCO_2 develops in these two settings of cardiac dysfunction, namely, circulatory failure and cardiac arrest (Fig. 14.8). Severe O_2 deprivation

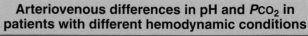

Causes of respiratory alkalosis	
Hypoxemia or Tissue Hypoxia	**Drugs and Hormones**
Decreased inspired O_2 tension	Respiratory stimulants (doxapram,
High altitude	nikethamide, ethamivan,
Bacterial or viral pneumonia	progesterone, medroxyprogesterone)
Aspiration of food, foreign body,	Salicylates
or vomitus	Nicotine
Laryngospasm	Xanthines
Drowning	Dinitrophenol
Cyanotic heart disease	Pressor hormones (epinephrine,
Severe anemia	norepinephrine, angiotensin II)
Left shift deviation of HbO_2 curve	
Hypotension	
Severe circulatory failure	
Pulmonary edema	
Pseudorespiratory alkalosis	
Central Nervous System Stimulation	**Miscellaneous**
Voluntary	Exercise
Pain	Pregnancy
Anxiety–hyperventilation syndrome	Gram-positive septicemia
Psychosis	Gram-negative septicemia
Fever	Hepatic failure
Subarachnoid hemorrhage	Mechanical hyperventilation
Cerebrovascular accident	Heat exposure
Meningoencephalitis	Recovery from metabolic acidosis
Tumor	Hemodialysis with acetate dialysate
Trauma	
Pulmonary Diseases with Stimulation of Chest Receptors	
Pneumonia	
Asthma	
Pneumothorax	
Hemothorax	
Flail chest	
Acute respiratory distress syndrome	
Cardiogenic and noncardiogenic	
pulmonary edema	
Pulmonary embolism	
Pulmonary fibrosis	

Figure 14.7   Causes of respiratory alkalosis.

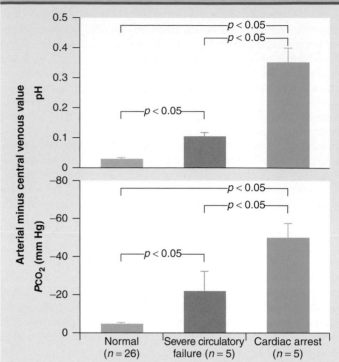

Figure 14.8   Arteriovenous differences in pH and P_{CO_2} in patients with different hemodynamic conditions.

prevails in the tissues in these two disorders, and it can be completely disguised by the reasonably preserved arterial O_2 values. Appropriate monitoring of acid-base composition and oxygenation in patients with advanced cardiac dysfunction requires mixed (or central) venous blood sampling in addition to the sampling of arterial blood.

Secondary Physiologic Response

Adaptation to acute hypocapnia is characterized by an immediate decrement in plasma HCO_3^- that results totally from nonrenal mechanisms and is explained principally by alkaline titration of the non-HCO_3^- body buffers (see second equation and Fig. 14.4). This adaptation is completed within 5 to 10 minutes of the onset of hypocapnia, and, if one assumes no further changes in $PaCO_2$, no additional detectable changes in acid-base equilibrium occur for a period of several hours.

Adaptation to chronic hypocapnia entails an additional, larger decrease in plasma HCO_3^- as a consequence of renal adjustments that reflect a dampening of H^+ secretion by the renal tubule.[7] Approximately 2 to 3 days are required for completion of the adaptation to chronic hypocapnia. Quantitative aspects of the secondary physiologic responses to acute and chronic hypocapnia are shown in Figure 14.4.

Clinical Manifestations

A rapid decrease in $PaCO_2$ to half normal values or lower is typically accompanied by numbness and paresthesias of the extremities, chest discomfort, circumoral numbness, lightheadedness, and mental confusion. Muscle cramps, increased deep-tendon reflexes, carpopedal spasm, and generalized seizures occur infrequently. Cerebral vasoconstriction and reduced cerebral blood flow have been well documented during acute hypocapnia; in severe cases, cerebral blood flow might reach values <50% of normal. Hypocapnia can have deleterious effects on the brain of premature infants, patients with traumatic brain injury, acute stroke, or general anesthesia, and after sudden exposure to very high altitude.[16] Long-term neurologic sequelae can develop when immature brains are exposed to $PaCO_2$ levels <15 mm Hg [2 kP] for even short periods. Furthermore, abrupt correction of hypocapnia in these patients leads to cerebral vasodilation, which might cause reperfusion injury or intraventricular hemorrhage.

The mechanisms of brain injury due to hypocapnia include cerebral ischemia; antioxidant-glutathione depletion caused by augmented production of cytotoxic excitatory amino acids; increases in anaerobic metabolism, cerebral oxygen demand, neuronal dopamine, and brain excitability; and seizure activity. If sepsis is present, the brain damage is enhanced by the release of lipopolysaccharide, interleukin-1β, and tumor necrosis factor α.[16]

The cardiovascular manifestations of respiratory alkalosis differ in passive and active hyperventilation. The induction of acute hypocapnia in anesthetized subjects (i.e., passive hyperventilation) results in a decrease in cardiac output, an increase in peripheral resistance, and a decrease in the systemic blood pressure. By contrast, active hyperventilation does not change, or might even increase, cardiac output and leaves systemic blood pressure virtually unchanged. The discrepant response of cardiac output during hyperventilation probably reflects the decrease in venous return caused by mechanical ventilation in passive hyperventilation and the reflex tachycardia consistently observed in active hyperventilation. Sustained hypocapnia induced by exposure to high altitude for several weeks results in a cardiac output equal to or higher than control values. Although acute hypocapnia does not lead to cardiac arrhythmias in normal volunteers, it appears that it contributes to the generation of both atrial and ventricular tachyarrhythmias in patients with ischemic heart disease; such arrhythmias are frequently resistant to standard forms of therapy. Chest pain and ischemic ST-T wave changes have been observed in acutely hyperventilating subjects with no evidence of fixed lesions on coronary angiography.

Diagnosis

Evaluation of the patient's history, a physical examination, and ancillary laboratory data are required to establish the diagnosis of respiratory alkalosis.[10,15] Careful observation can detect abnormal patterns of breathing in some patients, yet marked hypocapnia can occur without a clinically evident increase in respiratory effort. Arterial blood gas determinations are required to confirm the presence of hyperventilation.

The diagnosis of respiratory alkalosis, especially the chronic form, is frequently missed; physicians often misinterpret the electrolyte pattern of hyperchloremic hypobicarbonatemia as indicative of normal anion gap metabolic acidosis. If the patient's acid-base profile reveals hypocapnia in association with alkalemia, at least an element of respiratory alkalosis must be present. Yet hypocapnia might be associated with a normal or an acidic pH because of the concomitant presence of additional acid-base disorders. One should also note that mild degrees of chronic hypocapnia leave blood pH within the high-normal range. Once the diagnosis of respiratory alkalosis is made, a search for its cause should be carried out. The diagnosis of respiratory alkalosis can have important clinical implications; it often provides a clue to the presence of an unrecognized, serious disorder or signals the gravity of a known underlying disease.

Treatment

A synopsis of the management of respiratory alkalosis is presented in Figure 14.9. Accumulated evidence over the past few years indicates that the widely held view that hypocapnia poses little risk to health under most conditions is not accurate. In fact, substantial hypocapnia in hospitalized patients, whether spontaneous or deliberately induced, can be associated with transient or permanent damage in the brain as well as the respiratory and cardiovascular systems.[16] Furthermore, rapid correction of severe hypocapnia leads to vasodilation of ischemic areas resulting in reperfusion injury in the brain and lung. Consequently, severe hypocapnia in hospitalized patients must be prevented whenever possible, and, if present, abrupt correction should be avoided. Severe alkalemia caused by acute primary hypocapnia requires corrective measures that depend on whether serious clinical

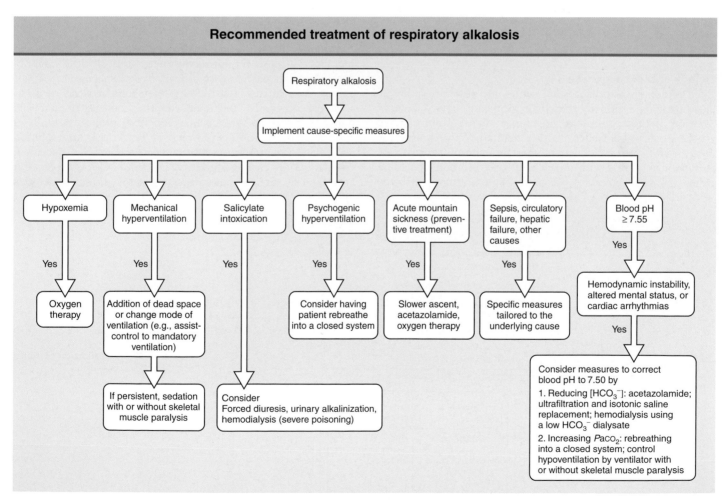

Figure 14.9   Recommended treatment of respiratory alkalosis.

manifestations are present. Such measures can be directed at reducing plasma bicarbonate concentration, increasing $PaCO_2$, or both. Even if baseline plasma bicarbonate is moderately decreased, reducing it further can be particularly rewarding in this setting, as this maneuver combines effectiveness with relatively little risk. For patients with the anxiety-hyperventilation syndrome in addition to reassurance or sedation, rebreathing into a closed system (e.g., a paper bag) might prove helpful by interrupting the vicious cycle that can result from the reinforcing effects of the symptoms of hypocapnia.

Respiratory alkalosis resulting from severe hypoxemia requires O_2 therapy. The oral administration of 250 to 500 mg acetazolamide can be beneficial in the management of signs and symptoms of high-altitude sickness, a syndrome characterized by hypoxemia and respiratory alkalosis.[15] Of course, patients undergoing mechanical ventilation lend themselves to an effective correction of hypocapnia (whether caused by maladjusted ventilator or other factors) by resetting the device.

MIXED ACID-BASE DISTURBANCES

Definition
Mixed acid-base disturbances are defined as the simultaneous presence of two or more acid-base disorders. Such association might include two or more simple acid-base disorders (e.g., metabolic acidosis and respiratory alkalosis), two or more forms of a simple disturbance having different time course or pathogenesis (e.g., acute and chronic respiratory acidosis or high anion gap and hyperchloremic metabolic acidosis, respectively), or a combination of the previous two forms.[17] The secondary or adaptive response to a simple acid-base disorder cannot be taken as one of the components of a mixed disorder.

Etiology and Pathogenesis
Mixed acid-base disturbances are commonly observed in hospitalized patients, especially those in critical care units.[18] Characterization of these disorders and proper identification of their pathogenesis can be challenging tasks and are a prerequisite for taking sound corrective action. Certain clinical settings are commonly associated with mixed acid-base disorders, including cardiorespiratory arrest, sepsis, drug intoxications, diabetes mellitus, and organ failure (especially renal, hepatic, and pulmonary failure). Patients with severe renal insufficiency or end-stage renal disease are prone to developing mixed acid-base disturbances of great complexity and severity.[19] Major relevant features of this state include the presence of metabolic acidosis of the high anion gap type, which is frequently accompanied by a component of hyperchloremic acidosis; inability to mount an appropriate secondary response to chronic respiratory acidosis or alkalosis; inability to respond to a load of fixed acids (e.g., lactic acid) or a primary loss of alkali (e.g., diarrhea) with the expected increase in net acid excretion; and inability to respond to an alkali load with bicarbonaturia despite the presence of an increased plasma HCO_3^- concentration. As a result, these patients are particularly vulnerable to the development of both extreme acidemia and extreme alkalemia.

A practical classification of mixed acid-base disorders recognizes three main groups of disturbances in accordance with the preceding definition (Fig. 14.10). Representative examples are depicted in Figure 14.11, and some of these mixed disorders are reviewed.

Metabolic Acidosis and Respiratory Acidosis
Clinical examples of metabolic acidosis combined with respiratory acidosis include untreated cardiopulmonary arrest, circulatory failure in patients with chronic obstructive pulmonary disease (COPD), severe renal failure associated with hypercapnic respiratory failure, various intoxications, and hypokalemic (or less frequently hyperkalemic) paralysis of respiratory muscles in patients with diarrhea or renal tubular acidosis (see Fig. 14.11, example 4, and Fig. 14.12).

Metabolic Alkalosis and Respiratory Alkalosis
Metabolic alkalosis combined with respiratory alkalosis might be encountered in patients with primary hypocapnia associated with chronic liver disease who develop metabolic alkalosis owing to a variety of causes, including vomiting, nasogastric drainage, diuretics, profound hypokalemia, and alkali administration (e.g., absorption of antacids or infusion of Ringer's lactate solution, alimentation solutions, or citrated blood products), especially in the context of renal insufficiency. This entity also is observed in critically ill surgical patients, particularly those undergoing

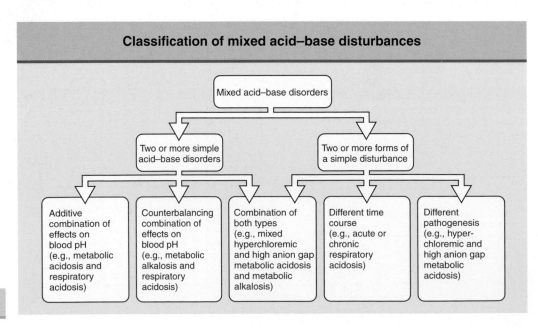

Figure 14.10 Classification of mixed acid-base disturbances.

Representative examples of mixed acid-base disorders

Type of Mixed Disorder	Example No.	pH	PaCO₂ (mm Hg)	HCO₃⁻ (mmol/l)	Na⁺ (mmol/l)	K⁺ (mmol/l)	Cl⁻ (mmol/l)	Anion gap (mmol/l)	Clinical Circumstances
Hyperchloremic and and high anion gap metabolic acidosis	1	7.12	16	5	137	3.6	114	18	Diabetic ketoacidosis with adequate salt and water balance
Mixed high anion gap metabolic acidosis and metabolic alkalosis	2	7.36	31	17	132	4.0	89	26	Alcoholic liver disease, vomiting, and lactic acidosis
	3	7.40	40	24	143	5.5	95	24	Diabetic ketoacidosis and lactic acidosis after bicarbonate therapy
Mixed high anion gap metabolic acidosis and respiratory acidosis	4	7.18	44	16	133	5.7	100	17	Hepatic, renal, and pulmonary failure
Metabolic alkalosis and respiratory acidosis	5	7.44	55	36	135	3.8	84	15	Chronic obstructive pulmonary disease and diuretics
Metabolic alkalosis and respiratory alkalosis	6	7.60	40	38	131	3.6	77	16	Congestive heart failure and diuretics
Acute or chronic respiratory acidosis	7	7.22	80	32	141	4.3	99	10	Chronic obstructive pulmonary disease and therapy with O₂-rich mixtures

Figure 14.11   Representative examples of mixed acid-base disorders. Anion gap is calculated as $[Na^+] - ([Cl^-] + [HCO_3^-])$.

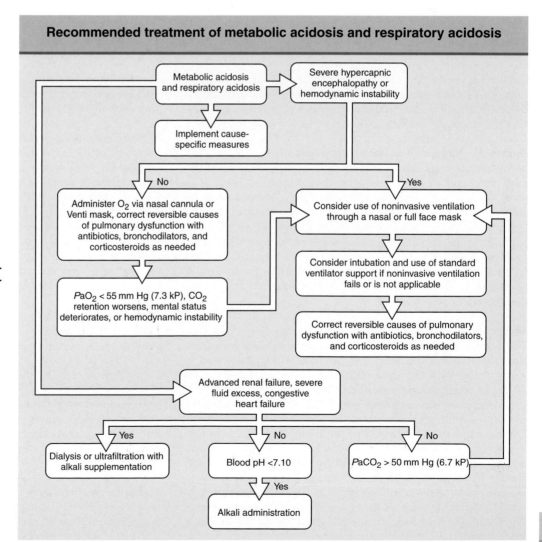

Figure 14.12 Recommended treatment of metabolic acidosis and respiratory acidosis.

175

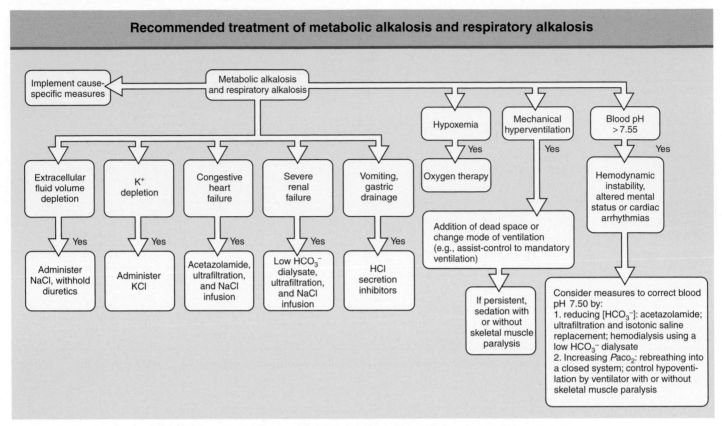

Figure 14.13 **Recommended treatment of metabolic alkalosis and respiratory alkalosis.**

mechanical ventilation, and in patients with respiratory alkalosis, caused by either pregnancy or heart failure, who experience metabolic alkalosis attributable to diuretics or vomiting (see Fig. 14.11, example 6, and Fig. 14.13).

Metabolic Alkalosis and Respiratory Acidosis
Metabolic alkalosis and respiratory acidosis represent one of the most frequently encountered mixed acid-base disorders. The usual clinical setting involves chronic lung disease caused by chronic bronchitis or emphysema in conjunction with diuretic therapy, but other causes of metabolic alkalosis (e.g., vomiting, administration of corticosteroids) might exist (see Fig. 14.11, example 5, and Fig. 14.14). Critically ill patients with respiratory failure caused by acute respiratory distress syndrome and, occasionally, those with profound hypokalemia also might develop this mixed disorder.

Metabolic Acidosis and Respiratory Alkalosis
The combination of metabolic acidosis and respiratory alkalosis, like respiratory acidosis and metabolic alkalosis, is characterized by normal or nearly normal blood pH; its two components exert offsetting effects on systemic acidity (Fig. 14.15). This disorder is commonly observed in patients hospitalized in intensive care units and, as such, is generally associated with high mortality rates. Primary hypocapnia might result from a variety of causes, including fever, hypotension, gram-negative septicemia, pulmonary edema, hypoxemia, and mechanical hyperventilation. The component of metabolic acidosis, in turn, might be attributable to lactic acidosis (e.g., complicating shock, hepatic failure) or renal acidosis. Salicylate intoxication represents another major cause of this mixed acid-base disorder. Stimulation of the ventilatory center in the brainstem accounts for the respiratory alkalosis, whereas the accelerated production of organic acids (including pyruvic, lactic, and keto acids) and, to a small extent, the accumulation of salicylic acid itself are responsible for the metabolic acidosis.

Metabolic Acidosis and Metabolic Alkalosis
Metabolic acidosis and metabolic alkalosis are typically observed in patients with alcoholic liver disease who develop fasting ketoacidosis or lactic acidosis in conjunction with metabolic alkalosis caused by vomiting, diuretics, or other causes (see Fig. 14.11, examples 2 and 3). Protracted vomiting or nasogastric suction superimposed on uremic acidosis, diabetic ketoacidosis, or metabolic acidosis caused by diarrhea might also generate this offsetting metabolic combination. A similar picture might develop after administration of alkali during cardiopulmonary resuscitation or as therapy for diabetic ketoacidosis.

Mixed Metabolic Acidosis
Pathogenetically disparate entities of metabolic acidosis coexist in patients with mixed metabolic acidosis. Mixed high anion gap metabolic acidosis in patients with diabetic or alcoholic ketoacidosis may be combined with lactic acidosis consequent to circulatory failure. Uremic patients with associated lactic acidosis or ketoacidosis are another example of mixed high anion gap acidosis. Representative cases of mixed hyperchloremic metabolic acidosis are seen in patients with renal tubular acidosis or those being treated with carbonic anhydrase inhibitors who also suffer substantial fecal losses of HCO_3^- caused by severe diarrhea. Coexistence of hyperchloremic and high anion gap metabolic acidosis occurs in patients with profuse diarrhea whose circulation becomes sufficiently compromised to generate, in turn, a high anion gap metabolic acidosis (as a result of renal failure or lactic acidosis). Patients with diabetic ketoacidosis, whose renal function

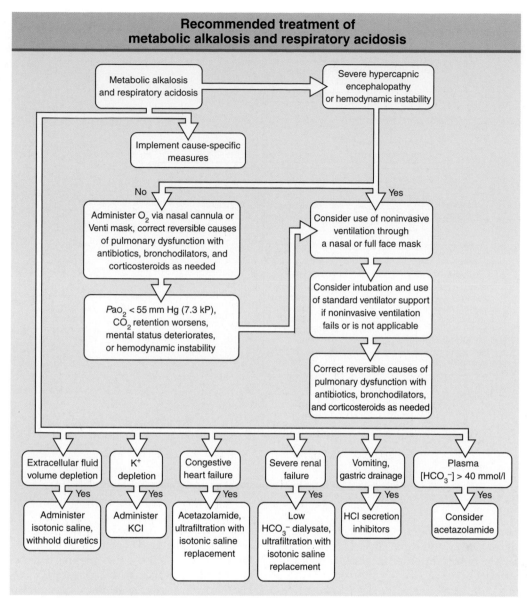

Figure 14.14   Recommended treatment of metabolic alkalosis and respiratory acidosis.

is maintained at reasonable levels by adequate salt and water intake, might develop an element of hyperchloremic metabolic acidosis because of preferential excretion of ketone anions and conservation of Cl^- (see Fig. 14.11, example 1).[20]

Mixed Metabolic Alkalosis

As in mixed metabolic acidosis, the simultaneous presence of several processes that each contribute to a primary increment in plasma HCO_3^- (including diuretic therapy, vomiting, mineralocorticoid excess, or severe potassium depletion) will give rise to mixed metabolic alkalosis.

Triple Disorders

The most frequent triple disorders comprise two cardinal metabolic disturbances in conjunction with either respiratory acidosis or respiratory alkalosis. A prime example of the former is illustrated by severely ill patients with COPD and CO_2 retention who might develop simultaneously metabolic alkalosis (usually caused by diuretics and a Cl^--restricted diet) and metabolic acidosis (commonly lactic acidosis caused by hypoxemia, hypotension, or sepsis). This type of triple disorder also might be

encountered during cardiopulmonary resuscitation when an element of metabolic alkalosis caused by alkali administration is superimposed on pre-existing respiratory acidosis and metabolic (lactic) acidosis. Patients with respiratory alkalosis caused by advanced congestive heart failure also might have diuretic-induced metabolic alkalosis and lactic acidosis from tissue hypoperfusion. Such triple acid-base disorders can also be seen in patients with chronic alcoholism who develop metabolic alkalosis from vomiting, lactic acidosis from volume depletion or ethanol intoxication, and respiratory alkalosis from hepatic encephalopathy or sepsis.

Less frequently, triple disorders encompassing two cardinal respiratory disturbances in combination with either metabolic acidosis or metabolic alkalosis are encountered. The typical presentation involves critically ill patients with chronic respiratory acidosis who experience an abrupt reduction in $PaCO_2$ because of mechanical ventilation and superimposed metabolic acidosis (usually lactic acidosis, reflecting circulatory failure) or metabolic alkalosis (e.g., as a result of gastric fluid loss, diuretics). In the last circumstance, extreme alkalemia might ensue because

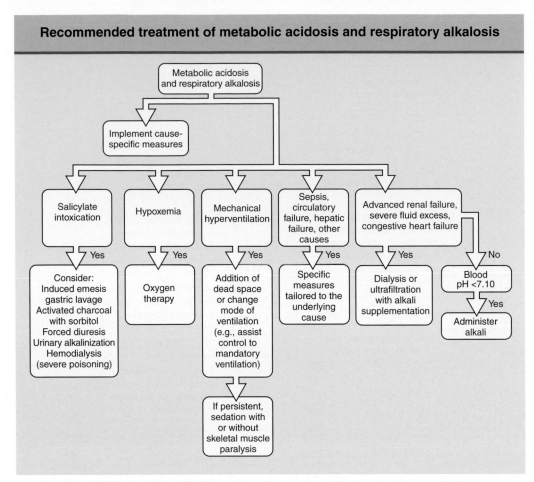

Figure 14.15 Recommended treatment of metabolic acidosis and respiratory alkalosis.

of the concomitant presence of hypocapnia and hyperbicarbonatemia. Even more infrequently, this same clinical setting might give rise to a quadruple acid-base disorder in which all four cardinal acid-base disturbances coexist.

Clinical Manifestations

As a general rule, the symptoms and signs of the underlying disease that give rise to the observed mixed acid-base disorder dominate the clinical picture. Yet, the development of severe abnormalities in either $PaCO_2$ (severe hypo- or hypercapnia) or systemic acidity (profound acidemia or alkalemia) might be responsible for the superimposition of additional clinical manifestations. On the one hand, profound hypocapnia might induce obtundation, generalized seizures, and, occasionally, even coma or death as a result of a critical reduction in cerebral blood flow and other mechanisms. Rarely, angina pectoris also might occur. On the other hand, severe hypercapnia might generate a profound encephalopathy with the classic features of pseudotumor cerebri, including headaches, obtundation, vomiting, and bilateral papilledema caused by increased intracranial pressure. Extreme acidemia results in depression of the central nervous system as well as the cardiovascular system.[7] Reduction in myocardial contractility and peripheral vascular resistance triggered by acidemia might result in severe hypotension. Finally, profound alkalemia might elicit paresthesias, tetany, cardiac dysrhythmias, or generalized seizures.

Diagnosis

The basic principles underlying the diagnosis of mixed acid-base disorders are identical to those required for the identification of

simple acid-base disturbances and include assessment of the accuracy of the acid-base data by ensuring that the available values for pH, $PaCO_2$, and plasma bicarbonate concentration satisfy the mathematical constraints of the Henderson-Hasselbach equation; obtaining a careful history and performing a complete physical examination; consideration of the plasma anion gap and other ancillary laboratory data; and knowledge of the quantitative aspects of the adaptive response to each of the four simple acid-base disturbances. Adherence to these principles cannot be overemphasized. Indeed, even experienced clinicians risk misdiagnosing the prevailing acid-base status by bypassing this systematic approach.

Normality of the acid-base parameters is not in itself sufficient to diagnose the presence of normal acid-base status; indeed, normal acid-base values might be the fortuitous result of mixed acid-base disorders (e.g., high anion gap acidosis treated with alkali infusion, diarrhea-induced metabolic acidosis in conjunction with vomiting-induced metabolic alkalosis). A given set of acid-base parameters is never diagnostic of a particular acid-base disorder, whether simple or mixed in nature, but rather is consistent with a range of acid-base abnormalities. What on the surface appears to be a clear-cut simple acid-base disorder might actually reflect the interplay of a number of coexisting acid-base disturbances. Information from the patient's history and findings from the physical examination frequently provide important insights into the prevailing acid-base status as well as useful clues to the differential diagnosis.

Blood parameters in diagnosis of mixed metabolic acid-base disorders					
Blood Composition	Normal	High Anion Gap Acidosis	High Anion Gap and Normal Anion Gap Acidosis	Metabolic Alkalosis	High Anion Gap Acidosis and Metabolic Alkalosis
pH	7.40	7.29	7.10	7.50	7.38
$Paco_2$ (mm Hg)	40	30	20	45	35
Bicarbonate (mmol/l)	24	14	6	34	20
Anion gap (mmol/l)	10	20	20	12	26
Δ Bicarbonate	0	−10	−18	+10	−4
Δ Anion gap	0	+10	+10	+2	+16

Figure 14.16 Blood parameters in diagnosis of mixed metabolic acid-base disorders.

A critical component of the diagnostic process is the examination of the plasma anion gap (Fig. 14.16). This derived parameter provides important insights into the nature of the prevailing changes in plasma HCO_3^- concentration. Occasionally, an elevated plasma anion gap might offer the first readily available clue to the presence of disordered acid-base status despite normal acid-base parameters. In the presence of a plasma HCO_3^- deficit ($\Delta[HCO_3^-]_p$), a normal or subnormal value for the plasma anion gap denotes that the entire decrease in HCO_3^- can be attributed to acidifying processes resulting in the loss of alkali (e.g., diarrhea, renal tubular acidosis) or to respiratory alkalosis. By comparison, with a high anion gap metabolic acidosis, there is usually a close reciprocal stoichiometry between the decrease in serum HCO_3^- and the increase in the anion gap, termed the Δ(anion gap). A reduction in serum HCO_3^- of 10 mmol/l is associated, therefore, with a Δ(anion gap) of 10 mmol/l. Addition of the value for the Δ(anion gap) to the prevailing level of serum HCO_3^- allows the derivation of the basal value of HCO_3^- existing before the development of the high anion gap metabolic acidosis. Appreciation of this reciprocal relationship between the $\Delta[HCO_3^-]_p$ and the Δ(anion gap) is important in distinguishing between a pure high anion gap metabolic acidosis and a mixed high and normal anion gap metabolic acidosis and in detecting a mixed high anion gap metabolic acidosis and metabolic alkalosis. Additional diagnostic insights are often obtained by examination of other laboratory data, including the serum levels of K^+, glucose, urea nitrogen, and creatinine; semi-quantitative measures for ketonemia or ketonuria; screening blood or urine for toxins; and estimation of the serum osmolar gap.

Mild acid-base disorders might pose particular diagnostic difficulty because of the considerable overlap of values for the simple disturbances near the normal range. In such circumstances, any of several simple disorders or a variety of mixed disturbances might fully account for the acid-base data under evaluation. Again, careful correlation of all available clinical information should guide the diagnostic process.

Treatment

The management of mixed acid-base disturbances is aimed at restoring the altered acid-base status by reversing all the elemental components present.[1,2,17,21] Thus, it encompasses the therapy of each simple acid-base disorder. Our recommendations for treatment of some common mixed acid-base disturbances are presented in Figures 14.12 through 14.15.

Given the nature of these different disorders and the variable response time to therapy of the individual components, it is crucial always to be aware of the effect that graded correction of a certain element might have on systemic acidity. The asynchronous reversal of the individual components might be used at times to therapeutic advantage, whereas on other occasions, such a practice might prove catastrophic. In this regard, patients featuring extreme acidemia caused by metabolic acidosis and respiratory acidosis or extreme alkalemia caused by metabolic alkalosis and respiratory alkalosis might derive prompt restitution of systemic acidity to safe levels by a rapid return of $Paco_2$ toward normal. By comparison, an asynchronous return of $Paco_2$ to normal values in a patient with profound metabolic acidosis and superimposed respiratory alkalosis might prove disastrous. Similarly, extreme caution should be exercised in treating patients with respiratory acidosis and metabolic alkalosis, one of the most commonly encountered mixed acid-base disorders. Although therapeutic measures intended to improve alveolar ventilation should be instituted, induction of an abrupt decrease in $Paco_2$ risks development of severe alkalemia. Therefore, aggressive measures should be taken to treat the element of metabolic alkalosis, making certain that reversal of the metabolic component does not lag behind the treatment of the respiratory element. In fact, because the ventilatory drive in patients with chronic respiratory acidosis depends in part on the prevailing acidemia, reversal of a complicating element of metabolic alkalosis regularly results in improved alveolar ventilation and consequently a decrease in $Paco_2$ and an increase in Pao_2 are realized.

REFERENCES

1. Adrogué HJ, Madias NE: Management of life-threatening acid-base disorders (part I). N Engl J Med 1998;338:26–34.
2. Adrogué HJ, Madias NE: Management of life-threatening acid-base disorders (part II). N Engl J Med 1998;338:107–111.
3. Adrogué HJ, Wesson DE: Overview of acid-base disorders. In Adrogué HJ, Wesson DE (eds): Blackwell's Basics of Medicine: Acid-base. Boston: Blackwell Science, 1994, pp 49–133.
4. Epstein SK, Singh N: Respiratory acidosis. Respir Care 2001;46:366–383.
5. Adrogué HJ, Rashad MN, Gorin AB, et al: Assessing acid-base status in circulatory failure: Differences between arterial and central venous blood. N Engl J Med 1989;320:1312–1316.
6. Adrogué HJ, Rashad MN, Gorin AB, et al: Arteriovenous acid-base disparity in circulatory failure: Studies on mechanism. Am J Physiol 1989;257:F1087–F1093.

7. Adrogué HJ, Madias NE: Respiratory acidosis. In Gennari FJ, Adrogué HJ, Galla JH, Madias NE (eds): Acid-base Disorders and Their Treatment. Boca Raton, FL: Taylor & Francis, 2005, pp 597–640.

8. Madias NE, Adrogué HJ: Influence of chronic metabolic acid-base disorders on the acute CO_2 titration curve. J Appl Physiol 1983;55:1187–1195.

9. Adrogué HJ, Madias NE: Influence of chronic respiratory acid-base disorders on acute CO_2 titration curve. J Appl Physiol 1985;58:1231–1238.

10. Adrogué HJ, Madias NE: Arterial blood gas monitoring: Acid-base assessment. In Tobin MJ (ed): Principles and Practice of Intensive Care Monitoring. New York: McGraw-Hill, 1998, pp 217–241.

11. Adrogué HJ, Tobin MJ: Management of respiratory failure. In Adrogué HJ, Tobin MJ (eds): Blackwell's Basics of Medicine, Vol. 6, Respiratory Failure. Boston: Blackwell Science, 1997, pp 311–331.

12. Amato MBP, Barbas CSV, Medeiros DM, et al: Effect of a protective-ventilation strategy on mortality in the acute respiratory distress syndrome. N Engl J Med 1998;338:347–354.

13. Cardenas VJ, Zwischenberger JB, Tao W, et al: Correction of blood pH attenuates changes in hemodynamics and organ blood flow during permissive hypercapnia. Crit Care Med 1996;24:827–834.

14. Adrogué HJ, Brensilver J, Cohen JJ, Madias NE: Influence of steady-state alterations in acid-base equilibrium on the fate of administered bicarbonate in the dog. J Clin Invest 1983;71:867–883.

15. Foster GT, Vaziri ND, Sassoon CSH: Respiratory alkalosis. Respir Care 2001;46:384–391.

16. Laffey JG, Kavanagh BP: Hypocapnia. N Engl J Med 2002;347:43–53.

17. Adrogué HJ, Madias NE: Mixed acid-base disorders. In Jacobson HR, Striker GE, Klahr S (eds): The Principles and Practice of Nephrology, 2nd ed. Philadelphia: Decker, 1995, pp 953–962.

18. Anderson LE, Henrich WL: Alkalemia-associated morbidity and mortality in medical and surgical patients. South Med J 1987;80:729–733.

19. Madias NE, Perrone RD: Acid-base disorders in association with renal disease. In Schrier SW, Gottschaid CW (eds): Diseases of the Kidney, 5th ed. Boston: Little, Brown, 1993, pp 2669–2699.

20. Adrogué HJ, Wilson H, Boyd AE, et al: Plasma acid-base patterns in diabetic ketoacidosis. N Engl J Med 1982;307:1603–1610.

21. Leung JM, Landow L, Franks M, et al: Safety and efficacy of intravenous Carbicarb in patients undergoing surgery: Comparison with sodium bicarbonate in the treatment of mild metabolic acidosis. Crit Care Med 1994;22:1540–1549 [erratum in Crit Care Med 1995,23:420].

CHAPTER
15

Introduction to Glomerular Disease: Pathogenesis and Classification

Richard J. Johnson, Jürgen Floege, Helmut G. Rennke, and John Feehally

INTRODUCTION

Numerous inflammatory and noninflammatory diseases affect the glomerulus and lead to alterations in glomerular permeability, structure, and function. Many glomerular diseases come under the generic title glomerulonephritis (GN), which implies that there is an immune pathogenesis. Not all glomerular disease is caused by GN and other causes need to be considered in its differential diagnosis. Particularly important are diabetic nephropathy and amyloidosis, as well as the hereditary nephropathies, most commonly Alport's syndrome.

GN may be primary, restricted in clinical manifestations to the kidney, or it may be part of a multisystem disease, most frequently systemic lupus or vasculitis. While the likelihood of a patient having GN can be estimated with varying degrees of confidence from the clinical setting and laboratory tests, it cannot ultimately be diagnosed without histologic examination of cortical renal tissue.

CLASSIFICATION

GN is classified by the different patterns of histologic injury seen on a renal biopsy sample examined by light microscopy, immunofluorescence, and electron microscopy (EM). This classification is not ideal since it cannot always be assumed that one histologic pattern has a single etiology or that it will have a single clinical presentation. Furthermore, one etiology may produce a variety of histologic patterns (for example, the varied glomerular disease seen in association with hepatitis B virus [HBV] infection or lupus).

It is more helpful to regard the renal biopsy appearance as a pattern rather than a disease: a pattern that may frequently have a number of clinical correlates and a number of putative etiologic agents and that may eventually prove to have more than one immune mechanism. Nevertheless, the classification of GN remains largely based on renal pathology, and the approach taken in this book chiefly subdivides GN on this basis.

HISTOPATHOLOGY

The full assessment of a renal biopsy requires light microscopy, electron microscopy, and examination for immune deposits of complement and immunoglobulin by immunofluorescence or immunoperoxidase.

Light Microscopy

In GN, the dominant, but not the only, histologic lesions are in glomeruli (Fig. 15.1). GN is described as focal (only some glomeruli are involved) or diffuse. In any individual glomerulus, injury may be segmental (affecting only part of any glomerulus) or global. There is a potential for sampling error in a renal biopsy: the extent of a focal lesion may be misjudged in a small biopsy specimen and sections through glomeruli may miss segmental lesions. Lesions may also be hypercellular due to either an increase in endogenous endothelial or mesangial cells (termed proliferative) and/or to an infiltration of inflammatory leukocytes (termed exudative). Severe acute inflammation may produce glomerular necrosis, which is often segmental. The walls of the glomerular capillaries can also be thickened by a number of processes, which include an increase in glomerular basement membrane (GBM) material and immune deposits. Methenamine silver staining is helpful because the silver stains basement membranes and other matrix black. It may, for example, reveal a double contour to the GBM because of the interposition of cellular material, or it may show increased mesangial matrix not easily seen with other techniques. Segmental sclerosis and scarring may also occur and are characterized by segmental capillary collapse with the accumulation of hyaline material and mesangial matrix and often with attachment of the capillary wall with Bowman's capsule (synechiae or adhesion formation).

Crescents are inflammatory collections of cells in Bowman's space. Crescents develop when severe glomerular injury results in local rupture of the capillary wall or Bowman's capsule allowing plasma proteins and inflammatory material to enter into Bowman's space. Crescents consist of proliferating parietal and visceral epithelial cells, infiltrating fibroblasts, and lymphocytes and monocytes/macrophages, often with local fibrin deposition. They are called crescents because of their appearance when the glomerulus is cut in one plane for histology. They are destructive and rapidly increasing in size and may lead to glomerular tuft occlusion (see Fig. 15.1). If the acute injury is stopped, the crescents may either resolve with restitution of normal morphology or heal by fibrosis, causing irretrievable loss of renal function. Crescents are most commonly observed with vasculitis, in Goodpasture's syndrome, and in severe acute GN of any etiology.

Abnormalities are not confined to the glomeruli in GN. Tubulointerstitial inflammation is common, the more so with acute and severe GN. In advanced GN, as glomeruli fail their associated tubules will atrophy, leading to interstitial fibrosis in a pattern no different from those of other progressive chronic renal diseases (see Chapter 68).

Immunofluorescence and Immunoperoxidase Microscopy

Indirect immunofluorescence and immunoperoxidase staining are both used to identify immune reactants (Fig. 15.2). It is routine to

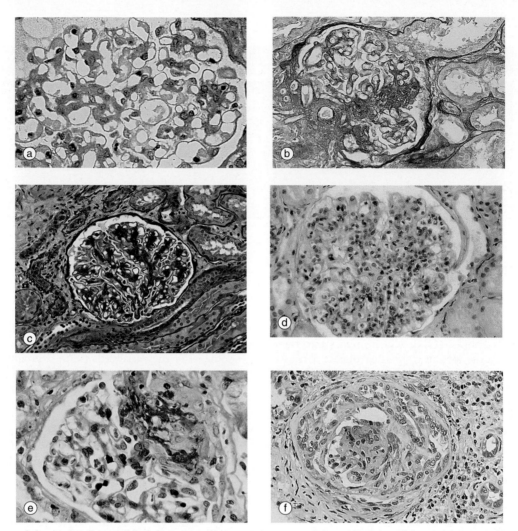

Figure 15.1 Pathology of glomerular disease: light microscopy. Characteristic patterns of glomerular disease illustrating the range of histologic appearances and the descriptive terms used. *a*, Normal glomerulus: minimal change disease. *b*, Segmental sclerosis: focal segmental glomerulosclerosis. *c*, Diffuse mesangial hypercellularity: IgA nephropathy. *d*, Diffuse endocapillary hypercellularity: poststreptococcal glomerulonephritis. *e*, Segmental necrosis: renal vasculitis. *f*, Crescent formation: antiglomerular basement membrane disease. (*a* and *b*, Hematoxylin and eosin; *c*, *d*, and *f*, periodic acid–Schiff; *e*, trichrome.)

look for the deposition of immunoglobulins IgG, IgA, and IgM, for components of both the classical and alternative pathways of complement (usually C3, C4, and C1q), and for the presence of fibrin, which is commonly observed in crescents and in capillaries in thrombotic disorders (such as hemolytic uremic syndrome and the antiphospholipid syndrome). Immune deposits may occur along the capillary loops or in the mesangium. They may be continuous (linear) or discontinuous (granular) along the capillary wall or in the mesangium.

Granular deposits in glomeruli are sometimes called immune complexes. This implies the deposition or local formation of an antigen-antibody complex in the glomerulus. However, in very few situations is the putative antigen known and only rarely is there definite evidence of antigen deposition along with antibody in human GN. The term immune complex harkens back to experimental models of GN where there is strong evidence of antigen-antibody complexes directly initiating glomerular injury. The more general term immune deposit is preferable.

Electron Microscopy
EM is valuable for defining the morphology of the basement membranes (abnormal in some forms of hereditary nephropathy, e.g., Alport's syndrome and thin basement membrane nephropathy

[see Chapter 45]), and also for identifying fibrils (e.g., in amyloidosis) or tubuloreticular intracellular structures (e.g., in lupus nephritis). EM is also useful for localizing the site of immune deposits (which are usually homogeneous and electron dense; Fig. 15.3). Electron-dense deposits are seen in the mesangium or along the capillary wall on the subepithelial or subendothelial side of the GBM. Uncommonly, the electron-dense material lies linearly within the GBM. The sites of immune deposits are helpful in the classification of the types of GN.

PATHOGENESIS OF GLOMERULAR INJURY

The type of glomerular injury depends not only on the initial immune response but also on the extent to which that response is perpetuated and provokes glomerular injury. It also depends on the extent to which the initial inflammation resolves without scarring or proceeds to glomerular destruction, either by rapid inflammation and necrosis or by slowly progressive glomerulosclerosis and tubulointerstitial fibrosis (Fig. 15.4).

Immune Glomerular Injury
Events involved in the initiation of glomerular disease are still poorly understood. Most glomerular diseases develop as a result

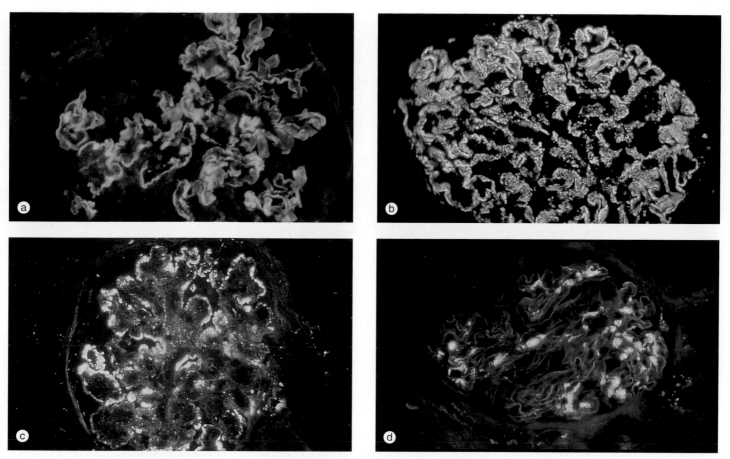

Figure 15.2   Pathology of glomerular disease: immunofluorescence microscopy. Common patterns of glomerular staining found by immunofluorescence. *a*, Linear capillary wall IgG: antiglomerular basement membrane disease. *b*, Fine granular capillary wall IgG: membranous nephropathy. *c*, Coarse granular capillary wall IgG: membranoproliferative glomerulonephritis type I. *d*, Granular mesangial IgA: IgA nephropathy.

of immune dysregulation, either an inappropriate immune response to self-antigens occurring through a failure of tolerance (autoimmunity) or an ineffectual response to a foreign antigen.

Autoimmunity

In health, a tension exists between the normal immune response to foreign antigen and tolerance, which is the cellular process that prevents an immune response to self-antigen. Tolerance develops because self-reactive T and B cells are clonally deleted during fetal and neonatal life, although small numbers survive outside the thymus. Under certain conditions, these peripheral self-reactive T and B cells can be stimulated to generate a cellular and humoral response to a self-antigen. Infection or toxins may play a role in initiating the response by releasing antigens from sequestered sites so they have access to T cells, by altering host proteins to make them more immunogenic, or by molecular mimicry, in which antibodies to an exogenous antigen (such as those present in an infecting organism) cross-react with a native protein. For example, recently it has been shown that oxidants, such as may occur with smoking or aging, can alter the GBM to expose the Goodpasture antigen from an otherwise cryptic site that may not only allow it to function as a neoantigen but also to be recognized by anti-GBM antibody.[1] Certain bacteria and viruses also express superantigens, which can activate T cells directly and may lead to polyclonal B cell expansion. Once there is an inflammatory response, the further release of antigens may result in the generation of additional autoantibodies, a process known as determinant spreading. Activation of T cells may be

further enhanced by the release of cytokines and lymphokines, and the conversion of normally innocuous endogenous renal cells) into antigen-presenting cells via the upregulated or *de novo* expression of HLA class II molecules.

Recently, a population of regulatory T cells (CD4$^+$CD25$^+$) has been shown to have a key role in controlling T cell responses and preventing the development of autoimmunity. These cells appear to be decreased in patients with anti-GBM disease at the time of presentation, and their lack may have a role in the loss of tolerance. Indeed, in experimental anti-GBM nephritis, the administration of these cells can reduce glomerular damage by blocking T cell–dependent renal injury.[2]

Genetic Background of Glomerulonephritis

Variations in HLA molecules and the T cell receptor are under strong genetic influence. For that reason, immunogenetic associations, particularly between HLA expression and various patterns of GN, have been studied in great detail, but none of the reported associations is absolutely specific. For example, while HRA-DR2 identifies a powerful relative risk of the development of Goodpasture's syndrome, it is still possible to develop the disease without HRA-DR2, and the vast majority of individuals with HRA-DR2 never develop this rare disease. Furthermore, the HLA associations often differ among racial groups with different distributions of HLA. This suggests that the associations so far identified are not the disease susceptibility genes themselves but are adjacent to them and associated by linkage disequilibrium and that there may be other susceptibility genes not yet identified,

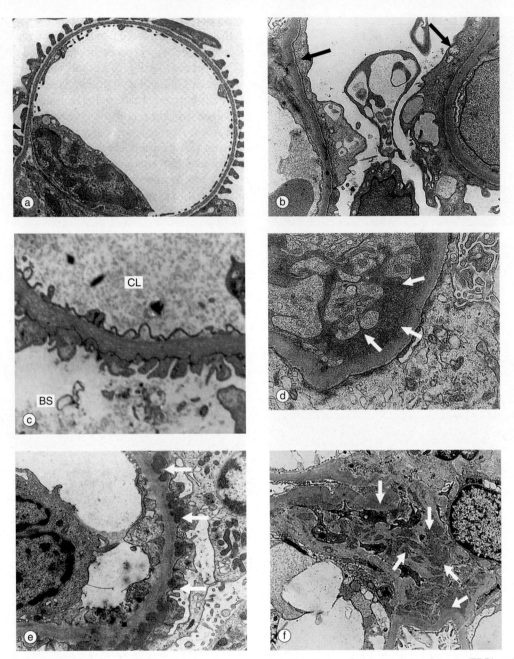

Figure 15.3   Ultrastructural pathology of glomerular disease. Some characteristic patterns of electron-dense deposits (EDD) and glomerular basement membrane (GBM) abnormalities seen in glomerular disease. *a*, Normal. *b*, Foot process effacement: minimal change disease (*arrows*). *c*, GBM thickening and splitting: Alport's syndrome. *d*, Subendothelial EDD (*arrows*): membranoproliferative glomerulonephritis type I. *e*, Subepithelial EDD (*arrows*): membranous nephropathy. *f*, Mesangial EDD (*arrows*): IgA nephropathy.

perhaps on remote chromosomes. It also suggests that environmental events may have great importance, acting on genetic background, in inducing GN. HLA associations have no practical diagnostic or therapeutic implications as yet, and HLA typing is not needed in the clinical management of GN.

Ineffectual Response to a Foreign Antigen

Some glomerular diseases may occur as a consequence of an inability to eliminate a foreign antigen. A classic example is HBV infection, in which infection, particularly in fetal or early life, results in tolerance and a chronic carrier state. Despite a strong humoral response, viral infection persists because the cell-mediated response required for elimination of HBV from the liver is impaired. The consequence is a state of persistent antigenemia

with circulating antigen-antibody complexes, which predisposes to glomerular injury.

Mechanisms of Immune-Complex Formation within the Glomerulus

In most cases of GN, there is immunoglobulin deposition in glomeruli, often codeposited with components of the complement cascade, which is presumed to represent immune-complex formation.[3]

Circulating immune complexes (CICs) may localize to the glomerulus by passive deposition from the circulation. Normally, complexes of antibody and foreign antigen engage complement and are cleared from the circulation by binding of the complex to the C3b receptors on erythrocytes; the immune complexes

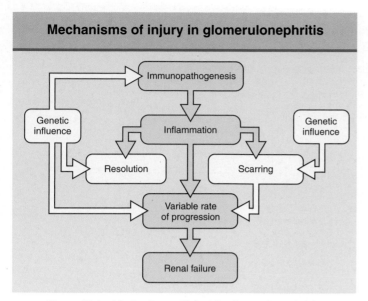

Mechanisms of injury in glomerulonephritis

Figure 15.4 Mechanisms of injury in glomerulonephritis.

are then removed and degraded during transit of the erythrocytes in the liver and spleen. If antigenemia persists or clearance of complexes is impaired (as in chronic liver disease or because of defective immune-complex binding by erythrocytes), immune complexes may deposit in the glomerulus by binding to Fc receptors on mesangial cells or by passive deposition in the mesangium or subendothelial space. Physical characteristics of the complexes may also favor deposition, including avidity, charge, and size. Measurement of CICs in patients with GN has not, however, shown close correlation with glomerular events, nor has analysis of CICs led to identification of many pathogenetic antigens.

A second mechanism for immune-complex localization involves local *in situ* formation. Antibody may bind directly to an intrinsic glomerular antigen. Alternatively, a nonglomerular antigen, such as a viral or food antigen, may first localize to a glomerular structure (planted antigen) followed by antibody binding. This situation may be more likely when the antigen has characteristics favoring binding to glomeruli (such as cationic antigens that can bind the anionic basement membrane) or when the antibody has low avidity (thereby favoring dissociation of the immune complexes in the circulation).

Identification of Antigens

Most of the specific antigens involved in human GN remain unknown. The best characterized antigen that is involved with autoimmunity is the α3 chain of type IV collagen, which is the target antigen in anti-GBM disease (Goodpasture's syndrome).[4] Recently, congenital membranous nephropathy (MN) in six children has been associated with the passive transfer of antibodies directed against neutral endopeptidase (NEP) present on the podocyte, as a consequence of alloimunization during pregnancy of a mother genetically lacking NEP.[5] The best example of a response to a foreign antigen is poststreptococcal GN, in which streptococcal antigens (glyceraldehyde-3-phosphate dehydrogenase [GAPDH]/ nephritis associated plasmin receptor and exotoxin B precursor/ zymogen) can be found in the glomerular deposits.[6] Another example is HBV-associated GN.

The failure to identify the antigens within immune deposits in GN may be due to the fact that the relevant antigens may not have been considered or the fact that the initiating antigen may

no longer be present and the immune deposits are being perpetuated by a secondary anti-idiotype antibody response directed against the original antibody. In some cases, an antigen may never have been present in the first place, the immunoglobulin being deposited not in response to antigen but for other reasons, possibly physicochemical (e.g., IgM deposits in focal segmental glomerulosclerosis [FSGS]).

Cell-Mediated Immune Mechanisms

In contrast to the immune-complex mechanisms discussed previously, certain glomerular diseases develop primarily through cell-mediated immunity. For example, a direct role for T cells in mediating proteinuria and crescent formation has been shown in experimental crescentic nephritis.[7] It is thought that T cells sensitized to endogenous or exogenous antigen present in the glomeruli recruit macrophages, resulting in a local delayed-type hypersensitivity reaction. In certain models, CD8+ T cells have also been shown to mediate crescent formation, for example, via perforins (enzymes that act similarly to the complement membrane attack complex). Cell-mediated immunity has also been incriminated in minimal change disease (MCD); here, it has been postulated to result from a T cell product that injures the glomerular epithelial cell and induces a permeability defect (see later discussion).

Effector Mechanisms

The course of glomerular injury is largely determined by the local inflammatory response. In immune-complex disease, the amount of inflammation is dependent on the amount, mechanism of formation, and biologic properties of the complexes as well as their site of deposition (see later discussion).

Complement

The complement system is an amplifying cascade of proteins that produces cell injury and promotes inflammation (Fig. 15.5). The central event in the complement cascade is the cleavage of C3, which leads to the production of the membrane attack complex and to C3 fragments, which are active in inflammation. Complement can be activated by immune complexes via the classical pathway, initiated by the binding of C1q to the Fc portion of antibody. Classical pathway activation typically occurs in diffuse proliferative lupus nephritis, cryoglobulinemia, and membranoproliferative GN type I. In this setting, both serum C3 and C4 are usually low. Complement can also be activated via the mannose-binding pathway initiated by a lectin (mannose-binding lectin), which has a similar structure to C1q. The role of the mannose-binding pathway in GN has not yet been clearly established.

Finally, the complement cascade can also be initiated via the alternative pathway, an amplification loop for C3 activation, which is independent of immune complexes but is triggered by polysaccharide antigens, polymeric IgA, injured cells, or endotoxins. This pathway appears to be activated in IgA nephropathy, membranoproliferative GN type II, and in some cases of poststreptococcal GN. Except for IgA nephropathy, in which serum C3 and C4 are usually normal, serum C3 is typically low, but C4 is normal. Nephritic factors are IgG autoantibodies that stabilize various convertases in the complement pathway and modify their action; they play a key role in the pathogenesis of membranoproliferative GN (see Chapter 20).

Activation of the complement pathway has several consequences. Leukocyte recruitment is facilitated by the chemotactic factor C5a, and C3b binding is important in the binding and

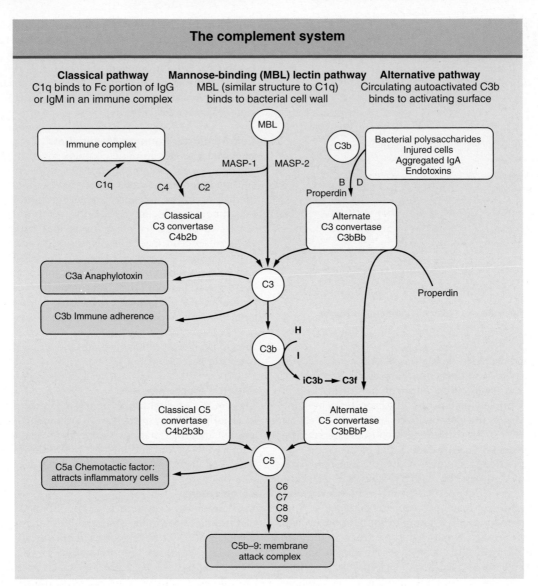

Figure 15.5   The complement system. The complement system is a self-amplifying cascade of proteins that generates a membrane attack complex, which is cytolytic; the cascade promotes inflammation by the activity of the fragments it produces. The amplifying cascades occur because activated fragments of the components combine to make convertase enzymes that degrade C3 and C5. The complement cascade is controlled in part by the very short active life of many of its components. There are also inhibitory regulatory proteins, most notably factors H and I inhibiting C3b. Activated fragments of any component are designated b, e.g., C3b; anaphylatoxic fragments are designated a, e.g., C5a. Inflammatory functions of complement components are shown in *green*. MASP, MBL-associated serine protease.

opsonization of the immune complexes by the infiltrating leuko-cytes. The terminal membrane attack complex of the cascade, C5b-9, inserts into cell membranes where it can kill cells or activate them to secrete cytokines, oxidants, and extracellular matrix. C5b-9 is thought to be particularly important in mediating injury to the glomerular epithelial cell in MN, a disease in which immune deposits and complement activation occur in the subepithelial space. Complement can also be activated in proteinuric urine as a consequence of amidation of C3 by ammonia, and this may have a role in mediating tubulointerstitial injury even in conditions not associated with immune-complex formation. Recent studies have emphasized the importance of local synthesis of complement components by the tubular cells as a mechanism that may augment this process.

Inflammatory Cells

Infiltration by inflammatory cells is largely determined by the site of immune deposits. Immune deposits with direct access to the

circulation (in particular those in subendothelial and basement membrane locations) are usually associated with a pronounced leukocyte accumulation. Mesangial deposits elicit an intermediate response, whereas immune deposits in the subepithelial space (such as in MN) generally are not associated with inflammatory cells.

Leukocyte infiltration is more severe in acute forms of GN such as membranoproliferative GN. With acute injury, the predominant infiltrating cells are neutrophils and monocytes, and in chronic injury, the predominant cells are monocytes/macrophages and T cells. The primary mechanism for attracting these cells is the secretion of chemokines and the expression of leukocyte adhesion molecules by local endothelial and resident cells; local release of complement activation fragments (C5a) is also important.

Intrinsic glomerular cells (epithelial, mesangial, and endothe-lial) may also be activated by the injury to become inflammatory-like cells. Mesangial cells, for example, can be activated to produce oxidants, proteases, cytokines (including chemokines and growth factors), vasoactive mediators and extracellular matrix; mesangial cell proliferation and matrix expansion are critical pathogenic features in IgA nephropathy.

Soluble Factors

The biology of these soluble factors is very complex, but already known to be important are cytokines, chemokines, growth factors, vasoactive mediators, reactive oxygen species, proteases, and proteins of the coagulation cascade. These factors variously promote the recruitment and activation of inflammatory cells, activate resident glomerular cells, directly cause tissue injury, stimulate production of matrix proteins (which forms the basis of scarring), and may either block or promote inflammation.

Mechanisms of Proteinuria

Proteinuria is a hallmark of glomerular disease. In the normal individual, minimal protein is filtered because of the charge and size selectivity of the glomerular capillary wall. Proteins, which are mainly negatively charged, are repelled by negative charges both within the GBM (mainly heparan sulfate proteoglycans) and on the surface of glomerular endothelial cells and glomerular epithelial cells (GECs; primarily sialoproteins). In addition, the slit diaphragms between the podocyte foot processes act as the primary site for the size barrier to protein filtration (Fig. 15.6).

The slit diaphragm consists of several transmembrane proteins that extend from adjacent interdigitating foot processes to form a zipper-like scaffold on the outer side of the GBM (Fig. 15.7). Recently, several genetic causes of nephrotic syndrome have been linked to mutations in genes associated with the slit diaphragm (see Chapter 17).[8] Mutations in the *NHPS1* gene, which codes for nephrin, are responsible for the autosomal recessive congenital nephrotic syndrome of the Finnish type that histologically resembles MCD. Mutations in *NHPS2*, which codes for podocin, is responsible for autosomal recessive steroid-resistant FSGS in children and rarely adults and may underlie up to 20% to 30% of sporadic steroid-resistant FSGS.[9] Autosomal dominant FSGS in children or adults is associated with mutations in *ACTN4*, which encodes the podocyte cytoplasmic protein α-actinin-4, as well as a gain-in-function mutation of *TRPC6*, which codes for a cation channel (TRPC6) present in the podocyte.[10] The cytoplasmic binding protein, CD2-associated protein (CD2AP), which interacts with nephrin and podocin, is also critical for the glomerular permeability barrier, as gene knockout mice lacking CD2AP develop nephrotic syndrome.

The key role for the GEC slit diaphragm in the permeability barrier to protein has renewed interest in the role for the podocyte in diseases associated with massive proteinuria. Foot process fusion, which was once viewed as a secondary consequence of proteinuria, is now recognized as a manifestation of podocyte injury rather than a cause of the proteinuria. The injury may be mediated by immune deposits with complement activation, such as in MN, or due to injury by an as yet unidentified toxin or cytokine such as occurs in MCD. Filtration is actually reduced at sites where the foot processes fuse (which may account for the reduction of the filtration coefficient K_f seen in nephrotic syndrome), but there are gaps where the GECs are detached from the GBM. It is at these sites that massive protein filtration occurs; structurally, the capillary wall defects are likely to correspond to the large pores noted in functional studies (Fig. 15.8).[11] The principal mechanisms responsible for proteinuria in the different patterns of glomerular disease are described and shown in Figure 15.9.

Minimal Change Disease and Focal Segmental Glomerulosclerosis

In MCD and FSGS, there are no deposits of immunoglobulin other than the nonspecific IgM deposits in scarred glomerular segments, and the disease does not appear to be mediated by immune-complex deposition (see Chapters 17 and 18). MCD may be mediated by T cells, in view of the rapid response to corticosteroids, the association with Hodgkin's lymphoma, and evidence of activation of the Th2 subset of T cells in the circulation. T cell hybridomas from patients with MCD have also been found to secrete a factor that provokes heavy proteinuria in rats.[12]

In some patients, focal and segmental sclerotic changes develop; the pathogenesis of segmental sclerosis is unclear, although an increase in protein trafficking across the GBM has been proposed[13] as a consequence of the increase in net ultrafiltration pressure that occurs secondary to the hypoalbuminemia and low oncotic

Figure 15.6 Proteins of the podocyte slit diaphragm involved in proteinuria. Several inherited glomerular diseases involve mutations of antigens associated with the slit diaphragm. These include nephrin (congenital nephrotic syndrome of the Finnish type), podocin (autosomal recessive focal segmental glomerulosclerosis [FSGS]), α-actinin, and TRPC6 (both associated with autosomal dominant FSGS). In addition, mutation of CD2-associated protein results in nephrotic syndrome in mice. (Adapted from Mundel P, Shankland SJ: Podocyte biology and response to injury. J Am Soc Nephrol 2002;13:3005–3015.)

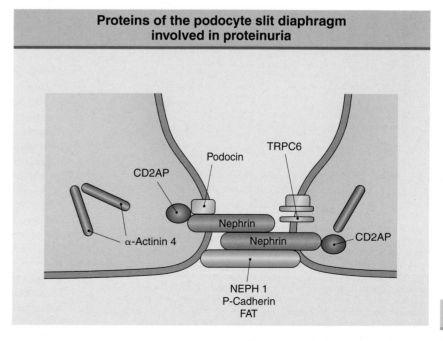

Proteins of the podocyte slit diaphragm involved in proteinuria

TRPC6
Podocin
CD2AP
Nephrin
α-Actinin 4
Nephrin
CD2AP
NEPH 1
P-Cadherin
FAT

Mechanisms of proteinuria

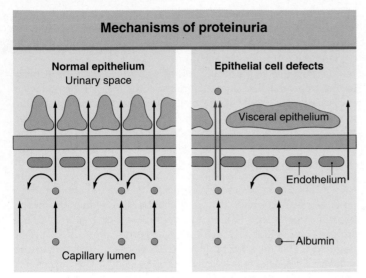

Figure 15.7 Mechanisms of proteinuria. Normally negatively charged proteins, such as albumin, are retarded by the negatively charged proteins in the endothelium (sialoglycoproteins) and basement membrane (heparan sulfate proteoglycans), as well as by a size barrier in the glomerular basement membrane (GBM) and at the slit diaphragm. In most proteinuric states, the podocytes are injured, leading to foot process swelling and injury to the slit diaphragm; in these situations, protein (albumin) can pass through the GBM and the gaps between the fused foot processes.

pressure[14] and/or podocyte loss with resulting formation of an adhesion between the capillary tuft and Bowman's capsule. It is not known whether FSGS represents part of the spectrum that includes MCD or whether they are separate entities. However, both conditions are characterized by generalized foot process fusion and massive proteinuria.

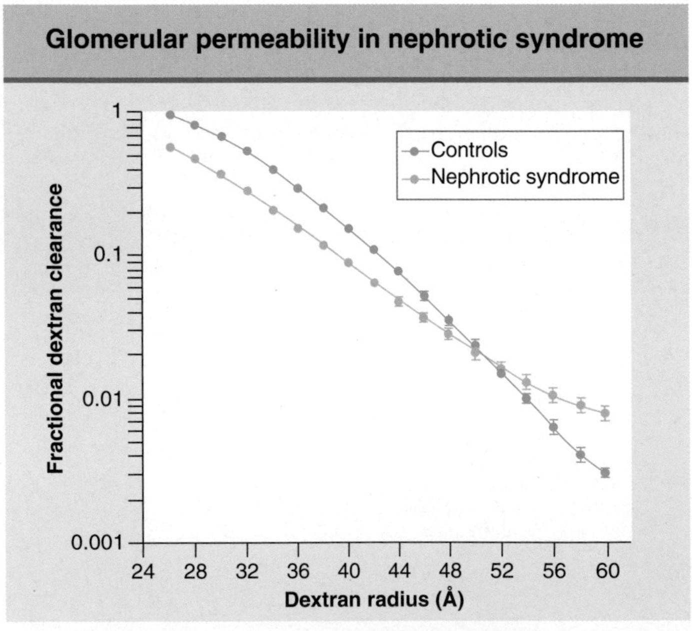

Glomerular permeability in nephrotic syndrome

Figure 15.8 Glomerular permeability in nephrotic syndrome. A dextran sieving curve showing the relative glomerular permeability of different-sized dextrans in normal subjects and nephrotic patients with membranous nephropathy and minimal change disease. Nephrotic subjects actually have a lower fractional dextran clearance for small dextrans (26–48 Å [2.6–4.8 nm]) but have an increased clearance for dextrans of larger molecular weight (52–60 Å [5.2–6.0 nm]). This is consistent with large pores appearing in the glomerular basement membrane. (Adapted from Myers BD, Guasch A: Mechanisms of proteinuria in nephrotic humans. Pediatr Nephrol 1994;8:107–112.)

A variant of FSGS is collapsing FSGS, in which there is proliferation of the normally quiescent podocyte, leading to collapse of the glomerular tuft, often in association with massive proteinuria. This entity can be either idiopathic or associated with infection (human immunodeficiency virus or parvovirus) or drugs (pamidronate, intravenous heroin, and other drugs). The pathogenesis may be due to production by the podocyte of growth factors (such as vascular endothelial growth factor) or to local inhibition of cell cycle proteins that normally maintain the podocyte in a nonproliferative state.[15]

Membranous Nephropathy

In MN (see Chapter 19), immune deposits are localized to the subepithelial space. Most experimental studies suggest that deposits are formed *in situ* by accretion of antibody to intrinsic or planted antigens on the GECs. In animal studies (passive Heyman nephritis), the intrinsic antigen (megalin) has been identified. In human studies, NEP has been identified as the antigen in congenital MN,[5] but the antigen(s) in childhood and adult cases remains unknown. Some cases of MN may be due to low avidity immune complexes, which may dissociate and then re-form at the subepithelial space; this may provide a mechanism for some MN due to viruses such as HBV. GEC injury is mediated by local complement activation with insertion of C5b-9 into the cell membrane of the GEC.[3]

Mesangial Proliferative Glomerulonephritis

IgA nephropathy (see Chapter 21) is the most common cause of mesangial proliferative GN. Here IgA deposits localize to the mesangium; the glomerular capillary wall is relatively spared. Marked proteinuria is not commonly a major feature of the clinical presentation. Mesangial cell injury may be mediated by binding of the IgA-containing immune complexes to Fcα or other IgA receptors on the mesangial cell, resulting in the release of chemokines and growth factors that provokes leukocyte infiltration and mesangial cell proliferation (driven primarily by platelet-derived growth factor) and mesangial matrix production (mediated by transforming growth factor β). While it had generally been thought that the mesangial cell population was a specialized cell that was strictly resident within the glomerulus, recent experimental studies suggest that mesangial cell progenitors may in part be bone marrow derived.[16] The role of these bone marrow–derived mesangial progenitors in mesangial diseases such as IgA nephropathy is not yet known.

Membranoproliferative Glomerulonephritis

In membranoproliferative GN, the immune deposits localize both to the mesangium and the subendothelial space (see Chapter 20). A similar pattern is observed in cryoglobulinemic GN in which the immune complexes contain a monoclonal IgM (type II) or polyclonal IgM (type III) that acts as a rheumatoid factor by binding to the IgG in the immune complex. In both cases, the disease is thought to occur by passive deposition from the circulation. When this pattern is seen in lupus nephritis, it may be facilitated by the binding of nucleosomes to the complexes (nucleosomes are cationic nuclear proteins that can interact with the negatively charged proteins within the glomerulus).

Studies in experimental models suggest that the intraglomerular immune complexes cause local complement activation with the generation of chemotactic factors (including C5a, chemokines, leukotrienes, and platelet-activating factor). Leukocyte adhesion molecules on endothelial cells are upregulated (intracellular adhesion molecule-1) or expressed *de novo* (E- and P-selectins).

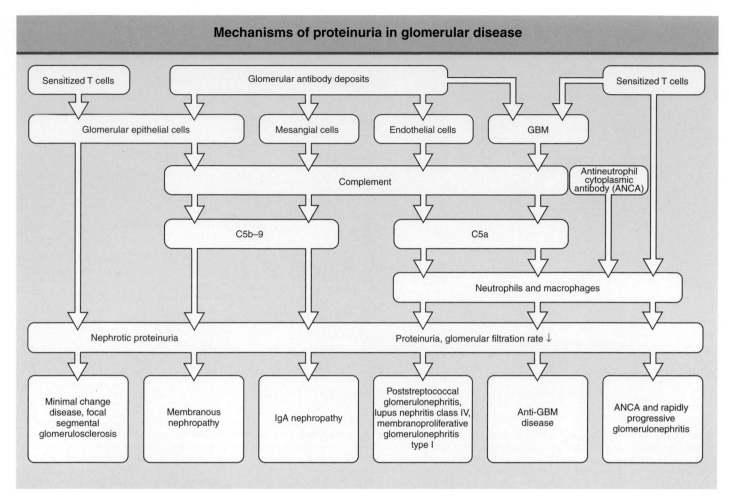

Figure 15.9 Mechanisms of proteinuria in glomerular disease. The main immune mechanisms involved in glomerular injury and the common glomerular diseases in which they occur. (Courtesy of Dr. William G. Couser.)

Proinflammatory cytokines (interleukin-1 and tumor necrosis factor α) are generated locally and augment the inflammatory response. Neutrophils, platelets, and monocytes/macrophages then localize in the glomerulus and release oxidants (particularly hypohalous acids generated by neutrophil myeloperoxidase) and proteases (elastase, cathepsin G, and metalloproteinases) that cause local cellular injury and GBM degradation.

Poststreptococcal Glomerulonephritis

Poststreptococcal GN has long been considered the human equivalent of acute serum sickness in rabbits. It is thought that certain nephritogenic strains of group A streptococcus release certain antigens, especially nephritis-associated plasmin receptor (recently identified as GAPDH) and zymogen into the circulation where they bind to antibody and localize to glomeruli.[6] The zymogen antigen is cationic and may preferably localize to the subepithelial space; the plasmin binding receptor protein also activates the alternative pathway of complement and may augment the inflammatory response independent of antibody. Activation of complement in the proximity of the endothelium leads to a brisk inflammatory reaction with local endothelial and mesangial cell proliferation and manifestations of the nephritic syndrome.

Pathogenesis of Crescent Formation

Crescent formation can occur with any severe glomerular injury, most notably in vasculitis (see Chapter 23), anti-GBM disease (see Chapter 22), and severe forms of immune complex GN (such as IgA nephropathy or poststreptococcal GN). The crescent is a proliferation of extracapillary cells within Bowman's space. There is evidence that crescent formation is initiated by cytokine-driven proliferation of the parietal and possibly the visceral GEC. Local breaks in the GBM or Bowman's capsule, mediated by activated leukocytes, are followed by macrophage infiltration, myofibroblast accumulation, and local fibrin deposition (Fig. 15.10). Most evidence suggests that crescent formation is a manifestation of cell-mediated rather than humoral immune mechanisms (see also Chapter 22).[7]

Pathogenesis of Progressive Renal Failure in Glomerular Disease

Two key processes characterize progressive renal failure: glomerulosclerosis and interstitial fibrosis. Although the original disease contributes to these processes, there is abundant evidence that progression is largely mediated by common nonimmunologic mechanisms.[17] These mechanisms are discussed in more detail in Chapter 68.

Glomerulosclerosis may be a direct consequence of the original glomerular injury, but in addition, a secondary form of FSGS may develop (see Chapter 18). It appears to be a consequence of reduced functioning nephron number, which is followed by glomerular capillary hypertension (in response to afferent arteriolar dysregulation) and hypertrophy (in response to cytokines and

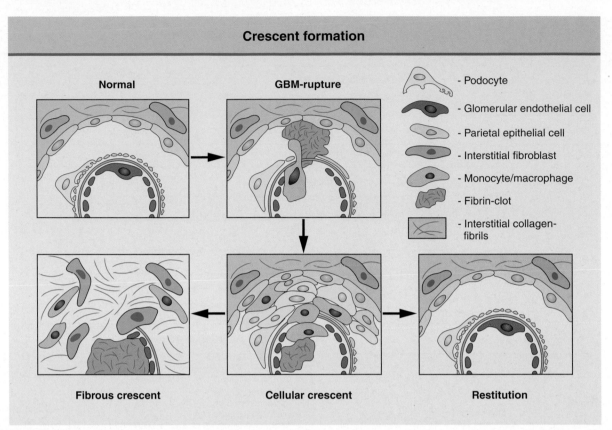

Figure 15.10 Crescent formation. In early crescent formation, cytokines and growth factors cross the glomerular basement membrane (GBM) to initiate proliferation of the parietal epithelial cells. Small breaks in the GBM occur secondary to injury from oxidants and proteases from neutrophil and macrophages, thus allowing the macrophage to enter Bowman's space where it can proliferate. Breaks in Bowman's capsule secondary to the periglomerular inflammation also occur, allowing the entrance of more inflammatory cells as well as fibroblasts. The proliferation of parietal and visceral epithelial cells and macrophages is associated with fibrin deposition, slowly choking the glomerular tuft until filtration becomes impossible. In the late stages, the crescent becomes fibrotic and the glomerulus end stage. Alternatively, in less severe cases, complete restitution of the glomerular tuft can occur.

growth factors). Death of glomerular endothelial cells results in capillary collapse and activation of the coagulation system. At the same time, progressive expansion of the capillary wall during glomerular hypertrophy results in denuded GBM since GEC hypertrophy and proliferation is ineffectual; the denuded GBM abuts Bowman's capsule, initiating synechiae formation, subsequent hyalin formation, and capillary collapse.[18] Mesangial cell proliferation also occurs and is associated with increased matrix synthesis. The result is a segmental and eventually global glomerulosclerosis.

Tubulointerstitial fibrosis also accompanies progressive glomerular disease and correlates with both renal function and prognosis. Tubulointerstitial fibrosis may occur via several different mechanisms. Proteinuria has been shown to activate tubular cells and induce toxicity, either directly or via the generation of oxidants (from iron proteins excreted in the urine) or from complement activation (which can be shown in proteinuric urine). Tubulointerstitial ischemia may also be involved in the pathogenesis of renal fibrosis, as a progressive loss of glomerular and peritubular capillaries can be shown in both experimental models and human disease.

There is growing understanding of the cellular responses involved in tubulointerstitial fibrosis.[19] The fibrotic process is characterized by early tubular cell proliferation with release of chemotactic factors, the recruitment of monocyte/macrophages and, to a lesser extent, T cells, the local stimulation and accumulation of fibroblast-like cells (myofibroblasts) with the synthesis and deposition of extracellular matrix, a progressive loss of the microvasculature, and the eventual apoptosis of tubular cells

resulting in a dense acellular fibrosis. Recently, it has been recognized that the myofibroblast may derive from a resident population of fibroblasts or by "transdifferentiation" from injured tubular cells.[20]

The mechanism by which tubulointerstitial fibrosis impairs renal function relates to the progressive loss of functioning nephrons. However, recently it has been recognized that glomeruli in some diseased nephrons may appear normal, but are nonfunctional due to tubulointerstitial fibrosis that causes a stricture or loss of the tubular lumen (resulting in atubular glomeruli).[21] Kriz and Lehir[18] have postulated that this may develop as a consequence of the glomerular capillary loop abutting Bowman's capsule, thereby "misdirecting" filtration into the interstitium, where it may lead to a local fibrotic response and effectively choke off the glomerulus.[18] It is thought that this may explain why tubulointerstitial fibrosis often correlates better with renal function than the severity of the glomerular lesion.

Resolution of Inflammation

While irreversible injury is common in GN because the result of the glomerular inflammation is fibrosis, it is striking that acute forms of the disease may sometimes resolve with little or no apparent permanent damage (poststreptococcal GN is the best example of this). There has been much interest in understanding the mechanisms involved in the dispersal and efflux of the leukocytes and in the proteolytic degradation of extracellular matrix. Recently, it has been shown that there are chemorepellants (such as Slit-1 and Robo) that may be expressed in glomeruli and counter the effects of chemotactic factors and may prevent or repel leukocytes from binding to the endothelium; these factors may be important in the recovery of glomeruli from acute inflammation.[22] Another key factor involved in the clearance of the inflammatory cells is apoptosis (programmed cell death). This process allows inflammatory or injured intrinsic cells to be consumed by a phagocytic cell rather than to necrose and liberate its injurious contents.[23] Research aimed at identifying these natural restorative mechanisms may provide insights into new approaches for therapy.

REFERENCES

1. Kalluri R, Cantley LG, Kerjasckhi D, Neilson EG: Reactive oxygen species expose cryptic epitopes associated with autoimmune Goodpasture syndrome. J Biol Chem 2000;275:20027–20032.
2. Wolf D, Hochegger K, Wolf AM, et al: CD4+CD25+ regulatory T cells inhibit experimental anti-glomerular basement membrane glomerulonephritis in mice. J Am Soc Nephrol 2005;16:1360–1370.
3. Couser WG: Pathogenesis of glomerular damage in glomerulonephritis Nephrol Dial Transplant 1998;13(Suppl 1):10–15.
4. Kalluri R, Wilson CB, Weber M, et al: Identification of the alpha 3 chain of type IV collagen as the common autoantigen in antibasement membrane disease and Goodpasture syndrome. J Am Soc Nephrol 1995;6:178–185.
5. Debiec H, Nauta J, Coulet F, et al: Role of truncating mutations in MME gene in fetomaternal alloimmuisation and antenatal glomerulopathies. Lancet 2004;364:1252–1259.
6. Yoshizawa N, Oshima S, Sagel I, et al: Role of a streptococcal antigen in the pathogenesis of acute poststreptococcal glomerulonephritis. J Immunol 1992;148:3110–3116.
7. Atkins RC, Nikolic-Patterson DJ, Song Q, et al: Modulators of crescentic glomerulonephritis. J Am Soc Nephrol 1996;7:2271–2278.
8. Antignac C: Molecular basis of steroid-resistant nephrotic syndrome. Nefrologia 2005;25(Suppl 2):25–28.
9. Ruf RG, Lichtenberger A, Karle SM, et al: Patients with mutations in NPHS2 (podocin) do not respond to standard steroid treatment of nephrotic syndrome. J Am Soc Nephrol 2004;15:722–732.
10. Winn MP, Conlon PJ, Lynn KL, et al: A mutation in the TRPC6 cation channel causes familial focal segmental glomerulosclerosis. Science 2005;308:1801–1804.
11. Myers BD, Guasch A: Mechanisms of proteinuria in nephrotic humans. Pediatr Nephrol 1994;8:107–112.
12. Koyama A, Fukisaki M, Kobayashi M, et al: A glomerular permeability factor produced by human T cell hybridomas. Kidney Int 1991;40:453–460.
13. Remuzzi G: A unifying hypothesis for renal scarring linking protein trafficking to the different mediators of injury. Nephrol Dial Transplant 2000;15(Suppl 6):58–60.
14. Johnson RJ: Have we ignored the role of oncotic pressure in the pathogenesis of glomerulosclerosis? Am J Kidney Dis 1997;29:147–152.
15. Eremina V, Quaggin SE: The role of VEGF-A in glomerular development and function. Curr Opin Nephrol Hypertens 2004;13:9–15.
16. Cornacchia F, Fornoni A, Plati AR, et al: Glomerulosclerosis is transmitted by bone marrow-derived mesangial cell progenitors. J Clin Invest 2001;108:1649–1656.
17. Brenner BM, Mackenzie HS: Nephron mass as a risk factor for progression of renal disease. Kidney Int Suppl 1997;63:S124–S127.
18. Kriz WR, Lehir M: Pathways to nephron loss starting from glomerular diseases—insights from animal models. Kidney Int 2005;67:404–419.
19. Eitner F, Floege J: Therapeutic targets for prevention and regression of progressive fibrosing renal diseases. Curr Opin Investig Drugs 2005;6:255–261.
20. Jinde K, Nikolic-Paterson DJ, Huang XR, et al: Tubular phenotypic change in progressive tubulointerstitial fibrosis in human glomerulonephritis. Am J Kidney Dis 2001;38:761–769.
21. Marcussen N: Tubulointerstitial damage leads to atubular glomeruli: Significance and possible role in progression. Nephrol Dial Transplant 2000;15:S74–S745.
22. Kanellis J, Garcia GE, Li P, et al: Modulation of inflammation by slit protein in vivo in experimental crescentic glomerulonephritis. Am J Pathol 2004;165:341–352.
23. Savill J: Apoptosis in resolution of inflammation. Kidney Blood Press Res 2000;23:173–174.

Introduction to Glomerular Disease: Clinical Presentations

Jürgen Floege and John Feehally

INTRODUCTION

Glomerular disease has clinical presentations that vary from the asymptomatic individual who is found to have hypertension, edema, hematuria and/or proteinuria at a routine medical assessment to a patient with a fulminant illness with acute renal failure (ARF) possibly associated with life-threatening extrarenal disease (Fig. 16.1). The most dramatic symptomatic presentations are uncommon. Asymptomatic urine abnormalities are much more common but less specific; they may also indicate a wide range of nonglomerular urinary tract disease.

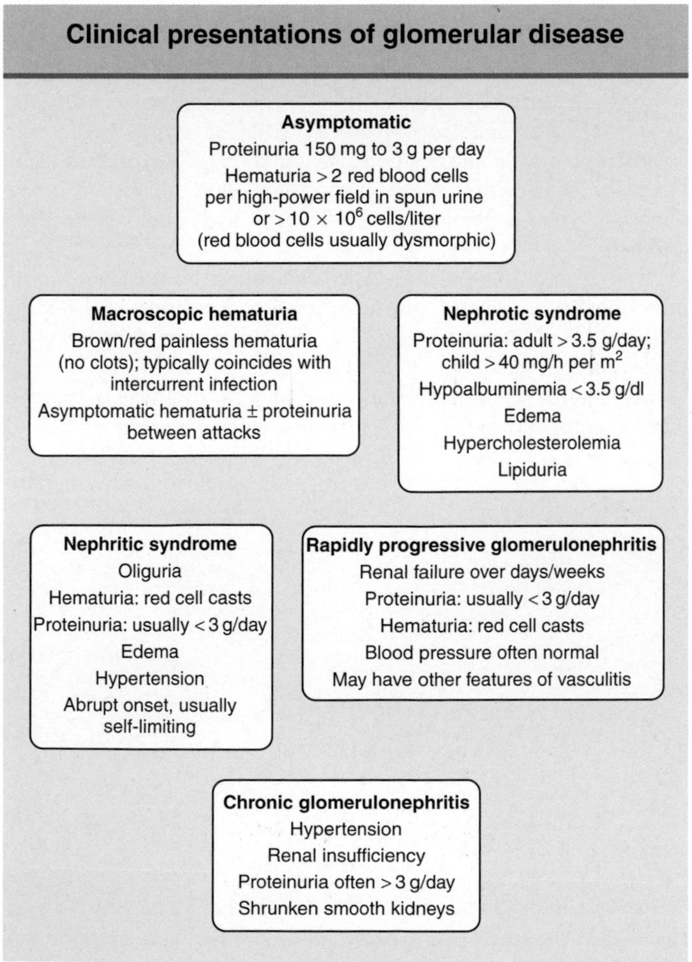

Clinical presentations of glomerular disease

Asymptomatic
Proteinuria 150 mg to 3 g per day
Hematuria > 2 red blood cells
per high-power field in spun urine
or > 10 × 10^6 cells/liter
(red blood cells usually dysmorphic)

Macroscopic hematuria
Brown/red painless hematuria
(no clots); typically coincides with
intercurrent infection
Asymptomatic hematuria ± proteinuria
between attacks

Nephrotic syndrome
Proteinuria: adult > 3.5 g/day;
child > 40 mg/h per m^2
Hypoalbuminemia < 3.5 g/dl
Edema
Hypercholesterolemia
Lipiduria

Nephritic syndrome
Oliguria
Hematuria: red cell casts
Proteinuria: usually < 3 g/day
Edema
Hypertension
Abrupt onset, usually
self-limiting

Rapidly progressive glomerulonephritis
Renal failure over days/weeks
Proteinuria: usually < 3 g/day
Hematuria: red cell casts
Blood pressure often normal
May have other features of vasculitis

Chronic glomerulonephritis
Hypertension
Renal insufficiency
Proteinuria often > 3 g/day
Shrunken smooth kidneys

Figure 16.1   Clinical presentations of glomerular disease.

CLINICAL EVALUATION OF GLOMERULAR DISEASE

The history, physical examination, and investigations are aimed at excluding nonglomerular disease, finding evidence of associated multisystem disease, and establishing renal function.

History

The majority of glomerular diseases do not lead to symptoms that patients will report. However, specific questioning may reveal edema, hypertension, foamy urine, and/or urinary abnormalities during prior routine testing (e.g., during routine medical examinations). Multisystem diseases associated with glomerular disease include diabetes, hypertension, amyloid, lupus, and vasculitis. Apart from the individual history suggesting either of these diseases, a positive family history may also be obtained in some cases. Other causes of familial renal disease may include Alport's syndrome (especially if associated with hearing loss), uncommon familial forms of IgA nephropathy, focal segmental glomerulosclerosis (FSGS), and hemolytic-uremic syndrome (HUS). Morbid obesity can be associated with FSGS. Certain drugs and toxins may cause glomerular disease, including minimal change disease (MCD; nonsteroidal anti-inflammatory agents [NSAIDs] and interferon), membranous nephropathy (penicillamine, NSAIDs, mercury present in skin-lightening creams), FSGS (pamidronate, heroin), or HUS (cyclosporine, tacrolimus, mitomycin C, oral contraceptives). Recent or persistent infection may also be associated with a variety of glomerular diseases (especially streptococcal infection, infective endocarditis, and certain viral infections; see Chapter 25).

Various malignancies are associated with glomerular disease, including lung, breast, and gastrointestinal carcinoma (membranous nephropathy), Hodgkin's disease (MCD), non-Hodgkin's lymphoma (membranoproliferative glomerulonephritis [MPGN]), and renal carcinoma (amyloid; see Chapter 26). Occasionally patients will present with the renal disease as the first manifestation of their tumor.

Physical Examination

The presence of dependent pitting edema suggests the nephrotic syndrome, heart failure, or cirrhosis. In the nephrotic subject, edema is often periorbital in the morning (Fig. 16.2), whereas the face is not affected overnight in edema associated with heart failure (because of orthopnea resulting from pulmonary congestion) or cirrhosis (because the patient cannot lie flat due to pressure on the diaphragm from ascites). As it progresses, edema of

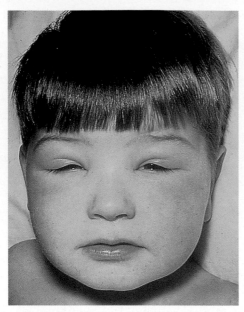

Figure 16.2 Nephrotic edema. Periorbital edema in the early morning in a nephrotic child. The edema resolves during the day under the influence of gravity.

genitals and abdominal wall becomes apparent, and accumulation of fluid in body spaces leads to ascites and pleural effusions. Edema is unpleasant; it leads to feelings of tightness in the limbs and a bloated abdomen. There are practical problems of clothes and shoes no longer fitting. Yet surprisingly, edema may become massive in nephrotic syndrome before patients seek medical help; fluid gains of 20% of normal body weight are by no means unusual (Fig. 16.3). The edema only becomes firm and stops pitting when long-standing. In children, fluid retention may also be striking with nephritic syndrome: A useful clinical sign to help to distinguish nephrotic from nephritic syndrome is the paper-thin, floppy ears (Heyman's sign) typical of nephrotic syndrome. Chronic hypoalbuminemia is also associated with loss of normal pink color under the nails, resulting in white nails or white bands if the nephrotic syndrome is transient (Muehrcke's bands, Fig. 16.4). Xanthelasmas may also be present as a result of the hyper-lipidemia associated with the nephrotic syndrome (Fig. 16.5).

The presence of pulmonary signs should suggest one of the pulmonary-renal syndromes (see Figs. 22.9 and 22.10). Palpable

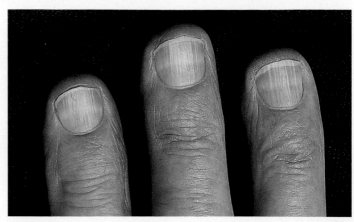

Figure 16.4 Muehrcke's bands in nephrotic syndrome. The white band grew during a transient period of hypoalbuminemia caused by the nephrotic syndrome.

purpura may be seen in vasculitis, systemic lupus, cryoglobulinemia, or endocarditis.

Laboratory Studies

Assessing renal function and careful examination of the urine (see Chapters 3 and 4) are critical. The quantity of urine protein and the presence or absence of dysmorphic red cells and casts will help to classify the clinical presentation (see Fig. 16.1).

Certain serologic tests are also helpful, including antinuclear and anti-DNA antibodies (lupus), cryoglobulins and rheumatoid factor (both suggestive of cryoglobulinemia), antiglomerular basement membrane (anti-GBM) antibodies (Goodpasture's syndrome), antineutrophilic cytoplasmic antibodies (ANCAs; vasculitis), and antistreptolysin O titer or streptozyme test (poststreptococcal glomerulonephritis [GN]). Serum and urine electrophoresis will detect monoclonal light chains or heavy chains (myeloma-associated amyloid or light-chain deposition disease).

Testing for the presence of ongoing bacterial or viral infections is also useful and includes blood cultures and testing for hepatitis B, hepatitis C, and human immunodeficiency virus (HIV) infection.

Measurements of systemic complement pathway activation by testing for serum C3, C4, and CH_{50} (50% hemolyzing dose of

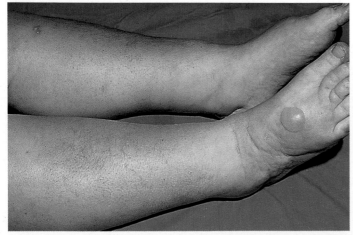

Figure 16.3 Nephrotic edema. Severe peripheral edema in nephrotic syndrome; note the blisters caused by intradermal fluid.

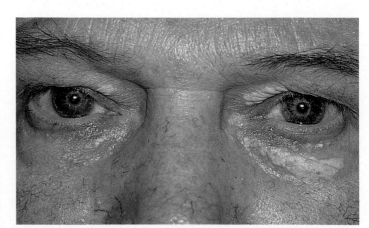

Figure 16.5 Xanthelasmas in nephrotic syndrome. These prominent xanthelasmas developed within a period of 2 months in a patient with recent onset of severe nephrotic syndrome and serum cholesterol of 550 mg/dl (14.2 mmol/l).

Hypocomplementemia in glomerular disease			
Pathway Affected	Complement Changes	Glomerular Diseases	Nonglomerular Diseases
Classical pathway activation	$C3 \downarrow$, $C4 \downarrow$, $CH_{50} \downarrow$ + C4 nephritic factor	Lupus nephritis (especially class IV), mixed essential cryoglobulinemia Membranoproliferative GN type I	
Alternative pathway activation	$C3 \downarrow$, C4 normal, $CH_{50} \downarrow$ + C3 nephritic factor	Poststreptococcal GN GN associated with other infection* endocarditis shunt nephritis hepatitis B Hemolytic-uremic syndrome Membranoproliferative GN type II	Atheroembolic renal disease

Reduced complement synthesis	Acquired
	Hereditary
	    C2 deficiency
	    Factor H deficiency
		
		Lupus nephritis
		Familial hemolytic-uremic syndrome
		Membranoproliferative glomerulonephritis
			Hepatic disease
			Malnutrition

Figure 16.6 Hypocomplementemia in glomerular disease. *Glomerulonephritis (GN) associated with visceral abscesses is generally associated with normal or increased complement (elevations occur because complement components are acute-phase reactants). CH_{50}, 50% hemolyzing dose of complement.

complement) is particularly helpful in limiting the differential diagnosis (Fig. 16.6).

Imaging

Ultrasonography is recommended in the workup to ensure the presence of two kidneys, to rule out obstruction or anatomic abnormalities, and to assess kidney size. Renal size is often normal in GN, although sometimes large kidneys (>14 cm) are seen in nephrotic syndrome associated with diabetes, amyloid, or HIV infection. Large kidneys can also occasionally be seen with any acute severe GN. The occurrence of small kidneys (<9 cm) suggests chronic renal disease and should limit enthusiasm for renal biopsy or aggressive immunosuppressive therapies.

Renal Biopsy

Renal biopsy is generally required to establish the type of glomerular disease and to guide treatment decisions. The principles and practice of renal biopsy are discussed in Chapter 6. There are some situations, however, where renal biopsy is not performed. If there are no unusual clinical features in nephrotic children, the probability of MCD is so high that corticosteroids can be initiated without biopsy (see Chapter 17). In acute nephritic syndrome, if all features point to poststreptococcal GN, especially in an epidemic, biopsy can be reserved for the minority who do not show early spontaneous improvement (see Chapter 25). In anti-GBM disease (see Chapter 22), the presence of lung hemorrhage and rapidly progressive renal failure with urinary red cell casts and high titers of circulating anti-GBM antibody establishes the diagnosis without the need for a biopsy, although a biopsy may still provide prognostic information. In patients with systemic features of vasculitis, a positive ANCA, negative blood cultures, and a tissue biopsy from another site showing vasculitis are sufficient to secure a diagnosis of renal vasculitis. Again, however, renal biopsy may provide important clues to disease activity and chronicity. Biopsy is also not generally performed in long-standing diabetes with characteristic findings suggestive of diabetic nephropathy and other evidence of microvascular complications of diabetes (see Chapter 29). Biopsy may also not be indicated in many patients with mild glomerular disease presenting with asymptomatic urine abnormalities as the prognosis is excellent and histologic findings will not alter management.

ASYMPTOMATIC URINE ABNORMALITIES

Urine testing that detects proteinuria or microscopic hematuria is often the first evidence of glomerular disease. The random nature of urine testing in most communities inevitably means that much mild glomerular disease remains undetected. In some countries, symptomless individuals may only have a urine test if they require medical approval for some key life event: to obtain life insurance, to join the armed forces, or sometimes for employment purposes. In other countries, for example, Japan, urinalysis is performed routinely in school or for employment. These different practices may partly account for the apparently variable incidence of certain diseases such as IgA nephropathy. Asymptomatic proteinuria and hematuria, and the combination of the two, increase in prevalence with age (Fig. 16.7).[1] Nevertheless, there is no evidence to justify routine population-wide screening for asymptomatic urine abnormalities, as renal biopsy and/or therapeutic intervention are rarely required when renal function is preserved. Screening, in particular for microalbuminuria, may be indicated for high-risk populations, for example, patients with diabetes, hypertension, or cardiovascular disease and those with a family history of renal disease.

Asymptomatic Microscopic Hematuria

Microscopic hematuria is defined as the presence of more than two red blood cells per high-power field in a spun urine sediment (3000 rpm for 5 minutes) or red blood cells $>10 \times 10^6$/l.

Microscopic hematuria is common in many glomerular diseases, especially IgA nephropathy and thin basement membrane nephropathy, although there are many other causes of hematuria (discussed further in Chapter 56). A glomerular origin should especially be considered if >5% of the red cells are acanthocytes (see Chapter 4) or if the hematuria is accompanied by red cell casts or proteinuria (Fig. 16.8).

Pathogenesis

Glomerular hematuria is thought to result from small breaks in the GBM that allow extravasation of red blood cells into the urinary space. This may occur in the peripheral capillary wall but more commonly occurs in the paramesangial basement membrane, particularly in diseases in which there is injury to the mesangium (mesangiolysis).

Urinary abnormalities in men of different ages

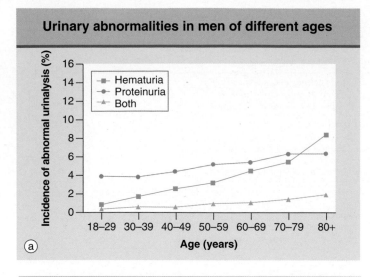

(a)

Urinary abnormalities in women of different ages

(b)

Figure 16.7   Prevalence of asymptomatic proteinuria and hematuria with age. Mass screening of a population of 107,192 adult men (*a*) and women (*b*) in Okinawa, Japan. Hematuria is more common in women. (Adapted from Iseki K, Iseki C, Ikemiya Y, Fukiyama K: Risk of developing end-stage renal disease in a cohort of mass screening. Kidney Int 1996;49:800–805.)

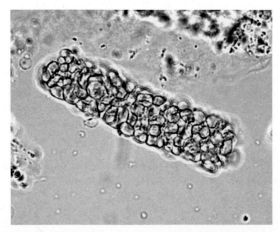

Figure 16.8   Red-cell cast. A red-cell cast typical of glomerular hematuria.

Evaluation

The evaluation of microscopic hematuria, which is discussed further in Chapter 56, begins with a thorough history. Urine culture should exclude urinary or prostatic infection. Phase contrast microscopy should follow in cases of persistent microhematuria to search for dysmorphic red cells and red cell casts. Any detectable proteinuria in the setting of asymptomatic microhematuria virtually excludes "urologic" bleeding and strongly suggests a glomerular origin. If this evaluation is nondiagnostic, renal imaging is performed to exclude anatomic lesions such as polycystic kidneys, stones, tumors, or arteriovenous malformations.

In those older than 40 years of age who have persistent isolated microhematuria without evidence of a glomerular origin (see previous discussion), cystoscopy is mandatory to exclude uroepithelial malignancy. In people younger than 40 years, such malignancy is so rare that cystoscopy is not recommended. If all the prior studies are negative, a glomerular etiology is likely.[2] The glomerular etiology can only be determined by renal biopsy, but this is rarely done since the prognosis is excellent in the setting of normal renal function, normal blood pressure, and low-grade proteinuria (<0.5 g/ day). However, repeated evaluation is mandatory.

Asymptomatic Non-nephrotic Proteinuria

The hallmark of glomerular disease is the excretion of protein in the urine. Normal urine protein excretion is <150 mg/24 h (consisting of 20 to 30 mg albumin, 10 to 20 mg of low molecular weight proteins that undergo glomerular filtration, and 40 to 60 mg of secreted proteins such as Tamm-Horsfall protein and IgA). Proteinuria is identified and quantified by dipstick testing or by assay in timed urine collections. The interpretation of these methods is discussed in Chapter 4.

Microalbuminuria is defined as the excretion of 30 to 300 mg albumin/day (equivalent to a urine albumin-to-creatinine (g/g) ratio of 0.03–0.3) and is detected by quantitative immunoassay or by special urine dipsticks, as this is below the sensitivity of the normal dipstick. This measurement is primarily used to identify diabetic subjects at risk of developing nephropathy and to assess cardiovascular risk, for example, in patients with hypertension.

Non-nephrotic proteinuria is usually defined as a urine protein excretion of <3.5 g/24 h, or a urine protein-to-creatinine (g/g) ratio of <3. Although nephrotic-range proteinuria is absolutely characteristic of glomerular disease, asymptomatic proteinuria (<3.5 g/24 h) is much less specific and may occur with a wide range of nonglomerular parenchymal diseases as well as with non-parenchymal renal and urinary tract conditions that must be excluded by clinical evaluation and investigation.

Selectivity of proteinuria is measured by the ratio of IgG and albumin clearances. Highly selective proteinuria, IgG-to-albumin clearance ratio <10% (i.e., loss of the glomerular charge barrier with an intact glomerular size barrier), is characteristic of MCD. In other nephrotic diseases, nonselective proteinuria (i.e., loss of both size and charge barriers) is more usual. Urine protein selectivity now rarely influences clinical decision making and need not be measured routinely.

Increased urine protein excretion may result from alterations in glomerular permeability or tubulointerstitial disease, although only in glomerular disease is it in the nephrotic range. It can also occur from increased filtration through normal glomeruli (overflow proteinuria).

Overflow Proteinuria

Overflow proteinuria is typical of urinary light-chain excretion. It is seen in myeloma but can occur in other settings (such as the release of lysozyme by leukemic cells) and should be suspected when the urine dipstick is negative for albumin despite detection of large amounts of proteinuria by other tests.

Tubular Proteinuria

Tubulointerstitial disease can also be associated with low-grade (usually <2 g/day) proteinuria. In addition to the loss of tubular proteins (such as α_1- or β_2-microglobulin), there will also be some albuminuria owing to impaired tubular reabsorption of filtered albumin. Tubular proteinuria accompanying glomerular (nonselective) proteinuria is an adverse prognostic sign in various glomerular diseases as it usually indicates advanced tubulointerstitial damage.

Glomerular Proteinuria

Glomerular proteinuria is further classified into that which is transient or hemodynamic (functional), that which is present only during the day (orthostatic), and that which is persistent or fixed.

Functional Proteinuria

Functional proteinuria refers to the transient non-nephrotic proteinuria that can occur with fever, exercise, heart failure, and hyperadrenergic or hyper-reninemic states. Functional proteinuria is benign; it is usually assumed to be hemodynamic in origin and to be the consequence of increases in single nephron flow or pressure.

Orthostatic Proteinuria

In children and young adults, low-grade glomerular proteinuria may be orthostatic, meaning that proteinuria is absent when urine is generated in the recumbent position. If there is no proteinuria in early morning urine, the diagnosis of orthostatic proteinuria can be made. The mechanism of orthostasis is not understood. Total urine protein in orthostatic proteinuria is usually <1 g/24 h; hematuria and hypertension are absent. Renal biopsy usually shows normal morphology or occasionally mild glomerular change. The prognosis is uniformly good and renal biopsy is not indicated.[3]

Fixed Non-nephrotic Proteinuria

Fixed non-nephrotic proteinuria is usually caused by glomerular disease. If GFR is preserved and proteinuria is <1 g/day, biopsy is not indicated but prolonged follow-up is necessary so long as significant proteinuria persists to rule out the possibility of the disease progressing. Previous studies indicate that the range of biopsy findings in these patients will be similar to those seen in nephrotic syndrome, although milder lesions are more common, particularly mesangial proliferative GN without immune deposits. Generally, no treatment is necessary.

Although controversial, many nephrologists will perform a renal biopsy in patients with normal GFR if non-nephrotic proteinuria exceeds 1 g/day, in particular if it persists after initiation of angiotensin-converting enzyme (ACE) inhibitor or angiotensin receptor blocker (ARB) therapy.

The evaluation of isolated asymptomatic proteinuria is summarized in Figure 16.9.

Asymptomatic Proteinuria with Hematuria

When asymptomatic hematuria and proteinuria coincide, there is a much greater risk of significant glomerular injury, hypertension, and progressive renal dysfunction. Minor histologic changes are less common. Renal biopsy is indicated even if urine protein is only 0.5 to 1 g/24 h if there is also persistent microscopic hematuria with casts.

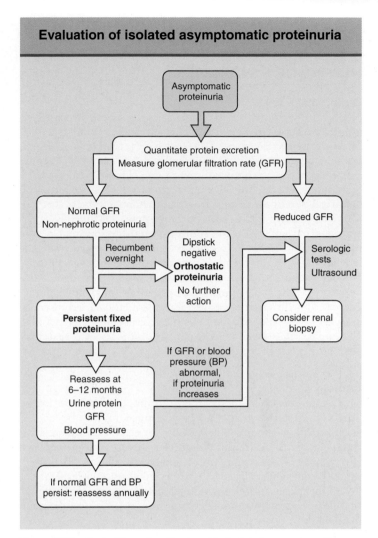

Evaluation of isolated asymptomatic proteinuria

Figure 16.9   Evaluation of patients with isolated asymptomatic proteinuria.

MACROSCOPIC HEMATURIA

Episodic painless macroscopic hematuria associated with glomerular disease is often brown or "smoky" rather than red, and clots are unusual. It must be distinguished from other causes of red or brown urine, including hemoglobinuria, myoglobinuria, porphyrias, consumption of food dyes, particularly beetroot, and intake of drugs, in particular rifampin (rifampicin).

Macroscopic hematuria caused by glomerular disease is observed primarily in children and young adults and is rare past the age of 40 years. Most cases are caused by IgA nephropathy, but hematuria may occur with other glomerular and nonglomerular renal diseases, including acute interstitial nephritis. Although macroscopic hematuria is typically painless, there may be an accompanying dull loin ache that may suggest other diagnoses such as stone disease or loin-pain hematuria syndrome. In IgA nephropathy, the frank hematuria is usually episodic, occurring within a day of an upper respiratory infection. There is a clear distinction between this history and the 2- to 3-week latency between an upper respiratory tract infection and hematuria that is highly suggestive of postinfectious (usually poststreptococcal) GN; furthermore, in poststreptococcal disease, there will usually be other features of nephritic syndrome. Macroscopic hematuria requires urologic evaluation including cystoscopy at any age unless the history (as shown previously) is characteristic of glomerular hematuria.

NEPHROTIC SYNDROME

Definition

Nephrotic syndrome is pathognomonic of glomerular disease. It is a clinical syndrome with a characteristic pentad (see Fig. 16.1).[4] Patients may be nephrotic with preserved renal function, but in many circumstances, progressive renal failure will become superimposed when nephrotic syndrome is prolonged.

Independent of the risk of progressive renal failure, the nephrotic syndrome has far-reaching metabolic effects that can influence the general health of the patient. Fortunately, some episodes of nephrotic syndrome are self-limiting and a few respond completely to specific treatment (e.g., corticosteroids in MCD). However, for most patients, it is a chronic condition. Not all patients with proteinuria >3.5 g/24 h will have a full nephrotic syndrome; some have a normal serum albumin and no edema. This difference presumably reflects the varied response of protein metabolism: Some patients sustain an increase in albumin synthesis in response to heavy proteinuria that may even normalize serum albumin.

Etiology

The major causes of nephrotic syndrome are shown in Figure 16.10. Proteinuria in the nephrotic range in the absence of edema and hypoalbuminemia has similar etiologies. The relative frequency of the different glomerular diseases varies with age (Fig. 16.11). Although predominant in childhood, MCD remains common at all ages.[5] There is an increased prevalence of FSGS in African Americans, and historical comparisons indicate that FSGS is becoming more common and MPGN less common in all adults.[6]

Hypoalbuminemia

Hypoalbuminemia is mostly a consequence of urinary losses. The liver responds by increasing albumin synthesis, but this compensatory mechanism appears to be blunted in nephrotic syndrome.[7] The end result is that serum albumin falls further. White bands in the nails (Muehrcke's bands) are a characteristic clinical sign of hypoalbuminemia (see Fig. 16.4). The increase in protein synthesis in response to proteinuria is not discriminating; as a result, proteins that are not being lost in the urine may actually increase in concentration in plasma. This is chiefly determined by molecular weight; large molecules will not spill into the urine and will increase in the plasma; smaller proteins, although synthesized to excess, will enter the urine and be diminished in the plasma. These variations in plasma proteins are clinically important in two areas: hypercoagulability and hyperlipidemia (see later discussion).

Edema

At least two major mechanisms are involved in the formation of nephrotic edema (Fig. 16.12).[8] In the first mechanism, which is more common in children with MCD, the edema appears to be the consequence of the low serum albumin producing a decrease in plasma oncotic pressure, which allows increased transudation of fluid from capillary beds into the extracellular space according to the laws of Starling. The consequent decrease in circulating blood volume (underfill) produces a secondary stimulation of the renin angiotensin system resulting in aldosterone-induced sodium retention in the distal tubule. This attempt to compensate for hypovolemia merely aggravates edema because the low oncotic pressure alters the balance of forces across the capillary wall in favor of hydrostatic pressure, forcing more fluid into the interstitial space rather than retaining it within the vascular compartment.

In many nephrotic patients, however, there appears to be a primary defect in the ability of the distal nephron to excrete

Common glomerular diseases presenting as nephrotic syndrome in adults		
Disease	**Associations**	**Serologic Tests Helpful in Diagnosis**
Minimal change disease	Allergy, atopy, NSAIDs, Hodgkin disease	None
Focal segmental glomerulosclerosis	African Americans	—
	HIV infection	HIV antibody
	Heroin, pamidronate	—
Membranous nephropathy	Drugs: gold, penicillamine, NSAIDs	—
	Infections: hepatitis B, C; malaria	Hepatitis B surface antigen, anti–hepatitis C virus antibody
	Lupus nephritis	Anti-DNA antibody
	Malignancy: breast, lung, gastrointestinal tract	—
Membranoproliferative glomerulonephritis (type I)	C4 nephritic factor	C3 ↓, C4 ↓
Membranoproliferative glomerulonephritis (type II)	C3 nephritic factor	C3 ↓, C4 normal
Cryoglobulinemic membranoproliferative glomerulonephritis	Hepatitis C	Anti–hepatitis C virus antibody, rheumatoid factor, C3 ↓, C4 ↓, CH_{50} ↓
Amyloid	Myeloma	Serum protein electrophoresis, urine immunoelectrophoresis
	Rheumatoid arthritis, bronchiectasis, Crohn's disease (and other chronic inflammatory conditions), familial Mediterranean fever	
Diabetic nephropathy	Other diabetic microangiopathy	None

Figure 16.10 Common glomerular diseases presenting as nephrotic syndrome in adults. HIV, human immunodeficiency virus; NSAIDs, nonsteroidal anti-inflammatory drugs.

Age-related variations in nephrotic syndrome					
	Prevalence (%)				
	Child	**Young Adult**		**Middle and Old Age**	
	(<15 years)	Whites	Blacks	Whites	Blacks
Minimal change disease	78	23	15	21	16
Focal segmental glomerulosclerosis	8	19	55	13	35
Membranous nephropathy	2	24	26	37	24
Membranoproliferative glomerulonephritis	6	13	0	4	2
Other glomerulonephritis	6	14	2	12	12
Amyloid	0	5	2	13	11

Figure 16.11   Age-related variations in nephrotic syndrome. (Data adapted from Cameron JS: Nephrotic syndrome in the elderly. Semin Nephrol 1996; 16:319–329; and Haas M, Meehan SM, Karison TG, Spargo BH: Changing etiologies of unexplained adult nephrotic syndrome: A comparison of renal biopsy findings from 1976–1979 and 1995–1997. Am J Kidney Dis 1997;30:621–631.)

sodium. As a result, there is an increased blood volume, suppression of renin angiotensin and vasopressin, and a tendency to hypertension rather than hypotension; the kidney is also relatively resistant to the actions of atrial natriuretic peptide. An elevated blood volume results (overfill), which, in association with the low plasma oncotic pressure, provokes transudation of fluid into the extracellular space and edema. The mechanism for the defect in sodium excretion remains unknown, although it has been hypothesized that inflammatory leukocytes in the interstitium, which are found in many glomerular diseases, may impair sodium excretion by producing angiotensin II and oxidants (the latter inactivates local nitric oxide, which is natriuretic).[9]

Metabolic Consequences of Nephrotic Syndrome
Negative Nitrogen Balance

The heavy proteinuria leads to marked negative nitrogen balance, usually measured in clinical practice by serum albumin. Nephrotic syndrome is a wasting illness, but the degree of muscle loss is masked by edema and not fully apparent until the

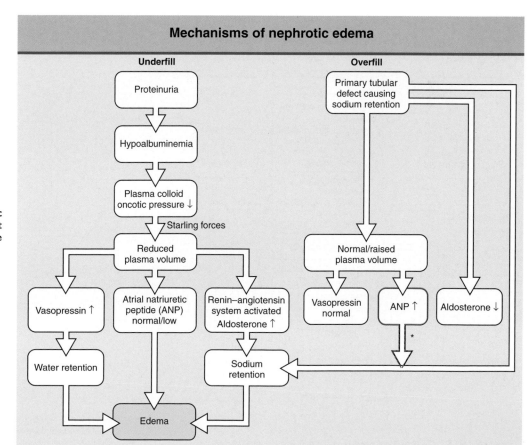

Figure 16.12   Mechanisms of nephrotic edema. *The kidney is relatively resistant to ANP in this setting, so ANP has little effect in countering sodium retention.

patient is rendered edema free. Loss of 10% to 20% of lean body mass is not uncommon. Albumin turnover is increased in response to the tubular catabolism of filtered protein rather than merely to urinary protein loss. Increasing protein intake does not improve albumin metabolism since the hemodynamic response to an increased intake is a rise in glomerular pressure, producing enhanced urine protein losses. A low-protein diet in turn will reduce proteinuria but also reduces the albumin synthesis rate and, in the longer term, may increase the risk of a worsening negative nitrogen balance.

Hypercoagulability

Multiple proteins of the coagulation cascade have altered levels in nephrotic syndrome; in addition, platelet aggregation is enhanced.[10] The net effect is a hypercoagulable state that is enhanced further by immobility, coincidental infection, and hemoconcentration if the patient has a contracted plasma volume (Fig. 16.13). Not only is venous thromboembolism common at any site, but spontaneous arterial thrombosis may occur. In adults, arterial thrombosis may occur in the context of atheroma, promoting coronary and cerebrovascular events in particular, but it also occurs in nephrotic children, in whom spontaneous thrombosis of major limb arteries is an uncommon but feared complication. Up to 10% of nephrotic adults and 2% of children will have a clinical episode of thromboembolism. Individual levels of coagulation proteins are not helpful in assessing the risk of thromboembolism, and serum albumin is mostly used as a surrogate marker. Thromboembolic events increase markedly if the serum albumin decreases to <2 g/dl.

The hypo- and dysproteinemia produce an increase in erythrocyte sedimentation rate (ESR). Values up to 100 mm/h are not unusual, so ESR loses its clinical value as a marker of an acute-phase response in nephrotic patients.

Renal vein thrombosis (see Chapter 61) is an important complication of nephrotic syndrome. At one time, it was thought that renal vein thrombosis could cause nephrotic syndrome; this is no longer considered true. Renal vein thrombosis is reported clinically in up to 8% of nephrotic patients, but when sought systematically (by ultrasonography or contrast venography), the frequency increases to 10% to 50%. It may be more common in membranous nephropathy than other disease patterns, although there is no explanation for this observation. Symptoms when the thrombosis is acute may include flank pain and hematuria; rarely, ARF can occur if the thrombosis is bilateral. However, often the thrombosis develops insidiously with minimal symptoms or signs because of the development of collateral blood supply. Pulmonary embolism is an important complication. Screening for renal vein thrombosis should not be routine in nephrotic patients.

Hyperlipidemia and Lipiduria

Hyperlipidemia is such a frequent finding in patients with heavy proteinuria that it is regarded as an integral feature of nephrotic syndrome.[11] Clinical stigmata of hyperlipidemia, such as xanthelasmas, may have a rapid onset (see Fig. 16.5). It is not uncommon for serum cholesterol to be >500 mg/dl (13 mmol/l), although serum triglyceride levels are highly variable. The lipid profile in nephrotic syndrome (Fig. 16.14) is known to be highly atherogenic in other populations. The presumption that coronary heart disease is increased in nephrotic syndrome owing to the combination of hypercoagulation and hyperlipidemia has been difficult to prove. Many patients who are nephrotic for more

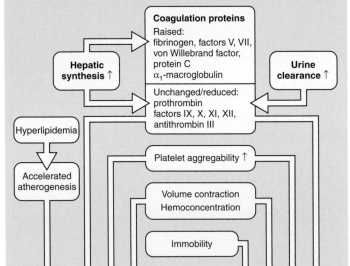

Figure 16.13   Coagulation abnormalities in nephrotic syndrome.

Coagulation abnormalities in nephrotic syndrome

Lipid abnormalities in nephrotic syndrome

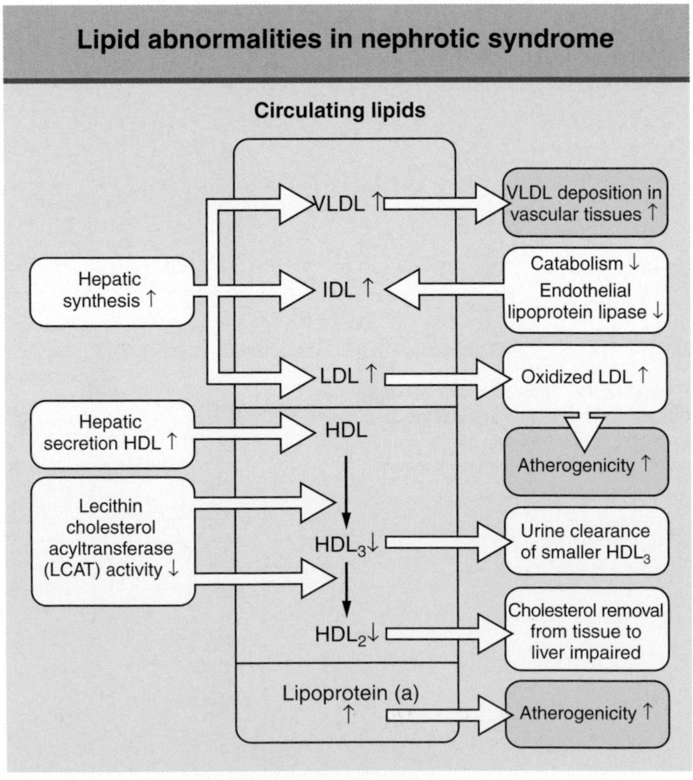

Figure 16.14   Lipid abnormalities in nephrotic syndrome. Changes in HDLs are more controversial than those in VLDLs. HDL, high-density lipoprotein; IDL, intermediate-density lipoprotein; VLDL, very-low-density lipoprotein.

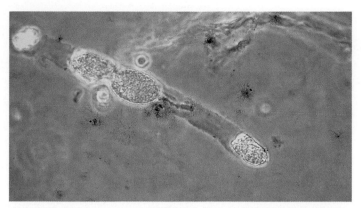

Figure 16.15   Fat in the urine. A hyaline cast containing oval fat bodies that are tubular epithelial cells full of fat. Oval fat bodies often appear brown in color.

than 5 to 10 years will develop additional cardiovascular risk factors, including hypertension and uremia, so it is difficult to separate these influences. However, it is now generally accepted that nephrotic patients do carry about a fivefold increased risk of coronary death, with the exception of those with MCD. Presumably this is because the transience of the nephrotic state before remission with steroid treatment does not subject the patient with minimal change to prolonged hyperlipidemia.

There is experimental evidence that hyperlipidemia contributes to progressive renal disease by various mechanisms, with protection afforded by lipid-lowering agents. However, although a meta-analysis suggests lipid lowering may slow the rate of progression of chronic renal disease,[12] there are not yet adequate prospective clinical studies to support the use of lipid-lowering agents with this goal in mind, and lipid-lowering drugs are chiefly indicated in nephrotic syndrome for cardiovascular reasons.

Several mechanisms account for the lipid abnormalities in nephrotic syndrome, including increased hepatic synthesis of low-density lipoprotein (LDL), very low density lipoprotein (VLDL), and lipoprotein (a) secondary to the hypoalbuminemia; defective peripheral lipoprotein lipase activity resulting in increased VLDL; and urinary losses of high-density lipoprotein (HDL; see Fig. 16.14).

Lipiduria, the fifth component of the nephrotic syndrome, is manifested by the presence of refractile accumulations of lipid in cellular debris and casts (oval fat bodies and fatty casts; Fig. 16.15). However, the lipiduria appears to be a consequence of the proteinuria and not of the plasma lipid abnormalities.

Other Metabolic Effects of Nephrotic Syndrome
Vitamin D–binding protein is lost in the urine, resulting in low plasma 25-hydroxyvitamin D levels, but free vitamin D is usually normal, and overt osteomalacia or uncontrolled hyperparathyroidism is very unusual in nephrotic syndrome in the absence of renal insufficiency. Thyroid-binding globulin is lost in the urine and total circulating thyroxine is reduced, but free thyroxine and thyroid-stimulating hormone are normal and there are no clinical alterations in thyroid status. Occasional cases of copper, iron, or zinc deficiency have been described as a consequence of the loss of binding proteins in the urine.

Drug binding may be altered by the decrease in serum albumin. Although most drugs do not require dose modifications, one important exception is clofibrate, which at normal doses in nephrotic patients produces a severe myopathy. Reduced protein binding may also reduce the dose of warfarin (Coumadin) required

to achieve adequate anticoagulation or the dose of furosemide required to achieve adequate fluid loss (see later discussion).

Infection
Nephrotic patients are prone to bacterial infection. Before steroids were shown to be effective in childhood nephrotic syndrome, sepsis was the most common cause of death and remains a major problem in the developing world. Primary peritonitis, especially that caused by pneumococci, is particularly characteristic of nephrotic children. It is less common with increasing age: By the age of 20 years, most adults have antibodies against pneumococcal capsular antigens. Peritonitis caused by both β-hemolytic streptococci and gram-negative organisms occurs, but staphylococcal peritonitis is not reported. Cellulitis, especially in areas of severe edema, is also common, most frequently caused by β-hemolytic streptococci.

There are several explanations for the increased risk of infection. Large fluid collections are sites for bacteria to grow easily; nephrotic skin is fragile, creating sites of entry; and edema may dilute local humoral immune factors. Loss of IgG and complement factor B (of the alternative pathway) in the urine impairs host ability to eliminate encapsulated organisms such as pneumococci. Zinc and transferrin are lost in the urine, and both are required for normal lymphocyte function. Neutrophil phagocytic function is impaired in nephrotic syndrome, and a number of *in vitro* T cell dysfunctions are described, although their clinical significance is uncertain.

Acute and Chronic Changes in Renal Function in Nephrotic Syndrome
Acute Renal Failure
Patients with nephrotic syndrome are also at risk for the development of ARF,[13] which can occur by a variety of mechanisms that are summarized in Figure 16.16. These include volume depletion and/or sepsis resulting in either prerenal azotemia or acute tubular necrosis[14]; transformation of the underlying disease (such as the development of crescentic nephritis in a patient with membranous nephropathy); development of bilateral renal vein thrombosis; increased disposition to azotemia from NSAIDs and ACE inhibitors or ARBs; and increased risk of allergic interstitial nephritis secondary to drugs, including diuretics. It has also been postulated that some patients develop ARF from intrarenal

Acute renal failure in nephrotic syndrome
Prerenal failure due to volume depletion
Acute tubular necrosis due to volume depletion and/or sepsis
Intrarenal edema
Renal vein thrombosis
Transformation of underlying glomerular disease, e.g., crescentic nephritis superimposed on membranous nephropathy
Adverse effects of drug therapy
Acute allergic interstitial nephritis secondary to various drugs, including diuretics
Hemodynamic response to nonsteroidal anti-inflammatory drugs and angiotensin-converting enzyme (ACE) inhibitors or angiotensin receptor blockers (ARBs)

Figure 16.16   Acute renal failure in nephrotic syndrome. Problems to consider when evaluating acute deterioration in renal function in nephrotic syndrome.

Proteinuria and prognosis in glomerular disease

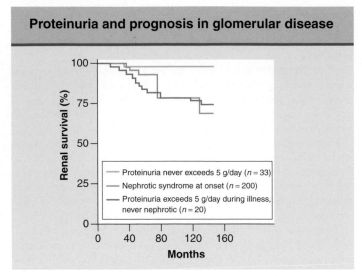

Figure 16.17 Proteinuria and prognosis in glomerular disease. The influence of heavy proteinuria on long-term renal function in 253 patients with primary glomerular disease at Manchester Royal Infirmary, United Kingdom. Heavy proteinuria at any time during long-term follow-up substantially worsens the prognosis even without frank nephrotic syndrome. (Courtesy of Dr. C. D. Short.)

edema with compression of tubules[15]; these patients, like nephrotic subjects with prerenal azotemia, may respond with diuresis to albumin infusions coupled with a loop diuretic.

Chronic Renal Insufficiency

With the exception of MCD, most causes of nephrotic syndrome are associated with some risk of the development of progressive renal failure. In this regard, one of the greatest risk factors for progression is the degree of proteinuria (see Chapter 68). Progression is uncommon if proteinuria is <2 g/day. The risk increases in proportion to the severity of the proteinuria (Fig. 16.17), with marked risk of progression when protein excretion is >5 g/day. This may be because proteinuria identifies patients with severe glomerular injury, but there is also experimental and clinical evidence that proteinuria, per se, may be toxic, especially to the tubulointerstitium.[16] In several experimental models, measures that reduce proteinuria, such as the use of ACE inhibitors, also prevent tubulointerstitial disease and progressive renal failure.

NEPHRITIC SYNDROME

In nephrotic syndrome, the glomerular injury manifests primarily as an increase in permeability of the capillary wall to protein. By contrast, in the nephritic syndrome, there is evidence of glomerular inflammation resulting in a reduction in GFR, non-nephrotic proteinuria, edema and hypertension (secondary to sodium retention), and hematuria with red-cell casts.

The classic nephritic syndrome presentation is that seen with acute poststreptococcal GN in children. These children usually present with rapid onset of oliguria, weight gain, and generalized edema over a few days. The hematuria results in brown rather than red urine, and clots are not seen. The urine contains protein, red cells, and red-cell casts. Since proteinuria is rarely in the nephrotic range, serum albumin is usually normal. Circulating volume increases with hypertension, and pulmonary edema follows without evidence of primary cardiac disease.

The distinction between typical nephrotic syndrome and nephritic syndrome is usually straightforward on clinical and

Differentiation between nephrotic syndrome and nephritic syndrome

Typical Features	Nephrotic	Nephritic
Onset	Insidious	Abrupt
Edema	++++	++
Blood pressure	Normal	Raised
Jugular venous pressure	Normal/low	Raised
Proteinuria	++++	++
Hematuria	May/may not occur	+++
Red-cell casts	Absent	Present
Serum albumin	Low	Normal/slightly reduced

Figure 16.18 Differentiation between nephrotic syndrome and nephritic syndrome.

laboratory grounds (Fig. 16.18) and the use of these clinical descriptions is particularly helpful in the approach to patients with suspected GN at first presentation, helping to narrow the differential diagnosis. However, the classification systems are imperfect and patients with certain glomerular disease patterns, for example, MPGN, may present with either a nephrotic or a nephritic picture.

Etiology

The primary glomerular diseases associated with the nephritic syndrome and the serologic tests helpful in diagnosis are shown in Figure 16.19. The classification is even more challenging than for nephrotic syndrome as some diseases are identified by histology (IgA nephropathy), others by serology and histology (ANCA-associated vasculitis and lupus nephritis), and others by etiology (postinfectious GN).

RAPIDLY PROGRESSIVE GLOMERULONEPHRITIS

Rapidly progressive GN (RPGN) describes the clinical situation in which glomerular injury is so acute and severe that renal function deteriorates over days or weeks. The patient may present as a uremic emergency, with nephritic syndrome that is not self-limiting but moves on rapidly to renal failure, or with rapidly deteriorating renal function when being investigated for extra-renal disease (many of the patterns of GN associated with RPGN occur as part of a systemic immune illness).

The histologic counterpart of RPGN is crescentic GN: The proliferative cellular response seen outside the glomerular tuft but within Bowman's space is known as a crescent because of its shape on histologic cross section (see Fig. 15.10). Typically, the glomerular tuft also shows segmental necrosis, or focal segmental necrotizing GN; this is particularly characteristic of the vasculitis syndromes.

The term RPGN is, therefore, often used to describe acute deterioration in renal function in association with a crescentic nephritis. Unfortunately, not all patients with a nephritic urine sediment and ARF will fit this syndrome. For example, ARF may also occur in milder forms of glomerular disease if complicated by accelerated hypertension, renal vein thrombosis, or acute tubular necrosis. This emphasizes the need to obtain histologic confirmation of the clinical diagnosis.

Common glomerular diseases presenting as nephritic syndrome		
Disease	Associations	Serologic Tests Helpful in Diagnosis
Poststreptococcal glomerulonephritis	Pharyngitis, impetigo	ASO titer, streptozyme antibody
Other postinfectious disease		
Endocarditis	Cardiac murmur	Blood cultures, C3 ↓
Abscess	—	Blood cultures, C3, C4 normal or increased
Shunt	Treated hydrocephalus	Blood cultures, C3 ↓
IgA nephropathy	Upper respiratory or gastrointestinal infection	Serum IgA ↑
Systemic lupus	Other multisystem features of lupus	Antinuclear antibody, anti–double-stranded DNA antibody, C3 ↓, C4 ↓

Figure 16.19 Common glomerular diseases presenting as nephritic syndrome.

Etiology

The primary glomerular diseases associated with RPGN and helpful serologic tests are shown in Figure 16.20. As with nephritic syndrome, different assessment methods are useful for different diseases causing RPGN.

CHRONIC RENAL INSUFFICIENCY

In most types of chronic GN, a proportion of patients (often between 25% and 50%) will have slowly progressive renal impairment. If no clinical event early in the course of the disease brings them to medical attention, patients may present late with established hypertension, proteinuria, and renal impairment. In very long standing GN, the kidneys shrink (but remain smooth and symmetrical). Renal biopsy at this stage is more hazardous and less likely to provide diagnostic material. Light microscopy often shows nonspecific features of end-stage kidney disease, consisting of focal or global glomerulosclerosis and dense tubulointerstitial fibrosis, and it may not be possible to define with confidence that a glomerular disease was the initiating renal injury, let alone define the pattern further. Immunofluorescence may be more helpful; in particular, mesangial IgA may be present in adequate amounts to allow a diagnosis of IgA nephropathy to be made. However, when renal imaging shows small kidneys, only rarely will biopsy be appropriate. For this reason, chronic GN has often been a presumptive diagnosis in patients presenting late with shrunken kidneys, proteinuria, and renal impairment. This is imprecise and in the past has led to an overestimate of the frequency of GN as a cause of end-stage renal disease in registry data. GN should only be diagnosed if there is confirmatory histologic evidence.

TREATMENT OF GLOMERULAR DISEASE

General Principles

Prior to any therapeutic decisions, it should always be ascertained that glomerular disease is primary and that no specific therapy is available. For example, treatment of an underlying infection or tumor may result in remission of GN. In the remaining cases, both general supportive treatment[17] (see Chapter 69) and disease-specific therapy should be considered. The former includes measures to treat blood pressure, reduce proteinuria, control edema, and address other metabolic consequences of nephrotic syndrome. If successful, these relatively nontoxic therapies can prevent the need for immunosuppressive drugs, which have multiple potential side effects. Supportive therapy is usually not necessary in steroid-sensitive MCD with rapid remission or in patients with IgA nephropathy, Alport's syndrome, or thin basement membrane nephropathy as long as they exhibit neither proteinuria nor hypertension.

Common glomerular diseases presenting as rapidly progressive glomerulonephritis		
Disease	Associations	Serologic Tests Helpful in Diagnosis
Goodpasture's syndrome	Lung hemorrhage	Anti–glomerular basement membrane antibody (occasionally antineutrophil cytoplasmic antibodies [ANCA] present)
Vasculitis		
Wegener's granulomatosis	Upper and lower respiratory involvement	Cytoplasmic ANCA
Microscopic polyangiitis	Multisystem involvement	Perinuclear ANCA
Pauci-immune crescentic glomerulonephritis	Renal involvement only	Perinuclear ANCA
Immune complex disease		
Systemic lupus erythematosus	Other multisystem features of lupus	Antinuclear antibody, anti–double-stranded DNA antibody, C3 ↓, C4 ↓
Poststreptococcal glomerulonephritis	Pharyngitis, impetigo	ASO titer, streptozyme antibody, C3 ↓, C4 normal
IgA nephropathy/Henoch-Schönlein purpura	Characteristic rash ± abdominal pain in HSP	Serum IgA ↑ (30%), C3 and C4 normal
Endocarditis	Cardiac murmur; other systemic features of bacteremia	Blood cultures, ANCA (occasionally) C3 ↓, C4 normal

Figure 16.20 Common glomerular diseases presenting as rapidly progressive glomerulonephritis. Note the overlap between the diseases in this figure and those in Figure 16.19. A number of glomerular diseases may present with either nephritic syndrome or rapidly progressive glomerulonephritis.

Hypertension

Hypertension is very common in GN; it is virtually universal as chronic GN progresses toward end-stage renal disease and is the key modifiable factor in preserving renal function (see also Chapter 69). Sodium and water overload is an important part of the pathogenetic process, and high-dose diuretics with moderate dietary sodium restriction are usually an essential part of the treatment. As in other chronic renal diseases, the aim of blood pressure control is not only to protect against the cardiovascular risks of hypertension but also to delay progression of the renal disease. The ideal target blood pressure is not finally established but in the Modification of Diet in Renal Disease (MDRD) study, patients with proteinuria (>1 g/day) had a better outcome if their blood pressure was reduced to 125/75 mm Hg rather than the previous standard of 140/90 mm Hg.[18,19] There are strong theoretical and experimental reasons for ACE inhibitors and ARBs to be first-choice therapy, and this is now well documented in clinical studies.[20–22] Nondihydropyridine calcium channel blockers may also have a beneficial effect on proteinuria as well as blood pressure. As in essential hypertension, lifestyle modification (salt restriction, weight normalization, regular exercise, and smoking cessation) should be an integral part of the therapy. If target blood pressure cannot be achieved with these measures, antihypertensive therapy should be stepped up according to current guidelines (see Chapter 34).

Treatment of Proteinuria

Besides hypertension, proteinuria represents the second key modifiable factor to preserve GFR (see also Chapter 69). Most studies suggest that the progressive loss of renal function observed in many glomerular diseases can largely be prevented if proteinuria can be reduced to levels <0.5 g/day. This may be because many of the measures to reduce protein excretion, such as the use of ACE inhibitors or ARBs, also reduce glomerular hypertension, which contributes to progressive renal failure. However, there is also increasing evidence that proteinuria or factors present in proteinuric urine per se may be toxic to the tubulointerstitium.[16] Finally, in nephritic patients, a reduction of proteinuria to a non-nephrotic range can induce serum proteins to rise, with alleviation of many of the metabolic complications of nephrotic syndrome.

Most of the agents used to reduce urinary protein excretion do so hemodynamically, either by blocking efferent arteriolar constriction (ACE inhibitors or ARBs) or by reducing preglomerular pressure (most other classes of antihypertensives). Some of the agents, such as ACE inhibitors and ARBs, may also have direct effects on reducing the increased glomerular capillary wall permeability. A consequence of this type of therapy is a reduction in GFR; however, in general, the decrease in GFR is of a lower magnitude than the decrease in protein excretion. The antiproteinuric agents of choice are ACE inhibitors and ARBs, which reduce proteinuria by an average of 40% to 50%, particularly if the patient is on dietary salt restriction. There is little clinical evidence to suggest that ACE inhibitors differ from ARBs in this respect. However, the combination of the two may result in additive antiproteinuric activity.[23] In addition, while other classes of antihypertensive agents will reduce proteinuria coincident with a decrease in systemic blood pressure (particularly the nondihydropyridine calcium channel blockers such as diltiazem), both ACE inhibitors and ARB usually reduce proteinuria independent of blood pressure. Dose should be increased slowly because symptomatic hypotension can develop in pateints taking ACE inhibitors and ARBs. This allows therapy in the normotensive proteinuric patient. Also, increasing the dose of ACE inhibitors or ARBs may further reduce proteinuria without

lowering blood pressure, an observation that may relate to the inefficacy of usual antihypertensive drug levels in blocking the stimulated intrarenal renin angiotensin system. Common side effects include hyperkalemia in patients with advanced renal failure, which may necessitate a loop diuretic and rarely should lead to cessation of the medication and cough in the case of ACE inhibitors, in which case ARBs should be used instead. Since ACE inhibitors and ARBs lower GFR (see previous discussion) a 10% to 20% increase in serum creatinine may be observed. Unless serum creatinine continues to increase, this moderate increase reflects the therapeutic effect of these medications and should not prompt withdrawal of them.

NSAIDs lessen proteinuria by reducing intrarenal prostaglandin production and dipyridamole through adenosine-mediated afferent arteriolar vasoconstriction. Given the safety of the therapies discussed previously, as well as the risk with NSAIDs of profound decreases in GFR, salt retention, and diuretic resistance, they are rarely used.

A low-protein diet will lessen proteinuria, but must be advised with great care because of the risk of malnutrition. Adequate compensation must be made for urine protein losses[24] and the patient must be carefully monitored for evidence of malnutrition (see Chapter 77).

Treatment of Hyperlipidemia

Treatment of hyperlipidemia in patients with glomerular disease should usually follow the guidelines that apply to the general population to prevent cardiovascular disease. It may also be that statin therapy protects from a decrease in GFR, although this is not firmly established. Dietary restriction alone has only modest effects on hyperlipidemia in glomerular disease, in particular in nephrotic syndrome. Side effects of some medications, for example, rhabdomyolysis provoked by fibrates, occur more frequently in patients with renal failure. The addition of bile acid sequestrants, such as cholestyramine, may lower LDL further and increase HDL but is usually not tolerated because of gastrointestinal effects.

Avoidance of Nephrotoxic Substances

Apart from NSAIDs, which may induce ARF, particularly in patients with pre-existing renal impairment and dehydration, other nephrotoxic substances such as radiocontrast agents, cytostatic drugs, and antibiotics (e.g., aminoglycoside antibiotics) should also be used with caution in patients with glomerular disease and renal impairment or nephrotic syndrome.

Special Therapeutic Issues in Patients with Nephrotic Syndrome
Treatment of Nephrotic Edema

In contrast to the lack of therapies in the past (Fig. 16.21), the mainstays of treatment nowadays are diuretics accompanied by moderate dietary sodium restriction (60 to 80 mmol/24 h). Nephrotic patients are diuretic resistant even if GFR is normal: Loop diuretics must reach the renal tubule to be effective and transport from the peritubular capillary requires protein binding, which is reduced in hypoalbuminemia; once the drug reaches the renal tubule, it will become 70% bound to protein present in the urine and, therefore, be less effective. Oral diuretics with twice-daily administration are usually preferred given the longer therapeutic effect compared to intravenous diuretics. However, in severe nephrosis, gastrointestinal absorption of the diuretic may be uncertain because of intestinal wall edema, and intravenous diuretic, by bolus injection or infusion, may be necessary to

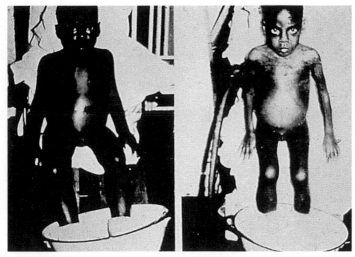

Figure 16.21 Treatment of nephrotic edema before the availability of diuretics. Edema in nephrotic syndrome was very difficult to treat: This child with anasarca, pictured in 1953, stands in a bowl while edema fluid drips out through small tubes placed through needles in the skin of the feet. This was nevertheless effective treatment: The two pictures of the same child were taken four days apart, during which time the child lost 4.5 kg (10 lb), or 18% of body weight. (Courtesy of Dr Robert Vernier.)

provoke an effective diuresis. Alternatively, combining a loop diuretic with a thiazide diuretic or with metolazone may overcome diuretic resistance. The characteristics of different diuretics are discussed in Chapter 7. Significant hypovolemia is not often a clinical problem provided that fluid removal is controlled and gradual. Daily weight is the best measurement of progress. Nephrotic children are much more prone to hypovolemic shock than adults. A stepwise approach to diuretic use is required, aiming at fluid removal in adults of no more than 2 kg daily, moving on to the next drug level if this is not achieved (Fig. 16.22).

Correction of Hypoproteinemia

In view of the problems associated with either increased protein administration or dietary protein restriction in nephrotic patients (see previous discussion), adequate dietary protein should be ensured (0.8 to 1 mg/kg/day) with a high carbohydrate intake to maximize utilization of that protein. When there is very heavy proteinuria, the amount of urinary protein loss should be added to dietary protein intake.

In the rare setting where proteinuria is so severe that the patient is dying of the complications of nephrotic syndrome, one may have to resort to nephrectomy to prevent continued protein losses. This may be done as a medical nephrectomy: the deliberate use of NSAIDs combined with ACE inhibitors and diuretic to lessen proteinuria by provoking ARF. If medical nephrectomy alone does not adequately reduce proteinuria, bilateral renal artery embolization can be considered. It may be a painful procedure and is not always as successful as might be expected (perhaps because of collateral arterial supply to the kidneys, which is not blocked by the embolization). A final alternative is bilateral nephrectomy, which carries significant mortality in these severely ill hypoproteinemic patients and is rarely used in adults, although it is a conventional part of management of infants with congenital nephrotic syndrome.

Treatment of Hypercoagulability

The risk of thrombotic events becomes progressively more important as serum albumin values decrease to <2.5 g/dl. Immobility

as a consequence of edema or intercurrent illness further aggravates the risk. Prophylactic low-dose anticoagulation (e.g., heparin 5000 units subcutaneously twice daily) is indicated at times of high risk such as relative immobilization in hospital and albumin levels between 2 and 2.5 g/dl. Full-dose anticoagulation with low molecular weight heparin or warfarin (Coumadin) should be considered if serum albumin decreases to <2 g/dl[25] and is mandatory if a thrombosis or pulmonary embolism is documented. Heparin is used for initial anticoagulation, but an increased dose may be needed since part of the action of heparin depends on antithrombin III, which is often reduced in the plasma in nephrotic patients. Warfarin (Coumadin; target international normalized ratio 2 to 3) is the long-term treatment of choice but should be manipulated with special care because of altered protein binding, which may require dose reductions.

Management of Infection

A high order of clinical suspicion for infection is vital in nephrotic patients. Especially in nephrotic children, ascitic fluid should be examined microscopically and cultured if there is any suspicion of systemic infection. Bacteremia is common even if clinical signs

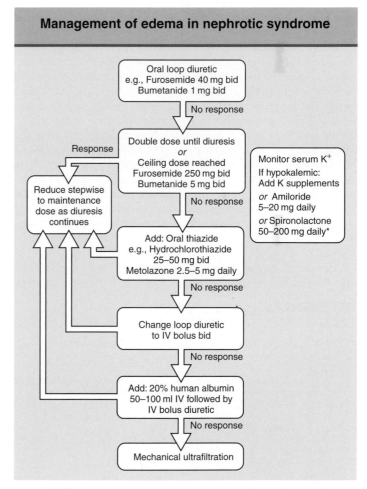

Figure 16.22 Management of edema in nephrotic syndrome. Edema is often diuretic resistant, but the response is not predictable. Therefore, stepwise escalation of therapy is appropriate until diuresis occurs. Even when there is anasarca, diuresis should not proceed faster than 2 kg/day in adults to minimize the risk of clinically significant hypovolemia. Mechanical ultrafiltration is rarely required for nephrotic edema unless there is associated renal insufficiency. *Spironolactone is less effective in nephrotic syndrome than in cirrhosis and is often poorly tolerated because of gastrointestinal side effects.

are localized. ESR is unhelpful, but an elevated C-reactive protein may be more informative. Parenteral antibiotics should be started once cultures are taken, and the regimen should include benzylpenicillin (to cover pneumococci). If repeated infections occur, serum immunoglobulins should be measured. If serum IgG is <600 mg/dl, there is evidence in an uncontrolled study that infection risk is reduced by monthly administration of intravenous immunoglobulin 10 to 15 g to keep the IgG levels >600 mg/dl.[26]

Disease-Specific Therapies

Specific treatments for glomerular diseases are discussed in the subsequent chapters; the general principles are discussed here. As most glomerular disease is thought to have an immune pathogenesis, treatment has generally consisted of immunosuppressive therapy aimed at blocking both the systemic and local effects. In the setting where glomerular disease results from an ineffectual elimination of a foreign antigen, treatment involves measures to eliminate this antigen whenever possible (such as antibiotics in endocarditis-associated GN or interferon-α for cryoglobulinemia associated with hepatitis C infection).

In general, the more severe and acute the presentation of GN, the more successful is immune treatment; there has been little success for immunosuppression in chronic GN. In situations where renal function is declining rapidly, there is little to lose and the toxicity of intensive regimens becomes acceptable for a short period but would be unacceptable if prolonged. Furthermore, the nonspecific nature of most immune treatments results in widespread interruption of immune and inflammatory events at multiple levels. In the acute situation, this broad-based attack is a virtue; in more indolent disease, more specific treatment is needed but is unavailable. Despite great increases in the understanding of immune mechanisms in glomerular disease since the 1970s, immune therapies have not yet become more specific and precise. The mainstays of treatment remain agents that were available in the 1960s: corticosteroids, azathioprine, and cyclophosphamide. Other newer immunosuppressive agents developed for use in transplantation, including cyclosporine, tacrolimus, mycophenolate, and rapamycin, or those developed in oncology, including rituximab, have emerging indications in glomerular disease.

The use of immunosuppressive therapies to treat GN has certain drawbacks. In many diseases, treatment is based on small series, and good prospective controlled trials are lacking. Because of both the rarity and the variable natural history of GN, proof of efficacy for a particular therapy often requires a multicenter approach with prolonged follow-up, which is logistically difficult. It should also be recognized that if sufficient glomerular damage is present, proteinuria and progressive deterioration of renal function may occur by nonimmune pathways that may not be responsive to immunosuppressive therapies. Unfortunately, good noninvasive markers to assess disease activity are missing in most clinical circumstances. Given the frequent uncertainty of the response to immunosuppressive therapy, it becomes mandatory to weigh the potential benefits against the risks of therapy.

Immunosuppression may be associated with reactivation of tuberculosis and hepatitis B infection and can also lead to a hyperinfection syndrome in patients with *Strongyloides* species infection. Therefore, high-risk patents should be screened for these diseases prior to embarking on therapy.

Alkylating agents, such as cyclophosphamide and chlorambucil, have considerable toxicity. In the short term, leukopenia is common, as is alopecia, although hair will regrow within a few months of discontinuing therapy. These agents can cause infertility (observed in adults with cumulative doses of cyclophosphamide >200 mg/kg and chlorambucil 10 mg/kg). There is also an increased incidence of leukemias (observed with total doses of cyclophosphamide >80 g and chlorambucil 7 g). Cyclophosphamide is also a bladder irritant, and treatment can result in hemorrhagic cystitis and bladder carcinoma, particularly after therapy lasting more than 6 months.[27] Irritation of the bladder is caused by a metabolite, acrolein. The effect can be minimized in patients receiving IV cyclophosphamide by enforcing a good diuresis and administering mesna. The dose of mesna (mg) should equal the dose of cyclophosphamide (mg); 20% is given intravenously with the IV cyclophosphamide, and the remaining 80% should be given in two equal oral doses at 2 and 6 hours by IV infusion at the same dose as the cyclophosphamide. Chlorambucil and cyclophosphamide also require dose reduction in the setting of renal insufficiency. Given all these concerns, oral treatment with these agents should ideally be limited to 12 weeks.

The modes of action and potential adverse effects of corticosteroids, azathioprine, and other immunosuppressives occasionally used in glomerular disease are discussed further in Chapter 90.

REFERENCES

1. Iseki K, Iseki C, Ikemiya Y, Fukiyama K: Risk of developing end-stage renal disease in a cohort of mass screening. Kidney Int 1996;49:800–805.
2. Topham PS, Harper SJ, Furness PN, et al: Glomerular disease as a cause of isolated microscopic haematuria. Q J Med 1994;87:329–336.
3. Springberg PD, Garrett LE, Thompson AL, et al: Fixed and reproducible orthostatic proteinuria. Results of a 20 year follow up study. Ann Intern Med 1982;97:516–519.
4. Orth SR, Ritz E: The nephrotic syndrome. N Engl J Med 1998;338:1201–1212.
5. Cameron JS: Nephrotic syndrome in the elderly. Semin Nephrol 1996;16:319–329.
6. Haas M, Meehan SM, Karison TG, Spargo BH: Changing etiologies of unexplained adult nephrotic syndrome: A comparison of renal biopsy findings from 1976–1979 and 1995–1997. Am J Kidney Dis 1997;30:621–631.
7. Kaysen G, Gambertoglio J, Felts J, Hutchison F: Albumin synthesis, albuminuria and hyperlipidemia in nephrotic syndrome. Kidney Int 1987;31:1368–1376.
8. Humphreys MH: Mechanisms and management of nephrotic edema. Kidney Int 1994;45:266–281.
9. Rodriguez-Iturbe B, Herrera-Acosta J, Johnson RJ: Interstitial inflammation, sodium retention and the pathogenesis of nephrotic edema. Kidney Int 2002;62:1379–1384.
10. Rabelink TJ, Zwaginga JJ, Koomans HA, Sixma JJ: Thrombosis and hemostasis in renal disease. Kidney Int 1994;46:287–296.
11. Wheeler DC, Bernard DB: Lipid abnormalities in nephrotic syndrome. Am J Kidney Dis 1994;23:331–346.
12. Fried LF, Orchard TJ, Kasiske BL: Effect of lipid reduction on the progression of renal disease: A meta-analysis. Kidney Int 2001;59:260–269.
13. Smith JD, Hayslett JP: Reversible renal failure in the nephrotic syndrome. Am J Kidney Dis 1992;19:201–213.
14. Jennette JC, Falk RJ: Adult minimal change glomerulopathy with acute renal failure. Am J Kidney Dis 1990;16:432–437.
15. Lowenstein J, Schacht RG, Baldwin DS: Renal failure in minimal change nephritic syndrome. Am J Med 1981;70:227–233.
16. Burton C, Harris KPG: The role of proteinuria in the progression of chronic renal failure. Am J Kidney Dis 1996;27:765–775.

17. Wilmer WA, Rovin BH, Hebert CJ, et al: Management of glomerular proteinuria: A commentary. J Am Soc Nephrol 2003;14:3217–3232.

18. Klahr S, Levey AS, Beck GJ, et al: The effects of dietary protein restriction and blood pressure control on the progression of chronic renal disease. N Engl J Med 1994;330:877–884.

19. National Health and Nutritional Examination Survey: The Sixth Report of the Joint National Committee on Prevention, Detection, Evaluation and Treatment of High Blood Pressure. Arch Intern Med 1997;157: 2413–2415.

20. Maschio G, Alberti D, Janin G, et al: Effect of the angiotensin-converting-enzyme inhibitor, benazepril, on the progression of chronic renal insufficiency. N Engl J Med 1996;334:939–945.

21. The GISEN Group: Randomised placebo-controlled trial of effect of ramipril on decline in glomerular filtration rate and risk of terminal renal failure in proteinuric, non-diabetic nephropathy. Lancet 1997;349: 1857–1863.

22. Jafar TH, Schmid CH, Landa M, et al: Angiotensin-converting enzyme inhibitors and progression of non-diabetic renal disease. A meta-analysis of patient-level data. Ann Intern Med 2001;135:73–87.

23. Nakao N, Yoshimura A, Morita H, et al: Combination treatment of angiotensin-II receptor blocker and angiotensin-converting enzyme inhibitor in non-diabetic renal disease [COOPERATE]: A randomised controlled trial. Lancet 2003;361:117–134.

24. Maroni BJ, Staffield C, Young VR, et al: Mechanisms permitting nephrotic patients to achieve nitrogen equilibrium with a protein restricted diet. J Clin Invest 1997;99:2479–2487.

25. Sarasin FP, Schifferli JA: Prophylactic oral anticoagulation in nephrotic patients with idiopathic membranous nephropathy. Kidney Int 1994;45: 578–585.

26. Ogi M, Yokoyama H, Tomosui N, et al: Risk factors for infection and immunoglobulin replacement therapy in adult nephrotic syndrome. Am J Kidney Dis 1994;24:427–436.

27. Talar-Williams C, Hijazi C, Walther M, et al: Cyclophosphamide-induced cystitis and bladder cancer in patients with Wegener's granulomatosis. Ann Intern Med 1996;124:477–484.

INTRODUCTION AND DEFINITIONS

Minimal change disease (MCD) is the cause of the nephrotic syndrome in about 90% of children aged younger than 10 years, about 50% to 70% of older children, and 10% to 15% of adults. It is defined by the absence of histologic glomerular abnormality, other than ultrastructural evidence of epithelial cell foot process fusion, in a patient presenting with nephrotic syndrome who is typically corticosteroid responsive. Corticosteroid-responsive or corticosteroid-sensitive nephrotic syndrome are the terms used to describe the disease occurring in children with nephrotic syndrome who respond to corticosteroids but have not had a renal biopsy to provide the histologic proof of MCD. The presence of the nephrotic syndrome is important because similar histopathologic appearances may be seen in patients with proteinuria in the absence of nephrotic syndrome. Such patients may have different conditions with different prognoses and requirements for management.

The relationship between MCD, focal segmental glomerulosclerosis (FSGS; see Chapter 18), and IgM nephropathy (see later discussion) is poorly defined. Corticosteroid responsiveness is a shared feature, although there is increasing steroid resistance as one moves from MCD to IgM nephropathy to FSGS (Fig. 17.1). The lesions may form part of a continuum, and some believe that FSGS develops in a proportion of patients with MCD, while others believe that they have different causes. Undoubtedly, some patients with FSGS behave as if they had MCD, and it is possible that the segmental lesions may be coincidental, especially in adults older than 40 years of age in whom sclerotic lesions become increasingly common. There have been some reports that increased expression of transforming growth factor β may distinguish between prognostic groups,[1] but more studies are needed to confirm these claims. Operationally a distinction is unnecessary, at least for the initial phase of management.

ETIOLOGY AND PATHOGENESIS

In a minority of patients with MCD, there is a clear association with a factor that appears to provoke the nephrotic syndrome (Fig. 17.2).

In normal glomeruli, the barrier to protein filtration is provided by a combination of size barriers and charge selectivity. Neutral molecules larger than 4 to 4.5 nm are excluded; although albumin molecules are smaller than this, they are excluded because they are anionic and are repelled by the negative charge on the epithelial cells and glomerular basement membrane (GBM; mainly

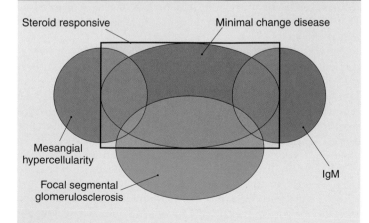

Histologic patterns and steroid responsiveness in diseases causing nephrotic syndrome

Steroid responsive   Minimal change disease

Mesangial hypercellularity

Focal segmental glomerulosclerosis

IgM

Figure 17.1 Histologic patterns and corticosteroid responsiveness in nephrotic syndrome. The interrelationships between corticosteroid responsiveness and minimal change disease, focal segmental glomerulosclerosis, mesangial hypercellularity, and mesangial IgM deposition.

Factors associated with the onset of nephrotic syndrome in minimal change disease
Drugs
Nonsteroidal anti-inflammatory drugs
Interferon-α
Lithium: rare (usually causes chronic interstitial nephritis)
Gold: rare (usually causes membranous nephropathy)
Allergy
Pollens
House dust
Insect stings
Immunizations
Malignancy
Hodgkin's disease
Mycosis fungoides
Chronic lymphocytic leukemia: uncommon (usually associated with membranoproliferative glomerulonephritis)

Figure 17.2 Factors associated with the onset of nephrotic syndrome in minimal change disease.

owing to heparan sulfate). In MCD, FSGS, and some other causes of the nephrotic syndrome, the clearance of small neutral molecules is actually less than normal, suggesting that the massive albumin filtration is primarily the result of loss of GBM surface charge.

Although the injury is manifested as a change in glomerular capillary permeability, it is probable that the underlying problem is toxic epithelial cell injury. There is increasing circumstantial evidence that a circulating factor is involved in the pathogenesis and that there may be an abnormality of cell-mediated immunity. The close clinical relationship between MCD and FSGS has led some to suggest a shared pathogenesis, but the increasing evidence of differences makes this less likely.

MCD is likely to be a systemic condition rather than an intrinsic disease of the kidney and an immune abnormality has been suspected for some time. In the precorticosteroid era, it was observed that the nephrotic syndrome often remitted in children who contracted measles, which is known to have powerful depressive effects on cell-mediated immunity. MCD is also associated with lymphomas (especially Hodgkin's disease) and atopy (up to 30% of children in some series) and responds to immunosuppressive drugs. There are also many reports of abnormal humoral and cellular immunity in patients with MCD during relapse and sometimes in remission as well, but not in those with other causes of nephrotic syndrome. Finally, an association has been reported with HLA-DR7 (in some ethnic groups), at least in corticosteroid-responsive individuals. There are many reports of MCD relapse following vaccination[2] or exposure to an allergen in sensitive individuals. As a result, patients with identified food allergies have been managed with exclusion diets with reported complete or partial remissions and relapse following reintroduction of the offending food. However, even if the relationship is real, it is possible that the allergic events merely trigger relapse, as may infections.

The histopathology does not give any clues to pathogenesis, although the absence of immune deposits implies that immune mechanisms are likely to be cellular rather than humoral. The characteristic podocyte foot process fusion likely represents a manifestation of podocyte injury and is believed to be responsible for proteinuria. However, this hypothesis is challenged by the observations of preserved foot processes in the early phase of some highly proteinuric states (e.g., recurrent FSGS after renal transplantation) and of podocyte foot process fusion in children with severe hypoalbuminemia, but no proteinuria, dying of kwashiorkor.[3] Reduced levels of dystroglycans (adhesion molecules believed to anchor podocytes to the GBM) have been reported in MCD but not in FSGS, with normalization following corticosteroid treatment.[4]

A circulating factor acting on podocytes has not yet been identified. Lymphocyte-derived cytokines were first proposed many years ago but remain elusive, although studies in which the supernatant from T cell hybridomas derived from these patients provokes proteinuria and foot process fusion when infused into rats are suggestive of such a mechanism.[5] Hemopexin, an acute phase reactant extracted from human plasma, is capable of inducing proteinuria in rats,[6] and in one small study, plasma hemopexin activity was increased in MCD patients in relapse with some evidence of an altered isoform.[7] Evidence of a circulating factor in humans is also supported by the observation that proteinuria resolved within days following transplantation from a cadaveric donor with MCD.[8] In view of the identification of mutations in several podocyte proteins in some patients with MCD and the occasional family with more than one affected individual, it has

been suggested that several of these may act as disease-modifying genes influencing response to treatment and possibly the risk of subsequently developing FSGS.

EPIDEMIOLOGY

MCD affects 2 to 7 per 100,000 children per annum, with a prevalence of 15 per 100,000, most commonly presenting between 2 and 7 years of age. It is also an important cause of the nephrotic syndrome in adults of all ages, although the incidence varies geographically: as low as 1 per million in the United Kingdom and up to 27 per million in the United States. It is more common in South Asians and Native Americans but is rarer in Africans, who are much more likely to have corticosteroid-resistant nephrotic syndrome and FSGS. Some data suggest that MCD has recently become less common in children[9] and adults.[10] Boys are twice as likely to be affected as girls, but the sex incidence is equal in adolescents and adults.

CLINICAL MANIFESTATIONS

Typically, patients present with edema that develops over a short period of time, with fluid retention exceeding 3% of the body weight and often very much more. Up to two thirds of presentations and relapses follow an infection, most commonly in the upper respiratory tract, but whether these are of causative significance is uncertain.

The clinical signs and symptoms are the same as those for the nephrotic syndrome from any cause (see Chapter 16), although the nephrotic syndrome is often of very rapid onset, increasing the risk of hypovolemia, particularly in children. Pleural effusions and ascites are common, particularly in children, who may present with abdominal pain, a symptom that may suggest peritonitis or herald hypovolemia. Pericardial effusions may occur, but pulmonary edema is uncommon except following treatment with albumin or with coexisting cardiac disease. Hepatomegaly is frequent in children, and this may be painful. The distribution of the edema is gravitational, but facial puffiness is common and genital swelling may be very uncomfortable, especially in men. Gross edema may predispose to ulceration and infection of dependent skin; striae often appear even without corticosteroids, and lacerations or needlestick punctures weep fluid profusely. Edema of the bowel may cause diarrhea with significant albumin loss from the gut. Other clinical features include white nails, sometimes in bands (Muehrcke's bands) correlating with periods of clinical relapse (see Fig. 16.4). Occasionally, xanthomata are associated with gross hyperlipidemia.

Microscopic hematuria is rare in MCD and although hypertension is not usually regarded as typical, it was a feature at presentation in 30% of 89 adults reported from Guy's Hospital, London, United Kingdom[11]; hypertension has also been described in 14% to 21% of children, when making comparisons with appropriate age- and sex-matched blood pressure reference ranges. This usually resolves during remission, especially in children. Hypertension is sometimes associated with expansion of the intravascular volume but may paradoxically be related to hypovolemia and stimulation of the renin angiotensin axis.

Before the introduction of corticosteroids, the morbidity and mortality of patients with MCD were high because of complications of the nephrotic syndrome, particularly infection. This continues to be a serious problem,[12] and six out of 389 children with MCD reported by the International Study of Kidney Disease in Children in 1984 died of sepsis.[13] Peritonitis is still a major cause of mortality in the developing world, mainly in children. *Streptococcus pneumoniae*, *Haemophilus influenzae*, and other encapsulated bacteria are commonly implicated. Children with persistent nephrotic syndrome should be immunized against *S. pneumoniae* and *H. influenzae* and given prophylactic oral penicillin.[14] Peritonitis is rare in adults, who usually have protective antibodies against these bacteria, and prophylactic antibiotics are not indicated.

The risk of thromboembolism is increased in MCD, as in all nephrotics (see Chapter 16). Venous thromboembolism may occur in the common sites, but nephrotic children occasionally have other catastrophic events such as intracerebral venous thrombosis. Arterial thrombosis is also a rare and feared complication that seems to affect children almost exclusively and may result in loss of limbs.

Renal function is generally preserved, but the creatinine is sometimes slightly elevated in adults. Acute renal failure is a complication particularly seen in adults. It may follow hypovolemia, which should be avoided especially during intensive diuretic treatment, but acute renal failure may also occur in patients who are volume replete (see also Chapter 16).

Non-nephrotic Proteinuria
Identical light microscopic appearances, but usually without the foot process effacement, may be found in adults and children investigated for asymptomatic proteinuria who never become nephrotic.

PATHOLOGY

Classically, MCD is associated with a completely normal appearance in the glomeruli on light microscopy and immunohistology. Podocyte (epithelial cell) foot process effacement seen with electron microscopy (Fig. 17.3) is the only abnormality, but this is a nonspecific finding. The presence of mesangial IgM is considered by some to define a separate entity (see later discussion). Hyaline casts obstructing tubules, foam cells, and occasionally appearances consistent with acute tubular necrosis may be seen, especially if acute renal failure is present at the time of biopsy.

Variants
Mild mesangial hypercellularity is now accepted as an infrequent finding (3% to 5%), and small amounts of mesangial IgG, and

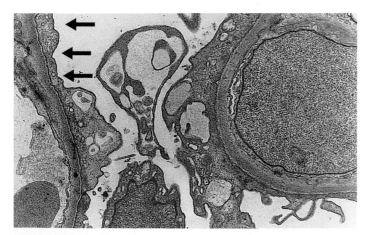

Figure 17.3   Podocyte foot process fusion in minimal change disease. The epithelial cells (*arrows*) are completely effaced along the glomerular basement membranes. (Electron micrograph ×6000.) The normal appearance of epithelial cell foot processes is shown in Figures 1.7 and 1.8 (see Chapter 1).

complement C3, and occasionally IgA are sometimes seen in patients whose clinical course is indistinguishable from classic MCD.

The glomerular tip lesion describes structural segmental changes adjacent to the tubular pole of Bowman's capsule, with protrusion into the tubular lumen. There is considerable controversy surrounding the prognostic significance of the glomerular tip lesion partly because it has been used in several contexts and is seen in other conditions as well as MCD, including membranoproliferative glomerulonephritis, IgA nephropathy, and renal allografts. The most important reason to recognize the lesion is to prevent a misdiagnosis of a proliferative glomerulonephritis.

While the presence of mesangial hypercellularity in MCD may be a better predictor of resistance to corticosteroid therapy and a poor clinical prognosis, attempts to correlate its significance in FSGS have yielded conflicting results.[15] Some consider mesangial hypercellularity to be an intermediate step in the evolution (progression) of MCD to FSGS.

IgM Nephropathy
Some patients presenting with the nephrotic syndrome have mesangial deposits of IgM, often with a minor degree of mesangial hypercellularity. Patients are more likely to have microscopic (and occasionally macroscopic) hematuria and are said to be less likely to respond to corticosteroids (50% compared with 90% for MCD).[16] Others challenge the existence of this condition, pointing out that IgM deposits, at least to some degree, are seen in MCD, FSGS, and mesangial proliferative glomerulonephritis in a similar proportion of patients.

DIAGNOSIS AND DIFFERENTIAL DIAGNOSIS

The clinical diagnosis of nephrotic syndrome is straightforward, with edema in the presence of heavy proteinuria, usually without microscopic hematuria on urine dipstick testing. Urine microscopy reveals hyaline casts and sometimes lipid casts. There is hypoalbuminemia and nephrotic range proteinuria (>3.5 g/24 h in adults or >40 mg/h/m² in children or a protein-to-creatinine ratio of >0.25 g/mmol [>2 mg protein/mg] creatinine on a spot urine) with hyperlipidemia. Hyponatremia and hemoconcentration may be seen, even before treatment. Elevated urea and creatinine concentrations occur more often in adults. Typically, IgG levels are low and IgM is increased. Serum complement levels are normal. In children, corticosteroid-responsive MCD is usually associated with selective proteinuria of smaller molecules including albumin and transferrin but not of larger molecules such as immunoglobulins and ferritin. A selectivity index is usually derived from the ratio of IgG clearance to albumin clearance:

$$\text{selectivity index} = \frac{[(\text{IgG})_u\,(\text{albumin})_s]}{[(\text{IgG})_s\,(\text{albumin})_u]},$$

where subscript u is concentration in urine and s is that in serum. If the selectivity index is <0.1, the proteinuria is highly selective, and if >0.2, it is nonselective. This is of limited clinical value since highly selective proteinuria is less common in adult MCD and does not influence a decision to treat with corticosteroids. However, highly selective proteinuria, when present, does indicate that MCD is more likely to be the diagnosis, and some argue that such patients should be given a trial of corticosteroids without a renal biopsy, especially if the risk of biopsy complications is high.

In children aged 1 to 12 years, renal biopsy is unnecessary unless the patient does not respond to corticosteroid treatment. In adults in whom there is a wide differential diagnosis for the nephrotic syndrome and corticosteroid responsiveness is less likely, a renal biopsy is required to establish the diagnosis. It has been argued that, in the absence of a specific contraindication to corticosteroid therapy, it is safer to give a therapeutic trial of corticosteroids and reserve a renal biopsy for the nonresponders. However, adults with corticosteroid-responsive nephrotic syndrome may take up to 12 weeks to respond, so the morbidity from corticosteroids does become significant, outweighing the risks of a renal biopsy.

NATURAL HISTORY

There is a tendency for patients with MCD to run a relapsing-remitting course, and this is more frequent in children. Those presenting younger are more likely to have a longer disease course before long-term remission occurs (Fig. 17.4). Relapse is common, affecting more than two thirds of children, and nearly 50% will relapse more than four times, usually following corticosteroid cessation or reduction. If relapse occurs during corticosteroid reduction, the patient is described as corticosteroid dependent. Long-term remission can be expected in 75% of initial responders who do not relapse within 6 months, while those who do relapse become nonrelapsing after an average of 3 years and 84% are in long-term remission after 10 years.[17] However, it is reassuring that <5% of children with MCD enter adulthood still having relapses, although the younger the age is at the onset of the first attack, the longer the child is likely to continue having relapses.[18] In general, increasing time since last relapse reduces the risk of further relapse, but occasionally adults will have a relapse after an interval of 10 years or more.

MCD does not progress to renal failure. However, a number of patients with this diagnosis are found to have FSGS on subsequent biopsies and they may develop progressive renal function loss. It is still unclear whether the focal nature of the disease resulted in the correct diagnosis being missed on the initial biopsy or whether evolution from MCD to FSGS does occur.

TREATMENT

Secondary MCD is treated according to the underlying cause and treatment of Hodgkin's disease generally induces remission. Withdrawal of nonsteroidal anti-inflammatory drugs is usually sufficient, and although corticosteroids are frequently given, there is little evidence that they modify the course of the nephrotic syndrome.

In primary cases, corticosteroid treatment induces remission in almost all patients with MCD. Before remission is achieved and in nonresponders, it is important that the general management of the nephrotic syndrome is optimal through control of edema, consideration of prophylactic measures for the thrombotic tendency and infection, control of hypertension, and, in the longer term, control of hyperlipidemia (see Chapter 16).

Although corticosteroids form the core of treatment, at least initially, there is considerable variation in dose and duration recommended, and individual regimens have not been compared in adequate controlled trials. The management guidelines described here are widely, but not universally, accepted. They are justified, where possible, by evidence from clinical trials.

Childhood Minimal Change Disease
Treatment of First Episode
Children should be treated with oral prednisolone 60 mg/m² or 1 mg/kg/day (up to 80 mg) or 2 mg/kg on alternate days (all calculated on the basis of estimated dry weight). About 75% respond within 2 weeks, 80% to 85% within 4 weeks, and >90% within 8 weeks.[16] Corticosteroids should be continued at the initial

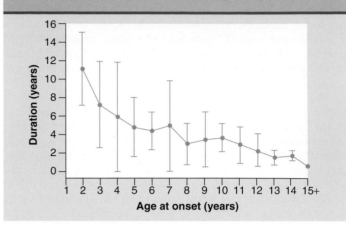

Figure 17.4 Long-term outcome in childhood-onset minimal change disease. The duration of disease is inversely related to the age of presentation. (Adapted from Trompeter RS, Lloyd BW, Hicks J, et al: Long-term outcome for children with minimal change nephrotic syndrome. Lancet 1985;1:368–370.)

dose for an additional 4 weeks once the urine is protein free and then switched to alternate-day dosing for 4 to 8 weeks (see later discussion) followed by subsequent tapering (e.g., reducing every 2 weeks by 15 mg/m² on alternate days until corticosteroid withdrawal is completed). Figure 17.5 shows the treatment algorithm for childhood MCD. The aim of this regimen is to keep patients on corticosteroids for 3 to 4 months since this appears to be associated with a lower 1-year relapse rate compared with children receiving corticosteroids for 2 months or less (19% and 64%, respectively).[19] If proteinuria persists for more than 4 weeks during corticosteroid treatment, there is some anecdotal evidence that increasing the corticosteroid dose or giving an intravenous pulse of methylprednisolone (1 g/1.73 m²) will improve the probability of inducing a remission. Reasons for treatment failure include noncompliance and poor absorption from an edematous bowel, and therefore in the presence of diarrhea, it is logical to give intravenous corticosteroids. Even in the absence of diarrhea, prescription of nonenteric-coated corticosteroid formulations is recommended since occasionally patients will absorb enteric-coated tablets inadequately. Increased appetite, hyperactivity, and mood swings may be particular problems in children taking high-dose corticosteroids.

Diagnosis and Treatment of Relapses
The urine should be (self-)tested daily during and after treatment. The rationale is that relapses should be treated based on proteinuria (usually requiring at least three or more dipstick measurements) for three consecutive days to initiate a further course of corticosteroids. The aim is to treat relapse early to avoid complications.

Management of relapsing children is intended to maintain the child in a non-nephrotic state with the lowest possible dose of corticosteroids. The first relapse is generally treated with a second induction course of corticosteroids, although a shorter course (about 2 weeks at full dose followed by 2 weeks of alternate-day treatment) is probably adequate.[20] Subsequent relapses may be treated similarly or by tapering the prednisolone to 15 mg/m² on alternate days and continuing for 12 to 18 months (assuming this dosage is above the corticosteroid threshold at which relapse occurs in that individual). Clearly, the acceptability of this approach depends on the corticosteroid threshold.

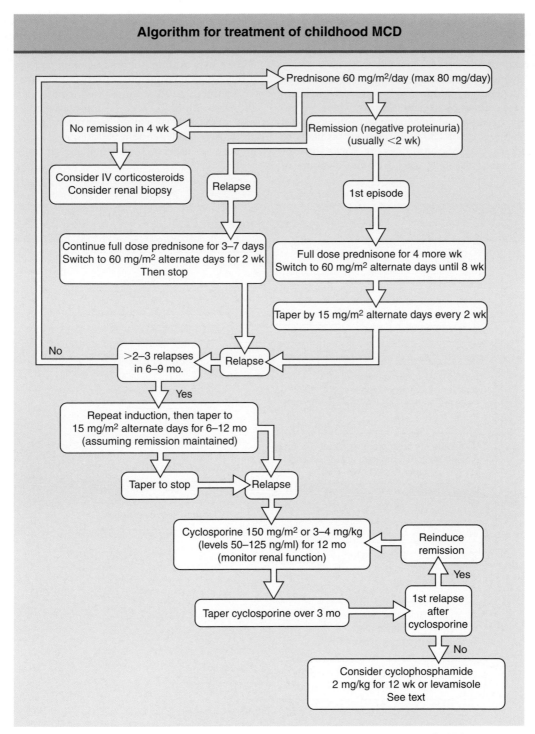

Figure 17.5 Algorithm for treatment of childhood minimal change disease (MCD).

Frequent Relapsers

There is even more variation in the management of frequent relapsers, with a paucity of controlled data, but generally second-line drugs are used to avoid corticosteroid toxicity, most commonly alkylating agents (cyclophosphamide and chlorambucil), levamisole, and cyclosporine. The decision as to when to use these treatments may be difficult. More than two or three relapses within 6 to 9 months might trigger second-line therapy, but this will depend on how quickly steroid-induced remission occurs and how steroids are tolerated. Usually the patient or parents are involved in the decision after considering the potential side effects of the second-line treatment selected.

Alkylating agents were historically used as first-line therapy, although other agents are now usually tried initially. This is mainly because of the potential side effects of alkylating agents (initially infection and alopecia and subsequently sterility,[21] hemorrhagic cystitis, and hematologic malignancy), which although probably minor, especially for a 3-month course, need to be balanced against the fact that MCD is usually self-limiting. In addition, the permanent remission rate is lower in children than in adults. A course of oral cyclophosphamide (2 to 2.5 mg/kg/day) is often effective, and some studies suggest that a 12-week course gives a 2-year remission rate of 60% versus 30% for an 8-week course.[22] Chlorambucil (0.2 mg/kg/day) for 2 months appears to have effects similar to those of cyclophosphamide and, apart from not provoking hemorrhagic cystitis, has the same range of adverse effects, although it is associated with a risk of seizures.[23] Some data suggest that frequent relapsers are more likely to have a long-term remission following an 8-week course of cyclophosphamide than corticosteroid-dependent children (75% versus 35%). There are few data on second courses of alkylating agents, which are not recommended partly because the maximum acceptable cyclophosphamide cumulative dose of 150 to 250 mg/kg[21] is likely to be exceeded and because the response rates are lower than for the initial course. During treatment with cyclophosphamide or chlorambucil, blood counts should be checked weekly and dose reductions made to avoid cytopenias. Herpes zoster infection carries a particular risk for nonimmune children who should receive hyperimmune immunoglobulin and probably valacyclovir if there is an unavoidable contact with active zoster.

Azathioprine has no proven role in the management of children with MCD and was ineffective in a randomized trial. It may perhaps have a place as a corticosteroid-sparing agent in corticosteroid-dependent children resistant to second-line treatments who have to be maintained on long-term alternate-day corticosteroids.

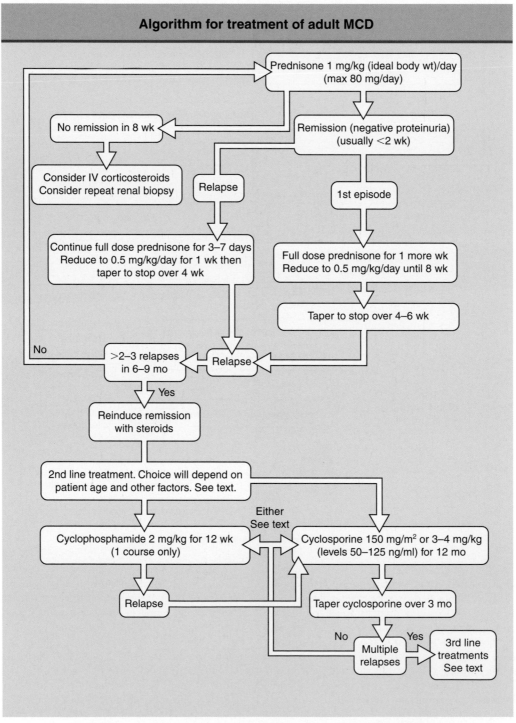

Figure 17.6 Algorithm for treatment of adult minimal change disease (MCD).

Cyclosporine (up to 150 mg/m^2 or 3 to 4 mg/kg/day with trough levels of 50 to 125 ng/ml) is usually effective in children with both corticosteroid-dependent and frequently relapsing nephrotic syndrome.[24] However, relapse is almost invariable within 3 months of stopping treatment. If there is no response, increasing the dose of cyclosporine is sometimes effective, but there is a risk of cyclosporine nephrotoxicity even with low-dose regimens and careful monitoring of blood levels, glomerular filtration rate, and blood pressure. The aim of therapy is that cyclosporine will maintain remission without corticosteroids until the underlying disease remits. The optimal duration of therapy is not established, but treatment for 1 year followed by its slow withdrawal is a well-used regimen.

Levamisole, an antihelminthic drug, has also been used successfully (2.5 mg/kg on alternate days for 3 months),[25,26] but most patients relapse within 3 months of stopping the drug. Nevertheless, as with cyclosporine, it may provide a relatively nontoxic alternative to corticosteroids until spontaneous remission of the condition eventually occurs.

Newer Agents

Patients not responding to the established treatments are increasingly being tried on newer agents, including tacrolimus and mycophenolate. The anecdotal and uncontrolled results published so far do not suggest that they are especially effective. Pending trial data, these should not be used as first- or second-line treatment.

Adult Minimal Change Disease

There are fewer good studies comparing different corticosteroid regimens in adults with MCD, and conventional treatment recommendations are extrapolated from successful approaches in children, although using slightly lower doses of oral prednisolone (1 mg/kg/day, up to 80 mg/day; Fig. 17.6). Response is often delayed in comparison with children, and 25% fail to remit after 3 to 4 months (Fig. 17.7).[11] The reasons for this are unclear. It has been suggested that many adults are often given a smaller dose of corticosteroids, a maximum of prednisolone 60 mg/day rather than 1 mg/kg/day, or it may be that a greater proportion of adults have FSGS, missed on the original biopsy, which is more likely to be corticosteroid resistant. The prednisolone should be reduced to a half dose 1 week after remission (the absence of protein on urine dipstick) for 4 to 6 weeks, followed by tailing off over an additional 4 to 6 weeks, aiming, as in children, for a total initial corticosteroid course of at least 4 months (although this principle is not evidence based).

Frequent Relapsers

Adults relapse less often than children (30% to 50%). Like children, some adults will develop transient non-nephrotic relapses. Treatment, initially a repeat course of corticosteroids, should await firm evidence of relapse with more than five consecutive days of proteinuria (>2+ on urine dipstick) and a

Steroid response in minimal change disease

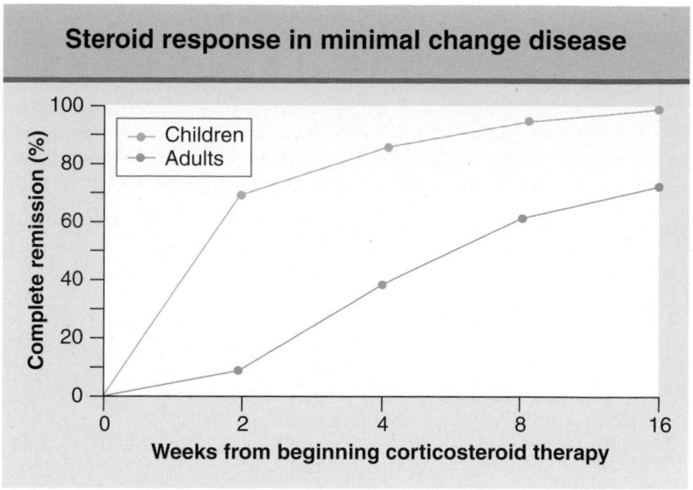

Figure 17.7 Corticosteroid response in adults and children with minimal change disease. Adults with the nephrotic syndrome and minimal change disease take longer to respond and are less likely to remit than children. (From Nolasco F, Cameron JS, Heywood EF, et al: Adult-onset minimal change nephrotic syndrome: A long term follow-up. Kidney Int 1986;29:1215–1223.)

significant weight gain and/or the development of edema. Frequently relapsing and corticosteroid-dependent patients should be treated with cyclophosphamide, which induces a permanent remission more often in adults than in children (75% and 66% at 2 and 5 years, respectively).[11] Although there are no satisfactory studies comparing 8- and 12-week courses in adults, a 12-week course may be logical by extension of the pediatric experience, especially since adults may be less susceptible to gonadal damage, and men can be given the opportunity to bank sperm prior to treatment.

For patients who relapse after cyclophosphamide treatment, cyclosporine (4 to 6 mg/kg/day) is also effective, but relapse usually follows dose reduction or withdrawal. It is worth considering as a short- to medium-term management strategy since there is evidence that remission eventually occurs in 50% to 75% of patients even without treatment.[11] However, careful monitoring is required since nephrotoxicity is common after more than 1 year of treatment.[27] Some nephrologists prefer to try this before cyclophosphamide, especially in younger adults. Several uncontrolled reports suggest that mycophenolate mofetil may also have a place in managing corticosteroid- and cyclosporine-dependent patients,[28-30] but tacrolimus does not appear to be more effective than cyclosporine.

Minimal Change Disease with Non-nephrotic Proteinuria

This should not be treated except for controlling hypertension if present (usually with an angiotensin-converting enzyme inhibitor or angiotensin II receptor antagonist), with long-term monitoring to detect increasing proteinuria or renal impairment, in which case a repeat biopsy is usually indicated.

REFERENCES

1. Strehlau J, Schachter AD, Pavlakis M, et al: Activated intrarenal transcription of CTL-effectors and TGF-beta1 in children with focal segmental glomerulosclerosis. Kidney Int 2002;61:90–95.
2. Abeyagunawardena AS, Goldblatt D, Andrews N, Trompeter RS: Risk of relapse after meningococcal C conjugate vaccine in nephrotic syndrome. Lancet 2003;362:449–450.
3. Golden MH, Brooks SE, Ramdath DD, Taylor E: Effacement of glomerular foot processes in kwashiorkor. Lancet. 1990;336:1472–1474.
4. Regele HM, Fillipovic E, Langer B, et al: Glomerular expression of dystroglycans is reduced in minimal change nephrosis but not in focal segmental glomerulosclerosis. J Am Soc Nephrol 2000;11:403–412.
5. Koyama A, Fujisaka M, Kobayashi M, et al: A glomerular permeability factor produced by human T cell hybridomas. Kidney Int 1991;40:453–460.
6. Cheung PK, Klok PA, Baller JF, Bakker WW: Induction of experimental proteinuria in vivo following infusion of human plasma hemopexin. Kidney Int 2000;57:4512–4520.

7. Bakker WW, van Dael CM, Pierik LJ, et al: Altered activity of plasma hemopexin in patients with minimal change disease in relapse. Pediatr Nephrol 2005;20:10410–10415.

8. Ali AA, Wilson E, Moorhead JF, et al: Minimal-change glomerular nephritis: Normal kidneys in an abnormal environment? Transplantation 1994;58:849–852.

9. Srivastava T, Simon SD, Alon US: High incidence of focal segmental glomerulosclerosis in nephrotic syndrome of childhood. Pediatr Nephrol 1999;13:13–18.

10. Haas M, Meehan SM, Karrison TG, Spargo BH: Changing etiologies of unexplained adult nephrotic syndrome: A comparison of renal biopsy findings from 1976–1979 and 1995–1997. Am J Kidney Dis 1997;30:521–531.

11. Nolasco F, Cameron JS, Heywood EF, et al: Adult-onset minimal change nephrotic syndrome: A long term follow-up. Kidney Int 1986;29:1215–1223.

12. Feinstein EI, Chesney RW, Zelikovic I: Peritonitis in childhood renal disease. Am J Nephrol 1988;8:247–265.

13. International Study of Kidney Disease in Children: Minimal change nephrotic syndrome in children: Deaths during the first 5 to 15 years' observation: Report of the International Study of Kidney Disease in Children. Pediatrics 1984;73:497–501.

14. Overturf GD: American Academy of Pediatrics: Committee on Infectious Diseases: Technical report: Prevention of pneumococcal infections, including the use of pneumococcal conjugate and polysaccharide vaccines and antibiotic prophylaxis. Pediatrics 2000;106:367–376.

15. Border WA: Distinguishing minimal change disease from mesangial disorders. Kidney Int 1988;34:419–434.

16. The primary nephrotic syndrome in children: Identification of patients with minimal change nephrotic syndrome from initial response to prednisone: A report of the International Study of Kidney Disease in Children. J Pediatr 1981;98:461–464.

17. Tarshish P, Tobin JN, Bernstein J, et al: Prognostic significance of the early course of minimal change nephrotic syndrome: Report of the International Study of Kidney Disease in Children. J Am Soc Nephrol 1997;8:769–776.

18. Trompeter RS, Lloyd BW, Hicks J, et al: Long-term outcome for children with minimal change nephrotic syndrome. Lancet 1985;1:368–370.

19. Hodson EM, Knight JF, Willis NS, Craig JC: Corticosteroid therapy for nephrotic syndrome in children (Cochrane Review). Cochrane Database Syst Rev 2001;2:CD001533.

20. Mendoza SA, Tune BM: Treatment of childhood nephrotic syndrome. J Am Soc Nephrol 1992;3:889–894.

21. Trompeter RS, Evans PR, Barratt TM: Gonadal function in boys with steroid-responsive nephrotic syndrome treated with cyclophosphamide for short periods. Lancet 1981;1:1177–1179.

22. Arbeitsgemeinschaft für Padiatrische Nephrologie: Cyclophosphamide treatment of steroid-dependent nephrotic syndrome: Comparison of eight weeks with 12 weeks course. Arch Dis Child 1987;62:1102–1106.

23. Latta K, von Schnakenburg C, Ehrich JH: A meta-analysis of cytotoxic treatment for frequently relapsing nephrotic syndrome in children. Pediatr Nephrol 2001;16:371–382.

24. Durkan AM, Hodson EM, Willis NS, Craig JC: Immunosuppressive agents in childhood nephrotic syndrome: A meta–analysis of randomized controlled trials. Kidney Int 2001;59:1919–1927.

25. British Association for Paediatric Nephrology: Levamisole for corticosteroid-dependent nephrotic syndrome in childhood. Lancet 1991;337:1555–1557.

26. Al-Saran K, Mirza K, Al-Ghanam G, Abdelkarim M: Experience with levamisole in frequently relapsing, steroid–dependent nephrotic syndrome. Pediatr Nephrol 2006;21:201–205.

27. Melocoton TL, Vanni ES, Cohen AS, Fine RN: Long-term cyclosporin A treatment of steroid-resistant nephrotic and steroid-dependent nephrotic syndrome. Am J Kidney Dis 1991;18:583–538.

28. Choi MJ, Eustace JA, Gimenez LF, et al: Mycophenolate mofetil treatment for primary glomerular diseases. Kidney Int 2002;61:1098–1114.

29. Day CJ, Cockwell P, Lipkin GW, et al: Mycophenolate mofetil in the treatment of resistant idiopathic nephrotic syndrome. Nephrol Dial Transplant 2002;17:2011–2113.

30. Bagga A, Hari P, Moudgil A, Jordan SC: Mycophenolate mofetil and prednisolone therapy in children with steroid-dependent nephrotic syndrome. Am J Kidney Dis 2003;42:114–120.

Focal Segmental Glomerulosclerosis: Genetic and Spontaneous Causes

Gerald B. Appel, Martin R. Pollak, and Vivette D'Agati

INTRODUCTION AND DEFINITION

Focal segmental glomerulosclerosis (FSGS), a histologic pattern of glomerular injury, defines a number of clinicopathologic syndromes that may be primary (idiopathic) or secondary to diverse etiologies.[1-4] Early in the disease process, the pattern of glomerular sclerosis is focal, involving a minority of glomeruli, and segmental, involving a portion of the glomerular tuft.[4,5] As the disease progresses, more diffuse and global glomerulosclerosis evolves. Alterations of the podocyte cytoarchitecture are the major ultrastructural findings. Although FSGS accounts for only a small percentage of cases of idiopathic nephrotic syndrome in children, it comprises as many as 35% of cases in adults.[3] It is a common cause of progressive renal disease and end-stage renal disease (ESRD) in certain populations.[6] Different pathogenetic mechanisms are clearly involved in the primary and various secondary forms of the disease.[5] It appears that the pattern of FSGS seen on biopsy represents a common pathway for a number of distinct entities with differing clinical courses and pathogenetic mechanisms. Although primary FSGS is potentially treatable and curable in many patients, the optimal type and duration of immunosuppressive therapy, as well as adjunctive therapy, remain controversial. Effective therapy to modify the course of many patients with secondary forms of FSGS exists as well.

ETIOLOGY AND PATHOGENESIS

Although FSGS was once thought to be a single disease entity, it has become clear that it represents a common phenotypic expression of diverse clinicopathologic syndromes with distinct etiologies (Fig. 18.1). Disorders as diverse as those associated with genetic mutations, circulating permeability factors or maladaptive responses involving glomerular hypertension/hyperfiltration can result in similar histologic and clinical manifestations within the FSGS disease spectrum.

Minimal Change Disease versus Focal Segmental Glomerulosclerosis

By definition, the etiology of idiopathic or primary FSGS is unknown. Clinical data in some patients support similar etiologic factors as those operant in minimal change disease (MCD; see Chapter 17).[3] Some FSGS patients who are initially steroid responsive and have what appears to be MCD on initial renal biopsy, will relapse and be found on repeat biopsy to have lesions of FSGS. In some FSGS patients, this may just represent a sampling error in the initial renal biopsy owing to failure to obtain glomeruli with diagnostic segmental lesions because these may be limited to the deep juxtamedullary glomeruli early in the disease. However, in other patients with well-documented repeated relapses of the nephrotic syndrome and multiple biopsies over many years, the FSGS pattern appears to have truly evolved from an initial MCD pattern. The relatedness of these two diseases is further supported by the observation that the nonsclerotic glomeruli of idiopathic FSGS resemble glomeruli from patients with MCD in that they exhibit minimal abnormalities by light

Etiologic classification of focal segmental glomerulosclerosis
Primary (Idiopathic) FSGS (see Fig. 18.2)
Secondary FSGS

1. Familial FSGS
    A. Mutations in α-actinin 4 (autosomal dominant)
    B. Mutations in podocin (autosomal recessive)
    C. Mutations in TRPC6 (autosomal dominant)

2. Virus associated
    A. HIV (HIV-associated nephropathy)
    B. Parvovirus B19

3. Drug toxicity
    A. Heroin (heroin nephropathy)
    B. Pamidronate
    C. Lithium
    D. Interferon-α

4. Secondary FSGS mediated by adaptive structural-functional responses
    A. Reduced renal mass
        Oligomeganephronia
        Unilateral renal agenesis
        Renal dysplasia
        Reflux nephropathy
        Sequela to cortical necrosis
        Surgical renal ablation
        Chronic allograft nephropathy
        Any advanced renal disease with reduction in functioning nephrons
 	
    B. Initially normal renal mass
        Hypertension
        Atheroemboli or other acute vaso-occlusive processes
        Obesity
        Cyanotic congenital heart disease
        Sickle cell anemia

Figure 18.1   Etiologic classification of focal segmental glomerulosclerosis (FSGS). HIV, human immunodeficiency virus.

microscopy and diffuse effacement of foot processes by electron microscopy.[5]

As in MCD, in FSGS there is evidence that loss of the glomerular capillary wall charge barrier allows negatively charged albumin to leak into Bowman's space. The alterations in glomerular capillary wall permeability may occur in response to lymphokine production or other circulating humoral mechanisms. Circulating permeability factors that promote *in vitro* permeability of glomeruli to albumin have been found in the plasma of some FSGS patients.[7] The presence of such permeability factors, although only partially defined biochemically, has been used to predict the recurrence of FSGS in transplanted FSGS patients.[8] The fact that some FSGS patients with recurrence of the nephrotic syndrome following transplantation achieve remissions of proteinuria and the nephrotic syndrome following plasma exchange or use of a protein A adsorption column supports the presence of a circulating factor in the pathogenesis of the proteinuria.[9,10]

While there are similarities between MCD and FSGS, the proteinuria in FSGS is often less selective than in MCD. This implies leakage of higher molecular weight macromolecules through "larger pores" in the glomerular basement membrane (GBM).[11] In some toxin-induced animal models of FSGS, such as puromycin or adriamycin nephrosis, nonselective proteinuria develops in conjunction with detachment of the visceral epithelial foot processes from the GBM. Rats injected with sera from patients with idiopathic collapsing FSGS developed proteinuria, glomerular tuft retraction, and podocyte damage, changes that were not seen in rats injected with sera from patients with other FSGS variants or normal controls.[12] The damage was lessened by removing IgG from the FSGS sera. This implies there may be more than one circulating factor involved in the proteinuria of FSGS patients: one related to IgG and a second independent one.

In idiopathic FSGS evaluated early in the course of the disease and in many secondary forms of FSGS, such as obesity-related focal sclerosis, there is initially a high glomerular filtration rate (GFR), supporting roles for hyperfiltration and increased intracapillary glomerular pressures as mediators of FSGS.[13] Likewise, in secondary forms of FSGS with reduced nephron numbers, maladaptive hemodynamic alterations may be associated with glomerular hyperfiltration and increased intraglomerular capillary pressures leading to proteinuria and the segmental glomerulosclerosis.[14] Glomerulomegaly (glomerular hypertrophy) is a common feature of these forms of secondary FSGS, as in patients with remnant kidneys or obesity.[15] Other factors such as intraglomerular coagulation and abnormalities of lipid metabolism may contribute to the glomerulosclerosis in these patients. Recently, secondary FSGS has been reported in nonobese, highly muscular patients with elevated body mass index due to bodybuilding.[16] Biopsies resemble obesity-related glomerulopathy with hypertrophied glomeruli and secondary FSGS, supporting a hyperfiltration mechanism.

Genetic Variants of Focal Segmental Glomerulosclerosis

The pathogenesis of secondary forms of FSGS may be very different from that of idiopathic FSGS. Indeed, various secondary forms clearly have different pathogenetic mechanisms that lead to the same FSGS phenotype. Several different genetic mutations are associated with a FSGS phenotype.[17–20] Most have been related to defects in structural proteins of the visceral epithelial cells and slit diaphragms (see Fig. 15.6). Defects in the *NPHS2* gene result in abnormalities in the encoded protein podocin, a

membrane protein associated with the podocyte slit diaphragm, which, through its interaction with nephrin and CD2AP, has an important role in maintaining glomerular capillary permselectivity.[17,19] *NPHS2* genetic mutations have been found in familial autosomal recessive FSGS in children with steroid-resistant nephrotic syndrome. Mutations in *NPHS2* have also been found in children and adults with sporadic steroid-resistant FSGS and less commonly in some patients who are steroid and cyclosporine responsive.[21–23] The incidence of these genetic abnormalities is much higher in patients with familial histories of FSGS and in children and young adults. Approximately 20% to 30% of sporadic childhood FSGS in fact results from *NPHS2* mutations. Using biopsy specimens of patients with *NPHS2* mutations, abnormal expression and/or localization of podocin was documented as well as changes in the distribution of nephrin, CD2AP, and α-actinin 4 with mislocalization to the podocyte cell body.[24] Thus, genetic *NPHS2* mutations result in major changes in the expression and distribution of both podocin and other structural podocyte proteins. Mutant missense podocin cDNA constructs transfected into human embryonic kidney cells as opposed to wild-type podocin do not localize to the plasma membrane.[25] There are attendant alterations in wild-type nephrin trafficking. Although mutations in both *NPHS1* (nephrin) alleles cause an extreme form of nephrosis (i.e., Finnish-type congenital nephrotic syndrome) rather than FSGS, this is likely due to the severity of the slit-diaphragm lesion, which leads to approximately 20 to 30 g of proteinuria present at birth in affected infants. Compound heterozygous mutations in small numbers of tested adults also have been linked to steroid-resistant FSGS.[23]

Defects in the α-actinin 4 gene lead to an autosomal dominant transmission of FSGS and subnephrotic proteinuria.[18–20] All disease-associated α-actinin 4 mutations identified to date show altered cellular localization and actin binding.[26] Mice that lack α-actinin 4 or carry disease-associated point mutations develop phenotypes similar to those in human FSGS.[27]

Recently, a genetic defect in the transient receptor potential cation 6 channel (TRPC6 channel) has also been found in autosomal dominant familial FSGS. This nonselective cation channel is also found in the podocytes and appears to associate with nephrin and podocin.[28,29] Of the TRPC6 mutations reported to date, some, but not all, cause the encoded channel to have increased current amplitude, consistent with a gain-of-function effect.

In cases of primary FSGS, a genetic predisposition may underlie a susceptibility for a "second-hit" phenomenon when patients' immune systems are stimulated by viral or other insults that lead to the initiation of the disease process. The known FSGS susceptibility genes account for only a fraction of familial cases. It is unclear to what extent these genetic variants contribute to sporadic FSGS and perhaps increase the susceptibility to secondary forms of FSGS as well.

Viral Induction of Focal Segmental Glomerulosclerosis

Although a number of studies have noted a relationship between prior viral infection with parvovirus or other viruses and FSGS, the data have been far from consistent.[30,31] In some studies, parvovirus B19 has been demonstrated in almost 80% of biopsies and >85% of the blood samples from patients with idiopathic collapsing FSGS. However, the incidence of parvovirus infection in the general population is high and the specificity of this viral pathogen for development of collapsing FSGS has not been confirmed.

On the contrary, there is a wealth of clinical, histologic, and experimental data on FSGS associated with human immunodeficiency virus (HIV) infection[32–34] (see Chapter 25). Mice transgenic for a noninfectious HIV genome (with deletion of gag and pol, but expressing the HIV regulatory genes) develop the typical histologic findings of HIV-associated nephropathy,[35] supporting a role for viral gene expression in the kidney. Transplantation experiments between transgenic kidneys and nontransgenic littermates have revealed that HIV-associated nephropathy expression is related to the renal transgene expression.[35] Normal wild-type kidneys do not develop nephropathy when transplanted into HIV transgenic mice. This argues against a systemic cytokine effect as causative in the disease process. Recent evidence suggests that podocytes and renal tubular epithelial cells can be infected by HIV and serve as a reservoir for the virus.[34]

Drug-Induced Focal Segmental Glomerulosclerosis

A number of drugs and medications have been associated with the FSGS phenotype, including heroin, lithium, pamidronate, and interferon-α. The abuse of heroin has been associated with the nephrotic syndrome and an FSGS pattern on biopsy.[36] Some patients have experienced remissions of the disease after discontinuation of the drug abuse. Pamidronate, a bisphosphonate used to prevent bone disease in myeloma and metastatic tumors, has been associated with collapsing FSGS in a number of series.[37,38] Some patients have biopsy specimens showing FSGS and others MCD. Patients have experienced stabilization of renal function and in some cases resolution of the nephrotic syndrome following discontinuation of pamidronate.

Structural Maladaptation Leading to Focal Segmental Glomerulosclerosis

Common secondary forms of FSGS are mediated by adaptive structural-functional responses.[39–41] These include a number of forms with congenital reduction of numbers of functioning nephrons (e.g., oligomeganephronia, unilateral renal agenesis, renal dysplasia) or acquired reduction of nephron numbers (e.g., reflux nephropathy, surgical renal ablation, chronic allograft nephropathy; see Fig. 18.1). Other secondary forms are associated with hemodynamic stress placed on an initially normal nephron population (e.g., obesity, hypertension, sickle cell disease associated FSGS). The biopsies of patients with these forms of secondary FSGS typically show glomerulomegaly. In a number of models of surgical reduction in renal mass, functional hypertrophy of remnant nephrons has been documented associated with high glomerular plasma flow and increased intraglomerular pressures. While these changes are initially "adaptive," the resultant hyperfiltration and increased glomerular pressure become "maladaptive" and serve as mechanisms for progressive glomerular damage.

Pathogenesis of Progressive Renal Failure in Focal Segmental Glomerulosclerosis

While much attention has been focused on the pathogenetic basis for proteinuria in FSGS, it is clear that the segmental and eventual global glomerulosclerosis in association with interstitial fibrosis underlie the progression to renal failure.[42–44] The etiology of the glomerulosclerosis and its progressive nature is only partially known and is discussed in detail in Chapters 15 and 68. Podocytes in some forms of FSGS, such as the collapsing variant, display a dysregulated phenotype with dedifferentiation, loss of their highly differentiated cytoarchitecture, proliferation, and apoptosis.[45] There is altered podocyte expression of cell cycle–related proteins (increased cyclin E, A, and B1, CDK2, p21) in some patients with FSGS,[46,47] which might contribute to either abnormal proliferation or apoptosis of podocytes. In renal biopsy specimens of patients with FSGS, the expression of transforming growth factor β1, thrombospondin 1, transforming growth factor β II receptor proteins mRNAs are all increased over controls, as are markers of the signaling pathway phosphorylated Smad2/Smad3 in the visceral glomerular epithelial cells.[48] Thus, there is increased expression of fibrogenic proteins with activation of the Smad signaling pathways in damaged podocytes, probably leading to an overproduction of extracellular matrix and progressive sclerosis.

EPIDEMIOLOGY

Studies of biopsied patients show an increasing prevalence of FSGS in both adults and children.[49] This has been documented in a number of different countries on different continents. In a Canadian study in children, this was documented in a catchment area where referrals were mandatory.[50] In some countries, such as Brazil, FSGS is currently the most common primary renal disease.[51] An analysis of the prevalence of ESRD in the United States caused by FSGS over a 21-year period shows an increase from 0.2% in 1980 to 2.3% in 2000.[6] Although some of this change in prevalence may relate to changes in biopsy practice or disease classification, it is likely there is a real increase in the frequency of FSGS.

Primary FSGS is slightly more common in males than females, and the incidence in both children and adults is higher in blacks than in Caucasians.[3] In the United States, FSGS is the most common cause of idiopathic nephrotic syndrome in adult African Americans.[6,52] African Americans had a fourfold greater risk of ESRD from FSGS than Caucasians. Nevertheless, even in a population almost entirely Caucasian in the United States, a clear increase in the incidence of FSGS has been documented over a 20-year period.[53] The incidence of ESRD due to FSGS in males of all races is 1.5 to 2 times higher than in females. In the United States, idiopathic FSGS is the most common primary glomerular disease detected on renal biopsy that leads to ESRD in all races.[6]

CLINICAL MANIFESTATIONS

Most patients with idiopathic FSGS present with either asymptomatic proteinuria or full nephrotic syndrome.[1–4] In children, the 10% to 30% with asymptomatic proteinuria are most commonly detected on routine check-ups and sports physical examinations, while in adults asymptomatic detection occurs at military induction examinations, routine gynecologic or obstetric check-ups, and insurance or employment physical examinations. The incidence of nephrotic range proteinuria at onset in children is 70% to 90%, while only 50% to 70% of adults with FSGS present with the nephrotic syndrome. Edema is, by far, the most common manifestation of FSGS. Secondary forms of FSGS associated with hyperfiltration, such as the remnant kidney and obesity-related glomerulopathy, typically have lower levels of proteinuria than classic idiopathic FSGS, and most such patients have subnephrotic proteinuria and normal serum albumins.[15]

Hypertension is found in 30% to 50% of children and adults with FSGS at the time of diagnosis. Microscopic hematuria is found in 25% to 75% of these patients, and a decreased GFR is noted at presentation in 20% to 30%.[1–4] Daily urinary protein excretion ranges from <1 to >30 g/day. Proteinuria is typically nonselective, that is, it contains not only albumin but also higher molecular weight proteins. Complement levels and other serologic tests are normal. Occasional patients will have glycosuria, aminoaciduria, phosphaturia, or a concentrating defect indicating functional tubular damage as well as glomerular injury.

A number of studies have evaluated the clinical presentation of various morphologic variants of FSGS. When patients with the glomerular tip lesion (see later discussion) were compared to cases of MCD and FSGS not otherwise specified (NOS), their clinical features were more similar to those of adults with MCD than to those with FSGS.[54] They presented with edema and the nephrotic syndrome (almost 90%). The tip lesion patients more closely resembled MCD patients than classic FSGS patients with respect to their abrupt clinical onset of disease, high frequency of the nephrotic syndrome, severity of proteinuria, and absence of chronic tubulointerstitial disease.[54] These patients had a short time from onset of clinical disease to renal biopsy, suggesting that the tip lesion may be more common in early stages of FSGS. Patients with the collapsing variant of FSGS often present with greater degrees of proteinuria, a higher elevation of their serum creatinine level, and full-blown nephrotic syndrome.[55–57]

DIAGNOSIS AND DIFFERENTIAL DIAGNOSIS

Prior to biopsy, patients with FSGS may be confused with any patient who has glomerular disease or the nephrotic syndrome with negative serologic tests. In children with FSGS, the majority of whom present with the nephrotic syndrome, the major differential will be between MCD and other variants of steroid-resistant nephrotic syndrome. In adults with subnephrotic proteinuria, the differential includes almost all glomerular diseases without positive serologic tests. In adults with the nephrotic syndrome, membranous nephropathy and MCD may present in an identical fashion. The findings of microhematuria, hypertension, and even reductions of the GFR do not help distinguish these entities, and only a renal biopsy will clarify the diagnosis.[58] Once the renal biopsy is performed, the differential is greatly narrowed. However, even then, the diagnosis may be problematic since the morphologic features are nonspecific and can occur in a variety of other conditions or superimposed on other glomerular processes.[4,5,59] Focal sclerosing lesions due to other glomerulopathies (e.g., segmental scarring due to lupus nephritis) must be excluded. Moreover, since the defining glomerular lesion of FSGS is focal, it may not be sampled on the renal biopsy. A large glomerular sample of >20 glomeruli for light microscopy increases the likelihood of identifying the diagnostic segmental lesions. Even after the diagnosis of FSGS is established, the primary (idiopathic) form must be distinguished from secondary forms (see Fig. 18.1).[4,5,59] A diagnosis of primary FSGS requires exclusion of all secondary forms of FSGS, including familial FSGS, HIV-associated nephropathy, and secondary FSGS caused by structural-functional adaptations mediated by intrarenal vasodilatation and increased glomerular capillary pressures and plasma flow rates. In general, many forms of structural-functional adaptive FSGS have lower levels of proteinuria than idiopathic FSGS, a lower incidence of hypoalbuminemia, and, on biopsy, lesser degrees of foot process effacement. In patients younger than 25 years of age and in those with a family history of FSGS, genetic screening to evaluate for podocin or other mutations may be useful.

PATHOLOGY

A classification of biopsies with FSGS into a number of histologic variants was proposed recently[60] (Fig. 18.2). This morphologic classification can be applied both to primary and secondary forms of FSGS listed in Figure 18.1. The classification requires that the nonspecific pattern of FSGS due to other glomerulopathies (e.g., hereditary nephritis, scarred glomerulonephritis) first be excluded by immunofluorescence (IF), electron microscopy, and clinical correlation. The remaining lesions are divided into morphologic variants based on light microscopic findings. These include (a) FSGS, classic or NOS; (b) a perihilar variant in which >50% of glomeruli with segmental lesions display perihilar hyalinosis and sclerosis; (c) a cellular variant associated with endocapillary hypercellularity, with or without sclerotic lesions; (d) a collapsing variant with at least one glomerulus having global collapse and overlying podocyte hyperplasia and hypertrophy; and (e) a tip lesion that has at least one glomerulus with segmental glomerular tuft involvement at the tubular pole. This is currently a working classification and remains to be validated by prospective series. Other more controversial histologic variants of FSGS include FSGS with diffuse mesangial hypercellularity and C1q nephropathy (see Chapter 27). Some believe that these are distinct disease entities with unique clinical pathologic features; others believe they are merely subgroups of general FSGS lesions.[61–63]

Classic Focal Segmental Glomerulosclerosis (Focal Segmental Glomerulosclerosis Not Otherwise Specified)

Classic FSGS, also called FSGS NOS, is the common generic form of FSGS. It is defined by discrete segmental solidifications of the glomerular tuft involving any portion of the tuft, either the vascular pole (perihilar) region or the periphery of the tuft[4,5,59] (Fig. 18.3). It requires that the other histologic variants described later be excluded. Glomerular capillaries are segmentally occluded by acellular matrix material, often with hyalinosis (plasmatic insudation of amorphous glassy material beneath the GBM), endocapillary foam cells, and wrinkling of the GBM (Fig. 18.4). While the segmental lesions have a predilection for the juxtamedullary glomeruli early in the disease process, more diffuse and global glomerular involvement develops over time. Glomerular lobules unaffected by segmental sclerosis appear normal by light microscopy except for mild podocyte swelling. Adhesions or synechiae to Bowman's capsule are common, and overlying viseral epithelial cells often appear swollen and form a cellular "cap" over the sclerosing segment. Patchy tubular atrophy and interstitial fibrosis are commensurate with the degree of glomerular sclerosis.

On IF, there is focal and segmental granular deposition of IgM, C3, and more variably C1 in the distribution of the

Morphologic variants of focal segmental glomerulosclerosis
1. FSGS, not otherwise specified (also known as classic FSGS)
2. FSGS, perihilar variant
3. FSGS, cellular variant
4. FSGS, collapsing variant (also known as collapsing glomerulopathy)
5. FSGS, tip variant

Figure 18.2 Morphologic variants of focal segmental glomerulosclerosis (FSGS).

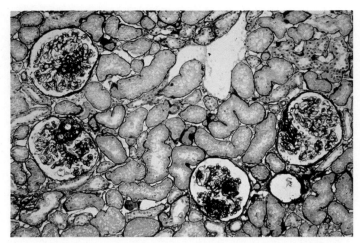

Figure 18.3 Focal segmental glomerulosclerosis not otherwise specified. A low-power view shows four glomeruli with discrete lesions of segmental sclerosis involving a portion of the tuft. The adjacent nonsclerotic capillaries are unremarkable. In this example, there is no evidence of tubulointerstitial injury (Jones methenamine silver; magnification ×100).

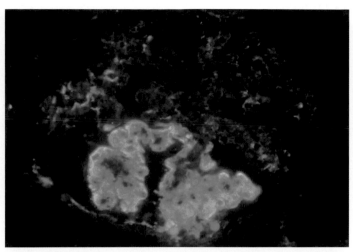

Figure 18.5 Focal segmental glomerulosclerosis not otherwise specified. The lesions of segmental sclerosis contain deposits of IgM corresponding to areas of increased matrix and hyalinosis. Weaker staining for IgM is also seen in the adjacent mesangium (immunofluorescence micrograph; magnification ×400).

segmental glomerular sclerosis (Fig. 18.5). Not all glomeruli with segmental sclerosing lesions contain these deposits.

On electron microscopy, segmental sclerosis lesions show wrinkling and retraction of the GBM, accumulation of inframembranous hyaline, and narrowing or occlusion of the glomerular capillary lumina (Fig. 18.6). Typical immune type electron-dense deposits are not found along the GBMs. Overlying the segmental sclerosis, there is usually complete effacement of foot processes and podocyte hypertrophy with focal microvillous transformation (the formation of slender cellular projections resembling villi along the surface of the podocytes). Adjacent nonsclerotic glomerular capillaries show only foot process effacement. Thus, despite the focal nature of the process at the light microscopic level, the podocyte alterations are diffuse at the electron microscopic level.

Perihilar Variant of Focal Segmental Glomerulosclerosis

The perihilar variant is defined as perihilar hyalinosis and sclerosis involving >50% of glomeruli with segmental lesions.[60] This

category requires that the cellular, tip, and collapsing variants be excluded. While this pattern may occur in primary FSGS, it is particularly common in the many secondary forms of FSGS mediated by adaptive structural-functional responses. In the setting of secondary FSGS due to adaptive responses, there is typically glomerular hypertrophy. The segmental lesions tend to be predominantly perihilar podocytes, often involving hypertrophied glomeruli (Fig. 18.7). Hypertrophy and hyperplasia are uncommon. Immunofluorescence reveals segmental deposits of IgM and C3 in areas of sclerosis and hyalinosis. There is variable foot process effacement.

Cellular Variant of Focal Segmental Glomerulosclerosis

The cellular variant is characterized by focal and segmental endocapillary hypercellularity that may mimic a form of focal proliferative glomerulonephritis.[64] Glomerular capillaries are segmentally occluded by endocapillary hypercellularity, including foam cells, infiltrating leukocytes, karyorrhectic debris, and hyaline (Fig. 18.8). There is often hyperplasia of the visceral epithelial cells,

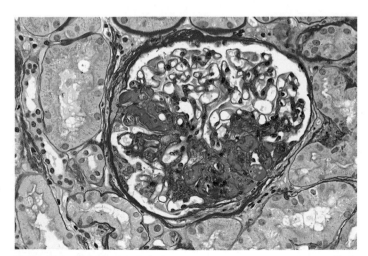

Figure 18.4 Focal segmental glomerulosclerosis not otherwise specified. The lesions of segmental sclerosis display increased extracellular matrix and hyalinosis. There is adhesion to Bowman's capsule without significant podocyte hypertrophy. The nonsclerotic capillaries have glomerular basement membranes of normal thickness and mild podocyte swelling (periodic acid–Schiff; magnification ×400).

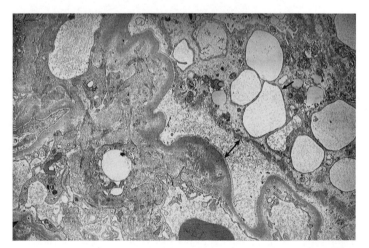

Figure 18.6 Focal segmental glomerulosclerosis not otherwise specified. An electron micrograph illustrates the lesion of segmental sclerosis with obliteration of the glomerular capillaries by increased extracellular matrix with wrinkled and retracted glomerular basement membranes. The overlying podocytes are detached with complete effacement of foot processes (*double-headed arrow*) and numerous electron lucent intracellular transport vesicles (*arrow*). (magnification ×2500).

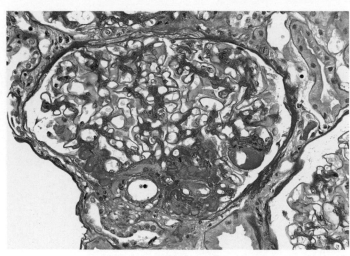

Figure 18.7 Focal segmental glomerulosclerosis (perihilar variant). A discrete lesion of segmental sclerosis and hyalinosis is located at the glomerular vascular pole (i.e., perihilar). The glomerulus is hypertrophied. The patient had secondary FSGS in the setting of solitary kidney due to contralateral renal agenesis (periodic acid–Schiff; magnification ×250).

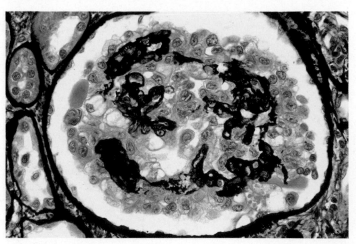

Figure 18.9 Focal segmental glomerulosclerosis (collapsing variant). There is global implosive collapse of the glomerular tuft with obliteration of capillary lumina. The overlying podocytes appear hypertrophied and hyperplastic with enlarged nuclei and nucleoli. There are no adhesions to Bowman's capsule (Jones methenamine silver; magnification ×400).

which may appear swollen and crowded, sometimes forming pseudocrescents. This variant requires that tip lesions and collapsing lesions be excluded. Immunofluorescence microscopy again shows focal and segmental glomerular positivity for IgM and C3. On electron microscopy, there is usually severe foot process effacement, correlating with the generally high levels of proteinuria.

Collapsing Variant of Focal Segmental Glomerulosclerosis

The collapsing variant is defined by at least one glomerulus with segmental or global collapse and overlying hypertrophy and hyperplasia of visceral epithelial cells (Fig. 18.9). In these areas, there is occlusion of glomerular capillary lumina by implosive wrinkling and collapse of the GBMs.[55–57] This lesion is more often global than segmental. Overlying podocytes display striking hypertrophy

and hyperplasia. They express proliferation markers, indicating cell-cycle engagement. Podocytes often contain prominent intracytoplasmic protein resorption droplets and may fill Bowman's space, forming pseudocrescents (Figs. 18.10 and 18.11). Although podocyte hyperplasia is found in both the collapsing and cellular variants of FSGS, collapsing glomerulopathy is distinguished by the absence of endocapillary hypercellularity. In fact, there is often an apparent reduction in the number of endocapillary cells in the collapsed tuft. Glomeruli with collapsing sclerosis usually lack the hyalinosis, endocapillary foam cells, and adhesions to Bowman's capsule found in FSGS NOS. However, a single biopsy specimen may show glomeruli with collapsing lesions side by side with sclerosing lesions of the usual NOS type. In collapsing FSGS, there is prominent tubulointerstitial disease, including tubular atrophy, interstitial fibrosis, interstitial edema, and inflammation. A common distinctive feature is the presence of dilated tubules forming microcysts that contain loose proteinaceous casts.

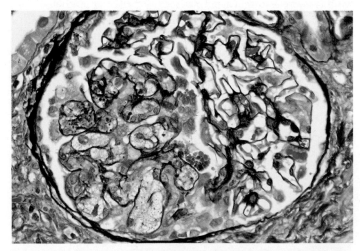

Figure 18.8 Focal segmental glomerulosclerosis (cellular variant). The glomerular capillary lumina are segmentally occluded by endocapillary cells, including foam cells, infiltrating mononuclear leukocytes, and pyknotic debris. The findings mimic a proliferative glomerulonephritis because of the hypercellularity and absence of extracellular matrix material. There are hypertrophy and hyperplasia of the overlying podocytes, some of which contain protein resorption droplets (Jones methenamine silver; magnification ×400).

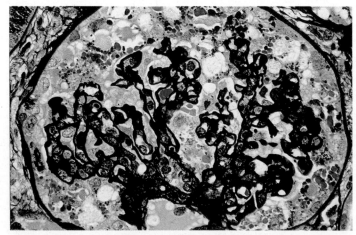

Figure 18.10 Focal segmental glomerulosclerosis (collapsing variant). In this example, the exuberant proliferation of visceral epithelial cells forms a pseudocrescent that obliterates the urinary space. The pseudocrescent lacks the spindle cell morphology, ruptures of Bowman's capsule, or pericellular matrix typically seen in true inflammatory crescents of parietal epithelial origin (Jones methenamine silver; magnification ×400).

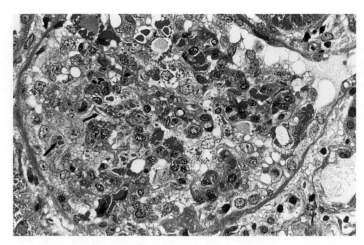

Figure 18.11 Focal segmental glomerulosclerosis (collapsing variant). The crescent-like proliferation of glomerular epithelial cells contains numerous intracytoplasmic vacuoles and trichrome–red protein resorption droplets (Masson trichrome; magnification ×400).

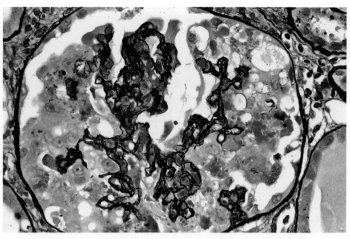

Figure 18.13 Focal segmental glomerulosclerosis (collapsing variant) due to pamidronate toxicity. The glomerular tuft is retracted, without appreciable increase in matrix material. The overlying podocytes are enlarged and hyperplastic (*arrows*) with numerous intracytoplasmic vacuoles and protein resorption droplets (Jones methenamine silver; magnification ×400).

The IF findings are similar to other forms of FSGS. On electron microscopy, there is typically severe foot process effacement affecting both collapsed and noncollapsed glomeruli (Fig. 18.12). The presence of endothelial tubuloreticular inclusions is helpful to identify collapsing glomerulopathy secondary to HIV-associated nephropathy. These inclusions are lacking in primary collapsing FSGS.

Collapsing glomerulopathy may occur as a primary form of FSGS.[55–57] This pattern is also commonly observed in secondary FSGS due to HIV infection, parvovirus B19 infection, interferon-α therapy, and pamidronate toxicity (Fig. 18.13).

Tip Lesion Variant of Focal Segmental Glomerulosclerosis

This variant is defined by the presence of at least one segmental lesion involving the tip domain (i.e., the outer 25% of the tuft next to the origin of the proximal tubule). The adhesion is either between the tuft and Bowman's capsule at the tubular lumen or neck or at the confluence of podocytes with parietal or tubular epithelial cells at the tubular lumen or neck. The proximal tubular pole must be identified in the defining glomerulus. In

some cases, the affected segment appears to herniate into the tubular lumen. The segmental lesions may be cellular or sclerosing in type (Figs. 18.14 and 18.15). Foam cells and hyalinosis are common. There is often podocyte hypertrophy and hyperplasia overlying the involved segment. Although initially peripheral, these lesions may evolve more centrally.[55] While the FSGS glomerular tip lesion may occur alone or with segmental lesions that are peripheral or indeterminate in location, the presence of perihilar sclerosis or collapsing sclerosis rules out the tip variant. In one recent study of FSGS tip lesions, biopsy specimens had glomerular tip lesions alone in 26% and glomerular tip lesions plus other peripheral FSGS lesions in the other 74%.[54] IF findings are similar to those of other biopsies with FSGS. Foot process effacement tends to be severe.

Other Variants of Focal Segmental Glomerulosclerosis

Two more controversial histologic variants often included with FSGS that may be distinct clinical entities include FSGS with diffuse mesangial hypercellularity and C1q nephropathy[61–63] (see also Chapter 27). FSGS with diffuse mesangial hypercellularity

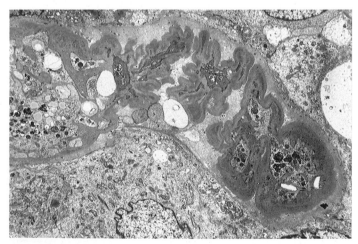

Figure 18.12 Focal segmental glomerulosclerosis (collapsing variant). On electron microscopy, there is tight collapse of the glomerular capillaries with corrugated glomerular basement membrane. The overlying podocytes appear detached and hypertrophied with complete loss of foot processes (magnification ×2500).

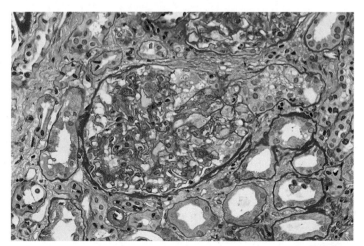

Figure 18.14 Focal segmental glomerulosclerosis (tip lesion variant). A cellular tip lesion displays engorgement of glomerular capillaries by foam cells and adhesion of the involved segment to the origin of the proximal tubule (tubular pole) (periodic acid–Schiff; magnification ×250).

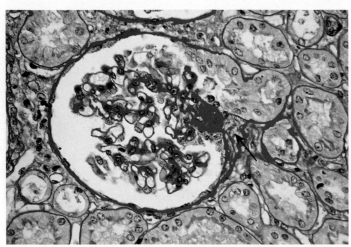

Figure 18.15 Focal segmental glomerulosclerosis (tip lesion variant). A sclerosing tip lesion forms an adhesion to the tubular pole (*arrow*) (periodic acid–Schiff; magnification ×250).

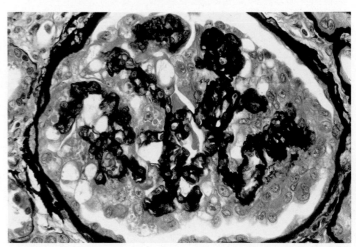

Figure 18.16 Human immunodeficiency virus–associated nephropathy. A globally collapsed glomerulus shows marked podocyte hypertrophy and hyperplasia (Jones methenamine silver; magnification ×400).

has lesions of FSGS on a background of generalized mesangial hypercellularity. On IF, there is diffuse mesangial positivity for IgM, with more variable mesangial staining for C3, and on electron microscopy, there is extensive foot process effacement without glomerular electron-dense deposits. This variant occurs almost exclusively in young children.

C1q nephropathy is an idiopathic glomerulopathy defined by dominant or codominant IF staining for C1q, mesangial electron-dense deposits, and light microscopic findings resembling FSGS or MCD with variable mesangial hypercellularity. In a recent study, 17 patients had a light microscopic appearance of FSGS (including six collapsing and two cellular) and three of MCD.[61] In addition to C1q staining, biopsies may show deposition of other immunoglobulins (particularly IgG) and complement components (C3), making exclusion of other clinical disease entities important (e.g., lupus nephritis and membranoproliferative glomerulonephritis). In C1q nephropathy, electron-dense deposits are typically located predominantly in the paramesangial region subjacent to the GBM reflection. There is variable foot process effacement. Whereas some investigators advocate that C1q nephropathy represents a subgoup of FSGS, others maintain that it should be considered a separate unrelated condition.[61–63]

Secondary Focal Segmental Glomerulosclerosis

Although the pathology of some secondary forms of FSGS resembles closely that of primary FSGS, there are several noteworthy differences. While the light microscopic findings in HIV-associated nephropathy are similar to those of idiopathic collapsing FSGS (Fig. 18.16), tubular microcysts are particularly common, and with advanced disease, they may almost completely replace the cortical parenchyma (Fig. 18.17).[65–67] At the ultrastructural level, a major difference is the abundance of tubuloreticular inclusions in the glomerular endothelial cells of HIV-associated nephropathy. These "interferon footprints" consist of 24-nm interanastomosing tubular structures located within dilated cisternae of endoplasmic reticulum (Fig. 18.18). Tubuloreticular inclusions are less frequent in patients treated with highly active antiretroviral therapy.

Many secondary forms of FSGS are mediated by adaptive structural-functional responses to either reduced numbers of functioning nephrons or hemodynamic stress placed on an initially normal nephron population. The biopsy specimens of patients with

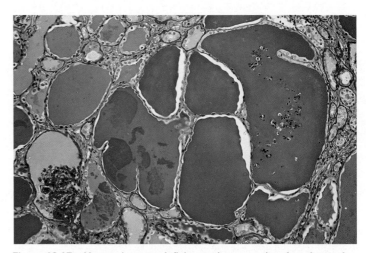

Figure 18.17 Human immunodeficiency virus–associated nephropathy. At low power, the renal parenchyma contains abundant tubular microcysts with proteinaceous casts. The glomerulus is collapsed with dilated urinary space (periodic acid–Schiff; magnification ×80).

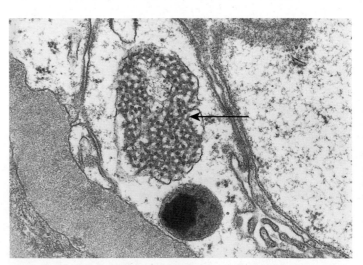

Figure 18.18 Human immunodeficiency virus–associated nephropathy. The glomerular endothelial cell pictured here contains a large intracytoplasmic tubuloreticular inclusion ("interferon footprint"; *arrow*) composed of interanastomosing tubular structures within a dilated cisterna of endoplasmic reticulum (electron micrograph; magnification ×15,000).

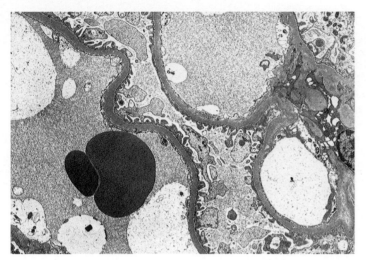

Figure 18.19 Secondary focal segmental glomerulosclerosis due to obesity. By light microscopy, this patient with morbid obesity had glomerular hypertrophy and predominantly perihilar lesions of segmental sclerosis and hyalinosis. The foot processes show mild effacement involving approximately 20% of the glomerular capillary surface area despite the presence of nephrotic-range proteinuria (electron micrograph). This mild degree of foot process effacement is less than that usually seen in primary FSGS (magnification ×2500).

these forms of secondary FSGS typically show glomerulomegaly and predominantly perihilar lesions of segmental sclerosis and hyalinosis. There is usually little if any podocyte hypertrophy or hyperplasia. In secondary FSGS resulting from loss of renal mass (such as due to reflux nephropathy or hypertensive arterio-nephrosclerosis), FSGS is usually seen on a background of extensive global glomerulosclerosis, tubular atrophy, interstitial fibrosis, and arteriosclerosis. In secondary FSGS related to sickle cell disease, there is glomerular hypertrophy and sclerosis in association with capillary congestion by sickled erythrocytes and double contours of the GBM resembling those seen in chronic thrombotic microangiopathy. Importantly, while IF changes in most forms of secondary FSGS are similar to those of primary FSGS, on electron microscopy, the degree of foot process fusion is generally milder, affecting <50% of the total glomerular capillary surface area (Fig. 18.19).

NATURAL HISTORY AND PROGNOSIS

The natural history of FSGS is as varied as the many forms of disease fitting under this histologic diagnostic umbrella.[1–4] Without therapy or response to therapy, the majority of patients with primary FSGS will experience a progressive increase in protein-uria and progression to renal failure. Only a minority of patients (5% to 25%) experiences a spontaneous remission of proteinuria and/or the nephrotic syndrome.[67] Both unresponsive children and adults have a similar course; most develop ESRD 5 to 20 years from presentation. Many series show approximately 50% of such patients reaching ESRD by 5 years (Fig. 18.20).

Certain epidemiologic, clinical, and histologic findings at the time of diagnosis help predict the long-term course of FSGS patients[1,3,5,68,69] (Fig. 18.21). While gender is no risk factor, African Americans, even when controlled for degree of protein-uria hypertension and other features, experience a more rapid progression to renal failure. At the time of biopsy, both an ele-vated serum creatinine and greater degrees of proteinuria pre-dict a more progressive course. Several studies have found that greater degrees of interstitial fibrosis correlate with a more

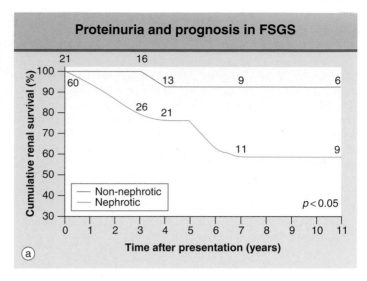

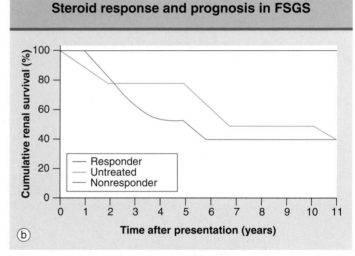

Figure 18.20 Prognosis in primary focal segmental glomerulosclerosis. *a,* The risk of developing renal failure is related to the extent of proteinuria. Those with nephrotic-range proteinuria are much more likely to develop renal failure than those with low-grade proteinuria. The figures indicate the number of at-risk patients at different time points. *b,* Steroid-responsive patients are significantly less likely to develop renal failure than nonresponders and untreated patients. (Adapted from Rydel JJ, Korbet SM, Borok RZ, Schwartz MM: Focal segmental glomerular sclerosis in adults: Presentation, course, and response to treatment. Am J Kidney Dis 1995;25:534–542.)

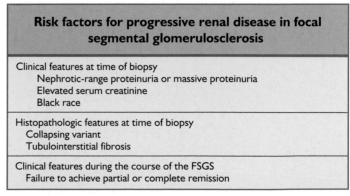

Risk factors for progressive renal disease in focal segmental glomerulosclerosis

Clinical features at time of biopsy
    Nephrotic-range proteinuria or massive proteinuria
    Elevated serum creatinine
    Black race

Histopathologic features at time of biopsy
    Collapsing variant
    Tubulointerstitial fibrosis

Clinical features during the course of the FSGS   Failure to achieve partial or complete remission

Figure 18.21 Risk factors for progressive renal disease in focal segmental glomerulosclerosis.

progressive course, whereas the degree of glomerulosclerosis has been much less consistent as a prognostic finding.[1–4]

Outcomes differ among the various histologic variants of FSGS. The cellular FSGS variant appears fairly responsive to immunosuppressive therapy, perhaps related to the early and relatively active stage of glomerular injury.[64] Of all the histologic variants, collapsing FSGS has had the most rapidly progressive course to renal failure and appears the least responsive to therapeutic intervention.[55–57] The course of idiopathic collapsing FSGS is very dependent on the findings at the time of biopsy: Patients with higher serum creatinine levels and more interstitial fibrosis fare poorly.[65] Patients with the glomerular tip lesion pattern of FSGS have the most favorable outcome, with higher rates of responsiveness to immunosuppressives than other patterns of FSGS and a better long-term prognosis. In one study of 47 tip lesion patients, 59% had a complete and 14% a partial remission with treatment at less than 2 years follow-up. Only one progressed to ESRD.[54] The course of C1q nephropathy and of FSGS with diffuse mesangial hypercellularity has been variable depending on associated clinical and histologic features.[61–63]

In all series, patients who experience a remission of proteinuria and the nephrotic syndrome have a far better renal survival than those who do not.[68,70] Recent studies confirm that even patients with a partial remission of the nephrotic syndrome have a lower rate of long-term renal failure.[71]

TREATMENT

There is still considerable debate over the appropriate treatment for patients with FSGS[1–4,70] (Fig. 18.22). In part, this relates to confusion between secondary and primary forms of the disease. New genetic and other secondary forms of FSGS that may not respond to immunosuppressive therapy are still being separated from the general idiopathic group.[28,29] Even after renal biopsy, it

is not always clear whether an obese person with glomerulomegaly and many segmentally sclerotic lesions has secondary or primary disease.[15] Moreover, the course of the disease is variable and only recently have clear prognostic features been defined. Finally, although the disease is common in adults, most well-designed trials have been conducted in young children. There are many therapeutic options with few randomized, controlled trials on which to base judgment.

In general, patients with a sustained remission of their nephrotic syndrome and with major reductions in proteinuria are unlikely to experience a loss of GFR over time.[70] Those with unremitting nephrotic syndrome are likely to progress to ESRD. In early studies of FSGS patients, only a small percentage (10% to 30%) of those treated with corticosteroids or other immunosuppressive agents experienced a remission of proteinuria. Moreover, the relapse rate after treatment was high.[3,70] Thus, many nephrologists considered FSGS to be resistant to therapy and did not advocate immunosuppressive treatment. Almost 20 years ago, an important study on FSGS in the Toronto region documented that almost all children in the study were treated with immunosuppressives and that 44% experienced a remission of proteinuria. Although the response rate for treated adults was similar (39%), most of the adults never received any immunosuppressive therapy.[68]

Use of Corticosteroids

In recent trials using longer (≥6 months) courses of prednisone, the results have been much more promising than in the past. Steroid therapy is usually with prednisone or prednisolone 1 mg/kg/day or 1.5 to 2 mg/kg every other day for an initial period of 4 to 8 weeks with subsequent tapering of the dose.[1–4,70] Initial response rates have ranged from 25% to 60%. In children with biopsy-documented FSGS or steroid-resistant nephrotic syndrome, as many as 20% to 25% will have a complete remission

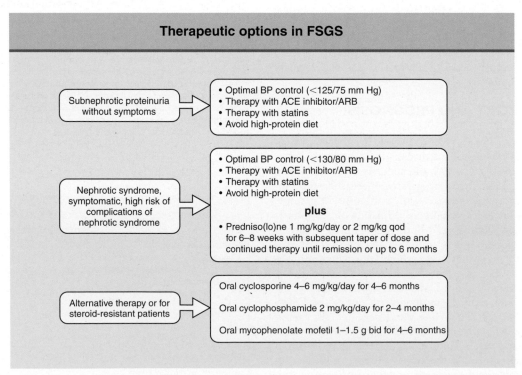

Figure 18.22 Therapeutic options in focal segmental glomerulosclerosis. For secondary FSGS treatment directed at the underlying cause (e.g., human immunodeficiency virus–associated nephropathy: treatment with highly active antiretroviral therapy; pamidronate nephrotoxicity: discontinue the medication; obesity-related glomerulopathy: weight loss). ACE, angiotensin-converting enzyme; ARB, angiotensin receptor blocker; BP, blood pressure.

with a short course of corticosteroids, but as many as 50% will remit with more intensive therapy. In adults, although there are no large or randomized, controlled trials, more prolonged use of corticosteroids has led to much higher remission rates of the nephrotic syndrome than in earlier studies.[70] It has been proposed that earlier studies used too short a treatment period for adults, with most studies using only a few months of therapy. Thus, an Italian study using >6 months of prednisone, cyclophosphamide, and/or azathioprine therapy found 60% of FSGS patients to have a complete remission of the nephrotic syndrome with an excellent long-term renal survival.[72,73] Other trials using ≥6 months of corticosteroid therapy have also documented complete remission rates of 32% to 44%, with additional patients experiencing partial remission of proteinuria. For example, an American study of >50 nephrotic adults with FSGS also showed a better than 50% response rate as well as long-term improvement in renal survival in the treated group.[74] The median duration of steroid treatment to achieve complete remission is 3 to 4 months, with most patients responding by 6 months. Most clinicians would treat all nephrotic FSGS patients and those at risk of progressive disease with a prolonged course (6 to 9 months) of daily or every other day corticosteroid therapy (starting with 60 mg/day prednisone or 120 to 150 mg every other day and tapering to lower doses after several months) or other immunosuppressive medication in the hopes of inducing a remission of the nephrotic syndrome and preventing eventual ESRD.

Other Immunosuppressive Agents

Children with idiopathic nephrotic syndrome are generally steroid resistant before a renal biopsy is performed and the diagnosis of FSGS is confirmed. For many years, either chlorambucil or cyclophosphamide was the treatment of choice for these children and for adults with steroid-resistant FSGS.[75] Repeated or prolonged corticosteroid use was associated with growth failure, cosmetic changes, risk of infection, hypertension, and aseptic necrosis of bones to mention only a few complications of therapy. Cytotoxic agents carried the risk of infertility, alopecia, marrow suppression and infection, hemorrhagic cystitis, and the long-term risk of malignancy. Attempts to avoid these toxicities led to a number of trials with other modalities. For example, one uncontrolled trial in children using combined intravenous pulse steroids and long-term immunosuppression with corticosteroids and cytotoxics found a 60% complete remission rate and a 16% partial remission rate of the nephrotic syndrome and a low rate of progression to renal failure.[76] In adults with FSGS treated with either oral cyclophosphamide or chlorambucil, pooled data show a high response rate for patients with steroid dependence or intolerance, but a <20% remission rate for those who are steroid resistant.[70]

A number of studies have used low-dose cyclosporine (4 to 6 mg/kg/day for 2 to 6 months) to treat steroid-resistant FSGS[77,78] (Fig. 18.23). Complete plus partial remission rates of 60% to 70% have been achieved with the use of cyclosporine versus 17% to 33% in the placebo group. The North American Collaborative Study of Cyclosporine in Nephrotic Syndrome randomized adult FSGS patients to either cyclosporine with low-dose corticosteroids or the same very low dose of corticosteroids alone for a 6-month period.[79] There was a much higher remission rate (12% complete and >70% complete and/or partial) in the group treated with cyclosporine. Despite relapses after the cyclosporine was discontinued, at the end of long-term follow-up, there were still significantly more remitters in the treated group. Moreover, despite initial worries about nephrotoxicity with the calcineurin inhibitor, the percentage of patients with reduction of GFR over

4 years was significantly less in the treated group. There has been more concern about potential nephrotoxicity in children, and it is unclear whether, in this trial, the low dose of cyclosporine (and corresponding serum levels) and short course of treatment (6 months) contributed to this beneficial result. Nevertheless, because there is a high relapse rate when the drug is discontinued, many clinicians use a 1-year course with slow taper in those patients who have a favorable reduction of proteinuria with cyclosporine.[3,70]

Although data are more limited with tacrolimus and there are no large controlled trials, the results have been similar. Since the major side effects of nephrotoxicity, hypertension, and hyperkalemia are the same for both drugs, choice may depend on cosmetic and other less severe adverse side effects (e.g., gum swelling, tremor). Tacrolimus has been effective in some patients who are resistant to or intolerant of cyclosporine.

Many clinicians believe that cyclosporine or tacrolimus are better second-line agents of treatment than are cytotoxic agents such as cyclophosphamide and chlorambucil. A recent multicenter German collaborative study compared the efficacy and safety of steroids plus cyclosporine to steroids plus chlorambucil in steroid-resistant adults with FSGS and the nephrotic syndrome.[80] Total and partial remission rates were similar (about 20% full and 40% to 50% partial remission) and the addition of chlorambucil to the regimen did not improve outcome. Whether cyclosporine is equivalent or superior to corticosteroids as first-line therapy for FSGS has never been documented. However, some clinicians use cyclosporine as first-line therapy in patients at high risk of corticosteroid complications, such as those with concurrent diabetes or morbid obesity.

Mycophenolate mofetil has been used in several uncontrolled series of FSGS patients.[81–83] In some, including those resistant to other therapies, there have been remissions of the nephrotic syndrome and major reductions in proteinuria. There is currently

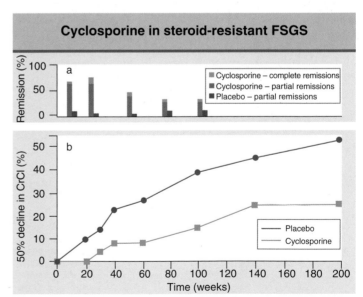

Figure 18.23 Cyclosporine in steroid-resistant focal segmental glomerulosclerosis (FSGS). A randomized, controlled trial of 6 months of treatment with prednisolone and either cyclosporine or placebo. *a*, Cyclosporine induces a partial or complete remission significantly more often than placebo. *b*, Cyclosporine treatment results in a lower rate of decline in renal function than placebo even after 4 years. (Adapted from Cattran D, Appel GB, Hebert L, et al: A randomized trial of cyclosporine in patients with steroid resistant focal segmental glomerulosclerosis: North America Nephrotic Syndrome Study Group. Kidney Int 1999;56:2220–2226.

a large multicenter National Institutes of Health trial in the United States comparing cyclosporine and a regimen of oral mycophenolate mofetil plus dexamethasone for steroid-resistant patients with FSGS.

Rapamycin has been used in several small series of patients with glomerular disease including FSGS patients.[84,85] In two series, it was associated with worsening of renal function, episodes of acute renal failure, and no remissions of the nephrotic syndrome.[84] In the third, which included >20 steroid-resistant FSGS patients, 19% experienced a complete remission, 38% a partial remission, and, hence, >50% a beneficial result.[85] Patients who responded to treatment had a shorter duration of their FSGS than resistant patients.

Plasma exchange, which is successful in treating some patients with recurrent FSGS in the renal allograft, has not proven useful in patients with disease in their native kidneys.[10] A study of low-density lipoprotein apheresis and prednisone in steroid- and cyclosporine-resistant children with primary FSGS achieved a remission in 7 of 11 patients. Unfortunately, the role of the individual components of treatment and the mechanisms of action is difficult to define in such uncontrolled trials.

Other Therapeutic Interventions

While the ideal immunosuppressive regimen to treat steroid-resistant patients with idiopathic FSGS and the nephrotic syndrome remains unclear, corticosteroids and other immunosuppressives are not indicated in the treatment of patients with subnephrotic levels of proteinuria and little damage shown on their renal biopsies. This group is less likely to have progressive disease and to benefit from immunosuppression. Most would treat all FSGS patients without contraindications with angiotensin-converting enzyme inhibitors and/or angiotensin receptor blockers as well as statins to reduce proteinuria and its consequences. Whether combination inhibitor/angiotensin receptor blocker therapy is superior to maximal doses of potent agents in each class used with diuretics remains to be proven.[86] Clearly, optimal blood pressure control itself is also critical to slow or prevent the progression of the disease (see also Chapter 69).

For patients with secondary forms of FSGS, attempts to treat the primary etiology of the FSGS should be the initial step in management. Patients with FSGS secondary to obesity and heroin nephropathy have had remissions of proteinuria after weight reduction or cessation of heroin use, respectively. In patients with HIV-associated nephropathy, therapy with highly active antiretroviral drugs and blockers of the renin angiotensin system has proven useful.[87,88] The role of immunosuppressives has not yet been documented in controlled, randomized trials in any form of secondary FSGS.[89] In all forms of secondary FSGS, use of blockers of the renin angiotensin system and other nonspecific methods to reduce proteinuria are also crucial to prevent progressive renal disease in this population. Strict attention to optimal blood pressure control and use of statins to reduce lipids may improve both renal and cardiovascular outcomes. In those patients with either primary idiopathic or secondary forms of FSGS who remain nephrotic, control of fluid retention and edema can be managed with salt restriction and diuretics (see Chapter 16).

TRANSPLANTATION

Idiopathic FSGS may recur in the transplanted kidney, where it presents with severe proteinuria and the nephrotic syndrome.[3,70,90,91] Children with FSGS and patients who manifested more severe proteinuria and a more rapid course to renal failure in their native kidneys are at greater risk of recurrence in the allograft. Those who have lost a prior allograft due to recurrent FSGS are at highest risk of recurrence. Recurrence in the allograft may be seen immediately after transplantation or years later. Plasma exchange has been used successfully to induce remissions of the proteinuria associated with recurrence, but the results are more favorable in children than in adults (see also Chapter 69).[10]

Analysis of the outcomes of renal transplantation in children with FSGS shows a profound effect of race.[92] Among African American children with FSGS, allograft survival was not different from that of non-FSGS patients. Among non–African American children with FSGS, the risk of allograft failure was 1.3 times higher than for other causes of ESRD. Nevertheless, for non–African American children, a transplant from a living-related donor gave a better allograft survival than that seen with transplants from cadaveric donors. While most patients with genetic forms of FSGS have not experienced a recurrence in the allograft, this is not universally true, especially when dealing with patients with compound heterozygote defects.[17-19]

REFERENCES

1. Chun MJ, Korbet SM, Schwatz MM, Lewis EJ: FSGS in nephrotic adults: Presentation, prognosis, and response to therapy of the histologic variants. J Am Soc Nephrol 2004;15:2169–2177.
2. Appel GB, Glassock RJ: Glomerular, vascular, and tubulointerstitial diseases. Nephrology Self-Assessment Program 2005;4:117–153.
3. Crew RJ, Appel GB: Focal segmental glomerulosclerosis. In Greenberg A, ed. The NKF Primer on Kidney Disease, 4th ed. Philadelphia, Elsevier, 2005, pp 178–182.
4. D'Agati V: Pathologic classification of focal segmental glomerulosclerosis. Semin Nephrol 2003;23:117–135.
5. D'Agati VD: Focal segmental glomerulosclerosis. In D'Agati V, Jennette JC, Silva FS, eds. Atlas of Nontumor Pathology: Nonneoplastic Kidney Diseases. Silver Spring, Md, American Registry of Pathology Press, 2005, pp 125–159.
6. Kitiyakara C, Eggers P, Kopp JB: Twenty-one year trends in ESRD due to FSGS in the United States. Am J Kidney Dis 2004;44: 815–825.
7. Savin VJ, McCarthy ET, Sharma M: Permeability factors in FSGS. Semin Nephrol 2003;23:147–161.
8. Savin VJ, Artero M, Sharma R, et al: Circulating factor associated with increased glomerular permeability to albumin in recurrent focal segmental sclerosis. N Engl J Med 1996;334:878–882.

9. Dantal J, Bigot E, Bogers W, et al: Effect of plasma protein absorption on protein excretion in kidney-transplant recipients with recurrent nephrotic syndrome. N Engl J Med 1994;330:7–11.
10. Matalon A, Markowitz GS, Joseph RE, et al: Plasmapheresis treatment of recurrent FSGS in adult transplant recipients. Clin Nephrol 2001; 56:271–278.
11. Fogo A: Animal models of FSGS: Lessons for pathogenesis and treatment. Semin Nephrol 2003;23:161–172.
12. Del Carmen Avila-Casado M, Perez-Torres I, Auron A, et al: Proteinuria in rats induced by serum from patients with collapsing glomerulopathy. Kidney Int 2004;66:133–143.
13. Verani RR: Obesity-associated focal segmental glomerulosclerosis: Pathologic features of the lesion and relationship with cardiomegaly and hyperlipidemia. Am J Kidney Dis 1992;20:629–634.
14. Floege J, Alpers CE, Burns MW, et al: Glomerular cells, extracellular matrix, and the development of glomerulosclerosis in the remnant kidney model. Lab Invest 1992;66:485.
15. Kambham N, Markowitz GS, Valeri AM, et al: Obesity related glomerulomegaly: An emerging epidemic. Kidney Int 2001;59:1498–1509.
16. Schwimmer JA, Markowitz GS, Valeri A, et al: Secondary FSGS in non-obese patients with increased muscle mass. Clin Nephrol 2003;60: 233–241.

17. Niaudet P: Podocin and nephrotic syndrome: Implications for the clinician. J Am Soc Nephrol 2004;15:832–834.
18. Pollak M: Inherited podocytopathies: FSGS and nephrotic syndrome from a genetic viewpoint. J Am Soc Nephrol 2002;13:3016–3023.
19. Tryggvason K, Patrakka K, Wartiovarra J: Hereditary proteinuria syndromes and mechanisms of proteinuria. N Engl J Med 2006;354:1387–1401.
20. Kaplan JM, Kim SH, North KN, et al: Mutations in ACTN4, encoding α-actinin-4, cause familial focal segmental glomerulosclerosis. Nat Genet 2000;24:251–256.
21. Caridi G, Bertelli R, DiDuca M, et al: Broadening the spectrum of diseases related to podocin mutations. J Am Soc Nephrol 2003;14: 1278–1286.
22. Ruf RG, Lichtenberger A, Karle SM, et al: Patients with mutations in NPHS2 (podocin) do not respond to standard steroid treatment of nephrotic syndrome. J Am Soc Nephrol 2004;15:722–732.
23. Weber S, Gribouval O, Esquivel EL, et al: NPHS2 mutation analysis shows genetic heterogeneity of steroid-resistant nephrotic syndrome and low post-transplant recurrence. Kidney Int 2004;66:571–579.
24. Nishibori Y, Liu L, Hosoyamada M, et al: Disease-causing missense mutations in NPHS2 gene alter normal nephrin trafficking to the plasma membrane. Kidney Int 2004;66:1755–1765.
25. Tsukoguchi H, Sudhakar A, Nguen T, et al: NPHS2 mutations in late onset focal segmental glomerulosclerosis. J Clin Invest 2002;110: 1659–1666.
26. Weins A, Kenlan P, Herbert S, et al: Mutational and biological analysis of alpha-actinin-4 in focal segmental glomerulosclerosis. J Am Soc Nephrol 2005;16:3694–3701.
27. Michaud J-L, Lemieux LI, Dube M, et al: FSGS in mice with podocyte-specific expression of mutant alpha-actinin-4. J Am Soc Nephrol 2003; 14:1200–1211.
28. Winn MP, Conlon PJ, Lynn KL, et al: A mutation in the TRPC6 cation channel causes familial focal segmental glomerulosclerosis. Science 2005;308:1801–1804.
29. Reiser J, Polu KR, Moller CC, et al: TRPC6 is a glomerular slit diaphragm-associated channel required for normal renal function. Nat Genet 2005;37:739–744.
30. Moudgil A, Nast CC, Bagga A et al: Association of parvovirus B19 infection with idiopathic collapsing glomerulopathy. Kidney Int 2001;59: 2126–2133.
31. Tanawattanacharoen S, Falk RJ, Jennette JC, Kopp JB: Parvovirus B19 DNA in kidney tissue of patients with focal segmental glomerulosclerosis. Am J Kidney Dis 2000;35:1166–1174.
32. Weiner NJ, Goodman JN, Kimmel PL: The HIV associated renal diseases: Current insights into pathogenesis and therapy. Kidney Int 2003,63:1618–1631.
33. Szczech L, Gupta SK, Habash R, et al: The clinical epidemiology and course of the spectrum of renal disease associated with HIV infection. Kidney Int 2004;66:1145–1157.
34. Bruggeman LA, Ross MD, Tanji N, et al: Renal epithelium is a previously unrecognized site of HIV-1 infection. J Am Soc Nephrol 2000;11: 2079–2087.
35. Bruggeman LA, Dikman S, Meng C, et al: Nephropathy in human immunodeficiency virus-1 transgenic mice is due to renal transgene expression. J Clin Invest 1997;199:84–92.
36. Llach F, Descoeudres C, Massry SG: Heroin associated nephropathy: Clinical and histological studies in 19 patients. Clin Nephrol 1979;11: 7–12.
37. Barri YM, Munshi NC, Sukumalchantra S, et al: Podocyte injury associated glomerulopathies induced by pamidronate. Kidney Int 2004;65:634–641.
38. Markowitz G, Appel GB, Fine P, et al: Collapsing focal segmental glomerulosclerosis following treatment with high dose pamidronate. J Am Soc Nephrol 2001;12:1164–1172.
39. Nagata M, Kriz W: Glomerular damage after uninephrectomy in young rats. II. Mechanical stress on podocytes as a pathway to sclerosis. Kidney Int 1992;42:148–160.
40. Rennke H, Klein PS: Pathogenesis and significance of non-primary focal and segmental glomerulosclerosis. Am J Kidney Dis 1989;13:443–455.
41. Rennke HG: How does glomerular epithelial cell injury contribute to progressive glomerular damage? Kidney Int 1994:45(Suppl):S58–S63.
42. Eddy AA: Expression of genes that promote renal interstitial fibrosis in rats with proteinuria. Kidney Int 1996;54(Suppl):S49–S54.
43. Eddy AA: Interstitial nephritis induced by protein-overload proteinuria. Am J Pathol 1989;135:719–733.
44. Kriz W, Hosser H, Hahnel B, et al: From segmental glomerulosclerosis to total nephron degeneration and interstitial fibrosis: A histopathologic study in rat models and human glomerulopathies. Nephrol Dial Transplant 1998;13:2781–2798.
45. Barisoni L, Kriz W, Mundel P, D'Agati V: The dysregulated podocyte phenotype: A novel concept in the pathogenesis of collapsing idiopathic FSGS and HIV associated nephropathy. J Am Soc Nephrol 1999;10: 51–61.
46. Wang S, Kim JH, Moon KC, et al: Cell-cycle mechanisms involved in podocyte proliferation in cellular lesion of FSGS. Am J Kidney Dis 2004;43:19–27.
47. Shankland SJ, Eitner F, Hudkins KL, et al: Differential expression of cyclin-dependent kinase inhibitors in human glomerular disease: Role in podocyte proliferation and maturation. Kidney Int 2000;58:674–683.
48. Kim JH, Kim BK, Moon KC, et al: Activation of the TGF-beta/Smad signaling pathway in focal segmental glomerulosclerosis. Kidney Int 2003;64:1715–1721.
49. Haas M, Meehan S, Karrison TG, Spargo BH: Changing etiologies of unexplained adult nephrotic syndrome: A comparison of renal biopsy findings from 1976–1979 and 1995–1997. Am J Kidney Dis 1997;30: 621–631.
50. Filler G, Young E, Geier P, et al: Is there really an increase in non-minimal change nephrotic syndrome in children? Am J Kidney Dis 2003;42:1107–1113.
51. Bahiense-Oliveira M, Saldanha LB, Andrade Mota EL, et al: Primary glomerular disease in Brazil: 1979–1999. Is the frequency of FSGS increasing? Clin Nephrol 2004;61:90–97.
52. Korbet SM: Treatment of focal segmental glomerulosclerosis. Kidney Int 2002;62:2301–2310.
53. Fervenza F, et al: Changing incidence of glomerular disease in the United States: A 30 year renal biopsy study. Clin J Am Soc Nephrol (in press).
54. Stokes MB, Markowitz GSM, Lin J, et al: Glomerular tip lesion: A distinct entity within the minimal change/focal segmental glomerulosclerosis spectrum. Kidney Int 2004;65:1690–1702.
55. Valeri A, Barisoni L, Appel GB, et al: Idiopathic collapsing FSGS: A clinicopathologic study. Kidney Int 1996;50:1734–1746.
56. Schwimmer JA, Markowitz GS, Valeri A, Appel GB: Collapsing glomerulopathy. Semin Nephrol 2003;23:209–219.
57. Detwiler RK, Falk RJ, Hogan SL, Jennette JC: Collapsing glomerulopathy: A clinically and pathologically distinct variant of focal segmental glomerulosclerosis. Kidney Int 1994;45:1416–1424.
58. Waldman M, Stokes MB, D'Agati VD, Appel GB: Adult minimal change disease: Clinical characteristics, treatment and outcomes (submitted)
59. D'Agati V: The many masks of focal segmental glomerulosclerosis. Kidney Int 1994;46:1223–1241.
60. D'Agati VD, Fogo AB, Bruijn JA, Jennette JC: Pathologic classification of focal segmental glomerulosclerosis: A working proposal. Am J Kidney Dis 2004;43:368–382.
61. Markowitz GS, Schwimmer JA, Stokes MB, et al: C1q nephropathy: A variant of focal segmental glomerulosclerosis. Kidney Int 2003;64: 1232–1240.
62. Jennette JC, Hipp CG: C1q nephropathy: A distinct pathologic entity usually causing nephrotic syndrome. Am J Kidney Dis 1985;6:103–110.
63. Schoeneman MJ, Bennett B, Greifer I: The natural history of focal segmental glomerulosclerosis with and without mesangial hypercellularity in children. Clin Nephrol 1978;9:45–54.
64. Schwartz MM, Evans J, Bain R, Korbet SM: Focal segmental glomerulosclerosis: Prognostic implication of the cellular lesion. J Am Soc Nephrol 1999;10:1900–1907.
65. Laurinavicius A, Hurwitz S, Rennke HG: Collapsing glomerulopathy in HIV and non–HIV patients: A clinicopathological and follow–up study. Kidney Int 1999;56:2203–2213.
66. D'Agati V, Appel GB: Renal pathology of human immunodeficiency virus infection. Semin Nephrol 1998;18:406–421.
67. Stirling CM, Mathieson P, Bolton-Jones JM, et al: Treatment and outcome of adult patients with primary focal segmental glomerulosclerosis in five UK renal units. Q J Med 2005;98:443–449.
68. Pei Y, Cattran D, Delmore T, et al: Evidence suggesting under-treatment of adults with idiopathic FSGS. Am J Med 1987;82:938–944.
69. Ingulli E, Tejani A: Racial differences in the incidence and renal outcome of idiopathic focal segmental glomerulosclerosis in children. Pediatr Nephrol 1991;5:393–397.
70. Matalon A, Valeri A, Appel GB: Treatment of focal segmental glomerulosclerosis. Semin Nephrol 2000;20:309–317.
71. Troyanov S, Wall CA, Miller JA, et al: Focal and segmental glomerulosclerosis: Definition and relevance of a partial remission. J Am Soc Nephrol 2005;16:1061–1068.
72. Ruf RG, Lichtenberger A, Karle SM, et al: Patients with mutations in NPHS2 do not respond to standard steroid treatment of nephrotic syndrome. J Am Soc Nephrol 2004;15:722–732.

73. Ponticelli C, Villa M, Banfi G, et al: Can prolonged treatment improve the prognosis of adults with FSGS? Am J Kidney Dis 1999;34:618–625.

74. Korbet SM: Treatment of primary focal and segmental glomerulosclerosis. Kidney Int 2002;62:2301–2310.

75. Ponticelli C, Passerini P: Other immunosuppressive agents for FSGS. Semin Nephrol 2003;23:242–248.

76. Tune BM, Kirpekor R, Sibley R, et al: IV methylprednisolone and oral alkylating agent therapy of prednisone resistant pediatric FSGS: Long-term follow up. Clin Nephrol 1995;43:83–88.

77. Klein M, Radhakrishnan J, Appel GB: Cyclosporin treatment of glomerular disease. Annu Rev Med 1999;50:1–15.

78. Lieberman KV, Tejani A, for the NY-NJ Pediatric Nephrology Study Group: A randomized double-blind trial of cyclosporine in steroid resistant FSGS in children. J Am Soc Nephrol 1996;7:56–63.

79. Cattran D, Appel GB, Hebert L, et al: A randomized trial of cyclosporine in patients with steroid resistant focal segmental glomerulosclerosis: North America Nephrotic Syndrome Study Group. Kidney Int 1999;56: 2220–2226.

80. Heering P, Braun N, Mullejans R, et al: Cyclosporin A and chlorambucil in the treatment of idiopathic focal segmental glomerulosclerosis. Am J Kidney Dis 2004;43:10–18.

81. Choi MJ, Eustace JA, Gimenez LF, et al: Mycophenolate mofetil treatment for primary glomerular disease. Kidney Int 2002;61:1098–1114.

82. Cattran DC, Wang MM, Appel GB, et al: Mycophenolate mofetil in the treatment of focal segmental glomerulosclerosis. Clin Nephrol 2005;62: 405–412.

83. Appel GB, Radhakrishnan J, Ginzler E: Use of mycophenolate mofetil in glomerular diseases. Transplantation 2005;80(Suppl 2):8265–8271.

84. Fervenza F, Fitzpatrick PM, Mertz J, et al: Acute rapamycin nephrotoxicity in native kidneys in patients with chronic glomerulopathies. Nephrol Dial Transplant 2004;19:1288–1292.

85. Tumlin JA, Miller D, Near M, et al: A prospective open-label trial of sirolimus in the treatment of focal segmental glomerulosclerosis. Clin J Am Soc Nephrol 2006;1:109–117.

86. Nakao N, Yoshimura A, Morita H, et al: Combined angiotensin receptor blocker and angiotensin converting enzyme therapy in non-diabetic renal disease (Cooperate Study): A randomized controlled trial. Lancet 2003;361:117–124.

87. Winston JA, Bruggeman LA, Ross MD, et al: Nephropathy and establishment of a renal reservoir of HIV type 1 during primary infection. N Engl J Med 2001;344:1979–1984.

88. Burns GC, Paul SK, Toth IR, Sivak SL: Effect of angiotensin converting enzyme inhibition in HIV associated nephropathy. J Am Soc Nephrol 1997;8:1140–1146.

89. Eustace JA, Nuermberger F, Chjoi M, et al: Cohort study of severe HIV associated nephropathy with corticosteroids. Kidney Int 2000;58: 1253–1260.

90. Artero M, Biava C, Amend W, et al: Recurrent focal glomerulosclerosis: Natural history and response to therapy. Am J Med 1992;92:375–383.

91. Vincenti F, Ghiggeri GM: New insights into the pathogenesis and the therapy of recurrent FSGS. Am J Transplant 2005;5:1179–1185.

92. Huang K, Ferris ME, Andreoni KA, Gipson DS: The differential effect of race among pediatric kidney transplant recipients with FSGS. Am J Kidney Dis 2004;43:1082–1090.

Membranous Nephropathy

William G. Couser

INTRODUCTION AND DEFINITION

Membranous nephropathy (MN) is a glomerular disease in which immune deposits of IgG and complement components develop predominantly or exclusively beneath podocytes on the subepithelial surface of the glomerular capillary wall. Deposition is associated with a marked increase in glomerular permeability to protein, which is manifested clinically as nephrotic syndrome.[1] The disease occurs in association with a variety of conditions, some of which are likely causal and some of which probably represent only associations (Fig. 19.1).[2] However, most occurrences (two thirds) are idiopathic, without obvious initiating events. MN is the most common cause of idiopathic nephrotic syndrome in white adults older than 60 years, and is rare in children.

The term membranous refers to thickening of the glomerular capillary wall, but the entity now referred to as MN was clearly defined only following the advent of immunofluorescence and electron microscopy as routine tools in the study of renal biopsies in the 1950s and 1960s. These techniques first revealed the presence early in the development of the disease of the diffuse, finely granular immune deposits in the subepithelial space that are now regarded as pathognomonic of MN. Consequently, MN is a pathologic diagnosis made when glomeruli exhibit these deposits without associated hypercellularity or inflammatory change.

ETIOLOGY AND PATHOGENESIS

Etiology

The pathogenesis of human MN is not known. However, the frequent occurrence of this lesion in autoimmune disorders such as lupus and type 1 diabetes, as well as its remarkable similarity to a lesion induced in rats with antibody to antigens expressed on the surface of the glomerular podocyte, have fueled speculation that the disease is caused by deposits of autoantibody to fixed components of the podocyte membrane.[3,4] A large number of agents appear to be capable of initiating this process in genetically susceptible individuals (see Fig. 19.1) and include viruses such as hepatitis B virus (HBV) and hepatitis C virus (HCV), drugs including gold, penicillamine, and nonsteroidal anti-inflammatory agents (NSAIDs), toxins such as hydrocarbons and formaldehyde, and a variety of chronic immune disorders such as lupus, thyroiditis, graft-versus-host disease, antiglomerular basement membrane (GBM) and antineutrophilic cytoplasmic antibody (ANCA)–positive crescentic glomerulonephritis (GN), and renal allografts. In about two thirds of patients, no obvious etiologic agent or condition can be identified.

Recently, there has been one well-documented case of congenital MN that was shown to be mediated by an antibody to an endogenous antigen (neutral endopeptidase [NEP]) on the glomerular podocyte. In this situation, the mother, who had a hereditary deficiency in NEP, became sensitized during pregnancy

Conditions and agents associated with membranous nephropathy		
Group	Common	Uncommon
Immune diseases	Systemic lupus erythematosus, type 1 diabetes mellitus	Rheumatoid arthritis, Hashimoto's disease, Graves' disease, mixed connective tissue disease, Sjögren's syndrome, primary biliary cirrhosis, bullous pemphigoid, small bowel enteropathy syndrome, dermatitis herpetiformis, ankylosing spondylitis, graft-versus-host disease, Guillain-Barré syndrome, bone marrow and stem cell transplantation, anti–glomerular basement membrane and antineutrophil cytoplasmic antibody–positive crescentic glomerulonephritis
Infectious or parasitic diseases	Hepatitis B	Hepatitis C, syphilis, filariasis, hydatid disease, schistosomiasis, malaria, leprosy
Drugs and toxins	Gold, penicillamine, nonsteroidal anti-inflammatory agents	Mercury, captopril, formaldehyde, hydrocarbons, bucillamine
Miscellaneous	Tumors, renal transplantation	Sarcoidosis, sickle cell disease, Kimura's disease, angiofollicular lymph node hyperplasia

Figure 19.1 Conditions and agents associated with membranous nephropathy. The list excludes conditions for which only a single case has been reported or where the lesions were atypical of membranous nephropathy. (Modified from Couser WG, Alpers CE: Membranous nephropathy. In Neilson EG, Couser WG [eds]: Immunologic Renal Diseases. Philadelphia: Lippincott Williams & Wilkins, 2001, pp 1029–1036.)

and passively transferred anti-NEP IgG to her infant at birth, resulting in a lesion of MN.[3]

Mechanisms of Immune Deposit Formation

Regardless of the initiating event(s), the disease appears to be mediated primarily by the Th2 humoral immune response, which leads to deposition of IgG and complement on the outer surface of the glomerular capillary wall. Experimental evidence suggests that this is unlikely to be the consequence of passive glomerular trapping of preformed immune complexes directly from the circulation. However, such deposits can be produced by local or *in situ* immune-complex formation involving antigens that could be exogenous or endogenous and could act in three ways.[5] First, exogenous antigens could localize on the subepithelial surface because of their cationic charge and small size; second, they could form immune complexes on the inner surface of the capillary wall that dissociate, traverse the GBM, and re-form in the subepithelial space; and finally, the antigens could be endogenous constituents of a subepithelial component of the capillary wall such as the podocyte membrane.[3] The total absence of deposits at subendothelial (and mesangial) sites in idiopathic MN, as well as the ability to duplicate the lesion with anti–podocyte antibodies, strongly favors the third or autoimmune explanation for the unique localization of deposits in this disease. In rat models of MN, which closely simulate the human disease (Heymann nephritis), the antigens responsible are components of the Heymann nephritis antigenic complex: a large (516-kd) glycoprotein, called megalin, bound to a smaller receptor-associated protein (RAP) expressed in the clathrin-coated pits of the podocyte foot processes.[4] While antibodies to small antigenic determinants on both molecules can form subepithelial immune-complex deposits, additional antigen-antibody systems involving an unidentified glycolipid antigen that activates complement and antibodies that neutralize complement regulatory proteins are required to induce proteinuria in animals. Once formed, these complexes of antigen and antibody are capped and shed from the cell surface, where they bind to underlying GBM, resist degradation, and persist for weeks or months as immune deposits detectable by immunofluorescence and electron microscopy (Fig. 19.2).[4,5]

However, other than the rare case of congenital MN due to antibody to NEP, such autoantibodies have not yet been identified in human MN, and the two exogenous antigen mechanisms have not been excluded (although in the authors' judgment they are unlikely), particularly in disease induced by foreign agents such as viruses.

Mechanism of Glomerular Injury

Based entirely on studies in animal models, the mechanism by which damage to the glomerular filtration barrier sufficient to cause proteinuria occurs appears to involve sublytic effects of complement C5b-9 (a multimer comprising several complement components and also known as the membrane attack complex) on the podocyte (Fig. 19.3).[4,6] Complement activation and cleavage of C5 generates the chemotactic factor C5a, which presumably is flushed by filtration forces into the urinary space and does not move backwards across the GBM to attract circulating inflammatory cells. The other product of C5 cleavage, C5b, combines with C6 to form a lipophilic complex that inserts into the lipid bilayer of the podocyte where C7, C8, and multiple C9 molecules are added to create a pore-forming complex, C5b-9 (see Figs. 19.2 and 19.3). The podocyte is resistant to lysis and endocytoses the C5b-9, transporting it intracellularly in multivesicular bodies and extruding it into the urinary space (see Fig. 19.2). However, the membrane insertion of C5b-9, although insufficient to cause cell lysis, does induce cell activation and signal transduction, with increased production of multiple potentially nephritogenic molecules, including oxidants, proteases, cytokines, growth factors, vasoactive molecules, and extracellular matrix (see Fig. 19.3).[6] Current evidence

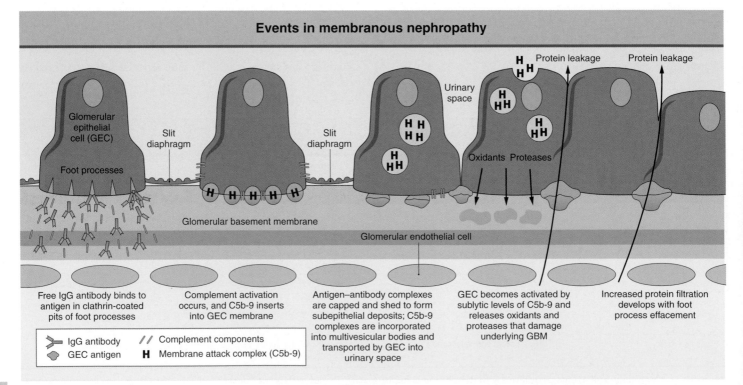

Figure 19.2 Events in a rat model of membranous nephropathy. Immune deposit formation, C5b-9 insertion, and podocyte activation lead to proteinuria (see text).

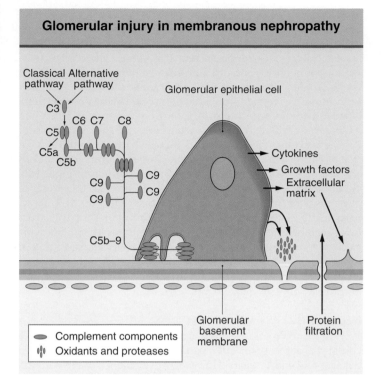

Glomerular injury in membranous nephropathy

Figure 19.3 Postulated mechanism of glomerular injury in membranous nephropathy. Antibodies against the podocytes induce complement activation via the classical or alternative pathway, leading to formation of C5b-9. Insertion of C5b-9 is insufficient to cause lysis but stimulates the podocyte to release a host of inflammatory mediators that damage the underlying glomerular basement membrane, leading to increased protein filtration.

is strongest for the role of podocyte-derived oxidants in producing the GBM damage that leads to increased protein filtration in MN, but an equivalent role for unique podocyte-derived proteases has not been excluded. During the period when antibody deposition, deposit formation, and complement activation are occurring, increased excretion of C5b-9 and of viable podocytes can be measured in the urine.[6,7]

Consequences of Injury Induced by C5b-9

The glomerular injury mediated by C5b-9 induces a nonselective proteinuria through loss of both the size- and the charge-selective properties of the glomerular capillary wall. The subsequent reduction in GFR that occurs in progressive MN has both glomerular and interstitial components. In the glomerulus, there is thickening of the GBM resulting from overproduction of several different extracellular matrix molecules, which are deposited between and around the immune deposits to form subepithelial "spikes." GBM spikes are characteristic of this disease when a biopsy is studied with silver-methenamine staining (see Fig. 19.5c). This appears to occur in part through upregulation of podocyte production of transforming growth factors (TGFs), TGF-β_2 and TGF-β_3, as well as increased expression of TGF-β receptors in response to C5b-9.[6] Podocyte cell number decreases due to apoptosis and cell detachment as the glomerulus expands secondary to increased pressures and flows. The podocyte itself has limited ability to proliferate and cover denuded areas due to overexpression of cyclin kinase inhibitors and cell cycle arrest.[8] In the interstitium, there is an increased macrophage infiltrate and overproduction of matrix by interstitial fibroblasts, leading to interstitial fibrosis.[2,9] The interstitial response is likely common to all nonselective proteinuric disorders and results from toxic effects of normal serum proteins, lipid-derived chemotactic factors, iron, intratubular C5b-9 activation, and other glomerular-derived mediators on the tubular cells (see also Chapter 69).[9] When nephrotic-range proteinuria persists, the consequence is glomerular sclerosis as well as interstitial fibrosis and progression to renal failure at a rate directly related to both the magnitude and the duration of increased protein filtration.

EPIDEMIOLOGY

The disease is uncommon in children, accounting for 2% to 12% (usually <5%) of pediatric patients undergoing biopsy for nephrotic syndrome. In adults, about 30% of all biopsies for idiopathic nephrotic syndrome reveal MN, and the disease accounts for about 50% of biopsied cases of idiopathic nephrotic syndrome in older white adults, a population in which MN remains the leading cause of idiopathic nephrotic syndrome.[1,2] There is some variation in these figures among different countries, with slightly lower numbers in the United Kingdom and higher numbers in Greece and Macedonia. The U.S. Renal Data System records 1392 patients with end-stage renal disease (ESRD) owing to established MN in 1991 to 1995, or about 0.5% of the total ESRD population.[10] However, if one includes patients with lupus MN and an estimated 5% of patients classified only as chronic GN, the total is probably twice that. Further, if only 50% of patients progress to renal failure, and another 20% to 30% are clinically silent, the real prevalence of this disease is probably around 2000 patients per year in the United States or about eight patients per million population per year.

There is a threefold increased risk of MN in patients with HLA-DR3, and associations with HLA-B8 and HLA-B18 have also been reported.[2] HLA-DR5, in addition to HLA-DR3, appears to increase the risk of progression. In Japan, MN is associated with HLA-DR2. Some white patients have a deletion of C4 with the HLA-B8-DR3 haplotype. Rare examples of familial MN have also been reported, usually presenting in brothers.

CLINICAL MANIFESTATIONS

Idiopathic Disease

MN is a disorder of insidious onset in which the only clinical manifestations of early disease are an increase in urine protein excretion and the consequences thereof. Most patients present with a gradual development of peripheral edema without other signs or symptoms. The disease has been reported in children younger than 1 year of age and in adults older than 90 years, but it is uncommon in patients younger than 30. MN is more common in men than women by about a 2 to 3:1 ratio, and individual peaks occur between ages 30 and 40 years and again between ages 50 and 60 years.[1,2]

About 80% of patients have overt nephrotic syndrome at the time of presentation, with urine protein excretion exceeding 3.5 g/day, reduced serum albumin levels, and elevated serum lipids, as well as fluid retention and edema (see Chapter 16). However, the disease likely develops over a period of several weeks or months before proteinuria of this magnitude occurs, and about 20% of patients are detected with asymptomatic non-nephrotic proteinuria (<3.5 g/day). Proteinuria is always nonselective and generally in the 5- to 15-g/day range. Urine protein excretion >15 g is more suggestive of minimal change disease, but this is not absolute. Day-to-day fluctuations in protein excretion are frequent in MN and likely reflect changes in protein intake, posture, exercise, and hemodynamic variables more than changes in the activity of the disease.

Microscopic hematuria may be seen in up to 50% of adults, but macroscopic hematuria and red blood–cell casts are extremely unusual and suggest a different diagnosis. Patients with active, ongoing glomerular immune deposit formation exhibit elevated levels of urinary C5b-9 excretion, and this may be a marker of active disease and suggest a worse prognosis.[2,6] Hypertension is not a common feature of MN. It has been reported in up to 30% of patients, but usually only with more advanced degrees of renal insufficiency.[1]

Patients with MN appear to have an increased incidence of renal vein thrombosis, above that seen in other nephrotic glomerular diseases. Prospective studies document renal vein thrombosis in up to 40% of patients.[1,2] However, there is no evidence that the presence of renal vein thrombi alters disease severity or renal function. Nonetheless, patients with renal vein thrombosis are at increased risk of thromboembolic phenomena, and prophylactic anticoagulation treatment is recommended for such patients (see later discussion).

Reduction in renal function develops slowly in MN, and renal function is usually well preserved at the onset of disease. Usually, nephrotic-range proteinuria precedes any fixed loss of glomerular filtration rate (GFR) by weeks or months, although some pre-renal azotemia may develop in patients who are hypoalbuminemic and have depleted extracellular fluid volume. Less than 20% of patients have a reduction in GFR at the time of initial diagnosis.[1,2,11,12]

The diagnostic studies that should be performed in patients with known or suspected MN are listed in Figure 19.4.

Common Secondary Causes

While the typical clinical features of MN are not unique or different from those of several other diseases that cause idiopathic nephrotic syndrome, about one third of patients have MN as a manifestation of some other systemic disease process. Several of these associations are sufficiently common to warrant separate mention.

Membranous Lupus Nephritis

The class V, or membranous, form of lupus nephritis may be indistinguishable from idiopathic MN clinically and even serologically.[13] This lesion accounts for about 20% of patients with lupus nephritis and often presents as nephrotic syndrome in young women who do not have other clinical or serologic manifestations of systemic lupus, although they usually develop these later. In patients with lupus MN, anti-DNA antibody levels and antinuclear antibody titers are often low, and the antibody is of very low avidity compared with that in patients with class IV lesions (diffuse proliferative lupus nephritis). Complement levels are also often normal. While the glomerular lesion of lupus MN closely mimics the idiopathic form of the disease, the presence of deposits of immunoglobulins other than IgG (i.e., IgA, IgM), particularly in the mesangium, as well as tubuloreticular structures seen by electron microscopy suggest lupus as an underlying etiology.[1,2,13] The natural history of lupus MN is similar to that of the idiopathic form of the disease, with about 85% renal survival at 10 years. Treatment generally is similar to that suggested for idiopathic MN (see also Chapter 24).

Hepatitis B

Worldwide there is a strong association between MN and a chronic carrier state for HBV, particularly in young males between the ages of 2 and 12 years. However, the incidence of HBV in MN varies widely in different parts of the world, from about 30% to 40% of adult patients in Asia to less than 1% in the United States.[14] In children, the rate is much higher, ranging from 20% to 64% in the United States to >80% in eastern Europe, Asia, and Africa. The presence of HBV antigens, particularly HBe antigen, in glomeruli, together with antibody to it, suggests that HBV antigens participate in *in situ* immune-complex formation, leading to disease development in patients who cannot clear antigens and remain in persistent antigen excess or exhibit low-avidity antibodies.[14]

Clinically, HBV MN presents like idiopathic MN with nephrotic syndrome. It occurs in patients who often have a

---

Diagnosis and management of patients with membranous nephropathy	
Patient Groups	**Test**
All patients	
General	Renal function (serum creatinine and creatinine clearance)
	Blood pressure
	Urine protein excretion (24-hour urine or urine protein-to-creatinine ratio)
	Serum albumin
	Serum cholesterol
	Urinalysis
	Renal biopsy
Associated disease	Hepatitis B (HBs antigen)
	Hepatitis C (HCV antibody)
	Antinuclear antibody, anti–double-stranded DNA (the hallmark of systemic lupus erythematosus)
	Complement C3, C4 (usually normal in idiopathic membranous nephropathy)
Selected patients	
With suspected thromboembolic events, flank pain, hematuria, acute renal failure	Renal vein angiography
With sudden decrease in renal function, development of active urine sediment	Anti–glomerular basement membrane and antineutrophilic cytoplasmic antibody
Older than 50 years of age	Cancer screening (see text)

Figure 19.4 Diagnosis and management of patients with membranous nephropathy.

history of viral hepatitis, laboratory evidence of low-grade chronic hepatitis, and evidence of HBs antigen, and often Hbe antigen, in the circulation. Complement levels are more often reduced in HBV MN than in the idiopathic form of the disease (30% to 50% of patients), and hematuria and hypertension are also more common.[14] The course is more benign than in idiopathic MN, with most children undergoing spontaneous remission within 5 years and only 10% to 20% of adults progressing to chronic renal failure. Treatment is generally supportive, with diuretics and angiotensin-converting enzyme (ACE) inhibitors to reduce protein excretion. In symptomatic or progressive disease, a trial of antiviral therapy with interferon-α is probably indicated (see also Chapter 25).[15] Many adults enter remission following antiviral therapy if renal function is well preserved. Corticosteroids are without obvious benefit to the glomerular lesion and may induce viral replication and worsen liver disease. Similar problems beset the use of cytotoxic drug therapy, including the immunosuppressive regimens required for transplantation. MN has also been reported with HCV infection, sometimes in the absence of cryoglobulins or rheumatoid factor, although this association is less well established than that with HBV.

Cancer

An association between MN and solid tumors is well established, particularly in adults older than 50 years, in whom the incidence of malignancy in MN in some reports has approached 20%.[1,16] The most common associated cancers are those of the lung, breast, kidney, and gastrointestinal tract, but cases of MN have been reported with most forms of cancer. In patients with cancer-associated MN, the nephrotic syndrome may precede clinical evidence of the tumor by 12 to 18 months.[1,2,16] A careful search for malignancy is, therefore, mandatory in older patients who present with MN. This should include chest radiography, colonoscopy, stool test for occult blood, mammography in women, and measurement of tumor markers such as CEA (carcinoembryonic antigen) and PSA (prostate-specific antigen). In patients with other signs suggesting cancer, such as unexplained weight loss or pain, an abdominal computed tomography scan is indicated. The glomerular lesion and nephrotic syndrome have been reported to resolve following successful resection of early tumors, although this does not always occur. Prognosis is generally determined more by the tumor than by the MN, and no form of immunosuppressive therapy has been shown to be useful in such patients.

Membranous Nephropathy in Renal Allografts

MN may recur occasionally in allografts; this usually occurs in patients with severe disease who progress from onset of symptoms to renal failure in ≤3 years. Recurrent MN generally appears in the first 6 to 12 months following transplantation.[17] More commonly, MN develops *de novo* in the allograft, where it accounts for up to 30% of transplant recipients with nephrotic syndrome. It is second only to transplant glomerulopathy as a cause of nephrotic syndrome in transplant recipients and generally presents ≥2 years following transplantation.[17] In patients with renal allografts and *de novo* MN, 60% are nephrotic and 40% have non-nephrotic proteinuria. As in idiopathic MN, the pathogenesis of the lesion is unknown, although some cases are associated with HCV infection. The presence of *de novo* MN does not appear to be a significant risk factor for allograft survival, and most such grafts are lost from chronic rejection. There are no data to document a benefit of disease-specific therapy in reducing proteinuria

or prolonging graft survival beyond the immunosuppressive regimen utilized for transplantation, but therapy to lower urine protein excretion (see later discussion) seems prudent.

Membranous Nephropathy and Rapidly Progressive Glomerulonephritis

A rare but well-documented event in MN is the superimposition of a crescentic glomerular lesion with sudden deterioration in renal function accompanied by an active urine sediment. This may occur from the development of either anti-GBM antibodies or ANCAs. Linear staining of the GBM may be difficult to distinguish from the very finely granular deposits that characterize uncomplicated MN. When this characterization does occur, treatment for anti-GBM disease or renal vasculitis, usually including steroids, cyclophosphamide, and plasma exchange (for anti-GBM disease; see Chapter 22), should be instituted.

PATHOLOGY

The pathologic features of MN evolve from the initial formation of subepithelial immune complexes of IgG and complement along the outer surface of the capillary wall without other morphologic abnormalities rendering the early disease indistinguishable from minimal change nephrotic syndrome by light microscopy alone. Changes occur first in the podocyte, then in glomerular barrier function leading to proteinuria, then in the renal interstitium (probably as a consequence of the proteinuria), and finally in the GBM itself, which becomes thickened (membranous) through the accumulation of additional matrix material along the outer surface, often in an irregular or spikelike pattern.[2,11]

Light Microscopy

In the earliest stages of the disease, the glomeruli and interstitium may be essentially normal by light microscopy, and the diagnosis can be made only by application of immunofluorescence and electron microscopy (Fig. 19.5a). However, the disease progresses early to a homogeneous thickening of the capillary wall, seen in light microscopy in sections stained with hematoxylin and eosin or with periodic acid–Schiff reagent (see Fig. 19.5b). By methenamine silver staining, early projections of the GBM between deposits may be detected in a characteristic spikelike configuration (see Fig. 19.5c).

In contrast to diseases in which similar quantities of immune deposits are formed along the subendothelial surface of the capillary wall or in the mesangium, no glomerular leukocyte infiltration occurs in MN. This is presumably because chemotactic products of complement activation follow filtration forces into the urinary space rather than diffusing backward into the capillary lumen, and the intervening GBM prevents immune adherence mechanisms from being operative. Although similar deposits at other sites may induce proliferation of glomerular endothelial and, particularly, mesangial cells, podocytes *in vivo* seem terminally differentiated and rarely proliferate.[6,18] As a result, the pathologic lesion of MN is characterized only by changes in podocytes and basement membrane without any associated glomerular hypercellularity.

The podocyte response to this form of injury does include effacement of foot processes, which is visible only by electron microscopy. A variety of molecules are upregulated in damaged or activated podocytes in experimental MN, including cysteine-rich acidic secreted protein (SPARC), desmin, platelet-derived growth factor, VEGF, TGF-β, TGF-β receptors, and several

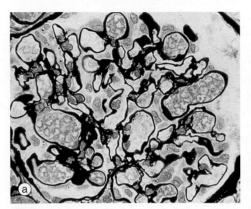
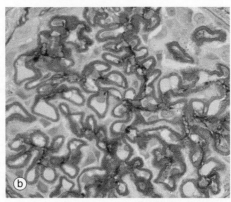
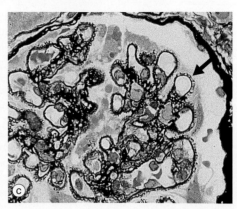

Figure 19.5   Light microscopy in membranous nephropathy (MN). *a*, Early MN: a glomerulus from a patient with severe nephrotic syndrome and early MN, exhibiting normal architecture and peripheral capillary basement membranes of normal thickness (methenamine silver ×400). *b*, Morphologically advanced MN: uniform increase in the thickness of the glomerular capillary walls throughout the glomerulus without any increase in glomerular cellularity (periodic acid–Schiff ×400). *c*, Morphologically more advanced MN (same patient as in *b*): discrete spikes of matrix emanating from the outer surface of the basement membrane (*arrow*) indicative of advanced MN are revealed by methenamine silver stain (×400). (Courtesy of C. E. Alpers.)

other cytokines.[6,18] There generally are no visible mesangial or endothelial cell abnormalities. The presence of significant mesangial hypercellularity suggests immune deposit formation in the mesangium and is more consistent with a secondary MN such as class V lupus nephritis (see previous discussion). In some patients with heavy proteinuria and progressive disease, glomeruli exhibit reduced podocyte numbers and areas of focal sclerosis that are similar to the appearance of idiopathic focal segmental glomerulosclerosis (see Chapter 18). These patients often have a more rapidly progressive course and a poor response to therapy. These sclerotic lesions may be a consequence of glomerular hypertrophy accompanied by an inability of the terminally differentiated podocytes to proliferate,[6] leading to areas of denuded GBM, attachment to Bowman's capsule, and subsequent capillary collapse (see Chapter 15).

As in all nephrotic glomerular diseases, interstitial changes predict renal function and outcome better than glomerular abnormalities do. The degree of interstitial change reflects the magnitude of proteinuria and its duration. Interstitial changes include a diffuse mononuclear cell infiltrate comprising T cells, monocytes, macrophages, and B cells. Tubular degeneration and atrophy and interstitial fibrosis (composed predominantly of type I collagen) evolve over time. In the experimental setting, a number of mediators are overexpressed in the interstitium, including osteopontin (a macrophage chemotactic and adhesive protein made by tubular cells), TGF-β (derived from tubular cells), macrophages, fibroblasts, and thrombospondin (an activator of TGF-β).[6]

Immunofluorescence Microscopy

The pattern of IgG staining in MN is characteristic and easily recognizable by immunofluorescence (Fig. 19.6). Positive staining for IgG marks the finely granular subepithelial deposits, which are present on the outer surface of all capillary loops.[2] The predominant IgG subclass in idiopathic MN is IgG$_4$. Staining in MN is positive only for IgG in an exclusively subepithelial distribution. Positive staining for IgA or IgM or significant staining in the glomerular mesangium suggests lupus as an underlying mechanism. Complement C3 is also present in about 50% of patients and usually reflects staining for C3c, a breakdown product of C3b that is rapidly cleared. Consequently, positive C3 staining likely reflects active, ongoing immune deposit formation and complement activation at the time of the biopsy, whereas the

absence of C3 suggests that the process of forming deposits has ceased. When looked for, staining for C5b-9 is generally present as well, which is consistent with the proposed pathogenetic role of C5b-9 in this disease (see previous discussion).[2,6] C1 and C4 are often absent, indicating activation of complement through the alternative pathway as a consequence of podocyte damage or downregulation of complement regulatory proteins expressed on the podocyte membrane.[19]

Electron Microscopy

The presence of subepithelial electron-dense deposits by electron microscopy parallels IgG staining. In idiopathic MN, immune deposit formation occurs only in a subepithelial distribution, and deposits are not seen in mesangial or subendothelial sites. These deposits in early stages of the disease process are homogeneous and may even be confluent in some areas with overlying podocyte foot process effacement and little change in the underlying GBM (stage I). As the disease persists, there is projection of basement membrane material up between the deposits to form subepithelial spikes that can be detected by light microscopy using a methenamine silver stain and are easily visible by electron

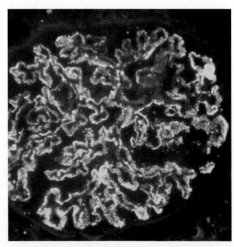

Figure 19.6   Immunofluorescence in membranous nephropathy. A glomerulus with diffuse, finely granular deposition of IgG along the outer surface of all capillary walls. The antibody is believed to represent autoantibody directed at some constituent of the podocyte membrane (original magnification ×400). (Courtesy of C. E. Alpers.)

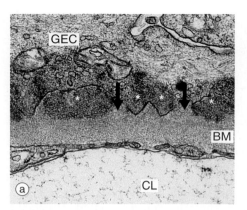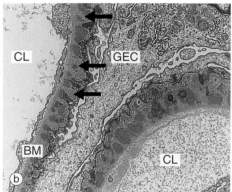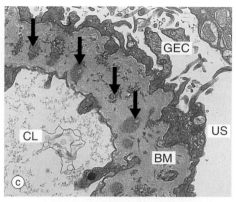

Figure 19.7   Electron microscopy in membranous nephropathy (MN). *a*, Early (stage II) disease: glomerular capillary wall with discrete electron-dense deposits on the subepithelial surface of the basement membrane (BM) corresponding to granular deposits of IgG detected by immunofluorescence microscopy (corresponding to the light micrograph in Fig. 19.6). There are diffuse, granular immune-complex deposits (*asterisks*) along the outer surface of the capillary wall with effacement of overlying podocyte foot processes. Small extensions of BM between deposits (*arrows*) are also evident and represent the projections that are seen as spikes by light microscopy with methenamine silver staining. *b*, More advanced disease (stage III): two glomerular capillary loops showing involvement of the BM by the immune-complex deposition. There is prominent membrane synthesis surrounding and incorporating these deposits into the BM (corresponding to the spikes seen on methenamine silver–stained histologic preparations). Overlying glomerular epithelial cells (GEC) continue to demonstrate widespread effacement of foot processes. *c*, Morphologically advanced MN (stage IV): the capillary BM is diffusely thickened; scattered electron-dense immune deposits (*arrows*) are present throughout its thickness in addition to scattered subepithelial deposits. Overlying GECs continue to demonstrate effacement of foot processes. CL, capillary lumen; US, urinary space (original magnification ×18,000). (Courtesy of C. E. Alpers.)

microscopy (stage II; Fig. 19.7a). Later, the spikes extend and the deposits may become surrounded by new basement membrane–like material (stage III; see Fig. 19.7b). In stage IV disease, the basement membrane is overtly thickened, the deposits incorporated in it become more lucent, and the spikes are less apparent (see Fig. 19.7c). This sequence of events, observed primarily by electron microscopy, has led pathologists to classify the glomerular changes into "stages" ranging from minimal change with only small deposits (stage I) through the evolution to thickened basement membrane with resolution of deposits (stage IV).[2,11] The extent to which individual patients will exhibit these sequential changes depends on the duration of the underlying immunopathologic process and its severity. Although these changes clearly reflect the severity and duration of disease, they do not correlate well with clinical manifestations or outcome.

DIFFERENTIAL DIAGNOSIS

The differential diagnosis of MN before biopsy is the differential diagnosis of acquired idiopathic nephrotic syndrome (see Chapter 16) and includes minimal change/focal segmental glomerulosclerosis, systemic lupus erythematosus, membranoproliferative GN types I and II, and dysproteinemias such as amyloid and light-chain deposition disease. The pathogenetic antibody is not known (and is likely to be present in the circulation only intermittently anyway), so there are no laboratory tests that establish the diagnosis. An outline of appropriate studies to perform in patients with known or suspected MN is presented in Figure 19.4.

The presence of hypocomplementemia is more suggestive of MN associated with lupus or HBV. MN is rare in children as a cause of idiopathic nephrotic syndrome (<5%) but is the most common cause in adults older than 50 years, particularly in white patients. MN is generally associated with lower levels of protein excretion than usually seen in minimal change disease, averaging about 10 g/day, and less hypertension than in focal glomerulosclerosis or membranoproliferative GN.[1,2,11] However, a definitive diagnosis can be made only with a diagnostic renal biopsy, which we believe is indicated in all patients with idiopathic nephrotic syndrome.

Once the diagnosis has been established, it is mandatory to look for other causes of MN, particularly HBV, systemic lupus, and malignancy (see Fig. 19.1). These disorders can usually be excluded by appropriate clinical and serologic evaluation.

NATURAL HISTORY AND PROGNOSIS

Before considering approaches to therapy, which remain controversial, it is imperative to understand the nature of untreated MN and its prognosis. Although not proven, it is likely that the onset of disease probably precedes development of overt nephrotic syndrome by weeks or months. In fact, it is probable that the period of ongoing antibody deposition that characterizes active disease has ceased in some patients by the time a diagnosis is made. This is made more likely by the observation that the fully developed lesion of MN requires weeks or months to resolve after the initiating pathogenetic process is abrogated. Therefore, the presence of nephrotic syndrome does not necessarily imply the presence of active immunologic disease, and the clinical course of MN in terms of proteinuria and renal function may be substantially dissociated from the initiating disease mechanism.

When MN is drug induced, the disease always resolves but can take years to do so. In idiopathic MN, spontaneous resolution occurs in >50% of children within 5 years, and 10-year renal survival exceeds 90%. Most children and most women will experience spontaneous remissions, and disease-specific therapy is rarely indicated unless there is a documented loss of GFR.[1,20–22]

In adult men, the prognosis is worse. In non-nephrotic patients, the outcome is generally good without disease-specific therapy with a 10-year renal survival rate of close to 100%.[21] When only patients with nephrotic syndrome and >3 years of follow-up are considered, about 50% of untreated patients develop progressive renal disease.[20] Another 25% of patients eventually have a spontaneous complete remission (normal protein excretion), usually within 3 to 5 years, and another 25% have partial remissions (<2 g/day proteinuria) with persistent proteinuria but no loss of GFR. About 25% of patients who enter remission suffer a subsequent relapse of nephrotic syndrome. For patients who exhibit partial remission or maintain normal GFR for >3 years, the prognosis is excellent.[20,21]

The mean time to doubling of serum creatinine in patients with progressive disease is about 30 months, but a subset of patients with a more rapidly progressive course can develop ESRD within ≤3 years. In this group of patients, there is an increased probability of recurrence of MN in the renal allograft. Since disease-specific therapy is generally associated with significant side effects, it is important to try to identify patients at substantial risk of progression to receive such treatment and to spare those patients who are likely to have a benign course independent of cytotoxic immunosuppressive therapy.[12,20,22] Figure 19.8 lists the factors that have been established or suggested to portend a poor prognosis in MN.[20–23]

Estimates of the predictive value of various prognostic factors in identifying patients whose disease will subsequently progress have been reported (see Fig. 19.8).[20,23,24] The best established clinical parameters are the presence of persistent proteinuria (>8 g for >6 months, >6 g for >9 months, or >4 g for >1 year) and increased serum creatinine at the time of diagnosis or during follow-up, which documents that progression is already in progress.[20,25] Urinary excretion of >250 mg/day of IgG (an index of urine protein selectivity) and >0.5 µg/min of β_2-microglobulin

(an index of tubular function that likely reflects severity of interstitial disease) are also strong predictors of progressive disease, with an established specificity of about 90%.[20,24]

THERAPY

Despite the fact that MN is a relatively common glomerular disease and has been subjected to multiple controlled trials of various steroid and immunosuppressive regimens, the therapy of MN is still controversial.[20,22,25] Some experienced investigators advocate no disease-specific treatment because of the relatively benign course, while others treat all patients with aggressive cytotoxic drug protocols. Multiple factors complicate interpretation of such studies. These include the limited number of patients or short duration of most studies, failure to measure or control for some as yet poorly defined variables such as etiologic and immunogenetic factors that are likely to affect prognosis (see Fig. 19.8), and inability to incorporate the likely benefits for nephrotic patients of current nonspecific therapies such as achieving good blood pressure control, utilization of modern lipid-lowering agents, and drugs or dietary manipulations that nonspecifically lower the level of urine protein excretion (such as protein restriction, ACE inhibitors, and angiotensin receptor blockers [ARBs]). The currently available therapeutic options for treating patients with MN are listed in Figure 19.9.

Treatment That Is Not Disease Specific
Non–disease-specific variables have been shown to affect the prognosis of all glomerular diseases adversely, including MN. These variables include elevated blood pressure, elevated serum lipid levels, tubular dysfunction, and urine protein excretion rates >2 to 3 g/day (see Fig. 19.8).

The importance of good blood pressure control, to values of ≤125/75 mm Hg, is stressed elsewhere in this book with suggested approaches to treatment (see Chapters 16 and 69). In nephrotic syndrome, sodium restriction and the use of agents that reduce intraglomerular as well as systemic blood pressure are of particular importance. Although hypertension is not a common initial sign in MN, patients who develop any degree of renal insufficiency or patients subjected to therapy with drugs such as steroids or cyclosporine may require careful attention to blood pressure control. Increased blood pressure increases the risk of progressive disease in MN two- or threefold. Therefore, combinations of dietary sodium restriction, diuretics, and long-acting ACE inhibitors or ARBs are appropriate for all patients.[21,22,25]

Increased lipid levels, including total cholesterol >220 mg/dl (5.7 mmol/l), low ratios of high-density lipoprotein (HDL) to low-density lipoprotein (LDL), or LDL cholesterol >190 mg/dl (4.94 mmol/l), contribute to an increased risk of coronary disease in nephrotic patients. Experimental data suggest that elevated lipids may also adversely affect renal function. Therefore, the judicious use of statins is also appropriate in patients with prolonged elevations in urine protein excretion and secondary hyperlipidemia.[25]

There is little question now that progression in all glomerular diseases is closely linked to the magnitude and duration of urine protein excretion, probably because of the adverse effects of proteinuria on the renal interstitium (see previous discussion).[26] Therefore, any measures that can lower levels of proteinuria, even if independent of an effect on the underlying disease process, are likely to slow the rate of progression in patients with more moderate disease. Several studies have documented the benefit of

Factors associated with progression of membranous nephropathy		
Factors	Predictor	Positive Predictive Value (%)*
Clinical Features		
Age	Older > younger	43
Sex	Male > female	30
HLA type	HLA/B18/DR 3/Bffl present	71
Hypertension	Present	39
Serum albumin	>1.5 g/dl	56
Serum creatinine	Above normal	61
Urine Protein		
Nephrotic syndrome	Present	32
Proteinuria	>8 g for >6 months	66
IgG excretion	>250 mg/day	80
β_2-Microglobulin excretion	>0.5 µg/min	79
C5b-9 excretion	>7 µg/mg creatinine	67
Biopsy Changes		
Focal sclerosis	Present	34
Tubulointerstitial disease	Present	48
Electron microscopy	Stages III, IV	67

Figure 19.8 Likelihood of progression of membranous nephropathy. Factors associated with increased likelihood of progression and their predictive value. (*Adapted from Reichert LJM, Koene RAP, Wetzels JFM: Prognostic factors in idiopathic membranous nephropathy [editorial review]. Am J Kidney Dis 1998;31:1–11 and Branten AJ, du Buf-Vereijken PW, Klasen IS, et al: Urinary excretion of beta2-microglobulin and IgG predict prognosis in idiopathic membranous nephropathy: A validation study. J Am Soc Nephrol 2005;16:169–174.)

Therapeutic options in membranous nephropathy
Non–Disease-Specific Therapy (All Patients)
Blood pressure control (125/75 mm Hg): sodium restriction drug therapy, angiotensin-converting enzyme (ACE) inhibitors or angiotensin II receptor antagonists (ARBs) preferred
Reduction in lipid levels
Reduction in urine protein excretion
Dietary protein restriction (0.8 g/kg/day): ACE inhibitors or ARBs, nonsteroidal anti-inflammatory agents (selected patients), anticoagulation (selected patients)
Disease-Specific Therapy (Selected Patients)

Low-dose steroids and cytotoxic drugs
    Oral cyclophosphamide (1.5–2 mg/kg/day) for 6–12 months
    Alternating monthly cycles of oral chlorambucil (0.1–0.2 mg/kg/day) and pulse steroids for 6 months
    Possibly mycophenolate mofetil 1g bid

Low-dose cyclosporine (2.5–5 mg/kg/day) for 12–24 months
Rituximab, IV immunoglobulin

Figure 19.9 Therapeutic options in membranous nephropathy. Therapies suitable for selected patients are discussed in the text.

moderate dietary protein restriction (usually 0.8 g/kg/day) in reducing proteinuria by 15% to 25% and slowing progression of renal disease without significant side effects or adverse changes in serum protein levels, especially in patients with urinary protein excretion between 2 and 10 g/day.[27] Some clinicians advocate adding back to the diet the amount of protein excreted in the urine, but the necessity for this is not established. Similarly, it is not known at what level of hypoalbuminemia protein restriction becomes detrimental.

An additional approach for reducing proteinuria in a nonspecific manner is through the effects of ACE inhibitors or ARBs, which exhibit their effects primarily by altering glomerular hemodynamics but may also have a direct effect on interstitial fibrotic processes. Some studies report that ACE inhibitors can lower protein excretion in early MN by an average of 35% without having adverse effects on blood pressure or GFR. However, in contrast to results in focal sclerosis, this effect does not appear to result in a clinically significant reduction in the rate of disease progression in MN.[20,28] The effect of ARBs is likely similar.[29] Some patients respond to the use of both an ACE inhibitor and an ARB together with a further reduction in proteinuria. These agents are generally employed in long-acting form and titrated to the maximal dose that can be tolerated without adversely affecting systemic blood pressure, GFR, or serum potassium levels. They should be used cautiously in older patients with possible renal vascular disease or significant renal insufficiency. ACE inhibitors may require several weeks to achieve maximal effects on proteinuria, and these effects may persist for weeks or months after the drug is discontinued, suggesting an effect on nonhemodynamic variables that modulate glomerular permeability to protein.

A third approach for reducing urine protein excretion nonspecifically is by judicious use of a nonsteroidal anti-inflammatory drug (NSAID). Such agents should probably be employed only in patients who have not achieved a reduction in proteinuria by 40% to 50% with dietary protein restriction and ACE inhibitors or ARBs, and great caution should be used in older patients and in those with renal insufficiency, hypertension, or upper gastrointestinal symptoms, including patients receiving steroid therapy. It must be kept in mind that NSAIDs can occasionally cause renal failure and rarely cause MN (see Fig. 19.1). However, drugs such as indomethacin or meclofenamate can sometimes reduce protein excretion by 30% to 50% and have been shown to have additive effects with ACE inhibitors, sometimes achieving reductions in protein excretion of >50%. Such a regimen is likely to be of benefit only at the expense of some reduction in GFR, although this is usually reversible on discontinuation of the drug.

A fourth nonspecific therapy to consider is the use of oral anticoagulants in severely nephrotic patients with MN. The apparent increased risk of renal vein thrombosis and thromboembolic phenomena in these patients is discussed earlier. Studies using decision analysis document a benefit of prophylactic anticoagulation in reducing fatal thromboembolic episodes in nephrotic patients without a concomitant excessive risk of bleeding.[30] In patients who are severely nephrotic (proteinuria >10 g/day and serum albumin <2.5 g/dl), subjected to intensive diuretic therapy, or placed at bed rest, prophylactic anticoagulant therapy should be employed if no contraindications are present.

The advent of better measures to reduce urinary protein excretion nonspecifically, as well as to control blood pressure and lower lipid levels, almost certainly means that the natural history of MN without disease-specific therapy is better than that discussed previously. However, there are a significant number of patients, particularly males older than age 50, who have persistent nephrotic syndrome with progressive loss of renal function despite vigorous application of all these nonspecific measures. These patients are candidates for treatment directed specifically at the underlying disease process.

Disease-Specific Therapy

As mentioned previously, the selection of patients for more aggressive therapy, and the efficacy of such therapy, remain topics of significant controversy.[20,24,25,31] The following summarizes what we regard as the most salient current information in this area.

Based on several controlled studies, there is a consensus that utilization of high-dose oral steroids alone is not beneficial in MN.[20,22,25] A more promising approach has been the use of oral steroids combined with cytotoxic drugs, usually alkylating agents. The best and most convincing studies of this approach have been those of Passerini and Ponticelli[32] and Ponticelli and Passerini,[33] who have studied primarily patients with nephrotic syndrome and normal renal function. They have employed a regimen of a

3-day course of methylprednisolone 1.0 g intravenously followed by high-dose (0.4 to 0.5 mg/kg/day) oral prednisone for 1 month alternating with 1 month of oral chlorambucil (0.2 mg/kg/day) for a total treatment period of 6 months. As expected, after 5 years of follow-up, renal function had deteriorated in about 50% of the control group but only 10% of the treated patients; progression to dialysis occurred in 4 of 39 in the control group and only 1 of 42 treated patients.[32] At 10 years, 88% of treated and only 47% of control patients had complete or partial remissions of nephrotic syndrome, and of the treated group, only 8% were in renal failure compared with almost 40% of controls.[33] Decision analysis of these data using an average 40-year-old patient with MN suggests a reduction in quality-adjusted life expectancy of only 4 years with this therapy compared to 11 years in untreated patients. The Italian group has treated all patients with MN, making the results even more impressive since many patients would likely have had a benign course without therapy.

Although the Ponticelli and Passerini studies provide strong evidence for the efficacy of combined steroid/cytotoxic drug therapy in MN, the protocol employed has not been widely used in the United States because of problems with bone marrow suppression and infection in chlorambucil-treated patients, particularly if any renal insufficiency is present.[20] More popular has been oral cyclophosphamide, usually 1.5 to 2.0 mg/kg/day, in combination with low-dose prednisone (0.5 mg/kg/day), for periods of 3 to 6 months. Ponticelli and colleagues[34] have compared chlorambucil and cyclophosphamide in their treatment regimen and found them to give comparable results. Using oral cyclophosphamide together with the Ponticelli steroid regimen, in 33 patients with normal renal function initially and evidence of tubular injury, du Buf-Vereijken and coworkers[20] reported a 97% 5-year renal survival, results comparable to those of Ponticelli and associates using chlorambucil. Whether similar results can be obtained if one waits for evidence of deterioration of renal function is uncertain, but renal survival rates of 93% at 5 years and 81% at 10 years have been reported by these same authors in a series of patients with a mean serum creatinine of 1.9 mg/dl at the time therapy was initiated, and some response has occurred in patients with creatinine levels as high as 5 mg/dl.[20] Other small studies in high-risk patients including some with mild to moderate renal insufficiency have shown similar benefits.[35–38] Patients who relapse following initial therapy have also responded to second courses.[38] Of interest, one controlled trial of intravenous cyclophosphamide in MN did not show any significant benefit. Whether azathioprine can be substituted for the more toxic cyclophosphamide after 3 months of therapy, as has been shown to be effective in lupus nephritis,[39] is unclear, but some have advocated this approach, particularly in younger patients and patients with renal insufficiency.[20] Meta-analysis of the existing literature describing the use of cytotoxic drugs in MN confirms a benefit in reducing proteinuria but not in preserving renal function, probably because of the relatively short-term nature of most such studies.[40]

In the author's judgment, the data cited and a host of other smaller studies do strongly suggest a benefit of combined low-dose prednisone and cytotoxic drug therapy in preserving renal function in MN in selected patients, although more and better data are clearly needed. The necessity for the steroids is not established. Although steroids alone do not appear beneficial, one study of oral cyclophosphamide without steroids also did not show a benefit. However, the benefits of current therapy are not dramatic, as they are, for example, in minimal change nephrotic syndrome, and the toxicity is significant with up to 50% of patients having infectious or bone marrow complications. Therefore, only patients at high risk of progression should be treated, and the search must continue for other more effective and less toxic alternatives (Fig. 19.10).

The best-studied alternative to steroid/cytotoxic drug therapy for MN is cyclosporine, usually employed in relatively low doses of 3.5 to 5 mg/kg/day adjusted to trough levels of 150 to 225 mg/l. Cyclosporine does reduce protein excretion in MN, usually by 30% to 50%, and some studies have reported a 60% to 70% rate of occasional complete or more commonly partial remission.[20,41] The disease often relapses after short (4 to 6 months) courses of cyclosporine, but more prolonged courses (1 to 2 years) may produce more permanent remissions. In patients who do respond, a stabilization of renal function has also been reported. In the authors' judgment, cyclosporine is a second choice to cytotoxic drug therapy because of the significantly lower incidence of complete remissions, the tendency to relapse when therapy is discontinued, the potential nephrotoxic effects of the drug itself, and the problems of hypertension and hyperkalemia encountered during treatment. Cyclosporine should not be used in patients with impaired renal function.

Among alternative therapies that have only preliminary data to support their use, mycophenolate mofetil (MMF; a significantly less toxic immunosuppressive agent than cyclophosphamide or

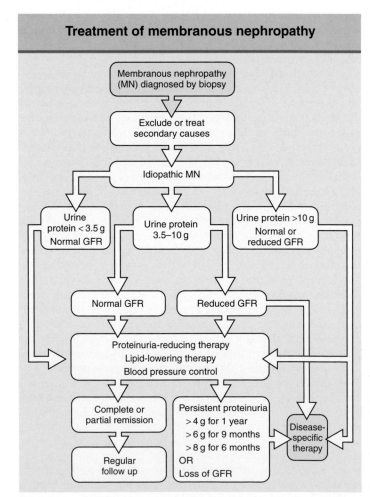

Figure 19.10 Algorithm for the treatment of membranous nephropathy. Details of possible therapies are discussed in the text. GFR, glomerular filtration rate.

chlorambucil) may be beneficial in some patients with MN, especially patients intolerant of, or dependent on, cyclophosphamide or cyclosporine.[42,43] Preliminary results suggest that some patients may respond to MMF used with steroids in a dose of 2 g/day for a year,[20] but insufficient data are available to establish a role for MMF in the treatment of MN. Another therapy with some promise is IV immunoglobulin. In one study from 1991, eight of nine patients had a complete or partial remission following IV immunoglobulin therapy, including four of five with normal GFR and three of four with some renal impairment,[44] but these observations have not been confirmed. More recent data are available on the use of Rituximab, an anti–B cell monoclonal antibody.[45] Given in four weekly infusions to eight patients with resistant MN, proteinuria was significantly reduced and renal function stabilized 1 year later. Preliminary data have also suggested that pentoxyfylline, a tumor necrosis factor α–suppressing agent, may also reduce proteinuria in MN.[46]

With these data in mind, the author's suggested approach to the treatment of idiopathic MN is illustrated in Figure 19.10 and outlined here. Patients with <1 g/day of proteinuria and normal renal function, particularly women and children, generally have an excellent prognosis and do not require therapy, although careful follow-up to ensure that the disease is not worsening is mandatory. In patients with proteinuria of 1 to 10 g/day, there is also no compelling need to initiate disease-specific therapy if renal function is well maintained. All patients should be treated aggressively using non–disease-specific therapy, as discussed previously, to control blood pressure, lower lipid levels, and attempt to reduce proteinuria by at least 50% (dietary protein restriction, ACE inhibitors and/or ARBs, and, possibly, NSAIDs [if GFR is normal]), and they should be followed for 6 months if GFR is stable. If there is any evidence of loss of GFR, and/or if proteinuria in excess of 8 g/day persists for >6 months (or 6 g for >9 months or 4 g for >1 year), despite maximal therapy to reduce proteinuria, then disease-specific therapy should be instituted. Measurements of urinary excretion of IgG and β_2-microglobulin may permit selection of higher risk patients without waiting to establish the persistence of nephrotic-range proteinuria or evidence of renal functional deterioration.[20] If initial levels of protein excretion exceed 10 g/day, other risk factors should be examined. For example, in a woman with normal GFR and normal blood pressure, a trial of nonspecific therapy is probably a reasonable initial approach. However, if the patient is male, has any reduction in GFR, has elevated IgG or

β_2-microglobulin excretion, or has any predictive signs of progression on biopsy such as focal glomerulosclerosis or interstitial fibrosis, disease-specific therapy is indicated if the serum creatinine is <3.5 mg/dl. There is little evidence that disease-specific therapy is efficacious in patients with serum creatinine levels >3.5 mg/dl.[20] Patients being treated with steroids and immunosuppressive agents for MN should also receive full treatment to control blood pressure and lipids and to reduce urinary protein excretion by other mechanisms.

If a course of steroid/cytotoxic drug therapy is indicated, the authors generally start with prednisone 0.5 mg/kg/day or 1 mg/kg on alternate days, together with cyclophosphamide 1.5 mg/kg/day. The patient's white blood cell count should be monitored weekly, and good hydration maintained, particularly if there is a reduction in GFR. Treatment should continue until a complete or partial remission (<2 g/day proteinuria) is achieved or for up to 6 months. In patients who do not achieve a complete or partial remission on this protocol, therapy can be changed to cyclosporine 3 to 6 mg/kg/day for 3 months if renal function is normal. The Ponticelli protocol of alternate monthly cycles of high-dose steroids and chlorambucil can be considered if the patient seems resistant and GFR remains >50 ml/min. MMF may be an alternative to steroids and cyclophosphamide or chlorambucil in patients who are intolerant or resistant to these drugs, but its long-term efficacy in MN is less well established. Trials of rituximab, IV immunoglobulin, or pentoxyfylline would be warranted only in very resistant patients.

In treating patients with MN, the long lag time between successful interruption of the immune response and a corresponding reduction in urine protein excretion must be kept in mind before declaring a patient resistant to therapy. This averages about 3 months but may be as long as a year. Adjunct therapy to be considered in patients receiving steroids and immunosuppressive drugs include cotrimoxazole (trimethoprim and sulfamethoxazole) sulfa for prophylaxis against *Pneumocystis carinii* pneumonia and bisphosphonates along with calcium and vitamin D to prevent steroid-induced osteopenia.

Finally, we must always remind ourselves as nephrologists that renal replacement therapy is effective and often safer than prolonged and repeated courses of very toxic immunosuppressive medication in patients with compromised renal function who are resistant to treatment. The issue of recurrence of MN or development of *de novo* MN in renal allografts is discussed in Chapter 96.

REFERENCES

1. Cattran DC: Idiopathic membranous glomerulonephritis. Kidney Int 2001;59:1983–1994.
2. Couser WG, Alpers CE: Membranous nephropathy. In Neilson EG, Couser WG, eds. Immunologic Renal Diseases. Philadelphia: Lippincott Williams & Wilkins, 2001, pp 1029–1036.
3. Ronco P, Debiec H: Molecular pathomechanisms of membranous nephropathy: From Heymann nephritis to alloimmunization. J Am Soc Nephrol 2005;16;1205–1213.
4. Kerjaschki D: Pathomechanisms and molecular basis of membranous glomerulopathy. Lancet 2004;364:1194–1196.
5. Nangaku M, Couser WG: Mechanisms of immune-deposit formation and the mediation of immune renal injury. Clin Exp Nephrol 2005;9:183–191.
6. Nangaku M, Shankland SJ, Couser WG: Cellular response to injury in membranous nephropathy. J Am Soc Nephrol 2005;16:1195–1204.
7. Yu D, Petermann A, Kunter U, et al: Urinary podocyte loss is a more specific marker of ongoing glomerular damage than proteinuria. J Am Soc Nephrol 2005;16:1733–1741.
8. Shankland SJ, Pippin JW, Couser WG: Complement (C5b-9) induces glomerular epithelial cell DNA synthesis but not proliferation in vitro. Kidney Int 1999;56:536–548.
9. Nangaku M, Pippin J, Couser WG: C6 inhibits chronic progressive renal disease in remnant kidney rats. J Am Soc Nephrol 2002;13:928–936.
10. U.S. Renal Data System: USRDS 2001 Annual Data Report. Atlas of End-Stage Renal Disease in the United States. Bethesda, MD: National Institutes of Health, National Institute of Diabetes and Digestive and Kidney Diseases, 2001.
11. Zucchelli IP, Cagnoli L, Pasquali C: Clinical and morphologic evolution of idiopathic membranous nephropathy. Clin Nephrol 1986;25:282–288.
12. Hogan SL, Muller KE, Jennette JC, Falk RJ: A review of therapeutic studies of idiopathic membranous glomerulopathy. Am J Kidney Dis 1995;25:862–868.
13. Austin HA, Illei GG: Membranous lupus nephritis. Lupus 2005;14:65–71.

14. Johnson RJ, Couser WG: Hepatitis B infection and renal disease: Clinical, immuno-pathogenetic and therapeutic considerations. Kidney Int 1990;37:663–676.

15. Conjeevaram HS, Hoofnagle JH, Austin HA, et al: Long-term outcome of hepatitis B virus-related glomerulonephritis after therapy with interferon alfa. Gastroenterology 1995;109:540–546.

16. Burstein DM, Korbet SM, Schwartz MM: Membranous glomerulonephritis and malignancy. Am J Kidney Dis 1993;22:5–17.

17. Couser W: Recurrent glomerulonephritis in the renal allograft: An update of selected areas. Exp Clin Transplant 2005;3:283–288.

18. Mundel P, Shankland SJ: Podocyte biology and response to injury. J Am Soc Nephrol 2002;13:3005–3015.

19. Cunningham PN, Quigg RJ: Contrasting roles of complement activation and its regulation in membranous nephropathy. J Am Soc Nephrol 2005;16:1214–1222.

20. du Buf-Vereijken PWG, Branten AJW, Wetzels JFM: Idiopathic membranous nephropathy: Outline and rationale of a treatment strategy. Am J Kidney Dis 2005;46:1012–1029.

21. Schieppati A, Mosconi L, Perna A, et al: Prognosis of untreated patients with idiopathic membranous nephropathy. N Engl J Med 1993;329:85–89.

22. Glassock RJ: The treatment of idiopathic membranous nephropathy: A dilemma or a conundrum? Am J Kidney Dis 2004;44(Suppl):S62–S66.

23. Reichert LJM, Koene RAP, Wetzels JFM: Prognostic factors in idiopathic membranous nephropathy [editorial review]. Am J Kidney Dis 1998;31:1–11.

24. Branten AJ, du Buf-Vereijken PW, Klasen IS, et al: Urinary excretion of beta2-microglobulin and IgG predict prognosis in idiopathic membranous nephropathy: A validation study. J Am Soc Nephrol 2005;16:169–174.

25. Cattran D: Management of membranous nephropathy: When and what for treatment. J Am Soc Nephrol 2005;16:1188–1194.

26. Perico N, Codreanu I, Schieppati A, Remuzzi G: Pathophysiology of disease progression in proteinuric nephropathies. Kidney Int Suppl 2005;94:S79–S82.

27. Klahr S, Levey A, Beck G, et al: The effects of dietary protein restriction and blood-pressure control on the progression of chronic renal disease. N Engl J Med 1994;330:877–884.

28. Praga M, Hernandez E, Montoyo C, et al: Long-term beneficial effects of angiotensin-converting enzyme inhibition in patients with nephrotic proteinuria. Am J Kidney Dis 1992;20:240–248.

29. Hilgers KF, Mann JF: ACE inhibitors versus AT(1) receptor antagonists in patients with chronic renal disease. J Am Soc Nephrol 2002;13:1100–1108.

30. Sarasin F, Schifferli J: Prophylactic oral anticoagulation in nephrotic patients with idiopathic membranous nephropathy. Kidney Int 1994;45:578–585.

31. Schieppati A, Perna A, Zamora J, et al: Immunosuppressive treatment for idiopathic membranous nephropathy in adults with nephrotic syndrome. Cochrane Database Syst Rev 2004;4:D004293.

32. Passerini P, Ponticelli C: Corticosteroids, cyclophosphamide, and chlorambucil therapy of membranous nephropathy. Semin Nephrol 2003:23;355–361.

33. Ponticelli C, Passerini P: Treatment of membranous nephropathy. Nephrol Dial Transplant 2001;16(Suppl 5):8–10.

34. Ponticelli C, Altieri P, Scolari F, et al: A randomized study comparing methylprednisolone plus chlorambucil versus methylprednisolone plus cyclophosphamide in idiopathic membranous nephropathy. J Am Soc Nephrol 1998;9:444–450.

35. Bruns FJ, Adler S, Fraley DS, Segel DP: Sustained remission of membranous glomerulonephritis after cyclophosphamide and prednisone. Ann Intern Med 1991;114:725–730.

36. Branten AJ, Wetzels JF: Short- and long-term efficacy of oral cyclophosphamide and steroids in patients with membranous nephropathy and renal insufficiency: Study Group. Clin Nephrol 2001;56:1–9.

37. Reichert LJ, Huysmans FT, Assman K, et al: Preserving renal function in patients with membranous nephropathy: Daily oral chlorambucil compared with intermittent monthly pulses of cyclophosphamide. Ann Intern Med 1994;121:328–334.

38. Branten JW, Reichert LJ, Koene AP, Wetzels JF: Oral cyclophosphamide versus chlorambucil in the treatment of patients with membranous nephropathy and renal insufficiency. Q J Med 1998;91:359–365.

39. Jayne D, Rasmussen N, Andrassy K, et al: European Vasculitis Study Group: A randomized trial of maintenance therapy for vasculitis associated with antineutrophil cytoplasmic antibodies. N Engl J Med 2003;349:36–44.

40. Imperiale TF, Goldfarb S, Berns JS: Are cytotoxic agents beneficial in idiopathic membranous nephropathy? A meta-analysis of the controlled trials. J Am Soc Nephrol 1995;5:1553–1558.

41. Cattran DC, Appel GB, Hebert LA, et al: North American Nephrotic Syndrome Study Group. Kidney Int 2001;59:1484–1490.

42. Choi MJ, Eustace JA, Gimenez LF, et al: Mycophenolate mofetil treatment for primary glomerular disease. Kidney Int 2002;61:1098–1108.

43. Briggs WA, Choi MJ, Scheel PJ: Successful mycophenolate mofetil treatment of glomerular disease. Am J Kidney Dis 1998;31:213–216.

44. Palla R, Cirami C, Panichi V, et al: Intravenous immunoglobulin therapy of membranous nephropathy: Efficacy and safety. Clin Nephrol 1991;35:98–102.

45. Ruggenenti P, Chiurchiu C, Brusegan V, et al: Rituximab in idiopathic membranous nephropathy: A one-year prospective study. J Am Soc Nephrol 2003;14:1851–1857.

46. Ducloux D, Bresson-Vautrin C, Chalopin JM: Use of pentoxifylline in membranous nephropathy. Lancet 2001;357:1672.

Membranoproliferative Glomerulonephritis and Cryoglobulinemic Glomerulonephritis

F. Paolo Schena and Charles E. Alpers

INTRODUCTION AND DEFINITION

Membranoproliferative glomerulonephritis (MPGN), or mesangiocapillary glomerulonephritis (GN), is characterized by diffuse proliferative lesions and widening of the capillary loops, often with a double contoured appearance. MPGN may be primary (idiopathic) or secondary to chronic infections, cryoglobulinemia, or systemic autoimmune disorders that result in aberrant immune complex formation. Based on the histomorphologic pattern, three types of MPGN can be described. Type I is characterized by the presence of immune deposits in the subendothelial space (capillary wall thickening) and in the mesangium. Type II, also known as dense deposit disease, is defined by the presence of dense deposits within the mesangium and in the basement membranes of the glomeruli, tubules, and Bowman's capsules. Type III, which is a variant of type I, is characterized by marked disruption (layering, fragmentation) of the glomerular basement membrane (GBM), with confluent subendothelial and subepithelial electron-dense deposits. This process is accompanied by alterations and remodeling of the lamina densa of the GBM and newly elaborated lamina densa–like material.

ETIOLOGY AND PATHOGENESIS

Although frequently idiopathic, the histologic diagnosis of MPGN should provoke a search for secondary causes (Fig. 20.1).[1] In children and young adults (younger than 30 years) with MPGN type II, the disease is often associated with the presence of nephritic factors, which are IgG or IgM autoantibodies that bind to and stabilize the C3 convertase of the alternative (C3bBb), classic (C4b2b), or common pathway (Fig. 20.2), thus resulting in continued complement activation with a

Etiology of membranoproliferative glomerulonephritis	
Type	**Secondary Causes**
MPGN Type I	
With mixed (type II or III) cryoglobulinemia	Hepatitis C virus (70%–90% of patients) Other infections: bacterial endocarditis, chronic hepatitis B viral infection Collagen vascular disease: systemic lupus erythematosus, Sjögren's syndrome Malignancy: chronic lymphocytic leukemia, non-Hodgkin's lymphoma
Without cryoglobulinemia	Bacterial infections: endocarditis, abscess, infected ventriculoatrial shunt Viral infections: hepatitis B, C, and G, human immunodeficiency virus, hantavirus Malarial (*Plasmodium malariae*) Collagen vascular disease (systemic lupus erythematosus–hypocomplementemic urticarial vasculitis) Hereditary complement deficiency (C1q, C2, C4, or C3) Acquired complement deficiency (presence of C4 nephritic factor) Chronic liver disease (especially associated with hepatitis B or C infection, chronic schistosomal infection, with splenorenal shunt for liver fibrosis, and with α_1-antitrypsin deficiency) Sickle cell disease Malignancy: chronic lymphocytic leukemia, lymphoma, thymoma, renal cell carcinoma
MPGN Type II	
Associated with C3 nephritic factor (C3 Nef)	With or without partial lipodystrophy and retinal abnormalities
Associated with factor H defect	Inherited mutations of factor H (deficiency) Autoantibodies to factor H
MPGN Type III	
Associated with or without terminal complement hephritic factor	Secondary causes similar to MPGN type I (hepatitis C or B, and others)

Figure 20.1   Etiology of membranoproliferative glomerulonephritis (MPGN).

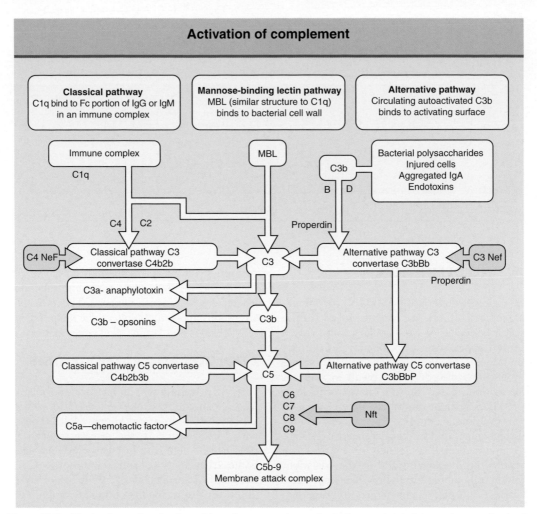

Figure 20.2 Mechanisms of activation of complement pathways including nephritic factors. See text for details.

depletion of various complement components. In older adults (older than 30 years), MPGN type I is frequently associated with cryoglobulinemia and hepatitis C virus (HCV) infection.

MPGN type I is most likely to occur in the setting of chronic immune-complex diseases, for example, when the host defenses cannot eliminate a foreign antigen effectively despite a humoral response. This may account for the MPGN observed with chronic blood-borne viral (HCV and hepatitis B virus [HBV]), bacterial (endocarditis, infected ventriculoatrial shunt), and malarial infection (*Plasmodium malariae*). A histologic pattern resembling MPGN can also be observed in chronic immune-complex diseases associated with collagen vascular diseases (such as lupus) or with malignancy (especially chronic lymphocytic leukemia). Chronic immune-complex disease and MPGN also occur if the host has a defect in clearing immune complexes, as in complement deficiency, or when the reticuloendothelial system is impaired, as occurs with liver or splenic disease. Hereditary deficiencies of the classic pathway of complement (C1q, C2, C4) and of C3 are associated with the development of MPGN in addition to predisposing to lupus and bacterial infections.

The pathogenesis of MPGN type I is believed to result from the glomerular deposition of immune complexes from the circulation that preferentially localize in the mesangium and subendothelial space of the capillary walls. Once localized, the immune complexes activate complement via the classic pathway, leading to the generation of chemotactic factors (C5a), opsonins (C3b),

and the membrane attack complex (C5b-9) as well as low C3 and C4 serum levels. In some patients, complement is activated by the C4 nephritic factor; in other cases, activation of complement may occur by the mannose-binding lectin pathway (see Fig. 20.2). Mannose-binding lectin, a lectin that binds IgG and activates the complement pathway, has been localized to the immune deposits of some patients with MPGN type I.[2] Complement activation results in the release of chemotactic factors that stimulate platelet and leukocyte accumulation (Figs. 20.2 and 20.3). Leukocytes release oxidants and proteases that mediate capillary wall damage and cause proteinuria and a fall in the glomerular filtration rate. Cytokines and growth factors released by both exogenous and endogenous glomerular cells lead to mesangial proliferation and matrix expansion.

The pathogenesis of MPGN type II (dense deposit disease) is intricately linked to continual overactivation of the alternative pathway of complement (see Fig. 20.2). This can occur in humans through the dysfunction of a constitutive inhibitor (factor H) or through the presence of an IgG or IgM autoantibody (C3 nephritic factor [C3Nef]) that binds the alternative pathway C3 convertase (C3bBb) and prevents its inactivation by factor H (see Fig. 20.2). Although patients with MPGN and hereditary deficiency of factor H (from homozygous or heterozygous factor H deficiency) have been described, most patients with MPGN type II have C3Nef. This factor activates C3 rapidly when added to serum, does not activate terminal components, and does not require properdin. The consequence is a low C3

Pathogenesis of membranoproliferative glomerulonephritis type I

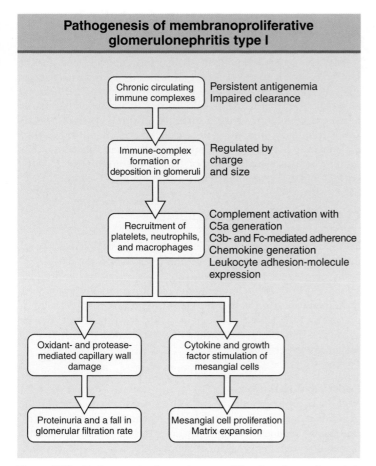

Figure 20.3 Pathogenesis of membranoproliferative glomerulonephritis type I.

level in the setting of normal classic (C2 and C4) and terminal (C5 through C9) components. C3c or C3d split products of C3 are present in the dense deposits. As yet, there have been no specific relationships between C3Nef levels, C3 levels in serum, or in deposits that predict disease outcome.[3–5]

MPGN type II may be associated with partial lipodystrophy (see later), often acutely and sometimes after a viral infection such as measles. The lipodystrophy results from complement-dependent loss of the adipocyte, mediated by activation of

complement on the adipocyte surface due to both the presence of C3Nef and the overproduction by the adipocyte of adipsin, a protein that is identical to factor D of the alternative pathway (see Fig. 20.2).

The pathogenesis of MPGN type III is similar to MPGN type I, except that certain characteristics of the immune complexes may also favor localization in the subepithelial space. The nephritic factor of the terminal pathway (NFt) may be present in this form. NFt activates C3 slowly, activates terminal components, and requires properdin (see Fig. 20.2). In addition to a depressed C3 level, there is a reduced level of properdin, depressed levels of C5, depressed levels of one or more of the other four terminal components, and elevated levels of C5b-9. NFt seems to be solely responsible for hypocomplementemia in MPGN type III. This rare disease has been found to map to chromosome 1q31-32 in an Irish family.[6]

Cryoglobulins are immunoglobulin that precipitate in the cold and can be categorized as types I through III (Fig. 20.4). The mixed cryoglobulinemias (types II and III) are the types most commonly associated with MPGN; these have been strongly associated with chronic HCV infection in 90% and 70% of patients, respectively. The non-HCV cases have been associated with other infections (chronic HBV, bacterial endocarditis), collagen vascular diseases (systemic lupus), and other immunologic disorders (notably poststreptococcal GN). Chronic lymphocytic leukemia may also be associated with cryoglobulinemia or MPGN; interestingly, some of these patients are also infected with HCV and have a circulating monoclonal IgM-κ. Chronic lymphocytic leukemia and lymphoma also have been associated with MPGN in the absence of cryoglobulinemia.[7]

The mechanism by which chronic HCV infection causes cryoglobulinemia is not entirely known. Most patients with HCV infection and cryoglobulinemia will have an IgM-κ monoclonal antibody that has intrinsic rheumatoid factor activity, and this rheumatoid factor can be found with anti-HCV IgG and HCV RNA in the cryoprecipitates. It has been postulated that the IgM is produced as a consequence of dysregulation of the B cell, which can also be infected with HCV. Cryoglobulinemia does not develop until many years (>10) after HCV infection, but by the time chronic active hepatitis or cirrhosis develops as many as 30% to 40% of patients will have circulating cryoglobulins. Most of these patients will not develop renal disease, but in some patients, particularly those in whom the

Classification of cryoglobulins		
Type	Composition	Associated Disease
I	Monoclonal IgG, IgA, or IgM	Multiple myeloma (IgG, IgM) Chronic lymphocytic leukemia Waldenström's macroglobulinemia (IgM) Idiopathic monoclonal gammopathy Lymphoproliferative disorders
II	Polyclonal IgG and monoclonal IgM (with rheumatoid factor activity)	Hepatitis C virus Neoplasms: chronic lymphocytic leukemia, diffuse lymphoma, B lymphocytic neoplasia Essential
III	Polyclonal IgG and polyclonal IgM	Infections: viral (hepatitis B and C, Epstein-Barr virus, cytomegalovirus), bacterial (endocarditis, leprosy, poststreptococcal glomerulonephritis), parasitic (schistosomiasis, toxoplasmosis, malaria) Autoimmune disorders: systemic lupus erythematosus, rheumatoid arthritis Lymphoproliferative disorders Chronic liver disease Essential

Figure 20.4 Classification of cryoglobulins.

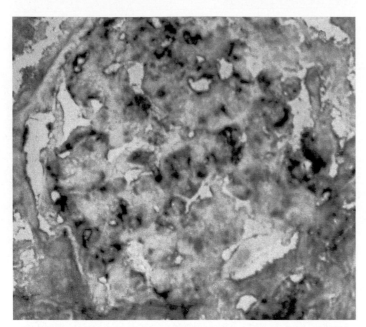

Figure 20.5 **Hepatitis C virus–related antigen (c22-3) in the capillary wall of a glomerulus from a patient with cryoglobulinemic membranoproliferative glomerulonephritis (light microscopy ×100).**

cryoglobulins have an affinity for fibronectin, the cryoglobulins containing HCV antigens will deposit in glomeruli (Fig. 20.5).[8]

Specific HCV-related proteins have been detected in glomerular and tubulointerstitial vascular structure in patients with cryoglobulinemic HCV-positive MPGN,[9] although difficulties with the antisera available to detect HCV have made such findings controversial. Glomerular HCV deposits display two different patterns: (1) a linear homogeneous deposition along glomerular capillary walls, including endothelial and subendothelial spaces; (2) a granular appearance with distinct deposits in mesangial and paramesangial areas. IgG, IgM, and C3 deposits display features comparable to those of HCV RNA and core protein deposits, thus indicating that in cryoglobulinemic HCV-positive MPGN, kidney deposits consist of HCV containing immune complexes that play a direct pathogenetic role in the renal damage.[10]

New mouse models will likely advance knowledge of the pathogenesis of MPGN: (1) an MPGN type I model, the transgenic TSLP (thymic stromal lymphopoietin) mouse model, which develops mixed cryoglobulinemia, and (2) an MPGN type II model, the factor H–deficient mouse.[11]

EPIDEMIOLOGY

In North America and Europe, MPGN (types I and II) characterizes less than 5% of all primary glomerulonephritides. It accounts for approximately 4% to 10% of primary renal causes of nephrotic syndrome in children and adults. The prevalence of MPGN I is decreasing in Europe, presumably because some chronic infections are becoming less common. In the Middle East (Saudi Arabia), South America (Peru), and Africa (Nigeria), MPGN remains one of the most common causes of nephrotic syndrome and may account for 30% to 40% of all cases because of the association of chronic bacterial, viral, and parasitic infections with MPGN type I. The disease may be familial in rare cases, and different histologic lesions may occur in family members (i.e., type I in one member and type III in another).

MPGN type II (dense deposit disease) accounts for less than 20% of cases of MPGN in children and a very low percentage of cases in adults.

MPGN occurs equally in males and females, and in the United States is relatively more common in Caucasians than in African Americans. Two distinct presentations of MPGN are particularly common. MPGN presenting in childhood (primarily between age 8 and 14 years) includes all three types of MPGN and is frequently idiopathic or associated with nephritic factors. By contrast, MPGN presenting in adults (typically older than age 18 years) is usually type I or III and is commonly associated with cryoglobulinemia and HCV infection (see Chapter 25).

CLINICAL MANIFESTATIONS

MPGN may present as microscopic hematuria and non-nephrotic proteinuria (35%), as nephrotic syndrome with minimally depressed renal function (35%), as a chronically progressive GN (20%), or with rapidly deteriorating renal function with proteinuria and red cell casts (10%). Systemic hypertension is present in 50% to 80% of patients, and, occasionally, it may be so severe that the presentation may be confused with that of malignant hypertension.

Pediatric Population

MPGN in children and young adults is usually idiopathic and presents as a primary kidney disease without systemic manifestations. In Japanese children diagnosed as a consequence of a urinalysis screening program at school, blood pressures, proteinuria, and serum creatinines were lower compared to subjects who were diagnosed after presenting with symptoms.[12] Thus, early identification of the disease by urinary screening may allow for early treatment.

MPGN type II affects both genders equally and is usually diagnosed in children who are between 5 and 15 years old.[5] Patients usually present with either hematuria, proteinuria, hematuria plus proteinuria, acute nephritic syndrome, or nephrotic syndrome.[5] Twenty percent to 25% of patients with MPGN type II may also manifest partial lipodystrophy that preferentially involves the face and upper body (Fig. 20.6a), may precede the renal disease by many years, and is mediated by complement-mediated destruction of adipose tissue with a high content of adipsin. Some patients with MPGN type II will also have mild visual field and color defects and prolonged dark adaptation with mottled retinal pigmentation (drusen bodies; see Fig. 20.6b), and sometimes deterioration of vision. Eye examinations, including dark adaptation, electroretinography, and electro-oculography, should be performed upon first presentation and periodically thereafter. Indocyanine green angiography of the retina may reveal dense deposits in the ciliary epithelial basement membrane (abnormal fluorescent dots) and choroidal neovascularization.[13,14]

Adult Population

MPGN in adults is also often limited to the kidney in its presentation but occasionally can be associated with systemic cryoglobulinemia. These patients, who usually have chronic HCV infection, may present with the triad of weakness, arthralgias, and purpura. The arthralgias are only rarely accompanied by arthritis, are usually symmetrical, and classically involve the knees, hips, and shoulders. The purpura (Fig. 20.7) is usually

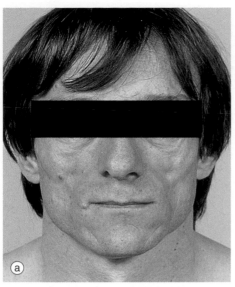
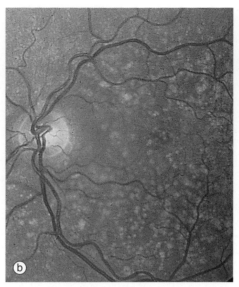

Figure 20.6 Membranoproliferative glomerulonephritis type II. *a*, Partial lipodystrophy; note the absence of subcutaneous fat from the face. *b*, Drusen bodies in the retina. (Courtesy of Dr. C. D. Short.)

painless, palpable, and nonpruritic, occurs in "crops" that last 4 to 10 days, and preferentially localizes to the extremities. Other manifestations may include ulcerative, vasculitic lesions that classically involve the lower extremities (see Fig. 20.7) and buttocks (Fig. 20.8), Raynaud phenomenon, digital necrosis (Fig. 20.9), peripheral neuropathy, hepatomegaly, and, rarely, signs of cirrhosis (clubbing, spider angiomata, ascites). Although most patients with cryoglobulinemia have a chronic waxing and waning course, occasionally patients may have a more fulminant

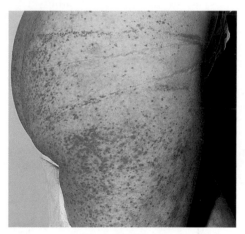

Figure 20.8 Purpura in a patient with hepatitis C virus–associated cryoglobulinemia. Purpuric lesions are present on the buttocks and thigh of the patient. Interestingly, note the presence of purpuric lesions along the superior and inferior elastic border of the undergarment line.

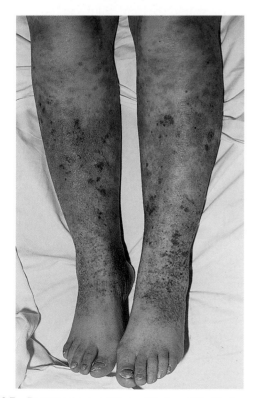

Figure 20.7 Purpura in a patient with hepatitis C virus–associated cryoglobulinemia. Raised purpuric lesions are present on the legs of this individual. The differential diagnosis of purpura and renal disease includes cryoglobulinemia, Henoch-Schönlein purpura, vasculitis, and endocarditis.

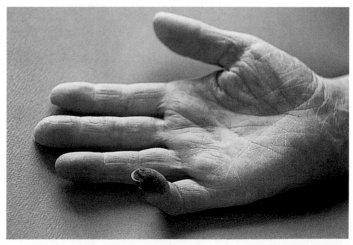

Figure 20.9 Necrosis of the distal portion of the little finger in a young woman with essential mixed cryoglobulinemia.

247

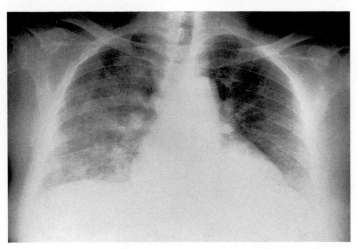

Figure 20.10 Chest radiograph showing nodular infiltrate in the lung secondary to cryoglobulinemic vasculitis in a patient with hepatitis C virus infection.

presentation, with congestive heart failure (from an HCV-induced cardiomyopathy), nodular infiltrates in the lung from deposition of cryoglobulins (Fig. 20.10), pulmonary hypertension, severe systemic hypertension, or mesenteric ischemia.

In view of the conditions associated with MPGN (see Fig. 20.1), signs of bacterial infection, viral infection, systemic lupus, malignancy, and chronic liver disease should be sought.

Laboratory Findings

MPGN is often associated with depressed complement levels (C3 and total hemolytic complement [CH_{50}]). In MPGN type I, and in cryoglobulinemic MPGN, the classical pathway is activated (low C3, low C4, and low CH_{50}); in type II, the alternative pathway is activated (low C3, normal C4, and low CH_{50}); and in type III, C3 is generally low in association with a depression of terminal complement components (C5 through C9). C3Nef activity is usually detected in plasma by the hemolytic test or the C3NeF IgG solid phase assay.[15] The presence of rheumatoid factors or cryoglobulins should prompt testing for anti-HCV antibody and HCV RNA. However, MPGN can be associated with HCV infection in the absence of cryoglobulinemia or rheumatoid factors.[16] Failure to detect the cryoglobulins may result from improper handling of specimens or occur because the cryoglobulinemia was transient; however, in some patients (especially in renal transplant recipients), tests for cryoglobulinemia may be persistently negative. Clinical or laboratory evidence of liver disease should prompt a search for causes of chronic liver disease, including HCV, HBV, and, if appropriate, rare entities such as schistosomiasis or α_1-antitrypsin deficiency.

PATHOLOGY

By light microscopy, MPGN type I is classically described as hypercellular, owing to both the influx of circulating leukocytes and intrinsic glomerular cell proliferation (typically mesangial cells), leading to a lobular appearance in some cases (Fig. 20.11a). Accumulation of extracellular material, predominantly matrix, contributes to the mesangial expansion that occurs in most cases of MPGN. The glomerular appearance can range from markedly hypercellular to predominantly sclerotic, which, in the latter case in its most advanced form, can manifest as nodules of accumulated mesangial matrix indistinguishable from the nodular mesangial sclerosis of severe diabetic nephropathy. Using the methenamine silver stain, a double contouring of the GBM can often be appreciated ("tram tracks") as a result of the interposition of mesangial cells, leukocytes, and/or endothelial cells in the capillary wall with the synthesis of new basement membrane material (Fig. 20.12). Monocytes and macrophages are commonly present in the glomerulus and the periglomerular areas.[1,17] MPGN type II is characterized by dense deposits

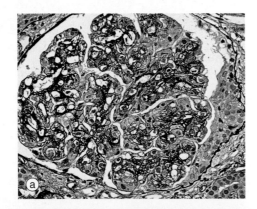

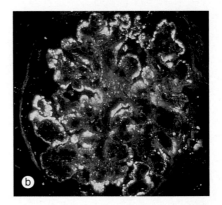

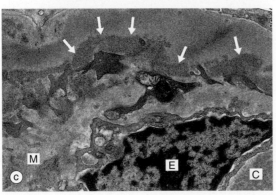

Figure 20.11 Pathology of membranoproliferative glomerulonephritis type I. *a,* Light microscopy shows a hypercellular glomerulus with accentuated lobular architecture and a small cellular crescent (methenamine silver). *b,* Immunofluorescence usually shows discrete, granular staining of the peripheral capillary wall for IgG (seen here) and C3, and occasionally for IgM and earlier complement components (C1q and C4). *c,* By electron microscopy, numerous subendothelial deposits are observed (*arrows*) between the duplicated basement membrane; these deposits extend into the mesangium (M). C, capillary lumen; E, endothelial cell nucleus.

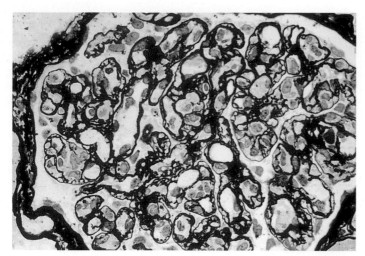

Figure 20.12 "Tram tracks" in membranoproliferative glomerulonephritis (MPGN) type I. By silver stain, a double contouring of the glomerular basement membrane can be observed in MPGN type I, resembling tram tracks.

within the mesangium and the basement membranes of the glomeruli, tubules, and Bowman's capsules, often visible with eosin and periodic acid–Schiff stains. The hallmark of MPGN type III is the interruption of lamina densa associated with subendothelial and subepithelial deposits, often confluent, and interspersed with multilayers of new lamina densa. Type I and III MPGN form a morphologic continuum and thus are not always separable by light microscopy.

Immunofluorescence in MPGN type I and III frequently shows the deposition of IgM, IgG, and C3 in a granular capillary wall distribution (see Fig. 20.11b), although the immunoglobulin deposits may be scant. Staining for C3 in a peripheral (lobular) pattern involving capillary walls and mesangial areas is the most constant and strongest pattern, while staining for classic complement components (C1q, C4) may also be seen in MPGN type I. In MPGN type II, the immunofluorescence pattern is positive for C3 but is negative for both classic complement pathway components and for immunoglobulins. The latter helps to distinguish it from other types of injury with an MPGN pattern. The C3 stain is not thought to bind the core material of

the dense deposits, but rather binds to an unidentified substrate at the surface of the dense deposits, which occasionally gives an appearance of tram tracks or mesangial rings.

By electron microscopy, discrete immune deposits can be observed in the subendothelial portions of the capillary walls and mesangial regions in MPGN type I, often in association with platelet and leukocyte infiltration (see Fig. 20.11c). The deposits are often discrete, but may be confluent in their involvement of the capillary wall. They can be small and sparse or large and numerous such that they are visible by light microscopy. In addition, a separation of the endothelium from the GBM can occasionally be observed, usually with some synthesis of new basement membrane material under the endothelial cells that have become detached from the original basement membrane. Between these layers (old and new) of basement membranes interposed cells of mesangial, endothelial, or leukocyte origin may be found, as well as immune deposits and matrix. In contrast, in MPGN type II, electron microscopy shows replacement of large sections of the GBM with an extremely electron-dense band of homogeneous material, the exact identity of which remains unknown (Fig. 20.13). Involvement of mesangial regions, Bowman's capsules, and tubular basement membranes by the deposits is common. Perhaps 15% of cases of MPGN demonstrate both subendothelial and subepithelial deposits that are associated with minute disruptions of the lamina densa and newly elaborated lamina densa–like material (MPGN type III). There can be a continuum of subepithelial deposits in MPGN I and III from none or scanty to numerous, making it difficult to separate all cases into type I (scanty or no subepithelial deposits) or type III (numerous deposits) categories. After a number of years of normocomplementemia, the type III lesions can disappear, but there is no evidence that this will inevitably occur.[18]

Cryoglobulinemic MPGN may appear histologically identical to MPGN type I by light, immunofluorescence, and electron microscopy. However, the cryoprecipitates can occasionally be observed by light microscopy as intracapillary hyaline-like deposits, and there is often a more pronounced infiltration of macrophages within capillary lumina. Electron microscopy may also show the highly organized tubular or finely fibrillar structures consisting of the precipitated cryoglobulins (Fig. 20.14).

DIAGNOSIS AND DIFFERENTIAL DIAGNOSIS

MPGN is diagnosed by renal biopsy in patients presenting with nephrotic or non-nephrotic proteinuria, especially when accompanied by microhematuria. By light microscopy, other entities may appear histologically similar, including poststreptococcal GN, the thrombotic microangiopathies, paraproteinemias, fibrillary GN, and several rare diseases (Fig. 20.15). Immunofluorescence and electron microscopy are critical for separating these diseases (see earlier). Systemic lupus usually can be eliminated by serologic testing.

Other useful tests are serum C3, C4, and CH_{50} levels. Low complement levels can also be observed in atheroembolic renal disease (low C3 with eosinophilia), in thrombotic microangiopathy, in chronic liver disease (because of decreased synthesis), and in several glomerular diseases including systemic lupus (low C3 and C4) and poststreptococcal GN (low C3). The detection of C3NeF activity in plasma suggests the presence of MPGN type II.

Once MPGN is diagnosed, careful evaluation for secondary causes should be conducted (see Fig. 20.1 and Chapter 25).

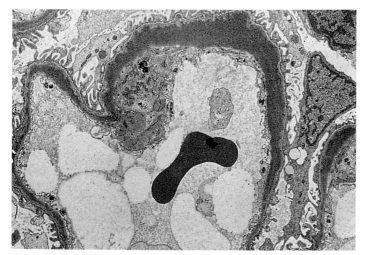

Figure 20.13 Electron microscopy of membranoproliferative glomerulonephritis type II. Dense material replaces sections of the glomerular basement membrane.

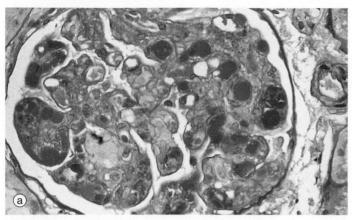
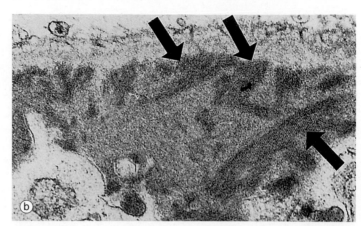

Figure 20.14   Pathology of cryoglobulinemic membranoproliferative glomerulonephritis (MPGN). *a,* Although cryoglobulinemic MPGN may histologically appear similar to MPGN type I (see Fig. 20.11), occasionally discrete precipitates of cryoglobulins may be found occluding individual capillary loops. *b,* In addition, electron microscopy shows organized fibrillar or tubular structures consistent with cryoglobulins (*arrows*). (*a,* Kim RY, Faktorovich EG, Kuo CY, Olson JL: Retinal function abnormalities in membranoproliferative glomerulonephritis type II. Am J Ophthalmol 1997;123:619–628, with permission. *b,* Reproduced with permission from Johnson RJ, et al: Membranoproliferative glomerulonephritis associated with hepatitis C virus infection. N Engl J Med 1993;328:465–470. Copyright © 1993 Massachusetts Medical Society. All rights reserved.)

Diseases that histologically resemble membranoproliferative glomerulonephritis
Paraproteinemias: especially fibrillary glomerulonephritis, light chain nephropathy
Thrombotic microangiopathies: hemolytic uremic syndrome, scleroderma, radiation nephropathy, malignant hypertension
Glomerulosclerois in liver diseases
Postinfectious glomerulonephritis
"Transplant" glomerulopathy
Rare diseases: collagen III glomerulopathy, C1q nephropathy, lipoprotein nephropathy

Figure 20.15   Diseases that histologically resemble membranoproliferative glomerulonephritis.

NATURAL HISTORY

Idiopathic MPGN in childhood has a relatively poor prognosis, with 40% to 50% of untreated patients progressing to renal failure over 10 years. Risk of progression is greater for those presenting with elevated creatinine, nephrotic proteinuria, severe hypertension, or a renal biopsy specimen showing more than 50% crescents or marked interstitial fibrosis. Renal failure may also be more likely to develop in patients with type II MPGN.

Idiopathic MPGN in adults also carries an unfavorable prognosis because 5 years after biopsy, 50% of patients either die or need renal replacement therapy (dialysis or transplantation). This proportion increases to 64% after 10 years.[19] The unfavorable outcome appears to be influenced by the severity of crescents (regardless of pathologic type[19]), the tubulointerstitial lesions, and interstitial fibrosis.

TRANSPLANTATION

The severity of crescent formation in native kidney biopsy specimens has predictive value for recurrence of disease in subsequent renal allografts.[20] MPGN recurs in renal transplant recipients with a frequency of 20% to 30% in type I and 80% to 90% in types II and III. Although the disease is often milder, it is associated with a reduced graft survival (see Chapter 96). Systemic activation of the complement system usually indicates more likely recurrence of the disease. Therapy of recurrent disease is usually supportive only. HCV-associated MPGN can also occur *de novo* or recur in renal transplant recipients and after liver transplantation. Cryoglobulinemia is frequently absent and complement levels may be normal.

TREATMENT

The initial treatment plan in MPGN is based on identifying the etiology, if possible, and on general supportive measures to reduce proteinuria and control blood pressure (see Chapter 69). Treatment plans for the various types of MPGN are discussed in the following sections (Fig. 20.16).

Idiopathic Disease in Childhood

Some studies that primarily used historical or nonrandomized controls have shown a beneficial role of alternate-day corticosteroids in childhood MPGN, particularly if administered within the first year of presentation.[21] While these data are not definitive, we recommend an initial treatment approach using alternate-day corticosteroids in this population. For children with MPGN with moderate proteinuria (<3 g/day) and normal renal function, we administer prednisone (40 mg/m^2 on alternate days) for 3 months. In patients with nephrotic syndrome and/or impaired renal function, the high dose of corticosteroids is administered for 2 years (40 mg/m^2 on alternate days). In case of reduction of proteinuria and/or improvement of renal function, prednisone is tapered to a maintenance dose of 20 mg on alternate days for 3 to 10 years.[21] Treatment may be associated with a reduction in hematuria (80%), partial or complete reduction of proteinuria (25%–40%), and better preservation of renal function (80% at 10 years versus 50% in historical controls). The most important side effects are exacerbation of hypertension, growth retardation, weight gain, and obesity. If no benefit is seen after 1 year of treatment, corticosteroids should be withdrawn and supportive therapy only continued. Responses to alternate-day corticosteroids are superior in children with type I MPGN, whereas children with type III

Suggested management of membranoproliferative glomerulonephritis	
Type	Treatment
All types	Supportive therapy following the recommendations discussed in Chapter 69
Idiopathic MPGN in children	Non-nephrotic proteinuria, normal renal function: follow with 3-month visits Normal renal function and moderate proteinuria (>3g/day): prednisone 40mg/m^2 on alternate days for 3 months Nephrotic or impaired renal function: prednisone 40 mg/m^2 on alternate days (80 mg maximum) for 2 years, tapering to 20mg on alternate days for 3–10 years
Idiopathic MPGN in adults	Non-nephrotic, normal renal function: follow with 3-month visits Nephrotic or impaired renal function: 6-month course of corticosteroid with/without cyctotoxic agents (cyclophosphamide) or other drugs used: cyclosporine, tacrolimus, mycophenolate mofetil Rapidly progressive renal failure with diffuse crescents: treat as for idiopathic rapidly progressive glomerulonephritis (see Chapter 23) In the presence of chronic renal failure or nephrotic proteinuria: ACE inhibitors
MPGN associated with hepatitis C virus or cryoglobulinemia	Non-nephrotic, normal renal function: treat with interferon-α (see Chapter 25) based on severity of liver disease (diagnosed by biopsy) Nephrotic syndrome, reduced renal function, or signs of cryoglobulinemia: pegylated interferon-α-2b (1 µg/kg weekly) and ribavirin (15 mg/kg/day) for 12 months, followed by a short-term course of low-dose corticosteroids; if relapse occurs, consider high-dose interferon-α (10 million U daily for 2 weeks, then every other day for 6 more weeks) Rapidly progressive renal failure or severe symptoms of vasculitis (heart failure, pulmonary disease): methylprednisolone 1g daily for 3 days, followed by oral prednisone 60 mg/daily with slow taper over 2–3 months Cyclophosphamide (2 mg/kg/day with adjustment for renal function) and cryofiltration may be added as adjunctive therapy; when the prednisone is reduced to 20 mg/day and the cyclophosphamide is discontinued, add interferon-α MPGN in the renal or liver transplant recipient: consider course of oral ribavirin (0.6–1 g/day)

Figure 20.16 Suggested management of membranoproliferative glomerulonephritis (MGPN).

MPGN are more likely to have a progressive reduction in renal function, slower reduction of serum C3, more persistent urinary abnormalities, and more frequent relapses.[22]

In children with MPGN type II, corticosteroids and calcineurin inhibitors lack efficacy. Removal of C3NeF from the serum through plasma exchange improved serum creatinine in only in a few cases.[23] The utility of immunosuppressive agents such as mycophenolate mofetil (MMF) has not been established. Plasma exchange is an effective therapy in patients with MPGN type II secondary to protein-inactivating mutations of factor H. This therapy replaces deficient factor H with normal factor H, correcting the complement defect.[5]

Idiopathic Disease in Adults

For patients with normal renal function and asymptomatic non-nephrotic range proteinuria, no specific therapy is necessary. Close follow-up every 3 to 4 months is recommended.[21] In patients with nephrotic syndrome and normal or impaired renal function, a 3- to 6-month course of corticosteroids (prednisone 1 mg/kg body weight per day) may be prescribed. If there is considerable reduction of proteinuria, corticosteroids may be continued at the minimal effective dose. If no response is observed within 3 months, corticosteroids should be stopped; treatment with cyclosporine, tacrolimus, or MMF has been recommended.[24] In nonresponders, antiplatelet agents have also been used to treat MPGN in adults; however, a re-analysis of the original trial suggests that these agents did not produce a long-term benefit.[21]

Hepatitis B Virus–Associated Membranoproliferative Glomerulonephritis

In HBV-associated MPGN, treatment with antivirals aimed at eradicating HBV (interferon, lamivudine) is the recommended initial treatment, and immunosuppressive agents are discouraged since they promote further HBV viral replication and occasional deterioration of hepatic function (see Chapter 25).

Hepatitis C Virus–Associated Disease and Cryoglobulinemia

Treatment options in mixed cryoglobulinemia with renal involvement include corticosteroids, cytotoxic drugs such as cyclophosphamide, and parenteral administration of interferon-α (IFN-α) alone or in association with ribavirin. Parenteral IFN-α often improves extrarenal manifestations in close association with reduced levels of viremia, but relapse is common after cessation of therapy.

As also discussed in Chapter 25, the current treatment of choice in patients with HCV-associated MPGN or cryoglobulinemic MPGN is pegylated IFN-α-2b (1 µg/kg weekly for 48 weeks) and ribavirin (15 mg/kg/day) for 6 to 12 months.[25–27] However, ribavirin may be associated with the development of hemolysis, and its toxicity is increased in the setting of renal insufficiency. Alternatively, high-dose IFN-α (10 million U/day for 2 weeks) followed by 10 million U three times weekly for an additional 6 weeks may result in negative HCV RNA and cryoglobulins, normal complement levels, and remission of the nephrotic syndrome.[28,29] However, high-dose IFN-α may cause severe influenza-like symptoms, depression or psychosis, the development of hypothyroidism, and, rarely, the development of proteinuria (with a minimal change type of lesion).

Cryofiltration, that is, double-filtration plasmapheresis with a cooling unit, has been introduced as a means to remove cryoglobulins.[30] If combined with IFN-α and low doses of corticosteroids in elderly patients, it may improve proteinuria and renal function. The major adverse effects of this combination therapy are bleeding and myelosuppression. Corticosteroids, immunosuppressive drugs, and, on occasion, plasmapheresis may exacerbate viremia and chronic HCV, but are still first-line intervention if renal involvement is severe.

In patients with acute exacerbation and/or rapidly progressive MPGN, an initial treatment protocol might include corticosteroids (methylprednisolone 1 g/day IV for 3 days followed by oral prednisone 60 mg/day with slow tapering over 2 to 3 months) and cytotoxic drugs (cyclophosphamide 2 mg/kg/day with adjustment for renal function) followed by the previously described antiviral therapy. Acute oliguric renal failure may also be reversed by cryofiltration and oral administration of prednisolone. Only preliminary data are currently available for rituximab, a CD20 antibody, and MMF (see Chapter 25).

Other Types of Membranoproliferative Glomerulonephritis

MPGN associated with other infections may evoke similar lesions. MPGN associated with α_1-antitrypsin deficiency has been reported to be cured by liver transplantation, which cures the genetic defect. MPGN associated with malignancy such as B cell lymphoma may respond to effective treatment of the underlying cancer.

REFERENCES

1. Rennke HG: Secondary membranoproliferative glomerulonephritis (clinical conference). Kidney Int 1995;47:643–656.
2. Lhotta K, Würzner R, König P: Glomerular deposition of mannose-binding lectin in human glomerulonephritis. Nephrol Dial Transplant 1999;14:881–886.
3. Ohi H, Watanabe S, Fujita T, Yasugi T: Significance of C3 nephritic factor (C3 NeF) in non-hypocomplementaemic serum from patients with membranoproliferative glomerulonephritis (MPGN). Clin Exp Immunol 1992;89:479–484.
4. Rodriguez de Cordoba S, Esparza-Gordillo J, Goicoechea de Jorge E, et al: The human complement factor H: Functional roles, genetic variations and disease associations. Mol Immunol 2004;41:355–367.
5. Appel GB, Cook HT, Hageman G, et al: Membranoproliferative glomerulonephritis type II (dense deposit disease): An update. J Am Soc Nephrol 2005;16:1392–1404.
6. Neary JJ, Conlon PJ, Croke D, et al: Linkage of a gene causing familial membranoproliferative glomerulonephritis type III to chromosome 1. J Am Soc Nephrol 2002;8:2052–2057.
7. Alpers CE, Cotran RS: Neoplasia and glomerular injury. Kidney Int 1986;30:465–473.
8. Fornasieri A, Armelloni S, Bernasconi P, et al: High binding of immunoglobulin M kappa rheumatoid factor from type II cryoglobulins to cellular fibronectin: A mechanism for induction of in situ immune complex glomerulonephritis? Am J Kidney Dis 1996;27:476–483.
9. Sansonno D, Gesualdo L, Manno C, et al: Hepatitis C virus–related proteins in kidney tissue from hepatitis C virus–infected patients with cryoglobulinemic membranoproliferative glomerulonephritis. Hepatology 1997;24:1237–1244.
10. Sansonno D, Lauletta G, Montrone M, et al: Hepatitis C virus RNA and core protein in kidney glomerular and tubular structures isolated with laser capture microdissection. Clin Exp Immunol 2005;140:498–506.
11. Smith KD, Alpers CE: Pathogenic mechanisms in membranoproliferative glomerulonephritis. Curr Opin Nephrol Hypertens 2005;14:396–403.
12. Kawasaki Y, Suzuki J, Nozawa R, Suzuki H: Efficacy of school urinary screening for membranoproliferative glomerulonephritis type I. Arch Dis Child 2002;86:21–25.
13. Kim RY, Faktorovich EG, Kuo CY, Olson JL: Retinal function abnormalities in membranoproliferative glomerulonephritis type II. Am J Ophthalmol 1997;123:619–628.
14. Parrat E, Arndt CF, Labalette P, et al: Retinochoroidal involvement of type II membranoproliferative glomerulonephritis: An angiographic study with indocyanine green. J Fr Ophthalmol 1997;20:430–438.
15. Schwertz R, Rother U, Anders D, et al: Complement analysis in children with idiopathic membranoproliferative glomerulonephritis: A long-term follow-up. Pediatr Allergy Immunol 2001;12:166–172.
16. Johnson RJ, Gretch DR, Couser WG, et al: Hepatitis C virus–associated glomerulonephritis. Effect of alpha-interferon therapy. Kidney Int 1994;46:1700–1704.
17. Gesualdo L, Grandaliano G, Ranieri E, et al: Monocyte recruitment in cryoglobulinemic membranoproliferative glomerulonephritis: A pathogenetic role for monocyte chemotactic peptide-I. Kidney Int 1997;51:155–163.
18. West CD, McAdams AJ: Membranoproliferative glomerulonephritis type III: Association of glomerular deposits with circulating nephritic factor–stabilized convertase. Am J Kidney Dis 1998;32:56–63.
19. Schmitt H, Bohle A, Reincke T, et al: Long-term prognosis of membranoproliferative glomerulonephritis type I: Significance of clinical and morphological parameters: An investigation of 220 cases. Nephron 1990;55:242–250.
20. Little MA, Dupont P, Campbell E, et al: Severity of primary MPGN, rather than MPGN type, determines renal survival and post-transplantation recurrence risk. Kidney Int 2006;69:504–511.
21. Levin A: Management of membranoproliferative glomerulonephritis: Evidence-based recommendations. Kidney Int 1999;55:S41–S46.
22. Braun MC, West CD, Strife CF: Differences between membranoproliferative glomerulonephritis types I and III in long-term response to an alternate-day prednisone regimen. Am J Kidney Dis 1999;34:1022–1032.
23. McGinley E, Watkins R, McLay A, Bulton-Jones JM: Plasma exchange in the treatment of mesangiocapillary glomerulonephritis. Nephron 1985;40:385–390.
24. Jones G, Juszczak M, Kingdon E, et al: Treatment of idiopathic membranoproliferative glomerulonephritis with mycophenolate mofetil and steroids. Nephrol Dial Transplant 2004;12:3160–3164.
25. Rossi P, Bertani T, Baio P, et al: Hepatitis C virus–related cryoglobulinemic glomerulonephritis: Long-term remission after antiviral therapy. Kidney Int 2003;63:2236–2241.
26. Bruchfeld A, Lindahl K, Stahle L, et al: Interferon and ribavirin treatment in patients with hepatitis C–associated renal disease and renal insufficiency. Nephrol Dial Transplant 2003;18:1573–1580.
27. Alric L, Plaisier E, Thébault S, et al: Influence of antiviral therapy in hepatitis C virus–associated cryoglobulinemic MPGN. Am J Kidney Dis 2004;43:617–623.
28. Daghestani L, Pomeroy C: Renal manifestations of hepatitis C infection. Am J Med 1999;106:347–354.
29. Sarac E, Bastacky S, Johnson JP: Response to high-dose interferon-α after failure of standard therapy in MPGN associated with hepatitis C virus infection. Am J Kidney Dis 1997;30:113–115.
30. Kiyomoto H, Hitomi H, Hosotani Y, et al: The effect of combination therapy with interferon and cryofiltration on mesangial proliferative glomerulonephritis originating from mixed cryoglobulinemia in chronic hepatitis C virus infection. Ther Apher 1999;3:329–333.

IgA Nephropathy and Henoch-Schönlein Nephritis

John Feehally and Jürgen Floege

INTRODUCTION AND DEFINITIONS

IgA Nephropathy

IgA nephropathy (IgAN) is a mesangial proliferative glomerulonephritis characterized by diffuse mesangial deposition of IgA. IgAN was first recognized when immunofluorescence techniques were introduced for the study of renal biopsy. It was described in 1968 by a Parisian pathologist, Jean Berger (it has also been called Berger's disease). Although its most common clinical presentation is visible hematuria provoked by mucosal infection, this is neither universal nor necessary for the diagnosis. IgAN is unique among glomerular diseases in being defined by the presence of an immune reactant rather than by any other morphologic feature found on renal biopsy, and the light microscopic changes are very variable. IgAN is the most prevalent pattern of glomerular disease seen in most Western and Asian countries where renal biopsy is widely practiced. At one time, the term *benign recurrent hematuria* was also used for IgAN, but it is now known to be an important cause of end-stage renal disease (ESRD). It is likely that IgAN is not a single entity but rather a common response to various injurious mechanisms.

Henoch-Schönlein Purpura

Henoch-Schönlein purpura (HSP) is a small-vessel vasculitis affecting the skin, joints, gut, and kidneys that predominantly affects children. It is defined by tissue deposition of IgA. HSP was described separately by Schönlein in 1837 and Henoch in 1874. Typically there is clinical involvement in the skin, gut, and kidneys. The nephritis associated with HSP is also characterized by mesangial IgA deposition; indeed, the renal histologic features of Henoch-Schönlein (HS) nephritis are indistinguishable from those of IgAN. HS nephritis is differentiated from IgAN by the extrarenal manifestations.

ETIOLOGY AND PATHOGENESIS

Although infective episodes precede HSP in up to 50% of cases, there is no evidence of a role for any specific antigen. The clinical association of visible hematuria with upper respiratory tract infection in IgAN indicates that the mucosa may be a site of entry for foreign antigens. An infectious source has long been suspected, and there have been occasional reports of IgAN in association with microbial infection, both bacterial (including *Campylobacter*, *Yersinia*, *Mycoplasma*, and *Haemophilus*) and viral (including cytomegalovirus, adenovirus, coxsackievirus, and Epstein-Barr virus). None, however, has been consistently implicated by finding microbial antigen in glomerular deposits. Food antigens have also been proposed (particularly gliadin) but their involvement is not proven. The mesangial IgA may represent a common immune response to a variety of foreign antigens, the original antigen having disappeared from the deposits by the time of the biopsy. Alternatively, it may be an autoimmune disease directed against mesangial antigens, or it may develop through an antigen-independent mechanism such as altered IgA glycosylation.[1]

The regular recurrence of IgAN and HS nephritis after renal transplantation strongly implies an abnormality in the host IgA immune system.

IgA Immune System

IgA is the most abundant immunoglobulin in the body and is chiefly concerned with mucosal defense. It has two subclasses, IgA1 and IgA2. Mucosal antigen challenge provokes polymeric IgA (pIgA) production by plasma cells of the mucosa-associated lymphoid tissue; the pIgA is then transported across epithelium into mucosal fluids. The function of circulating IgA is less clear; it is bone marrow derived and mostly monomeric IgA1 (mIgA1). Circulating IgA1 is cleared by the liver through hepatocyte asialoglycoprotein receptors and Kupffer cell Fcα receptors.

The mesangial IgA in IgAN is predominantly pIgA1. The clinical association with mucosal infection originally suggested that the mesangial pIgA1 comes from the mucosal immune system. In IgAN, however, pIgA1 production is downregulated in the mucosa and upregulated in the bone marrow. Moreover, the pIgA response to systemic immunization with common antigens is increased, whereas the response to mucosal immunization is impaired. Impaired mucosal IgA responses allowing enhanced antigen challenge to the marrow could be the primary abnormality in IgAN, although this remains unproven. Similarly attractive, yet still unproven, is the hypothesis that some mucosal IgA-producing plasma cells translocate to the bone marrow in IgAN; this could also explain the defective glycosylation of IgA1 in IgAN (see later discussion). Tonsillar pIgA1 production is also increased, although IgAN can occur after tonsillectomy and the tonsil is a very minor source of IgA production compared to the mucosa or marrow. Hepatic clearance of IgA is reduced, possibly as a consequence of the altered molecular characteristics of IgA in IgAN (see later discussion).

Serum IgA levels are increased in one third of patients with IgAN and HSP. There are elevations in both mIgA and pIgA. High serum IgA *per se* is not, however, sufficient to cause IgAN; high circulating levels of monoclonal IgA (in myeloma) or polyclonal

IgA (in acquired immunodeficiency syndrome [AIDS]) only infrequently provoke mesangial IgA deposition.

Circulating macromolecular IgA is characteristic of IgAN. It is often described as IgA immune complexes, although the antigen is only rarely identified. There are circulating IgA rheumatoid factors (IgA against the constant domain of IgG) in 30% of those with IgAN and 55% of those with HSP. IgA-fibronectin complexes, at one time thought to be diagnostic for IgAN, are a function of the general increase in serum IgA. Studies *in vitro* indicate that IgA production by mononuclear cells is exaggerated in IgAN and that these cells show abnormal patterns of cytokine production. The direct relevance of these observations to events *in vivo* is uncertain, however.

IgA Glycosylation

IgA1 carries distinctive O-linked sugars at its hinge region; IgA2 has no hinge and carries no such sugars. There is good evidence that circulating IgA1 in IgAN and HS nephritis has abnormal O-linked hinge-region sugars with reduced galactosylation and sialylation.[2] It has recently been shown that mesangial IgA1 in IgAN has the same abnormalities of O-glycosylation.[3,4] The altered glycosylation may promote mesangial IgA1 deposition by predisposing to the formation of circulating IgA1 immune complexes or by directly modifying IgA1 interactions with matrix proteins and mesangial cell and/or monocyte Fc receptors. It may also impair IgA1 clearance by inhibiting IgA1 interactions with hepatic IgA receptors (Fig. 21.1).

Glomerular Injury Following IgA Deposition

Polymeric IgA deposition in the mesangium is typically followed by mesangial proliferative glomerulonephritis (GN). In animal models, codeposition of IgG and complement is necessary for inflammation, but this is not mandatory in human disease. Circulating anti–mesangial IgG has been associated with disease activity in IgAN; this remains unconfirmed, however. Complement deposits are usually C3 and properdin without C1q and C4. The extent to which IgA engages inflammatory cells in the circulation and especially in the kidney will also determine the intensity of inflammation. Fc receptors for IgA (Fcα receptors) on myeloid and mesangial cells may play a key role.

The mechanisms of mesangial proliferative GN have been studied in detail in animal models, particularly anti-Thy 1 nephritis in the rat. These studies[5] have shown the key role of cytokines and growth factors in mesangial cell proliferation (particularly the B and D isoforms of platelet-derived growth factor[5,6] [PDGF] and basic fibroblast growth factor) and in the subsequent matrix production and sclerosis (particularly transforming growth factor β [TGF-β]). Studies of renal biopsies in human IgAN also support a role for PDGF and TGF-β. These mechanisms are not unique to IgAN but are likely to be involved in all forms of mesangial proliferative GN, including those without IgA deposition. Clinical trials based on these pathogenetic insights, in particular with respect to PDGF, are currently being planned.[6]

Animal Models of IgA Nephropathy

Animal IgA does not have the same characteristics as human IgA1, and some animals also have IgA clearance mechanisms distinct from those in humans. It follows that animal models, even if they provoke mesangial IgA deposits, are not particularly informative about the mechanisms that underlie human mesangial pIgA1 deposition, although they have provided many insights into events after IgA deposits have developed. There is no animal model in existence for HSP.

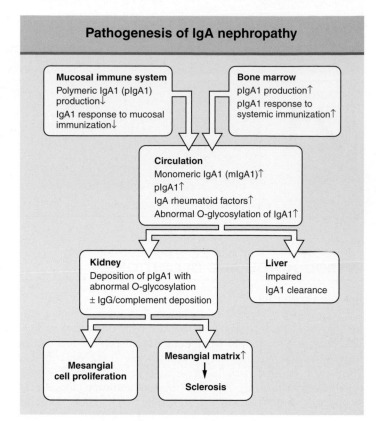

Figure 21.1   Pathogenesis of IgA nephropathy. Abnormalities in IgA immunity leading to mesangial IgA deposition and injury.

Relationship Between IgA Nephropathy and Henoch-Schönlein Purpura

Despite some differences in age of onset and natural history of IgAN and HS nephritis,[7] there is much evidence to support a close pathogenetic link between the two conditions. Monozygotic twins who developed IgAN and HSP respectively at the same time have been reported. The evolution of IgAN into HSP in the same patient is described in both adults and children, and HSP patients with ESRD receiving a renal transplant may experience recurrent disease in the form of IgAN. Many of the abnormalities of IgA production and handling reported in IgAN are also detected in HSP.

IgA antineutrophil cytoplasmic antibody (IgA-ANCA) has been proposed as a marker of the systemic features that differentiate HSP from IgAN. Circulating IgA-ANCA has been described in HSP, although findings are not consistent. IgA-ANCA is not found in IgAN.

EPIDEMIOLOGY

IgAN is the most prevalent pattern of glomerular disease in most countries where renal biopsy is widely used as an investigative tool. However, there is striking geographic variation (Fig. 21.2). Genetic variations may be important. For example, in North America IgAN is less common in African Americans than Caucasians of European origin. It is also very uncommon among black South Africans. In New Zealand, IgAN is much less common among Polynesians than among Caucasians of European origin, even though Polynesians have an increased prevalence of many other renal diseases. Perceived prevalence of IgAN may also be influenced by attitudes to the investigation of microscopic hematuria. A country with an active program of routine urine testing will inevitably identify

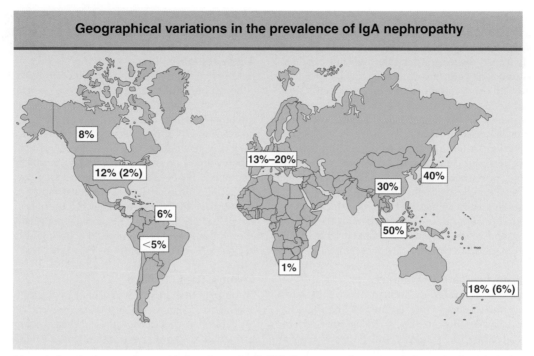

Figure 21.2 Geographic variations in the prevalence of IgA nephropathy (IgAN). Percentages of patients with glomerular disease who have IgA nephropathy. The figures in parentheses are percentages of glomerular disease in minority racial groups: among African Americans in the United States and among Polynesians in New Zealand.

more individuals with urine abnormalities, but IgAN will be identified only if renal biopsy is performed. Even then, the prevalence of IgAN will be underestimated; a study of kidney donors suggests that the prevalence of IgAN with mesangioproliferative changes and glomerular C3-deposits in the general population in Japan may be 1.6%.[8]

In children, HSP is usually diagnosed on clinical grounds without biopsy confirmation of tissue IgA deposition. Transient urine abnormalities are very common in the acute phase. However, only those with persistent urine abnormalities or with more overt renal disease will come to renal biopsy. Therefore, the incidence of HS nephritis is almost certainly underestimated with many unidentified mild and transient cases. There is no information on geographic variations in HSP.

Genetic Basis of IgA Nephropathy

Urine abnormalities increase in frequency among the relatives of those with IgAN, although only in a few pedigrees is IgAN found in multiple generations. One very large pedigree has been described in Kentucky, and other large families have been found in Italy. However, >90% of all cases of IgAN appear to be sporadic.

Encouraging recent work has identified a region on chromosome 6 that in familial IgAN shows much promise as a disease susceptibility gene; further characterization is awaited.[9]

Many studies have sought genes associated with disease in sporadic IgAN without consistent findings. A deletion allele (D) in the angiotensin-converting enzyme (ACE) gene increases serum and tissue ACE levels and has been associated with risk of progression of IgAN,[10] although these findings are not confirmed in all studies. The link is unlikely to be specific for IgAN: an association between increased rate of progression of chronic renal failure and DD genotype has been found in patients with other causes of renal failure.[9] Other reported associations with candidate gene polymorphisms await confirmation. As yet, these studies have had no impact on clinical management.

CLINICAL MANIFESTATIONS OF IgA NEPHROPATHY

The wide range of clinical presentations of IgAN varies in frequency with age (Fig. 21.3). No clinical pattern is pathognomonic of IgAN. In populations of Caucasian descent, it is more common in males than in females by a ratio of 3:1, whereas the ratio approaches 1:1 in most Asian populations.

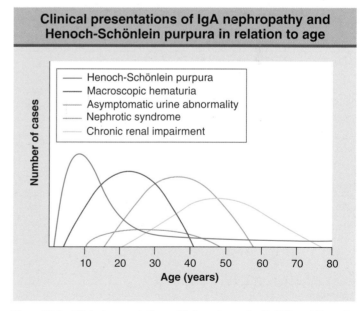

Figure 21.3 Clinical presentations of IgA nephropathy (IgAN) and Henoch-Schönlein purpura (HSP) in relation to age at diagnosis. HSP is most common in childhood but may occur at any age. Macroscopic hematuria is very uncommon after the age of 40 years. The importance of asymptomatic urine abnormality as the presentation of IgAN will depend on attitudes to routine urine testing and renal biopsy. It is uncertain whether those presenting late with chronic renal impairment have a disease distinct from that of those presenting younger with macroscopic hematuria. Data from patients presenting in Leicester, United Kingdom, 1980 to 1995.

Macroscopic Hematuria

In 40% to 50% of cases, the clinical presentation is episodic macroscopic hematuria, most frequently in the second and third decades of life. The urine is usually brown rather than red and clots are unusual. There may be loin pain due to renal capsular swelling. Hematuria usually follows intercurrent mucosal infection, commonly in the upper respiratory tract (the term *synpharyngitic hematuria* has been used) or occasionally in the gastrointestinal tract. Hematuria is usually visible within 24 hours of the onset of the symptoms of infection, differentiating it from the 2- to 3-week delay between infection and subsequent hematuria in postinfectious (for example, poststreptococcal) GN. The macroscopic hematuria resolves spontaneously in the course of a few days. There is persistent microscopic hematuria between attacks. Most patients have only a few episodes of frank hematuria. These become less frequent and resolve over a few years at most. Such episodes are sometimes associated with acute renal impairment.

Asymptomatic Hematuria and Proteinuria

Asymptomatic urine testing identifies 30% to 40% of patients with IgAN in most reported series. Microscopic hematuria with or without proteinuria (usually <2 g/24 h) is noted. The number of patients identified in this way will depend on local attitudes to urine screening as well as the use of renal biopsy in patients with isolated microscopic hematuria. Most patients with IgAN are asymptomatic and would only be identified when there is population-based urine screening.

Proteinuria and Nephrotic Syndrome

It is rare for proteinuria to occur without microscopic hematuria. Nephrotic syndrome is uncommon, occurring in only 5% of all patients with IgAN. Nephrotic syndrome may occur early in the course of the disease, with minimal glomerular change or with active mesangial proliferative GN. Alternatively, it may occur as a late manifestation of advanced chronic glomerular scarring.

Acute Renal Failure

Acute renal failure is very uncommon in IgAN (<5% of all cases), although one study reports that it may be the presentation in up to 27% of those older than 65 years.[11] It develops by three distinct mechanisms. There may be acute severe immune injury with necrotizing GN and crescent formation (crescentic IgA nephropathy); this may be the first presentation of IgAN or it may develop superimposed on established, less aggressive disease. Rapid deterioration in IgAN may occur in pregnancy due to crescentic transformation. Alternatively, acute renal failure can occur with mild glomerular injury when heavy glomerular hematuria leads to tubule occlusion by red cells. Finally, especially in elderly patients, chronic IgAN will predispose to acute renal failure from a variety of non–IgA-related conditions (see Chapter 63).

Chronic Renal Failure

Some patients already have renal impairment and hypertension when first diagnosed. These patients tend to be older, and it is probable that they have long-standing disease that previously remained undiagnosed because the patient neither had frank hematuria nor underwent routine urinalysis. Hypertension is common as in other chronic glomerular disease; accelerated hypertension occurs in 5% of patients.

Clinical Associations with IgA Nephropathy

Although IgAN is clinically restricted to the kidney in most cases, there are associations with other conditions, particularly with a number of immune and inflammatory diseases (Fig. 21.4). Their relationship to abnormalities of the IgA immune system is not always clear.

Diseases reported in association with IgA nephropathy			
Disease	Common	Reported	Rare
Rheumatic and autoimmune disease	Ankylosing spondylitis Rheumatoid arthritis Reiter syndrome Uveitis	Behçet's syndrome* Takayasu's arteritis† Myasthenia gravis	Sicca syndrome
Gastrointestinal disease	Celiac disease	Ulcerative colitis	Crohn's disease Whipple's disease
Hepatic disease	Alcoholic liver disease Nonalcoholic cirrhosis Schistosomal liver disease		
Lung disease	Sarcoid		Pulmonary hemosiderosis
Skin disease	Dermatitis herpetiformis		
Malignancy		IgA monoclonal gammopathy	Bronchial carcinoma Renal carcinoma Laryngeal carcinoma Mycosis fungoides Sézary syndrome
Infection	Human immunodeficiency virus, hepatitis B (in endemic areas)	Brucellosis	Leprosy
Miscellaneous		Wiskott-Aldrich syndrome‡	

Figure 21.4 Diseases reported in association with IgA nephropathy (IgAN): common, reported, and rare. Rare associations have been made in one or two reported cases only. In a disease as common as IgAN, it is therefore uncertain whether they are truly related. *Behçet's syndrome: a systemic vasculitis typified by orogenital ulceration and chronic uveitis. †Takayasu's arteritis: a systemic vasculitis involving the aorta and its major branches, most often found in young women. ‡Wiskott-Aldrich syndrome: an X-linked disorder in which increased serum IgA is associated with the triad of recurrent pyogenic infection, eczema, and thrombocytopenia.

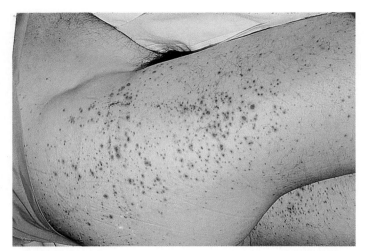

Figure 21.5   Henoch-Schönlein purpura. The rash is a palpable purpuric vasculitis on the lower limbs spreading on extensor surfaces to the buttocks and occasionally to the upper limbs. Histology shows leukocytoclastic vasculitis with IgA deposits in blood vessel walls.

Mesangial IgA deposition is a frequent finding in autopsy studies in chronic liver disease. Although particularly associated with alcoholic cirrhosis, it can occur in other chronic liver disease, including that caused by hepatitis B and schistosomiasis. It is thought to be a consequence of impaired clearance of IgA by the Kupffer cells (which express Fcα receptors) and hepatocytes (which express the asialoglycoprotein receptor). Only a small minority of patients have any clinical evidence of renal disease other than microscopic hematuria, although occasional patients will develop ESRD.

A number of case reports have associated IgAN with human immunodeficiency virus/AIDS. The polyclonal increase in serum IgA, which is a feature of AIDS, has been cited as a predisposing factor. Autopsy studies indicate, however, that IgAN is not unduly common in large populations of AIDS patients.[12]

CLINICAL MANIFESTATIONS OF HENOCH-SCHÖNLEIN PURPURA

HSP is most prevalent in the first decade of life but may occur at any age. A palpable purpuric rash, which may be recurrent, occurs on extensor surfaces (Fig. 21.5). There may be polyarthralgia (usually without joint swelling) and abdominal pain caused by gut vasculitis. This may be severe, with bloody diarrhea if

intussusception develops. In practice, the diagnosis is made by clinical criteria in the great majority of children in whom HSP is a self-limiting illness. In adults, clinical features include purpura, arthritis and gastrointestinal symptoms in 95%, 60%, and 50% of patients, respectively.[13] Renal involvement in adults with HSP is not different from isolated IgAN. Tissue confirmation of IgA deposition by renal or skin biopsy is necessary to establish the diagnosis.

Much renal involvement in HSP is transient. Urine abnormalities are noted during the acute presentation, but may disappear. Of those referred to a nephrologist, asymptomatic urine abnormality is still the most frequent clinical manifestation. Nephrotic syndrome occurs in 20% to 30% of patients. Acute renal failure may develop as a result of crescentic GN.

PATHOLOGY

The respective renal histopathologies in IgAN and HS nephritis may be indistinguishable from each other (Fig. 21.6).

Immune Deposits
Diffuse mesangial IgA, shown in Figure 21.6b, is the defining hallmark. C3 is codeposited in up to 90% of cases. IgG in 40% and IgM in 40% of cases may also be found in the same distribution. IgA also deposits sometimes along capillary loops (a pattern more common in HS nephritis); in IgAN, this pattern is associated with a worse prognosis. C5b-9 is found with properdin but not C4, indicating alternative complement pathway activation. Disappearance of IgA deposits after prolonged clinical remission has been documented in both children and adults.

Light Microscopy
Light microscopic changes are remarkably variable and do not correlate topographically with the IgA deposits. They can vary from almost normal glomerular architecture, diffuse mesangioproliferative GN (see Fig. 21.6a) to focal segmental GN or, in rare cases, focal segmental necrotizing GN with extracapillary proliferation. Typical cases are characterized by an increase in mesangial cells and mesangial matrix with normal-appearing peripheral glomerular basement membranes (GBMs). Focal segmental or global glomerular sclerosis indicates that the disease has been ongoing for some time already. In addition to glomerular changes, the preglomerular arterial vessels often exhibit wall hyalinosis and subintimal fibrosis even in cases of only mild arterial hypertension. In long-standing disease, tubulointerstitial inflammation leads to interstitial fibrosis and tubular atrophy in a pattern no different

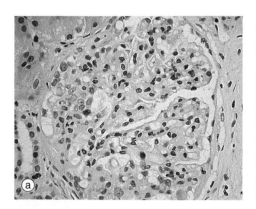
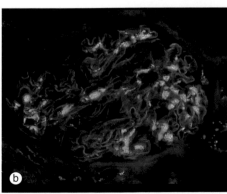
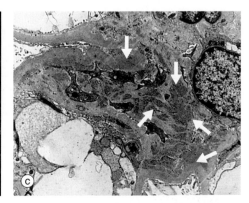

Figure 21.6   Renal pathology in IgA nephropathy. *a,* Light microscopy: diffuse mesangial hypercellularity (hematoxylin-eosin ×300). *b,* Immunofluorescence microscopy: diffuse mesangial IgA (indirect immunofluorescence with fluorescein isothiocyanate–anti-IgA ×300). *c,* Electron microscopy: mesangial electron-dense deposits. The deposits are shown by *arrows* (electron micrograph ×16,000). (*a* and *c,* Courtesy of Prof. P. Furness.)

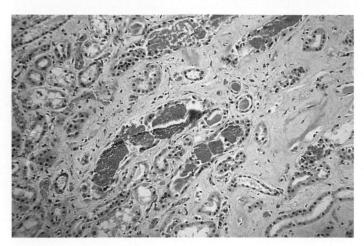

Figure 21.7   Acute renal failure in IgA nephropathy. Tubular occlusion by red cells (hematoxylin-eosin ×300). This appearance may be associated with only minor glomerular changes.

from other progressive glomerular disease. Occasionally, IgAN and minimal change nephrotic syndrome coincide (see later under Nephrotic Syndrome), in which case, light microscopy is normal, but there are mesangial IgA deposits.

Classification of the morphology is of some value in predicting prognosis, although there is no universal agreement as to the ideal classification. The classifications of both Haas[14] and Lee and colleagues[15] are most widely used, but each has some limitations as a prognostic indicator.[16]

Two distinct patterns of injury are seen in acute renal failure. There may be tubular occlusion by red cells with acute tubular epithelial injury in macrohematuria-associated acute renal failure (Fig. 21.7). Alternatively, glomerular injury may be the cause of acute renal failure with necrotizing GN and cellular crescent formation. Such crescentic IgAN may develop on a histologic background of established chronic renal injury due to IgAN, or may be the first presentation of IgAN. It is not uncommon to see small numbers of crescents in patients with stable renal function and no other pathologic evidence of severe glomerular inflammation; the term crescentic IgAN should not be used for such cases, in which the prognosis is often favorable.

Electron Microscopy

Electron-dense deposits correspond to the mesangial (or capillary loop) IgA, as shown in Figure 21.6c. Typically, electron-dense deposits are confined to mesangial and paramesangial areas, but, in addition, subepithelial and subendothelial deposits are also seen. Up to one third of patients will have some focal thinning of the GBM. Occasionally there will be extensive GBM thinning, suggesting a coincident diagnosis of thin membrane nephropathy (see Chapter 45).

DIFFERENTIAL DIAGNOSIS

The diagnosis of IgAN or HS nephritis requires identification of mesangial IgA in the glomeruli. It cannot be made, therefore, without a renal biopsy, no matter how suggestive the clinical presentation may be. Serum IgA is often increased, and there may be IgA in cutaneous blood vessels in IgAN, and in both affected and unaffected skin in HSP. Neither finding, however, is reliable enough to support the diagnosis without a renal biopsy. Serum complement components are normal.

Mesangial IgA occurs in other conditions (Fig. 21.8) that can usually be differentiated on clinical, serologic, and histologic criteria. None of the light microscopic features are of themselves diagnostic of IgAN.

Hematuria

Nonglomerular causes of hematuria, particularly stones and neoplasia, must be excluded by appropriate investigations (see Chapter 56). In its most characteristic clinical setting (recurrent macroscopic hematuria coinciding with mucosal infection in a male in the second or third decade of life), the diagnosis can be strongly suspected. Such a diagnosis, however, cannot be made without a biopsy since recurrent macroscopic hematuria also occurs in other glomerular diseases, particularly in children and young adults.

Nephrotic Syndrome

Patients with IgAN occasionally develop nephrotic syndrome, which is indistinguishable from that in minimal change disease. There is a sudden onset of nephrosis, with biopsy evidence of glomerular epithelial cell foot process effacement and a prompt complete remission of proteinuria in response to corticosteroids. Only hematuria and mesangial IgA deposits persist after treatment. This pattern occurs particularly in children. These patients are usually regarded as having two separate common glomerular diseases, IgAN and minimal change disease.[17]

Other patients with IgAN may develop nephrotic syndrome with more structural glomerular damage and lack the response to corticosteroids. The clinical differential diagnosis includes common causes of nephrotic syndrome appropriate for the age of the patient (see Chapter 16).

Chronic Renal Disease: Hypertension, Proteinuria, Renal Impairment

In this context, IgAN will be clinically indistinguishable from many forms of chronic renal disease. The renal biopsy may be diagnostic, by identifying mesangial IgA, even when structural damage is so advanced on light microscopy that it has the nonpecific features of end-stage kidney disease.

Acute Renal Failure

In acute renal failure, renal biopsy should be performed unless there is rapid improvement in renal function over 2 to 3 days in response to supportive care and vigorous hydration. Renal biopsy may be required to differentiate the tubular occlusion and acute tubular necrosis, which occasionally follow heavy glomerular

---

Differential diagnosis of IgA nephropathy: conditions associated with mesangial IgA deposition
IgA nephropathy
Henoch-Schönlein nephritis
Lupus nephritis*
Alcoholic liver disease
IgA monoclonal gammopathy
Schistosomal nephropathy

Figure 21.8   Differential diagnosis of IgA nephropathy: conditions associated with mesangial IgA deposition. *Distinguishing lupus nephritis (especially International Society of Nephrology/Renal Pathology Society classes II and III) may cause difficulty. The finding of C1q deposition is useful. It indicates classical pathway involvement found in lupus nephritis.

hematuria, from crescentic IgAN, or other coincidental causes of acute renal failure (see Fig. 21.7).

Differential Diagnosis of Henoch-Schönlein Purpura

In children the diagnosis of HSP is usually made based on clinical criteria. Confirmatory evidence of tissue IgA deposition will not be obtained unless persistence of renal disease results in a renal biopsy. In adults, the differential diagnosis is much wider and includes other forms of systemic vasculitis requiring diagnosis by clinical, serologic, and histologic characteristics (see Chapter 23).

NATURAL HISTORY

Natural History of IgA Nephropathy

The overall prognosis of IgAN has now been defined in long-term natural history studies.[18] Although the evidence shows clinical remission (disappearance of hematuria and proteinuria) in up to one third of patients with mild disease, large studies with prolonged follow-up indicate a slow attrition. By 20 years, one fourth of patients will have ESRD, and a further 20% will have progressive impairment of renal function. It is, however, important to appreciate that these natural history data are based on studies initiated >20 years ago; it is possible that long-term prognosis has improved significantly since then with more active and widespread supportive therapy.

Although an active approach to the investigation of microscopic hematuria will increase the size of the cohort of patients found to have IgAN, it will include more with a good prognosis, thus altering the perceived risk of disease progression. Episodes of macroscopic hematuria do not confer a worse prognosis. This may indicate that such episodes only occur early in the natural history of the disease and that patients doing less well from the point of diagnosis in fact were only identified at a later stage in their disease. This is also suggested by the adverse influence on outcome of advancing age at diagnosis.

The risk of renal failure is not uniform. As in any chronic glomerular disease, the presence of hypertension, proteinuria, and renal impairment at presentation, as well as histologic evidence of glomerular and interstitial fibrosis, identifies at the time of diagnosis those with a poor prognosis[18] (Fig. 21.9). Hyperuricemia and increased body mass index are also independent risk factors for progression. However, during follow-up, only hypertension and proteinuria are reliable predictors of risk of progression. Some evidence suggests geographic variation in risk of progression. A Canadian study indicates risk of progression is negligible when proteinuria remains <0.2 g/24 h with normal blood pressure.[19] However, in contrast, a study from Hong Kong suggests that among those presenting with isolated microscopic hematuria, as many as 44% may subsequently develop proteinuria, hypertension, or renal impairment over a 7-year follow-up.[20]

Natural History of Henoch-Schönlein Nephritis

This is less well defined than IgAN. Observations are restricted to those referred for renal biopsy. This therefore excludes the majority of patients with minor transient renal involvement who have an excellent prognosis. The renal prognosis is worse in adults than children. In adults, up to 40% will have chronic kidney disease or ESRD 15 years after biopsy. One series reports an increased mortality due to lung and gastrointestinal malignancy.[13]

Prognostic markers at presentation in IgA nephropathy	
Clinical	Histopathologic
Poor Prognosis	
Hypertension	Glomerular sclerosis
Renal impairment	Tubular atrophy
Severity of proteinuria	Interstitial fibrosis
Hyperuricemia	Capillary loop IgA deposits
Increasing age	Crescents (controversial)
Gross obesity	
Duration of preceding symptoms	
Good Prognosis	
Recurrent macroscopic hematuria	
No Impact on Prognosis	
Gender	Intensity of IgA deposits
Serum IgA level	

Figure 21.9 Prognostic markers at presentation in IgA nephropathy. None of the clinical or histopathologic adverse features, except capillary loop IgA deposits, are specific to IgA nephropathy.

TRANSPLANTATION

Recurrent IgA Nephropathy

There is no evidence from transplant registry data that transplant outcome is inferior if IgAN is the primary renal disease. Nevertheless, mesangial IgA deposits recur in the donor transplant kidney in up to 60% of patients with IgAN.[21] They may occur within days or weeks, but the risk increases with the duration of the transplant. The deposits seem benign in the short term and are not often associated initially with light microscopic changes. Graft failure due to recurrent IgAN, associated with proteinuria and hypertension, occurs in about 5% of cases within 5 years but significantly worsens the prognosis of grafts from 10 years onward or in case of repeated transplantation. In pooled series, recurrent IgAN is 30% in living related transplants versus 23% in cadaveric grafts,[21] but this does not affect graft survival and living related donation should not be discouraged. However, any urinary abnormality in a potential related donor requires thorough evaluation including, if necessary, a renal biopsy. Recurrence of crescentic IgAN with rapid graft failure occurs uncommonly and is generally resistant to treatment.

In a few unwitting experiments, cadaver kidneys with IgA deposits have been transplanted into recipients without IgAN. In all cases, the IgA rapidly disappeared, supporting the concept that abnormalities in IgAN lie in the IgA immune system and not in the kidney.

Recurrent Henoch-Schönlein Nephritis

HSP can recur as isolated IgA deposits in the graft (about 50% of transplants), full-blown yet isolated IgAN, or rarely as a full recurrence of systemic involvement including a rash. The characteristics of renal recurrence are apparently similar to those of recurrent primary IgAN.[21] Delaying transplantation once ESRD is reached does not reduce the risk of recurrence.

TREATMENT

Although specific early treatment intervention might influence the IgA immune system abnormalities that underlie IgAN, the mechanisms of chronic disease progression are unlikely to be unique. It is probable, therefore, that studies of such IgAN patients will provide information applicable to many forms of chronic GN for which IgAN is the paradigm.

The balance of risk against benefit for immunosuppressive therapy is often unfavorable in IgAN, except in the unusual circumstance of crescentic IgAN.

The need for randomized, controlled trials of adequate power to answer questions about the prevention of chronic renal failure in IgAN is pressing. It is disappointing, despite the prevalence of IgAN and consensus about its definition and natural history, that there are so few such studies.[22,23] They are shown in Figure 21.10. Patients with HSP have been excluded from almost all treatment studies, so it is uncertain whether any strategies developed for IgAN are applicable to HS nephritis.

TREATMENT OF IgA NEPHROPATHY

Treatment recommendations are summarized in Figure 21.11.

Reduction of IgA Production

Tonsillectomy reduces the frequency of episodic hematuria when tonsillitis is the provoking infection. A long-term retrospective study from Japan suggests tonsillectomy may reduce the risk of renal failure,[24] but this is not supported by a German study.[25] The lack of controlled trials is particularly important as the natural history is for macroscopic hematuria to become less frequent with time, independent of any specific treatment. Tonsillectomy may be indicated in the occasional patient with recurrent ARF with macroscopic hematuria induced by tonsillitis. There is no role for prophylactic antibiotics. Dietary gluten restriction, used to reduce mucosal antigen challenge, has not been shown to preserve renal function.

Prevention and Removal of IgA Deposits

The ideal treatment for IgAN would remove IgA from the glomerulus and prevent further IgA deposition. This remains a

Randomized controlled trials* in IgA nephropathy			
Treatment	Country/Year	Study Group	Outcome
Phenytoin	Australia/1980	Adults	No benefit
Corticosteroids	Hong Kong/1986	Adults: nephritic	16 weeks of treatment No benefit: response in subgroup with minimal change
	US/1992	Children: low-grade proteinuria	12 weeks of treatment No benefit
	Italy/1999 and 2004	Adults: proteinuria	6 months of treatment Proteinuria lessened, renal function preserved
	Japan/2000	Adults: low-grade proteinuria	Proteinuria lessened, histology at 12 months improved
	Japan/2003	Adults: progressive	Proteinuria lessened, no benefit on renal function
Corticosteroids/azathioprine	Japan/1999	Children: low-grade proteinuria	2 years of treatment Proteinuria lessened, renal function unchanged, less glomerulosclerosis
Cyclophosphamide	UK/2001	Adults: proteinuria, progressive	Renal failure delayed
	Singapore/1991	Adults: proteinuria, progressive	Renal failure delayed
Mycophenolate mofetil	Belgium/2003	Adults: proteinuria, progressive	No benefit
	US/2005	Adults: proteinuria, progressive	No benefit
	Hong Kong/2005	Adults: proteinuria, progressive	Proteinuria lessened
Dipyridamole/warfarin	Australia/1990	Adults: proteinuria, progressive	Proteinuria lessened, no benefit on renal function
	Hong Kong/1987	Adults: proteinuria	No benefit
	Singapore/1989	Adults: proteinuria, progressive	Renal function preserved
ACE inhibitors	Italy/1994	Adults: proteinuria, normotensive	Proteinuria reduced
	Australia/1995	Adults: proteinuria, hypertensive	Proteinuria reduced: glomerular filtration rate no different at 1 year
	Hong Kong/1999	Adults: proteinuria, hypertensive	No benefit
	Spain/2005	Adults: proteinuria, hypertensive	Renal failure delayed
Fish oil	Australia/1989	Adults: proteinuria, progressive	No benefit
	Hong Kong/1990	Adults: advanced renal impairment	No benefit
	Sweden/1994	Adults: proteinuria, progressive	No benefit
	US/1994	Adults: proteinuria, progressive	Renal failure delayed: proteinuria unchanged

Figure 21.10 Randomized controlled trials in IgA nephropathy. ACE, angiotensin-converting enzyme. *These are reviewed in references 22 and 23.

Treatment recommendations for IgA nephropathy
Recurrent macroscopic hematuria (preserved renal function)   Aggressive hydration (no role for antibiotics or tonsillectomy)

Macroscopic hematuria with acute renal failure
    Renal biopsy mandatory if persistent acute renal failure (see text)
    Acute tubular necrosis: supportive measures only
    Crescentic IgAN
        Induction: prednisolone 0.5–1 mg/kg/day for up to 8 weeks; cyclophosphamide 2 mg/kg/day for up to 8 weeks (no evidence favoring oral or intravenous
            route—follow local practice)
        Maintenance: prednisolone in reducing dosage, azathioprine 2.5 mg/kg/day

Proteinuria <1 g/24 h (±microscopic hematuria)   No specific treatment
Nephrotic syndrome (with minimal change on light microscopy)   Prednisolone 0.5–1 mg/kg/day (children 60 mg/m²/day) for up to 8 weeks

Non-nephrotic proteinuria >1 g/24 h (±microscopic hematuria)
    ACE inhibitor and/or ARB (maximize dosage or combine to achieve target blood pressure and proteinuria < 0.5 g/day); for additional measures,
        see Chapter 69
    If proteinuria still >1 g/24 h on maximal supportive therapy and GFR <70 ml/min, consider fish oil—12 g/daily for 6 months. If further progression of renal
        failure, consider prednisolone (40 mg/day decreasing to 10 mg by 2 years) + azathioprine (1.5 mg/kg/day)

Hypertension
    ACE inhibitor and ARB are agents of first choice. If proteinuria <1 g/24 h, target blood pressure is 130/80 mm Hg; if proteinuria >1 g/24 h target blood
        pressure is 125/75 mm Hg

Transplantation   No special measures required

Figure 21.11   Treatment recommendations for IgA nephropathy. ACE, angiotensin-converting enzyme; ARB, angiotensin receptor blocker.

remote prospect, while the pathogenesis remains incompletely understood.

Altering Immune and Inflammatory Events That Follow IgA Deposition
Rapidly Progressive Renal Failure Associated with Crescentic IgA Nephropathy

In this uncommon situation, the risk-benefit balance is most strongly placed in favor of intensive immunosuppressive therapy since, untreated, there will be rapid progression to ESRD. Treatment has often combined plasma exchange with prednisolone and cyclophosphamide.[26] Early clinical response is favorable, as in other crescentic nephritis. Medium-term results, however, are disappointing: one half of the reported patients have reached ESRD within 12 months.[26] A subset of patients with circulating IgG-ANCA may have a more favorable response to immunosuppressive therapy similar to that seen in other ANCA-positive crescentic nephritis.[27] There have been no controlled trials of treatment, so it is not possible to be certain which elements of the regimen (corticosteroids, cyclophosphamide, or plasma exchange) are mandatory.

Early Treatment with Immunosuppressive or Anti-inflammatory Regimens
Corticosteroids   Corticosteroids have been given in two short-term randomized, controlled trials: one in nephrotic adults and one in children with low-grade proteinuria. Neither trial showed benefit. Among the nephrotic adults, however,[28] there was a small

group with very minor histologic changes that responded rapidly to treatment. Nephrotic syndrome may occur in this setting when minimal change disease and IgAN coincide, in which case the nephrotic syndrome will be fully and promptly steroid responsive. A trial of high-dose corticosteroid therapy is therefore justified in IgAN when there is nephrotic syndrome associated with minimal glomerular injury.

Despite the generally negative outcome of the two short-term studies, uncontrolled data have favored the use of prolonged administration of alternate-day steroids, and this approach is further supported by a randomized, controlled trial suggesting that 6 months of intravenous pulse methylprednisolone plus alternate-day corticosteroids in adults with low-grade proteinuria may protect renal function during long-term follow-up.[29]

Another controlled trial using smaller doses of corticosteroids in patients with non-nephrotic proteinuria showed some reduction in protein excretion but no protection of renal function.[30]

Corticosteroids combined with azathioprine have also been used in a 2-year randomized trial in children with early disease[31] in whom proteinuria lessened and glomerulosclerosis was avoided, although there was no effect on renal function.

Cyclophosphamide   Cyclophosphamide has been used in combination with warfarin and dipyridamole in two randomized, controlled trials, the results of which are not mutually consistent. Both showed modest reduction in proteinuria, but only one preserved renal function. Cyclophosphamide followed by azathioprine combined with prednisolone preserved renal function in a controlled trial in patients with a poor prognosis.[32] Many physicians regard the toxicity of cyclophosphamide as unacceptable in young adults with IgAN.

Mycophenolate Mofetil Mycophenolate mofetil has been used in three controlled trials in high-risk patients. Two trials in Caucasian patients failed to demonstrate any benefit, whereas a short-term study in Chinese patients noted reduced proteinuria. Whether racial effects indeed underlie these discrepant results remains to be clarified.[33]

Dipyridamole and Warfarin These have also been given in two controlled trials that showed mutually inconsistent results. There was no benefit in one and preserved renal function in the other.

Cyclosporine Cyclosporine has been used in one controlled trial. There was a reversible decrease in proteinuria. This went in parallel with a decrease in creatinine clearance, suggesting that the changes were a hemodynamic effect of cyclosporine rather than an immune-modulating effect.

Pooled Human Immunoglobulin Pooled human immunoglobulin has given encouraging preliminary results in IgAN with an aggressive clinical course: proteinuria lessened, deterioration in glomerular filtration rate (GFR) slowed, and histologic activity lessened on repeat renal biopsies.[34] No controlled trial is yet available for this approach.

Treatment of Slowly Progressive IgA Nephropathy

There is little evidence to indicate that the events of progressive glomerular injury are unique to IgAN. Treatments available are nonspecific approaches for chronic glomerular disease (see also Chapter 69), of which IgAN is the most common and most easily defined.

Hypertension

There is compelling evidence of the benefit of lowering blood pressure (BP) in the treatment of chronic progressive glomerular disease such as IgAN. In IgAN, there is also evidence that casual clinic BP readings underestimate BP load as judged by ambulatory BP monitoring and echocardiographic evidence of increased left ventricular mass.[35] Two prospective, controlled trials strongly support the use of ACE inhibitors and in particular the combination of ACE inhibitors with angiotensin receptor blockers (ARB) in IgAN as first-choice hypotensive agents to minimize proteinuria as well as BP.[36,37] Low target BPs (<130/80 mm Hg if proteinuria <1 g/24 h, 125/75 mm Hg if proteinuria >1 g/24 h) are recommended from a number of large studies of chronic progressive renal disease. In a randomized study of IgAN, achieving a mean BP of 129/70 mm Hg prevented the decrease in renal function over 3 years seen in those achieving mean BPs of 136/76 mm Hg.[38]

It is unfortunate that available randomized, controlled trials of corticosteroids, immunosuppressive agents, and fish oil in IgAN have not controlled BP rigorously to these low targets and have not uniformly used ACE inhibitors and ARBs; it is therefore not possible to be certain whether the apparent benefits in these trials would be sustained if tight BP control with renin-angiotensin blockade is maintained. Inconsistencies in the outcomes of the immunosuppressive trials may in part be explained by differences in achieved BP and variable use of renin-angiotensin blockade.

Fish Oil

The favorable effects of supplementing the diet with omega-3 fatty acids in the form of fish oil include reductions in eicosanoid and cytokine production, changes in membrane fluidity and rheology, and reduced platelet aggregability. These features should significantly reduce the adverse influence of many mechanisms thought to affect progression of chronic glomerular disease.

A randomized, controlled trial provides convincing evidence of protection from 2 years of treatment with fish oil in patients with proteinuria and increasing serum creatinine.[39] It is, however, surprising that fish oil did not significantly reduce proteinuria, a major risk factor for progression. A further study showed no advantage for high- over low-dose fish oil.[40] However, other smaller controlled trials have shown no benefit,[41] although severity of renal impairment before treatment was not equivalent in all these studies. Fish oil treatment does not have the drawbacks associated with immunosuppressive treatment. It is safe apart from a decrease in blood coagulability, which is not usually a practical problem, and an unpleasant taste, with flatulence, which may make compliance difficult. Some fish oil preparations contain significant amounts of cholesterol, necessitating close surveillance if such treatment is initiated. A further confirmatory study of fish oil would be of great value.

Recommendation

The treatment of IgAN with proteinuria >1 g/24 h remains controversial. Physicians are increasingly using corticosteroids when there is preserved renal function (GFR >70 ml/min) and fish oil when there is renal impairment (GFR <70 ml/min). However, in these authors' opinion, the case is not yet made for either of these therapies. Tight control of BP with ACE inhibitors and ARB should be the first line of treatment. Fish oil or corticosteroids should only be considered if proteinuria >1 g/24 h persists on maximal ACE inhibitor/ARB therapy with BP <125/75 mm Hg. Azathioprine (or even cyclophosphamide) combined with corticosteroids should be reserved for desperate cases, in which all other measures have failed, and this treatment option needs to be well balanced against its associated risks.

Transplant Recurrence

There is no evidence that newer immunosuppressive agents have modified the frequency of recurrent IgA deposits or are of value in recurrent disease. Most clinicians therefore just optimize supportive care in such instances. When crescentic IgAN recurs with rapidly deteriorating graft function, treatment as for primary crescentic IgAN has been used, although evidence of its success is sparse.

TREATMENT OF HENOCH-SCHÖNLEIN NEPHRITIS

Many patients have transient nephritis during the early phase of HSP, which spontaneously remits and requires no treatment. There are no prospective, randomized, controlled trials to guide the treatment of HS nephritis. Most therapeutic studies of IgAN exclude those with HSP, so it is uncertain whether a number of potential treatments have a role in HS nephritis. Treatment recommendations are summarized in Figure 21.12.

Rapidly Progressive Renal Failure Caused by Crescentic Nephritis

Crescentic nephritis is more common in HS nephritis than in IgAN, particularly early in the course of HSP. There is little

Treatment recommendations for Henoch-Schönlein nephritis
Crescentic nephritis: regimen as for crescentic IgA nephropathy (see Fig. 21.11)
All other Henoch-Schönlein nephritis (including nephrotic syndrome): no specific treatment, supportive measures only
Hypertension: ACE inhibitor and ARB are agents of first choice; target blood pressure: 130/80 mm Hg *if* proteinuria <1 g/24 h, 125/75 mm Hg *if* proteinuria >1 g/24 h
Transplantation: cadaveric donor may be preferable to living related donor in children (controversial)

Figure 21.12 Treatment recommendations for Henoch-Schönlein nephritis. ACE, angiotensin-converting enzyme; ARB, angiotensin receptor blocker.

specific information on treatment in adults or children, but regimens based on those for other forms of systemic vasculitis are widely used. These have included corticosteroids and cyclophosphamide, with the addition of plasma exchange or pulse methylprednisolone in some cases. There have been no controlled trials and HS nephritis has usually been excluded from trials of severe nephritis in systemic vasculitis. It is not possible to define the best regimen on available evidence.

Active Henoch-Schönlein Nephritis Without Renal Failure

There is little information about less aggressive HS nephritis. Corticosteroids alone have never been shown to be beneficial. It has been proposed, but not confirmed, that early use of corticosteroids in HSP may prevent nephritis.[42] Promising findings with combination therapy of corticosteroids, cyclophosphamide, and antiplatelet agents have only been reported in small nonrandomized studies.[43] A nonrandomized study reported that prednisolone/azathioprine preserved renal function and improved histologic appearances, but relied on historical controls.[44] There are very few patients with HS nephritis included in the promising studies of immunoglobulin.

Slowly Progressive Renal Failure

While the renal histology and clinical course of slowly progressive HS nephritis and IgAN may be indistinguishable, patients with HS nephritis have not been included in studies of fish oil. Tight BP control with ACE inhibitors or ARB is recommended for proteinuric HS nephritis as for IgAN.

Transplant Recurrence

No treatment is known to reduce the risk of recurrence. There is some evidence that recurrence is more common and more likely to lead to graft loss in children receiving live donor kidneys than cadaver kidneys,[45] although this is not confirmed in adults.[46] If crescentic HS nephritis recurs, intensive immunosuppression may be justified as for primary disease. This, however, has not been thoroughly evaluated.

REFERENCES

1. Barratt J, Feehally J, Smith AC: Pathogenesis of IgA nephropathy. Semin Nephrol 2004;24:197–217.
2. Allen AC, Bailey EM, Barratt J, et al: Analysis of IgA1 O-glycans in IgA nephropathy by fluorophore assisted carbohydrate electrophoresis. J Am Soc Nephrol 1999;10:1763–1771.
3. Allen AC, Bailey EM, Brenchley PEC, et al: Mesangial IgA1 in IgA nephropathy exhibits aberrant O-glycosylation: Observations in three patients. Kidney Int 2001;60:969–973.
4. Hiki Y, Odani H, Takahashi M, et al: Mass spectrometry proves underglycosylation of glomerular IgA1 in IgA nephropathy. Kidney Int 2001;59:1077–1085.
5. Johnson RJ: The glomerular response to injury: Mechanisms of progression or resolution. Kidney Int 1994;45:1769–1782.
6. Floege J, van Roeyen C, Ostendorf T: PDGF-D: A novel mediator of mesangioproliferative glomerulonephritis. Drugs Future 2004;29: 179–184.
7. Davin JC, ten Berge IJ, Weening J: What is the difference between IgA nephropathy and Henoch-Schönlein purpura nephritis? Kidney Int 2001;59:823–834.
8. Suzuki K, Honda K, Tanabe K, et al: Incidence of latent mesangial IgA deposition in renal allograft donors in Japan. Kidney Int 2003;63: 2286–2294.
9. Gharavi AG, Yan Y, Scolari F, et al: IgA nephropathy, the most common glomerulonephritis, is linked to 6q22-23. Nat Genet 2000;26:354–357.
10. Hsu SI, Ramirez B, Winn MP, et al: Evidence for genetic factors in the development and progression of IgA nephropathy. Kidney Int 2000;57: 1818–1835.
11. Rivera F, Lopez-Gomez JM, Perez-Brea MF, et al: Clinicopathologic correlations of renal pathology in Spain. Kidney Int 2004;66:898–904.
12. Cohen AH: Human immunodeficiency virus and IgA nephropathy. Nephrology 1997;3:51–54.
13. Pillebout E, Thervet E, Hill G, et al: Henoch-Schönlein purpura in adults: Outcome and prognostic factors. J Am Soc Nephrol 2002;13: 1271–1278.
14. Haas M: Histologic classification of IgA nephropathy: A clinicopathologic study of 244 cases. Am J Kidney Dis 1997;29:829–842.
15. Lee SM, Rao VM, Franklin WA, et al: IgA nephropathy: Morphological predictors of progressive renal disease. Hum Pathol 1982;13:314–322.
16. Feehally J: Predicting prognosis in IgA nephropathy. Am J Kidney Dis 2001;38:881–883.
17. Clive DM, Galvanek EG, Silva FG: Mesangial immunoglobulin-A deposits in minimal change nephrotic syndrome: A report of an older patient and a review of the literature. Am J Nephrol 1990;10:31–36.
18. D'Amico G: Natural history of IgA nephropathy and factors predictive of disease outcome. Semin Nephrol 2004;24:179–196.
19. Bartosik L, Lajoie G, Sugar L, Cattran DC: Predicting progression in IgA nephropathy. Am J Kidney Dis 2001;38:728–735.
20. Szeto CC, Lai FM, To KF, et al: Natural history of immunoglobulin A nephropathy presenting with hematuria and minimal proteinuria. Am J Med 2001;110:434–437.
21. Floege J: Recurrent IgA nephropathy after renal transplantation. Semin Nephrol 2004;24:287–291.
22. Feehally J: IgA nephropathy and Henoch-Schönlein purpura. In Brady HR, Wilcox CS, eds. Therapy in Nephrology and Hypertension, 2nd ed. Philadelphia: WB Saunders, 2003, pp 165–177.
23. Floege J, Eitner F: Present and future treatment options in IgA-nephropathy. J Nephrol 2005;18:354–361.
24. Hotta OF, Miyazaka M, Furuta T, et al: Tonsillectomy and steroid pulse therapy significantly impact on clinical remission in patients with IgA nephropathy. Am J Kidney Dis 2001;38:36–43.
25. Rasche FM, Schwarz A, Keller F: Tonsillectomy does not prevent a progressive course in IgA nephropathy. Clin Nephrol 1999;51:147–152.
26. Roccatello D, Ferro G, Cesano D, et al: Steroid and cyclophosphamide in IgA nephropathy. Nephrol Dial Transplant 2000;15:833–835.
27. Haas M, Jafri J, Bartosh SM, et al: ANCA-associated crescentic glomerulonephritis with mesangial IgA deposits. Am J Kidney Dis 2000;36: 709–718.
28. Lai KN, Lai FM, Ho CP, et al: Corticosteroid therapy in IgA nephropathy with nephrotic syndrome: A long-term controlled trial. Clin Nephrol 1986;26:174–180.
29. Pozzi C, Andrulli S, Del Vecchio L, et al: Corticosteroid effectiveness in IgA nephropathy: Long-term results of a randomized, controlled trial. J Am Soc Nephrol 2004;15:157–163.
30. Katafuchi R, Ikeda K, Mizumasa T, et al: Controlled, prospective trial of steroid treatment in IgA nephropathy: A limitation of low-dose prednisolone therapy. Am J Kidney Dis 2003;41:972–983.

31. Yoshikawa N, Ito H, Sakai T, et al: A controlled trial of combined therapy for newly diagnosed severe childhood IgA nephropathy. J Am Soc Nephrol 1999;10:101–109.

32. Ballardie FW, Roberts IDS: Controlled prospective trial of prednisolone and cytotoxics in progressive IgA nephropathy. J Am Soc Nephrol 2002; 13:142–148.

33. Floege J: Mycophenolate mofetil alleviates persistent proteinuria in IgA nephropathy. Nature Clin Pract Nephrol 2006;2:16–17.

34. Rostoker G, Desvaux-Belghiti D, Pilatte Y, et al: High-dose immunoglobulin therapy for severe IgA nephropathy and Henoch-Schönlein purpura. Ann Intern Med 1994;120:476–484.

35. Stefanski A, Schmidt KG, Waldherr R, Ritz E: Early increase in blood pressure and diastolic left ventricular malfunction in patients with glomerulonephritis. Kidney Int 1995;54:926–931.

36. Praga M, Gutierrez E, Gonzalez E, et al: Treatment of IgA nephropathy with ACE inhibitors: A randomized and controlled trial. J Am Soc Nephrol 2003;14:1578–1583.

37. Nakao N, Yoshimura A, Morita H, et al: Combination treatment of angiotensin-II receptor blocker and angiotensin-converting enzyme inhibitor in non-diabetic renal disease [COOPERATE]: A randomised controlled trial. Lancet 2003;361:117–134.

38. Kanno Y, Okada H, Saruta T, Suzuki H: Blood pressure reduction associated with preservation of renal function in hypertensive patients with IgA nephropathy: A 3-year follow-up. Clin Nephrol 2000;54: 360–365.

39. Donadio JV, Grande JP, Bergstralh EJ, et al: The long-term outcome of patients with IgA nephropathy treated with fish oil in a controlled trial. J Am Soc Nephrol 1999;10:1772–1777.

40. Donadio JV, Larson TS, Bergstralh EJ, Grande JP: A randomised trial of high-dose compared with low-dose omega-3 fatty acids in severe IgA nephropathy. J Am Soc Nephrol 2001;12:791–799.

41. Dillon JJ: Fish oil therapy for IgA nephropathy: Efficacy and interstudy variability. J Am Soc Nephrol 1997;8:1739–1744.

42. Mollica F, LiVolti S, Garozzo R, et al: Effectiveness of early prednisone treatment in preventing the development of nephropathy in anaphylactoid purpura. Eur J Pediatr 1992;151:140–144.

43. Oner A, Tinaztepe K, Erdogan O: The effect of triple therapy on rapidly progressive type of Henoch-Schönlein nephritis. Pediatr Nephrol 1995; 9:6–10.

44. Foster BJ, Bernard C, Drummond KN, Sharma AK: Effective therapy for Henoch-Schönlein purpura nephritis with prednisone and azathioprine: A clinical and histopathologic study. J Pediatr 2000;136:370–375.

45. Hasegawa A: Fate of renal grafts with recurrent Henoch-Schönlein purpura nephritis in children. Transplant Proc 1989;21:2130–2133.

46. Meulders Q, Pirson Y, Cosyns J-P, et al: Course of Henoch-Schönlein nephritis after renal transplantation. Transplantation 1994;48: 1179–1186.

Antiglomerular Basement Membrane Disease and Goodpasture's Disease

Richard G. Phelps and A. Neil Turner

INTRODUCTION

The syndrome of renal failure and lung hemorrhage was associated with the name of Ernest Goodpasture by Stanton and Tange in their description of nine cases in 1958.[1,2] All nine patients presented with pulmonary hemorrhage and acute renal failure and died within hours or days, largely as a result of massive pulmonary hemorrhage. These features had been prominent in the case of a young man who died during the influenza pandemic of 1919, whose postmortem findings were memorably reported by Goodpasture[1]: "The lungs gave the impression of having been injected with blood through the bronchi so that all the air spaces were filled" (Fig. 22.1).

It is almost certain that the patients described by Goodpasture[1] and Stanton and Tange[2] had different diseases but with similar dominant clinical features. Several diseases are now recognized as being associated with alveolar hemorrhage and rapidly progressive glomerulonephritis (RPGN). Nevertheless, this remains a striking clinical entity with relatively few causes and few pathogenetic mechanisms.

Because the first recognized mechanism was antiglomerular basement membrane (anti-GBM) antibody formation and deposition, Goodpasture's name is firmly associated with anti-GBM disease (Goodpasture's disease), even though this is responsible for only a proportion of patients with Goodpasture's syndrome of lung hemorrhage and RPGN. The terminology used in this chapter is defined in Figure 22.2.

ETIOLOGY AND PATHOGENESIS

Autoimmunity to a Component of the Glomerular Basement Membrane

Goodpasture's disease is caused by autoimmunity to a specific component of the GBM that has been identified as the carboxyl terminal, noncollagenous (NC1) domain of a type IV collagen chain, α_3(IV)NC1, also known as the Goodpasture antigen.[3,4] Type IV collagen is an essential constituent of all basement membranes. In most tissues, it is composed of trimers comprising two α_1 and one α_2 chains, but there are also four tissue-specific chains, α_3 through α_6.[5,6] Three of these, α_3 through α_5, are found in GBM as well as in the basement membranes of the alveolus, the cochlea, parts of the eye (including corneal basement membrane and Bruch's membrane), the choroid plexus of the brain, and some endocrine organs.

All patients with RPGN, lung hemorrhage, and anti-GBM antibodies have antibodies to α_3(IV)NC1, usually binding

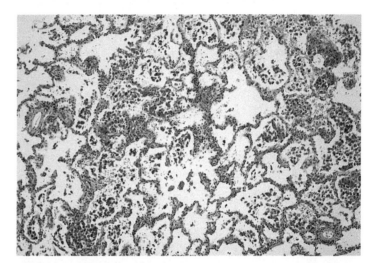

Figure 22.1 Alveolar hemorrhage in a patient with Goodpasture's disease. Open lung biopsy. (Courtesy of Dr. E. Mary Thompson.)

predominantly to a single or a very restricted set of epitopes. Some patients also have antibodies to other basement membrane constituents, including other collagen IV chains, usually in low titer.

Predisposing Factors

As is mostly the case in autoimmune disease, both environmental and genetic factors appear to be important in etiology. Genetic influences are apparent from reports of the disease occurrence in siblings and twins and from the strong association between Goodpasture's disease and HLA class II alleles. One of the alleles contributing to the DR2 specificity, HLA-DRB1*1501, is carried by 64% to 91% of patients but only 20% to 31% of controls. There is a less pronounced but significant association with HLA-DR4 alleles, and 90% to 97% of patients carry DRB1*1501 or DR4. DR1 and DR7 confer strong and dominant protection.[7]

Precipitating Factors

Reports of the temporal and geographic clustering of cases suggest an environmental trigger.[8] No specific infectious agent has been consistently identified. Hydrocarbon exposure has been linked to disease onset in several striking case reports, but in some cases such exposure may simply trigger pulmonary hemorrhage in patients who already have the disease. Furthermore, exposures of this kind are very common in the modern world. Similarly,

Definition of terms

Term	Definition	Pathogenesis
Pulmonary renal syndrome	Renal and respiratory failure	Many causes (see Fig. 22.9)
Goodpasture's syndrome	RPGN and alveolar hemorrhage	Several causes (see Fig. 22.10)
Anti-GBM disease	Disease associated with antibodies specific for (any) components of the GBM	Most important are Goodpasture's and Alport's syndrome post-transplant anti-GBM disease
Goodpasture's disease	Disease associated with autoantibodies specific for $\alpha_3(IV)NCl$ May include RPGN, lung hemorrhage, or both	Autoimmunity to $\alpha_3(IV)NCl$
Alport's syndrome post-transplant anti-GBM disease	Glomerulonephritis associated with anti-GBM antibodies developing after renal transplantation in patients with Alport's syndrome	Immunity to foreign collagen IV chains not expressed in Alport's syndrome patients (usually α_3 or $\alpha_5(IV)NCl$)

Figure 22.2 Definition of terms. GBM, glomerular basement membrane; RPGN, rapidly progressive glomerulonephritis.

cigarette smoking may precipitate pulmonary hemorrhage in patients who already have circulating autoantibodies, but whether it plays a role in causation is less clear.

Intriguingly, there are several instances where renal trauma or inflammation (Fig. 22.3) has preceded the development of the disease. These may alter $\alpha_3(IV)NC1$ turnover and metabolism qualitatively or quantitatively, providing an opportunity for self-tolerance to be broken. A possible qualitative change is the accessibility of relevant epitopes within the basement membrane, which is increased, for example, by exposure to reactive oxygen species likely to be abundant in inflamed glomeruli. The quantity of $\alpha_3(IV)NC1$ presented to T cells may be greater where there has been damage to the basement membrane, as occurs in systemic small-vessel vasculitis (see Chapter 23); some features suggest that the anti-GBM response may be a secondary phenomenon in most of these patients.[9,10] The association with membranous nephropathy is interesting as the thickened GBM in that disease contains increased amounts of the tissue-specific type IV collagen chains, including the α_3 chain, which bears the Goodpasture antigen. The same could apply to a recently suggested possible association with long-standing type 1 diabetes mellitus (reviewed by Turner and Rees[11]).

Mechanisms of Renal Injury

Several lines of evidence support a direct role for anti-$\alpha_3(IV)NC1$ autoantibodies (Fig. 22.4) in the pathogenesis of Goodpasture's disease.[12] Antibodies eluted from the kidneys of patients who had died of Goodpasture's disease rapidly bind to the GBM and cause glomerulonephritis (GN) when injected into monkeys.[13] Furthermore, the deposited antibodies are predominantly IgG1 and are complement fixing. Experimental models have shown that contributions to renal injury mediated by such antibodies come from complement and from neutrophil and macrophage infiltration. However, T cells are essential for driving autoantibody production by T cell–dependent B cells, and in experimental renal disease, they are critical in producing glomerular crescents,[14] which are a usual feature of Goodpasture's disease.

Agents that downregulate inflammation by inhibiting interleukin (IL)-1 or tumor necrosis factor α (TNF-α) or inhibit recruitment of inflammatory cells by blockade of adhesion molecules or chemoattractants suppress injury in experimental models of anti-GBM disease. There is supportive evidence in humans and in experimental animals that the severity of renal injury may be increased by proinflammatory cytokines or by stimuli likely to elicit them, such as bacteremia.[14]

Conditions and events associated with the presentation of Goodpasture's disease

Possibly Induce Autoimmune Response and Disease
Systemic small-vessel vasculitis affecting glomeruli
Membranous nephropathy
Lithotripsy of renal stones
Urinary obstruction
Precipitate Pulmonary Hemorrhage
Cigarette smoke
Hydrocarbon exposure
Pulmonary infection
Fluid overload

Figure 22.3 Conditions and events associated with the presentation of Goodpasture's disease.

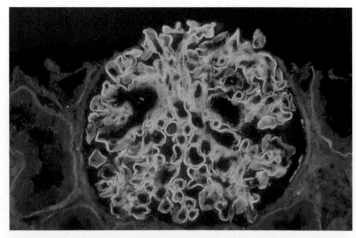

Figure 22.4 Autoantibodies to the Goodpasture antigen bound to a normal glomerulus. Shown by direct immunofluorescence in a patient with lung hemorrhage and hematuria. (Courtesy of Dr. Richard Herriot.)

Crescent formation is seen in aggressive inflammatory GN. The mechanism by which it is believed to occur is described in Chapter 15 (see Fig. 15.10).

Pulmonary Hemorrhage

Lung hemorrhage in Goodpasture's disease (but not in small-vessel vasculitis, the other major cause of Goodpasture's disease) only occurs if there is an additional insult to the lung, which is usually cigarette smoke. However, infection, fluid overload, toxicity from inhaled vapors or other irritants, and the effects of systemic administration of some cytokines are also possibilities. This is probably because the alveolar capillary endothelial cell provides more of a barrier between circulating immunoglobulin and the underlying basement membrane than the diaphragm-free fenestrations of the glomerular capillary endothelial cell.

In the glomerulus, antibodies have direct access to the GBM because of the fenestrations of glomerular endothelium. Other sites at which the Goodpasture antigen is found are not involved in Goodpasture's disease, except possibly the choroid plexus, where the endothelium is again fenestrated and, more rarely, the eye.

EPIDEMIOLOGY

Goodpasture's disease is rare, with an estimated incidence in Caucasian populations of between 0.5 and 0.9 cases per million per annum.[11] The incidence in Black and South Asian populations appears to be lower. The incidence in other racial groups is uncertain because of sparse reports, but is probably also very low. There is a slight male predominance. Most are young men in their second and third decades, with a smaller peak incidence in the sixth and seventh decades, but cases in both sexes and at all ages are reported.

Lung hemorrhage is more common in younger male patients, but it is unclear whether this reflects age-related susceptibility or demographic differences in smoking.

CLINICAL MANIFESTATIONS

The principal clinical manifestations of Goodpasture's disease arise from lung hemorrhage and/or RPGN.[11] Between 50% and 75% of patients present with acute symptoms of lung hemorrhage and are found to be in a state of advanced renal failure. Usually symptoms are confined to the preceding few weeks or months, but very rapid progression (over days) or much slower progression (over many months) may occur. A lack of systemic symptoms, other than those related to anemia, is typical, although it is common for an apparently minor infection to trigger the clinical presentation.

Pulmonary Hemorrhage

Lung hemorrhage may occur with renal disease or in isolation. Presenting symptoms may include cough, hemoptysis, exertional dyspnea, and fatigue. Hemorrhage into alveolar spaces occurs and may result in marked iron-deficiency anemia and exertional dyspnea, even in the absence of hemoptysis. Depending on the degree and chronicity of lung hemorrhage, examination findings may include pallor, scattered dry inspiratory crackles, signs of consolidation, or respiratory distress. Recent pulmonary hemorrhage is usually apparent on a chest radiograph (Fig. 22.5), typically appearing as central shadowing that may traverse fissures and give rise to the appearance of an air bronchogram. However, even pulmonary hemorrhage sufficient to reduce the hemoglobin concentration may cause only minor or transient radiographic changes, and these cannot be confidently distinguished from other causes of alveolar shadowing (notably edema, infection) by radiologic appearances alone. The most sensitive indicator of recent pulmonary hemorrhage is an increased uptake of inhaled carbon monoxide (D_LCO). Patients with lung hemorrhage are usually current cigarette smokers.

In isolated lung disease, progressive alveolar or fibrotic disease or pulmonary hemosiderosis may be suspected, although at least hematuria is usually present. This may continue for months or in rare cases recurrently for years before significant renal disease occurs.

Glomerulonephritis

Patients with GN may notice dark or red urine, but sometimes progression to oliguria is so rapid that this phase, if it occurs, is missed. In one third to one half of patients, GN occurs in the absence of lung hemorrhage. In this subgroup, because systemic symptoms are generally not prominent, progression is silent

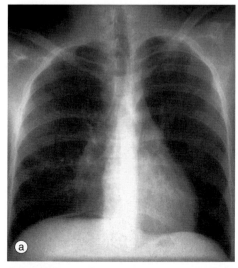 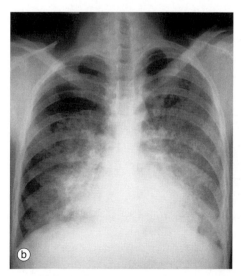

Figure 22.5 Pulmonary hemorrhage. *a,* Chest radiograph of a patient with lung hemorrhage. *b,* Radiograph taken 4 days later shows the evolution of alveolar shadowing caused by lung hemorrhage.

unless disease is signaled by hematuria, and presentation is often late with renal failure.

Whatever the early pattern of disease, once significant renal impairment has occurred further deterioration in renal function is usually rapid. Presentation at the time of, or very shortly after, acceleration of the disease process, is common, and patients may demonstrate very rapid loss of renal function and life-threatening lung hemorrhage. Urinalysis always reveals hematuria (even in almost all patients with apparently isolated pulmonary disease), usually modest proteinuria, and on microscopy, dysmorphic red cells and red-cell casts. The kidneys are generally of normal size, but may be enlarged. Hematuria may be substantial or associated with loin pain in acute disease. In a small minority of patients with a subacute presentation, proteinuria is in the nephrotic range, and the rate of progression of the disease is slow.

PATHOLOGY

Renal biopsy is essential as it provides diagnostic and prognostic information. Typical appearances are of diffuse proliferative GN with variable degrees of necrosis, crescent formation, glomerulosclerosis, and tubular loss (Fig. 22.6). The degree of crescent formation and tubular loss correlates with renal prognosis. Characteristically, the crescents all appear to be of similar age and cellularity. When biopsied earlier in the disease, changes may be limited to focal and segmental mesangial expansion, with or without necrosis. This progresses to hypercellularity and then to more general changes including fractures of the GBM and Bowman's capsule, neutrophils in the glomeruli, and glomerular capillary thrombosis.[15]

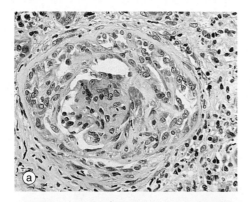

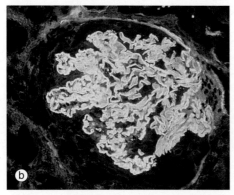

Figure 22.6 Renal biopsy in Goodpasture's disease. *a*, Glomerulus from a patient with Goodpasture's disease showing a recent, mostly cellular crescent. *b*, Direct immunofluorescence study showing ribbon-like linear deposition of IgG along the glomerular basement membrane. The glomerular tuft is slightly compressed by cellular proliferation, forming a crescent (*arrows*). (Courtesy of Dr. Richard Herriot.)

Conditions associated with linear binding of immunoglobulin to the GBM
Specific Binding to the GBM
Goodpasture's syndrome
Alport's syndrome after renal transplantation
Nonspecific Binding to the GBM
Diabetes
Cadaver kidneys
Light-chain disease
Fibrillary glomerulopathy
Systemic lupus erythematosus (possibly specific but not considered directly pathogenic)

Figure 22.7   Conditions associated with linear binding of immunoglobulin to the glomerular basement membrane (GBM).

Immunohistology

In the presence of severe glomerular inflammation, linear deposition of immunoglobulin along the GBM is pathognomonic. The immunoglobulin is usually IgG, sometimes (10% to 15%) with IgA or IgM, but very rarely IgA alone is detected. Linear deposition of C3 is detectable in about 75% of biopsies. Linear immunofluorescence with anti-immunoglobulin reagents is occasionally seen in other conditions (Fig. 22.7), usually without glomerular inflammation. In most instances, the deposited immunoglobulin is less abundant than in Goodpasture's disease and is either nonspecifically deposited or bound to GBM components other than type IV collagen chains.

Circulating IgG anti-GBM antibodies are almost invariably present, even in the rare instances where only IgM or IgA has been reported to be bound to the GBM. They may be detected and quantified using immobilized Goodpasture antigen in an immunoassay. The titer of anti-GBM antibody at presentation correlates with the severity of nephritis. Treatment and relapse are often mirrored by changes in titer.

Pathology in Other Tissues

Pathologic changes in lung tissue can be difficult to interpret because the changes in Goodpasture's disease, including immunoglobulin deposition, are often patchy and may be missed. Frequently, the only findings are mild, chronic inflammation and hemosiderin-laden macrophages, which are consistent with other more common pathologic diagnoses. This makes negative bronchoscopic or open lung biopsies unhelpful in excluding the diagnosis.

Other tissues in which $\alpha_3(IV)NC1$ is expressed are rarely available for pathologic analysis, but if antibody is deposited in other sites, then pathology is rarely associated with it. A number of case reports describe neurologic syndromes, particularly convulsions, which might be related to antibody deposition in the choroid plexus (Fig. 22.8) but may have other explanations in patients with acute renal failure. Other reports have described retinal detachment, in one instance with antibody deposition, but again this is rare.

DIFFERENTIAL DIAGNOSIS

Diagnosis of Goodpasture's disease in patients who present with Goodpasture's syndrome does not usually present difficulties once

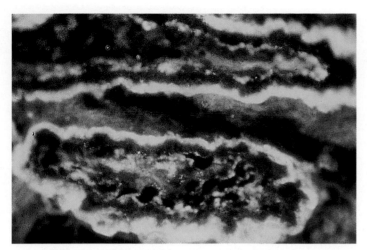

Figure 22.8   Direct immunofluorescence study showing binding of IgG to the choroid plexus of a patient who died of Goodpasture's disease. (Courtesy of Dr. Stephen Cashman.)

the possibility has been raised, although the urgency is often not appreciated. Direct immunofluorescence on renal tissue and assay for circulating anti-GBM antibodies are the most rapid techniques, and renal biopsy is always indicated as outlined in the Pathology section. Diagnosis is often delayed when patients present with subacute disease affecting the lung or the kidney in isolation. Patients with subacute lung hemorrhage may never report hemoptysis and may present as cases of diffuse lung disease, of which there are many causes.

Detection of Antiglomerular Basement Membrane Antibodies

Detection of tissue-deposited, anti-GBM antibodies is usually achieved by direct immunohistology using antibodies that are specific for different classes of immunoglobulin. The technique is very sensitive for detecting anti-GBM antibody production, as the GBM selectively adsorbs and concentrates low levels of circulating antibody from the circulation. However, in some circumstances, GBM may also adsorb antibody nonspecifically (see Fig. 22.7). Detection of anti-GBM antibodies in serum requires solid-phase enzyme-linked immunosorbent assays (ELISAs) or radioimmunoassays based on preparations of human or animal GBM or recombinant antigen. The quality of these assays is variable. Confirmation of the specificity of anti-GBM antibodies may be obtained by Western blotting of serum onto solubilized human GBM or recombinant α_3(IV)NC1, usually at a reference laboratory. Indirect immunohistology is too insensitive for reliable diagnostic use.

False-positive results may be encountered in various assays, particularly in sera from patients with inflammatory diseases that often exhibit increased nonspecific binding. This places greater emphasis on the purity of antigen used for anti-GBM assays. False-negative results are usually encountered in patients with low titers of antibodies in association with isolated lung disease or with very early or subacute renal disease. However, low titers may occasionally be associated with anti-GBM disease that occurs after renal transplantation in patients with Alport's syndrome (see later discussion).

In very advanced disease, linear antibody deposition may not be seen because of extensive destruction of GBM structure. Otherwise, deposited immunoglobulin remains detectable by direct immunohistology for some months after circulating immunoglobulin ceases to be detectable by ELISA.

Patients with Antiglomerular Basement Membrane Antibodies and Other Diseases
Antineutrophil Cytoplasmic Antibody and Systemic Small-Vessel Vasculitis

Anti-GBM antibodies are sometimes detected in patients with sera that contains antineutrophil cytoplasmic antibody (ANCA), especially in those ANCA with specificity for myeloperoxidase (see Chapter 23). Such double-positive patients may have a clinical course and response to treatment more typical of vasculitis than of Goodpasture's disease and have possibly developed anti-GBM antibodies secondary to vasculitic glomerular damage.[8–10] Some patients have symptoms and signs in other organs suggesting systemic vasculitis. Anti-GBM titers tend to be lower in ANCA-positive anti-GBM antibody–positive patients than in patients with anti-GBM antibodies alone. Recovery of renal function may be more likely if ANCAs are present, even if patients are dialysis dependent when treatment is started, although some recent observations have failed to detect the differences described in early reports.

Membranous Nephropathy

Anti-GBM antibodies are occasionally identified in patients with membranous nephropathy, usually coincident with an accelerated decline in renal function and the formation of glomerular crescents.[5,16,17] In approximately two thirds of the two dozen or so published reports, there was evidence of evolution from pre-existing nephrotic syndrome and in about half, a previous kidney biopsy specimen showed typical membranous nephropathy. Progression to end-stage renal disease (ESRD) has usually been rapid, but the diagnosis has rarely been made at an early enough stage to expect intensive treatment to be successful. Three patients with Goodpasture's disease later developed typical membranous nephropathy.

Differential Diagnosis of Goodpasture's Syndrome

A wide variety of conditions may cause simultaneous pulmonary and renal disease. The term pulmonary-renal syndrome implies failure of both organs, the most common cause being fluid overload in a patient with renal failure of any cause. This may resemble Goodpasture's syndrome, particularly if there is hematuria and pre-existing cardiac dysfunction. However, a number of diseases may mimic Goodpasture's syndrome (pulmonary hemorrhage with RPGN) to varying degrees by causing acute renal failure with acute lung disease (Fig. 22.9). Diseases associated with the syndrome fall into two pathogenetic classes: those characterized by systemic vasculitis and those associated with anti-GBM antibodies (Goodpasture's disease; Fig. 22.10).

These diseases can sometimes be confidently differentiated clinically, but usually serology and renal biopsy are required. Renal biopsy also provides valuable prognostic information.

NATURAL HISTORY

There is some variability in the pattern of early disease. Most patients present acutely with lung hemorrhage and/or advanced renal failure and report that the illness developed over only weeks or a few months. However, there are several reports of patients presenting with mild respiratory symptoms or incidental microscopic hematuria and with disease progressing much more slowly over months or years. It is unclear to what extent these reports indicate differences in clinical course or earlier detection, as patients with slowly progressive or static disease may abruptly develop the full acute syndrome.

Nonimmune causes of pulmonary renal syndrome

With Pulmonary Edema
Acute renal failure with hypervolemia
Severe cardiac failure
Infective
Severe bacterial pneumonia (e.g., *Legionella*) with renal failure
Hantavirus infection
Opportunistic infections in the immunocompromised
Other
Acute respiratory distress syndrome with renal failure in multiorgan failure
Paraquat poisoning
Renal vein/inferior vena cava thrombosis with pulmonary emboli

Figure 22.9   Nonimmune causes of pulmonary renal syndrome.

Causes of Goodpasture's syndrome (lung hemorrhage and rapidly progressive glomerulonephritis)

Diseases Associated with Antibodies to the GBM (20%–40% of cases)
Goodpasture's disease (spontaneous anti-GBM disease)
Diseases associated with Systemic Vasculitis (60%–80% of cases)
Wegener's granulomatosis (common)
Microscopic polyangiitis
Systemic lupus erythematosus
Churg-Strauss syndrome
Henoch-Schönlein purpura
Behçet's syndrome
Essential mixed cryoglobulinemia
Rheumatoid vasculitis
Drugs: penicillamine, hydralazine, propylthiouracil

Figure 22.10   Causes of Goodpasture's syndrome (lung hemorrhage and rapidly progressive glomerulonephritis). GBM, glomerular basement membrane.

Once RPGN has developed, renal function is rapidly and often irretrievably destroyed. Progression is often much more rapid than in RPGN occurring in other contexts such as microscopic polyangiitis, perhaps because more glomeruli are simultaneously affected. Consequently, there is a much narrower window of opportunity for effective treatment.

Although a severe exacerbation of lung disease commonly coincides with deterioration of renal function, the natural history of isolated lung disease critically depends on continued exposure to irritants.

TREATMENT

Immunosuppressive Regimens
Before the introduction of immunosuppressive treatment, most patients died shortly after the development of renal impairment or pulmonary hemorrhage.[17] Nowadays pulmonary hemorrhage can usually be arrested within 24 to 48 hours. Renal function can

be protected if impairment is mild, and in some circumstances even severe renal impairment can be reversed. However, dialysis-dependent patients rarely recover kidney function despite immunosuppression and should probably only be immunosuppressed if pulmonary hemorrhage occurs.

A chart recording treatment of a patient with Goodpasture's disease is shown in Figure 22.11. Recommended treatment for acute severe disease is shown in Figure 22.12. The regimen was devised to reduce levels of circulating pathogenic antibodies as rapidly as possible and to curtail their contribution to the rapid glomerular destruction that can occur during acute severe disease and is very effective. Once the disease is controlled, immunosuppression can usually be tapered off over 3 months and subsequent relapse is uncommon. The immune response is also self-limiting if renal function is supported, with antibodies disappearing over 1 to 2 years.

In RPGN where there is no evidence of an infective cause, immunosuppressive therapy should be started immediately, sometimes before the renal biopsy findings are available. If therapy is stopped after a few days, the patient will have incurred very little risk (as long as pulsed high-dose corticosteroids are avoided), but sometimes has a great deal to gain from earlier treatment.

Plasma Exchange and Immunosuppression
Only one element, plasma exchange, has been tested in a randomized, controlled trial, but the regimen dramatically improved the outlook for patients when it was introduced in the 1970s. The trial[18] suggested some additional benefit of plasma exchange, but the interpretation was complicated by the fact that the recipient group had less severe disease at presentation. It showed that milder disease can be effectively treated with corticosteroids and cyclophosphamide alone, although the overall outcomes for all

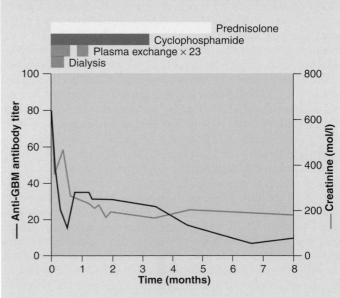

Response to immunosuppressive treatment in a patient with Goodpasture's disease

Prednisolone
Cyclophosphamide
Plasma exchange × 23
Dialysis

Figure 22.11   Response to immunosuppressive treatment in a patient with Goodpasture's disease. The patient required dialysis for renal disease but had no lung hemorrhage. The good response to treatment was unusual but not unique. The renal biopsy showed 85% of glomeruli contained recent (mostly cellular) crescents, suggesting very acute disease, which may be indicative of a more favorable response to treatment. GBM, glomerular basement membrane.

Treatment regimen for acute Goodpasture's disease	
Prednisolone	I mg/kg/24 h orally. Reduce at weekly intervals to achieve one sixth of this dose by 8 weeks. For a starting daily dose of 60 mg, use weekly reductions to 45, 30, 25, 20, and 15 mg; then 2 weekly to 12.5 and 10 mg. Maintain this dose to 3 months; then taper to stop by 4 months.
Cyclophosphamide	3 mg/kg/24 h orally, rounded down to the nearest 50 mg. Patients >55 years receive a reduced dose of 2.5 mg/kg.
Plasma exchange	Daily exchange of 1 volume of plasma for 5% human albumin for 14 days or until the circulating antibody is suppressed. In the presence of pulmonary hemorrhage or within 48 hours of an invasive procedure, 300 to 400 mL of fresh-frozen plasma is given at the end of each treatment or according to coagulation tests.
Monitoring	Daily blood count during plasma exchange and while antibody titer remains elevated. At least twice weekly during first month, weekly thereafter. If white blood cell count decreases to $<3.5 \times 10^9/l$, stop cyclophosphamide until the count recovers. Resume at lower dose if cessation has been necessary. Baseline DLCO, with further measurements as indicated. Daily coagulation tests during plasma exchange to monitor for significant depletion of clotting factors. Initially, daily checks of renal and hepatic function, glucose.
Prophylaxis against complications of treatment	Oral antifungal lozenges or rinse; proton pump inhibitor. Cotrimoxazole prophylaxis against *Pneumocystis carinii*. Avoid nonessential lines, catheters.

Figure 22.12   Treatment regimen for acute Goodpasture's disease.

patients were not as good as have been described with more intensive regimens.[18]

Historical evidence suggests that treatment with corticosteroids alone, or corticosteroids with azathioprine, is less effective. Plasma exchange is only of value if accompanied by adjunctive immunosuppressive therapy. Immunoadsorption to protein A also lowers anti-GBM antibodies rapidly; it does not deplete complement components or clotting factors, and a few reports suggest that it is as effective as plasma exchange, albeit more expensive.

Lung hemorrhage occurring alone tends to be relapsing and remitting, so there have been many reports of treatments (including bilateral nephrectomy) that may help. Use of pulse methylprednisolone is particularly popular. High doses of corticosteroids fail to alter the underlying pathogenetic immune response and put the patient at increased risk of infective and other complications. Therefore, administration of these drugs alone is not recommended. Seriously ill patients should be treated with moderate doses of corticosteroids plus plasma exchange and cyclophosphamide.

Anecdotal experience in other acute severe diseases suggests that daily administration of cyclophosphamide may be more rapidly and consistently effective than pulse administration, and this remains our usual practice. Patients unable to take the drug orally can be given daily intravenous therapy at the usual oral dose. Dose does not need to be reduced in severe renal failure, but reductions for older patients are important (see Fig. 22.12), and close monitoring of leukocyte counts is imperative in all patients.

Results from all series show that recovery of renal function is unlikely if at the time it is commenced, the patient is oliguric, has a very high proportion of glomeruli with circumferential crescents, or has a serum creatinine level of >5.5 to 6.5 mg/dl (about 500 to 600 μmol/l).[19] This is a notably different experience from that encountered in systemic vasculitis or idiopathic RPGN (see Chapter 23), in which renal disease of apparently similar severity (judged by histology and creatinine level) can be salvaged by similar treatment protocols.[20] It has led to the suggestion that immunosuppressive treatment should be withheld from patients in whom the chance of recovery is slight to protect them from the risks of the treatment itself. This is considered further in the following.

Supportive Treatment
The most likely cause of death in the first few days is respiratory failure caused by lung hemorrhage. Lung hemorrhage may be precipitated or exacerbated by the following factors.

- Fluid overload
- Smoking and other pulmonary irritants possibly including high fractional inspired oxygen concentrations
- Local or distant infection
- Anticoagulation used during dialysis or plasma exchange
- The thrombocytopenia, defibrination, and depletion of clotting factors that may occur as a consequence of plasma exchange

It is therefore sensible to ensure correct fluid balance, prohibit smoking, use the lowest fractional inspired oxygen concentration that gives adequate oxygenation, and minimize the use of heparin.

Plasma exchange should be monitored by daily blood counts and coagulation tests, and if pulmonary hemorrhage occurs, diminished clotting factor levels should be replenished by administering fresh frozen plasma or clotting factor preparations at the end of each plasma exchange session.

After the first few days, the major cause of morbidity and mortality is infection. Infection carries the added risk of potentiating glomerular and lung inflammation and injury so precautions to reduce the risk of infection, such as minimizing the number of indwelling cannulae, are particularly important. The neutrophil count should be monitored and if leukopenia <3.5 $\times 10^9/l$ or neutropenia develops, cyclophosphamide should be discontinued and resumed at a lower dose when the neutrophil count recovers, if necessary with the assistance of granulocyte colony–stimulating factor.

Monitoring Effect of Treatment on Disease Activity
The effect of treatment on the renal disease may be monitored by following serum creatinine levels. Indicators of recent pulmonary hemorrhage include hemoptysis, decreases in hemoglobin concentration, chest radiograph changes, and increases in the D_LCO, the latter being the most sensitive. Any worsening of symptoms during treatment may indicate inadequate immunosuppression, but frequently it is a consequence of intercurrent infection exaggerating immunologic injury, or fluid overload or other factors precipitating pulmonary hemorrhage.

Monitoring anti-GBM titers during and particularly 24 hours after the last planned plasma exchange treatment is useful for confirming effective suppression of autoantibodies. They should be undetectable within 8 weeks, but without treatment remain detectable for an average of 14 months.

Duration of Treatment and Relapses

Steroid treatment may be gradually reduced and cyclophosphamide discontinued at 3 months. In contrast with the treatment of small-vessel vasculitis, it is not usually necessary to continue immunosuppression for longer than this. Longer treatment is appropriate for patients who are both anti-GBM antibody positive and ANCA positive (see later discussion). Late increases in anti-GBM level may predict clinical relapse, although antibodies are generally permanently suppressed in patients who have completed the immunosuppressive regimen. If there is recurrence, success has been achieved by treating as at first presentation.

Electing Not to Treat

Advanced renal failure, frequently already established at presentation, is generally not salvaged by any current treatment.[17,19,21] Furthermore, the immunosuppressive regimen outlined carries significant risks, the plasma exchange element is expensive, and careful monitoring is required. For these reasons, it may be reasonable not to commence potentially dangerous immunosuppression in patients who present with advanced renal failure without pulmonary hemorrhage. The decision not to treat is strengthened if the renal biopsy specimen shows widespread glomerulosclerosis and tubular loss and the patient is dialysis dependent at presentation (Fig. 22.13). The risk of developing late pulmonary hemorrhage in these circumstances seems to be very low, but warrants particular care to avoid the major precipitating factors, smoking, and pulmonary edema, in at least the first few months.

However, patients who are dialysis dependent should be treated if the renal biopsy specimen changes are unexpectedly mild or very recent (highly cellular crescents, even if 100% of glomeruli are involved) as several reports describe good outcomes in these circumstances even after prolonged oliguria.

Treatment of Double-Positive Patients

Patients with ANCA and anti-GBM antibodies (double-positive patients) may have other extrarenal disease requiring treatment (see Fig. 22.13). There is conflicting evidence as to whether their renal prognosis is the same as, or better than, that of other patients with anti-GBM antibodies. Earlier series suggested a better prognosis, but this has not been confirmed in two recent reports.[9,10] However, the risk of missing serious disease in other organs makes it difficult to completely withhold treatment in these circumstances, unless the patient is well with minimal evidence of systemic inflammation and/or is at exceptional risk from immunosuppression. Double-positive patients should receive an immunosuppressive regimen similar to that given for small-vessel vasculitis with continuing immunosuppression with azathioprine after 3 months of cyclophosphamide (see Chapter 23).

In contrast to advanced renal failure where treatment is unlikely to lead to recovery of renal function, even severe pulmonary hemorrhage is likely to respond to treatment with full or nearly full recovery of lung function.

TRANSPLANTATION

Renal transplantation in patients who have had Goodpasture's disease carries the additional risk of disease recurrence. Recurrence with consequent loss of the graft has been reported and appears more likely when circulating anti-GBM antibodies are still detectable at the time of transplantation. For this reason, it is reasonable to delay transplantation until circulating anti-GBM antibodies have been undetectable for 6 months and to monitor graft function, urinary sediment, and circulating anti-GBM antibody levels to detect recurrent disease (see Chapter 96). Biopsies of well-functioning grafts sometimes show linear deposition of immunoglobulin on the GBM without clinical or histologic disease or apparently an adverse prognosis.

ALPORT'S SYNDROME POST-TRANSPLANT ANTI– GLOMERULAR BASEMENT MEMBRANE DISEASE

Patients with Alport's syndrome have mutations in a gene encoding one of the tissue-specific type IV collagen chains, usually α_5. Because these chains assemble with each other during biosynthesis, the resulting phenotype in the case of most mutations has all the tissue-specific chains (α_3 through α_5) missing from the basement membranes, where they are normally coexpressed. Altered expression may lead to absent or inadequate immunologic tolerance to these proteins and to the preservation of the capacity to mount a powerful (allo) immune response to the type IV collagen chains expressed in a normal donor kidney after renal

Factors influencing decision to treat or not treat aggressively in Goodpasture's disease		
	Factors Favoring Aggressive Treatment	Factors Against Aggressive Treatment
Pulmonary	Present	Absent hemorrhage
Oliguria	Absent	Present
Creatinine	<5.5 mg/dl (approximately 500 μmol/l)	>5.5–6.5 mg/dl (approximately 500–600 μmol/l) and ANCA negative Severe damage on kidney biopsy No desire for early kidney transplantation
Other factors	Creatinine >500–600 μmol/l *but* Rapid and recent progression ANCA positive Glomerular damage less severe than expected Crescents recent, nonfibrous Early renal transplantation desired	
Associated disease	Absent	Unusually high risk from immunosuppression

Figure 22.13 Factors influencing decision to treat or not treat aggressively in Goodpasture's disease. ANCA, antineutrophilic cytoplasmic antibody.

transplantation. Most Alport's syndrome patients accommodate renal transplants with conventional immunosuppression without developing anti-GBM nephritis. However, the development of low titers of anti-GBM antibodies is shown by the fact that many such patients have linear deposition of IgG on the GBM of the transplanted kidney (by direct immunofluorescence).

A minority of patients (up to about 5%) develop RPGN clinically indistinguishable from Goodpasture's syndrome but without pulmonary hemorrhage. This is more likely if they have a large gene deletion causing the disease rather than a point mutation, with the inference that their immune system has never been exposed to the mature protein. Typically, graft function is lost despite treatment for presumed acute rejection. Disease is usually encountered some months or longer after a first renal transplant, after weeks in a second, and after days in a third.[22] In the past, the diagnosis has only rarely been appreciated before glomeruli have been largely destroyed.

Experience with regrafting patients who have lost kidneys to Alport's post-transplant anti-GBM disease is limited and generally depressing. However, regrafting has been successful in two cases known to us and in two further cases in the literature. If the disease is recognized early, there are sound theoretical reasons for treating with the regimen recommended for Goodpasture's syndrome, but there are few data on its effectiveness. There is good evidence that both T- and B-lymphocyte–mediated mechanisms are important.[22]

In contrast to spontaneous Goodpasture's syndrome, the specificity of anti-GBM antibodies in Alport's post-transplant anti-GBM disease is not always to $\alpha_3(IV)NC1$. In many patients, possibly in most, the autoantibodies are specific for $\alpha_5(IV)NC1$, encoded by the gene usually implicated in causation of the disease.[23] This is important because immunoassays for anti-GBM antibodies have usually been optimized for detection of the anti-$\alpha_3(IV)NC1$ antibodies of spontaneous Goodpasture's syndrome, and they may have very low sensitivity for anti-$\alpha_5(IV)NC1$ antibodies. In the absence of widely available assays for these uncommon antibodies, renal biopsy with immunohistology is the only reliable method of diagnosis.

REFERENCES

1. Goodpasture EW: The significance of certain pulmonary lesions in relation to the etiology of influenza. Am J Med Sci 1919;158:863–870.
2. Stanton MC, Tange JD: Goodpasture's syndrome (pulmonary haemorrhage associated with glomerulonephritis). Aust N Z J Med 1958;7:132–144.
3. Saus J, Wieslander J, Langeveld J, et al: Identification of the Goodpasture antigen as the α3(IV) chain of collagen IV. J Biol Chem 1988;263:13374–13380.
4. Turner N, Mason PJ, Brown R, et al: Molecular cloning of the human Goodpasture antigen demonstrates it to be the α3 chain of type IV collagen. J Clin Invest 1992;89:592–601.
5. Kashtan CE, Michael AF: Alport syndrome. Kidney Int 1996;50:1445–1463.
6. Aumailley M: Structure and supramolecular organization of basement membranes. Kidney Int 1995;49:54–57.
7. Phelps RG, Rees AJ: The HLA complex in Goodpasture's disease: A model for analyzing susceptibility to autoimmunity. Kidney Int 1999;56:1638–1654.
8. Bolton WK: Goodpasture's syndrome. Kidney Int 1996;50:1753–1766.
9. Rutgers A, Slot M, van Paassen P, et al: Coexistence of anti-glomerular basement membrane antibodies and myeloperoxidase-ANCAs in crescentic glomerulonephritis. Am J Kidney Dis 2005;46:253–262.
10. Levy JB, Hammad T, Coulthart A, et al: Clinical features and outcome of patients with both ANCA and anti-GBM antibodies. Kidney Int 2004;66:1535–1540.
11. Turner AN, Rees AJ: Antiglomerular basement membrane disease. In Davison AM, Cameron S, Grunfeld JP, et al, eds. Oxford Textbook of Clinical Nephrology. Oxford: Oxford University Press, 2005, pp 579–600.
12. Phelps RG, Turner AN: Goodpasture's syndrome: New insights into pathogenesis and clinical picture. J Nephrol 1996;9:111–117.
13. Lerner RA, Glassock RJ, Dixon FJ: The role of antiglomerular basement membrane antibody in the pathogenesis of human glomerulonephritis. J Exp Med 1967;126:989–1004.
14. Feehally J, Savill J, Floege J, Turner AN: Glomerular injury and glomerular response. In Davison AM, Cameron S, Grunfeld JP, eds. Oxford Textbook of Clinical Nephrology. Oxford: Oxford University Press, 2005, pp 363–388.
15. Heptinstall RH: Schönlein-Henoch syndrome: Lung hemorrhage and glomerulonephritis. In Heptinstall RH, ed. Pathology of the Kidney. Boston: Little Brown, 1983, pp 761–791.
16. Thitiarchakul S, Lal SM, Luger A, Ross G: Goodpasture's syndrome superimposed on membranous nephropathy: A case report. Int J Artif Org 1995;18:763–765.
17. Turner AN, Rees AJ: Anti-glomerular basement membrane antibody disease. In Brady HR, Wilcox N, eds. Therapy in Nephrology and Hypertension: A Companion to Brenner and Rector's The Kidney. Philadelphia: WB Saunders, 1999, pp 152–157.
18. Johnson JP, Moore JJ, Austin HA, et al: Therapy of anti-glomerular basement membrane antibody disease: Analysis of prognostic significance of clinical, pathologic and treatment factors. Medicine (Baltimore) 1985;64:219–227.
19. Levy JB, Turner AN, Rees AJ, Pusey CD: Long-term outcome of anti-glomerular basement membrane antibody disease treated with plasma exchange and immunosuppression. Ann Intern Med 2001;134:1033–1042.
20. Hind CRK, Paraskevakou H, Lockwood CM, et al: Prognosis after immunosuppression of patients with crescentic nephritis requiring dialysis. Lancet 1983;1:263–265.
21. Flores JC, Taube D, Savage COS, et al: Clinical and immunological evolution of oliguric anti-GBM nephritis treated by haemodialysis. Lancet 1986;1:5–8.
22. Browne G, Brown PA, Tomson CR, et al: Retransplantation in Alport post-transplant anti-GBM disease. Kidney Int 2004;65:675–681.
23. Brainwood D, Kashtan C, Gubler MC, et al: Targets of alloantibodies in Alport anti-glomerular basement membrane disease after renal transplantation. Kidney Int 1998;53:762–766.

Renal and Systemic Vasculitis

J. Charles Jennette and Ronald J. Falk

INTRODUCTION

The kidneys are targets for a variety of systemic vasculitides, especially those that affect small vessels.[1–5] This is not surprising given the large number and variety of renal vessels. Vasculitis involving the kidneys can produce a wide variety of clinical manifestations depending in large measure on the type of renal vessel affected. As demonstrated in Figures 23.1 through 23.3, vasculitides can be categorized as large-vessel vasculitis, medium-sized vessel vasculitis, and small-vessel vasculitis. The categorization of systemic vasculitides is controversial. For the purposes of the discussion in this chapter, the Chapel Hill Consensus Conference definitions are used (see Fig. 23.3).[4]

A number of the vasculitides listed in Figure 23.2 are covered elsewhere in the book and are not reviewed in detail here except in the context of differential diagnosis: for example, cryoglobulinemic vasculitis (see Chapter 25), Henoch-Schönlein purpura (see Chapter 21), and anti-glomerular basement membrane (GBM) disease (see Chapter 22). Nephrologists most often encounter patients with small-vessel vasculitis; thus, these receive the most attention in this chapter.

Small-Vessel Vasculitis

Small-vessel vasculitis is necrotizing polyangiitis that affects predominantly vessels smaller than arteries, including capillaries, venules, and arterioles; however, arteries also may be involved. The most common renal targets for small-vessel vasculitides are the glomeruli, and, therefore, the most common clinical renal manifestations are those of glomerulonephritis (GN).

Medium-Sized Vessel Vasculitis

Medium-sized vessel vasculitis is necrotizing arteritis that affects predominantly major visceral arteries and may involve any renal arteries, although the interlobar arteries and arcuate arteries are affected most often. Inflammation and necrosis of arteries may result in thrombosis or rupture, which causes renal infarction and hemorrhage, respectively.

Large-Vessel Vasculitis

Large-vessel vasculitis is chronic granulomatous arteritis that affects predominantly the aorta and its major branches. When there is renal involvement, the ostia of the renal arteries and the main renal arteries are most often affected. The most common clinical renal manifestation is renovascular hypertension.

SMALL-VESSEL PAUCI-IMMUNE VASCULITIS

Wegener's granulomatosis, Churg-Strauss syndrome, and microscopic polyangiitis share an indistinguishable form of necrotizing small-vessel vasculitis that affects capillaries, venules, arterioles, and small arteries.[1–4] Some patients, however, have no evidence of involvement of arteries, even though they have involvement of glomerular capillaries, causing GN; pulmonary alveolar capillaries, causing pulmonary hemorrhage; or dermal venules, causing purpura. These so-called pauci-immune small-vessel vasculitides are distinguished from clinically and histologically similar forms of immune-complex small-vessel vasculitis, such as cryoglobulinemic vasculitis and Henoch-Schönlein purpura, by the absence or paucity of immune-complex deposits in vessel walls. The diagnosis for the specific subtypes of pauci-immune small-vessel vasculitides can be made based on the accompanying syndrome.[4]

- Wegener's granulomatosis occurs in association with necrotizing granulomatous inflammation, which most often affects the respiratory tract.
- Churg-Strauss syndrome is vasculitis occurring in association with asthma, eosinophilia, and necrotizing granulomatous inflammation.
- Microscopic polyangiitis is pauci-immune systemic vasculitis occurring in the absence of evidence of Wegener's granulomatosis or Churg-Strauss syndrome, that is, in the absence of asthma and eosinophilia and with no evidence of necrotizing granulomatous inflammation.

Microscopic polyangiitis, Wegener's granulomatosis, and, less frequently, Churg-Strauss syndrome also share an indistinguishable pattern of GN that is the expression of the vasculitis in glomerular capillaries.[1,2] The GN usually has necrosis and crescent formation and an absence or paucity of immunoglobulin deposition and is often designated pauci-immune crescentic GN. When pauci-immune crescentic GN occurs in the apparent absence of systemic vasculitis, it is sometimes referred to as renal vasculitis, renal-limited vasculitis, or idiopathic rapidly progressive GN (RPGN).

Pathogenesis

Wegener's granulomatosis, microscopic polyangiitis, Churg-Strauss syndrome, and isolated pauci-immune crescentic GN are all associated with the presence in serum of autoantibodies against components of the cytoplasm of neutrophils: circulating antineutrophil cytoplasmic antibodies (ANCA).[6–9] The most common antigen specificities of ANCA in patients with vasculitis and GN are for proteinase 3 (PR3) and myeloperoxidase (MPO).

The strong association of ANCA with a distinctive form of small-vessel vasculitis raises the possibility that ANCA are involved in the pathogenesis. The observation that ANCA titers correlate with disease activity is more suggestive; however, this is not a very tight correlation.[7,8] Even more supportive of a pathogenetic link is the observation that administration of certain

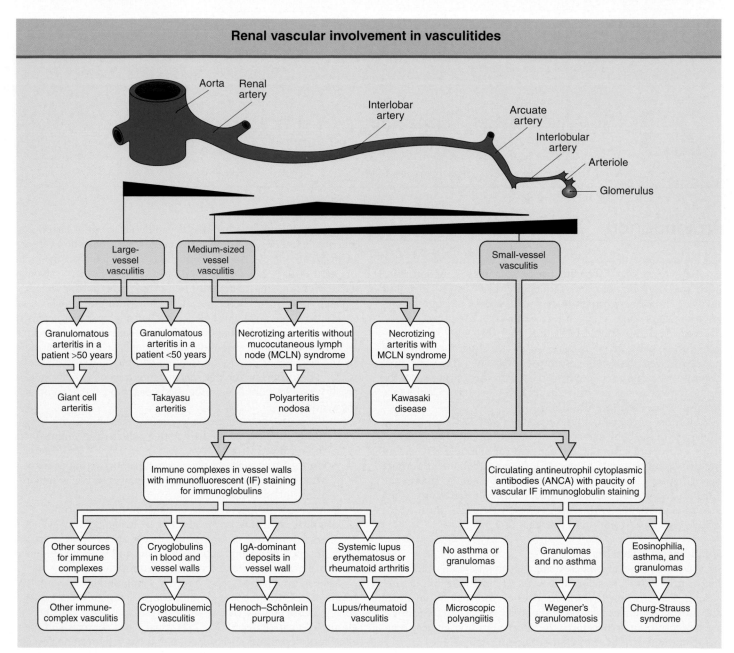

Figure 23.1 Renal vasculitis: the predominant distribution of renal vascular involvement by a variety of vasculitides. The heights of the trapezoids represent the relative frequency of involvement of different portions of the renal vasculature by the three major categories of vasculitis. (Adapted from Jennette JC, Falk RJ: Renal involvement in systemic vasculitis. In Greenberg A, Cheung AK, Coffman TM, et al, eds. National Kidney Foundation nephrology primer, 4th ed. Philadelphia: WB Saunders, 2005, pp 226–233.)

drugs, such as propylthiouracil, hydralazine, and penicillamine, can induce ANCA in the circulation concurrent with the development of pauci-immune crescentic GN and small-vessel vasculitis.[10] Most compelling of all is the report of a neonate who developed GN and pulmonary hemorrhage apparently caused by transplacental passage of MPO-ANCA IgG.[11]

The ability of ANCA IgG to cause pauci-immune necrotizing and crescentic GN and vasculitis has been demonstrated in a mouse model. Wild-type or immunodeficient mice that receive anti-MPO antibodies intravenously develop pauci-immune focal necrotizing GN with crescents.[12] This GN is mediated by neutrophil activation and can be prevented by neutrophil depletion.[13] A rat model of pauci-immune necrotizing and crescentic GN has been developed by immunizing rats with human MPO

resulting in the development of antibodies that cross react with rat MPO and are able to induce pauci-immune glomerular necrosis and crescents.[14]

A number of *in vitro* observations suggest mechanisms by which ANCA can cause vascular injury. Priming of neutrophils by cytokines, as would occur with a viral infection, causes neutrophils to increase expression of ANCA antigens on their surfaces where they are accessible to interact with ANCA. Cytokine-primed neutrophils that are exposed to ANCA release IgG from granules, release toxic oxygen metabolites, and kill cultured endothelial cells.[15–17] ANCA-antigen complexes adsorb onto endothelial cells where they could participate in *in situ* immune-complex formation.[18] ANCA activation of neutrophils is mediated by both F(ab)′$_2$ binding to neutrophils and Fc receptor

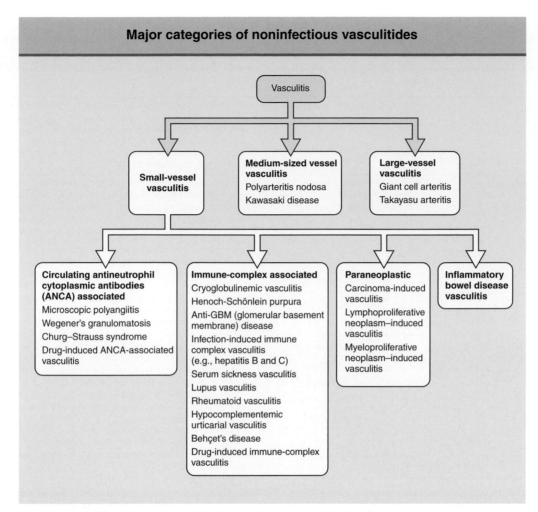

Figure 23.2   The major categories of noninfectious vasculitis. Not included are vasculitides that are known to be caused by direct invasion of vessel walls by infectious pathogens, such as rickettsial vasculitis and neisserial vasculitis.

engagement.[19,20] Neutrophils that have been activated by ANCA adhere to endothelial cells and release mediators of inflammation and cell injury.[14,16,17,21] If these events occurred *in vivo*, they would lead to vasculitis as a result of neutrophils adhering to, penetrating, and destroying vessel walls (Fig. 23.4).[22]

Thus, the clinical and the experimental animal data support the hypothesis that ANCA can activate neutrophils and cause vasculitis, especially if there is a concurrent synergistic proinflammatory stimulus. The requirement for a synergistic inflammatory process may be reflected in the very frequent association of the onset of ANCA small-vessel vasculitis with a flulike syndrome.[23] A flulike syndrome is a manifestation of high levels of circulating cytokines that could serve as priming factors for neutrophils.

Epidemiology

Wegener's granulomatosis, microscopic polyangiitis, and Churg-Strauss syndrome usually begin during the fifth, sixth, and seventh decades of life, although they may occur at any age. There is a slight male predominance. Caucasians have a disproportionately greater incidence than African Americans. In Europe, microscopic polyangiitis has a prevalence of approximately 2.5/100,000, Wegener's granulomatosis 2.5/100,000, and Churg-Strauss syndrome 1/100,000.[24] Although not fully documented, there is a suspicion that Wegener's granulomatosis is more frequent in colder

compared to warmer climates, whereas microscopic polyangiitis has the opposite trend.[24]

Clinical Manifestations

The clinical manifestations of Wegener's granulomatosis, microscopic polyangiitis, and Churg-Strauss syndrome are extremely varied because they are influenced by the sites of involvement, and the activity versus the chronicity of involvement. All three categories of vasculitis share features caused by the small-vessel vasculitis, and patients with Wegener's granulomatosis and Churg-Strauss syndrome have the additional features that define each of these syndromes.[2,4,5,7,8,23,25,26]

Renal involvement is very common in Wegener's granulomatosis and microscopic polyangiitis, and less frequent in Churg-Strauss syndrome (Fig. 23.5).[2] The most common renal manifestations are caused by glomerular involvement and include hematuria, proteinuria, and renal failure. The renal failure often has the characteristics of RPGN in patients with Wegener's granulomatosis and microscopic polyangiitis but usually is less severe in those with Churg-Strauss syndrome. Wegener's granulomatosis and microscopic polyangiitis also can present as a subacute or chronic nephritis. A cohort of >300 pauci-immune crescentic GN patients evaluated at the time of renal biopsy had a mean age of 56 ± 20 years (range, 2 to 92), male-to-female ratio of 1.0:0.9, mean serum creatinine of 6.5 ± 4.0 (range, 0.8

	Names and definitions of vasculitis adopted by the Chapel Hill Consensus Conference on the nomenclature of systemic vasculitis	
Category	Type	Definition
Large-vessel vasculitis	Giant cell (temporal) arteritis	Granulomatous arteritis of the aorta and its major branches, with a predilection for the extracranial branches of the carotid artery. Often involves the temporal artery. Usually occurs in patients older than 50 and often is associated with polymyalgia rheumatica.
	Takayasu arteritis	Granulomatous inflammation of the aorta and its major branches. Usually occurs in patients younger than 50.
Medium-sized vessel vasculitis	Polyarteritis nodosa (classic polyarteritis nodosa)	Necrotizing inflammation of medium-sized or small arteries without glomerulonephritis or vasculitis in arterioles, capillaries, or venules.
	Kawasaki disease	Arteritis involving large, medium-sized, and small arteries and associated with mucocutaneous lymph node syndrome. Coronary arteries are often involved. Aorta and veins may be involved. Usually occurs in children.
Small-vessel vasculitis	Wegener's granulomatosis	Granulomatous inflammation involving the respiratory tract and necrotizing vasculitis affecting small to medium-sized vessels, e.g., capillaries, venules, arterioles, and arteries. Necrotizing glomerulonephritis is common.
	Churg-Strauss syndrome	Eosinophil-rich and granulomatous inflammation involving the respiratory tract and necrotizing vasculitis affecting small to medium-sized vessels; associated with asthma and blood eosinophilia.
	Microscopic polyangiitis (microscopic polyarteritis)	Necrotizing vasculitis with few or no immune deposits affecting small vessels, i.e., capillaries, venules, or arterioles. Necrotizing arteritis involving small and medium-sized arteries may be present. Necrotizing glomerulonephritis is very common. Pulmonary capillaritis often occurs.
	Henoch-Schönlein purpura	Vasculitis with IgA-dominant immune deposits affecting small vessels, i.e., capillaries, venules, or arterioles. Typically involves skin, gut, and glomeruli and is associated with arthralgias or arthritis.
	Essential cryoglobulinemic vasculitis	Vasculitis with cryoglobulin immune deposits, affecting small vessels, i.e., capillaries, venules, or arterioles; associated with cryoglobulins in serum. Skin and glomeruli are often involved.
	Cutaneous leukocytoclastic angiitis	Isolated cutaneous leukocytoclastic angiitis without systemic vasculitis or glomerulonephritis.

Figure 23.3   Names and definitions of vasculitis adopted by the Chapel Hill Consensus Conference on the nomenclature of systemic vasculitis. Note that all three categories affect arteries, but only small-vessel vasculitis has a predilection for vessels smaller than arteries. (Adapted from Jennette JC, Falk RJ: Pathogenesis of the vascular and glomerular damage in ANCA-positive vasculitis. Nephrol Dial Transplant 1998;13[Suppl 1]:16–20.)

to 22.1 mg/dl), and proteinuria of 1.94 ± 2.95 (range, 0.11 to 18.00 g/dl).[27]

Generalized nonspecific manifestations of systemic inflammatory disease often are present, such as fever, malaise, anorexia, weight loss, myalgias, and arthralgias. As noted earlier, many patients trace the origin of their disease to a flulike illness.[23]

Cutaneous involvement is frequent. Purpura is a common manifestation of Wegener's granulomatosis, microscopic polyangiitis, and Churg-Strauss syndrome (Fig. 23.6). The purpura is most common on the lower extremities and tends to occur as recurrent crops. The purpura may be accompanied by small areas of ulceration. Nodular cutaneous lesions are much more frequent in Wegener's granulomatosis and Churg-Strauss syndrome than in microscopic polyangiitis. Nodules can be caused by dermal or subcutaneous arteritis and by the necrotizing granulomatous inflammation.

Upper and lower respiratory tract involvement is most common in Wegener's granulomatosis and Churg-Strauss syndrome but also occurs in those with microscopic polyangiitis. All three categories can have pulmonary hemorrhage caused by hemorrhagic capillaritis. Wegener's granulomatosis and Churg-Strauss syndrome also can have pulmonary injury caused by necrotizing granulomatous inflammation, which may be detected radiographically as nodular or cavitary lesions. By definition, patients with microscopic polyangiitis do not have granulomatous respiratory tract lesions.[4]

Manifestations of upper respiratory tract disease include subglottic stenosis, sinusitis, rhinitis, otitis media, and ocular inflammation. These features are most common in Wegener's granulomatosis but may occur in Churg-Strauss syndrome and microscopic polyangiitis. The upper respiratory tract inflammation in microscopic polyangiitis is caused by angiitis alone, without granulomatous inflammation. Destruction of bone, for example, resulting in septal perforation and saddle nose deformity, appears to require necrotizing granulomatous inflammation and, therefore, does not occur in microscopic polyangiitis.

Cardiac disease is identified in approximately 50% of patients with Churg-Strauss syndrome but in <20% of patients with Wegener's granulomatosis or microscopic polyangiitis. Manifestations range from transient heart block and ventricular hypokinesis that respond to immunosuppressive treatment to infarction and severe life-threatening myocarditis. Pericarditis and endocarditis also may occur.

Peripheral neuropathy, usually with a mononeuritis multiplex pattern, is the most common neurologic manifestation and is most frequent in Churg-Strauss syndrome. Central nervous system involvement is less common and includes vasculitis within the meninges. Gastrointestinal involvement typically causes abdominal pain and blood in the stool, with mesenteric ischemia and, rarely, intestinal perforation. Vasculitis in the pancreas and liver can mimic pancreatitis and hepatitis symptomatically.

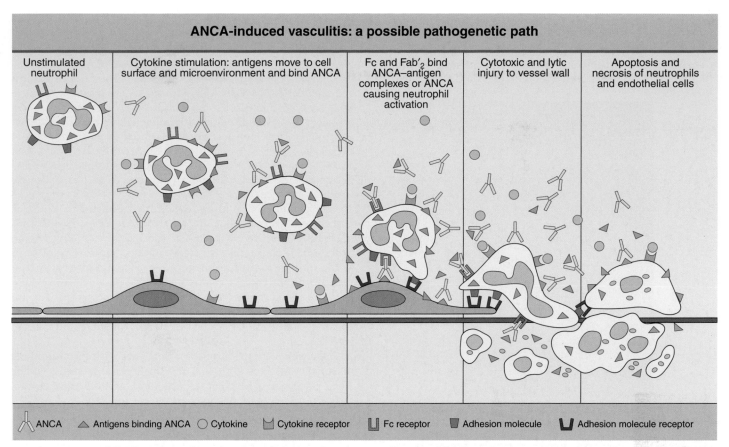

Figure 23.4 Vasculitis induced by antineutrophil cytoplasmic antibodies (ANCA): a hypothetical sequence of pathogenetic events. (Adapted with permission from Jennette JC, Falk RJ: Pathogenesis of the vascular and glomerular damage in ANCA-positive vasculitis. Nephrol Dial Transplant 1998;13[Suppl 1]:16–20.)

Antineutrophil Cytoplasmic Autoantibodies

Serologic testing for ANCA is a useful diagnostic procedure for pauci-immune small-vessel vasculitis and pauci-immune crescentic GN but should be interpreted in the context of other patient characteristics.[7,8,28–31] Laboratory testing for ANCA should include both indirect immunofluorescence microscopy assay (IFA) and enzyme immunoassay (EIA).[30]

IFA using normal human neutrophils as substrate produces two major staining patterns: cytoplasmic (c-ANCA), where staining occurs diffusely throughout the cytoplasm, and peripheral (p-ANCA; Fig. 23.7). By EIA, most c-ANCA have specificity for PR3 (PR3-ANCA) and most p-ANCAs have specificity for MPO (MPO-ANCA). For adequate diagnostic accuracy, all serologic testing for ANCA should include an immunochemical analysis for antigen specificity, such as an EIA.[30] Although positive results are rare in completely healthy individuals, approximately one fourth of patients with other inflammatory renal diseases (especially lupus) will have a false-positive IFA result (usually with a p-ANCA pattern) and approximately 5% will have a false-positive EIA result (usually at low titer).[31]

ANCA testing has good sensitivity for pauci-immune small-vessel vasculitis and GN (80% to 90%). The specificity and

	Frequency of Involvement (%)				
Organ System	Microscopic Polyangiitis	Wegener's Granulomatosis	Churg-Strauss Syndrome	Henoch-Schönlein Purpura	Cryoglobulinemic Vasculitis
Kidney	90	80	45	50	55
Skin (cutaneous)	40	40	60	90	90
Lungs	50	90	70	>5	>5
Ear, nose, and throat	35	90	50	>5	>5
Musculoskeletal system	60	60	50	75	70
Neurologic system	30	50	70	10	40
Gastrointestinal system	50	50	50	60	30

Organ system involvement in small-vessel vasculitis

Figure 23.5 Organ system involvement in small-vessel vasculitis. (Modified from Jennette JC, Falk RJ: Small vessel vasculitis. N Engl J Med 1997;337: 1512–1523.)

predictive value depend on the patient population.[29] Although ANCA are most frequent in patients with pauci-immune crescentic GN, approximately one fourth to one third of patients with anti-GBM crescentic GN and one fourth of patients with idiopathic immune-complex crescentic GN are ANCA positive.[27,32]

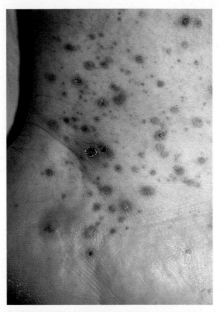

Figure 23.6 Cutaneous vasculitis. Ankle of a patient with small-vessel vasculitis, showing purpura and a few small ulcers.

Patients with concurrent ANCA and anti-GBM antibodies have a worse prognosis than patients with ANCA alone.

Figure 23.8 provides an estimate of the relative frequencies of PR3-ANCA/c-ANCA and MPO-ANCA/p-ANCA in the different clinical phenotypes of pauci-immune small-vessel vasculitis and crescentic GN. PR3-ANCA/c-ANCA are most prevalent in Wegener's granulomatosis and MPO-ANCA/p-ANCA are most prevalent in renal-limited pauci-immune crescentic GN. Patients with microscopic polyangiitis have a more even distribution of PR3-ANCA/c-ANCA and MPO-ANCA/p-ANCA. These data make it clear that ANCA antigen specificity cannot be used to determine the clinicopathologic phenotype of pauci-immune small-vessel vasculitis.

Changes in ANCA titers over time correlate to a degree with disease activity but are not infallible markers and thus must be interpreted with much caution.[7,8,30,33,34] In general, titers usually decrease with treatment and increase prior to or at the time of disease recurrence. An increase in ANCA titer should prompt careful evaluation of the patient for corroborating evidence of exacerbation, but most physicians do not modify treatment based on an increase in titer without accompanying clinical or laboratory evidence for increased disease activity.

Approximately 10% to 20% of patients with pauci-immune necrotizing and crescentic GN and small-vessel vasculitis will be ANCA negative. The clinical, pathologic, and outcome characteristics of these patients are no different from those of ANCA-positive patients.[35]

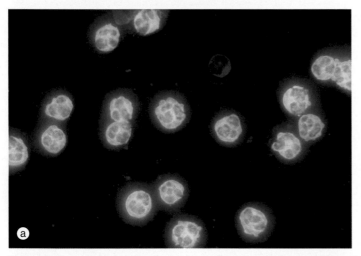
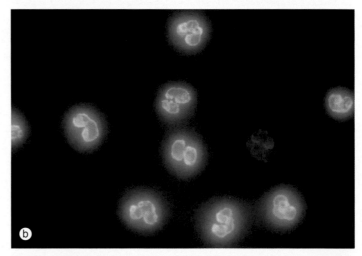

Figure 23.7 Indirect immunofluorescence for antineutrophil cytoplasmic antibodies (ANCA). Staining pattern of alcohol-fixed normal human neutrophils. *a*, Cytoplasmic pattern caused by ANCA with specificity for proteinase 3. *b*, Perinuclear pattern caused by ANCA with specificity for myeloperoxidase (anti-IgG, original magnification ×250).

Antineutrophil cytoplasmic antibodies (ANCA) in small-vessel vasculitis			
	Frequency (%)		
	Proteinase 3 (PR3/c-ANCA)	Myeloperoxidase (MPO/p-ANCA)	Negative
Wegener's granulomatosis	70	25	5
Microscopic polyangiitis	40	50	10
Churg-Strauss syndrome	10	60	30
Pauci-immune glomerulonephritis	20	70	10

Figure 23.8 Antineutrophil cytoplasmic antibodies (ANCA) in small-vessel vasculitis. Approximate frequency of ANCA with specificity for proteinase 3 (PR3/c-ANCA) and for myeloperoxidase (MPO/p-ANCA) in patients with different categories of pauci-immune small-vessel vasculitis and crescentic glomerulonephritis.

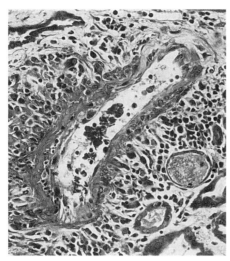

Figure 23.9 Necrotizing arteritis in an interlobular artery from a patient with antineutrophil cytoplasmic antibody–associated small-vessel vasculitis. There is segmental fibrinoid necrosis with adjacent perivascular leukocyte infiltration (hematoxylin-eosin, original magnification ×50).

ANCA may sometimes be positive with other inflammatory conditions, which may need to be considered in the differential diagnosis, including inflammatory bowel disease, rheumatoid disease, chronic inflammatory liver disease, bacterial endocarditis, and cystic fibrosis.[7] In this setting, specificity of the ANCA may not be against PR3 or MPO but against other neutrophil antigens including lactoferrin, cathepsin G, and antibactericidal/permeability-increasing protein.

Pathology

The basic shared acute vascular lesion of the pauci-immune small-vessel vasculitides is segmental fibrinoid necrosis, often accompanied by leukocyte infiltration and leukocytoclasia (leukocyte fragmentation; Figs 23.9 and 23.10).[1,2,36,37] The earliest vasculitic lesions have infiltrating neutrophils that are quickly replaced by predominantly mononuclear leukocytes. The acute necrotizing lesions evolve into sclerotic lesions and may be complicated by thrombosis.

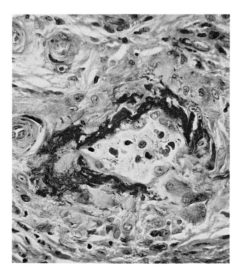

Figure 23.10 Necrotizing arteritis in an interlobular artery from a patient with antineutrophil cytoplasmic antibody–associated small-vessel vasculitis. The fibrinoid necrosis is accentuated by the red staining of the trichrome stain (Masson trichrome, original magnification ×100).

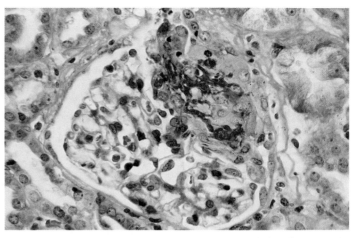

Figure 23.11 Segmental glomerular necrosis and crescent formation in a patient with antineutrophil cytoplasmic antibody–associated small-vessel vasculitis. The fibrinoid material is red. The uninvolved segments appear normal (Masson trichrome, original magnification ×150).

These focal necrotizing lesions can affect many different vessels, thus causing many different signs and symptoms, for example, involvement of glomerular capillaries causing nephritis, alveolar capillaries causing pulmonary hemorrhage, dermal venules causing purpura, upper respiratory tract mucosal venules causing rhinitis and sinusitis, abdominal visceral arteries causing abdominal pain, and epineural arteries causing mononeuritis multiplex.

The shared glomerular lesion of the pauci-immune small-vessel vasculitides is a necrotizing GN, usually with resultant crescent formation (Figs. 23.11 and 23.12).[1,2,36,37] Early mild lesions have segmental fibrinoid necrosis with or without an adjacent small crescent (see Fig. 23.11). Severe acute lesions may have essentially global necrosis with large circumferential crescents (see Fig. 23.12). In a cohort of 181 renal biopsy specimens from patients with ANCA-associated GN, 89.5% had glomerular crescent that on average affected 49% of glomeruli, with half having crescents in ≥50% of glomeruli.[27] Non-necrotic segments within segmentally injured glomeruli (see Fig. 23.11) and glomeruli without necrosis typically have slight or no histologic abnormalities.

As mentioned previously, approximately one fourth of patients with anti-GBM crescentic GN and one fourth of patients with immune complex–mediated crescentic GN will be

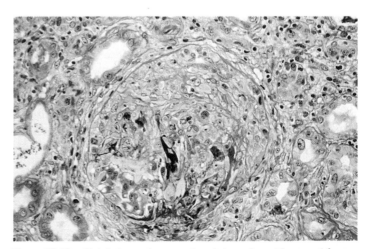

Figure 23.12 Global glomerular necrosis and circumferential crescent formation in a glomerulus from a patient with antineutrophil cytoplasmic antibody–associated small-vessel vasculitis (Masson trichrome, original magnification ×150).

Clinical differences between polyarteritis nodosa and microscopic polyangiitis		
Clinical Feature	Polyarteritis Nodosa	Microscopic Polyangiitis
Microaneurysms by angiography	Yes	No (?rare)
Rapidly progressive nephritis	No	Yes (very common)
Pulmonary hemorrhage	No	Yes
Renovascular hypertension	Yes (10%–33%)	No
Peripheral neuropathy	Yes (50%–80%)	Yes (10%–20%)
Positive hepatitis B serology	Uncommon	No
Positive antineutrophil cytoplasmic antibody	Rare	Frequent
Relapses	Rare	Frequent

Figure 23.17 **Clinical differences between polyarteritis nodosa and microscopic polyangiitis.** (Modified from Lhote F, Guillevin L: Polyarteritis nodosa, microscopic polyangiitis, and Churg-Strauss syndrome. Clinical aspects and treatment. Rheum Dis Clin North Am 1995;21:911–947.)

Kawasaki disease causes necrotizing arteritis but is distinguished from polyarteritis nodosa by the presence of the mucocutaneous lymph node syndrome.

Natural History

The natural history of polyarteritis nodosa is difficult to determine because most of the early studies of outcome grouped polyarteritis nodosa together with microscopic polyangiitis. Polyarteritis nodosa with multisystem involvement has a very poor prognosis without therapy. Polyarteritis nodosa usually is treated with corticosteroids and cytotoxic drugs, such as cyclophosphamide.[62] The 10-year survival rate with appropriate treatment is approximately 80%. Approximately 15% of patients who enter remission develop a relapse, which is much less frequent than microscopic polyangiitis. Relapse is more likely if treatment is delayed.

Treatment

Polyarteritis nodosa in patients with no evidence of hepatitis B virus infection is treated with corticosteroids and cytotoxic drugs, usually cyclophosphamide.[60–63] The regimens vary and include treatment approaches similar to those described earlier for microscopic polyangiitis and Wegener's granulomatosis. However, in patients with no risk factors for poor outcome (such as age older than 50 years, cardiac involvement, gut involvement, or renal involvement), corticosteroids alone may be adequate and are less toxic therapy than corticosteroids combined with cytotoxic agents.

Aggressive immunosuppressive therapy without initial antiviral therapy is contraindicated in patients with hepatitis B virus–associated polyarteritis nodosa because of potential adverse effects on the outcome of the hepatitis B virus infection. Short-term steroid treatment combined with antiviral agents and possibly plasma exchange should precede more extensive immunosuppression in such patients.[61,64]

KAWASAKI DISEASE

Definition

Kawasaki disease is an acute febrile illness that usually occurs in young children, often younger than 1 year old.[4,66–68] The mucocutaneous lymph node syndrome is the characteristic clinical presentation of Kawasaki disease. This includes fever (usually 38° to 40°C), erythema of the oropharyngeal mucosa, polymorphous erythematous rash, erythema of the palms and soles, and indurative edema of the extremities, followed by desquamation, conjunctivitis, and nonsuppurative lymphadenopathy. Necrotizing arteritis is a complication of Kawasaki disease that is present in some but not all patients. Clinically significant renal involvement is very rare; therefore, Kawasaki disease is rarely encountered by nephrologists.

Pathogenesis

The occasional occurrence of Kawasaki disease as an endemic or epidemic disease suggests that the cause may be an infectious agent or an environmental toxin. Both cell-mediated and antibody-mediated mechanisms have been incriminated, including a possible role for antiendothelial antibodies.[68] At the current time, the etiology and pathogenesis of Kawasaki disease are unproven.

Epidemiology

Kawasaki disease usually occurs in children younger than 5 years old and has a peak incidence in the first year of life. It was first described in Japan, but it occurs worldwide. The disease is more common in Asians and Polynesians than in Caucasians and Blacks. In Japan, the incidence is 50/100,000 children younger than 5 years old, with 50% of the children younger than 2 years old.[69] Kawasaki disease occasionally occurs in an endemic or epidemic pattern but usually is sporadic.

Clinical Manifestations

The mucocutaneous syndrome is the characteristic clinical manifestation of Kawasaki disease.[4,68] This includes fever (usually 38° to 40°C), mucosal inflammation, swollen red tongue (strawberry tongue), polymorphous erythematous rash, indurative edema of the extremities, erythema of palms and soles, desquamation from the tips of digits, conjunctival injection, and enlarged lymph nodes.

The frequency of active arteritic lesions peaks during the first week of the illness and is markedly reduced after 1 month. Arteritis most often manifests as cardiac disease. Thrombosis of inflamed coronary arteries in patients with Kawasaki disease is the most common cause of childhood myocardial infarction. Clinically significant renal disease is uncommon. This is somewhat surprising because autopsy reveals arteritis in renal vessels in up to three fourths of patients.[66]

Pathology

The arteritis of Kawasaki disease involves small and medium-sized arteries. The acute histologic lesion is necrotizing inflammation

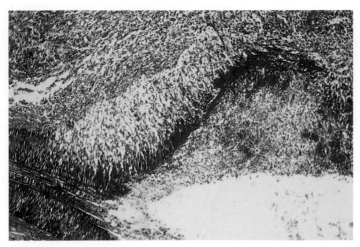

Figure 23.18 Kawasaki disease arteritis affecting a renal interlobar artery in a young child. The artery wall is intact on the far left. The remainder of the wall has extensive edema, infiltration by mononuclear leukocytes, and a band of fuchsinophilic (red) fibrinoid material roughly at the junction between the inflamed intima and muscularis (Masson trichrome, original magnification ×25).

with less fibrinoid necrosis and more edema than is usually observed with polyarteritis nodosa (Fig. 23.18).[65] Aneurysm (pseudoaneurysm) formation and thrombosis may occur.

The most frequent site of arteritis is the coronary arteries, followed by the renal arteries.[66] Arteritis most often affects interlobar arteries, occasionally arcuate arteries, and only rarely interlobular arteries.

Differential Diagnosis

Kawasaki disease has sometimes been misdiagnosed as childhood polyarteritis nodosa. The differentiation of Kawasaki disease from polyarteritis nodosa is very important because corticosteroid treatment may increase the risk of coronary artery aneurysms in Kawasaki disease. Arteritis in a child younger than 5 should always raise the possibility of Kawasaki disease. The presence or absence of the mucocutaneous lymph node syndrome is the basis for distinguishing between Kawasaki disease and other forms of arteritis.[4]

Natural History

Kawasaki disease usually is self-limited with an uneventful recovery if treated promptly with intravenous gamma globulins.[67,68] Recurrence is rare. Only about 1% of patients develop severe arteritic complications, usually affecting the coronary arteries.

Treatment

Aspirin and intravenous gamma globulin are the standard therapy for Kawasaki disease.[67,68] Corticosteroid treatment may increase the risk of adverse coronary artery complications, although the data supporting this are limited.

TAKAYASU ARTERITIS AND GIANT CELL ARTERITIS

Takayasu arteritis and giant cell arteritis affect the aorta and its major branches.[4,65,70] Giant cell arteritis has a predilection for the extracranial branches of the carotid artery but can affect arteries in almost any organ. Takayasu arteritis has a predilection for major arteries supplying the extremities. Both diseases cause chronic vascular inflammation, often with a granulomatous appearance that may include multinucleated giant cells. Giant cell arteritis, but not Takayasu arteritis, is associated with polymyalgia rheumatica.

Pathogenesis

The etiology and pathogenesis of giant cell arteritis and Takayasu arteritis are unknown. Because of the histologic changes and the nature of the infiltrating leukocytes, cell-mediated immune mechanisms are incriminated. The inciting antigen or autoantigen has not been identified.

Epidemiology

Takayasu arteritis is seen most frequently in Asia. Giant cell arteritis is most frequent in individuals of northern European ancestry. Takayasu arteritis has a female-to-male ratio of approximately 9:1, and giant cell arteritis has a female-to-male ratio of 4:1. Takayasu arteritis usually is diagnosed in those between the ages of 10 and 20 years and is very rare after 50 years of age. Giant cell arteritis is very rare before age 50 years.

Clinical Manifestations

In addition to nonspecific constitutional symptoms such as fever, arthralgias, and weight loss, the major clinical manifestations of Takayasu arteritis and giant cell arteritis are caused by arterial narrowing and resultant ischemia.[70]

The major clinical manifestations of Takayasu arteritis are reduced pulses (95% of patients), vascular bruits, claudication, and renovascular hypertension. Renovascular hypertension is a major cause for morbidity and mortality and results from renal ischemia caused by renal artery stenosis or aortic coarctation.[70,71] Reduced aortic elasticity and impairment of carotid artery baroreceptors also may play a role in some patients.

Headache is the most common presenting symptom in patients with giant cell arteritis. Temporal artery tenderness, nodularity, or decreased pulsation is present in about half of patients. Additional common symptoms include blindness, deafness, jaw claudication, tongue dysfunction, extremity claudication, and reduced pulses. More than half of patients with giant cell arteritis have polymyalgia rheumatica, which is characterized by stiffness and aching in the neck and the proximal muscles of the shoulders and hips. Clinically significant renal disease is much rarer in giant cell arteritis than in Takayasu arteritis. There are case reports of necrotizing and crescentic GN associated with giant cell arteritis, but these may represent examples of Wegener's granulomatosis or microscopic polyangiitis with temporal artery involvement.

Pathology

The aortitis and arteritis of Takayasu arteritis and giant cell arteritis cannot be confidently distinguished from each other by pathologic examination.[65] Both are characterized in the active phase by inflammation with a predominance of mononuclear leukocytes, often with scattered multinucleated giant cells (Fig. 23.19). The chronic phase is characterized by progressive fibrosis that may cause severe narrowing of vessels, with resultant ischemia. Major renal arteries are often found to be involved at autopsy in both Takayasu arteritis and giant cell arteritis patients. However, clinically significant renal disease is relatively common in Takayasu arteritis but rare in giant cell arteritis. A glomerular lesion characterized by nodular mesangial matrix expansion and mesangiolysis may occasionally be a component of Takayasu arteritis.[72]

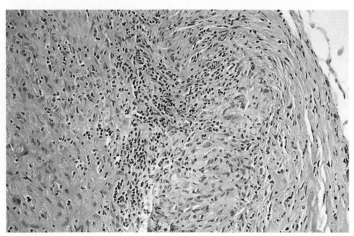

Figure 23.19 Severe giant cell arteritis affecting a main renal artery. This caused marked renal atrophy and renovascular hypertension (hematoxylin-eosin, original magnification ×50).

Differential Diagnosis

There is a great deal of overlap between the clinical manifestations and pathologic features of Takayasu arteritis and giant cell arteritis. The age of the patient and the presence or absence of polymyalgia rheumatica are the best features for discriminating between these two vasculitides.

Giant cell arteritis also has been called temporal arteritis. This is a misleading designation because all patients do not have temporal artery involvement and patients with other types of vasculitis, such as polyarteritis nodosa, Wegener's granulomatosis, and microscopic polyangiitis, can have involvement of the temporal arteries. Some of the reported examples of necrotizing GN associated with temporal arteritis probably represent Wegener's granulomatosis or microscopic polyangiitis with temporal artery involvement.

Treatment

Corticosteroids are the usual treatment for giant cell arteritis and Takayasu arteritis, for example, initial daily therapy with 0.5 to 1 mg/kg prednisolone for 1 to 2 months followed by tapering over several months. More prolonged treatment may be dictated by persistent disease activity. Cytotoxic agents such as cyclophosphamide may be required in patients with recalcitrant disease.

Management of renal disease is not an issue with typical giant cell arteritis, although rare patients have ischemic renal manifestations. Renovascular hypertension is the major renal problem caused by Takayasu arteritis.[70,71] When bilateral renal artery involvement occurs, angiotensin-converting enzyme inhibitors may precipitate renal failure in patients with Takayasu arteritis.[73] When medical management fails, the renovascular hypertension in patients with Takayasu arteritis may be controlled by bypass surgery or angioplasty.[71] The management of renovascular hypertension is covered in Chapter 61.

REFERENCES

1. Jennette JC, Falk RJ: The pathology of vasculitis involving the kidney. Am J Kidney Dis 1994;24:130–141.
2. Jennette JC, Falk RJ: Small vessel vasculitis. N Engl J Med 1997;337:1512–1523.
3. Jennette JC, Falk RJ: Renal involvement in systemic vasculitis. In Greenberg A, Cheung AK, Coffman TM, et al, eds. National Kidney Foundation Nephrology Primer, 4th ed. Philadelphia: WB Saunders, 2005, pp 226–233.
4. Jennette JC, Falk RJ, Andrassy K, et al: Nomenclature of systemic vasculitides: The proposal of an international consensus conference. Arthritis Rheum 1994;37:187–192.
5. Samarkos M, Loizou S, Vaiopoulos G, Davies KA: The clinical spectrum of primary renal vasculitis. Semin Arthritis Rheum 2005;35:95–111.
6. Jennette JC, Falk RJ: Anti-neutrophil cytoplasmic autoantibodies: Discovery, specificity, disease associations and pathogenic potential. Adv Pathol Lab Med 1995;8:363–377.
7. Savige J, Davies D, Falk RJ, et al: Antineutrophil cytoplasmic antibodies (ANCA) and associated diseases. Kidney Int 2000;57:846–862.
8. Savage CO: ANCA-associated renal vasculitis. Kidney Int 2001;60:1614–1627.
9. Franssen CF, Stegeman CA, Kallenberg CG, et al: Antiproteinase 3- and antimyeloperoxidase-associated vasculitis. Kidney Int 2000;57:2195–2206.
10. Choi HK, Merkel PA, Walker AM, Niles JL: Drug-associated antineutrophil cytoplasmic antibody-positive vasculitis: Prevalence among patients with high titers of antimyeloperoxidase antibodies. Arthritis Rheum 2000;43:405–413.
11. Schlieben DJ, Korbet SM, Kimura RE, et al: Pulmonary-renal syndrome in a newborn with placental transmission of ANCAs. Am J Kidney Dis 2005;45:758–761.
12. Xiao H, Heeringa P, Hu P, et al: Antineutrophil cytoplasmic autoantibodies specific for myeloperoxidase cause glomerulonephritis and vasculitis in mice. J Clin Invest 2002;110:955–963.
13. Xiao H, Heeringa P, Liu Z, et al: The role of neutrophils in the induction of glomerulonephritis by anti-myeloperoxidase antibodies. Am J Pathol 2005;167:39–45.
14. Little MA, Smyth CL, Yadav R, et al: Antineutrophil cytoplasm antibodies directed against myeloperoxidase augment leukocyte-microvascular interactions in vivo. Blood 2005;106:2050–2058.
15. Falk RJ, Terrell RS, Charles LA, Jennette JC: Anti-neutrophil cyto-plasmic autoantibodies induce neutrophils to degranulate and produce oxygen radicals in vitro. Proc Natl Acad Sci U S A 1990;87:4115–4119.
16. Savage CO, Gaskin G, Pusey CD, Pearson JD: Myeloperoxidase binds to vascular endothelial cells, is recognized by ANCA and can enhance complement dependent cytotoxicity. Adv Exp Med Biol 1993;336:121–123.
17. Ewert BH, Jennette JC, Falk RJ: Anti-myeloperoxidase antibodies stimulate neutrophils to damage human endothelial cells. Kidney Int 1992;41:375–383.
18. Vargunam M, Adu D, Taylor CM, et al: Endothelium myeloperoxidase-antimyeloperoxidase interaction in vasculitis. Nephrol Dial Transplant 1992;7:1077–1081.
19. Kettritz R, Jennette JC, Falk RJ: Cross-linking of ANCA-antigens stimulates superoxide release by human neutrophils. J Am Soc Nephrol 1997;8:386–394.
20. Williams JM, Ben Smith A, Hewins P, et al: Activation of the G(i) heterotrimeric G protein by ANCA IgG F(ab')2 fragments is necessary but not sufficient to stimulate the recruitment of those downstream mediators used by intact ANCA IgG. J Am Soc Nephrol 2003;14:661–669.
21. Calderwood JW, Williams JM, Morgan MD, et al: ANCA induces beta2 integrin and CXC chemokine-dependent neutrophil-endothelial cell interactions that mimic those of highly cytokine-activated endothelium. J Leukoc Biol 2005;77:3–43.
22. Jennette JC, Falk RJ: Pathogenesis of the vascular and glomerular damage in ANCA-positive vasculitis. Nephrol Dial Transplant 1998;13(Suppl 1):16–20.
23. Falk RJ, Hogan S, Carey TS, Jennette JC: Clinical course of anti-neutrophil cytoplasmic autoantibody-associated glomerulonephritis and systemic vasculitis: The Glomerular Disease Collaborative Network. Ann Intern Med 1990;113:656–663.
24. Mahr A, Guillevin L, Poissonnet M, Ayme S: Prevalences of polyarteritis nodosa, microscopic polyangiitis, Wegener's granulomatosis, and Churg-Strauss syndrome in a French urban multiethnic population in 2000: A capture-recapture estimate. Arthritis Rheum 2004;51:92–99.
25. Duna GF, Galperin C, Hoffman GS: Wegener's granulomatosis. Rheum Dis Clin North Am 1995;21:949–986.
26. Lhote F, Guillevin L: Polyarteritis nodosa, microscopic polyangiitis, and Churg-Strauss syndrome: Clinical aspects and treatment. Rheum Dis Clin North Am 1995;21:911–947.

27. Jennette JC: Rapidly progressive crescentic glomerulonephritis. Kidney Int 2003;63:1164–1177.

28. Hagen EC, Daha MR, Hermans J, et al: Diagnostic value of standardized assays for anti-neutrophil cytoplasmic antibodies in idiopathic systemic vasculitis: EC/BCR Project for ANCA Assay Standardization. Kidney Int 1998;53:743–753.

29. Jennette JC, Wilkman AS, Falk RJ: Diagnostic predictive value of ANCA serology. Kidney Int 1998;53:796–798.

30. Savige J, Gillis D, Davies D, et al: International consensus statement on testing and reporting of antineutrophil cytoplasmic antibodies (ANCA). Am J Clin Pathol 1999;111:507–513.

31. Lim LC, Taylor JG III, Schmitz JL, et al: Diagnostic usefulness of antineutrophil cytoplasmic autoantibody serology: Comparative evaluation of commercial indirect fluorescent antibody kits and enzyme immunoassay kits. Am J Clin Pathol 1999;111:363–369.

32. Rutgers A, Slot M, van Paassen P, et al: Coexistence of anti-glomerular basement membrane antibodies and myeloperoxidase-ANCAs in crescentic glomerulonephritis. Am J Kidney Dis 2005;46:253–262.

33. Segelmark M, Phillips BD, Tuttle R, et al: Monitoring PR3-ANCA for the detection of relapses in small vessel vasculitis. Clin Diagn Lab Immunol 2003;120:321–318.

34. Han WK, Choi HK, Roth RM, et al: Serial ANCA titers: Useful tool for prevention of relapses in ANCA-associated vasculitis. Kidney Int 2003; 63:1079–1085.

35. Eisenberger U, Fakhouri F, Vanhille P, et al: ANCA-negative pauci-immune renal vasculitis: Histology and outcome. Nephrol Dial Transplant 2005;20:1392–1399.

36. Hauer HA, Bajema IM, Hagen EC, et al: Long-term renal injury in ANCA-associated vasculitis: An analysis of 31 patients with follow-up biopsies. Nephrol Dial Transplant 2002;17:587–596.

37. Vizjak A, Rott T, Koselj-Kajtna M, et al: Histologic and immunohistologic study and clinical presentation of ANCA-associated glomerulonephritis with correlation to ANCA antigen specificity. Am J Kidney Dis 2003;41:539–549.

38. Little MA, Pusey CD: Glomerulonephritis due to antineutrophil cytoplasm antibody-associated vasculitis: An update on approaches to management. Nephrology 2005;10:368–376.

39. Bajema IM, Hagen EC, Hermans J, et al: Kidney biopsy as a predictor for renal outcome in ANCA-associated necrotizing glomerulonephritis. Kidney Int 1999;56:751–1758.

40. Hauer HA, Bajema IM, van Houwelingen HC, et al: Determinants of outcome in ANCA-associated glomerulonephritis: A prospective clinico-histopathological analysis of 96 patients. Kidney Int 2002;62:732–742.

41. Hogan SL, Falk RJ, Chin H, et al: Predictors of relapse and treatment resistance in ANCA small vessel vasculitis. Ann Intern Med 2005;143: 621–631.

42. Bacon PA: Therapy of vasculitis. J Rheumatol 1994;21:788–790.

43. Nachman PH, Hogan SL, Jennette JC, Falk RJ: Treatment response and relapse in ANCA-associated microscopic polyangiitis and glomerulonephritis. J Am Soc Nephrol 1996;7:33–39.

44. Jayne D: Update on the European Vasculitis Study Group trials. Curr Opin Rheumatol 2001;13:48–55.

45. Pusey CD, Rees AJ, Evans DJ, et al: Plasma exchange in focal necrotizing glomerulonephritis without anti-GBM antibodies. Kidney Int 1991;40:757–763.

46. Jayne DR, Davies MJ, Fox CJ, et al: Treatment of systemic vasculitis with pooled intravenous immunoglobulin. Lancet 1991; 337:1137–1139.

47. Jayne D, Rasmussen N, Andrassy K, Bacon P, et al: A randomized trial of maintenance therapy for vasculitis associated with antineutrophil cytoplasmic autoantibodies. N Engl J Med 2003;349:36–44.

48. Klemmer PJ, Chalermskulrat W, Reif MS, et al: Plasmapheresis therapy for diffuse alveolar hemorrhage in patients with small-vessel vasculitis. Am J Kidney Dis 2003;42:1149–1153.

49. Guillevin L, Cordier JF, Lhote F, et al: A prospective, multicenter, randomized trial comparing steroids and pulse cyclophosphamide versus steroids and oral cyclophosphamide in the treatment of generalized Wegener's granulomatosis. Arthritis Rheum 1997;40:2187–2198.

50. Jayne DR: Conventional treatment and outcome of Wegener's granulomatosis and microscopic polyangiitis. Cleve Clin J Med 2002;69(Suppl 2):SII110–SII115.

51. De Groot K, Rasmussen N, Bacon PA, et al: Randomized trial of cyclophosphamide versus methotrexate for induction of remission in early systemic antineutrophil cytoplasmic antibody-associated vasculitis. Arthritis Rheum 2005;52:2461–2469.

52. Booth A, Harper L, Hammad T, et al: Prospective study of TNFalpha blockade with infliximab in anti-neutrophil cytoplasmic antibody-associated systemic vasculitis. J Am Soc Nephrol 2004;15:717–721.

53. Aries PM, Hellmich B, Both M, et al: Lack of efficacy of rituximab in Wegener's granulomatosis with refractory granulomatous manifestations. Ann Rheum Dis 2006;65:853–858.

54. Joy MS, Hogan SL, Jennette JC, et al: A pilot study using mycophenolate mofetil in relapsing or resistant ANCA small vessel vasculitis. Nephrol Dial Transplant 2005;20:2725–2732.

55. Wegener's Granulomatosis Etanercept Trial (WGET) Research Group: Etanercept plus standard therapy for Wegener's granulomatosis. N Engl J Med 2005;352:351–361.

56. Stegeman CA, Cohen Tervaert JW, Sluiter WJ, et al: Association of chronic nasal carriage of *Staphylococcus aureus* and higher relapse rates in Wegener's granulomatosis. Ann Intern Med 1994;120:12–17.

57. de Groot K, Reinhold-Keller E, Tatsis E, et al: Therapy for the maintenance of remission in sixty-five patients with generalized Wegener's granulomatosis. Methotrexate versus trimethoprim/sulfamethoxazole. Arthritis Rheum 1996;39:2052–2061.

58. Rostaing L, Modesto A, Oksman F, et al: Outcome of patients with anti-neutrophil cytoplasmic antibody-associated vasculitis following cadaveric kidney transplantation. Am J Kidney Dis 1997;9:96–102.

59. Nachman PH, Segelmark M, Westman K, et al: Recurrent ANCA-associated small vessel vasculitis after transplantation: A pooled analysis. Kidney Int 1999;56:1544–1550.

60. Gayraud M, Guillevin L, le Toumelin P, et al: Long-term followup of polyarteritis nodosa, microscopic polyangiitis, and Churg-Strauss syndrome: Analysis of four prospective trials including 278 patients. Arthritis Rheum 2001;44:666–675.

61. Guillevin L, Lhote F, Leon A, et al: Treatment of polyarteritis nodosa related to hepatitis B virus with short term steroid therapy associated with antiviral agents and plasma exchanges: A prospective trial in 33 patients. J Rheumatol 1993;20:289–298.

62. Guillevin L: Treatment of classic polyarteritis nodosa in 1999. Nephrol Dial Transplant 1999;14:2077–2079.

63. Lhote F, Guillevin L: Polyarteritis nodosa, microscopic polyangiitis, and Churg-Strauss syndrome: Clinical aspects and treatment. Rheum Dis Clin North Am 1995;21:911–947.

64. Janssen HL, van Zonneveld M, van Nunen AB, et al: Polyarteritis nodosa associated with hepatitis B virus infection: The role of antiviral treatment and mutations in the hepatitis B virus genome. Eur J Gastroenterol Hepatol 2004;16:801–807.

65. D'Agati V, Jennette JC, Silva FG: Antineutrophil cytoplasmic autoantibody-associated pauci-immune glomerulonephritis and vasculitis, and other vasculitides. In Non-Neoplastic Renal Disease. Silver Springs, Md: ARP Press, 2005, pp 385–423.

66. Naoe S, Takahashi K, Masuda H, Tanaka N: Kawasaki disease. With particular emphasis on arterial lesions. Acta Pathol Jpn 1991;41:785–797.

67. Newburger JW, Takahashi M, Burns JC, et al: The treatment of Kawasaki syndrome with intravenous gammaglobulin. N Engl J Med 1986;315:341–347.

68. Burns JC, Glode MP: Kawasaki syndrome. Lancet 2004;364:533–544.

69. Watts RA, Scott DG: Epidemiology of the vasculitides. Semin Respir Crit Care Med 2004;25:455–464.

70. Maksimowicz-McKinnon K, Hoffman GS: Large-vessel vasculitis. Semin Respir Crit Care Med 2004;25:569–579.

71. Lagneau P, Michel JB: Renovascular hypertension and Takayasu's disease. J Urol 1985;134:876–879.

72. Yoshimura M, Kida H, Saito Y, et al: Peculiar glomerular lesions in Takayasu's arteritis. Clin Nephrol 1985;24:120–127.

73. Rapoport M, Averbukh Z, Chaim S, et al: Takayasu aortitis simulating bilateral renal-artery stenoses in patients treated with ACE inhibitors [letter]. Clin Nephrol 1991;36:156.

Lupus Nephritis

Gerald B. Appel and J. Stewart Cameron

INTRODUCTION AND DEFINITIONS

Lupus nephritis is a serious, but treatable, feature of systemic lupus erythematosus (lupus) that contributes significantly to patient morbidity and mortality.[1-4] Lupus itself is defined by a combination of clinical and laboratory features usually in combination with antibodies directed against one or more nuclear component, particularly double-stranded DNA (dsDNA). It is best regarded as a syndrome in which a number of different immune disturbances lead to a similar clinical picture in which immune complex–mediated damage plays a major component. The criteria of the American College of Rheumatology (ACR) for defining lupus have proven useful both for recruitment of patients into controlled trials and for epidemiologic studies (Fig. 24.1). Use of the ACR criteria excludes many patients with lupus-like conditions who should also be recognized and treated. Some patients, for example, those with membranous lupus nephropathy, may not fulfill four ACR criteria for a number of years into the course of the disease despite clear renal involvement. Some patients who fulfill fewer than four of the ACR criteria will have antiphospholipid antibodies (APAs) with associated thromboses, that is, the antiphospholipid syndrome rather than immune-complex deposition causing their renal disease.

American College of Rheumatology criteria for the diagnosis of lupus
The presence of four or more of the following criteria gives 96% sensitivity and specificity for the diagnosis of lupus:
1. Malar rash
2. Discoid rash
3. Photosensitivity
4. Oral ulcers
5. Nonerosive arthritis
6. Pleuropericarditis
7. Renal disease (proteinuria and/or granular casts)
8. Neurologic disorder (seizures or psychosis in the absence of precipitating circumstances)
9. Hematologic disorder (hemolytic anemia, leukopenia/lymphopenia, thrombocytopenia)
10. Positive LE cell preparation, raised anti-DNA antibody, anti-Sm present, false-positive antitreponemal test)
11. Positive fluorescent antinuclear antibody test

Figure 24.1   American College of Rheumatology criteria for the diagnosis of lupus.

ETIOLOGY AND PATHOGENESIS

Origins of Autoimmunity

Autoimmunity in lupus is probably the consequence of rather diverse pathogenetic events (see later discussion). In contrast to organ-specific autoimmunity such as antiglomerular basement membrane nephritis (see Chapter 22), lupus patients typically exhibit a wide variety of autoantibodies directed against nucleic acids and proteins concerned with intracellular transcriptional and translational machinery.[5] The main targets are nucleosomes (DNA histone) or even quaternary antigens on the chromatin itself, small nuclear ribonucleoproteins, and small cytoplasmic nuclear ribonucleoproteins. Polyclonal hyperactivity of the B cell system or defects of T cell autoregulation are likely primary events in lupus.[2,3,6-9] One hypothesis is that some autoreactive T cells survive thymic deletion and persist into adult life in a suppressed state, with the emergence of clones of autoreactive cells and autoantibodies and tissue damage if this suppression fails. A second hypothesis is that presentation of self-antigen (such as histone-derived peptides) to a mature immune system is capable of inducing germline mutations resulting in the production of new autoantibodies that are not adequately suppressed. A variant of this hypothesis is that viral or bacterial peptides contain sequences that are similar or identical to those of native antigens with which they cross-react: so-called antigenic mimicry. A third hypothesis is that there is nonspecific polyclonal B cell stimulation via superantigens, the resultant B cell repertoire including pathogenetic autoantibodies that again fail to be suppressed. A potential role of microorganisms in lupus flares would also explain the finding of type I interferonemia in lupus patients since not only immune complexes containing nucleic acid but also viral nucleic acid and CpG DNAs are potent interferon inducers. Activation of Toll-like receptors, components of the innate immune system, will also contribute to the net response and may result from DNA and RNA species as well as lipopolysaccharide.

Genetic factors are important in lupus with racial predilections, familial clustering, and monozygotic twins showing 25% concordance. In addition, healthy relatives of lupus patients may show antinuclear and other autoantibodies. Only weak major histocompatibility complex associations have been noted, but clear associations with genetic deficiencies of certain complement components, and FcγRIIIa receptor polymorphisms exist. Although certain medications may precipitate a lupus syndrome, such as hydralazine and procainamide, in general, renal disease is uncommon in these patients. Excess sun exposure, female hormones, and gender can influence the onset and course of the disease.

Spontaneous lupus has been studied in a number of animal models including mice such as the NZB B/W F1 hybrid and MRL-lpr.[2,6-9] Both have primary defects that lead to B cell proliferation, including defects in the Fas/APO-1-ligand system, which has a role in apoptosis. It is assumed in these animals that defective apoptosis leads to defective clonal deletion of self-reactive lymphocyte clones. In addition, lupus can be provoked in animal models by injecting autoantibodies against DNA or phospholipids or by inducing graft-versus-host disease, or by injection of peptides derived from the Smith (Sm) antigen.

Pathogenesis of Renal Injury

Patients with lupus nephritis typically have autoantibodies directed against dsDNA, Sm antigen, and C1q, but the pathogenetic role of these autoantibodies and the immune complexes derived from them has been debated.[5] Aggregates of immunoglobulin and complement components are present at the sites of glomerular damage and along the tubules in the majority of patients with active nephritis. Whether most are derived from precipitation of circulating immune complexes or from *in situ* formation is still unclear.[2] Deficiencies in the handling of immune complexes and other foreign antigens have been described at times in association with inheritance of specific HLA haplotypes (A1, DR3, B8) or Fc receptor polymorphisms (FcγRIIIa). Anti-dsDNA antibody has been eluted from human nephritic kidneys along with dsDNA and histone, and in animals, infusion of anti-dsDNA antibodies can cause proteinuria and renal disease. In some instances, dsDNA-dsDNA antibody components fix to DNA receptors on endothelial cells, while in others, histones appear to mediate binding to matrix and cells. The interstitial cellular infiltrates in lupus have an excess of CD8+ cytotoxic T lymphocytes over CD4 helper T lymphocytes, which differentiates them from patients with primary glomerulonephritis.

It remains unclear why only some lupus patients develop clinical renal disease and why only some of those develop severe proliferative lupus nephritis. Those with active nephritis typically have high titers of circulating anti-dsDNA antibodies. They also have high-avidity antibodies that activate complement strongly. Cationic antibodies and antibodies against C1q appear to be more frequent in patients with severe nephritis.

EPIDEMIOLOGY

The incidence, prevalence, and mortality of lupus are three to four times higher in African American females than in Caucasians, whereas the disease appears relatively rare in Africans, except perhaps in urban areas.[3,4] In the United Kingdom, lupus is twice as frequent in persons of East Asian descent as it is in Caucasians. The incidence of lupus in Asia is very variable and may depend more on ascertainment than true geographic differences. Gender is a major risk factor for the development of lupus with approximately 90% of adult patients being female. Although lupus is uncommon before puberty, childhood cases are well recognized.

CLINICAL MANIFESTATIONS

Lupus can affect virtually any organ (Fig. 24.2) and typically follows a course with periods of illness (flares) followed by periods of remission. Disease activity can be assessed reliably and reproducibly using the Systemic Lupus Erythematosus Disease Activity Index (SLEDAI), the British Isles Lupus Assessment Group (BILAG), or the Systemic Lupus Activity Measure (SLAM).

Renal Manifestations

Only 30% to 50% of patients with lupus have abnormalities of the urine or renal function early in their course[1-4,10] (see Fig. 24.2). Up

Most frequent clinical manifestations in patients with lupus		
Percent*	Site	Manifestation
100	—	Fever, weight loss
95	Musculoskeletal	Arthralgias, synovitis, arthritis
80	Serosa	Pleuritis, pericarditis
75	Skin	"Butterfly" facial rash, photodermatosis, alopecia
50	Hematologic	Anemia, leukopenia, thrombocytopenia, thromboses
50	Kidney	Proteinuria (100%), nephrotic syndrome (45%–65%)
		Granular casts (30%), red-cell casts (10%)
		Microhematuria (80%), macrohematuria (1%–2%)
		Reduced renal function (40%–80%), RPGN (30%), ARF (1%–2%)
		Hypertension (15%–50%)
		Hyperkalemia (15%)
		Tubular abnormalities (usually asymptomatic; 60%–80%)

Figure 24.2 Most frequent clinical manifestations in patients with lupus. *Percentage of patients. ARF, acute renal failure; RPGN, rapidly progressive glomerulonephritis.

to 60% of young adults and a greater percentage of children may develop abnormalities later. The dominant features are proteinuria, urinary sediment changes with microhematuria and erythrocyte casts, hypertension, and progressive renal dysfunction. The clinical findings correlate with histologic findings on biopsy (see later discussion). Renal tubular manifestations are also seen, including renal tubular acidosis (RTA) accompanied by either hypokalemia (type 1 RTA) or less commonly, in more severely affected patients, hyperkalemia (type 4 RTA). Some of the former patients may show nephrocalcinosis.

Extrarenal Manifestations

Many patients with lupus nephritis present with nonspecific complaints of malaise, low-grade fever, poor appetite, and weight loss. Patients may have alopecia, oral or nasal ulcerations, arthralgias or nondeforming arthritis, and various dermal findings including photosensitivity, Raynaud's phenomenon, and the classic "butterfly" facial rash.[1-4,10] Livedo reticularis is seen in up to 15% of cases and when associated with miscarriages or thrombocytopenia should suggest the presence of APA.[11-13] Neuropsychiatric involvement is one of the most serious extrarenal findings and can present with a variety of manifestations, including headache, which may be persistent and often migrainous; chorea; nerve palsies; frank coma; and psychoses. Serositis can present as pleuritis or pericarditis and affects up to 40% of patients. Pulmonary hypertension may result from multiple pulmonary emboli or intravascular coagulation in association with APA. Libman-Sacks endocarditis is usually detected with clinical findings and echocardiography. Splenomegaly and lymphadenopathy are present in about one fourth of patients.

Hematologic abnormalities are common in lupus patients and include anemia, leukopenia, and thrombocytopenia. The anemia may be due to impaired erythropoiesis, autoimmune hemolysis, or bleeding. Thromboses when present should prompt a search for APA and other procoagulant abnormalities.

DIAGNOSIS AND DIFFERENTIAL DIAGNOSIS

The diagnosis of lupus is usually obvious in a young female with systemic manifestations, nephritis, and the presence of serologic markers of disease. However, some patients, especially those with membranous lupus nephropathy, may present with renal disease as their initial manifestation. About 50% of lupus patients are initially suspected of having another disease prior to the correct diagnosis. The presence of four or more of the ACR criteria (see Fig. 24.1) carries 96% sensitivity and specificity for lupus.

Nephritis has been reported in a minority of patients with mixed connective tissue disease. Although the differential diagnosis can be difficult clinically, analysis for the presence of anti-Ro and anti-La antibodies and the absence of anti-dsDNA antibodies is helpful. Rheumatoid arthritis can be associated with mesangial proliferative glomerulonephritis, in particular IgA nephropathy, or renal disease due to AA amyloidosis. Although they rarely have the systemic manifestations of lupus patients, some older lupus patients will present with joint deformities typical of rheumatoid arthritis. Henoch-Schönlein purpura (HSP) may present with rash, systemic symptoms, arthritis, and nephritis. In contrast to the dominant or codominant IgA deposits of HSP, most lupus patients have a predominance of IgG and the presence of C1q on biopsy. Vasculitis, especially antineutrophil cytoplasmic antibody (ANCA)–positive rapidly progressive glomerulonephritis and cryoglobulinemia may be confused with lupus until the serologic and renal biopsy results confirm the correct diagnosis (see Chapters 20 and 23). Some patients will have the presence of ANCA as well as positive antinuclear antibody (ANA) or anti-dsDNA. If the renal biopsy does not have immune deposits they should be treated as other pauci-immune glomerulonephritis patients. Bacterial endocarditis with or without renal involvement (see Chapter 25) can also mimic lupus and is diagnosed based on bacteriologic findings.

Immunologic Tests in Lupus

A firm diagnosis of lupus nephritis should not be made without the presence of some ANA in the serum. ANA, particularly those against dsDNA, are present in up to 90% of untreated lupus patients.[5] Although a variety of tests for anti-dsDNA antibodies are available, most centers now rely on enzyme-linked immunosorbent assay. The presence of various patterns of ANA (e.g., diffuse, speckled) is not reliable in distinguishing lupus from similar rheumatologic diseases. Most lupus-like patients with negative ANA tests have no clinical renal disease. Many of the latter will be found to have APA.

Sm antibodies are strongly associated with the diagnosis of lupus and the presence of nephritis, but are present in only about 30% of patients. Hypocomplementemia is found at presentation in more than three fourths of untreated lupus patients. C3 and C4 either are mutually depressed or the C4 is preferentially depressed in lupus patients as opposed to patients with postinfectious glomerulonephritis and idiopathic membranoproliferative glomerulonephritis in which C3 is often preferentially depressed.

From one third to one half of lupus patients will have APA.[11–13] The double misnomer lupus anticoagulant activity is based on the presence of APA, directed mainly against the

β_2-globulin phospholipid carrier protein. These antibodies prolong phospholipid-dependent coagulation studies *in vitro* (activated partial thromboplastin time [APTT] and kaolin clotting time [KCT]) but *in vivo* are associated with thrombosis. The prolonged APTT and KCT are not corrected by mixing with normal plasma. The mechanisms for the thrombotic tendency remain unclear. APA have been associated with renal arterial, venous, and glomerular capillary thrombosis, Libman-Sacks endocarditis, cerebral thromboses, thrombocytopenia, pulmonary hypertension, frequent miscarriages, and livedo reticularis. Despite *in vitro* prolongation of the APTT and KCT, it is safe to do needle biopsies in the presence of APA. In contrast, prolonged APTT and KCT, which correct with admixture with normal plasma, suggest a true anticoagulant and require fresh-frozen plasma prior to biopsy.

PATHOLOGY

Lupus nephritis is pleomorphic and may affect every structure of the kidney. Adjacent glomeruli may show different degrees of involvement, and over time glomerular lesions may transform. Until recently, the World Health Organization (WHO) classification of lupus nephritis, last modified in 1995, was extensively accepted and used (Fig. 24.3).[14] More recently, a newer 2004 modification has led to the International Society of Nephrology (ISN)/Renal Pathology Society (RPS) classification, which refines and clarifies some of the deficiencies of the older WHO classifications[15] (see Fig. 24.3). As in the WHO classification, the ISN classification is based on light microscopy (LM) glomerular alterations integrated with immunofluorescence (IF) and electron microscopy (EM) findings. Several recent studies have confirmed the greater reproducibility of the new ISN classification versus the older WHO classification of lupus nephritis as well as its predictive value.[16] Moreover, the value of dividing ISN class IV into segmental lesions and global diffuse lesions has already been confirmed.

Pathology of Lupus Nephritis According to the International Society of Nephrology Classification

ISN class I (Fig. 24.4) denotes normal glomeruli by LM but with mesangial immune deposits by IF and EM. ISN class II (Fig. 24.5), mesangial proliferative lupus nephritis, is defined as pure mesangial hypercellularity (more than three mesangial cells in areas away from the vascular pole in 3-μm thick histologic sections) by LM with mesangial immune deposits. ISN class III (Fig. 24.6), focal lupus nephritis, is defined as focal segmental and/or global endocapillary and/or extracapillary glomerulonephritis affecting <50% of the total glomeruli sampled. ISN class IV (Fig. 24.7), diffuse lupus nephritis, has diffuse segmental and/or global endocapillary and/or extracapillary glomerulonephritis affecting ≥50% of glomeruli. Both class III and class IV have subendothelial immune deposits. The ISN classification subdivides lupus nephritis class IV into diffuse segmental versus diffuse global proliferation to facilitate future studies addressing possible differences in outcome and pathogenesis between these subgroups. Class IV-S is used if >50% of affected glomeruli have segmental lesions, while class IV-G is used if >50% of affected glomeruli have global lesions. Both class III and class IV may have active (proliferative), inactive (sclerosing), or combined active and inactive lesions subclassified as A, C, or A/C, respectively. ISN class V (Fig. 24.8), membranous lupus nephritis, is defined by subepithelial immune deposits. While the membranous alterations may be present alone or on a background of mesangial

293

Comparison of the WHO classification of lupus nephritis (LN) (1995) with the new ISN/PRS (2004) classification			
WHO, 1995		**ISN/RPS, 2004**	
Class	Definition	Class	Definition
I	Normal glomeruli (by LM, IF, EM)	I	Minimal mesangial LN Normal glomeruli by LM, but mesangial immune deposits by IF
II	Purely mesangial disease IIa: Normocellular mesangium by LM but mesangial deposits by IF and/or EM IIb: Mesangial hypercellularity with mesangial deposits by IF and/or EM	II	Mesangial proliferative LN Mesangial hypercellularity with mesangial immune deposits
III	Focal segmental proliferative glomerulonephritis (<50%)	III	Focal LN III (A): Purely active lesions: focal proliferative LN III (A/C): Active and chronic lesions: focal proliferative and sclerosing LN III (C): Chronic inactive lesions with glomerular scars: focal sclerosing LN
IV	Diffuse proliferative glomerulonephritis (50%)	IV	Diffuse LN IV-S (A) or IV-G (A): Purely active lesions: diffuse segmental (S) or global (G) proliferative LN IV-S (A/C) or IV-G (A/C): Active and chronic lesions: diffuse segmental or global proliferative and sclerosing LN IV-S (C) or IV-G (C): inactive with glomerular scars: diffuse segmental or global sclerosing LN
V	Membranous glomerulonephritis Va: pure membranous Vb: associated mild mesangial proliferation Vc: associated focal proliferative disease Vd: associated diffuse proliferative disease	V	Membranous LN
		VI	Advanced sclerosing LN 90% of glomeruli globally sclerosed without residual activity

Figure 24.3 Comparison of the World Health Organization (WHO) classification of lupus nephritis (LN) (1995) with the new International Society of Nephrology (ISN)/Renal Pathology Society (2004) classification. In the ISN classification, the distribution of hypercellularity is assessed as mesangial, endocapillary, or extracapillary (crescentic) and as focal (with <50% glomerular involvement) versus diffuse (with >50% glomeruli affected). The distribution of immune deposits by immunofluorescence (IF) and electron microscopy (EM) is judged as mesangial, subepithelial, and/or subendothelial. LM, light microscopy.

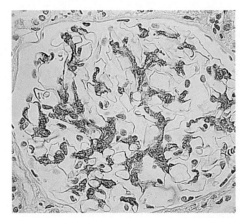

Figure 24.4 International Society of Nephology/Renal Pathology Society class I minimal mesangial lupus nephritis. Light microscopy is normal, but immunoperoxidase shows C1q localization (associated with IgG and C3) throughout the mesangial area.

classification, class VI (Fig. 24.9), advanced sclerosing lupus nephritis, is defined by global glomerular sclerosis affecting >90% of glomeruli.

On IF, IgG is almost always the dominant immunoglobulin, and early complement components such as C4 and especially C1q are usually present along with C3. The presence of all three immunoglobulins, IgG, IgA, and IgM, along with the two

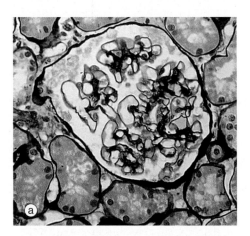

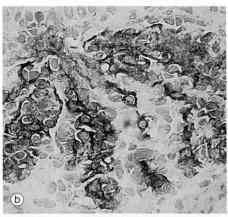

Figure 24.5 International Society of Nephrology/Renal Pathology Society class II lupus nephritis (mesangial disease). *a,* Mesangial expansion but little increase in tuft cellularity; the peripheral capillary walls are normal (silver methenamine stain). *b,* Extensive mesangial IgG deposits shown by immunoperoxidase; the aggregates are just beginning to invade peripheral capillary walls.

hypercellularity and immune deposits, patients with additional true focal or diffuse proliferative lesions and subendothelial immune-complex deposition are no longer classified as Vc or Vd, as in the older WHO classification. These would be classified as V + III and V + IV under the ISN classification. Under the ISN

complement components C1q and C3 is known as "full-house" staining (after the poker hand!). It is highly suggestive of lupus nephritis, as is strong C1q staining. Fibrin is often present in the glomerular tuft and especially in crescents.

On EM, the distribution of immune deposits corresponds to that of IF. Some electron-dense deposits have an organized substructure known as "fingerprinting" corresponding to the presence of curvilinear microtubular or fibrillar structures composed of bands ranging from 10 to 15 nm in diameter.

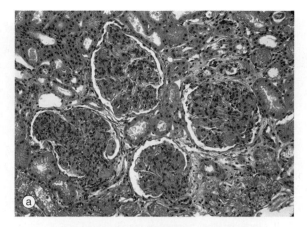

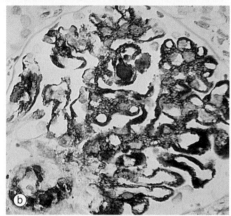

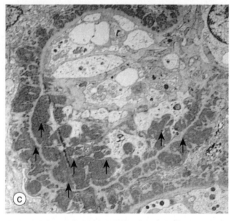

Figure 24.7 International Society of Nephrology/Renal Pathology Society class IV lupus nephritis. *a,* active diffuse proliferative lupus nephritis. *b,* By immunoperoxidase staining, there are dense irregular aggregates of IgG along the peripheral capillary walls. *c,* Electron microscopy reveals the immune aggregates as electron-dense deposits (*arrows*) predominantly in the subendothelial location.

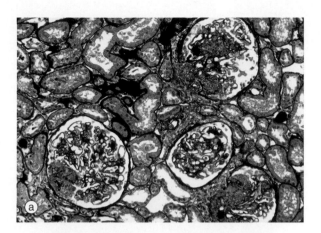

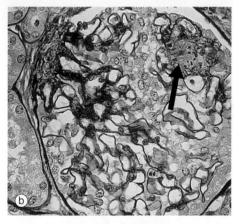

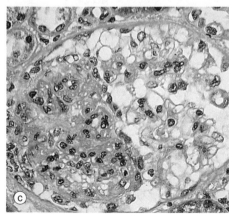

Figure 24.6 International Society of Nephrology/Renal Pathology Society class III focal proliferative lupus nephritis. *a,* Low power showing focal and segmental proliferative lesion: active (class III A) with <50% glomeruli affected (hematoxylin and eosin). *b,* An area of focal necrosis containing cellular debris, karyorrhexis (*arrow*) is surrounded by an area of cellular proliferation (silver methenamine/hematoxylin eosin). *c,* A major focal and segmental proliferative lesion affecting almost half of the glomerular capillary tuft (hematoxylin/ lissamine green).

Tubuloreticular inclusions, 24-nm interanastomosing tubular structures located in the dilated cisternae of the endoplasmic reticulum of renal endothelial cells, are often found in biopsies of patients with lupus nephritis.

Tubulointerstitial and Vascular Disease

Although most classifications of lupus nephritis are based on the degree of glomerular involvement, histologic and clinical involvement of other renal compartments is not rare in lupus

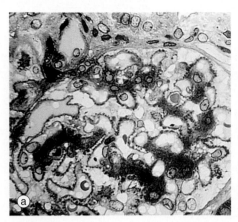
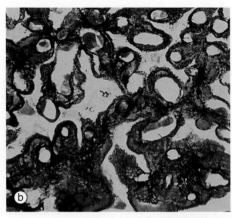
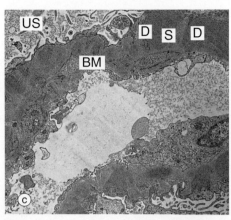

Figure 24.8 International Society of Nephrology/Renal Pathology Society class V: membranous lupus. *a*, A thick (~0.5 μm) araldite-embedded section stained with toludine blue, showing not only the extra-membranous material in dark blue, but also the presence of mesangial deposits, which are common in lupus membranous nephropathy. *b*, A silver methenamine–stained section showing some double contouring of the silver-positive basement membrane and subendothelial-desposited material as well as the characteristic silver-positive spikes of basement membrane–like material. *c*, An electron microphotograph showing the predominantly subepithelial electron-dense deposits (D) separated by protrusions of basement membrane material (spikes [S]). BM, basement membrane.

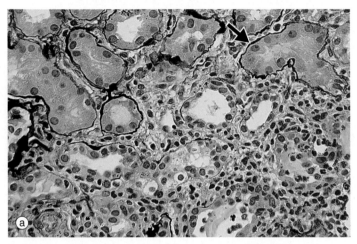
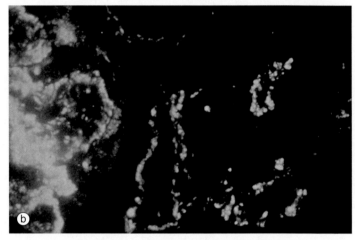

Figure 24.9 Interstitial lupus nephritis. *a*, Interstitial infiltrate invading and destroying tubules (tubulitis). The tubular basement membrane (TBM), stained black with silver (*arrow*), is digested (see the lower half of *a*). *b*, Immunofluorescence showing aggregates of C3 in the TBM (*right*) as well as within the glomerulus (*left*). Such TBM aggregates are common in lupus nephritis, being found in 60% to 65% of biopsy specimens overall and with increasing frequency from class II (20%) to class IV (75%).

patients.[2,17,18] In about 50% of patients with nephritis, predominantly those with proliferative glomerular lesions, immune aggregates are found along the tubular basement membranes. Interstitial infiltrates mainly of CD4+ and CD8+ T lymphocytes and monocytes are commonly found. In active disease, infiltration and invasion of the tubules (tubulitis) are found, while in chronic disease, the interstitium is expanded by fibrosis and sparser infiltrates. Interstitial inflammation has been correlated with renal dysfunction and hypertension, while immune deposition along the tubular basement membrane correlates better with the presence of a high anti-dsDNA titer and depressed serum complement level. In some patients, tubulointerstitial nephritis is seen in the absence of glomerular disease and may produce acute renal failure or renal tubular acidosis.

A number of vascular lesions may be seen in lupus patients[18] (Fig. 24.10). True vasculitis is extremely rare. More commonly, there are vascular immune deposits seen by IF or EM or a fibrinoid noninflammatory necrotizing lesion of the vessels in patients with severe proliferative nephritis or a thrombotic microangiopathy. The latter is most often found in patients who are APA positive with prior evidence of coagulation events.

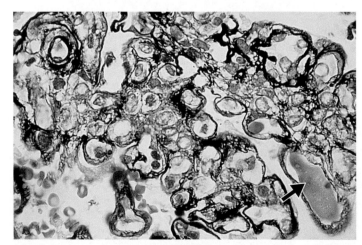

Figure 24.10 Vascular damage in lupus nephritis. Thrombus (*arrow*) occludes a glomerular capillary loop in this class IV biopsy. Such a thrombus contains platelets and cross-linked fibrin as well as immunoglobulins and thus has some characteristics of true thrombus. Note also the subepithelial aggregates, spike formation, and double contouring of the capillary walls, all typical of class IV and active class III biopsies (silver methenamine/hematoxylin).

Transformation of Histologic Appearance and Silent Lupus Nephritis

Serial biopsy specimens show that transformation of histologic glomerular class is quite frequent.[4] Some patients with increased clinical activity will transform from a more benign or less proliferative class (ISN class II or V) to a more proliferative lesion (ISN class III or IV). This is often heralded by increasing proteinuria and active urinary sediment. With successful treatment, other patients will transform from a proliferative class (ISN class III or IV) to a more predominant membranous pattern (ISN class V).

Extremely uncommon patients have active proliferative lupus nephritis on biopsy but no clinical or urinary sediment changes to indicate active disease and normal anti-dsDNA and serum complement levels.[2] If the urine sediment is carefully checked, most patients with proliferative lesions will have microhematuria and often erythrocyte casts.

Clinical Histopathologic Correlations and Other Correlates of Outcome

In general, the clinical correlates of the new ISN classification system are similar to those of the older WHO classification system.

ISN class I patients usually have no evidence of clinical renal disease. Likewise, ISN class II patients may have an elevated anti-DNA antibody titer or low serum complement, but, in general, urinary sediment is inactive, hypertension is infrequent, the glomerular filtration rate (GFR) is preserved, and proteinuria is rarely >1 g/24 h. Patients with either class I or II biopsy specimens have an excellent renal prognosis unless they transform to another pattern. An exception to this presentation is lupus patients who present with minimal change nephrotic syndrome or lupus podocytopathy.[19] They have the sudden onset of nephrotic syndrome with renal biopsy specimens showing only class I or II changes along with extensive foot process effacement.

Patients with active ISN class III A or A/C often have microhematuria, hypertension, and proteinuria. Up to one third of patients will have the nephrotic syndrome and up to one quarter an elevated serum creatinine at renal biopsy. Patients with focal glomerular scarring (ISN class IIIC) have hypertension and reduced renal function but without active urinary sediment. Patients with mild proliferation in only a few glomeruli generally respond well to therapy with <5% progressing to renal failure over 5 years of follow-up. Others with more glomerular involvement or with necrotizing features and crescent formation have a prognosis similar to that of class IVA patients. In one study, patients with severe focal proliferative class III lesions actually fared worse than those with diffuse proliferative class IV lesions.[20]

Patients with ISN class IVA classically have high serologic activity along with active urinary sediment, hypertension, and heavy proteinuria. The GFR is usually reduced. Class IV diffuse proliferative disease still carries the worst renal prognosis in most series, although this is greatly influenced by prognostic features such as racial background, socioeconomic factors, and renal features at presentation. Patients with segmental diffuse proliferative class IVS fare worse than those with diffuse global involvement class IVG.

ISN class V patients typically present with proteinuria and features of the nephrotic syndrome. However, at biopsy, up to 40% will have subnephrotic proteinuria and up to 20% less than 1 g/24 h of proteinuria. Patients with ISN class V typically have less clinical renal and serologic activity. Some develop what appears to be idiopathic nephrotic syndrome before developing other features of lupus. ISN class V patients are predisposed to thrombotic complications such as renal vein thrombosis and pulmonary emboli.[18] Ten-year renal survival rates in class V patients are 75% to 85%.

Advanced sclerotic lupus nephritis, ISN class VI, is usually the result of burnt-out class III or IV lupus nephritis. Many patients will, nevertheless, have persistent microhematuria and some proteinuria along with hypertension and a decreased GFR.

Other Histologic Prognostic Factors

Some investigators have found that features of reversible (active) or irreversible (chronic) damage on biopsy can predict the course of lupus nephritis patients. Those with a higher activity index or chronicity index score (calculated by scoring on each biopsy specimen the various histologic features of activity and chronicity and adding the scores) were more likely to progress to renal failure.[3,4] Other groups have not been able to confirm that such classifications are either reproducible or accurate in predicting prognosis.[21] However, most studies do confirm the poor prognosis of patients whose biopsies show extensive glomerulosclerosis and/or interstitial fibrosis.[2,17,22] Likewise, patients with high degrees of both activity and chronicity on biopsy specimens (activity index score >7 + chronicity index score >3) fare badly as do those with the combination of cellular crescents and interstitial fibrosis on biopsy. Likewise, certain histologic features found on repeat renal biopsy at 6 months predict 5-year progression to renal failure including ongoing inflammation with cellular crescents and macrophages in the tubular lumens, persistent immune deposits (especially C3), and persistent subendothelial and mesangial deposits.[23] The finding of both crescents and interstitial fibrosis persisting on the 6-month biopsy led to a very poor renal outcome.

NATURAL HISTORY

The clinical course of lupus can no longer be considered separately from the results of treatment. Fifty years ago, few patients with severe grade IV nephritis survived more than a year or two, and half of those with even less severe forms of nephritis used to die within 5 years. However, spontaneous remissions of lupus nephritis can occur: in the 1960s, 68 unbiopsied patients with lupus and proteinuria (some nephrotic) were left untreated; in 16 cases (28%), the proteinuria became intermittent or disappeared spontaneously.

In most patients today, there is a gratifying response to early treatment, followed by relatively quiescent disease under continuing immunosuppression that can be tapered off eventually without further relapse (Fig. 24.11). Another common pattern is the quiescent patient who suddenly relapses. The frequency of relapse depends not only on the underlying disease but on the intensity and duration of immunosuppression.

End-stage renal disease (ESRD) now affects 8% to 15% of patients with lupus nephritis. Rare patients with ESRD may regain enough renal function to terminate dialysis. A renal biopsy is often useful to determine whether the disease is still active and potentially treatable or chronic with irreversible renal scarring. In dialysed lupus patients, fatal infections are the usual cause of death. Infection also remains the most commonly reported cause of early death in those without ESRD, although retrospective reports may not reflect current practice. Extrarenal disease is the next most common cause of early death, particularly affecting the central nervous system or lung. Overall, however, almost half of

Survival in lupus and lupus nephritis

Period	5-Year Survival (percent)*		
	All Lupus	Lupus Nephritis	Class IV Nephritis
1953–1969	49	44	17
1970–1979	82	67	55
1980–1989	86	82	80
1990–1995	92	82	82

Figure 24.11 Survival in lupus and lupus nephritis. Five-year actuarial survival for lupus, lupus nephritis, and World Health Organization class IV nephritis over the past 40 years. *Weighted mean of published series.

all lupus deaths are the result of excess cardiovascular mortality, often later in the course of the disease and particularly from premature myocardial ischemia.

Apart from the histological outcome predictors discussed previously, there has been considerable controversy over which epidemiologic and clinical features influence outcome in lupus nephritis.[24–27] Some suggested adverse prognostic findings include African American descent, high activity on the biopsy specimen, presence of crescents, high baseline serum creatinine or greater baseline proteinuria, younger age (younger than 24 years old), hypertension, delay in therapy, and low socioeconomic status. Of these, African American descent has been a universal predictor of poorer outcome in multiple series.[24–27] Most ongoing studies now stratify patients according to racial background to avoid biased results.

The principal useful predictor among laboratory tests is anemia, with thrombocytopenia, hypocomplementemia, and increased DNA binding at onset all correlated with a poorer outcome.

TREATMENT

In recent years, it is clear that disease activity can be suppressed in the majority of patients. However, the toxicity of the regimens used has often limited the utility of treatment regimens. It is useful to divide the treatment of patients with lupus nephritis with other than minor disease into an induction and a maintenance phase. The induction phase of treatment typically deals with severe, acute life-threatening disease, often affecting many systems and usually near the onset of disease; here the threat of the disease is paramount. Then follows the maintenance treatment and long-term management of chronic, more or less indolent disease. Here protection from the side effects of treatment while preventing relapse becomes increasingly important.

Use of the older WHO and the current ISN/RPS biopsy classification (see Fig. 24.3) can also serve as a guide to therapy.[3,4] In general, patients with ISN class I and II need no therapy directed at the kidney. Whether treatment with corticosteroids or other immunosuppressive agents at this point might prevent subsequent evolution to severe disease in the future is unknown. The majority of patients will have a benign long-term outcome, and the potential toxicity of any immunosuppressive regimen will negatively alter the risk-to-benefit ratio of treatment. An exception is the group of recently described lupus patients with minimal change syndrome or lupus podocytopathy (see previous discussion). These patients respond to a short course of high-dose corticosteroids in a fashion similar to patients with minimal change disease.[19]

It is in the groups of patients with active focal proliferative lupus nephritis (ISN class IIIA and IIIA/C), active diffuse proliferative lupus nephritis (ISN class IV A and IV A/C), and membranous lupus (ISN class V) that immunosuppression is most widely used.

Treatment of Proliferative Lupus Nephritis: Induction Phase
Corticosteroids

Many clinicians treat all patients with active proliferative lupus nephritis with high doses of corticosteroids. These have typically been used alone in the past and more commonly with other immunosuppressives in recent studies. High-dose oral regimens (e.g., prednisone starting dose 60 mg/day) as well as pulsed intravenous methylprednisolone infusions (0.5–1.0 g/day for 1 to 3 days) followed by lower doses of oral corticosteroids have been used since early nonrandomized data did suggest a benefit from higher treatment doses. Both oral and intravenous regimens carry a significant risk of side effects. Cosmetic effects, risk of gastrointestinal ulceration, hypertension, psychoses, and an enhanced risk of infectious complications have all led to attempts to minimize prolonged courses of corticosteroid therapy in lupus patients. Some small trials suggested that intravenous pulsed therapy is either more effective or less toxic than high-dose oral therapy.

Cytotoxic Agents

Cytotoxic agents in conjunction with corticosteroids play a major role in most induction therapies for lupus nephritis.[28,29] Cyclophosphamide is a powerful inhibitor of B cells as well as other phases of the immune response. Whether oral therapy or intravenous-pulse cyclophosphamide is more effective in treating the nephritis remains inconclusive,[29] but the latter is presumed to produce less toxicity.

Trials at the National Institutes of Health (NIH) in the United States initially established a role for intravenous pulses of cyclophosphamide every third month in preventing renal failure in patients with diffuse proliferative lupus nephritis. Subsequent randomized, controlled trials in patients with severe proliferative lupus nephritis[30] established that six pulses of intravenous cyclophosphamide (0.5 to 1 g/m^2) on consecutive months followed by follow-up pulses every third month along with low-dose corticosteroids were effective and prevented relapses better than a shorter regimen limited to six doses. A subsequent controlled trial established that pulsed cyclophosphamide when given with monthly pulses of methylprednisolone leads to better long-term GFR than either regimen alone.[31] Long-term follow-up of these patients showed that the regimen of intravenous pulsed cyclophosphamide plus methylprednisolone had no more side effects than the regimen using pulses of cyclophosphamide alone. This in part may have been due to fewer relapses and greater initial efficacy of the prior regimen leading to less need for retreatment in the follow-up period. Nevertheless, side effects were significant (see later discussion) in both therapeutic arms of this study.[31] A recent study used intravenous cyclophosphamide to induce remissions in 59 patients with severe lupus nephritis, almost one half of whom were African American, with a mean serum creatinine of 1.6 mg/dl (140 μmol/l) and an average urinary protein-to-creatinine ratio >5.[32] With six to eight monthly intravenous doses, 83% had a remission, with a mean creatinine reduction from 1.59 to 0.97 mg/dl (140 to 85 μmol/l), mean urinary protein-to-creatinine ratio decreasing from 5.1 to 1.7, and correction of hypertension and serologic abnormalities. It is clear that cyclophosphamide is effective in induction therapy, and studies using newer agents have focused on achieving this high induction response rate with fewer side effects.

A recent trial by the Euro-Lupus Group tried to decrease the risk of side effects from cyclophosphamide therapy without sacrificing efficacy.[33] This study randomized 90 patients with diffuse or focal proliferative or membranous plus proliferative disease to receive either a standard six monthly pulses of cyclophosphamide followed by infusions every third month or to a shorter treatment course consisting of 500 mg intravenously every 2 weeks for six total doses and then switching to azathioprine maintenance therapy. Both regimens were equally effective in various renal and extrarenal outcomes. The shorter regimen had less toxicity with significantly fewer and less severe infections as a complication of treatment. This trial was largely performed in Caucasians and may not be applicable to all populations at high risk of poor renal outcomes.

Mycophenolate Mofetil

Several recent controlled trials have examined the role of mycophenolate mofetil (MMF) in the induction of remission of severe lupus nephritis.[34–36] One in a Chinese population evaluated 42 patients randomized to receive either 12 months of oral MMF (2 g/day for 6 months followed by 1 g/day for 6 months) or 6 months of oral cyclophosphamide (2.5 mg/kg/day) followed by oral azathioprine (1.5 mg/kg/day) for 6 months.[34] Both groups received concomitant tapering doses of corticosteroids. At 12 months, the number of complete or partial remissions and relapses was not different between the regimens. There were fewer infections in the MMF arm, and all mortality was in the cyclophosphamide group (0 versus 10%). Longer follow-up confirmed the long-term benefits of the MMF group.[37] A second trial, also in a Chinese population, evaluated 46 patients treated with either pulse intravenous cyclophosphamide or MMF for 6 months.[35] Patients treated with MMF had greater reductions in proteinuria, hematuria, anti-DNA antibody titer, and greater improvement found on renal biopsy.

Another trial examined 140 patients with proliferative lupus nephritis.[36] One half was randomized to intravenous cyclophosphamide monthly pulses and one half to MMF in conjunction with a fixed tapering dose of corticosteroids as induction therapy over 6 months. The study included >50% African Americans and allowed crossover at 3 months for treatment failures. Complete remissions at 6 months were significantly more common in the MMF arm as were complete plus partial remissions. Side effect profile was better in the MMF group. At 3 years, there were no significant differences in numbers of patients with renal failure, ESRD, or mortality. A large international multicenter trial of induction therapy with either MMF or monthly intravenous cyclophosphamide is under way and should help to resolve present uncertainties.[38] In the meantime, we recommend MMF as the first choice for a cytotoxic agent during the induction phase (Fig. 24.12).

Other Agents

A number of other therapeutic interventions have been directed at blockade of specific areas of the immune response in attempts to induce remissions in patients with lupus nephritis. Plasma exchange has been added to other induction therapies, for example, cyclophosphamide, in several controlled, randomized trials. There has been no benefit in terms of renal or patient survival or in reduction of proteinuria or improvement of GFR. Intravenous gamma globulin has given encouraging results as adjunct therapy for patients with severe lupus and nephritis, although it has not been studied in adequately powered controlled trials. A major problem is that there is no standard preparation of intravenous IgG, even from a single manufacturer, and hence no dose can be recommended generally. Moreover, a decrease in GFR may be seen during administration that is not always reversible.

For patients with life-threatening resistant disease, small pilot studies have used total lymphoid irradiation and marrow ablation with or without reconstitution with allogenic stem cells. These approaches are experimental at this time and have potentially high toxicity.

Early studies of monoclonal antibodies directed against B and T cell costimulation (anti–CD 40 ligand) have proved unsuccessful, in part due to lack of efficacy and in part due to thrombotic complications. New trials using CTLA4Ig to block T and B cell

Figure 24.12 Treatment of severe proliferative lupus nephritis (International Nephrology Society [ISN] class III A or IIIA/C or ISN class IVA or IV A/C). ACE, angiotensin-converting enzyme; ARB, angiotensin receptor blocker; MMF, mycophenolate mofetil.

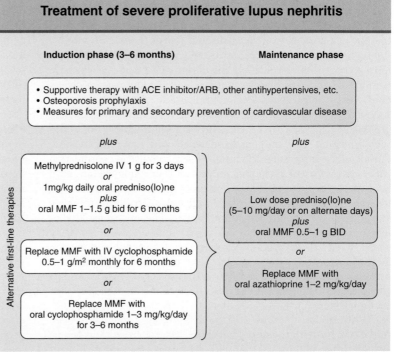

Treatment of severe proliferative lupus nephritis

Induction phase (3–6 months)   Maintenance phase

- Supportive therapy with ACE inhibitor/ARB, other antihypertensives, etc.
- Osteoporosis prophylaxis
- Measures for primary and secondary prevention of cardiovascular disease

plus   *plus*

Methylprednisolone IV 1 g for 3 days
or
1mg/kg daily oral predniso(lo)ne
plus
oral MMF 1–1.5 g bid for 6 months

Low dose predniso(lo)ne
(5–10 mg/day or on alternate days)
plus
oral MMF 0.5–1 g BID

or

Replace MMF with IV cyclophosphamide
0.5–1 g/m² monthly for 6 months

or

Replace MMF with
oral azathioprine 1–2 mg/kg/day

or

Replace MMF with
oral cyclophosphamide 1–3 mg/kg/day
for 3–6 months

Alternative first-line therapies

costimulation are under way. In uncontrolled, nonrandomized trials of small numbers of patients, rituximab, a monoclonal antibody directed against CD19 and CD20 B cells, has proven useful in inducing remissions in some patients with severe lupus nephritis including some who have failed cyclophosphamide or MMF therapy.[39] It is currently being studied in a multicenter, controlled, randomized U.S. trial.[40] Other new medications that block other areas of the immune response such as anti-BLyS are being studied as well.

Treatment of Proliferative Lupus Nephritis: Maintenance Therapy

In most patients, acute renal disease will come under control by 3 months of therapy. By 6 months, almost all responders will have improving serologic markers (anti-DNA antibody titer, serum complement), improvement of GFR, and a decrease in proteinuria. Persistent but decreasing levels of proteinuria or some urinary sediment abnormalities at 6 months are not rare and do not indicate disease activity. The challenges once remission has been induced is to avoid relapse and flares of disease activity, to avoid smoldering activity leading to chronic irreversible renal scarring, and to prevent long-term side effects of therapy. A number of agents have been studied in maintenance regimens for lupus nephritis patients after induction therapy.

Corticosteroids are a major component of treatment in the maintenance phase of lupus nephritis therapy. There are no studies that exclude the use of steroids in maintenance therapy. To minimize the side effects of long-term corticosteroids, the dose should be limited (e.g., predniso(lo)ne 5 to 15 mg/day) and osteoporosis prophylaxis should be given concomitantly (see Fig. 24.12). Both daily and alternate-day regimens have been used.

A number of meta-analyses unequivocally favor the additional benefit of using a cytotoxic agent during the maintenance phase of lupus nephritis therapy. In long-term trials at the NIH, there was less renal scarring in those who received an additional cytotoxic agent. More than 10 to 15 years of follow-up regimens of either intravenous cyclophosphamide, oral cyclophosphamide, or oral cyclophosphamide plus oral azathioprine showed less progression of renal scarring than regimens using either prednisone or azathioprine alone.

While oral cyclophosphamide has been used for induction therapy in a number of trials, its use for longer than 3 to 6 months should be avoided due to toxicity. Alopecia is especially unpleasant for the young lupus population. Bladder toxicity, which can include hemorrhagic cystitis, bladder scarring, and bladder cancer, occurs rarely with intravenous cyclophosphamide administered with adequate hydration. However, intravenous cyclophosphamide, like prolonged daily oral treatment, carries a considerable dose- and age-dependent risk of gonadal damage and early menopause. Timing of the intravenous cyclophosphamide pulse in coordination with the menstrual cycle and the use of leuprolide acetate have been attempted, but infertility remains a major complication in all women older than the age of 30 and especially those receiving longer than a 6-month induction course. The oncogenic risk of regimens including alkylating agents may not be evident for many years. Clearly, the risk of infection and marrow suppression increases with the extended use of more aggressive immunosuppression. Chlorambucil is rarely used in lupus patients because its gonadal and oncogenic properties, if anything, are greater than cyclophosphamide.

Azathioprine in doses of 1 to 2.5 mg/kg/24 h has proven remarkably safe in the very long term. Macrocytosis, leukopenia at high doses, and interaction with allopurinol making it difficult to use in patients with gout are all potential side effects along with the ever-present risk of infection from immunosuppression. Pancreatitis and hepatotoxicity are rare side effects of treatment. Azathioprine has only a small oncogenic potential, and pregnancy during maintenance azathioprine is relatively safe. Two recent studies used azathioprine successfully as maintenance therapy after induction with a short or long course of cyclophosphamide.[32,33]

MMF has been used to maintain remission after induction therapy with the drug in a number of lupus trials.[32,37] Moreover, in a one study, azathioprine and MMF both proved superior in maintaining remissions and preventing mortality or ESRD than did continued intravenous cyclophosphamide every third month.[32] Major side effects (including hospitalized days, amenorrhea, and severe infections) were all significantly less in the group receiving the oral agents. MMF therapy carries the risk of immunosuppression and infection and gastrointestinal side effects. At present, MMF is far more expensive than azathioprine therapy.

Cyclosporine has been used with limited success as monotherapy for maintenance of remissions in patients with proliferative lupus nephritis. It has a greater role in the treatment of membranous lupus in reducing proteinuria and in combination with other medications to maintain remission of proliferative lupus. Nephrotoxicity, hypertension, hyperuricemia, and hyperkalemia are all potential adverse side effects. Tacrolimus has similar toxicities and has been used in limited trials in lupus nephritis.

Several studies have been conducted with a designer molecule composed of a polyglycol platform and four DNA side chains, LJP 394, to try to prevent flares of lupus nephritis.[41] Although anti-DNA antibody titers decreased, it still remains unclear whether the drug can actually prevent flares of disease activity.

A summary of disease-specific maintenance treatments is given in Figure 24.12 for both induction and maintenance phases of treatment of severe proliferative lupus nephritis. General renoprotective measures such as the use of angiotensin-converting enzyme inhibitors and/or angiotensin receptor blockers, the use of statins for both their lipid-lowering and pleiotropic effects, and optimal blood pressure control can all reduce morbidity in the lupus nephritis population. Other agents used to treat extrarenal findings in lupus patients, including nonsteroidal drugs, antimalarial drugs, androgens, and fish oils, have not shown benefit in nephritis. The majority of patients will be maintained in remission by such treatment, but in a few cases, the initial disease is so severe that it does not come under control and/or frequent early relapses are seen. An approach to the management of such patients is summarized in Figure 24.13.

Membranous Lupus Nephropathy

In the past, investigators reported very different renal survival rates for different populations with membranous lupus nephropathy. In part this was due to problems with the WHO classification since renal survival in WHO class Va and Vb (see Fig. 24.3) was 75%, 59% for Vc patients, and 18% for Vd patients >5 years.[42] Moreover, patients with subnephrotic proteinuria and pure membranous lupus nephropathy do extremely well regardless of treatment options, and no consensus of management has emerged yet for this group of patients.

In a controlled trial, 42 patients with lupus WHO class Va and Vb only were randomized to receive either monthly pulses of intravenous cyclophosphamide, oral cyclosporine, or oral prednisone for 1 year.[43] The patients had preserved GFR, but a mean proteinuria of almost 6 g/day. At the last follow-up, there were more complete and partial remissions in the cyclophosphamide

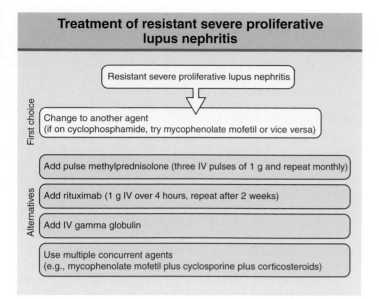

Figure 24.13   Treatment of resistant severe proliferative lupus nephritis.

and cyclosporine groups than in the prednisone group. Remissions occurred more quickly in the cyclosporine group, but there were fewer relapses in the cyclophosphamide group. Patients who relapsed or failed to respond to cyclosporine could subsequently be brought into remission with intravenous cyclophosphamide. In a 140-patient induction trial in the United States, 27 patients had pure membranous lupus nephropathy.[44] Remissions, relapses, and courses were similar in the patients treated with oral MMF and intravenous cyclophosphamide induction therapy. Azathioprine

along with corticosteroids has also been successful in some populations with membranous lupus.

Thus, for patients with membranous nephropathy who have subnephrotic levels of proteinuria and a preserved GFR, we recommend (Fig. 24.14) either a short course of cyclosporine or corticosteroids along with angiotensin-converting enzyme inhibitor and/or angiotensin receptor blocker and a statin. For fully nephrotic patients and those at higher risk of progressive disease, there are multiple treatment options: a course of oral cyclosporine, monthly intravenous pulses of cyclophosphamide, MMF, or azathioprine plus corticosteroids. In all these options, the course will have to be at least 6 months and avoiding side effects is paramount.

Remissions and Relapses

Achieving a remission of lupus nephritis predicts an improved long-term outcome. In one study, the 5-year patient and renal survival rates were 95% and 94%, respectively, for the group achieving remission and only 69% and 45%, respectively, for the group not achieving remission.[24]

Predictors of remission included lower baseline serum creatinine, lower baseline urinary protein excretion, better renal histologic class by the WHO/ISN classification, lower chronicity index, stable GFR after 4 weeks of therapy, and Caucasian race.

The relapse rate for lupus nephritis has ranged from 35% to almost 60%, depending on which population is studied, what criteria for relapse are used, and what maintenance therapy is used.[45-47] Elevation of the anti-DNA antibody titer and decline in the serum complement levels may presage relapse. However, a number of patients maintain elevated anti-DNA antibody titers for years without relapse, and most clinicians prefer not to treat serologic activity alone in the absence of clinical disease activity. A

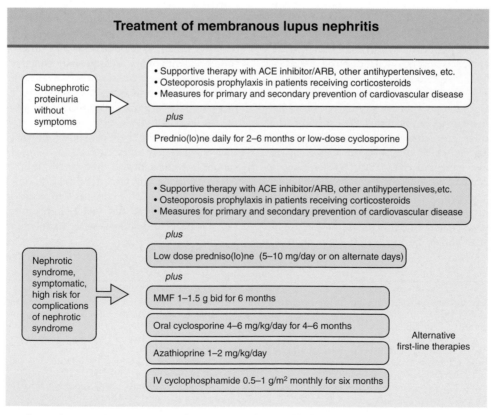

Figure 24.14   Treatment of membranous lupus nephritis (International Society of Nephrology class V). ACE, angiotensin-converting enzyme; ARB, angiotensin receptor blocker; MMF, mycophenolate mofetil.

major value of a normal anti-DNA titer is to permit safe reduction of treatment during the chronic phase of maintenance therapy.

When Can Treatment for Lupus Nephritis Be Stopped?

The goal of long-term management in patients with lupus nephritis is suppression of disease with minimum side effects of treatment. While normal results from immunologic tests and urinary sediment examination may be helpful, a repeat renal biopsy will be useful in some patients to clarify whether a slow decrease in GFR is the result of persistent active glomerular disease or of secondary sclerosis.

While some patients will relapse many years after remission and disease quiescence, it is often possible to stop treatment entirely in many patients after ≥5 years when the disease process has apparently "burned out." Stable GFR, lack of proteinuria, and normal immunologic tests predict successful discontinuation of immunosuppressives. It is clear that results will be different for populations of different backgrounds and different initial presentations.

Antiphospholipid Antibodies and Atherosclerotic and Other Complications

A significant percentage of lupus patients will have some form of APA detectable.[11-13,29,48] Very high titer IgG isotypes increase the likelihood of thrombotic episodes. Prophylactic anticoagulation is generally not given since many patients remain antibody positive without ever having a coagulation event. If thrombosis occurs, therapy with warfarin is instituted as long as the APA persists. Many clinicians aim for an international normalized ratio of 2.5 to 3.0 to prevent further clotting but also to avoid excessive anticoagulation with bleeding episodes that require discontinuation of the anticoagulation and carry the highest risk of subsequent thrombosis. Disappearance of APA is unusual despite complete clinical remissions with immunosuppressives and normalization of the anti-DNA antibody titer and other immunologic markers.

Lupus patients with the nephrotic syndrome, and especially those with membranous lupus and heavy proteinuria, are at risk of renal vein thrombosis.[18] Anticoagulation in such patients is discussed in Chapter 19.

As the treatment and survival of lupus patients have improved,[49] active organ involvement by lupus itself and infectious complications of treatment are being replaced by atherosclerotic complications as leading causes of morbidity and mortality.[50,51] Patients with lupus have increased risk of atherosclerotic complications when compared to age-matched controls and greater atherosclerotic plaque burden. Patients with active lupus have abnormalities of numerous cardiovascular risk factors including hyperlipidemia, hypertension, and systemic inflammation. Reduction of atherosclerotic risk should be focused on tight control of

blood pressure (to 130/80 mm Hg), use of statins to correct lipid abnormalities, and suppression of active inflammatory disease activity.

Pregnancy in some lupus patients has been associated with flares of lupus activity either in the third trimester or shortly after delivery (see Chapter 42). Recent studies suggest that oral contraceptive use is not associated with increased severe or mild/moderate flares of disease activity.[52] The use of hormone replacement therapy has only been associated with a small increase in the incidence of mild to moderate flares of disease.[53]

Osteoporosis and avascular necrosis of bone have become important long-term health issues for many lupus patients. Minimizing the use of corticosteroids, especially the maintenance dose, and use of vitamin D and calcium supplements along with other agents to reduce bone loss is important.

End-Stage Renal Disease and Renal Transplantation

No more than 10% to 15% of lupus patients develop ESRD and lupus comprises only 1% to 2% of all patients with ESRD. Many patients will have inactive "burnt out" disease by the time they reach ESRD. Some who develop irreversible renal failure rapidly may still have active disease and require vigorous treatment while on renal replacement therapy. Survival of lupus patients on dialysis is comparable to other primary renal diseases. Some patients with antiphospholipid syndrome require anticoagulation to prevent arteriovenous fistulas or graft clotting.

Transplantation in lupus patients, whether from cadaveric or living donors, can be performed with only a few extra precautions. Cross matching donors with lupus patients may be difficult because the sera may contain antilymphocyte autoantibodies, rendering a false-positive cross match. These can usually be "absorbed out" in testing and, in general, do not influence the course of the allograft. Immunosuppression, rejection episodes or graft loss, and infectious complications are similar compared to nonlupus patients. Many clinicians prefer to wait until a patient has been maintained on 6 to 12 months of dialysis to be certain that the lupus is not active at the time of transplantation. For those patients who are clinically inactive but retain serologic activity with an elevated anti-DNA antibody titer, starting transplant immunosuppressives in a prophylactic fashion several weeks to a month before transplantation using a live donor may suppress the serologic activity.

Thrombosis may be a problem following transplantation, especially in patients with APA.[11,54,55] Renal transplant arterial and venous as well as intraglomerular thromboses have been reported. Anticoagulation shortly after transplantation should be reserved for those APA-positive patients with a previous thrombotic event, but in such cases, it may yield good results. Recurrent disease in the allograft in patients with lupus nephritis is discussed in Chapter 96.

REFERENCES

1. Waldman M, Appel GB: Update on the treatment of lupus nephritis. Kidney Int 2006;70:1403–1412.
2. Cameron JS: Lupus nephritis. J Am Soc Nephrol 1999;10:413–424.
3. D'Agati V, Appel GB: Lupus nephritis: Pathology and pathogenesis. In Wallace DJ, Hahn BH (eds): Dubois' Lupus Erythematosus, 7th ed., 2006.
4. Appel GB, Radhakrishnan J, D'Agati V: Secondary glomerular diseases. In Brenner B (ed): The Kidney. Philadelphia, Elsevier, 2004.
5. Waldman M, Madaio MP: Pathogenic autoantibodies in lupus nephritis. Lupus 2005;141:19–24.
6. Lipsky PE: Systemic lupus erythematosus: An autoimmune disease of B cell hyperactivity. Nat Immunol 2001;2:764–766.
7. Jacobi AM, Diamond B: Balancing diversity and tolerance: Lessons from patients with systemic lupus erythematosus. J Exp Med 2005;202:341–344.
8. Davidson A, Diamond B: Autoimmune diseases. N Engl J Med 2001;345:340–350.
9. Goodnow CC: Pathways for self tolerance and the treatment of autoimmune diseases. Lancet 2001;357:2115–2121.
10. Schwartz MM, Korbet SM: Lupus Nephritis. Oxford: Oxford University Press, 1999, pp 159–184.
11. Joseph R, Radhakrishnan J, Appel GB: Anticardiolipin antibodies and renal disease. Curr Opin Hypertens Nephrol 2001;10:175–181.

12. Nzerue CM, Hewan-Lowe K, Pierangeli S, Harris EN: "Black swan in the kidney." Renal involvement in the antiphospholipid antibody syndrome. Kidney Int 2002;62:733–744.
13. Tektonidou MG, Sotsiou F, Nakopoulu L, et al: Antiphospholipid syndrome nephropathy in patients with SLE and antiphospholipid antibodies: prevalence, clinical associations, and long-term outcome. Arthritis Rheum 2004;50:2569–2579.
14. Churg J, Bernstein J, Glassock R: Renal Disease: Classification and Atlas of Glomerular Diseases, 2nd ed. New York: Igaku-Shoin, 1995, p 152.
15. Weening JJ, D'Agati VD, Appel GB, et al: The classification of glomerulonephritis in systemic lupus nephritis revisited. Kidney Int 2004;65:521–530.
16. Mittal B, Hurwitz S, Rennke H, Singh AK: New categories of class IV lupus nephritis: Are there clinical, histologic and outcome differences? Am J Kidney Dis 2004;44:1050–1059.
17. Hill GS, Delahousse M, Nochy D, et al: Proteinuria and tubulointerstitial lesions in lupus nephritis. Kidney Int 2001;60:1893–1903.
18. Appel GB: Renal vascular involvement in SLE. In Lewis EJ, Schwartz M, Korbet SM (eds): Lupus Nephritis. Oxford, UK: Oxford University Press, 1999, pp 241–262.
19. Dube GK, Markowitz GS, Radhakrishnan J, et al: Minimal change disease in SLE. Clin Nephrol 2002;57:120–126.
20. Najafi CC, Korbet SM, Lewis EJ, et al: Significance of histologic patterns of glomerular injury upon long-term prognosis in severe lupus glomerulonephritis. Kidney Int 2001;59:2156–2163.
21. Schwartz MM: The Holy Grail: Pathological indices in lupus nephritis. Kidney Int 2000;58:1354–1355.
22. Austin HA 3rd, Boumpas DT, Vaughan EM, Balow JE: High-risk features of lupus nephritis: Importance of race and clinical and histological factors in 166 patients. Nephrol Dial Transplant 1995;10:1620–1628.
23. Hill GS, Delahousse M, Nochy D, et al: Predictive power of the second renal biopsy in lupus nephritis: Significance of macrophages. Kidney Int 2001;59:304–316.
24. Korbet SM, Lewis EJ, Schwartz MM, et al: Factors predictive of outcome in severe lupus nephritis. Lupus Nephritis Collaborative Study Group. Am J Kidney Dis 2000;35:904–914.
25. Chan TM: Preventing renal failure in patients with severe lupus nephritis. Kidney Int 2005;67(Suppl 94):S116–119.
26. Barr RG, Seliger S, Appel GB, et al: Prognosis in proliferative lupus nephritis: The role of socio-economic status and race/ethnicity. Nephrol Dial Transplant 2003;18:2039–2046.
27. Dooley MA, Hogan S, Jennette C, Falk R: Cyclophosphamide therapy for lupus nephritis: Poor renal survival in black Americans. Glomerular Disease Collaborative Network. Kidney Int 1997;51:1188–1195.
28. Cameron JS: What is the role of long-term cytotoxic agents in the treatment of lupus nephritis? J Nephrol 1993;6:172–176.
29. Contreras G, Roth D, Pardo V, et al: Lupus nephritis: A clinical review for the practicing nephrologist. Clin Nephrol 2002;57:95–107.
30. Gourley MF, Austin HA 3rd, Scott D, et al: Methylprednisolone and cyclophosphamide, alone or in combination, in patients with lupus nephritis. A randomized, controlled trial. Ann Intern Med 1996;125:549–557.
31. Illei GG, Austin HA, Crane M, et al: Combination therapy with pulse cyclophosphamide plus pulse methylprednisolone improves long-term renal outcome without adding toxicity in patients with lupus nephritis. Ann Intern Med 2001;135:248–257.
32. Contreras G, Pardo V, Leclercq B, et al: Sequential therapies for proliferative lupus nephritis. N Engl J Med 2004;350:971–980.
33. Houssiau FA, Vasconcelos C, D'Cruz D, et al: Immunosuppressive therapy in lupus nephritis: The Euro-Lupus Nephritis Trial, a randomized trial of low-dose versus high-dose intravenous cyclophosphamide. Arthritis Rheum 2002;46:2121–2131.
34. Chan TM, Li FK, Tang CS, et al: Efficacy of mycophenolate mofetil in patients with diffuse proliferative lupus nephritis. Hong Kong-Guangzhou Nephrology Study Group. N Engl J Med 2000;343:1156–1162.
35. Hu W, Liu Z, Chen H, et al: Mycophenolate mofetil vs cyclophosphamide therapy for patients with diffuse proliferative lupus nephritis. Chin Med J (Engl) 2002;115:705–709.
36. Ginzler EM, Dooley MA, Aranow C, et al: Mycophenolate mofetil or intravenous cyclophosphamide for lupus nephritis. N Engl J Med 2005;353:2219–2228.
37. Chan TM, Tse KC, Tang CS, et al: Long-term study of mycophenolate mofetil as continuous induction and maintenance treatment for diffuse proliferative lupus nephritis. J Am Soc Nephrol 2005;16:1076–1084.
38. Sinclair A, Appel GB, Dooler MA, et al: The Aspreva Lupus Management-ALMS trial. J Am Soc Nephrol 2005;16:528A.
39. Sfikakis PP, Boletis JN, Lionaki S, et al: Remission of proliferative lupus nephritis following B cell depletion therapy is proceeded by down regulation of the T cell co-stimulatory molecule CD40 ligand: An open label trial. Arthritis Rheum 2005;52:501–513.
40. Leandro MJ, Cambridge G, Edwards JC, et al: B cell depletion in the treatment of patients with systemic lupus erythematosus: A longitudinal analysis of 24 patients. Rheumatology (Oxford) 2005;44:1542–1545.
41. Alarcon-Segovia D, Tumlin JA, et al: LJP 394 for the prevention of renal flare in patients with SLE: Results from a randomized, double-blind, placebo-controlled study. Arthritis Rheum 2003;48:442–454.
42. Sloane RP, Schwartz MM, Korbet SM, et al: Long-term outcome in systemic lupus erythematosus membranous glomerulonephritis. J Am Soc Nephrol 1996;7:299–305.
43. Austin HA, Balow JE: Long-term observation in a clinical trial of prednisone, cyclosporine, and cyclophosphamide for membranous lupus nephropathy. J Am Soc Nephrol 2004;15:54A.
44. Radhakrishnan J, Ginzler E, Appel GB: Mycophenolate mofetil versus IV cyclophosphamide for severe lupus nephritis: Subgroup analysis of patients with membranous lupus. J Am Soc Nephrol 2005;16:8A.
45. Illei GG, Takada K, Parkin D, et al: Renal flares are common in patients with severe proliferative lupus nephritis treated with pulse immunosuppressive therapy: Long-term followup of a cohort of 145 patients participating in randomized controlled studies. Arthritis Rheum 2002;46:995–1002.
46. Mosca M, Bencivelli W, Neri R, et al: Renal flares in 91 SLE patients with diffuse proliferative glomerulonephritis. Kidney Int 2002;61:1502–1509.
47. Ponticelli C, Moroni G: Flares in lupus nephritis: Incidence, impact on renal survival and management. Lupus 1998;7:635–638.
48. Moroni G, Ventura D, Riva P, Panzeri P: Antiphospholipid antibodies are associated with an increased risk for chronic renal insufficiency in patients with lupus nephritis. Am J Kidney Dis 2004;43:28–36.
49. Bono L, Cameron JS, Hicks JA: The very long-term prognosis and complications of lupus nephritis and its treatment. Q J Med 1999;92:211–218.
50. Roman MJ, Shanker BA, Davis A, et al: Prevalence and correlates of accelerated atherosclerosis in systemic lupus erythematosus. N Engl J Med 2003;349:2399–2406.
51. Bruce IN, Urowitz MB, Gladman DD, et al: Risk factors for coronary heart disease in women with systemic lupus erythematosus: The Toronto Risk Factor Study. Arthritis Rheum 2003;48:3159–3167.
52. Petri M, Kim MY, Kalunian KC, et al: Combined oral contraceptives in women with SLE. N Engl J Med 2005;353:2550–2558.
53. Buyon JP, Petri MA, Kim MY, et al: The effect of combined estrogen and progesterone hormone replacement therapy on disease activity in SLE: A randomized trial. Ann Intern Med 2005;142:953–962.
54. Stone JH, Amen WJ, Criswell LA: Antiphospholipid antibody syndrome in renal transplantation: Occurrence of clinical events in 96 consecutive patients with SLE. Am J Kidney Dis 1999;34:1040–1047.
55. Radhakrishnan J, Williams G, Appel GB, et al: Renal transplantation in anticardiolipin antibody positive SLE patients. Am J Kidney Dis 1994;23:286–289.

Glomerular Diseases Associated with Infection

Bernardo Rodríguez-Iturbe, Emmanuel A. Burdmann, Vuddhidej Ophascharoensuk, and Rashad S. Barsoum

GENERAL CHARACTERISTICS OF GLOMERULAR DISEASES ASSOCIATED WITH INFECTION

Glomerulonephritis (GN) may occur in a variety of diseases caused by bacterial, viral, fungal, and helminthic pathogens (Fig. 25.1). Some infection-related glomerulonephritides are subclinical and transient; others are chronic and lead to end-stage renal disease (ESRD). The majority of renal diseases associated with infection are immune complex related (Fig. 25.2). Antigen load, charge, and size and the characteristics of the host antibody response and efficiency of disposal of the nephritogenic immune complexes are factors that define the characteristics of the renal lesion. Therefore, the duration and severity of the infection, the effectiveness of treatment, and the existence of comorbid conditions are, to a large extent, responsible for the histologic appearance and course of GN. Not surprisingly, pathologic patterns of glomerular damage and their corresponding clinical manifestations vary in different stages of the natural history of some infectious diseases. For example, the initial, serum sickness–like, clinical presentation of hepatitis B virus (HBV) may be associated with self-limited acute mesangioproliferative GN, while the chronic carrier state may be associated with membranous nephropathy in children and with membranoproliferative (mesangiocapillary) GN (MPGN) in adults. Alternatively, different infectious diseases, such as visceral bacterial abscesses and hepatitis C virus (HCV) infection, may present with nephrotic syndrome resulting from histologically similar MPGN.

The histologic patterns and the most typical infectious disease associated with them are shown in Figure 25.2. Mesangial proliferative GN is usually acute and self-limited. Microscopic hematuria and non-nephrotic proteinuria are present in association with

deposits of IgG, IgM, and C3. Serum complement may be transiently decreased. Diffuse proliferative GN is also acute and self-limited if the infection is eradicated. IgG, IgM, and C3 deposits are prominent in the mesangium and glomerular capillaries and electron-dense deposits are present in mesangial, subendothelial, and subepithelial locations. The immune complexes deposited in the glomeruli may or may not contain bacterial antigens, and cryoglobulins may be present. The clinical presentation is the acute nephritic syndrome. MPGN is the usual pattern of GN resulting from chronic infections. The clinical presentation is frequently that of the nephrotic syndrome with microscopic hematuria and variable degrees of hypertension. Complement may be low or normal. Immunoglobulins and C3 deposits are usually found and, if liver disease is present (as in *Schistosoma mansoni* infection), IgA may be a predominant component of the immune deposits. Membranous nephropathy (MN) is associated with chronic infections. Infection-related MN generally presents as the nephrotic syndrome.

Infections may also be associated with renal disease via mechanisms that do not involve immune complexes (see Fig. 25.2). Focal segmental glomerulosclerosis with glomerular collapse (collapsing glomerulopathy) may occur with human immunodeficiency virus (HIV) or parvovirus B19 infection and usually presents as a sudden, massive nephrotic syndrome with rapid progression to chronicity. Vasculitis may develop in association with viral (especially HBV and HIV) or bacterial (rarely *Streptococcus*) infections, the hemolytic-uremic syndrome (from verotoxin-producing *Escherichia coli* or *Shigella* species; see Chapter 28), and amyloidosis from chronic infections such as tuberculosis, leprosy, and schistosomiasis. Interstitial nephritis manifested as acute renal failure may be associated with several viral (especially Epstein-Barr virus) or

Some infectious agents associated with renal disease
Bacterial: *Streptococcus* (group A, *Streptococcus viridans*), *Staphylococcus* (*aureus, epidermidis*), *Salmonella* (*typhi, paratyphi*), *Escherichia coli, Leptospira, Treponema pallidum, Neisseria* species, *Mycobacterium leprae, Yersinia enterocolitica, Coxiella burnettii, Brucella abortus, Listeria monocytogenes*
Viral: Hepatitis A, B, and C, human immunodeficiency virus, varicella-zoster, parvovirus B19, cytomegalovirus, mumps, influenza, Epstein-Barr virus, coxsackievirus, and enteric cytopathic human orphan (ECHO) virus
Fungus: *Histoplasma capsulatum, Candida*
Protozoal: *Plasmodium* (*falciparum, malariae, vivax*, and *ovale*); *Trypanosoma, Toxoplasma*
Helminthic: *Schistosoma* (*mansoni, haematobium*), *Wuchereria bancrofti, Trichinella spiralis*, filaria (*Onchocerca volvulus*, Loa loa)

Figure 25.1 Some infectious agents associated with renal disease.

Major renal syndromes associated with infection				
Type	Time Course	Clinical Presentation	Other	Examples
Mesangial proliferative GN IgM, C3 dominant IgA dominant	Acute Acute or chronic	Subclinical, microhematuria, non-nephrotic proteinuria	Coexistent liver disease is frequent in IgA dominant cases	Acute typhoid fever, acute malaria
Diffuse proliferative GN IgM; IgG, C3 C3 only	Acute	Renal dysfunction, hypertension, proteinuria, edema	Occasionally with crescents or thrombi	Endocarditis- or pneumococcal pneumonia–associated GN Poststreptococcal GN
Membranoproliferative GN type I (± cryoglobulinemia)	Chronic	Nephrotic or non-nephrotic, GFR decreased	Occasionally with sclerosis	Hepatitis C virus–associated GN, schistosomal GN (class III), quartan malaria nephropathy
Membranous	Chronic	Nephrotic syndrome	Occasionally with mesangial deposits	Hepatitis B virus–associated GN, syphilis
Focal segmental glomerulosclerosis	Acute or chronic	Nephrotic syndrome, GFR decreased		HIV or parvovirus B19 infection
Vasculitis	Acute or chronic	Hypertension, GFR decreased, systematic symptoms		Hepatitis B virus–associated vasculitis, HIV–associated vasculitis, vasculitis associated with poststreptococcal GN
Amyloid	Chronic	Nephrotic syndrome		Leprosy, kala-azar, schistosomiasis
Hemolytic-uremic syndrome	Acute	Acute renal failure, low platelet count, anemia		*Escherichia coli* 0157:H7 infection, shigellosis
Interstitial nephritis	Acute	Acute renal failure, microhematuria		Epstein-Barr virus, Legionnaires' disease, leptospirosis, kala-azar, Hantavirus

Figure 25.2 Major renal syndromes associated with infection. GFR, glomerular filtration rate; GN, glomerulonephritis; HIV, human immunodeficiency virus.

bacterial (especially *Legionella*) infections and also may be due to antibiotic therapy. Certain viruses, especially within the Hantavirus family, can also induce a hemorrhagic fever–renal failure syndrome in which infection of the interstitial capillaries and tubules leads to an acute renal failure (see Chapter 59).

PATHOGENESIS OF INFECTION-RELATED GLOMERULAR DISEASE

GN results from both humoral and cell-derived mediators released in response to immune complexes localizing in glomeruli. Immune-complex formation consisting of a bacterial or viral antigen and its corresponding antibody may occur in the circulation and be subsequently deposited in the glomeruli or, alternatively, may occur *in situ*, within the glomerulus (see Chapter 15). The deposition of circulating complexes occurs on reaching an appropriate antigen-to-antibody ratio that favors precipitation and their pathogenic potential depends on the characteristics of the immune complex and the efficiency of their removal (see Chapter 15).

Deposited or locally formed immune complexes activate the complement system, resulting in the generation of the chemotactic factor C5a and the expression of chemokines and leukocyte adhesion molecules that stimulate leukocyte infiltration, as well as proliferation and matrix expansion by glomerular cells (see Chapter 15). Whereas clearance of the immune complexes with resolution of injury may occur, progression to ESRD may also result if the infection is not controlled and the immune process continues. In the event extensive nephron loss occurs, renal disease may progress even if the infection is controlled (see Chapter 68).

Several studies suggest that infection-related GN, as well as immune complex–associated GN, may occur more frequently and have a worse prognosis in conditions in which there is difficulty clearing the infection and/or immune complexes. These conditions include HIV infection, infections acquired in the neonatal period (when tolerance is often induced such as is observed with HBV infection), chronic liver disease, and chronic alcoholism (increased infection risk and reduced clearance of immune complexes).

BACTERIAL INFECTIONS

Poststreptococcal Glomerulonephritis
History and Epidemiology
The observation of dark, scanty urine in the convalescent period of scarlet fever is more than two centuries old. The postulate that the disease had an allergic, serum sickness–like etiology, made by Bela Schick nearly a century ago, was a landmark observation that opened the field of immune-mediated renal disease.

The incidence of poststreptococcal GN (PSGN) has decreased in the industrialized countries as shown by reports from the United States, Europe, and China. Furthermore, PSGN, traditionally a disease of children, is now affecting debilitated elderly individuals, particularly alcoholics, diabetics, and intravenous drug users. In Italy, for example, the disease is now more common after the age of 60 (0.9 patients per million population) than before this age (0.4 patients per million population).[1]

Nevertheless, PSGN continues to have a worldwide distribution. It is a frequent cause of acute renal failure in pediatric intensive care units in developing countries and is the most common cause of acute GN in children, and cluster cases repeatedly occur in aboriginal groups, particularly in Australia and in Latin American communities with poor socioeconomic conditions.

The reasons for the changes in epidemiology are not entirely, clear but may be related to increased accessibility to early medical care and antibiotic treatment in industrialized countries. The lack of proper sanitation conditions prevalent in underdeveloped countries may predispose to a Th1 type of response (characteristic of PSGN) in contrast with the Th2 type of response that tends to result in minimal change disease in the industrialized countries with high hygiene standards.[2] Another factor that may have contributed to the decline in acute PSGN in industrialized countries is the widespread use of fluorination of water since fluoride exposure reduces the expression of virulence factors with potential pathogenetic roles in cultures of *Streptococcus pyogenes*.[3]

The observation that epidemics of PSGN occur in some areas (such as the Red Lake Indian Reservation in Minnesota, Port of Spain in Trinidad, and Maracaibo in Venezuela), but not in others with similar socioeconomic characteristics, has suggested a potential genetic predisposition, although none has been identified. PSGN is more common in males (2:1) and usually affects children 2 to 14 years old. Traditionally, only certain nephritogenic strains of group A *S. pyogenes* result in GN. In the tropics and southern United States, PSGN usually follows streptococcal impetigo of M types 47, 49, 55, and 57. Throat infections with streptococcus types 1, 2, 4, and 12 are also nephritogenic.[4] More recently, ingestion of unpasteurized milk contaminated with group C

Streptococcus (*Streptococcus zooepidemicus*) has caused clusters of cases and at least one large epidemic.[5] The risk of nephritis in epidemics may range from 5% in throat infections to as high as 25% in M type 49 pyoderma. The risk of PSGN is reduced by early antibiotic treatment.[4]

Pathogenesis

Several putative nephritogenic streptococcal antigens have been studied over the years.[6] The two major antigens currently investigated are nephritis-associated plasmin receptor, which was identified as glyceraldehyde-3-phosphate dehydrogenase (GAPDH)[7] and a cationic (pK >8.0) streptococcal antigen, which was identified as the cationic proteinase streptococcal pyrogenic exotoxin B (SPEB) and its more immunogenic precursor zymogen.[8] GAPDH and SPEB have been identified in renal biopsy specimens of acute PSGN, and antibody titers to both these antigens have been demonstrated in the vast majority of convalescent sera. GAPDH has been localized in areas of the glomeruli with plasmin-like activity, suggesting a local direct mechanism of glomerular inflammatory damage, but it is not colocalized with complement or immunoglobulins.[9] In contrast, SPEB is colocalized with both complement and IgG, suggesting a participation in the immune-mediated glomerular damage.[10] Furthermore, SPEB is the only putative streptococcal nephritogen that so far has been demonstrated in the subepithelial electron-dense deposits known as "humps" (Fig. 25.3), the most typical histologic lesion of acute PSGN.[10] Interestingly, recent back-to-back studies[10] have shown that, at least in patients from Latin America and Central Europe, SPEB, but not GAPDH, is usually detectable in renal biopsy specimens of acute PSGN patients and, correspondingly, increased serum antibody titers to SPEB, but not GAPDH, were present. These results are in direct contrast with the results found in Japanese patients by Yoshizawa and colleagues.[7]

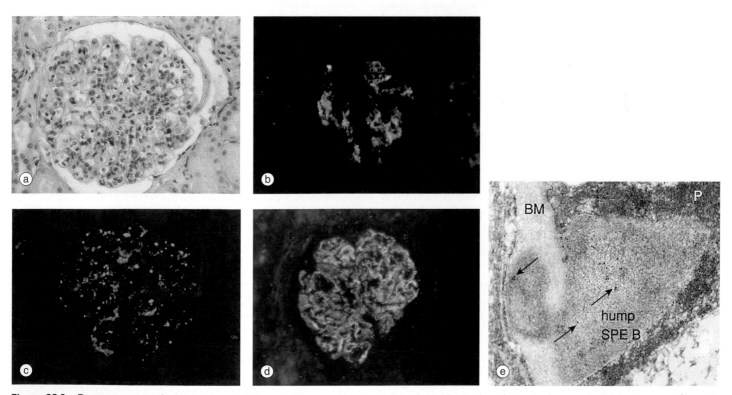

Figure 25.3 **Poststreptococcal glomerulonephritis.** *a*, A diffuse proliferative and exudative glomerulonephritis can be seen by light microscopy. Immunofluorescence with antibodies to IgG showing the mesangial (*b*), starry sky (*c*), and garland (*d*) patterns. *e*, Immune electron microscopy showing the characteristic subepithelial electron-dense deposits (humps) inside which streptococcal pyrogenic exotoxin B (SPEB) is demonstrated (*arrows*) (immunogold staining). BM, basement membrane; P, podocyte. (From Batsford SR, Mezzano S, Mihatsch M, et al: Is the nephritogenic antigen in post-streptococcal glomerulonephritis pyrogenic exotoxin B [SPE B] or GAPDH? Kidney Int 2005;68:1120–1129.)

These contrasting results raise the interesting possibility that different streptococcal fractions are capable of inducing acute nephritis in different ethnic groups.

According to the current paradigm, persistent streptococcal infection results in antigenemia and the development of circulating immune complexes that primarily deposit in the subendothelial and mesangial locations to initiate an inflammatory cascade with local complement activation and the recruitment of neutrophils and monocytes/macrophages. Subepithelial immune deposits (humps) develop due to the presence of cationic antigens (e.g., zymogen) and/or the dissociation of immune complexes in the subendothelial space with transit and reformation on the outer aspect of the glomerular basement membrane. A role for cell-mediated immunity is supported by the presence of CD4 (helper) T lymphocytes in the glomeruli. Cytokines and vasoactive mediators also contribute to the local inflammation and injury. Urinary MCP-1 correlates with the severity of proteinuria in the acute phase of PSGN.[11]

Several issues remain unresolved. First, the identity of the nephritogenic antigen remains a matter of debate. Second, the role of *in situ* formation of immune complexes is debated (in contrast with the traditional circulating immune-complex pathogenesis) since the subepithelial electron dense deposits, such as the humps seen in PSGN, are typical of the *in situ* formation of immune deposits induced by cationic antigens such as SPEB. Third, the mechanisms of complement activation are unclear since immune complex disease should result in activation of the classic complement pathway, yet, in most cases, C4 levels are normal and only C3 is found in the deposits. This could be explained by the presence of antigens (such as GAPDH) that activate the alternative pathway. In some patients, C3Nef IgG antibodies have been demonstrated in sera that are capable of activating the alternative complement pathway. More recently, it has been proposed that the mannose-binding lectin complement pathway is activated by *N*-acetyl glucosamine residues in the bacterial cell wall.[12]

Finally, the role of autoimmune mechanisms remains to be clarified.[6] Rheumatoid factors (especially IgG rheumatoid factor) and cryoglobulins are found in the serum of one third of patients in the first week of the disease. Anti-IgG deposits have been shown in one third of the renal biopsies and in the eluate from the kidney in a fatal case. Anti-IgG reactivity may result from the loss of sialic acid from autologous IgG due to streptococcal neuraminidase (sialidase) or from binding of the Fc fragment of IgG to type II Fc receptors in the streptococcal wall. Additional manifestations of autoimmune reactivity include antineutrophil cytoplasmic antibodies (ANCA), particularly in severe cases, and rarely, anti-DNA reactivity and autoimmune hemolytic anemia.

Pathology

Renal biopsy shows a diffuse endocapillary GN with proliferation of mesangial and endothelial cells (see Fig. 25.3). Glomerular and interstitial infiltration of monocytes and lymphocytes is present, and glomerular accumulation of neutrophils is common and is termed exudative GN. Glomerular immune deposits of C3 (100% of the cases), IgG (62%), IgM (76%), properdin, and the terminal membrane attack complex C5b-C9 (85% of the cases, usually codeposited with C3) have been shown in glomerular capillary loops and in the mesangium. A seminal work by Sorger described three patterns of immunofluorescence in the glomeruli and their clinical correlations: the *mesangial pattern* of irregular and heavy immune deposits, the *starry-sky pattern* of deposits scattered in mesangium and in capillary walls and the *garland pattern* formed by gross deposits in the capillary loops

(see Fig. 25.3).[13] The garland pattern is clinically relevant because it is associated with heavy proteinuria and a large number of electron-dense subepithelial immune deposits. Ultrastructural studies demonstrate the subepithelial humps, which are typical although not pathognomonic of PSGN, as they may also be observed in postinfectious GN of other etiologies (classically endocarditis-associated GN secondary to staphylococcal infection), cryoglobulinemia, and lupus nephritis.

GN resolves by apoptosis of the excess cells, a mechanism that is stimulated by SPEB. Residual renal injury is common, and biopsy specimens years later show variable degrees of focal glomerulosclerosis and mesangial expansion even in the absence of clinical disease. The clinical significance of these changes is undetermined.

Clinical Manifestations

Most patients give a history of a streptococcal infection. The incubation period is classically longer after skin infections (several weeks) than after throat infections (2 weeks). However, the infection is often resolved at presentation. The acute nephritic syndrome is observed in the vast majority of overt cases and usually lasts less than 2 weeks. Hypertension is found in 80% of patients. Edema occurs in 80% to 90% of cases and is the chief complaint in 60%; yet ascites is distinctly unusual.[4] Primary sodium retention is the cause of expanded intravascular volume, hypertension, and edema. Plasma renin activity and aldosterone are reduced and endothelin-1 is increased.[4,14] Hematuria is universal and in 30% of cases is macroscopic.

The nephrotic syndrome may occur at the onset in 2% of the children and 20% of adults. A rapidly progressive course, resulting from extracapillary crescent formation, occurs in <1% of the patients. Azotemia occurs in 25% to 40% of the children and in as many as 83% of the adults.

Positive cultures for *Streptococcus* are obtained in 10% to 70% of the cases during epidemics and in about 20% to 25% of sporadic cases. Antistreptolysin O (ASO) titers are increased in more than two thirds of patients with PSGN following throat infections, and anti-DNAse B titers are elevated in 73% of postimpetigo cases[8] (increases in this context mean two or more dilutions above the mean titer in the general population). The streptozyme panel (which measures antibodies to four antigens: anti-DNAse B, antihyaluronidase, ASO, and antistreptokinase) is more sensitive and is positive in >80% of subjects. Antibody tests to GAPDH and SPEB/zymogen, while more sensitive and specific,[8] are not clinically available.

Serum C3 levels are decreased in >90% of patients in the first week of disease and return to normal in less than 2 months. C4 levels are frequently, but not always normal. The terminal complement complexes (C5b-C9) are elevated in samples taken within 30 days from onset and return to normal with the improvement of GN. Serum IgG and IgM are elevated in 80% of the cases, and, in contrast with another poststreptococcal disease, rheumatic fever, IgA is normal. Cryoglobulins and elevated rheumatoid factor are present in up to one third of patients, and rare patients may have low titers of anti-DNA and ANCAs.[4]

It is important to note that subclinical disease, manifested by microscopic hematuria and decrease in serum complement, occurs four to five times more frequently than clinically overt disease and prospective studies in families have shown that 38% of the siblings of index cases of sporadic PSGN develop the disease.[4] Occasionally, whole families have various manifestations of PSGN; it is thus important to inquire about a history of streptococcal infections and signs of nephritic syndrome among family members.

Management

Renal biopsy is not routinely indicated in PSGN but may be required to confirm the diagnosis when it presents with unusual clinical features, such as nephrotic proteinuria, decreased C3 levels lasting for more than a month (suggests lupus or hypocomplementemic MPGN), or increasing azotemia (suggests crescentic GN).

Management includes the treatment of streptococcal infection with penicillin even if no persistent infection is present in order to decrease antigenic load (1.2 million units of benzylpenicillin in adults or half this dose in small children or, alternatively, oral phenoxyethyl or phenoxymethyl penicillin G 125 mg, every 6 hours for 7 to 10 days) or in persons allergic to penicillin, erythromycin (250 mg every 6 hours in adults, and 40 mg/kg in children, for 7 to 10 days). Rapid high-sensitivity streptococcal tests are useful if positive, but the culture confirmation of negative results is generally advised. However, a recent report indicates that the decision not to treat, based only on a negative test, was not associated with increased incidence of poststreptococcal complications.[15] Preventive antibiotic treatment is justified in populations at risk during epidemics and in siblings of index cases who usually show evidence of streptococcal infection within 2 to 3 weeks after the presentation of the index case; over one third will develop nephritis.[4] Prevention of new cases of PSGN in high-risk communities has been achieved by treating household members of index cases with penicillin.[16]

The treatment of the acute nephritic syndrome includes restriction of fluid and sodium intake and the use of loop diuretics to treat circulatory congestion. Oral long-acting calcium antagonist is usually sufficient to control hypertension, but parenteral hydralazine may be required. Nitroprusside is needed in exceptional cases with hypertensive encephalopathy. Dialysis (either hemodialysis or peritoneal dialysis) is required in 25% to 30% of adults but seldom in children.

Anecdotal reports suggest that the rare patients with crescentic GN associated with PSGN may benefit from pulse methylprednisolone therapy, and if spontaneous improvement is not observed in 2 weeks, this therapy may be tried. The prognosis of crescentic PSGN is significantly better than those from other etiologies, but a complete recovery may be expected in less than half of the cases.

Prognosis

The immediate prognosis of PSGN is excellent in children, but the elderly patient has a high incidence of azotemia (60% to 70%), congestive heart failure (40%), nephrotic proteinuria (20%), and significant early mortality (25%).[17]

While symptomatic GN resolves within a few weeks, mild proteinuria (<500 mg/day) may persist for several months and microscopic hematuria for up to 1 year without worsening the long-term prognosis.

The long-term prognosis is worse in adults compared to children and also for patients with persistent severe proteinuria. The prognosis of subclinical PSGN is excellent. However, other issues are more controversial: in most studies in which the follow-up extends for 10 to 15 years, the incidence of proteinuria is 4% to 13%, but the range extends from 1.4% to 46%. The incidence of hypertension ranges from that seen in the general population in the same geographic area to about twice that risk. Abnormal renal biopsy findings are relatively frequent, but they do not necessarily mean progressive renal disease. Several characteristics increase the likelihood of subsequent development of abnormal renal function, proteinuria, and hypertension; among them are older age at the time of the acute attack and presentation with proteinuria in the nephrotic range. These patients should be followed closely. A particularly severe prognosis is found in older patients with massive proteinuria; more than two thirds of this subgroup of patients develops chronic renal failure. Despite discrepancies in reported data, which may reflect population differences and dissimilar characteristics of the studies, the follow-up studies of PSGN, taken collectively, indicate that ESRD occurs in <1% of the children followed for one to two decades after the acute attack. Our usual practice in children with complete recovery is to have a follow-up visit 1 year after discharge following the acute attack.

A significantly worse long-term prognosis has been reported in alcoholic patients with PSGN and in a specific outbreak of PSGN resulting from consumption of cheese contaminated with *Streptococcus zooepidemicus*. In the later study, a re-evaluation done after 5.4 years in which 54 of 56 patients were adults, arterial hypertension was present in 30%, reduced creatinine clearance in 49%, and microalbuminuria in 22%.[18] Specific communities have a worse long-term prognosis, which has suggested that if PSGN develops in patients who have other independent risk factors for chronic renal failure, such as low birth weight, diabetes, or features of the metabolic syndrome, their long-term prognosis is significantly worsened.[19]

Endocarditis-Associated Glomerulonephritis

Community-acquired native-valve endocarditis in the United States and Western Europe has an incidence of 1.7 to 6.2 cases per 100,000 person-years, and, as determined by population-based surveys, its incidence remained unchanged in the past three decades.[20] The more significant changes observed in the epidemiology are the emergence of health care–associated infective endocarditis and, particularly in this category, the predominance of staphylococcal etiology. Among these patients, chronic hemodialysis patients represent the most important subgroup with 20 to 60 times the incidence in the general population.[21]

The complication of embolic nonsuppurative GN in bacterial endocarditis was noted more than 90 years ago by Löhlein. In subsequent years, the embolic component was questioned and the immune complex etiology was emphasized. In the 1970s and 1980s, immune complex GN was observed primarily in patients with rheumatic or congenital heart disease with subacute bacterial endocarditis caused by *Streptococcus viridans*. One third of patients with bacterial endocarditis develop azotemia and the risk increases with age, a history of hypertension, thrombocytopenia, and prosthetic valve infection.[22]

Pathogenesis and Pathology

The pathogenesis of endocarditis-associated GN is similar to that proposed for PSGN. Type III cryoglobulins (i.e., polyclonal) are present in 50% of subjects and may be found in glomeruli. Some bacteria (classically methicillin-resistant *Staphylococcus aureus*) express superantigens that can also activate T cells directly and lead to a polyclonal gammopathy and immune complex GN.[23]

In a recent survey of 62 of 354 patients with infective endocarditis in whom renal tissue was available for study, biopsy and autopsy material demonstrated GN in 26%, of which many cases were characterized by vasculitis without glomerular immunoglobulin deposition. Other pathologies included localized infarcts in 31%, half of which were septic, and interstitial nephritis, mostly attributable to antibiotics, in 10%. Cortical necrosis was found in 10% of the cases.[24] These findings are in contrast with earlier literature that indicated that immune-complex GN was the more common renal lesion associated with endocarditis. The most common glomerular pathology is diffuse proliferative GN.

Less commonly, focal GN, membranous nephropathy, and MPGN type I may be found. Crescent formation is found in about half of the proliferative GN forms. Widespread deposition of IgM, IgG, and C3 and electron-dense subendothelial, mesangial, and subepithelial deposits (which resemble poststreptococcal humps), are usually evident. In subacute endocarditis, focal segmental proliferative lesions with fibrinoid necrosis or capillary thrombi and mesangial immune deposits may be present. Tubulointerstitial cellular infiltration and variable degrees of atrophy and fibrosis may be seen. Intense eosinophilic infiltration should suggest another diagnosis such as acute interstitial nephritis, secondary to antibiotics.[24]

Clinical Manifestations and Diagnosis

The clinical picture includes fever, arthralgias, anemia, and purpura. However, occasionally infective endocarditis can present as apparently primary renal disease with abnormal renal function or abnormal urinalysis.

Classic findings in endocarditis, such as Osler's nodes, Janeway lesions, and splinter hemorrhages, are seldom seen. The renal manifestations usually are microscopic hematuria and mild proteinuria, with or without mild azotemia. A rapidly progressive clinical course or nephrotic syndrome are unusual.

Abnormal serologic tests include decreased C3 and C4 levels (consistent with activation of the classical complement pathway), high titers of rheumatoid factor, circulating immune complexes, and type III cryoglobulins.[25] These serologic findings are observed in 50% of subjects with subacute bacterial endocarditis and in higher percentages in patients with endocarditis-associated GN, although complement levels may be normal in superantigen-mediated GN.[23] Cytoplasmic ANCA has been reported in rare cases with subacute endocarditis and GN.

The differential diagnosis includes antibiotic-associated acute renal failure or interstitial nephritis and embolism. Embolism may originate from the left side of the heart or from the right if the foramen ovale is patent. Microscopic or large emboli may occlude small or large vessels, the latter observed with fungal or *Haemophilus* endocarditis. Large emboli may produce flank pain, hematuria, and pyuria, while the microemboli produce local infarcts and microabscesses that give the kidney the classic "flea-bitten" appearance. Interstitial nephritis is often associated with fever, eosinophilia, and eosinophiluria. Unfortunately, endocarditis-associated GN may also present with fever, and eosinophiluria can complicate crescentic nephritis of any etiology. Antibiotic treatment for 4 to 6 weeks usually results in complete eradication of endocarditis with correction of serologic abnormalities, but microscopic hematuria, proteinuria, and elevation of serum creatinine may persist for months after eradication of the infection.[26] Normalization of C3 levels during therapy correlates with a good outcome. In cases with crescentic GN, pulse steroid therapy as well as plasma exchange have been used in addition to effective antibiotic therapy, but the value of these treatments remains undefined. The overall mortality of bacterial endocarditis is 20% and increases to 36% in the patients who develop renal failure.[23,25,26]

Shunt Nephritis

Atrioventricular shunts may become infected in about 30% of cases. GN may develop in 0.7% to 2% of the infected atrioventricular shunts in an interval of time ranging from 2 months to many years after insertion.[27] The infective organisms are usually *Staphylococcus epidermidis* and *S. aureus* and less frequently *Propionibacterium acne*, diphtheroids, *Pseudomonas*, or *Serratia*

species.[28] In contrast with atrioventricular shunts, ventriculoperitoneal shunts are rarely complicated with GN.

The clinical picture includes insidious low-grade fever, arthralgias, weight loss, anemia, skin rash, hepatosplenomegaly, hypertension, and signs of increased intracranial pressure. The renal manifestations are microscopic hematuria (90%) and proteinuria, frequently massive and with the full nephrotic syndrome in 25% of the cases. Serologic findings include signs of infection, high rheumatoid factor titers, cryoglobulinemia, and decreased serum C3, C4, and CH50 levels. Positive proteinase 3 ANCA titers may be found.[29]

Renal histology shows MPGN type I in nearly 60% of the cases and non-IgA mesangial proliferative GN in about one third of the patients. There are IgM, IgG, and C3 deposits in the glomerular capillary and mesangium. The pathogenesis of these lesions involves the deposition of immune complexes and activation of the classic and alternative complement pathways.

Treatment requires antibiotic therapy and the prompt removal of the infected atrioventricular shunt; the latter is usually replaced by a ventriculoperitoneal shunt. Delay in diagnosis and in removal of the shunt worsens the prognosis of the renal lesion. In the event that dialysis is required, hemodialysis is the preferred modality since peritonitis complicating chronic peritoneal dialysis carries the risk of meningitis in patients with a ventriculoperitoneal shunt. Complete recovery occurs in more than half of the patients, while persistent urinary abnormalities have been found in 22% and ESRD in 6% of the patients.[27]

Glomerulonephritis Associated with Other Bacterial Infections

Osteomyelitis and intra-abdominal, pelvic, pleural, and dental abscesses can be associated with GN. A common feature in these conditions is that infection is usually present for several months before it is properly diagnosed and treated. The clinical presentation of renal disease may vary from mild urinary abnormalities to rapidly progressive GN, but the most frequent presentation is the nephrotic syndrome. Unlike other infection-associated GN, complement levels are often normal. A polyclonal gammopathy is frequently present, which may relate to the fact that many of the organisms (especially methicillin-resistant *S. aureus*) contain superantigens.[22] Renal histology reveals MPGN, diffuse proliferative GN, or mesangioproliferative GN (Fig. 25.4). Crescents may be present. Treatment is directed to eradicate the existing infection. Complete recovery of renal function may be expected only if treatment is started early.

Congenital and secondary (or early latent) syphilis may be associated with GN.[30] In congenital syphilis, patients present with anasarca 4 to 12 weeks after birth. Nephrotic syndrome occurs in 8% of the patients and may be the primary clinical manifestation (as opposed to the more classic triad of rhinitis, osteochondritis, and rash). In acquired syphilis, renal involvement occurs in 0.3% of all patients. Adults may present with the nephrotic syndrome or occasionally with an acute nephritic picture. Serologic tests for syphilis are positive (rapid plasmin reagin, VDRL, and fluorescent treponemeal antibody absorption test). MN is the most common form of renal pathology in children and adults. However, other histologic patterns can be observed, particularly in adults, including diffuse proliferative GN, with or without crescents, MPGN, and mesangioproliferative GN. *Treponema* antigens have been identified in the immune deposits. The glomerular disease generally responds to the treatment of syphilis, although complete remission may not occur for 4 to 18 months.

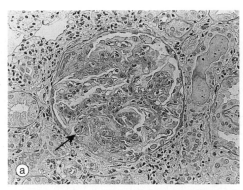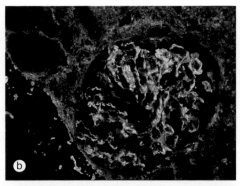

Figure 25.4   Glomerulonephritis (GN) associated with infection from methicillin-resistant *Staphylococcus aureus*. *a*, Membranoproliferative GN with early crescent formation is seen on light microscopy (*arrow*). *b*, Immunofluorescence demonstrates IgG in a capillary wall and a mesangial pattern. (Courtesy of M. Kobayashi, Ibaraki, Japan.)

Acute typhoid fever (*Salmonella typhi* infection) is characterized by fever, splenomegaly, and gastrointestinal symptoms.[31] Severe cases may develop shock and acute renal failure as a part of disseminated intravascular coagulation or hemolytic-uremic syndrome, but these complications are rare.[32] Overt manifestations of GN occur in 2% of the cases, but microscopic hematuria and mild proteinuria may be present in 25% of the cases (Fig. 25.5). Diagnosis requires the culture of the organisms from blood or stools or rising antibody titers in the Widal test. A specific type of GN resulting from *Salmonella* infection is that occurring in patients with schistosomiasis and coexisting *Salmonella* infection of the urinary tract (see later discussion).

Leprosy (*Mycobacterium leprae* infection) may be associated with GN, interstitial nephritis, or amyloidosis.[33] In a recent review of autopsy findings, the incidence of amyloidosis was 4% to 31%, GN 5% to 14%, and interstitial nephritis 4% to 54%.[34] GN is manifested clinically in <2% of the patients but may be present in 13% to 70% of renal biopsies. It remains controversial whether GN is more common in lepromatous leprosy than in tuberculoid leprosy. Urinary abnormalities consistent with GN often accompany the episodes of erythema nodosum leprosum. The clinical manifestations are usually nephrotic syndrome, less frequently acute nephritic syndrome, and, more rarely, rapidly progressive GN.

The most commonly observed lesions are MPGN and diffuse proliferative GN. Immunofluorescence demonstrates IgG, C3, IgM, IgA, and fibrin deposits. Response of glomerular disease to treatment of leprosy is variable. Prednisolone (40 to 50 mg/day) has been used in short courses to treat erythema nodosum leprosum associated with acute renal failure. AA amyloidosis

was very frequent in the early investigations, but is reported in approximately 2% of the cases of leprosy in recent studies and is much more common in lepromatous leprosy than in tuberculoid leprosy. Other renal abnormalities associated with leprosy include interstitial nephritis and tubular functional defects without histologic lesions.

Acute pneumonia due to *Streptococcus pneumoniae* infection may be associated with microhematuria and proteinuria. Most of the cases reported correspond to the preantibiotic era when effective treatment was unavailable. GN in pneumococcal infection is immune complex–mediated, with mesangioproliferative or diffuse proliferative histology, and with immunofluorescent and electron-dense deposits similar to those observed with poststreptococcal GN. Pneumococcal antigen (particularly type 14) has been demonstrated in the immune deposits, and the bacterial capsular antigen is capable of activating the alternative complement pathway. Rarely, pneumococcal pneumonia can also be associated with hemolytic uremic syndrome due to unmasking of the Thomsen-Friedenreich antigen in glomeruli by pneumococcal neuraminidase, which then elicits an immune response.[35]

Gastroenteritis due to *Campylobacter jejuni* may be associated with mesangioproliferative or diffuse proliferative GN. There are also reports of GN with other bacterial infections including those due to *E. coli*, *Yersinia*, *Meningococcus*, and *Mycoplasma pneumoniae*.

VIRAL INFECTIONS

GN may result from several viral infections (see Fig. 25.1). The most common are those associated with hepatitis B and C viruses

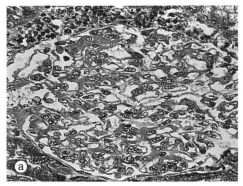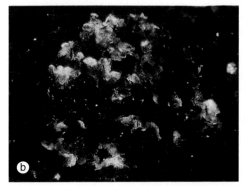

Figure 25.5   Glomerulonephritis (GN) in typhoid fever. *a*, Mesangial proliferative GN. *b*, Immunofluorescent staining demonstrates granular deposition of *Salmonella typhi* Vi antigens in the capillary wall. (Courtesy of V. Boonpucknavig, Bangkok, Thailand.)

and HIV. Rarely, GN may follow yellow fever, mumps, measles, herpes, or varicella. Pathogenetic mechanisms include deposition or *in situ* formation of exogenous (viral) immune complexes, autoantibody formation directed to endogenous antigen modified by viral injury, virus-induced release of proinflammatory cytokines, chemokines, adhesion molecules, growth factors, and direct cytopathic effects of viral proteins.[36]

Hepatitis-Associated Glomerulonephritis
Hepatitis A Virus–Associated Renal Disease
Renal failure associated with severe hepatitis A virus infection may be due to interstitial nephritis or acute tubular necrosis. Rarely, immune complex–related diffuse proliferative GN with Ig and C3 deposits and the clinical picture of nephritic or nephrotic syndrome may develop, at times with renal insufficiency. Recovery of GN usually coincides with the improvement of hepatitis.

Hepatitis B Virus–Associated Renal Disease
Acute HBV infection may be associated with a short-lived serum sickness–like syndrome: urticaria or maculopapular rash, neuropathy, arthralgia or arthritis, microscopic hematuria, and non-nephrotic proteinuria.[37] A renal biopsy specimen, if obtained, shows a mesangial proliferative GN, and the clinical picture resolves spontaneously as the hepatitis improves. Acute HBV infection may resolve uneventfully, but in 10% of adults and in the vast majority of children, the patients become chronic carriers. Vertical (mother to infant at birth) transmission is responsible for about 50% of the chronic carrier states in China and Southeast Asia, whereas horizontal transmission among children and young adults is more important in the Middle East, India, and Africa.[38] In Europe and the United States, the prevalence is lower, and most carriers acquire the infection as adults as a consequence of drug abuse, blood transfusions, or sexual relations.

HBV carriers present the most important renal syndromes associated with HBV infection: MN, MPGN, polyarteritis nodosa, and IgA nephropathy.[38]

Membranous Nephropathy MN is most frequent in Asian populations. The association with the carrier state of HBV surface antigen (HBsAg) is well established (Fig. 25.6). Typically, the patient is 2 to 12 years of age, almost always male, with nephrotic syndrome, microscopic hematuria, and normal renal function. Other clinical presentations include asymptomatic proteinuria and, rarely, chronic renal failure.[38] History and clinical evidence of

hepatitis are often missing and hepatic enzymes may be normal, but HBsAg and anti-HBV core antigen antibodies are present. HBV early antigen (HBeAg) has been found in 80% of the cases, and liver biopsy reveals chronic persistent hepatitis. The clinical course of hepatitis in children is usually favorable, resolving spontaneously, frequently in association with the appearance of anti-HBe antibodies in circulation. In contrast, resolution is uncommon in adults, who have more severe pathologic changes in the liver (chronic active hepatitis or cirrhosis) and often progress to chronic renal disease.[39] Circulating immune complexes are present in the majority of patients and C3 and C4 levels are decreased in 20% to 50%. Renal pathology demonstrates MN with granular deposits of IgG, IgM, and C3 in the capillary wall. Electron microscopy shows subepithelial as well as mesangial and subendothelial immune deposits, in contrast with idiopathic MN in which the mesangial and subendothelial locations are frequently absent. Virus-like particles have been identified in various areas of the glomeruli.

The pathogenesis of the HBV-related MN is thought to be due to passive trapping of immune complexes or to the formation of *in situ* immune complexes involving HBeAg and anti-HBe antibody. Since anti-HBe antibodies are cationic, charge-driven penetration into the basement membrane would favor the otherwise inaccessible subepithelial location.

Membranoproliferative Glomerulonephritis MPGN is the most common glomerular lesion in adult patients with HBV infection. HBsAg and anti-HBs antibodies are universally present. At the time of presentation, patients often have no history of liver disease but have abnormal transaminases. However, liver biopsy specimens, if obtained, often show chronic active or chronic persistent hepatitis and occasionally cirrhosis. Hypertension is present in 54% of the cases and renal failure in 20%. Microscopic hematuria is frequently present.[38]

The pathogenesis of HBV-MPGN involves mesangial and subendothelial deposition of HBsAg and anti-HBs antibodies immune complexes. Renal histology is similar to MPGN type I with prominent subendothelial deposits and mild proliferation. Occasionally, histology resembles type III cryoglobulinemia, with coexisting subepithelial and mesangial deposits.

Mesangioproliferative Glomerulonephritis with IgA Deposits Several reports have emphasized the frequency with which HBV DNA is demonstrated in biopsies of IgA nephropathy.[40] The relationship between these entities may be incidental since the association is reported in countries with a high incidence of both diseases and the prevalence of the HBsAg carrier state among patients with this lesion is lower than in MN and MPGN.

Treatment of Hepatitis B Virus–Associated Glomerulonephritis
Antiviral treatment is recommended for both HBV-MN and HBV-MPGN in adults. In general the response rate is greater for HBV-MN than HBV-MPGN because, in the former, clinical remission generally occurs with clearance of HBeAg and the appearance of anti-HBe antibodies, whereas in the latter, remission correlates with actual cure of the viral infection (disappearance of HBVsAg and development of anti-HBs antibodies). Interferon (IFN)-α (5 million units daily for 6 months) resulted in seroconversion in 8 of 15 patients (from HBeAg to anti-HBe) with clinical remission of their nephrotic syndrome; however, all responding patients had HBV-MN. Lamivudine (100 mg orally once daily for 52 weeks) has been used as initial treatment of

Association of hepatitis B infection with membranous nephropathy			
Presence of Hepatitis B Virus Surface Antigen	North America, Western Europe, Australia	Eastern Europe, South America	Asia, Africa
General carrier rate (%)	0.1–1	1–5	>5
Frequency in membranous nephropathy (%)			
Children	20–64	80	80–100
Adults	>5	15–20	30–45

Figure 25.6 Association of hepatitis B virus infection with membranous nephropathy. (Adapted from Johnson RJ, Couser WG: Hepatitis B infection and renal disease: Clinical immunopathogenetic and therapeutic considerations [editorial review]. Kidney Int 1990;37:663–676.)

chronic HBV, and a recent study showed the efficacy of lamivudine in the improvement of proteinuria, normalization of alanine transaminase levels, disappearance of HBV DNA, and stabilization of renal function in HBV-MN.[41] Pegylated IFN-α may also be useful in the treatment for HBV-associated GN.[42] Steroid treatment is contraindicated because it is ineffective and may delay or prevent seroconversion and accelerate the progression of liver disease.

The prevailing view has been that treatment is not required for children with HBV-MN. The reason for this opinion was that the majority of children are likely to undergo spontaneous remission. However, clearance of HBV DNA and HBeAg has been achieved in about half of the children in controlled studies, with a higher incidence of resolution of the proteinuria in the treated group. Since there have been reports that HBV-MN may progress to ESRD even in children, a definite recommendation is difficult to make at present, and it seems reasonable to evaluate individual cases and prescribe antiviral treatment when proteinuria is severe or there is evidence of progression of renal disease.

Polyarteritis Nodosa

HBV-related vasculitis (HBV-polyarteritis nodosa [PAN]) is observed primarily in adult males who acquire HBV infection from drug abuse or transfusion and is usually observed during the convalescent phase of a mild attack of hepatitis. It is almost never observed in children and is rare in areas of the world where HBV infection is acquired at birth or in childhood, as in Asia.[43] The typical patient with HBV-PAN presents with signs of serum sickness preceding and during a mild or asymptomatic attack of hepatitis. Unlike HBV-associated serum sickness, which resolves spontaneously with clearing of the HBVsAg, in these patients the disease progresses to involve numerous organs. Arteritis of small and medium-sized arteries may be manifested by symptoms of myocardial ischemia, mesenteric angina, Churg-Strauss pulmonary syndrome with asthma and eosinophilia, cerebral ischemia, or mononeuritis multiplex. Renal vasculitis is manifested by microhematuria, nephrotic or non-nephrotic proteinuria, renin-dependent hypertension, and renal failure.

The pathogenesis of HBV-associated PAN is thought to be the deposition of HBsAg–anti-HBs immune complexes in the arterial wall that results in a subsequent inflammatory reaction with the activation of complement.[43] The vessels often show a predominance of IgM and HBsAg, suggesting that the injury is mediated by HBsAg/IgM complexes. Serologic tests reveal HBsAg and anti-HBV core antigen antibodies. Serum complement is usually normal and ANCAs are negative.

Diagnosis requires detection of circulating HBsAg in association with either biopsy or angiographic evidence of vasculitis. Biopsy studies demonstrate vascular lesions, which are typically panmural and in different stages of development. Variable degrees of fibrinoid necrosis, fibrin deposition, and leukocyte infiltration are present. HBsAg, IgM, and occasionally IgG are deposited in the vessel wall. Angiographic studies demonstrating narrow segments and saccular or fusiform aneurysms in celiac or renal arteries have higher diagnostic yield than biopsies.

Liver biopsy demonstrates chronic active or persisting hepatitis or, rarely, acute hepatitis. The renal biopsy, in addition to the arteriolar lesions, may show relatively preserved glomeruli with variable degrees of collapse in the glomerular tuft, likely resulting from ischemic changes. In contrast with idiopathic microscopic polyangiitis, necrotizing lesions with crescent formation are rare. Mesangial proliferative GN, diffuse proliferative GN, MPGN, or MN have all been reported.

The treatment of HBV-PAN historically involves both steroids (typically pulse steroids) and cytotoxic agents (classically cyclophosphamide), and this is associated with a marked increase in short-term survival; however, long-term studies demonstrated accelerated progression of liver disease in these patients. Recent studies suggest that excellent long-term results may be obtained with a short course of steroids (prednisone 1 mg/kg/day for 2 weeks) and plasma exchange (9 to 12 exchanges over 3 weeks) followed by IFN-α therapy and/or lamivudine.[44]

Hepatitis C Virus–Associated Renal Disease

Renal disease in HCV patients is usually MPGN manifested by proteinuria (mild or massive), microhematuria and mild to moderate renal insufficiency. Cryoglobulinemic MPGN and MPGN type I secondary to HCV infection is discussed in detail in Chapter 20. HCV infection may be the major cause of MPGN in Southern Europe, the United States, and Japan.[45] In both cryoglobulinemic (about 90% of the patients with mixed cryoglobulinemia have anti-HCV antibodies and 50% of HCV patients have cryoglobulinemia) and noncryoglobulinemic HCV-associated MPGN, the findings are similar, but leukocytic infiltration and immune aggregates are less conspicuous in the latter. IgM, IgG, and C3 deposits are frequently present. Interestingly, recent investigations have shown that HCV infection may cause significant tubulointerstitial injury, manifested by HCV in perinuclear areas of tubulointerstitial and infiltrating cells in association with genomic and replicative HCV RNA in renal tissues.[46]

Occasional patients manifest signs of a severe vasculitis, including rapidly progressive GN. The disease is observed in adults with long-standing HCV infection (>10 years) and is more common in women.

Chronic disease is usually treated with IFN-α (3 to 5 million U three times weekly for 12 to 18 months) or pegylated IFN-α (1 μg/kg weekly for 48 weeks). A recent report indicates that the combined use of pegylated IFN-α and ribavirin given for 18 ± 10 months achieved HCV RNA clearance for at least 6 months in 12 of 18 patients.[47] However, ribavirin is contraindicated in patients with creatinine clearance <50 ml/min due to an increased frequency of ribavirin-induced hemolysis.

In patients with ESRD, serious adverse effects (pulmonary edema, cerebral hemorrhage, pancreatitis, cardiomyopathy, diplopia) observed with IFN therapy are more common than in other patients. They occur in an average of 26% of the patients (range, 0% to 51%). Preliminary data suggest that ribavirin, at reduced doses,[48] anti-CD20 monoclonal antibody treatment (rituximab),[49] and mycophenolate mofetil[50] may be useful in the treatment of HCV associated with renal disease.

A potentially useful strategy may be the pretransplant treatment of HCV-positive recipients. Administration of IFN-α for 1 year prior to transplantation resulted in a higher percentage of HCV RNA negatives at the time of transplantation (67% versus 29% in the untreated group) and a reduction in the number of post-transplantation *de novo* GN cases (6.7% versus 19%).[51] If there are signs of severe vasculitis or rapid progression, antiviral agents are often withheld and the renal disease is treated with pulse methylprednisolone with or without cyclophosphamide and plasma exchange. IFN-α is generally not administered until the prednisone dose is reduced to ≤20 mg/day and the patient is off cytotoxic therapy, as there are data showing that efficacy may be retarded when cytotoxic therapy is used or prednisone doses are high.

Other Hepatitis C Virus–Associated Glomerulonephritis

HCV infection may be associated with other glomerular diseases with or without cryoglobulinemia. Patients with MN (HCV-MN) have been described in which HCV antigens have been identified in the subepithelial immune deposits. The association has been reported in Spain, Japan, and the United States, especially in renal transplant recipients. The clinical and histologic findings are similar to those observed in idiopathic MN except that HCV RNA and anti-HCV antibodies are positive.

Other reported associations include fibrillary GN, focal glomerulosclerosis (especially in African Americans), and thrombotic microangiopathy with anticardiolipin antibodies (especially following renal transplantation).

Human Immunodeficiency Virus–Associated Renal Disease

HIV infection is associated with a number of renal syndromes, including HIV-associated nephropathy (HIVAN), immune-complex GN, thrombotic microangiopathies, vasculitis, acute renal failure, and electrolyte disorders. In addition, HIVAN may coexist with nephropathies caused by concomitant infection with HBV or syphilis (MN), HCV (MPGN with cryoglobulinemia), or diabetes. Furthermore, a variety of drugs used in the management of HIV infection can also cause renal dysfunction[52] (Fig. 25.7). Recent data indicate that 1.5% (range, 0.3% to 3.4%) and 0.4% (range, 0% to 1%) of dialysis patients have HIV infection and acquired immunodeficiency syndrome, respectively.[53] HIV infection is the third leading cause of ESRD in African Americans between the ages of 20 and 64 years.[54]

Human Immunodeficiency Virus–Associated Nephropathy

HIVAN is the most frequent renal manifestation of HIV infection (see also Chapter 18). In African Americans, the incidence ranges from 3.5% (biopsy findings in proteinuric patients) to 12% (autopsy findings).[55] The disease is caused by infection of renal cells with HIV-1 virus. Not only HIV-1 mRNA and DNA have been demonstrated in human tubular and glomerular cells, but, in addition, there is evidence of active viral replication in the renal tissue. Therefore, the kidney may be an active reservoir, as well as the target, for HIV. Transgenic mice, expressing a gag/pol deleted HIV genome, develop a renal lesion similar to HIVAN with proteinuria and azotemia. Cross-transplantation experiments have shown that renal transgene expression is a key factor in the development of HIVAN.[56] The mechanism of penetration of HIV-1 is still unclear since the viral receptors and coreceptors (CD4$^+$, CXCR4, CCR5) are not constantly present in renal cells.

HIVAN is usually a late manifestation of HIV infection but occasionally may be the initial manifestation of HIV-1 infection. The patients are usually Black, and the clustering of cases with chronic renal failure in uninfected relatives suggests common environmental or inherited factors that predispose to renal disease. The clinical picture typically includes proteinuria in the nephrotic range and progressive azotemia. Peripheral edema is uncommon, and the relative rarity of hypertension has led to the speculation that salt wasting may be part of HIVAN.[57] The urinary sediment frequently presents tubular epithelial cells and ultrasonography shows echogenic kidneys of large or normal size.

The need for biopsy is emphasized by the fact that only 50% of the cases suspected to be HIVAN are actually confirmed by the renal biopsy. The typical lesion is a collapsing focal segmental glomerulosclerosis (see Chapter 18).

Treatment with drugs of the highly active antiretroviral therapy (HAART) group markedly reduces the risk of HIVAN as well as its progression and are likely responsible for the fact that the numbers of patients with ESRD caused by HIV has remained steady since 1995, while the prevalence of HIV in the general population has risen steadily.[55,58] Angiotensin-converting enzyme inhibitors have

Renal syndromes associated with antiretroviral agents		
Type of Agent	Drug (Trade Name)	Clinical Syndrome (Histology)
Nucleoside reverse transcriptase inhibitors	Abacavir*	Acute renal failure (acute interstitial nephritis)
	Didanosine,[†] Lamivudine,[†] Stavudine[†]	Fanconi syndrome Fanconi syndrome Fanconi syndrome
Nucleotide reverse transcriptase inhibitors	Tenofovir fumarate[†]	Fanconi syndrome, nephrogenic diabetes insipidus, acute renal failure (proximal tubule damage)
Other reverse transcriptase inhibitors	Delavirdine[‡] Efavirenz[‡] Nevarapine[‡]	
Protease inhibitors	Indavidir[‡]	Renal colic, urolithiasis, urinary tract obstruction, acute and chronic renal failure (interstitial nephritis, intratubular drug crystals)
	Nelfinavir[‡] Ritonavir[‡]	Renal colic Acute renal failure
HIV-1 fusion inhibitor	Enfurvirtide	Membranoproliferative GN

Figure 25.7 Renal syndromes associated with antiretroviral agents. *No dose adaptation with glomerular filtration rate reduction needed. [†]Dose adaptation with glomerular filtration rate reduction needed. [‡]Data about requirements of dose adaptation with reduced glomerular filtration rate reduction not available. GN, glomerulonephritis; HIV, human immunodeficiency virus. (Modified from Daugas E, Rougier P, Hill G: HAART-related nephropathies in HIV-infected patients. Kidney Int 2005;67:393–403.)

been shown to prevent deterioration of renal function in patients with a creatinine level <2 mg/dl. Oral prednisone treatment results in a decrease in serum creatinine levels in some patients, but relapse is common after suspension of the therapy.

The mortality of HIV patients with ESRD in dialysis programs has drastically improved from a mean survival of 1 to 3 months in the pre-HAART era to the present figures of first-year survivals of 74%, not too different from the general population of ESRD patients.[59] Recent data indicate that comparable results can be obtained with peritoneal and hemodialysis. Similarly, transplantation has been performed in HIV-infected patients in recent years, and short-term data indicate that survival may be similar to noninfected patients. HIV-1 seropositive patients without a history of opportunistic infections, CD4 T cell counts >200/mm^3, and undetectable viral loads, had 1-year graft and patient survival rates similar to those in the database of the United Network for Organ Sharing.[60]

Human Immunodeficiency Virus–Associated Immune Complex Glomerulonephritides

Glomerulonephritides resulting from immune complexes containing HIV gp120 or p24 are characterized by mesangial, subepithelial, and subendothelial deposits, at times so intense that they acquire a lupus-like appearance. The histologic picture is that of membranoproliferative GN and less frequently membranous nephropathy. The clinical presentation can vary from microscopic hematuria to renal failure. Proteinuria may be in the nephrotic range, but hypercholesterolemia is usually absent. In contrast with HIVAN, hypertension is common. Hypocomplementemia and cryoglobulinemia are present in 30% to 50% of the cases.

Patients with HIV-associated immune complex nephropathies usually progress rapidly to renal failure, and co-infection with HCV results in a particularly aggressive form of renal disease.

Human Immunodeficiency Virus–Associated Thrombotic Microangiopathy

HIV infection may occasionally induce the hemolytic-uremic syndrome (see also Chapter 28). Hypertension, hemolytic anemia, thrombocytopenia, and neurologic manifestations are part of the clinical picture. The disease is thought to be due to endothelial cell injury. The characteristic renal lesions are thrombi in arterioles and glomerular capillaries and signs of mesangiolysis. The prognosis is poor, and very few HIV patients who develop thrombotic microangiopathy survive for more than 2 years. Fortunately, this manifestation of HIV infection has become very unusual since the introduction of HAART.

Other Virus Infection–Associated Glomerular Diseases

Severe cytomegalovirus (CMV) infection in healthy individuals is rare. Associations described with IgA nephropathy and transplant glomerulopathy do not appear to have a causal relationship. There have been rare reports in both adults and neonates of an immune complex GN with diffuse proliferative changes and granular immune deposits containing CMV antigens. CMV infection can also involve the kidneys in renal transplant recipients and is generally manifested by tubular cells and macrophages in the interstitium with characteristic intracytoplasmic, "owl-like" inclusions; while there is some evidence that this may be a cause of tubular dysfunction, there is no evidence that this results in glomerular injury. Only exceptionally, CMV infection may be complicated by collapsing glomerulopathy and ESRD in patients not infected with HIV.[61]

Parvovirus B19 infection is a cause of aplastic crisis in patients with sickle cell disease and has been implicated in rare cases of nephrotic syndrome that sometimes develop 3 days to 7 weeks after the aplastic crises.[62] Histology during the acute phase shows diffuse proliferative GN or MPGN and later a collapsing FSGS, with similarities to heroin nephropathy and HIVAN.[63] A few cases of GN have been associated with acute parvovirus B19 infection in adults who do not have sickle cell disease; clinically helpful signs include the presence of a transient rash, arthralgias or arthritis, and anemia. There is also serologic evidence of increased antibodies to parvovirus B19 in collapsing glomerulosclerosis and its DNA has been demonstrated in kidney tissue of FSGS (see also Chapter 18).[64]

Other viruses, particularly those causing upper respiratory infections, may result in transient proteinuria and a mesangioproliferative histology. This suggests that mild proteinuria, which is often present in acute febrile illnesses may not always be due to alterations in glomerular permeability caused by changes in intrarenal hemodynamics from fever, but rather due to undiagnosed, transient, and mild GN. Mumps, for example, can be associated with transient microscopic hematuria and non-nephrotic proteinuria with normal renal function in up to 25% of patients. Biopsy specimen reveals mesangial proliferative GN with IgM, IgA, and C3 deposits and mumps antigens in the mesangium. Measles may infrequently be associated with endocapillary proliferative GN and viral antigen has been identified in the glomeruli. Anecdotal reports suggest that measles infection may result in remission of the nephrotic syndrome in minimal change

disease. Varicella infection can rarely be associated with nephrotic syndrome and histologic changes similar to those described with mumps. Varicella antigens have been demonstrated in the capillary walls and mesangium. Adenovirus and influenza A and B infections may also be associated with transient microhematuria, proteinuria, and complement depression in 3% of the cases. Biopsy findings include MPGN with immune deposits, predominantly C3 and to a lesser degree IgM and IgG. Upper respiratory infections with coxsackievirus B-5 and A-4 strains are sometimes associated with microhematuria and mild proteinuria and diffuse proliferative GN. Dengue hemorrhagic fever may be caused by four serotypes of the family Flaviviridae. The clinical manifestations, reflecting increased vascular permeability, include muscular pains, gastrointestinal symptoms, and, in severe cases, bleeding manifestations and shock. Acute renal failure may accompany the severe cases and in some less severely ill patients, acute endocapillary GN with mesangial proliferation may develop and may be manifested by microhematuria and proteinuria. Intense granular deposits of IgG, IgM, and C3 in mesangial areas and to a lesser degree in capillary walls are usually present.

Mild renal abnormalities can also be observed with acute Epstein-Barr virus (EBV) infection, with microhematuria and proteinuria in 10% to 15% of cases. Acute interstitial nephritis is probably the most common renal complication, but diffuse proliferative and MPGN may also occur. Replicating EBV was localized not only to infiltrating macrophages, but also to proximal tubular cells that were shown to express the CD21 receptor for EBV. It was suggested that EBV might be a major cause of chronic interstitial nephritis.[65]

PARASITIC INFECTIONS

Malaria-Associated Renal Disease

Malaria, caused by a protozoan of the genus *Plasmodium* and acquired through the sting of infected *Anopheles* mosquitoes, is a major world health problem, with 300 to 500 million cases and 1.5 to 2.7 million deaths each year (Fig. 25.8). About 90% of the cases occur in Africa, India, Southeast Asia, and Latin America.[66] Malaria can also be acquired by blood transfusions (prevalence among blood donors in a teaching hospital in Nigeria was 32%),[67] and bites by infected vectors introduced in aircraft ("airport malaria").

Infestation with *Plasmodium falciparum* is usually associated with heavy parasitemia because it invades red blood cells of any age; in contrast, *Plasmodium vivax* and *Plasmodium ovale* infect only young red cells and *Plasmodium malariae* infects aging erythrocytes. Antigen-monocyte interactions occur with increased expression of intracellular adhesion molecule-1 and CD14, interaction with T helper 1 (Th1) and Th2 cytokines and secretion of tumor necrosis factor α. Infected red cells express surface antigens (Pf155/RESA) that favor Th2 lymphocyte responses. *P. falciparum* also activates the alternative pathway of complement and the intrinsic coagulation cascade.[68]

Fluid and electrolyte disturbances and acute renal failure are common, especially with *P. falciparum*. Malarial acute renal failure has mortality ranging from 15% to 45%.[66]

Acute transient GN may occur in *P. ovale*, *P. vivax* infections, and *P. falciparum* infections. In the latter, acute nephritic and nephrotic syndromes are occasionally seen. Mesangial proliferation, finely granular deposition of IgM, and C3 and electron-dense deposits are present (Fig. 25.9). Patients present with microscopic hematuria, mild proteinuria, and often hypocomplementemia (low C3 and C4 levels), and circulating immune complexes.

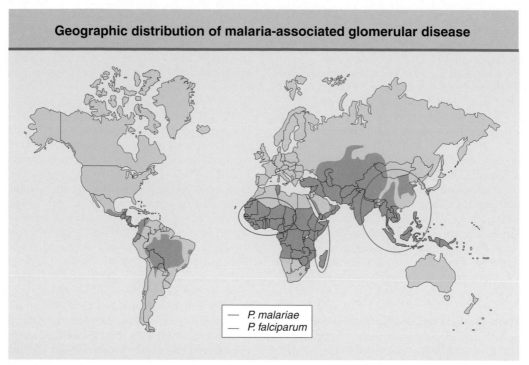

Geographic distribution of malaria-associated glomerular disease

— *P. malariae*
— *P. falciparum*

Figure 25.8   Geographic distribution of malaria-associated glomerular disease. Although malaria is endogenous to many areas of the world (*shaded orange*), the major areas where malaria-associated glomerular disease has been reported (*ringed*) and their respective species are shown.

Chronic GN is characteristic of *P. malariae* infections, although recently some cases have been associated with *P. vivax*, primarily in West Africa and Nigeria. The clinical syndrome is nonspecific, apart from the clinical features of quartan malaria. The patients are usually children (peak age 6 to 8 years) or young adults with heavy proteinuria and overt nephrotic syndrome. Serum complement is normal, cholesterol is normal because of the associated nutritional deficiency, and hypertension is a late finding. The characteristic lesion is MPGN with coarsely granular IgG, IgM, and C3 deposits and subendothelial electron-dense material, and intramembranous lacunae (due to reabsorption of immune complexes) are typical biopsy specimen characteristics of quartan malaria nephropathy (Fig. 25.10). Crescent formation is rare. The reason why this chronic nephropathy is observed with *P. malariae* and not with

P. falciparum may relate to the mechanism of infection. *P. falciparum* may infect all red blood cells (RBCs), so the symptoms are often severe and the patient is more likely to seek medical attention early. In contrast, *P. malariae* only infects senescent RBCs and the clinical manifestations are often more subdued and infection more indolent. *P. malariae* infection also results in a Th2 response as opposed to *P. falciparum* infection, which is mediated primarily by a Th1 response. Because parasitemia is more prolonged, the host may have more time to stimulate humoral and cell-mediated responses and patients also have liver congestion and splenomegaly (tropical splenomegaly). Despite successful treatment of the malaria, chronic renal failure usually develops in 3 to 5 years. The progressive course of renal disease of quartan malaria is unmodified by steroids and immunosuppressive agents. The

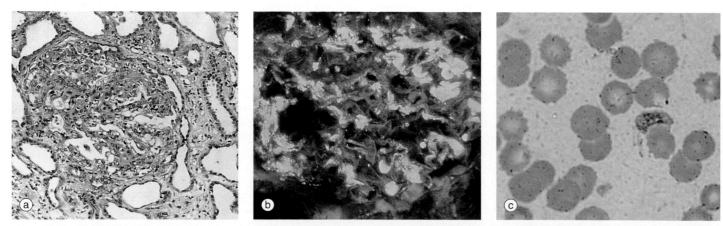

Figure 25.9   Glomerulonephritis (GN) associated with *Plasmodium falciparum* malaria. *a*, Light microscopy shows a mesangioproliferative GN. *b*, Immunofluorescence may reveal *P. falciparum* antigens in a mesangial pattern. *c*, Peripheral blood smear confirms acute *P. falciparum* infection, with banana-shaped gametocytes and multiple ring forms in erythrocytes. (*a*, From Barsoum RS: Malarial nephropathies. Nephrol Dial Transplant 1998;13:1588–1597; *b* and *c*, courtesy of V. Boonpucknavig, Bangkok, Thailand.)

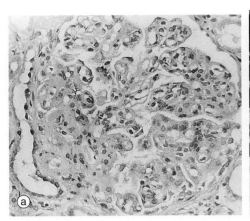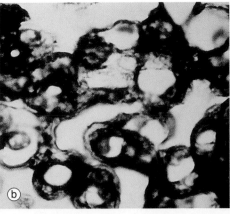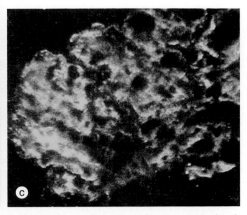

Figure 25.10 Quartan malarial nephropathy. *a*, Light microscopy shows a sclerosing membranoproliferative glomerular nephropathy. *b*, This is associated with a double contour of the basement membrane shown by silver stain. *c*, Malarial antigens detected by glomerular immunofluorescence in a child with quartan malarial nephropathy. (From Barsoum RS: Malarial nephropathies. Nephrol Dial Transplant 1998;13:1588–1597.)

progression to chronicity may be favored by genetic factors, yet undefined, and possibly by the coexistence of malnutrition, EBV infection, and autoimmune reactivity.

Renal Disease Associated with Schistosomiasis
This topic is dealt with in detail in Chapter 53.

Other Parasitic Infestations
Renal involvement has been reported in filarial infections. *Onchocerca volvulus* infection ("river blindness") is associated usually with MPGN, Loa loa infections induce MN or proliferative glomerulonephritides, and *Wuchereria bancrofti* and *Brugia malayi* may induce mesangial GN, MPGN, or diffuse proliferative GN.

Microfilariae have been found in the glomerular capillaries. Except in the case of onchocercosis, filarial antigens have not been demonstrated in glomeruli. Antifilarial treatment does not improve the nephrotic syndrome, and treatment with the antifilarial drug diethylcarbamazine may exacerbate proteinuria. Visceral leishmaniasis (kala-azar) frequently presents with microhematuria and interstitial nephritis or diffuse proliferative GN or MN. The pathogenesis of interstitial nephritis is uncertain. Trichinosis may occasionally present with MPGN, manifested clinically with microhematuria and non-nephrotic proteinuria. Immune deposits are present in mesangium and capillary walls, but specific antigens have not been demonstrated in the glomeruli. GN has also been rarely reported with trypanosomiasis and with congenital toxoplasmosis.

REFERENCES

1. Coppo R, Gianoglio B, Porcellini MG, Maringhini S: Frequency of renal diseases and clinical indications for renal biopsies in children (Report of the Italian National registry of Renal Biopsies in Children). Nephrol Dial Transplant 1998;13:293–297.
2. Johnson RJ, Hurtado A, Merszei J, et al: Hypothesis: Dysregulation of immunologic balance resulting from hygiene and socioeconomic factors may influence the epidemiology and cause of glomerulonephritis worldwide. Am J Kidney Dis 2003;42:575–581.
3. Thongboonkerd V, Luengpailin J, Cao J, et al: Fluoride exposure attenuates expression of *Streptococcus pyogenes* virulence factors. J Biol Chem 2002;277:16599–16605.
4. Rodriguez-Iturbe B: Epidemic poststreptococcal glomerulonephritis. (Nephrology Forum). Kidney Int 1984;25:129–136.
5. Balter S, Benin A, Pinto SW, et al: Epidemic nephritis in Nova Serrana, Brazil. Lancet 2000;355:1776–1780.
6. Rodríguez-Iturbe B: Nephritis-associated streptococcal antigens: Where are we now? J Am Soc Nephrol 2004;15:1961–1962.
7. Yoshizawa N, Yamakami K, Fujino M, et al: Nephritis-associated plasmin receptor and acute poststreptococcal glomerulonephritis: Characterization of the antigen and associated immune response. J Am Soc Nephrol 2004;15:1785–1793.
8. Parra G, Rodrìguez-Iturbe B, Batsford S, et al: Antibody to streptococcal zymogen in the serum of patients with acute glomerulonephritis: A multicentric study. Kidney Int 1998;54:509–517.
9. Oda T, Yamakami K, Omasu F, et al: Glomerular plasmin-like activity in relation to nephritis-associated plasmin receptor in acute poststreptococcal glomerulonephritis. J Am Soc Nephrol 2005;16:247–254.
10. Batsford SR, Mezzano S, Mihatsch M, et al: Is the nephritogenic antigen in post-streptococcal glomerulonephritis pyrogenic exotoxin B (SPE B) or GAPDH? Kidney Int 2005;68:1120–1129.
11. Oshawa I, Ohi H, Endo M, et al: Evidence of lectin complement pathway activation in poststreptococcal glomerulonephritis. Kidney Int 1999;56: 1158–1159.
12. Besbas N, Ozaltin F, Catal F, et al: Monocyte chemoattractant protein-1 and interleukin-8 levels in children with acute poststreptococcal glomerulonephritis. Pediatr Nephrol 2004;19:864–868.
13. Sorger K, Balun J, Hubner FK, et al: The garland type of acute postinfectious glomerulonephritis: Morphological characteristics and follow-up studies. Clin Nephrol 1983;20:17–26.
14. Nicolaidon P, Georgouli H, Matsinos Y, et al: Endothelin-1 in children with acute poststreptococcal glomerulonephritis and hypertension. Pediatr Int 2003;45:35–38.
15. Webb KH, Needham CA, Kurtz SR: Use of a high-sensitivity rapid strep test without culture confirmation of negative results: 2 years' experience. J Family Pract 2000;49:34–36.
16. Johnston F, Carapetis J, Patel MS, et al: Evaluating the use of penicillin to control outbreaks of acute poststreptococcal glomerulonephritis. Pediatr Infect Dis J 1999;18:327–332.
17. Melby PC, Musik WD, Luger AM, Khanna R: Poststreptococcal glomerulonephritis in the elderly: Report of a case and review of the literature. Am J Nephrol 1987;7:235–240.
18. Sesso R, Pinto WL: Five-year follow-up of patients with epidemic glomerulonephritis due to *Streptococcus zooepidemicus*. Nephrol Dial Transplant 2005;20:1808–1812.
19. White AV, Hoy WE, McCredie DA: Childhood post-streptococcal glomerulonephritis as a risk for chronic renal disease in later life. Med J Aust 2001;174:492–496.
20. Tlevjeh IM, Steckelberg JM, Murad HS, et al: Temporal trends in infective endocarditis: A population-based study in Olmsted County, Minnesota. JAMA 2005;293:3022–3028.

21. Hoen B: Infective endocarditis: A frequent disease in dialysis patients. Nephrol Dial Transplant 2004;19:1360–1362.

22. Conlon PJ, Jefferies F, Krigman HR, et al: Predictors of prognosis and risk of acute renal failure in bacterial endocarditis. Clin Nephrol 1998; 49:96–101.

23. Yoh K, Kobayashi M, Yamaguchi N, et al: Cytokines and T cell responses in superantigen-related glomerulonephritis following methicillin-resistant *Staphylococcus aureus* infection. Nephrol Dial Transplant 2000;15: 1170–1174.

24. Majumdar A, Chowdhary S, Ferreira MAAS, et al: Renal pathological findings in infective endocarditis. Nephrol Dial Transplant 2000;15: 1782–1787.

25. Agarwal A, Clemens J, Sedmark DD, et al: Subacute bacterial endocarditis masquerading as type III essential mixed cryoglobulinemia. J Am Soc Nephrol 1997;8:1971–1976.

26. Badour LM, Wilson WR, Bayer AS, et al: Infective endocarditis. Diagnosis, antimicrobial therapy and management of complications. Circulation 2005;111:3167–3184.

27. Haffner D, Schinderas F, Aschoff A: The clinical spectrum of shunt nephritis. Nephrol Dial Transplant 1997;12:1143–1148.

28. Balogun RA, Palmisano J, Kaplan AA, et al: Shunt nephritis from *Propionibacterium acnes* in a solitary kidney. Am J Kidney Dis 2001; 38:E18.

29. Iwata Y, Ohta S, Kawai K, et al: Shunt nephritis with positive titers for ANCA specific for proteinase 3. Am J Kidney Dis 2004;43:E11–E16.

30. Hunte W, Ghraoui F, Cohen RJ: Secondary syphilis and nephrotic syndrome. J Am Soc Nephrol 1993;3:1351–1355.

31. Chugh KS, Sakhuja V: Glomerular disease in the tropics. Am J Nephrol 1990;10:437–450.

32. Albaqali A, Ghuloom A, Al Arrayed A, et al: Hemolytic uremic syndrome in association with typhoid fever. Am J Kidney Dis 2003;41:709–713.

33. Nakayama EE, Ura S, Fleury RN, Soares V: Renal lesions in leprosy: A retrospective study of 199 autopsies. Am J Kidney Dis 2001;38:26–30.

34. Lomonte C, Chiarulli G, Cazzato F, et al: End-stage renal disease in leprosy. J Nephrol 2004;17:302–305.

35. Krysan DJ, Flynn JT: Renal transplantation after *Streptococcus pneumoniae*-associated hemolytic uremic syndrome. Am J Kidney Dis 2001;37:E15.

36. Barbiano De Belgioso G, Ferrario F, Landriani N: Virus-related glomerular diseases: Histological and clinical aspects. J Nephrol 2002;15:469–479.

37. Bhimma R, Coovadia HM: Hepatitis B virus-associated nephropathy. Am J Nephrol 2004;24:198–211.

38. Johnson RJ, Couser WG: Hepatitis B infection and renal disease: Clinical immunopathogenetic and therapeutic considerations [editorial review]. Kidney Int 1990;37:663–676.

39. Lai KN, Lai FM-M: Clinical features and natural course of hepatitis B-related glomerulopathy in adults. Kidney Int 1991;40:S40–S45.

40. Wang N-S, Wu Z-L, Zhang Y-E, Liao L-T: Existence and significance of hepatitis B virus DNA in kidneys of IgA nephropathy. World J Gastroenterol 2005;11:712–716.

41. Tang S, Lai FM, Lui YH, et al: Lamivudine in hepatitis B-associated membranous nephropathy. Kidney Int 2005;68:1750–1758.

42. Lau GK, Piratvisuth T, Luo KX, et al. and the Peginterferon Alfa-2a HBeAg-Positive Chronic Hepatitis B Study Group: Peginterferon Alfa-2a, lamivudine, and the combination for HBeAg-positive chronic hepatitis B. N Engl J Med 2005;352:2682–2695.

43. Guillevin L, Lhote F, Cohen P, et al: Polyarteritis nodosa related hepatitis B virus: A prospective study with long-term observation of 41 patients. Medicine (Baltimore) 1995;74:238–253.

44. Erhardt A, Sagir A, Guillevin L, et al: Successful treatment of hepatitis B virus associated polyarteritis nodosa with a combination of prednisolone, alpha interferon and lamivudine. J Hepatol 2000;33:677–683.

45. Meyers CM, Seef LB, Stehman-Breen CO, Hoofnagle JH: Hepatitis C and renal disease: An update. Am J Kidney Dis 2003;42:631–657.

46. Kasuno K, Ono T, Matsumori A, et al: Hepatitis C virus-associated tubulointerstitial injury. Am J Kidney Dis 2003;41:767–775.

47. Alric L, Plaisier E, Thébault S, et al: Influence of antiviral therapy in hepatitis C virus-associated cryoglobulinemic MPGN. Am J Kidney Dis 2004;43:617–623.

48. Tan AC, Brouwer JT, Glue P: Safety of interferon and ribavirin therapy in hemodialysis patients with chronic hepatitis C: Results of a pilot study. Nephrol Dial Transplant 2001;16:193–195.

49. Rovatello D, Baldovio S, Rossi D, et al: Long term effects of anti-CD20 monoclonal antibody treatment of cryoglobulinemic glomerulonephritis. Nephrol Dial Transplant 2004;19:3054–3061.

50. Reed MJ, Alexander GJ, Thiru S, Smith KG: Hepatitis C-associated glomerulonephritis: A novel therapeutic approach. Nephrol Dial Transplant 2001;16:869–871.

51. Cruzado JM, Casanovas-Taltavull T, Torres J, et al: Pretransplant interferon prevents hepatitis C virus-associated glomerulonephritis in renal allografts by HCV-RNA clearance. Am J Transplant 2003;3:357–360.

52. Daugas E, Rougier P, Hill G: HAART-related nephropathies in HIV-infected patients. Kidney Int 2005;67:393–403.

53. Gupta SK, Eustace JA, Winston JA, et al: Guidelines for the management of chronic kidney disease in HIV-infected patients: Recommendations of the HIV Medicine Association of the Infectious Disease Society of America. Clin Infect Dis 2005;40:1559–1585.

54. U.S. Renal Data System: USRDS 2003 Annual Data Report: Atlas of End Stage Renal Disease in the United States. Bethesda, MD. National Institutes of Health, National Institute of Diabetes and Digestive and Kidney Diseases, 2003.

55. Lu T-C, Ross M: HIV-associated nephropathy. Mt Sinai J Med 2005;72: 193–198.

56. Bruggeman LA, Dikman S, Meng C, et al: Nephropathy in human immunodeficiency virus-1 transgenic mice is due to transgene expression. J Clin Invest 1997;100:84–92.

57. Laradi A, Mallet A, Beaufils H, et al: HIV-associated nephropathy: Outcome and prognosis factors. Groupe d' Etudes Nephrologiques d'Ile de France. J Am Soc Nephrol 1998;9:2327–2335.

58. Lucas GM, Eustace JA, Sozio S, et al: Highly active antiretroviral therapy and the incidence of HIV-1-associated nephropathy: A 12 year cohort study. AIDS 2004;18:541–546.

59. Ahuja TS, Grady J, Khan S: Changing trends in the survival of dialysis patients with human immunodeficiency virus in the United States. J Am Soc Nephrol 2002;13:1889–1893.

60. Roland ME, Stock PG: Review of solid-organ transplantation in HIV-infected patients. Transplantation 2003;75:425–429.

61. Tomlinson L, Borskin Y, McPhee I, et al: Acute cytomegalovirus infection complicated by collapsing glomerulopathy. Nephrol Dial Transplant 2003;18:187–189.

62. Takeda S, Takaeda C, Takazura E, Haratake J: Renal involvement induced by human parvovirus B19 infection. Nephron 2001;89:280–285.

63. Moudgil A, Nast CC, Bagga A, et al: Association of parvovirus B19 infection with idiopathic collapsing glomerulopathy. Kidney Int 2001; 59:2126–2133.

64. Kakazawa T, Tomosugi N, Sakamoto K, et al: Acute glomerulonephritis after human parvovirus B19 infection. Am J Kidney Dis 2001;35:E31.

65. Becker JL, Miller F, Nuovo GJ, et al: Epstein-Barr virus infection of renal proximal tubular cells: Possible role in chronic interstitial nephritis. J Clin Invest 1999;104:1673–1681.

66. Barsoum RS: Malarial acute renal failure. J Am Soc Nephrol 2000;11: 2147–2154.

67. Okocha EC, Ibeh CC, Ele PU, Ibeh NC: The prevalence of malaria parasitaemia in blood donors in a Nigerian teaching hospital. J Vector Borne Dis 2005;42:21–24.

68. Barsoum RS: Malarial nephropathies. Nephrol Dial Transplant 1998;13: 1588–1597.

Renal Amyloidosis and Glomerular Diseases with Monoclonal Immunoglobulin Deposition

Pierre M. Ronco, Pierre Aucouturier, and Bruno Moulin

INTRODUCTION

Because the renal plasma flow represents 20% of the total plasma flow and the glomerulus is the renal filtering unit continuously exposed to plasma proteins, the glomerulus is the first structure in the body in which abnormal proteins or proteins with a peculiar affinity for constituents of the capillary wall become deposited. The resulting diseases include amyloidosis, nonamyloid monoclonal immunoglobulin deposition disease (MIDD), and other plasma cell dyscrasia–related glomerulopathies. In most cases, the nephritogenic protein is a monoclonal immunoglobulin subunit.

These diseases can be classified into two categories by electron microscopy (Fig. 26.1). The first category includes diseases with fibril formation, mainly amyloidosis, and diseases with microtubule formation, including cryoglobulinemic (see Chapter 20) and immunotactoid glomerulonephritis. The second category is characterized by nonorganized electron-dense granular deposits. They are localized along basement membranes in most tissues, especially in the kidney, and define a disease now called MIDD. In some cases, monotypic immune complex–like deposits are observed in the setting of proliferative glomerulonephritis. In addition to immunglobulins, a large number of other precursor proteins can result in renal amyloid deposits (Fig. 26.2).

Glomerular diseases with tissue deposition or precipitation of monoclonal immunoglobulin components	
Immunoglobulin Deposits	Glomerular Disease

Organized
    Fibrillar
    Microtubular
	Amyloidosis (AL, AH)
	Cryoglobulinemia; immunotactoid glomerulonephritis

Nonorganized: granular	Monoclonal immunoglobulin deposition disease: light-chain, heavy-chain, and light-plus heavy-chain deposition diseases Immune complex–like proliferative glomerulonephritis

Figure 26.1   Glomerular diseases with tissue deposition or precipitation of monoclonal immunoglobulin components.

RENAL AMYLOIDOSIS

General Characteristics of Amyloidosis
Definition
Amyloidosis is a general term for a family of diseases defined by morphologic criteria. The diseases are characterized by the deposition in extracellular spaces of a proteinaceous material with well-defined morphologic and ultrastructural features. Amyloid deposits are typically composed of a feltlike array of 7.5- to 10-nm-wide rigid, linear, nonbranching, aggregated fibrils of indefinite length.[1] One amyloid fibril is made of two twisted 3-nm-wide filaments, each having a regular antiparallel β-pleated sheet configuration. The β-sheets are perpendicular to the filament axis.

Amyloid Precursor–Based Classification
Amyloidoses include various conditions that differ essentially by the nature of the precursor protein that yields the main component of fibrils, and are classified accordingly (see Fig. 26.2).[2] The propensity for forming amyloid seems related to the ability of this precursor to adopt a β-pleated sheet conformation. The amyloidogenic potential is enhanced by an overproduction or an impaired clearance of the precursor or by genetically transmitted mutations.

Renal amyloidoses include immunoglobulin light chain (AL) and systemic secondary (AA) amyloidoses. Other precursors, such as transthyretin, fibrinogen, and lysozyme, are responsible for rare familial cases.

Other Components of All Amyloid Fibrils
Glycosaminoglycans (GAGs) have been found tightly associated to amyloid fibrils. GAGs are polysaccharide chains made of repeating hyaluronic acid/hexosamine units normally linked to a protein core, thus forming proteoglycans, an important constituent of extracellular matrices. Proteoglycans, mostly of the heparan sulfate type, might induce and stabilize the β-pleated amyloid structure.

Another constituent of all amyloid deposits is the serum amyloid P component (SAP). SAP is remarkably resistant to proteolytic digestion, suggesting that coating of amyloid fibrils with SAP could result in their protection from catabolism. The high affinity of SAP toward amyloid was exploited for diagnosing, locating, and monitoring the extent of systemic amyloidosis using scintigraphy with [¹²³I]-SAP.

Classification of amyloidoses				
Amyloid Protein	Precursor	Distribution	Type	Syndrome or Involved Tissues
AA	Serum amyloid A	Systemic	Acquired	Secondary amyloidosis, reactive to chronic infection of inflammation, including hereditary periodic fever (FMF, TRAPS, HIDS, FCU, and MWS)
AApoAI	Apolipoprotein A-I	Systemic	Hereditary	Liver, kidney, heart
AApoAII	Apolipoprotein A-II	Systemic	Hereditary	Kidney, heart
Aβ	Aβ protein precursor	Localized / Localized	Acquired / Hereditary	Sporadic Alzheimer's disease, aging / Prototypical hereditary cerebral amyloid angiopathy, Dutch type
Aβ2M	β2-microglobulin	Systemic	Acquired	Chronic hemodialysis
ABri	ABri protein precursor	Localized or systemic?	Hereditary	British familial dementia
ACys	Cystatin C	Systemic	Hereditary	Icelandic hereditary cerebral amyloid angiopathy
AFib	Fibrinogen Aα chain	Systemic	Hereditary	Kidney
AGel	Gelsolin	Systemic	Hereditary	Finnish hereditary amyloidosis
AH	Immunoglobulin heavy chain	Systemic or localized	Acquired	Primary amyloidosis, myeloma associated
AL	Immunoglobulin light chain	Systemic or localized	Acquired	Primary amyloidosis, myeloma associated
ALys	Lysozyme	Systemic	Hereditary	Kidney, liver, spleen
APrP	Prion protein	Localized / Localized	Acquired / Hereditary	Sporadic (iatrogenic) CJD, new variant CJD / Familial CJD, GSSD, FFI
ATTR	Transthyretin	Systemic	Hereditary / Acquired	Prototypical FAP / Senile heart, vessels

Figure 26.2   Classification of amyloidoses. Entries in *italic* type indicate amyloid types with kidney involvement. The following proteins may also cause amyloidosis: calcitonin, islet-amyloid polypeptides, atrial natriuretic factor, prolactin, insulin, lactadherin, keratoepithelin, and Danish amyloid protein (which comes from the same gene as ABri and has an identical N-terminal sequence). CJD, Creutzfeldt-Jakob disease; FAP, familial amyloidotic polyneuropathy; FCU, familial cold urticaria; FFI, fatal familial insomnia; FMF, familial Mediterranean fever; GSSD, Gerstmann-Straussler-Scheinker disease; HIDS, hyper-IgD syndrome; MWS, Muckle-Wells syndrome; TRAPS, tumor necrosis factor receptor–associated periodic syndrome. (Adapted from Westermark G, Benson MD, Buxbaum JN, et al: Amyloid fibril protein nomenclature. Amyloid 2002;9:197–200 and Merlini G, Bellotti V: Molecular mechanisms of amyloidosis. N Engl J Med 2003;349:583–596.)

General Mechanisms of Fibrillogenesis

Amyloidogenesis seems to involve a nucleation-dependent polymerization process. Formation of an ordered nucleus is the initial and limiting step, followed by addition of monomers, leading to elongation of the fibrils.[3] Fibrillogenesis may be the consequence of several mechanisms of processing the amyloid precursor, including partial proteolysis and conformational modifications. Conformational changes lead to a soluble, partially folded intermediate whose subsequent ordered self-assembly results in fibril formation. Phagocytic cells, in particular macrophages, have a central role in the disease by providing the intralysosomal processing of the precursor. In AL-amyloidosis, the variable domain of the light chain V_L is the main component, which indicates partial proteolysis of the light-chain precursor.

Pathology

The unique conformation of fibrils is responsible for peculiar tinctorial properties. On light microscopy, the deposits are extracellular, eosinophilic, and metachromatic. After Congo red staining, they appear faintly red (Fig. 26.3a) and show the characteristic apple-green birefringence under polarized light (see Fig. 26.3b). Metachromasia is also observed with Crystal violet, which stains the deposits red. Treatment with permanganate before the Congo red procedure may help to discriminate AA fibrils, which are sensitive to permanganate oxidation, from AL amyloid, which is resistant.

In the kidney, the earliest lesions are located in the mesangium (see Fig. 26.3a), along the glomerular basement membrane, and in the blood vessels. Within the mesangium, deposits are primarily associated with the mesangial matrix and subsequently increase irregularly by spreading from lobule to lobule and then invading the whole mesangial area. Amyloid deposits may also infiltrate the glomerular basement membrane or be localized on both sides of it. When subepithelial deposits predominate, spikes similar to those seen in membranous glomerulopathy may be observed. Advanced amyloid typically produces a nonproliferative, noninflammatory glomerulopathy, which is responsible for a marked enlargement of the kidney. The amyloid deposits replace the normal glomerular architecture, with a consequent loss of cellularity. When glomeruli become massively sclerotic, the deposits may be difficult to demonstrate by Congo red staining, and electron microscopy may then be helpful. The latter is also required at very early stages, which may not be detected by light microscopy examination in patients presenting with the nephrotic syndrome. Except in fibrinogen Aα-chain, which characteristically does not affect renal vessels, the media of the blood vessels is prominently involved at early stages. Vascular involvement may predominate and occasionally occurs alone, particularly in AL-amyloidosis. Deposits may

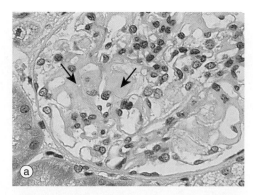

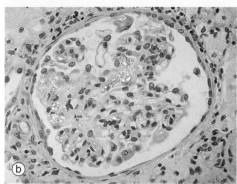

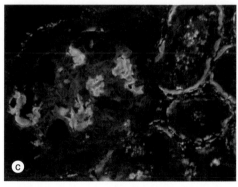

Figure 26.3   Amyloidosis. *a*, Amyloid deposits (*arrows*) in a glomerulus (hematoxylin-eosin, ×312). *b*, Congo red staining. Apple-green birefringence under polarized light (×312). *c*, Immunofluorescence with anti–κ antibody. Note glomerular and tubular deposits (×312). (Courtesy of Dr. Béatrice Mougenot.)

also affect the tubules and the interstitium, leading to atrophy and disappearance of the tubular structures and to interstitial fibrosis.

Because of the heterogeneity of amyloidotic diseases, immunohistology with specific antisera should be routinely performed (see Fig. 26.3c). Immunohistochemical classification of amyloid type is possible in most cases. However, immunohistology with sera directed against immunoglobulin chains may be more difficult to interpret than that with anti-AA antiserum, perhaps because of the absence or inaccessibility of light-chain epitopes. A genetic cause should be sought in all patients with amyloidosis in whom confirmation of the amyloid precursor cannot be obtained by immunohistochemistry.[4] On electron microscopy, amyloid deposits are characterized by randomly oriented, nonbranching fibrils with an 8- to 15-nm diameter (Fig. 26.4).

Immunoglobulin-Associated Amyloidosis (AL and AH)

Free immunoglobulin subunits, mostly light chains, secreted by a single clone of B cells, are the cause of the most frequent and severe amyloidosis affecting the kidney. Studies on the mechanisms

of AL-amyloidogenesis are made particularly difficult by the unique degree of structural heterogeneity of the precursor: each monoclonal light chain is different from all others, so each patient is a unique case. The involvement of an immunoglobulin heavy chain in amyloidosis is exceptional.[5]

Pathogenesis

Determinant factors are borne by the precursor light chain. In AL-amyloidosis, a striking overrepresentation of the λ isotype, which is two- to fourfold more frequent than the κ isotype, is observed. A homology family of light-chain variable regions, the $V_{\lambda VI}$ variability subgroup, is found only in amyloid-associated monoclonal immunoglobulins and is overrepresented in AL-amyloidosis.

Amyloidogenicity is frequently associated with certain physico-chemical features such as the presence of low molecular mass light-chain fragments in the patient's urine, and low isoelectric point (pI). An analysis of nearly 200 light-chain sequences identified 12 positions in κ-chains and 12 in λ-chains where certain residues were significantly associated with amyloidosis. Four structural risk factors were shown to define most fibril-forming κ light chains.[6] Because of their high dimerization constants, light chains from patients with AL-amyloidosis may also behave as an antibody with affinity for extracellular structures.

The tropism of organ involvement may also be influenced by the germ line gene used for the light-chain variable region (V_L). Patients expressing monoclonal light chain of the $V_{\lambda VI}$ subgroup are more likely to present with dominant renal involvement, whereas those with other λ light chains seem to develop dominant cardiac and multisystem disease.[7] Patients with κ light chains are more likely to have dominant hepatic involvement.

In addition, organ-specific environmental factors are most likely to be involved. For example, the kidney contains high concentrations of urea that were shown to enhance fibril formation by reducing the nucleation lag time.

Amyloid light chains may contribute directly to the pathogenesis, independent of extracellular fibril deposition. In the heart and the kidney at least, the infiltration alone does not correlate well with clinical manifestations. Light chains from amyloid patients incubated with cultured human mesangial cells induce a macrophage-like phenotype, whereas those from light-chain

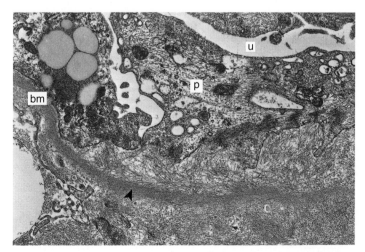

Figure 26.4   Electron micrograph of amyloid deposits invading glomerular basement membrane. Randomly oriented fibrils are located on both sides of the basement membrane (bm) and the lamina densa is attenuated (*arrowhead*) (×10,000). p, podocyte; u, urinary space. (Courtesy of Dr. Béatrice Mougenot.)

deposition disease (LCDD) patients induce a myofibroblastic phenotypic transformation.[8]

Epidemiology

The incidence of AL-amyloidosis is nine per million per year. Fewer than one of four patients with AL-amyloidosis is considered to have an overt immunoproliferative disease, which usually is a multiple myeloma, although other forms such as Waldenström's macroglobulinemia are not exceptional. Amyloid deposits are found in approximately 10% of all patients with myeloma and in 20% of those with pure light-chain myeloma. In fact, the true prevalence of myeloma depends on the criteria used for its diagnosis. Epidemiologic characteristics of primary amyloidosis, that is, amyloidosis without overt immunoproliferative disease, and myeloma are not significantly different. The median age at diagnosis is 64 years in patients with primary amyloidosis,[9] with a slight predominance of male patients.

Clinical Manifestations

The main clinical symptoms at presentation are weakness and weight loss (Fig. 26.5). Except for bone pain, there is no difference in the incidence of initial symptoms in patients with and without myeloma. Nephrotic syndrome, orthostatic hypotension, and peripheral neuropathy are more frequent in patients with AL-amyloidosis without myeloma than in those with associated myeloma.[10] Renal insufficiency occurs usually in the presence of marked kidney enlargement and is usually not associated with hypertension. Proteinuria, mainly composed of albumin, occurs in the absence of microscopic hematuria. When present, the hematuria should prompt examination for a bleeding lesion in the urinary tract. Renal manifestations may also include renal tubular acidosis (mostly as a part of Fanconi syndrome; see Chapter 59) and polyuria-polydipsia (resulting from urinary concentration

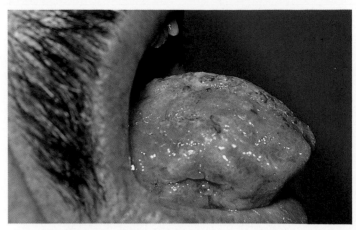

Figure 26.6 Macroglossia in a patient with AL-amyloidosis. (Courtesy of Dr. S. Aractinji.)

defect), when amyloid deposits occur around proximal tubules and Henle's loops (or collecting ducts), respectively.

AL-amyloidosis may infiltrate almost any organ other than the brain and, therefore, can be responsible for a wide variety of clinical manifestations. Restrictive cardiomyopathy is found at presentation in up to one third of patients and causes death in about one half. Infiltration of the ventricular walls and the septum may be recognized by echocardiography. Amyloid may also induce arrhythmias and the sick sinus syndrome. Amyloid deposits in the coronary arteries may result in angina pectoris and myocardial infarction. Blood levels of cardiac troponins and N-terminal pro-brain natriuretic peptide are sensitive markers of myocardial dysfunction and powerful predictors of overall survival in patients with AL-amyloidosis.

Involvement of the gastrointestinal tract is also common and can cause motility disturbances, malabsorption, hemorrhage, or obstruction. Macroglossia (Fig. 26.6) may interfere with eating and obstruct airways. Abnormalities of hepatic function remain generally mild. Hyposplenism, commonly associated with splenomegaly, is occasionally found. Peripheral nerve involvement is usually responsible for a painful sensory polyneuropathy followed later by motor deficits. Autonomic neuropathy causing orthostatic hypotension, lack of sweating, gastrointestinal disturbances, bladder dysfunction, and impotence may occur alone or together with peripheral neuropathy. Orthostatic hypotension is one of the major hampering complications of AL-amyloidosis, with some patients being bedridden. Skin involvement may take the form of purpura, characteristically around the eyes (Fig. 26.7); ecchymoses; papules; nodules; and plaques, occurring usually on the face and upper trunk. AL-amyloidosis may also infiltrate articular structures and mimic rheumatoid or an asymmetrical seronegative synovitis. Infiltration of the shoulders may produce severe pain and swelling (shoulder pad sign).

A rare but potentially serious manifestation of AL-amyloidosis is an acquired bleeding diathesis that may be associated with deficiency of factor X and sometimes also factor IX, or with increased fibrinolysis. It should be systematically sought before any biopsy of a deep organ. Widespread vascular deposits may also be responsible for bleeding. Partial thromboplastin (PT) and activated partial thromboplastin time (aPTT) measurements as well as determination of bleeding times may be required to assess bleeding diathesis.

On average, monoclonal light chains can be detected by immunoelectrophoresis in 73% of the urine samples, and the λ isotype is twice as frequent as the κ, contrasting with the 1:2 ratio of λ to κ observed in patients with multiple myeloma alone.

Clinical and laboratory features at presentation in 474 patients with proven AL-amyloidosis	
Features	Percentage
Initial symptoms	
Fatigue	62
Weight loss	52
Pain	5
Purpura	15
Gross bleeding	3
Physical findings	
Hepatomegaly	24
Palpable spleen	5
Lymphadenopathy	3
Macroglossia	9
Laboratory findings	
Increased plasma cells (bone marrow 6%)	56*
Anemia (hemoglobin <10 g/dl)	11
Elevated serum creatinine (1.3 mg/dl) (>155 μmol/l)	45
Elevated alkaline phosphatase	26
Hypercalcemia (>11 mg/dl) (>2.75 mmol/l)	2
Proteinuria (1.0 g/24 h)	55
Urine light chain	73†
κ chain	23
λ chain	50

Figure 26.5 Clinical and laboratory features at presentation in 474 patients with proven AL-amyloidosis. *Fifteen percent of patients having a myeloma. †Of 429 patients. (From Kyle RA, Gertz MA: Primary systemic amyloidosis: Clinical and laboratory features in 474 cases. Semin Hematol 1995;32:45–59.)

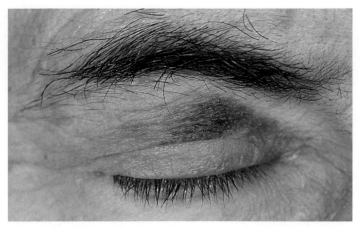

Figure 26.7 Skin involvement in AL-amyloidosis. Noninfiltrated purpuric macule of the superior eyebrow, very typical of AL-amyloidosis. (Courtesy of Dr. S. Aractinji.)

With the use of more sensitive immunochemical techniques, a monoclonal immunoglobulin is found in the serum and/or the urine in nearly 90% of patients. The combination of immunochemical techniques and serum-free light-chain assay detects an abnormal result in 99% of patients.[11]

Diagnosis

AL-amyloidosis should be considered in any patient who presents with nephrotic-range proteinuria with or without renal insufficiency, nondilated cardiomyopathy, peripheral neuropathy, hepatomegaly, or autonomic neuropathy, whether or not a paraprotein can be detected in the serum or urine (Fig. 26.8). Particular vigilance should be maintained in patients with multiple myeloma or monoclonal gammopathy of undetermined significance (MGUS), especially of the λ isotype. Initial investigation should confirm the diagnosis of amyloidosis on tissue biopsy, and this should be followed by investigations to establish the type of amyloid present and the extent of organ involvement.

All patients require immunofixation of serum and urine in an attempt to demonstrate the presence of a monoclonal light chain. A bone marrow specimen is necessary because 10% of patients will not have a demonstrable monoclonal light chain by immunofixation, and a clone of plasma cells detected in the bone marrow by immunohistochemistry is strong supportive evidence of AL-amyloidosis. Immunonephelometric quantitation of free light chains is a useful complement to immunofixation because it shows remarkable specificity and sensitivity.[11]

Histologic diagnosis may be achieved by biopsies of various tissues. Biopsy of an affected organ is usually diagnostic, but less invasive alternatives should be preferred first. Biopsies of salivary glands or subcutaneous abdominal fat yield positive results in 80% to 90% of cases. Rectal biopsy is diagnostic in >80% of cases, provided that the biopsy specimen contains submucosal vessels in which early deposits are located. Bone marrow biopsy should also be stained with Congo red for the presence of amyloid, and involvement of the bone marrow (observed in about 50% of patients) is strongly suggestive of the AL type. Evaluation of adequate specimens in experienced laboratories is necessary to maintain high diagnostic sensitivity and specificity.

It is not always easy to be certain that amyloidosis is of the AL type because immunohistochemical staining for immunoglobulin light chains may not be diagnostic (due to loss of epitopes), and the presence of a monoclonal component is strong but not conclusive

evidence of the AL type. Extreme caution is required when patients have an intact monoclonal immunoglobulin in the serum without evidence of circulating free light chains in the serum or urine. In those cases, hereditary forms of amyloidosis should be considered because they may produce clinical syndromes indistinguishable from AL and coexist with MGUS.[4] In cases of doubt, DNA analysis and/or amyloid fibril sequencing by mass spectrometry may be necessary.

Natural History and Treatment

AL-amyloidosis is among the most severe complications of plasma cell proliferative disorders. Median survival is about 10 months. Cardiac involvement responsible for congestive heart failure and arrhythmia account for at least 40% of deaths.

Therapy is aimed at annihilating the plasma cell clone. All patients with AL-amyloidosis deserve a trial of chemotherapy because of the improved survival of responders. In the latter, gradual regression of AL-amyloid deposits is possible.[12] However, the results of chemotherapy in AL-amyloidosis are difficult to document because there is no easy way to measure the amount of amyloid in a patient. Investigators have long recognized that resolution of the nephrotic syndrome does not necessarily reflect that of amyloid deposits and that the progressive deposition of amyloid can occur in the presence of improved clinical and laboratory findings. Scintigraphy after the injection of [^{123}I]-SAP component may be helpful for monitoring the extent of systemic amyloidosis, but this technique is available in a few centers only.[12] The definition of a response in amyloidosis should be hematologic and organ based. A complete hematologic response is defined by negativity of serum and urine for a monoclonal protein by immunofixation, normal free light-chain ratio by the

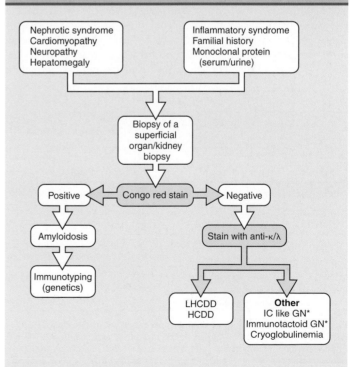

Figure 26.8 Algorithm of diagnostic procedures in AL-amyloidosis and monoclonal immunoglobulin deposition disease. *No extrarenal manifestation. GN, glomerulonephritis; IC, immune complex.

serum free light-chain assay,[13] and <5% plasma cells in the bone marrow. Criteria for organ response and organ disease progression have been recently reviewed.[14]

To date, physicians treating patients with AL-amyloidosis are facing a dilemma because clinical benefit from conventional chemotherapy does not occur for many months after the underlying plasma cell clone has been suppressed. Therefore, patients who receive slow-acting conventional chemotherapy regimens (e.g., low-dose melphalan and prednisone) often do not live long enough to derive benefit.[15] On the other hand, more intensive chemotherapy (e.g., high-dose melphalan with peripheral blood stem cell transplantation [PBSCT]) is associated with much greater treatment-related toxicity than seen in patients with myeloma because of multiple organ involvement that may be clinically latent. However, this treatment can result in reversal of the clinical manifestations of AL-amyloidosis in up to 60% of patients who survive the procedure. A summary of available clinical trials[15–20] is shown in Figure 26.9. The role of PBSCT in treatment of AL-amyloidosis is far from settled,[21] in the absence of data from well-designed, randomized, controlled trials that would compare benefit-to-risk ratios of high-dose therapy and an effective conventional therapy like melphalan and high-dose pulsed dexamethasone. Such a trial enrolling 100 patients has just been closed in France.[22] Preliminary data analysis suggests that high-dose chemotherapy and the melphalan/high-dose dexamethasone regimens are not different in terms of hematologic and clinical response and median survival. However, early transplant-related mortality within the first 100 days was 24% after intensive chemotherapy, whereas mortality was only 10% in the group receiving conventional therapy.

Dialysis and Transplantation

Most studies of the clinical course and outcome of patients on dialysis include both AL- and AA-amyloidosis. The patient's survival rate is low, but it compares favorably with that of patients not requiring dialysis: from 66% to 72% at 1 year, it decreases to 30% to 44% at 5 to 6 years. No difference in survival was observed at any time between patients with AL- and AA-amyloidosis. The survival rate of patients treated with continuous ambulatory peritoneal dialysis (PD) is similar to that of patients on hemodialysis (HD).

Cardiac amyloid is the most important predictor of poor survival in patients with AL-amyloidosis undergoing dialysis,[23] and cardiac deaths represent the main cause of mortality in such patients. The management of patients with AL-amyloid on HD is also often complicated by permanent hypotension, gastrointestinal hemorrhage, chronic diarrhea, and difficulties in the creation and maintenance of vascular accesses. It has, therefore, been suggested that PD could have several advantages over HD in the management of end-stage renal amyloidosis, including avoiding vascular access and deleterious effects on blood pressure. However, PD may induce protein loss in the dialysate and thus enhance malnutrition.

Renal transplantation is limited by the severity of heart involvement and the recurrence of deposits in the transplanted kidney. There are a few case reports and small series reported in the literature of renal transplantation in AL-amyloidosis. Renal transplantation may be considered in patients whose underlying clonal plasma cell disease has remitted following chemotherapy.

Epidemiology and Specific Features of AA-Amyloidosis
Epidemiology
AA-amyloidosis develops in 5% of patients with sustained elevation of serum amyloid A protein (SAA). Patients at risk are those with a long duration of chronic inflammatory disease (median, about 10 years), high magnitude of acute phase SAA response, homozygosity for SAA1 isotype, familial Mediterranean fever (FMF) trait (heterozygosity for variant pyrin), and a family history of AA amyloidosis.

An important epidemiologic aspect of AA-amyloidosis is the changing spectrum of underlying diseases. Pyogenic and granulomatous infections, especially tuberculosis, account for far fewer cases nowadays than in the older series. This is because of the efficacy of antibiotic treatments, which shows that amyloidosis can be efficiently prevented when its cause is suppressed. In contrast, the prevalence (currently about 70%) of amyloid linked to autoimmune inflammatory diseases, such as rheumatoid arthritis and juvenile chronic arthritis, has increased dramatically. AA-amyloidosis in patients with Hodgkin's disease

Outcome in previously untreated AL-amyloidosis						
Regimen	Series (ref. no.)	No. of Patients	Response (% all patients)*	TRM[†]	Overall Survival (median)	Comments
MP	Kyle et al.,[15] 1997	77	28	Not reported	18 mo	Risk of MDS
	Gertz et al.,[16] 1999	52	27	Not reported	29 mo	
M-HDD	Palladini et al.,[17] 2004	46	67	None	Not reached	Patients ineligible for PBSCT
HDD-IFN	Dhodapkar et al.,[18] 2004	93	53 (of evaluable hematologic) 45 (of evaluable organ)	7%	31 mo	
PBSCT	Comenzo and Gertz,[19] 2002	148	39 (62% of evaluable)	21%–39%[‡]	60%–70% at 1 yr	Selected patients
	Skinner et al.,[20] 2004	312	40	13%	54 mo	Selected patients

Figure 26.9 Outcome in previously untreated AL-amyloidosis. HDD-IFN, high-dose pulsed dexamethasone with maintenance dexamethasone/interferon-α; IDM, intermediate-dose melphalan; MDS, myelodysplastic syndrome; M-HDD, melphalan and high-dose pulsed dexamethasone; MP, melphalan and prednisone; PBSCT, peripheral blood stem cell transplantation; VAD, vincristine, Adriamycin, dexamethasone. *Response criteria have varied but generally include response of either plasma cell dyscrasia and/or organ dysfunction. [†]Treatment-related mortality (TRM) is defined as death during treatment or within 100 days from completing treatment. Note that the reported TRM in PBSCT studies did not include deaths during mobilization and re-infusion of peripheral blood progenitor cells. [‡]Twenty-one percent average of four single-center studies; 39% average of two multicenter studies. (Adapted from Guidelines Working Group of UK Myeloma Forum; British Committee for Standards in Haematology, British Society for Haematology: Guidelines on the diagnosis and management of AL amyloidosis. Br J Haematol 2004;125:681–700.)

has virtually disappeared with more efficient treatment of the hematologic disease. In contrast, hereditary AA-amyloidoses associated with familial recurrent fever syndromes account for an increasing part, of about 10% of cases, in recent series.

Clinical Manifestations

There are a number of clinical manifestations of AA-amyloidosis (Fig. 26.10).[24,25] The main target organ is the kidney, which is affected in almost all patients with AA-amyloidosis. Renal dysfunction may be acute with nephrotic syndrome or very insidious. Proteinuria is absent in about 5% of cases. Gastrointestinal disturbances (including diarrhea, constipation, and malabsorption) and hepatosplenomegaly are the next most common manifestations. In contrast with AL-amyloidosis, congestive heart failure, peripheral neuropathy, macroglossia, and carpal tunnel syndrome occur infrequently. The reason for the differential distribution of AA and AL tissue deposits is not understood.

Diagnosis

The optimal method for diagnosing AA-amyloidosis remains controversial. Although kidney biopsy is positive in about 100% of symptomatic patients, less invasive biopsy procedures should be attempted first. Biopsies of accessory salivary glands, abdominal fat, and rectal mucosa yield positive results in 50% to 80% of patients. Immunohistochemical staining using antibodies to SAA is required to confirm that Congo red positive amyloid deposits are of the AA type. SAP scintigraphy shows early

accumulation of amyloid in spleen while bones are not affected (contrary to AL-amyloid).

Natural History and Treatment

Survival time of patients with AA-amyloidosis is usually longer than in AL-amyloidosis (see Fig. 26.10). As in AL-amyloidosis, an elevated serum creatinine and a low serum albumin are strong adverse prognostic indicators. Main causes of death are infections and dialysis-related complications but not cardiac complications.

Amyloid load and clinical outcome in AA amyloidosis are dependent on circulating concentrations of SAA.[26] Estimated survival at 10 years was 90% in patients whose median SAA was under 10 mg/l, and 40% among those whose median SAA exceeded this value. These data emphasize the fact that underlying inflammatory diseases must be treated as vigorously as possible and SAA (preferentially to C-reactive protein) levels must be monitored monthly and maintained at a target value of <5 mg/l. In patients with inflammatory arthritis, the new anti–tumor necrosis factor-α therapy may help to achieve this goal.

Series of renal transplantation in AA-amyloidosis mostly concern patients with rheumatic diseases and come from Scandinavia. Amyloid deposits recur in about 10% of the grafts. Infection is the main cause of early deaths.

Familial Mediterranean Fever and Other Hereditary Recurrent Fever Syndromes

FMF represents both a particular type of AA-amyloidosis and the most frequent cause of familial amyloidosis. Colchicine has proved to be efficient both in the prevention and treatment of this type of amyloidosis. FMF is usually transmitted as an autosomal recessive disorder and occurs most commonly in Sephardic Jews and Armenians. It is caused by mutations of the gene (MEFV) encoding a protein called pyrin or marenostrin.[27] Clinically there are two independent phenotypes. In the first, brief, episodic, febrile attacks of peritonitis, pleuritis, or synovitis occur in childhood or adolescence and precede the renal manifestations. In the second, renal symptoms precede and may be the only manifestation of the disease for a long time. The attacks are accompanied by dramatic elevations of acute-phase reactants, including SAA. Amyloid deposits are responsible for severe renal lesions with prominent glomerular involvement, leading to end-stage renal disease at a young age, and for early deaths. Colchicine can prevent the development of proteinuria, may occasionally reverse the nephrotic syndrome and may prevent the decline in renal function in patients with non-nephrotic proteinuria. It is less effective in preventing progression in patients with nephrotic syndrome or renal insufficiency. The minimal daily dose of colchicine for prevention of amyloidosis is 1 mg, and patients with clinical evidence of amyloidotic kidney disease and kidney transplant recipients should receive daily doses of 1.5 to 2 mg.

The recent identification of genes responsible for syndromes of periodic fever with amyloidosis has opened the way to a molecular diagnosis of hereditary AA-amyloidosis. These syndromes include the tumor necrosis factor receptor–associated periodic syndrome, the Muckle-Wells syndrome, and the familial cold autoinflammatory syndrome. Only one case of systemic AA amyloidosis has been reported in the hyperimmunoglobulinemia D with periodic fever syndrome.

Characteristics of patients with secondary AA-amyloidosis		
Characteristics	Series I*	Series 2†
Number of patients	75	64
Age, yr (range)	57 (18–81)	56 (14–80)
Male-to-female ratio	0.8	1.5
Presenting clinical syndrome (%)	Proteinuria/renal failure (65) Gastrointestinal disturbance (5) Hepatosplenomegaly (4)	Proteinuria/renal failure (91) Gastrointestinal disturbance (22) Goiter (9) Neuropathy/carpal tunnel (3)
Source of tissue for diagnosis (%)	Rectum (60) Kidney (15)	Rectum (50) Kidney (38) Stomach/small bowel (23) Marrow (19)
Causes of death (%)	Renal failure (49) Bronchopneumonia (19) Cardiac disorder (11)	Uremia/dialysis complications (68) Sepsis (9) Cardiac disorder (9)
Survival	~40% at 3 yr	~40% at 3 yr (median, 24.5 mo)

Figure 26.10 Characteristics of patients with secondary AA-amyloidosis. *From Browning MJ, Banks RA, Tribe CR, et al: Ten years' experience of an amyloid clinic—a clinicopathological survey. Q J Med 1985;215: 213–227. †Gertz MA, Kyle RA: Secondary systemic amyloidosis: Response and survival in 64 patients. Medicine (Baltimore) 1991;70:246–256.

Therapeutic Prospects in Amyloidotic Diseases

Amyloid deposits exist in a state of dynamic turnover that is accessible to new therapeutic strategies.

Decreasing Amyloid Precursor Synthesis

Curing the underlying disease has proved to be extremely effective, as shown in FMF and infection/inflammation–related-AA amyloidosis. This objective must be envisioned, at least theoretically, in all forms of amyloidosis.

Preventing Amyloid Fibril Deposition

RAGE, a receptor for advanced glycation end products, is also a receptor for the amyloidogenic form of serum amyloid A. AA-amyloid deposition that occurs in the spleen of mice injected with amyloid-enhancing factor and silver nitrate is inhibited by a soluble form of RAGE or by blocking antibodies.[28] Small sulfated compounds can interfere with experimental mouse AA-amyloidosis, probably by competing with the interaction between the amyloid precursor and proteoglycans. One of these compounds is currently being used in clinical trials in patients with AA-amyloidosis.

Dissolving Amyloid Fibrils

A competitive inhibitor of SAP binding to amyloid fibrils has been developed.[29] This palindromic compound crosslinks and dimerizes SAP molecules, leading to their very rapid clearance by the liver, and thus produces a marked depletion of circulating human SAP, which in turn removes SAP from amyloid deposits. This drug may provide a new therapeutic approach to both systemic amyloidosis and diseases associated with local amyloid including Alzheimer's disease. It is currently being tested in animal models and clinical trials.

Immunotherapeutic Perspectives

The immune system may be manipulated in order to recognize amyloid fibrils as harmful foreign entities. Therapeutic vaccinations were performed in mouse models of Alzheimer disease with remarkable success. In AL-amyloidosis, an anti–light-chain monoclonal antibody specific for an amyloid-related conformational epitope accelerated the clearing of amyloid in the mouse.[30] Although we are still far from applicable human immunotherapy, such experimental approaches might lead to future developments.

MONOCLONAL IMMUNOGLOBULIN DEPOSITION DISEASE

History and Definition

It was known from the late 1950s that nonamyloidotic forms of glomerular disease "resembling the lesion of diabetic glomerulosclerosis" could occur in multiple myeloma. The presence of monoclonal light chains in these lesions was recognized by Randall and colleagues.[31]

In clinical and pathologic terms, light-chain, light- and heavy-chain-, and heavy-chain deposition disease (LCDD, LHCDD, and HCDD, respectively) are similar and may therefore be referred to as MIDD. They differ from amyloidosis in that the deposits lack affinity for Congo red and do not have a fibrillar organization. The distinction also relates to different pathophysiology of amyloid, which implicates one-dimensional elongation of a pseudocrystalline structure, and MIDD, which would rather involve a one-step precipitation of immunoglobulin chains.

Epidemiology

LCDD is found in 5% of myeloma patients at autopsy, while the prevalence of AL-amyloidosis is about 11%. LCDD and HCDD may occur in a wide range of ages (28 to 94 years) with a male preponderance (Fig. 26.11). More than 20 patients with HCDD

	Clinical, histologic, and laboratory features in patients with monoclonal immunoglobulin deposition disease	
Characteristics	LCDD/LHCDD	HCDD
Male-to-female ratio	1.7	0.8
Age, yr (range)	57 (28–94)	57 (26–79)
Hypertension (%)	53	90
Renal failure (serum creatinine ≥130 μmol/l) (1.47 mg/dl)	93	83
Nephrotic syndrome* (%)	36	46
Hematuria (%)	45	89
Nodular glomerulosclerosis (%)	31–100	96
Multiple myeloma (%)	53	24
Monoclonal protein (blood or urine) (%)	88	58†

Figure 26.11 Clinical, histologic, and laboratory features in patients with monoclonal immunoglobulin deposition disease. HCDD, heavy-chain deposition disease; LCDD, light-chain deposition disease; LHCDD, light- and heavy-chain deposition disease. *Proteinuria ≥3 g/day. †Including two cases with only free κ chain.

have been reported so far, but the disease is most likely under-diagnosed.

Pathogenesis

That light-chain deposition involves unusual light-chain properties is supported by the absence of a detectable monoclonal component in the serum and urine in 10% to 20% of patients with LCDD, the recurrence of the disease in the transplanted kidney, the biosynthesis of abnormal light chains by bone marrow plasma cells, and the fact that discrete changes in the V_L sequence were responsible for light-chain deposition in a mouse experimental model. However, light-chain deposition does not mean pathogenicity. Singular properties of light chain are most likely required for completion of the pathogenetic process leading to kidney fibrosis.

The following properties of light-chain variable domains may contribute to MIDD pathogenesis.[32] The first is the restricted usage of three κ germline genes, with an apparent overrepresentation of the rare $V_{\kappa IV}$ variability subgroup. Second, size abnormalities of light chains have been documented in about one third of patients by bone marrow biosynthesis experiments. Third, unusual amino acid substitutions have been identified in primary structures of LCDD light chains, mostly in peptide loops corresponding to parts of the molecules normally implicated in antigen binding. In particular, hydrophobic residues could strongly modify the light-chain conformation or be responsible for hydrophobic interactions between V domains or between V domains and extracellular matrix proteins. Fourth, when pathogenic light chains could not be detected in the serum and urine, they seemed to be N-glycosylated in all tested cases. Thus, glycosylation might increase the light-chain propensity to precipitate in tissues. However, as in AL-amyloidosis, extrinsic conditions may also contribute to aggregation of the light chain. The same light chain can form granular aggregates or amyloid fibrils depending on the environment, and different partially folded intermediates of the light chain may be responsible for amorphous or fibrillar aggregation pathways.[33]

A deletion of the first constant domain C_H1 was found in the deposited or circulating heavy chain in the 11 patients with γ-HCDD in whom testing was done.[32,34] In the blood, the deleted heavy chain was either associated with light chains or circulated in small amounts as a free unassembled subunit.[35] It is likely that the C_H1 deletion facilitates the secretion of free heavy chains that are rapidly cleared from the circulation by organ deposition. The variable V_H domain also is required for tissue precipitation.

A striking feature of LCDD and HCDD is the dramatic accumulation of extracellular matrix. Nodules are made of normal matrix constituents. A role for transforming growth factor β is supported by its strong expression in glomeruli of MIDD patients and by *in vitro* experiments using cultured mesangial cells.[36] Incubation of mesangial cells with light chains from patients with LCDD induces specific cell changes, whereas light chains toxic to tubules have no effect.[37] Light chains responsible for LCDD or AL-amyloidosis are endocytosed by cultured mesangial cells through a yet unidentified caveolae-associated receptor; their different pathologic effects result from distinct cellular trafficking.[38]

Clinical Manifestations

MIDD is a systemic disease with immunoglobulin chain deposition in a variety of organs leading to various clinical manifestations but visceral immunoglobulin chain deposits may be totally asymptomatic and found only at autopsy.[32]

Renal Manifestations

Renal involvement is a constant feature of MIDD, and renal symptoms, mostly proteinuria and renal failure, often dominate the clinical presentation (see Fig. 26.11).[32,34] In 18% to 53% of LCDD patients, albuminuria is associated with the nephrotic syndrome. However, in about one fourth, it is <1 g/day, and these patients exhibit mainly a tubulointerstitial syndrome. Albuminuria is not correlated with the existence of nodular glomerulosclerosis, at least initially, and may occur in the absence of significant glomerular lesions as detected by light microscopy. Hematuria is more frequent than one would expect for a nephropathy in which cell proliferation is usually modest.

The high prevalence, early appearance, and severity of renal failure are other salient features of LCDD. In most cases, renal function declines rapidly, which is a main reason for referral. Renal failure occurs with comparable frequency in patients with either low or heavy protein excretion and may present in the form of a subacute tubulointerstitial nephritis or a rapidly progressive glomerulonephritis, respectively. The prevalence of hypertension is variable, but it must be interpreted according to associated medical history. Renal features of patients with HCDD are basically similar to those seen in LCDD and LHCDD (see Fig. 26.11).

Extrarenal Manifestations

Liver and cardiac involvement occur in about one fourth of patients with LCDD and LHCDD. Liver deposits are constant. They are either discrete and confined to the sinusoids and basement membranes of biliary ductules without associated parenchymal lesions or massive with marked dilatation and multiple ruptures of sinusoids, resembling peliosis. Hepatomegaly with mild alterations of liver function tests are the most usual symptoms, but patients may also develop life-threatening hepatic insufficiency and portal hypertension.

Cardiac involvement is also frequent and may be responsible for cardiomegaly and severe heart failure. Arrhythmias, conduction disturbances, and congestive heart failure are seen. Echocardiography and catheterization may reveal diastolic dysfunction and reduction in myocardial compliance similar to that found in cardiac amyloid.

Deposits may also occur along the nerve fibers and in the choroid plexus, as well as in the lymph nodes, bone marrow, spleen, pancreas, thyroid gland, submandibular glands, adrenal glands, gastrointestinal tract, abdominal vessels, lungs, and skin. They may be responsible for peripheral neuropathy (20% of the reported cases), gastrointestinal disturbances, pulmonary nodules, amyloid-like arthropathy, and sicca syndrome. Extrarenal deposits are less common in patients with HCDD.

Hematologic Findings

Myeloma is diagnosed in about 50% of the patients with LCDD or LHCDD and in about 25% of those with HCDD. MIDD, like AL-amyloidosis, is often the presenting disease that leads to the discovery of myeloma at an early stage. MIDD may occasionally complicate Waldenström's macroglobulinemia, chronic lymphocytic leukemia, and nodal marginal zone lymphoma. It often occurs in the absence of a detectable malignant process, even after prolonged (>10 years) follow-up. A monoclonal bone marrow plasma cell population is then easily detectable by immunohistologic examination.

Pathology
Light Microscopy

MIDD should not be considered a purely glomerular disease. In fact, tubular lesions may be more conspicuous than the glomerular damage. Tubular lesions are characterized by the deposition of a refractile, eosinophilic, periodic acid–Schiff (PAS)-positive, ribbon-like material along the outer part of the tubular basement membrane. The deposits predominate around the distal tubules, the loops of Henle, and, in some instances, around the collecting ducts whose epithelium is flattened and atrophied. Typical myeloma casts are only occasionally seen in pure forms of MIDD. In advanced stages, a marked interstitial fibrosis including refractile deposits is frequently associated with tubular lesions.

Glomerular lesions are much more heterogeneous. Nodular glomerulosclerosis is the most characteristic (Fig. 26.12a); it is found in 30% to 100% of patients with LCDD. Expansion of the mesangial matrix was observed in all cases of HCDD, with nodular glomerulosclerosis in almost all of them. Mesangial nodules are composed of PAS-positive, membrane-like material and are often accompanied by mild mesangial hypercellularity. Lesions resemble diabetic nodular glomerulosclerosis, but some characteristics are distinctive: the distribution of the nodules is fairly regular in a given glomerulus, the nodules are often poorly argyrophilic, and exudative lesions as fibrin caps and extensive hyalinosis of the efferent arterioles are not observed. In occasional cases with prominent endocapillary cellularity and mesangial interposition, the glomerular features mimic membranoproliferative glomerulonephritis. Milder forms of LCDD simply show an increase in mesangial matrix and sometimes in mesangial cells, and a modest thickening of the basement membranes, which are abnormally bright and rigid. Glomerular lesions may not be detected by light microscopy but require ultrastructural examination. These lesions may represent early stages of glomerular disease or be induced by light chains with a weak pathogenic potential. Their diagnosis would be unrecognized without the immunostaining results.

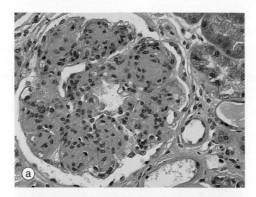

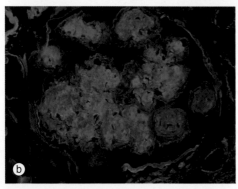

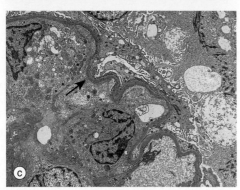

Figure 26.12 Light-chain deposition disease. *a,* Nodular glomeruloscle-rosis with mesangial matrix accumulation (Masson's trichrome, ×312). *b,* Bright staining of mesangial nodules and tubular basement membranes with anti-κ antibody (immunofluorescence, ×312). *c,* Electron micrograph showing a layer of dense granular deposits (*arrow*) under the endothelium along the glomerular basement membrane (×2500). (Courtesy of Dr. Béatrice Mougenot).

Arteries, arterioles, and peritubular capillaries all may contain PAS-positive deposits in close contact with their basement membranes. Deposits do not show the staining characteristics of amyloid, but they may be associated with Congo red–positive amyloid deposits in approximately 10% of patients.[34]

Immunohistology

A key step in the diagnosis of the various forms of MIDD is immunohistologic examination of the kidney. All biopsy specimens show evidence of monotypic light chain (mostly κ; see Fig. 26.12b) and/or heavy-chain fixation along tubular basement membranes. This criterion is required for the diagnosis of MIDD.

The tubular deposits stain strongly (see Fig. 26.12b) and predominate along the loops of Henle and the distal tubules, but they also often are detected along the proximal tubules. In contrast, the pattern of glomerular immunohistology displays marked heterogeneity. In patients with nodular glomerulosclerosis, deposits of monotypic immunoglobulin chains are usually found along the peripheral glomerular basement membranes and, to a lesser extent, in the nodules themselves (see Fig. 26.12b). The staining in glomeruli is typically weaker than that observed along the tubular basement membranes. This may not be a function of the actual amount of deposited material because several cases have been reported in which glomerular immunohistology was negative despite the presence of large amounts of granular glomerular deposits by electron microscopy. Local modifications of deposited light chains thus might change their antigenicity. In patients without nodular lesions, glomerular staining occurs mainly along the basement membrane, but it may involve the mesangium in some cases. A linear staining usually decorates Bowman's capsule. Deposits are frequently found in vascular walls and interstitium.

In patients with HCDD, immunofluorescence immuno-histology with anti–light-chain antibodies is negative despite typical nodular glomerulosclerosis. Monotypic deposits of γ, α, or μ heavy chains may be identified. Any γ subclass may be observed. Analysis of the kidney biopsy with monoclonal antibodies specific for the constant domains of the γ heavy chain allowed identification of a deletion of the C_H1 domain in all tested cases. In most cases of HCDD, especially when a γ1 or γ3 chain is involved, complement components including C1 could be demonstrated in a granular or pseudolinear pattern. Complement deposits were often associated with signs of complement activation in serum.

Electron Microscopy

The most characteristic ultrastructural feature is the presence of finely to coarsely granular electron-dense deposits along the outer (interstitial) aspect of the tubular basement membranes. In the glomerulus, they predominate in a subendothelial position along the glomerular basement membrane and are located mainly along and in the lamina rara interna (see Fig. 26.12c). They can also be found in mesangial nodules, Bowman's capsule, and the wall of small arteries between the myocytes. Nonamyloid fibrils have been reported in a few patients with LCDD or HCDD.

Diagnosis

The diagnosis of MIDD must be suspected in any patient with the nephrotic syndrome or rapidly progressive tubulointerstitial nephritis, or with echocardiographic findings indicating diastolic dysfunction and the presence of a monoclonal immunoglobulin component in the serum and/or the urine (see Fig 26.8). The same combination is also seen in AL-amyloidosis, but the latter is more often associated with the λ light chain isotype. Since sensitive techniques including immunofixation fail to identify a monoclonal immunoglobulin component in 10% to 20% of patients with LCDD/LHCDD and about 40% of patients with HCDD (see Fig. 26.11), renal biopsy plays an essential role in the diagnosis of MIDD and the associated dysproteinemia.

The definitive diagnosis is made by the immunohistologic analysis of tissue from an affected organ, in most cases the kidney, using a panel of immunoglobulin chain–specific anti-bodies, including anti–κ and anti–λ light-chain antibodies to stain the non–Congo-philic deposits. When the biopsy stains for a single heavy-chain isotype and does not stain for light-chain isotypes, the diagnosis of HCDD should be suspected.

The diagnosis of the plasma cell dyscrasia relies on bone marrow aspiration and bone marrow biopsy with cell morpho-logic evaluation and, if necessary, immunophenotyping with anti-κ and anti-λ antisera to demonstrate monoclonality.

Outcome and Treatment

The outcome of MIDD remains uncertain, mainly because extrarenal deposits of light chains can be totally asymptomatic or cause severe organ damage that leads to death. Survival from onset of symptoms varies from 1 month to 10 years. In the largest series of patients with LCDD as yet reported,[39] 36 of the 63 (57%) patients reached uremia, 37 of those patients (59%) died during follow-up and patient survival was only 66% at 1 year and 31% at 8 years, although 54 patients (86%) were treated by chemotherapy. Multivariate analysis showed that the only variables independently associated with renal survival were age and degree of renal insufficiency at presentation[39] or the time of renal biopsy.[34] Those independently associated with a worse patient survival were age, initial creatinine level, associated multiple myeloma, and extrarenal light-chain deposition.[34,39] Survival of the uremic patients treated with dialysis was not different from that of the patients not reaching uremia. Renal and patient survivals were significantly better in patients with pure MIDD (mean, 22 and 54 months, respectively), compared to those who presented with cast nephropathy (mean, 4 and 22 months, respectively).[34]

Treatment

As in AL-amyloidosis, treatment should be aimed at reducing immunoglobulin production. Clearance of the light-chain deposits has been unequivocally demonstrated in a few patients after intensive chemotherapy with syngeneic bone marrow transplantation or blood stem cell autografting. Disappearance of nodular mesangial lesions and light chain deposits was also reported after long-term chemotherapy. These observations demonstrate that fibrotic nodular glomerular lesions are reversible, and they argue for intensive chemotherapy in patients with severe visceral involvement.

In a recent retrospective study of 11 patients (younger than 65 years) with LHCDD treated by high-dose therapy with the support of autologous blood stem cell transplantation, no treatment-related death occurred.[40] A decrease in the monoclonal immunoglobulin level was observed in eight patients, with complete disappearance from serum and urine in six cases. Improvement in manifestations related to deposits was observed in six patients, and histologic regression was documented in cardiac, hepatic, and skin biopsies. Reversal of dialysis dependency and sustained improvement in renal function were also occasionally noted. Whether high-dose chemotherapy with blood stem cell transplantation provides benefits compared to conventional chemotherapy including high-dose dexamethasone remains to be established. The former should be preferred in LCDD patients with overt myeloma, while the latter is the only therapy for those older than the age of 70 years.

As with AL-amyloidosis, monitoring of light-chain production should rely on free light-chain assay, particularly in those patients without a blood and urine monoclonal component.

Kidney transplantation has been performed in a few patients with MIDD. Recurrence of the disease is usually observed. Therefore, kidney transplantation should not be an option for LCDD patients unless measures have been taken to reduce light-chain production.[41]

Renal Diseases Associated with Monoclonal Immunoglobulin Deposition Disease
Myeloma Cast Nephropathy

The association of monoclonal light chain deposits, mostly along renal tubular basement membranes, with typical myeloma cast nephropathy is more frequent than reported initially. It was found in 11 of 34 (32%) patients with MIDD.[34] Nodular glomerulosclerosis is, however, infrequent (<10%), and some ribbon-like tubular basement membranes are seen in less than half of the patients. In addition, one third of the patients do not have granular-dense deposits on electron microscopy.

AL-Amyloidosis

Amyloid deposits are found in one or more organs in about 7% of LCDD patients. Because amyloid deposits are focal, the true incidence of the association may be markedly underestimated. Although this association may result from peculiar light chains endowed with intrinsic properties that make them prone to form both fibrillar and nonfibrillar deposits depending on the environment,[33] one cannot exclude the possibility that the coexisting diseases are induced by different variant clones.

NONAMYLOID FIBRILLARY AND IMMUNOTACTOID GLOMERULOPATHIES

Definition

Fibrillary and immunotactoid glomerulopathy are characterized, respectively, by fibrillar and microtubular deposits in the mesangium and the glomerular capillary loops (Fig. 26.13). These deposits do not have a β-pleated sheet organization and, therefore, are readily distinguishable from amyloid by the larger thickness of fibrils and lack of Congo red staining. Whether fibrillar and immunotactoid glomerulopathies are totally distinct entities remains the subject of considerable debate.

For Korbet and colleagues,[42] immunotactoid glomerulopathy is a unifying term for glomerular deposition of either amyloid-like fibrils (12 to 22 nm) or larger microtubules (>30 nm) in patients for whom an associated systemic disease including cryoglobulinemia and lymphoproliferative disorders has been excluded. For others,[43–46] the distinction between nonamyloid fibrillary and immunotactoid glomerulopathy may be of great clinical and pathophysiologic interest in the context of protein dyscrasias (see Fig. 26.13).

Epidemiology

The incidence of glomerulopathy with nonamyloid deposition of fibrillary or microtubular material in a nontransplant adult biopsy population is estimated at around 1% (equivalent to that of antiglomerular basement membrane disease). It is most likely underestimated because of the insufficient attention given to atypical reactions with histochemical stains for amyloid and the lack of immuno-ultrastructure studies of most biopsy specimens.

Clinical Manifestations

The characteristics of fibrillary and immunotactoid glomerulopathies are described in Figure 26.13 in comparison to AL-amyloid. Patients with immunotactoid and fibrillary glomerulopathies have a mean age of 55 to 60 years (extreme: 19 to 86) with a male-to-female ratio that varies from one series to another. They usually present with the nephrotic syndrome, microscopic hematuria, and mild to severe renal failure. In most recent series,[45,46] there was no significant difference between immunotactoid and fibrillary glomerulopathy patients in serum creatinine level, incidence of nephrotic syndrome, microscopic hematuria, hypertension, and renal failure. Extrarenal manifestations are uncommon and may involve the lung, skin, and peripheral nervous system.

		Immunologic and clinical characteristics of fibrillary and immunotactoid glomerulopathies	
Characteristics	Amyloidosis (AL Type)	Fibrillary Glomerulopathy	Immunotactoid Glomerulopathy
Congo red staining	Yes	No	No
Composition	Fibrils	Fibrils	Microtubules
Fibril or microtubule size	8–15 nm	12–22 nm	>30 nm*
Organization in tissues	Random (β-pleated sheet)	Random	Parallel arrays
Immunoglobulin deposition	Monoclonal LC (mostly λ)	Usually polyclonal (mostly IgG4), occasionally monoclonal (IgG1, IgG4)	Usually monoclonal (IgGκ or IgGλ)
Glomerular lesions	Deposits spreading from the mesangium	MPGN, CGN, MP	Atypical MN, MPGN
Renal presentation	Severe NS, absence of hypertension and hematuria	NS with hematuria, hypertension; RPGN	NS with microhematuria and hypertension
Extrarenal manifestations (fibrillar deposits)	Systemic deposition disease	Pulmonary hemorrhage	Microtubular inclusions in leukemic lymphocytes
Association with LPD	Yes (myeloma)	Uncommon	Common (CLL, NHL, MGUS)
Treatment	Melphalan + dexamethasone; intensive therapy with blood stem cell autograft	Corticosteroids ± cyclophosphamide (crescentic GN)	Treatment of the associated LPD

Figure 26.13 Immunologic and clinical characteristics of fibrillary and immunotactoid glomerulopathies. CGN, crescentic glomerulonephritis; CLL, chronic lymphocytic leukemia; GN, glomerulonephritis; LC, light chain; LPD, lymphoproliferative disorder; MGUS, monoclonal gammopathy of undetermined significance; MN, membranous nephropathy; MP, mesangial proliferation; MPGN, membranoproliferative glomerulonephritis; NHL, non-Hodgkin's lymphoma; NS, nephrotic syndrome; RPGN, rapidly progressive glomerulonephritis. *Mean diameter of the substructures did not differ between fibrillary glomerulonephritis (15.8 ± 3.5 nm) and immunotactoid glomerulopathy (15.2 ± 7.3 nm) in Bridoux et al.[45] series.

Pathology

Immunotactoid Glomerulopathy

Renal biopsy shows either membranous glomerulonephritis (often associated with segmental mesangial proliferation; Fig. 26.14) or lobular membranoproliferative glomerulonephritis. By immunohistology, coarse granular deposits of IgG and C3 are observed along capillary basement membranes and in mesangial areas. In a recent series of 23 patients where diagnosis was based on ultrastructural appearance of the deposits, IgG deposits were monotypic in 13 of 14 patients with immunotactoid glomerulopathy (κ, seven cases; λ, six cases), and in only one of nine patients with fibrillary glomerulopathy.[45] However, a circulating monoclonal immunoglobulin was detected by immunoelectrophoresis or immunoblotting in only six of the 14 patients with immunotactoid glomerulopathy.

On electron microscopy, the distinguishing morphologic features of immunotactoid glomerulopathy are the presence of organized deposits of large, thick-walled microtubules, typically >30 nm in diameter, at times arranged in parallel arrays (see Fig. 26.14c).

Of the 14 patients with immunotactoid glomerulopathy reported by Bridoux and associates,[45] six had a chronic lymphocytic leukemia, one a small lymphocytic B cell lymphoma, and three an MGUS. Intracytoplasmic crystal-like immunoglobulin inclusions were found in four patients with chronic lymphocytic leukemia and in the lymphoma patient.[45] They showed the same microtubular organization and contained the same IgG subclass and light-chain isotype as renal deposits.

Fibrillary Glomerulopathy

Mesangial proliferation and aspects of membranoproliferative glomerulonephritis are predominantly reported in series of fibrillary glomerulopathy. Glomerular crescents are present in about 30% of the biopsy specimens. Immunofluorescence studies mainly show IgG deposits of the γ4-isotype with a predominant mesangial localization. Monotypic deposits containing mostly IgGκ are detected in no more than 15% of patients.

On electron microscopy, fibrils are randomly arranged and their diameter varies between 12 and 22 nm. Of note, the fibril size alone is not sufficient to distinguish nonamyloidotic fibrillary glomerulonephritis from amyloid.[45]

Diagnosis

Diagnosis of immunotactoid and fibrillary glomerulopathies relies on electron microscopy examination, which must be systematically performed in patients with atypical membranous nephropathy or membranoproliferative glomerulonephritis, as well as in those with monotypic deposits in glomeruli. Renal biopsies from such patients with glomerular disease should be routinely examined with anti–κ and anti–λ light-chain antibodies.

In patients with immunotactoid glomerulopathy, a careful search for a lymphoproliferative disease is needed. Association of immunotactoid and fibrillary glomerulopathy with hepatitis C virus or human immunodeficiency virus infection has also been reported.

Outcome and Treatment

Patients with fibrillary glomerulopathy usually respond poorly to corticosteroids and cytotoxic drugs, with an incidence of end-stage renal disease of 50%. By contrast, in those with immunotactoid glomerulopathy, corticosteroid and/or chemotherapy were associated with partial or complete remission of the nephrotic syndrome in most cases, with a parallel improvement of the hematologic parameters.[45] In the largest series,[45] patient survival was found to be similar in both types of glomerulopathies. The incidence of chronic renal failure and end-stage renal failure tended to be lower in the immunotactoid glomerulopathy group, but the difference was not significant. Renal

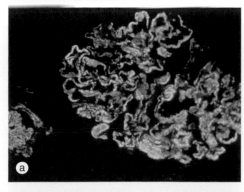

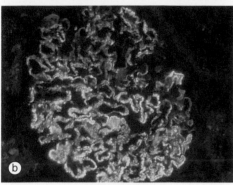

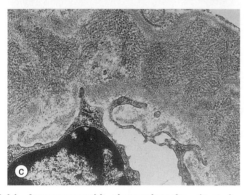

Figure 26.14 Immunotactoid glomerulopathy. Atypical membranous nephropathy showing exclusive staining of the deposits with anti-γ (*a*) and anti-κ (*b*) antibodies (immunofluorescence, ×312). *c*, Electron micrograph of glomerular basement membrane showing microtubular structure of the subepithelial deposits (uranyl acetate and lead citrate, ×20,000). (Courtesy of Dr. Béatrice Mougenot.)

transplantation has been performed in only a few patients, and recurrent disease occurred in several of them.[47]

GLOMERULAR LESIONS ASSOCIATED WITH WALDENSTRÖM'S MACROGLOBULINEMIA

In Waldenström's macroglobulinemia, symptomatic renal disease is much less common than in multiple myeloma. Glomerulonephritis with intracapillary thrombi of aggregated IgM, considered almost specific for Waldenström's macroglobulinemia, is the most frequent renal morphologic finding, but it has become a rare entity probably because of the increased efficacy of chemotherapy. It is associated with variable degrees of proteinuria and normal or slightly altered renal function. It is characterized by PAS-positive, Congo red–negative endomembranous deposits that are sometimes so voluminous as to occlude the capillary lumens. By immunohistology, thrombi and deposits stain with anti-IgM and with anti-κ. Some of these patients have cryoglobulinemia. Others have high amounts of circulating IgM, suggesting that hyperviscosity could favor IgM deposition in glomerular capillaries where ultrafiltration further increases the protein concentration. Treatment by intensive plasma exchange and alkylating agents is then indicated.

Renal amyloidosis, mostly of the AL type, is uncommon but may be found in patients presenting with massive proteinuria. Since renal biopsy may be hazardous in patients with Waldenström's macroglobulinemia, who frequently have increased bleeding time, it is wise to search for amyloid deposits first by a less invasive tissue biopsy.

OTHER TYPES OF GLOMERULONEPHRITIS

In some patients, glomerular deposition of monoclonal IgG can produce a proliferative glomerulonephritis that mimics immune-complex glomerulonephritis on light and electron microscopy.[48] Proper recognition of this entity requires confirmation of monoclonality by staining for the γ heavy-chain subclasses. Tissue fixation of complement was observed in 90% of cases, and 40% of patients had hypocomplementemia. Clinical presentation included renal insufficiency in 80%, proteinuria in 100%, nephrotic syndrome in 44%, and microhematuria in 60%. A monoclonal serum protein with the same heavy- and light-chain isotype as that of the glomerular deposits was identified in 50% of cases. No patient had overt myeloma or lymphoma at presentation or over the course of follow-up.

REFERENCES

1. Glenner GG: Amyloid deposits and amyloidosis: The β-fibrilloses. N Engl J Med 1980;302:1283–1292.
2. Westermark G, Benson MD, Buxbaum JN, et al: Amyloid fibril protein nomenclature. Amyloid 2002;9:197–200.
3. Merlini G, Bellotti V: Molecular mechanisms of amyloidosis. N Engl J Med 2003;349:583–596.
4. Lachmann HJ, Booth DR, Booth SE, et al: Misdiagnosis of hereditary amyloidosis as AL (primary) amyloidosis. N Engl J Med 2002;346: 1786–1791.
5. Eulitz M, Weiss DT, Solomon A: Immunoglobulin heavy-chain-associated amyloidosis. Proc Natl Acad Sci U S A 1990;87:6542–6546.
6. Stevens FJ: Four structural risk factors identify most fibril-forming kappa light chains. Amyloid 2000;7:200–211.
7. Comenzo RL, Zhang Y, Martinez C, et al: The tropism of organ involvement in primary systemic amyloidosis: Contributions of Ig V_L germ line gene use and clonal plasma cell burden. Blood 2001;98:714–720.
8. Keeling J, Teng J, Herrera GA: AL-amyloidosis and light-chain deposition disease light chains induce divergent phenotypic transformations of human mesangial cells. Lab Invest 2004;84:1322–1338.
9. Kyle RA, Gertz MA: Primary systemic amyloidosis: Clinical and laboratory features in 474 cases. Semin Hematol 1995;32:45–59.
10. Kyle RA, Greipp PR: Amyloidosis (AL): Clinical and laboratory features in 229 cases. Mayo Clin Proc 1983;58:665–683.
11. Katzmann JA, Abraham RS, Dispenzieri A, et al: Diagnostic performance of quantitative kappa and lambda free light chain assays in clinical practice. Clin Chem 2005;51:878–781.
12. Hawkins PN: Studies with radiolabelled serum amyloid P component provide evidence for turnover and regression of amyloid deposits in vivo. Clin Sci (Lond) 1994;87:289–295.
13. Lachmann HJ, Gallimore R, Gillmore JD, et al: Outcome in systemic AL amyloidosis in relation to changes in concentration of circulating free immunoglobulin light chains following chemotherapy. Br J Haematol 2003;122:78–84.
14. Gertz MA, Comenzo R, Falk RH, et al: Definition of organ involvement and treatment response in immunoglobulin light chain amyloidosis (AL): A consensus opinion from the 10th International Symposium on Amyloid and Amyloidosis. Am J Hematol 2005;79: 319–328.

15. Kyle RA, Gertz MA, Greipp PR, et al: A trial of three regimens for primary amyloidosis: Colchicine alone, melphalan and prednisone, and melphalan, prednisone, and colchicine. N Engl J Med 1997;336:1202–1207.

16. Gertz MA, Lacy MQ, Lust JA, et al: Prospective randomized trial of melphalan and prednisone versus vincristine, carmustine, melphalan, cyclophosphamide, and prednisone in the treatment of primary systemic amyloidosis. J Clin Oncol 1999;17:262–267.

17. Palladini G, Perfetti V, Obici L, et al: Association of melphalan and high-dose dexamethasone is effective and well tolerated in patients with AL (primary) amyloidosis who are ineligible for stem cell transplantation. Blood 2004;103:2936–2938.

18. Dhodapkar MV, Hussein MA, Rasmussen E, et al: Clinical efficacy of high-dose dexamethasone with maintenance dexamethasone/alpha interferon in patients with primary systemic amyloidosis: results of United States Intergroup Trial Southwest Oncology Group (SWOG) S9628. Blood 2004;104:3520–3526.

19. Comenzo RL, Gertz MA: Autologous stem cell transplantation for primary systemic amyloidosis. Blood 2002;99:4276–4282.

20. Skinner M, Sanchorawala V, Seldin DC, et al: High-dose melphalan and autologous stem-cell transplantation in patients with AL amyloidosis: An 8-year study. Ann Intern Med 2004;140:85–93.

21. Working Group of UK Myeloma Forum; British Committee for Standards in Haematology, British Society for Haematology: Guidelines on the diagnosis and management of AL amyloidosis. Br J Haematol 2004; 125:681–700.

22. Jaccard A, Moreau P, Leblond V, et al: Best therapy for primary amyloidosis, a not-yet-solved question. Blood 2004;104:2990–2991.

23. Gertz MA, Kyle RA, O'Fallon WM: Dialysis support of patients with primary systemic amyloidosis. A study of 211 patients. Arch Intern Med 1992;152:2245–2250.

24. Browning MJ, Banks RA, Tribe CR, et al: Ten years' experience of an amyloid clinic—a clinicopathological survey. Q J Med 1985;215:213–227.

25. Gertz MA, Kyle RA: Secondary systemic amyloidosis: Response and survival in 64 patients. Medicine (Baltimore) 1991;70:246–256.

26. Gillmore JD, Lovat LB, Persey MR, et al: Amyloid load and clinical outcome in AA amyloidosis in relation to circulating concentration of serum amyloid A protein. Lancet 2001;358:24–29.

27. Dode C, Pecheux C, Cazeneuve C, et al: Mutations in the MEFV gene in a large series of patients with a clinical diagnosis of familial Mediterranean fever. Am J Med Genet 2000;92:241–246.

28. Yan SD, Zhu H, Zhu A, et al: Receptor-dependent cell stress and amyloid accumulation in systemic amyloidosis. Nat Med 2000;6:643–651.

29. Pepys MB, Herbert J, Hutchinson WL, et al: Targeted pharmacological depletion of serum amyloid P component for treatment of human amyloidosis. Nature 2002;417:254–259.

30. Hrncic R, Wall J, Wolfenbarger DA, et al: Antibody-mediated resolution of light chain-associated amyloid deposits. Am J Pathol 2000;157: 1239–1246.

31. Randall RE, Williamson WC Jr, Mullinax F, et al: Manifestations of systemic light chain deposition. Am J Med 1976;60:293–299.

32. Ronco PM, Alyanakian MA, Mougenot B, Aucouturier P: Light chain deposition disease: A model of glomerulosclerosis defined at the molecular level. J Am Soc Nephrol 2001;12:1558–1565.

33. Khurana R, Gillespie JR, Talapatra A, et al: Partially folded intermediates as critical precursors of light chain amyloid fibrils and amorphous aggregates. Biochemistry 2001;40:3525–3535.

34. Lin J, Markowitz GS, Valeri AM, et al: Renal monoclonal immunoglobulin deposition disease: The disease spectrum. J Am Soc Nephrol 2001; 12:1482–1492.

35. Moulin B, Deret S, Mariette X, et al: Nodular glomerulosclerosis with deposition of monoclonal immunoglobulin heavy chains lacking C_{H1}. J Am Soc Nephrol 1999;10:519–528.

36. Zhu L, Herrera GA, Murphy-Ullrich JE, et al: Pathogenesis of glomerulosclerosis in light chain deposition disease. Am J Pathol 1995;147: 375–385.

37. Russell W, Cardelli J, Harris E, et al: Monoclonal light chain-mesangial cell interactions: Early signaling events and subsequent pathologic effects. Lab Invest 2001;81:689–703.

38. Teng J, Russell WJ, Gu X, et al: Different types of glomerulopathic light chains interact with mesangial cells using a common receptor but exhibit different intracellular trafficking patterns. Lab Invest 2004;84: 440–445.

39. Pozzi C, D'Amico M, Fogazzi GB, et al: Light chain deposition disease with renal involvement: clinical characteristics and prognostic factors. Am J Kidney Dis 2003;42:1154–1163.

40. Royer B, Arnulf B, Martinez F, et al: High dose chemothcrapy in light chain or light and heavy chain deposition disease. Kidney Int 2004;65: 642–648.

41. Leung N, Lager DJ, Gertz MA, et al: Long-term outcome of renal transplantation in light-chain deposition disease. Am J Kidney Dis 2004;43:147–153.

42. Korbet SM, Schwartz MM, Lewis EJ. Current concepts in renal pathology. The fibrillary glomerulopathies. Am J Kidney Dis 1994;23: 751–765.

43. Fogo A, Qureshi N, Horn RG: Morphologic and clinical features of fibrillary glomerulonephritis versus immunotactoid glomerulopathy. Am J Kidney Dis 1993;22:367–377.

44. Alpers CE: Immunotactoid (microtubular) glomerulopathy: An entity distinct from fibrillary glomerulonephritis. Am J Kidney Dis 1992;19: 185–191.

45. Bridoux F, Hugue V, Coldefy O, et al: Fibrillary glomerulonephritis and immunotactoid (microtubular) glomerulopathy are associated with distinct immunologic features. Kidney Int 2002;62:1764–1775.

46. Rosenstock JL, Markowitz GS, Valeri AM, et al: Fibrillary and immunotactoid glomerulonephritis: Distinct entities with different clinical and pathologic features. Kidney Int 2003;63:1450–1461.

47. Pronovost PH, Brady HR, Gunning ME, et al: Clinical features, predictors of disease progression and results of renal transplantation in fibrillary immunotactoid glomerulopathy. Nephrol Dial Transplant 1996;11:837–842.

48. Nasr SH, Markowitz GS, Stokes MB, et al: Proliferative glomerulonephritis with monoclonal IgG deposits: A distinct entity mimicking immune-complex glomerulonephritis. Kidney Int 2004;65:85–96.

Other Glomerular Disorders, Including Congenital Nephrotic Syndrome

Richard J. Glassock

INTRODUCTION

This chapter provides a description of several glomerular diseases, not necessarily related to each other. Although uncommon, each must be recognized and differentiated from other more common glomerular disorders in order to plan an appropriate course of therapy, to estimate the prognosis for progression to end-stage renal disease (ESRD), to determine whether a familial disorder is present, or to determine the risk of a recurrence in the transplanted kidney. Appropriately, emphasis is placed on diagnosis and management.

MESANGIAL PROLIFERATIVE GLOMERULONEPHRITIS (WITHOUT IgA DEPOSITS)

Mesangial proliferative glomerulonephritis (MesPGN) encompasses a very heterogeneous collection of disorders of diverse and largely unknown etiology and pathogenesis that have in common a histologic pattern by light microscopy of glomerular injury characterized by mesangial proliferation (Fig. 27.1).[1–3] As the name implies, it is noted for a diffuse and global increase in mesangial or axial hypercellularity, often accompanied by an increase in mesangial matrix. Although the mesangial cells may be primarily involved in the proliferative response, other cells (e.g., monocytes) that are trafficking through the mesangial regions of the glomerulus

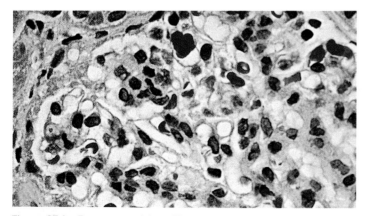

Figure 27.1 Pure mesangial proliferative glomerulonephritis. Note the increase in mesangial cellularity, the delicate peripheral capillary walls, and the absence of sclerosis or parietal epithelial cell proliferation (hematoxylin-eosin, ×410). (Adapted from Churg J, Bernstein J, Glassock R, eds. Renal Disease: Classification and Atlas of Glomerular Disease. New York: Igaku-Shoin, 1995, p 93.)

but are normally not resident in the glomerulus may also contribute to the hypercellularity of the mesangial regions.

For the purpose of this discussion, other forms of cellular proliferation that occur within the mesangial zones but are more focally and segmentally distributed are not included. These focal and segmental forms of proliferative GN may be a part of the evolutionary stages of an initially pure MesPGN, but they very often signify the presence of systemic disease processes. These processes include systemic lupus erythematosus (SLE), Henoch-Schönlein purpura, infective endocarditis, microscopic polyangiitis, Goodpasture's disease, mixed connective tissue disease, and IgA nephropathy. These topics are covered here or in other chapters. Occasionally, a lesion of focal and segmental proliferative GN is discovered in the absence of any recognizable multisystem disease process and in the absence of IgA deposits (i.e., idiopathic focal and segmental proliferative GN). Such patients have a clinical presentation, course, and response to treatment that are similar to those described for pure MesPGN, but they are not discussed further in this section.

In pure MesPGN, the peripheral capillary walls are thin and delicate without obvious deposits, reduplication, focal disruptions, or cellular necrosis. The visceral and parietal epithelial cells, while occasionally enlarged, have not undergone proliferation. Crescents and segmental sclerosis should be absent in the pure disease. In addition, large deposits staining with periodic acid–Schiff or fuchsin in the mesangium should not be observed. The presence of these deposits suggests IgA nephropathy (see Chapter 21) or lupus nephritis (see Chapter 24), respectively. The tubulointerstitium and vasculature are usually normal, unless reduced renal function or hypertension is present or the patient is of advanced age.

On immunofluorescence microscopy, the heterogeneity of the lesion is dramatically displayed and a wide variety of patterns is observed (Fig. 27.2). Most commonly, diffuse and global IgM and C3 deposits are found scattered throughout the mesangium in a granular pattern (so-called IgM nephropathy), but isolated C3, C1q, or even IgG deposits may also be seen.[4] If IgA is the predominant immunoglobulin deposited, then a diagnosis of IgA nephropathy can be made with confidence. Not uncommonly, no immunoglobulin deposits are found at all.

On electron microscopy, the number of mesangial cells are increased, with an occasional infiltrating monocyte or polymorphonuclear leukocyte. The amount of mesangial matrix is commonly diffusely increased. Electron-dense deposits with the mesangium can be seen in many cases, particularly those with immunoglobulin (IgG, IgM, or IgA) deposits on immunofluorescence microscopy. Very large mesangial or paramesangial electron-dense deposits suggest IgA nephropathy even if immunofluorescence microscopy is

Immunofluorescence microscopy patterns in mesangial proliferative glomerulonephritis	
Pattern	Associated Disorders
Predominantly mesangial IgA deposits	IgA nephropathy (± IgM, C3)
Predominantly mesangial IgG deposits	Often associated with systemic lupus (± IgM, C3)
Predominantly mesangial IgM deposits	IgM nephropathy (± C3)
Mesangial C1q deposits	C1q nephropathy (± IgG, IgM, C3)
Isolated mesangial C3 deposits	Often associated with resolving poststreptococcal glomerulonephritis
Negative for immunoglobulin or complement deposits	Idiopathic mesangial proliferative glomerulonephritis

Figure 27.2 Immunofluorescence microscopy patterns in mesangial proliferative glomerulonephritis.

not available. Subendothelial and/or subepithelial deposits are not seen. If present, they suggest a postinfectious etiology or underlying lupus nephritis. Large numbers of tubuloreticular inclusions and deposits of multiple immunoglobulin classes identified by immunofluorescent or immunoperoxidase techniques also suggest underlying lupus nephritis.

The clinical presentation of MesPGN is varied, although persistent or recurring microscopic or macroscopic hematuria with mild proteinuria is most common. Nephrotic syndrome with heavy proteinuria is a less frequent initial presentation but is seen more frequently in association with diffuse mesangial IgM deposits (IgM nephropathy)[2] or C1q deposits (C1q nephropathy).[4,5] These entities are described later. Pure MesPGN is a rather uncommon lesion (<5%) in patients diagnosed with idiopathic nephrotic syndrome.[2,3] Renal function and blood pressure are usually normal, at least initially. Serologic studies are generally unrewarding. Serum C3 and C4 complement components and hemolytic complement activity (CH50) are normal. Assays for fluorescent antinuclear antibody (ANA), antineutrophil cytoplasmic autoantibody, anti–glomerular basement membrane (anti-GBM) autoantibody, and cryoimmunoglobulins are negative. Nevertheless, these studies should be performed in most patients to exclude known causes. MesPGN can also be a finding in resolving postinfectious (poststreptococcal) GN. Isolated C3 deposits with scanty subendothelial and/or subepithelial (humplike) deposits on electron microscopy may be seen in this situation.

IgM Nephropathy

IgM nephropathy[2] is characterized by diffuse and generalized glomerular deposits of IgM often accompanied by C3. Mesangial electron-dense deposits are also observed. On light microscopy, a picture of pure MesPGN is observed. Patients may present with recurring hematuria and proteinuria, the latter in the nephrotic range in as many as 50% of patients. Persisting abnormalities and a poor response to corticosteroids and/or immunosuppressive therapy are often seen. As many as 50% of patients will eventually progress to typical focal and segmental glomerulosclerosis and, if unresponsive to corticosteroids, will slowly develop chronic kidney disease and ESRD. The etiology and pathogenesis are unknown.

C1q Nephropathy

C1q nephropathy is characterized by diffuse deposits of C1q, often accompanied by IgG, IgM, or both.[4,5] C3 deposits are observed less

frequently. These immunopathologic features resemble those seen in lupus nephritis; however, these patients have none of the clinical features of SLE and do not develop SLE even after prolonged follow-up.[5] In addition to MesPGN other morphologic lesions, including focal and segmental glomerulosclerosis, are observed by light microscopy. Nephrotic-range proteinuria, often with hematuria, is observed. Males predominate and African Americans are commonly affected. Serum C3 components, ANA and anti–double-stranded DNA antibodies are consistently normal or negative. The response to treatment is poor and progression to ESRD may occur. The existence of both entities, that is, IgM and C1g nephropathy is disputed by some renal pathologists.

Mesangial Proliferative Glomerulonephritis Associated with Minimal Change Disease

MesPGN may also be a part of the spectrum of minimal change disease/focal segmental glomerulosclerosis (FSGS) lesions (see also Chapters 17 and 18). Distinct mesangial hypercellularity superimposed on a lesion of minimal change disease (diffuse foot process effacement seen on electron microscopy) may point to a greater likelihood for corticosteroid unresponsiveness and an eventual evolution to the FSGS lesion.

Natural History of Mesangial Proliferative Glomerulonephritis

The natural history of MesPGN is quite varied, undoubtedly the result of pathogenic and etiologic heterogeneity. Fortunately, in many patients, a benign course ensues, especially if hematuria and scant proteinuria (<1 g/day) are the principal features. Persisting nephrotic syndrome has a less favorable prognosis, and such patients may evolve into FSGS (see Chapter 18) and accompanying progressive renal insufficiency.[3]

Treatment of Mesangial Proliferative Glomerulonephritis

The treatment of pure MesPGN, unaccompanied by other underlying diseases or lesions such as SLE, C1q nephropathy, IgM nephropathy, minimal change lesion, or IgA nephropathy has not been well defined.[2,3] No prospective, randomized, controlled trials of treatment have been or likely will be performed due to the uncommon nature of the disorder. As the prognosis for patients with isolated hematuria or hematuria combined with mild proteinuria is generally benign, no treatment other than management of hypertension is needed. For those patients with nephrotic syndrome, with or without impaired renal function, a more aggressive approach is often recommended, especially in the presence of diffuse IgM deposits, because many such patients will eventually progress to FSGS. As a result, even in the absence of controlled trials, an initial course of corticosteroid therapy may be justified in most patients with nephrotic-range proteinuria (e.g., prednisone 60 mg/day or 120 mg every other day for 2 to 3 months followed by lowered doses, on an alternate-day regimen, for 2 to 3 additional months). About 50% of patients so treated will experience a decrease in proteinuria to subnephrotic levels, and occasionally complete remissions will occur. However, relapses of proteinuria are common when corticosteroids are tapered or discontinued. Such relapsing, partially corticosteroid-responsive patients might benefit from the addition of cyclophosphamide, chlorambucil, or even cyclosporine or mycophenolate mofetil to the regimen, although information on the therapeutic efficacy and safety of these agents in pure MesPGN is quite limited and no randomized, prospective clinical trials have yet been conducted.

Patients with persistent treatment-unresponsive nephrotic syndrome will almost invariably progress to ESRD over a period of several years, nearly always accompanied by the development of superimposed lesions of FSGS. While transplantation is not contraindicated, those patients who do progress to ESRD rapidly and who develop superimposed FSGS may have a high risk of recurrence of proteinuria and FSGS in the transplanted kidney.

GLOMERULONEPHRITIS WITH RHEUMATIC DISEASE

Several so-called collagen-vascular diseases other than SLE may be complicated by GN (Fig. 27.3). This section covers the glomerulonephritides that accompany rheumatoid arthritis, mixed connective tissue disease,[6] dermatomyositis/polymyositis, acute rheumatic fever, scleroderma, and relapsing polychondritis. IgA nephropathy may also be seen in association with the seronegative spondyloarthropathies.

Rheumatoid Arthritis

A wide variety of glomerular, tubulointerstitial, and vascular lesions of the kidney may complicate rheumatoid arthritis (Fig. 27.4). Renal abnormalities, including abnormal urinalyses (hematuria, leukocyturia, proteinuria), and reduced renal function are quite common in patients with rheumatoid arthritis, particularly those with severe or long-standing disease. Membranous nephropathy (see Chapter 19) is the most common glomerular lesion encountered. This may be owing to the underlying disease itself or to its therapy (parenteral or oral gold or penicillamine). The presence of HLA-DR3 increases the risk of developing membranous nephropathy in a patient with rheumatoid arthritis, which itself is strongly associated with HLA-DR4.

The course of membranous nephropathy in association with rheumatoid arthritis, in the absence of drugs, is similar to that of the idiopathic disease, although spontaneous remissions appear to be less likely to occur. By comparison, membranous nephropathy associated with drugs used to treat rheumatoid arthritis is most likely to remit following discontinuance of the drug therapy.[7] Such remissions may take many months to occur. Nevertheless, 60% to 80% of patients with drug-induced membranous nephropathy in a setting of rheumatoid arthritis will remit within a year of discontinuance of treatment.

Secondary amyloidosis is found in 5% to 20% of patients with rheumatoid arthritis undergoing renal biopsy. Such amyloidosis has

Collagen-vascular (rheumatic) diseases associated with glomerular lesions
Systemic lupus erythematosus (see Chapter 24)
Rheumatoid arthritis
Mixed connective tissue disease
Rheumatic fever
Ankylosing spondylitis
Reiter's syndrome
Dermatomyositis/polymyositis
Scleroderma
Relapsing polychondritis
Systemic or renal limited polyangiitis (see Chapter 23)

Figure 27.3   Collagen-vascular (rheumatic) diseases associated with glomerular lesions.

Renal disease in rheumatoid arthritis
Glomerular Lesions That May Be Direct Complications of the Disease
Membranous nephropathy
Mesangial proliferative GN (± IgA or IgM deposits)
Diffuse proliferative GN   Necrotizing and crescentic GN (rheumatoid vasculitis)
Amyloidosis (AA type)
Glomerular Lesions Associated with Agents Used in the Treatment of Rheumatoid Arthritis
Gold: membranous nephropathy, minimal change disease, acute tubular necrosis
Penicillamine: membranous nephropathy, crescentic GN, minimal change disease
Nonsteroidal anti-inflammatory agents: acute tubulointerstitial nephritis (TIN) with minimal change disease, acute tubular necrosis, minimal change disease without TIN
Cyclosporine: chronic vasculopathy and tubulointerstitial nephropathy, focal and segmental glomerulosclerosis (?)
Azathioprine/6-mercaptopurine: acute interstitial nephritis
Pamidronate: focal segmental glomerulosclerosis

Figure 27.4   Renal disease in rheumatoid arthritis.

the tinctorial and immunohistochemical properties of AA-amyloid, and the serum amyloid A–associated protein is greatly increased in rheumatoid arthritis. However, an increase in the serum concentration of serum amyloid–associated protein is not sufficient for the induction of amyloidosis. Other factors, including a genetic predisposition, appear to play a role. Secondary amyloidosis in rheumatoid arthritis may also involve the heart, gastrointestinal tract, and nerves. Nephrotic syndrome and progressive renal failure are common. The use of nonsteroidal anti-inflammatory drugs (NSAIDs) may also produce tubulointerstitial nephritis, minimal change disease, and nephrotic syndrome[8] (see also Chapter 17). A severe, necrotizing polyangiitis may sometimes complicate the course of long-standing rheumatoid arthritis (rheumatoid vasculitis).[8] The patients may have profound reduction in C3 levels, striking elevation of rheumatoid factors, and marked polyclonal hypergammaglobulinemia. Renal involvement in rheumatoid vasculitis is relatively uncommon for poorly understood reasons.

Mixed Connective Tissue Disease

Mixed connective tissue disease is characterized by features that overlap with those of SLE, scleroderma, and polymyositis. Typically, the serum of such patients contains high-titer autoantibodies to extractable nuclear antigens (ribonucleoprotein-extractable nuclear antigen, U1 ribonucleoprotein antigen). Low titers of anti–double-stranded DNA antibody may also be found. Renal disease, originally thought to be quite rare, is found in 10% to 50% of patients, most frequently membranous nephropathy and MesPGN.[9] Treatment with corticosteroids is generally quite effective, but some patients may progress to chronic renal insufficiency. Patients with severe GN may respond to treatment regimens similar to those used in the treatment of lupus nephritis (see Chapter 24).

Polymyositis/Dermatomyositis

These related collagen-vascular diseases are characterized by inflammatory lesions in muscle, variably by skin lesions, and often include Raynaud's phenomenon.[10] Occasionally, patients develop proteinuria and hematuria secondary to MesPGN with IgM deposits. Acute renal failure may rarely supervene when severe muscle injury and myoglobinuria are present. Treatment with corticosteroids may, at least in part, ameliorate the renal manifestations in concert with improvement in the muscle and skin manifestations.

Acute Rheumatic Fever

Acute rheumatic fever secondary to a pharyngeal infection with a rheumatogenic strain of group A β-hemolytic streptococci is seldom accompanied by renal disease.[11] Poststreptococcal GN and acute rheumatic fever almost never coexist because of the distinct difference between nephritogenic and rheumatogenic strains of streptococci. In addition, cutaneous streptococcal infections are never associated with acute rheumatic fever sequelae. Nevertheless, on rare occasions, MesPGN has been associated with acute rheumatic fever.[11] It usually manifests with hematuria with scant proteinuria and often resolves with appropriate treatment and control of acute rheumatic fever.

Ankylosing Spondylitis and Reiter Syndrome (Seronegative Spondyloarthropathies)

The seronegative spondylo- and oligoarticular arthropathies may from time to time be associated with mesangial IgA deposition. Clinical manifestations are usually mild and nonprogressive. Secondary (AA) amyloidosis may complicate long-standing ankylosing spondylitis.

Scleroderma (Systemic Sclerosis)

Scleroderma is a heterogeneous disorder of unknown etiology and pathogenesis characterized by uncontrolled expansion of connective tissue in the skin and other visceral organs. There is also a marked tendency to produce vascular thickening and narrowing. Clinical manifestations vary from increased connective tissue in localized patches of skin (morphea) to diffuse and generalized disease (systemic sclerosis). The latter pattern leads to thickening of the skin of the face and hands, telangiectasia, Raynaud's phenomenon, tendon friction rubs, and sclerodactyly. A characteristic pattern of blood vessel abnormalities is seen in the nailbeds.

Visceral involvement in the systemic form causes interstitial pulmonary fibrosis, loss of esophageal and other gastrointestinal motility, restrictive cardiomyopathy, and renal disease. Limited forms of the disease (CREST syndrome: *c*alcinosis, *R*aynaud's phenomenon, *e*sophageal dysmotility, *s*clerodactyly, and *t*elangiectasia) also occur but are seldom associated with renal disease. The disorder is seen more frequently in females, with an onset usually in young adults. Approximately 90% of patients will have a speckled pattern of fluorescent ANA; 20% will have detectable antibody to topoisomerase I (Scl-70). Anticentromere antibody is strongly associated with the CREST syndrome. Anti-DNA polymerase is associated with a poor prognosis and a high prevalence of renal involvement. Rarely, the visceral abnormalities may occur in the absence of cutaneous lesions (scleroderma *sine* scleroderma).

Renal involvement in scleroderma can be quite varied and may vary from a low-grade proteinuria and slight impairment of glomerular filtration rate and a more marked reduction in renal blood flow leading to a greatly elevated filtration fraction owing to a mild MesPGN, to severe acute renal failure. The latter clinical phenomenon is referred to as scleroderma renal crisis and consists of severe (hyper-reninemic) hypertension, encephalopathy, systolic and diastolic congestive heart failure, and acute renal failure. There is often an accompanying microangiopathic hemolytic anemia with schistocytes in the peripheral smear and greatly elevated serum lactic dehydrogenase levels. Occasionally, acute renal failure may develop in the absence of hypertension. Acute renal failure results from primary involvement of the arcuate and interlobular arteries (Fig. 27.5) and may be superimposed on lesions of malignant hypertension (such as fibrinoid necrosis of the afferent arterioles) and by ischemic glomerular changes such as wrinkling of the capillary wall and thickening of the basal lamina. The prognosis of scleroderma crisis has remarkably improved with the use of angiotensin-converting enzyme (ACE) inhibitors. In one study, ACE inhibitor treatment was associated with better patient survival at 1 year (75% versus 15%) and with significant preservation or recovery of renal function.[12] Transplantation may be a reasonable treatment option, but progression of disease in other visceral organs may limit life expectancy.

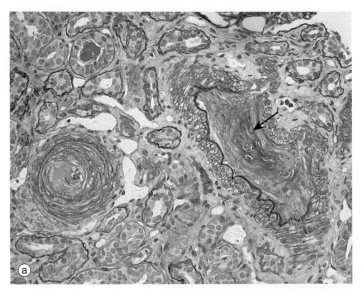 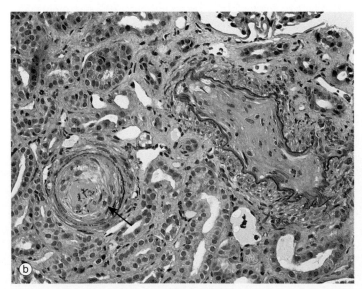

Figure 27.5 Systemic sclerosis. Two interlobular arteries, one transversally, one tangentially cut, show a pronounced subendothelial thickening with weakly periodic acid–Schiff-positive mucinous material and myofibroblasts (*arrow*) (*a*). Fragmented erythrocytes (schistocytes) can be seen in the Goldner elastica stain in red (*arrow*) (*b*). The process is limited to the intima as the lamina elastica interna is preserved. Surrounding tubules are collapsed and have atrophic epithelia due to postarteriolar ischemia. (Courtesy of H. J. Groene, Heidelberg, Germany.)

Relapsing Polychondritis

Polychondritis is a chronic relapsing disorder characterized by destructive inflammation of cartilage (ear, nose, trachea, costal cartilage) and may be associated with crescentic GN, MesPGN, or membranous nephropathy. Lesions of cartilage may lead to deformities (saddle nose, floppy ears, tracheal collapse/stenosis), and the renal disease may be severe and progressive, leading to renal failure. Aggressive management of progressive disease with steroids and cytotoxic agents (cyclophosphamide) is indicated to control both the systemic and renal manifestations.

GLOMERULONEPHRITIS ASSOCIATED WITH MALIGNANCY

Many malignant disorders and their treatment may be complicated by the development of glomerular lesions.[13] Furthermore, the treatment of glomerular disease with certain agents may give rise to neoplasia. Malignant neoplasms may also be associated with a wide variety of fluid, electrolyte, acid-base, divalent ion, tubulointerstitial, and vascular disorders, including direct invasion of the renal parenchyma by neoplastic cells.

The glomerular lesions commonly observed in association with neoplastic processes are listed in Figure 27.6. Membranous nephropathy is the most common lesion (see also Chapter 19). Approximately 7% to 10% of patients found to have membranous nephropathy by renal biopsy (most often for the evaluation of nephrotic syndrome) will be found to have an underlying malignancy. Most patients are adults older than the age of 50; however, because of the increasing frequency of malignancy with age, the association between membranous nephropathy and neoplasia may be more apparent than real. Some epidemiologic studies suggest that the prevalence of malignancy is no higher in patients with membranous nephropathy than in age-matched controls.

Major glomerular lesions associated with neoplastic disease	
Glomerular Disease	**Commonly Associated Malignancy**
Membranous nephropathy	Colon, breast, stomach, and lung cancer
Minimal change disease	Hodgkin's lymphoma, pancreatic cancer, mesothelioma, prostate cancer
Focal segmental glomerulosclerosis	Leukemia, lymphoma
Membranoproliferative glomerulonephritis (GN)	Chronic lymphocytic leukemia, lymphoma (some associated with hepatitis C virus)
IgA nephropathy	Lung carcinoma
Crescentic GN/systemic vasculitis	Lung carcinoma
Systemic amyloidosis AL type	Multiple myeloma, Waldenström's macroglobulinemia
Systemic amyloidosis AA type	Carcinoma (especially renal)
Cryoglobulinemic GN	Chronic lymphocytic leukemia (often hepatitis C associated)
Light chain nephropathy	Lymphoma, myeloma
Fibrillary (immunotactoid) GN	Lymphoma
Hemolytic-uremic syndrome	Gastric cancer, mucin-producing cancer

Figure 27.6 Major glomerular lesions associated with neoplastic disease.

Notwithstanding these observations, remissions (albeit temporary) can be achieved by surgical removal or chemotherapy of the neoplastic disease, and relapses may develop with recurrence of tumor. Tumor neoantigens or antibodies have rarely been detected within the glomerular deposits, suggesting an immune pathogenesis. In about one third of patients, the neoplastic disorder is already evident before the development of glomerular lesions; in about one third, it is discovered concomitantly with the onset of glomerular disease, and in about one third of patients, the neoplastic process is detected after the diagnosis of glomerular disease.

Less frequent lesions observed in patients with neoplasia include minimal change lesion, FSGS, proliferative GN (including crescentic GN), thrombotic microangiopathy, monoclonal immunoglobulin deposition diseases, and amyloidosis. Minimal change disease may be associated with lymphoma (particularly Hodgkin's disease) and certain other cancers (pancreas, mesothelioma, prostate). Membranoproliferative GN (MPGN) may be associated with chronic lymphocytic leukemia and lymphoma. FSGS may also occasionally be encountered in patients with underlying malignancy, including leukemia and lymphoma. IgA deposits and crescentic GN may be associated with lung cancer. Vasculitis accompanied by crescentic GN, often resembling Henoch-Schönlein purpura, has been reported to occur with several malignancies, most notably lung cancer.

Systemic amyloidosis (AL type) may affect the kidney and produce nephrotic syndrome and renal failure in 10% to 15% of patients with multiple myeloma and rarely in association with Waldenström's macroglobulinemia (see Chapter 26). Carcinomas, including renal cell carcinoma, are also rarely complicated by amyloidosis, which is usually of the AA variety. Monoclonal immunoglobulin deposition disease (see Chapter 26) may accompany lymphomas and leukemias. Light-chain nephropathy, in which deposits of either κ or γ light chain are found in the glomerular capillaries and tubular basement membranes, may occur in association with a variety of neoplastic lymphoproliferative states (see also Chapter 26).

Thrombotic microangiopathies, including hemolytic-uremic syndrome, producing renal cortical necrosis or glomerular lesions resembling MPGN may be seen in association with disseminated cancer (carcinoma of the stomach) and other mucin-producing carcinomas. It may also appear secondary to treatment with certain antineoplastic agents, especially mitomycin (mitomycin C; see also Chapter 28).

Interferon treatment, used in the management of certain malignancies, may rarely cause minimal change disease in association with interstitial nephritis. Finally, cyclophosphamide therapy of glomerular disease, particularly if prolonged high-dose therapy is involved, may result in a variety of malignancies including leukemias, B cell lymphomas, and bladder cancers. Azathioprine increases the risk of papillomavirus-associated squamous cell carcinoma of the cervix and/or vulva and also certain skin cancers.[14]

CONGENITAL NEPHROTIC SYNDROME

According to the common usage of the term congenital nephrotic syndrome, this disorder is defined as the presence of nephrotic syndrome at the time of birth or the discovery of nephrotic syndrome in infants younger than 3 months of age. As such, congenital nephrotic syndrome can arise consequent to a number of disorders (Fig. 27.7).

Classic Finnish-Type Congenital Nephrotic Syndrome

The Finnish type of congenital nephrotic syndrome is the most common form, seen in about 1.2/10,000 live births in Finland

Causes of congenital nephrotic syndrome
Idiopathic (primary) focal segmental glomerulosclerosis (FSGS) or FSGS due to mutations of podocyte proteins, including classic Finnish-type nephrotic syndrome (see Chapter 18)
Diffuse Mesangial Sclerosis
With pseudohermaphroditism/gonadoblastoma (Denys-Drash syndrome, Frasier syndrome)
With microcephaly/microcoria (Galloway-Mowat syndrome, Pierson-Zenker syndrome)
Idiopathic
Genetic Disorders
Lowe syndrome
Mucopolysaccharidoses
Nail-patella syndrome
Sialic acid storage disease
Congenital Infections
Cytomegalovirus
Syphilis
Rubella
Toxoplasmosis
Hepatitis B

Figure 27.7   Causes of congenital nephrotic syndrome.

(see also Chapter 18). Congenital nephrotic syndrome is also occasionally observed in families of non-Finnish extraction. The Finnish form is an autosomal recessive disorder due to mutations of *NHPS1* gene that codes for nephrin, a critical protein component of the slit diaphragm.[15] A detailed description of the genetics and pathogenesis of the Finnish-type congenital nephrotic syndrome is given in Chapter 18.

Children with the Finnish type of congenital nephrotic syndrome are born prematurely and often have a very large placenta, sometimes giving rise to a difficult delivery. Raised levels of α-fetoprotein occur in the amniotic fluid and are sometimes also observed in maternal plasma, which may be an indication of the development of congenital nephrotic syndrome *in utero*. These observations may lead to the consideration of early termination of pregnancy.

Children with congenital nephrotic syndrome may be markedly edematous at birth or develop severe anasarca within a few days of delivery. Ascites, delayed development, severe erythrocytosis, and spontaneous vascular thromboses are also common. Pathologically diffuse foot process effacement and cystic dilatations of the proximal tubule accompanied by mesangial sclerosis are commonly seen (Fig. 27.8). Later, diffuse mesangial sclerosis is the most common pathology. The permeability abnormality due to nephrin deficiency responsible for the Finnish type of congenital nephrotic syndrome may cause alterations in podocyte attachment to the GBM leading to progressive capillary collapse and sclerosis (see also Chapter 18).

Children with classic Finnish-type congenital nephrotic syndrome usually develop progressive renal failure within the first year of life. Aggressive therapy (see later discussion) may permit some infants to survive long enough to receive a successful renal transplant. Other than transplantation, no treatments are effective. Interestingly, the disease may recur in the transplanted kidney in about 25% of patients, which has recently been shown to be mediated by an immune response to the nephrin in the normal transplanted kidney[16] (similar to the situation in Alport's syndrome; see Chapters 22 and 45).

Denys-Drash and Frasier Syndromes

Diffuse mesangial sclerosis and male pseudohermaphroditism (Denys-Drash syndrome) is a relatively uncommon cause of congenital nephrotic syndrome in infants. Such patients have a high frequency of developing Wilms' tumors. Karyotyping will detect the abnormality in phenotypic females.[17] Frasier syndrome consists of XY gonadal dysgenesis, gonadoblastoma, and a high frequency of Wilms' tumor.[18] Mutations of the Wilms' tumor suppressor gene (*WT-1*) are responsible for both syndromes.[17,18] The nephropathy in both syndromes also almost invariably evokes progressive renal failure, and bilateral nephrectomies must be performed prior to renal transplantation to avoid the emergence of Wilms' tumor. There is no effective treatment; however, aggressive treatment with angiotensin inhibition may delay the onset of renal failure. Diffuse mesangial sclerosis may also occur in the absence of systemic or developmental abnormalities. This

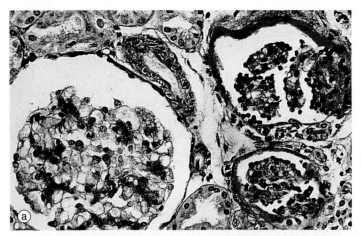
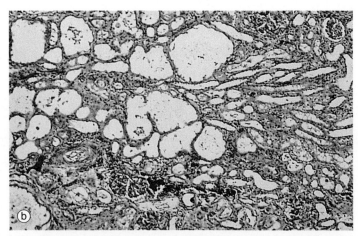

Figure 27.8   Congenital nephrotic syndrome Finnish type. *a,* Diffuse mesangial thickening and partially collapsed glomeruli (periodic acid–Schiff, ×260). *b,* Microcystic dilatation of the tubules (hematoxylin-eosin, ×150). (Adapted from Churg J, Bernstein J, Glassock R, eds. Renal Disease: Classification and Atlas of Glomerular Disease. New York: Igaku-Shoin, 1995, p 422.)

idiopathic form behaves in a similar fashion to the forms associated with pseudohermaphroditism and nephroblastoma.

Galloway-Mowat Syndrome

Galloway-Mowat syndrome is an autosomal recessive disorder that includes microcephaly, developmental retardation, seizures, hiatal hernia, and renal disease.[19] The precise genetic abnormality remains unknown. The GBM abnormalities are similar to those found in the nail-patella syndrome (see Chapter 45). No treatment is successful, and nearly all patients progress to ESRD within 3 to 5 years. A closely related syndrome with the additional features of large corneas, microcoria (small unreactive pupils), and posterior lenticonus (Pierson-Zenker syndrome) has also been described.[19] Deficiency of laminin β2 and mutations in the *LAMB2* gene on chromosome 3p14–p22 may be responsible for the clinical expression of the Pierson-Zenker syndrome.[20]

Infection-Related Congenital Nephrotic Syndrome

Several congenital infections may be associated with the development of nephrotic syndrome in early infancy. Most important among these infections are congenital syphilis and cytomegalovirus infection. Renal biopsy shows membranous nephropathy or proliferative GN, sometimes with immune deposits containing the microbial antigen. Treatment of the basic disease with appropriate antimicrobials or antiviral agents will often result in improvement.

Other Rare Causes of Congenital Nephrotic Syndrome

Recently an autosomal recessive steroid-resistant nephrotic syndrome (sometimes manifest at birth or in early infancy) has been associated with mutations in *NHPS2* which codes podocin.[21] Mutations in *ACTN4*, which codes the cytoplasmic protein α-actinin 4, or a gain-in-function mutation of *TRPC6*, which codes for a cation channel,[22] have been associated with an autosomal dominant familial focal segmental glomerulosclerosis. Both of these mutations target podocyte proteins and likely alter podocyte function. Several cases of congenital membranous nephropathy have also been described in which antibodies to a podocyte antigen, neutral endopeptidase, were transferred by the mother (who lacked this antigen and was sensitized by the baby) to the baby during birth[23] (see also Chapter 19). Unilateral renal arterial stenosis in the newborn has also been reported to cause congenital nephrotic syndrome.

Management of Nephrotic Syndrome in Newborns and Infants

In the past, most children with congenital nephrotic syndrome died within the first 6 months of life. However, increased survival is being observed with an aggressive regimen of daily intravenous albumin, early use of oral or intravenous diuretics, the use of ACE inhibitors or angiotensin receptor blockers (the latter less effective in Finnish-type congenital nephrotic syndrome), as well as vitamin D supplements (along with magnesium and calcium), thyroxine replacement, anticoagulants (heparin and warfarin), and antibiotics (as indicated).[24]

When severe nephrotic syndrome supervenes that produces a serious threat to the patient's life (usually from profound protein malnutrition), "medical nephrectomy" can be considered. This consists of high doses of an ACE inhibitor, such as enalapril, plus high doses of an NSAID, such as indomethacin. However, if this approach is not successful, surgical bilateral nephrectomy between 6 and 10 months of age with the institution of peritoneal dialysis could be attempted until the child reaches a size and weight (usually 8 to 9 kg) when renal transplantation can be performed. Recurrence of nephrotic syndrome in the graft may develop in some patients, particularly those with the Finnish type of congenital nephrotic syndrome, due to complete absence of nephrin in the diseased kidneys. The recipient may develop antibodies or cell-mediated immunity to the native nephrin in the transplanted kidney.[16]

OTHER UNCOMMON DISORDERS

Lipoprotein Glomerulopathy

Lipoprotein glomerulopathy is believed to be caused by an abnormality in lipoprotein metabolism[25] and is characterized by extensive deposits of apolipoprotein A, B, and E in the glomeruli, leading to greatly expanded capillaries filled with pale-staining, meshlike substance having the appearance of lipid "thrombi" (Fig. 27.9). Clinically, heavy proteinuria with nephrotic syndrome may be present. Apolipoprotein B and E levels are increased in plasma in association with a type III hyperlipoproteinemia. The apolipoprotein E usually shows a heterozygous E2/E3 or E2/E4 phenotype, but homozygosity for apolipoprotein E2 or E3 has also been observed. Homozygous apolipoprotein E2 is also seen in familial type III hyperlipoproteinemia. Low low-density

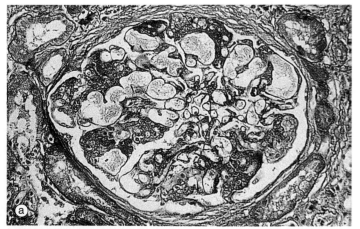
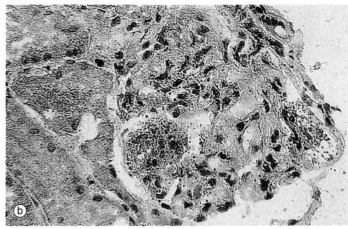

Figure 27.9   Lipoprotein glomerulopathy. *a,* Dilated capillary lumina containing a pale-stained, meshlike or granular substance (trichrome stain, ×260). *b,* The granules stain positively with oil red O and antilipoprotein E antisera (oil red O, ×260). (Adapted from Churg J, Bernstein J, Glassock R, eds. Renal Disease: Classification and Atlas of Glomerular Disease. New York: Igaku-Shoin, 1995, p 457.)

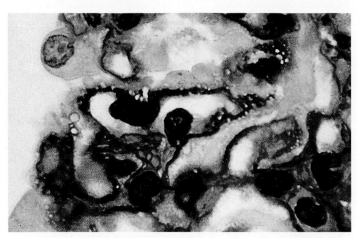

Figure 27.10 Lecithin-cholesterol acyltransferase deficiency. Note the irregular thickened glomerular capillary walls containing clear vacuoles, which are characteristic of the lesion (periodic acid–Schiff, ×1000). (Adapted from Churg J, Bernstein J, Glassock R, eds. Renal Disease: Classification and Atlas of Glomerular Disease. New York: Igaku-Shoin, 1995, p 453.)

lipoprotein receptor binding and high heparin affinity may explain some of the pathogenetic processes in lipoprotein glomerulopathy. The disease can be associated with psoriasis[26]; otherwise, there are no distinctive clinical features. Familial cases have strongly suggested a hereditary abnormality. The disorder may recur in the renal transplant. Treatment with benzfibrate or fenofibrate may be effective.[27,28]

Lecithin-Cholesterol Acyltransferase Deficiency

Lecithin-cholesterol acyltransferase (LCAT) deficiency is an autosomal recessive disorder.[29] The mutations are on the *LCAT* gene located on chromosome 16q22.[29] The clinical characteristics include corneal opacities (misty deposits, also known as "fish eye"); normocytic, normochromic anemia; premature atherosclerosis; low high-density lipoprotein and α-lipoprotein levels; and elevated low-density lipoproteins. Proteinuria (including the nephrotic syndrome), hypertension, and progressive renal failure are the main renal manifestations. On light microscopy, the glomeruli reveal foam cells, intimal hyperplasia, and thickening of the basement membrane with effacement of the foot processes (Fig. 27.10). Progressive renal failure is the rule; however, it is of slow and insidious onset and is usually first detected by the fourth

decade of life. Treatment is generally ineffective, but theoretically an inhibitor of hepatic acyl-coenzyme A–cholesterol acyltransferase activity might be of benefit.[30]

Collagen III Glomerulopathy

Collagen III glomerulopathy (also known as collagenofibrotic glomerulopathy) is a systemic disorder with prominent renal manifestations that may be a *forme fruste* of nail-patella syndrome (see Chapter 45) since the glomerular abnormalities are similar.[31,32] Nevertheless, patients with collagen III glomerulopathy lack the typical skeletal abnormalities observed in the nail-patella syndrome. An autosomal recessive pattern is observed. Clinically, patients present with proteinuria and slowly progressive renal failure. Patients may be of any age and males predominate. On light microscopy, the glomeruli are enlarged with a marked expansion of the mesangial matrix with weakly periodic acid–Schiff-positive material (Fig. 27.11). Conventional immunofluorescence microscopy is negative, but antisera to collagen type III will strongly react with the glomerular deposits. Electron microscopy shows bundles spirally arranged and frayed fibrillar deposits (Congo red negative) with periodicity characteristic of collagen. Similar deposits may be found in the spleen, liver, myocardium, and thyroid in fatal cases. No treatment is effective, and there are no data yet on recurrent disease, but due to the systemic nature of the disease, such recurrences would be likely.

Fibronectin Glomerulopathy

Fibronectin glomerulopathy is a rare autosomal dominant fibrillary glomerular disease with onset usually in early adolescence with proteinuria, microhematuria, hypertension, distal (type IV) renal tubular acidosis, and slowly progressive renal failure.[33,34] The gene responsible for the disorder maps to chromosome 1q32 near markers D1S2872 and D1S2891.[35] Most patients reach ESRD between the second and sixth decades of life. The renal pathology usually reveals an enlarged, hyperlobular, and normocellular glomerulus with a homogeneous or fibrillar material (on periodic acid–Schiff staining) in the mesangium and subendothelium (Congo red negative). Electron microscopy shows randomly oriented fibrils (12 to 16 nm wide and 120 to 170 nm long). Immunofluorescence is negative for antibody and complement components but will stain brightly using an antifibronectin antibody. The pathogenesis of the disease is unknown, although mice "knocked out" for uteroglobin develop a similar lesion.

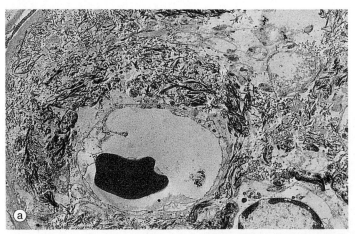

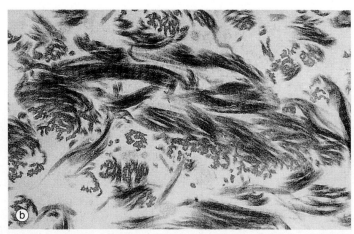

Figure 27.11 Electron microscopy of collagen III glomerulopathy (collagenofibrotic glomerulopathy). *a*, Fine fibrils occur in the mesangial and subendothelial areas (×3000). *b*, These fibrils are randomly oriented with typical periodicity and average 30 nm in diameter. The fibrils are strongly positive for staining with periodic acid–Schiff stain and react with anticollagen III antibodies (×15,000). (Adapted from Churg J, Bernstein J, Glassock R, eds. Renal Disease: Classification and Atlas of Glomerular Disease. New York: Igaku-Shoin, 1995, pp 441–443.)

However, preliminary studies in humans have not documented any linkage to the uteroglobulin or fibronectin genes. There is no known effective treatment.

Nephropathic Cystinosis

Late-onset adult cystinosis is a variant of typical pediatric cystinosis in which the mutations in the *CTNS* gene result in a milder phenotype. These patients may present with glomerular disease during the teenage years. Nephrotic syndrome may occur, and the glomerular lesions resemble FSGS except that crystals of cystine are found in glomerular and tubular epithelial cells.[36] Patients with cystinosis may also have blonde hair, photophobia, hypothyroidism, corneal deposits, rickets, and Fanconi syndrome (see also Chapter 47).

Miscellaneous Storage Diseases and Other Unusual Glomerular Lesions

A variety of diseases associated with storage of abdominal lipids or carbohydrates in tissue may provoke glomerular lesions; these include Hurler's syndrome (type I mucopolysaccharidoses), von Gierke's disease (glycogen storage disease), Gaucher's disease, Refsum's disease, nephrosialidosis, and I-cell disease (mucolipidosis type II). Juvenile malabsorption of vitamin B_{12} with megaloblastic anemia (Imerslund syndrome) can be associated with prolonged glomerular proteinuria, but progressive renal disease does not develop. Asphyxiating thoracic dystrophy (Jeune's syndrome) is associated with glomerular, tubular, and interstitial abnormalities. Hereditary osteolysis causing arthralgias and deformities of wrists and ankles can be accompanied by chronic GN. The nail-patella syndrome and Fabry's disease are discussed in Chapter 45.

"Idiopathic" Nodular Glomerulosclerosis

An intercapillary nodular expansion of the mesangium encroaching on the glomerular capillary lumens is characteristically called the Kimmelstiel-Wilson lesion and is most commonly associated with diabetes mellitus and proliferative diabetic retinopathy (see Chapter 29). However, in recent years, a small group of patients has been described in whom a similar or identical lesion is seen in the absence of any features of diabetes mellitus or other known causes of a similar lesion (such as κ light chain nephropathy [see Chapter 26], chronic thrombotic microangiopathy, monoclonal immunoglobulin deposition diseases, fibrillary GN, and fibronectin glomerulopathy). Thus, idiopathic nodular glomerulosclerosis is a diagnosis of exclusion. The first examples of this new disorder were recognized by Alpers and Biava[37] in 1989, and approximately 40 additional cases have been subsequently reported.[38–40] While some of these patients may have had intermittent manifestation of diabetes or only mild abnormalities of glucose homeostasis, such as an abnormal glucose tolerance test, most have not had any features conventionally used to define the presence of diabetes mellitus (i.e., normal fasting blood sugar and hemoglobin A1c measurements). Thus, the intercapillary nodular lesion does not appear to require prolonged abnormal glucose homeostasis for its generation.

The clinical features are nonspecific and nondiagnostic. Patients with idiopathic nodular glomerulosclerosis are usually older (average age about 70 years), and nephrotic syndrome is a common presentation. A heavy smoking history and long-standing hypertension is very frequently present, but the role of these abnormalities in the pathogenesis of the lesion is unknown.

The pathology includes typical intercapillary nodular glomerulosclerosis with thickening of the glomerular basement membranes and varying degrees of arteriolonephrosclerosis and hyalinosis. These lesions are identical to those described in the diabetes-associated Kimmelstiel-Wilson lesions. No electron-dense or organized deposits are seen on electron microscopy. The GBM and tubular basement membrane may "stain" with IgG and albumin on immunofluorescence. Neovascularization can be seen within the nodules.

The prognosis is poor and relates to the persistence of nephrotic-range proteinuria. Most patients will progress to ESRD, sometimes quite rapidly. The 50% renal survival point in those who continue to smoke heavily is about 1 year after diagnosis. There is no known effective therapy, other than angiotensin inhibition to reduce the proteinuria. Stopping smoking may be beneficial and should be urged for all patients with this diagnosis.

REFERENCES

1. Churg J, Bernstein J, Glassock R, eds.: Renal disease: Classification and Atlas of Glomerular Disease. New York: Igaku-Shoin, 1995.
2. Cohen AH, Border WA, Glassock R: Nephrotic syndrome with glomerular mesangial IgM deposits. Lab Invest 1978;38:610–619.
3. Alexopoulos E, Papagianni A, Stangou M, et al: Adult onset idiopathic nephrotic syndrome associated with pure diffuse mesangial hypercellularity. Nephrol Dial Transplant 2000;15:981–987.
4. Jennette C, Falk R: C1q nephropathy. In Massry S, Glassock R, eds. Textbook of Nephrology, 3rd ed. Baltimore: Williams & Wilkins, 1995, pp 749–752.
5. Sharman A, Furness P, Feehally J: Distinguishing C1q nephropathy from lupus nephritis. Nephrol Dial Transplant 2004;19:1420–1426.
6. Samuels B, Lee JC, Engleman EP, Hopper J: Membranous nephropathy in patients with rheumatoid arthritis: Relationship to gold therapy. Medicine (Baltimore) 1978;57:319–327.
7. Cohen IM, Swerdlin AHR, Steenberg S, Stone RA: Mesangial proliferative GN in mixed connective tissue disease. Clin Nephrol 1980;13:93–96.
8. Whelton A: Nephrotoxicity of nonsteroidal anti-inflammatory drugs: Physiological functions and clinical implications. Am J Med 1999;106:13S–24S.
9. Geirsson AJ, Sturfelt G, Truedsson L: Clinical and serological features of severe vasculitis in rheumatoid arthritis: Prognostic implications. Ann Rheum Dis 1987;46:727–733.
10. Valenzuela OF, Reiser W, Porush JG: Idiopathic polymyositis and glomerulonephritis. J Nephrol 2001;14:120–124.
11. Gibney R, Reinecke H, Bannayan G, Stein J: Renal lesions in rheumatic fever. Ann Intern Med 1981;94:322–326.
12. Steen VD, Constantino JP, Shapiro AP, Medsger TA: Outcome of renal crisis in systemic sclerosis: Relation to availability of angiotensin converting enzyme inhibitors. Ann Intern Med 1991;114:249–250.
13. Alpers CE, Cotran R: Neoplasia and glomerular injury. Kidney Int 1986;30:465–473.
14. Penn I: Cancers in cyclosporine-treated versus azathioprine-treated patients. Transplant Proc 1996;28:876–878.
15. Tryggvason K: Unraveling the mechanism of glomerular ultrafiltration: Nephrin, a key component of the slit diaphragm. J Am Soc Nephrol 1999;10:2440–2445.
16. Patrakka J, Rhotsalainen V, Reponen P, et al: Recurrence of nephrotic syndrome in kidney grafts of patients with congenital nephrotic syndrome of the Finnish type: Role of nephrin. Transplantation 2002;73:394–403.
17. Niaudet P, Gubler MC: WT1 and glomerular diseases. Pediatr Nephrol 2006 (in press).
18. Wang NJ, Song HR, Schamen NC, et al: Frasier syndrome comes full circle: Genetic studies performed in an original patient. J Pediatr 2005;146:843–844.
19. Zenker M, Tralau T, Lennert T, et al: Congenital nephrosis, mesangial sclerosis and distinct eye abnormalities with microcoria: An autosomal recessive syndrome. Am J Med Genet 2004;130:138–145.
20. Zenker M, Aigner T, Wendler O, et al: Human laminin beta2 deficiency causes congenital nephrosis with mesangial sclerosis and distinct eye abnormalities. Hum Mol Genet 2004;13:2625–2632.
21. Boute N, Gribouval O, Roselli S, et al: NHPS2, encoding the glomerular protein, podocin, is mutated in autosomal recessive steroid-resistant nephrotic syndrome. Nat Genet 2000;24:349–354.

22. Kaplan JM, Kim SH, North KN, et al: Mutations in ACTN4, encoding alpha-actinin-4, cause familial focal segmental glomerulosclerosis. Nat Genet 2000;24:251–256.

23. Debiec H, Guigonis V, Mougenot B, et al: Antenatal membranous glomerulonephritis due to anti-neutral endopeptidase (NEP) antibodies. N Engl J Med 2002;346:2053–2060.

24. Savage JM, Jefferson JA, Maxwell AP, et al: Improved prognosis for congenital nephrotic syndrome of the Finnish type in Irish families. Arch Dis Child 1999;80:466–469.

25. Saito T, Oikawa S, Sato H, et al: Lipoprotein glomerulopathy: Renal lipoidosis induced by novel apolipoprotein E variants. Nephron 1999; 83:193–201.

26. Chang CF, Lin CC, Chen JY, et al: Lipoprotein glomerulopathy associated with psoriasis vulgaris: A report of 2 cases with apolipoprotein E3/3. Am J Kidney Dis 2003;42:E18–E23.

27. Arai T, Yamashita S, Yamane M, et al: Disappearance of intraglomerular lipoprotein thrombi and marked improvement of nephrotic syndrome by benzfibrate treatment in a patient with lipoprotein glomerulopathy. Atherosclerosis 2003;169:293–299.

28. Ieiri N, Hotta O, Taguma Y: Resolution of typical lipoprotein glomerulopathy by intensive lipid-lowering therapy. Am J Kidney Dis 2003;41: 244–249.

29. Calabresi L, Pisciotta L, Cosantin A, et al: The molecular basis of lecithin: cholesterol acyltransferase deficiency syndromes: A comprehensive study of molecular and biochemical findings in 13 unrelated Italian families. Arterioscler Thromb Vasc Biol 2005;25:1972–1978.

30. Vaziri N, Liang K: ACAT inhibition reverses LCAT deficiency and improves plasma HDL in chronic renal failure. Am J Physiol Renal Physiol 2004;287:F1038–F1043.

31. Ikeda K, Yokayama H, Tomosugi N, et al: Primary glomerular fibrosis: A new nephropathy caused by diffuse intraglomerular increase in atypical collagen III fibers. Clin Nephrol 1990;33:155–159.

32. Yasuda T, Imai H, Nakamoto Y, et al. Collagenofibrotic glomerulopathy: A systemic disease. Am J Kidney Dis 1999;33:123–127.

33. Strumf EH, Banfi G, Krapg R, et al: Glomerulopathy associated with predominant fibronectin deposits: A newly recognized hereditary disease. Kidney Int 1995;48:163–170.

34. Gemperle O, Neuweiler J, Reutter FW, et al: Familial glomerulopathy with giant fibrillar (fibronectin-positive) deposits: A 15 year follow-up in a large kindred. Am J Kidney Dis 1996;28:668–675.

35. Vollmer M, Jung M, Ruschendorf F, et al: The gene for human fibronectin glomerulopathy maps to 1q32, in the region of the regulation of complement activation gene cluster. Am J Hum Genet 1998;63:1724–1731.

36. Pabico RC, Panner BJ, McKenna BA, Bryson MF: Glomerular lesions in patients with late onset cystinosis with massive proteinuria. Renal Physiol 1980;3:347–354.

37. Alpers CE, Biava CG: Idiopathic lobular glomerulonephritis (nodular mesangial sclerosis). A distinct diagnostic entity. Clin Nephrol 1989;32: 68–74.

38. Herzenberg AM, Holden JK, Singh S, Magil AB: Idiopathic nodular glomerulosclerosis. Am J Kidney Dis 1999;34:560–564.

39. Markowitz GS, Lin J, Valeri AM, et al: Idiopathic nodular glomerulosclerosis as a distinct clinicopathologic entity linked to hypertension and smoking. Hum Pathol 2002;33:826–835.

40. Navaneethan DS, Singh S, Choudry W: Nodular glomerulosclerosis in a non-diabetic patient: Case report and review of the literature. J Nephrol 2005;18:613–615.

Thrombotic Microangiopathies, Including Hemolytic Uremic Syndrome

Piero Ruggenenti, Michele Ceruti, and Giuseppe Remuzzi

INTRODUCTION

Thrombotic microangiopathy (TMA) is characterized by an acute syndrome of microangiopathic hemolytic anemia, thrombocytopenia, and variable signs of organ injury due to platelet thrombosis in the microcirculation.[1] Depending on the distribution of the lesions—kidney or central nervous system—two pathologically identical but clinically distinct entities are described: hemolytic uremic syndrome (HUS) and thrombotic thrombocytopenic purpura (TTP). The former usually affects young children and is characterized by acute renal failure (ARF) and absent or minimal neurologic abnormalities. The latter occurs in adults and is characterized by severe neurologic involvement in most cases and variable renal involvement. In some patients, features of HUS and TTP may coexist. The mechanisms behind the different organ involvement of TMA are not clearly understood. Injury to the endothelium is an important and likely inciting factor of the events leading to microvascular thrombosis. This is suggested by data showing that most agents associated with TMA such as exotoxins, endotoxins, autoantibodies, immune complexes, and certain drugs are toxic to endothelial cells (Fig. 28.1).

CLINICAL AND LABORATORY SIGNS

TMA is characterized by thrombocytopenia, often with purpura, but rarely with severe bleeding, microangiopathic hemolytic anemia, ARF that may be associated with anuria, neurologic deficits, and fever. Thrombocytopenia and hemolytic anemia are the key laboratory abnormalities. Thrombocytopenia is caused by platelet aggregation in the microcirculation while hemolytic anemia is due to mechanical fragmentation of erythrocytes during their passage through the narrowed vessels. Thrombocytopenia is usually more severe in TTP than in HUS. At the onset of TTP, platelet counts may be $<20 \times 10^9$ cells/l. In HUS, values between 30×10^9 and 100×10^9 cells/l are frequent; however, normal values may also be detected. Anemia is usually severe with hemoglobin concentrations <6.5 mg/dl in about 40% of cases. Hyperbilirubinemia (mainly indirect), reticulocytosis, circulating free hemoglobin, and low haptoglobin levels are usually present. The serum lactate dehydrogenase (LDH) level is extremely high, reflecting hemolysis but also, in some patients, diffuse tissue infarction. Both platelet count and serum LDH are useful parameters for both diagnosis and response to treatment. Fragmented red blood cells (schistocytes) with the typical appearance of a helmet in the peripheral smear (Fig. 28.2) and a negative Coombs' test (with the exception of neuraminidase-associated

TMA) are needed to confirm the microangiopathic nature of hemolysis. Shigatoxin (Stx)-associated HUS is often associated with leukocytosis with a left shift, while leukocytes are usually normal in atypical HUS and TTP. Hypocomplementemia (low serum C3 levels) is occasionally present. Prothrombin time (PT) and partial thromboplastin time (PTT), factor V, factor VIII, and fibrinogen are normal in most cases. ARF is usually associated with mild proteinuria (usually 1 to 2 g/day) and few red blood cells and casts on urinary sediment. Seizure and coma may occur in TTP and, much less frequently, HUS.

DIAGNOSIS AND DIFFERENTIAL DIAGNOSIS

The diagnosis of TMA is based on the preceding clinical and laboratory findings. Renal biopsy is indicated when the diagnosis is

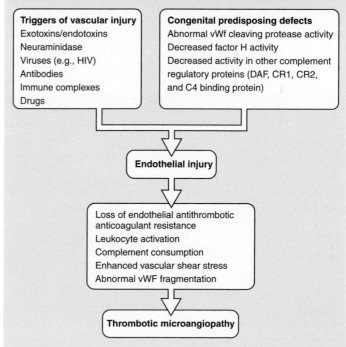

Etiology and pathogenesis of microangiopathy

Triggers of vascular injury
Exotoxins/endotoxins
Neuraminidase
Viruses (e.g., HIV)
Antibodies
Immune complexes
Drugs

Congenital predisposing defects
Abnormal vWf cleaving protease activity
Decreased factor H activity
Decreased activity in other complement regulatory proteins (DAF, CR1, CR2, and C4 binding protein)

Endothelial injury

Loss of endothelial antithrombotic anticoagulant resistance
Leukocyte activation
Complement consumption
Enhanced vascular shear stress
Abnormal vWF fragmentation

Thrombotic microangiopathy

Figure 28.1 A suggested sequence of events leading to thrombotic microangiopathy in predisposed subjects exposed to triggers of endothelial injury. HIV, human immunodeficiency virus; vWf, von Willebrand factor.

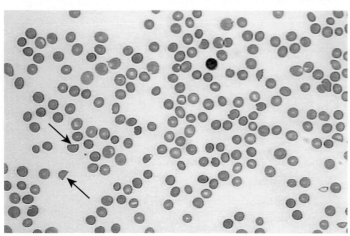

Figure 28.2 Peripheral blood smear from a patient with hemolytic uremic syndrome. The presence of fragmented red blood cells with the appearance of a helmet (*arrows*) is pathognomonic for microangiopathic hemolysis in patients with no evidence of heart valvular disease.

uncertain and thrombocytopenia is not severe. In case of thrombocytopenia, microangiopathic hemolytic anemia, and ARF, the differential diagnosis includes systemic vasculitis, malignant hypertension, disseminated intravascular coagulation (DIC), and, where present, Hantavirus infection. Other conditions that can cause a HUS-like picture include scleroderma and radiation injury. Vasculitis is usually characterized by other systemic symptoms such as cutaneous rash and arthralgias; the platelet count is usually normal and neurologic involvement is predominantly peripheral rather than central. Patients with malignant hypertension have a history of high blood pressure, very high systolic/diastolic blood pressure at the time of evaluation, and typical retinal lesions. DIC is usually associated with sepsis, shock, and obstetric complications; patients typically have consumption of all the components of coagulation cascade, including fibrinogen, factor V, and factor VIII, with subsequent prolongation of PT and PTT. Hantavirus infection causes high fever, lumbar pain, ARF, and thrombopenia but usually no hemolysis.

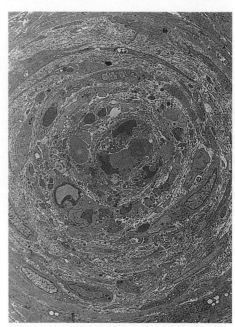

Figure 28.4 Electron micrograph of a renal arteriole in hemolytic uremic syndrome. The vascular lumen is completely occluded by thrombi. There is marked intimal edema with consequent separation of myointimal cells.

PATHOLOGY

The histologic lesions of TMA consist of vessel (capillary and arteriole) wall widening on electron microscopy, with swelling and detachment of the endothelial cells from the basement membrane and the accumulation of fluffy material in the subendothelium (Fig. 28.3), intraluminal platelet thrombi, and partial or complete obstruction of vessel lumina (Fig. 28.4). These lesions are similar to those seen in other renal diseases such as scleroderma, malignant nephrosclerosis, chronic transplant rejection, and calcineurin inhibitor nephrotoxicity. In HUS, microthrombi are present primarily in the kidneys, while in TTP they mainly involve the brain, where thrombi may repeatedly form and resolve, producing intermittent neurologic deficits. In pediatric patients, particularly in those younger than 2 years of age, and in those with HUS secondary to gastrointestinal infection with Stx-producing strains of *Escherichia coli*, the glomerular injury is predominant (Figs. 28.5

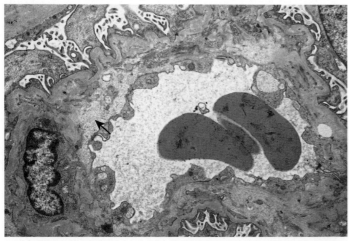

Figure 28.3 Electron micrograph of a glomerular capillary in hemolytic uremic syndrome. The endothelium is detached from the glomerular basement membrane; the subendothelial space is widened and occupied by electron-lucent fluffy material and cell debris (*arrow*). Beneath the endothelium is a thin layer of newly formed glomerular basement membrane.

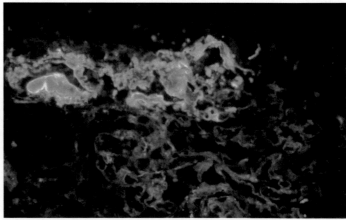

Figure 28.5 Glomerulus with its vascular pole from a patient with shigatoxin-associated hemolytic uremic syndrome. Strong staining with fluorescein-labeled antifibrinogen antibody occurs in the glomerulus and in the arteriolar wall.

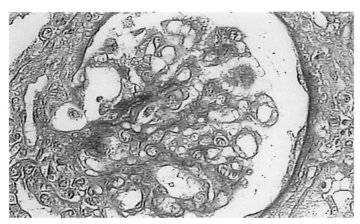

Figure 28.6 Glomerulus from a patient with shigatoxin-associated hemolytic uremic syndrome. A marked thickening of the glomerular capillary wall occurs with many double contours.

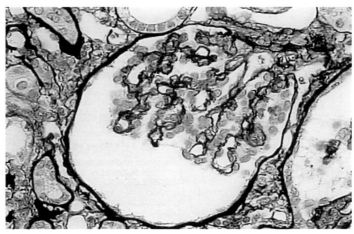

Figure 28.8 Glomerulus from a patient with atypical hemolytic uremic syndrome with predominant vascular involvement. Severe ischemic changes have occurred. Note the shrinkage of the glomerular tuft and marked thickening and wrinkling of the capillary wall.

and 28.6). Thrombi and infiltration by leukocytes are common in the early phases of the disease and usually resolve after 2 to 3 weeks. Patchy cortical necrosis may be present in severe cases; crescent formation is uncommon. In idiopathic and familial forms and in adults, the injury mostly involves arteries and arterioles (Fig. 28.7) with secondary glomerular ischemia and retraction of the

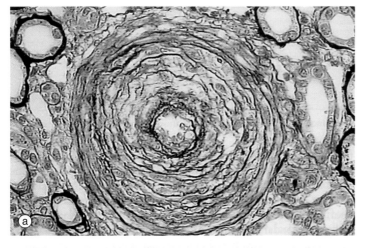

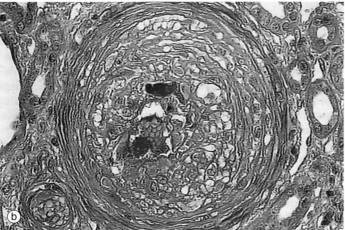

Figure 28.7 Interlobular artery in a case of hemolytic uremic syndrome with severe vascular involvement. *a*, The vascular lumen is almost completely occluded. Changes include myointimal proliferation and reduplication of the lamina elastica. *b*, Thrombotic material and erythrocytes can be seen in the lumen and within the vascular wall.

glomerular tuft (Fig. 28.8). The prognosis is good in the patients with predominant glomerular involvement, but it is more severe in those with predominant preglomerular injury. Focal segmental glomerulosclerosis may be a long-term sequela of acute cases of HUS and is usually seen in children with long-lasting hypertension and progressive chronic renal function deterioration.

The typical pathologic changes of TTP are the thrombi that occlude capillaries and arterioles in many organs and tissues. These thrombi consist of fibrin and platelets, and their distribution is widespread. They are most commonly detected in kidneys, pancreas, heart, adrenals, and brain. Compared to HUS, pathologic changes of TTP are more extensively distributed, probably reflecting the more systemic nature of the disease.

CLINICAL FEATURES, MECHANISMS, AND MANAGEMENT OF SPECIFIC FORMS OF THROMBOTIC MICROANGIOPATHY

Differentiation of the various forms of TMA is important to predict disease outcome and to establish the correct therapeutic approach based on different clinical presentations (Figs. 28.9 through 28.11).

Thrombotic Microangiopathy Associated with Infectious Diseases

Shigatoxin-Associated Hemolytic Uremic Syndrome

Stx-associated HUS is the most frequent form of TMA.[1] It is associated with infection by certain strains of *E. coli* (mostly O157:H7 serotype) or *Shigella dysenteriae* type 1 that produce a powerful exotoxin. The human disease is caused by two distinct *E. coli* exotoxins, Stx-1 and Stx-2, almost identical to the toxin produced by *S. dysenteriae* type 1.

It is also referred to as D+ HUS because ARF is preceded by diarrhea. The overall incidence rate is estimated to be 2.1 cases per 100,000 persons per year, with a peak incidence in children younger than 5 years old (6.1/100,000 per year), although no age group is exempt. *E. coli* O157:H7 infection is most frequent in the warm summer months. Illness follows Stx *E. coli* infection a few days later. HUS complicates enteric infection with *E. coli* O157:H7 infection in about 3% to 7% of sporadic cases and ≥20% of the epidemic form. HUS is usually diagnosed 6 days after the onset of diarrhea. Humans may be infected from contaminated milk and meat and fecally contaminated water or

HELLP Syndrome

In the HELLP syndrome there is evidence of microangiopathic hemolysis and liver injury in addition to hypertension and renal dysfunction. The syndrome is most common in white multiparous women with a history of poor pregnancy outcome. It usually occurs in the late third trimester, including the intrapartum period. Occasionally, after an uncomplicated pregnancy, symptoms may also arise within 24 to 48 hours postpartum. Diagnosis is based on laboratory findings of hemolysis (defined as fragmented erythrocytes in the circulation and serum LDH of 600 U/l), elevated liver enzymes (serum glutamic-oxaloacetic transaminase >70 U/l), and low platelets (platelet count <100 × 10³/mm³). Overt DIC is reported in 25% of cases. Intrahepatic hemorrhage, subcapsular liver hematoma, and liver rupture are rare but life-threatening complications. The maternal and perinatal mortality rates range from 0% to 24% and from 7.7% to 60%, respectively. Most of the perinatal deaths are related to abruptio placentae, intrauterine asphyxia, and extreme prematurity. As many as 44% of the infants are growth retarded. Delivery is the only definitive therapy. Hydralazine is the first-choice drug to control pregnancy-induced hypertension, and magnesium sulfate is used to prevent and treat convulsions. Both peritoneal dialysis and hemodialysis have been used to treat ARF. Platelet transfusions are needed for clinical bleeding.

In approximately 5% of patients with HELLP syndrome, symptoms and laboratory abnormalities do not improve after delivery. These more often include central nervous system abnormalities associated with renal and cardiopulmonary dysfunction and activation of coagulation. Uncontrolled studies suggest that plasma exchange may help recovery in patients with persistent evidence of disease ≥72 hours after delivery. Plasma therapy is ineffective during pregnancy and may increase fetal and maternal risk when used to delay delivery. Preliminary evidence suggests that, postpartum, corticosteroids may hasten disease recovery and, antepartum, postpone delivery and reduce the mother's need for blood products.

Postpartum Hemolytic Uremic Syndrome

Postpartum HUS manifests within 6 months from normal delivery. The clinical course is usually fulminant. Supportive care, including dialysis, transfusions, and careful fluid management, remains the most important form of treatment. Whether plasma therapy improves survival or limits renal sequelae has not been established. Antiplatelet agents, heparin, and antithrombotic therapy may enhance the risk of bleeding and have no proven efficacy. Full recovery of renal function is very uncommon. The mortality rate has ranged from 50% to 60% in the various reports. Patients who survive the acute phase of the disease have residual renal dysfunction and hypertension.

Systemic Disease–Associated Thrombotic Microangiopathy
Antiphospholipid Syndrome, Scleroderma, Malignant Hypertension

Plasma therapy should always be attempted in TMA associated with systemic diseases even though its efficacy is poorly defined.[33] In the antiphospholipid syndrome, oral anticoagulation remains the only treatment of proven efficacy to prevent and treat micro- and macrovascular thrombosis, even if concomitant thrombocytopenia may increase the risk of bleeding. Blood pressure control is fundamental in TMA associated with scleroderma crisis and malignant hypertension.

Human Immunodeficiency Virus–Associated Thrombotic Microangiopathy

HUS and TTP are both possible complications of acquired immune deficiency syndrome (AIDS) that may account for as much as 30% of hospitalized TMA patients in cities where AIDS is epidemic.[34] Plasma therapy is the only feasible approach in these forms, although the prognosis is poor. Uncontrolled series show that the survival rate of human immunodeficiency virus–infected patients with TTP and without AIDS is comparable to that of idiopathic TTP.

Malignancy-Associated Thrombotic Microangiopathy

TMA may spontaneously arise in patients with advanced cancer. It complicates almost 6% of cases of metastatic carcinoma with gastric cancer, which accounts for about 50% of all cases of malignancy-associated TMA. The prognosis is extremely poor, and most patients die within a few weeks. Therapy is minimally effective. Administration of blood products to correct symptomatic anemia often results in exacerbation of the syndrome, with rapid worsening of hemolysis, deterioration of renal function, and pulmonary edema.[1,2]

Drug-Associated Thrombotic Microangiopathy

Different drugs have been associated with TMA,[35] including mitomycin C, ticlopidine, clopidogrel, quinine, interferon, calcineurin inhibitors, and estrogen-containing oral contraceptives (Fig. 28.12). Discontinuing the offending drug is fundamental. The efficacy of plasma therapy is unclear; it seems ineffective

Drug-associated thrombotic microangiopathy
Drugs Used in Cancer Therapy
Mitomycin C*
Tamoxifen*
Bleomycin*
Cisplatin*
Gemcitabine
Deoxycorfomycin
Methyl-CCNU
Daunorubicin
Cytosine arabinoside
Neocarcinostatin
Other Drugs
Ticlopidine/clopidogrel*
Quinine*
Interferon-α*
Calcineurin inhibitors*
OKT3*
Oral contraceptives
Penicillin
Rifampin
Metronidazole

Figure 28.12 Drug-associated thrombotic microangiopathy (TMA). *Drugs most commonly involved in drug-associated TMA.

with some drugs such as mitomycin C and very important with others such as quinine.

Mitomycin and Anticancer Drugs

TMA, more commonly resembling HUS, is described in 2% to 10% of cancer patients treated with mitomycin C. Disease manifestation is dose related since renal dysfunction rarely occurs in patients given a cumulative dose lower than 30 mg/m^2. Patients who develop mitomycin C–associated TMA are usually in remission from their malignancy; thus, they significantly differ from the very ill patients who develop TMA as a complication of advanced tumor. The fatality rate is about 70% and median time to death is about 4 weeks. Patients surviving the acute phase often remain on chronic dialysis or die later of recurrence of the tumor or metastases. The possibility of preventing the disease by giving steroids during mitomycin treatment has been suggested and needs to be confirmed in prospective controlled trials. Plasma exchange is usually attempted, but its effectiveness is unproved. Platinum- and bleomycin-containing combinations have also been reported to induce HUS.

Antiplatelet Drugs

TMA has been reported in one case per 1600 to 5000 patients treated with ticlopidine. Neurologic abnormalities dominate the clinical picture and usually occur within a few weeks of treatment. The overall survival rate is 67% and is improved by early treatment withdrawal and plasma therapy. Generation of an autoantibody against ADAMTS13 may be involved in the pathogenesis of ticlopidine-associated TTP.[15] ADAMTS13 activity recovered after discontinuation of ticlopodine and plasma exchange. Eleven cases have been reported during treatment with clopidogrel.[16] The disease occurred within 2 weeks of therapy in 10 patients. All patients had neurologic involvement and were treated with plasma exchange: eight fully recovered, two had relapses but rapidly recovered after retreatment with plasma exchange, and one died. Half the patients were concomitantly treated with cholesterol-lowering drugs, and clinicians should be aware of this possible complication.

Quinine

Quinine is one of the most common drugs associated with TMA.[36] It is generally used to treat muscle cramps but is also contained in beverages or nutrition health products (e.g., tonic water, herbal preparations). TMA typically occurs in patients sensitized by prior exposure to quinine and rapidly follows re-exposure to the drug. Quinine-dependent antiplatelet, antierythrocyte, antigranulocyte, antilymphocyte, and antiendothelial antibodies may be involved in the pathogenesis of the disease. Predominant severe renal impairment is present, and hemodialysis is required in most cases. Despite a previous article that reported a good outcome,[37] recent work has showed a high rate of death and chronic renal failure (4 and 7 of 17 patients, respectively).[36] Cessation of quinine and institution of plasma therapy should be provided as early as possible. Avoidance of future quinine use is necessary to prevent recurrences.

Interferon-α

TMA associated with interferon-α is characterized by predominant renal impairment.[35] Recovery of the disease is common in cases of early discontinuation of the drug and prompt supportive therapy. However, kidney prognosis is usually poor, with ESRD reported in about 42% of cases. Because of the few cases reported, it is not possible to evaluate the effectiveness of specific therapies such as plasma exchange or infusion.

Organ Transplantation–Associated Thrombotic Microangiopathy

Post-transplantation HUS is reported with increasing frequency.[38] In renal transplants, HUS may develop for the first time in patients who have not previously had the disease (*de novo* post-transplantation HUS) or may affect patients whose primary cause of ESRD was HUS (recurrent post-transplantation HUS). Treatment of post-transplantation HUS rests on relief of symptoms, removal of the inciting factor(s), and plasma therapy. No other approach has proved effective.

De Novo Post-transplantation Hemolytic Uremic Syndrome

This form affects both renal and nonrenal transplant recipients and is usually triggered by immunosuppressive drugs such as calcineurin inhibitors and OKT3 or, less frequently, by viral infections (human immunodeficiency virus, parvovirus B19) and in renal transplant recipients by acute vascular rejection.[38] A particular form of *de novo* post-transplantation HUS may affect the recipients of a bone marrow transplant, usually in cases of graft-versus-host disease (GVHD) or of intensive GVHD prophylaxis, including total body irradiation. Drug withdrawal or dose reduction and plasma therapy achieved a high success rate (84%) in *de novo* cyclosporine- and tacrolimus-associated forms. A similar response rate, but in smaller studies, has been described with intravenous IgG infusion given with the rationale to neutralize hypothetical circulating cytotoxic or platelet agglutinating factors. Once remission is achieved, possible immunosuppression treatments may include a decreased dose of cyclosporine or tacrolimus, a change from cyclosporine to tacrolimus or vice versa, or the avoidance of calcineurin inhibitors by using mycophenolate mofetil or sirolimus. However, some cases of HUS have also been reported with sirolimus. Monoclonal anti–interleukin-2 receptor antagonists may also be a valid option to maintain adequate immunosuppression while avoiding the toxic effects of calcineurin inhibitors. The outcome of *de novo* forms occurring in the setting of viral infection is strongly influenced by the response to the treatment of the underlying disease. The outcome of *de novo* forms complicating bone marrow transplantation is very poor, with a mortality rate close to 90%.[38] In addition to the severity of HUS, infection, progressive GVHD, or relapse of the underlying disease may account for these discouraging results.

Recurrent Post-transplantation Hemolytic Uremic Syndrome

The reported recurrence rate of HUS after transplantation is 25% to 50% (see also Chapter 96). Patients with idiopathic and, above all, genetic forms of TMA are at high risk of post-transplantation recurrence; in contrast, Stx-associated HUS does not recur. Older age at onset of HUS, short duration between HUS onset and ESRD, and transplant from living donors confer an increased risk of post-transplantation recurrence.[38] Recurrent forms usually do not respond to any type of therapy and are associated with graft loss in most of cases. Preliminary data suggest that patients with allograft loss because of recurrent HUS may be successfully retransplanted without the use of calcineurin inhibitors.

REFERENCES

1. Ruggenenti P, Noris M, Remuzzi G: Thrombotic microangiopathy, hemolytic uremic syndrome, and thrombotic thrombocytopenic purpura. Kidney Int 2001;60:831–846.
2. Noris M, Remuzzi G: Hemolytic uremic syndrome. J Am Soc Nephrol 2005;16:1035–1050.
3. Rizzoni G, Claris-Appiani A, Edefonti A: Plasma infusion for hemolytic uremic syndrome in children: Results of a multicenter controlled trial. J Pediatr 1988;112:284–290.
4. Loirat C, Sonsino E, Hinglais N, et al: Treatment of the childhood haemolytic uraemic syndrome with plasma. A multicentre randomized controlled trial. The French Society of Paediatric Nephrology. Pediatr Nephrol 1988;2:279–285.
5. Dundas S, Murphy J, Soutar RL, et al: Effectiveness of therapeutic plasma exchange in the 1996 Lanarkshire *Escherichia coli* O157:H7 outbreak. Lancet 1999;354:1327–1330.
6. Carter AO, Borczyk AA, Carlson JA, et al: A severe outbreak of *Escherichia coli* O157:H7–associated hemorrhagic colitis in a nursing home. N Engl J Med 1987;317:1496–1500.
7. Remuzzi G, Galbusera M, Salvadori M, et al: Bilateral nephrectomy stopped disease progression in plasma-resistant hemolytic uremic syndrome with neurological signs and coma. Kidney Int 1996;49:282–286.
8. McGraw ME, Lendon M, Stevens RF, et al: Haemolytic uraemic syndrome and the Thomsen Friedenreich antigen. Pediatr Nephrol 1989;3:135–139.
9. Furlan M, Robles R, Lammle B: Partial purification and characterization of a protease from human plasma cleaving von Willebrand factor to fragments produced by in vivo proteolysis. Blood 1996;87:4223–4234.
10. Lammle B, Kremer Hovinga J, Studt JD: Thrombotic thrombocytopenic purpura. Hematol J 2004;5:S6–S11.
11. Remuzzi G, Galbusera M, Noris M: Von Willebrand factor cleaving protease (ADAMTS13) is deficient in recurrent and familial thrombotic thrombocytopenic purpura and hemolytic uremic syndrome. Blood 2002;100:778–785.
12. Moake JL: Thrombotic microangiopathies. N Engl J Med 2002;347:589–600.
13. Remuzzi G: Is ADAMTS-13 deficiency specific for thrombotic thrombocytopenic purpura? No. J Thromb Haemost 2003;1:632–634.
14. Moake JL: Thrombotic thrombocytopenic purpura and the hemolytic uremic syndrome. Arch Pathol Lab Med 2002;126:1430–1433.
15. Tsai HM, Rice L, Sarode R, et al: Antibody inhibitors to von Willebrand factor metalloproteinase and increased binding of von Willebrand factor to platelets in ticlopidine-associated thrombotic thrombocytopenic purpura. Ann Intern Med 2000;132:794–799.
16. Bennett CL, Connors JM, Carwile JM, et al: Thrombotic thrombocytopenic purpura associated with clopidogrel. N Engl J Med 2000;342:1773–1777.
17. Bell WR, Braine HG, Ness PM, Kickler TS: Improved survival in thrombotic thrombocytopenic purpura-hemolytic uremic syndrome. Clinical experience in 108 patients. N Engl J Med 1991;325:398–403.
18. Rock GA, Shumak KH, Buskard NA, et al: Comparison of plasma exchange with plasma infusion in the treatment of thrombotic thrombocytopenic purpura. Canadian Apheresis Study Group. N Engl J Med 1991;325:393–397.
19. Byrnes JJ, Moake JL, Klug P, Periman P: Effectiveness of the cryosupernatant fraction of plasma in the treatment of refractory thrombotic thrombocytopenic purpura. Am J Hematol 1990;34:169–174.
20. Gutterman L, Kloster B, Tsai H: Rituximab therapy for refractory thrombotic thrombocytopenic purpura. Blood Cells Mol Dis 2002;28:385–391.
21. Fakhouri F, Vernant JP, Veyradier A, et al: Efficiency of curative and prophylactic treatment with rituximab in ADAMTS13-deficient thrombotic thrombocytopenic purpura: A study of 11 cases. Blood 2005;106:1932–1937.
22. Joszi M, Manuelian T, Heinen S, et al: Attachment of the soluble complement regulator factor H to cell and tissue surfaces: Relevance for pathology. Histol Histopathol 2004;19:251–258.
23. Noris M, Ruggenenti P, Perna A, et al: Hypocomplementemia discloses genetic predisposition to hemolytic uremic syndrome and thrombotic thrombocytopenic purpura: Role of factor H abnormalities. Italian Registry of Familial and Recurrent Hemolytic Uremic Syndrome/Thrombotic Thrombocytopenic Purpura. J Am Soc Nephrol 1999;10:281–293.
24. Taylor CM: Complement factor H and the haemolytic uraemic syndrome. Lancet 2001;358:1200–1202.
25. Caprioli J, Bettinaglio P, Zipfel PF, et al: The molecular basis of familial hemolytic uremic syndrome: Mutation analysis of factor H gene reveals a hot spot in short consensus repeat 20. J Am Soc Nephrol 2001;12:297–307.
26. Stratton JD, Warwicker P: Successful treatment of factor H-related haemolytic uraemic syndrome. Nephrol Dial Transplant 2002;17:684–685.
27. Remuzzi G, Ruggenenti P, Codazzi D, et al: Combined kidney and liver transplantation for familial haemolytic uraemic syndrome. Lancet 2002;359:1671–1672.
28. Remuzzi G, Ruggenenti P, Colledan M, et al: Hemolytic uremic syndrome: A fatal outcome after kidney and liver transplantation performed to correct factor H gene mutation. Am J Transplant 2005;5:1146–1150.
29. Constantinescu AR, Bitzan M, Weiss LS, et al: Non-enteropathic hemolytic uremic syndrome: Causes and short-term course. Am J Kidney Dis 2004;43:976–982.
30. Noris M, Brioschi S, Caprioli J, et al: Familial haemolytic uraemic syndrome and an MCP mutation. Lancet 2004;362:1542–1547.
31. Dragon-Durey MA, Loirat C, Cloarec S, et al: Anti-factor H autoantibodies associated with atypical hemolytic uremic syndrome. J Am Soc Nephrol 2005;16:555–563.
32. Weiner CP: Thrombotic microangiopathy in pregnancy and the postpartum period. Semin Hematol 1987;24:119–129.
33. Ruggenenti P, Galli M, Remuzzi G: Hemolytic uremic syndrome, thrombotic thrombocytopenic purpura, and antiphospholipid antibody syndromes. In Neilson EG, Couser WG, eds. Immunologic Renal Diseases, 2nd ed. Philadelphia: Lippincott Williams and Wilkins, 2001, pp 1179–1208.
34. Thompson CE, Damon LE, Ries CA, et al: Thrombotic microangiopathies in the 1980s: Clinical features, response to treatment, and the impact of the human immunodeficiency virus epidemic. Blood 1992;80:1890–1895.
35. Pisoni R, Ruggenenti P, Remuzzi G: Drug-induced thrombotic microangiopathy: Incidence, prevention and management. Drug Saf 2001;24:491–501.
36. Kojouri K, Vesely SK, George JN: Quinine-associated thrombotic thrombocytopenic purpura-hemolytic uremic syndrome: Frequency, clinical features, and long-term outcomes. Ann Intern Med 2001;135:1047–1051.
37. Gottschall JL, Neahring B, McFarland JG, et al: Quinine-induced immune thrombocytopenia with hemolytic uremic syndrome: Clinical and serological findings in nine patients and review of literature. Am J Hematol 1994;47:283–289.
38. Ruggenenti P: Post-transplant hemolytic-uremic syndrome. Kidney Int 2002;62:1093–1104.

CHAPTER
29
Pathogenesis, Clinical Manifestations, and Natural History of Diabetic Nephropathy

Eberhard Ritz

DEFINITIONS

Diabetic nephropathy (DN) is the leading cause of end-stage renal disease (ESRD) in most Western societies. It can develop in the course of both type 1 and type 2 diabetes.

Type 1 diabetes is an autoimmune disease characterized by antibody- and cell-mediated destruction of pancreatic islets. Circulating C peptide is absent indicating failure of insulin production; all patients with type 1 diabetes eventually require treatment with insulin. Type 1 diabetes may occur at any age but is common in childhood, usually presenting prior to the age of 30 years.

Type 2 diabetes is characterized by a combination of insulin resistance and qualitative or quantitative insulin deficiency. It may represent a component of the metabolic syndrome, a potentially prediabetic state comprising insulin resistance, visceral obesity, hypertension, and dyslipidemia with high triglycerides and low amounts of high-density lipoprotein. For a long period, insulin resistance is compensated by increased insulin secretion. Recent data document a gradual decline in pancreatic β-cell function, culminating in hyperglycemia and ultimately insulin requirement in 40% to 50% of patients with type 2 diabetes. Type 2 diabetes is typically a disease of older adults, although it is increasingly seen in children.

Overt diabetic nephropathy is characterized by persistent albuminuria (>300 mg/24 h or >200 μg/min) on at least two occasions separated by 3 to 6 months. This is equivalent to total proteinuria >500 mg/24 h. Patients invariably develop hypertension, a progressive increase in proteinuria, and a predictable and relentless decrease in glomerular filtration rate (GFR). A major clinical problem is the association of DN as a microvascular complication of diabetes with other *microvascular* (e.g., retinopathy, neuropathy) and *macrovascular* complications (mainly coronary heart disease and peripheral artery disease).

PATHOGENESIS OF DIABETIC NEPHROPATHY

Hemodynamic Changes

Hyperfiltration is common in early diabetes, and this can be corrected with good glycemic control. The mechanism for the increased GFR may involve glucose-dependent effects on afferent arteriolar dilation, mediated by a range of vasoactive mediators including insulin-like growth factor I (IGF-I), nitric oxide, prostaglandins, and/or glucagon. Hyperfiltration may predict the development of DN[1] especially in type 1 diabetes. However, this was not found in all studies.

In experimental models, hyperfiltration was the result of afferent arteriolar dilatation with concomitant efferent vasoconstriction causing an increase in glomerular hydrostatic pressure. Measures that reduce the glomerular pressure, such as reduction of the systemic blood pressure, low protein diet (which blocks the afferent arteriolar dilation), or angiotensin-converting enzyme (ACE) inhibitors (which block angiotensin II [Ang II]–mediated constriction of the efferent arteriole; Fig. 29.1) as well as blockade of vascular endothelial growth factor[2] reduce the development of glomerular damage and proteinuria.

Renal Hypertrophy

The early hyperfiltration is associated with glomerulomegaly and renal organomegaly. The size of the kidney may increase by several centimeters. Glomerular enlargement is associated with an increase in the number of capillary loops and in the filtration surface area. Most of the changes in the glomeruli are due to hypertrophy, whereas the tubular epithelial cells undergo both proliferation and an increase in cellular size.

Experimentally, such renal hypertrophy can be largely prevented by intensified insulin therapy and resultant normoglycemia. The mechanism by which elevated plasma glucose levels cause hypertrophy appears to be stimulation of several growth factors within the kidney, including IGF-I, epidermal growth factor, platelet-derived growth factor, vascular endothelial growth factor (VEGF), and transforming growth factor β (TGF-β). Proliferation and hypertrophy may also be initiated by decreased antiproliferative factors, such as "secreted protein, acidic and rich in cysteine" (SPARC).

The role of TGF-β in diabetic renal hypertrophy has been most studied. It is overexpressed in glomeruli and the tubulointerstitium of both experimental and human DN. Both glucose and glucose derived advanced glycation end products (AGEs) stimulate the production of TGF-β in a variety of cell types. Hyperglycemia also induces the expression of thrombospondin, a potent activator of latent TGF-β. In turn, TGF-β stimulates protein synthesis (hypertrophy) in numerous cell types, but prevents cell proliferation and division. Treatment of diabetic mice with neutralizing anti–TGF-β antibodies attenuated diabetes-related renal hypertrophy, extracellular matrix accumulation, and preserved renal function.

Mesangial Expansion and Nodule Formation

The hallmark of DN is mesangial expansion, eventually culminating in the development of nodular diabetic glomerulosclerosis (the Kimmelstiel-Wilson nodule) or diffuse glomerulosclerosis (see later discussion). Mesangial expansion correlates better than glomerular basement membrane (GBM) thickness with the

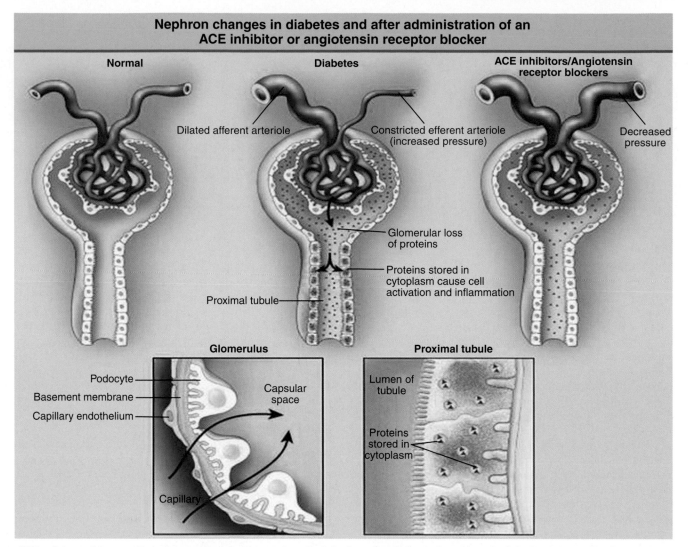

Nephron changes in diabetes and after administration of an ACE inhibitor or angiotensin receptor blocker

Normal

Diabetes

ACE inhibitors/Angiotensin receptor blockers

Dilated afferent arteriole

Constricted efferent arteriole (increased pressure)

Decreased pressure

Glomerular loss of proteins

Proteins stored in cytoplasm cause cell activation and inflammation

Proximal tubule

Glomerulus

Podocyte

Basement membrane

Capillary endothelium

Capsular space

Capillary

Proximal tubule

Lumen of tubule

Proteins stored in cytoplasm

Figure 29.1 **Schematic comparison of a normal nephron, a nephron in diabetic nephropathy, and a nephron in diabetic nephropathy after administration of angiotensin-converting enzyme (ACE) inhibitor/angiotensin receptor blocker (ARB).** Note afferent vasodilation and efferent angiotensin II–mediated vasoconstriction in diabetes causing glomerular hypertension, which is relieved by ACE inhibitor/ARB treatment. Note also protein leakage into the filtrate and tubular loading with endocytosed protein causing an inflammatory reaction promoting interstitial fibrosis. This is reversed by ACE inhibitor/ARB treatment.

subsequent development of renal failure. The early mesangial lesion is characterized by variable increases in mesangial cell number with an increased deposition of several extracellular matrix components, including type IV and V collagen, laminin, and fibronectin. Later, there is a general loss of mesangial cellularity, and the homogeneous acellular nodules consist primarily of type VI collagen.

The mesangial expansion is mediated by direct effects of both glucose and glucose-induced AGEs. In experimental models, mesangial changes can largely be prevented by tight glycemic control or the use of AGE inhibitors such as aminoguanidine. The effects may be mediated by TGF-β, given its known propensity to stimulate mesangial matrix synthesis and decrease its degradation via reduced activity of matrix metalloproteinases. There is also evidence that glycation makes matrix components more resistant to degradation. Angiotensin II directly stimulates TGF-β production by mesangial and tubular epithelial cells; ACE inhibitors reduce renal expression of TGF-β and its receptors in diabetic rodents.

Development of Proteinuria

Widening of the GBM is associated with an accumulation of type IV collagen and a net reduction in negatively charged

heparin sulfate proteoglycans. This combination disrupts both GBM structure and its electrostatic charge properties and is thought to contribute to abnormal permselectivity and leakage of proteins. Depletion of negative charges would permit the polyanionic albumin molecules to escape into the glomerular filtrate (selective albuminuria). In more advanced stages, the texture of the basal membrane is deranged, thus creating gaps and holes that were thought to allow high molecular weight serum proteins to escape into the filtrate as well (nonselective proteinuria). However, recent insights into podocyte function and their slit membrane as well as interaction of podocytes with intraglomerular cells[3] have led to the concept that the podocyte is a prime player in the genesis of proteinuria. For instance, the expression of one permeability controlling protein, nephrin, is abnormally low[4] and is restored by administration of angiotensin receptor blockers (ARBs). In addition, both experimental and biopsy controlled human studies showed that DN is associated with progressive loss of podocytes.

Tubulointerstitial Fibrosis

The two most important structural changes that correlate with progression in DN are the degree of mesangial expansion and the severity of the tubulointerstitial disease. Tubulointerstitial changes come early[5] and correlate not only with current renal function, but also with prognosis.[6] The potential mechanisms for the development of tubulointerstitial fibrosis are similar to those postulated for tubulointerstitial fibrosis and in other progressive renal diseases (see Chapter 68) and include release of growth factors, in particular TGF-β, and cytokines from the glomerulus and direct or indirect effects of proteinuria. Overload of proximal tubular epithelial cells with proteins, particularly modified proteins, changes cell phenotype, activates the proinflammatory switch nuclear factor κB, and induces the secretion of various cytokines and chemokines.[7] An important mechanism may also be renal ischemia and hypoxia[8] induced by the progressive hyalinosis of the afferent and efferent arterioles and possibly loss of peritubular capillaries.

Hyperglycemia and Diabetic Nephropathy
Role of Glucose Control
Poor glycemic control and duration of disease are the two major risk factors for the development of DN. Evidence of the role of tight glycemic control in retarding the development of DN includes

- Studies suggesting that with good glycemic control (reflected by an average HbA1$_c$ of 7.0%), only 9% of type 1 diabetic subjects will develop ESRD after 25 years as opposed to the historical prevalence of 40%.[9]
- Results from the Diabetes Control and Complications Trial that showed a remarkable reduction in progression from normoalbuminuria to microalbuminuria and other microvascular complications, specifically retinopathy, in patients with type 1 diabetes with tight glycemic control.[10] At least for cardiovascular sequelae, the benefit of early aggressive reduction of glycemia persisted despite later deterioration of the glycemic control.[11]
- Studies in which euglycemia following isolated transplantation of the pancreas was associated with a regression of the diabetic glomerulosclerosis after 10 years.[12]
- Evidence from the United Kingdom Diabetes Prospective Study that reducing HbA1c by ~0.9% in subjects with type 2 diabetes reduces the risk of development of microvascular complications including nephropathy.[13]

The mechanisms by which hyperglycemia induces DN are complex and may involve not only effects of elevated glucose levels *per se*, but also the generation of glycated proteins and alcohol sugars (polyols) as a consequence of hyperglycemia.

Direct Effects of Glucose: Role of Protein Kinase C
In cell culture studies, glucose induces cell hypertrophy, extracellular matrix synthesis, and TGF-β production in a variety of cell types. Many of the adverse effects of hyperglycemia have been attributed to activation of protein kinase C (PKC), a family of serine-threonine kinases that regulate diverse vascular functions, including contractility, blood flow, cellular proliferation, and vascular permeability. Activity of PKC, especially the membrane-bound form, is increased in the retina, aorta, heart, and glomeruli of diabetic animals, probably because of the *de novo* synthesis of diacylglycerol, a major endogenous activator of PKC. In short- and long-term studies in diabetic rats, an orally effective PKC-β-selective inhibitor ameliorated glomerular hyperfiltration, albuminuria, and renal TGF-β overexpression and extracellular matrix accumulation.[14] PKC-α may represent an additional therapeutic target, since albuminuria was virtually absent in diabetic PKC-α knockout mice.[15]

Effects of Advanced Glycation End Products
Chronic hyperglycemia can lead to the nonenzymatic glycation of amino acids and proteins (Maillard or browning reaction). Glucose binds nonenzymatically to amino residues forming glycated Schiff bases, with later rearrangement to form a more stable but still reversible Amadori product. Over time, these products undergo rearrangement including crosslinking to become irreversible AGEs (Fig. 29.2). Both circulating and tissue proteins as well as lipids and nucleic acids may thus be glycated. A classic example is hemoglobin (Hb) that initially forms the Amadori product HbA1$_c$, but ultimately AGE-Hb is generated. Although primarily observed in diabetes, AGEs also accumulate in aging and in renal failure.

The concentration of AGEs is increased in the sera of diabetic patients with nephropathy. AGEs have also been localized to diabetic glomeruli by immunohistochemistry. AGEs bind to a variety of cell types, including the macrophage and mesangial cell. They mediate a variety of cellular actions, including expression of adhesion molecules, cell hypertrophy, extracellular matrix synthesis, epithelial to mesenchymal transdifferentiation of tubular cells, and the inhibition of nitric oxide synthesis. AGEs injected *in vivo* induce albuminuria and glomerulosclerosis.[16] Among several binding sites, the most important is the putative receptor RAGE (receptor for AGE),[17] a pattern recognition receptor. It is present in tubular cells and to a lesser extent in glomeruli. One of the actions of RAGE is activation of nuclear factor κB, but it may also be involved in the clearance of AGEs. sRAGE, the soluble extracellular domain of RAGE, acts as a decoy receptor and ameliorates experimentally the renal lesions in diabetes.

Administration of aminoguanidine, an inhibitor of AGE formation, to animals with diabetes reduces AGE deposition, mesangial matrix expansion, and albuminuria, but has inconsistent effects on

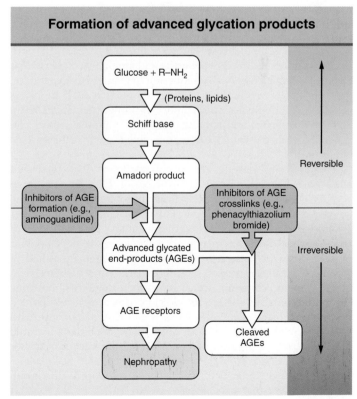

Formation of advanced glycation products

Glucose + R–NH$_2$

(Proteins, lipids)

Schiff base

Amadori product

Inhibitors of AGE formation (e.g., aminoguanidine)

Inhibitors of AGE crosslinks (e.g., phenacylthiazolium bromide)

Advanced glycated end-products (AGEs)

AGE receptors

Cleaved AGEs

Nephropathy

Reversible

Irreversible

Figure 29.2 Mechanism of formation of advanced glycation end products.

GBM thickening. Preliminary clinical studies suggest beneficial effects on retinopathy, lipids, and proteinuria. The clinical experience with this compound has been disappointing and riddled with side effects. Newer, more specific agents have been developed that may be more potent at blocking AGE formation. Furthermore, phenacylthiazolium bromide is a novel compound that cleaves covalent, AGE-derived protein crosslinks and provides a conceptual basis for the reversal of AGE-mediated tissue damage, which until now has been regarded as irreversible.

Effect of Sorbitol (the Polyol Pathway)

Hyperglycemia-induced generation of polyols has also been suggested to mediate some of the complications of diabetes. In tissues where glucose uptake is independent of insulin, such as in the lens, retina, and kidney, chronic hyperglycemia results in increased tissue levels of glucose. The excess glucose is subsequently reduced to sorbitol by aldose reductase. Accumulation of sorbitol is accompanied by an increase in intracellular osmolality, a depletion of free myoinositol, loss of Na^+,K^+ adenosine triphosphatase activity, and increased consumption of the enzyme cofactors NADPH (reduced nicotinamide adenine dinucleotide phosphate) and NAD^+ (oxidized nicotinamide adenine dinucleotide), leading to changes in cellular redox potential. The role of polyols in diabetic complications has been assessed using aldose reductase inhibitors, such as sorbinil, tolrestat, and ponalrestat. They have shown promise in preventing diabetic cataracts and improving or stabilizing diabetic neuropathy. Aldose reductase inhibitors also blunt hyperfiltration and have a mild effect on reducing albuminuria in both experimental and human diabetes. However, overall, the experience of treatment with aldose reductase inhibitors on DN has been somewhat disappointing and treatment was associated with hypersensitivity reactions and liver function abnormalities. Therefore, it is unlikely that these agents will have a major role in the management of DN.

Renin Angiotensin System and Diabetic Nephropathy

In rats with streptozotocin-induced diabetes, treatment with ACE inhibitors reduced proteinuria and ameliorated glomerular changes in association with a reduction in glomerular hydrostatic pressure.[18] More recently, it has been shown that ACE inhibitors also reduce tubulointerstitial injury in experimental diabetes. Studies in humans also suggest that ACE inhibitors retard DN progression in patients with type 1 and type 2 diabetes (see Chapter 30).

Paradoxically, despite the strong evidence that the renin angiotensin system (RAS) is involved in DN, plasma renin activity is low, although it may be inappropriately high for the increased extracellular volume and exchangeable sodium that accompany DN. This has raised the possibility that activation of the intrarenal RAS may play a critical role in the development of DN. Sites of local RAS activation have been identified in glomeruli and renal vessels during experimental diabetes.[19] In rats transgenic for renin, renal injury is accelerated following the induction of diabetes. In addition, prorenin levels (which may reflect increased synthesis) are elevated in patients with DN. Specific prorenin/renin receptors have been demonstrated in the kidney[20]; binding of prorenin to the receptor causes nonenzymatic activation of prorenin to yield renin activity and locally produce Ang II.[21] It has been proposed that renin inhibitors interfere specifically with such local Ang II generation, a hypothesis susceptible to testing with the renin inhibitor aliskiren. Further complexity is introduced by the observation that in diabetes, chymase is strikingly expressed in the kidney, an enzyme that generates Ang II but is not inhibited by ACE inhibitors.[22]

In addition to Ang II's hemodynamic effects to increase systemic and glomerular pressures, to mediate proteinuria, and to induce renal vasoconstriction, it also has nonhemodynamic effects and mediates cell proliferation, hypertrophy, matrix expansion, and cytokine (TGF-β) synthesis. Therefore, ACE inhibitors and ARBs could act by hemodynamic as well as by nonhemodynamic actions.

Much recent interest has focused on aldosterone. Aldosterone accelerates progression in renal damage models independently of Ang II.[23] In DN, aldosterone escape has been linked to progression of proteinuria and blockade of the mineralocorticoid receptor by spironolactone lowered proteinuria, a surrogate marker for progression (see Chapter 30).

Other vasoactive agents may also be involved in the pathogenesis of DN, including alterations in systemic or intrarenal production of endothelin, nitric oxide, the kallikrein-kinin system, and natriuretic peptides.

Genesis of Hypertension in Diabetic Nephropathy

Danish diabetologists were the first to show that lowering of blood pressure attenuates the rate of progression.[24,25] Understanding the pathogenesis of hypertension in DN is important for rational selection of antihypertensive agents:

- The important role of *sodium retention and hypervolemia* explains why dietary sodium restriction and diuretics are so effective in DN.
- The activation of the *intrarenal RAS(s)* despite suppressed systemic RAS explains the unique efficacy of ACE inhibitors and ARBs in DN.[26–28]
- The activation of the *sympathetic nerve system* and its role in the genesis of renal hypertension presumably explains why β-blockers are so effective in lowering blood pressure and retarding progression in diabetic patients with renal disease.[24,25]

EPIDEMIOLOGY

In most Western countries, DN has become the leading cause of ESRD. According to the U.S. Renal Data System (www.USRDS.org), in 2003, in 43% of incident patients or 334 ppm (per million population per year) DN was the primary diagnosis, an increase by 238% compared to 1990. The proportion of diabetics among patients with ESRD varies considerably between countries, but is consistently on the rise in all countries. Prevention and management of diabetes and its renal complications are thus an immense global challenge.[29] In patients admitted for renal replacement therapy, we found diabetes in 49%, but classic features of DN were observed in only 60% of these (i.e., large kidneys, proteinuria exceeding 1 g/24 h with or without retinopathy); 13% exhibited an atypical presentation with ischemic nephropathy and in 27% of the cases a known primary renal disease (e.g., polycystic kidney disease, analgesic nephropathy, glomerulonephritis) coexisted with diabetes. Often the diagnosis of diabetes had not been made at the time of admission because hyperglycemia often disappears when patients lose weight secondary to anorexia from renal failure (so-called diabetic nephropathy without diabetes). This may explain why at least 5% of patients develop apparent *de novo* diabetes after the start of dialysis.

The great majority, in our experience >90%, of patients entering ESRD with diabetes as a comorbid condition suffer

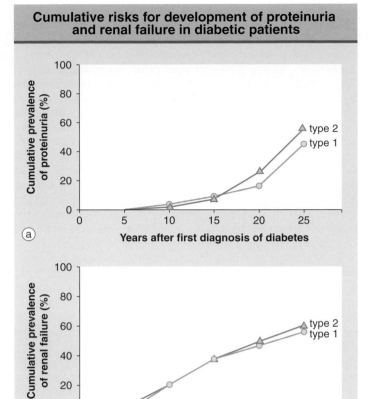

Cumulative risks for development of proteinuria and renal failure in diabetic patients

Figure 29.3 Cumulative risks for development of proteinuria and progression to renal failure in patients with type 1 and type 2 diabetes.[30]

from type 2 diabetes. In the past, few patients with type 2 diabetes had a chance to live long enough to develop nephropathy. Today, with better treatment of hypertension and of coronary heart disease, an increasing proportion of patients with type 2 diabetes survive and are exposed to the risk of developing DN and ESRD. The proportion of patients with type 1 and type 2 diabetes who develop proteinuria and elevated serum creatinine is related to the duration of diabetes. As shown in Figure 29.3, the cumulative risks of developing proteinuria and progressing are practically superimposable in type 1 and type 2.[30]

Risk Factors for the Development of Diabetic Nephropathy

On the one hand, only between 30% and 40% of patients with type 1 diabetes and 10% to 20% of those with type 2 diabetes develop nephropathy. On the other hand, nephropathy may develop in some patients despite good glycemic control, but it may fail to develop in others despite years of severe hyperglycemia. These findings suggest that factors other than glycemia, specifically hereditary and environmental factors, also contribute to the development of DN.

The prevalence of nephropathy among diabetic patients varies between different racial and ethnic groups such that it is relatively increased in African Americans, Native Americans, Mexican Americans, Polynesians, Australian Aborigines, and urbanized Indo-Asian immigrants in the United Kingdom when compared to Caucasians. Although barriers to care seem likely to account for some of these interpopulation differences, genetic factors are also likely to contribute.

Familial clustering of DN has been reported in both type 1 and type 2 diabetes and in both Caucasian and non-Caucasian populations. In a type 1 diabetic patient who has a first-degree relative with diabetes and nephropathy, the risk of developing DN is 83%. The frequency is only 17% if he or she has a first-degree relative with diabetes but without nephropathy.[31] In type 2 diabetes, familial clustering has been well documented in Pima Indians,[32] and a familial determinant is also suggested by the observation that albumin excretion rates are higher in offspring of patients with type 2 diabetes with nephropathy. The risk is particularly high in the offspring if the mother had been hyperglycemic during pregnancy, presumably because this causes reduced formation of nephrons (nephron underdosing) in the offspring[33] as shown in experimental studies.[34] Low birth weight and nephron underdosing are also associated with hypertension, metabolic syndrome, and, although the data are somewhat controversial on this point, DN. The hypothesis has been proposed that nephron underdosing[35] leads to compensatory glomerular hypertrophy and increased single-nephron GFR, thus aggravating glomerular injury if a renal insult such as diabetes occurs.

Gene polymorphisms may also contribute to familial clustering. A recent study suggested a genetic predisposition to DN due to a polymorphism in the carnosinase gene causing cumulation of carnosine with antioxidant properties.[36] Several studies also suggested some detrimental effect of the double deletion (DD) polymorphism of the ACE genotype on disease progression,[37] although the finding has not been uniformly confirmed.[38]

In addition to genetic factors, shared environmental influences also contribute to the familial and racial clustering of diabetic renal disease. For instance, tobacco smoking promotes both the onset and progression of DN in addition to accelerating cardiovascular disease.[39]

In diabetic patients, the risk of ESRD increases progressively with increasingly higher baseline blood pressure values, even when they are still within the normal range.[40] Further risk factors are albumin excretion rates in the upper normal range,[41] marked insulin resistance, male gender, and onset of type 1 diabetes before the age of 20.

CLINICAL MANIFESTATIONS AND NATURAL HISTORY

DN constitutes a part of a generalized microvascular syndrome, which is further modulated by macrovascular disease (Fig. 29.4).

Evolution of Diabetic Nephropathy

One of the earliest changes of renal function in diabetes is an increase in GFR, or hyperfiltration (Fig. 29.5), which is observed in many patients with type 1 diabetes and in a lower percentage of those with type 2 diabetes. It is paralleled by an increase in renal size. The next observable change is the development of microalbuminuria. Persistent microalbuminuria, as noted by repeated testing, is associated with changes in both glomerular structure (mesangial expansion and basement membrane thickening) and permeability and thus is sometimes referred to as incipient nephropathy. These changes occur in 30% to 50% of patients with type 1 diabetes within 5 to 10 years after onset of diabetes and may be present in 20% to 30% of those with type 2 diabetes at initial diagnosis, presumably because of a considerable duration of undiagnosed diabetes. Diabetic patients with persistent microalbuminuria are at markedly increased risk of developing overt DN, which is heralded by the development of proteinuria

Major microvascular and macrovascular complications in patients with diabetic nephropathy
Microvascular Complications
Retinopathy
Polyneuropathy including autonomic neuropathy (gastroparesis, diarrhea/obstipation, detrusor paresis, painless myocardial ischemia, erectile impotence, supine hypertension/orthostatic hypotension)
Macrovascular Complications
Coronary heart disease, left ventricular hypertrophy, congestive heart failure
Cerebrovascular disease
Peripheral artery occlusive disease
Combined Microvascular and Macrovascular Complications
Diabetic foot (neuropathic, vascular)

Figure 29.4 Major microvascular and macrovascular complications in patients with diabetic nephropathy.

around 15 years after disease onset. This progresses to proteinuria in the nephrotic range, hypertension, and progressive renal insufficiency.[42]

Mogensen[43] proposed a scheme of the different stages of DN (see Fig. 29.5) that is valid in type 1 diabetes, but less reliable in type 2 diabetes. An early stage of renal hyperfunction is followed by a stage of clinical latency that may last up to 20 years. It is subsequently followed in a very well defined time frame by the stages of microalbuminuria progressing to that of overt nephropathy and renal failure.

Hypertension and Diabetic Nephropathy

The typical frequencies of associated hypertension and microvascular complications in those with type 1 diabetes are given in Figure 29.6. If hypertension develops in a patient with type 1 diabetes, it is almost always of renal parenchymal origin. In contrast, in patients with type 2 diabetes, hypertension often precedes the onset of diabetes, let alone DN, by years and decades, since it often is the consequence of the metabolic syndrome rather than DN (Fig. 29.7). In these patients, hypertension does not indicate the presence of DN. As shown in Figure 29.8, at the time when type 2 diabetes is diagnosed, an abnormal blood pressure and/or an abnormal circadian blood pressure profile are found in 79% of patients.[44] If patients with type 2 diabetes ultimately develop nephropathy, the prevalence of hypertension increases further and the degree of blood pressure elevation is greater, but generally the relationship between hypertension and nephropathy is much less close than in type 1 diabetes.[45]

In DN, it has been well documented that the nocturnal blood pressure decrease is frequently attenuated (nondipping). Recently, it has also been found that in patients with type 1 diabetes, nondipping even precedes the onset of microalbuminuria.[46] Furthermore, the blood pressure response to exercise tends to be exaggerated, even when the blood pressure is normal under basal conditions.

The prediabetic blood pressure is related to onset and progression of DN. Nelson and associates[47] showed that hypertension prior to the onset of type 2 diabetes predicts the development of proteinuria 5 years after type 2 diabetes has been diagnosed. Diminished compliance of the central arteries in diabetes has been known for decades. The stiffening of the aorta increases the peak systolic pressure and decreases the diastolic pressure, resulting in an increased blood pressure amplitude. The great blood pressure amplitude explains why isolated systolic hypertension is so common in patients with type 2 diabetes.

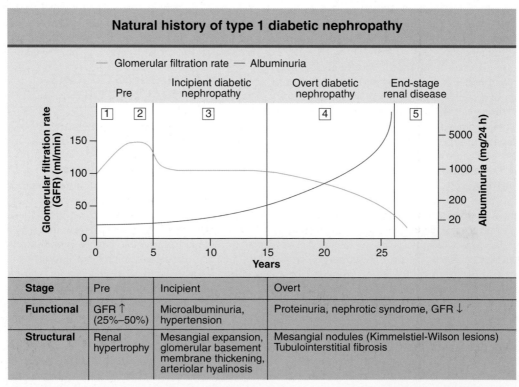

Stage	Pre	Incipient	Overt
Functional	GFR ↑ (25%–50%)	Microalbuminuria, hypertension	Proteinuria, nephrotic syndrome, GFR ↓
Structural	Renal hypertrophy	Mesangial expansion, glomerular basement membrane thickening, arteriolar hyalinosis	Mesangial nodules (Kimmelstiel-Wilson lesions) Tubulointerstitial fibrosis

Figure 29.5 Natural history of type 1 diabetic nephropathy. Functional and structural manifestations of diabetic nephropathy. Numbers 1 through 5 indicate the stages of nephropathy defined by Mogensen.[43]

Albuminuria in type I diabetics and the development of hypertension, retinopathy, and neuropathy				
Urine Albumin Excretion Status	Prevalence of Hypertension (> 140/90 mm Hg) (%)	Prevalence of Proliferative Retinopathy (%)*	Prevalence of Diabetes-Related Blindness (%)	Prevalence of Neuropathy (%)
Normoalbuminuria	20	12	1	21
Microalbuminuria	40	28	6	31
Macroalbuminuria	80	58	11	50

Figure 29.6   Albuminuria in type I diabetics and the development of hypertension, retinopathy, and neuropathy. *Background retinopathy is found in >90% of patients with nephropathy.

Hypertension in diabetes mellitus	
Type I diabetes	Renoparenchymal hypertension
Type 2 diabetes	Primary hypertension (metabolic syndrome) + superimposed renoparenchymal hypertension + high blood pressure amplitude (systolic hypertension)

Figure 29.7   Hypertension in diabetes mellitus.

Blood pressure at the time of diagnosis of type 2 diabetes[55]	
Ambulatory 24-hour blood pressure >130/80 mm Hg	60%
<15% dipping of blood pressure at nighttime	61%
Abnormal according to first or second criterion	79%
Only 21% of patients have normal blood pressure profile	

Figure 29.8   Blood pressure at the time of diagnosis of type 2 diabetes. (From the sixth report of the Joint National Committee on prevention, detection, evaluation, and treatment of high blood pressure. Arch Intern Med 1997;157: 2413–2446.)

Extrarenal Complications Associated with Diabetic Nephropathy

Renal complications develop on average 15 to 20 years after the onset of diabetes at a time when the patient is also at high risk of developing microvascular and macrovascular complications (see Fig. 29.4).

Diabetic retinopathy is present in virtually all patients with type 1 diabetes with nephropathy.[25] In contrast, only 50% to 60% of proteinuric patients with type 2 diabetes suffer from retinopathy.[48] Consequently, the absence of retinopathy does not exclude the diagnosis of DN in patients with type 2 diabetes. The risk of blindness because of severe proliferative retinopathy is substantially higher in diabetic patients with nephropathy. Retinopathy tends also to progress more rapidly, so that frequent ophthalmologic examination, that is, at yearly or half-yearly intervals, is clearly indicated in patients with DN.

Many patients with DN also have polyneuropathy. Sensory polyneuropathy is an important aspect of the diabetic foot. Motor and sensory neuropathy may cause areflexia, wasting, and sensory disturbances such as paresthesia, anesthesia, and impaired perception of vibration and pain, but the most vexing clinical problems are the result of autonomic polyneuropathy. Because cardiac innervation is defective, pain and angina are frequently absent when the patient has ischemic heart disease and myocardial infarction. Further consequences of autonomic polyneuropathy are gastroparesis, that is, delayed emptying of gastric contents into the gut, and diarrhea or constipation (often alternating with each other). These problems are caused by impaired intestinal innervation, often complicated by intestinal bacterial overgrowth because of stasis. Finally, urogenital abnormalities are frequent such as erectile impotence or detrusor paresis with delayed and incomplete emptying of the bladder.

The major macrovascular complications are stroke, coronary heart disease, and peripheral vascular disease. These complications are again up to fivefold more frequent in diabetic patients with than without DN.

Survival in Patients with Diabetic Nephropathy

The onset of DN is a turning point in the life of a diabetic patient. The presence of DN greatly increases mortality in both type 1 and type 2 diabetes. Compared to the background population, patients with type 1 diabetes without proteinuria have only a slightly, namely, two- to threefold elevated mortality; in contrast, mortality is increased by a factor of 20 to 200 in patients with proteinuria.[49] In patients with type 2 diabetes, mortality is equally amplified by the presence of albuminuria/proteinuria[50] (Fig. 29.9).

The major increase in risk starts when microalbuminuria has developed, but a higher risk (Fig. 29.10) is found even in the upper normal range of albuminuria.[41] It is not certain why microalbuminuria is linked with cardiovascular death, but it is widely thought that the presence of microalbuminuria reflects generalized endothelial cell dysfunction, thus increasing the risk of atherosclerosis. Its presence is also associated with many

United Kingdom Prospective Diabetes Study	
Progression of Diabetic Nephropathy	
Normoalbuminuria to microalbuminuria	2% per year
Microalbuminuria to macroalbuminuria	2.8% per year
Macroalbuminuria to elevated serum creatinine*	2.3% per year
Annual Death Rate	
Normoalbuminuria	0.7%
Microalbuminuria	2.0%
Macroalbuminuria	3.5%
Elevated serum creatinine*	12.1%
Macroalbuminuria: more likely to die of cardiovascular causes than to develop end-stage renal disease	

Figure 29.9   United Kingdom Prospective Diabetes Study. *>2 mg/dl (176 μmol/l). (Modified from Adler AI, Stevens RJ, Manley SE, et al: Development and progression of nephropathy in type 2 diabetes: The United Kingdom Prospective Diabetes Study (UKPDS 64). Kidney Int 2003;63: 225–232.)

Normoalbuminuric patients with type 2 diabetes: rising albumin excretion increases renal and cardiovascular risk events		
	Relative Risk of Progression to	
Albuminuria (mg/24 h)	Microalbuminuria	Cardiovascular Event
0–10	1	1
10–20	2.34	1.9
20–30	12.4	9.8

Figure 29.10 Normoalbuminuric patients with type 2 diabetes: rising albumin excretion increases renal and cardiovascular risk events. (Modified from Adler AI, Stevens RJ, Manley SE, et al: Development and progression of nephropathy in type 2 diabetes: The United Kingdom Prospective Diabetes Study (UKPDS 64). Kidney Int 2003;63:225–232.)

cardiovascular risk factors, such as elevated blood pressure, dyslipoproteinemia, increased platelet aggregation, increased C-reactive protein concentration, and others. An added risk factor is presumably the association of microalbuminuria with autonomic polyneuropathy,[51] which predicts death from myocardial infarction or arrhythmia (sudden death). Further cardiac abnormalities associated with microalbuminuria are cardiac hypertrophy and impaired left ventricular diastolic function.

The prognosis is particularly grim in diabetic patients with overt proteinuria, that is, with clinically manifest DN[49] in whom the risk of cardiovascular death is higher by a factor of 12 (see Fig. 29.9).

RENAL PATHOLOGY

Following the onset of diabetes, kidney weight increases by an average of 15%. Renal size remains increased until overt nephropathy is established. In most patients with type 1 diabetes, there is a sustained increase in glomerular volume and glomerular capillary luminal volume. Although atrophic ischemic glomeruli are present, some of the nonfunctioning glomeruli fill up with material staining with periodic acid–Schiff (PAS), thus preserving their increased dimensions. These changes are accompanied by hypertrophy of the interstitium.

In patients with a duration of diabetes >10 years, irrespective of whether nephropathy is present, GBM thickening up to three times the normal range of 270 to 359 nm is an almost universal feature (Fig. 29.11). In advancing DN, there is a consistent correlation between GBM thickness and fractional mesangial volumes with the urinary albumin excretion rate.

Nodular glomerular intercapillary lesions in advanced DN were described in 1936 by Kimmelstiel and Wilson (Fig. 29.12). The nodules are located in the central regions of peripheral glomerular lobules as well-demarcated eosinophilic and PAS positive masses (see Fig. 29.12c and d). When not acellular, they contain pyknotic nuclei. It is suggested that they result from microaneurysmal dilatation of the associated capillary followed by mesangiolysis and laminar organization of the mesangial debris with lysis of the center of the lobule. Foam cells often surround the nodules. These appearances are pathognomonic for diabetes, but are reported in only 10% to 50% of biopsies in both type 1 and type 2 diabetes. Nodules are also seen in membranoproliferative glomerulonephritis (see Chapter 20),

amyloid and in light-chain deposition disease (see Chapter 26); specific stains and immunofluorescence findings, respectively, will clarify the diagnosis. When there are no nodules seen, specific staining should be used to exclude amyloid.

The diffuse glomerular lesion is more frequent than the nodular lesion, with an incidence of >90% for patients with type 1 diabetes of >10 years' duration and an incidence of 25% to 50% in patients with type 2 diabetes. It comprises an increase of mesangial matrix extending to involve the capillary loops (see Fig. 29.12b). In contrast to nodular lesions, which are of little functional significance, the degree of diffuse glomerulosclerosis correlates with the clinical manifestations of worsening renal function. Accumulation of mesangial matrix is the feature most consistently associated with progression.[52] In more severe disease, the capillary wall thickening and mesangial expansion lead to capillary narrowing (see Fig. 29.11b) and hyalinization, with accompanying periglomerular fibrosis.

Arteriolar lesions are prominent in diabetes, with hyaline material progressively replacing the entire wall structure and involving both the afferent and efferent vessels. The latter is highly specific for diabetes.

The tubules and the interstitium may show a variety of nonspecific changes, including tubular cell vacuolization and tubulointerstitial fibrosis. These features are not universally found in patients with microalbuminuric type 2 diabetes.[53] In a proportion of patients with type 2 diabetes, the kidney has an appearance more suggestive of glomerular ischemia or tubulointerstitial disease.

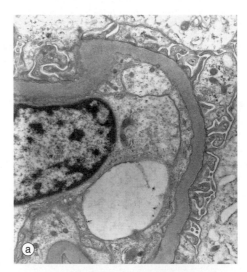

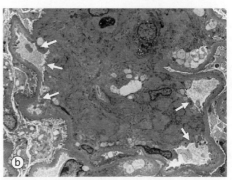

Figure 29.11 Electron microscopy of structural changes in diabetic nephropathy. a, Glomerular basement membranes are diffusely thickened. b, The expanded mesangium encroaches on the capillary spaces (arrows).

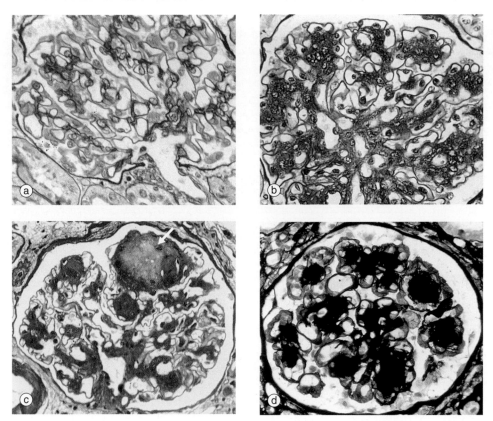

Figure 29.12 Light microscopy of structural changes in diabetic nephropathy. *a*, Normal glomerulus (periodic acid–Schiff). *b*, Diffuse glomerular lesion: widespread mesangial expansion (periodic acid–Schiff). *c*, Nodular lesion: as well as mesangial expansion, there is a typical Kimmelstiel-Wilson nodule at the top of the glomerulus (*arrow*) (periodic acid–Schiff). *d*, Nodular lesion: methenamine silver staining showing the marked nodular expansion of mesangial matrix.

DIAGNOSIS

The diagnosis of DN is based on the detection of proteinuria. In addition, many patients will also have hypertension and retinopathy. The main diagnostic procedures to establish the diagnosis of DN are summarized in Figure 29.13 and include

- Determination of albuminuria or of proteinuria
- Measurement of blood pressure
- Measurement of serum creatinine concentration and measurement or estimation of GFR
- Ophthalmologic examination

Measurement of Albuminuria/Proteinuria

Microalbuminuria is defined as the excretion of 30 to 300 mg/h albumin in at least two of three consecutive nonketotic sterile urine samples (Fig. 29.14). There is substantial intraindividual day-to-day variation (coefficient of variation 30% to 50%). In this range of albumin concentrations, albumin is normally not detected by nonspecific tests for protein (e.g., Biuret reaction). Albumin can be detected, however, using specific techniques such as dipstick, enzyme-linked immunosorbent assay, nephelometry, and radioimmunoassay. If 24-hour urine collections are not possible, the albumin concentration can be determined in spot urine or better morning urine samples. The normal range is 20 to 200 mg/min or 20 to 200 mg/ml.

A recently recognized methodologic problem is the fact that these assays, which are based on immunologic methods, may miss nonimmunoreactive albumin that is detected by high-performance liquid chromatography.[54] This may turn out to allow even earlier detection of nephropathy, but does not yet have clinical implications.

The definition of the normal range of albumin excretion is somewhat arbitrary because the risk of progression and of cardiovascular events (see Fig. 29.10) is definitely higher even in the upper quantiles of normal albumin excretion.[41]

The main advantage of searching for microalbuminuria early in the course of diabetes is that it predicts a high renal risk and thus allows targeted intervention: 80% of patients with type 1 diabetes with microalbuminuria go on to develop clinical nephropathy. In patients with type 2 diabetes, the proportion is closer to 40%. It also predicts a high cardiovascular risk. Therefore, the American Diabetes Association (www.diabetes.org) and other societies recommend annual screening of all patients.[55]

The measurement of urinary albumin concentration is a specific indicator of DN only if confounding factors such as fever, physical exercise, urinary tract infection, nondiabetic renal disease, hematuria from other causes, heart failure, uncontrolled hypertension, or uncontrolled hyperglycemia have been excluded.

By definition, clinically overt DN (macroalbuminuria) is present if the rate of albumin excretion exceeds 300 mg/day. At this point, usually serum proteins other than albumin are excreted in the urine as well (nonselective proteinuria; see Fig. 29.14).

Measurement of Blood Pressure

When measuring the blood pressure in a diabetic patient, one should be aware of several problems:

- In overweight patients with type 2 diabetes, the size of the cuff has to be adapted to the upper arm circumference.

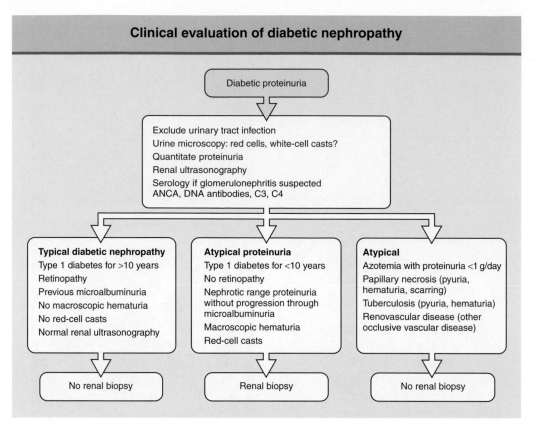

Figure 29.13 **Clinical evaluation of diabetic renal disease.** ANCA, antineutrophil cytoplasmic antibody.

When this exceeds 32 cm, cuffs of 18 cm width are indicated.

- For unknown reasons, the prevalence of white coat hypertension is lower in diabetic patients with DN.
- Patients with severe autonomic polyneuropathy tend to develop orthostatic hypotension, namely, a decrease of systolic blood pressure by >20 mm Hg in the upright position. It is therefore advisable to measure blood pressure in the upright position at regular intervals.
- In diabetic patients with sclerosis or calcification of the radial and brachial arteries, pseudohypertension may occasionally occur, that is, spuriously elevated blood pressure values despite normotension by intra-arterial blood pressure measurements. Suspicion of this condition should be raised if a discrepancy is found between modest target organ damage, for example, left ventricular hypertrophy and very high measured blood pressure values. Such patients tend to develop marked hypotension even with relatively modest antihypertensive medication.

- The circadian blood pressure profile tends to be abnormal in early stages[46] and even a paradoxical increase in the nighttime blood pressure is not rare. In the diabetic patient with nephropathy, it has been shown that a nighttime increase in blood pressure is independently associated with a 20-fold higher mortality and a higher risk of renal failure.[56] Occasional measurements of ambulatory blood pressure are particularly useful to assess the efficacy of antihypertensive treatment.

Measurement of Serum Creatinine and Estimation of Glomerular Filtration Rate

In clinical practice, the serum creatinine concentration is most frequently used to assess renal function, but it may be grossly misleading in wasted patients when muscle mass is low. This problem is particularly frequent in elderly female patients with type 2 diabetes. Therefore, the Kidney Disease Outcome Quality Initiative (KDOQI) guidelines recommend that the GFR be estimated according to the MDRD or Cockcroft-Gault formula (see Chapter 3).

Indications for Renal Biopsy

Further investigation including a renal biopsy should be considered (see Fig. 29.13)

- If retinopathy is not present in type 1 diabetes (absence of retinopathy does not exclude DN in type 2 diabetes)
- If the onset of proteinuria has been sudden and rapid, particularly if in type 1 diabetes, and the duration of the disease is <5 years or if the evolution has been atypical, for example, without transition through usual stages,

Urinary albumin excretion rate (UAER)		
	UAER	
Condition	24-hr (mg/day)	Overnight (µg/min)
Normoalbuminuria	>30	>20
Microalbuminuria	30–300	20–200
Overt nephropathy	>300	>200

Figure 29.14 **Urinary albumin excretion rate.** Levels of 24-hour and overnight urinary albumin excretion are diagnostic for microalbuminuria and overt diabetic nephropathy.

particularly the development of nephrotic syndrome without previous microalbuminuria

- If macroscopic hematuria is present or an active urinary sediment is found that is suggestive of an active glomerulonephritis, such as acanthocytes and red-cell casts; the sediment in DN typically is unremarkable apart from some occasional erythrocytes
- If the decline of renal function is exceptionally rapid (Fig. 29.15) or if renal dysfunction is found without significant proteinuria (first, of course, renovascular disease must be excluded)

If the preceding criteria are applied, the chances of detecting renal pathology other than diabetic nephropathy are high (certainly exceeding 50%).

Additional Evaluations in the Diabetic Patient with Impaired Renal Function

When seeing a diabetic patient with renal failure, one should

- Assess the cause of renal failure (acute versus chronic, diabetic glomerulosclerosis and nephropathy versus alternative causes of renal failure)
- Assess the rate of progression and the magnitude of proteinuria
- Monitor the patient for clinical evidence of the extrarenal microvascular and macrovascular complications listed in Figure 29.4

The majority of diabetic patients with heavy proteinuria and/or renal failure suffer from DN. Renal ischemia or atherosclerotic renal artery stenosis and cholesterol microembolism are much more common in diabetic patients than was previously assumed, however. In 10% to 20% of patients, often with small kidneys and low GFR, no albuminuria and small contracted kidneys are detected,[57] while in patients with typical DN, the kidneys are usually enlarged. In the past, urinary tract infection frequently led to purulent papillary necrosis and intrarenal abscess formation. This has now become rare, presumably due to the frequent use of antibiotics and better management of urinary tract infection. There is no doubt, however, that if urinary tract infections occur, they are more severe in the diabetic compared to the nondiabetic patient. Glomerulonephritis, particularly membranous nephropathy, was thought to be more common in diabetic patients than in the general population,[58,59] but this has not been confirmed.[60,61] The clinician should suspect the presence of nondiabetic renal disease if a nephritic urinary sediment is found and if urinary abnormalities and/or renal dysfunction occur early in the course of type 1 diabetes. In this case, renal biopsy is indicated (see previous discussion).

Diabetic patients with nephropathy are particularly prone to develop acute renal failure after administration of nonsteroidal

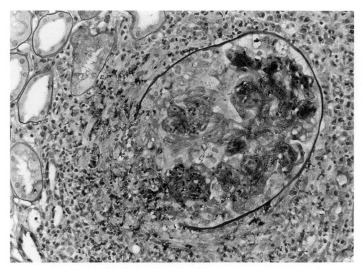

Figure 29.15 Glomerulonephritis superimposed on diabetic nephropathy. A glomerulus showing a cellular crescent with rupture of Bowman's capsule superimposed on nodular diabetic nephropathy. The patient, known to have diabetic nephropathy, presented with rapidly deteriorating renal function and red-cell casts in the urine.

anti-inflammatory agents or radiocontrast. The risk is similar for ionic and nonionic radiocontrast media, but it has recently been described that the renal risk is less for dimeric radiocontrast media.[62] The risk can be reduced considerably by attention to preventive measures including administration of fluid as well as temporary omission of diuretics and possibly ACE inhibitors (see also Chapter 64). To reduce the risk of radiocontrast, it has been proposed to adjust the dose in proportion to the reduction of renal function.

The diabetic patient with advanced renal failure usually has a much higher burden of microvascular and macrovascular complications (see Fig. 29.4) than the diabetic patient with no or with early stages of DN.

The major clinical problem is accelerated and premature atherosclerosis, frequently causing coronary heart disease: This may take the form of myocardial infarction (often silent), angina pectoris, or ischemic cardiomyopathy. There is also an excess frequency of cerebrovascular disease and peripheral artery disease, particularly in smokers. Even the asymptomatic diabetic patient with advanced renal impairment must therefore be monitored at regular intervals for timely detection of the preceding complications (ophthalmologic examination at half-yearly intervals, yearly cardiac and angiologic status including imaging of the carotid artery, foot inspection preferably at each visit).

REFERENCES

1. Amin R, Turner C, van Aken S, et al: The relationship between microalbuminuria and glomerular filtration rate in young type 1 diabetic subjects: The Oxford Regional Prospective Study. Kidney Int 2005;68: 1740–1749.
2. de Vriese AS, Tilton RG, Elger M, et al: Antibodies against vascular endothelial growth factor improve early renal dysfunction in experimental diabetes. J Am Soc Nephrol 2001;12:993–1000.
3. Wolf G, Chen S, Ziyadeh FN: From the periphery of the glomerular capillary wall toward the center of disease: Podocyte injury comes of age in diabetic nephropathy. Diabetes 2005;54:1626–1634.
4. Doublier S, Salvidio G, Lupia E, et al: Nephrin expression is reduced in human diabetic nephropathy: Evidence for a distinct role for glycated albumin and angiotensin II. Diabetes 2003;52:1023–1030.
5. Katz A, Caramori ML, Sisson-Ross S, et al: An increase in the cell component of the cortical interstitium antedates interstitial fibrosis in type 1 diabetic patients. Kidney Int 2002;61:2058–2066.
6. Gilbert RE, Cooper ME: The tubulointerstitium in progressive diabetic kidney disease: More than an aftermath of glomerular injury? Kidney Int 1999;56:1627–1637.
7. Ozdemir AM, Hopfer U, Erhard P, et al: Processing advanced glycation end product-modified albumin by the renal proximal tubule and the early pathogenesis of diabetic nephropathy. Ann N Y Acad Sci 2005; 1043:625–636.
8. Nangaku M: Chronic hypoxia and tubulointerstitial injury: A final common pathway to end-stage renal failure. J Am Soc Nephrol 2006; 17:17–25.

9. Krolewski AS, Laffel LM, Krolewski M, et al: Glycosylated hemoglobin and the risk of microalbuminuria in patients with insulin-dependent diabetes mellitus. N Engl J Med 1995;332:1251–1255.

10. The effect of intensive treatment of diabetes on the development and progression of long-term complications in insulin-dependent diabetes mellitus. The Diabetes Control and Complications Trial Research Group. N Engl J Med 1993;329:977–986.

11. Nathan DM, Cleary PA, Backlund JY, et al: Intensive diabetes treatment and cardiovascular disease in patients with type 1 diabetes. N Engl J Med 2005;353:2643–2653.

12. Fioretto P, Steffes MW, Sutherland DE, et al: Reversal of lesions of diabetic nephropathy after pancreas transplantation. N Engl J Med 1998; 339:69–75.

13. Intensive blood-glucose control with sulphonylureas or insulin compared with conventional treatment and risk of complications in patients with type 2 diabetes (UKPDS 33). UK Prospective Diabetes Study (UKPDS) Group. Lancet 1998;352:837–853.

14. Koya D, Haneda M, Nakagawa H, et al: Amelioration of accelerated diabetic mesangial expansion by treatment with a PKC beta inhibitor in diabetic db/db mice, a rodent model for type 2 diabetes. FASEB J 2000; 14:439–447.

15. Menne J, Park JK, Boehne M, et al: Diminished loss of proteoglycans and lack of albuminuria in protein kinase C-alpha-deficient diabetic mice. Diabetes 2004;53:2101–2109.

16. Vlassara H, Striker LJ, Teichberg S, et al: Advanced glycation end products induce glomerular sclerosis and albuminuria in normal rats. Proc Natl Acad Sci U S A 1994;91:11704–11708.

17. Bierhaus A, Humpert PM, Morcos M, et al: Understanding RAGE, the receptor for advanced glycation end products. J Mol Med 2005;83: 876–886.

18. Zatz R, Dunn BR, Meyer TW, et al: Prevention of diabetic glomerulopathy by pharmacological amelioration of glomerular capillary hypertension. J Clin Invest 1986;77:1925–1930.

19. Anderson S, Jung FF, Ingelfinger JR: Renal renin-angiotensin system in diabetes: Functional, immunohistochemical, and molecular biological correlations. Am J Physiol 1993;265:F477–F486.

20. Nguyen G, Burckle CA, Sraer JD: Renin/prorenin-receptor biochemistry and functional significance. Curr Hypertens Rep 2004;6:129–132.

21. Ichihara A, Hayashi M, Kaneshiro Y, et al: Inhibition of diabetic nephropathy by a decoy peptide corresponding to the "handle" region for nonproteolytic activation of prorenin. J Clin Invest 2004;114:1128–1135.

22. Huang XR, Chen WY, Truong LD, et al: Chymase is upregulated in diabetic nephropathy: Implications for an alternative pathway of angiotensin II–mediated diabetic renal and vascular disease. J Am Soc Nephrol 2003;14: 1738–1747.

23. Greene EL, Kren S, Hostetter TH: Role of aldosterone in the remnant kidney model in the rat. J Clin Invest 1996;98:1063–1068.

24. Mogensen CE: Progression of nephropathy in long-term diabetics with proteinuria and effect of initial anti-hypertensive treatment. Scand J Clin Lab Invest 1976;36:383–388.

25. Parving HH, Andersen AR, Smidt UM, et al: Early aggressive antihypertensive treatment reduces rate of decline in kidney function in diabetic nephropathy. Lancet 1983;1:1175–1179.

26. Lewis EJ, Hunsicker LG, Bain RP, et al: The effect of angiotensin-converting-enzyme inhibition on diabetic nephropathy. The Collaborative Study Group. N Engl J Med 1993;329:1456–1462.

27. Lewis EJ, Hunsicker LG, Clarke WR, et al: Renoprotective effect of the angiotensin-receptor antagonist irbesartan in patients with nephropathy due to type 2 diabetes. N Engl J Med 2001;345:851–860.

28. Brenner BM, Cooper ME, de Zeeuw D, et al: Effects of losartan on renal and cardiovascular outcomes in patients with type 2 diabetes and nephropathy. N Engl J Med 2001;345:861–869.

29. Ritz E, Rychlik I, Locatelli F, et al: End-stage renal failure in type 2 diabetes: A medical catastrophe of worldwide dimensions. Am J Kidney Dis 1999;34:795–808.

30. Hasslacher C, Ritz E, Wahl P, et al: Similar risks of nephropathy in patients with type I or type II diabetes mellitus. Nephrol Dial Transplant 1989;4:859–863.

31. Seaquist ER, Goetz FC, Rich S, et al: Familial clustering of diabetic kidney disease. Evidence for genetic susceptibility to diabetic nephropathy. N Engl J Med 1989;320:1161–1165.

32. Nelson RG, Knowler WC, Pettitt DJ, et al: Diabetic kidney disease in Pima Indians. Diabetes Care 1993;16:335–341.

33. Nelson RG, Morgenstern H, Bennett PH: Intrauterine diabetes exposure and the risk of renal disease in diabetic Pima Indians. Diabetes 1998;47: 1489–1493.

34. Amri K, Freund N, Van Huyen JP, et al: Altered nephrogenesis due to maternal diabetes is associated with increased expression of IGF-II/mannose-6-phosphate receptor in the fetal kidney. Diabetes 2001;50: 1069–1075.

35. Zandi-Nejad K, Luyckx VA, Brenner BM: Adult hypertension and kidney disease: The role of fetal programming. Hypertension 2006;47:502–508.

36. Janssen B, Hohenadel D, Brinkkoetter P, et al: Carnosine as a protective factor in diabetic nephropathy: Association with a leucine repeat of the carnosinase gene CNDP1. Diabetes 2005;54:2320–2327.

37. Marre M, Jeunemaitre X, Gallois Y, et al: Contribution of genetic polymorphism in the renin-angiotensin system to the development of renal complications in insulin-dependent diabetes: Genetique de la Nephropathie Diabetique (GENEDIAB) study group. J Clin Invest 1997;99:1585–1595.

38. Schmidt S, Ritz E: Angiotensin I converting enzyme gene polymorphism and diabetic nephropathy in type II diabetes. Nephrol Dial Transplant 1997;12(Suppl 2):37–41.

39. Ritz E, Ogata H, Orth SR: Smoking: A factor promoting onset and progression of diabetic nephropathy. Diabetes Metab 2000;26(Suppl 4):54–63.

40. Hsu CY, McCulloch CE, Darbinian J, et al: Elevated blood pressure and risk of end-stage renal disease in subjects without baseline kidney disease. Arch Intern Med 2005;165:923–928.

41. Rachmani R, Levi Z, Lidar M, et al: Considerations about the threshold value of microalbuminuria in patients with diabetes mellitus: Lessons from an 8-year follow-up study of 599 patients. Diabetes Res Clin Pract 2000;49:187–194.

42. Cooper ME: Pathogenesis, prevention, and treatment of diabetic nephropathy. Lancet 1998;352:213–219.

43. Mogensen CE: How to protect the kidney in diabetic patients with special reference to NIDDM. Diabetes 1997;56(Suppl 2):104–111.

44. Keller CK, Bergis KH, Fliser D, et al: Renal findings in patients with short-term type 2 diabetes. J Am Soc Nephrol 1996;7:2627–2635.

45. Ritz E, Orth SR: Nephropathy in patients with type 2 diabetes mellitus. N Engl J Med 1999;341:1127–1133.

46. Lurbe E, Redon J, Kesani A, et al: Increase in nocturnal blood pressure and progression to microalbuminuria in type 1 diabetes. N Engl J Med 2002;347:797–805.

47. Nelson RG, Pettitt DJ, Baird HR, et al: Pre-diabetic blood pressure predicts urinary albumin excretion after the onset of type 2 (non-insulin-dependent) diabetes mellitus in Pima Indians. Diabetologia 1993;36:998–1001.

48. Gall MA, Rossing P, Skott P, et al: Prevalence of micro- and macroalbuminuria, arterial hypertension, retinopathy and large vessel disease in European type 2 (non-insulin-dependent) diabetic patients. Diabetologia 1991;34:655–661.

49. Borch-Johnsen K, Nissen H, Salling N, et al: The natural history of insulin-dependent diabetes in Denmark: 2. Long-term survival—who and why. Diabet Med 1987;4:211–216.

50. Adler AI, Stevens RJ, Manley SE, et al: Development and progression of nephropathy in type 2 diabetes: The United Kingdom Prospective Diabetes Study (UKPDS 64). Kidney Int 2003;63:225–232.

51. Standl E, Schnell O: A new look at the heart in diabetes mellitus: From ailing to failing. Diabetologia 2000;43:1455–1469.

52. Fioretto P, Steffes MW, Sutherland DE, et al: Sequential renal biopsies in insulin-dependent diabetic patients: Structural factors associated with clinical progression. Kidney Int 1995;48:1929–1935.

53. Fioretto P, Mauer M, Brocco E, et al: Patterns of renal injury in NIDDM patients with microalbuminuria. Diabetologia 1996;39:1569–1576.

54. Polkinghorne KR, Su Q, Chadban SJ, et al: Population prevalence of albuminuria in the Australian Diabetes, Obesity, and Lifestyle (AusDiab) study: Immunonephelometry compared with high-performance liquid chromatography. Am J Kidney Dis 2006;47:604–613.

55. The sixth report of the Joint National Committee on prevention, detection, evaluation, and treatment of high blood pressure. Arch Intern Med 1997;157:2413–2446.

56. Nakano S, Ogihara M, Tamura C, et al: Reversed circadian blood pressure rhythm independently predicts endstage renal failure in non-insulin-dependent diabetes mellitus subjects. J Diabetes Complications 1999;13: 224–231.

57. MacIsaac RJ, Tsalamandris C, Panagiotopoulos S, et al: Nonalbuminuric renal insufficiency in type 2 diabetes. Diabetes Care 2004;27:195–200.

58. Amoah E, Glickman JL, Malchoff CD, et al: Clinical identification of non-diabetic renal disease in diabetic patients with type I and type II disease presenting with renal dysfunction. Am J Nephrol 1988;8:204–211.

59. Parving HH, Gall MA, Skott P, et al: Prevalence and causes of albuminuria in non-insulin-dependent diabetic patients. Kidney Int 1992;41:758–762.

60. Waldherr R, Ilkenhans C, Ritz E: How frequent is glomerulonephritis in diabetes mellitus type II? Clin Nephrol 1992;37:271–273.

61. Olsen S, Mogensen CE: How often is NIDDM complicated with non-diabetic renal disease? An analysis of renal biopsies and the literature. Diabetologia 1996;39:1638–1645.

62. Aspelin P, Aubry P, Fransson SG, et al: Nephrotoxic effects in high-risk patients undergoing angiography. N Engl J Med 2003;348:491–499.

Prevention and Treatment of Diabetic Nephropathy

Eberhard Ritz

INTRODUCTION

The major therapeutic approaches for diabetic nephropathy that have been investigated include

- intensive glycemic control
- antihypertensive treatment with a particular focus on agents that interrupt the RAS
- restriction of dietary protein

Less investigated, but highly effective is the cessation of smoking.

Diabetic nephropathy (DN) evolves through several stages (see Fig. 29.5) which are clinically defined by the levels of urinary albumin excretion: normoalbuminuria, microalbuminuria (incipient DN), and macroalbuminuria (overt DN) that affect the choice of therapeutic interventions. A summary of preventive and therapeutic approaches is shown in Figure 30.1 and is discussed in detail here.

GLYCEMIC CONTROL IN DIABETES

The evidence that good glycemic control can slow progression, particularly in the early phases of DN, is based on numerous retrospective observational studies and a prospective study that showed that the rate of increase in albuminuria correlated with glycated hemoglobin over a mean period of approximately 10 years in both patients with type 1 and type 2 diabetes.[1]

In the Stage of Normoalbuminuria

The importance of strict glycemic control in the prevention of microalbuminuria in type 1 diabetes was best shown in the Diabetes Control and Complications Trial (DCCT): patients were randomized to intensive insulin therapy (consisting of at least three injections daily or the use of an insulin pump) or conventional therapy (two injections daily).[2] Over a 9-year period, patients on intensive therapy (mean HbA1c levels of 7.0%) had a 35% to 45% lower risk of developing microalbuminuria compared to the control group (mean HbA1c of 9%; Fig. 30.2). Similar findings were reported in a small Scandinavian study.[3] A drawback of such intensified therapy is the risk of hypoglycemic episodes.

The effect of intensive insulin therapy in type 2 diabetes was studies in the Kumamoto trial[4] and the UK Prospective Diabetes Study (UKPDS).[5] In the 6-year Kumamoto trial investigating 110 relatively young (mean age of 50 years) nonobese Japanese patients with type 2 diabetes, intensive insulin therapy reduced

Management of type 1 diabetes		
Stage	**Assessment**	**Management**
Normoalbuminuric/ normotensive	Screen yearly for micro-albuminuria; assess cardiovascular risk factors	Optimize glycemic control (target HbA1c <7%) Systolic BP target <130mmHg Add lipid lowering agent
Persistent microalbuminuria/ normotensive	Close monitoring of lipids, blood pressure (BP), glycemic control, and urinary albumin excretion	Add angiotensin-converting enzyme (ACE) inhibitor or angiotensin receptor blocker (ARB)
Persistent microalbuminuria/ hypertensive	Follow urinary albumin excretion, creatinine clearance, BP	Titrate ACE inhibitor or combine with ARB, aim for BP <130/85 mm Hg; consider addition of a diuretic or a low-sodium diet; perhaps add another antihypertensive
Proteinuria	Monitor urinary protein, BP, lipids, creatinine clearance	Aggressive BP control, aim for <125/75 mm Hg; possibly add lipid-lowering drugs, low-protein diet
Declining glomerular filtration rate (GFR)	Prepare for dialysis or transplant	Initiate dialysis when GFR is 10–12 ml/min (usually equating to a creatinine clearance of <15 ml/min or a serum creatinine of >6 mg/dl)

Figure 30.1   Management of type 1 diabetes. A similar strategy can be used in patients with type 2 diabetes with increased emphasis on management of cardiovascular risk factors. In all diabetic patients with early or overt nephropathy, there should be continued and possibly increased surveillance for other diabetic micro- and macrovascular complications.

the risk of onset of microalbuminuria by 62% (primary prevention). Furthermore, analysis of the HbA1c levels showed that below an apparent threshold of 6.5% microalbuminuria did not worsen (normal range, 4.8% to 6.4%).

The UKPDS has explored the effect of intensification of glycemic control with oral antidiabetic agents or insulin over 10 years in a large cohort of newly diagnosed patients with type 2 diabetes.[5] There was a 0.9% difference in HbA1c (7.0% versus 7.9%) between the intensified and conventionally treated groups; after 9 years of treatment, the development of microalbuminuria and proteinuria was lower by 25% to 30% and doubling of serum creatinine was lower by 50%.

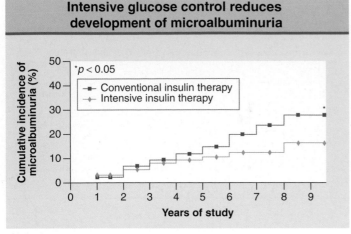

Intensive glucose control reduces development of microalbuminuria

Figure 30.2 Diabetes Control and Complications Trial. Intensive glucose control was associated with a decreased risk of the subsequent development of microalbuminuria in type I diabetes. (Adapted from Diabetes Control and Complications Trial Research Group: The effect of intensive treatment on the development and progression of long-term complications in insulin-dependent diabetes mellitus. N Engl J Med 1993;329:977–986.)

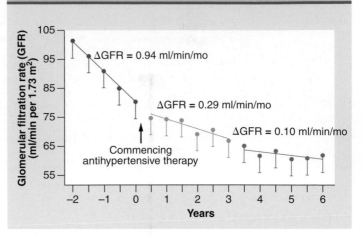

Control of blood pressure retards progression of type 1 diabetic nephropathy

Figure 30.3 Control of blood pressure reduces the risk for progression in type I diabetic neuropathy. (Adapted from Parving H-H, Andersen AR, Smidt VM, et al: Effect of anti-hypertensive treatment on kidney function in diabetic nephropathy. BMJ 1987;294:1443–1447.)

In the Stages of Microalbuminuria and Overt Diabetic Nephropathy

The evidence that intensified insulin therapy slows progression in patients with type 1 or type 2 diabetes and microalbuminuria remains controversial. Only a small number of patients entering the DCCT had microalbuminuria at baseline. Fewer patients progressed to frank albuminuria under intensive insulin treatment, but this did not reach statistical significance.[2] However, several small Scandinavian studies reported that in microalbuminuric patients with type 1 diabetes, intensive glucose control caused slower progression to DN.

One potential reason why it may be difficult to show a benefit of glucose control in patients with incipient or established DN is that the results are confounded by the effects of hypertension. It is of interest that a study from Guy's Hospital found that intensive glycemic control is of benefit in DN, provided blood pressure (BP) is well controlled.[6] However, these results must be interpreted with caution since they were not obtained as part of a prospective study.

ANTIHYPERTENSIVE THERAPY IN DIABETIC NEPHROPATHY

Hypertension, in the past defined as BP >140/90 mm Hg, classically develops within 2 to 5 years after the onset of microalbuminuria (see Fig. 29.5) and is usually associated with volume expansion and salt sensitivity. More recently, it has been shown that even before this stage, BP increases progressively within the range of normal values and that a change in the circadian BP pattern precedes the onset of microalbuminuria.[7] Major benefit from the control of systemic hypertension, that is, reduction of proteinuria and slowing progression to renal failure, has been documented in numerous studies in both type 1 and type 2 diabetes. The observation of a progressive slowing of progression with time by antihypertensive therapy, is illustrated in Figure 30.3.[8,9]

Controlled prospective evidence that BP lowering attenuates progression was provided by the Modification of Diet in Renal Disease (MDRD) study mainly on nondiabetic patients with renal disease.[10] The rate of progression was lower in patients randomized to intensified BP control (mean arterial pressure, 92 mm Hg) than in patients randomized to ordinary BP control (mean arterial pressure, 107 mm Hg)). This observation, as well as others, led the Seventh Joint National Committee[11] and other societies to recommend low targets for instituting antihypertensive therapy in diabetic patients: 130/85 mm Hg for diabetic patients and 125/75 mm Hg for those with proteinuria >1 g/24 hr.

Apart from lowering BP, a second issue is whether certain antihypertensive agents confer specific renoprotective effects in DN above and beyond BP lowering, particularly whether additional benefit is achieved by blockade of the renin angiotensin system (RAS) with ACE inhibitors or angiotensin receptor antagonists (ARBs), including patients who are normotensive. This issue has recently become very controversial,[12] but controlled head-on comparisons in prospective studies with nearly identical achieved BP values showed undisputedly a relatively small, but significant, additional benefit from blocking the RAS.[13–18] On a practical level, this issue is less relevant since even when the RAS is blocked, lowering BP provides additional benefit.[15] Consequently, both BP lowering and RAS blockade are needed. Furthermore, to achieve the recommended goal BP values in diabetic patients with impaired renal function, several classes of antihypertensive agents will usually be needed (typically four to five agents), which, by necessity, will include drugs blocking the RAS.

ANGIOTENSIN-CONVERTING ENZYME INHIBITORS OR ANGIOTENSIN RECEPTOR BLOCKERS IN DIABETIC NEUROPATHY

Angiotensin-Converting Enzyme Inhibitors in the Stage of Normoalbuminuria

The observation that ACE inhibitors slow progression in microalbuminuric patients with type 1 diabetes[19] has led to consideration that they may also be of benefit in diabetic patients prior to the development of microalbuminuria. In the EURODIAB Controlled Trial of Lisinopril in Insulin Dependent Diabetes (EUCLID) study, presumably underpowered to recognize the renal effect, no evidence of a beneficial role for the ACE inhibitor lisinopril was

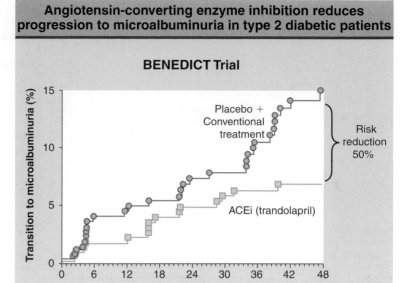

Figure 30.4 Angiotensin-converting enzyme inhibition reduces progression to microalbuminuria in type 2 diabetic patients: the Bergamo Nephrologic Diabetes Complications (BENEDICT) Trial.[23]

observed in normoalbuminuric patients with type 1 diabetes, despite evidence that it reduced the development of retinopathy.[20] A recent 3-year study noted that the ACE inhibitor perindopril retarded the increase in albuminuria that was observed in the placebo treated group.[21]

In a cohort of patients with type 2 diabetes with or without hypertension, enalapril retarded the development of microalbuminuria.[22] In normoalbuminuric patients with type 2 diabetes, the BENEDICT study recently documented that the ACE inhibitor trandolapril reduced the onset of microalbuminuria by approximately 50% (Fig. 30.4), and despite identical BP, this could not be achieved with the calcium channel blocker verapamil.[23] Whether this finding will ultimately translate into long-term renoprotection remains to be determined.

Angiotensin-Converting Enzyme Inhibitors in the Stage of Microalbuminuria and Normal Blood Pressure

The experimental observation that ACE inhibitors lower glomerular pressure and prevent glomerular damage in diabetic rats independent of effects on systemic hypertension (see Chapter 29) led to a large number of clinical studies to explore the role of ACE inhibition in normotensive patients with type 1 diabetes with early renal disease. These studies documented that ACE inhibitors will decrease albuminuria and retard the development of proteinuria in type 1 diabetes. However, it is not always clear whether the effect was independent of BP because most studies compared ACE inhibitors to placebo. As a consequence, systemic BP was mostly lower in the ACE-treated groups. In a recent meta-analysis of 12 placebo-controlled trials in 698 normotensive patients with type 1 diabetes with microalbuminuria treated with ACE inhibitors, the majority for >2 years, treatment was associated with a 60% reduction in progression to macroalbuminuria and a threefold increase in regression to normoalbuminuria.[19]

Although most patients with type 2 diabetes with microalbuminuria are hypertensive, some will be normotensive, particularly in the Asian population. Studies comparing ACE inhibitors to placebo have also suggested a benefit, particularly in decreasing the risk of developing proteinuria. Treatment with enalapril for 5 years was not only associated with a reduced risk of developing

proteinuria, but was also associated with stabilization of renal function. By contrast, the placebo-treated group had a 13% decline in renal function.[24] In Indo-Asian normotensive (<140/ 90 mm Hg) and microalbuminuric patients with type 2 diabetes, the reduction in albuminuria by enalapril occurred independently of a discernible difference in BP between the ACE inhibitor– and placebo-treated groups.[25]

Angiotensin-Converting Enzyme Inhibitors in the Stage of Microalbuminuria or Proteinuria and Hypertension

Most studies have shown that ACE inhibitors can reduce proteinuria of any etiology by 40% to 50%. So it is not surprising that most studies have documented that ACE inhibitors will reduce proteinuria in patients with type 1 or type 2 diabetes as compared with standard antihypertensive therapy using diuretics and β-blockers. However, there is also evidence that, in addition to reducing proteinuria, ACE inhibitors may slow the deterioration of renal function.

In the Collaborative Study on type 1 diabetic subjects with proteinuria (>500 mg/day), captopril treatment (25 mg three times daily) was compared to placebo. As shown in Figure 30.5, captopril was superior to placebo in reducing the risk to progress to end-stage renal disease (ESRD).[16] Captopril treatment was associated with a slowing of the deterioration of renal function over the 3-year period (11% versus 17% decline in creatinine clearance per year) and a 50% reduction in the proportion of patients reaching ESRD. Remission of nephrotic syndrome also occurred in seven of 42 nephrotic patients on captopril but in only one of 66 controls, and this was associated with lower BP in the captopril group.[26]

In patients with type 2 diabetes, microalbuminuria, and hypertension, ACE inhibitors are also more potent at reducing proteinuria than conventional therapy with diuretics and β-blockers. ACE inhibitors are also superior to other antihypertensive agents: in most studies, ACE inhibitors are more potent than particularly dihydropyridine calcium channel blockers in reducing proteinuria and stabilizing renal function.

While numerous studies clearly document the benefit of ACE inhibitors in normotensive and hypertensive microalbuminuric patients with type 1 and type 2 diabetes, there has been much discussion of the extent to which this effect is independent of

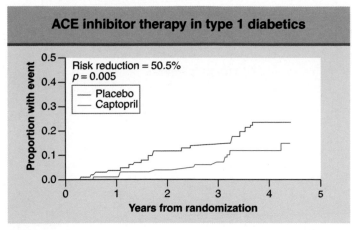

Figure 30.5 The Collaborative Study. Treatment with captopril was superior to placebo in reducing the risk of proteinuric patients with type 1 diabetes to progress to end-stage renal disease. (Adapted from Lewis EJ, Hunsicker LG, Bain RP, Rohde RD: The effect of angiotensin-converting-enzyme inhibition on diabetic nephropathy. The Collaborative Study Group. N Engl J Med 1993;329:1456–1462.)

BP-lowering effects. For example, in the Collaborative Study,[16] there was clearly less benefit in patients with type 1 diabetes with normal BP and relatively preserved renal function. The concept that the first priority is aggressive BP lowering rather than ACE inhibition *per se* is further supported by the Appropriate Blood Pressure Control in Diabetes study.[27] Patients were randomized to ordinary (achieved mean BP, 137/81 mm Hg) or intensified (128/75 mm Hg) BP control with either enalapril or nisoldipine.

Less progression from microalbuminuria to proteinuria was seen with intensified BP control, irrespective of whether an ACE inhibitor or calcium channel blocker was used.

Angiotensin Receptor Blockers in Diabetic Nephropathy

Experimental studies had suggested that ARBs have beneficial effects similar to those of ACE inhibitors. This has recently been confirmed in patients with early stages of DN, most with microalbuminuria. The Diabetics Exposed to Telmisartan and Enalapril (DETAIL) study[28] was designed to prove the noninferiority of the ARB telmisartan compared to the ACE inhibitor enalapril. The study documented marked attenuation of the loss of measured glomerular filtration rate (GFR), which was similar with both drugs. After 5 years, the rate of loss of GFR was no more than would be expected in individuals of advanced age. Comparison of this outcome to that in the Irbesartan in Diabetic Nephropathy Trial (IDNT)[17] or Reduction of Endpoints in Non-insulin Dependent Diabetes Mellitus with the Angiotensin II Antagonist Losartan (RENAAL)[18] Trial (Fig. 30.6) shows that the chances to halt progression are much greater early on in the course of DN than when treatment is started in later stages.

In hypertensive patients with type 2 diabetes with microalbuminuria (IRMA-2 study),[14] the ARB irbesartan reduced the development of overt proteinuria in a dose-dependent manner with increased regression to normoalbuminuria in the ARB-treated group compared to the placebo group treated with alternative antihypertensive agents (see Fig. 30.6).

The RENAAL[18] and IDNT[17] studies (see Fig. 30.6) addressed patients with type 2 diabetes with overt nephropathy. The RENAAL study involved predominantly hypertensive patients

Studies evaluating angiotensin receptor blockers in incipient and overt diabetic nephropathy

Study	Population	Design	Follow-up	Blood Pressure (mean [mm Hg])	Primary Endpoint	Secondary Endpoints
RENAAL (n = 1513)	Type 2 diabetes Hypertension (97%) Macroproteinuria	Losartan (L) 50–100 mg Placebo (P)	3.4 y	L 140/74 P 142/74	Risk reduction L vs. P: • Composite of doubling of sCr, ESRD and death: 16% ↓ • Doubling of sCr: 25% ↓ • ESRD: 28% ↓ • Death: similar	Risk reduction L vs. P: • Cardiovascular: similar • Hospitalization for heart failure (HF): 32% ↓
IDNT (n = 1715)	Type 2 diabetes Hypertension Macroproteinuria	Irbesartan (I) 300 mg Amlodipine (A) 10 mg Placebo (P)	2.6 y	I 140/77 A 141/77 P 144/80	Risk reduction of composite of doubling of sCr, ESRD, and death: • 20% ↓ I vs. P, 23% ↓ I vs. A Doubling of sCr: • 33% ↓ I vs. P, 37% ↓ I vs. A ESRD: • 23% ↓ I vs. both groups	Risk reduction I vs. P: • Cardiovascular: similar • Hospitalization for HF: 23% ↓
IRMA-2 (n = 590)	Type 2 diabetes Hypertension Microalbuminuria	Placebo (P) I 150 mg I 300 mg	2 y	P: 144/83 I 150: 143/83 I 300: 141/83	Hazard ratios for time to onset of overt nephropathy: • I 150 vs. P: 0.61, P = 0.08 • I 300 vs. P: 0.30, P < 0.001	Changes in level of albuminuria • +2% P • −24% I 150 • −38% I 300 Regression to normoalbuminuria • 21% P • 24% I 150 • 34% I 300

Figure 30.6 Studies evaluating angiotensin receptor blockers in incipient and overt diabetic nephropathy. ESRD, end-stage renal disease; IDNT, Irbesartan in Diabetic Nephropathy Trial; IRMA-2, Irbesartan MicroAlbuminuria Type 2 Diabetes Trial; RENAAL, Reduction of Endpoints in Non-insulin Dependent Diabetes Mellitus with the Angiotensin II Antagonist Losartan Trial; sCr, serum creatinine.

with type 2 diabetes with proteinuria and impaired renal function. Losartan was compared to conventional antihypertensive treatment that included a significant number of subjects receiving dihydropyridine calcium channel blockers. Losartan treatment reduced the risk of progression to ESRD by 28% in association with a reduction in proteinuria of 35%. The IDNT study was performed in a similar population and compared irbesartan with amlodipine or conventional treatment. With respect to reducing the number of subjects reaching the primary endpoint, a composite of doubling of serum creatinine, ESRD, and mortality, irbesartan was superior to both conventional treatment and amlodipine therapy. The BP difference between conventional and irbesartan treatment was no more than 4 mm Hg, and no difference in achieved BP was present between amlodipine and irbesartan therapy.

Combined Angiotensin-Converting Enzyme Inhibitors and Angiotensin Receptor Blockers

With new targets for BP in diabetic subjects, particularly those with proteinuria, combinations of antihypertensive drugs have been investigated to optimize BP control. A number of antihypertensive drug classes have been shown to reduce proteinuria and/or cardiovascular events in high-risk populations.[29] Of particular interest is the combination of ACE inhibitors and ARBs. The Candesartan and Lisinopril Microalbuminuria (CALM) study demonstrated that the combination of the ACE inhibitor lisinopril and the ARB candesartan achieved greater reduction of urinary albumin excretion in hypertensive, microalbuminuric patients with type 2 diabetes.[30] The achieved BP was lower in the combination group, however, rendering interpretation difficult. Similar benefit has also been reported in proteinuric diabetic patients. In a Danish study,[31] superior reduction of proteinuria was achieved with the ACE inhibitor/ARB combination compared to the respective monotherapies despite titrating the patients to achieve identical BP values. This observation points to additional benefit from combining the two antihypertensive classes, at least when submaximal doses are used.

If the goal of reduction of proteinuria is not achieved with conventional doses of ACE inhibitors or ARBs, an alternative strategy to combination is dose escalation of the single agent.[32] Several studies showed that doses higher than those licensed for BP lowering cause additional reduction in proteinuria.[33]

A simple maneuver to increase the efficacy of RAS blockade is to put the patient on low salt intake (i.e., <6 g sodium chloride/day) and/or diuretics; the rationale is that mild salt depletion increases the efficacy of RAS blockade.

A further maneuver to increase the efficacy of RAS blockade may be additional blockade of the mineralocorticoid receptor. It has been shown that the progressive loss of GFR despite RAS blockade in patients with DN is correlated with increased concentrations of aldosterone in plasma and urine.[34] In renal damage models, aldosterone aggravates renal damage independent of angiotensin II.[35] It is therefore of interest that addition of spironolactone to ACE inhibitors or ARBs lowers proteinuria in diabetic patients.[36] If the serum creatinine concentration is elevated, this approach is hazardous, however, because of the risk of hyperkalemia.

TREATMENT GOALS DURING ANTIHYPERTENSIVE THERAPY

Blood-Pressure Lowering

The guidelines of the American Diabetes Association (www.diabetes.org) recommend a target BP of <130/80 mm Hg for diabetic patients. In patients with DN, multiple antihypertensive drugs will usually be necessary to reach these targets.

Renin Angiotensin System Blockade

Although proportionally greater benefit is obtained from BP lowering *per se*, additional BP-independent benefit is also obtained from the blockade of the RAS.[37]

Reduction of Proteinuria

A novel treatment target is to reduce proteinuria as well as BP to a specified level. Given the important independent role of proteinuria in progression,[38] in proteinuric patients with type 2 diabetes, protein excretion should be lowered to at least <1 g/24 h, optimally <0.3 g/24 h. It is therefore justified to increase the dose of ACE inhibitor or ARB further in patients with persisting major proteinuria even when the target BP has been reached.[39]

Cardiovascular Protection

An additional consideration concerning the choice of antihypertensive therapy relates to its role in providing cardioprotection. Diabetic patients with persistent microalbuminuria are at increased risk of all-cause mortality, especially cardiovascular disease, and the risk is dramatically elevated in diabetic patients with overt proteinuria[40] (see Fig. 29.9). Therefore, it is critical to monitor and treat other cardiovascular risk factors. A recent study documented that intensified multifactorial treatment of high-risk diabetic patients aimed at treating the entire spectrum of renal and cardiovascular risk factors caused a dramatic reduction of progression of renal disease and cardiovascular events.[41]

DIETARY PROTEIN INTAKE

In addition to its ability to alleviate uremic symptoms, several studies involving small numbers of patients have suggested that protein restriction may also slow the progressive loss of renal function in patients with DN. A meta-analysis of the various trials in diabetic subjects concluded that there was a beneficial effect on GFR and albuminuria with modest (0.5 to 0.85 g/kg/day) protein restriction, but this analysis must be criticized on several accounts.[42] In contrast, in the large, multicenter MDRD study of mostly nondiabetic patients with renal disease, the effects of dietary protein restriction were inconclusive,[10] although subgroup analysis suggested that patients with heavy proteinuria did benefit. Although a sufficiently large long-term prospective study would be needed to establish the safety, efficacy, and compliance with protein restriction in DN, the American Diabetes Association recommends that nonpregnant diabetic patients should restrict their protein intake to 0.8 g/kg ideal body weight per day. In patients with advanced renal failure, concern about malnutrition tempers the enthusiasm for protein restriction. On the whole, the relatively modest benefit from protein restriction, if any, is vastly inferior to what can be achieved by BP lowering and blockade of the RAS.

LIPID LOWERING

Hyperlipidemia accelerates renal injury in experimental models, and some, but not all, studies suggested that statins retard the progression of incipient and overt DN,[43] but these findings have not been universal.

Based on controlled evidence, there is no doubt that statins are indicated for cardiovascular protection in early stages of renal dysfunction, although the outcome of a controlled study in diabetics on hemodialysis was negative.[44]

CESSATION OF SMOKING

In diabetic patients, smoking is a predictor of microalbuminuria and of progressive loss of renal function,[45] and there is suggestive evidence that cessation of smoking improves the renal prognosis,[46] in addition to the beneficial effect on cardiovascular outcome, but unfortunately compliance with medical advice concerning this risk factor is limited.

OUTLOOK

Finally, a source of optimism are recent reports that it is not only possible to halt progression, but even to reverse existing glomerulosclerosis in animal experiments,[47] and this has been shown in diabetic patients with nephropathy after isolated pancreas transplantation as well.[48] Additionally, various studies using new approaches to DN (e.g., sulodexide, thiazolidiones, renin inhibitors) are ongoing.

MANAGEMENT OF DIABETICS WITH ADVANCED OR END-STAGE RENAL DISEASE

Once DN advances to chronic kidney disease (CKD) stages 3 through 5, patients ideally should be treated in a multidisciplinary DN clinic, comprising nephrologists, diabetologists, podiatrists, dietitians, and specialist renal and diabetes nurses. In addition to

measures aimed at delaying progression (see previous discussion) and comprehensive care of cardiovascular disease, controlling the various consequences of renal failure becomes an important issue (see Chapter 70).

DN is the leading cause of ESRD in most countries (Fig. 30.7). As discussed in Chapter 80, whereas the mean estimated GFR at the start of dialysis is 7 to 8 ml/min/1.73 m^2, in most dialysis populations, a higher threshold is usually used in diabetics (serum creatinine >6 mg/dl [530 μmol/l] or a creatinine clearance of <15 ml/min), as they tend to tolerate uremia poorly and are frequently troubled by sodium retention and fluid overload. The renal replacement choices for diabetic subjects with ESRD are similar to those for patients with other primary renal diseases, namely, peritoneal dialysis, hemodialysis, or transplantation, including combined kidney pancreas transplantation (see Chapter 98). Selection of the mode of dialysis is discussed in Chapter 80; advantages and disadvantages of each technique are outlined in Figure 30.8. A clear difference in outcome between peritoneal dialysis and hemodialysis has not been observed consistently. In diabetic patients eligible for kidney transplantation, 2-year survival is up to four times better for the transplanted patient compared to staying on dialysis, even when the patients are matched for similar health.[49] Five-year patient survival rate after transplantation is approximately 70%, which is worse than for nondiabetic transplant patients, but it compared favorably to a 5-year survival rate of <35% in diabetic dialysis patients. Unfortunately, many diabetics

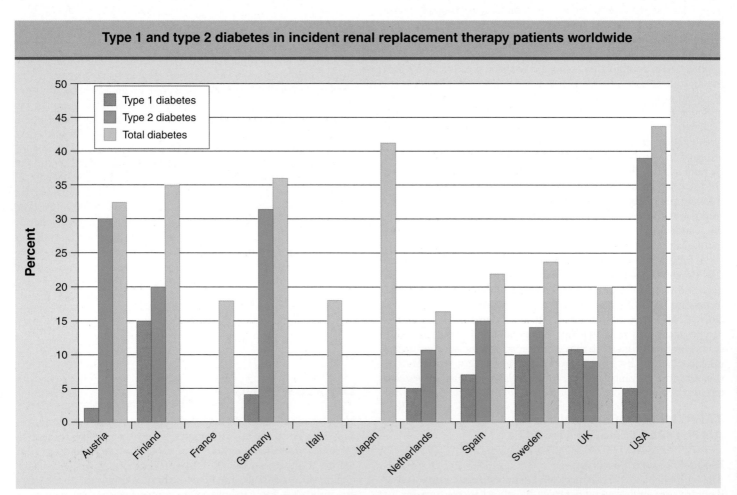

Figure 30.7 Worldwide representation of type 1 and 2 diabetes in incident renal replacement therapy patients in different countries. (Data from the ERA-EDTA registry (2003); Takashi Akiba: An overview of regular dialysis treatment in Japan as of Dec 31, 2004, published by the Japanese Society of Dialysis Therapy in 2005; U.S. Renal Data System, 2005 [www.usrds.org].)

Comparison of dialysis options for the diabetic patient

Parameters	Peritoneal Dialysis		Hemodialysis	
	Advantages	Disadvantages	Advantages	Disadvantages
Technique	No need for vascular access, better preservation of residual renal function	Low technique survival rate, high hospitalization rate, higher rate of infections	Better technique survival rate, lower hospitalization and infection rate	Frequent difficulty in obtaining good vascular access
Blood pressure	Good control, slow ultrafiltration, and fewer episodes of cardiovascular instability			Diffult control, more frequent hypotensive episodes (in particular, in patients with autonomic neuropathy)
Nutritional factors	Fewer dietary restrictions	Excessive weight gain, poor nutrition		Difficulty with fluid and dietary restrictions
Biochemical and metabolic control	Steady-state biochemical parameters	Worsening of blood glucose control and hyperlipidemia, increased insulin requirement	Efficient solute and water extraction	
Social factors	Maintains independence		Better medical surveillance	In most diabetics, cannot be performed at home

Figure 30.8   Comparison of dialysis options for the diabetic patient.

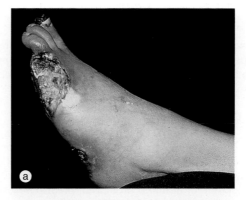

Prevention of diabetic foot complications

Identification of patients at risk

Education about foot care

Regular examination of the feet at clinic

Provision of appropriate footwear

Provision of podiatry services

Figure 30.9   The diabetic foot. *a*, Gangrenous ulcers in a diabetic caused by a combination of large- and small-vessel disease and neuropathy. *b*, Prevention of diabetic foot complications.

are excluded from transplantation because of the presence of comorbid conditions, particularly vascular disease or advanced age.

Search for Extrarenal Complications Caused by Microangiopathy and Macroangiopathy

As discussed in Chapter 29, even the asymptomatic diabetic patient with advanced CKD must be monitored at regular intervals for timely detection of micro- and macrovascular complications (ophthalmologic examination at half-yearly intervals, yearly cardiac and angiologic status including imaging of the carotid artery, foot inspection preferably at each visit). In particular, problems related to the diabetic foot are a major cause of hospital admission and nontraumatic amputation (Fig. 30.9). Diabetic microangiopathy of the foot is frequently complicated by diabetic and/or uremic polyneuropathy, both of which respond poorly to conventional treatments (see Chapter 76). Measures to prevent diabetic foot complications are shown in Figure 30.9. The situation is further aggravated by an increased risk in diabetics of soft tissue infections, in particular staphylococcal ones.

Cardiac Problems in the Diabetic Patient

Heart disease including myocardial infarction and angina pectoris, pathologic coronary angiography or the necessity for interventions is more frequent in diabetic (46%) than nondiabetic patients (32%) with renal failure.[50] If the diabetic patient on dialysis develops an acute coronary syndrome, the chances of survival are very poor.[51]

The cardiac mortality rate is 42% at 1 year and 75% at 5 years. The risk of an adverse cardiac outcome in the diabetic patient with ischemic heart disease is amplified because of the frequent coexistence of more severe left ventricular hypertrophy,[50] congestive heart failure,[52] disturbed sympathetic innervation,[53] and microvascular disease.[54]

A particular dilemma concerns the diagnosis of coronary heart disease (see also Chapter 71), and the best approach is still to proceed directly to coronary angiography if there is a suspicion of coronary heart disease, for example, left ventricular dilatation on echocardiography, regional contraction abnormalities on echocardiography, sudden deterioration of cardiac function with pulmonary edema, arrhythmia, or an increase in troponin T concentration. Treatment issues in patients with significant coronary disease and/or heart failure are discussed in Chapter 71.

Hypertension

At any given level of GFR, BP tends to be higher in diabetic compared to nondiabetic patients with CKD. As discussed, ACE inhibitors or ARBs are obligatory unless there are contraindications, for example, an acute increase in serum creatinine of ≥30% (in this case, assess for renal artery stenosis, hypovolemia, congestive heart failure) or hyperkalemia resistant to corrective maneuvers such as administration of loop diuretics, dietary potassium restriction, or correction of metabolic acidosis. An increase in serum creatinine of 10% to 20% is expected and should not deter from the administration of ACE inhibitors or ARBs. However, in patients with CKD stage 5, the introduction of ACE inhibitors may lower GFR to such an extent that acute dialysis becomes necessary. At this stage of renal dysfunction, these drugs are therefore no longer the antihypertensive medication of first choice. In the IDNT trial,[17] administration of ARBs extended the time until patients required dialysis. Therefore, the widely practiced habit of withdrawing ACE inhibitors or ARBs in advanced renal failure does not make sense, unless there has been an abrupt recent increase in serum creatinine (see also Chapter 69).

Because of their marked propensity to retain salt, patients with diabetic nephropathy are prone to develop hypervolemia and edema. Therefore, dietary salt restriction and administration of loop diuretics are usually indicated.

Glucose Control

Advancing CKD causes insulin resistance, impaired glucose tolerance, and hyperglycemia because a circulating factor interferes with the action of insulin. Since the insulin inhibitor is dialyzable, insulin resistance diminishes after the start of dialysis. At the same time, the half-life of insulin is prolonged, predisposing the patient to develop hypoglycemic episodes. This risk is further compounded by anorexia and by cumulation of most sulfonylurea compounds (with the exception of gliquidone or glimerpiride). Close monitoring of glycemia in diabetics with advanced CKD is therefore advisable. In the treatment of these patients, there is an increasing tendency to use short-acting insulins with or without a basis of long-acting insulin quite liberally to prevent catabolism and malnutrition. Insulin administration is obligatory during intercurrent illness, infection, surgery, or myocardial infarction.

Malnutrition

Diabetic patients with renal failure are often severely catabolic and tend to develop malnutrition (see also Chapter 77). This risk is particularly high during periods of intercurrent illness and fasting, but may also be the result of ill-advised recommendations to restrict protein intake. Anorectic obese patients with type 2 diabetes and advanced renal failure often undergo massive weight loss, leading to normalization of fasting glucose and even of glycemia after a glucose load. Low muscle mass because of wasting is an important reason for misjudging the severity of renal failure, leading, for example, to a delayed start of renal replacement therapy. Therefore, creatinine clearances should be measured or at least an estimate using the Cockroft-Gault or MDRD algorithm should be obtained.

Anemia

Patients with DN tend to have more severe anemia than nondiabetic patients (see also Chapter 72). There is some evidence that anemia is associated with more severe diabetic retinopathy and that reversal of anemia causes regression of retinopathy.[55] The role of anemia and its reversal by erythropoeisis stimulating agents in patients with peripheral artery disease is unclear.

Hyperparathyroidism and Bone Disease

Diabetic patients undergoing dialysis develop secondary hyperparathyroidism at a slower rate than nondiabetics and exhibit a predisposition to adynamic bone disease (see also Chapter 74). They also appear to accumulate aluminum more readily and are more susceptible to aluminum-induced bone disease. Aluminum-containing phosphate binders should always be avoided in the diabetic patient with advanced CKD.

REFERENCES

1. Gilbert RE, Tsalamandris C, Bach LA, et al: Long-term glycemic control and the rate of progression of early diabetic kidney disease. Kidney Int 1993;44:855–859.
2. The effect of intensive treatment of diabetes on the development and progression of long-term complications in insulin-dependent diabetes mellitus. The Diabetes Control and Complications Trial Research Group. N Engl J Med 1993;329:977–986.
3. Reichard P, Nilsson BY, Rosenqvist U: The effect of long-term intensified insulin treatment on the development of microvascular complications of diabetes mellitus. N Engl J Med 1993;329:304–309.
4. Ohkubo Y, Kishikawa H, Araki E, et al: Intensive insulin therapy prevents the progression of diabetic microvascular complications in Japanese patients with non-insulin-dependent diabetes mellitus: A randomized prospective 6-year study. Diabetes Res Clin Pract 1995;28:103–117.
5. Intensive blood-glucose control with sulphonylureas or insulin compared with conventional treatment and risk of complications in patients with type 2 diabetes (UKPDS 33). UK Prospective Diabetes Study (UKPDS) Group. Lancet 1998;352:837–853.
6. Alaveras AE, Thomas SM, Sagriotis A, et al: Promoters of progression of diabetic nephropathy: The relative roles of blood glucose and blood pressure control. Nephrol Dial Transplant 1997;12(Suppl 2): 71–74.
7. Lurbe E, Redon J, Kesani A, et al: Increase in nocturnal blood pressure and progression to microalbuminuria in type 1 diabetes. N Engl J Med 2002;347:797–805.
8. Mogensen CE: Progression of nephropathy in long-term diabetics with proteinuria and effect of initial anti-hypertensive treatment. Scand J Clin Lab Invest 1976;36:383–388.
9. Parving HH, Andersen AR, Smidt UM, et al: Reduced albuminuria during early and aggressive antihypertensive treatment of insulin-dependent diabetic patients with diabetic nephropathy. Diabetes Care 1981;4: 459–463.
10. Klahr S, Levey AS, Beck GJ, et al: The effects of dietary protein restriction and blood-pressure control on the progression of chronic renal disease. Modification of Diet in Renal Disease Study Group. N Engl J Med 1994;330:877–884.
11. Chobanian AV, Bakris GL, Black HR, et al: Seventh report of the Joint National Committee on Prevention, Detection, Evaluation, and Treatment of High Blood Pressure. Hypertension 2003;42:1206–1252.

12. Casas JP, Chua W, Loukogeorgakis S, et al: Effect of inhibitors of the renin-angiotensin system and other antihypertensive drugs on renal outcomes: Systematic review and meta-analysis. Lancet 2005;366:2026–2033.
13. Jafar TH, Schmid CH, Landa M, et al: Angiotensin-converting enzyme inhibitors and progression of nondiabetic renal disease. A meta-analysis of patient-level data. Ann Intern Med 2001;135:73–87.
14. Parving HH, Lehnert H, Brochner-Mortensen J, et al: The effect of irbesartan on the development of diabetic nephropathy in patients with type 2 diabetes. N Engl J Med 2001;345:870–878.
15. Pohl MA, Blumenthal S, Cordonnier DJ, et al: Independent and additive impact of blood pressure control and angiotensin II receptor blockade on renal outcomes in the irbesartan diabetic nephropathy trial: clinical implications and limitations. J Am Soc Nephrol 2005;16:3027–3037.
16. Lewis EJ, Hunsicker LG, Bain RP, Rohde RD: The effect of angiotensin-converting-enzyme inhibition on diabetic nephropathy. The Collaborative Study Group. N Engl J Med 1993;329:1456–1462.
17. Lewis EJ, Hunsicker LG, Clarke WR, et al: Renoprotective effect of the angiotensin-receptor antagonist irbesartan in patients with nephropathy due to type 2 diabetes. N Engl J Med 2001;345:851–860.
18. Brenner BM, Cooper ME, de Zeeuw D, et al: Effects of losartan on renal and cardiovascular outcomes in patients with type 2 diabetes and nephropathy. N Engl J Med 2001;345:861–869.
19. ACE Inhibitors in Diabetic Nephropathy Trialist Group: Should all patients with type 1 diabetes mellitus and microalbuminuria receive angiotensin-converting enzyme inhibitors? A meta-analysis of individual patient data. Ann Intern Med 2001;134:370–379.
20. Randomised placebo-controlled trial of effect of ramipril on decline in glomerular filtration rate and risk of terminal renal failure in proteinuric, non-diabetic nephropathy. The GISEN Group (Gruppo Italiano di Studi Epidemiologici in Nefrologia). Lancet 1997;349:1857–1863.
21. Kvetny J, Gregersen G, Pedersen RS: Randomized placebo controlled trial of perindopril in normotensive, normoalbuminuric patients with type 1 diabetes mellitus. QJM 2001;94:89–94.
22. Ravid M, Brosh D, Levi Z, et al: Use of enalapril to attenuate decline in renal function in normotensive, normoalbuminuric patients with type 2 diabetes mellitus. A randomized, controlled trial. Ann Intern Med 1998;128:982–988.
23. Ruggenenti P, Fassi A, Ilieva AP, et al: Preventing microalbuminuria in type 2 diabetes. N Engl J Med 2004;351:1941–1951.

24. Ravid M, Savin H, Jutrin I, et al: Long-term stabilizing effect of angiotensin-converting enzyme inhibition on plasma creatinine and on proteinuria in normotensive type II diabetic patients. Ann Intern Med 1993;118:577–581.

25. Ahmad J, Shafique S, Abidi SM, et al: Effect of 5-year enalapril therapy on progression of microalbuminuria and glomerular structural changes in type 1 diabetic subjects. Diabetes Res Clin Pract 2003;60:131–138.

26. Hebert LA, Bain RP, Verme D, et al: Remission of nephrotic range proteinuria in type I diabetes. Collaborative Study Group. Kidney Int 1994;46:1688–1693.

27. Schrier RW, Estacio RO, Esler A, et al: Effects of aggressive blood pressure control in normotensive type 2 diabetic patients on albuminuria, retinopathy and strokes. Kidney Int 2002;61:1086–1097.

28. Barnett AH, Bain SC, Bouter P, et al: Angiotensin-receptor blockade versus converting-enzyme inhibition in type 2 diabetes and nephropathy. N Engl J Med 2004;351:1952–1961.

29. Bakris GL, Williams M, Dworkin L, et al: Preserving renal function in adults with hypertension and diabetes: A consensus approach. National Kidney Foundation Hypertension and Diabetes Executive Committees Working Group. Am J Kidney Dis 2000;36:646–661.

30. Mogensen CE, Neldam S, Tikkanen I, et al: Randomised controlled trial of dual blockade of renin-angiotensin system in patients with hypertension, microalbuminuria, and non-insulin dependent diabetes: The Candesartan and Lisinopril Microalbuminuria (CALM) study. BMJ 2000; 321:1440–1444.

31. Rossing K, Jacobsen P, Pietraszek L, et al: Renoprotective effects of adding angiotensin II receptor blocker to maximal recommended doses of ACE inhibitor in diabetic nephropathy: A randomized double-blind crossover trial. Diabetes Care 2003;26:2268–2274.

32. Weinberg AJ, Zappe DH, Ashton M, et al: Safety and tolerability of high-dose angiotensin receptor blocker therapy in patients with chronic kidney disease: A pilot study. Am J Nephrol 2004;24:340–345.

33. Rossing K, Schjoedt KJ, Jensen BR, et al: Enhanced renoprotective effects of ultrahigh doses of irbesartan in patients with type 2 diabetes and microalbuminuria. Kidney Int 2005;68:1190–1198.

34. Schjoedt KJ, Andersen S, Rossing P, et al: Aldosterone escape during blockade of the renin-angiotensin-aldosterone system in diabetic nephropathy is associated with enhanced decline in glomerular filtration rate. Diabetologia 2004;47:1936–1939.

35. Greene EL, Kren S, Hostetter TH: Role of aldosterone in the remnant kidney model in the rat. J Clin Invest 1996;98:1063–1068.

36. Sato A, Hayashi K, Naruse M, et al: Effectiveness of aldosterone blockade in patients with diabetic nephropathy. Hypertension 2003;41:64–68.

37. Jafar TH, Stark PC, Schmid CH, et al: Progression of chronic kidney disease: The role of blood pressure control, proteinuria, and angiotensin-converting enzyme inhibition: A patient-level meta-analysis. Ann Intern Med 2003;139:244–252.

38. Remuzzi G, Benigni A, Remuzzi A: Mechanisms of progression and regression of renal lesions of chronic nephropathies and diabetes. J Clin Invest 2006;116:288–296.

39. de Zeeuw D, Remuzzi G, Parving HH, et al: Proteinuria, a target for renoprotection in patients with type 2 diabetic nephropathy: Lessons from RENAAL. Kidney Int 2004;65:2309–2320.

40. Adler AI, Stevens RJ, Manley SE, et al: Development and progression of nephropathy in type 2 diabetes: the United Kingdom Prospective Diabetes Study (UKPDS 64). Kidney Int 2003;63:225–232.

41. Gaede PH, Jepsen PV, Larsen JN, et al: The Steno-2 study. Intensive multifactorial intervention reduces the occurrence of cardiovascular disease in patients with type 2 diabetes]. Ugeskr Laeger 2003;165:2658–2661.

42. Pedrini MT, Levey AS, Lau J, et al: The effect of dietary protein restriction on the progression of diabetic and nondiabetic renal diseases: A meta-analysis. Ann Intern Med 1996;124:627–632.

43. Tonolo G, Ciccarese M, Brizzi P, et al: Reduction of albumin excretion rate in normotensive microalbuminuric type 2 diabetic patients during long-term simvastatin treatment. Diabetes Care 1997;20:1891–1895.

44. Wanner C, Krane V, Marz W, et al: Atorvastatin in patients with type 2 diabetes mellitus undergoing hemodialysis. N Engl J Med 2005;353:238–248.

45. Ritz E, Ogata H, Orth SR: Smoking: A factor promoting onset and progression of diabetic nephropathy. Diabetes Metab 2000;26(Suppl 4):54–63.

46. Sawicki PT, Didjurgeit U, Muhlhauser I, et al: Smoking is associated with progression of diabetic nephropathy. Diabetes Care 1994;17:126–131.

47. Adamczak M, Gross ML, Krtil J, et al: Reversal of glomerulosclerosis after high-dose enalapril treatment in subtotally nephrectomized rats. J Am Soc Nephrol 2003;14:2833–2842.

48. Fioretto P, Steffes MW, Sutherland DE, et al: Reversal of lesions of diabetic nephropathy after pancreas transplantation. N Engl J Med 1998;339:69–75.

49. Wolfe RA, Ashlay VB, Milford EL, et al: Comparison of mortality in all patients on dialysis, patients on dialysis awaiting transplantation and recipients of first cadaveric transplants. N Engl J Med 1999;34:1722–1730.

50. Foley RN, Culleton BF, Parfrey PS, et al: Cardiac disease in diabetic end-stage renal disease. Diabetologia 1997;40:1307–1312.

51. Herzog CA, Ma JZ, Collins AJ: Poor long-term survival after acute myocardial infarction among patients on long-term dialysis. N Engl J Med 1998;339:799–805.

52. Foley RN, Parfrey PS, Sarnak MJ: Epidemiology of cardiovascular disease in chronic renal disease. J Am Soc Nephrol 1998;9:S16–S23.

53. Standl E, Schnell O: A new look at the heart in diabetes mellitus: from ailing to failing. Diabetologia 2000;43:1455–1469.

54. Amann K, Ritz E: Microvascular disease—the Cinderella of uraemic heart disease. Nephrol Dial Transplant 2000;15:1493–1503.

55. Sinclair SH, DelVecchio C, Levin A: Treatment of anemia in the diabetic patient with retinopathy and kidney disease. Am J Ophthalmol 2003; 135:740–743.

CHAPTER

31 Normal Blood Pressure Control and the Evaluation of Hypertension

Friedrich C. Luft, William J. Lawton, and Gerald F. DiBona

NORMAL BLOOD PRESSURE CONTROL

Systemic arterial blood pressure (BP), or the pressure of the blood within the arteries exerted against the arterial wall, is produced by the contraction of the left ventricle (producing blood flow) and by the resistance of the arteries and arterioles. Systolic blood pressure (SBP), or maximum BP, occurs during left ventricular systole. Diastolic blood pressure (DBP), or minimum BP, occurs during ventricular diastole. The difference between SBP and DBP is the pulse pressure.[1] The mean arterial pressure (MAP) is clinically defined as the DBP + one third of the pulse pressure.

Blood flow (Q) is defined by Ohm's law and varies directly with the change in pressure (P) across a blood vessel and inversely with the resistance R (defined as Q = P/R). Rearrangement shows that pressure varies directly with blood flow and resistance (P = QR). Ohm's law suffices for an overall view of the circulation. However, for a more detailed picture of the resistance to flow in any given vessel, the relationship of Hagen-Poiseuille should be applied where

$$Q = \Delta P \times (\pi\, r^4/8\, L) \times (1/\eta).$$

Here r is the radius of the pipe, L is its length, and η is the coefficient of viscosity. Thus, as the lumen of a vessel decreases, the pressure will increase to the fourth power of the radius for the same blood flow. In other words, a 50% reduction in radius will require a 16-fold increase in pressure to maintain equivalent flow.

Normal BP control can be related to cardiac output and the total peripheral resistance and is dependent on the heart, the blood vessels, the extracellular volume, the kidneys, the nervous system, humoral factors, and cellular events at the membrane and within the cell (Fig. 31.1). The stroke volume (liters/minute) and the heart rate determine the cardiac output. In turn, the stroke volume is dependent in part on intravascular volume regulated by the kidneys as well as on myocardial contractility. The latter is a complex function involving sympathetic and parasympathetic control of heart rate, intrinsic activity of the cardiac conduction system, complex membrane transport and cellular events requiring influx of calcium, which lead to myocardial fiber shortening and relaxation, and the effects of humoral substances (e.g., catecholamines) in stimulating heart rate and myocardial fiber tension.

The regulation of the total peripheral resistance also involves complex interactive mechanisms, including baroreflexes and sympathetic nervous system activity, response to neurohumoral substances and endothelial factors, myogenic responses and intercellular events mediated by receptors and mechanisms for signal transduction.[2] For example, there are two major neural reflex arcs. Baroreflexes are derived from high-pressure baroreceptors in the aortic arch and carotid sinus and low-pressure cardiopulmonary baroreceptors in ventricles and atria. These receptors respond to stretch (high pressure) or filling pressures (low pressure) and send tonic inhibitory signals to the brainstem (nucleus tractus solitarius). If BP increases and tonic inhibition increases, inhibition of sympathetic efferent outflow occurs and decreases vascular resistance and heart rate. However, if BP decreases, less tonic inhibition ensues from the baroreflexes and both heart rate and peripheral vascular resistance increase, thereby increasing BP. In addition, the neural control of renal function produces alterations in renal blood flow, glomerular filtration rate (GFR), excretion of sodium, and water, and release of renin and other vasoactive substances. These factors, in turn, have effects on the regulation of intravascular volume, vascular resistance, and BP.[3]

Numerous vasoactive substances have effects on blood vessels, the heart, the kidneys, and the central nervous system (CNS) and often serve to counterbalance one another. Some of these substances and membrane and cellular events are shown in Figures 31.2 and 31.3. The renin angiotensin system (RAS) is an extremely important effector system that regulates both volume and peripheral vascular resistance. Renin is an enzyme that cleaves angiotensinogen to generate angiotensin (Ang) I, which is converted by angiotensin-converting enzyme (ACE) to Ang II. Ang II, in turn, constricts vascular smooth muscle; stimulates aldosterone secretion; potentiates sympathetic nervous system activity; stimulates salt and water reabsorption in the proximal tubule; stimulates prostaglandin, nitric oxide, and endothelin release; and increases thirst and is a growth factor. When present in excess, Ang II can induce remodeling, inflammation, and vasculopathy. Aldosterone mediates changes in sodium channels in distal renal tubular epithelium, leading to sodium retention and potassium excretion. The hormone may also function as a growth factor and exerts complex genomic and nongenomic events via the mineralocorticoid receptor in vascular cells and in the heart.

Renin and aldosterone are commonly measured in patients with hypertension. Plasma concentrations of both are inversely related to salt intake and are influenced by various medications. Aldosterone is measured by radioimmunoassay. Plasma renin is measured as plasma renin activity based on the generation of Ang I in the presence of Ang I–degrading enzyme inhibitors or as plasma renin concentration by immunoassay (involving either

Some factors involved in the regulation of blood pressure

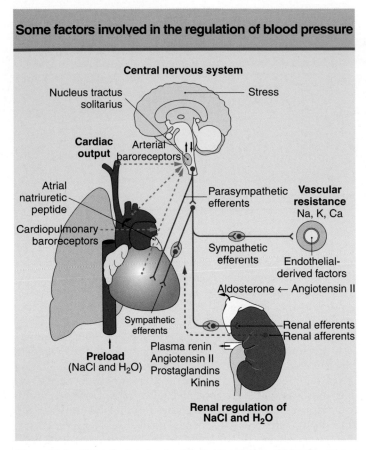

Figure 31.1 **Some factors involved in the regulation of blood pressure.**

Cellular events linked to the activity of vasoactive substances

Membrane sodium transport: Na^+-K^+-ATPasep; Na^+-Li^+ countertransport
Na^+-H^+ exchange; Na^+-Ca^{2+} exchange; Na^+-K^+-$2Cl^-$ transport; passive Na^+ transport
Potassium channels
Cell volume and intracellular pH changes
Calcium channels
Signal transduction via G proteins, cyclic nucleotides, inositol phosphates, protein kinases
Rho-Rho-kinase signaling

Figure 31.3 **Cellular events linked to the activity of vasoactive substances.**

Vasoactive substances that modulate blood pressure

Vasoactive Substances

Group	Compound	Effect
Catecholamines	Norepinephrine, epinephrine, dopamine	Adrenergic receptors (α_1, α_2, β_1, β_2) causing protein phosphorylation and increased intracellular calcium via G proteins linked to ion channels or second messengers (cyclic nucleotides, phosphoinositide hydrolysis)
Renin angiotensin system	Angiotensin II	Angiotensin receptors (AT1, AT2, AT4) causing increased intracellular calcium and protein phosphorylation via second messenger, phosphoinositide hydrolysis, and activated protein kinases. Aldosterone stimulation
Arachidonic acid products	Prostaglandins: prostaglandin E, prostacyclin, thromboxanes. Lipoxygenase enzyme products: leukotrienes, hydroxyeicosatetraenoates	
Endothelium-derived factors	Endothelium-derived relaxing factor (nitric oxide). Endothelins (ET-1, ET-2, ET-3). Urotensin II	Increased levels of cylic guanosine monophosphate cause activation of protein kinases. G proteins activate phospholipase C and L-type calcium channels. Class 2 G protein–coupled receptor
Kallikrein–kinin system	Bradykinin	
Natriuretic peptides (NPs)	Atrial, brain, and C-type NPs	Activation of three receptor types; further effects mediated by cGMP
Other substances	Acetylcholine, adenosine, insulin, neuropeptide Y, serotonin, sex hormones (estrogens, progesterone, androgens), glucocorticoids, other mineralocorticoids, substance P, vasopressin, renalase	

Figure 31.2 **Vasoactive substances that modulate blood pressure.**

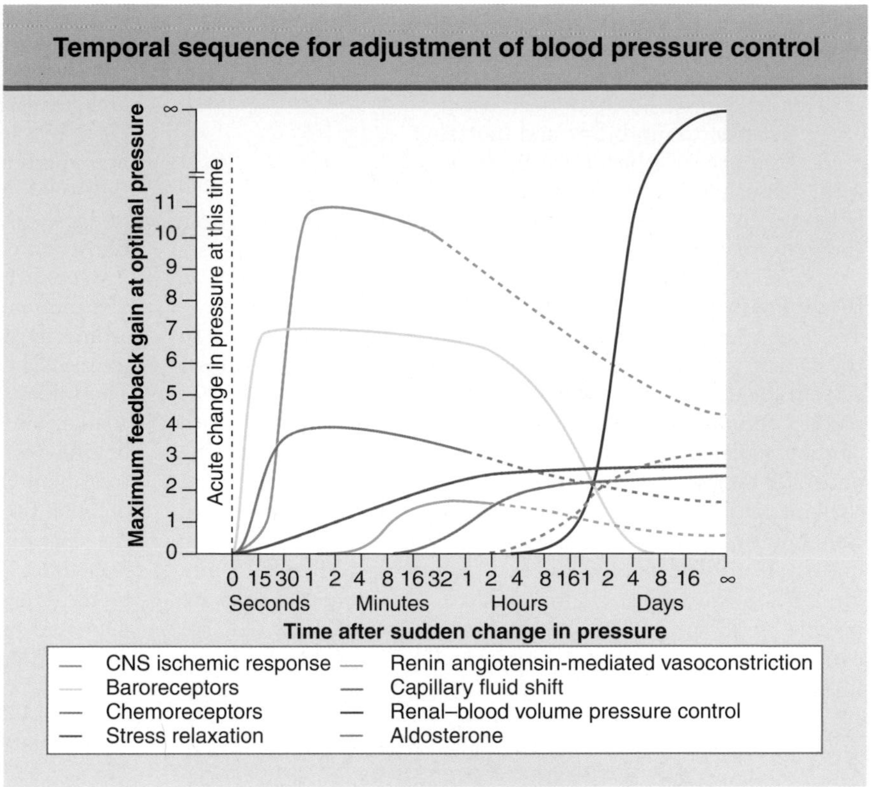

Figure 31.4 Temporal sequence for adjustment of blood pressure control. Degree of activity, expressed as feedback gain, of several arterial pressure control systems at various times after a sudden change in arterial pressure. Note the infinite gain of the renal-volume mechanism for pressure control. CNS, central nervous system. (From Guyton AC, Hall JE: Dominant role of the kidneys in long-term regulation of arterial pressure and in hypertension: The integrated system for pressure control. In Guyton AC, Hall JE, eds: Textbook of Medical Physiology, 10th ed. Philadelphia: WB Saunders, 2000, pp 221–234.)

an immunoradiometric assay using a second developing antibody bearing radioactive iodine or a chemoluminometric assay using an acridinium-labeled second antibody).

The second major effector system is the sympathetic nervous system. Nerve endings release norepinephrine. This potent neurotransmitter is a vasoconstrictor via α-adrenergic receptor–mediated mechanisms. Vascular cells, renal cells, and many other cells (e.g., adipocytes) are innervated. Epinephrine increases heart rate, stroke volume, and systolic BP (SBP) via α- and β-adrenoceptors. The hormone is released from the adrenal medulla. The evidence that increased sympathetic tone has long-term influences on cardiovascular regulation and that disturbed sympathetic tone may cause hypertension is compelling. In the kidneys, sympathetic nerves are important mediators of renin release. Furthermore, innervation of each individual nephron has an important bearing on sodium reabsorption. Thus, the sympathetic nervous system regulates both effective circulating fluid volume and peripheral vascular resistance.

Prostaglandin E and prostacyclin act to counterbalance vasoconstriction by Ang II and norepinephrine. Additional vascular cell–derived vasoconstrictor substances, such as urotensin, are being investigated. Two endothelium-derived factors have opposite effects on the blood vessels: nitric oxide is a vasodilator, whereas the endothelins are vasoconstrictors. The kallikrein-kinin system produces vasodilator kinins that, in turn, may stimulate prostaglandins and nitric oxide. Natriuretic peptides induce vasodilation, induce natriuresis, and inhibit other vasoconstrictors (renin-angiotensin, sympathetic nervous system, and endothelin). Renalase is a recently discovered flavin adenine dinucleotide–dependent amine oxidase that is secreted by the kidney, circulates in the blood, and modulates cardiac function and systemic BP. It acts by metabolizing catecholamines, and its discovery should facilitate our understanding of sympathetic regulation.[4] Postreceptor intracellular signaling events are also important regulatory sites of peripheral vascular resistance. For

instance, recent studies have revealed important roles for the small guanosine triphosphatase Rho and its effector, Rho-associated kinase (Rho kinase) in Ca^{2+}-independent regulation of smooth muscle contraction. The Rho-Rho-kinase pathway modulates the level of phosphorylation of the myosin light chain of myosin II, mainly through inhibition of myosin phosphatase, and contributes to agonist-induced Ca^{2+} sensitization in smooth muscle contraction. Rho-Rho-kinase mechanisms also participate in a variety of the cellular functions of nonmuscle cells, such as stress-fiber formation, cytokinesis, and cell migration. A specific pharmacologic Rho-kinase inhibitor (fasudil) has been developed that may have utility in treated cerebral artery spasm and other forms of severe vascular constriction.[5]

Guyton and Hall[1] have analyzed the temporal sequence for adjustment of BP. In their analysis, CNS mechanisms (e.g., baroreflexes) provide regulation of the circulation within seconds to minutes. Other mechanisms, such as the renin angiotensin aldosterone system and fluid shifts, occur over minutes to hours. Only the kidneys have the ability for long-term adjustments in BP, predominantly through regulation of extracellular volume (Fig. 31.4).[1] This framework served for over 40 years but does not appear to be strictly true. Indeed, recent evidence indicates that long-term afferent baroreflex stimulation via an electrical device can lower BP chronically in several different animal models.[6] The critical role for the kidney in the long-term control of BP received strong support from kidney cross-transplantation experiments. Nevertheless, precisely such experiments have recently shown that both intrarenal and extrarenal mechanisms are involved.[7]

DEFINITION OF HYPERTENSION

Concepts

BP is distributed as a continuum in the general population in a gaussian fashion. Thus, any definition of hypertension is necessarily arbitrary. Since hypertension is usually asymptomatic, patients do not "suffer" from hypertension, only from the sequelae or the treatments. In defining hypertension, three conceptual approaches have been used:

1. Relation to morbidity and mortality
2. Excess over arbitrary cutoff points
3. Thresholds for therapeutic benefit

Schemes to define hypertension have attempted to take these three approaches into account.

Blood Pressure in Relation to Morbidity and Mortality

The first approach defines hypertension by relating BP levels to the risk of morbidity and mortality, which therefore provides a system for the initiation of antihypertensive therapy. Numerous studies demonstrate that the association of SBP and DBP with cardiovascular and renal complications is continuous over the entire BP range.[8] Data from observational studies involving more than one million individuals have indicated that death from both ischemic heart disease and stroke increases progressively and linearly from BP levels as low as 115 mm Hg SBP and 75 mm Hg DBP upward (Figs. 31.5 and 31.6). The increased risks are present in all age groups ranging from 40 to 89 years old. For every 20-mm Hg SBP or 10-mm Hg DBP increase in BP, the mortality from both ischemic heart disease and stroke doubles. Based on these data, the Joint National Committee (JNC)-7 report introduced a new classification that includes the term *prehypertension* for those with BP ranging from 120 to 139 mm Hg SBP and/or 80 to 89 mm Hg DBP.[9] The designation prehypertensive identifies persons in whom early intervention (lifestyle) could reduce BP or avoid further increases.

Elevation of Blood Pressure by Arbitrary Cut Points

A second approach defines hypertension using the frequency distribution within a population. This statistical approach will arbitrarily designate values above a certain percentile as hypertensive. This method is used in defining hypertension in children. The values for defining hypertension will vary depending on age, gender, and race.[10] This frequency distribution method is not helpful for determining a value for initiating antihypertensive treatment but is useful in epidemiologic studies, for example, defining the prevalence of hypertension in various age groups or the changing prevalence of hypertension in a given population over time. For example, the prevalence of hypertension in adults in the United States, defined as BP of ≥140/90 mm Hg, has increased progressively from 11% of the population in 1939 to 31% in 2000.

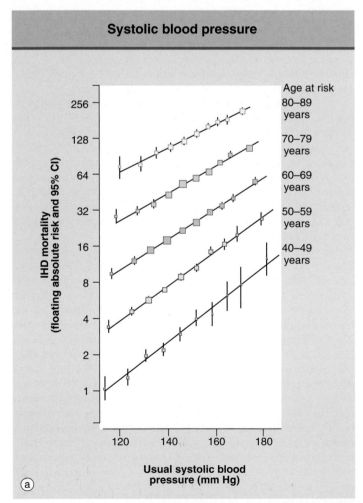

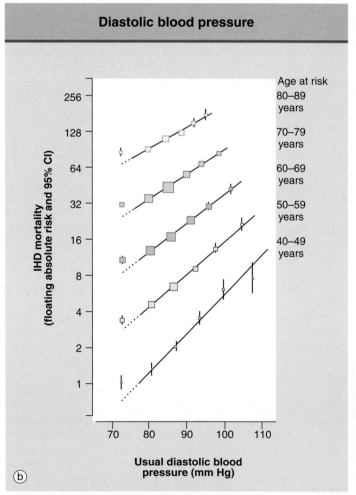

Figure 31.5 Ischemic heart disease (IHD) mortality rate in each decade of age versus usual blood pressure at the start of that decade. *a*, Systolic blood pressure. *b*, Diastolic blood pressure. Floating absolute risk corrects for the absolute death rate within a particular community. The size of the squares correlates inversely with the variance of the data collected for that data point. CI, confidence interval. (From Lewington S, Clarke R, Qizilbash N, et al: Prospective Studies Collaboration: Age-specific relevance of usual blood pressure to vascular mortality: A meta-analysis of individual data for one million adults in 61 prospective studies. Lancet 2002;360:1903–1913.)

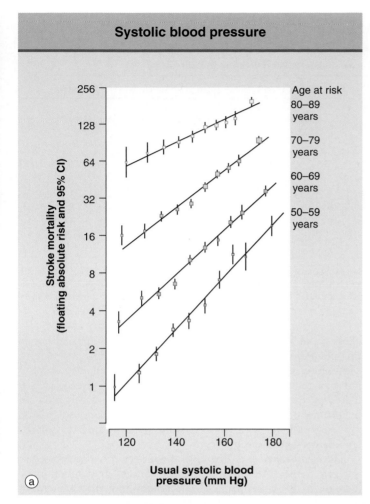

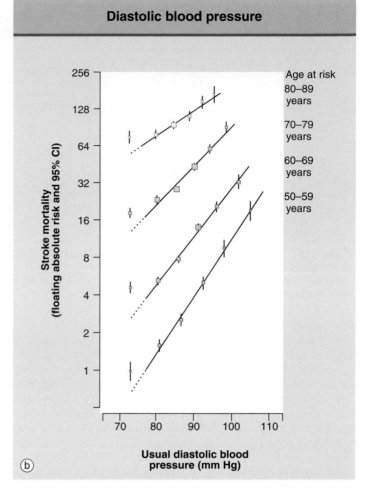

Figure 31.6 **Stroke mortality rate in each decade of age versus usual blood pressure at the start of that decade.** *a*, Systolic blood pressure. *b*, Diastolic blood pressure. Floating absolute risk corrects for the absolute death rate within a particular community. The size of the squares correlates inversely with the variance of the data collected for that data point. CI, confidence interval. (From Lewington S, Clarke R, Qizilbash N, et al: Prospective Studies Collaboration: Age-specific relevance of usual blood pressure to vascular mortality: A meta-analysis of individual data for one million adults in 61 prospective studies. Lancet 2002;360:1903-1913.)

Threshold of Therapeutic Benefit

The third concept for defining hypertension involves an understanding of data from randomized trials that have demonstrated reductions in mortality and morbidity. As a result of these clinical trials, consensus has been reached on intervention levels for moderate and severe hypertension but not for lower levels of hypertension. The HOT Study (Hypertension Optimal Treatment) showed benefits of lowering BP to 138/83 mm Hg. However, for diabetic persons in that study, the values may be lower. Progression of renal disease has also been a clinical endpoint. For nephrologists the level of BP control in diabetic and nondiabetic renal disease is particularly important. The Renoprotection in Patients with Nondiabetic Chronic Renal Disease (REIN-2) Trial, African American Study of Kidney Disease and Hypertension (AASK) Trial, and the Modification of Diet in Renal Disease Study were all designed to evaluate the effect of lower BP on kidney disease, not cardiovascular disease.[11] The variable outcomes from these trials may be a consequence of differences in levels of proteinuria, antihypertensive agents, and duration of follow-up.

Operational Definitions
European Society of Hypertension and Joint National Committee

The European Society of Hypertension (ESH) divided normotension into three categories, namely optimum (<120/<80 mm Hg),

normal (120 to 129/80 to 84 mm Hg), and high-normal (130 to 139/85 to 89) mm Hg (Fig. 31.7). Hypertension was divided into mild (140 to 159/90 to 99 mm Hg), moderate (160 to 179/100 to 109 mm Hg), and severe (>180/>110 mm Hg).[12] The ESH also gave values for automated 24-hour BP measurements, divided into daytime and nighttime. In the United States, the JNC 7 defined hypertension for individuals 18 years of age and older.[9] The committee settled on normal (<120/80 mm Hg), prehypertension (120 to 139/80 to 89 mm Hg), stage 1 hypertension (140 to 159/90 to 99 mm Hg), and stage 2 hypertension, given in Figure 31.8. For children, the JNC considers that BP at the 95th percentile or higher at each age is elevated.

Clinicians assign hypertensive patients into a category of overall risk based not only on BP. Age, gender, and ethnicity cannot be altered and are important risk factors. However, cholesterol, high-density lipoprotein (HDL) cholesterol, smoking, control of diabetes, and left ventricular hypertrophy are readily modified (Figs. 31.9 and 31.10).[13] Any degree of decreased renal function is now recognized as an important independent cardiovascular risk factor.[14] The same is true for proteinuria, starting with the barely detectable amount of >6 mg/day albumin. Figure 31.11 gives the JNC 7 recommendations for follow-up and management of BP findings in a given individual.

European Society of Hypertension consensus classification (Sendai, Japan, 2001)					
Conventional Blood Pressure Measurement*		**Ambulatory Blood Pressure Measurement†**			
Category	Boundaries	Measurement	P95‡	Normotension	Hypertension
Normotension		Ambulatory			
Optimum	<120/<80	24-h	132/82	<130/<80	>135/85
Normal	120–129/80–84	Daytime	138/87	>135/<85	>140/90
High-normal	130–139/85–89	Nighttime	123/74	<120/<70	>125/75
Hypertension		Self-recorded			
Grade I (mild)	140–159/90–99	Morning	136/85	<135/85	>140/90
Subgroup borderline	140–149/90–94	Evening	138/86	<135/85	>140/90
Grade II (moderate)	160–179/100–109	Both	137/85	<135/85	>140/90
Grade III (severe)	>180/>110				
Isolated systolic hypertension	>140/<90				
Subgroup borderline	140–149/<90				

Figure 31.7 European Society of Hypertension consensus classification (Sendai, Japan, 2001). Blood pressure readings are in mm Hg. *Consensus classification proposed by the European Society of Hypertension/European Society of Cardiology guidelines.[12] †Classification proposed at the Eighth International Consensus Conference on Ambulatory Blood Pressure Measurement (Sendai, Japan, October 2001). ‡Mean of 95th percentiles in subjects who on conventional blood pressure measurement were normotensive in large-scale studies.

Special Definitions

Borderline Hypertension—Prehypertension

Despite lack of uniform agreement, borderline hypertension is most usefully defined as BP between 130 to 139/85 to 89 mm Hg that may decrease to levels below this with rest. Estimates of borderline hypertension have ranged between 16% and 30% of the adult population. Although some individuals with borderline hypertension will progress to fixed hypertension, the frequency with which this occurs is not clear. Some estimates indicate only 12% develop sustained hypertension during a 20-year follow-up. However, weight gains of 15 to 20 lb (6.8 to 9.1 kg) in this group may be associated with a higher risk of developing fixed or sustained hypertension. Some of these individuals have been shown to have a high cardiac output and increased catecholamine turnover. Borderline hypertension may represent an exaggeration of normal physiologic responses to stress. Individuals with borderline pressures may have a greater frequency of obesity, abnormal lipids, and other cardiovascular risk factors and need to be followed closely. Since all BP is labile, the term labile hypertension is not helpful and should not be used.

White Coat Hypertension

White coat hypertension is defined as that seen in individuals in whom BP levels are normal during usual daily activities but hypertensive in a clinical setting. Normal pressures outside the physician's office have been determined by measurement with standard techniques or by ambulatory BP recordings. White coat hypertensives are more likely to be young women with a lower body weight, although this phenomenon can be seen at all ages including the elderly. The white coat phenomenon is seen less frequently when a nurse or technician takes the BP rather than a physician. Estimates of white coat hypertension are approximately 20% of hypertensive persons. Guidelines have been prepared to assist in assessing patients with isolated clinic hypertension or isolated ambulatory hypertension.[15]

The significance and prognosis of white coat hypertension are unclear. Some studies show that the office- or clinic-induced increase in BP is benign. Other studies show that white coat hypertension is characterized by increases in left ventricular mass index at levels intermediate between normotensive and persistently hypertensive persons.[16] White coat hypertensive patients have impaired diastolic function and higher levels of catecholamines, plasma renin activity, aldosterone, and low-density lipoprotein (LDL) cholesterol. There is also some evidence that subjects with white coat hypertension may be at increased risk of developing persistent hypertension.[16] Thus, each patient with white coat hypertension needs evaluation for cardiovascular risk factors and correction of these, if present, as well as continued follow-up.

Persistent Hypertension

Persistent hypertension, also called sustained hypertension, defines individuals whose BP levels are elevated both inside and outside the clinic setting, including at home and during usual daily activities. It should be noted that office BP readings are frequently higher in sustained hypertensives compared to their ambulatory BP.

Pseudohypertension

Pseudohypertension has been defined as "a condition in which the cuff pressure is inappropriately higher when compared to the intra-arterial pressure because of excessive atheromatosis and/or medial hypertrophy in the arterial tree."[17] The presence of pseudohypertension can be suspected by the Osler maneuver. The BP cuff is inflated above the SBP (detected by auscultation). If either the brachial or radial artery remains palpable, when pulseless, the patient is considered to be Osler maneuver positive. In general, patients with pseudohypertension have intra-arterial DBP measurements 10 to 15 mm Hg below indirect BP cuff diastolic measurements. None of the definitions specifically address the SBP. If a patient is suspected

JNC 7 classification of blood pressure for adults (2003)		
BP Classification	SBP (mm Hg)	DBP (mm Hg)
Normal	<120	and <80
Prehypertension	120–139	or 80–89
Stage 1 hypertension	140–159	or 90–99
Stage 2 hypertension	≥160	or ≥100

Figure 31.8 The Joint National Committee 7 classification of blood pressure for adults (2003). BP, blood pressure; DBP, diastolic blood pressure; SBP, systolic blood pressure.

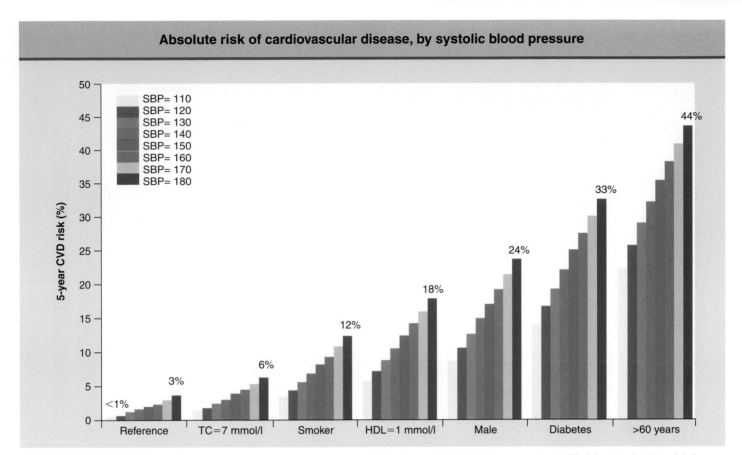

Figure 31.9 Absolute risk of cardiovascular disease over 5 years in patients by systolic blood pressure at specified levels of other risk factors. Reference category is a nondiabetic, nonsmoking woman aged 50 years with total cholesterol (TC) of 4 mmol/l (155 mg/dl) and high-density lipoprotein (HDL) level of 1.6 mmol/l. Risks are given for systolic blood pressure (SBP) levels of 110, 120, 130, 140, 150, 160, 170, and 180 mm Hg. In the other categories, additional risk factors are added consecutively, for example, the diabetes category is a diabetic 50-year-old male cigarette smoker with a total cholesterol of 7 mmol/l (270 mg/dl) and HDL of 1 mmol/l (39 mg/dl). CVD, cardiovascular disease.

of having pseudohypertension, confirmation by intra-arterial pressure measurement should be considered with decision of treatment based on the intra-arterial findings.

Isolated Systolic Hypertension Arteriosclerosis, characterized by remodeling and stiffening of large elastic arteries, is the most significant manifestation of vascular aging.[18] The increased stiffening is believed to originate from a gradual mechanical senescence of the elastic network, alterations in crosslinking of extracellular matrix components, fibrosis, and calcification of elastic fibers (medial elastocalcinosis). The stiffening of large arteries reduces their capacitance and accelerates pulse wave velocity, thus contributing to a widening of pulse pressure and to the increased prevalence of isolated systolic hypertension (ISH) with age. Perhaps as a consequence, the increase in SBP continues throughout life, in contrast to DBP that increases until age 50 years and decreases later in life (Fig. 31.12). Diastolic hypertension is more common before the age of 50 years, either alone or in combination with elevated SBP. After age 50 years, SBP is more important than DBP.

ISH is defined as SBP of ≥140 mm Hg and DBP <90 mm Hg. Others have defined ISH as SBP >160 mm Hg and DBP <90 mm Hg. The prevalence of ISH increases with age and affects most individuals older than age 60 years. In the Framingham study, elevations in SBP determined a greater risk of both heart attacks and strokes compared to elevations of DBP. Indeed, JNC 7 assigned SBP a higher level of importance than DBP.[9] Several clinical trials have clearly demonstrated that treatment of

hypertension significantly reduces the cardiovascular event rate.[19] Nevertheless, controversy exists as to the choice of antihypertensive agents. Elderly hypertensive patients should be treated aggressively to the same target blood pressures identified for younger patients. However, it is appropriate to initiate treatment with lower doses of antihypertensive agents and to bring the pressure down more slowly, monitoring for orthostatic hypotension, impaired cognition, and electrolyte abnormalities.

Accelerated Hypertension/Hypertensive Crises Accelerated hypertension is severe diastolic hypertension (usually >120 mm Hg) in the presence of grade III retinopathy (arteriolosclerotic changes of arteriolar narrowing and nicking plus hypertensive changes of flame-shaped hemorrhage and soft exudates).[20] In the past, malignant hypertension referred to severe diastolic hypertension and grade IV retinopathy (grade III plus papilledema). Since the prognosis for untreated severe hypertension with grade III or IV retinopathy is so poor, there is little clinical rationale for using the two terms separately. Accelerated malignant hypertension is preferred for severe diastolic hypertension with fundoscopic findings as noted previously and usually represents a hypertensive urgency, requiring treatment and decrease of BP within hours. Hypertensive emergencies are clinical conditions in which severe hypertension must be lowered within minutes. Emergencies include acute dissection of the aorta, acute left ventricular failure, intracerebral hemorrhage, and crises caused by pheochromocytoma, drug abuse, and eclampsia.

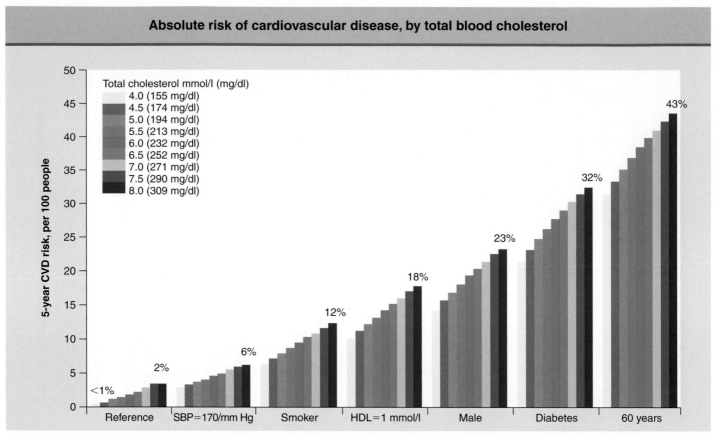

Absolute risk of cardiovascular disease, by total blood cholesterol

Figure 31.10 **Absolute risk of cardiovascular disease over 5 years in patients by blood total cholesterol at specified levels of other risk factors.** Reference category is a 50-year-old nonsmoker, nondiabetic woman with systolic blood pressure of 110 mm Hg, high-density lipoprotein (HDL) level of 1.6 mmol/l (62 mg/dl). Risks are given for total cholesterol (TC) concentrations of 4.0, 4.5, 5.0, 5.5, 6.0, 6.5, 7.0, 7.5, and 8.0 mmol/l. In each of the other categories, additional risk factors are added consecutively, for example, the HDL = 1 mmol/l category is a 50-year-old female cigarette smoker with systolic blood pressure of 170 mm Hg and HDL of 1 mmol/l (39 mg/dl). SBP, systolic blood pressure. Derived from data presented in the references cited.

Recommendations for follow-up based on the initial blood pressure measurements for adults		
Initial Blood Pressure (mm Hg)*		
Systolic	Diastolic	Follow-up Recommended
>130	>85	Recheck in 1 year
130–139	85–89	Recheck in 1 year; provide information about lifestyle modification
140–159	90–99	Confirm within 2 months
160–179	100–109	Evaluate or refer to source of care within 1 month
≥180	≥110	Evaluate or refer to source of care immediately or within 1 week, depending on clinical situation

Figure 31.11 **Recommendations for follow-up based on the initial blood pressure measurements for adults.** *If systolic and diastolic categories are different, follow recommendations for the shorter time for follow-up. The schedule for follow-up should be modified according to reliable information about past blood pressure measurements, other cardiovascular risk factors, or target organ disease.

Hypertension in Children Hypertension in children is defined by average SBP and/or DBP at or above the 95th percentile for gender and age, measured on at least three occasions. The identification of causes of hypertension in children varies depending on the published series. Most prepubertal hypertension is thought to have renal causes, although some children may have BP levels above the 95th percentile because of an earlier growth spurt and large size. In postpubertal children, mild hypertension is likely to be primary hypertension, while more severe hypertension is usually of renal cause. Primary aldosteronism and thyroid disease seem rare.

Hypertension in Pregnancy Hypertension may occur in >5% of all pregnancies and, over 5 years, in approximately 5% of women taking oral contraceptives. Usual definitions include the following[1]:
- Chronic hypertension: Hypertension diagnosed before the 20th week of gestation or present before pregnancy or persisting 6 weeks postpartum.[2]
- Preeclampsia: Elevated BP with proteinuria that occurs after 20 weeks of gestation in a previously normotensive woman (usually a primigravida).[3]

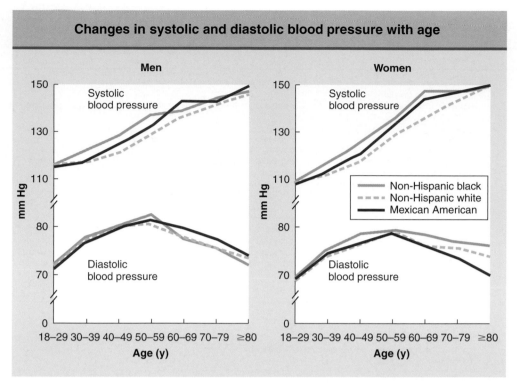

Figure 31.12 **Changes in systolic and diastolic blood pressure with age.** Systolic blood pressure and diastolic blood pressure by age and race or ethnicity for men and women older than 18 years of age in the U.S. population. Data from NHANES III, 1988 to 1991. (Burt VL, Whelton P, Roccella EJ, et al: Prevalence of hypertension in the US adult population: Results from the Third National Health and Nutrition Examination Survey, 1988–1991. Hypertension 1995;23:305–313.)

- Eclampsia: Seizures not due to other causes in a woman with preeclampsia.[4]
- Preeclampsia superimposed on chronic hypertension: BP increases of 30/15 mm Hg (systolic/diastolic) with the appearance of proteinuria in a woman with chronic hypertension who previously had no proteinuria.[5]
- Transient (gestational) hypertension: BP elevations during pregnancy or occurring in the first 24 hours postpartum, with no other signs of preeclampsia (no proteinuria) or pre-existing hypertension; this may be due to latent chronic hypertension and usually recurs in other pregnancies.[21]

BP in normal pregnancy usually falls during the first and middle trimester. Average sitting SBPs are between 100 and 105 mm Hg, lying SBP is 115 mm Hg, and DBP is 55 mm Hg. BP then returns toward prepregnant levels during the third trimester. This reduction in BP also occurs in women with pre-existing hypertension.

Classification by Cause of Hypertension

Although a large number of causes are recognized for hypertension, the etiology in 90% to 95% of patients with hypertension is unknown. These patients are considered to have essential or primary hypertension (see Chapter 32). Figure 31.13 shows the more common causes of secondary hypertension. The more common causes of secondary hypertension are renal parenchymal disease (2% to 6% of all hypertensives), renovascular hypertension (1% to 4%), all endocrine hypertension (1%, primary aldosteronism, pheochromocytoma, Cushing's syndrome), drug induced (1%, including oral contraceptives), and coarctation of the aorta (0.1% to 1.0%). An often overlooked category is hypertension

related to medication such as the use of decongestants or sympathomimetic agents.

EVALUATION OF HYPERTENSION

Proper Measurement of Blood Pressure

Arterial BP is usually measured using the cuff-based sphygmomanometer in which the arterial pressure is recorded by detecting sounds that are generated (auscultatory method) or by recording vascular pulsations (oscillometric method) following decompression of a compressed artery. Guidelines for blood pressure measurement are given in Figure 31.14. Unfortunately, if not properly used, the method can be unreliable and inaccurate. The most common reason for inaccuracy is an inappropriate cuff size as the accuracy of these measurements is influenced by the size of the inflatable bladder relative to the girth of the compressed limb. In order to provide uniform compression of the underlying artery, the length of the bladder should be at least 80% of the upper arm circumference and the width of the bladder should be at least 40% of the upper arm circumference. A simple bedside maneuver to check the appropriateness of the cuff size consists of aligning the cuff so that its long axis is parallel to the long axis of the arm. The cuff is positioned so that its inner surface faces outward. The bladder width should then be sufficient to encircle half of the upper arm circumference. If the bladder width encompasses less than half the upper arm, a larger cuff must be selected. No change in cuff size is necessary if the cuff encircles more than half the upper arm since large cuffs on thin limbs do not produce considerable errors in the BP measurement. For purists, accepted bladder dimensions for

Common causes of secondary hypertension	
Condition/Disorder	**Disease**
Renal disorders	Renal parenchymal disease: acute and chronic glomerular diseases, chronic tubulointerstitial disease, polycystic kidney disease, obstructive uropathy Renovascular disease: renal artery stenosis caused by atherosclerosis or fibromuscular dysplasia; arteritis; extrinsic compression of the renal artery Other renal causes: renin-producing tumors, renal sodium retention (Liddle syndrome)
Endocrine disorders	Adrenocortical disorders: primary aldosteronism, congenital adrenal hyperplasia, Cushing's syndrome Adrenomedullary tumors: pheochromocytoma (also extra-adrenal chromaffin tumor) Thyroid disease: hyperthyroidism, hypothyroidism Hyperparathyroidism: hypercalcemia Acromegaly Carcinoid tumors
Exogenous medications and drugs	Oral contraceptives, sympathomimetics, glucocorticoids, mineralocorticoids, nonsteroidal anti-inflammatory drugs, calcineurin inhibitors, tyramine-containing foods and monoamine oxidase inhibitors, erythropoietin, ergot alkaloids, amphetamines, herbal remedies, licorice (mimics primary aldosteronism), ethanol, cocaine and other illicit drugs, abrupt withdrawal of clonidine
Pregnancy	Preeclampsia and eclampsia
Coarctation of the aorta	
Neurologic disorders	Sleep apnea Increased intracranial pressure: brain tumors Affective disorders Spinal cord injury: quadriplegia, paraplegia, Guillain-Barré syndrome Baroreflex dysregulation
Psychosocial factors	
Intravascular volume overload	
Systolic hypertension	Loss of elasticity of aorta and great vessels Hyperdynamic cardiac output: hyperthyroidism, aortic insufficiency, anemia, arteriovenous fistula, beri-beri, Paget's disease of the bone

Figure 31.13 Common causes of secondary hypertension.

varying arm sizes are given in Figure 31.15. Another potential error relates to the auscultatory method, which relies on the ability to hear the Korotkoff sounds. The human ear has a sound threshold of about 16 Hz. The Korotkoff sounds occur at slightly above this level (25 to 50 Hz). Thus, the human ear is almost deaf to the sounds it must hear to measure BP. The bell-shaped stethoscope head should be used to measure BP. Interestingly, many physicians and most nurses are not equipped with a bell-shaped stethoscope head.

The oscillometric method is based on the principle of plethysmography to detect pulsatile pressure changes in a nearby artery. When an arm cuff is inflated, pulsatile pressure changes in an underlying artery produce periodic pressure changes in the inflated cuff. The oscillometric method thus measures periodic pressure changes, oscillations, in an inflated cuff as an indirect measure of pulsatile pressure in an underlying artery.

There are three types of sphygmomanometer in use worldwide. Due to environmental concerns, the standard mercury manometer has largely been abandoned.[22] The second type of manometer in wide use is the aneroid manometer. There are also numerous semiautomatic oscillometric electronic recording manometers. The manufacturers must ensure accuracy, and in many countries, the local hypertension societies have arranged for certification of these devices. The technical capabilities of the devices have increased greatly; however, room for improvement remains. Physicians must be aware that many patients purchase devices and measure their own BP. These devices should be inspected and checked by the physician.

Variability of Blood Pressure
Wake-Sleep Cycle and Office Versus Home Blood Pressure
BP varies considerably in individual subjects and may vary significantly throughout the day. This variation causes considerable difficulties in identifying individuals who are hypertensive, especially in terms of the preceding classification schemes. The differing BP values are due to both biologic variation (variations of pressures within a given individual) and variation in the measurement itself. Errors in measurement can be minimized by attention to the proper technique for recording BP, as noted previously. Biologic variation is addressed by repeated BP measurement at a given visit (at least two pressures taken at least 30 seconds apart or additional BP measurements if there is a 5-mm Hg difference between repeated measures). In addition, in most patients with milder forms of hypertension, repeated measurements during different clinic visits over time are recommended to approach the true BP.

Readings of BP at home, and outside the clinic or office setting, are recommended in order to assess the degree of hypertension and BP control during treatment. The instruments used at home must be checked against a standard on a regular basis, and the techniques for correct BP measurement must be taught to the patient. Levels measured at home are generally lower than those measured in the clinic or office. Patients should be discouraged from very frequent home BP measurement and from frequent adjustment of medications. Therapeutic chaos may ensue resulting in unnecessary emergency department visits and hospitalizations for uncontrolled hypertension or dizzy spells. It is worthwhile to ask the

Guidelines for measurement of blood pressure	
Factors	Important Features
Patient factors	Caffeine should not be taken for up to 1 hour before the blood pressure measurement. Cigarettes should not be smoked for at least 15 minutes prior to the blood pressure reading. The standard measurement should be made with the patient seated comfortably, arm supported, and the cuff must be at the level of the heart; the arm should be bared. On an initial examination, blood pressure should also be checked in the supine position after 5 minutes of rest, in the standing position after 2 minutes, and in both arms in patients who are diabetic, older than 65 years, or receiving antihypertensive therapy. Use the higher value if the arms have differing blood pressures. If sequential pressures are taken in the same position, at least 30 seconds must elapse between blood pressure readings. In patients younger than 30 years of age, check blood pressure in one leg. To establish a diagnosis of hypertension, obtain blood pressure readings on three different occasions, at least 1 week apart.
Equipment	The length of the bladder with the cuff should encircle at least 80% of the arm. The width of the cuff should be equal to two thirds of the distance from the antecubital space to the axilla and be 40% of the arm circumference. The best cuff for most adults is the 15-cm-wide cuff with a bladder of 33–35 cm in length. The distal edge of the cuff should be 2.5 cm above the antecubital fossa In extremely obese patients, blood pressure may be more accurate when measured in the forearm, palpating and auscultating the radial artery. For infants, ultrasound equipment may need to be used.
Technique	The initial systolic blood pressure should be checked by palpating the disappearance of the radial or brachial pulse prior to auscultation and the cuff then deflated. The second blood pressure check requires cuff inflation 20–30 mm Hg above the palpable systolic level. Deflate the cuff at a rate of 2–4 mm Hg per second. Record the Korotkoff sound I (appearance of sound) as the systolic pressure and record the Korotkoff sound V (the last sound before complete disappearance of sound) as the more reproducible diastolic pressure. If the sounds do not disappear, record the muffled sound (phase IV) as the diastolic. The sounds may be augmented by having the patient raise the arm and by opening and closing the hand 10 times before inflating the pressure. Do not stop between systolic and diastolic readings; deflate the cuff, wait at least 30 seconds, and then reinflate. On each occasion, record at least two readings. If the readings vary by more than 5 mm Hg, take additional readings until two are within 5 mm Hg. In children, the same standards apply for cuff size; Korotkoff sound V should be used. If the child is uncooperative, the systolic blood pressure may be determined by palpation.

Figure 31.14   Guidelines for measurement of blood pressure.

Accepted bladder dimensions for varying arm sizes			
Patient	Arm Circumference Range at Midpoint (cm)	Bladder Width (cm)	Bladder Length (cm)
Newborn	6	3	6
Infant*	6–15	5	15
Child*	16–21	8	21
Small adult	22–26	10	24
Adult	27–34	13	30
Large adult	35–44	16	38
Adult thigh	45–52	20	42

Figure 31.15   Accepted bladder dimensions for varying arm sizes. *To approximate a bladder width-to-arm circumference ratio of 0.4 more closely in children, additional cuffs are available. There is some overlap in the recommended ranges for arm circumference in order to limit the number of cuffs. It is suggested that the larger cuff is used if it is available. (From Perloff D, Grim C, Flack J, et al: Human blood pressure determination by sphygmomanometry. Circulation 1993;88:2460–2470.)

patient to keep a daily calendar and to measure BP under controlled conditions only twice daily, for instance, while sitting quietly in the mornings and evenings. If three fourths of the measurements achieve goal or better, office control is generally also achieved.

Biologic variation during the day is related to physical and mental activity and emotional factors. There is also diurnal variation with a decrease in BP during sleep (averaging 20%) secondary to a decrease in sympathetic activity; similar reductions in BP occur after hospital admission and bed rest. The normal diurnal pattern includes an increase in BP before awakening that has been associated with increased incidence of myocardial infarction, stroke, and sudden death in the first few hours after awakening. The usual pattern is for individuals to decrease their BP during sleep and these are referred to as dippers. Some individuals fail to reduce their BP during sleep and these have been labeled nondippers. The failure to decrease BP during sleep has been associated with increased incidence of left ventricular hypertrophy and raises the possibility of secondary hypertension.

Ambulatory Blood Pressure
Due to the variability in BP that occurs throughout the day, home BP and ambulatory BP monitoring is available to enable hyperten-

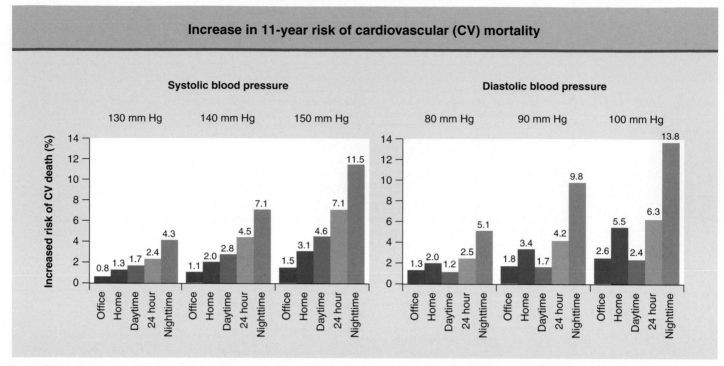

Figure 31.16 Increase in 11-year risk of cardiovascular (CV) mortality for 10-mm Hg increase in office, home, and ambulatory blood pressure (BP) at various initial BP values. (From Sega R, Facchetti R, Bombelli M, et al: Prognostic value of ambulatory and home blood pressures compared with office blood pressure in the general population: Follow-up results from the Pressioni Arteriose Monitorate e Loro Associazioni (PAMELA) study. Circulation 2005;111:1777–1783.)

sion to be defined more clearly. Home BP monitoring is advised for all patients and may help to identify white coat hypertension and borderline hypertension and may also help monitor response to therapy. The last includes identifying hypotension as well as hypertension. The instructions to each patient must be individualized, but home BP monitoring may be advised two to three times per day while the patient is awake. These BP values must be self-recorded and reviewed. The absolute value of 24-hour ambulatory BP measurement remains uncertain. The prognostic value of ambulatory and home BP compared to office BP in the general population and follow-up results were recently reported from the Pressioni Arteriose Monitorate e Loro Associazioni (PAMELA) study.[23] A total of 2051 persons were observed for 10 years. In the PAMELA population, risk of death increased more with a given increase in home or ambulatory BP than office BP. The overall ability to predict death, however, was not greater for home and ambulatory than for office BP, although it was somewhat increased by the combination of office and outside-of-office values. SBP was almost invariably superior to DBP, and night BP was superior to day BP (Fig. 31.16).

Ambulatory BP monitoring is recommended for certain indications beyond the information available from home BP recording (Fig 31.17). Ambulatory BP monitoring uses a noninvasive system. The BP is determined by auscultation using either oscillometry, which measures variations in pressure within the cuff, or by a microphone placed under the cuff and over the brachial artery. The

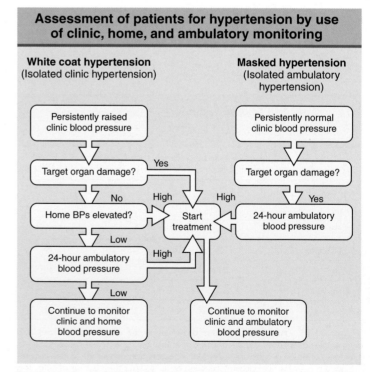

Figure 31.17 Guidelines for assessment of patients by use of clinic, home, and ambulatory monitoring of blood pressure.

ambulatory BP device can be programmed to record at frequent intervals during the daytime (e.g., every 10 minutes) and less frequently at night during sleep (e.g., every 30 minutes). The ambulatory BP equipment might not provide accurate readings in patients with large upper arms owing to obesity or increased musculature, and the equipment may be inaccurate during vigorous activity. The equipment generally records BP during a 24-hour period. Although most patients adjust to the repetitive measurements throughout the day, some patients may have a startle response with each BP recording. Most patients are able to sleep, although some have their sleep disturbed by the BP recording, and, therefore, determination of nocturnal fall in BP is inaccurate. Indications for ambulatory BP are shown in Figure 31.18.[24]

There are disadvantages to using the ambulatory BP equipment. Trained personnel must place the monitoring equipment. Calibration of ambulatory BP equipment with a mercury manometer must be recorded at the beginning and end of the ambulatory BP session. Three to six readings must be taken at each time and the SBP and DBP measurements must both agree within 5 mm Hg. The end calibration is critical to ensure proper functioning of the ambulatory BP monitor throughout the 24-hour period. The cuff inflation may interfere with activities, work, or sleep. The cuff may cause discomfort or skin irritation or it may malfunction and fail to deflate, causing pain and interruption of recording. The data correlating ambulatory BP with target organ disease are limited. Standards for assessment of data and their use in decisions for therapy are limited. In addition, equipment is expensive and its use is limited by lack of reimbursement by health insurance systems in a number of countries, including the United States and some European countries.

Risk Factors for Hypertension

A number of factors are known to be associated with an increased risk of primary hypertension.[25] These are discussed in detail in Chapter 32 (see Fig. 32.8).

Physical Factors, Genetics, and Congenital Factors

Hypertension is more common in men and postmenopausal women than in premenopausal women, is more common with increasing age, and is more common in African Americans than Caucasians. Hypertension is also more likely to occur in the subject with a high basal blood pressure and/or pulse and in those who show a marked increase in BP with cold pressor test or exercise. There are also congenital factors (increased risk of hypertension with low birth weight) as well as genetic factors since the risk of having hypertension is increased in those who have one or both parents or first-degree relatives with hypertension. However, while association studies have identified a number of genes with small (if any) effect on BP, in general, the results have been disappointing. This contrasts with a number of hereditary hypertension syndromes that are known to be mediated by specific mutations. Most of these disorders result in physiologic abnormalities in which there is increased sodium reabsorption, particularly in the distal nephron (see Chapter 46). However, there are five known genes causing pheochromocytoma, as well as an autosomal-dominant hypertension and brachydactyly syndrome, which is not a salt-sensitive condition. The latter disease is caused by a chromosomal rearrangement and the precise mechanisms have not been elucidated.[26]

Obesity and Physical Inactivity

One of the major risk factors for hypertension is obesity (especially truncal), which is all the more significant given the current epidemic of obesity. This condition often progresses into full-blown metabolic syndrome in which there is dyslipidemia, hyperuricemia, and insulin resistance. Another risk factor is physical inactivity. The odds ratio for a sedentary or physically unfit individual being hypertensive compared to the most physically fit individuals has ranged from 1.06 to 1.52. Thanks to recent studies, we now know the number of METs (metabolic equivalents) in both men and women that have a bearing on cardiovascular risk and overall survival.[27,28] One MET represents an oxygen consumption of 3.5 ml/kg/min, which for an ideal 70-kg person would be a VO_2 of about 250 ml/min. In persons with a normal hemoglobin, this amount translates into a cardiac output of 5 l/min and a DO_2 of 1000 ml/min, precisely as Adolph Fick predicted. Walking requires about 2 METs, while jogging at a 10-km/h rate represents about 8 METs. A huge body of evidence supports the notion that were the METs increased in the population, cardiovascular health would be greatly increased as well.

Dietary Factors

Considerable attention has been given to many dietary factors. The importance of obesity cannot be overemphasized. Gastric banding and bypass have been clearly shown to be effective, while lifestyle interventions have been generally disappointing. The pharmacologic treatment of obesity is being actively developed. Precisely what is driving the current obesity epidemic across the world is unclear but probably multifactorial. Some

Indications for ambulatory blood pressure determinations
White coat hypertension
Evaluation of apparent drug resistance
Hypotensive symptoms
Autonomic dysfunction
Episodic hypertension
Evaluation of nocturnal decreases in blood pressure, as a prognostic factor for target organ disease (left ventricular hypertrophy, ischemic optic neuropathy)
Evaluation of blood pressure changes in patients with paroxysmal nocturnal dyspnea and nocturnal angina
Carotid sinus syncope
Pacemaker syndromes
Safety of withdrawing antihypertensive medication
Assess 24-hour blood pressure control on once-daily medication
Borderline hypertension with target organ damage
Evaluation of antihypertensive drug therapy in clinical trials

Figure 31.18   Indications for ambulatory blood pressure determinations.

authorities have suggested that the acceleration of the obesity epidemic may be due in part to the introduction of fructose-based sweeteners and sugars that may induce features of the metabolic syndrome through a uric acid–dependent pathway.[29]

A strong association also exists between sodium intake and BP. Most populations studied consume between 100 and 200 mmol sodium per day (2.5 to 5 g sodium or 6 to 12 g salt). In a reanalysis of 47,000 individuals, a difference of sodium intake of 100 mmol/day was associated with differences in SBP in the range of 5 to 10 mm Hg. Potassium has also been inversely associated with BP such that a 60-mmol/day (2.3-g/day) increased excretion of urinary potassium has been related to approximately 3 mm Hg lower SBP. These epidemiologic data come from the INTERSALT study, which includes data from countries across four continents. In addition, an inverse relationship has been identified between intake of calcium and BP. Also, societies that consume diets with low fat and low protein of animal origin plus a high fiber content tend to have lower BP and a low prevalence of hypertension. The relationship of dietary modification to treatment of hypertension is discussed in Chapter 33.

Behavioral Factors

Increased alcohol consumption has been associated with hypertension in numerous studies. This relationship is seen with alcohol consumption of three drinks or more per day (approximately 40 g ethanol). This roughly corresponds to 24 oz (720 ml) of beer, 10 oz (300 ml) of wine, or 2 oz (60 ml) of 100-proof whiskey per day. Nicotine causes an increase in both SBP and DBP that may last for 15 to 30 minutes. If BP is taken >30 minutes after a cigarette, smokers may have normal BP. However, the repeated pressor effects likely contribute to elevated pressure in individuals who typically smoke one pack per day. Caffeine will increase BP in individuals who do not take caffeine or use it infrequently. However, tolerance to caffeine develops and BP generally does not increase in individuals who regularly use caffeine. Recent evidence suggests that caffeine may protect from diabetes.[30] Finally, psychological stress is also known to predispose individuals to develop hypertension.

Evaluation for Primary Versus Secondary Hypertension

Some authorities advocate assessment of patients with primary hypertension in terms of their plasma renin activity (renin profiling).[31] The notion is to treat patients with low plasma renin activity with drugs aimed at volume reduction and those with higher values with drugs aimed at peripheral vascular resistance. Although a 24-hour urine collection for sodium excretion is helpful information, the collection is not mandatory, nor must all medication be discontinued prior to a renin measurement. According to renin profiling, patients with plasma renin activity <0.65 ng/ml/h are more likely to have volume-related hypertension, while those with values >0.65 ng/ml/h have more predominant vasoconstriction. Systematic drug rotation studies have shown that the rank order of response to different drugs indeed varies substantially among patients.[32] In support of renin profiling, two broad patterns of response emerged. ACE inhibitors, ARBs, and β-blockers were useful primarily in hypertensive patients with higher renin values. These patients are generally younger Caucasians. Calcium channel blockers and diuretics were more useful in low-renin hypertension, which is commonly observed in Afro Caribbeans, African Americans, and older Caucasians.

The medical history, physical examination, and a limited number of laboratory tests provide critical information in deciding which individuals require further evaluation for secondary hypertension and target organ disease (Figs. 31.19 and 31.20). All hypertensive persons should be assessed for cardiovascular risk factors, including total cholesterol, HDL- and LDL-cholesterol, fasting triglycerides, renal function and proteinuria (according to Kidney Disease Outcomes Quality Initiative classification), and the presence of diabetes mellitus or the metabolic syndrome. If the history, physical examination, or screening laboratory studies suggest secondary hypertension, additional studies are warranted. If renal parenchymal disease is suspected, quantitative studies to assess GFR and urinary protein excretion should be performed. Renal ultrasonography is useful to evaluate renal size and echogenicity (to help assess chronicity) as well as evaluate for obstructive uropathy. Renal artery stenosis should be suspected by the presence of severe hypertension (≥ medication classes for control) with abnormal renal function or with asymmetric renal size. If primary aldosteronism is suspected due to hypokalemia, the ratio of plasma aldosterone to plasma renin activity may be useful. If the ratio is >25 to 30 and plasma aldosterone is >20 ng/dl, the diagnosis should be pursued further. The extended results of patients undergoing operation have been published.[33] Resolution of hypertension after adrenalectomy for primary aldosteronism was independently associated with a lack of family history of hypertension and preoperative use of two or fewer antihypertensive agents. Further evaluation for other forms of secondary hypertension is listed in Figure 31.20.

Evaluation for primary versus secondary hypertension			
Classification	Medical History	Physical Examination	Laboratory Studies
General information and evaluation of target organs	Duration and course of hypertension Prior work-up and treatment Diet/lifestyle: salt intake, tobacco, caffeine	Evaluation of volume status, optic fundi, heart, lungs, peripheral vessels, and nervous system	Complete blood count, fasting glucose, lipid profile (includes HDL, LDL, cholesterol, triglyceride), uric acid Consider echocardiogram
Primary (essential or idiopathic) or secondary?	Family history: hypertension, cardiovascular and renal diseases Symptoms of target organ disease (related to eyes, central nervous system, cardiorespiratory, and peripheral vascular)	See Figure 31.20	

Figure 31.19   Evaluation for primary versus secondary hypertension. HDL, high-density lipoprotein; LDL, low-density lipoprotein.

Evaluation of secondary hypertension

Target Organ/System	Medical History	Physical Examination	Laboratory Studies
Kidney Renal parenchymal	History of renal disease (including glomerulonephritis, nephrotic syndrome, calculi, urinary tract infection) Symptoms include nocturia, frequency, dysuria, hesitancy, urgency, incomplete emptying, dribbling, hematuria, pyuria, flank pain	Tenderness in costovertebral angles; palpable kidneys	Blood urea nitrogen, serum creatinine; urinalysis, urine culture if indicated; 24-h urine for protein and creatinine clearance if indicated; consider microalbuminuria measurement, or random urine protein-to-creatinine ratio
Renovascular hypertension		Epigastric bruit; other vascular bruits	Renal ultrasonography with duplex Doppler flow study; consider angiography or magnetic resonance angiography
Endocrine Primary aldosteronism	Muscle weakness, cramps		Serum potassium: consider serum aldosterone-to-plasma renin activity ratio; 24-h urine aldosterone, Na, K, creatinine
Cushing's syndrome	Weight gain, cosmetic changes	Body habitus: body fat, striae	Morning serum cortisol after dexamethasone suppression
Pheochromocytoma	Headaches; vasomotor symptoms, (inappropriate sweating, pallor); cardiac symptoms (awareness, tachycardia, palpitations)	Paroxysmal or intermittent hypertension (50% of patients) catecholamines, vanillylmandelic acid (VMA)	Single voided urine for metanephrine and creatinine; consider 24-h urine for (VMA), metanephrines; if positive, proceed with magnetic resonance imaging or thin-section computed tomography of the adrenals
Carcinoid	Flushing		24-h urine 5-hydroxyindoleacetic acid excretion
Hyperthyroidism	Weight loss, tachycardia, palpitations, sweating, heat intolerance	Palpable thyroid	Total and free thyroxine
Hypothyroidism	Weight gain, dry skin, cold intolerance, hair loss		Thyroid-stimulating hormone, total and free thyroxine
Hyperparathyroidism	Nausea, vomiting, bone pain, nephrolithiasis		Serum calcium, intact parathyroid hormone
Acromegaly	Change in size of head, hands, or feet (adult)	Appearance	GH level (see Fig.36.11)
Medication	Review of prescribed and over-the-counter medications (especially oral contraceptives, nonsteroidal anti-inflammatory drugs, sympathomimetic agents [cold and allergy drugs], illicit or recreational drugs, including alcohol, herbal remedies)		
Coarctation of the aorta	Onset or detection of hypertension in childhood or adolescence	Simultaneous palpation of radial and femoral arteries to detect pulse lag in femorals; leg blood pressure	Chest radiograph for heart size, configuration of aorta, rib notching; consider aortography
Neurologic disorders Sleep apnea	Obesity; weight gain; daytime somnolence; snoring, poor sleep habits (frequent awakening, not rested on arising); early morning headache	Obesity; narrowed airway in hypopharynx; redundant pharyngeal tissue	Formal sleep study (polysomnography)
Increased intracranial pressure	Headache; neurologic symptoms	Papilledema	↑ Cerebrospinal fluid pressure
Affective disorders[†] Spinal cord injury[†]			
Psychosocial factors	Family and support structure, occupation, education, stressors		
Volume overload	Excess salt and water intake (may be iatrogenic with excess parenteral fluid)	Increased jugular venous distention, pulmonary rales, presacral and peripheral edema, hepatomegaly	Chest radiograph
Isolated systolic hypertension		Pseudohypertension (positive Olser's maneuver); cardiac and vascular examination (evaluate for aortic insufficiency, arteriovenous fistula)	

Figure 31.20 History, physical examinaion, and initial laboratory evaluation for secondary hypertension. A more detailed discussion is provided in other relevant chapters. Pregnancy-associated hypertension is discussed in Chapters 41 and 42.

REFERENCES

1. Guyton AC, Hall JE: Dominant role of the kidneys in long-term regulation of arterial pressure and in hypertension: The integrated system for pressure control. In Guyton AC, Hall JE, eds. Textbook of Medical Pysiology, 10th ed. Philadelphia: WB Saunders, 2000, pp 221–234.

2. Izzo JL Jr, Black HR, eds: Hypertension Primer, 3rd ed. Dallas: Council on High Blood Pressure Research, American Heart Association, 2003, pp 3–78.

3. DiBona GF: Functionally specific renal sympathetic nerve fibers: Role in cardiovascular regulation. Am J Hypertens 2001;14:163S–170S.

4. Xu J, Li G, Wang P, et al: Renalase is a novel, soluble monoamine oxidase that regulates cardiac function and blood pressure. J Clin Invest 2005;115:1275–1280.

5. Fukata Y, Amano M, Kaibuchi K: Rho-Rho-kinase pathway in smooth muscle contraction and cytoskeletal reorganization of non-muscle cells. Trends Pharmacol Sci 2001;22:32–39.

6. Lohmeier TE, Hildebrandt DA, Warren S, et al: Recent insights into the interactions between the baroreflex and the kidneys in hypertension. Am J Physiol Regul Integr Comp Physiol 2005;288:R828–R836.

7. Crowley SD, Gurley SB, Oliverio MI, et al: Distinct roles for the kidney and systemic tissues in blood pressure regulation by the renin-angiotensin system. J Clin Invest 2005;115:1092–1099.

8. Lewington S, Clarke R, Qizilbash N, et al: Prospective Studies Collaboration: Age-specific relevance of usual blood pressure to vascular mortality: A meta-analysis of individual data for one million adults in 61 prospective studies. Lancet 2002;360:1903–1913.

9. Chobanian AV, Bakris GL, Black HR, et al, Joint National Committee on Prevention, Detection, Evaluation, and Treatment of High Blood Pressure. National Heart, Lung, and Blood Institute; National High Blood Pressure Education Program Coordinating Committee. Seventh report of the Joint National Committee on Prevention, Detection, Evaluation, and Treatment of High Blood Pressure. Hypertension 2003; 42:1206–1252.

10. Cruickshank JK, Mzayek F, Liu L, et al: Origins of the "black/white" difference in blood pressure: Roles of birth weight, postnatal growth, early blood pressure, and adolescent body size: The Bogalusa Heart Study. Circulation 2005;111:1932–1937.

11. Levey AS, Mulrow CD: An editorial update: What level of blood pressure control in chronic kidney disease? Ann Intern Med 2005;143: 79–81.

12. Staessen JA, Wang J, Bianchi G, Birkenhager WH: Essential hypertension. Lancet 2003;361:1629–1641.

13. Jackson R, Lawes CM, Bennett DA, et al: Treatment with drugs to lower blood pressure and blood cholesterol based on an individual's absolute cardiovascular risk. Lancet 2005;365:434–441.

14. Klausen K, Borch-Johnsen K, Feldt-Rasmussen B, et al: Very low levels of microalbuminuria are associated with increased risk of coronary heart disease and death independently of renal function, hypertension, and diabetes. Circulation 2004;110:32–35.

15. Pickering TG, Gerin W, Schwartz AR: What is the white-coat effect and how should it be measured? Blood Press Monit 2002;7:293–300.

16. Ohkubo T, Kikuya M, Metoki H, et al: Prognosis of "masked" hypertension and "white-coat" hypertension detected by 24-h ambulatory blood pressure monitoring 10-year follow-up from the Ohasama study. J Am Coll Cardiol 2005;46:508–515.

17. Mansoor GA: A practical approach to persistent elevation of blood pressure in the hypertension clinic. Blood Press Monit 2003;8:97–100.

18. Dao HH, Essalihi R, Bouvet C, Moreau P: Evolution and modulation of age-related medial elastocalcinosis: Impact on large artery stiffness and isolated systolic hypertension. Cardiovasc Res 2005;66:307–317.

19. Sander GE: Hypertension in the elderly. Curr Hypertens Rep 2004;6: 469–476.

20. Elliot WJ: Clinical features and management of selected hypertensive emergencies. J Clin Hypertens (Greenwich) 2004;6:587–592.

21. Sibai B, Dekker G, Kupferminc M: Pre-eclampsia. Lancet 2005;365: 785–799.

22. Jones DW, Frohlich ED, Grim CM, et al: Mercury sphygmomanometers should not be abandoned: An advisory statement from the Council for High Blood Pressure Research, American Heart Association. Hypertension 2001;37:185–186.

23. Sega R, Facchetti R, Bombelli M, et al: Prognostic value of ambulatory and home blood pressures compared with office blood pressure in the general population: follow-up results from the Pressioni Arteriose Monitorate e Loro Associazioni (PAMELA) study. Circulation 2005; 111:1777–1783.

24. O'Brien E, Asmar R, Beilin L, et al: European Society of Hypertension Working Group on Blood Pressure Monitoring: Practice guidelines of the European Society of Hypertension for clinic, ambulatory and self blood pressure measurement. J Hypertens 2005;23:697–701.

25. Franklin SS, Pio JR, Wong ND, et al: Predictors of new-onset diastolic and systolic hypertension: The Framingham Heart Study. Circulation 2005;111:1121–1127.

26. Luft FC: Present status of genetic mechanisms in hypertension. Med Clin North Am 2004;88:1–18.

27. Morris CK, Myers J, Froelicher VF, et al. Nomogram based on metabolic equivalents and age for assessing aerobic exercise capacity in men. J Am Coll Cardiol 1993;22:175–182

28. Gulati M, Black HR, Shaw LJ, et al: The prognostic value of a nomogram for exercise capacity in women. N Engl J Med 2005;353:468–475.

29. Nakagawa T, Tuttle KR, Short RA, Johnson RJ: Hypothesis: Fructose-induced hyperuricemia as a causal mechanism for the epidemic of the metabolic syndrome Nat Clin Pract Nephrol 2005;1:80–86.

30. van Dam RM, Hu FB. Coffee consumption and risk of type 2 diabetes: A systematic review. JAMA 2005;294:97–104.

31. Laragh JH, Sealey JE: Relevance of the plasma renin hormonal control system that regulates blood pressure and sodium balance for correctly treating hypertension and for evaluating ALLHAT. Am J Hypertens 2003;16:407–415.

32. Mackenzie IS, Brown MJ: Genetic profiling versus drug rotation in the optimisation of antihypertensive treatment. Clin Med 2002;2:465–473.

33. Sawka AM, Young WF, Thompson GB, et al: Primary aldosteronism: Factors associated with normalization of blood pressure after surgery. Ann Intern Med 2001;135:258–261.

Essential Hypertension

Richard J. Johnson, George L. Bakris, and Bernardo Rodríguez-Iturbe

DEFINITION

Essential (or primary) hypertension is defined as a blood pressure (BP) of >140/90 mm Hg without an identifiable cause. Several readings on different occasions and times are necessary to document the BP as being elevated because of substantial variability in BP. This variability in BP results from a circadian rhythm that generates the most significant increase in BP in early morning hours (6 to 10 AM). BP decreases at bedtime with recumbency or sleep, secondary to a decrease in sympathetic nervous system (SNS) tone and reduced activity of other neuroendocrine systems. There are also minute-to-minute variations in BP (Fig. 32.1). Transient elevations in BP, reaching 150 mm Hg systolic, occur in the majority of normotensive subjects on any given day.[1] However, BP that is repeatedly ≥140/90 mm Hg is considered elevated. Details on the method and interpretation of BP measurements, including the use of ambulatory BP monitoring, can be found in Chapter 31.

Hypertension is classified according to severity (Fig. 32.2).[2] Stages in hypertension have been adapted by both the Joint National Committee and European Society of Hypertension and European Society of Cardiology guidelines to allow a prognosis to be associated with different levels of BP elevation. The prognosis has been adapted from epidemiologic studies that demonstrate a linear relationship between the risk of cardiovascular events and sustained elevations of arterial pressure.

If only the systolic BP is elevated (systolic BP >140 and diastolic BP <90 mm Hg), it is called isolated systolic hypertension. Borderline hypertension (defined as BP between 130 and 139/85 and 89 mm Hg) is classified as prehypertension in

Classification of blood pressure			
BP Classification	Systolic BP (mm Hg)		Diastolic BP (mm Hg)
Normal	<120	and	<80
Prehypertension	120–139	or	80–89
Stage 1 hypertension	140–159	or	90–99
Stage 2 hypertension	≥160	or	≥100

Figure 32.2   Classification of blood pressure (BP). Shown is the BP classification according to the seventh report of the Joint National Committee on Prevention, Detection, Evaluation and Treatment of High Blood Pressure: the JNC 7 report.[2]

the United States and high normal by the European Guidelines and is further classified as white coat hypertension if an increase of >20 mm Hg systolic pressure is noted only in the physician's office.

Other terms used to describe certain clinical presentations of severe hypertension include malignant and accelerated. Malignant hypertension refers to elevated BP associated with severe end-organ damage and suggests irreversible injury. With improvements in treatment, this condition is only rarely observed. Accelerated hypertension refers to elevated BP, which is difficult to control and also may be associated with organ injury.

ETIOLOGY/PATHOGENESIS

Before we discuss the current hypotheses on etiology, it is necessary to discuss two major mediator systems involved in hypertension.

The renin angiotensin system (RAS) is one of the most important mechanisms by which the host regulates blood volume and pressure. Angiotensinogen, released primarily from the liver, is converted by renin to angiotensin I, which is further degraded in the presence of angiotensin-converting enzymes (ACEs) or chymases (such as present in the human heart) to angiotensin II (Ang II; Fig. 32.3). Most of the actions of Ang II are mediated by the AT1 receptor and include stimulating vascular smooth muscle contraction and hypertrophy, increasing cardiac contractility, stimulating the SNS in the central and peripheral nervous systems, increasing thirst and vasopressin release, and stimulating aldosterone synthesis. Stimulation of the AT1 receptor by Ang II causes renal vasoconstriction (especially of the efferent arteriole and vasa rectae), a decrease in renal blood flow, and an increase in renal vascular resistance. Ang II increases sodium reabsorption, not only through aldosterone but also by direct effects on the proximal tubules and by increasing the sensitivity of the tubuloglomerular feedback response (see Chapter 2). In addition

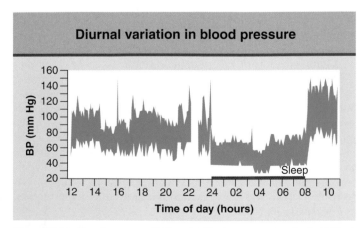

Figure 32.1   Blood pressure (BP) variability in a normotensive individual. In most normal individuals, systolic blood pressure reaches 150 mm Hg at least once per day. (From Bevan AT, Honour AJ, Stott FH: Direct arterial pressure recording in unrestricted man. Clin Sci 1969;36:329–344.)

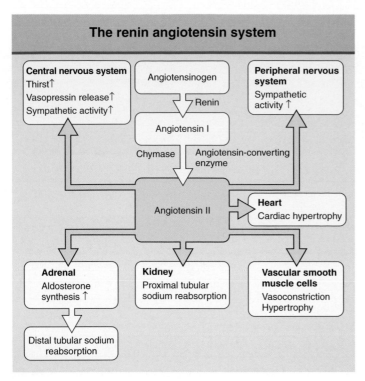

Figure 32.3   The renin angiotensin system.

to the systemic RAS, a local RAS is present in blood vessels, the heart, and the kidney that causes local effects (such as tissue remodeling) independent of circulating renin or angiotensinogen levels.

The role of the RAS in essential hypertension is complex. Whereas plasma renin activity is elevated in 20% of patients, renin activity is either normal (50%) or low (30%) in the majority. However, in many of the patients with normal renin activity, the plasma renin may be inappropriately high in relation to the total body sodium. This is indicated by the observations that saline depletion or infusion results in blunted changes in renin levels in these patients and that BP in these patients frequently responds to ACE inhibitors. Sealey and colleagues[3] have suggested that the reason for the widely varying renin levels may be nephron heterogeneity within individual kidneys, in which there are some ischemic nephrons making excess renin and other hyperfiltering nephrons in which renin secretion is suppressed. According to these authors, the increased renin released from the ischemic nephrons enters the circulation and leads to Ang II generation, which causes inappropriate vasoconstriction and sodium reabsorption in the other hyperfiltering nephrons. This results in sodium retention and the development of hypertension.

Sympathetic Nervous System

Guyton and colleagues[4] suggested that much of the short-term arterial pressure control is mediated by the central and autonomic nervous systems. High-pressure baroreceptors in the carotid sinus and aortic arch respond to acute elevations in pressure by causing a reflex vagal bradycardia and inhibition of sympathetic output from the central nervous system (CNS); the opposite occurs when BP suddenly decreases. Low-pressure cardiopulmonary receptors in the atria and ventricles likewise respond to increases in atrial filling by increasing heart rate (via inhibition of the cardiac SNS), increasing atrial natriuretic peptide release, and inhibiting vasopressin release. These reflexes are largely controlled centrally,

particularly in the nucleus tractus solitarius of the dorsal medulla. This vasomotor center also receives input from the limbus and hypothalamus in response to emotional or psychological stress.

Stimulation of the SNS results in peripheral vasoconstriction, an increase in heart rate, release of norepinephrine from the adrenals, and an increase in systemic BP. The increase in SNS activity also has a role in mediating vascular hypertrophy and stiffness. Renal efferent sympathetics are also activated and cause intrarenal vasoconstriction, with a decrease in renal blood flow and an increase in renal vascular resistance. The renal SNS directly stimulates sodium reabsorption and renin release from the juxtaglomerular apparatus.

The SNS is often hyperactive in essential hypertension, particularly in young or borderline hypertensive patients.[5] Many patients with newly diagnosed hypertension have elevated plasma norepinephrine levels, with increased heart rate and cardiac indices. These patients often show increases in BP with stress, exercise, or emotion. Such subjects may have elevated plasma renin levels reflecting β-adrenergic stimulation of renin secretion. These patients may also have increased vascular reactivity, increased systemic vascular resistance, and low blood volume.

The mechanisms involved in the stimulation of the SNS in hypertension have been studied intensely. A defect in baroreceptor sensitivity has been postulated and may contribute to the increased BP variability noted in some hypertensive patients. An increase in SNS response to emotional or work-related stress may also be a contributing factor. Hyperactivity of the SNS has been reported in African Americans, in obesity, in insulin resistance, and with the use of certain drugs (nicotine, alcohol, cyclosporine, cocaine) associated with hypertension. Furthermore, there may be a subset of patients in which compression of the lateral medulla by cranial nerves and/or vessels may result in increased SNS activity and hypertension; in some of these patients, selective decompression may ameliorate the hypertension. Finally, activation of the CNS/SNS may result from renal afferent sympathetics from hypertensive kidneys. Indeed, in several experimental models of hypertension, renal sympathectomy can cause a reduction in BP.[6]

Hypotheses on the Etiology of Hypertension

When hypertension was first discovered in the early 1800s, most cases were associated with glomerulonephritis or chronic kidney disease. The discovery that hypertension could occur in the absence of clinically evident kidney disease by Mahomed in the 1870s led to the recognition of the entity known today as essential hypertension. Disputes developed at that time as to whether the BP in these patients was increased due to a blood toxin such as lead or uric acid (Mahomed's hypothesis) or due to systemic vascular disease (arteriolosclerosis; the hypothesis of Gull and Sutton) or kidney disease (George Johnson's hypothesis). Goldblatt in the 1930s combined these hypotheses by proposing that hypertension resulted from arteriolar disease, but only if the arteriolar disease was in the kidney. He hypothesized that the arteriolar disease led to renal ischemia with the release of substances such as renin that would increase BP. However, his hypothesis was rejected in the 1950s when several groups reported that some cases (<10%) of essential hypertension did not have renal arteriolosclerosis; in addition, the arteriolosclerosis was considered a consequence of hypertension, as opposed to its cause.

The next major hypothesis was put forth by Guyton and colleagues,[4] who proposed that hypertension results from a physiologic defect in renal sodium handling such that higher BPs are required to excrete sodium for any given salt load (Fig. 32.4).

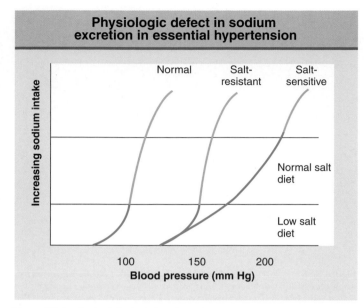

Figure 32.4   A physiologic defect in sodium excretion in essential hypertension. Evidence suggests that in patients with essential hypertension a higher blood pressure is required to excrete an individual sodium load. In salt-resistant hypertension, the pressure natriuresis curve has a rightward but parallel shift; with salt-sensitive hypertension, it is both a shift to the right as well as a change in slope. (Adapted from Guyton AC, Coleman TG, Cowley AV Jr, et al: Arterial pressure regulation. Overriding dominance of the kidneys in long-term regulation and in hypertension. Am J Med 1972;52:584–594.)

This was best illustrated by the pressure-natriuresis curve, in which increasing sodium intake results in an increase in pressure associated with prompt excretion of the salt load. Patients with hypertension demonstrate a defect in the pressure-natriuresis curve, either with a parallel rightward shift (resulting in a salt-resistant form of hypertension since the change in pressure is similar for changing sodium load) or with a change in the slope (resulting in a salt-sensitive form of hypertension in which BP increases more for the same sodium load). Evidence supporting a renal defect came from studies in genetically hypertensive rats in which the propensity for hypertension could be transferred by renal transplantation to nonhypertensive rats and vice versa. Epidemiologic studies also linked dietary sodium content with the prevalence of hypertension in various populations, and intervention studies with salt restriction or loading have shown that the BP response in many hypertensive patients is salt sensitive. The observation that Liddle syndrome and other rare causes of hypertension involve defects in renal sodium excretion are also consistent with this pathway. This led Lifton and colleagues[7] to hypothesize that the primary mechanism for essential hypertension may likely be the expression of genetic polymorphisms that favor sodium retention by the kidney in a westernized society in which we are all ingesting excessive (often >10 g/d) amounts of salt. Nevertheless, while some genetic polymorphisms in sodium transport are associated with essential hypertension, it has been difficult to demonstrate a strong role for genetics in essential hypertension.

Low Nephron Number Hypothesis

Congenital mechanisms may also contribute to hypertension. Barker[8] observed a marked increased risk for hypertension, obesity, and diabetes in subjects with low birth weights. Mothers of low birth weight infants frequently have conditions such as hypertension, obesity, preeclampsia, or malnutrition, and these maternal factors are also associated with an increased risk for hypertension in the progeny. Brenner and colleagues[9] postulated that the reason might be that low birth weight infants usually have kidneys that did not fully develop, resulting in low nephron number.[8] A low nephron number may predispose to renal injury over time with an impairment in sodium excretion. Consistent with this hypothesis, experimental studies have demonstrated that maternal malnutrition predisposes to small babies, low nephron number, and the future predisposition for hypertension. Furthermore, a recent study reported that humans with essential hypertension dying in motor vehicle accidents have nearly 50% fewer nephrons than age- and sex-matched controls.[10] While this mechanism is attractive, it cannot be the only risk factor, for while low birth weight infants have a 25% risk of developing hypertension as an adult, high birth weight infants have a 20% risk.[11] Thus, it is likely that other mechanisms are also contributory in the pathogenesis of hypertension.

Renal Vasoconstriction and Acquired Renal Injury as Mechanisms for Hypertension

We have proposed that hypertension may involve two phases (Fig. 32.5).[12] Early hypertension is mediated by renal vasoconstriction induced by an exogenous mechanism, such as endothelial dysfunction (with impaired endothelial nitric oxide generation or bioavailability), a hyperactive SNS, or activation of the RAS. Renal vasoconstriction could be induced by other mechanisms, including hyperuricemia, cyclosporine use, chronic hypokalemia, or systemic hypoxia. Evidence that each of these mechanisms is associated with the development of hypertension is extensive. Experimentally, each of these mechanisms also results in hypertension. The intrarenal vasoconstriction results in sodium

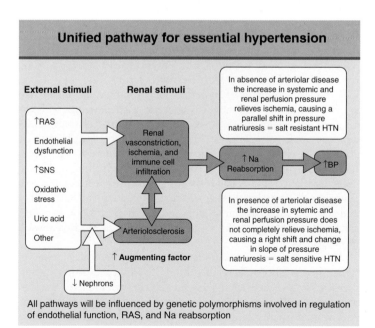

Figure 32.5   Unified pathway for essential hypertension. Hypertension may be hypothesized as occurring in two phases. The first phase is mediated by renal vasoconstriction due to external stimuli such as a hyperactive sympathetic nervous system (SNS), hyperuricemia, endothelial dysfunction, or an activated renin angiotensin system (RAS). This results in a salt resistant form of hypertension. While hypertension may remain salt resistant, we hypothesize that in many patients, progressive renal microvascular disease and tubulointerstitial inflammation will develop, with a switch to a salt sensitive phenotype and an increased risk of microalbuminuria. BP, blood pressure.

retention and an increase in BP. As BP increases, intrarenal perfusion pressure increases until renal ischemia is relieved. This results in a parallel shift in pressure natriuresis resulting in a salt resistant form of hypertension.

The continued intrarenal vasoconstriction leads to the recruitment of leukocytes that express oxidants and Ang II.[12] These changes lead to local inactivation of nitric oxide and perpetuate the intrarenal vasoconstriction. The afferent arteriole becomes progressively diseased from both the effects of the hypertension as well as direct stimulation of vascular smooth muscle cell proliferation by Ang II and other mediators, resulting in renal arteriolosclerosis. At this point, the hypertension becomes driven by the structural changes in the kidney. Because the arteriolar lesions are not uniform, the increase in BP results in some areas of the kidney being hyperperfused and other regions being underperfused. This nephron heterogeneity results in some ischemic nephrons continuing to produce renin, while others have suppressed expression.[3] The inability of the increase in BP to adequately relieve the ischemia leads to a change in the slope of the pressure natriuresis curve, resulting in salt sensitive hypertension.

Consistent with the hypothesis is the observation that early hypertension is often associated with a hyperactive SNS and with endothelial dysfunction, with low blood volumes, and with a salt resistant form of hypertension. In contrast, older hypertensive subjects often have prominent renal arteriolosclerosis, evidence of subtle renal injury such as the presence of microalbuminuria, and a salt sensitive form of hypertension. Furthermore, this pathway can be demonstrated experimentally in animals. Blocking the intrarenal inflammation and arteriolar injury will prevent the salt sensitive phase. Treatment of the arteriolopathy and tubulointerstitial injury with vascular remodeling agents such as vascular endothelial growth factor also ameliorates the salt sensitivity and reduces in BP in the cyclosporine model.

Potential Role of Hyperuricemia and Fructose in the Development of Hypertension

Recently, the role of uric acid in the pathogenesis of hypertension has been reevaluated.[13] An elevated serum uric acid is an independent predictor of hypertension in numerous studies and is also common when subjects present with new-onset hypertension, especially in adolescence (Fig. 32.6).[14] Experimental hyperuricemia also causes hypertension. The mechanism is complex. Uric acid enters endothelial cells where it inactivates local nitric oxide. In the rat, this results in systemic and renal vasoconstriction and a salt resistant form of hypertension. Over time, renal arteriolar disease develops secondary to both direct and indirect effects of uric acid, and the hypertension becomes salt sensitive. Studies to verify these pathways in humans are still in process.

Uric acid becomes a candidate to account for the epidemic of hypertension since it is readily altered by diet and other means. Thus, a Western diet rich in fatty meats is known to increase serum uric acid, and epidemiologic studies have linked hyperuricemia and/or gout with the epidemics of obesity and hypertension observed both in developing and industrialized nations, in studies of immigrants, and with rural to urban movement. Interestingly, uric acid is increased by fructose ingestion. In the past 40 years, there has been a marked increase in the ingestion of sweeteners, primarily table sugar (sucrose, which contains 50% fructose) and high fructose corn syrup (55% fructose). The increase in total fructose intake correlates directly with the epidemic of hypertension and obesity. Feeding fructose to rats also causes hypertension and

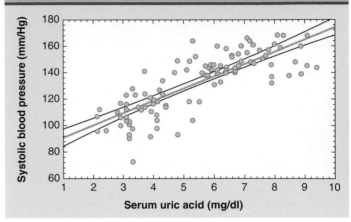

Figure 32.6 Relationship of serum uric acid with systolic BP in normal adolescents and adolescents with essential hypertension. The *orange line* indicates the best fit. The *red lines* show the 95% confidence internal. (From Feig DI, Johnson RJ: Hyperuricemia in childhood primary hypertension. Hypertension 2003;42:247–252.)

the metabolic syndrome. The observation that uric acid blocks endothelial nitric oxide bioavailability provides a mechanism since low nitric oxide will predispose an animal to hypertension (see previous discussion) and to be insulin resistant (since nitric oxide is required for insulin-dependent glucose delivery to skeletal muscle). Interestingly, the treatment of fructose-fed rats with allopurinol (which lowers uric acid) resulted in improvement of BP, insulin resistance, and lower body weights.[15]

In addition to linking uric acid with fatty meats and sugar intake associated with westernization, uric acid is increased by low levels of lead or cadmium ingestion, both of which are also associated with hypertension. Furthermore, an elevated uric acid in preeclampsia is associated with intrauterine growth retardation and the future development of hypertension among the progeny. Since uric acid inhibits endothelial cell growth and function, the diffusion of uric acid into the fetal circulation could be a mechanism for a low nephron number.[16]

How Does Salt Retention Lead to Hypertension?

An acute infusion of saline administered to animals with experimentally induced hypertension will initially increase blood volume and cardiac output, but the increase in cardiac output is transient and is replaced by an increase in the systemic vascular resistance, a process that Guyton and colleagues[4] termed autoregulation. It is thought that this may underlie the process by which the renal defect in sodium excretion leads to the high systemic vascular resistance observed in essential hypertension. Several mechanisms could account for this.

First, the normal response to a salt load is an inhibition of the SNS. However in salt sensitive hypertensive patients, the SNS is not inhibited but may even be activated with a salt load.[6] A possible explanation is that, in the setting of tubulointerstitial injury and intrarenal ischemia, the salt load will trigger an intense tubuloglomerular feedback signal with activation of the renal afferent SNS that subsequently triggers the CNS response. Indeed, there is evidence that renal afferent nerves activate CNS sympathetic activity in both experimental hypertension and chronic renal disease.[6]

Second, sodium retention may result in the release of substances that raise systemic vascular resistance. Circulating

Na$^+$-K$^+$-adenosine triphosphatase (ATPase) inhibitors as well as nitric oxide synthase inhibitors have been documented in some patients with essential hypertension. One Na$^+$-K$^+$-ATPase inhibitor has been identified as ouabain-like and is derived from the adrenals. Blaustein and Hamlyn[17] have suggested that these substances, which are presumably secreted in an attempt to facilitate sodium excretion, may have the adverse consequence of increasing intracellular sodium and thus facilitating sodium-calcium exchange in the vascular smooth muscle cell. This would lead to an increase in intracellular calcium and stimulate vascular smooth muscle contraction, vasoconstriction, and an increase in vascular resistance. Vasopressin has also been implicated in African American hypertensives since vasopressin V$_{1A}$ receptor antagonists lower BP by as much as 10 mm Hg in the presence of a high-salt diet and clonidine, both of which suppress the SNS.[18]

A third mechanism is the loss of a vasodepressor substance. A lipid-like vasodepressor factor, termed medullipin, is expressed by interstitial cells in the renal medulla and juxtamedullary region. Release of this factor into the circulation appears to depend on medullary blood flow, which could be impaired in the setting of renal vasoconstriction that occurs in essential hypertension.[19]

Finally, the increase in pressure associated with sodium retention could lead to damage of the systemic capillaries, resulting in microvascular rarefaction (which has been observed in forearms and nail beds of patients with essential hypertension), and thereby increase peripheral vascular resistance.

EPIDEMIOLOGY

Essential hypertension is epidemic. In the United States, the prevalence has increased from 5% to 11% of the population in the early 1900s to 31% (65 million people) today (Fig. 32.7). The increase in prevalence, which has also been observed in Europe, cannot be completely accounted for by the increasing life expectancy in the population. Similarly, hypertension was practically absent outside Europe and North America until the 1930s, but has subsequently increased to prevalence rates of 20% to 30% in conjunction with adaptation of the Western diet and lifestyle. The increase in hypertension correlates with

Risk factors for essential hypertension	
Genetic	Family history Polymorphisms (adducin, endothelial nitric oxide synthase, angiotensinogen, β-adrenoreceptor, protein β3)
Congenital	Low birth weight, low nephron number, maternal hypertension, maternal preeclampsia, maternal malnutrition
Physical	Obesity, older age, African American, African Caribbean, increased heart rate (>83 beats/min), increased emotional stress
Diet/toxin	Increased sodium intake, low potassium intake, low dairy products intake, heavy alcohol intake, low level lead or cadmium intoxication
Metabolic (laboratory-based parameters)	Elevated uric acid, insulin resistance, elevated hematocrit
Other	Low socioeconomic status, urban vs rural

Figure 32.8   Major risk factors for essential hypertension.

increasing frequencies of obesity, type 2 diabetes, and chronic kidney disease, suggesting a strong interrelationship.

There are several major risk factors for hypertension (Fig. 32.8). First, the risk of essential hypertension increases with age, with a 65% prevalence in the population at age 65, and 75% at age 75. This age-related increase in prevalence of hypertension has been observed in most Western countries but has not been uniformly observed in all populations. Second, hypertension is more common in men, although the prevalence in women approaches that of men in the postmenopausal years. Certain racial groups are also at increased risk, particularly African Americans. Obesity, insulin resistance, hyperuricemia and/or gout, and sleep apnea are also associated with increased risk, as are low socioeconomic status and increased stress at work. Certain physical features, such as increased heart rate or an increased BP response to exercise, are also predictive, as is increased hematocrit.

Genetic factors also contribute. While the inheritance patterns do not follow classic mendelian genetics for a single gene locus, there is evidence that as much as 30% of hypertension may have a genetic basis due to the cumulative effect of multiple susceptibility genes (the polygene hypothesis). In this regard, an increased risk of hypertension has been noted with certain genetic polymorphisms involving vasoactive mediators (angiotensinogen, endothelial nitric oxide synthase, prostacyclin synthase, the β$_2$-adrenoceptor and G protein β3) or mediators controlling renal sodium transport (for example, α-adducin and 11β-hydroxysteroid dehydrogenase type 2).[20]

Maternal factors also influence the risk of hypertension. Hypertension is more likely to occur if the mother has a history of hypertension, obesity, preeclampsia, or malnutrition. These risk factors are all associated with intrauterine growth retardation and low birth weight babies, both of which appear to predispose to future hypertension, as well as diabetes and obesity.

Dietary and other environmental factors may contribute to the risk of hypertension. Obesity (with or without features of insulin resistance and the metabolic syndrome) is the most salient risk factor for hypertension. Obesity is increasing in both developing and industrialized countries and parallels the increase in hypertension in these countries. Epidemiologic and interventional studies have linked salt intake with hypertension, although the

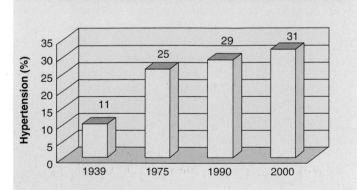

Prevalence of essential hypertension in the United States

Figure 32.7   Epidemic of hypertension. The prevalence of essential hypertension (defined as BP >140/90 mm Hg) in the United States has been increasing from 11% in 1939 to 31% today. Data from a study in Chicago in 1939 (Robinson SC, Brucer M: Arch Intern Med 1939;64:409–444), the Hypertension Detection and Followup Program, and the National Health and Nutrition Examination Survey III.

relationship is best demonstrated in older subjects and in African Americans. Diets low in calcium/dairy products or potassium are also associated with a higher prevalence of hypertension. Increasing potassium intake lowers BP in both experimental and human studies. Finally, certain toxins, most notably low level lead or cadmium intoxication, are associated with increased frequency of essential hypertension.

CLINICAL MANIFESTATIONS AND DIAGNOSIS

Evaluation of a patient with hypertension should include a careful history and physical examination to document the presence of hypertension, to evaluate risk factors for essential hypertension, to evaluate for potential secondary causes of hypertension, and to evaluate for end-organ damage.

To document the presence of hypertension, BP should be repeatedly measured on at least three occasions to confirm persistent hypertension using the techniques described in Chapter 31. Documentation that hypertension is present in the home or outside the clinic should be obtained with home BP monitoring. This may help in the identification of hypertension that occurs only in the physician's office (white coat hypertension) or more rarely in identifying masked hypertension in which increases in BP occur only outside the physician's office. Documentation of these latter two conditions often can be verified with 24-hour ambulatory BP monitoring (see Fig. 31.17 and Chapter 31 for a list of indications). Both white coat and masked hypertension are no longer considered benign as they are associated with some end-organ disease (including left ventricular hypertrophy and microalbuminuria) and increased cardiovascular risk. These patients need assessment of risk factors and more frequent evaluation of their BP.

The medical history should include questions related to the history and duration of hypertension in the patient. A family history of hypertension and cardiovascular and renal disease should be sought. The history should identify risk factors (e.g., obesity, diabetes, physical activity, alcohol, smoking, diet, emotional or work-related stress, use of over-the-counter and prescribed medications) and any hypertension-related morbidity.

Hypertension is usually asymptomatic. On rare occasions, some patients may complain of headache (classically occipital and pulsatile), although most studies have not been able to document a strong relationship unless the person has stage II hypertension. Hypertensive encephalopathy may rarely occur with mental status changes and/or seizures. In patients with malignant hypertension, there may also be visual changes (from papilledema), and patients are at acute risk of myocardial infarction and congestive heart failure with pulmonary edema, dissection, stroke, and renal failure. Last, it should be noted that the Hypertension Optimal Treatment trials demonstrated that those with hypertension whose diastolic pressure was lowered to <85 mm Hg reported better memory and general improvement in well-being than before their BP was decreased.

Physical examination should include careful attention to the cardiovascular system. Measurement of BP in both arms and a careful cardiac examination including measurement of the pulse is mandatory. Attention should be focused on both the large vessels (by both palpation and listening for bruits) and the retina to grade the severity of disease in the microvasculature (Fig. 32.9).

Laboratory tests should include hematocrit, electrolytes, urea nitrogen and creatinine, calcium and phosphate, fasting lipid profile (cholesterol and triglycerides), uric acid, C-reactive protein, and urinalysis, including a spot urine albumin-to-creatinine ratio for microalbuminuria. A chest radiograph and electrocardiogram should also be obtained to assess cardiac size and the presence of left ventricular hypertrophy and to look for aortic dilatation (Fig. 32.10).

Additional tests that may be helpful under certain circumstances include a 24-hour urine collection to assess creatinine clearance and sodium and potassium levels. The latter is an indication of how much sodium and potassium the patient is ingesting, as the urinary excretion will correlate closely with intake if the patient is in steady state (the desirable values are <100 mmol/l Na$^+$ and >100 mmol/l K$^+$ in 24 hours). Testing for microalbuminuria and performing echocardiography to look for concentric left ventricular hypertrophy (Fig. 32.11) may provide additional evidence of end-organ damage. Echocardiography is not recommended for

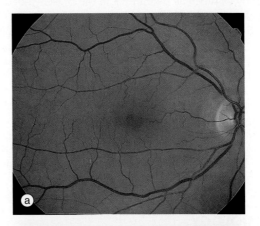

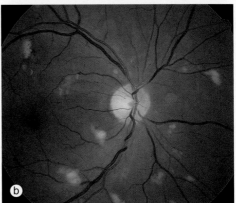

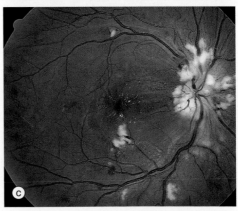

Figure 32.9 Different grades of hypertensive retinopathy. *a*, Mild hypertensive retinopathy, with arteriolar narrowing and arteriovenous nicking. *b*, Moderate hypertensive retinopathy, with cotton wool spots (nerve fiber layer infarcts) and arteriovenous nicking. *c*, Malignant hypertension with papilledema, cotton wool spots, macular yellow exudates (star formation pattern), and retinal hemorrhages. (Gift of J. Kinyoun, University of Washington.)

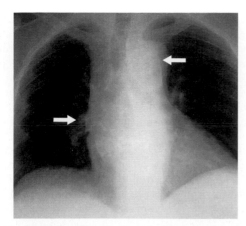

Figure 32.10   Chest radiograph of aortic dilatation in a patient with essential hypertension. Dilatation of the aortic arch (*arrow*) and ascending aorta (noted by the mediastinal convexity, *arrow*) is present. (Gift of D. Godwin, University of Washington.)

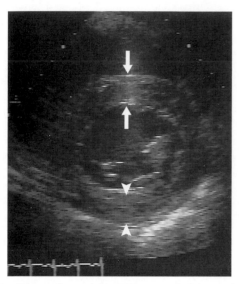

Figure 32.11   Echocardiogram showing concentric left ventricular hypertrophy. Septal thickness (*between large arrows*) and posterior wall thickness (*between arrowheads*) are increased (to 16 mm) in a patient with essential hypertension (normal is ≤11 mm). (Gift of A. Pearlman, University of Washington.)

routine use in people with hypertension due to its cost. It is, however, recommended in people with coronary artery disease with other risk factors.[21]

The major secondary causes include renal parenchymal disease, renal artery stenosis, adrenal hyperplasia or tumors (such as primary aldosteronism), medications such as sympathomimetics, illicit drugs such as cocaine, and heavy alcohol use. A more complete list is provided in Chapter 31. If a secondary cause is suspected, then further studies such as aldosterone-to-renin ratios, radiographic studies, and urinary catecholamines should be performed, as discussed in Chapter 31.

PATHOLOGY

Essential hypertension has a characteristic renal biopsy specimen (benign nephrosclerosis) in which there is preferential involvement of the preglomerular arterial vessels, primarily the afferent arteriole and interlobular artery. The classic arterial lesion, which is observed in 90% of biopsy cases, is termed arteriolosclerosis and consists of the replacement of smooth muscle cells of the

media in the afferent arteriole by connective tissue (Fig. 32.12). Often there is also accumulation of hyaline material (plasma proteins) in the subintima (hyalinosis). In association with arteriolar disease, there is often evidence of glomerular and tubulointerstitial ischemia with shrinkage of the glomerular tuft, tubular atrophy, and interstitial fibrosis. Occasionally biopsies show evidence of glomerulosclerosis and severe tubulointerstitial injury (termed decompensated nephrosclerosis).[22] In cases of malignant hypertension, the arterial lesion is more of a proliferative arteriolopathy, occasionally with fibrinoid necrosis. Concentric layers of connective tissue and cells may give an onion-skin appearance to the intima, which may progress to a total obliteration of the lumen. In these severe cases, fibrinoid necrosis may also be seen in the glomerulus.

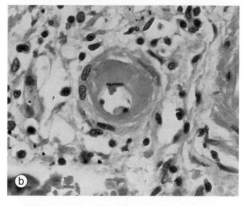

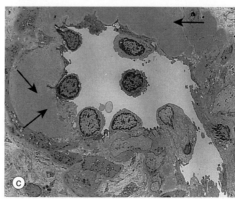

Figure 32.12   Renal biopsy findings in essential hypertension. *a*, A granular pitted kidney of benign nephrosclerosis. *b*, Arteriolosclerosis with subintimal hyalinosis. *c*, Electron micrograph showing hyalinosis with the accumulation of insudate plasma proteins in the subendothelium of an arteriole (*arrows*). (*a*, Gift from Harvard Medical School; *b* and *c*, courtesy of C. E. Alpers, University of Washington.)

NATURAL HISTORY

Hypertension commonly develops after the age of 40, but is observed with increasing frequency in adolescents and young adults. Early hypertension is often salt resistant, whereas salt sensitivity is increasing severe and more frequent in older hypertensive subjects and in African Americans. The sudden worsening of hypertension should make one consider secondary causes, especially renal artery stenosis.

The major long-term risk of hypertension is cardiovascular disease. Hypertension is the most common cause of congestive heart failure and stroke, and the second most common cause of end-stage renal disease in the westernized world. Increased systolic, diastolic, and pulse pressure all confer risk, although the systolic BP and the pulse pressure appear to be the more important determinants for the risk of the hypertensive complications, especially for stroke and renal disease.

The cardiovascular and cerebrovascular morbidity and mortality increase linearly with increments in BP from 120/80 mm Hg upward (Fig. 32.13).[23] This increased risk is dependent on age (increases with age), sex (greater in males), ethnic origin (greater in African Americans and other associated risk factors (e.g., diabetes) and is associated with both atherosclerotic and hypertensive (pressure-related) disease. Atherosclerotic complications include myocardial infarction, thrombotic stroke, peripheral vascular disease, and aortic aneurysm; hypertensive complications include congestive heart failure, hemorrhagic stroke, aortic dissection, and bleeding cerebral aneurysms. In addition to an increased prevalence of hypertension, African Americans also have 80% greater stroke mortality and 50% more heart disease.

Hypertensive heart disease often begins with concentric left ventricular hypertrophy associated with supernormal systolic function. Over time, impaired diastolic dysfunction may occur, as manifested by slow diastolic filling, which reflects decreased diastolic relaxation. This may progress to congestive heart failure. Nearly 90% of patients with heart failure have a history of hypertension.

Renal Disease

Most patients with newly diagnosed essential hypertension will have either stage 1 (glomerular filtration rate [GFR] >90 ml/min per 1.73 m^2) or stage 2 chronic kidney disease (GFR 60 to 90 ml/min per 1.73 m^2) with increased renal vascular resistance.[24] Despite relatively normal renal function, a renal biopsy specimen, if obtained, usually shows arteriolosclerosis and hyalinosis (see Fig. 32.12).

Prior to effective antihypertensive agents, proteinuria developed in up to 40% of patients and as many as 18% developed renal insufficiency over time. Currently, microalbuminuria occurs in 15% to 30% of patients, and fewer patients develop non-nephrotic, or, rarely, nephrotic-range proteinuria. The development of microalbuminuria is associated with salt sensitivity, the loss of nocturnal dipping in BP, and increased target organ damage (especially left ventricular hypertrophy).

An elevated serum creatinine develops in 10% to 20% of patients, and the risk is greater in African Americans, the elderly, and those with higher systolic BP (systolic BP >160 mm Hg).[25,26] In 2% to 5%, progression to renal failure will occur over the subsequent 10 to 15 years (Figs. 32.14 and 32.15). Despite the relative infrequency for hypertension to progress to end-stage renal

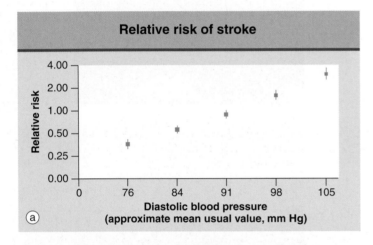

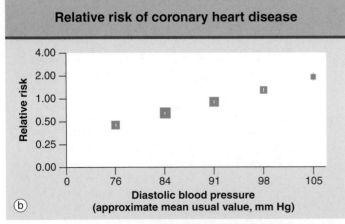

Figure 32.13 **Relative risks of stroke (*a*) and coronary heart disease (*b*) increase with increased diastolic blood pressure.** The stroke data are from seven prospective observational studies and 843 events; the coronary heart disease data are from nine studies and 4856 events. Sizes of squares are proportional to the number of events in each category; the vertical lines indicate 95% confidence intervals. (Adapted from MacMahon S, Peto R, Cutler J, et al: Blood pressure, stroke, and coronary heart disease. Part I, Prolonged differences in blood pressure: Prospective observational studies corrected for the regression dilution bias. Lancet 1990;335:765–774.)

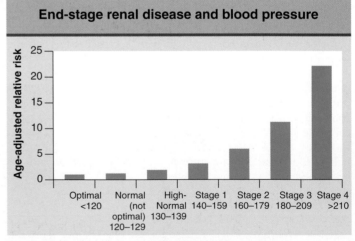

Figure 32.14 **End-stage renal disease and blood pressure.** Incidence of end-stage renal disease related to baseline blood pressure in the MRFIT study. Mean follow-up was 16 years. Systolic BP for each category is shown below. (Adapted from Klag MJ, Whelton PK, Randall BL, et al: Blood pressure and end-stage renal disease in men. N Engl J Med 1996;334:13–18.)

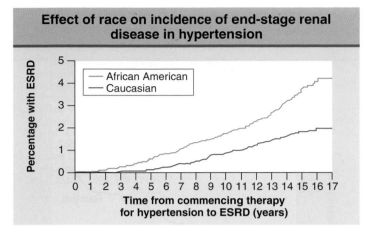

Effect of race on incidence of end-stage renal disease in hypertension

Figure 32.15 Effect of race on incidence of end-stage renal disease (ESRD) in hypertension. The rate of end-stage renal disease in African American and Caucasian hypertensive veterans. Kaplan-Meier estimates of the rates of end-stage renal disease in hypertensives. (From Perry HM Jr, Miller JP, Fornoff JR, et al: Early predictors of 15-year end-stage renal disease in hypertensive patients. Hypertension 1995;25:587–594.)

disease, the large population of hypertensive patients means that hypertension remains the second most common cause of end-stage renal disease after diabetes in the United States. Furthermore, virtually all diabetic subjects have hypertension when they start dialysis. The risk of renal failure secondary to hypertension is threefold greater in African Americans.[27]

Effect of Antihypertensive Therapy on the Natural History of Hypertensive Cardiovascular Disease and Renal Disease Progression

According to a recent report, only 59% of subjects with hypertension in the United States are on treatment and only 34% have their BP under adequate (<140/90 mm Hg) control.[2] Although there has been significant reduction in the age-adjusted death rate for stroke and coronary artery disease since the early 1980s as a result of better BP control (and better treatment of other risk factors such as hyperlipidemia), heart disease and stroke remain the first and third leading causes of death in the United States. This emphasizes the importance of identifying and treating patients with hypertension.

Antihypertensive therapy has been shown to reduce cardiovascular and cerebrovascular complications in patients with moderate to severe hypertension (diastolic BP >105 mm Hg) and in patients with mild hypertension and associated cardiovascular risk factors (Fig. 32.16). The risk reduction has been most significant for stroke and congestive heart failure, but also occurs for myocardial infarction.[28] Several epidemiologic studies have also demonstrated a benefit in treating mild hypertension.[29,30]

Antihypertensive therapy also reduces the risk of progression of renal disease[31,32] and may even be associated with some recovery of renal function in patients presenting with BP values in excess of 180/110 mm Hg. Clinical trials in African Americans[32] and in nondiabetic, proteinuric renal disease[33] demonstrate that lowering systolic BP to 130 to 139 mm Hg using an ACE inhibitor as one of the BP-lowering agents reduces the risk of end-stage

Outcome in clinical trials according to first-line therapy for hypertension

Outcome	Drug regimen	Dose	No. of trials	Relative risk (95% confidence interval)
Stroke	Diuretics	High	9	
	Diuretics	Low	4	
	β-blockers		4	
	Hypertension and Detection Followup Program (HDFP)	High	1	
Coronary heart disease	Diuretics	High	11	
	Diuretics	Low	4	
	β-blockers		4	
	HDFP	High	1	
Congestive artery failure	Diuretics	High	9	
	Diuretics	Low	3	
	β-blockers		2	
Total mortality	Diuretics	High	11	
	Diuretics	Low	4	
	β-blockers		4	
	HDFP	High	1	
Cardiovascular mortality	Diuretics	High	11	
	Diuretics	Low	4	
	β-blockers		4	
	HDFP	High	1	

Figure 32.16 Outcome in clinical trials according to first-line therapy for hypertension. Effect of antihypertensive therapy on stroke, coronary artery disease, congestive heart failure, and total and cardiovascular mortality. Data are taken from a meta-analysis of randomized, placebo-controlled clinical trials in hypertension according to first-line therapy. The total numbers of participants were 24,294 (active treatment) and 23,926 (placebo). (From Psaty BM, Smith NL, Siscovick DS, et al: Health outcomes associated with antihypertensive therapies used as first-line agents. A systematic review and meta-analysis. JAMA 1997;277:739–745.)

Nonpharmacologic Prevention and Treatment of Hypertension

Brian Rayner, Karen E. Charlton, Estelle V. Lambert, and Wayne Derman

Over the past few decades, lifestyles have undergone substantial changes. A combination of increased fat and refined carbohydrate intake and a reduction in physical activity has resulted in an epidemic of obesity, type 2 diabetes mellitus, and hypertension. This is a worldwide phenomenon, which is particularly evident in the United States.

Adoption of healthy lifestyles by all individuals is critical for the prevention of high blood pressure (BP) and is an indispensable part of the management of those with hypertension according to the Seventh Report of the Joint National Committee on Prevention, Evaluation, and Treatment of High Blood Pressure (JNC 7).[1] Lifestyle interventions lower BP, enhance efficacy of antihypertensive therapy, and lower overall cardiovascular risk factors. The lifestyle changes that are widely agreed to lower BP and cardiovascular risk are (1) smoking cessation, (2) weight reduction, (3) moderation of alcohol intake, (4) physical exercise, (5) reduction of salt intake, (6) increase in fruit and vegetable intake, and (7) a decrease in saturated and total fat intake.[1,2]

Interventions may have similar efficacy to single drug therapy (Fig. 33.1); however, lifestyle changes should not unnecessarily delay the initiation of drug therapy, especially in patients at higher cardiovascular risk.[2]

PREVENTION

The prevention of hypertension has been as elusive as the identification of the multiple causes for hypertension itself. Despite this obstacle, the importance of primary prevention has been underscored by the recognition that treatment of hypertension is expensive, control of BP in hypertensive individuals does not restore cardiovascular risk to normal, and the majority of hypertensive individuals are not receiving adequate treatment. It therefore becomes important to identify the modifiable factors influencing increases in BP as well as those individuals who are most susceptible to these factors, especially obesity and lifestyle-behavioral factors (smoking, alcohol consumption, and dietary intake of sodium and potassium).

Another clue to the increased susceptibility for the development of hypertension is the BP level itself. The JNC 7 acknowledged this fact by the creation of a new category of BP designated prehypertension (120 to 139/80 to 89 mm Hg).[1] In earlier studies, individuals with this level of BP were found to have an increased prevalence of early vascular damage and an increased risk of the development of hypertension. Reports from the Framingham Study indicate that these levels of BP are associated with an

Lifestyle modifications for the prevention and management of hypertension (Joint National Committee guidelines[1])		
Modification	Recommendation	Average Systolic BP Reduction Range Achieved with Intervention*
Weight reduction	Maintain normal body weight (BMI = 18.5–24.9 kg/m²)	5–20 mm Hg/10 kg
DASH eating plan	Adopt a diet rich in fruits, vegetables, and low-fat dairy products with reduced content of saturated and total fat	8–14 mm Hg
Dietary sodium restriction	Reduce dietary sodium intake to 100 mmol/day (2.4 g sodium or 6 g sodium chloride).	2–8 mm Hg
Aerobic physical activity	Regular aerobic physical activity (e.g., brisk walking) at least 30 min/day, most days of the week	4–9 mm Hg
Moderation of alcohol consumption	Men: limit to 2 drinks[†] per day; women and lighter-weight persons: limit to 1 drink per day	2–4 mm Hg

Figure 33.1   Lifestyle modifications for the prevention and management of hypertension (Joint National Committee 7 guidelines[1]). BMI, body mass index; BP, blood pressure; DASH, Dietary Approaches to Stop Hypertension. *Effects are dose and time dependent. [†]One drink = ½ oz or 15 ml ethanol (e.g., 12 oz of beer, 5 oz of wine, 1.5 oz of 80-proof whiskey).

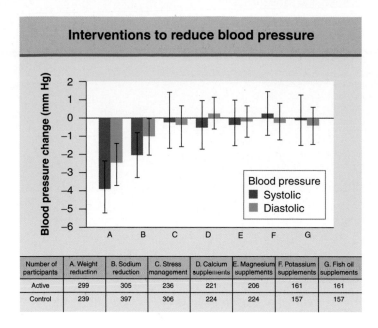

Figure 33.2 Interventions to reduce blood pressure. Net mean changes in systolic and diastolic blood pressure (baseline minus follow-up) with various interventions in patients with high-normal levels of blood pressure. (Adapted Trials of Hypertension Prevention Collaboration Research Group: The effects of nonpharmacologic interventions on blood pressure of persons with high-normal levels. JAMA 1992;267:1213–1220.)

Number of participants	A. Weight reduction	B. Sodium reduction	C. Stress management	D. Calcium supplements	E. Magnesium supplements	F. Potassium supplements	G. Fish oil supplements
Active	299	305	236	221	206	161	161
Control	239	397	306	224	224	157	157

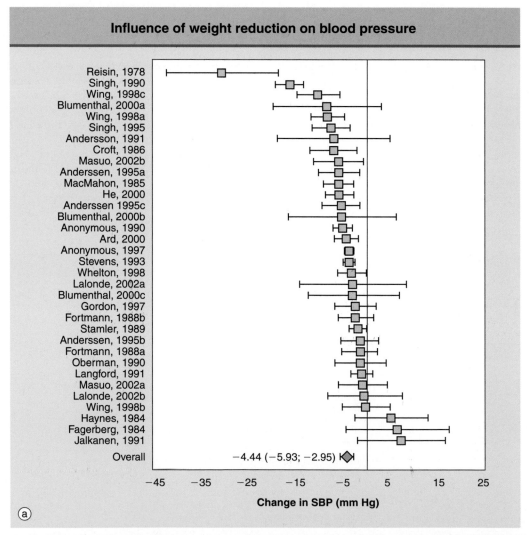

Figure 33.3 Influence of weight reduction on blood pressure. A meta-analysis of randomized, controlled trials. *Squares* represent average net changes in systolic blood pressure (SBP) (*a*) in individual trials (or trial strata), with 95% confidence intervals; pooled estimates from meta-analysis are depicted as a *diamond*. Suffixes (a, b, c) denote different strata from the same trial.

increased risk of cardiovascular events when compared to those with optimal levels (<120/80).[3] The JNC 7 recommends lifestyle changes in all patients in prehypertensive category to prevent the development of hypertension and reduce their cardiovascular risk.[1]

The contributions of body weight, physical inactivity, and dietary factors to the prevalence of hypertension in Finland, Italy, The Netherlands, the United Kingdom, and the United States has been quantified in a metaregression analysis.[4] Being overweight made the largest contribution to hypertension, with population-attributable risk percentages (PAR%) between 11% (Italy) and 25% (United States). PAR% was 5% to 13% for physical inactivity, 9% to 17% for high sodium intake, 4% to 17% for low potassium intake, and 4% to 8% for low magnesium intake. The impact of alcohol was small (2% to 3%) in all populations. PAR% varied among populations for inadequate intake of calcium (2% to 8%), magnesium (4% to 8%), coffee (0% to 9%), and fish fatty acids (3% to 16%).

WEIGHT LOSS

Obesity has now reached epidemic proportions in the United States, as well as in many other developed and developing countries. Sixty-five percent of the U.S. adult population are either overweight (body mass index [BMI] = 25.0 to 29.9) or obese (BMI = 30).[5]

Obese individuals have a threefold increased prevalence of hypertension. Possible mechanisms for obesity-induced hypertension

include overactivity of the sympathetic nervous system, hyperinsulinemia (which may increase renal sodium reabsorption), hyperuricemia, and sleep apnea. Abdominal or visceral obesity is a greater predictor of both hypertension and cardiovascular disease risk as compared to a predominant lower body fat distribution. Abdominal obesity is defined as a waist circumference >88 cm in women and >102 cm in men. These reference values were developed in Caucasian populations, and differing criteria may be appropriate in other ethnic groups.

In obese hypertensives or those with high-normal BP, weight loss of as little as 4 to 5 kg is often associated with a significant reduction in BP. Weight loss is, in fact, one of the most effective nonpharmacologic interventions to reduce BP (Fig. 33.2).[6] A meta-analysis of weight loss and BP trials has demonstrated that a weight reduction of 5.1 kg, by means of energy restriction, increased physical activity, or both, reduced systolic BP by 4.44 mm Hg and diastolic BP by 3.57 mm Hg (Fig. 33.3).[7] A rule of thumb is that for every kilogram of weight loss, a corresponding BP reduction of 1.05 mm Hg and 0.92 mm Hg for systolic and diastolic, respectively, is observed. In order to minimize risk of relapse (regain in weight) and for weight loss to be sustainable, an initial target should be 5% to 10 % of current weight, or 1 to 2 BMI units. Marked oscillations in weight should be avoided as it is associated with an increased risk of developing hypertension in obese, normotensive subjects.[8] Diets that are not sustainable should be avoided.

A randomized trial of the effectiveness of four popular diets on sustained weight loss and cardiovascular disease risk reduction

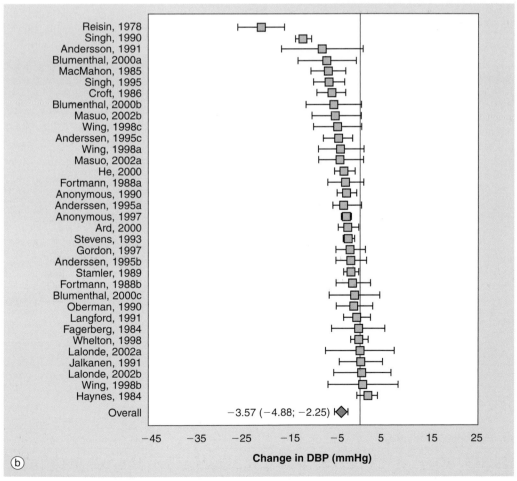

Figure 33.3, cont'd *Squares* represent average net changes in diastolic blood pressure (DBP) (*b*) in individual trials (or trial strata), with 95% confidence intervals; pooled estimates from meta-analysis are depicted as a *diamond*. Suffixes (a, b, c) denote different strata from the same trial. (Modified from Neter JE, Stam BE, Kok FJ, et al: Influence of weight reduction on blood pressure. A meta-analysis of randomized controlled trials. Hypertension 2003;42:878–884.)

concluded that a variety of diets can similarly reduce weight and BP, but only a minority of individuals can sustain high dietary adherence.[9] High-protein diets such as the Atkins diet, often advocated for weight loss by the media and lay public, have no place in hypertensive patients with renal disease.

Weight reduction should be accompanied by recommendations to increase physical activity unless contraindicated. Bariatric surgery, pharmacologic interventions for weight loss (e.g., sibutramine and orlistat), and the use of very low calorie (liquid) diets or meal replacement diets may be useful to achieve weight loss in some patients, but always as an adjunct rather than a substitute for lifestyle modification.

PHYSICAL ACTIVITY

There is now a well-established link between regular physical activity and lowered risk of all-cause mortality and morbidity. Physical inactivity is associated with at least a 1.5- to twofold higher risk of hypertension and coronary heart disease.[10] These studies corroborate existing public health recommendations suggesting that 30 minutes of moderate to vigorous physical activity on most days is protective.

Exercise Training Dose Response
In a meta-analyses of more than 68 studies, representing >1500 patients, the effect of exercise training on BP in normotensive subjects has been shown to reduce 3.0 ± 1 and 1.7 ± 1 mm Hg systolic and diastolic BP, respectively.[11] Furthermore, changes in BP associated with exercise training are even more marked in those who are already hypertensive (7.8 ± 3.5 and 5.8 ± 2.0 mm Hg for systolic and diastolic, respectively). Weekly accumulated exercise dose and BP response have been studied after 8 weeks of exercise training in hypertensive patients. It was found that BP response to an increasing dose of physical activity was sigmoidal with a peak effect at 90 minutes, after which there was no further improvement.[12] Investigators concluded that a relatively modest amount of exercise was needed to reduce BP in patients with hypertension (>30 min/wk).

Fagard[11] found no benefit of increasing exercise intensity on BP reduction with exercise training, as long as intensity ranged between 40% and 70% of maximal, age-predicted heart rate. This contrasts with the acute effects of exercise on the attenuation of postexercise BP. Exercise of higher intensity (75% maximum) was associated with a more marked and prolonged reduction in BP in the postexercise window compared to lower-intensity exercise (50% maximum).[13]

Putative Mechanisms
The mechanisms underlying both the acute and chronic effects of exercise on BP control are not fully understood. In the acute postexercise period, the reduction in BP has been linked to a sympathetic inhibition and increased release of vasodilator substances.[14] Mechanisms that have been implicated in the effect of chronic exercise on BP control include reductions in vascular resistance secondary to neurohumoral and structural adaptations.

Antihypertensive Medication and Guidelines for Exercise
Exercise guidelines exist for patients with hypertension (Fig. 33.4).[15] In relation to antihypertensive agents, β-blockers decrease exercise tolerance and are therefore not ideal. Angiotensin-converting enzyme inhibitors, angiotensin II receptor blockers, and calcium channel blockers may be better suited for these patients or athletes with hypertension. β-Blockers and diuretics alter thermoregulation in hot environments and may provoke hypoglycemia. Patients using these medications should be educated about exercising in the heat, clothing, the role of adequate hydration, and methods to prevent hypoglycemia.[16–18]

For patients undergoing supervised exercise training, the monitoring of postexercise BP may be helpful so that medications may be adjusted appropriately, considering the likelihood of postexercise hypotension. Particular care should be taken with patients planning to exercise in a hot environment.

DIET

Salt Intake
Epidemiologic studies demonstrate that the prevalence of hypertension and its associated cardiovascular consequences are directly related to the level of dietary salt intake in societies throughout the world in whom the intake is above 50 to 100 mmol/day (Fig. 33.5).[19] In societies where habitual intake is below that range,

Practical guidelines for exercise in patients with hypertension
All apparently healthy individuals should undergo pre-exercise screening to determine health risk status. The American College of Sports Medicine (ACSM) recognizes that two or more of the following risk factors increase the risk associated with exercise and individuals should undergo pre-exercise graded exercise testing. Risk factors include male gender (older than age 45 years) or female (older than 55 years); serum cholesterol concentrations >5.2 mmol/l; impaired glucose tolerance or diabetes mellitus, smoking; obesity (body mass index ≥30); inactivity; and family history of cardiovascular disease.
Patients with uncontrolled hypertension should embark on exercise training only after evaluation and initiation of therapy. Furthermore, patients should not participate in an exercise training session if resting systolic blood pressure is >200 mm Hg or diastolic blood pressure is >115 mm Hg.
Many patients with hypertension are overweight and should therefore be encouraged to follow a program that combines both exercise training and restricted calorie intake.[16]
Type of exercise: this should be predominantly endurance physical activity including walking, jogging, cycling, swimming, or dancing. This should be supplemented by resistance exercise that can be prescribed according to the ACSM or American Heart Association guidelines.[17]
Frequency of exercise: most or preferably every day.
Intensity of exercise: moderate intensity at 40%–60% of VO_2 peak.
Duration of exercise: >30 minutes of continuous or accumulated moderate physical activity daily.

Figure 33.4 Practical guidelines for exercise in patients with hypertension. (Adapted from Pescatello LS, Franklin BA, Farquhar WB, et al: American College of Sports Medicine. American College of Sports Medicine position stand. Exercise and hypertension. Med Sci Sports Exerc 2004;36:533–553.)

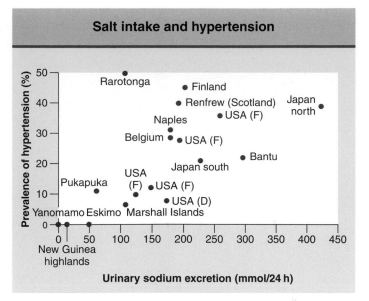

Figure 33.5 **Relationship of salt intake with frequency of hypertension in different populations.** D, data from Dahl. F, data from the Framingham Study. (Adapted from MacGregor GA: Sodium is more important than calcium in essential hypertension. Hypertension 1985;7:628–637.)

BP-increasing effects of sodium. However, a prospective study of 1173 men and 1263 women in Finland found that coronary heart disease, cardiovascular disease, and all-cause mortality all increased significantly with increasing 24-hour urinary sodium excretion, independently of other cardiovascular risk factors, including BP.[21]

Not all individuals respond similarly to high salt intakes: the concept of sodium sensitivity, whereby a decrease in BP is observed during periods of salt restriction, accompanied by an increase in BP with sodium chloride loading, is well described.[22,23] Since there is no quick and easy way to predict whether an individual is sodium sensitive, the classification has remained in the research domain rather than being of practical or clinical importance.

However, it is useful to identify which groups are most likely to be sensitive to high salt intakes. Epidemiologic studies have shown a higher frequency of sodium sensitivity in the following demographic groups:

- African Americans
- Elderly people
- Obese (not in all studies)
- Insulin-dependent diabetic subjects
- Patients on cyclosporine
- Renal insufficiency

Sodium sensitivity is observed in 75% of hypertensive African Americans compared to about 50% of Caucasian hypertensives[23] and increases with age in both the normotensive and hypertensive population (Fig. 33.7).[24] There is convincing motivation for universal sodium restriction in all older people. A randomized, controlled trial in British people aged 60 to 78 years who were not receiving antihypertensive medication found that a modest salt restriction from 10 g to 5 g per day resulted in an impressive reduction of BP of 7.2/3.2 mm Hg over a 4-week period.[25] Importantly, unlike studies in younger subjects, similar decreases in BP were seen for both normotensive and hypertensive subjects. The findings are

hypertension is rare. It is also evident that salt plays a role in the age-related increase in BP (Fig. 33.6).[20] Cross-sectional observations demonstrate that such age-related increases in BP are most commonly observed in industrialized societies, that is, those featuring habitual salt intake >120 mmol/day.[19] By comparison, in societies in which the usual salt intake is much lower, such age-related increases in BP have not been reported.

It has been argued for decades that a high salt intake may not be detrimental in subjects who are not sensitive to the

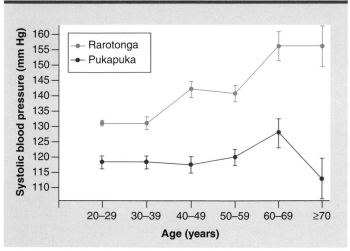

Figure 33.6 **Blood pressure changes with age and salt intake.** The increase in systolic blood pressure with age correlates with a higher sodium intake in two Polynesian populations. In men of Rarotonga Island in Polynesia, where the sodium intake averages 130 mmol/day, systolic blood pressure increases with age. In contrast, it remains constant in men from Pukapuka Island, in which the sodium intake averages 50 to 70 mmol/day. (Adapted from Prior IAM, Evans JG, Harvey HB, et al: Sodium intake and blood pressure in two Polynesian populations. N Engl J Med 1968;279: 515–520.)

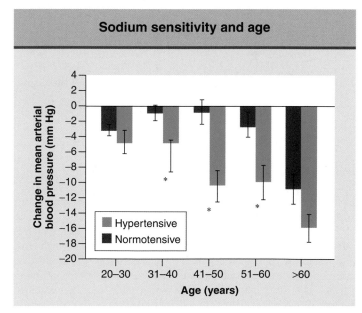

Figure 33.7 **Increase in magnitude of sodium sensitivity with increasing age.** Sodium sensitivity (determined by a standardized test evaluating the change in blood pressure from a volume-expanded to a contracted state) increases proportionally with age in both hypertensive and normotensive subjects (bars indicate standard error of the mean; *P < 0.05). (Adapted from Weinberger MH, Fineberg NS: Sodium and volume sensitivity of blood pressure: Age and pressure change over time. Hypertension 1991;18:67–71.)

consistent with predictions that a reduction in sodium intake of 50 mmol/d (about 3 g salt) in older people would lower the population's systolic BP by an average of 5 mm Hg.[26] This magnitude of BP reduction is similar to trials of drug therapy with thiazide diuretics in this age group, in which a 36% reduction in the 5-year incidence of stroke has been estimated.

Putative mechanisms for salt sensitivity are alterations in circulating levels of (or renal responses to) atrial natriuretic factor, kallikrein, prostaglandins, and nitric oxide; increased levels of norepinephrine; abnormal suppression of both renin and aldosterone; genetic mechanisms; and acquired renal microvascular and tubular injury.[23,27]

The JNC 7 guidelines recommend a salt intake of <100 mmol/ day (2.4 g sodium or 6 g sodium chloride).[1] If an individual is prepared to give up salt added to food and to avoid eating salt-rich processed foods, salt intake can be reduced from the average intake of around 9 g (144 mmol or 3310 mg sodium) to about 6 g/day. To reduce sodium intake further requires bread intake to be limited, as well as portion sizes of foods that are relatively high in natural sodium, such as meat, milk, and eggs.

Despite these recommendations, a systematic review of the long-term effects of advice to restrict dietary sodium in adults, with and without hypertension, reported disappointingly small reductions in BP (average of 1.1/0.6 mm Hg) at 13 to 60 months of follow-up.[28] These long-term results undoubtedly reflect subjects' inability to comply with dietary advice to reduce salt intake. However, it may be possible to improve dietary compliance with regular patient contact, periodic diet history taking (preferably by a dietitian), ongoing education/counseling sessions, and even the use of occasional 24-hour urinary sodium analyses to quantify actual salt intake.

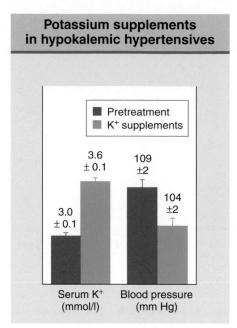

Figure 33.8 Potassium supplementation lowers blood pressure in hypokalemic hypertensive patients. Treatment with potassium chloride (60 mmol/day potassium for 6 weeks) resulted in an increase in serum potassium and a decrease in mean arterial pressure in hypertensive patients taking thiazide diuretics. (Redrawn from Kaplan N, Carnegie A, Risking P, et al: Potassium supplementation in hypertensive patients with diuretic-induced hypokalemia. N Engl J Med 1985;312:746–749.)

Potassium Intake

One of the confounding factors of the relationship of sodium intake to BP has been the inverse relationship between the intakes of sodium and potassium. Typically, societies with a high salt intake are relatively deficient in potassium (and calcium) consumption, while in those groups who habitually consume little salt, the potassium (and calcium) intakes are quite high. These disparate groups also differ in other factors such as physical activity and the degree of industrialization (acculturation) of the society, as well as in racial and genetic characteristics. Therefore, intervention studies are useful to clarify the effect of potassium intake on BP.

In normotensive subjects with an average potassium intake >1.95 g/day (50 mmol/day), further potassium supplementation appears to have no significant effect on BP. However, among hypertensive individuals who are potassium deficient as the result of diuretic treatment or a low dietary potassium intake, potassium supplementation has been observed to lower BP (Fig. 33.8).[29] The Dietary Approaches to Stop Hypertension (DASH) diet, which is beneficial to lower BP, is high in potassium because of its high fruit and vegetable content (Fig. 33.9).[30] It is not clear which of these components or combination thereof was responsible for this observation. The mechanisms by which a low potassium diet leads to sodium retention is complex and poorly understood, but may relate to stimulation of intrarenal angiotensin II and endothelin, inhibition of intrarenal nitric oxide and prostaglandins, and the induction of renal ischemia. Experimental hypokalemia also induces endothelial dysfunction. Overall, it appears to be beneficial to optimize potassium intake in hypertensive humans, being careful to avoid the risk of hyperkalemia in subjects with renal impairment or in other

susceptible individuals. If renal function is normal, optimal potassium intake is 80 to 120 mmol/day.

Calcium Intake

Cross-sectional population surveys of self-reported nutrient intake suggest an inverse relationship between calcium intake and blood pressure. However, this relationship is more convincing at low levels of calcium consumption (i.e., in groups who habitually consume calcium intakes of 300 to 600 mg/day). It has been suggested that there may be a threshold of dietary calcium intake (700 to 800 mg/day) above which any further potential blood pressure–lowering effect of calcium may not be seen. A meta-analysis of randomized calcium supplementation trials (mostly with 1 or 1.5 g calcium/day) has demonstrated only small reductions in systolic BP (–0.9 to –1.7 mm Hg), which are of little public health importance.[31]

Magnesium Intake

A weak inverse relationship has been reported between dietary magnesium intake and blood pressure, although the weight of evidence is minimal. Moreover, there have been few convincing interventional data to support a recommendation for magnesium supplementation for the reduction of blood pressure. A meta-analysis of 20 randomized clinical trials[32] demonstrated that the pooled estimate of the effect of magnesium supplementation on both systolic and diastolic BP was small and insignificant. Benefits were seen only in the few trials that included doses in the higher range of 20 to 40 mmol/day. Magnesium has been shown to influence cardiac function and rhythm; therefore, the JNC 7 has recommended an adequate intake of magnesium pending more definitive information.[1] The optimal levels of magnesium intake are not yet clearly established.

			Dietary Approaches to Stop Hypertension (DASH) diet*	
Food Group	Daily Servings	Serving Sizes	Examples and Notes	Significance to the DASH Diet Pattern
Grains and grain products	7–8	1 slice bread $1/2$ cup dry cereal $1/2$ cup cooked rice, pasta, or cereal	Whole-wheat bread, muffin, pita bread, bagel, cereals, oatmeal	Major sources of energy and fiber
Vegetables	4–5	1 cup raw, leafy vegetables $1/2$ cup cooked vegetables $1/2$ cup cooked vegetables 6 oz vegetable juice	Tomatoes, potatoes, carrots, peas, squash, broccoli, turnip greens, kale, spinach, artichokes, green beans, sweet potatoes	Rich sources of potassium, magnesium, and fiber
Fruits	4–5	1 medium fruit $1/4$ cup dried fruit 6 oz fruit juice $1/2$ cup fresh, frozen, or canned fruit	Apricots, bananas, dates, oranges, orange juice, grapefruit, grapefruit juice, mangoes, melons, peaches, pineapples, prunes, raisins, strawberries, tangerines	Important sources of potassium, magnesium, and fiber
Lowfat or nonfat dairy foods	2–3	8 oz milk 1 cup yogurt 1.5 oz cheese	Skim or low-fat (2%) milk, skim or low-fat buttermilk, nonfat or low-fat yogurt, nonfat or low-fat cheeses	Major sources of calcium and protein
Meats, poultry, and fish	≤2	3 oz cooked meats, poultry, or fish	Select only lean meats; trim away visible fats; broil, roast, or boil instead of frying; remove skin from poultry	Rich sources of protein and magnesium
Nuts, seeds, and legumes	4–5 wk	1.5 oz 1/3 cup nuts $1/2$ oz or 2 tablespoons seeds $1/2$ cup cooked legumes	Almonds, mixed nuts, peanuts, walnuts, sunflower seeds, kidney beans, lentils, split peas	Rich sources of energy, magnesium, potassium, protein, and fiber

Figure. 33.9   Dietary Approaches to Stop Hypertension (DASH) diet. The DASH eating plan shown is based on 2000 kcal/day (8400 kJ/day). Depending on energy needs, the number of daily servings in a food group may varies from those listed. (Adapted from the Sixth Report of the Joint National Committee on Prevention, Detection, Evaluation, and Treatment of High Blood Pressure.)

Dietary Fats and Sugars

There is little information to support the use of increased dietary fat intake for reduction of blood pressure. A meta-analysis of omega-3 fatty acid studies found that marine fish oils have an independent hypotensive effect,[33] possibly as a result of increased synthesis of prostacyclin (a vasodilator) and reduced synthesis of thromboxane (a vasoconstrictor) from the long-chain eicosapentaenoic fatty acid. However, the amounts of fish oil required for this effect have shown to be not tolerable by most subjects. A minimum of 3 g/day may be needed for a significant reduction in blood pressure,[33] which is equivalent to about 10 portions of oily fish per week or nine to 10 fish oil capsules per day. Side effects of eructation (belching) and fishy taste are associated with such high levels of intake. Concerns over the dioxin and polychlorinated biphenyl content (environmental pollutants that have carcinogenic potential and, being fat soluble, can accumulate in the body) of some fish oil supplements also raise questions about the safety of very large doses. At present, it is prudent to advise individuals with hypertension to consume 200 to 400 g of oily fish per week (about three portions of at least 100 g [3 to 4 oz] in weight). Suitable oily fish with a high omega-3 fatty acid content include herring, kippers, mackerel, pilchards, sardines, salmon, trout, sprats, dogfish, fresh tuna (canned variety has much lower omega-3 levels), swordfish, whitebait, conger eel, and crab. It is important to closely monitor the lipid profiles of hypertensive subjects and to encourage avoidance of a high total dietary fat intake, particularly from sources of saturated and trans-polyunsaturated fats (mostly found in hard margarines, confectionery, and manufactured cookies and cakes).

There has also been the recognition recently that the acceleration of the obesity and hypertension epidemic correlates with an increasing intake of fructose present in table sugar (sucrose) and sweeteners (especially high-fructose corn syrup).[34] Fructose feeding to animals rapidly induces hypertension and the metabolic syndrome. Experimental studies have recently linked the mechanism to uric acid–induced endothelial dysfunction.[35]

Dietary Approaches to Stop Hypertension Diet

The DASH randomized, controlled trial provided unequivocal evidence that nonpharmacologic methods can reduce BP as much as some antihypertensive drugs.[30] Subjects fed a diet rich in fruit and vegetables for 8 weeks had a greater reduction in systolic and diastolic BP (2.8 and 1.1 mm Hg, respectively) than subjects on a typical American control diet. Subjects randomized to the DASH diet, rich in fruit, vegetables, and low-fat dairy products and with a reduced saturated and total fat intake (see Fig. 33.9), had an even greater reduction in both systolic and diastolic BP (5.5 and 3.0 mm Hg, respectively). The effects of the 8-week DASH diet were greatest in the hypertensive African American subgroup, in which a BP reduction of 13.2/6.1 mm Hg was demonstrated.[36] Increased efficacy of the DASH diet in African Americans may reflect a greater response to the higher potassium, calcium, and magnesium content of the diet (sodium intake remained unchanged) in subjects who have habitually low or inadequate intake of these nutrients.

The follow-up DASH sodium study investigated the additional benefits of salt restriction over and above the merits of the DASH diet.[37] Reducing sodium intake from a high (150 mmol/day) to either an intermediate (100 mmol/day) or low (65 mmol/day) intake resulted in a stepwise reduction in BP, which was approximately twice as great in subjects on the control than on the DASH diet (Fig. 33.10). Sodium restriction from high to low intake in

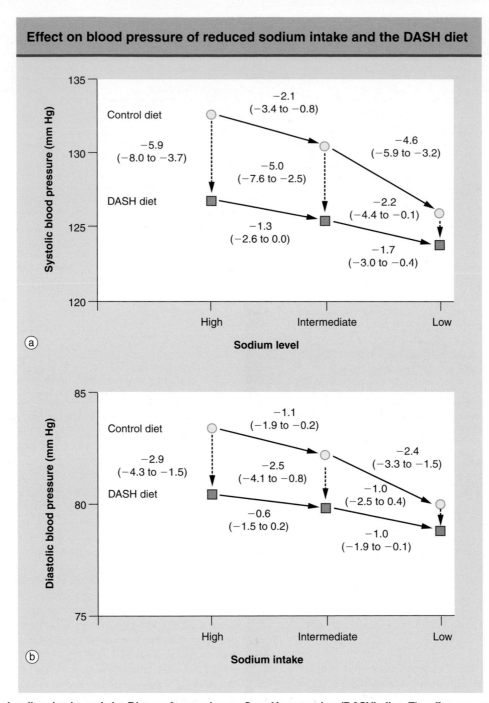

Figure 33.10 **Reduced sodium intake and the Dietary Approaches to Stop Hypertension (DASH) diet.** The effect on systolic blood pressure (a) and diastolic blood pressure (b) (Redrawn from Sacks FM, Svetky LP, Vollmer WM, et al, for the DASH-Sodium collaborative research group. Effects on blood pressure of reduced dietary sodium and the dietary approaches to stop hypertension [DASH] diet. N Engl J Med 2001;344:3–10.)

those following the DASH diet resulted in a relatively small additional decrease in BP (3.0 and 1.6 mm Hg for systolic and diastolic BP, respectively). Thus, the greatest benefits in sodium restriction are seen in those with a poor diet (i.e., typical westernized high-fat, low nutrient diet). Individuals who consume a large quantity of fruit and vegetables, together with low-fat diary products, may be able to tolerate higher amounts of salt.

The DASH diet, based on a 2000-kJ dietary intake, would provide, on average, 64 g of protein (if only one meat serving of 90 g/day is included), between 1070 and 2570 mg sodium and between 1935 and 3295 mg potassium per day, depending on food

choices (see Fig. 33.9). The calculated sodium content presumes that no salt is added to foods at the table nor in cooking and does not include any salty snacks. Despite this, the upper range for estimation of sodium content exceeds the recommended maximum reference limit of 2.4 g/day.

SMOKING

Smoking greatly increases overall noncardiovascular and cardiovascular morbidity and mortality, and all hypertensives should be advised to quit. Nicotine patches or buspirone therapy is safe in hypertensives and should be considered, where necessary, to facilitate abstinence from smoking. However, the cessation of smoking may not lower BP.[38] Nevertheless, smoking may interfere with the beneficial effects of antihypertensive agents such as β-blockers.[39]

MODERATION OF ALCOHOL CONSUMPTION

There is a linear relationship between alcohol consumption, BP levels, and the prevalence of hypertension in populations.[40] In Japan, alcohol intake >300 g/week (about three drinks per day) was associated with significantly greater increases of BP over a 7-year period, and baseline BP was higher in drinkers consuming 200 g/wk.[41] Heavy drinking is associated with increased risk of stroke, an increase in BP after alcohol withdrawal, and attenuation of antihypertensive efficacy.[2] Paradoxically, alcohol has a J-shaped relationship with coronary heart disease with moderate consumption having the lowest risk. In a major epidemiologic study, modest alcohol consumption was protective against a first myocardial infarction.[42] Alcohol probably increases BP through activation of the sympathetic nervous system and protects against myocardial infarction by increasing high-density lipoprotein, lowering fibrinogen, and inhibiting platelet aggravation. The JNC 7 guidelines recommend limiting alcohol consumption to no more than two drinks per day (24 oz of beer, 10 oz of wine, or 3 oz of 80-proof whiskey) in most men, and no more than one drink per day in women or lighter weight men (see Fig. 33.1).

MODERATION OF CAFFEINE CONSUMPTION

Caffeine is by far the most widely used psychoactive substance worldwide. In a survey undertaken by the National Coffee Association, 54% of U.S. adults drink coffee daily. Caffeine stimulates the cardiovascular system through the blockade of vascular adenosine receptors.[43] In a recent meta-analysis of randomized, controlled studies of caffeine tablet and coffee ingestion, BP increases appeared to be greater for caffeine tablets (systolic: 4.16 mm Hg; diastolic 2.41 mm Hg) than for coffee (systolic: 1.22 mm Hg; diastolic 0.49 mm Hg), despite similar caffeine (total g) intake.[44] The JNC 7 guidelines are silent on the issue of caffeine, but it seems sensible that regular modest coffee consumption is safe, but the pharmacologic ingestion of caffeine and the use of "smart drinks" (that are supplemented with caffeine) should be avoided.

STRESS REDUCTION

Accumulating evidence indicates that chronic psychosocial stress is an important contributor to the development and maintenance of hypertension. For example, in a longitudinal study of job strain and ambulatory BP among 215 men, an effect of systolic BP of past exposure and current exposure was shown.[45] Men with 50% lifetime and current exposure to job strain had a 10.7-mm Hg and 15.4-mm Hg higher work and home ambulatory systolic BP than controls, respectively. It seems intuitive that stress reduction should assist in the control in BP. More recently, the INTERHEART study showed that stress was associated with a twofold increase in the risk of the first myocardial infarction.[42] However, the efficacy of stress reduction approaches for hypertension have shown either negative results or heterogeneity of effects on BP.[46] As a result, the JNC 7 does not recommend stress reductions techniques for the management of hypertension.[2] However, recent evidence suggests that transcendental meditation and control of respiration have important effects on BP as an adjunct to pharmacologic therapy.[47,48]

FEASIBILITY OF ADOPTING LIFESTYLE MODIFICATIONS

The question of whether patients are able to comply with advice to make multiple lifestyle changes has been addressed in a number of trials. The Prevention of Myocardial Infarction Early Remodeling (PREMIER) trial evaluated the effects of implementing JNC 7 lifestyle recommendations and the feasibility of implementing the DASH diet in the outpatient setting.[49] Adults with above-optimal BP or untreated stage 1 hypertension were randomly assigned to one of three groups for 6 months. The advice only (i.e., control) group had a single 30-minute individual session with a dietitian and were given printed educational materials. The established guidelines group had JNC recommendations (i.e., weight loss, exercise, and restriction of sodium and alcohol intake) as their goals, while the established plus DASH groups were also advised to consume a DASH diet. Both intervention groups had an identical contact pattern of 18 face-to-face contacts and were encouraged to lose weight by increasing activity and lowering energy intake. At 6 months, the established and established plus DASH groups had significantly reduced both systolic and diastolic BP in comparison with the advice only group. Surprisingly, the addition of the DASH diet to lifestyle modification resulted in an incremental decrease of BP of only 0.6/0.9 mm Hg (1.7/1.6 mm Hg in hypertensive individuals). These results suggested that combined lifestyle interventions on BP do not appear to be additive. However, participants purchased their own foods in the PREMIER study, instead of being provided with foods as in the DASH[30] and DASH sodium[37] studies. Indeed, the average fruit and vegetable intake of research subjects in the original DASH study was 9.6 servings fruit/vegetables per day, whereas reported intake of these foods increased from 4.8 to 7.8 servings per day in the PREMIER Trial (confirmed by an increase in urinary potassium of 105% in DASH study versus only 28% in PREMIER trial). It can be concluded that in the outpatient setting, even highly motivated individuals cannot meet DASH dietary goals unless their meals are provided. Similarly in the DASH sodium study, the BP-lowering effect attributable to sodium reduction was –6.7/–3.5 mm Hg from high to low sodium on control diet, whereas in meta-analyses of 40 sodium-restriction trials in which participants prepared their own low-salt meals, this effect was only –2.54/–1.96 mm Hg.[50]

In the Trials of Hypertension II study, the problems of sustainability of dietary intervention and the need for regular counseling were demonstrated.[51] The effect of adding sodium restriction to weight loss appeared to offer no further decrease in BP. Analyzing the change in urinary sodium excretion as an indication of compliance with dietary advice, adherence to lower dietary sodium was poor over the long term. At 36 months of follow-up, mean urinary sodium was 40.4 mmol/24 h lower than baseline in the sodium-restricted group and only 21% achieved the target of <80 mmol/24 h. A higher attendance at counseling sessions was associated with a greater reduction in urinary sodium. At 36 months, a decrease of 84 mmol/day of sodium from baseline levels could only be achieved in those who attended ≥80% of the counseling sessions. In summary, the sustainability of long-term lifestyle interventions remains problematic, but it appears that regular and long-term counseling can improve adherence.

REFERENCES

1. Chobanian A, Bakris GL, Black HR, et al: The seventh report of the Joint National Committee on Prevention, Detection, Evaluation, and Treatment of High Blood Pressure. The JNC 7 Report. JAMA 2003; 289:2560–2582.
2. Guidelines Committee: 2003 European Society of Hypertension–European Society of Cardiology guidelines for the management of arterial hypertension. J Hypertens 2003;21:1011–1053.
3. Vasan RS, Larson MG, Leip EP, et al: Impact of high-normal blood pressure on the risk of cardiovascular disease. N Engl J Med 2001;345:1291–1297.
4. Geleijnse JM, Kok FJ, Grobbee DE: Impact of dietary and lifestyle factors on the prevalence of hypertension in Western populations. Eur J Public Health 2004;14:235–239.
5. Hedley AA, Ogden CL, Johnson CL, et al: Overweight and obesity among US children, adolescents, and adults, 1999–2002. JAMA 2004;291: 2847–2850.
6. Trials of Hypertension Prevention Collaboration Research Group: The effects of nonpharmacologic interventions on blood pressure of persons with high normal levels. JAMA 1992;267:1213–1220.
7. Neter JE, Stam BE, Kok FJ, et al: Influence of weight reduction on blood pressure. A meta-analysis of randomized controlled trials. Hypertension 2003;42:878–884.
8. Schulz M, Liese AD, Boeing H, et al: Associations of short-term weight changes and weight cycling with incidence of essential hypertension in the EPIC-Potsdam Study. J Hum Hypertens 2005;19:61–67.
9. Dansinger ML, Gleason JA, Griffith JL, et al: Comparison of the Atkins, Ornish, Weight Watchers and Zone diets for weight loss and heart disease risk reduction. JAMA 2005;293:43–53.
10. Farrell SW, Kampert JB, Kohl HW 3rd, et al: Influences of cardiorespiratory fitness levels and other predictors on cardiovascular disease mortality in men. Med Sci Sports Exerc 1998;30:899–905.
11. Fagard RH: Exercise characteristics and the blood pressure response to dynamic physical training. Med Sci Sports Exerc 2001;33:S484–S492.
12. Ishikawa-Takata K, Ohta T, Tanaka H: How much exercise is required to reduce blood pressure in essential hypertensives: A dose-response study. Am J Hypertens 2003;16:629–633.
13. Quinn J: Twenty-four hour, ambulatory blood pressure responses following acute exercise: Impact of exercise intensity. Hum Hypertens 2000;14: 547–553.
14. Halliwill J: Mechanisms and clinical implications of post-exercise hypotension in humans. Exerc Sports Sci Rev 2001;29:65–70.
15. Pescatello LS, Franklin BA, Farquhar WB, et al: American College of Sports Medicine. American College of Sports Medicine position stand. Exercise and hypertension. Med Sci Sports Exerc 2004;36:533–553.
16. Carroll S, Duffield M: What is the relationship between exercise and metabolic abnormalities? A review. Sports Med 2004;34:371–418.
17. Pollock ML, Franklin BA, Balady GJ, et al: AHA Science Advisory. Resistance exercise in individuals with and without cardiovascular disease: benefits, rationale, safety, and prescription: An advisory from the Committee on Exercise, Rehabilitation, and Prevention, Council on Clinical Cardiology, American Heart Association. Circulation 2000;101:828–833.
18. Franklin BA, Gordon S, Timmis GC: Exercise prescription for hypertensive patients. Ann Med 1991;23:279–287.
19. MacGregor GA: Sodium is more important than calcium in essential hypertension. Hypertension 1985;7:628–637.
20. Prior IAM, Evans JG, Harvey HB, et al: Sodium intake and blood pressure in two Polynesian populations. N Engl J Med 1968;279:515–520.
21. Tuomilehto J, Jousilahti P, Rastenyte D, et al: Urinary sodium excretion and cardiovascular mortality in Finland: A prospective study. Lancet 2001;357:848–851.
22. Kawasaki T, Delea CS, Bartter FC, Smith H: The effect of high-sodium and low-sodium intakes on blood pressure and other related variables in human subjects with idiopathic hypertension. Am J Med 1978;64:193–198.
23. Weinberger MH: Salt sensitivity of blood pressure in humans. Hypertension 1996;27:481–490.
24. Weinberger MH, Fineberg NS: Sodium and volume sensitivity of blood pressure: Age and pressure change over time. Hypertension 1991;18:67–71.
25. Cappuccio FP, Markandu ND, Carney C, et al: Double-blind randomised trial of modest salt restriction in older people. Lancet 1997;350:850–854.
26. Law MR, Frost CD, Wald NJ: By how much does dietary salt reduction lower blood pressure? III. Analysis of data from trials of salt reduction. BMJ 1991;302:819–824.
27. Johnson RJ, Herrera-Acosta J, Schreiner GF, Rodriguez-Iturbe B: Mechanisms of disease: Subtle acquired renal injury as a mechanism of salt-sensitive hypertension. N Engl J Med 2002;346:913–923.
28. Hooper L, Bartlett C, Smith GD, Ebrahim S: Systematic review of long term effects of advice to reduce dietary salt intake in adults. BMJ 2002; 325:628–637.
29. Kaplan N, Carnegie A, Risking P, et al: Potassium supplementation in hypertensive patients with diuretic-induced hypokalemia. N Engl J Med 1985;312:746–749.
30. Appel L, Moore T, Obarzanek et al: A clinical trial of the effects of dietary patterns on blood pressure. N Engl J Med 1997;336:1117–1124.
31. Griffith LE, Guyatt GH, Cook RJ, et al: The influence of dietary and nondietary calcium supplementation on blood pressure: An updated meta-analysis of randomized controlled trials. Am J Hypertens 1999;12:84–92.
32. Jee SH, Miller ER, Guallar E, et al: The effect of magnesium supplementation on blood pressure: A meta-analysis of randomised clinical trials. Am J Hypertens 2002;15:691–696.
33. Appel LJ, Miller ER, Seidler AJ, Whelton PK. Does supplementation of diet with fish oil reduce blood pressure? A meta-analysis of controlled clinical trials. Arch Intern Med 1993;153:429–438.
34. Nakagawa T, Tuttle KR, Short RA, Johnson RJ: Hypothosis: Fructose-induced hyperuricemia as a causal mechanism for the epidemic of the metabolic syndrome. Nat Clin Pract Nephrol 2005;1:80–86.
35. Nakagawa T, Hu H, Zharikov S, et al: A causal role for uric acid in fructose-induced metabolic syndrome. Am J Physiol Renal Physiol 2006;290:F625–F631.
36. Svetky LP, Simons-Morton D, Vollmer WM, et al: Effects of dietary patterns on blood pressure: Subgroup analysis of the Dietary Approaches to Stop Hypertension (DASH) randomised controlled trial. Arch Intern Med 1999;159:285–293.
37. Sacks FM, Svetky LP, Vollmer WM, et al, for the DASH-Sodium collaborative research group. Effects on blood pressure of reduced dietary sodium and the dietary approaches to stop hypertension (DASH) diet. N Engl J Med 2001;344:3–10.
38. Omvik P: How smoking affects blood pressure. Blood Press 1996;5:71–77.
39. Medical Research Council Working Party. MRC trial on treatment of mild hypertension: Principal results. Medical Research Council. BMJ 1985; 291:97–104.
40. Puddey IB, Beilin LJ, Rakey V. Alcohol, hypertension, and the cardiovascular system: A critical appraisal. Addict Biol 1997;2:159–170.
41. Yoshita K, Miura K, Morikawa Y, et al: Relationship of alcohol consumption to 7-year blood pressure change in Japanese men. J Hypertens 2005; 23:1485–1490.
42. Yusuf S, Hawken S, Ôunpuu S, et al on behalf of the INTERHEART Study Investigators. Effect of potentially modifiable risk factors associated with myocardial infarction in 52 countries (the INTERHEART study): Case-control study. Lancet 2004;364:937–950.
43. Smits P, Boekema P, de Abreu R, et al: Evidence for an antagonism between caffeine and adenosine in the human cardiovascular system. J Cardiovasc Pharmacol 1987;10:13–143.
44. Marlies N, Uiterwaal CSPM, Arends LR, et al: Blood pressure response to chronic intake of coffee and caffeine: A meta-analysis of randomized controlled trials. J Hypertens 2005;23:921–928.
45. Schnall PL, Schwartz JE, Landsbergis PA, et al: A longitudinal study of job strain and ambulatory blood pressure: Results from a three-year follow-up. Psychosomatic Med 1998;60:697–706.
46. Ebrahim S, Smith G: Lowering blood pressure: A systematic review of sustained effects of non-pharmacological interventions. J Pub Health Med 1998;20:441–448.
47. Parati G, Izzo JL, Gavish B: Respiration and blood pressure. In Izzo JL, Black HR (eds): Hypertension Primer, 3rd ed. Council for High Blood Pressure Research, Dallas, American Heart Association, 2003, pp 117–120.
48. Schneider RH, Alexander CN, Stagers F, et al: A randomized controlled trial of stress reduction in African Americans treated for hypertension for over one year. Am J Hypertens 2005;18:88–98.
49. Writing Group of the PREMIER Collaborative Research Group: Effects of comprehensive lifestyle modification on blood pressure control: Main results of the PREMIER clinical trial. JAMA 2003;289:2083–2093.
50. Geleijnse JM, Kok FJ, Grobbee DE: Blood pressure response to changes in sodium and potassium intake: A metaregression analysis of randomised trials. J Hum Hypertens 2003;17:471–480.
51. Kumanyika SK, Cook NR, Cutler JA, et al: Sodium reduction for hypertension prevention in overweight adults: Further results from the Trials of Hypertension Prevention Phase II. J Hum Hypertens 2005;19:33–45.

Pharmacologic Treatment of Hypertension

Nitin Khosla and George L. Bakris

INTRODUCTION

Appropriate treatment of an asymptomatic disease associated with a high risk of cardiovascular and renal complications is difficult. This is apparent in the treatment of hypertension. Historically, awareness, detection, and treatment of hypertension have been poor. Moreover, while the awareness of high blood pressure has improved, the percentage of patients whose blood pressure is controlled to ≤140/90 mm Hg has remained relatively unchanged (Fig. 34.1).

This failure to achieve adequate blood pressure control is evidenced by a flattened downward trend in cardiovascular mortality and stroke as well as an increased incidence of heart failure.[1] This trend in mortality and heart failure, along with the increased incidence of end-stage renal disease (ESRD; Fig. 34.2), suggests that we need to be more aggressive in achieving blood pressure control. Our ability to lower but inadequately achieve the recommended arterial pressure goals has led to more people living longer but with a substantially greater morbidity. In addition to increased morbidity associated with both ESRD and heart failure, the subsequent loss in productivity translates into a major financial burden to society. Inadequate arterial pressure lowering is more sobering in the context of the overwhelming data that show achieving goal blood pressure (e.g., levels <130/80 mm Hg) in certain high-risk populations does lead to a preservation of renal function.

This chapter addresses the approach and pharmacologic management of patients with essential hypertension. Many of the concepts put forth are adopted from the seventh report of the Joint National Committee (JNC 7) on Detection, Evaluation, Treatment, and Prevention of High Blood Pressure, as well as the recommendations of the American Diabetes Association and the National Kidney Foundation. The new classification system for hypertension is considered, and mechanisms of antihypertensive drug action are put into the context of rational drug combinations to maximally reduce blood pressure, minimize side effects, maintain organ function, and reduce morbidity and mortality. High-risk populations for renal disease progression and reduction of proteinuria as a goal of therapy are also discussed.

WHO SHOULD RECEIVE PHARMACOLOGIC THERAPY?

The National Health and Nutrition Examination Survey (NHANES 1999 to 2000) documented that many patients are either undertreated or not treated for their elevated blood pressure.[2] While lifestyle modifications, especially weight loss and reduced dietary sodium intake, significantly contribute to blood pressure reduction, most people fail to follow consistently such recommendations. Thus, antihypertensive agents are required to reduce arterial pressure adequately in the majority of patients.

A high systolic pressure (≥140 mm Hg) in the absence of an elevated diastolic pressure is associated with a higher cardiovascular and renal event rate compared to diastolic hypertension alone, especially in the older patients.[1,3] Therefore, a more aggressive approach to the treatment of hypertension, both diastolic and isolated systolic, is recommended to reduce cardiovascular and renal morbidity and mortality. In light of the NHANES III findings, this more aggressive approach to hypertension may appear unachievable. Nevertheless, increasing patient awareness, together with a more diligent effort by physicians, including the early use of multiple medications, may allow attainment of blood pressure within the recommended goals.

CLASSIFICATION OF HYPERTENSION

One of the main reasons for the publication of JNC 7 was to simplify the classification system of hypertension (see Fig. 32.2). First, the stages of hypertension were pared down to just two stages. The primary benefit of streamlining the stages is that it allows for the easy identification of patients who should be started on more than one drug at the beginning of treatment (e.g., stage 2 hypertensives). The other major difference between the new

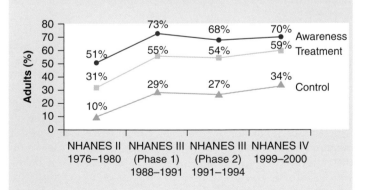

Hypertension awareness, treatment, and control in the United States, 1976–2000

Figure 34.1 The awareness, treated, and controlled percentage of the hypertensive population surveyed by National Health and Nutrition Examination Survey (NHANES) over time. Note that there was no improvement in the number controlled or treated. (Adapted from Chobanian AV, Bakris GL, Black HR, et al: The seventh report of the Joint National Committee on Prevention, Detection, Evaluation, and Treatment of High Blood Pressure: The JNC 7 report. JAMA 2003;289:2560–2572.)

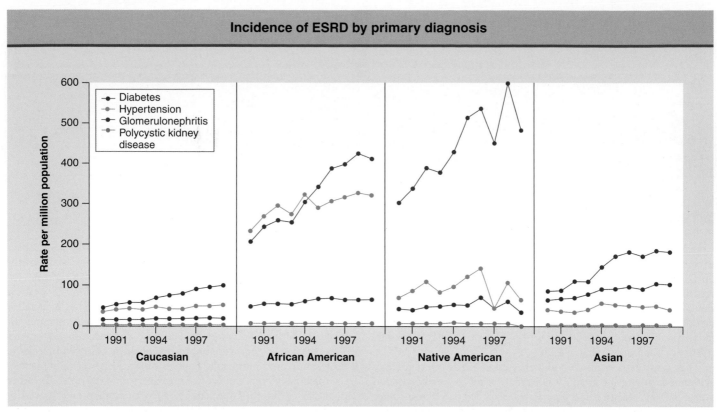

Figure 34.2   The incidence of end-stage renal disease (ESRD) by primary diagnosis adjusted for age and race.

classification system and the previous systems is the creation of a prehypertension group. With the emergence of the knowledge that the risk of cardiovascular mortality doubles with every 20/10-mm Hg increase in blood pressure over 115/75 mm Hg, special attention has been placed on patients in the prehypertensive range.[4] The focus in these patients is to encourage lifestyle modifications to both delay the onset of hypertension and, in a small subset of patients, prevent hypertension entirely.

GOAL OF ANTIHYPERTENSIVE THERAPY

The goal of treating hypertension is to reduce morbid events, such as renal failure, stroke, and cardiovascular mortality. All mortality trials, to date, demonstrate that blood pressure needs to be reduced to levels <140/90 mm Hg to achieve this benefit.[1,3,5] However, previous studies call into question whether this level of pressure is low enough for patients with significant comorbidities. An analysis of participants with diabetes, renal disease, or coronary heart disease in the Multiple Risk Factor Intervention Trial found that after adjustment for risk factors and clinical state, the group with lower arterial pressures had the greatest reduction in cardiovascular events.[6] In the Modification of Diet in Renal Disease (MDRD) Trial, patients with renal insufficiency and proteinuria randomized to a mean arterial pressure of <92 mm Hg manifested significantly slower rates of decline in renal function compared to those randomized to mean pressures between 102 and 106 mm Hg.[7] Moreover, the subgroup of African Americans randomized to the lower blood pressure had far better renal outcomes in this trial.[8] The ACE-Inhibition in Progressive Renal Disease study group also looked at patients with nondiabetic renal disease and found that patients who achieved a systolic

blood pressure of 110 to 129 mm Hg had the lowest rate of renal disease progression. The subgroup of patients that derived the greatest benefit were those with >1 g of proteinuria per day.[9]

However, the evidence to support a lower blood pressure goal is not as strong in those patients with <1 g of proteinuria per day. The African American Study of Kidney Disease (AASK), which randomized patients with hypertensive kidney disease (glomerular filtration rate [GFR] 20 to 65 ml/min) to a mean arterial pressure of <92 mm Hg or 102 to 107 mm Hg, found that patients with <300 mg of proteinuria per day derived no additional benefit from achieving the lower blood pressure goal.[10] However, in this same study, those with >50% reduction in proteinuria from baseline at 6 months had a 72% risk reduction for progression to ESRD at 5 years.[11]

While the evidence suggests a lower blood pressure goal in patients with nondiabetic kidney disease with proteinuria, it also supports a lower blood pressure target in all those with diabetes, regardless of proteinuria status. A recent meta-analysis that compared 33,395 patients with diabetes and 125,314 without diabetes found that achieving a lower blood pressure led to large reductions in cardiovascular events in diabetics compared to nondiabetics.[12] Furthermore, evidence from *post hoc* analyses of numerous studies among those with diabetes support the notion that arterial pressure should be reduced to levels well below 130/80 mm Hg to slow or prevent progression of nephropathy, a fact incorporated into all guidelines.[1,13–16] A summary of these recommendations and specific agents that should be used in certain populations is presented Figures 34.3 and 34.4.

Finally, a discussion of the blood pressure J curve in the context of cardiovascular events is important for perspective. Since its inception in 1979, the concept that reducing diastolic blood pressure to levels <85 mm Hg was associated with a paradoxical

Recommended blood pressure goals based on risk profile			
	JNC 7	NKF	ADA
No CV risk factors, target-organ damage, or clinical CV disease	<140/90 mm Hg		
No target-organ damage or clinical CV disease and at least one CV risk factor (not diabetes)	<140/90 mm Hg		
Target-organ damage or clinical CV disease	<130/80 mm Hg		
Diabetes mellitus	<130/80 mm Hg	<130/80 mm Hg	<130/80 mm Hg
Nondiabetic renal disease	<130/80 mm Hg	<130/85 mm Hg	

Figure 34.3   Recommended blood pressure goals based on risk profile. ADA, American Diabetes Association; CV, cardiovascular; JNC 7, Joint National Committee 7; NKF, National Kidney Foundation.

increase in cardiovascular mortality has been controversial. A J curve exists among patients with established symptomatic coronary artery disease or unstable angina or those who are in the immediate postmyocardial infarction period.[17] However, a *post hoc* analysis of trials in kidney disease that have randomized subjects to different levels of blood pressure control demonstrate no significant increase in cardiovascular events among those with renal insufficiency and diastolic blood pressures of <85 mm Hg compared to the group randomized to higher diastolic blood pressures.[8,18] Likewise, recent *post hoc* analyses of both the Reduction of Endpoints in NIDDM with the Angiotesin II Antagonist Losartan (RENAAL) trial and Irbesartan Diabetic Nephropathy Trial (IDNT) studies showed no J curve for cardiovascular mortality related to blood pressure lowering except in the IDNT when systolic pressure was lowered to <115 mm Hg, where the presence of heart failure, rather than myocardial infarction, drove the events.[19,20] Last, evidence of the absence of a J curve in the general population comes from the Hypertension Optimal Treatment (HOP) trial. This trial did not have a higher cardiovascular event rate in the group randomized to a diastolic blood pressure of 80 mm Hg.[21] Thus, each patient needs to be evaluated in the context of these observations.

The J curve should not serve as a deterrent for failing to lower blood pressure to recommended levels. In the absence of any clear evidence of coronary disease or unstable angina, patients who are at higher risk of renal disease and those with diabetes should have their blood pressures aggressively reduced to levels recommended for these populations (see Fig. 34.4).[1]

OVERVIEW OF ANTIHYPERTENSIVE DRUG MECHANISMS

The JNC has been updating its recommendations since the early 1970s. The current report (JNC 7) recommends tailoring therapy for individual groups of patients to reduce morbidity and mortality related to cardiovascular and renal causes by the least intrusive means possible. This tailored therapy approach considers individual patients based on their risk factor profile as well as their comorbidities.[1]

There are three primary neurohumoral systems responsible for maintaining arterial pressure in humans that must be understood before treating patients with hypertension: (1) the sympathetic nervous system, (2) the renin angiotensin aldosterone system (RAAS), and (3) arginine vasopressin in African Americans. Historically, many studies have described the state of the RAAS system as a predictor of antihypertensive drug efficacy. For example, when the RAAS is not activated, as in African Americans and the elderly, antihypertensive agents that lower pressure by mechanisms that do not affect this system have greater efficacy (e.g., calcium antagonists or diuretics).

This aforementioned observation led to the avoidance of certain antihypertensive agents such as angiotensin-converting enzyme (ACE) inhibitors that may be clearly indicated but are not used because they do not lower blood pressure in these groups. In fact, numerous studies attest to the antihypertensive efficacy of ACE inhibitors in African Americans when used in higher doses.[10,22] Moreover, one ACE inhibitor, trandolapril, has a U.S. Food and Drug Administration (FDA) indication for use in African Americans to lower arterial pressure starting at double the normal initiating dose.[23] Additionally, several prospective clinical trials demonstrate that use of either an ACE inhibitor or an angiotensin receptor blocker (ARB) with a diuretic is very efficacious in African Americans not only for reducing blood pressure but also for reducing progression of nephropathy.[10,24,25]

To understand how to select or add antihypertensive medications for a given patient, the mechanisms by which a drug lowers pressure must be understood. The pharmacologic mechanisms and renal sites of action for the different drug classes are shown in Fig. 34.5. The principal positive and adverse effects for each of the antihypertensive drug classes are summarized in Figure 34.6.

High-risk groups that require aggressive blood pressure reduction to protect against renal disease progression		
Patient Groups	Desired BP Goal	Data Supporting Agents in Specific Antihypertensive Cocktail
Patients with type 2 diabetes	<130/80 mm Hg	ACE inhibitors or angiotensin II receptor blockers
Patients with renal insufficiency (>1.4 mg/dl)	<130/80 mm Hg	ACE inhibitors

Figure 34.4   High-risk groups that require aggressive blood pressure reduction to protect against renal disease progression. Antihypertensive cocktail refers to the concept that more than one antihypertensive agent must be used to control blood pressure to the prescribed levels. Moreover, the agents selected should have complementary effects on mechanisms that reduce pressure. ACE, angiotensin-converting enzyme; BP, blood pressure.

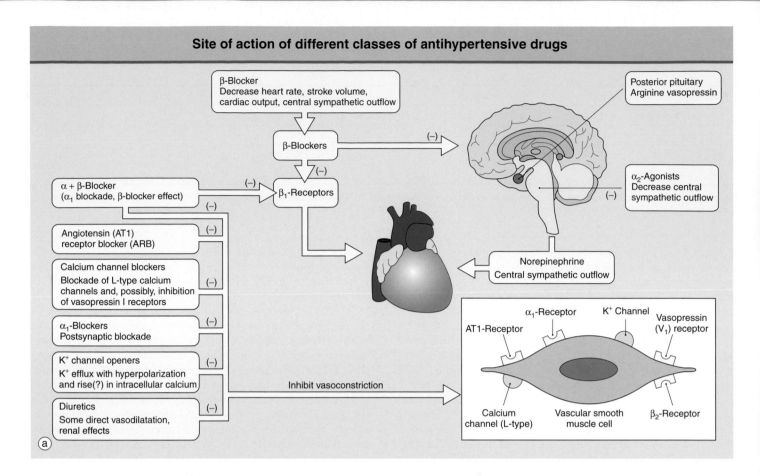

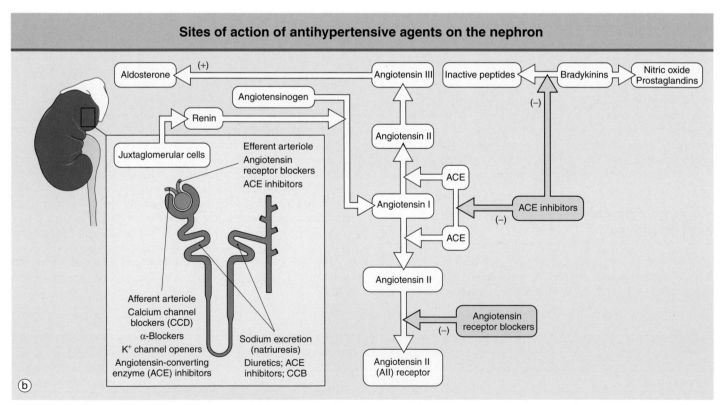

Figure 34.5 Site of action and effects of different classes of antihypertensive agents. *a,* Site of action by different classes of antihypertensive medications. *b,* The effects of various antihypertensive agents on the nephron. Inhibition of effect (–); potentiation of effect (+). CCB, calcium channel blocker.

Common side effects associated with various classes of antihypertensive drugs	
Drug Class	Side Effects
ACE inhibitors	Cough, hyperkalemia
Angiotensin II receptor blockers (ARB)	Much less frequent hyperkalemia compared to ACE inhibitors

Calcium channel blockers
    DHPCCB
    Non-DHPCCB
	
	Pedal edema, headache
	Constipation (verapamil), headache (diltiazem)

Diuretics	Frequent urination, hyperglycemia, hyperlipidemia, hyperuricemia, sexual dysfunction
Central α-agonists	Sedation, dry mouth, rebound hypertension, sexual dysfunction
α-Blockers	Pedal edema, orthostatic hypotension, dizziness
β-Blockers	Fatigue, bronchospasm, hyperglycemia, sexual dysfunction
[K$^+$] Channel openers	Hypertrichosis (minoxidil); lupus-like reactions, and pedal edema (hydralazine)

Figure 34.6   Common side effects associated with various classes of antihypertensive drugs. ACE, angiotensin-converting enzyme; ARB, angiotensin II receptor antagonists; DHPCCB, dihydropyridine calcium channel blocker; non-DHPCCB, nondihydropyridine calcium channel blocker.

SELECTION OF INITIAL DRUG THERAPY

The goal of lowering arterial pressure is to prevent the development of target organ damage (i.e., myocardial infarction, renal failure, stroke) and to achieve target blood pressure in a timely fashion. One of the major changes in JNC 7 compared to its predecessors is that it calls for the aggressive use of combination therapy.[26] After a discussion of the role of combination therapy, we classify approaches to antihypertensive therapy in the uncomplicated and complicated patient.

Combination Therapy

Combination therapy is an ideal way to lower blood pressure and to halt the progression of renal disease. Lower than therapeutic doses of two different drugs are combined in a single pill to reduce arterial pressure to the same level as a higher dose of an individual component. In this way, they are not only additive for blood pressure reduction but also have lower side effect profiles. Moreover, many fixed-dose combinations act to counteract each other's side effects. For example, ACE inhibitors markedly reduce pedal edema associated with dihydropyridine calcium channel blockers (CCBs) as well as reduce the risk of new-onset diabetes by diuretics.[27]

In the early 1960s, fixed-dose combination antihypertensive therapy was introduced with a reserpine/thiazide diuretic combination. Since then, there have been many new fixed-dose combinations introduced (Fig. 34.7). Because of their convenient once-daily dosing schedule, these agents are of particular use in high-risk populations that require aggressive reduction of blood pressure. Thus, the physician may now select agents with complementary modes of action that minimize side effects and maximize compliance to achieve better rates of blood pressure control. A detailed discussion of this topic is beyond the scope of this chapter but is reviewed elsewhere.[28,29]

Uncomplicated Patients

An uncomplicated patient is one with an absence of comorbid conditions, such as dyslipidemia, obesity, and surrogate markers of target-organ disease. Such patients are distinctly rare thus far in the 21st century. The JNC 7 committee reviewed long-term, randomized, double-blind controlled trials available up to 2003 and found that diuretics should be the cornerstone of therapy for most patients.[1] Diuretics can be the sole agents used in patients with mild hypertension (e.g., those with stage 1 hypertension), but JNC 7 recommends the initiation of combination therapy at the onset of treatment for stage 2 hypertension (>160 mm Hg systolic or >99 mm Hg diastolic). Specifically, it recommends

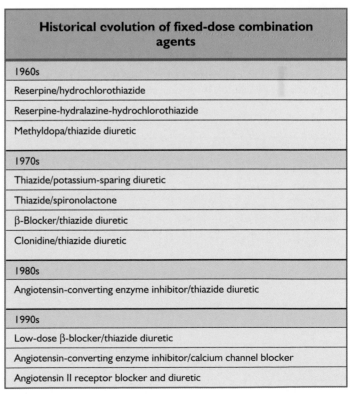

Historical evolution of fixed-dose combination agents
1960s
Reserpine/hydrochlorothiazide
Reserpine-hydralazine-hydrochlorothiazide
Methyldopa/thiazide diuretic
1970s
Thiazide/potassium-sparing diuretic
Thiazide/spironolactone
β-Blocker/thiazide diuretic
Clonidine/thiazide diuretic
1980s
Angiotensin-converting enzyme inhibitor/thiazide diuretic
1990s
Low-dose β-blocker/thiazide diuretic
Angiotensin-converting enzyme inhibitor/calcium channel blocker
Angiotensin II receptor blocker and diuretic

Figure 34.7   Historical evolution of fixed-dose combination agents.

combining a thiazide diuretic with an ACE inhibitor or ARB as the initial combination therapy.

Complicated Patients

A complicated patient has compelling indications such as diabetes and/or heart failure, ischemic heart disease, chronic kidney disease, recurrent stroke, or evidence of surrogate markers of end-organ disease, such as left ventricular hypertrophy (LVH) or microalbuminuria, that put them at an increased risk of a cardiovascular event.[1] These comorbid conditions mandate tailoring antihypertensive therapy to reduce cardiovascular risk optimally and renal disease progression. The effects of various antihypertensive agents on these surrogate markers of target-organ damage are shown in Figure 34.8. Four prominent risk factors associated with a high cardiovascular mortality (LVH, microalbuminuria, diabetes, and renal dysfunction) and the special populations of the obese and the elderly are discussed in more detail.

The Heart Outcomes Prevention Evaluation (HOPE) study randomized >9000 participants who were considered complicated (high risk) because of age and vascular disease and/or diabetes to either ramipril or placebo. Ramipril reduced the risk of cardiovascular events by 22% overall.[30] Given that diseases of the heart are the leading cause of death in the United States (accounting for 28% of deaths in 2003),[31] blockade of the RAAS should be considered as an option for first-line therapy in hypertension and the first agent to be added to diuretic therapy to achieve target blood pressure.

Left Ventricular Hypertrophy

LVH results from chronic increases in arterial pressure causing cardiac myocyte hypertrophy and remodeling of the coronary resistance vessels. This leads to perivascular fibrosis of the intramyocardial arteries and arterioles. Over time, these changes in the myocardium contribute to the development of ventricular wall stiffness and diastolic dysfunction.[32]

LVH is an independent risk factor for predicting an adverse cardiovascular event.[33] In the Framingham study, there was a significant relationship between the presence of LVH and high cardiovascular morbidity and mortality.[34] Previous studies have

suggested that regression of hypertrophy is associated with improved prognosis in hypertensives.[35,36] This was also observed in the Treatment of Mild Hypertension Study with nutritional hygienic measures such as weight loss, reduced salt and alcohol intake, and exercise, although the presence of a diuretic added to the benefit.[37]

The most important factor responsible for left ventricular regression is prolonged reduction of systolic blood pressure. However, there are pharmacologic differences in the degree of LVH regression. A meta-analysis of randomized, controlled trials revealed that ACE inhibitors were the most efficacious for regressing LVH followed by calcium antagonists, diuretics, and β-blockers.[32] In contrast, direct vasodilators such as minoxidil and hydralazine that work through opening $[K^+]$ channels, do not reduce LVH.[32] This is thought to result from profound sympathetic stimulation and subsequent increase in cardiac workload. Thus, if these agents are used to lower arterial pressure, they should always be used in the presence of a β-blocker to reduce sympathetic activity and a diuretic to counteract their effect on sodium retention. It should be noted that minoxidil has been implicated in the development of myocardial fibrosis and, hence, should be either avoided or used with agents such as spironolactone, ACE inhibitors, or ARBs to the reduce the risk of such a development.[38]

ARBs act by blocking AT_1 receptors and are considered as substitute therapy if ACE inhibitors cannot be tolerated. In the Losartan Intervention for Endpoint trial, losartan was markedly superior to atenolol in terms of regressing LVH and for reducing cardiovascular mortality in patients with hypertension and LVH.[39,40] Losartan was also found to significantly reduce the frequency of developing diabetes.[39] These studies suggest that ARBs and ACE inhibitors should be first-line therapy for hypertensive subjects with LVH, especially if they have risk factors for the development of diabetes.

Microalbuminuria

The emergence of recent data has made it clear that microalbuminuria is not only a marker of increased cardiovascular risk, but also a target of therapy.[40–44] Microalbuminuria, which is below

Pharmacologic effects by different classes of antihypertensive agents on surrogate markers of cardiovascular disease

	Central α-Agonists	α-Blockers	α,β-Blockers	Vasodilator	β-Blockers	ACE Inhibitors	ARB	CCB	Diuretics
Metabolic									
Cholesterol LDL	→	→	→	→	→ ↑*	→	→	→	→ ↑
HDL	→	↑	→	→	→↓	→	→	→	→
Insulin resistance	→	↓	→ ↑	→ ↑	→ ↑	↓	↓	→	→ ↑
Glucose control	→	→	→	→	→ ↓	→ ↑	→	= ↓ →	→ ↓
Cardiovascular									
Left ventricular hypertrophy	↓	↓	↓	→ ↑	↓	↓	↓	↓	→ ↓
Renal									
Microalbuminuria	→	→	→ ↓	→ ↑	→ ↓	↓ ↓	↓ ↓	↓ →†	→ ↓

Figure 34.8 Pharmacologic effects by different classes of antihypertensive agents on surrogate markers of cardiovascular disease. ACE, angiotensin-converting enzyme; ARB, angiotensin receptor blocker; CCB, calcium channel blocker; HDL, high-density lipoprotein; LDL, low-density lipoprotein; →, no effect; ↑, increase; ↓, decrease. *Only β-blockers with intrinsic sympathomimetic activity; only when used in high doses (e.g., 480 mg/day diltiazem, 480 mg/day verapamil, 90 mg/day nifedipine). †Only nonhydropyridine calcium channel blockers (CCBs, verapamil, diltiazem).

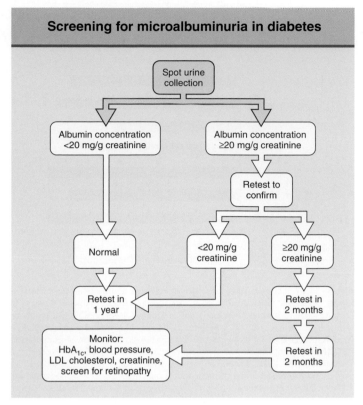

Screening for microalbuminuria in diabetes

Figure 34.9 Screening for microalbuminuria in diabetes. HbA$_{1c}$, hemoglobin A$_{1c}$; LDL, low-density lipoprotein.

the detectable range with conventional dipstick methodology, is defined as an abnormal urinary excretion rate of albumin in the range of 20 to 200 μg/min or 30 to 299 mg/day[45] (Fig. 34.9). The low prevalence of microalbuminuria in those without diabetes or kidney disease and the uncertainty of the significance of its modification in these groups do not make it cost-effective for routine screening in this population.[46,47] However, microalbuminuria can serve as a marker of the duration of blood pressure control in these patients.

The merits of normalizing or reducing the level of albuminuria have been clearly demonstrated by the results of several recent *post hoc* analyses. Data from both RENAAL and IDNT have clearly demonstrated that early reductions in proteinuria retard the progression of renal disease and lead to significant reductions in the incidence of ESRD in diabetic patients.[48,49] Similar findings were reported in a nondiabetic population in AASK. In this trial, the effect was seen even in people with low levels of proteinuria.[50]

Because there are established renoprotective and cardiovascular-protective effects of lowering microalbuminuria in diabetic patients with antihypertensive regimens containing either an ACE inhibitor or ARB, one of these agents should be part of the antihypertensive regimen used in patients with microalbuminuria.[13,14,51] The data are especially compelling for ACE inhibitors. These agents reduce albuminuria by reducing intraglomerular pressure and decreasing glomerular membrane permeability. The substudy of HOPE, the Microalbuminuria, Cardiovascular, and Renal Outcomes HOPE, looked at whether the addition of the ACE inhibitor ramipril to the current regimen of patients with diabetes can lower the risk of cardiovascular events and overt nephropathy in patients with microalbuminuria. Of 3577 participants with diabetes randomized

to ramipril or placebo, 1140 were considered to have microalbuminuria. Ramipril lowered the risk of the primary outcome (myocardial infarction, stroke, or cardiovascular death) by >21%. Of 295 participants who developed an albumin-to-creatinine ratio of >36 mg/mmol, 117 (7%) participants on ramipril and 149 (8%) on placebo developed overt nephropathy (relative risk 24% [3% to 40%, $P = 0.027$). Ramipril lowered the risk of overt nephropathy in participants who did and did not have baseline microalbuminuria and led to a lower albumin-to-creatinine ratio.[52]

ARBs are thought to have similar renal benefits. In a recent study, 590 type 2 diabetics were randomly assigned to either irbesartan (150 or 300 mg/day) or placebo and followed for 2 years. The primary endpoint was the time from baseline to first detection of overt nephropathy (urine albumin excretion >200 μg/min and at least a 30% increase from baseline on two consecutive visits). This endpoint occurred with significantly higher frequency in the placebo group compared to the irbesartan group (14.9% versus 9.7% and 5.2%, respectively, with 150 and 300 mg irbesartan) and was not related to significant differences in blood pressure.[53] The effects of various classes of antihypertensive drugs on intrarenal hemodynamic and membrane permeability as they relate to the development of albuminuria are summarized in Figure 34.10.

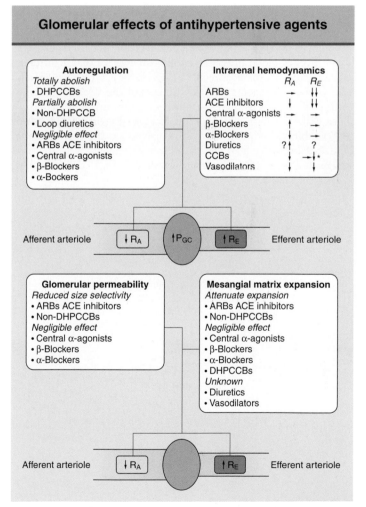

Glomerular effects of antihypertensive agents

Figure 34.10 Glomerular effects of antihypertensive agents. *Some evidence exists to suggest that verapamil may reduce efferent arteriolar tone. ACE, angiotensin-converting enzyme; ARB, angiotensin II receptor antagonist; CCBs, calcium blockers; DHPCCBs, dihydropyridine calcium channel blockers; non-DHPCCBs, nondihydropyridine calcium channel blockers.

DIABETES

Hypertension may account for up to 75% of all diabetes mellitus–related complications, including nephropathy and ESRD.[54] Additionally, a large number of these patients have cardiovascular events prior to progressing to ESRD. Reduction of hypertension has proven beneficial not only for reducing renal disease progression, but also for reducing cardiovascular morbidity and micro-angiopathic complications.

An important observation is that what is considered normotensive in people without diabetes is actually hypertensive in diabetics. JNC 7 recognized this fact by placing diabetics in the higher risk group and recommending a target blood pressure goal of <130/80 mm Hg.[1] Analysis of data from a variety of studies found that the lower the blood pressure was in diabetics, the slower that renal function is lost and the longer it takes for patients to require renal replacement therapy[7,55] (Fig. 34.11). Additionally, in the HOT study, in which 1501 diabetic subjects were randomized to three different levels of diastolic blood pressure control (<90, <85, and <80 mm Hg), those who achieved the lowest blood pressure goal experienced the lowest rate of cardiovascular events. Although there was only a 4-mm Hg difference in the achieved diastolic blood pressure between the intensively treated group and the other groups, this resulted in a significantly lower cardiovascular event rate in the diabetic subgroup and a greater preservation of renal function.[21]

The choice of the antihypertensive agents to use in diabetics, although important, is not a one-time decision since achieving this lower level of blood pressure requires an average of 3.2 different antihypertensive medications[13,14] (Fig. 34.12). However, specific antihypertensive agents, such as blockers of the RAAS and nondihydropyridine CCBs, have properties that are more beneficial in those diabetics with nephropathy. Captopril reduced the risk of the combined endpoint of death, dialysis or transplantation in type 1 diabetics by 50% compared to other agents used to attain similar levels of blood pressure control.[56] Both the RENAAL

Number of antihypertensive agents needed to achieve target systolic BP goals

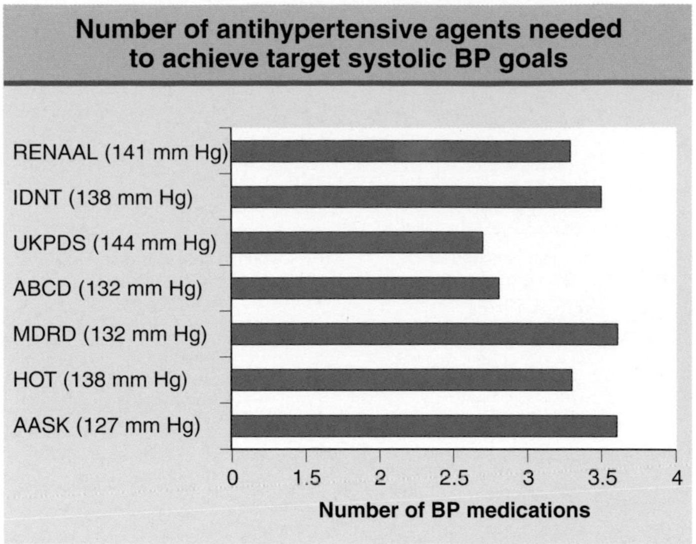

Figure 34.12 The number of antihypertensive agents used for intensive blood pressure (BP) goal. ABCD, Appropriate Blood Pressure Control in Diabetes; AASK, African American Study of Kidney Disease; HOT, Hypertension Optimal Treatment; IDNT, Irbesartan Diabetic Nephropathy Trial; MDRD, Modification of Diet in Renal Disease Trial; RENAAL, Reduction of Endpoints in NIDDM with the Angiotensin II Antagonist Losartan; UKPDS, UK Prospective Diabetes Study. (Data from Staessen JA, Wang JG, Thijs L: Cardiovascular prevention and blood pressure reduction: A quantitative overview updated until 1 March 2003. J Hypertens 2003;21:1055–1076; Lea J, Greene T, Hebert L, et al: The relationship between magnitude of proteinuria reduction and risk of end-stage renal disease: Results of the African American Study of Kidney Disease and hypertension. Arch Intern Med 2005;165:947–953; Jafar TH, Stark PC, Schmid CH, et al: Proteinuria as a modifiable risk factor for the progression of non-diabetic renal disease. Kidney Int 2001;60:1131–1140; Elliott WJ: Hypertensive emergencies. Crit Care Clin 2001;17:435–451.)

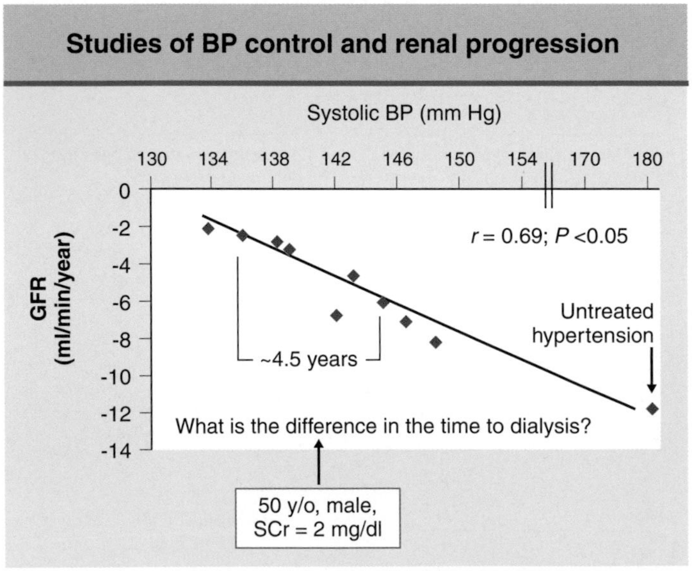

and the IDNT showed that ARBs reduced the risk of attaining the primary combined endpoint of doubling of serum creatinine, dialysis, or transplantation or death compared to placebo or amlodipine, despite similar levels of blood pressure control (relative risk, 16%; $P = 0.02$ and relative risk, 19%; $P = 0.03$, respectively).[57,58] In addition, initial data have suggested that nondihydropyridine CCBs reduce albuminuria and have additive antialbuminuric effects with ACE inhibitors independent of further reductions in blood pressure.[55] However, the results of the recent completed Bergamo Nephrologic Diabetes Complications Trial have suggested that nondihydropyridine CCBs do nothing to further decrease proteinuria when combined with ACE inhibitors.[59]

In the past, the use of certain classes of antihypertensive medications, such as thiazides and β-blockers, has been avoided in diabetics because of concerns about unfavorable metabolic profiles. However, recent studies have demonstrated these medications can be quite effective and safe in diabetics. The Antihypertensive and Lipid-Lowering Treatment to Prevent Heart Attack Trial showed that in 33,357 patients at high risk of cardiovascular events, there was no difference in cardiovascular outcomes in patients treated with thiazides, ACE inhibitors, or calcium antagonists.[60] Furthermore, a *post hoc* analysis showed no differences between the treatment groups in terms of renal outcomes.[61] Both the cardiovascular and renal results were found to be independent of diabetic status. Concerns over masking the manifestations of hypoglycemia in type 1 diabetics and a negative metabolic profile have prevented the use of β-blockers in diabetics. However, JNC 7 states that these concerns should not preclude their use in diabetic patients. In fact, one β-blocker, carvedilol, has demonstrated cardiovascular risk

Studies of BP control and renal progression

Figure 34.11 Achieved systolic blood pressure (SBP) in clinical trials of renal disease progression in relation to the calculated or measured decrease in glomerular filtration rate (GFR).[47] Given a linear progression in decrease of kidney function, it is estimated that a man with a serum creatinine (SCr) of 2 mg/dl (177 μmol/l) would require dialysis 4.5 years earlier if SBP was 145 mm Hg rather than 135 mm Hg.

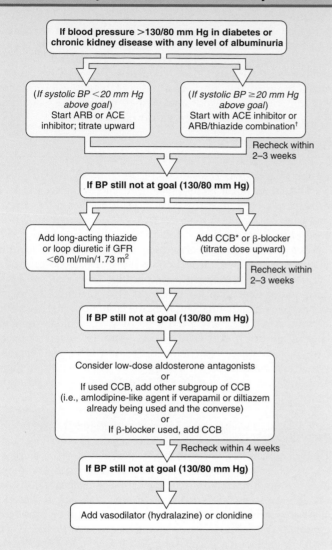

Figure 34.13 Clinical approach to managing hypertension in a diabetic or a patient with chronic kidney disease. All subjects with diabetes mellitus or renal insufficiency should be instructed on lifestyle modifications (see Chapter 33). Antihypertensive therapy is initiated if blood pressure is >130/80 mm Hg. If BP is <150/100 mm Hg, angiotensin-converting enzyme (ACE) inhibitors can be used alone; otherwise use a combination renin angiotensin aldosterone system inhibitor with a thiazide diuretic. Chlorthalidone with a longer half-life may provide better BP control compared to hydrochlorothiazide.[103,104] ARB, angiotensin receptor blocker. *If proteinuria is present (>300 mg/day), a nondihydropyridine calcium channel blocker (CBB) is preferred. †If estimated glomerular filtration rate (GFR) is <50 ml/min, a loop diuretic such as furosemide used twice daily is preferred for BP control.

reduction with neutral metabolic effects and β-blockers are particularly useful in lowering blood pressure if the patient has a baseline pulse rate >84 bpm. At pulse rates lower than this, there is little effect on blood pressure when used in combination with ACE inhibitors. Figure 34.13 shows a recommended paradigm for treating hypertension in diabetics.

RENAL DYSFUNCTION

The available data show that aggressive blood pressure reduction (<130/80 mm Hg) is needed to maximally slow progression

of renal disease, especially among patients with an elevated serum creatinine ≥1.4 mg/dl.[1,3,14,62] ACE inhibitors clearly slow progression of diabetic nephropathy to a greater extent than other antihypertensive agents, assuming blood pressure reduction to levels around 140/90 mm Hg. To assess the effect of ACE inhibitors in nondiabetic renal disease, a meta-analysis was performed that analyzed pooled individual patient data. It found that ACE inhibitors reduced the risk of ESRD and doubled serum creatinine by 31% and 30%, respectively, adjusting for baseline variables, decrease in systolic blood pressure, and decrease in urinary protein excretion.[63]

In spite of the evidence from many long-term clinical trials, there is a general fear by clinicians to use ACE inhibitors in such patients. This is because the initiation of ACE inhibitors often is followed by an increase in serum creatinine. While this may be a concern, it should only be worrisome if the serum potassium increases or if the creatinine continues to increase after a month of therapy (Fig. 34.14).

It is common to see reductions of 5% to 15% GFR in people within 1 to 4 weeks of ACE inhibitor therapy initiation.[64] Long-term clinical trials have confirmed that this reduction in renal function plateaus within a month.[64] Moreover, after ACE inhibitors were discontinued after 10 years of therapy, GFR returned to baseline.[65] This return to baseline GFR has not been reported with other classes of antihypertensive agents studied. It should be noted that the increase in serum creatinine is most commonly seen in individuals who are overdiuresed or volume depleted. However, because of the benefits of ACE inhibition in subjects with renal dysfunction, an increase in creatinine should

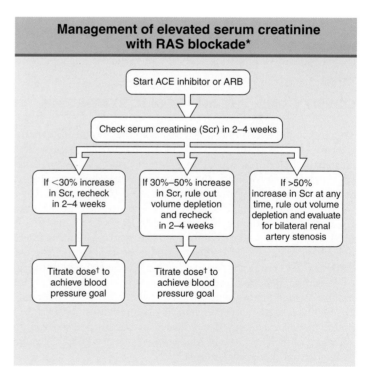

Figure 34.14 Management of elevated serum creatinine (SCr) in subjects receiving inhibitors of the renin angiotensin system (RAS). Shown is an algorithm for the use of an angiotensin-converting enzyme (ACE) inhibitor and angiotensin receptor blocker (ARB) in subjects with modest renal insufficiency (baseline creatinine <3.0 mg/dl [264 μmol/l]). As noted, a mild (<30%) increase in serum creatinine is usually acceptable if the creatinine values remain stable over time. *Algorithm only applies to people with a baseline creatinine ≤3.0 mg/dl and age younger than 70. †Required moderate to high dose of ACE inhibitor or ARB to achieve goal blood pressure.

be tolerated under certain circumstances. A review of 12 randomized clinical trials using ACE inhibitors in patients with pre-existing renal insufficiency found that a strong association existed between acute increases in serum creatinine of up to 30% that stabilized within the first 3 to 4 months of ACE inhibitor therapy with long-term preservation of renal function.[13] Thus, a useful clinical recommendation is that serum creatinine and potassium be checked in the first 7 to 14 days after initiation of ACE inhibitor therapy in anyone with a serum creatinine of ≥1.4 mg/dl, and a withdrawal of the ACE inhibitor in such patients should occur only when the increase in creatinine exceeds 30% above baseline within the first 3 to 4 months of therapy or if hyperkalemia develops (i.e., serum potassium ≥5.6 mmol/l) in a patient who is euvolemic.[13]

Diuretics may need to be withdrawn or the dose significantly reduced for short periods to promote euvolemia. If the serum creatinine has increased >30%, it should be rechecked within 1 week. If the creatinine continues to increase or hyperkalemia is present, then ACE inhibitors should be stopped and the patient assessed for bilateral renal arterial disease. Failure to follow this recommendation may lead to chronic irreversible renal failure.

Thus, while any class of antihypertensive agent may be used to achieve target blood pressure to preserve renal function, the following should be kept in mind. First, blood pressure will never be adequately controlled in patients with renal insufficiency without adequate volume control. In people with compromised GFR, this necessitates the use of a loop diuretic. Second, various combinations of medications will be needed to achieve blood pressure reduction, although these antihypertensive "cocktails" should contain an ACE inhibitor. If side effects are noted with the ACE inhibitor, an ARB may be substituted to ensure renal protection and blood pressure reduction. However, while animal studies clearly demonstrate similar efficacy between ACE inhibitors and ARBs in regard to renal preservation, clinical trials have only demonstrated their equivalence in diabetic renal disease.[57,66]

OBESITY AND THE METABOLIC SYNDROME

The metabolic syndrome is a condition that promotes atherosclerosis and increases the risk of cardiovascular events. The National Cholesterol Education Program Adult Treatment Panel III states that to establish the diagnosis of metabolic syndrome, at least three of the following criteria need to be present: (1) a waist circumference >102 cm (40 inches) for men or >88 cm (37 inches) for women; (2) triglyceride levels ≥150 mg/dl; (3) HDL cholesterol <40 mg/dl for men and <50 mg/dl for women; (4) blood pressure ≥130/85 mm Hg; or (5) fasting glucose ≥110 mg/dl.[67] Using similar criteria, it has been estimated that 50 to 75 million people in the United States may exhibit significant manifestations of this syndrome by 2010.[68] These components are highly related. Hypertension has been well established as a metabolic disorder and is predictive of insulin resistance.[69] In addition, as many as 50% of hypertensives have comorbid insulin resistance and hyperinsulinemia.[70]

The cornerstone of therapy in people with the metabolic syndrome is lifestyle modification.[1] Most patients with the metabolic syndrome will have either prehypertension or stage 1 hypertension. For those patients with documented hypertension, pharmacologic therapy should be instituted, but only after consideration is given to the specific properties of the different classes of medications. High-dose thiazide diuretics may worsen insulin resistance, and β-blockers may confer an increased risk of

general side effects in patients with the metabolic syndrome.[71,72] Conversely, ACE inhibitors and ARBs reduce blood pressure through vasodilatation, which may actually improve insulin resistance by increasing insulin-mediated glucose uptake. A recent meta-analysis suggests that this effect correlates with a reduction in the risk of developing diabetes by 27% for ACE inhibitors and 23% for ARBs.[73] Taken all together, the data suggest that ACE inhibitors or ARBs should be coupled with aggressive lifestyle modifications as the initial treatment of hypertension in those with the metabolic syndrome. Other medications should be added on as needed to achieve target blood pressure.

ELDERLY

Isolated systolic hypertension increases in prevalence as people age. The almost linear increase seen with increasing age is related to increasing arterial stiffness that leads to decreased arterial compliance. The net effect of this is an increase in systolic blood pressure and a decrease in diastolic blood pressure.[74] The importance of treating isolated systolic hypertension in older patients was explored in a meta-analysis of placebo-controlled trials. A 10-mm Hg increase in systolic blood pressure was significantly and independently correlated with increases by nearly 10% in the risk of all fatal and nonfatal complications, except for coronary events.[5] At any given level of systolic blood pressure, the risk of death rose with lower diastolic blood pressure, thereby suggesting that pulse pressure (difference between systolic and diastolic blood pressure) was an important predictor of cardiovascular risk. Antihypertensive therapy reduced the risk of stroke by 33% and of coronary events by 23%.

The second Swedish Trial in Old Patients with Hypertension study looked at whether the newer antihypertensive agents were better than the older antihypertensive agents in elderly patients. The trial randomized patients to conventional therapy (diuretics, β-blockers, or both), ACE inhibitors, or CCBs and found that there was no difference in reducing cardiovascular morbidity and mortality between the treatment groups.[75] As such, diuretics, unless comorbidities suggest otherwise, should still be considered first-line therapy. The clinician should be aware of problems such as volume depletion and hypokalemia. Of note, two meta-analyses have questioned the use of β-blockers in the elderly, citing evidence that, except in subjects with coronary artery disease, these agents did not reduce cardiovascular morbidity or mortality when used alone.[76,77]

Last, a long-term, 14-year, follow-up of the Systolic Hypertension in the Elderly Program (SHEP) trial noted that new-onset diabetes was associated with a higher cardiovascular event rate similar to those who already had diabetes.[78] Note, however, that new-onset diabetes related to diuretics was not associated with a significant increase in mortality.

REFRACTORY HYPERTENSION

Failure to adequately reduce blood pressure may be a result of multiple factors including secondary causes of hypertension and noncompliance.[1] However, a very common cause of uncontrolled blood pressure is related to concomitant use of over-the-counter medications, the two most prevalent types being nonsteroidal anti-inflammatory agents, such as ibuprofen, and sympathomimetics, such as a pseudoephedrine, in cold preparations. Additionally, oral contraceptive and steroid medications will blunt the antihypertensive effect of most agents. In prospective studies, only CCBs and, to a lesser degree, diuretics, maintain their antihypertensive effects in the presence of these symptom-relieving medications.

Sexual Dysfunction

A common cause of refractory hypertension in males is noncompliance secondary to the development of impotence. Almost all medications have been implicated in causing impotence; however, the incidence is highest for the central α_2-agonists, diuretics, and β-blockers. However, in most cases, with the exception of the central α_2-agonists and possibly β-blockers, the drug is only the indirect cause of the problem.[79]

The primary problem of impotence relates to abnormal vascular homeostasis within the penile circulation that dampens intrapenile blood pressure. Thus, when blood pressure is dramatically reduced and maintained at lower levels, there is a period of readjustment. In many cases, impotence resolves on its own, but it may take as long as 4 to 6 months.[79] Thus, all patients, including diabetics without neuropathy, should be encouraged to stay on their medications if arterial pressure is controlled because the problem should resolve. In those who have persistent erectile dysfunction, prostaglandin inhibitors can be used with success.

MALIGNANT HYPERTENSION/ HYPERTENSIVE CRISES

Malignant hypertension was the term originally used to classify patients who presented with severely increased blood pressure and signs or symptoms of acute target-organ damage.[80] Such patients were unlikely to survive a year. The dramatic advancements in therapy and a correspondingly improved prognosis for afflicted patients have led to the evolution of the terms hypertensive urgency and hypertensive emergency. The terminology of malignant hypertension is now replaced by emergent (requiring treatment in minutes) or urgent (requiring treatment in hours) hypertensive crises. Nearly all authorities have accepted the revised terminology.[1,81]

Hypertensive emergency, as defined by JNC 7, is a severely increased blood pressure (>180/120 mm Hg) with signs and symptoms of acute end-organ damage, that is, encephalopathy, intracranial hemorrhage, chest pain, myocardial infarction, aortic dissection, pulmonary edema, eclampsia, or microscopic hematuria with acute renal failure. Patients must be hospitalized and treated immediately with parenteral drug therapy. Patients sometimes present with very high blood pressures, but without evidence of acute target organ damage; this situation is considered hypertensive urgency and need not be treated either in the hospital setting or using intravenous medication. A physician taking care of a patient with elevated blood pressures needs to be able to distinguish between these two situations for two major reasons. The route of administration of drug therapy is different (parenteral therapy is typical for emergencies, whereas oral therapy can be given for urgencies), and hospitalization (usually in the intensive care unit) is frequently necessary for hypertensive emergencies, but rarely required for hypertensive urgencies.

A common presentation of severe hypertension is that of an asymptomatic patient who is seen for an unrelated complaint, with a normal physical examination and stable (if not normal) laboratory results. This patient is not having a hypertensive crisis and requires only a prescription for an antihypertensive drug and an appointment for follow-up within 24 to 48 hours.[82] In such cases, every effort should be made to ensure that the patient is seen as scheduled and that the blood pressure has been lowered out of a potentially dangerous range.

In most clinical settings, the typical history involves a hypertensive person who discontinued treatment or reduced therapy without having the blood pressure checked thereafter. In a large series from New York City, not having a primary care physician (available to refill antihypertensive medication prescriptions) was the single most important risk factor for presenting to a hospital emergency department with severely increased blood pressure.[83] Occasionally, withdrawal of antihypertensive medications, especially drugs such as clonidine, or ingestion of substances that increase blood pressure, is responsible for hypertensive emergency. Public health data from Georgia suggests that nonadherence to chronic antihypertensive therapy (due to lack of a primary care physician or funds to pay for antihypertensive medications) is the primary reason for hypertensive emergencies in the United States today.

Hypertensive crises are more likely to occur in patients with certain forms of secondary hypertension, particularly renovascular disease or pheochromocytoma. Crises are rare in patients with mineralocorticoid excess states (e.g., primary hyperaldosteronism), perhaps because blood pressure increases more gradually or because renin secretion tends to be suppressed as a result of chronic volume expansion.[84] An evaluation for secondary causes of hypertension is a routine part of the care of a person with a hypertensive crisis and is typically undertaken after the patient is stable. The structural compensatory changes and the attendant functional shift of the autoregulatory range explain why chronically hypertensive patients can often tolerate very high blood pressures without problems and why normotensive patients or those with only a recent onset or rapidly increasing blood pressure can develop hypertensive crises at relatively lower blood pressure levels.

The organ systems that require special attention during the initial evaluation of the patient in a hypertensive crisis include the neurologic, ophthalmologic, cardiac, renal, and peripheral vasculature. The patients with either new hemorrhages/exudates or papilledema represent a hypertensive emergency. High-grade retinopathy and a hypertensive emergency in general are extremely unusual in patients with primary hyperaldosteronism. The presence of an abdominal bruit (with both systolic and diastolic components) suggests the presence of renovascular hypertension.[85] The radiofemoral pulse delay due to a coarctation of the aorta should not be missed on clinical examination. Occasionally, palpation of a pheochromocytoma can initiate a typical episode and suggest the diagnosis. Assessment of renal function is crucial. It is important to compare the presenting serum creatinine with a recent measurement of the patient's renal function because acute deterioration in renal function in the presence of very high blood pressure is classified as a hypertensive crisis. The presence of gross or microscopic hematuria at presentation is consistent with acute renal damage due to very high blood pressures. Red-cell casts and significant proteinuria generally mean that acute glomerulonephritis is the cause of the increased blood pressure and subsequent crisis.

Most authorities suggest that in most true hypertensive emergencies (with the exception of aortic dissection and some neurologic crises), the mean arterial pressure should be reduced only 10% to 15% during the first hour. Gradually thereafter, a diastolic blood pressure target between 100 and 110 mm Hg (or a reduction of 25% compared to the initial baseline, whichever is higher) is appropriate. Reduction of blood pressure to <90 mm Hg diastolic or even by as little as 35% of the initial mean arterial pressure, has been associated with major organ dysfunction, coma, and death, even in recent years.[86]

The goal in a hypertensive crisis is to lower the patient's blood pressure gradually over 6 to 24 hours. An intravenously administered medication with a short duration of action is usually used for this purpose since the hypotensive effect of the drug can be promptly reversed if the response is excessive (Fig. 34.15). With a short-acting, intravenous drug, the clinician has much tighter control over both the rates of blood pressure decrease and the ultimate blood pressure target. For many years, sodium nitroprusside was the standard intravenously administered drug for all hypertensive crises. Nitroprusside has an onset of action within 2 to 3 minutes and serum half-life of 1 to 2 minutes, may be easily titrated, is inexpensive, and has a long record of effectiveness in treating hypertensive crises of nearly all types. Limitations of nitroprusside therapy include the need for invasive monitoring (an arterial line is required in many hospitals) and its metabolic products (thiocyanate and cyanide), which contraindicate its use in pregnancy, and accumulate when nitroprusside is used in patients with renal or hepatic dysfunction. Nitroprusside is typically begun at 0.3 µg/kg/min and increased by 0.2 to 1.0 µg/kg/min every 3 to 5 minutes until the blood pressure reaches the target range. Once the effective dose of nitroprusside has been found, an oral medication should also be started.

Two other drugs approved in the United States in hypertensive crises are being increasingly used; neither has potentially toxic metabolites. Nicardipine, a dihydropyridine calcium channel blocker, may have a special role in patients with coronary disease or after cardiac surgery.[87] Fenoldopam mesylate, a dopamine-1 agonist, was approved in 1997. The drug acts on receptors that are located in the renal and splanchnic arteries with lesser density in the coronary and cerebral arteries. However, intravenous fenoldopam does not cross the blood-brain barrier and has no central nervous system activity because it is a poorly lipid-soluble molecule. In clinical trials against nitroprusside, fenoldopam demonstrates beneficial renal effects (increased diuresis, natriuresis, and creatinine clearance) over nitroprusside.[88] Fenoldopam probably is most useful for blood pressure reduction in patients with renal impairment and those undergoing vascular surgery.[89] In addition, fenoldopam is not associated with any thiocyanate toxicity and is not degraded by light. Both nicardipine and fenoldopam are more expensive than nitroprusside, but often can be given with just a blood pressure cuff to monitor the effects outside an intensive care unit. The total cost of care may be lower with either of these than with nitroprusside, which in most hospitals is used only in an intensive care unit with an arterial line in place. However, no outcome studies have yet had sufficient power to demonstrate the potential benefits of these agents against the time-tested standard nitroprusside. The adverse effects are similar to any vasodilator, which include headache, flushing, dizziness, tachycardia, or bradycardia. Of note, two important adverse effects were noted during the fenoldopam studies. One is the T-wave flattening on the electrocardiogram in all leads except aVR without evidence of myocardial ischemia. It has been speculated that acute reductions in blood pressure might be responsible for this finding. This also occurs with nitroprusside. The second adverse effect is increased intraocular pressure, which has been attributed in part to diminished drainage of aqueous humor. Thus,

Treatment of hypertensive emergencies and urgencies			
Hypertensive Emergencies*			
Medications	Mechanism	Dose (onset of action)	Side Effects
Vasodilators			
Sodium nitroprusside	↑ Cyclic GMP Blocks cell $[Ca^{2+}]$	0.25–10 µg kg/min (immediate)	Nausea, severe hypotension, thiocyanate toxicity (check levels every 48 hours especially in renal failure)
Nitroglycerin	↑ Nitrate receptors	5–100 µg/min (2–5 min)	Headache, vomiting, methemoglobinemia, tachyphylaxis
Hydralazine	Opens $[K^+]$ channels	10 mg IV/IM every 4–6 h (15–30 min)	Hypotension, reflex sympathetic stimulation, exacerbates angina, myocardial infarction
Diazoxide	Direct acting	50–150 mg every 5 min or 15–30 mg/min (2–4 min)	Nausea, flushing, reflex sympathetic stimulation, exacerbates angina, myocardial infarction
Fenoldopam	Dopamine 1 receptor agonist	0.1–0.3 µg/kg/min (>5 min)	Tachycardia, headache, nausea, flushing
Nicardipine	CCB	5–15 mg every hour IV (1–5 min)	Hypotension, tachycardia, nausea, vomiting, phlebitis
Enalaprilat	ACE inhibitor	0.625–1.25 mg every 6 h (15–30 min)	Severe hypotension, delayed excretion in renal failure
Labetalol	α,β-Blocker	20-to-80 mg IV bolus every 10 min or 0.5–2.0 mg/min infusion (5–10 min)	Nausea, hypotension, asthma, congestive heart failure, formication
Hypertensive Urgencies†			
Medications	Mechanism	Dose (onset of action)	Side Effects
Captopril	ACE inhibitor	25 mg every 1–2 h (15–30 min)	Angioedema, acute renal failure
Clonidine	Central α_2-agonist	0.1–0.2 mg every 1–2 h (30–60 min)	Hypotension, sedation, dry mouth
Labetalol	α,β-Blocker	200–400 mg every 2–3 h (30–120 min)	Heart block, bronchoconstriction, orthostatic hypotension
Nifedipine	CCB	Used frequently in hypertensive emergency; however, has potential for abrupt hypotension with risk of stroke, angina, myocardial infarction, or sudden death	

Figure 34.15   Treatment of hypertensive emergencies and urgencies. * Goal is to decrease BP in minutes. †Goal is to decrease BP within hours. CCB, calcium channel blocker; GMP, guanosine monophosphate.

cautious administration of fenoldopam, if at all, in patients with glaucoma or high intraocular pressures has been recommended. Fenoldopam is typically begun at 0.1 µg/kg/min and increased at 20-minute intervals by 0.1 to 0.2 µg/kg/min, with a maximum dose of 1.5 µg/kg/min.

Other intravenously administered antihypertensive drugs are most useful only in specific clinical situations. Nimodipine (either oral or intravenous) has been associated with improved outcomes after subarachnoid hemorrhage, but its use in acute stroke is controversial. Its beneficial effects may be more related to preserving neurons in peril by limiting calcium influx into ischemic cells rather than to its hypotensive effects. The usual dose is 60 mg (two 30-mg capsules) every 4 hours for 21 days after the neurologic event. Nitroglycerin is useful in the setting of angina pectoris, coronary artery bypass surgery, or neurosurgery, but is now being replaced in some hospitals by nicardipine. It has the disadvantages of being unstable in solution, adhering to the intravenous line, leading to tolerance during prolonged administration and causing profound headaches. It is typically begun at 5 µg/min, and the dose is increased every 3 to 5 minutes by 5 to 10 µg/min, as needed. Phentolamine is a nonselective α-antagonist and is very useful in pheochromocytoma and other catecholamine excess states. It is typically delivered in 2- to 5-mg minibolus injections to minimize precipitous decreases in blood pressure.

The choice of drugs for the treatment of hypertensive urgency is currently much broader than for emergencies since almost all antihypertensive drugs lower blood pressure effectively and reasonably rapidly (see Fig. 34.15). The drug of choice should be effective, quick acting, and unlikely to cause alterations in mental status or to produce hypotension. Nifedipine, clonidine, labetalol, and captopril are often used. The dangers of short-acting nifedipine were highlighted in 1996.[90] The issue with nifedipine capsules is not that they are ineffective in lowering BP, but that their effects are somewhat unpredictable. The FDA declined to approve this approach to treatment. Several other dihydropyridine calcium antagonists have been reported to be effective in treating hypertensive urgencies. As might be expected from their pharmacokinetics, both nicardipine and nicardipine have a slightly longer onset of action and are less likely to cause the precipitous decreases in blood pressure seen occasionally with nifedipine.

Although clonidine effectively controls blood pressure, there is a significant risk of hypertensive urgency in those patients who are nonadherent given the danger of rebound hypertension associated with clonidine withdrawal. In Brazil, oral captopril is a common drug for hypertensive urgencies; it is typically given in a 12.5- to 25-mg dose, crushed to hasten absorption. ACE inhibitors must be used with caution because they can cause or exacerbate renal impairment in the occasional patient with critical renal artery stenosis. Parenteral hydralazine has been reformulated and typically is the first parental drug given in obstetrics for hypertensive urgencies. Minoxidil has been used effectively, when patients present with uncontrolled hypertension but are already taking a diuretic and a β-blocker. Recent reviews suggest that each of these drugs is effective in approximately 85% to 95% of hypertensive urgencies with an approximate equal tolerability.

The unanswered question is whether it is necessary to give any particular antihypertensive medication to most people with hypertensive urgency. Many emergency departments have standard operating procedures that prohibit release of patients into the community with blood pressures >180/110 mm Hg. Primarily medicolegal concerns rather than medical and therapeutic principles generate these policies.

HYPERTENSION IN PREGNANCY

General treatment recommendations for hypertension in pregnancy are discussed in Chapters 41 and 42. For hypertensive crises, the first choice of antihypertensive therapy is complicated because there are two patients who must be considered, the mother and the baby. Drugs with teratogenic potential (e.g., nitroprusside, ACE inhibitors, ARBs) are contraindicated. Although most obstetricians prefer $MgSO_4$ and methyldopa for inpatient and outpatient treatment of hypertension, respectively, parenteral hydralazine or labetalol is the typical drug chosen for initial treatment of preeclampsia.

SCLERODERMA RENAL CRISIS

Scleroderma renal crisis is defined as a new onset of accelerated hypertension and/or rapidly progressive renal failure and is deemed a medical emergency. It requires hospitalization and parenteral drug therapy, occurs in 10% to 25% of patients with scleroderma (systemic sclerosis), and is associated with diverse outcomes. Diffuse skin involvement, rapid progression of skin thickening, new-onset anemia, disease duration of <4 years, the presence of anti-RNA polymerase antibody, new cardiac, events such as congestive heart failure and pericardial effusion, and use of high corticosteroids may be predictors of scleroderma renal crisis. When associated with thrombocytopenia, hyperreninemia, and hemolytic anemia, it carries the poorest prognosis. The vascular changes of intima proliferation, medial thinning, and increased collagen deposition in the adventitial layer of the small renal arteries result in decreased renal blood flow, hypertension, and progressive renal impairment. Interestingly, many patients may initially present in a renal crisis as a manifestation of their disease. The mainstay of treatment is an ACE inhibitor or an ARB and additional agents (i.e., nondihydropyridine CCB or other vasodilators, as necessary) to control blood pressure. This treatment slows the progression to ESRD.[91] The fact that scleroderma renal crisis is declining in frequency is consistent with the observation that renal disease has been superseded by cardiopulmonary complications as the leading cause of death in systemic sclerosis.

NEWER AGENTS

Renin Inhibitors

Renin catalyzes the first and rate-limiting step of the RAAS and has high specificity for its substrate angiotensinogen; renin inhibitors offer the potential for blocking this complex hormonal system at its initial point of activation, with a low likelihood of side effects. Because renin inhibitors prevent the formation of both angiotensin (Ang) I and Ang II, they may offer a therapeutic profile distinct from both ACE inhibitors and ARBs. Renin inhibitors also do not affect kinin metabolism and hence would not be expected to cause dry cough or angioneurotic edema, which are characteristic side effects of ACE inhibitors. ARBs increase levels of Ang II, an effect that does not occur with renin inhibitors.[92]

A wide variety of potential renin inhibitors have been developed over the past 20 years, but low potency, poor bioavailability, and short duration of action after oral administration in humans meant that these compounds were not clinically useful drugs.[92] Aliskiren is the first in a new class of orally effective, nonpeptide, low molecular weight renin inhibitors for the treatment of hypertension.[93]

Oral administration of aliskiren to sodium-depleted marmosets caused complete inhibition of renin and sustained reductions in arterial blood pressure. In humans, once-daily oral doses of aliskiren of up to 640 mg are well tolerated and caused dose dependent and sustained RAAS inhibition in healthy volunteers. Moreover, a recent study in 226 patients with mild to moderate hypertension showed that aliskiren 300 mg/day lowered blood pressure with the efficacy and tolerability similar to those of the ARB losartan at twice the recommended daily dose.

Endothelin Receptor Antagonist

While the use of the endothelin receptor antagonist bosentan has been primarily used to treat pulmonary hypertension, endothelin receptor antagonists have also been used as antihypertensive agents, but their relative antihypertensive potency has been weak.[94,95] The new endothelin A receptor antagonist darusentan has found a place for treatment of resistant hypertension. It is a relatively more potent agent for blood pressure reduction.[96] A recent study of 115 people already receiving three different antihypertensive agents who were still not at the blood pressure goal showed that addition of darusentan significantly lowered blood pressure and increased the percentage of people at the blood pressure goal. Sixty-one percent of these people had diabetes and/or chronic kidney disease and 76 received darusentan. At baseline, mean systolic blood pressure was 146.6 ± 14.8 mm Hg and mean diastolic blood pressure was 80.0 ± 12.3 mm Hg. In this study, those treated with darusentan showed a placebo-corrected change from baseline systolic pressure of –11.6 ± 3.3 mm Hg after 10 weeks. Changes in mean ambulatory 24-hour placebo-corrected systolic pressure were –9.2 ± 2.2 mm Hg. In addition, 49% of darusentan-treated versus 28% of placebo-treated subjects achieved JNC 7 systolic blood pressure goals. Darusentan was well tolerated. The most frequent adverse event was peripheral edema (17%). This agent has promise for use in resistant hypertension.[97]

Selective Aldosterone Receptor Antagonists

While the diuretic spironolactone has been used since the 1960s for the treatment of hypertension, renewed interest has been given to aldosterone antagonists with the approval of eplerenone for treatment of hypertension in 1997 and its added efficacy in a heart failure outcome trial.[98] Eplerenone is a selective aldosterone receptor antagonist that lacks the side effect of gynecomastia.[99,100] Eplerenone has an antihypertensive efficacy similar to amlodipine and reduces cardiovascular mortality and morbidity in patients with heart failure and renal insufficiency.[101] Just as with spironolactone, serum potassium must be followed closely when using eplerenone because levels rise in a dose-dependent fashion. This effect is more pronounced in patients with impaired renal function. Aldosterone receptor blockade has found its way into treatment of African American patients with refractory hypertension.[102] The mechanism behind its efficacy is still unclear, but its clinical benefit on blood pressure lowering is definite.

REFERENCES

1. Chobanian AV, Bakris GL, Black HR, et al: The seventh report of the Joint National Committee on Prevention, Detection, Evaluation, and Treatment of High Blood Pressure: The JNC 7 report. JAMA 2003; 289:2560–2572.
2. Hajjar I, Kotchen TA: Trends in prevalence, awareness, treatment, and control of hypertension in the United States, 1988–2000. JAMA 2003;290:199–206.
3. Perry HM Jr, Miller JP, Fornoff JR, et al: Early predictors of 15-year end-stage renal disease in hypertensive patients. Hypertension 1985;25:587–594.
4. Lewington S, Clarke R, Qizilbash N, et al: Age-specific relevance of usual blood pressure to vascular mortality: A meta-analysis of individual data for one million adults in 61 prospective studies. Lancet 2002;360:1903–1913.
5. Staessen JA, Wang JG, Thijs L: Cardiovascular prevention and blood pressure reduction: A quantitative overview updated until 1 March 2003. J Hypertens 2003;21:1055–1076.
6. Stamler J, Vaccaro O, Neaton JD, Wentworth D: Diabetes, other risk factors, and 12-year cardiovascular mortality for men screened in the Multiple Risk Factor Intervention Trial. Diabetes Care 1993;16: 434–444.
7. Sarnak MJ, Greene T, Wang X, et al: The effect of a lower target blood pressure on the progression of kidney disease: Long-term follow-up of the modification of diet in renal disease study. Ann Intern Med 2005; 142:342–351.
8. Lazarus JM, Bourgoignie JJ, Buckalew VM, et al: Achievement and safety of a low blood pressure goal in chronic renal disease. The Modification of Diet in Renal Disease Study Group. Hypertension 1997;29:641–650.
9. Jafar TH, Stark PC, Schmid CH, et al: Progression of chronic kidney disease: The role of blood pressure control, proteinuria, and angiotensin-converting enzyme inhibition: A patient-level meta-analysis. Ann Intern Med 2003;139:244–252.
10. Wright JT Jr, Bakris G, Greene T, et al: Effect of blood pressure lowering and antihypertensive drug class on progression of hypertensive kidney disease: Results from the AASK trial. JAMA 2002;288: 2421–2431.
11. Lea J, Greene T, Hebert L, et al: The relationship between magnitude of proteinuria reduction and risk of end-stage renal disease: Results of the African American Study of Kidney Disease and hypertension. Arch Intern Med 2005;165:947–953.
12. Turnbull F, Neal B, Algert C, et al: Effects of different blood pressure-lowering regimens on major cardiovascular events in individuals with and without diabetes mellitus: Results of prospectively designed overviews of randomized trials. Arch Intern Med 2005;165: 1410–1419.
13. Bakris GL, Williams M, Dworkin L, et al: Preserving renal function in adults with hypertension and diabetes: A consensus approach. National Kidney Foundation Hypertension and Diabetes Executive Committees Working Group. Am J Kidney Dis 2000;36:646–661.
14. K/DOQI clinical practice guidelines on hypertension and antihypertensive agents in chronic kidney disease. Am J Kidney Dis 2004;43: 1–290.
15. European Society of Hypertension-European Society of Cardiology Committee: 2003 European Society of Hypertension-European Society of Cardiology guidelines for the management of arterial hypertension. J Hypertens 2003;21:1011–1053.
16. Lind L, Lithell H, Pollare T: Is it hyperinsulinemia or insulin resistance that is related to hypertension and other metabolic cardiovascular risk factors? J Hypertens Suppl 1993;11:S11–S16.
17. Farnett L, Mulrow CD, Linn WD, et al: The J-curve phenomenon and the treatment of hypertension: Is there a point beyond which pressure reduction is dangerous? JAMA 1991;265:489–495.
18. Estacio RO, Jeffers BW, Gifford N, Schrier RW: Effect of blood pressure control on diabetic microvascular complications in patients with hypertension and type 2 diabetes. Diabetes Care 2000;23(Suppl 2): B54–B64.
19. De Zeeuw D, Remuzzi G, Parving HH, et al: Albuminuria, a therapeutic target for cardiovascular protection in type 2 diabetic patients with nephropathy. Circulation 2004;110:921–927.
20. Berl T, Hunsicker LG, Lewis JB, et al: Impact of achieved blood pressure on cardiovascular outcomes in the Irbesartan Diabetic Nephropathy Trial. J Am Soc Nephrol 2005;16:2170–2179.
21. Hansson L, Zanchetti A, Carruthers SG, et al: Effects of intensive blood-pressure lowering and low-dose aspirin in patients with hypertension: Principal results of the Hypertension Optimal Treatment (HOT) randomised trial. HOT Study Group. Lancet 1998;351: 1755–1762.

22. Bakris GL, Smith DH, Giles TD, et al: Comparative antihypertensive efficacy of angiotensin receptor blocker-based treatment in African-American and white patients. J Clin Hypertens (Greenwich) 2005;7:587–595.

23. Weir MR, Gray JM, Paster R, Saunders E: Differing mechanisms of action of angiotensin-converting enzyme inhibition in black and white hypertensive patients. The Trandolapril Multicenter Study Group. Hypertension 1995;26:124–130.

24. Ruilope LM, Rosei EA, Bakris GL, et al: Angiotensin receptor blockers: Therapeutic targets and cardiovascular protection. Blood Press 2005;14:196–209.

25. Bakris GL, Smith DH, Giles TD, et al: Comparative antihypertensive efficacy of angiotensin receptor blocker-based treatment in African-American and white patients. J Clin Hypertens (Greenwich) 2005;7:587–595.

26. Chobanian AV, Bakris GL, Black HR, et al: Seventh report of the Joint National Committee on Prevention, Detection, Evaluation, and Treatment of High Blood Pressure. Hypertension 2003;42:1206–1252.

27. Weir MR, Rosenberger C, Fink JC: Pilot study to evaluate a water displacement technique to compare effects of diuretics and ACE inhibitors to alleviate lower extremity edema due to dihydropyridine calcium antagonists. Am J Hypertens 2001;14:963–968.

28. Epstein M, Bakris G: Newer approaches to antihypertensive therapy. Use of fixed-dose combination therapy. Arch Intern Med 1996;156:1969–1978.

29. Bakris GL: Protecting renal function in the hypertensive patient: Clinical guidelines. Am J Hypertens 2005;18:112S–119S.

30. Yusuf S, Sleight P, Pogue J, et al: Effects of an angiotensin-converting-enzyme inhibitor, ramipril, on cardiovascular events in high-risk patients. The Heart Outcomes Prevention Evaluation Study Investigators. N Engl J Med 2000;342:145–153.

31. Hoyert DL, Kung HC, Smith BL: Deaths: Preliminary data for 2003. Natl Vital Stat Rep 2005;53:1–48.

32. Devereux RB: Do antihypertensive drugs differ in their ability to regress left ventricular hypertrophy? Circulation 1997;95:1983–1985.

33. de Simone G, Verdecchia P, Pede S, et al: Prognosis of inappropriate left ventricular mass in hypertension: The MAVI Study. Hypertension 2002;40:470–476.

34. Levy D, Garrison RJ, Savage DD, et al: Prognostic implications of echocardiographically determined left ventricular mass in the Framingham Heart Study. N Engl J Med 1900;322:1561–1566.

35. Muiesan ML, Salvetti M, Rizzoni D, et al: Association of change in left ventricular mass with prognosis during long-term antihypertensive treatment. J Hypertens 1995;13:1091–1095.

36. Verdecchia P, Schillaci G, Borgioni C, et al: Prognostic significance of serial changes in left ventricular mass in essential hypertension. Circulation 1998;97:48–54.

37. Neaton JD, Grimm RH Jr, Prineas RJ, et al: Treatment of Mild Hypertension Study. Final results. Treatment of Mild Hypertension Study Research Group. JAMA 1993;270:713–724.

38. Mesfin GM, Piper RC, DuCharme DW, et al: Pathogenesis of cardiovascular alterations in dogs treated with minoxidil. Toxicol Pathol 1989;17:164–181.

39. Dahlof B, Devereux RB, Kjeldsen SE, et al: Cardiovascular morbidity and mortality in the Losartan Intervention for Endpoint Reduction in Hypertension Study (LIFE): A randomised trial against atenolol. Lancet 2002;359:995–1003.

40. Ibsen H, Olsen MH, Wachtell K, et al: Reduction in albuminuria translates to reduction in cardiovascular events in hypertensive patients: Losartan intervention for endpoint reduction in hypertension study. Hypertension 2005;45:198–202.

41. Mogensen CE: Microalbuminuria predicts clinical proteinuria and early mortality in maturity-onset diabetes. N Engl J Med 1984;310:356–360.

42. Kistorp C, Raymond I, Pedersen F, et al: N-terminal pro-brain natriuretic peptide, C-reactive protein, and urinary albumin levels as predictors of mortality and cardiovascular events in older adults. JAMA 2005;293:1609–1616.

43. Asselbergs FW, Diercks GF, Hillege HL, et al: Effects of fosinopril and pravastatin on cardiovascular events in subjects with microalbuminuria. Circulation 2004;110:2809–2816.

44. Bakris GL: Clinical importance of microalbuminuria in diabetes and hypertension. Curr Hypertens Rep 2004;6:352–356.

45. Eknoyan G, Hostetter T, Bakris GL, et al: Proteinuria and other markers of chronic kidney disease: A position statement of the National Kidney Foundation (NKF) and the National Institute of Diabetes and Digestive and Kidney Diseases (NIDDK). Am J Kidney Dis 2003;42:617–622.

46. Boulware LE, Jaar BG, Tarver-Carr ME, et al: Screening for proteinuria in US adults: A cost-effectiveness analysis. JAMA 2003;290:3101–3114.

47. Lydakis C, Efstratopoulos A, Lip GY: Microalbuminuria in hypertension: Is it up to measure? J Hum Hypertens 1997;11:695–697.

48. De Zeeuw D, Remuzzi G, Parving HH, et al: Proteinuria, a target for renoprotection in patients with type 2 diabetic nephropathy: Lessons from RENAAL. Kidney Int 2004;65:2309–2320.

49. Hunsicker LG, Atkins RC, Lewis JB, et al: Impact of irbesartan, blood pressure control, and proteinuria on renal outcomes in the Irbesartan Diabetic Nephropathy Trial. Kidney Int Suppl 2004;92:S99–S101.

50. Lea J, Greene T, Hebert L, et al: The relationship between magnitude of proteinuria reduction and risk of end-stage renal disease: Results of the African American Study of Kidney Disease and Hypertension. Arch Intern Med 2005;165:947–953.

51. Ravid M, Lang R, Rachmani R, Lishner M: Long-term renoprotective effect of angiotensin-converting enzyme inhibition in non-insulin-dependent diabetes mellitus. A 7-year follow-up study. Arch Intern Med 1996;156:286–289.

52. Moller DE: Potential role of TNF-alpha in the pathogenesis of insulin resistance and type 2 diabetes. Trends Endocrinol Metab 2000;11:212–217.

53. Parving HH, Lehnert H, Brochner-Mortensen J, et al: The effect of irbesartan on the development of diabetic nephropathy in patients with type 2 diabetes. N Engl J Med 2001;345:870–878.

54. Coresh J, Astor BC, Greene T, et al: Prevalence of chronic kidney disease and decreased kidney function in the adult US population: Third National Health and Nutrition Examination Survey. Am J Kidney Dis 2003;41:1–12.

55. Bakris GL: Progression of diabetic nephropathy. A focus on arterial pressure level and methods of reduction. Diabetes Res Clin Pract 1998;39(Suppl):S35–S42.

56. Lewis EJ, Hunsicker LG, Bain RP, Rohde RD: The effect of angiotensin-converting-enzyme inhibition on diabetic nephropathy. The Collaborative Study Group. N Engl J Med 1993;329:1456–1462.

57. Lewis EJ, Hunsicker LG, Clarke WR, et al: Renoprotective effect of the angiotensin-receptor antagonist irbesartan in patients with nephropathy due to type 2 diabetes. N Engl J Med 2001;345:851–860.

58. Parving HH, Brenner BM, Cooper ME, et al: [Effect of losartan on renal and cardiovascular complications of patients with type 2 diabetes and nephropathy]. Ugeskr Laeger 2001;163:5514–5519.

59. Ruggenenti P, Fassi A, Ilieva AP, et al: Preventing microalbuminuria in type 2 diabetes. N Engl J Med 2004;351:1941–1951.

60. Major outcomes in high-risk hypertensive patients randomized to angiotensin-converting enzyme inhibitor or calcium channel blocker vs diuretic: The Antihypertensive and Lipid-Lowering Treatment to Prevent Heart Attack Trial (ALLHAT). JAMA 2002;288:2981–2997.

61. Rahman M, Pressel S, Davis BR, et al: Renal outcomes in high-risk hypertensive patients treated with an angiotensin-converting enzyme inhibitor or a calcium channel blocker vs a diuretic: A report from the Antihypertensive and Lipid-Lowering Treatment to Prevent Heart Attack Trial (ALLHAT). Arch Intern Med 2005;165:936–946.

62. Bakris GL, Williams M, Dworkin L, et al: Preserving renal function in adults with hypertension and diabetes: A consensus approach. National Kidney Foundation Hypertension and Diabetes Executive Committees Working Group. Am J Kidney Dis 2000;36:646–661.

63. Jafar TH, Stark PC, Schmid CH, et al: Proteinuria as a modifiable risk factor for the progression of non-diabetic renal disease. Kidney Int 2001;60:1131–1140.

64. Bakris GL, Barnhill BW, Sadler R: Treatment of arterial hypertension in diabetic humans: Importance of therapeutic selection. Kidney Int 1992;41:912–919.

65. Hansen KW, Poulsen PL, Christiansen JS, Mogensen CE: Determinants of 24-hour blood pressure in IDDM patients. Diabetes Care 1995;18:529–535.

66. Parving HH, Lehnert H, Brochner-Mortensen J, et al: [Effect of irbesartan on the development of diabetic nephropathy in patients with type 2 diabetes]. Ugeskr Laeger 2001;163:5519–5524.

67. American Diabetes Association: Summary of Revisions for the 2004 Clinical Practice Recommendations. Diabetes Care 2004;27:S3.

68. Hansen KW, Poulsen PL, Mogensen CE: [Evidence-based reduction of complications of type 2 diabetes following intensive antihypertensive treatment]. Ugeskr Laeger 1999;161:4764.

69. Lind L, Lithell H, Pollare T: Is it hyperinsulinemia or insulin resistance that is related to hypertension and other metabolic cardiovascular risk factors? J Hypertens Suppl 1993;11:S11–S16.

70. McLaughlin T, Abbasi F, Lamendola C, et al: Carbohydrate-induced hypertriglyceridemia: An insight into the link between plasma insulin and triglyceride concentrations. J Clin Endocrinol Metab 2000;85:3085–3088.

71. UK Prospective Diabetes Study Group: Efficacy of atenolol and captopril in reducing risk of macrovascular and microvascular complications in type 2 diabetes: UKPDS 39. BMJ 1998;317:713–720.

72. Krentz AJ, Nattrass M: Insulin resistance: A multifaceted metabolic syndrome. Insights gained using a low-dose insulin infusion technique. Diabet Med 1996;13:30–39.

73. Abuissa H, Jones PG, Marso SP, O'Keefe JH Jr: Angiotensin-converting enzyme inhibitors or angiotensin receptor blockers for prevention of type 2 diabetes a meta-analysis of randomized clinical trials. J Am Coll Cardiol 2005;46:821–826.

74. Staessen J, Amery A, Fagard R: Isolated systolic hypertension in the elderly. J Hypertens 1990;8:393–405.

75. Hansson L, Lindholm LH, Ekbom T, et al: Randomised trial of old and new antihypertensive drugs in elderly patients: Cardiovascular mortality and morbidity the Swedish Trial in Old Patients with Hypertension-2 study. Lancet 1999;354:1751–1756.

76. Messerli FH, Grossman E, Goldbourt U: Are beta-blockers efficacious as first-line therapy for hypertension in the elderly? A systematic review. JAMA 1998;279:1903–1907.

77. Wink K: Are beta-blockers efficacious as first-line therapy for hypertension in the elderly? Curr Hypertens Rep 2003;5:221–224.

78. Kostis JB, Wilson AC, Freudenberger RS, et al: Long-term effect of diuretic-based therapy on fatal outcomes in subjects with isolated systolic hypertension with and without diabetes. Am J Cardiol 2005;95:29–35.

79. Jaffe A, Chen Y, Kisch ES, et al: Erectile dysfunction in hypertensive subjects. Assessment of potential determinants. Hypertension 1996;28:859–862.

80. Schottstaedt MF, Sokolow M: The natural history and course of hypertension with papilledema (malignant hypertension). Am Heart J 1953;45:331–362.

81. Kaplan NM: Management of hypertensive emergencies. Lancet 1994;344:1335–1338.

82. Zeller KR, Von Kuhnert L, Matthews C: Rapid reduction of severe asymptomatic hypertension. A prospective, controlled trial. Arch Intern Med 1989;149:2186–2189.

83. Shea S, Misra D, Ehrlich MH, et al: Predisposing factors for severe, uncontrolled hypertension in an inner-city minority population. N Engl J Med 1992;327:776–781.

84. Oka K, Hayashi K, Nakazato T, et al: Malignant hypertension in a patient with primary aldosteronism with elevated active renin concentration. Intern Med 1997;36:700–704.

85. Mann SJ, Pickering TG: Detection of renovascular hypertension. State of the art: 1992. Ann Intern Med 1992;117:845–853.

86. Elliott WJ: Hypertensive emergencies. Crit Care Clin 2001;17:435–451.

87. Vincent JL, Berlot G, Preiser JC, et al: Intravenous nicardipine in the treatment of postoperative arterial hypertension. J Cardiothorac Vasc Anesth 1997;11:160–164.

88. Pilmer BL, Green JA, Panacek EA, et al: Fenoldopam mesylate versus sodium nitroprusside in the acute management of severe systemic hypertension. J Clin Pharmacol 1993;33:549–553.

89. Oparil S: Treating multiple-risk hypertensive populations. Am J Hypertens 1999;12(Suppl):121S–129S.

90. Grossman E, Messerli FH, Grodzicki T, Kowey P: Should a moratorium be placed on sublingual nifedipine capsules given for hypertensive emergencies and pseudoemergencies? JAMA 1996;276:1328–1331.

91. Chang K, Sauereisen S, Dlutowski M, et al: A cost-effective method to characterize variation in clinical practice. Eval Health Prof 1999;22:184–196.

92. Stanton A, Jensen C, Nussberger J, O'Brien E: Blood pressure lowering in essential hypertension with an oral renin inhibitor, aliskiren. Hypertension 2003;42:1137–1143.

93. Gradman AH, Schmieder RE, Lins RL, et al: Aliskiren, a novel orally effective renin inhibitor, provides dose-dependent antihypertensive efficacy and placebo-like tolerability in hypertensive patients. Circulation 2005;111:1012–1018.

94. Bonderman D, Nowotny R, Skoro-Sajer N, et al: Bosentan therapy for inoperable chronic thromboembolic pulmonary hypertension. Chest 2005;128:2599–2603.

95. Krum H, Viskoper RJ, Lacourciere Y, et al: The effect of an endothelin-receptor antagonist, bosentan, on blood pressure in patients with essential hypertension. Bosentan Hypertension Investigators. N Engl J Med 1998;338:784–790.

96. Nakov R, Pfarr E, Eberle S: Darusentan: An effective endothelin A receptor antagonist for treatment of hypertension. Am J Hypertens 2002;15:583–589.

97. Black HR, El Shahawy M, Weiss R, et al: Darusentan antihypertensive effect in patients with resistant systolic hypertension. Submitted 2006.

98. Pitt B, Williams G, Remme W, et al: The EPHESUS trial: Eplerenone in patients with heart failure due to systolic dysfunction complicating acute myocardial infarction. Eplerenone Post-AMI Heart Failure Efficacy and Survival Study. Cardiovasc Drugs Ther 2001;15:79–87.

99. Sica DA: Current concepts of pharmacotherapy in hypertension. Eplerenone: A new aldosterone receptor antagonist: Are the FDA restrictions appropriate? J Clin Hypertens (Greenwich) 2002;4:441–445.

100. White WB, Carr AA, Krause S, et al: Assessment of the novel selective aldosterone blocker eplerenone using ambulatory and clinical blood pressure in patients with systemic hypertension. Am J Cardiol 2003;92:38–42.

101. White WB, Duprez D, St Hillaire R, et al: Effects of the selective aldosterone blocker eplerenone versus the calcium antagonist amlodipine in systolic hypertension. Hypertension 2003;41:1021–1026.

102. Calhoun DA, Nishizaka MK, Zaman MA, Harding SM: Aldosterone excretion among subjects with resistant hypertension and symptoms of sleep apnea. Chest 2004;125:112–117.

Renovascular Hypertension

Stephen C. Textor and Marc A. Pohl

INTRODUCTION AND GENERAL PRINCIPLES

Renovascular hypertension (RVH), usually due to renal artery (RA) stenosis, is the most common secondary form of hypertension. Reduced perfusion of the kidney can increase arterial pressure and threaten the viability of the kidney.

High blood pressure in patients with RA stenosis frequently evokes the assumption that the stenosis is the cause of the hypertension. However, some patients with RA stenosis, particularly those with atherosclerotic renovascular disease, are not hypertensive,[1,2] and in others, the hypertension is not due to the RA stenosis but rather due to concomitant essential hypertension. Therefore, there are several scenarios for patients with RA stenosis and hypertension: (1) true RVH, in which RA stenosis is the sole cause of the hypertension; (2) pure essential hypertension in which RA stenosis is present, but does not contribute to the hypertension at all; (3) essential hypertension with superimposed RA stenosis producing a renovascular contribution to the underlying essential hypertension; and (4) RA stenosis in concert with renal parenchymal damage (e.g., arteriolar nephrosclerosis) wherein the elevated arterial pressure may be driven by the pathophysiologic factors characteristic of renal parenchymal hypertension.[3] Final proof that a patient has RVH rests with the demonstration that the hypertension, presumed to be renovascular, is eliminated or improved by removing the stenosis by surgical or endovascular revascularization or by removing the kidney distal to the stenosis. In practice, this rarely can be separated entirely from consideration of preservation of renal function beyond an atherosclerotic lesion, which is discussed in Chapter 61.

DEFINITION, ETIOLOGY, AND EPIDEMIOLOGY

RVH may be defined as a syndrome of elevated blood pressure (systolic and diastolic) produced by a variety of conditions that interfere with arterial circulation to kidney tissue. The majority of patients with RVH have significant main RA stenosis with concomitant reduced renal perfusion pressure. Figure 35.1 provides a more complete list of lesions that can produce the syndrome of RVH by impairing renal blood supply. Many of these are rare but underscore the point that the final common pathway depends on reduced renal perfusion pressure rather than on a specific pathologic lesion. Other rarely encountered clinical conditions associated with the syndrome of RVH include unilateral renal trauma with associated intrarenal or perirenal hematoma, unilateral ureteral obstruction, atrophic pyelonephritis, and a congenitally hypoplastic kidney. These conditions are additional examples of two-kidney hypertension. Occasionally,

atheroembolic renal disease produces the syndrome of RVH of one-kidney hypertension (see Fig. 35.1) variety. Of all the lesions or clinical conditions that may produce the syndrome of RVH, main RA disease is by far the most likely condition.

There are two broad categories of RA disease: fibromuscular dysplasia (FMD) and atherosclerotic renal vascular disease (ASRVD). FMD is most common among young females. Medial fibroplasia is the most prevalent of the subtypes observed. This diagnosis should be considered in anyone with early-onset, severe hypertension, but occasionally it is discovered incidentally during angiography for other reasons. FMD often responds well to either surgical or endovascular revascularization. These lesions usually arise beyond the first several centimeters of the RA and may be associated with more distal branch disease (Fig. 35.2).

Atherosclerotic disease of the RAs (Fig. 35.3) is the most common cause of RVH.[4] These lesions most often arise in the first 1 to 2 cm of the RA and may comprise an extension of a large aortic plaque. RA stenosis from atherosclerotic disease often represents a manifestation of systemic vascular disease and with involvement of other vascular beds including coronary, cerebrovascular, peripheral vascular, and aortic sites.

The prevalence of ASRVD appears to be increasing. This likely reflects demographic trends in the United States and other Western

Lesions producing the syndrome of renovascular hypertension by impairing renal blood supply	
Type	Lesions
Two-kidney hypertension: implies contralateral (nonaffected) kidney is present	Unilateral atherosclerotic renal artery disease Unilateral fibrous and fibromuscular disease: medial fibromuscular dysplasia, intimal fibroplasia, periarterial fibroplasia Renal artery aneurysm Arterial embolism Arteriovenous fistula (congenital and traumatic) Segmental arterial occlusion (traumatic) Pheochromocytoma compressing the renal artery Metastatic tumor (compressing the renal parenchyma)
One-kidney hypertension: implies ischemia of total renal mass	Stenosis to a solitary functioning kidney Bilateral arterial stenosis Aortic coarctation Vasculitis (polyarteritis nodosa and Takayasu's disease)

Figure 35.1 Lesions producing the syndrome of renovascular hypertension by impairing renal blood supply.

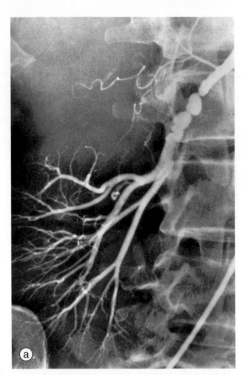
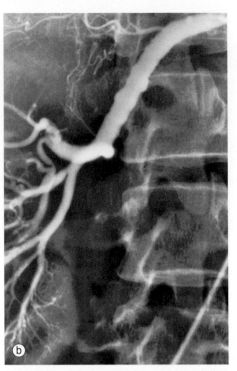

Figure 35.2 **Fibromuscular dysplasia.** *a*, Selective renal arteriogram illustrating the beaded appearance of fibromuscular dysplasia with multiple webs characteristic of medial fibroplasia in a 39-year-old woman. *b*, Selective injection of the same renal artery after technically successful percutaneous renal transluminal angioplasty. (Courtesy of Michael McKusick, M.D., Mayo Clinic.)

countries. Since the early 1970s, mortality rates from stroke and coronary artery disease have been decreasing steadily, associated with lengthening life spans. The age group of those older than 65 years is the most rapidly expanding group in the United States. As a consequence, more people are surviving to ages when atherosclerotic vascular disease in the visceral abdominal vessels can reach critical levels, producing RVH when the kidney is affected. Hence, atherosclerotic RA stenosis is the single most common cause of secondary resistant hypertension in patients older than 50 years of age,[5] and many of these patients have predominantly severe systolic hypertension with wide pulse pressures. Traditionally, the

level of diastolic blood pressure (DBP) and the magnitude of reduction of DBP have been central to definitions of RVH. The notion that isolated systolic hypertension, wide pulse pressure, and/or disproportionate increases in systolic blood pressure (SBP) with minimal increases in DBP could be renovascular in origin has received little attention. One recent study reported that in patients with ASRVD, RA angioplasty and stent placement produced a substantial reduction in SBP, particularly in patients with high baseline SBP.[6] The therapeutic yield of surgical or endovascular renal revascularization in this aging atherosclerotic population with ASRVD is a subject of current interest.

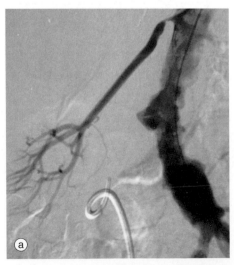
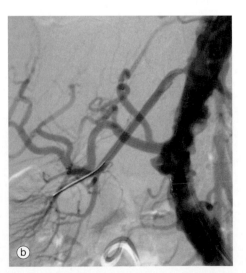

Figure 35.3 **Proximal renal artery stenosis secondary to atherosclerosis.** Before (*a*) and after (*b*) successful percutaneous angioplasty. (From Textor SC, Canzanello VJ: Radiographic evaluation of the renal vasculature. Curr Opin Nephrol Hypertens 1996;5:541–551.)

PATHOPHYSIOLOGY

The presence of a vascular stenotic lesion does not establish its role in regulating arterial pressure. The cross-sectional area of the stenotic lesion must be severely reduced before any measurable change in either blood flow or perfusion pressure can be detected (Fig. 35.4), usually in the range of 75% to 80%.[7] Lesions with less luminal compromise are unlikely to have hemodynamic significance.

When critical levels of stenosis develop and reduce renal perfusion pressure, multiple mechanisms are activated in the kidney to restore renal blood flow. Central to this process is the release of renin from the juxtaglomerular apparatus, leading to activation of the renin angiotensin aldosterone system. This is mediated in part by stimulation of neuronal nitric oxide synthase 1 and cyclooxygenase-2 in the macula densa. Blockade of the renin angiotensin system (RAS) at the time of placement of an experimental RA lesion prevents the development of hypertension.[8] Without blockade of this system, systemic arterial pressures increase until renal perfusion is restored. Studies in experimental models and humans indicate that additional mechanisms contribute to long-term elevation of blood pressure in the presence of RA stenosis, including intrarenal activation of the sympathetic nervous system, impairment of nitric oxide generation, and release of endothelin, as well as hypertensive microvascular injury to the nonstenosed kidney.[8]

Mechanisms responsible for sustained RVH differ depending on whether one or both kidneys are affected by vascular lesions, either pathologic or created in animal models using clips (Fig. 35.5). A nomenclature has evolved regarding this phenomenon, in which one clip is present with a normal contralateral or unclipped kidney (so-called 1-clip–2-kidney hypertension) as distinct from a situation in which the entire renal mass is affected with no contralateral kidney (1-clip–1-kidney hypertension). Both of these situations depend on impaired renal perfusion and initial activation of the RAS with sodium retention. However, the presence of a normal contralateral kidney has important consequences, as it responds to elevated arterial pressures by excreting the excess

sodium due to an intact pressure natriuresis mechanism (see Chapter 2). Because the nonstenotic kidney effectively functions to eliminate the excess sodium, the level of perfusion to the stenotic side remains reduced, leading to sustained activation of the RAS. This sequence of events, producing angiotensin II–dependent hypertension and secondary aldosteronism with hypokalemia, is summarized in Figures 35.4b and 35.5a.

By contrast, the model of 1-clip–1-kidney hypertension represents a model in which the entire renal mass is exposed to poststenotic pressures. There is no normal or nonstenotic kidney to counteract increased systemic pressures. As a result, sodium is retained and blood volume expanded, which eventually feeds back to inhibit the RAS (see Fig. 35.5b). Therefore, hypertension is typically not angiotensin dependent unless removal of volume is achieved that reduces renal perfusion pressure and activates the RAS.

Understanding the fundamental differences between these forms of RVH has clinical implications. Many diagnostic studies used to evaluate the functional significance of RA lesions depend on comparisons of the physiologic response of the two kidneys, which may give a false impression if both kidneys are involved. Furthermore, diagnostic tests that depend on differences in physiologic responses to alterations in sodium status (such as measuring renal vein renins following sodium depletion) may be problematic, as high levels of angiotensin II and aldosterone stimulate sodium reabsorption in both the stenotic and nonstenotic kidney. This accounts in part for the less frequent use of such tests in recent years.

Complicating the understanding of the pathophysiologic mechanisms of RVH is the element of its natural history. Rarely is it known at which point critical levels of stenosis develop. In experimental models, the relative importance of pressor mechanisms, including measurable activation of the RAS, changes with time. Levels of circulating plasma renin decrease, as does the responsiveness of blood pressure to short-term blockade of the renin system. Several mechanisms have been proposed to explain such changes, including a slowly developing pressor action of angiotensin II, a transition to alternate pressor

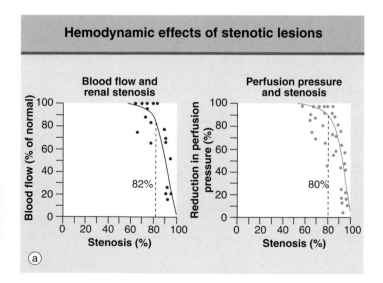

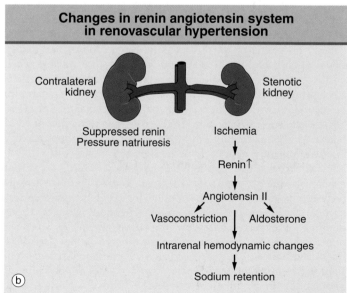

Figure 35.4 **Hemodynamic effects of stenotic lesions.** *a*, Changes in blood flow and arterial pressure across a carefully quantitated arterial lesion are barely detectable until cross-sectional area diminishes by 75% to 80%. *b*, When critical levels of renal artery stenosis occur, a sequence of steps activating the renin angiotensin system, among others, leads to increase both in arterial pressure and in retention of sodium by the stenotic kidney. (From Textor SC: Pathophysiology of renovascular hypertension. Urol Clin North Am 1984;11:373–381.)

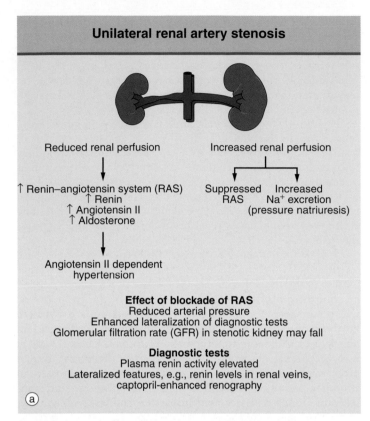

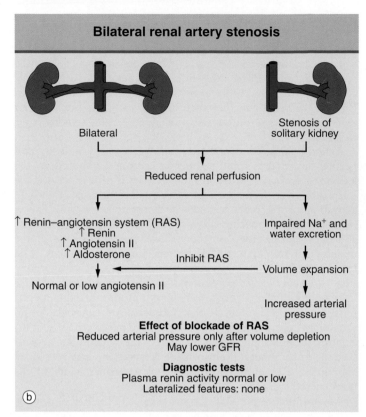

Figure 35.5 **Pathogenesis of renovascular hypertension in one-kidney versus two-kidney model.** *a*, In unilateral stenosis with two kidneys, opposing forces between the stenotic kidney, which has reduced perfusion pressures, and the nonstenotic contralateral kidney, which has increased perfusion pressures, result in laboratory and clinical features of angiotensin-dependent hypertension. *b*, In unilateral stenosis with a solitary functioning kidney (or in a patient with bilateral critical renal artery stenosis), reduced perfusion pressure to the stenotic kidney(s) in the absence of a normal kidney excreting sodium leads to sodium and volume retention, ultimately associated with hypertension without persistent activation of the renin angiotensin system.

mechanisms, and intrinsic renal injury to the nonstenotic kidney, which ultimately sustains hypertension despite reversal of the vascular lesion.[8] Experimentally, this translates into a time limit for reversibility of RVH.

There are several clinical correlates of this experimental time course. First, it is not yet known how to identify when revascularization will fail to benefit blood pressure with certainty, although a brief duration of hypertension suggests a more favorable response to intervention. As a result, many of the diagnostic studies that depend on lateralization of effects have only modest predictive value when negative. As a general rule, they are reliable when positive, meaning that high-grade lateralization accurately predicts a benefit with revascularization. A negative test, however, may also be associated with a beneficial outcome in the majority of cases. Second, clinical extrapolations from experimental models of RVH relate mainly to alterations in SBP and DBP. The pathophysiology of predominantly systolic hypertension in patients with atherosclerotic RA stenosis is not well understood. Third, coexistent intrarenal disease, that is, arteriolar nephrosclerosis, usually dictates the outcome of intervention for relief of hypertension, particularly for patients with ASRVD.[9] In these patients, a long duration of hypertension allows the development of arteriolar nephrosclerosis in the contralateral unaffected kidney (see Figs. 35.4b and 35.5a). Thus, old age and a long duration of hypertension, for example, >3 to 5 years, predict a poorer outcome of intervention in this patient population. Most of these elderly patients with ASRVD also have impaired renal function owing to arteriolar nephrosclerosis in addition to main RA stenosis. For younger patients with FMD who are unlikely to have arteriolar nephrosclerosis of aging and who usually have a normal overall glomerular filtration rate (GFR), a favorable response to RA intervention may be achieved despite a longer (>5 years) duration of hypertension.

Relationship to Ischemic Renal Disease

Activation of pressor mechanisms producing RVH can occur without loss of renal size or function. However, the more common clinical scenario involves both increasing severity of hypertension and deteriorating renal function, often with loss of renal size. Hence, the decision to consider renal revascularization most commonly combines consideration of both the likelihood of salvage or preservation of function and the benefits regarding blood pressure control. It should be emphasized that mechanisms underlying parenchymal renal damage may differ from those responsible for generating hypertension. Improved blood pressure control after revascularization may be achieved without appreciable benefits to the function of the kidney. For more discussion on ischemic nephropathy, see Chapter 61.

CLINICAL MANIFESTATIONS

Renovascular disease leads to elevation of arterial pressure fundamentally indistinguishable from that resulting from other causes, particularly essential hypertension. In the 1970s, a cooperative study of RVH compared clinical characteristics of patients with surgically proven RVH with those of patients identified as having essential hypertension. Some of these were statistically more prevalent, such as the identification of an abdominal bruit, hypokalemia, and absence of a family history of hypertension. (Fig. 35.6). Studies of resistant hypertension

Clinical characteristics of renovascular hypertension

Clinical Features	Essential Hypertension (%)	Renovascular Hypertension (%)
Duration: <1 year	12	24
Age at onset >50 years	9	15
Family history of hypertension	71	46
Grade 3 or 4 retinopathy	7	15
Abdominal bruit	9	46
Blood urea nitrogen >20 mg/l	8	16
Potassium <3.4 mmol/l	8	16
Urinary casts	9	20
Proteinuria	32	46

Figure 35.6 Clinical characteristics of renovascular hypertension. Clinical features that differ (*P* <0.05) between closely matched groups of 131 patients with essential and renovascular hypertension. These features underscore the potential severity of hypertension in candidates for surgery, but none allows clinical discrimination with confidence. (From Simon N, Franklin SS, Bleifers KH, Maxwell MH: Clinical characteristics of renovascular hypertension. JAMA 1972; 220:1209–1218.)

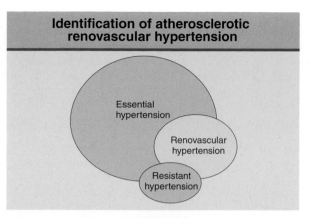

Identification of atherosclerotic renovascular hypertension

Figure 35.7 Identification of atherosclerotic renovascular hypertension. Venn diagram indicates that many patients with renovascular hypertension are indistinguishable from patients with essential hypertension. A subset develops problematic or resistant hypertension, which brings them to clinical attention and consideration for renal revascularization.

indicate that elevated cholesterol, azotemia, body mass index, and smoking offer positive clues.[10] In practical terms, none of these features is of sufficient sensitivity or specificity to offer diagnostic precision. Recent reports indicate that RVH may rarely be associated with nephrotic-range proteinuria. This may regress with correction of the vascular lesions.[11] Hence, the finding of proteinuria does not exclude this diagnosis.

The severity of RVH may span a wide range. Acute occlusion of a RA may only gradually produce an increase in pressure or it may produce accelerated-phase hypertension rapidly. Before the current era of antihypertensive agents, 30% of Caucasian patients appearing in an emergency department with accelerated hypertension (defined as severe hypertensive retinopathy [see Chapter 32] with or without malignant hypertension) were ultimately found to have RVH.[12] Patients with RVH may have labile blood pressures, with loss of normal circadian patterns of blood pressure control. Syndromes of polydipsia and accelerated hypertension, sometimes attributed to the dipsogenic actions of angiotensin II, with hyponatremia and hypokalemia also have been observed.

Current antihypertensive medications have changed the clinical presentation of RVH. Most recent consensus documents regarding hypertension emphasize the need for effective population-wide blood pressure control, while limiting the number and expense of diagnostic studies. As a result, most patients with identified hypertension simply are treated and subjected to few laboratory investigations. For those who reach acceptable blood pressure control without adverse effects, no further studies are performed. The introduction of orally active antihypertensive agents that block the RAS, beginning with captopril, improved medical therapy of RVH. Initial studies indicated that satisfactory blood pressure control can be achieved in >86% of patients with RVH compared with <50% with previously available drugs.[4] In recent years, widespread application of angiotensin-converting enzyme (ACE) inhibitors and angiotensin receptor blockers (ARBs) for indications other than hypertension, for example, congestive cardiac failure,

diabetic nephropathy, and other proteinuric renal disease, increases the exposure of individuals with undetected RA stenosis to these drugs.[13,14] Hence, many, if not most, cases of true RVH are not detected (Fig. 35.7) unless hypertension becomes more difficult to treat or renal dysfunction ensues.

One result of these changes has been the emergence of distinctive clinical syndromes that merit evaluation in patients at risk of RVH. These are summarized in Figure 35.8 and are discussed in further detail in Chapter 61. The overall result of these developments is that patients reaching consideration for evaluation and renal revascularization are a subset of the patient population with RVH. This subset is characterized generally by more severe hypertension, decreasing renal function, propensity for rapid volume accumulation manifested as flash pulmonary edema, and, occasionally, advanced renal failure.

Comorbid Disease Risk

Many of the entities leading to RVH (see Fig. 35.1) may appear as isolated lesions in the kidney. FMD may involve other vascular sites, particularly the carotid circulation. Both sites are involved in approximately 15% of patients. Hence, young patients presenting with spontaneous carotid artery dissection or occlusion should be considered at risk of FMD of the kidney and vice versa.

Atherosclerotic disease of the RAs is highly correlated with disease both in the coronary and peripheral vasculature. Series of

Clinical syndromes associated with renovascular hypertension

Early or late onset of hypertension (<30 or >50 years)
Acceleration of treated essential hypertension
Deterioration of renal function in treated essential hypertension
Acute renal failure during treatment of hypertension
Flash pulmonary edema
Progressive renal failure

Figure 35.8 Clinical syndromes associated with renovascular hypertension. These syndromes should alert the clinician to the possible contribution of renovascular hypertension in a given patient. The last three are the most common in patients with bilateral disease, many of whom are treated for essential hypertension until these characteristics appear (see text).

patients undergoing coronary angiography indicate that between 20% and 30% of patients will have some degree of RA stenosis, the severity of which is generally correlated with the severity and extent of coronary disease. The majority of these patients with coexisting ASRVD and coronary artery disease have mild to moderate degrees of RA stenosis (50% to 75%) of minimal hemodynamic significance. Screening renal aortography at the time of formal coronary angiography is a widespread clinical practice, particularly by interventional cardiologists, but the benefit of imaging the RAs at the time of coronary angiography is unclear. Although many of these patients with concomitant coronary artery disease and ASRVD have hypertension, the likelihood that these patients truly have RVH has usually not been thoroughly explored prior to the time of coronary angiography. Intervening on hemodynamically insignificant lesions by RA angioplasty or stenting has become a widespread clinical practice,[15] the benefit of which remains to be determined. One follow-up study of patients with incidentally detected RA lesions during coronary angiography indicates that the presence of RA lesions is an independent risk factor for mortality, which may reach 30% over 4 years in high-risk groups.[16] However, this does not necessarily imply that revascularization will reduce mortality risk. Series of patients undergoing evaluation for lower extremity peripheral vascular disease may have identifiable RA stenosis in >50% of cases. Whether the RA lesions in such patients participate in progressive vascular disease and warrant revascularization when detected incidentally is controversial (see later discussion).

NATURAL HISTORY

A central issue in managing RVH is the likelihood that vascular stenosis will progress. Since many cases of RA stenosis are never detected prior to initiating antihypertensive therapy, one must consider whether medical therapy assigns such patients to progressive loss of kidney function, which may not be detected until it is beyond recovery. Most of the lesions identified in Figure 35.1 do not progress, although some forms of FMD appear to induce more severe hemodynamic limitations with age. Occasional instances of thrombosis and occlusion of the kidney are described in these latter patients, primarily under conditions of markedly reduced arterial blood flow.

Atherosclerotic lesions can progress to more severe stenosis, although the factors regulating this process are not well understood. Retrospective studies using serial angiograms (obtained for other reasons) indicate rates of clinical progression approaching 40% to 50% over 4 to 5 years, with 16% of the most severe lesions producing total occlusion. Prospective studies using Doppler ultrasonography in patients with incidentally detected RA lesions indicate that progression overall approaches 31% over 3 years, varying considerably by the degree of initial stenosis. In this series, nine of 295 vessels (3%) produced total occlusion.[17]

How often changes in apparent vascular stenosis translate into clinical worsening of either blood pressure control or renal function is controversial. Follow-up studies of patients with incidentally detected, high-grade RA stenosis (>70%) treated without revascularization show that <10% require later revascularization for intractable hypertension.[18] These observations are consistent with a recent report that few patients with incidental RA stenosis progressed later to end-stage renal disease.[19] Determining the rate of clinical disease progression is important because decisions regarding vascular intervention may depend heavily on estimating the likelihood of losing renal parenchymal viability during medical therapy of RVH.

DIAGNOSIS

Several screening studies have been proposed to identify patients with RVH. Some of these depend on identifying activation of the RAS, such as renin-sodium profiling, and many depend on side-to-side comparisons of kidneys, assuming that one kidney is unaffected. Under the best of circumstances, these studies are rarely >80% sensitive or specific. As a result, their value as predictors depends greatly on the pretest probability of renovascular disease.[20,21] Furthermore, most of the functional tests related to activation of the RAS depend heavily on the test conditions, including sodium intake and concurrent antihypertensive medications, many of which affect levels of plasma renin activity. As a result, many clinicians no longer use these tests extensively.

Fundamentally, the *sine qua non* of RVH is identification of a stenotic vascular lesion affecting the RAs. Conventional angiography remains the reference standard to identify the anatomy of the renal vasculature, but it is commonly performed only after a less invasive procedure has increased the level of probability that such a lesion is present. In many cases, percutaneous transluminal renal angioplasty (PTRA) with or without stenting is performed at the same time as diagnostic angiography.

Various imaging methods of the renal vasculature provide different types of information regarding blood supply and parenchymal renal function (Fig. 35.9). Noninvasive vascular studies most commonly employed include renography (usually captopril- or enalapril-enhanced renography), RA duplex ultrasonography, or magnetic resonance angiography (MRA) (see Chapter 5). It should be emphasized that these methods provide different information and may differ in availability and reliability between institutions. Figure 35.10 illustrates an example of a captopril-enhanced renogram in a patient with RA stenosis. No direct image of the vessel is presented, but the study provides a view of the rate of isotope appearance and washout, reflecting the sequence of renal blood flow and filtration. The study provides functional information regarding the size and excretory capacity of the kidney as well as emphasizing the role of angiotensin II in maintaining GFR. Some studies emphasize the potential for predicting benefit from renal revascularization based on changes induced by the ACE inhibitor. This test has a high negative predictive value when completely normal. It may be argued that many intrinsic renal abnormalities may change these curves, particularly in the presence of reduced GFR (serum creatinine >2.0 mg/dl or 176 μmol/l). Several studies indicate that a completely normal captopril renogram effectively excludes the presence of hemodynamically significant RA stenosis.[22] This observation underscores the central issue related to noninvasive testing: the most important consideration is the negative predictive value of the study. In effect, a clinician performs such a study as a prelude to further studies. A positive result will lead commonly to subsequent angiography. The real goal and merit of noninvasive testing is to allow the physician to discontinue further invasive testing. Hence, the practical value of such studies should be assessed by the degree of confidence that a negative study provides that no important lesion is being overlooked by not proceeding further.

RA duplex scanning is applied widely to identify and to follow hemodynamic effects of vascular lesions serially. It is relatively inexpensive and requires no contrast. It is most effective in detecting lesions of the main RA near the origin. The reliability of this method depends on the skill and dedication of the ultrasonography technician, however, and on the body habitus of the patient in many instances. Duplex ultrasonography does not provide functional information regarding the kidney beyond the

Relative value of imaging methods for evaluating the renal vasculature					
Methods	Images of Vessels	Tissue Perfusion	Function (GFR)	Advantages	Disadvantages
Contrast angiography	+++	++	±	Nephrography estimates volume of viable tissue; the gold standard	Risk of catheter-induced injuries and contrast nephropathy
Captopril renography	−	+++	++	Change in GFR might estimate reversibility of the lesion; widely available, noninvasive; totally normal renogram effectively excludes significant vascular disease	
Duplex ultrasonography	++	++	−	Precise measurement of flow velocity, suitable for serial studies, relatively inexpensive	Produces little functional information, is not suitable for accessory vessels
Magnetic resonance angiography	++	++	±	Nontoxic in advanced renal failure	Accuracy limited to proximal vessels, angiography produces little functional information, not suitable for accessory vessels
Spiral computed tomographic angiography	+++	+	±	Provision of three types of images, examination of venous structures, might be useful for evaluating transplant donors	High contrast requirement

Figure 35.9   Relative value of imaging methods for evaluating the renal vasculature. The available techniques vary in their ability to image the renal vessels, assess tissue perfusion, and measure glomerular filtration rate (GFR).

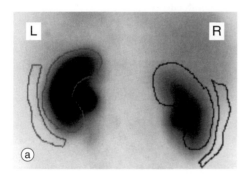

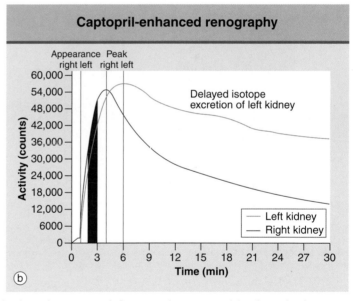

Figure 35.10   Captopril-enhanced renography. *a,* Scan in a patient with newly developing hypertension. *b,* Renogram demonstrates delayed arrival and excretion of isotope (MAG3) in the affected left kidney. L, left; R, right.

vascular lesion, although many important structural features including the size of the kidney and presence of ureteral obstruction may be determined.

MRA offers the potential to provide both structural vascular imaging and functional information. Particularly with gadolinium contrast enhancement, the main RAs may be visualized with confidence in many patients (Fig. 35.11). While expensive, MRA imaging offers the ability of examining the aorta and RAs with confidence in patients with significant renal failure without risk of contrast-induced nephropathy or atheroembolic complications associated with catheter-induced injuries.

Using these methods, clinicians now evaluate patients at risk of renovascular disease with greater confidence than ever before. It is prudent to determine exactly the question to be addressed

with such studies beforehand: Is there justification for proceeding further if the test is suggestive of vascular stenosis? Is the patient a candidate clinically for revascularization, and will a negative test allow conclusion of vascular studies? In some instances, it may be sufficient to answer the question "Is bilateral disease present?"

TREATMENT

The overall goal of hypertension therapy is to reduce morbidity and mortality by the least intrusive means possible. In RVH, this means balancing the risks and benefits of many potential means of treating the disorder, ranging from medical therapy to surgical or endovascular repair.

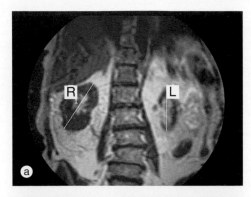

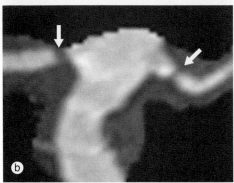

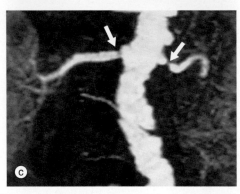

Figure 35.11   Magnetic resonance angiogram in renal failure. Angiogram of an elderly woman with renal failure (serum creatinine 2.5 mg/dl) and severe hypertension. *a,* Severe discrepancy in kidney size with a small left kidney. *b,* Gadolinium-enhanced aortography illustrating high-grade, bilateral renal artery stenotic lesions (*arrows*). *c,* Extensive aortic and iliac disease, bilateral renal artery stenoses (*arrows*), and markedly diminished filtration on the left side. L, left; R, right.

Medical Therapy

Most patients with RA stenosis and RVH are treated initially with conventional antihypertensive medications (see Chapter 34).[23] Treatment should include addressing all modifiable cardiovascular risk factors, including promoting weight loss, smoking cessation, and control of hyperlipidemia with statin therapy. Current guidelines for satisfactory blood pressure control target levels <140/90 mm Hg. The effectiveness of agents that interfere with the RAS, such as ACE inhibitors and ARBs, as well as the dihydropyridine class of calcium channel blockers to control BP have considerably reduced the clinical need to evaluate patients for RVH. Furthermore, even successful renal revascularization rarely leads to withdrawal of all antihypertensive medications in the current era (so-called cure of hypertension). Most patients with ASRVD have pre-existing essential hypertension and will therefore require some antihypertensive drug therapy even after successful revascularization. Hence, it may be questioned whether the costs and risks of renal revascularization are warranted at all in patients whose blood pressures and kidney function are stable on an acceptable regimen of current antihypertensive medications.

Adverse Consequences of Medical Therapy

Studies of critical stenosis of the RA indicate that reduction of arterial pressures poses the potential for reduction of renal blood flow below levels needed to sustain glomerular filtration. Because of the gradient across the stenotic lesion, RA pressures may decrease below those needed for autoregulation, considered to be about 60 mm Hg in humans. Such a reduction in blood flow can develop with many antihypertensive drugs, including β-blockers and sodium nitroprusside. Under these circumstances, rates of renal blood flow may decrease so far as to allow complete occlusion, as discussed in Chapter 61. In this respect, antihypertensive agents acting by blockade or interruption of the RAS can prevent the effects of angiotensin II at the efferent arteriole. When preglomerular pressures are reduced for any reason, intrarenal activation of angiotensin II preserves transcapillary filtration pressures at the glomerulus, allowing continued urine formation despite marginal blood flow. Removal of angiotensin II under these conditions allows abrupt cessation of glomerular filtration and urine formation (Fig. 35.12). Such a decrease in filtration produces a syndrome of acute functional renal insufficiency, first described clinically with ACE inhibitors.[24] The decrease in GFR is apparent clinically only under conditions in which the entire renal mass is affected, for example, bilateral RA stenosis or stenosis to a solitary functioning kidney. These principles are important for the nephrologist because removal of the efferent actions of angiotensin II and reduction of transcapillary filtration pressure are primary pathways by which the advantages of ACE inhibition accrue in other renal diseases characterized by glomerular hyperfiltration, such as diabetic nephropathy.

Whether the effects of ACE inhibitors and ARBs on GFR in renovascular hypertensive patients are beneficial or detrimental is a matter of controversy. Some of the diagnostic studies to identify functionally important RA stenosis employ ACE inhibitors to magnify differences between kidneys, for example, captopril-enhanced renography and captopril-stimulated renal vein renin determinations. It may be argued that identifying a decrease in GFR with an ACE inhibitor allows early detection of critical stenotic lesions in time for renal revascularization. Conversely, some have proposed that administration of an ACE inhibitor to patients with RA stenosis poses the hazard of a pharmacologic nephrectomy, with the potential for inducing irreversible renal parenchymal injury through ischemia.[25] Although the decrease in GFR induced by ACE inhibitors is usually reversible, occasionally patients do not recover renal function. Hence, ACE inhibitors must be recognized as a double-edged sword in RVH. They have unique properties, allowing more effective blood pressure control than previously possible, but at the same time, this class of medication has the potential for early loss of filtration pressure in patients with critical levels of RA stenosis.

Clinical experience with ACE inhibitors is reassuring in this regard. Monitoring studies both in clinical use and in large, prospective trials in patients at high risk of undetected RA stenosis, such as the trials of congestive heart failure, indicate that clinically important loss of GFR is not common. Most of these trials excluded patients with significant renal dysfunction, however. Postmarketing surveys of >15,000 prescriptions in the United Kingdom after the release of enalapril indicated few, but significant, adverse experiences. Most often, these were patients with pre-existing renal dysfunction who were taking potassium-sparing

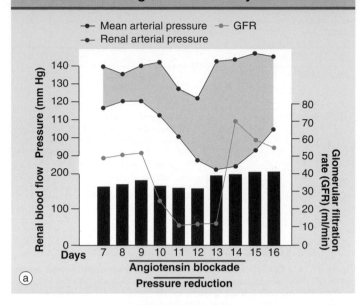

Systemic pressure reduction and angiotensin blockade in a dog with renal artery constriction

(a)

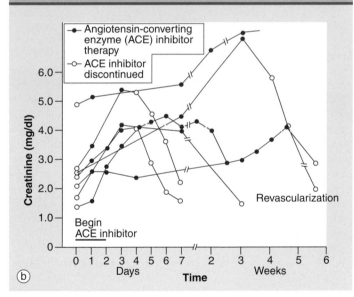

Patients with bilateral renal artery stenosis and angiotensin blockade

(b)

Figure 35.12 **Systemic pressure reduction and angiotensin blockade in renal artery constriction.** *a,* In a dog with renal artery stenosis, arterial pressures were reduced with sodium nitroprusside and the intravenous angiotensin II antagonist Sar-1-Ala-8-angiotensin was used to block the renin angiotensin system. Despite preservation of renal blood flow (*red bars*), glomerular filtration rate (GFR) fell. Such a decrease in GFR reflects its dependence on angiotensin II at the efferent arteriole under these conditions. *b,* In patients with bilateral renal artery stenosis or a stenotic solitary kidney, acute functional renal insufficiency can develop during administration of angiotensin-converting enzyme (ACE) inhibitors. In most cases, discontinuing the ACE inhibitors is associated with rapid improvement of the renal function.

diuretics and had other known atherosclerotic disease.[26,27] Taken together, the clinician caring for patients with complex hypertension should recognize both hyperkalemia and increasing creatinine values during treatment with ACE inhibitors or ARBs (Fig. 35.13) as a sign of potentially critical RA stenosis, which may be considered for alternative therapy and/or renal revascularization.

Difficult-to-Control Hypertension and/or Declining Renal Function during Medical Therapy

Further diagnostic and therapeutic maneuvers may be warranted in patients requiring more complex medical regimens (usually three drugs or more) whose blood pressures remain unsatisfactorily controlled. As noted previously, these patients are likely to have associated cardiovascular disease and other comorbid risk. Such patients may benefit materially from renal revascularization regarding both level of blood pressure control and stabilization of renal function.

Renal Revascularization

Restoring the renal blood supply is a rational goal of treating hypertension related to renovascular disease. Few conditions are more rewarding to treat than hypertension in a young person with fibromuscular dysplasia in whom a permanent cure is achievable. Revascularization offers such a patient relief from a lifelong regimen of antihypertensive medications and cardiovascular risk associated with high blood pressure. In practice, however, cures are infrequent. More often, renal revascularization allows improved blood pressure control and stabilization of the kidney circulation. Most institutions are limited in available expertise regarding vascular intervention and tend to favor either surgical or endovascular intervention, depending on local experience.

Percutaneous Transluminal Renal Angioplasty and Stenting

In many institutions, PTRA is the method of choice for both fibromuscular and atherosclerotic lesions of the RAs. Fibromuscular lesions are located away from the orifice of the aorta and often respond well to PTRA alone. Atherosclerotic lesions vary in location and may not be separable from a plaque arising from within the aorta at the ostium. Such ostial lesions have lower rates of technical success with simple angioplasty. Recent

Guidelines for limiting renal toxicity with ACE inhibitors	
Recognize predisposing condition	Widespread atherosclerotic disease Associated renal artery stenosis Impaired pretreatment renal function Solitary functioning kidney Activated renin angiotensin system Low sodium intake Diuretic therapy Other volume losses: vomiting, diarrhea Vasodilator administration Low cardiac function: hypotension, hyponatremia Other agents affecting kidney function, e.g., nonsteroidal anti-inflammatory agents
Monitor effects of initiating ACE inhibitor therapy	Serum creatinine: measure over the first days and at weeks 2 and 4, especially in high-risk subjects Elevated serum potassium: withhold potassium supplements, withhold potassium-sparing agents, and use low-potassium diet
Manage volume	Temporarily withhold diuretics Dose titrate both diuretics and ACE inhibitor Liberalize sodium intake/replace volume, consider rechallenge with ACE inhibitor after volume repletion

Figure 35.13 **Guidelines for limiting renal toxicity with angiotensin-converting enzyme (ACE) inhibitors.**

Technical success and clinical effect of percutaneous transluminal renal angioplasty (PTRA)

	1989–1995 (%)	1981–1987 (%)
Patients	1359	691
Arteries	1664	—
Fibromuscular disease		
Cured	42	53
Improved	36	38
Cured plus improved	78	91
Failed	21	8
Atherosclerotic renovascular disease		
Cured	14	18
Improved	51	48
Cured plus improved	65	67
Failed	34	32

Figure 35.14 Technical success and clinical effect of percutaneous transluminal renal angioplasty (PTRA). Summary of 17 reports of PTRA comprising >2000 patients, beginning in 1981. (Adapted from Aurell M, Jensen G: Treatment of renovascular hypertension. Nephron 1997;75:373–383, and Ramsey LE, Waller PC: Blood pressure response to percutaneous transluminal angioplasty for renovascular hypertension: An overview of published series. BMJ 1990;300: 569–572.)

Complications of percutaneous transluminal renal angioplasty (PTRA)

Type	Complications
Total (63/691 or 9.1%)	—
Fatal (3/691)	Cholesterol embolism Cerebral hemorrhage Bowel infarction
Most frequent	Cholesterol embolism Contrast-associated nephrotoxicity Renal artery dissection Renal artery thrombosis/occlusion Segmental renal infarction Hematoma at puncture site
Classified as indirect	Cerebrovascular accident Myocardial infarction Anterior spinal artery thrombosis Branchial artery thrombosis Bowel infarction

Figure 35.15 Complications of percutaneous transluminal renal angioplasty (PTRA). (Adapted from Ramsey LE, Waller PC: Blood pressure response to percutaneous transluminal angioplasty for renovascular hypertension: An overview of published series. BMJ 1990;300:569–572.)

developments favor the use of endovascular stents in such cases, with higher rates of both immediate and secondary patency achieved.[28] The use of stents is expanding, although the long-term patency rates and incidence of restenosis are not yet known with certainty.

Figure 35.14 summarizes 17 reported series assessing technical success and clinical effect of PTRA in patients with RVH.[29,30] When technically successful, PTRA offers stabilization of renal function and improved blood pressure control. Results in these studies are highly variable, in part depending on definitions of blood pressure change and length of follow-up. Cure of hypertension is unusual in any of these series, even in patients with FMD. It is more common in FMD than in patients with ASRVD of the RAs. More recent series (after 1989) generally acknowledge a higher failure rate with PTRA in FMD. Restenosis rates before the introduction of stents were 12% to 24% at 1 year, sometimes leading to repeat procedures. Antihypertensive medication requirements commonly decrease but rarely disappear entirely in patients with atherosclerotic disease, presumably because of pre-existing essential hypertension. The overall benefits of PTRA may be overstated somewhat as a result of the convention of omitting patients from analysis for whom PTRA could not be achieved for technical reasons (10% to 20% of patients).[31–33]

Complications

Reviews of PTRA and stenting vary widely regarding the incidence of minor and major complications. These likely reflect varying practice between centers and individual operators. Large reviews emphasize this disparity and are summarized in Figure 35.15. Among those complications with greatest prevalence are contrast nephrotoxicity, which is usually reversible, and atheroembolism, from which patients commonly do not recover. Particularly in patients with a badly diseased aorta, some degree of atheroembolism is unavoidable. Recent reviews suggest that between 7.5% and 9% of individuals have a major complication related to the procedure.[34] Occasionally, these produce arterial

dissection, including aortic dissection and segmental renal infarction. These may progress to overt renal insufficiency. While such occurrences are not common, renal function only rarely recovers.

Surgical Revascularization

Prior to introduction of PTRA, surgical revascularization was the standard treatment for RVH. Procedures were developed in the 1960s that for the first time allowed vascular bypass to the kidneys with grafts to the aorta. A summary of results of surgical revascularization for RVH is shown in Figure 35.16.[35] Blood pressure responses were consistently better in patients with FMD compared with those with atherosclerosis, and the former group had no surgical mortality due to the procedure. Many developments have improved surgical outcomes, including preoperative screening of the coronary and carotid circulation in high-risk patients. Such procedures nonetheless involve major vascular surgery and carry considerable risk, cost, and morbidity. This is especially true in older patients with widespread comorbid disease risk. As a result, surgical intervention for renovascular disease

Blood pressure outcome for surgical revascularization in renovascular hypertension

Outcome (%)	Fibromuscular Disease (N = 575)	Atherosclerosis of Renal Arteries (N = 631)
Cured	62	37
Improved	26	46
Cured plus improved	89	84
Failed	10	15

Figure 35.16 Blood pressure outcome for surgical revascularization in renovascular hypertension. A summary of results for >1200 patients. Follow-up procedures and definitions of blood pressure cure varied greatly between series. Surgical mortality was 1.3% to 5.8% in patients with stenosis from atherosclerosis and nil in those with fibromuscular disease. (Adapted from Stanley JC, David M: Hume Memorial Lecture. Surgical treatment of renovascular hypertension. Am J Surg 1997;174:102–110.)

commonly is reserved for patients refractory to medical therapy in whom PTRA fails or may not offer adequate therapy for associated aortic disease.[36] In many institutions, advances in medical therapy have made surgical revascularization no longer a first choice for blood pressure control. Revascularization now is undertaken both for improved blood pressure control and in the hope of preserving renal function by restoring blood supply to compromised kidneys. As a result, surgical series now more commonly include patients with more advanced renal failure, combined renal and aortic disease, and widespread vascular disease. Despite these caveats, it must be emphasized that successful surgical revascularization offers durable restoration of kidney blood supply and long-term survival (81% at 5 years) with which newer techniques must be compared.[37]

While restoration of blood flow and salvage of kidney function is the primary objective, occasional cases of RVH present with either total occlusion or nonfunction of one kidney. In such cases, the pressor role of the nonfunctioning kidney may be relieved by nephrectomy. Results from a recent series indicate that improved blood pressures can be obtained in such instances without detectable loss of renal function. Estimates of renal function in this group were 11% in the removed kidney and 89% in the contralateral kidneys.[38] With the introduction of laparoscopic techniques for nephrectomy, such an approach may offer clinical benefits in selected cases with less morbidity than a standard operative nephrectomy.

Complications

In most cases, surgical revascularization requires hospitalization and care comparable with other aortic surgery. The primary immediate causes of morbidity and mortality are related to coronary and cerebrovascular events. In most cases, risk stratification and therapy for associated coronary and cerebrovascular diseases should be performed first.

Outcomes of Renal Revascularization

In many patients, successful renal revascularization leads to improved blood pressure control and reduced morbidity and mortality in the long term. Antihypertensive medication requirements decrease, although rarely are they eliminated entirely. Most series report stabilization of renal function, meaning that average serum creatinine levels do not change. This interpretation may be misleading. Some patients experience a marked improvement in renal function, while others have a clinically significant loss of renal function. In most series, this occurs in up to 18% to 20% of patients treated either with PTRA or surgery. Although group average values do not change, a substantial number of patients experience adverse effects on renal function that must be considered before undertaking vascular intervention of any kind, particularly when blood pressure control is the primary concern.[39] The benefits of modestly improved blood pressure control should not be understated. Treatment trials in hypertension based on blood pressure differences of 10 to 15 mm Hg between treatment and placebo groups established major differences in cardiovascular endpoints, including overall mortality. Early series of medically treated versus surgically treated patients with RVH underscored the high risks of uncontrolled blood pressure in the medical group.

There are few prospective data comparing medical therapy with renal revascularization in the current era. Most of the literature regarding endovascular procedures for renal revascularization consists of observational reports that are frequently limited by poorly standardized methods of blood pressure measurement and drug therapy. Three recent, prospective, randomized trials comparing medical therapy with angioplasty report only modest benefits attributable to PTRA. The major features of these prospective, randomized, controlled trials are summarized in Figure 35.17.[31–33] These studies are small but do underscore the effectiveness of current drug regimens and the relative infrequency of cure in patients with atherosclerotic renal arterial stenosis. All these excluded many patients with progressive renal dysfunction, accelerated hypertensive disease, or recent cardiovascular events.

The largest of these studies was published in 2000 as the DRASTIC study (Dutch Renal Artery Stenosis Intervention Cooperative Study Group). It included 106 patients with relatively resistant hypertension randomized either to medical therapy or PTRA. The lack of difference in blood pressure after 1 year between patients treated with PTRA and treated medically led the authors to conclude that "angioplasty has little advantage over antihypertensive drug therapy."[31] This study was analyzed under intention-to-treat statistical rules, in which 22 of 50 patients assigned to medical therapy (44%) crossed over to the PTRA arm due to uncontrolled blood pressure levels at 3 months. Despite their inclusion in the medical arm, many authorities reviewing these data might argue that this group offers compelling evidence of medical treatment failure in some instances and the benefit of renal revascularization for such individuals. The available data suggest that effective blood pressure control achieved by any means is the central determinant of cardiovascular outcomes.

Three randomized prospective studies comparing medical treatment and PTRA (with and without stents)			
Study	Number of Subjects	Features	Outcome
Webster et al.[31]	N = 55, unilateral = 27	Randomized, prospective, single center	Lower BP in the PTRA group with bilateral renal artery stenosis; no difference in BP in the unilateral renal artery stenosis group; no difference in renal function or survival
Plouin et al.[32]	N = 49, all unilateral	Multicenter evaluation with ambulatory BP monitoring at 6 months; no ACE inhibitors	No difference in BP; fewer BP medication requirements in PTRA group, but more complications; crossover in medication: 7/26 (27%)
Van Jaarsveld et al.[33]	N = 106	Multicenter, office, and automated BP, lateralization studies (scan, renal vein renin)	No difference in BP at 12 months; crossover in medication: 22/50

Figure 35.17 Three randomized prospective studies comparing medical treatment and percutaneous transluminal renal angioplasty (PTRA) (with and without stents).[31–33] ACE, angiotensin-converting enzyme; BP, blood pressure.

Integrated Approach to Treating Renovascular Hypertension

The aging demographics of the United States and other Western countries favor more patients developing critical levels of RA stenosis than ever before. Critical to the management of such patients is the recognition of distinctive clinical syndromes of renovascular disease, linking acceleration of hypertension with deteriorating renal function and, occasionally, episodic circulatory congestion (flash pulmonary edema). Many patients can be managed by medical means. It must be emphasized that evaluating such patients is an ongoing process that must be reviewed at regular intervals. When progressively more complex antihypertensive regimens become required and/or renal function deteriorates, consideration should be given to identification and correction of critical vascular lesions affecting the kidneys.

Figure 35.18 is an algorithm by which such patients can be managed. This scheme emphasizes the need to evaluate whether the patient is a candidate for renal vascularization based on clinical features, including age, other diseases, and whether stable blood pressure and kidney function can be achieved using medical therapy. If the patient is not a candidate for revascularization, there is little to be gained from extensive diagnostic studies. Conversely, if blood pressure control and stable renal function are not achieved by a reasonable effort with medical therapy, one is justified in beginning a systematic evaluation of the renal vasculature with the objective of vascular intervention if a significant lesion is identified. Evaluation for surgery or angioplasty should be considered for patients resistant to therapy, either by virtue of inadequate blood pressure control or unstable renal function, and who are candidates for renal vascularization should a stenotic lesion be found. The latter is a highly individual judgment based on comorbid disease risk, age, and so on. If the patient is a candidate for further evaluation, a noninvasive study, such as MRA, may allow exclusion of a high-grade lesion or bilateral disease. In cases of atherosclerotic disease, invasive angiography should be limited mainly to patients in whom revascularization is anticipated, often at the same procedure. This approach limits the hazards of vessel instrumentation and contrast nephrotoxicity to a single procedure. With the introduction of stent-supported angioplasty, surgical reconstruction is often limited to patients with technically challenging vascular lesions and/or associated aortic disease needing additional reconstruction.

Even with successful revascularization, medical therapy and follow-up remain essential. Balancing the potential risks and benefits of medical therapy versus primary revascularization remains a complex challenge. This is particularly true in view of other causes of morbidity and mortality in patients with atherosclerotic vascular disease. Most often, management decisions are based on considerations of preserving renal function and avoiding adverse effects of progressive vascular disease.

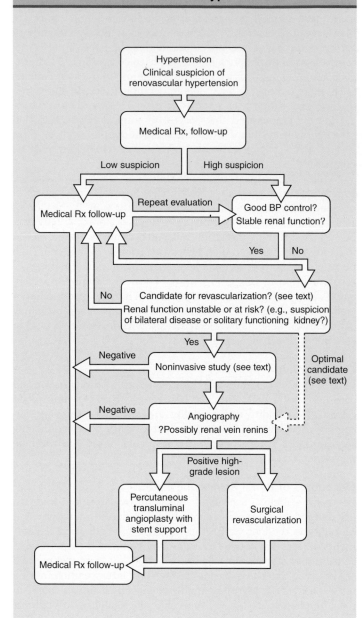

Algorithm for management of patients with renovascular hypertension

Figure 35.18 Clinical algorithm for management of patients with renovascular hypertension. Initiation of the algorithm depends on the index of suspicion for the possible role of renovascular disease in aggravating hypertension and/or declining renal function and the success of medical therapy (see text).

REFERENCES

1. Eyler WR, Clark MD, Garman JE, et al: Angiography of the renal areas including a comparative study of renal artery stenosis in patients with and without hypertension. Radiology 1962;78:879–892.
2. Dustan HP, Humphries AW, deWolfe VG, et al: Normal arterial pressure in patients with renal arterial stenosis. JAMA 1964;187:1028–1029.
3. Smith MC, Rahman M, Dunn MJ: Hypertension associated with renal parenchymal disease. In Schrier RW (ed): Diseases of the Kidney and Urinary Tract, 7th ed. Philadelphia: Lippincott Williams & Wilkins, 2001, pp 1363–1397.
4. Safian RD, Textor SC: Medical progress. Renal-artery stenosis. N Engl J Med 2001;344:431–442.
5. Anderson GH Jr, Blakeman N, Streeten DH: The effect of age on prevalence of secondary forms of hypertension in 4429 consecutively referred patients. J Hypertens 1994;12:609–615.
6. Burket MW, Cooper CJ, Kennedy DJ, et al: Renal artery angioplasty and stent placement: Predictors of a favorable outcome. Am Heart J 2000;139:64–71.
7. Textor SC: Pathophysiology of renovascular hypertension. Urol Clin North Am 1984;11:373–381.
8. Romero JC, Feldstein AE, Rodriguez-Porcel MG, Cases-Amenos A: New insights into the pathophysiology of renovascular hypertension. Mayo Clin Proc 1997;72:251–260.
9. Vertes V, Grauel JA, Goldblatt H: Renal arteriography, separate renal-function studies, and renal biopsy in human hypertension. N Engl J Med 1964;270:656–659.
10. Krijnen P, van Jaarsveld BC, Steyerberg EW, et al: A clinical prediction rule for renal artery stenosis. Ann Intern Med 1998;129:705–711.

11. Chen R, Novick AC, Pohl M: Reversible renin mediated massive protein-uria successfully treated by nephrectomy. J Urol 1995;153:133–134.

12. Davis BA, Crook JE, Vestal RE, Oates JA: Prevalence of renovascular hypertension in patients with grade III or IV hypertensive retinopathy. N Engl J Med 1979;301:1273–1276.

13. Maschio G, Alberti D, Janin G, et al: Effect of the angiotensin-converting-enzyme inhibitor benazepril on the progression of chronic renal insufficiency. The Angiotensin-Converting-Enzyme Inhibition in Progressive Renal Insufficiency Study Group. N Engl J Med 1996;334:939–945.

14. Lewis EJ, Hunsicker LG, Clarke WR, et al: Renoprotective effect of the angiotensin-receptor antagonist irbesartan in patients with nephropathy due to type 2 diabetes. N Engl J Med 2001;345:851–860.

15. Murphy TP, Soares G, Kim M: Increase in utilization of percutaneous renal artery interventions by medicare beneficiaries, 1996–2000. AJR Am J Roentgenol 2004;183:561–568.

16. Conlon PJ, Athirakul K, Kovalik E, et al: Survival in renal vascular disease. J Am Soc Nephrol 1998;9:252–256.

17. Caps MT, Perissinotto C, Zierler RE, et al: Prospective study of athero-sclerotic disease progression in the renal artery. Circulation 1998;98:2866–2872.

18. Chabova V, Schirger A, Stanson AW, et al: Outcomes of atherosclerotic renal artery stenosis managed without revascularization. Mayo Clin Proc 2000;75:437–444.

19. Leertouwer TC, Pattynama PM, Berg-Huysmans A: Incidental renal artery stenosis in peripheral vascular disease: A case for treatment? Kidney Int 2001;59:1480–1483.

20. Wilcox CS: Non-invasive evaluation of renovascular disease. Tech Vasc Intervent Radiol 1999;2:60–64.

21. Mann SJ, Pickering TG: Detection of renovascular hypertension. State of the art: 1992. Ann Intern Med 1992;117:845–853.

22. Wilcox CS: Ischemic nephropathy: Noninvasive testing. Semin Nephrol 1996;16:43–52.

23. Pohl MA: Medical management of renovascular hypertension. In Novick AC, Scoble J, Hamilton G (eds): Renal Vascular Disease. London: WB Saunders, 1996, pp 339–349.

24. Hricik DE, Browning PJ, Kopelman R, et al: Captopril-induced func-tional renal insufficiency in patients with bilateral renal-artery stenoses or renal-artery stenosis in a solitary kidney. N Engl J Med 1983;308:373–376.

25. Jackson B, Matthews PG, McGrath BP, Johnston CI: Angiotensin con-verting enzyme inhibition in renovascular hypertension: Frequency of reversible renal failure. Lancet 1984;1:225–226

26. Speirs CJ, Dollery CT, Inman WH, et al: Postmarketing surveillance of enalapril. II: Investigation of the potential role of enalapril in deaths with renal failure. BMJ 1988;297:830–832.

27. Textor SC: Renal failure related to angiotensin-converting enzyme inhibitors. Semin Nephrol 1997;17:67–76.

28. van de Ven PJ, Kaatee R, Beutler JJ, et al: Arterial stenting and balloon angioplasty in ostial atherosclerotic renovascular disease: A randomised trial. Lancet 1999;353:282–286.

29. Aurell M, Jensen G: Treatment of renovascular hypertension. Nephron 1997;75:373–383.

30. Ramsay LE, Waller PC: Blood pressure response to percutaneous transluminal angioplasty for renovascular hypertension: An overview of published series. BMJ 1990;300:569–572.

31. Webster J, Marshall F, Abdalla M, et al: Randomised comparison of percutaneous angioplasty vs continued medical therapy for hypertensive patients with atheromatous renal artery stenosis. Scottish and Newcastle Renal Artery Stenosis Collaborative Group. J Hum Hypertens 1998;12:329–335.

32. Plouin PF, Chatellier G, Darne B, Raynaud A: Blood pressure outcome of angioplasty in atherosclerotic renal artery stenosis: A randomized trial. Essai Multicentrique Medicaments vs Angioplastie (EMMA) Study Group. Hypertension 1998;31:823–829.

33. van Jaarsveld BC, Krijnen P, Pieterman H, et al: The effect of balloon angioplasty on hypertension in atherosclerotic renal-artery stenosis. Dutch renal artery stenosis intervention cooperative study group. N Engl J Med 2000;342:1007–1014.

34. Leertouwer TC, Gussenhoven EJ, Bosch JL, et al: Stent placement for renal arterial stenosis: Where do we stand? A meta-analysis. Radiology 2000;216:78–85.

35. Stanley JC, David M: Hume Memorial Lecture. Surgical treatment of renovascular hypertension. Am J Surg 1997;174:102–110.

36. Hallett JW Jr, Textor SC, Kos PB, et al: Advanced renovascular hyper-tension and renal insufficiency: Trends in medical comorbidity and surgical approach from 1970 to 1993. J Vasc Surg 1995;21:750–759.

37. Steinbach F, Novick AC, Campbell S, Dykstra D: Long-term survival after surgical revascularization for atherosclerotic renal artery disease. J Urol 1997;158:38–41.

38. Kane GD, Textor SC, Schirger A, Garovic V: Predictors of cure in patients undergoing nephrectomy for pressor kidney [abstract]. J Am Soc Nephrol 2001;345:485A.

39. Textor SC, Wilcox CS: Renal artery stenosis: A common, treatable cause of renal failure? Annu Rev Med 2001;52:421–442.

INTRODUCTION

The true incidence and prevalence of hypertension with endocrine etiology is unknown. In the past, endocrine forms of hypertension were thought to account for <1% of all cases of hypertension. However, an endocrine cause of hypertension may remain undiagnosed because physicians consider these conditions rare and therefore unlikely. Access to the specialized tests required for diagnosis may be limited. Recent reports have identified primary aldosteronism in 2% to 12% of newly diagnosed cases of hypertension.

Endocrine hypertension may occur in the absence of readily observed signs, symptoms, or abnormalities in routine biochemical tests. However, certain features should trigger a simple screen (Fig. 36.1). First, these include a positive family history of conditions with inherited forms, including pheochromocytoma,

neurofibromatosis, multiple endocrine neoplasia, and aldosteronism. Second, refractory hypertension (i.e., blood pressure that is resistant to concurrent administration of two or three antihypertensive drugs of different classes) warrants consideration of secondary hypertension provided iatrogenic factors and noncompliance have been ruled out. The differential diagnoses will include endocrine, renal, and renovascular disease.

Third, symptoms and signs may be present. Hypokalemia, if sufficiently severe, may cause weakness, polyuria, and cardiac arrhythmia. Hyperadrenergic symptoms occur with pheochromocytoma. Changes in temperature tolerance, body weight, hair and skin condition, and bowel habit are clues in thyroid dysfunction or hypercortisolism. Thyroid disease, Cushing's syndrome, and acromegaly are associated with typical changes in body habitus. Abnormal sweating occurs in pheochromocytoma, thyrotoxicosis, and acromegaly.

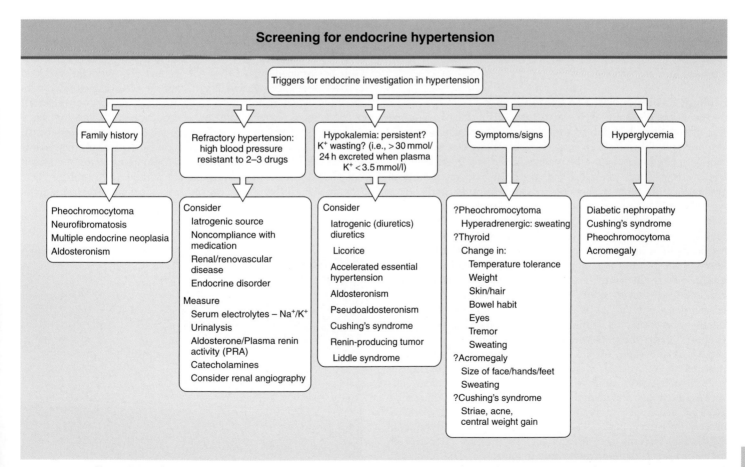

Figure 36.1 **Screening for endocrine hypertension.** Clinical observations suggesting endocrine investigation in hypertension.

Fourth, hypokalemia and diabetes mellitus are hallmarks of endocrine pathologies in hypertension. Hypokalemia is common to primary aldosteronism, pseudoaldosteronism, renin-secreting tumor, Cushing's disease, and accelerated hypertension of any cause. Therefore, concurrent high blood pressure and hypokalemia should prompt consideration of possible endocrine or other secondary causes of hypertension. Hyperglycemia, although most commonly due to diabetes without other endocrine abnormality, is common to Cushing's syndrome, pheochromocytoma (especially when epinephrine levels are increased), and acromegaly. Also, it is not uncommon in primary aldosteronism, presumably partly as a result of the hypokalemia.

Diagnosing endocrine forms of hypertension often offers the chance of cure, of altering an otherwise catastrophic natural history (e.g., in pheochromocytoma), and of applying highly specific and effective therapies that ameliorate other elements of the disease beyond control of blood pressure. Aldosteronism is addressed in Chapter 37. The following sections address other types of endocrine hypertension.

CUSHING'S SYNDROME

Introduction and Definition
This syndrome of sustained glucocorticoid excess is most commonly pituitary adrenocorticotropic hormone (ACTH)–dependent (Cushing's disease); is less frequently the result of cortisol overproduction from an adrenal adenoma, carcinoma, or other rare adrenal lesion; and may be secondary to ectopic ACTH or corticotropin secretion.[1] It also can be the result of exogenous glucocorticoid administration. The incidence of endogenous Cushing's syndrome is five to 10 cases per million population per year. Cushing's disease and cortisol-secreting adrenal tumors are four times more common in women than men. Approximately 0.5% of patients with bronchogenic carcinoma develop ectopic ACTH syndrome, which is more common in men than women.

Etiology, Pathogenesis, and Epidemiology
Hypertension, present in 80% of patients with Cushing's syndrome (less often when it is due to exogenous synthetic glucocorticoid administration), results from an increase in both cardiac output and total peripheral resistance. The reasons underlying these hemodynamic changes are complex and uncertain.[2] Cortisol-induced stimulation of renal mineralocorticoid receptors and hence excessive sodium retention is the favored explanation by some authors. However, the balance of evidence is against this being a mineralocorticoid type of hypertension except where there is overproduction of mineralocorticoid hormones (aldosterone, 11-deoxycorticosterone, and corticosterone). Alternatively, hypertension may result from elevated cortisol from an adrenal tumor with reduced activity of the renal enzyme 11β-hydroxysteroid dehydrogenase type 2 (which normally inactivates cortisol, thereby preventing its stimulatory action on mineralocorticoid receptors) or by the presence of extremely high levels of plasma cortisol, as in ectopic ACTH syndrome. Inhibition of vasodilator nitric oxide by cortisol is currently favored as one contributor to the hypertension, along with enhanced pressor responsiveness to catecholamines and angiotensin II (Ang II), heightened cardiac inotropic sensitivity to β-adrenergic stimulation, and, perhaps, increased plasma volume.[2] The sympathetic nervous and the renin angiotensin systems are, if anything, suppressed even though circulating levels of renin substrate are increased. The possibility that elevated levels of vasoconstrictor hormones (vasopressin, endothelin-1, thromboxane, erythropoietin, and insulin) or subnormal concentrations of vasodilator systems (kallikrein-kinins and prostaglandins) levels contribute to the hypertension of Cushing's syndrome has been raised, but the evidence is frail.[2] There is no lack of cardiac natriuretic peptide production as gauged by elevated plasma levels of atrial natriuretic peptide (ANP), although impairment in biologic responses to ANP have been documented[3] and could, in theory, contribute to the hypertension. Successful treatment of Cushing's disease or removal of an underlying adrenal adenoma usually results in a reduction of blood pressure and partial return of the previously impaired nocturnal fall in arterial pressure, although hypertension remains in a sizable minority of patients, especially the elderly and where there has been long-standing elevation of blood pressure.

Clinical Manifestations
Clinical features in Cushing's disease result from elevated circulating levels of pro-opiomelanocortin hormones including ACTH (increased pigmentation) and cortisol (central adiposity, muscle wasting and weakness, plethoric facies, purple striae [Fig. 36.2], easy bruising, osteoporosis, psychological problems) with, in some patients, androgen effects (hirsutism, acne, virilization), which may be striking in those with adrenal adenoma or carcinoma.[1] Ectopic ACTH syndrome due to small cell bronchogenic carcinoma or other tumors (e.g., bronchial or thymic carcinoid) presents typically as a wasting disease often with hyperpigmentation and hypokalemia. Hypertension is often associated with left ventricular hypertrophy, which can be disproportionate to the blood pressure,[4] and frank cardiac failure is occasionally the presenting feature.[5]

Differential Diagnosis
Pseudo-Cushing's syndrome, wherein clinical features of Cushing's syndrome exist with some evidence of hypercortisolism, can occur with a sustained high intake of alcohol (by inducing reduced cortisol metabolism due to hepatic damage and augmented cortisol secretion, which is perhaps a direct stimulatory effect of ethanol), in depression (which can be diagnostically challenging since patients with Cushing's syndrome are not infrequently depressed), and in obesity where the plasma clearance rate of cortisol is increased leading to a slightly elevated production rate of cortisol, but plasma levels of the hormone are normal.[1] A careful physical examination differentiates obesity from Cushing's syndrome in all but a few patients.

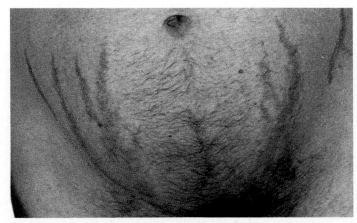

Figure 36.2 Striae and central obesity of Cushing's syndrome.

Diagnosis

Step 1 is to determine whether the patient has Cushing's syndrome. An elevated urinary free cortisol excretion (or early morning cortisol-to-creatinine ratio) and absence of suppression of 8 AM plasma cortisol after a low dose of dexamethasone (1 mg at midnight) are the commonly used tests.

Step 2 is to uncover the underlying cause of the Cushing's syndrome. Key investigations may include radiography (computed tomography [CT]) and magnetic resonance imaging (MRI) scanning of the pituitary and adrenals especially, but also of the thorax, abdomen, and pelvis when ACTH-producing carcinoid tumors are suspected), plasma ACTH (which is suppressed in cortisol-secreting adrenal tumors but is elevated, often to extreme levels, in the ectopic ACTH syndrome), the high-dose dexamethasone test (which partially suppresses ACTH in cases of pituitary tumors but not in patients with ectopic ACTH syndrome), the corticotropin-releasing hormone test, and simultaneous bilateral inferior petrosal sinus sampling for ACTH measurements. The latter test is useful in differentiating Cushing's disease from ectopic ACTH syndrome when the previously listed tests give equivocal results.

Natural History

Untreated, Cushing's syndrome has a 50% 5-year mortality rate relating in large part to a remarkably high level of cardiovascular risk due to hypertension along with glucose intolerance and insulin resistance, hyperlipidemia, obesity, and perhaps also hyperhomocysteinemia and elevated fibrinogen levels.[6,7] The prognosis after treatment, as noted later, is dependent on the underlying lesion and is good for Cushing's syndrome due to adrenocortical adenoma or pituitary microadenoma but is bad for adrenal carcinoma or ACTH-producing small cell bronchogenic carcinoma.

Treatment

Cushing's disease treated by selective removal of a pituitary microadenoma in a surgical center with extensive experience gives a cure rate of 80% to 90%, and around 50% for pituitary macroadenomas.[1] Cushing's syndrome due to an adrenal adenoma is almost always cured by unilateral adrenalectomy, but when the underlying lesion is adrenal carcinoma, most patients are dead within 2 years of the diagnosis. When Cushing's syndrome results from ectopic ACTH syndrome due to small cell bronchogenic carcinoma, the prognosis is poor. If the ACTH-producing tumor is benign and can be located, however, removal usually leads to cure. After cure of Cushing's syndrome, approximately 30% of patients are said to have persistent hypertension.[8]

Guidance on how best to manage the hypertension due to Cushing's syndrome receives little assistance from the sparse literature, and there is no good evidence to support the use of any class of antihypertensive drug over another. Potassium-losing diuretics can exacerbate both hypokalemia and glucose intolerance, whereas potassium-sparing diuretics, usually in combination, may correct hypokalemia and reduce edema while lowering the blood pressure.

PHEOCHROMOCYTOMA

Introduction and Definition

This disorder has challenged and fascinated clinicians since its first description by Frankel in 1886. Clinical manifestations can mimic a wide spectrum of other disorders; hence, the diagnosis is frequently delayed or missed altogether, sometimes with fatal

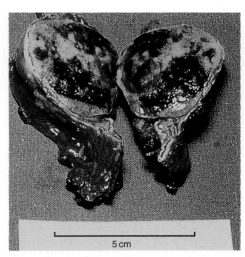

Figure 36.3 Large adrenal pheochromocytoma with areas of hemor-rhagic necrosis.

consequences. Accordingly, the challenge to "think of it" by Manger and Gifford,[9] authors of the classic text on the topic, is apt.

The term pheochromocytoma refers to a dusky tumor whose cells take on a brownish color when stained with chromium salts. Such tumors arise most commonly within the adrenal glands (Fig. 36.3), but approximately 10% are extra-adrenal (paraganglioma). Although the majority are benign tumors, around 10% metastasize to regional lymph nodes and beyond. Histologic features are not a reliable guide to malignant behavior. The tumors can secrete a wide variety of hormones but most characteristically produce norepinephrine, epinephrine, and dopamine, with quite different patterns occurring in different patients. Few paragangliomas produce epinephrine. Very high dopamine production is frequently associated with malignancy or a large tumor mass.

Etiology, Pathogenesis, and Epidemiology

The prevalence of pheochromocytoma in patients with hypertension in general medical outpatient clinics is 0.1% to 0.6%.[10] Since as many people die with unsuspected pheochromocytoma as die with a firm diagnosis,[11] however, the prevalence may be considerably higher.

Pheochromocytomas can be sporadic or familial. Whereas the former are usually unicentric and unilateral, familial pheochromocytomas are often multicentric and bilateral. Familial pheochromocytomas are the result of a germline mutation in one of five genes: the RET gene leading to multiple endocrine neoplasia type 2; the von Hippel-Lindau (VHL) gene, which causes the von Hippel-Lindau syndrome; the neurofibromatosis type 1 (NF1) gene resulting in von Recklinghausen's disease; and the genes encoding the B and D subunits of mitochondrial succinate dehydrogenase (SCHB and SDHD), which are associated with familial paragangliomas and pheochromocytomas. Clinical features of syndromes associated with pheochromocytoma are described in Figure 36.4. For patients with apparently sporadic pheochromocytomas, an underlying germline mutation of the genes mentioned may be present in around 20% of cases and should be considered in younger patients (younger than 50 years) and those with multifocal or extra-adrenal tumors.[10,12] Patients found to harbor a germline mutation need to be identified for appropriate guidance of medical management for them and their families.

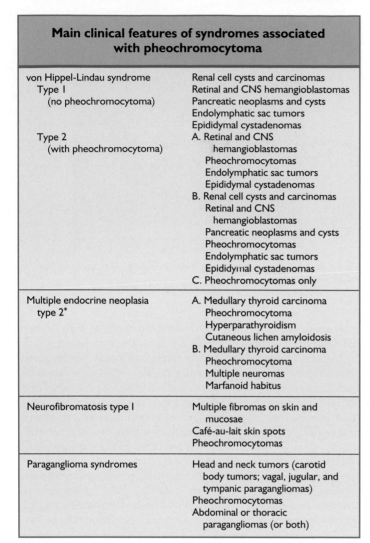

Main clinical features of syndromes associated with pheochromocytoma

von Hippel-Lindau syndrome Type I (no pheochromocytoma)	Renal cell cysts and carcinomas Retinal and CNS hemangioblastomas Pancreatic neoplasms and cysts Endolymphatic sac tumors Epididymal cystadenomas

Type 2
(with pheochromocytoma)
	A. Retinal and CNS
	    hemangioblastomas
	    Pheochromocytomas
	    Endolymphatic sac tumors
	    Epididymal cystadenomas
	B. Renal cell cysts and carcinomas
	    Retinal and CNS
	      hemangioblastomas
	    Pancreatic neoplasms and cysts
	    Pheochromocytomas
	    Endolymphatic sac tumors
	    Epididymal cystadenomas
	C. Pheochromocytomas only

Multiple endocrine neoplasia
type 2*
	A. Medullary thyroid carcinoma
	    Pheochromocytoma
	    Hyperparathyroidism
	    Cutaneous lichen amyloidosis
	B. Medullary thyroid carcinoma
	    Pheochromocytoma
	    Multiple neuromas
	    Marfanoid habitus

Neurofibromatosis type I	Multiple fibromas on skin and mucosae Café-au-lait skin spots Pheochromocytomas

Paraganglioma syndromes	Head and neck tumors (carotid
	    body tumors; vagal, jugular, and
	    tympanic paragangliomas)
	Pheochromocytomas
	Abdominal or thoracic
	    paragangliomas (or both)

Figure 36.4 Main clinical features of syndromes associated with pheochromocytoma. CNS, central nervous system. *A third type of MEN type 2 consists of familial medullary thyroid carcinoma only (without pheochromocytoma).

Clinical Manifestations

Clinical features reflect episodic or continuous overproduction of catecholamines and depend in part on which catecholamine dominates. Symptoms may include headache, sweating, palpitations, anxiety, pallor, and upset in almost any bodily function[13] (Fig. 36.5). Hypertension and/or diabetes mellitus, with or without symptoms, may be the initial manifestation. Alternatively, pheochromocytoma may present as a tumor mass, usually an enlarging primary lesion in the abdomen or a paraganglioma in the neck, ear, thorax, or abdomen. Occasionally, a metastatic lesion may be the presenting sign. Physical examination may reveal labile (66%) or persistent (33%) hypertension, sometimes with reciprocal changes in blood pressure and heart rate when the tumor secretes norepinephrine predominantly.[14] The patient may have cool, mottled extremities and a low-grade fever with tachycardia and postural hypotension. Patients may also present as an emergency with severe hypertension with or without heart failure and a variety of symptoms attributable to high plasma catecholamines. This can occur after minor or major trauma, at the time of delivery, or apparently spontaneously owing to sudden release of catecholamines from, or hemorrhage into, the tumor. Pheochromocytoma in pregnancy presents particular difficulties in diagnosis and management.[15]

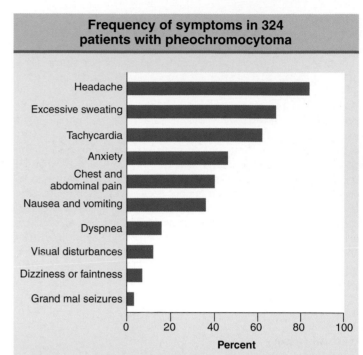

Frequency of symptoms in 324 patients with pheochromocytoma

Figure 36.5 Frequency of symptoms in 324 patients with pheochromocytoma. (Adapted from Ross ZJ, Griffith DN: The clinical presentation of phaeochromocytoma. Q J Med 1989;71:485–494.)

Diagnosis

Diagnosis of pheochromocytoma is based on clinical suspicion but demands biochemical confirmation (Fig. 36.6). Current evidence is that plasma free metanephrines provide the best biochemical test for diagnosing or excluding pheochromocytoma,[16] and the levels are relatively independent of renal function[17] while also providing some guidance regarding tumor size and location.[18] When plasma free metanephrines are not available, plasma or urinary catecholamines or their other metabolites may be used and typically are five- to 10-fold greater than normal. When catecholamine levels are at the upper limits of normal, a suppression test using clonidine (which suppresses plasma norepinephrine into the normal range if there is no pheochromocytoma but fails to do so in patients harboring a pheochromocytoma)[19] is useful.

Once a firm biochemical diagnosis is secured, the lesion must be localized (see Fig. 36.6). Imaging of a pheochromocytoma requires realization that the tumor, like the clinical syndrome itself, may mimic other lesions.[20] An MRI or CT scan of the abdomen and pelvis, concentrating first on the adrenals, is successful in the vast majority of patients, but additional investigations may be required if no lesion is detected. Such investigations may include selective venous sampling from the great veins to detect where there is a step up in catecholamine levels, metaiodobenzyl-guanidine (MIBG) scanning, indium 111–labeled octreotide scanning, measurements of plasma free metanephrines coupled with vena caval sampling, and positron emission tomography scanning.[21] Removal of a pheochromocytoma-containing adrenal can result in compensatory medullary hyperplasia in the contralateral adrenal, giving a false-positive MIBG scan; hence, interpretation must be cautious.[22]

Treatment

Once the tumor has been localized, the patient should be prepared for surgery with a collaborative team approach by the surgeon, anesthesiologist, and physician. Blockade of α-adrenoceptors,

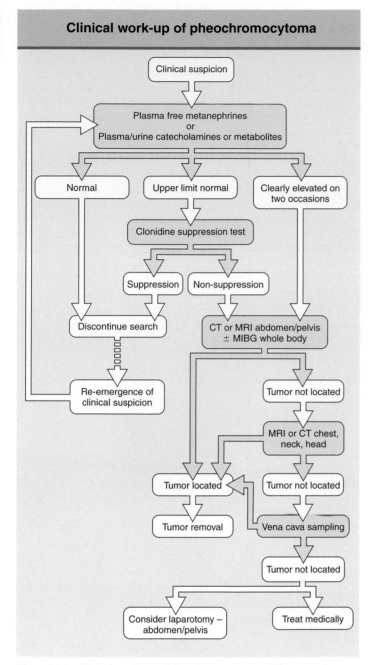

Figure 36.6 Clinical work-up of pheochromocytoma. CT, computed tomography; MIBG, metaiodobenzyl-guanidine; MRI, magnetic resonance imaging.

usually with phenoxybenzamine, with the later addition of β-blockade if necessary to control blood pressure and tachycardia, should be implemented for some weeks prior to surgery. Alternative drugs that have been used successfully prior to surgery include prazosin (α-blocker) and labetalol (combined α,β-blocker). A laparoscopic approach to surgical removal of adrenal pheochromocytomas and some extra-adrenal tumors has gained widespread acceptance, but the laparoscopic approach should be converted to open adrenalectomy for difficult dissection, invasion, adhesions, or surgical inexperience.[23] Laparoscopic surgery has also been used successfully for hereditary bilateral or recurrent pheochromocytoma.[24]

Hypotension and hypoglycemia are potential postoperative problems. In most cases, surgical removal of pheochromocytoma returns plasma catecholamine levels to normal while restoring

to normal previously suppressed central sympathetic outflow. Whereas blood pressure often improves with removal of the pheochromocytoma, in some patients it remains elevated, especially in those whose hypertension had been persistent as opposed to episodic. These subjects require long-term antihypertensive therapy.

For malignant pheochromocytoma, consideration should be given to aggressive surgical resection, particularly when there is a single metastatic lesion. Symptoms should be controlled with α- and β-blocking agents as needed, and radiation can be useful for bony metastases. Chemotherapy, usually with cyclophosphamide, vincristine, and dacarbazine, should be considered for those with surgically inaccessible metastases producing symptoms that cannot be controlled by α- and β-blockade. Progression of malignant pheochromocytoma is extremely variable, with survival over decades in some cases. Median survival is approximately 5 years.

RENIN-SECRETING TUMOR

Introduction and Definition

Primary reninism was the term proposed by Jerome Conn in 1972 for the clinical syndrome, first described in 1967[25] (with approximately 50 cases reported by 2000), of hypertension with hypokalemia due to high levels of active renin secreted by a tumor. Criteria for the diagnosis include an elevated plasma renin or prorenin level (or both), which decreases on removal of the tumor, and demonstration of renin within the tumor. Most cases are due to benign renal juxtaglomerular cell tumors ranging from 5 mm to 6 cm in diameter, but they occasionally occur with nephroblastomas, renal cell carcinomas, and extrarenal neoplasms (bronchial or pancreatic carcinoma, ovarian tumors, carcinoma of ileum or colon, soft-tissue sarcomas, orbital hemangiopericytoma).

Etiology and Pathogenesis

This syndrome of autonomous overproduction of renin illustrates the pathophysiologic significance of primary overactivity of the renin angiotensin system.[26] Renin secretion by the tumor results in sustained high circulating levels of Ang II, which, in the long term, increase arterial pressure to levels beyond those seen for the same level of Ang II during short-term infusions of the octapeptide, a phenomenon explained by the incremental, slow pressor action of Ang II. Hyperaldosteronism results from adrenal glomerulosa stimulation by Ang II giving rise to hypokalemia, while the high Ang II levels also induce hyponatremia in a minority of patients (via stimulation of thirst and antidiuretic hormone secretion together with a direct renal water-retaining action of the peptide) and, along with the hypertension, may give proteinuria.[25]

Clinical Manifestations

Patients are slightly more likely to be female than male, are often (75%) younger than the age of 30 years, presenting usually with severe, sometimes malignant, occasionally paroxysmal, hypertension (average 206/131 mm Hg), hypokalemia (<3.0 mmol/l in approximately 70% of cases), proteinuria (>0.4 g/day in around 50% of patients), and, in a minority of patients, hyponatremia.[26] The glomerular filtration rate is normal or high. Not surprisingly, the blood pressure may decrease substantially with the first dose of angiotensin-converting enzyme (ACE) inhibitor or angiotensin receptor blocker (ARB).

Pathology

Renin-secreting tumors are encapsulated, tan or grayish-yellow in color with scattered hemorrhages. On histologic examination, the tumors consist largely of polygonal or spindle cells in close contact with capillary and sinusoidal vessels and contain cytoplasmic renin granules.[26]

Diagnosis and Differential Diagnosis

Patients presenting with hypertension and hypokalemia together with elevated renin (and prorenin) and aldosterone levels may harbor a renin-secreting tumor, among which a renal juxtaglomerular cell tumor is most common. A schema for working up the diagnosis is given in Figure 36.7. Renal artery stenosis or occlusion must first be ruled out by CT or MRI angiography or renal arteriography. These investigations also might reveal a radiolucent, relatively avascular, usually peripheral juxtaglomerular cell tumor (Fig. 36.8).[27] CT and MRI scans, showing an isodense or hypodense lesion with little or no enhancement after injection of contrast, have proved helpful in the provisional localization of these tumors. Bilateral, simultaneous renal vein sampling may enable lateralization of the tumor. Since renal blood flow to the culprit kidney is not impaired, however, a renin ratio of ~1.2:1 between the two renal veins should not necessarily be expected, in contrast to the situation of unilateral renal artery stenosis in which reduced blood flow to the stenosed kidney plus renin oversecretion contribute to an often high renin ratio. Selective segmental renal vein renin sampling has proved helpful in localizing the tumor in some patients. When no renal lesion can be visualized and lateralization of renin secretion is not evident, an extrarenal renin-secreting lesion must be considered and sought by appropriate radiographic investigations and venous sampling for renin measurements.

Apart from renal artery stenosis or occlusion, it is vital in the differential diagnosis to exclude other rare renin-producing lesions noted here as well as Wilms' tumor, renal carcinoma, neuroblastoma, hepatocellular carcinoma, and pheochromocytoma, which can either themselves secrete renin or, alternatively, stimulate

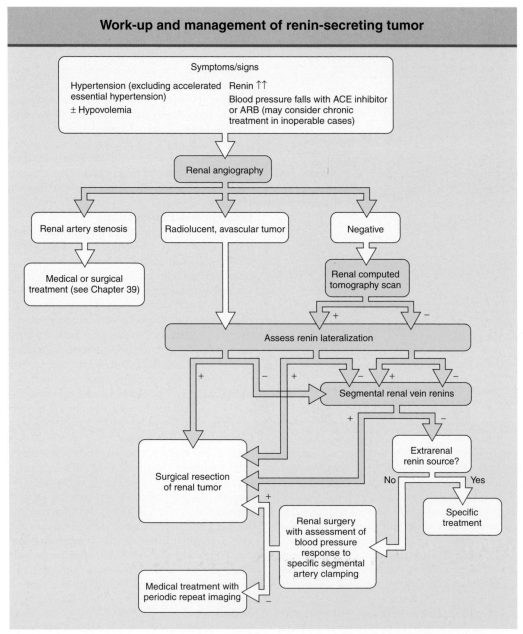

Figure 36.7 Work-up and management of renin-secreting tumor. ACE, angiotensin-converting enzyme; ATRA, angiotensin II receptor antagonist.

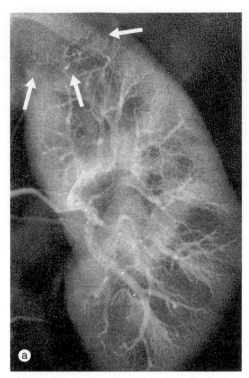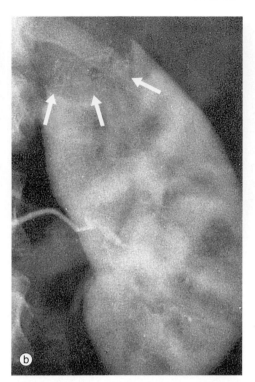

Figure 36.8 **Renin-secreting tumor.** Left renal angiography arterial (*a*) and nephrogram (*b*) phases revealing a 2.5-cm juxtaglomerular cell tumor with a circumscribed and relatively avascular appearance at the upper pole (*arrows*). (Adapted from Lam ASC, Bédard YC, Buckspan MB, et al: Surgically curable hypertension associated with reninoma. J Urol 1982;128:572–575.)

renal renin production. A careful clinical history and physical examination together with selected radiography and, occasionally, selective venous sampling for measurements of renin should, in most instances, differentiate these disorders from a juxtaglomerular cell tumor.

Treatment

Preoperative control of arterial pressure is based on an ACE inhibitor or ARB, introduced with caution to avoid first-dose hypotension. Provided the blood pressure is controlled and hypokalemia corrected, anesthesia presents no particular problem since intraoperative hemodynamics during removal of a juxtaglomerular cell tumor are quite stable. For juxtaglomerular cell tumors, local excision, where possible, is advisable to preserve nephrons. Where doubt exists, an intraoperative frozen section will differentiate a benign juxtaglomerular cell tumor from malignant lesions and guide surgery. Removal of a juxtaglomerular cell tumor results in the return of renin and aldosterone levels to normal. Blood pressure decreases rapidly, but not always to normal if there is a background of essential hypertension or when there is hypertensive vascular damage.

ACROMEGALY

Definition and Epidemiology

Acromegaly is caused by excessive circulating growth hormone (GH) usually from a pituitary tumor. Acromegaly is rare with a prevalence of 40 cases per million. Hypertension appears to be more common in acromegaly than the general population with an estimated 35% of subjects with a diastolic blood pressure >100 mm Hg[28] and with higher frequencies in female and older patients. Uncertainty over the exact prevalence (between 17.5%

and 57% in over 20 different reports) reflects variation in definitions of hypertension and the stage of the disease.[28,29] Acromegalic patients who have additional hypopituitarism or advanced cardiac disease may tend to have blood pressure reduction masking prior hypertension.

The pathogenesis of hypertension in acromegaly is complex but appears to be due to sodium retention and volume expansion associated with an inappropriate response of hormonal systems to counteract these effects. Total exchangeable sodium, total body water, and extracellular fluid volume are increased. Volume expansion should suppress plasma renin levels (as in primary aldosteronism), but, although levels are low, they are not consistent with the sodium status. Aldosterone levels are also normal or only slightly suppressed. Plasma ANP, which should be elevated in the volume-expanded state, remains normal in acromegaly. The kidneys are enlarged and glomerular filtration rate is increased, but sodium balance is not corrected unless the patient is cured of the acromegaly. Other mechanisms may also contribute to the hypertension, including the presence of circulating endogenous Na+-K+-ATPase (digoxin-like substances), GH-induced vascular hypertrophy resulting in decreased vascular compliance, effects on the sympathetic nervous system, and undefined genetic factors.

Clinical Manifestations

Acromegaly is characterized by enlargement of the skull (Fig. 36.9), hands (Fig. 36.10), and feet. Other symptoms result from local effects of an expanding pituitary tumor and include visual field defects and headache. Signs and symptoms include headache (40%), excessive sweating (50%), loss of libido (35%), amenorrhea (45%), carpal tunnel syndrome (25%), diabetes mellitus (19%), and visual field defects (5%).[28,30,31] Thyroid enlargement occurs in 50% of subjects and thyrotoxicosis in 6%.

449

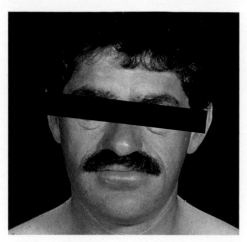

Figure 36.9 Facial features of acromegaly with enlargement of brow, nose, and jaw.

Tests for acromegaly
Plasma growth hormone
Plasma growth hormone responses to glucose tolerance test
Plasma insulin-like growth factor I
Lateral skull X-ray
Magnetic resonance imaging of the pituitary fossa
Visual field measurements
Assessment of other pituitary functions, e.g., thyroid function tests, thyroid-stimulating hormone, prolactin level, ACTH, and cortisol

Figure 36.11   Tests for acromegaly.

Hirsutism occurs in 24% of women and galactorrhea in 10%. Increasing size of the feet or hands (ring size) in the adult may also be helpful clues.

Diagnosis

Clinical suspicion should be raised by symptoms and signs. Figure 36.11 indicates appropriate tests. Elevated plasma GH, especially in response to an oral glucose tolerance test, is strongly suggestive of the diagnosis. Visual field assessment and MRI of the pituitary fossa are necessary to define the tumor and to exclude supratentorial extension. Most patients with acromegaly have a GH-secreting pituitary adenoma. Rarely, pancreatic or hypothalamic tumors release GH-releasing hormone with secondary GH excess. Breast and bronchial tumors can also produce growth hormone.

Treatment

Transsphenoidal adenomectomy is the treatment of choice. Irradiation and drug therapy are valuable when complete removal of

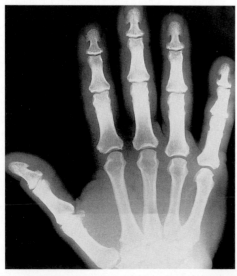

Figure 36.10   Radiograph of the hand in acromegaly. "Arrowhead" distal phalanges, expanded joint spaces, and increased soft tissue can be seen.

tumor tissue is not possible (in approximately one third of cases) and when surgery is contraindicated. Dopaminergic agents, such as bromocriptine or cabergoline, and the somatostatin analogue octreotide, reduce plasma GH in acromegaly. Bromocriptine may induce tumor shrinkage and improves the diabetic state in the majority of patients. Irradiation therapy may not exert its full effect for months or years. Hypopituitarism may occur late after treatment and necessitate endocrine replacement for ACTH, thyroid-stimulating hormone (TSH), and/or gonadotropin deficiency. Hence, regular monitoring of pituitary function is required after treatment.

Management of Hypertension in Acromegaly

Surgical removal of the pituitary adenoma with normalization of GH levels may reduce blood pressure to some extent, but the majority of patients will continue to require antihypertensive therapy. For example, in one series of 44 subjects undergoing surgery, only 14 had their diastolic blood pressure reduced to <100 mm Hg, and only five (11% of the total group) had diastolic blood pressures reduced to <90 mm Hg.

Antihypertensive treatment generally includes a diuretic, given the volume-expanded state. Additional antihypertensive agents are frequently required, and both calcium channel blockers and ACE inhibitors have been reported to be useful. β-Blockers (e.g., propranolol) may also be used, although theoretically such agents may increase GH hormone concentration.

HYPOTHYROIDISM

Definition and Epidemiology

Hypothyroidism results from deficient production of thyroid hormones, whether through inadequate TSH secretion (from hypothalamic or pituitary lesions) or impaired functioning of the thyroid itself (loss or atrophy of the gland, autoimmune destruction, iodine deficiency, antithyroid agents, or hereditary defects in hormone synthesis).[32] It is estimated that hypertension is 1.5 to two times more common in hypothyroid patients than in the general population.[33]

The pathogenesis of the hypertension is multifactorial and associated with both increased total body sodium and increased peripheral vascular resistance. Even within euthyroid subjects, serum free thyroxine index (FTI) is lower and TSH is higher in hypertensive than normotensive subjects and FTI also independently predicts the blood pressure response to increments in dietary sodium in both normotensive and hypertensive subjects.[34] Hypothyroidism is associated with increased aortic stiffness, which is reversed by hormone replacement therapy.[35] Observations of short-term hypothyroidism have confirmed increases in arterial pressure, plasma catecholamines, aldosterone, and cortisol, all reversible with thyroid hormone treatment.[36] The relationship between plasma catecholamine levels and blood pressure is steepened in hypothyroidism. The catecholamine levels of hypothyroid subjects also show more variability within a 24-hour period, and this is also associated with more variability in blood pressure and heart rate during this period. This suggests underdamping of swings in sympathetic activity in the hypothyroid state.[37]

Hypertension develops despite a low cardiac output. Thyroid replacement therapy corrects the electrolyte, hemodynamic, and hormone changes and cures the hypertension in most patients.

Clinical Features

Any organ system can be affected in primary hypothyroidism; therefore, symptoms and signs can be protean. The onset of clinical abnormalities is usually gradual, and diagnosis may not be made until gross hypothyroidism is established. Common clinical features include weakness, dry skin, lethargy, slow slurred speech, sensation of cold, thick tongue, facial puffiness (Fig. 36.12), coarse hair, failing memory, constipation, and weight gain with reduced appetite. Coronary heart disease is common. Whereas abnormal lipid metabolism may be the major etiologic factor, concomitant hypertension may accelerate the atherogenic process.

Diagnosis

Hypothyroidism should be considered in any patient with hypertension. Since the clinical manifestations of hypothyroidism are often difficult to elicit, especially in the elderly, thyroid function tests, including TSH when FTI is equivocal, should be performed. In patients with primary hypothyroidism in whom normotension

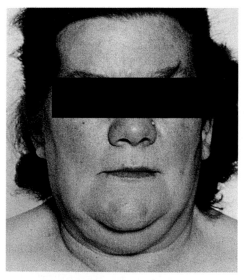

Figure 36.12 Hypothyroid facies.

is not achieved by full thyroxine replacement therapy, it is likely that essential hypertension (which afflicts approximately 20% of the population) is a concomitant disorder. For those with gross or long-standing hypothyroidism, replacement thyroxine therapy should be cautious to minimize the chances of exacerbating or developing symptoms of myocardial ischemia.

HYPERTHYROIDISM

Definition and Epidemiology

Hyperthyroidism and thyrotoxicosis may result from Graves' disease, and less commonly, toxic multinodular goiter, toxic adenoma, a high iodine intake, trophoblastic tumor, and (rarely) excessive pituitary TSH secretion. Hypertension is common in hyperthyroidism, with a prevalence of 60% in toxic adenoma and approximately 30% in Graves' disease.

Clinical Features

The clinical features depend on the underlying cause of the hyperthyroidism, severity of the disorder, rapidity of onset, age of the patient, and concomitant disease. Abnormalities may be evident in the cardiovascular system (tachyarrhythmias, heart failure), skin (increased sweating, increasing pigmentation with vitiligo), eyes (lid lag, exophthalmos), nervous system (hypertension, nervousness), alimentary system (increased appetite yet weight loss, diarrhea), and muscles (proximal weakness).

Hypertension in hyperthyroidism is associated with elevated systolic blood pressure and normal or low diastolic pressure. It may be observed both in postpartum thyrotoxicosis and neonatal thyrotoxicosis. Elevation of diastolic pressure is unusual unless there is concomitant essential hypertension.

The hemodynamic characteristics in hypertension of thyrotoxicosis are an increased cardiac output, increased myocardial contractility, tachycardia, decreased peripheral vascular resistance, and an expanded blood volume. These indices return to normal in most patients on achieving the euthyroid state. Interestingly, catecholamine levels tend to be low (inversely to hypothyroid hypertension), and there is no heightened activity of the sympathetic system. The renin angiotensin system tends to be activated and the aldosterone levels increased in hyperthyroidism, and this may contribute to the development of systolic hypertension.

Suspicion of hyperthyroidism should be high in the elderly patient with hypertension and a high pulse pressure, particularly if there is also atrial fibrillation. Such patients are liable to develop cardiac failure, in which case the increased systolic arterial pressure will diminish, masking previous hypertension. Hypertension with a high pulse pressure, while typical of hyperthyroidism, is observed in many elderly essential hypertensives due to the loss of the compliance of the aorta with aging and also in the rare patient with coarctation of the aorta.

Diagnosis and Treatment

Diagnosis of hyperthyroidism is confirmed by measuring thyroid function tests, including TSH. β-Blockers are often effective first-line therapy for hyperthyroidism-associated hypertension. Treatment of hyperthyroidism, whether by antithyroid drugs, surgery, or radioiodine, will often normalize the increased systolic arterial pressure, although this is by no means invariable in the elderly in whom there may be concomitant essential hypertension.

REFERENCES

1. Stewart PM: The adrenal cortex. In Larsen PR, Kronenberg HM, Melmed S, Polonsky KS (eds): Williams Textbook of Endocrinology, 10th ed. Philadelphia: Saunders, 2003, pp 491–551.
2. Whitworth JA, Williamson PM, Mangos G, Kelly JL: Cardiovascular consequences of cortisol excess. Vasc Health Risk Manage 2005;1:291–299.
3. Sala C, Ambrosi B, Morganti A: Blunted vascular and renal effects of exogenous atrial natriuretic peptide in patients with Cushing's disease. J Clin Endocrinol Metab 2001;86:1957–1961.
4. Sugihara N, Shimizu M, Kita Y, et al: Cardiac characteristics and post-operative courses in Cushing's syndrome. Am J Cardiol 1992;69:1475–1480.
5. Hersbach FMRJ, Bravenboer B, Koolen JJ: Hearty hormones. Lancet 2001;358:468.
6. Tauchmanova L, Rossi R, Biondi B, et al: Patients with subclinical Cushing's syndrome due to adrenal adenoma have increased cardiovascular risk. J Clin Endocrinol Metab 2002;87:4872–4878.
7. Mancini T, Kola B, Mantero F, et al: High cardiovascular risk in patients with Cushing's syndrome according to 1999 WHO/ISH guidelines. Clin Endocrinol 2004;61:768–777.
8. Baid S, Nieman LK: Glucocorticoid excess and hypertension. Curr Hypertens Rep 2004;6:493–499.
9. Manger WM, Gifford RW (eds): Clinical and Experimental Pheochromocytoma. Cambridge: Blackwell Science, 1996.
10. Lenders JWM, Eisenhofer G, Mannelli M, et al: Phaeochromocytoma. Lancet 2005;366:665–675.
11. McNeil AR, Blok BH, Koelmeyer TD, et al: Phaeochromocytomas discovered during coronial autopsies in Sydney, Melbourne and Auckland. Aust NZ J Med 2000;30:648–652.
12. Neumann HPH, Bausch B, McWhinney SR, et al: Germ-line mutations in nonsyndromic pheochromocytoma. N Engl J Med 2002;346:1459–1466.
13. Ross ZJ, Griffith DN: The clinical presentation of phaeochromocytoma. Q J Med 1989;71:485–494.
14. Richards AM, Nicholls MG, Espiner EA, et al: Arterial pressure and hormone relationships in phaeochromocytoma. J Hypertens 1983;1:373–379.
15. Manger WM: The vagaries of pheochromocytomas. Am J Hypertens 2005;18:1266–1270.
16. Lenders JW, Pacak K, Walther MM, et al: Biochemical diagnosis of pheochromocytoma. Which test is best? JAMA 2002;287:1427–1434.
17. Eisenhofer G, Huysmans F, Pacak K, et al: Plasma metanephrines in renal failure. Kidney Int 2005;67:668–677.
18. Eisenhofer G, Lenders JWM, Goldstein DS, et al: Pheochromocytoma catecholamines phenotypes and prediction of tumor size and location by use of plasma free metanephrines. Clin Chem 2005;51:735–744.
19. Bravo EL, Tarazi RC, Fouad FM, et al: Clonidine-suppression test. A useful aid in the diagnosis of pheochromocytoma. N Engl J Med 1981;305:623–626.
20. Blake MA, Kalra MK, Maher MM, et al: Pheochromocytoma: An imaging chameleon. Radiographics 2004;24(Suppl 1):S87–S99.
21. Pacak K, Goldstein DS, Doppman JL, et al: A "pheo" lurks: Novel approaches for locating occult pheochromocytoma. J Clin Endocrinol Metab 2001;86:3641–3646.
22. Burt MG, Allen B, Conaglen JV. False positive ^{131}I-metaiodobenzylguanide scan in the postoperative assessment of malignant phaeochromocytoma secondary to medullary hyperplasia. N Z Med J 2002;115:18.
23. Shen WT, Sturgeon C, Clark OH, et al: Should pheochromocytoma size influence surgical approach? A comparison of 90 malignant and 60 benign pheochromocytomas. Surgery 2004;136:1129–1137.
24. Nambirajan T, Leeb K, Neumann HP, et al: Laparoscopic adrenal surgery for recurrent tumours in patients with hereditary phaeochromocytoma. Eur Urol 2005;47:622–626.
25. Robertson PW, Klidjian A, Harding LK, et al: Hypertension due to a renin-secreting tumor. Am J Med 1967;43:963–976.
26. Lindop GBM, Leckie BJ, Mimran A: Renin-secreting tumors. In Robertson JIS, Nicholls MG (eds): The Renin-Angiotensin System. London: Gower Medical, 1993, pp 54.1–54.12.
27. Lam ASC, Bédard YC, Buckspan MB, et al: Surgically curable hypertension associated with reninoma. J Urol 1982;128:572–575.
28. Davies DL, Connell JMC, Reid R, Fraser R: Acromegaly: The effects of growth hormone on blood vessels, sodium homeostasis and blood pressure. In Robertson JIS (ed): Handbook of Hypertension: Clinical Hypertension. Amsterdam: Elsevier, 1992, pp 545–575.
29. Vitale G, Pivonello R, Auriemma RS, et al: Hypertension in acromegaly and in the normal population: Prevalence and determinants. Clin Endocrinol 2005;63:470–476.
30. Nabarro JDM: Acromegaly. Clin Endocrinol 1987;26:481–512.
31. Jadresic A, Banks LM, Child DG, et al: The acromegaly syndrome. Q J Med 1982;51:189–204.
32. Larsen PR, Ingbar SH: The thyroid gland. In Wilson JD, Foster DW (eds): Williams' Textbook of Endocrinology. Philadelphia: Saunders, 1992, pp 357–487.
33. Bing RF: Thyroid disease and hypertension. In Robertson JIS, ed. Handbook of Hypertension: Clinical Hypertension. Amsterdam: Elsevier, 1992, pp 576–593.
34. Gumieniak O, Perlstein TS, Hopkins PN, et al: Thyroid function and blood pressure homeostasis in euthyroid subjects. J Clin Endocrinol Metab 2004;89:3455–3461.
35. Dernellis J, Panaretou M: Effects of thyroid replacement therapy on arterial blood pressure in patients with hypertension and hypothyroidism. Am Heart J 2002;143:718–724.
36. Fommei E, Iervasi G: The role of thyroid hormone in blood pressure homeostasis: Evidence from short-term hypothyroidism in humans. J Clin Endocrinol Metab 2002;87:1996–2000.
37. Richards AM, Nicholls MG, Espiner EA, et al: Hypertension in hypothyroidism: Arterial pressure and hormone relationships. Clin Exp Hypertens 1985;7:1499–514.

Endocrine Causes of Hypertension: Aldosterone

I. David Weiner and Charles S. Wingo

INTRODUCTION

Recent advances have refined our ability to identify aldosterone-induced hypertension, with the recognition that primary hyperaldosteronism is more common than previously recognized. Effective diagnostic strategies are available and treatment regimens are highly efficacious.

ETIOLOGY/PATHOGENESIS

Aldosterone is a steroid hormone produced under normal circumstances by the zona glomerulosa of the adrenal glands. The enzyme aldosterone synthase, which is encoded by the gene *CYP11B2*, is the rate-limiting enzyme in adrenal aldosterone production.

Many factors regulate adrenal gland aldosterone synthesis. Figure 37.1 summarizes those known to either stimulate or inhibit aldosterone synthesis. The factors accepted as physiologically important include angiotensin II (Ang II), which stimulates aldosterone production through activation of the AT1 receptor, and atrial natriuretic peptide (ANP) and hypokalemia, which inhibit aldosterone production.[1]

Aldosterone regulates blood pressure through a number of mechanisms. These include effects on the kidneys, vasculature, central nervous system, and other endocrine hormones. No single effect is sufficient to explain the hypertension that occurs in primary hyperaldosteronism; taken together, they explain why primary hyperaldosteronism causes refractory hypertension. Figure 37.2 summarizes these various mechanisms.

Aldosterone has multiple renal effects that regulate blood pressure. First, aldosterone stimulates renal sodium chloride retention by increasing expression of the thiazide-sensitive sodium-chloride cotransporter in the distal convoluted tubule, the amiloride-sensitive epithelial sodium channel in the collecting duct, and the chloride-reabsorbing protein pendrin in the cortical collecting duct.[2–4] There are also acute effects of aldosterone on sodium reabsorption in these segments that may not require protein synthesis.[5]

Second, aldosterone alters blood pressure through generation of hypokalemia. Aldosterone increases sodium reabsorption, which enhances potassium secretion. In addition, aldosterone increases extrarenal cellular potassium uptake by stimulating the ubiquitous Na^+-K^+-ATPase, further decreasing extracellular potassium.[6] As discussed in Chapters 9 and 33, potassium depletion leads to hypertension through a variety of mechanisms.

Aldosterone has multiple effects on the vasculature. Aldosterone increases both basal vascular tone and vascular reactivity to circulating vasoconstrictors, including norepinephrine, epinephrine, Ang II, and vasopressin.[7,8] It decreases flow-mediated vasodilatation perhaps due to decreased nitric oxide production resulting from decreased endothelial nitric oxide synthase expression.[9] In the central nervous system, aldosterone stimulates central

Factors that regulate aldosterone release	
Stimulatory	**Inhibitory**
Angiotensin II	*Atrial natriuretic peptide*
Adrenocorticotropic hormone	*Hypokalemia*
Acetylcholine	Calcitonin gene-related peptide
Adenosine triphosphate	Dopamine
Bradykinin	Nitric oxide
Cholecystokinin	Platelet-derived growth factor
β-Endorphin	Somatostatin
Endothelin	Unsaturated fatty acids
Enkephalins	Transforming growth factor β
Epidermal growth factor	
Hyperkalemia	
Melanocyte stimulating hormone	
Neuropeptide Y	
Neurotensin	
Norepinephrine	
Parathyroid hormone	
Prolactin	
Serotonin	
Substance P	
Vasoactive intestinal peptide	
Vasopressin	

Figure 37.1 Factors that regulate aldosterone release. Those stimuli that exert significant effects on aldosterone release under most clinical circumstances are noted in *italics*. Stimuli listed in *italic* are those that are clinically most relevant; otherwise these stimuli are listed in alphabetical order. (Data from Quinn SJ, Williams GH: Regulation of aldosterone secretion. Annu Rev Physiol 1988;50: 409–426; and Spat A, Hunyady L: Control of aldosterone secretion: A model for convergence in cellular signaling pathways. Physiol Rev 2004;84:489–539.)

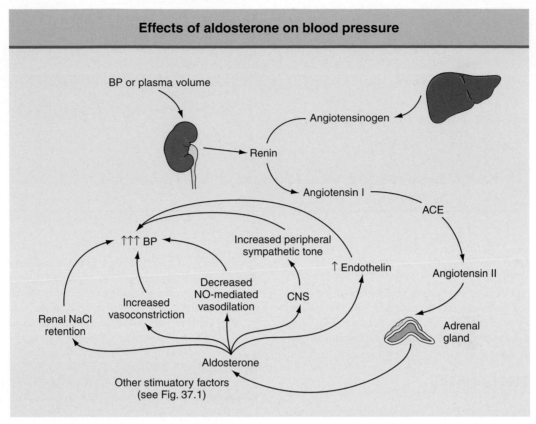

Effects of aldosterone on blood pressure

Figure 37.2   Effects of aldosterone on blood pressure (BP). ACE, angiotensin-converting enzyme; CNS, central nervous system; NO, nitric oxide.

nervous system–mediated sympathetic nervous tone, which further increases blood pressure.[10] Finally, aldosterone induces perivascular fibrosis and increases expression of other vasoconstrictive hormones, such as endothelin.[11]

Aldosterone mediates its physiologic and pathophysiologic effects predominantly through activation of the mineralocorticoid receptor (MR).[12] The MR is located in the inactive state in the cytoplasm; aldosterone binding to MR promotes a conformational change and translocation to the nucleus where it regulates gene transcription.

Cortisol is a naturally synthesized glucocorticoid with an affinity for the MR similar to that of aldosterone, but is present in plasma at approximately 100-fold greater levels than aldosterone. The enzyme 11β-hydroxysteroid dehydrogenase type 2 (11β-HSD2) is expressed in the aldosterone-sensitive distal nephron and collecting duct, metabolizes cortisol to cortisone, which binds to MR poorly, thereby preventing glucocorticoid-dependent activation of the MR.[13] Either the genetic deficiency or ingestion of inhibitors of 11β-HSD can result in excessive activation of the MR and the development of severe hypertension.[13] Aldosterone also has nongenomic (MR independent) effects, but its specific role in mineralocorticoid-dependent blood pressure regulation remains unclear at present.[14,15]

Primary hyperaldosteronism can result from either unilateral or bilateral adrenal disease. Typically, unilateral disease results from adenoma formation and bilateral disease from hyperplasia. This association is not absolute, and approximately 10% of those with primary hyperaldosteronism exhibit either bilateral aldosterone-producing adenoma (APA), which may be microscopic, or unilateral hyperplasia.

EPIDEMIOLOGY

The exact incidence of primary hyperaldosteronism varies with the patient population and the diagnostic criteria used. Early studies suggested that primary hyperaldosteronism was rare, with an incidence <1% to 2%.[16] In general, these studies recognized only severe cases of excessive aldosterone release. More accurate definitions have led to the recognition that primary hyperaldosteronism is relatively common. Patients with refractory hypertension, typically defined as hypertension not adequately controlled despite the use of appropriate doses of at least three antihypertensive medications, including a diuretic, have a high likelihood of having primary hyperaldosteronism, with rates typically of 20% to 40% and as high as 67% in some studies.[17] Some studies (Fig. 37.3) have found a 1% to 2% incidence of hyperaldosteronism in the normotensive population and a progressive increase in the incidence in patients with the severity of the hypertension.[18]

CLINICAL MANIFESTATIONS

Patients with primary hyperaldosteronism frequently have characteristics suggestive of secondary hypertension, such as onset of hypertension between ages 20 and 39, or in the elderly, worsening hypertension control or the need for multiple medications for blood pressure control. It may also present in those 40 to 50 years old and may not be diagnosed for many years because of the slow progression of the worsening of hypertension.[19] Figure 37.4 summarizes characteristics of those with primary hyperaldosteronism. It is important to recognize that both hypokalemia and

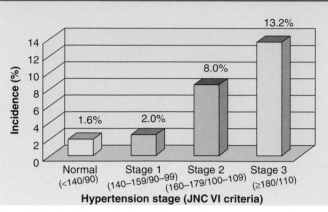

Incidence of primary hyperaldosteronism in patients with differing degrees of hypertension

Figure 37.3 Incidence of primary hyperaldosteronism in patients with differing degrees of hypertension, as defined by Joint National Committee (JNC) VI criteria.[18] Blood pressure level in mm Hg is shown in parentheses.

metabolic alkalosis, once thought to be a hallmark of primary hyperaldosteronism, are absent in the majority of patients.

PATHOLOGY

Primary hyperaldosteronism can result from either an APA (Fig. 37.5) or hyperplasia of the zona glomerulosa. In general, APAs are unilateral and are large enough (>1 cm) to be identified by imaging modalities such as computed tomography (CT) scanning (Fig. 37.6). However, APA may also be microscopic and may be bilateral. Hyperplasia is typically bilateral, but may develop asynchronously in the two adrenal glands, and it may be unilateral. The factors that lead to either APA or hyperplasia development are not well understood.

Typical characteristics at time of diagnosis of primary hyperaldosteronism	
Sex (female/male)	43%/57%
Age, yr (range)	52.2 ± 1.3 (29–74)
Hypertension duration (yrs)	10 ± 1.4
Number (range) of hypertensive medications	2.4 ± 0.1 (0–4)
Percentage requiring >3 medications	53.7%
Blood pressure controlled on current medical regimen	20.4%
Neither hypokalemic nor ≥3 medications	52%
Plasma aldosterone (ng/dl) <15 15–40 >40	37% 54% 9%
Plasma renin activity (ng Ang I/ml/hr)	0.3 ± 0.04

Figure 37.4 Typical characteristics at time of diagnosis of primary hyperaldosteronism. Data from Stowasser M, Gordon RD, Gunasekera TG, et al: High rate of detection of primary aldosteronism, including surgically treatable forms, after "non-selective" screening of hypertensive patients. J Hypertens 2003;21:2149–2157.

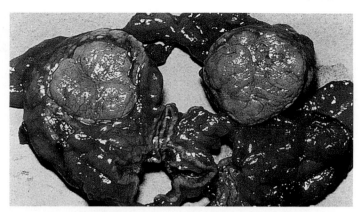

Figure 37.5 Adrenal adenoma. An aldosterone-producing adrenal adenoma with typical cholesterol-rich yellow appearance.

DIAGNOSIS AND DIFFERENTIAL DIAGNOSIS

The diagnosis of primary hyperaldosteronism should be considered in patients who have either refractory hypertension or spontaneous or easily provoked hypokalemia. Compliance with the medical regimen may be important to verify. It is important to emphasize that hypokalemia, although classically associated with primary hyperaldosteronism, is present in only a minority of patients with this condition. The lack of hypokalemia should not prevent consideration of this diagnosis.

Evaluation of the patient with suspected primary hyperaldosteronism is directed at identifying those who have autonomous aldosterone release and then at identifying whether treatment should be based on a medical or surgical approach. Multiple diagnostic algorithms are in use; Figure 37.7 shows a diagnostic algorithm that we favor.

The first step is to identify that the patient has autonomous aldosterone release. Because the predominant physiologic mechanism that increases adrenal aldosterone release is Ang II, evidence of Ang II–independent aldosterone release has been used as evidence of autonomous aldosterone release, and, therefore, of primary hyperaldosteronism. Because Ang II cannot be assayed for routine clinical use, renin has been used as a surrogate. A randomly obtained measure of the ratio of plasma aldosterone-renin (ARR,

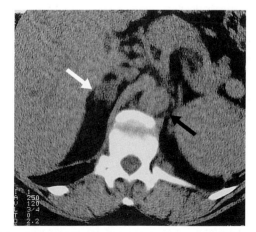

Figure 37.6 Adrenal adenoma by computed tomography scan. A normal linear image of the left adrenal (*black arrow*) and expansion of the right adrenal with a 2-cm aldosterone-producing adenoma (*white arrow*).

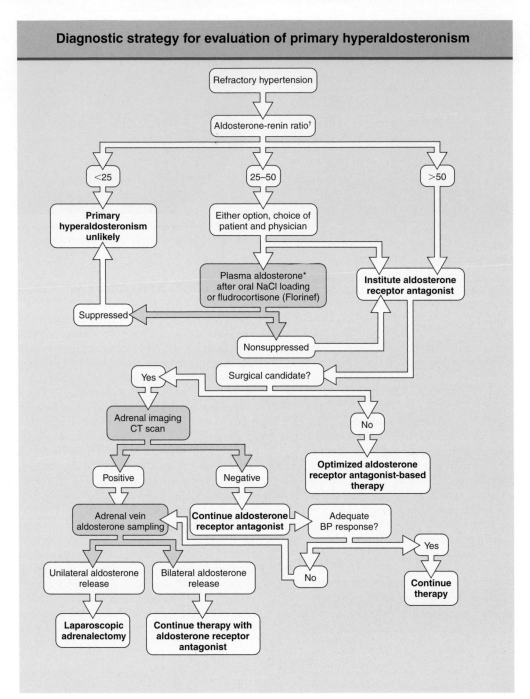

Figure 37.7 **Diagnostic strategy for evaluation of primary hyperaldosteronism.** ARR, aldosterone-renin ratio; BP, blood pressure; CT, computed tomography. *A 24-hour urine aldosterone excretion can also be used. †Calculated using plasma renin activity.

aldosterone-renin ratio) is obtained and provides an index of the extent to which Ang II is stimulating aldosterone production. If this ratio is elevated, then there is significant Ang II–independent aldosterone release, thereby providing evidence of autonomous aldosterone production and confirming primary hyperaldosteronism. Some investigators recommend confirming this diagnosis by examining either a plasma aldosterone or urinary aldosterone excretion rate while the patient is consuming a high-salt diet. If the ARR is more than five times the upper limit of normal, confirmatory tests may not be necessary because this group of patients appears to almost uniformly respond to MR blocker treatment with substantial improvements in blood pressure.[20] If the ARR is more than 2.5 and less than five times

normal, then confirmatory tests may be helpful, unless the patient is willing to undergo a diagnostic trial with an MR antagonist.

When evaluating the ARR, the clinician needs to be aware that two different renin assays are in routine clinical use. One measures renin activity, assayed as the rate of conversion of angiotensinogen to Ang I, and the second measures the amount of immunoreactive renin. While these two techniques yield results that correlate well with each other, the units and the numerical values obtained differ dramatically. For the plasma renin activity, the normal range is 1.9 to 3.7 ng Ang I/ml/h, and the lower level of detectability is 0.2 ng Ang I/ml/h in most clinical laboratories. For the direct renin assay, the normal range is typically 13 to 44 IU/ml, and lower level of detectability is approximately 6 to

8 IU/ml. Thus, the absolute values are approximately 10-fold greater with the direct renin assay than with the plasma renin activity. Accordingly, the normal ARR in individuals who do not have primary hyperaldosteronism is approximately 10:1 using the plasma renin activity assay and approximately 1:1 using the direct renin assay. It is important to recognize that because of technical reasons, the direct renin assay is less sensitive than plasma renin activity when renin levels are low.

The effects of common medicines that the patient may be taking on the ARR are typically mild and easily predictable.[21,22] β-Adrenergic receptor antagonists (β-blockers) suppress renin release, typically by approximately 50%. However, they generally will not result in a completely suppressed renin measurement and generally do not interfere with diagnosing primary hyperaldosteronism.[22] ACE inhibitors and angiotensin receptor blockers (ARBs), along with diuretics, can increase renin release in normal individuals, but in the patient with primary hyperaldosteronism, renin release remains suppressed. Other antihypertensive medications typically have little effect on the ARR measurement.

Once a diagnosis of primary hyperaldosteronism is made, the clinician should determine, for patients who are fit for surgery, whether there is unilateral autonomous aldosterone release, in which case adrenalectomy may be curative. Because approximately 90% of patients with unilateral aldosterone release have an APA, a CT scan, using an approximate distance of 3 mm between image planes, is the next diagnostic step (see Fig. 37.6). A conventional abdominal CT scan is typically performed with a 1-cm distance between image planes and may fail to identify small adrenal adenomas. Magnetic resonance imaging may be useful in those who cannot undergo CT scanning. Ultrasonography typically does not image the adrenal glands adequately to be a primary imaging modality.

If an adrenal adenoma is identified, then one should determine whether the adenoma is an APA or whether it is a nonfunctional adenoma that is present in approximately 5% of the adult population. Direct assessment of adrenal aldosterone release is generally recommended to differentiate between an APA and a nonfunctional adenoma. The most direct assessment is with adrenal vein aldosterone sampling.

Occasional patients may have unilateral autonomous aldosterone release but not have an adenoma detectable on CT scan. These patients may have either unilateral adrenal hyperplasia or micronodular APA. The optimal approach to identifying this subset of patients is not known, but we recommend considering this diagnosis in those patients in whom the response to MR antagonists, such as spironolactone and eplerenone, is inadequate. In this case, we consider proceeding to adrenal vein sampling despite a negative CT scan to identify whether the patient has surgically treatable unilateral autonomous adrenal aldosterone release.

Many other diagnostic tests have been suggested in the evaluation of primary hyperaldosteronism. The postural stimulation test and the saline suppression test may be helpful in the differentiation between bilateral adrenal hyperplasia and an APA. These tests require discontinuation of medications that affect the renin angiotensin system, including diuretics, β-blockers, ACE inhibitors, and ARBs, before testing. Because of the difficulty in controlling blood pressure in many of these patients, this may be difficult to perform, which limits the utility of these tests. Another diagnostic strategy takes advantage of the observation that functional adrenal adenomas frequently produce abnormal steroid metabolites. Assessment of 18-hydroxysteroid metabolites may be helpful; if elevated, they suggest the diagnosis of an APA.[23] A limitation in both of the sets of diagnostic strategies, however, is that they are best at differentiating adrenal hyperplasia from functional adenomas. However, in 10% to 20% of cases of primary hyperaldosteronism, there is unilateral adrenal hyperplasia, bilateral APAs, or a renin-responsive unilateral APA. In each of these instances, these indirect diagnostic strategies can fail to identify correctly whether unilateral or bilateral aldosterone release is present. Each of these diagnostic strategies has sensitivity and specificity of 70% to 80%. Accordingly, their use is not generally recommended.

Rare patients with an elevated ARR have glucocorticoid-remediable aldosteronism (GRA; see Chapter 46). In this condition, there is crossover between the *CYP11B1* and *CYP11B2* genes, resulting in a chimeric gene resulting in aldosterone synthase expression being regulated by adrenocorticotropic hormone (ACTH), and excessive aldosterone release.[24,25] GRA should be considered in the patient in whom primary hyperaldosteronism is due to bilateral autonomous aldosterone release and either the blood pressure does not respond well to aldosterone receptor antagonists or the patient is intolerant of these medications. It can be clinically identified by demonstrating that dexamethasone administration, which suppresses ACTH release, decreases aldosterone levels.[26] If GRA is identified, administration of glucocorticoids in the minimal dose necessary to suppress ACTH release can dramatically improve blood pressure control.

NATURAL HISTORY

The natural history of primary hyperaldosteronism has not been extensively studied because, once diagnosed, almost all patients are treated with either MR antagonists or adrenalectomy. Although there are case reports of remission of primary hyperaldosteronism, these all follow adrenal venography and may reflect complications related to the venography. As a result, treatment is almost universally recommended.

TREATMENT

Patients with an APA who are acceptable surgical candidates should undergo laparoscopic adrenalectomy by an experienced surgeon. Laparoscopic adrenalectomy is associated with a shortened hospital stay, decreased postoperative morbidity, decreased costs, and a quicker return to normal health. Patients with an APA who undergo laparoscopic adrenalectomy have a 30% to 60% chance of hypertension cure.[27–29] Patients most likely to experience cure of their hypertension are younger than 50 years of age and have few family members with essential hypertension. Those not cured have a >95% chance of improvement in their blood pressure.[28,29] Lack of cure may be associated with microvascular renal disease, presumably related to the pre-existing hyperaldosteronism and hypertension, that then perpetuates the hypertension.

Those with primary hyperaldosteronism who are either not candidates for surgical adrenalectomy or who have bilateral aldosterone production should be treated with MR antagonists. Figure 37.8 summarizes characteristics of the two major MR antagonists currently available: spironolactone and eplerenone. Both are highly efficacious. Their major difference relates to their side effect profiles and their costs. Spironolactone has partial affinity for both androgenic and progesterone receptors, resulting in dose-related side effects. For example, gynecomastia occurs in approximately 7% of men treated with ≤50 mg/day,

Comparison of currently available aldosterone-receptor antagonists

Medication	Dose Range (mg/day)	Common Side Effects	Relative Cost[l]
Spironolactone	25–400	Gynecomastia Breast pain (mastodynia) Impotence Decreased libido Menstrual irregularities	~1x
Eplerenone	25–200	Generally well tolerated Gynecomastia or abnormal vaginal bleeding in <2%	~5–10x

Figure 37.8 Comparison of currently available aldosterone-receptor antagonists.

but in 52% of those treated with ≥150 mg/day.[30] Eplerenone has affinity for the MR that is similar to that of spironolactone, but more than 100-fold less affinity for androgenic and progesterone receptors than does spironolactone.[31] Accordingly, the incidence of side effects related to androgenic or progesterone receptor

activation, such as gynecomastia, gynecodynia (breast pain), vaginal bleeding, and impotence, is greatly reduced. The use of eplerenone may be limited by its substantially higher cost.

Those treated with an MR antagonist generally experience a dramatic improvement in their blood pressure control. Many patients will be very responsive, enabling use of low doses, 25 to 50 mg/day, as initial therapy. Blood pressure, both systolic and diastolic, frequently decreases by approximately 25 mm Hg over a period of a few weeks to months. The dose of the aldosterone receptor antagonists can be increased as necessary; we do not routinely recommend changes more than every 2 to 4 weeks. Hypokalemia and metabolic alkalosis, if present, improve. Potassium supplements can be tapered rapidly with improvement of hypokalemia. With time, blood pressure can be controlled in many patients with an MR antagonist and a single alternative agent. We typically use ACE inhibitors in management of these patients. The renin activity, which is suppressed at time of initial diagnosis, typically increases after starting aldosterone receptor antagonist therapy. Synergistic use of an ACE inhibitor may prevent development of a renin-stimulated, Ang II–dependent component of hypertension. However, many medicine combinations can be used successfully in conjunction with an aldosterone receptor antagonist.

REFERENCES

1. Quinn SJ, Williams GH: Regulation of aldosterone secretion. Annu Rev Physiol 1988;50:409–426.
2. Verlander JW, Hassell KA, Royaux IE, et al: Deoxycorticosterone upregulates PDS (Slc26a4) in mouse kidney: Role of pendrin in mineralocorticoid-induced hypertension. Hypertension 2003;42:356–362.
3. Kim GH, Masilamani S, Turner R, et al: The thiazide-sensitive Na-Cl cotransporter is an aldosterone-induced protein. Proc Natl Acad Sci USA 1998;95:14552–14557.
4. Blazer-Yost BL, Liu X, Helman SI: Hormonal regulation of ENaCs: Insulin and aldosterone. Am J Physiol 1998;274:C1373–C1379.
5. Wingo CS, Kokko JP, Jacobson HR: Effects of in vitro aldosterone on the rabbit cortical collecting tubule. Kidney Int 1985;28:51–57.
6. Bia MJ, DeFronzo RA: Extrarenal potassium homeostasis. Am J Physiol 1981;240:F257–F268.
7. Finch L, Haeusler G: Vascular resistance and reactivity in hypertensive rats. Blood Vessels 1974;11:145–158.
8. Berecek KH, Stocker M, Gross F: Changes in renal vascular reactivity at various stages of deoxycorticosterone hypertension in rats. Circ Res 1980;46:619–624.
9. Nishizaka MK, Zaman MA, Green SA, et al: Impaired endothelium-dependent flow-mediated vasodilation in hypertensive subjects with hyperaldosteronism. Circulation 2004;109:2857–2861.
10. Gomez-Sanchez EP: Brain mineralocorticoid receptors: Orchestrators of hypertension and end-organ disease. Curr Opin Nephrol Hypertens 2004;13:191–196.
11. Gumz ML, Popp MP, Wingo CS, Cain BD: Early transcriptional effects of aldosterone in a mouse inner medullary collecting duct cell line. Am J Physiol Renal Physiol 2003;285:F664–F673.
12. Fuller PJ, Young MJ: Mechanisms of mineralocorticoid action. Hypertension 2005;46:1227–1235.
13. Rogerson FM, Fuller PJ: Mineralocorticoid action. Steroids 2000;65:61–73.
14. Funder JW: Non-genomic actions of aldosterone: Role in hypertension. Curr Opin Nephrol Hypertens 2001;10:227–230.
15. Funder JW: The nongenomic actions of aldosterone. Endocr Rev 2005;26:313–321.
16. Ganguly A: Primary aldosteronism. N Engl J Med 1998;339:1828–1834.
17. Eide IK, Torjesen PA, Drolsum A, et al: Low-renin status in therapy-resistant hypertension: A clue to efficient treatment. J Hypertens 2004;22:2217–2226.
18. Mosso L, Carvajal C, Gonzalez A, Barraza A, et al: Primary aldosteronism and hypertensive disease. Hypertension 2003;42:161–165.
19. Stowasser M, Gordon RD, Gunasekera TG, et al: High rate of detection of primary aldosteronism, including surgically treatable forms, after "non-selective" screening of hypertensive patients. J Hypertens 2003;21:2149–2157.
20. Benchetrit S, Bernheim J, Podjarny E: Normokalemic hyperaldosteronism in patients with resistant hypertension. Isr Med Assoc J 2002;4:17–20.
21. Seiler L, Rump LC, Schulte-Monting J, et al: Diagnosis of primary aldosteronism: Value of different screening parameters and influence of antihypertensive medication. Eur J Endocrinol 2004;150:329–337.
22. Mulatero P, Rabbia F, Milan A, et al: Drug effects on aldosterone/plasma renin activity ratio in primary aldosteronism. Hypertension 2002;40:897–902.
23. Ulick S, Blumenfeld JD, Atlas SA, et al: The unique steroidogenesis of the aldosteronoma in the differential diagnosis of primary aldosteronism. J Clin Endocrinol Metab 1993;76:873–878.
24. Lifton RP, Dluhy RG, Powers M, et al: A chimaeric 11 beta-hydroxylase/aldosterone synthase gene causes glucocorticoid-remediable aldosteronism and human hypertension. Nature 1992;355:262–265.
25. Pascoe L, Curnow KM, Slutsker L, et al: Glucocorticoid-suppressible hyperaldosteronism results from hybrid genes created by unequal crossovers between CYP11B1 and CYP11B2. Proc Natl Acad Sci USA 1992;89:8327–8331.
26. Dluhy RG, Lifton RP: Glucocorticoid-remediable aldosteronism. Endocrinol Metab Clin North Am 1994;23:285–297.
27. Weinberger MH, Grim CE, Hollifield JW, et al: Primary aldosteronism: Diagnosis, localization, and treatment. Ann Intern Med 1979;90:386–395.
28. Sawka AM, Young WF Jr, Thompson GB, et al: Primary aldosteronism: Factors associated with normalization of blood pressure after surgery. Ann Intern Med 2001;135:258–261.
29. Meyer A, Brabant G, Behrend M: Long-term follow-up after adrenalectomy for primary aldosteronism. World J Surg 2005;29:155–159.
30. Jeunemaitre X, Chatellier G, Kreft-Jais C, et al: Efficacy and tolerance of spironolactone in essential hypertension. Am J Cardiol 1987;60:820–825.
31. Lim PO, Young WF, Macdonald TM: A review of the medical treatment of primary aldosteronism. J Hypertens 2001;19:353–361.

Neurogenic Hypertension, Including Hypertension Associated with Stroke or Spinal Cord Injury

Venkatesh Aiyagari, Sean Ruland, and Philip B. Gorelick

INTRODUCTION

It has been recognized for quite some that there is an intimate relationship between the nervous system and control of blood pressure. For example, there is a subset of individuals with essential hypertension in which hypertension appears to be primarily driven by sympathetic activation (see Chapter 32).[1] These patients frequently have an elevated heart rate and increased cardiac output and some show increased levels of plasma and urine catecholamine levels and a high rate of norepinephrine turnover.[2] Importantly, these patients respond better to α- and β-blockers and are relatively resistant to treatment with diuretics and angiotensin-converting enzyme (ACE) inhibitors (Fig. 38.1).[1,3]

There is also evidence that a hyperactive sympathetic nervous system may be an early precursor for sustained normokinetic hypertension (see Chapter 32). Tachycardia, for example, is a strong predictor of future hypertension. Long-standing sympathetic stimulation has been thought to lead to a downregulation of the β-receptors and an upregulation of α_1-receptors leading to peripheral vasoconstriction; catecholamine-induced renal injury may also predispose to the development of salt sensitivity.[4]

Features of neurogenic essential hypertension
Young male
Mild hypertension
Tachycardia

Abnormal catecholamine metabolism
  Increased plasma catecholamines
  Increased catecholamine turnover
  Decreased catecholamine uptake
  Increased sympathetic neuronal firing rate

Associated conditions such as
  Sleep apnea
  Obesity
  Insulin resistance
  Anxiety
  Alcoholism

Response to treatment
  Good response to β-blockers and central α-agonists (such as clonidine)
  Poor response to diuretics
  Perhaps less effective response with ACE inhibitors

Figure 38.1   Features of neurogenic essential hypertension.

While debate continues in relation to the role of the sympathetic nervous system overactivity in essential hypertension, it is well accepted that hypertension following different types of neurologic insults is driven largely by the sympathetic nervous system response. Patients with acute neurologic injuries have been noted to have an immediate elevation of blood pressure that has been thought to be part of a teleologic response to maintain cerebral perfusion in the setting of brain ischemia or increased intracranial pressure. Certain forms of chronic hypertension such as those associated with spinal cord injury or neurovascular compression syndromes also have a clear neurologic basis.

PHYSIOLOGY AND PATHOPHYSIOLOGY

Neural Control of Blood Pressure

The results of several experiments have established that the brainstem, especially the ventral medulla, is a key area in the maintenance of blood pressure (Fig. 38.2). The neuronal groups that are thought to be important include the nucleus tractus solitarius, which receives inhibitory baroreceptor afferents, and adrenergic and serotoninergic neuronal groups in the rostral ventrolateral medulla (RVLM) and rostral ventromedial medulla, which are the source of excitatory descending bulbospinal pressor pathways. In addition, there appears to be a depressor center located in the caudal ventrolateral medulla composed of γ-aminobutyric acid (GABA)–containing neurons that receives afferents from the nucleus tractus solitarius and projects to the rostral ventral medulla. It has been postulated that the inhibitory GABA-containing neurons are tonically active, and reduced activity of these neurons leads to hypertension.[5–7]

The ultimate effector units are the sympathetic neurons located in the intermediolateral cell column of the spinal cord and the para-sympathetic neurons found in the dorsal motor nucleus of the vagus and nucleus ambiguus located in the medulla. In addition, afferent impulses from the limbic system, cerebral cortex and hypothalamus also directly or indirectly project to the intermediolateral cell column of the spinal cord and influence blood pressure regulation.

Cerebrovascular Autoregulation

Cerebral perfusion pressure (CPP) is traditionally defined as the difference between the mean arterial blood pressure (MAP) and the intracranial pressure (ICP). Therefore, in the face of increased ICP, systemic blood pressure needs to be higher in order to maintain a constant CPP.

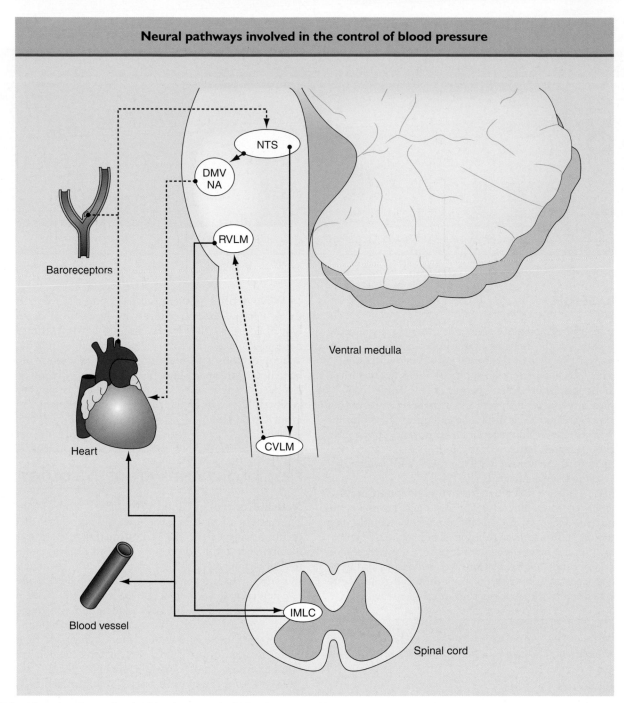

Neural pathways involved in the control of blood pressure

Figure 38.2 Neural pathways involved in the control of blood pressure. The ventral medulla has a key role in generating both excitatory (*solid line*) and inhibitory (*dotted line*) pathways, largely via the rostral ventrolateral medullary neurons (RVLM) and nucleus tractus solitarius (NTS), respectively. Ultimate effector control is provided by sympathetic activation originating in the intermediolateral cell column (IMLC) and parasympathetic action via the nucleus ambiguus (NA) and dorsal motor nucleus of the vagus nerve (DMV). CVLM, caudal ventrolateral medullary neurons.

Under normal conditions, cerebral blood flow (CBF) of the adult brain is 50 ml/100 g/min. CBF is regulated by the relationship between CPP and cerebrovascular resistance (CVR):

$$CBF = CPP/CVR.$$

Cerebrovascular autoregulation is the physiologic regulatory mechanism that maintains a constant blood flow over a wide range of CPPs. Normally, changes in CPP over a wide range have little effect on CBF. This is secondary to changes in CVR. An increase in CPP produces vasoconstriction and a decrease produces vasodilation. The normal range for autoregulation in human subjects is 60 to 150 mm Hg. In chronically hypertensive individuals, the cerebral arterioles develop medial hypertrophy and lose the ability to dilate effectively at lower pressures. This leads to a shift of the autoregulatory curve to the right.[8] In these individuals, a rapid reduction of blood pressure may lead to a drop in CBF even though the blood pressure might still be within the "normal" range. However, with effective control of hypertension for several months, the normal range for autoregulation can be re-established.[9]

Above the upper limit of autoregulation, there is breakthrough vasodilation leading to damage of the blood-brain barrier and cerebral edema. Below the lower limit of autoregulation, decreases in CPP lead to a decrease in CBF. Under these circumstances, increased extraction of oxygen and glucose maintains normal cerebral metabolism and brain function. When the CBF decreases to <20 ml/100 g/min, the increase in oxygen extraction is no longer able to supply the metabolic needs of the brain, leading to impairment of brain function.

SPECIFIC SYNDROMES

Hypertension Following Stroke
Epidemiology
Hypertension is the most important modifiable risk factor for stroke. A 5 mm lower diastolic pressure together with a 9 mm lower systolic pressure confers a 33% lower risk of stroke, and a 10 mm lower diastolic pressure together with an 18 to 19 mm lower systolic pressure confers more than a 50% reduction in stroke risk.[10] Combined data from 40 trials of antihypertensive agents have demonstrated that a 10% reduction in systolic blood pressure lowers stroke risk by one third.[11] Among patients who have already had a stroke, the results of the Perindopril Protection Against Recurrent Stroke Study (PROGRESS) showed a significant reduction of total stroke recurrence by 28% and a reduction of major coronary and vascular events by 26% over a 4-year follow-up period. This effect was achieved with an average net reduction in blood pressure by 9/4 (systolic/diastolic) mm Hg. This beneficial effect was present even in the subgroup with a normal initial blood pressure.[12] Thus, it is universally accepted that in the long run, reduction in blood pressure is effective in the primary prevention of stroke and also significantly improves outcomes in patients who have had a stroke.

However, the management of blood pressure in the immediate aftermath of a stroke is controversial.[13] A very high proportion of patients have elevated blood pressure immediately after a stroke, and blood pressure has been shown to spontaneously decrease over 7 to 10 days to the prestroke baseline in most patients. Most studies have shown that patients with increased blood pressure have higher mortality. However, it is uncertain whether the increased blood pressure directly contributes to poor outcome and whether immediate lowering of blood pressure will lead to better outcomes. There are no well-designed, controlled clinical trials that help answer questions such as how soon after a stroke blood pressure should be lowered, how fast, and by how much. In the following sections, we discuss the management of blood pressure in acute ischemic stroke, intracerebral hemorrhage (ICH), and subarachnoid hemorrhage (SAH).

Pathophysiology
Elevated blood pressure is seen in about one third to two thirds of all patients after a stroke. The cause of this increase in blood pressure and the subsequent decrease has not been determined. Some of the postulated causes are listed in Figure 38.3. An understanding of certain alterations of cerebrovascular physiology is essential in order to understand the pros and cons of treating hypertension in these patients (Fig. 38.4).

In patients with an ischemic stroke, there is evidence to suggest that vascular occlusion leads to a central core of irreversibly ischemic brain. This core is surrounded by an ischemic penumbra where blood flow is reduced but brain tissue is still viable. Usually, after 2 to 3 days, neurons in this ischemic penumbra either recover completely or undergo infarction. However, in the first few days, perfusion in this zone is marginal and a further decrease in blood flow by reduction in blood pressure might convert the ischemic zone to irreversible infarction. In

Postulated causes of hypertension after stroke
Pre-existing hypertension
White coat effect
Stress of hospitalization
Cushing reflex*
Catecholamine and cortisol release
Lesion of brainstem or hypothalamus
Nonspecific response to brain damage

Figure 38.3   Postulated causes of hypertension after stroke. *A hypothalamic response to ischemia consisting of hypertension with bradycardia.

Pros and cons of acute treatment of hypertension in stroke		
	Pros	**Cons**
Acute ischemic stroke	Might lower mortality Might decrease stroke progression Might decrease hemorrhagic transformation (especially after t-PA) Might decrease cerebral edema formation Might be helpful for systemic reasons (e.g., associated myocardial ischemia) Patients likely to be more compliant with antihypertensive use if treatment is initiated in the hospital	Decreases on its own No proven benefit Ongoing ischemia around the infarct (ischemic penumbra) Altered autoregulation due to Chronic hypertension Ischemia Large-vessel stenosis might have resulted in reduction of perfusion Chance of propagating thrombus Anecdotal case reports and trial results demonstrating deterioration with decrease in blood pressure Principle of do no harm (*primum non nocere*)
Acute intracerebral hemorrhage	Might lower mortality Might decrease hematoma expansion Might decrease cerebral edema formation Might be helpful for systemic reasons (e.g., associated myocardial ischemia) Patients likely to be more compliant with antihypertensive use if treatment is initiated in the hospital	Decreases on its own No proven benefit There may be a zone of ischemia around an intracerebral hematoma Chronically hypertensive patients require higher perfusion pressure due to shift of autoregulatory curve ICP may be elevated and lowering BP reduces what could be marginal CPP Principle of do no harm (*primum non nocere*)
Aneurysmal subarachnoid hemorrhage	Might decrease rebleeding rate Might help if there is cardiac ischemia (stunned myocardium)	No proven benefit ICP may be elevated and lowering BP reduces what could be marginal CPP Might lead to cerebral ischemia in the presence of vasospasm

Figure 38.4   Pros and cons of acute treatment of hypertension in stroke. BP, blood pressure; CPP, cerebral perfusion pressure; ICP, intracranial pressure; t-PA, tissue plasminogen activator.

addition, autoregulation is impaired in the setting of cerebral ischemia. Finally, hypotension might theoretically promote stasis and propagation of thrombus in the setting of vascular occlusion. On the other hand, hypertension might increase hemorrhagic transformation of the infarcted area and worsen edema formation. The risk of hemorrhagic transformation is particularly high when treatment with thrombolytic agents has been instituted, and this circumstance is discussed later. At times it might be difficult to distinguish between hypertensive encephalopathy, where lowering blood pressure is clearly indicated, and ischemic stroke with hypertension. It is important to remember that hypertensive encephalopathy is a syndrome of global neurologic dysfunction, usually with papilledema, and focal neurologic deficits are usually less prominent. On the other hand, in an acute ischemic stroke, the focal neurologic deficit is more prominent and alterations of consciousness are less common early on except with brainstem strokes. Last, a significant proportion of patients with stroke may have associated conditions such as myocardial infarction or aortic dissection where lowering blood pressure is warranted.

In patients with ICH, the considerations are slightly different. It is well recognized that hematoma expansion can occur in about one third of patients with ICH in the first 24 hours.[14] It seems intuitive to think that lowering blood pressure might decrease hematoma expansion; however, the evidence in support of this is not conclusive. Early studies had postulated that there may be a zone of ischemia around the hematoma, and lowering blood pressure might lead to neuronal death in this ischemic zone. However, recent studies do not support the existence of such a perihematomal ischemic zone. Last, increased ICP due to the ICH or associated hydrocephalus might lead to a decrease in CPP. In such a situation, where increased blood pressure may be maintaining optimal cerebral perfusion, lowering blood pressure is not warranted.

In patients with aneurysmal SAH, the considerations are again different. Immediately after aneurysmal rupture, there is a significant risk of rebleeding. In order to decrease the rebleeding risk, most neurosurgeons recommend tight control of blood pressure. A significant proportion of patients with SAH have associated myocardial dysfunction (stunned myocardium). A high systemic blood pressure might worsen myocardial function in such situations. However, one also needs to be cognizant of the CPP, which might become insufficient to maintain optimal cerebral perfusion when systemic blood pressure is lowered in the face of increased ICP due to hydrocephalus or an associated ICH. In the latter half of the first week and in the second week after SAH, many patients develop vasospasm of the intracranial arteries. This is often associated with altered autoregulation and cerebral ischemia. Reduction of blood pressure may lead to worsening of cerebral ischemia, and induced hypertension might improve cerebral perfusion. Therefore, once the aneurysmal rupture has been definitively treated with surgical clipping or coiling, blood pressure is usually maintained at a normal or slightly elevated level in these patients.

Diagnosis and Treatment

There is no firm evidence to help answer questions such as what the threshold should be at which blood pressure reduction should be instituted, when treatment should be started, how fast and by how much blood pressure should be lowered, and whether previously hypertensive patients should continue or stop taking their previous antihypertensives immediately after a stroke. Recommendations for treating blood pressure in different clinical situations outlined in Figure 38.5 reflect our personal preference.

Acute Ischemic Stroke

While several case reports document worsening of the neurologic deficit in patients with stroke after an abrupt severe decline in blood pressure, data from large clinical trials have not been conclusive. The Intravenous Nimodipine West European Stroke Trial showed that >20% reduction of diastolic blood pressure on day 2 was associated with a worse outcome.[15] In the Glycine Antagonist in Neuroprotection International Trial, however, early decrease in blood pressure had no effect on outcome.[16] The Acute Candesartan Cilexitil Evaluation in Stroke Survivors trial randomized 342 patients within 72 hours of a stroke if they were conscious, had a motor paresis, and were hypertensive (occasional blood pressure ≥200/110 mm Hg or median of two measurements in 30 minutes ≥180/105 mm Hg). The combined endpoint of total mortality, cerebral complications and cardiovascular complications at the end of 3 months was reduced by 47.5% for patients treated with candesartan (4 to 16 mg) initiated within 72 hours after stroke as compared to those in whom it was instituted 7 days later. However, this difference in outcome was not associated with any difference in blood pressure.[17]

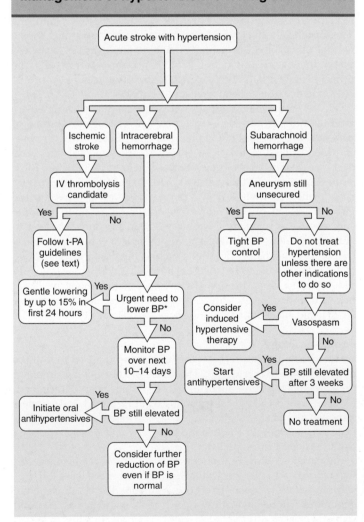

Figure 38.5   Management of hypertension following acute stroke. t-PA, tissue plasminogen activator. *Indication for treatment includes systolic blood pressure (BP) >220 mm Hg or diastolic BP >120 mm Hg for ischemic stroke, mean arterial BP >130 mm Hg for cerebral hemorrhage, and the presence of associated conditions such as aortic dissection or myocardial infarction.

Currently, the American Stroke Association (ASA) and the European Stroke Initiative (EUSI) recommend withholding antihypertensive treatment immediately after an ischemic stroke unless the systolic blood pressure is >220 mm Hg or the diastolic blood pressure is >120 mm Hg. The ASA recommends lowering blood pressure by 10% to 15%, while the EUSI suggests a target blood pressure of 180/100 to 105 mm Hg in hypertensive patients and 160 to 180/90 to 100 mm Hg in normotensive individuals. In patients who are candidates for treatment with intravenous tissue plasminogen activator (t-PA), systolic blood pressure should not be >185 mm Hg or diastolic blood pressure >110 mm Hg at the time of treatment. For the first 24 hours after treatment with t-PA, systolic blood pressure should be maintained at <180 mm Hg and diastolic blood pressure at <105 mm Hg.[18]

Intracerebral Hemorrhage

While a few small studies suggest that treatment of hypertension might be associated with better outcomes, a decrease in mean arterial pressure (MAP) by >20% or <110 mm Hg has also been shown to be associated with impaired autoregulation.[19] A small controlled study of 14 hypertensive patients with a small to moderate–sized ICH within 24 hours showed that treatment with nicardipine or labetalol to reduce MAP by 15% up to a lower limit of ~120 mm Hg produced no change in cerebral blood flow.[20] The American Heart Association recommends maintaining MAP at <130 mm Hg and CPP >70 mm Hg. Immediately after surgical evacuation of ICH, MAP should be kept at <110 mm Hg.[21] Since ICH is more likely to be associated with increased ICP compared to ischemic stroke, MAP and CPP goals rather than systolic or diastolic goals might be more appropriate in this setting.

Subarachnoid Hemorrhage

As discussed previously, prior to definitive treatment of the ruptured aneurysm, systolic blood pressure is usually kept at <140 to 160 mm Hg, although there is no conclusive evidence that higher blood pressures increase rebleeding rate. In patients with suspected elevation of ICP, it is important to monitor ICP and keep the CPP >70 mm Hg. After the ruptured aneurysm has been protected, aggressive treatment of blood pressure should be avoided and in the setting of cerebral vasospasm, systolic blood pressure is usually elevated until the neurodeficits resolve, generally up to a systolic blood pressure of 200 to 220 mm Hg.

Cerebrovascular Effects of Antihypertensive Agents

When choosing to treat hypertension in a patient with intracranial pathology, the clinician has several options. Different classes of antihypertensive agents have different direct effects on the CBF, ICP, and autoregulation. The ideal drug to choose would be one that does not increase ICP or decrease blood flow to ischemic regions. In addition, when treating hypertension in the acute setting, drugs that can be given intravenously, have a short half-life, and do not cause sedation are preferable. In the chronic phase after a stroke, there is no clear evidence favoring one class of antihypertensive agent over another.

The advantages and disadvantages of various classes of antihypertensive agents in the acute setting of stroke are summarized in Figure 38.6. Commonly used treatments include intermittent intravenous boluses of labetalol or hydralazine or infusions of agents such as nicardipine, esmolol, nitroprusside, and labetalol. β-Adrenergic antagonists such as esmolol and combined α- and β-adrenergic receptor antagonists like labetalol do not increase ICP or affect cerebral autoregulation. They are suitable for treatment of hypertension in the setting of cerebral ischemia or increased ICP. However, bradycardia secondary to increased ICP is a relative contraindication. Vasodilators like hydralazine, sodium nitroprusside, and nitroglycerin cause cerebral arterial dilation and venodilation and can theoretically increase ICP and cause a cerebral steal phenomenon in patients with cerebral ischemia. However, they may be used in patients with small- and moderate-sized ICH and in patients with SAH if increased ICP is not a concern. Calcium channel blockers have varying effects on

Preferred antihypertensive agents in the treatment of stroke-associated hypertension				
Drug	Mechanism of Action	Intravenous Dose	Advantages	Disadvantages
Labetalol	α_1-, β_1-, and β_2-receptor antagonist	Test dose 5 mg, then 20-to-80-mg bolus every 10 mins up to 300 mg; IV infusion 0.5–2 mg/min	Does not lower CBF 20-to-80 mg Does not increase ICP	May exacerbate bradycardia
Esmolol	β_1-receptor antagonist	500-µg/kg bolus, then 50–300 mg/kg/min	Does not lower CBF Does not increase ICP	May exacerbate bradycardia
Sodium nitroprusside	Vasodilator	0.25–10 µg/kg/min	Potent antihypertensive	May increase ICP Can cause cerebral steal Potential for cyanide toxicity
Nitroglycerin	Vasodilator	5–100 µg/kg/min	Can be helpful for concomitant cardiac ischemia	May increase ICP Can cause cerebral steal
Hydralazine	Vasodilator	2.5-to-10-mg bolus	Can be given as IV bolus when labetalol is contraindicated due to bradycardia	May increase ICP Can cause cerebral steal
Nicardipine	L-type calcium channel blocker	5–15 mg/h	Does not decrease CBF	May increase ICP Long duration of action
Enalaprilat	ACE inhibitor	0.625–1.25 mg every 6 hrs	Does not decrease CBF	Variable response Long duration of action

Figure 38.6   Preferred antihypertensive agents in the treatment of stroke-associated hypertension. ACE, angiotensin-converting inhibitor; CBF, cerebral blood flow; ICP, intracranial pressure.

cerebral autoregulation. Nifedipine can lead to drastic reduction in blood pressure and is not recommended. Nimodipine is used routinely in patients with SAH as it has been shown to improve outcome, possibly due to a neuroprotective effect. Nicardipine has been used in patients with acute ICH without any change in CBF and is often used in patients with SAH. ACE inhibitors such as perindopril and the angiotensin receptor blocker (ARB) candesartan have been used in patients with cerebral ischemia and have no effect on CBF. However, short-acting parenteral forms of these drugs are not available. ACE inhibitors and ARBs also have been shown to shift the lower limit of cerebral autoregulation toward lower blood pressure in rats and humans. However, these agents have a long half-life, which is not desirable in treating hypertension in the acute phase. Similarly, due to its long half-life and sedative effect the α_2-adrenergic agonist is not preferred. The recommended doses of these agents are summarized in Figure 38.6.

Hypertension Following Carotid Endarterectomy and Endovascular Procedures
Definition and Epidemiology
Hemodynamic disturbances such as hypotension, bradycardia, and hypertension are seen frequently following carotid endarterectomy (CEA) and endovascular procedures such as angioplasty or stenting. Hypertension develops in about 10% to 40% of such cases. It may be associated with a rare but serious consequence known as carotid hyperperfusion (or reperfusion) syndrome in about 10% of patients within the first week following surgery or angioplasty/stenting.[22–24] The syndrome manifests as transient or permanent contralateral neurologic signs, ipsilateral pulsatile headache, seizures, and ICH, or reversible cerebral edema.

Pathophysiology
Pre-existing hypertension, baroreceptor impairment following surgical manipulation, and elevated catecholamine levels after cerebral hypoperfusion during intraoperative cross-clamping have all been postulated to contribute to postoperative hypertension. Postoperative hypertension may, in turn, contribute to cerebral hyperperfusion. Although the mechanism responsible for carotid hyperperfusion syndrome is not known, it may be due to impaired autoregulation from chronic vasodilation of the distal vascular bed ipsilateral to a hemodynamically significant internal carotid artery stenosis.[25] Other postulated mechanisms for this syndrome include activation of the trigeminovascular axon reflex and derangement of the carotid baroreceptors.[26]

Diagnosis and Treatment
Patients at risk of development of this syndrome can be identified by various techniques that demonstrate preoperative hypoperfusion and impaired autoregulation or postoperative hyperperfusion.[27] Classically, hyperperfusion has been defined by >100% postoperative increase in CBF compared to preoperative flow. However, the increase in blood flow may only be approximately 20% compared to the contralateral side.[28] An intraoperative ipsilateral increase in cerebral oxygen saturation after unclamping the internal carotid artery can also identify patients at risk of developing this syndrome.[29]

Due to the risk of developing carotid hyperperfusion syndrome following carotid endarterectomy or stenting, all patients should have continuous intraoperative and postoperative blood pressure monitoring. Most authors advocate strict blood pressure control (systolic blood pressure <120 mm Hg) from the time of intraoperative internal carotid artery unclamping or angioplasty.

Elevated blood pressure should be treated with agents such as labetalol or clonidine. Vasodilators such as nitroglycerin and sodium nitroprusside should probably be avoided.[28]

Hypertension and Neurovascular Compression Syndromes
Definition and Epidemiology
In 1979, Jannetta and Gendell[30] reported that some patients with essential hypertension may have elevated blood pressure secondary to compression of the lower brainstem by vascular loops of the vertebral artery or posterior inferior cerebellar artery and that microvascular decompression of the ninth or 10th cranial nerves could lower the blood pressure. Since then, neuroimaging studies in selected patients with essential hypertension have reported a variable but common prevalence of this phenomenon.[31,32] Laxity of intracranial supporting tissue associated with aging has been postulated as a mechanism by which a vascular loop might come into abnormally close contact with mediating neural structures. Additionally, genetic factors have been suggested but the responsible gene has not been elucidated.[33] However, other studies have found an equal prevalence of vascular loops in patients with and without hypertension, which calls into question the existence of this mechanism of hypertension.

Pathophysiology
Pulsatile compression on the RVLM in the medulla from an abnormal vascular loop has been proposed to lead to increased sympathetic efferent activity. Increased blood pressure in animal models has been induced by experimental pulsatile compression of the RVLM but not the surrounding regions. Additionally, higher circulating plasma norepinephrine levels have been demonstrated in patients with essential hypertension and magnetic resonance imaging (MRI) evidence of pulsatile compression of the RVLM compared to those with essential hypertension and no MRI evidence of RVLM compression.[34]

Jannetta and some other investigators have shown favorable effects on arterial blood pressure following surgical decompression. Reduced plasma and urine norepinephrine levels and muscle sympathetic nerve activity have also been documented following microvascular decompression for cranial neuralgias in patients with essential hypertension noted to have compression of the RVLM by an abnormal vascular loop.[31,34,35]

Diagnosis and Treatment
Despite the observed benefits of surgical decompression in selected case series, the theory of neurovascular medullary compression as a cause of hypertension has not been universally accepted. Even where vascular compression can be demonstrated, surgical decompression has not been universally shown to decrease the elevated blood pressure. The risk-to-benefit ratio is not known, and, in addition, the efficacy of such treatment in leading to long-term control of blood pressure has not been proven. In the absence of definitive evidence that vascular compression of the medulla causes hypertension that can be treated by surgical decompression, the authors do not recommend screening for this entity or surgical decompression in hypertensive patients where a vascular loop compressing the RVLM has been incidentally found. A multicenter trial is being currently conducted to evaluate the efficacy of microvascular decompression in patients with persistent severe hypertension despite being on at least three antihypertensive medicines and having failed at least three different medication regimens in whom other causes of hypertension have been ruled out.[35]

Hypertension Following Spinal Cord Injury
Definition and Epidemiology

Venous thromboembolism, pressure sores (decubitus ulcers), infections, and gut immotility are well-known causes of morbidity and mortality after spinal cord injury. Autonomic dysreflexia is another perhaps underappreciated consequence occurring in up to 70% of case series. If unrecognized, it can result in serious sequelae such as posterior leukoencephalopathy, ICH, SAH, seizures, arrhythmia, pulmonary edema, and retinal hemorrhage and result in coma and even death.[36]

Pathophysiology and Diagnosis

The spinal cord lesion is typically above the sixth thoracic spinal nerve level. Immediately after the injury, there is initial loss of supraspinal sympathetic control similar to the initial period of muscular flaccidity. This often leads to hypotension and bradycardia (spinal shock). Subsequently, after a few weeks to months, there is extrajunctional sprouting of the α-receptors, denervation hypersensitivity, and impaired presynaptic uptake of norepinephrine. In addition, there may be derangement of spinal glutaminergic interneurons. Noxious stimuli below the neurologic level of the lesion trigger a spinal reflex arc that results in increased sympathetic tone and hypertension.[37] The most common inciting events are urinary overdistention and fecal impaction. However, it may be secondary to precipitants including sympathomimetic medications or sildenafil citrate used for sperm retrieval.[38]

Clinical symptoms include pulsatile headache, blurred vision, nasal congestion, nausea, and sweating above the spinal nerve level. The flushed sweaty skin above the lesion level is due to brainstem parasympathetic activation. At and below the lesion, the skin remains pale, cool, and dry. Heart rate can be quite variable from bradycardia to tachycardia. The hallmark physical finding is elevated blood pressure. However, as blood pressure may normally be quite low after spinal cord injury, baseline blood pressure readings may be within the normal range and be elevated for a given individual, making clinical suspicion and reliance on other clinical signs and symptoms paramount in the diagnosis if baseline blood pressure is not known.[37]

Treatment

Although vigilant preventive measures to decrease the incidence of autonomic dysreflexia such as proper bowel, bladder, and skin care are the primary treatment, clinical recognition and expeditious treatment initiation of elevated blood pressure are paramount to avoid the potentially severe consequences. Placing the patient upright to precipitate orthostatic blood pressure lowering and removal of any possible noxious stimuli such as binding clothing or devices are the initial treatment steps. Checking for urinary overdistention and changing, flushing, or inserting a new catheter if the patient receives intermittent catheterization is important.

Pharmacologic treatment with rapid-acting, short-lived agents may be indicated for systolic blood pressure elevation ≥150 mm Hg persisting after the preceding interventions. Caution should be taken to avoid nitrate-containing agents for patients using sildenafil or similar agents within the preceding 24 hours as concomitant nitrate use may result in precipitous hypotension.

If the bladder is empty and the blood pressure is <150 mm Hg, fecal disimpaction with topical anesthetic should be attempted. If dysreflexia is refractory or associated with severe clinical presentation, other precipitants should be sought and hospitalization may be indicated.[39]

Last, up to 90% of pregnant women with upper spinal cord injury experience autonomic dysreflexia during labor and delivery. Appropriate epidural or spinal anesthesia techniques can ameliorate the risk.[40]

REFERENCES

1. Grassi G, Mancia G: Neurogenic hypertension: Is the enigma of its origin near the solution? Hypertension 2004;43:154–155.
2. Schlaich MP, Lambert E, Kaye DM, et al: Sympathetic augmentation in hypertension: Role of nerve firing, norepinephrine reuptake, and angiotensin neuromodulation. Hypertension 2004;43:169–175.
3. Mann SJ: Neurogenic essential hypertension revisited: The case for increased clinical and research attention. Am J Hypertens 2003;16:881–888.
4. Egan BM: Neurogenic mechanisms initiating essential hypertension. Am J Hypertens 1989;2:357S–362S.
5. Chalmers J: Volhard Lecture. Brain, blood pressure and stroke. J Hypertens 1998;16:1849–1858.
6. Colombari E, Sato MA, Cravo SL, et al: Role of the medulla oblongata in hypertension. Hypertension 2001;38:549–554.
7. Talman WT: Cardiovascular regulation and lesions of the central nervous system. Ann Neurol 1985;18:1–13.
8. Strandgaard S, Olesen J, Skinhoj E, Lassen NA: Autoregulation of brain circulation in severe arterial hypertension. BMJ 1973;1:507–510.
9. Strandgaard S: Autoregulation of cerebral blood flow in hypertensive patients. The modifying influence of prolonged antihypertensive treatment on the tolerance to acute, drug-induced hypotension. Circulation 1976;53:720–727.
10. MacMahon S, Peto R, Cutler J, et al: Blood pressure, stroke, and coronary heart disease. Part 1, Prolonged differences in blood pressure: Prospective observational studies corrected for the regression dilution bias. Lancet 1990;335:765–774.
11. Lawes CM, Bennett DA, Feigin VL, Rodgers A: Blood pressure and stroke: An overview of published reviews. Stroke 2004;35:1024.
12. PROGRESS Collaborative Group: Randomised trial of a perindopril-based blood-pressure-lowering regimen among 6,105 individuals with previous stroke or transient ischaemic attack. Lancet 2001;358:1033–1041.
13. Powers WJ: Acute hypertension after stroke: the scientific basis for treatment decisions. Neurology 1993;43:461–467.
14. Brott T, Broderick J, Kothari R, et al: Early hemorrhage growth in patients with intracerebral hemorrhage. Stroke 1997;28:1–5.
15. Ahmed N, Nasman P, Wahlgren NG: Effect of intravenous nimodipine on blood pressure and outcome after acute stroke. Stroke 2000;31:1250–1255.
16. Aslanyan S, Fazekas F, Weir CJ, et al, GAIN International Steering Committee and Investigators. Effect of blood pressure during the acute period of ischemic stroke on stroke outcome: A tertiary analysis of the GAIN International Trial. Stroke 2003;34:2420–2425.
17. Schrader J, Luders S, Kulschewski A, et al: Acute Candesartan Cilexetil Therapy in Stroke Survivors Study Group: The ACCESS Study: Evaluation of Acute Candesartan Cilexetil Therapy in Stroke Survivors. Stroke 2003;34:1699–1703.
18. Klijn CJ, Hankey GJ, American Stroke Association and European Stroke Initiative: Management of acute ischaemic stroke: New guidelines from the American Stroke Association and European Stroke Initiative. Lancet Neurol 2003;2:698–701.
19. Kuwata N, Kuroda K, Funayama M, et al: Dysautoregulation in patients with hypertensive intracerebral hemorrhage. A SPECT study. Neurosurg Rev 1995;18:237–245.
20. Powers WJ, Zazulia AR, Videen TO, et al: Autoregulation of cerebral blood flow surrounding acute (6 to 22 hours) intracerebral hemorrhage. Neurology 2001;57:18–24.
21. Broderick JP, Adams HP Jr, Barsan W, et al: Guidelines for the management of spontaneous intracerebral hemorrhage: A statement for healthcare professionals from a special writing group of the Stroke Council, American Heart Association. Stroke 1999;30:905–915.
22. Qureshi AI, Luft AR, Sharma M, et al: Frequency and determinants of postprocedural hemodynamic instability after carotid angioplasty and stenting. Stroke 1999;30:2086–2093.

23. Wade JG, Larson CP Jr, Hickey RF, et al: Effect of carotid endarterectomy on carotid chemoreceptor and baroreceptor function in man. N Engl J Med 1970;282:823–829.

24. Wong JH, Findlay JM, Suarez-Almazor ME: Hemodynamic instability after carotid endarterectomy: Risk factors and associations with operative complications. Neurosurgery 1997;41:35–43.

25. Yoshimoto T, Houkin K, Kuroda S, et al: Low cerebral blood flow and perfusion reserve induce hyperperfusion after surgical revascularization: Case reports and analysis of cerebral hemodynamics. Surg Neurol 1997;48:132–139.

26. van Mook WN, Rennenberg RJ, Schurink GW, et al: Cerebral hyperperfusion syndrome. Lancet Neurol 2005;4:877–888.

27. Hosoda K, Kawaguchi T, Shibata Y, et al: Cerebral vasoreactivity and internal carotid artery flow help to identify patients at risk for hyperperfusion after carotid endarterectomy. Stroke 2001;32:1567–1573.

28. Karapanayiotides T, Meuli R, Devuyst G, et al: Postcarotid endarterectomy hyperperfusion or reperfusion syndrome. Stroke 2005;36:21–26.

29. Ogasawara K, Konno H, Yukawa H, et al: Transcranial regional cerebral oxygen saturation monitoring during carotid endarterectomy as a predictor of postoperative hyperperfusion. Neurosurgery 2003;53:309–315.

30. Jannetta PJ, Gendell HM: Clinical observations on etiology of essential hypertension. Surg Forum 1979;30:431–432.

31. Jannetta PJ, Segal R, Wolfson SK Jr: Neurogenic hypertension: Etiology and surgical treatment. I. Observations in 53 patients. Ann Surg 1985;201:391–398.

32. Morimoto S, Sasaki S, Miki S, et al: Neurovascular compression of the rostral ventrolateral medulla related to essential hypertension. Hypertension 1997;30:77–82.

33. Morimoto S, Sasaki S, Itoh H, et al: Sympathetic activation and contribution of genetic factors in hypertension with neurovascular compression of the rostral ventrolateral medulla. J Hypertens 1999;17:1577–1582.

34. Morimoto S, Sasaki S, Takeda K, et al: Decreases in blood pressure and sympathetic nerve activity by microvascular decompression of the rostral ventrolateral medulla in essential hypertension. Stroke 1999;30:1707–1710.

35. Levy EI, Scarrow AM, Jannetta PJ: Microvascular decompression in the treatment of hypertension: Review and update. Surg Neurol 2001;55:2–10; discussion 10–1.

36. Valles M, Benito J, Portell E, Vidal J: Cerebral hemorrhage due to autonomic dysreflexia in a spinal cord injury patient. Spinal Cord 2005;43:738–740.

37. Blackmer J: Rehabilitation medicine: 1. Autonomic dysreflexia. CMAJ 2003;169:931–935.

38. Sheel AW, Krassioukov AV, Inglis JT, Elliott SL: Autonomic dysreflexia during sperm retrieval in spinal cord injury: influence of lesion level and sildenafil citrate. J Appl Physiol 2005;99:53–58.

39. Consortium for Spinal Cord Medicine: Acute management of autonomic dysreflexia: Individuals with spinal cord injury presenting to health-care facilities. J Spinal Cord Med 2002;25(Suppl 1):S67–S88.

40. Ribes Pastor MP, Vanarase M: Peripartum anaesthetic management of a parturient with spinal cord injury and autonomic hyperreflexia. Anaesthesia 2004;59:94.

Hypertension in African Americans

John M. Flack, Samar A. Nasser, and Shannon M. O'Connor

DEFINITION

African American men and women have an earlier onset, higher incidence and prevalence, greater severity, and excess cardiovascular-renal target organ damage (i.e., stroke, left ventricular hypertrophy (LVH), renal insufficiency) for any given blood pressure (BP) level compared with Caucasians. This observation has caused some to hypothesize that there should be race-specific BP levels for the diagnosis and treatment of hypertension. The seventh report of the Joint National Committee on Prevention, Detection, Evaluation, and Treatment of High Blood Pressure (JNC 7) recommends a minimal target BP of <130/80 mm Hg for individuals with diabetes mellitus and/or chronic kidney disease (estimated glomerular filtration rate [GFR] <60 ml/min/1.73m² or a spot albumin-to-creatinine ratio of >200 mg/g).[1] These conditions all disproportionately affect African Americans. Therefore, when JNC 7 criteria are applied for risk stratification, many African Americans have target BP levels <130/80 mm Hg. The International Society on Hypertension in Blacks (ISHIB) recommends target BP levels <130/80 mm Hg for high-risk hypertensives with conditions such as metabolic syndrome, LVH, heart failure, and coronary heart disease.[2]

EPIDEMIOLOGY

The age-adjusted hypertension prevalence in the adult U.S. population is 28.7%.[3] The age-adjusted rate of hypertension in African Americans is 33.5% versus 28.9% for Caucasians and 20.7% in Mexican Americans. The African American excess of hypertension relative to Caucasians is greater in women than men. Although it is widely perceived that African Americans have the highest hypertension rates in the world, persons in Spain, Finland, and Germany all have higher rates of hypertension.[4] Interestingly, hypertension was rare in Blacks living in Africa prior to 1940, but with industrialization and the introduction of Western diet and culture, there has been a steady increase in prevalence of hypertension, particularly in the larger cities. There is also an escalating east-west prevalence gradient of hypertension risk in Blacks, being lowest in Africa, intermediate in the Caribbean, and highest in the urban Midwestern United States.[5]

There is also an increased frequency of hypertension-related complications in African Americans.[6] Overall, African Americans have a higher prevalence of hypertension-related target organ damage (stroke, LVH, and renal disease),[7] which in part may relate to the onset of hypertension at an earlier age than in Caucasians. In addition to an excess of pressure-related cardiovascular morbidity and mortality, African Americans have a marked (~4.5-fold) increased risk of developing renal failure secondary to hypertension.

PATHOGENESIS OF HYPERTENSION IN AFRICAN AMERICANS

There are numerous theories for the excess prevalence of hypertension among African Americans, some of which are based on the unproven belief that hypertension in African Americans is a distinct entity from hypertension in the Caucasian population. Figure 39.1 lists physiologic tendencies of the African American hypertensive. None of these characteristics are, however, unique to the African American hypertensive, but rather represent quantitative, not qualitative, differences between African Americans and other racial/ethnic groups.

Several factors predispose to the increased frequency of hypertension in the African American population. These include lower socioeconomic status, a diet higher in sodium and lower in potassium, obesity, insulin resistance, and physical inactivity.[8] Physical inactivity, especially among African American women, is a very likely contributor to the excess prevalence and incidence of hypertension. Low birth weight and/or prematurity have recently been recognized as augmenting cardiovascular-renal disease risk including the risk of hypertension.[9]

Physiologic characteristics associated with, but not unique to, hypertensive African Americans
Salt sensitivity
Obesity
High prevalence of coexisting cardiovascular disease risk factors in addition to increased blood pressure (i.e., insulin resistance, diabetes mellitus, smoking, dyslipidemia)
Decreased renal vasodilator hormones (e.g., reduced urinary kallikrein excretion)
Increased urinary protein excretion
Suppressed renin levels; possibly increased intrarenal angiotensin II
Decreased renal natriuretic capacity
High renal vascular resistance
Reduced renal blood flow
Increased peripheral vascular resistance
Excess blood pressure–related target organ damage (i.e., left ventricular hypertrophy, stroke, renal insufficiency)
Increased frequency of the double deletion (DD) genotype of the angiotensin-converting enzyme (ACE-DD)

Figure 39.1 Physiologic characteristics associated with, but not unique to, hypertensive African Americans.

Abnormal Diurnal Blood Pressure Variation

Normally BP falls ~10% to 20% from daytime (6 AM to 10 PM) levels during the night (12 AM to 6 AM). Individuals with lesser reductions in nocturnal BP have been classified as nondippers. Nondipping BP has been linked to higher levels of pressure-related target-organ injury and is more common in African Americans. Even among normotensives, approximately 30% of African Americans are nondippers.[10] Nevertheless, a number of dietary, physiologic, and environmental exposures appear to influence the magnitude of the nocturnal decline in BP (Fig. 39.2). Importantly, factors that lessen the nocturnal decline tend, in general, to be disproportionately prevalent in African Americans. However, the magnitude of the nocturnal fall in BP can be augmented, for example, by increased dietary intake of potassium.[11] Nondipping BP status also has been linked to salt sensitivity and renal progression.

Plasma Volume and Salt Sensitivity

Some studies have suggested that African American hypertensives are plasma volume expanded, but the evidence is not consistent.[12,13] In contrast, salt sensitivity is disproportionately manifest in African Americans, particularly among hypertensives. Salt sensitivity is defined as a rise in BP occurring during salt administration and/or a fall in BP occurring when salt is restricted. The excess prevalence of salt sensitivity among African Americans may relate to the increased frequency of obesity in the African American population, as it has been demonstrated in both Caucasians and African Americans that obesity is linked to salt sensitivity and that weight loss ameliorates salt sensitivity, at least among overweight Caucasian adolescents.[14] Salt sensitivity is associated with lesser reduction in nocturnal BP as well as microalbuminuria, other pressure-related target-organ injury, and greater antihypertensive medication requirements.

Sympathetic Nervous System

African Americans manifest higher α- but diminished β-adrenergic sympathetic nervous system (SNS) tone compared to Caucasians.[15] Obesity appears to play a role in heightened SNS tone in African American women. Interestingly, lean African American men appear to have SNS tone equivalent to that of overweight individuals of other race/sex groups.[16] There is no consistent pattern of racial difference in basal SNS tone. Nevertheless, stress-induced augmentation of SNS tone appears to be greater in African Americans than Caucasians, and the increase in peripheral arterial resistance appears to be greater in African Americans.[15]

Vascular Function

Most studies demonstrate more depressed endothelium-dependent and endothelium-independent vascular responses in African Americans compared to Caucasians,[17,18] which may contribute to target-organ ischemia/injury as well as modify vascular responsiveness to antihypertensive drugs.

Possible Mechanisms of Excessive Renal Injury in African Americans

It has been hypothesized that African Americans have defective renal autoregulation of glomerular filtration, in which inappropriately low tone of the afferent (preglomerular) arteriole leads to excessive transmission of systemic BP to the renal glomerulus. Indeed, an exaggerated increase in GFR, consistent with vasodilation of the afferent glomerular arteriole, has been shown during dietary salt loading in African Americans when compared with Caucasians.[19] In apparently healthy African Americans, the local renin angiotensin system (RAS) in the kidney appears to be more active than in similar Caucasians.[20] A number of conditions can lead to abnormal renal autoregulation including high sodium diet, reduced renal mass, proteinuria, and diabetes mellitus.[21] Other potential predisposing conditions may include obesity/metabolic syndrome, elevated uric acid, low-grade lead toxicity, and higher plasma transforming growth factor β (TGF-β) levels, all of which are increased in frequency in the African American.[22]

Hypertensive African Americans have higher renal vascular resistance and lower renal blood flow for the same level of BP, when compared with Caucasians. Glomeruli from African Americans are also larger, which may reflect a higher frequency of low birth weight and a congenital reduction in nephron number.[23] In turn, low birth weight and/or premature delivery appears to predispose to higher BP and endothelial dysfunction in childhood and cardiovascular diseases later in life including hypertension and diabetes mellitus. The reduction in nephron number may predispose to altered autoregulation with increased transmission of systemic BP into the glomerulus, thereby predisposing to renal injury (Fig. 39.3). A pervasive physiologic insult, like obesity, that is more common in African American than Caucasian women, may plausibly contribute to the excess renal injury observed in this population.[24]

Renin Angiotensin Aldosterone Kinin System

Hypertension in the African American has been characterized as a type of low-renin hypertension. As discussed previously, the evidence that this may be due to plasma volume expansion remains questionable. We have hypothesized that suppressed circulating renin levels may represent overactivity of the vasoconstrictive, proliferative, antinatriuretic arm of the renin angiotensin aldosterone kinin (RAAK) system with underactivity of the vasodilatory, antiproliferative natriuretic arm.[25] We have termed this imbalance RAAK system disequilibrium. Activation of the local RAS with intrarenal angiotensin II (Ang II) generation, perhaps via reduced blood flow, renal ischemia, and/or obesity could both suppress the systemic RAS and also potentially increase intraglomerular pressure, thereby predisposing to pressure-related renal injury. Further, hypertensive African Americans have lower urinary levels

Factors influencing the nocturnal decrease in blood pressure	
Magnitude	
Greater	Lesser
Increased potassium intake	Sleep apnea
Nocturnal administration of Aspirin Melatonin	Evening/night shift work
	Low socioeconomic status
	Male sex
	Obesity
	Postmenopausal
	Increased sodium intake
	Salt sensitivity
	Increased sympathetic nervous system activity

Figure 39.2 Factors influencing the nocturnal decrease in blood pressure.

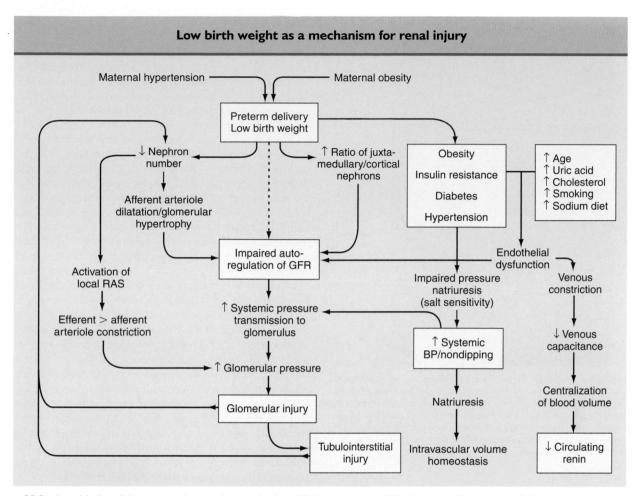

Figure 39.3 **Low birth weight as a mechanism for renal injury.** BP, blood pressure; GFR, glomerular filtration rate; RAS, renin angiotensin system.

of various natriuretic and vasodilatory substances, including kallikrein, nitric oxide metabolites, and dopamine.

Support for this hypothesis includes evidence of greater activation of the local renal RAS in apparently healthy African American compared to Caucasian adults.[19] Dietary sodium loading has also been reported to increase vascular generation of Ang II despite suppressing circulating renin in African Americans; the reverse was observed with sodium restriction.[26] Dietary sodium loading also depresses endothelium-dependent vascular function in the African American.[27] These studies significantly challenge the pervasive beliefs regarding the relationship of dietary sodium, circulating renin, and activity of the local RAS.

Endothelin

Endothelin-1 can induce vascular smooth muscle cell contraction and hypertrophy and stimulate Ang II synthesis while suppressing renin synthesis. Endothelin levels are elevated in hypertensive African Americans compared to normotensive and hypertensive African Americans and Caucasians.[28] In salt-sensitive hypertension, such as in African American patients, the endothelin response is exaggerated as a response to increased sympathetic activity.[29] Thus, endothelin may have a role in hypertension and related target organ damage, particularly in salt-sensitive African American hypertensives.

Transforming Growth Factor β

TGF-β1 is a fibrogenic cytokine induced by Ang II that is thought to have a major role in renal fibrosis and scarring.

TGF-β1 may also influence BP indirectly via stimulation of endothelin-1 from endothelial cells, by stimulation of renin from juxtaglomerular cells, and by inhibition of nitric oxide, a potent vasodilator. African Americans have higher serum levels than Caucasians, particularly those who are hypertensive or have kidney disease.[30] This increased TGF-β activity has been associated with an increased frequency of certain TGF-β isoforms within the African American population.[30] Among persons with renal disease, use of renin-angiotensin system modulators significantly lowers TGF-β1 levels.[31]

CLINICAL MANIFESTATIONS

Virtually all forms of pressure-related target organ injury are more common in African Americans than in Caucasians, including renal insufficiency/end-stage renal disease (ESRD), LVH, heart failure, retinopathy, and stroke. The risk of renal injury, as well as the risk of all other target organ damage, is directly related to the degree of BP elevation.

The increased risk of progression of renal disease in hypertensive African Americans has led some investigators to speculate that African Americans with hypertension and progressive renal disease may have renal lesions other than classic hypertensive (arteriolosclerotic) renal disease. In the African American Study for Kidney Disease and Hypertension (AASKD), however, the great majority of renal biopsies demonstrated classic but advanced hypertensive injury, with arteriolosclerosis of the afferent arteriole

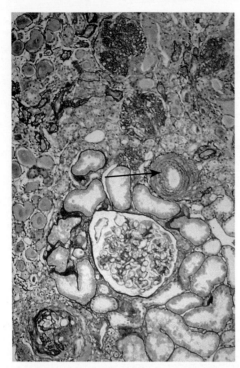

Figure 39.4 Renal histology in an African American with essential hypertension. Thickening of the interlobular artery (*arrow*) with severe global glomerulosclerosis and patchy tubulointerstitial fibrosis is shown. (From Fogo A, Breyer J, Smith M, and the AASK Pilot Study Investigators: Accuracy of the diagnosis of hypertensive nephrosclerosis in African Americans: A report from the African American Study of Kidney Disease Trial. Kidney Int 1997;51:244–252, with permission of Blackwell Science Ltd.)

and interlobular artery, focal and sometimes global glomerulosclerosis, and tubulointerstitial fibrosis (Fig. 39.4).[32]

DIFFERENTIAL DIAGNOSIS

In patients with hypertension and renal insufficiency, etiologies other than essential hypertension should be considered. Renovascular hypertension was once considered to have a lower prevalence in African Americans than in Caucasians. However, recent data derived from renal artery duplex scanning from the Cardiovascular Health Study cohort (persons >65 years) have documented approximately an 8% prevalence of critical renal artery stenosis in both African Americans and Caucasians.[33] Moreover, in a consecutive surgical series of hypertensive African Americans with critical renal artery stenosis, 13 of 23 (57%) patients with ischemic nephropathy experienced a >20% decline in serum creatinine.[34] In these patients, a beneficial BP response to surgical revascularization was obtained in 74%, with a mean improvement in estimated GFR from 34 to 43 ml/min per 1.73 m^2 ($P < 0.001$). These data emphasize the need to consider renovascular hypertension in appropriately selected African American hypertensives.

NATURAL HISTORY

African Americans with hypertension have a higher absolute risk of cardiac mortality, stroke, and ESRD compared with their sex- and age-matched Caucasian counterparts. This occurs, in part, because of a greater prevalence of extreme BP elevations, longer duration of BP elevations, frequent loss of the normal nocturnal dipping of BP, and an apparent increased target organ sensitivity to pressure-related injury at a given BP level.

TREATMENT

Lifestyle modifications, including dietary sodium and fat reduction, weight loss, and increased physical activity all lower BP and should be part of the management of the hypertensive African American (see Chapter 33). Some African Americans may be able to reduce or even avoid antihypertensive medication if such interventions are undertaken.

The level of BP control should be determined by the application of criteria for risk stratification using guidelines such as the JNC 7 or ISHIB reports.[1,2] Race, *per se*, should not be used to solely determine the target BP level nor should it be used to determine the selection of antihypertensive drugs needed to attain target BP levels. While multiple antihypertensive drug studies have reported that African Americans typically manifest lower group average BP responses to angiotensin-converting enzyme (ACE) inhibitors and angiotensin receptor blockers (ARBs), we believe that the racial differences in group average BP responses should not form the basis of blanket recommendations to favoring or avoiding drugs based on an individual's race. The rationale for this position is as follows: (1) while average BP responses may favor one racial group, the distribution of individual BP responses overlaps considerably for each antihypertensive; (2) antihypertensive monotherapy only rarely achieves BP therapeutic targets of <140 mm Hg systolic and therefore most hypertensive patients will require more than one antihypertensive drug to control their BP to target or lower levels; (3) there are virtually no reported racial differences in hypertensive patients during treatment with multiple antihypertensive drugs, particularly if one of the agents is either a diuretic or calcium antagonist, and (4) African Americans with specific target-organ indications for certain drugs less often receive them, possibly because of the avoidance, for example, of RAS antagonists, because of their lesser group BP-lowering efficacy. Therefore, the focus should be on the use of enough antihypertensive drugs that have been selected to maximize BP-lowering efficacy and reduce target organ damage rather than focusing on what a single antihypertensive drug will accomplish in regards to lowering BP.

Unfortunately physicians increase antihypertensive drug regimens only ~13% to 26% of the time in subjects with BP above target levels.[35–37] However, data from the Antihypertensive and Lipid-Lowering Treatment to Prevent Heart Attack Trial (ALLHAT)[37] also documented that African Americans were even less likely than Caucasians to have their antihypertensive drug therapy intensified when their BP was above goal levels and were also more likely to have characteristics (e.g., target-organ injury, reduced kidney function) linked to any treatment resistance. Figures 39.5 and 39.6 display the recommended considerations in the evaluation and treatment of hypertensive African Americans.

Diuretics

Diuretics are effective BP-lowering agents in African Americans and Caucasians and remain the most favored drug class in the recent JNC 7 report. In the setting of *ad libitum* (physiologically high) dietary sodium intake, diuretics lower BP robustly, and, importantly, augment the antihypertensive efficacy of virtually all other antihypertensive drug classes. It is critical to select the diuretic that is most appropriate for the level of kidney function. Thiazide diuretics are minimally effective when the GFR is <45 ml/min per 1.73 m^2, although chlorthalidone will lower BP at lower levels of GFR (perhaps down to 30 ml/min per 1.73 m^2). Loop diuretics or metolazone are a better choice when kidney function is reduced to <40 to 45 ml/min per 1.73 m^2. These

Therapeutic considerations when treating African American hypertensive patients

Risk Factor	Treatment Factors
High blood pressure (BP) levels	More monotherapy failures
Longer duration of hypertension	More short-term risk from rapid BP reduction; however, long-term benefits of BP normalization are greater
High burden of target organ damage	Need slow but aggressive BP control (>130/85 mm Hg); favor drugs with human data for target organ protection
Obesity	More likely to be salt sensitive; leading to higher BP medication requirements; lower sodium intake; titrate upward with angiotensin-converting enzyme (ACE) inhibitors
Glomerular hyperfiltration	Aggressive BP control; favor ACE inhibitors, possibly angiotensin receptor blocker (ARB)
Reduced natriuretic capacity	More often need diuretics, especially in complex drug regimens; premium on reducing dietary sodium intake

Figure 39.5 Therapeutic considerations when treating African American hypertensive patients. ARB, angiotensin receptor blocker.

Recommendations for the evaluation and treatment of hypertension in African Americans

Clinical/Diagnostic Evaluation	Action
Thorough, cost-efficient search for historical, biochemical evidence of pressure-related target organ injury	The presence of pressure-related target organ damage increases cardiovascular risk at a given electrocardiographic/echocardiographic blood pressure (BP) level and influences treatment initiation levels and the on-treatment target BP. Target-organ injury is also associated with a lesser longitudinal BP response to pharmacologic therapy.
Avoid utilization of race as the sole, or even predominant, criterion for drug selection	The previously reported racial differences are of insufficient magnitude to guide selection choices for individual patients; emphasize lifestyle modification in the context of cultural beliefs and preferences
Gradually lower BP over many weeks to months to the appropriate target	Give drugs for at least 4–6 weeks to manifest full BP-lowering effect after initiation of treatment and use dose titration; otherwise may risk greater drug-related side effects as well as inaccurate validation of the self-fulfilling prophecy that "these drugs do not work"
Expect the majority of patients with stage 2 hypertension (>160/100 mm Hg) ultimately to fail monotherapy	In this BP range, it is now recommended to consider initiating treatment with combination drug therapy; titrate the drug dose up over time and, ultimately, add additional agents if BP is not controlled

Figure 39.6 Recommendations for the evaluation and treatment of hypertension in African Americans.

agents are useful in complex antihypertensive drug regimens (more than two drugs) because they antagonize the drug-induced enhanced sodium retention/salt sensitivity and limit plasma volume expansion that likely undermines the decrease in BP occurring as a consequence of expansion of venous capacitance. It should be appreciated, however, that sometimes one diuretic is not enough to control plasma volume expansion. The combined used of thiazides and aldosterone antagonists in hypertensives with reasonably well-preserved renal function (GFR >50 ml/min per 1.73 m²) or the combined use of low-dose metolazone plus furosemide in patients with reduced renal function (GFR <40 to 45 ml/min per 1.73 m²) can appreciably augment BP lowering.

Aldosterone antagonists are highly effective BP-lowering agents in African Americans that are likely underutilized.[38] Amiloride, an inhibitor of the epithelial sodium channel, also lowers BP effectively and safely alone as well as in combination with spironolactone in hypertensive African Americans.[39]

β-Blockers
β-Blockers lower BP in African Americans, although they are relatively less effective than monotherapy with either diuretics or calcium antagonists. As with other drugs that have their effects via the RAS system, consumption of dietary sodium in amounts typical of many African Americans (and Caucasians) attenuates their BP-lowering efficacy. β-Blockers as well as combined αβ-blockers appear to be particularly efficacious in severe hypertensives, most often in combination with diuretics. However, the combination of a β-blocker with a calcium antagonist that lowers heart rate (such as verapamil or diltiazem) should be avoided.

Angiotensin-Converting Enzyme Inhibitors
ACE inhibitors are the preferred agents in African Americans with diabetes, depressed kidney function, and/or proteinuric renal disease. In a report from the AASKD,[40] initial therapy with ramipril, an ACE inhibitor, slowed the loss of renal function and reduced proteinuria more effectively than amlodipine, a dihydropyridine calcium antagonist, in nondiabetic African Americans with reduced kidney function. The difference was observed despite <2 mm Hg difference in BP and with both groups receiving a similar number (mean, 2.75) of antihypertensive agents. The advantage of ACE inhibitors was most evident in patients with proteinuria. This observation replicates what has been observed in other studies of ACE inhibitors in non–African American populations with reduced kidney function.

ACE inhibitors have several positive features. While ACE inhibitors do not affect fasting glucose levels, they do lessen insulin resistance and also lower the risk of developing diabetes mellitus,[41] an effect of considerable potential importance in a diabetes-prone group such as African Americans. ACE inhibitors also lower the risk of both microvascular and cardiovascular complications and the risk of heart failure.[41]

However, the BP-lowering effect of ACE inhibitors is affected by dietary sodium intake. When sodium intake is low, ACE inhibitors lower BP to the same degree as calcium antagonists; however, when sodium intake is high, the antihypertensive effect of ACE inhibitors is attenuated much more than that of calcium antagonists.[42] The risk of both angioedema and cough, although low in absolute terms, is also higher in African Americans than Caucasians.

Angiotensin Type I Receptor Blockers
Angiotensin type I receptor blockers (ARBs) are well-tolerated antihypertensive agents that are similar to ACE inhibitors in being antiproteinuric and renoprotective. Like ACE inhibitors, ARBs

lower BP less effectively in African Americans than Caucasians and are also less effective than diuretics in BP lowering in African Americans; however, the combination of an ARB with a diuretic markedly enhances BP responses.[38]

ARBs can be considered for ACE inhibitor–intolerant patients and may be particularly beneficial in diabetic nephropathy; the latter is disproportionately increased in the African American. The Irbesartan Diabetic Nephropathy Trial compared irbesartan, an ARB, with amlodipine and placebo.[43] Amlodipine and irbesartan lowered BP to a similar degree, but irbesartan provided greater renoprotection (30% less doubling of serum creatinine and lowered proteinuria to a greater degree). Heart failure incidence was also lower with irbesartan compared with the placebo and amlodipine groups. However, the rates of death due to cardiovascular disease, nonfatal myocardial infarction, and stroke tended to be higher in the irbesartan compared to the amlodipine group. The Reduction of Endpoints in Noninsulin Dependent Diabetes with the Angiotensin II Antagonist Losartan (RENAAL) study[44] compared the ARB losartan to an antihypertensive regimen not containing ARBs or ACE inhibitors (placebo). BP was lowered slightly more in the losartan group (140/74 versus 142/74 mm Hg) and both proteinuria and the composite endpoint of doubling of serum creatinine, ESRD, or death were also lower. There were fewer cases of new heart failure and a borderline significant trend toward fewer myocardial infarctions in the losartan group compared to placebo. Background therapy with calcium antagonists did not attenuate the benefits of losartan treatment. Similar clinical endpoint data for ARBs in persons with nondiabetic renal insufficiency are not currently available. A *post hoc* analysis[45] stratified by race of the Losartan Intervention for Endpoint Reduction (LIFE) trial that enrolled hypertensives with LVH found that African Americans and Caucasians had similar levels of BP lowering. However, among Caucasians, losartan was superior to atenolol in preventing the primary composite endpoint (cardiovascular death, stroke, myocardial infarction), while in African Americans, atenolol was superior to losartan. The explanation(s) for these divergent study results is unclear.

Calcium Antagonists

Calcium antagonists have long been considered a preferred monotherapy for achieving BP control in hypertensive African Americans. Monotherapy with these agents lowers BP to a similar degree as diuretics but is more effective than other antihypertensive drug classes, particularly when dietary sodium is not restricted, in African Americans. The BP-lowering potency of the calcium antagonists, as with the diuretics, is minimally affected by physiologically high levels of dietary salt consumption.[42] Unfortunately, the dihydropyridine calcium antagonists, and to a lesser extent verapamil and diltiazem, disrupt renal GFR autoregulation and, in the setting of elevated systemic BPs, can lead to

excess transmission of systemic pressures to the glomerulus. However, there are scant long-term clinical endpoint data regarding renal outcomes with the rate-limiting calcium antagonists. The data with the calcium antagonists in the RENAAL trial suggested that when an ARB is used in combination with a dihydropyridine calcium antagonist, there is no attenuation of the clinical benefit attributable to the ARB. There is no reason to avoid these agents, even the dihydropyridines, in hypertensive patients with depressed renal function and/or proteinuria, as long as they are combined with either an ACE inhibitor or ARB.

α_1-Adrenoceptor Antagonists

The α_1-adrenoceptor antagonists lower BP effectively in African Americans, although the dose required to achieve a given level of BP control appears to be slightly higher than in Caucasians. These agents may be useful in African Americans, mostly in combination with other antihypertensive drugs. They not only lower BP but also improve glucose tolerance, lessen insulin resistance, and favorably affect all lipoproteins (lowering cholesterol and triglycerides and raising HDL). The α_1-adrenoceptor antagonists also favorably influence the fibrinolytic system. These agents can, however, cause orthostatic hypertension, especially in diabetics and when combined with either diuretics or sympatholytic drugs. In addition, the doxazosin arm of the ALLHAT trial was discontinued because an interim analysis showed that, compared with chlorthalidone, the doxazosin group had higher rates of stroke, cardiovascular events, and heart failure.[46] Interestingly, there was no difference between the doxazosin and chlorthalidone treatment arms on the primary endpoint of fatal or nonfatal MI. Systolic BP lowering was ~3 mm Hg less with doxazosin. It seems more likely that doxazosin was not as effective as diuretics in lowering cardiovascular events as opposed to actually increasing the rate of these events. Thus, the most logical utilization of doxazosin in hypertension treatment is as an add-on drug.

Other Antihypertensive Agents

Central adrenergic inhibitors effectively lower BP in African Americans and may be used as first-line drug therapy; however, they are best reserved as add-on therapy. Typically, central adrenergic inhibitors are associated with bothersome side effects, such as dry mouth, depression, and orthostatic hypotension. Clonidine, however, is an excellent agent for use in true hypertensive urgencies. Direct vasodilators such as minoxidil and hydralazine are not suitable for use as monotherapy. These drugs are most often reserved for use as adjunctive treatments for hypertension. Direct vasodilators activate the sympathetic nervous system leading to bothersome tachycardia and also promote profound salt and water retention, necessitating that the patient be treated with a diuretic, usually a loop diuretic, and either a β-blocker or a rate-limiting calcium antagonist.

REFERENCES

1. Chobanian AV, Bakris GL, Black HR, et al: Seventh Report of the Joint National Committee on Prevention, Detection, Evaluation, and Treatment of High Blood Pressure. JNC 7. Hypertension 2003;42:1206–1252.
2. Douglas JG, Bakris GL, Epstein M, et al: Management of high blood pressure in African Americans: Consensus statement of the Hypertension in African Americans Working Group of the International Society on Hypertension in Blacks. Arch Intern Med 2003;163:25–41.
3. Hajjar I, Kotchen TA: Trends in prevalence, awareness, treatment, and control of hypertension in the United States, 1988–2000. JAMA 2003;290:99–206.
4. Cooper RS, Wolf-Maier K, Luke A, et al: An international comparative study of blood pressure in populations of European vs. African descent. BMC Med 2005;3:2.
5. Cooper R, Rotimi C, Ataman S, et al: The prevalence of hypertension in seven populations of West African origin. Am J Public Health 1997;87:55–56.
6. Burt V, Whelton P, Roccella E, et al: Prevalence of hypertension in the US adult population. Results from the Third National Health and Nutrition Examination Survey, 1988–1991. Hypertension 1995;25:305–313.
7. Flack JM, Neaton JD, Daniels B, Esunge P: Ethnicity and renal disease: Lessons from multiple risk factor intervention trial and the treatment of mild hypertension study. Am J Kidney Dis 1993;21(Suppl)1–40.

8. Liu K, Ruth KJ, Flack JM, et al: Blood pressure in young blacks and whites: Relevance of obesity and lifestyle factors in determining differences—the CARDIA study. Circulation 1996;93:60–66.
9. Curhan GC, Chertow GM, Willett WC, et al: Birth weight and adult hypertension and obesity in women. Circulation 1996;94:1310–1315.
10. Muna W, Kingue S, Kim KS, Adams-Campbell LL: Circadian rhythm of hypertensives in a Cameroon population: A pilot study. J Hum Hypertens 1995;9:797–800.
11. Wilson DK, Sica DA, Miller SB: Effects of potassium on blood pressure in salt-sensitive and salt-resistant black adolescents. Hypertension 1999;34:181–186.
12. Chrysant SG, Danisa K, Kem DC, et al: Racial differences in pressure, volume and renin interrelationships in essential hypertension. Hypertension 1979;1:136–141.
13. Messerli FH, DeCarvalho JG, Christie B, Frohlich ED. Essential hypertension in black and white subjects. Hemodynamic findings and fluid volume state. Am J Med 1979;67:27–31.
14. Rocchini AP, Key J, Bondie D, et al: The effect of weight loss on the sensitivity of blood pressure to sodium in obese adolescents. N Engl J Med 1989;321:580–585.
15. Ray CA, Monahan KD: Sympathetic vascular transduction is augmented in young normotensive blacks. J Appl Physiol 2002;92:651–656.
16. Abate NI, Mansour YH, Tuncel M, et al: Overweight and sympathetic overactivity in black Americans. Hypertension 2001;38:379–383.
17. Stein CM, Lang CC, Nelson R, et al: Vasodilation in black Americans: Attenuated nitric oxide-mediated responses. Clin Pharmacol Ther 1997;62:436–443.
18. Houghton JL, Philbin EF, Strogatz DS, et al: The presence of African American race predicts improvement in coronary endothelial function after supplementary L-arginine. J Am Coll Cardiol 2002;39:1314–1322.
19. Parmer J, Stone RA, Cervenka JH, et al: Renal hemodynamics in essential hypertension. Hypertension 1994;24:752–757.
20. Price DA, Fisher ND, Lansang MC, et al: Renal perfusion in blacks: Alterations caused by insuppressibility of intrarenal renin with salt. Hypertension 2002;40:86–89.
21. Palmer BF: Impaired renal autoregulation: Implications for the genesis of hypertension and hypertension-induced renal injury. Am J Med Sci 2001;321:388–400.
22. Johnson RJ, Segal MS, Srinivas TR, et al: Essential hypertension, progressive renal disease and uric acid: A pathogenetic link? J Am Soc Nephrol 2005;16:1909–1919.
23. Mackenzie H, Lawler E, Brenner B: Pathogenesis and pathophysiology of essential hypertension. Congenital oligonephropathy. The fetal flaw in essential hypertension? Kidney Int 1996;49:S30–S34.
24. Hall JE, Henegar JR, Dwyer TM, et al: Is obesity a major cause of chronic kidney disease? Adv Ren Replace Ther 2004;11:41–54.
25. Flack JM, Mensah GA, Ferrario CM: Using angiotensin converting enzyme inhibitors in African American hypertensives: A new approach to treating hypertension and preventing target-organ damage. Curr Med Res Opin 2000;16:66–79.
26. Boddi M, Poggesi L, Coppo M, et al: Human vascular renin-angiotensin system and its functional changes in relation to different sodium intakes. Hypertension 1998;31:836–842.
27. Cardillo C, Campia U, Kilcoyne CM, et al: Improved endothelium-dependent vasodilation after blockade of endothelin receptors in patients with essential hypertension. Circulation 2002;105:452–456.
28. Ergul S, Parish DC, Puett D, Ergul A: Racial differences in plasma endothelin-1 concentrations in individuals with essential hypertension. Hypertension 1996;28:652–655.
29. Elijovich F, Laffer CL, Amador E, et al: Regulation of plasma endothelin by salt in salt-sensitive hypertension. Circulation 2001;16:263–268.
30. August P, Suthanthiran M: Transforming growth factor-beta and progression of renal disease. Kidney Int Suppl 2003;87:S99–S104.
31. Sharma K, Eltayeb BO, McGowan TA, et al: Captopril-induced reduction of serum levels of transforming growth factor beta-1 correlated with long-term renoprotection in insulin-dependent diabetic patients. Am J Kidney Dis 1999;34:818–823.
32. Fogo A, Breyer J, Smith M, and the AASK Pilot Study Investigators: Accuracy of the diagnosis of hypertensive nephrosclerosis in African Americans: A report from the African American Study of Kidney Disease Trial. Kidney Int 1997;51:244–252.
33. Hansen KJ, Edwards MS, Craven TE, et al: Prevalence of renovascular disease in the elderly: A population-based study. J Vasc Surg 2002;36:443–451.
34. Deitch JS, Hansen KJ, Craven TE, et al: Renal artery repair in African Americans. J Vasc Surg 1997;26:465–473.
35. Okonofua EC, Simpson KN, Jesri A, et al: Therapeutic inertia is an impediment to achieving the Healthy People 2010 blood pressure control goals. Hypertension 2006;47:345–351.
36. Berlowitz DR, Ash AS, Hickey EC, et al: Inadequate management of blood pressure in a hypertensive population. N Engl J Med 1998;339:1957–1963.
37. Cushman WC, Ford CE, Cutler JA, et al: Success and predictors of blood pressure control in diverse North American settings: The antihypertensive and lipid lowering treatment to prevent heart attack trial (ALLHAT). J Clin Hypertens 2002;4:393–404.
38. Flack JM, Oparil S, Pratt JH, et al: Efficacy and tolerability of eplerenone and losartan in hypertensive black and white patients. J Am Coll Cardiol 2003;41:1148–1155.
39. Saha C, Eckert GJ, Ambrosius WT, et al: Improvement in blood pressure with inhibition of the epithelial sodium channel in blacks with hypertension. Hypertension 2005;46:481–487.
40. Agodoa LY, Appel L, Bakris GL, et al: Effect of ramipril vs. amlodipine on renal outcomes in hypertensive nephrosclerosis. JAMA 2001;285:2719–2728.
41. The Heart Outcomes Prevention Study Investigators: Effects of an angiotensin converting enzyme inhibitor, ramipril, on cardiovascular events in high-risk patients. N Engl J Med 2000;342:145–153.
42. Weir MR, Hall PS, Berhrens MT, Flack JM: Salt and blood pressure responses to calcium antagonism in hypertensive patients. Hypertension 1995;25:1339–1344.
43. Lewis EJ, Hunsicker LG, Clarke WR, et al: Renoprotective effect of the angiotensin receptor antagonist irbesartan in patients with nephropathy due to type 2 diabetes. N Engl J Med 2001;345:851–860.
44. Brenner BM, Cooper ME, De Zeeuw D, et al: Effects of losartan on renal and cardiovascular outcomes in patients with type 2 diabetes and nephropathy. N Engl J Med 2001;345:861–869.
45. Julius S, Alderman MH, Beevers G, et al: Cardiovascular risk reduction in hypertensive black patients with left ventricular hypertrophy: The LIFE study. J Am Coll Cardiol 2004;43:1047–1055.
46. ALLHAT Collaborative Research Group: Major cardiovascular events in hypertensive patients randomized to doxazosin vs. chlorthalidone: The antihypertensive and lipid lowering treatment to prevent heart attack trail (ALLHAT). JAMA 2000;283:1967–1975.

Renal Physiology in Normal Pregnancy

Chris Baylis and John M. Davison

INTRODUCTION

There are profound changes in renal function in normal pregnancy, which lead to marked alterations from the nonpregnant physiologic norm. An appreciation and understanding of these alterations are essential in order to recognize both normal and compromised pregnancies.

ANATOMY

The kidney increases 1 to 2 cm in length and in volume by up to 70% in normal pregnancy because of increases in both vascular and interstitial fluid compartments. The most striking anatomic change is dilation of the calyces, renal pelvis, and ureter (more prominent on the right side), and by the third trimester, about 80% of women show evidence of hydronephrosis[1] (Fig. 40.1). A consequence of the ureteral dilation is urinary stasis, which predisposes pregnant women with asymptomatic bacteriuria to develop ascending infection (acute symptomatic pyelonephritis). Very rarely the anatomic changes may be extreme and precipitate the overdistention syndrome, with massive dilation,

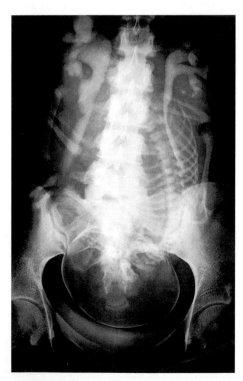

Figure 40.1 Hydronephrosis in normal pregnancy. Intravenous urogram at 36 weeks' gestation. Note bilateral hydronephrosis, more marked on the right side.

recurrent severe flank pain, increasing serum creatinine, hypertension, or even reversible acute renal failure.[2]

SYSTEMIC HEMODYNAMICS

There are significant alterations in systemic hemodynamics in normal pregnancy. A plasma (and extracellular fluid) volume expansion occurs while red cell volume also increases leading to a large increase in blood volume that correlates with clinical outcome and birth weight. Interestingly, subsequent pregnancies tend to be more successful than the first, with bigger babies and larger plasma volume increases. Women with twins and triplets have proportionately greater increments, and those with poorly growing fetuses, as in preeclampsia or where there is a history of poor reproductive performance, have correspondingly poor plasma volume responses. The increase in plasma volume (maximum increase ~1.25 liters) takes place progressively up to 32 to 34 weeks, after which there is little further change. The plasma volume expansion has a hemodilutional effect, causing decreases in hematocrit: the physiologic anemia of normal pregnancy.[3]

Cardiac output is significantly increased by the fifth gestational week, initially caused by a 10% to 20% increase in heart rate (80 to 90 bpm) with stroke volume >20% enhanced by the eighth week. Cardiac output increases of 40% to 50% are well established by the 24th week. Left atrial and left ventricular end-diastolic dimensions increase, suggesting an associated increase in venous return. There is also a progressive increase in aortic valve orifice area. Despite the 40% to 50% increase in cardiac output, systemic blood pressure substantially decreases in normal pregnancy (representative values are shown in Figs. 40.2 and 40.3).[4] The physiologic decrease in blood pressure results from a profound reduction in systemic vascular resistance of unknown cause, although the loss of responsiveness to vasoconstrictor agents (e.g., angiotensin II, arginine vasopressin [AVP]) certainly contributes.[5] Inhibition of angiogenic factors in preeclampsia causes vasoconstriction, suggesting that these factors, such as vascular endothelial growth factor may contribute importantly to the normal gestational vasodilation via stimulation of endothelial nitric oxide and prostaglandins.[6] The combination of increased cardiac output and peripheral vasodilation means that organ blood flow increases in pregnancy, with the most dramatic changes occurring in the kidney and skin circulation throughout gestation and in the uterus in the second part of the pregnancy.[4] In the third trimester, the enlarged uterus compresses surrounding tissues and can influence hemodynamic measurements, so that attention should be paid to maternal posture during hemodynamic monitoring. In the supine position, there is partial obstruction of the inferior vena cava and decreased venous return, reducing cardiac output and causing a decrease in blood pressure, the supine hypotensive syndrome of

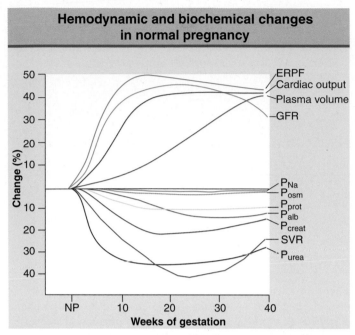

Figure 40.2 Alterations induced by normal pregnancy. Increments and decrements in hemodynamic and biochemical parameters shown as percentage of change from nonpregnant baseline. ERPF, effective renal plasma flow; GFR, glomerular filtration rate; NP, nonpregnant; SVR, systemic vascular resistance.

pregnancy. It is important to be aware of these postural effects when measuring blood pressure in late pregnant women.[4]

RENAL HEMODYNAMICS

There are striking changes in renal hemodynamics in normal pregnancy with an increase in glomerular filtration rate (GFR) and consequent decrease in serum creatinine detectable very early.[7]

Changes in some common indices during pregnancy

	Nonpregnant	Pregnant
Hematocrit (%)	41	33
Plasma protein (g/dl)	7.0	6.0
Plasma osmolality (mOsm/kg)	285	275
Plasma sodium (mmol/l)	140	135
Plasma creatinine (mg/dl, μmol/l)	0.8 (73)	0.5 (45)
Blood urea nitrogen (mg/dl)	12.7	9.3
Plasma urea (mmol/l)	4.5	3.3
pH units	7.40	7.44
Arterial PCO_2 (mm Hg)	40	30
Plasma bicarbonate (mmol/l)	25	20
Plasma uric acid (mg/dl, μmol/l)	4.0 (240)	3.2 (190) early 4.3 (260) late
Systolic BP (mm Hg)	115	105
Diastolic BP (mm Hg)	70	60

Figure 40.3 Changes in some common indices during pregnancy. BP, blood pressure. (Mean values compiled from references 7–9, 15, 23.)

The GFR increases ~25% by 4 weeks after the last menstrual period, and a robust early increase in GFR is invariably associated with a good obstetric outcome (see Fig. 40.3). Longitudinal studies in normal pregnant women show that GFR (measured by inulin or 24-hour creatinine clearance) increases by a maximum of ~50% by mid-pregnancy, which is maintained until the last few weeks of the pregnancy when values begin to decrease but remain above the nonpregnant level (see Figs. 40.2 and 40.4).[8] These marked increases in GFR mean that serum creatinine decreases to ~0.4 to 0.5 mg/dl (36 to 45 μmol/l) and values considered normal for nonpregnant conditions of 0.7 to 0.8 mg/dl (63 to 72 μmol/l) are a cause for concern in normal pregnancy (see Fig. 40.3). The increase in renal plasma flow (RPF) of ~60% is slightly more pronounced than the increase in GFR (see Fig. 40.2), so that the filtration fraction (FF) decreases (see later discussion). At the end of pregnancy, the RPF decreases proportionally more than the GFR, that is, FF increases to the nonpregnant value.[8,9]

A similar pattern of renal hemodynamic change occurs during pregnancy in some animals, including the rat, in which GFR increases to a maximum of 30% to 40% above the virgin value by midterm, with a late return toward the nonpregnant value close to term (22 days). Glomerular micropuncture studies have shown that the increase in GFR is paralleled by increases in single nephron GFR secondary to increased glomerular plasma flow.[10] Because the preglomerular and postglomerular resistance vessels dilate in parallel, glomerular plasma flow increases without a change in glomerular blood pressure. As shown in Figure 40.5, the glomerular blood pressure remains unchanged throughout the pregnancy despite marked alterations in preglomerular vascular resistance. Similar conclusions have been reached using an indirect modeling approach in normal pregnant women.[7,9] Whole-kidney GFR, RPF, and plasma protein concentrations were measured, and, in addition, polydisperse neutral dextran was infused for determination of dextran sieving curves. This approach allows

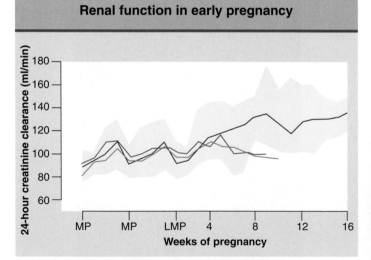

Figure 40.4 Renal function in early pregnancy. Changes in 24-hour creatinine clearance measured weekly before conception and through to uncomplicated spontaneous abortion in two women. The *blue line* represents the mean and the *yellow area* shows the range for nine women with successful obstetric outcome. LMP, last menstrual period; MP, menstrual period. (Modified from Lindheimer MD, Davison JM, Katz AI: The kidney and hypertension in pregnancy: Twenty exciting years. Semin Nephrol 2001;21:173–189; Baylis C, Davison JM: The renal system. In Chamberlain G, Broughton Pipkin F (eds): Clinical Physiology in Obstetrics, 3rd ed. Oxford: Blackwell Science, 1998, pp 263–307; Milne JEC, Lindheimer MD, Davison JM: Glomerular heteroporous membrane modelling in third trimester and postpartum before and during amino acid infusion. Am J Physiol 2002;282:F170–F175.)

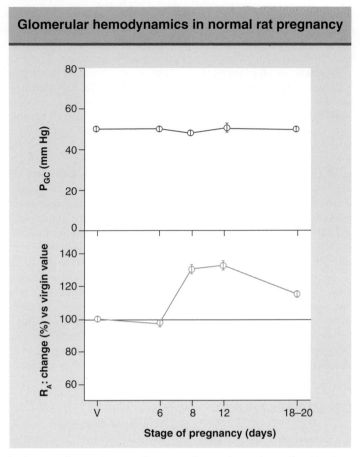

Figure 40.5   Glomerular hemodynamics in normal rat pregnancy. Summary of mean glomerular capillary blood pressure (P_{GC}; *upper panel*) and preglomerular arteriolar resistance (R_A; *lower panel*) in Munich Wistar rats in the virgin state (V) and throughout normal pregnancy.[10–12]

(with certain reasonable assumptions) modeling of glomerular hemodynamics. In pregnant women, there is a decrease in plasma protein concentration that contributes slightly to the increased GFR. As in the rat, the majority of the gestational increase in GFR in normal women is due to increased RPF with no change in glomerular blood pressure. The constancy of glomerular blood pressure during sustained renal vasodilation has important implications for the long-term effects of pregnancy on renal function, as discussed later.

It is often assumed that a change in FF reflects a change in glomerular blood pressure, but this is not always the case since FF is also determined by Kf, the product of water permeability of the glomerular wall and total glomerular capillary surface area.[8] Both glomerular wall water permeability and filtration pressure are very high, and thus filtration proceeds rapidly. In fact, in some situations, not all the available filtration surface area is used so that filtration ceases (because the driving pressure is exhausted) before the end of the glomerulus. This state is known as filtration pressure equilibrium. When plasma flow increases during filtration pressure equilibrium, a proportional increase in GFR occurs with no change in FF. This is seen in the normal pregnant rat.[10] In contrast, FF decreases during normal pregnancy in women as RPF is increasing.[8] Most likely this reflects the fact that humans are closer than rats to filtration pressure disequilibrium, a situation in which the entire glomerular capillary surface area available for filtration is used, leaving a positive driving pressure at the end of the glomerulus. At filtration pressure disequilibrium, GFR becomes less dependent on plasma flow; thus, an increase in plasma flow (with no change in the other determinants of

filtration) leads to a disproportionately smaller increase in GFR, with a decrease in FF (see reference 11 for a fuller explanation).

Despite the prolonged renal vasodilatation, the renal vasculature remains fully responsive to various stimuli during pregnancy. For example, in the rat, the intrinsic renal autoregulatory ability remains intact[12] and the tubuloglomerular feedback component of renal autoregulation is reset to recognize the elevated GFR as normal.[13] Both pregnant rats and women exhibit a marked additional renal vasodilation in response to amino acid infusion,[14,15] demonstrating substantial renal vasodilatory reserve in normal pregnancy. The cause of the gestational increase in GFR remains uncertain, although studies in the pseudopregnant rat have shown that the fetoplacental unit is not necessary,[16] indicating that a maternal stimulus must initiate the gestational renal hemodynamic changes. A number of vasoactive factors have been evaluated as possible mediators of the renal vasodilation,[10] and while there are no clinical data, animal studies have implicated a role for nitric oxide.[17,18] Recent studies have suggested a key role for the ovarian hormone relaxin, which may signal increased renal nitric oxide production in pregnancy, possibly via an endothelin type B receptor mechanism.[19,20] Of note, the renal vasodilatory signal of pregnancy is remarkably robust since women with single kidneys (organ donors) and transplant recipients, who have already undergone significant compensatory renal hypertrophy and vasodilation, are able to exhibit further increases in RPF and GFR in pregnancy.[7,8]

Glomerular hypertension associated with renal vasodilatation is considered a primary pathogenic stimulus to progressive renal injury in chronic renal disease.[21] As discussed previously, normal pregnancy is also a state of chronic renal vasodilation; however, glomerular blood pressure remains normal. This may account for the findings that repetitive pregnancies in women and rats with normal renal function have no long-term adverse effects on glomerular function or structure.[22] Pregnancy will increase the rate of loss of renal function in some women with underlying renal disease (see Chapter 42), but the available evidence suggests that this is not by a hemodynamically mediated action.[7,22]

Abnormal Renal Hemodynamics

A woman may lose up to 50% of her renal function and still maintain serum creatinine <1.5 mg/dl (130 μmol/l) because of hyperfiltration in remaining nephrons, but if there is more severe compromise, then further glomerular damage will cause serum creatinine to increase.[7,23,24] Pregnancy in the presence of impaired renal function has a marked adverse effect on obstetric outcome (discussed in Chapter 42).

In preeclampsia, both RPF and GFR decrease, although absolute values may remain above the nonpregnant range. A decrease in ultrafiltration coefficient (Kf) of around 50% in combination with reduced RPF is the most likely mechanism for the hypofiltration.[23] The endothelium is targeted at an early stage in preeclampsia and the glomerulus is not spared, with the vascular endothelial cell dysfunction (glomerular endotheliosis) resulting in the loss of glomerular barrier size and charge selectivities (see Chapter 41).

RENAL TUBULAR FUNCTION IN PREGNANCY

There is an enormous plasma volume expansion in normal pregnancy and resultant small decrements in plasma concentration of many solutes (see Fig. 40.2). Nevertheless, the large increase in GFR means that the filtered load of most plasma constituents will increase during pregnancy.[7,8] Increments in excretion are seen for some substances, but this is limited by increases in tubular reabsorption, preventing depletion. Often intake also increases, with net retention leading to positive balance for many of the key constituents. The renal handling of a number of solutes is altered in normal pregnancy.

Uric Acid

Uric acid, an endpoint of purine metabolism, is freely filtered at the glomerulus, extensively reabsorbed in the proximal tubule with further downstream reabsorption and possibly some active secretion, such that only ~10% of filtered load is excreted. Plasma uric acid concentration decreases during early pregnancy by ~25% (see Fig. 40.3), which may reflect a decrease in net tubular reabsorption.[8] As the pregnancy advances, fractional excretion of uric acid decreases leading to an increasing plasma uric acid concentration, attaining levels close to the nonpregnant mean. Uric acid concentrations are significantly higher in preeclamptic pregnancy, and above a critical level of 6 mg/dl (350 μmol/l), there is excess perinatal mortality in hypertensive patients (see Chapter 41). It must be borne in mind, however, that physiologic variability is such that some healthy women have high plasma uric acid levels without problems, so that uric acid values must be interpreted in the clinical context.

Glucose

Excretion of glucose increases soon after conception to approximately 10 times the nonpregnant value and remains high throughout pregnancy, although the glycosuria is very variable.[8] The glycosuria is not related to changes in plasma glucose and

reflects decreased tubular reabsorption. In the nonpregnant individual, there is usually complete renal reabsorption of glucose, mostly in the proximal tubule, where there is a very high capacity for glucose transport. This maximum transport capacity (T_{max}) is not usually reached until plasma glucose increases to values in excess of 200 to 300 mg/dl (11 to 17 mmol/l). The glycosuria of pregnancy is due to a decrease in T_{max} and/or the inability of the renal tubules to cope with the increased filtered glucose load and does not reflect a metabolic disturbance.

Water-Soluble Vitamins and Amino Acids

Nicotinic acid, ascorbic acid, and folic acid are all excreted in increased amounts during pregnancy,[7] which emphasizes the need for adequate vitamin supplementation.

Urinary excretion of most amino acids increases in pregnancy, probably as a result of decreased tubular reabsorption.[24] There are distinct patterns with glycine, histidine, threonine, serine, and alanine excretion increasing early and remaining elevated throughout pregnancy. Excretion of lysine, cystine, taurine, phenylalanine, valine, leucine, and tyrosine also increase in early pregnancy but later decline. Glutamic acid, methionine, and ornithine are excreted in slightly greater amounts than before pregnancy, isoleucine excretion is unchanged, and arginine excretion decreases, consistent with decreases in plasma arginine in normal pregnancy.

Acid-Base Balance

The generation of hydrogen ion increases in pregnancy due to an increased basal metabolism and greater food intake, but despite this, the blood concentration of hydrogen ions decreases; thus plasma pH increases slightly (see Fig. 40.3). This mild alkalemia is respiratory in origin since pregnant women normally hyperventilate, leading to a primary decrease in arterial PCO_2 and secondary compensatory decreases in plasma bicarbonate concentration (see Fig. 40.3). A mild chronic respiratory alkalosis is a normal feature of pregnancy.

Potassium

Potassium excretion decreases, and there is a slow cumulative net potassium retention in pregnancy, which is distributed between the enlarging maternal tissues and the developing fetus. The decrease in potassium excretion occurs in spite of the mild alkalosis and high aldosterone values of normal pregnancy and is at least partly due to the potent antimineralocorticoid action of progesterone[25] (see later discussion).

Calcium

Calcium excretion increases two to three times during pregnancy due to the increased filtered load and despite some increase in tubular reabsorption. The increased calcium excretion in pregnancy could predispose to the formation of calcium stones, but increased magnesium and citrate, acidic glycoproteins and nephrocalcin serve to inhibit calcium oxalate stone formation so that the incidence of stone formation is not increased in normal pregnancy.[26]

Protein

Increased urinary total protein excretion in pregnancy should not be considered abnormal until it exceeds 500 mg in 24 hours,[7–9,15] although many classifications and definitions of the hypertensive disorders of pregnancy still define >300 mg/24 hours as abnormal.[27] There is usually a small increment in albumin excretion during the third trimester. Increased total protein and albumin excretion may continue into the puerperium, with truly nonpregnant levels not restored until 5 to 6 months after delivery. The gestational changes are related to alterations in glomerular perm and charge selectivity as well as tubular function. In clinical practice, urine protein >300 mg/24 hours roughly correlates with 30 mg/dl in a random urine, but given the problems with dipstick tests, many still prefer a 24-hour or some timed quantitative determination. Use of random urine protein-to-creatinine ratios ≥30 mg/μmol is, however, a clinically useful alternative.[8,27]

Sodium

A massive, cumulative volume expansion occurs during pregnancy with an associated gradual retention of sodium of ~900 mmol, distributed between the products of conception and maternal extracellular space. This positive sodium balance develops despite a ~30% increase in filtered load and reflects an increase in tubular reabsorption that allows net additional sodium retention of ~2 to 3 mmol/day.[3] Nevertheless, it is normal for sodium excretion to increase in pregnancy, reflecting the marked increase in sodium intake. Lithium clearance studies in women have indicated enhanced sodium reabsorption in the proximal tubule and distal nephron segments in late pregnancy, while animal studies have been contradictory.[28] The reason for the net renal sodium retention in pregnancy is not known. As shown in Figure 40.6 there are many factors operating to both increase and decrease sodium excretion, and exactly how the normal balance of net retention is achieved remains a mystery. Several antinatriuretic systems are activated in normal pregnancy.[29] Renin, angiotensin, and aldosterone levels are all markedly increased, and the renin angiotensin system (RAS) can be appropriately regulated around these new set points when changes occur in extracellular fluid volume. In addition to stimulating aldosterone release, physiologic levels of angiotensin II act directly on the proximal tubule to increase sodium reabsorption. However, a marked refractoriness develops to the vascular actions of angiotensin II in normal pregnancy,[29] which may blunt angiotensin II–dependent net sodium retention. The high aldosterone levels of pregnancy will

certainly promote renal sodium retention in the distal tubule and collecting duct. The very high levels of deoxycorticosterone (from 21-hydroxylation of progesterone) may also exert mineralocorticoid actions to promote sodium retention.[30] Estrogens increase markedly during human pregnancy and may directly induce renal sodium retention and/or act indirectly by enhancing the conversion of progesterone to deoxycorticosterone.[30] In addition to hormonal factors, the increased ureteral pressure and the decrease in systemic blood pressure both decrease sodium excretion.

The concentrations of several natriuretic agents also increase in pregnancy. Progesterone increases by 10 to 100 times, and these levels exert a marked antimineralocorticoid action by competing with aldosterone for the mineralocorticoid receptor.[30] Plasma atrial natriuretic peptide (ANP) levels are also moderately elevated.[31] In addition to natriuretic factors, the large increase in GFR leads to increased filtration of sodium (despite the small decrease in plasma sodium concentration), which will also increase sodium excretion. Decreases in plasma albumin concentration and the increment in effective renal plasma flow during pregnancy will also enhance sodium excretion by inhibiting sodium reabsorption.[10]

Despite the many conflicting stimuli, net sodium retention and marked plasma volume expansion are normal in pregnancy. In the normal nonpregnant steady state, plasma volume expansion and renal sodium retention cannot coexist. However, pregnancy is not a steady state, and the volume-sensing and regulatory systems are dramatically readjusted throughout pregnancy to accommodate and maintain the volume expansion (see later discussion).

OSMOREGULATION

There is a very early decrease in plasma osmolality (P_{osm}) by ~10 mOsmol/kg below the nonpregnant norm due to a reduction in plasma sodium and associated anions (see Fig. 40.3). Whereas a decrease in P_{osm} of this magnitude would completely suppress release of the antidiuretic hormone AVP in nonpregnant individuals, in pregnancy, the osmotic thresholds for AVP release, as well as thirst, are reduced to recognize the reduced plasma osmolality as normal.[32] Figure 40.7 demonstrates the resetting of the relationship between plasma AVP and P_{osm} during normal pregnancy. The placental hormone human chorionic gonadotropin (which stimulates the release of ovarian relaxin)[33] may have a role in this reduction in the osmotic threshold for AVP release.[32] Plasma volume status is a separate, nonosmotic determinant of AVP release, and this system is also reset to recognize the massively expanded plasma volume as normal. The metabolic clearance rate of AVP has increased four times by mid-pregnancy due to the release of cystine aminopeptidase (vasopressinase) from the placenta,[32] so the rate of AVP production must also be accelerated. Despite these marked alterations, the urinary concentrating and diluting capacity remains good, although there is a slight reduction in the maximum urine concentration in the second part of pregnancy.[32]

VOLUME REGULATION

As discussed previously, there is a continual sodium retention and cumulative volume expansion in pregnancy that reflects complex readjustments of the various volume regulatory systems. These readjustments also permit volume expansion without increases in blood pressure; in fact, blood pressure decreases substantially as

Factors influencing sodium excretion during pregnancy	
Antinatriuretic	Natriuretic
Aldosterone	↑ Glomerular filtration rate
Angiotensin II	Progesterone
Estrogen	Atrial natriuretic peptide
Deoxycorticosterone	Nitric oxide
Supine posture	Prostaglandins
Upright posture	
Decreased blood pressure	
Increased ureteral pressure	
Placental shunting	

Figure 40.6 Factors influencing sodium excretion during pregnancy.

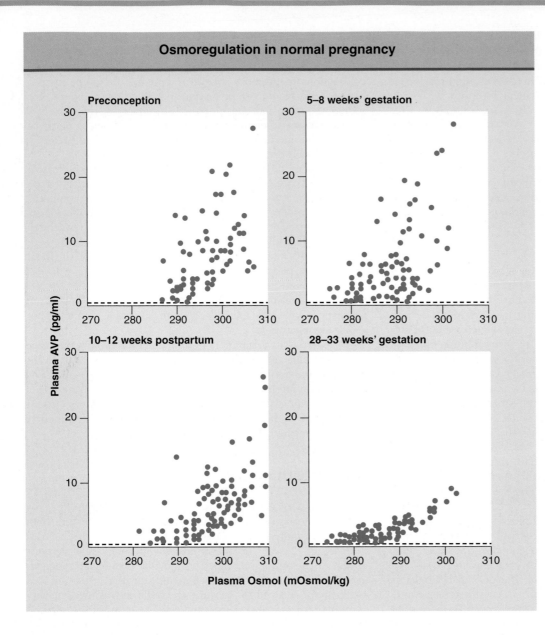

Figure 40.7 Osmoregulation in normal pregnancy. Relationship between plasma arginine vasopressin concentration (AVP) and plasma osmolarity (Osmol) during several 5% saline infusions in eight women before and during pregnancy. Each point represents an individual plasma measurement. There is a marked decrease in osmotic threshold for AVP release (abscissal intercept) during pregnancy. Values for the osmotic threshold for thirst (not shown) were always 2 to −5 mOsmol/kg above AVP release thresholds and 10 mOsmol/kg lower in pregnancy.[7,31,33]

pregnancy proceeds (see Fig. 40.3). What happens to volume perception/regulatory systems in pregnancy can be considered in terms of the effective circulating volume.[34,35] The RAS is an antinatriuretic system activated by volume depletion, and the increase in plasma renin activity, angiotensin, and aldosterone concentrations of normal pregnancy suggests an underfill signal, despite the absolute increase in plasma volume. Schrier[34] has suggested that the primary event in pregnancy is peripheral vasodilation that generates an underfill signal that leads to renal sodium retention. In contrast to the RAS, as discussed previously, both osmotic and nonosmotic control of AVP release is reset in a manner indicating that the expanded volume of pregnancy is sensed as normal. The tubuloglomerular feedback system is suppressed by volume expansion in the nonpregnant state but is reset in pregnant rats to recognize the expanded volume and increased GFR as normal.[13] Plasma ANP increases slightly in late pregnant women, but this is unlikely to reflect a physiologic response to volume expansion since even greater increases in ANP are seen in volume-contracted, preeclamptic pregnancies.[31,36] Thus volume regulation in pregnancy remains an enigma.

IMPACT OF MATERNAL HEMODYNAMIC CHANGES ON FETAL PROGRAMMING

There is strong evidence that women with normal pregnancies who have suboptimal increases in plasma volume are more likely to deliver small for gestational age babies. Fetal growth restriction is often seen in preeclamptic pregnancies in which volume contraction usually occurs.[37] Reductions in uterine blood flow (as occur in preeclampsia or when volume expansion is inadequate) and maternal (and thence fetal) malnutrition have been implicated in the pathogenesis of fetal growth restriction. There is considerable epidemiologic as well as animal evidence suggesting that adverse events *in utero* that lead to fetal growth restriction can program the offspring for the later development of hypertension, other cardiovascular events, and chronic kidney disease, at least in part due to reduction in nephron number.[38,39] Thus, optimal maternal systemic and renal hemodynamic changes have a huge impact not only on fetal well-being but on the long-term health of the offspring.

REFERENCES

1. Brown MA: Urinary tract dilatation in pregnancy. Am J Obstet Gynecol 1990;164:641–643.
2. Khauna N, Nguyn H: Reversible acute renal failure in association with bilateral ureteral obstruction and hydronephrosis in pregnancy. Am J Obstet Gynecol 2001;184:239–240.
3. Brown M, Gallery EDM: Volume homeostasis in normal pregnancy and preeclampsia: Physiology and clinical implications. Clin Obstet Gynecol 1994:8:287–310.
4. de Swiet M: The cardiovascular system. In Chamberlain G, Broughton Pipkin F (eds): Clinical Physiology in Obstetrics, 3rd ed. Oxford: Blackwell Science, 1998, pp 33–70.
5. Magness RR, Gant NF: Normal vascular adaptations in pregnancy. Potential clues for understanding pregnancy induced hypertension. In Walker JJ, Gant NF (eds): Hypertension in Pregnancy. London: Chapman & Hall Medical, 1997, pp 5–26.
6. Maynard SE, Min J-Y, Merchan J, et al: Excess placental soluble fms-like tyrosine kinase (sFlt1) may contribute to endothelial dysfunction, hypertension and proteinuria in preeclampsia. J Clin Invest 2003;111:649–658.
7. Lindheimer MD, Davison JM, Katz AI: The kidney and hypertension in pregnancy: Twenty exciting years. Semin Nephrol 2001;21:173–189.
8. Baylis C, Davison JM: The renal system. In Chamberlain, G, Broughton Pipkin F (eds): Clinical Physiology in Obstetrics, 3rd ed. Oxford: Blackwell Science, 1998, pp 263–307.
9. Roberts M, Lindheimer MD, Davison JM: Altered glomerular perm-selectivity to neutral dextran and heteroporous membrane modeling in human pregnancy. Am J Physiol 1996;270:F338–F343.
10. Baylis C: Glomerular filtration and volume regulation in gravid animal models. Clin Obstet Gynecol 1994:8:235–264.
11. Baylis C: Glomerular filtration dynamics. In Lote CJ (ed): Advances in Renal Physiology. London: Croom Helm, 1986, pp 33–83.
12. Reckelhoff JF, Yokota S, Baylis C: Renal autoregulation in mid-term and late pregnant rats. Am J Obstet Gynecol 1992;166:1546–1550.
13. Baylis C, Blantz RC: Tubuloglomerular feedback activity in virgin and pregnant rats. Am J Physiol 1985;249:F169–F173.
14. Baylis C: Effect of amino acid infusion as an index of renal vasodilatory capacity in pregnant rats. Am J Physiol 1988;254:F650–F656.
15. Milne JEC, Lindheimer MD, Davison JM: Glomerular heteroporous membrane modelling in third trimester and post-partum before and during amino acid infusion. Am J Physiol 2002;282:F170–F175.
16. Baylis C: Glomerular ultrafiltration in the pseudopregnant rat. Am J Physiol 1982;243:F300–F305.
17. Danielson LA, Conrad KP: Nitric oxide mediates renal vasodilation and hyperfiltration during pregnancy in chronically instrumented, conscious rats. J Clin Invest 1995;96:482–490.
18. Baylis C, Engels K: Adverse interactions between pregnancy and a new model of systemic hypertension produced by chronic blockade of EDRF in the rat. Clin Exp Hypertens 1992;B11:117–129.
19. Danielson LA, Sherwood OD, Conrad KP: Relaxin is a potent renal vasodilator in conscious rats. J Clin Invest 1999;103:525–533.
20. Conrad KP, Jeyabalan A, Danielson LA, et al: Role of relaxin in the maternal renal vasodilation of pregnancy. Ann NY Acad Sci 2005;1041:147–154.
21. Brenner BM: Nephron adaptation to renal injury or ablation. Am J Physiol 1985;249:F324–F337.
22. Baylis C: Glomerular filtration rate (GFR) in normal and abnormal pregnancies. Semin Nephrol 1999;9:133–139.
23. Moran P, Lindheimer MD, Davison JM: The renal response to preeclampsia. Semin Nephrol 2004;24:588–595.
24. Hytten FE, Cheyne GA: The aminoaciduria of pregnancy. J Obstet Gynaecol Br Commonw 1972;79:424–432.
25. Lindheimer MD, Richardson DA, Ehrlich EN, Katz AI: Potassium homeostasis in pregnancy. J Reprod Med 1987;32:517–520.
26. Eberts EG, Cunningham FG: Symptomatic nephrolithiasis complicating pregnancy. Obstet Gynecol 2000;96:753–756.
27. Roberts JM, Pearson GD, Cutler, JA, Lindheimer MD: Summary of NHLBI Group on Research on Hypertension during Pregnancy. Hypertens Pregnancy 2003;22:109–127.
28. Atherton JC, Beilinska A, Davison JM, et al: Sodium and water reabsorption in the proximal and distal nephron in conscious pregnant rats and third trimester women. J Physiol 1988;396:457–470.
29. August P, Lindheimer M: Pathophysiology of preeclampsia. In Laragh JH, Brenner BM (eds): Hypertension: Pathophysiology, Diagnosis and Management, 2nd ed. New York: Raven Press, 1995, pp 2407–2426.
30. MacDonald PC, Cutter S, MacDonald SC, et al: Regulation of extra-adrenal steroid 21hydroxylase activity: Increased conversion of plasma progesterone during estrogen treatment of women pregnant with a dead fetus. J Clin Invest 1982;69:469–474.
31. Irons DW, Baylis PH, Davison JM: Effect of atrial natriuretic peptide on renal hemodynamics and sodium excretion during human pregnancy. Am J Physiol 1996;271:F239–F242.
32. Lindheimer MD, Davison JM: Osmoregulation, the secretion of arginine vasopressin and its metabolism during pregnancy (minireview). Eur J Endocrinol 1995;132:133–143.
33. Randeva HS, Jackson A, Karteris E, Hillhouse EW: hCG production and activity during pregnancy. Fetal Matern Med Rev 2001;12:191–208.
34. Schrier RW: Pathogenesis of sodium and water retention in high-output and low-output cardiac failure, nephrotic syndrome, cirrhosis and pregnancy. Part 11. N Engl J Med 1988;319:1127–1134.
35. Durr JA, Lindheimer MD: Control of volume and body tonicity. In Lindheimer MD, Roberts JM, Cunningham FG (eds): Chesley's Hypertensive Disorders in Pregnancy, 2nd ed. Stamford CT: Appleton & Lange, 1999, pp 103–166.
36. Irons DW, Baylis PH, Davison JM: Effect of atrial natriuretic peptide on renal hemodynamics and sodium excretion during human pregnancy. Am J Physiol 1996;271:F239–F242.
37. Chesley LC, Lindheimer MD: Renal hemodynamics and intravascular volume in normal and hypertensive pregnancy. In Rubin PC (ed): Hypertension: Hypertension in Pregnancy. Amsterdam: Elsevier, 1988, pp 10–38.
38. Zandi-Nejad K, Luyckx VA, Brenner BM: Adult hypertension and kidney disease: The role of fetal programming. Hypertension 2006;47:502–508.
39. Godfrey KM, Barker DJ: Fetal programming and adult health. Public Health Nutr 2001;4:611–624.

URINALYSIS

For many young women, pregnancy is the first occasion that they have urinalysis and microscopy performed; hematuria, proteinuria, and pyuria may be detected, either related to or coincidental to the pregnancy.

Hematuria

Microscopic hematuria can be detected at some time during pregnancy in about 20% of women, but is persistent in only half of those and usually disappears after delivery, when, if still present, it can be investigated further. Persistent microscopic hematuria with normal blood pressure may be present in lupus nephritis, sickle cell trait, thin basement membrane disease, IgA nephropathy, polycystic kidneys, or with renal calculi. The most common cause of gross hematuria in pregnancy is hemorrhagic bacterial cystitis. A less common cause is renal calculi, and rarely it may be caused by bladder or renal neoplasms.

Proteinuria

The urinary excretion of protein increases during pregnancy owing to an increase in glomerular filtration rate (GFR; see Chapter 40), so that the 24-hour excretion of protein, normally <150 mg/day, may reach 300 mg/day. The pregnancy-induced increase in GFR usually produces more substantial increases in protein excretion in patients with pre-existing proteinuria. Patients with a history of glomerulonephritis in whom prepregnant levels of protein excretion are <1 g/24 h may excrete 2 to 6 g/24 h during a normal pregnancy because of glomerular hyperperfusion, without any other sign of exacerbation of the nephritis. In such women, plasma uric acid levels are unchanged if preeclampsia is not present. The development of new and significant proteinuria during pregnancy is almost always associated with the development of preeclampsia and therefore needs thorough investigation including the measurement of blood pressure, liver function tests, and serum uric acid level. In the absence of urinary tract infection or preeclampsia, isolated proteinuria in pregnancy usually reflects new-onset glomerular disease, for example, primary glomerulonephritis such as IgA nephropathy or focal segmental glomerulosclerosis or a systemic disease such as systemic lupus. If proteinuria is persistently detected by dipstick (≥1, corresponding to ~100 mg/dl), the ratio of protein to creatinine in a random urine sample should be measured. A ratio >0.3 mg protein/mg creatinine, which corresponds to a protein excretion of >300 mg/24 h, is needed to confirm proteinuria.

Pyuria

Isolated leukocyturia (pyuria) is common in normal pregnancy because of contamination by vaginal secretions. It requires no action other than ensuring that it disappears by 3 months postpartum.

RENAL BIOPSY

Percutaneous renal biopsy is usually avoided during pregnancy because of the fear of bleeding from the biopsy site, but it is not clear that the risk of hemorrhage is actually greater than in the nonpregnant state.[1] Renal biopsy is not usually required for the diagnosis and management of preeclampsia. Renal biopsy is indicated, however, if there is reason to suspect a renal disorder that may be treated successfully, especially in early pregnancy, while permitting the pregnancy to continue. Diseases in this category include lupus nephritis, minimal change nephrotic syndrome, immune-mediated interstitial nephritis, crescentic glomerulonephritis, and some forms of vasculitis including Wegener's granulomatosis. Percutaneous biopsy of the kidney may be performed using ultrasound localization in the usual prone position or with the patient lying on her right side.

KIDNEY SIZE AND HYDRONEPHROSIS

The volume, weight, and size of the kidneys increase in gestation, with renal lengths increasing by about 1 cm as measured by ultrasonography.[2] The collecting systems of both kidneys are normally dilated during pregnancy (see Chapter 40, Fig. 40.1), most marked on the right. The dilatation is probably caused by hormonal changes of pregnancy and also by ureteral obstruction by the pregnant uterus. Because ureteral dilatation is so common during normal gestation, it may be difficult to diagnose frank urinary obstruction. An unusual syndrome of late pregnancy is characterized by abdominal pain, marked hydronephrosis, and a variable increase in serum creatinine, managed successfully by the placement of ureteral stents.[2] Because physiologic hydronephrosis is so common, pregnant women are particularly susceptible to ascending pyelonephritis as a result of bladder infections. In the immediate puerperium, a rare occurrence is massive hematuria, usually from the right ureter, which subsides spontaneously and has been attributed to decompression of the partially obstructed right collecting system.

483

URINARY INFECTION AND ASYMPTOMATIC BACTERIURIA

Urinary frequency, sometimes accompanied by dysuria, is common during the latter half of pregnancy, even when the urine is not infected, because of pressure on the bladder from an enlarged pregnant uterus.

Urinary Tract Infection

One percent to 2% of pregnancies are complicated by urinary tract infections that may present as cystitis or acute pyelonephritis. Urinary stasis and anatomic displacement of the ureters during pregnancy contribute to pathogenesis. In pregnancy, quantitative urine cultures should be obtained in women with persistent leukocyturia (more than two to three white blood cells per high-power field in spun sediment) and/or symptoms of cystitis. If there are $>10^5$ bacteria of a single species per milliliter of urine, significant bacteriuria is present. Acute pyelonephritis or cystitis can be diagnosed, even with 10^2 bacteria/ml, if accompanied by clinical symptoms. Acute pyelonephritis is a very serious complication during pregnancy and usually presents between 20 and 28 weeks of gestation with fevers, loin pain, and dysuria. Bacteremia, usually accompanying pyelonephritis, can progress to endotoxic shock, disseminated intravascular coagulation, and acute renal failure. Pregnant women with acute pyelonephritis should be admitted to hospital and treated with intravenous antibiotics and hydration. Intravenous cephalosporins or gentamicin should be given for 24 to 48 hours or until the patient is afebrile, followed by oral antibiotics for 10 to 14 days.

Asymptomatic Bacteriuria

Asymptomatic bacteriuria complicates 2% to 7% of pregnancies and may occur without pyuria. It is frequently associated with a reduction in the concentrating ability of the kidney. The organisms associated with asymptomatic bacteriuria are shown in Figure 41.1. Reagent strip testing for asymptomatic bacteriuria is associated with a high false-negative rate, and quantitative urine culture should be used to rule out significant bacteriuria.

Asymptomatic bacteruria has been associated with an increased risk of premature delivery and low birth weight. Treatment of asymptomatic bacteriuria during pregnancy reduces these complications and improves perinatal morbidity and mortality.[3] Without treatment, asymptomatic bacteriuria will persist in >80% of women and may progress to symptomatic urinary tract infection or acute pyelonephritis. Screening for asymptomatic bacteriuria with a urine culture is recommended during the first prenatal visit

Safety of antibiotics commonly used to treat urine infection in pregnancy	
Category of Drug	Antibiotic
A. Drugs taken by large numbers of pregnant women without any proven fetal harm	Amoxicillin, ampicillin Cefalexin, cephalothin Nalidixic acid Nitrofurantoin Penicillins
B1. Drugs taken by a limited number of pregnant women without proven fetal harm; animal studies show no increase in fetal damage	Aztreonam Ceftazidime, cefotaxime, cefaclor Amoxicillin/clavulanic acid Floxacillin (flucloxacillin) Piperacillin
B2. As B1, but animal data are unavailable	Vancomycin
B3. As B1, but animal studies show an increase in fetal damage	Ciprofloxacin, norfloxacin, ofloxacin Imipenem, trimethoprim
C. Drugs whose pharmacologic effects are suspected of causing fetal harm	Sulfonamides Cotrimoxazole Fusidic acid
D. Drugs that are proven to cause fetal harm	Tetracyclines Gentamicin and other aminoglycosides Chloramphenicol

Figure 41.2   Safety of antibiotics commonly used to treat urinary tract infection in pregnancy.

and is only repeated in high-risk women such as those with a history of recurrent urinary infections or urinary tract anomalies. If asymptomatic bacteriuria is found, prompt treatment is warranted, usually with a cephalosporin for at least 3 to 7 days, Treatment with a single dose of fosfomycin can also be used. Antibiotics useful in treating urinary infections during pregnancy are listed in Figure 41.2. Trimethoprim-sulfamethoxazole (cotrimoxazole) is contraindicated in early pregnancy because of its association with birth defects. Tetracycline and chloramphenicol are also contraindicated. Use of quinolones is discouraged during pregnancy because of some evidence of teratogenicity in animals. Women treated for asymptomatic bacteriuria should give a repeat urine culture 2 weeks after therapy to ensure that bacteriuria has been eradicated. Suppressive therapy with nitrofurantoin or cephalexin is recommended for those patients with bacteriuria that persists after two courses of therapy. Prolonged suppressive treatment of bacteriuria reduces the incidence of pyelonephritis.[4]

RENAL CALCULI

Although intestinal absorption and urinary excretion of calcium are increased during pregnancy, there is no evidence that the risk of nephrolithiasis is increased. Women who have had kidney stones can be reassured that pregnancy is not likely to increase stone formation. The management of symptomatic stone disease in pregnancy is discussed further in Chapter 42.

HYPERTENSIVE DISORDERS OF PREGNANCY

Hypertensive disorders of pregnancy can be considered in three categories:

1. Gestational hypertension, including preeclampsia-eclampsia
2. Chronic or pre-existing hypertension of any cause
3. Preeclampsia superimposed on chronic hypertension

Organisms most commonly responsible for asymptomatic bacteriuria in pregnancy
Escherichia coli (>70% of infections)
Klebsiella species
Proteus species (particularly in diabetic women or urinary tract obstruction)
Enterococci
Staphylococci, especially *Staphyloccocus saprophyticus*
Pseudomonas
Streptococci

Figure 41.1   Organisms most commonly responsible for asymptomatic bacteriuria in pregnancy.

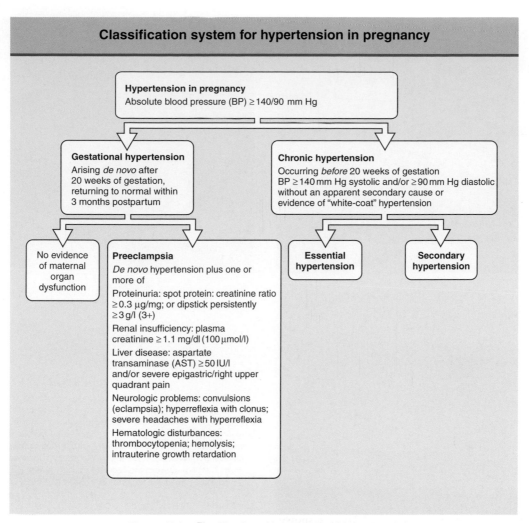

Classification system for hypertension in pregnancy

Hypertension in pregnancy
Absolute blood pressure (BP) ≥140/90 mm Hg

Gestational hypertension
Arising *de novo* after
20 weeks of gestation,
returning to normal within
3 months postpartum

Chronic hypertension
Occurring *before* 20 weeks of gestation
BP ≥140 mm Hg systolic and/or ≥90 mm Hg diastolic
without an apparent secondary cause or
evidence of "white-coat" hypertension

No evidence
of maternal
organ
dysfunction

Preeclampsia
De novo hypertension plus one or
more of
Proteinuria: spot protein: creatinine ratio
≥0.3 μg/mg; or dipstick persistently
≥3 g/l (3+)
Renal insufficiency: plasma
creatinine ≥1.1 mg/dl (100 μmol/l)
Liver disease: aspartate
transaminase (AST) ≥50 IU/l
and/or severe epigastric/right upper
quadrant pain
Neurologic problems: convulsions
(eclampsia); hyperreflexia with clonus;
severe headaches with hyperreflexia
Hematologic disturbances:
thrombocytopenia; hemolysis;
intrauterine growth retardation

**Essential
hypertension**

**Secondary
hypertension**

Figure 41.3   Classification of hypertension in pregnancy.

Figure 41.3 illustrates the various hypertensive disorders of pregnancy and the criteria used to make the distinction. Preeclampsia (pure or superimposed, categories 1 and 3) poses the greatest threat to fetal survival and is the disorder most often associated with severe maternal complications (including fatalities; Fig. 41.4). The majority of women in the second category have essential hypertension, and their pregnancies usually remain uncomplicated and end successfully. On occasion, however, the high blood pressure is due to specific causes including pheochromocytoma, Cushing's syndrome, renal artery stenosis, and/or primary renal disease,[5,6] and some of these women with secondary forms of hypertension do poorly during gestation. Thus, pheochromocytoma, although rare, may present for the first time during gestation and is especially lethal when unsuspected, whereas when diagnosed, it can be managed to a successful outcome, either surgically or pharmacologically (with α-blockade) depending on the stage of pregnancy.[5] Cushing's syndrome has been associated with exacerbations of hypertension during pregnancy and poor fetal outcomes. Finally, both angioplasty and stent placement have been successfully performed on pregnant women with renal artery stenosis.[5]

GESTATIONAL HYPERTENSION

Pregnant women with blood pressure >140/90 mm Hg, without proteinuria, and whose blood pressure was lower before pregnancy are described as having gestational hypertension. There is a range

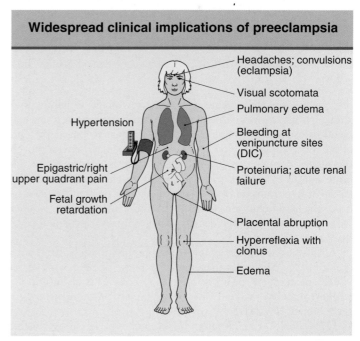

Widespread clinical implications of preeclampsia

Headaches; convulsions
(eclampsia)

Visual scotomata

Pulmonary edema

Hypertension

Bleeding at
venipuncture sites
(DIC)

Epigastric/right
upper quadrant pain

Proteinuria; acute renal
failure

Fetal growth
retardation

Placental abruption

Hyperreflexia with
clonus

Edema

Figure 41.4   Widespread clinical implications of preeclampsia. DIC, disseminated intravascular coagulation. (Adapted from Brown MA: Pregnancy-induced hypertension: Pathogenesis and management. Aust N Z J Med 1991; 21:257–273.)

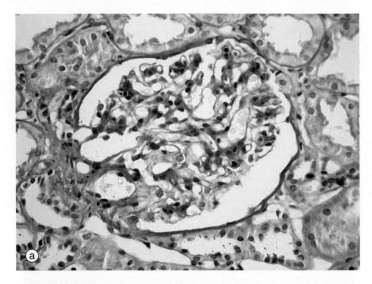

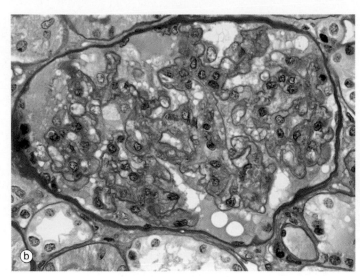

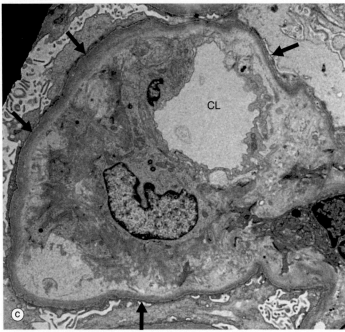

Figure 41.5 Glomerular endotheliosis. *a*, Normal glomerulus (periodic acid–Schiff, light microscopy ×40). *b*, Glomerulus from a patient with preeclampsia (periodic acid–Schiff, light microscopy ×40). Note occlusion of capillary lumina by swollen endothelial cells. *c*, Electron microscopy. Glomerular basement membrane (*arrows*) is separated from the reduced capillary lumen (CL) by swollen endothelial cell cytoplasm (original magnification ×7500). (Courtesy of Prof. P. Furness.)

of possible etiologies. Some hypertensive women, usually with a strong family history of essential hypertension, have a normal blood pressure throughout most of the pregnancy, but at the end of the third trimester, blood pressure tends to increase to approach the higher prepregnant level. Usually there is no protein in the urine and the blood uric acid is not elevated. There is evidence that transient hypertension of pregnancy occurs in women destined to have essential hypertension later in life (analogous to women with gestational hyperglycemia who eventually develop type 2 diabetes).

A substantial proportion of women (approximately 30%) with gestational hypertension have an early phase of preeclampsia, in which proteinuria has not yet appeared. This subgroup of patients may have some evidence of glomerular endotheliosis on renal biopsy (Fig. 41.5).[7]

Occasionally, the elevated blood pressure has a psychiatric cause such as an anxiety or panic disorder. A rare group of patients have activating mineralocorticoid receptor mutations that result in an exaggerated sensitivity to the usually weak mineralocorticoid effect of progesterone.[8] They manifest salt-sensitive hypertension,

accompanied by hypokalemia, but virtually undetectable aldosterone levels, most marked during pregnancy as progesterone levels rise.

The administration of large amounts of intravenous saline during a cesarean section can sometimes result in postpartum hypertension and edema that disappears in a few days when the large salt load is excreted.

PREECLAMPSIA

Definition

Preeclampsia is the most frequently encountered renal complication of pregnancy. It is characterized by the new onset of hypertension and proteinuria, usually after 20 weeks of pregnancy, and is commonly associated with edema and hyperuricemia. Blood pressure >140/90 mm Hg during pregnancy is required to make the diagnosis.[9] It was previously recommended that an increase in systolic blood pressure >30 mm Hg and/or diastolic >15 mm Hg from baseline values was sufficient to define hypertension; however, epidemiologic data indicate that outcomes are similar whatever the magnitude of the increase, provided blood pressure remains <140/90 mm Hg. Nevertheless, the U.S. National High Blood Pressure Education Program still recommends that women with blood pressure <140/90 mm Hg who have experienced a 30- and/or 15-mm Hg increase in systolic and/or diastolic levels, respectively, should be managed as high-risk patients. Proteinuria is defined as urine protein-to-creatinine ratio >0.3 μg/mg, which is sufficiently reliable to avoid the need for 24-hour urine collection. Finally, although serum uric acid is not included in the formal definition of preeclampsia, uric acid >4.5 mg/dl (270 μmol/l) may be used to diagnose preeclampsia, especially in patients with preexisting renal disease or hypertension (see Chapter 42). Preeclampsia is considered severe with urine protein-to-creatinine ratio >5 μg/mg, blood pressure >160/110 mm Hg, evidence of HELLP syndrome (*h*emolysis, *e*levated *l*iver enzymes, *l*ow *p*latelet syndrome), evidence of central nervous system dysfunction, or the presence of intrauterine fetal growth restriction (Fig. 41.6).

Epidemiology

Preeclampsia complicates approximately 5% of all pregnancies. It is about twice as common in first pregnancies as in multigravidas. Preeclampsia is also common in multigravidas who have a new partner, suggesting that prior exposure to paternal antigens may be protective.[10] However, recent evidence from a large Norwegian birth registry suggests that prolonged interpregnancy interval, rather than primipaternity, may account for this increase in risk for reasons that are unclear. Other predisposing factors include pre-existing hypertension, chronic renal disease, obesity, diabetes mellitus, thrombophilias (factor V Leiden, antiphospholipid syndrome, and antithrombin III deficiency), and multiple gestation (Fig. 41.7). It occurs more frequently in women whose mothers had preeclampsia and in women whose fathers were products of a preeclamptic pregnancy, perhaps because the placenta itself is a creation of both the mother and the father.[10] The incidence of preeclampsia is also higher in women who live in high altitudes,

Risk factors for the development of preeclampsia
Preeclampsia in prior pregnancy
Family history of preeclampsia
Nulliparity
Multiple gestation
Molar pregnancies
Older maternal age
Obesity
Preexisting hypertension
Preexisting chronic kidney disease
Diabetes mellitus
Thrombopohilia (antithrombin III deficiency, protein C or S deficiency, factor V Leiden, antiphospholipid antibody syndrome)
Trisomy 13 fetus
Fetal hydrops
High altitude

Figure 41.7   Risk factors for the development of preeclampsia.

suggesting that hypoxia may contribute to the development of the syndrome.

Pathogenesis

Preeclampsia occurs only in the presence of the placenta, even when there is no fetus (as in hydatidiform mole) and usually remits when the placenta is delivered. The placenta in preeclampsia is often abnormal, with evidence of hypoperfusion and ischemia. Preeclampsia is characterized by widespread systemic vascular endothelial dysfunction and microangiopathy in the mother, but not in the fetus. It is currently thought that preeclampsia is due to a circulating factor or factors produced by the diseased placenta that induce maternal vascular endothelial dysfunction.[11]

Abnormal Placentation in Preeclampsia

The characteristic placental lesion in preeclampsia is a diminution in endovascular invasion by cytotrophoblasts and a decrease in remodeling of the uterine spiral arterioles.[12] The hypothesis that defective trophoblastic invasion with accompanying uteroplacental hypoperfusion may lead to preeclampsia is supported by animal and human studies. Placentas from pregnancies with advanced preeclampsia often have numerous placental infarcts and sclerotic narrowing of arterioles.[10] Uteroplacental blood flow is usually diminished and uterine vascular resistance increased in preeclamptic women. Placental ischemia induced by mechanical constriction of the uterine arteries or aorta produces hypertension, proteinuria, and, variably, glomerular endotheliosis in several animal species.[13] However, placental ischemia alone, as seen in many cases of intrauterine growth restriction, does not appear to be sufficient to produce preeclampsia.

Preeclampsia Factor

The search for a circulating factor that causes the maternal syndrome of preeclampsia has been an area of intense investigation. Increased sensitivity to the vasopressor effects of angiotensin is a feature of preeclampsia, perhaps due to increased plasma concentrations of angiotensin I/bradykinin B2 receptor heterodimers.[10] Circulating concentrations of agonistic antibodies to the angiotensin I receptor have been reported in women with preeclampsia[14] and

Criteria for the diagnosis of severe preeclampsia
In patients with preeclampsia, **severe preeclampsia** can be diagnosed if any one of the following criteria is present:
Blood pressure $\geq$160 mm Hg systolic or $\geq$110 mm Hg diastolic or higher on two separate occasions at least 6 h apart
Proteinuria Random urine protein: creatinine ratio $\geq$5 μg/mg or proteinuria >5 g/24 h
Oliguria <500 ml in 24 h
Cerebral or visual disturbances such as cerebrovascular accident, seizures, and visual loss
Pulmonary edema
Epigastric or right upper quadrant pain
Hepatocellular injury (serum transaminases at least twice normal)
Serum lactate dehydrogenase: >600 IU/l
Thrombocytopenia: <100 × 10^9/l
Fetal growth restriction (birth weight lower than 10th percentile for the gestational age)

Figure 41.6.   Criteria for the diagnosis of severe preeclampsia. (Adapted from ACOG Practice Bulletin. Diagnosis and management of preeclampsia and eclampsia. Number 33, January 2002. Obstet Gynecol 2002;99:159–167.)

are also encountered in other examples of vascular injury such as vascular rejection, suggesting that they may be secondary to the generalized microangiopathy of preeclampsia.

Reactive free oxygen radicals may have a causal role in preeclampsia.[11] In some but not all studies, markers of oxidative stress are elevated in women with preeclampsia. Decreased intake of the antioxidant vitamin C and low circulating ascorbic acid levels are associated with an increased risk of preeclampsia. However, a randomized therapeutic trial of antioxidants (vitamins C and E) in pregnant women did not prevent preeclampsia, suggesting that oxidant stress is unlikely to be the primary mediator.[15] "Export" of fragments of trophoblastic material from the diseased placenta into the circulation has also been suggested as a possible cause for the generalized microangiopathy of preeclampsia.[11]

Circulating Antiangiogenic Factor

Recently, it has been found that sFlt-1 (soluble FMS-like tyrosine kinase-1, also referred to as sVEGFR-1) production is increased in the placenta in preeclamptic women.[16] sFlt-1 is a secreted protein, a splice variant of the VEGF (vascular endothelial growth factor) receptor Flt-1 lacking the transmembrane cytoplasmic domain of the membrane-bound receptor. It is a potent circulating antagonist to VEGF and placental growth factor (PlGF; Fig. 41.8). Both VEGF and PlGF are made by the placenta and circulate in high concentrations during pregnancy. VEGF is also synthesized by glomerular podocytes and vascular endothelial cells. Circulating sFlt-1 levels are greatly increased in women with established preeclampsia and prior to the onset of clinical symptoms, whereas free PlGF levels are decreased.[17] When administered to pregnant and nonpregnant rats, sFlt-1 produces hypertension, proteinuria, and glomerular endotheliosis resembling the human syndrome of preeclampsia. The glomerular lesion in these experimental animals, consisting of severe glomerular endothelial swelling and loss of endothelial fenestrae with relatively preserved foot processes in association with heavy proteinuria, is striking in its resemblance to human preeclampsia (see Fig. 41.5).[16,18]

The possibility that an antagonist of VEGF and PlGF might play a role in preeclampsia has a sound physiologic basis. As well as being potent promoters of angiogenesis, VEGF and PlGF are known to induce the synthesis of nitric oxide and vasodilating prostacyclins in endothelial cells, decreasing vascular tone and blood pressure. VEGF, synthesized in large amounts by glomerular podocytes, may be important in maintaining the health and healing of glomerular vascular endothelial cells, so that its absence induces proteinuria and glomerular endotheliosis.[19] The organs targeted in preeclampsia, such as the glomerulus or the hepatic sinusoids, have fenestrated endothelia. VEGF induces endothelial fenestrae *in vitro* and even a 50% decrease in VEGF production in the glomerulus in mice leads to glomerular endotheliosis and loss of glomerular endothelial fenestrae.[19] Antagonists of VEGF, used in cancer therapy, sometimes produce hypertension, proteinuria, and reversible posterior leukoencephalopathy, hallmarks of preeclampsia/eclampsia.[10] Furthermore, exogenous VEGF and PlGF can reverse the antiangiogenic effects of preeclamptic blood *in vitro*.[16] Thus,

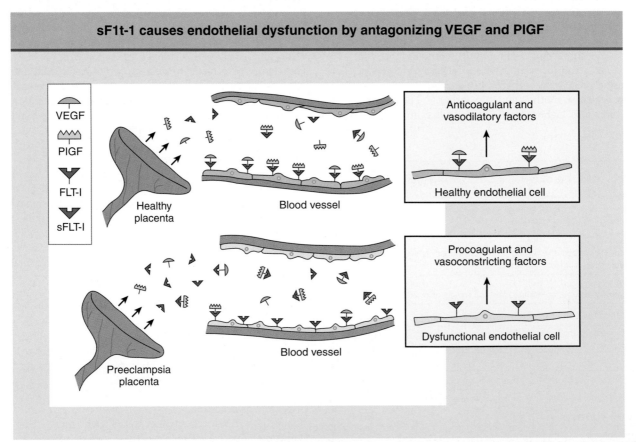

Figure 41.8 **Soluble FMS-like tyrosine kinase-1 (sFlt-1) causes endothelial dysfunction by antagonizing vascular endothelial growth factor (VEGF) and placental growth factor (PlGF).** There is mounting evidence that VEGF and possibly PlGF are required to maintain endothelial health in several tissues including the kidney and perhaps the placenta. In normal pregnancy, the placenta produces modest concentrations of VEGF, PlGF, and sFlt-1. In preeclampsia, excess placental sFlt-1 binds circulating VEGF and PlGF and prevents their interaction with endothelial cell surface receptors. This results in endothelial cell dysfunction, including decreased prostacyclin and nitric oxide production and release of procoagulant proteins such as von Willebrand factor, endothelin, cellular fibronectin (cFN), and thrombomodulin (TM). (From Karumanchi SA, Maynard SE, Stillman IE, et al: Preeclampsia: A renal perspective. Kidney Int 2005;67:2101–2113.)

the antiangiogenic effects of sFlt-1 may account for many of the manifestations of preeclampsia, including the unique glomerular changes.

The concentration of circulating sFlt-1 starts to increase near the end of the second trimester in women destined to have preeclampsia, 4 to 5 weeks before clinical manifestations of this syndrome, such as hypertension and proteinuria, are first detected.[17] By the time clinically overt preeclampsia has developed, plasma sFlt-1 is two to four times higher than is found in normal pregnancy at the same stage of gestation. The concentration of sFlt-1 in plasma is higher in patients with severe preeclampsia than in those with milder disease.[20] There is also a modest but significant decrease in circulating free PlGF levels in the first trimester in women who later develop preeclampsia, but from mid-pregnancy on, the concentration of PlGF in plasma decreases at the time when sFlt-1 levels are rising.[20] Since unbound PlGF is freely filtered, urinary PIGF levels may prove to be a predictor of subsequent preeclampsia.[20] Women carrying trisomy 13 fetuses have an increased risk of preeclampsia.[10] They also have high circulating concentrations of sFlt-1, perhaps not surprising since the gene for Flt-1/sFlt-1 is located on chromosome 13.

In addition to sFlt-1, recent studies have identified another circulating factor produced by ischemic placenta in the preeclamptic patient. Soluble endoglin is a coreceptor for transforming growth factor-β (TGF-β) that is anti-angiogenic and rises in the circulation beginning 2 to 3 months prior to the development of preeclampsia[21]; together with sFlt-1 it can induce a lesion in animals similar to preeclampsia but which also has features of HELLP syndrome.

Role of sFlt-1 and Soluble Endoglin

The likely role of sFlt-1 and soluble endoglin in the pathogenesis of preeclampsia is summarized in Figure 41.9. Overproduction of sFlt-1could explain susceptibility to preeclampsia in multiple gestation, hydatiform mole, trisomy 13, and, possibly, first

pregnancy. Alternatively, preeclampsia could follow sensitization of the maternal vascular endothelium to the antiangiogenic effects of sFlt-1. Such sensitization might occur in obesity, preexisting hypertension or renal disease, and diabetes. The average sFlt-1 level in the serum of obese patients with preeclampsia is lower than that in thinner preeclamptic patients.[17]

Hypoxia is known to increase the production of sFlt-1 by placental trophoblasts,[10] so that placental ischemia might trigger preeclampsia. Placental ischemia is common but not universal in preeclampsia. Placental infarction unaccompanied by preeclampsia is a common finding in mothers with sickle cell anemia and with intrauterine growth restriction. Placental overproduction of sFlt-1, whatever its cause, might itself decrease angiogenesis locally and result in placental ischemia, thereby initiating a vicious cycle leading to even more sFlt-1 production.

These three factors may all contribute in varying degree to the pathogenesis of preeclampsia: (1) a change in the balance of circulating factors controlling angiogenesis/antiangiogenesis attributable to placental overproduction of sFlt-1, soluble endoglin, and underproduction of PlGF, (2) increased vascular endothelial sensitivity to such factors,[22] and (3) placental ischemia. It is not surprising that in human pregnancy, characterized initially by rapid angiogenesis localized to the placenta, followed as pregnancy terminates by regression of blood vessel growth, there should sometimes occur systemic manifestations of a derangement of this process.

Pathology

Preeclampsia is associated with a unique and specific glomerular appearance, referred to as glomerular endotheliosis (see Fig. 41.5). On light microscopy, the glomerular capillary lumens are narrowed and appear bloodless, and the glomeruli are enlarged. Unlike other thrombotic microangiopathies, the endotheliosis of preeclampsia is usually not accompanied by prominent capillary thrombi. Immunofluorescence may reveal deposition of fibrinogen

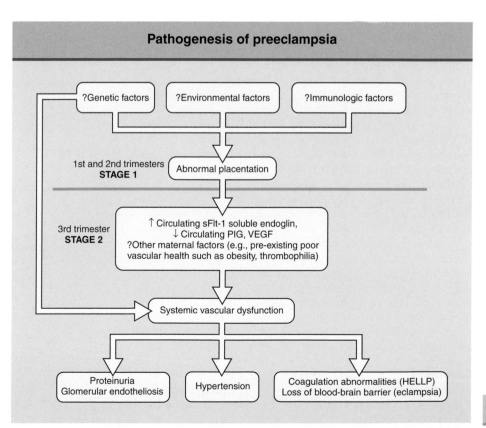

Figure 41.9 Summary of the pathogenesis of preeclampsia. PlGF, placental growth factor; sFlt-1, soluble FMS-like tyrosine kinase-1; VEGF, vascular endothelial growth factor.

derivatives, especially when signs of systemic thrombotic microangiopathy are prominent. There are no immune deposits in the glomeruli and serum complement levels are normal. Electron microscopy shows relative preservation of the podocyte foot processes despite heavy proteinuria, but there is loss of endothelial fenestrae, and endothelial cells become swollen and separated from the basement membrane by electron-lucent material.[18] Mild glomerular endotheliosis has been noted in up to 30% of patients with pregnancy-induced hypertension without proteinuria,[7,23] suggesting that some cases of pregnancy-induced hypertension may reflect an earlier or milder form of preeclampsia. The glomerular changes usually disappear within 8 weeks of delivery, coinciding with resolution of the hypertension and proteinuria. Focal segmental glomerulosclerosis is said to accompany the generalized glomerular endotheliosis of preeclampsia in up to 50% of cases.[10] Although this change has been taken by some to suggest there was kidney disease prior to pregnancy, it seems possible that it is the consequence of the preeclamptic process itself since similar changes may develop rapidly when glomerular endotheliosis is induced in animals.[19]

Clinical Manifestations

Preeclampsia is the most frequently encountered renal complication of pregnancy. It is characterized by the new onset of hypertension and proteinuria, usually during the last trimester of pregnancy, and is commonly associated with edema and hyperuricemia. Preeclampsia is characterized by widespread vascular endothelial dysfunction and microangiopathy in the mother, but not in the fetus. The predominant target organ may be the brain (seizures or eclampsia), the liver (HELLP syndrome), or the kidney (glomerular endotheliosis and proteinuria; see Fig. 41.4). Severe preeclampsia is also associated with intrauterine growth retardation and small-for-gestational-age babies.

Hypertension

During normal pregnancy, peripheral vascular resistance and systemic arterial blood pressure are decreased, but in preeclampsia these changes are reversed. Increased peripheral vascular resistance rather than increased cardiac output is the chief cause of hypertension.[10] As in other forms of hypertension, sympathetic activation is prominent, and there is an exaggerated response to infusions of angiotensin II and other hypertensive stimuli.[10]

In preeclampsia, the renin angiotensin aldosterone system (RAS) is suppressed,[24] suggesting that vasoconstriction, increased peripheral vascular resistance, and renal sodium and water retention are initial events, resulting in an increased effective circulating blood volume and subsequent RAS suppression. This is consistent with the observation that, although total plasma volume is slightly decreased, the hypertension of preeclampsia is exacerbated by salt loading and at least partly ameliorated by diuretics and salt deprivation.[10] A comparable decrease in total plasma volume with an increase in peripheral vascular resistance and arterial blood pressure can be produced by the infusion into normal subjects of norepinephrine and other vasoconstrictors. The vasoconstriction of preeclampsia appears to be mediated by alterations in several vasoactive molecules, including the vasoconstrictors norepinephrine, endothelin, and perhaps thromboxane, and the vasodilators prostacyclin and perhaps nitric oxide.

Edema

Sudden weight gain, with edema of the feet, hands, and face, is a common presenting symptom in preeclampsia. Women with preeclampsia excrete a much smaller percentage of an intravenous saline load than do normal pregnant women.[10] Since there is RAS suppression, this implies primary renal retention of salt and water. The edema of preeclampsia thus resembles the overfill edema of acute glomerulonephritis or of acute ischemic renal failure with volume overload.

A generalized increase in capillary permeability is unlikely to explain preeclamptic edema since the concentration of protein in interstitial fluid from preeclamptic patients is not elevated.[10] Hypoalbuminemia is common and may contribute to edema formation in some patients.

Renal Function, Proteinuria, and the Urinary Sediment

Abnormalities of renal function in preeclampsia are summarized in Figure 41.10. GFR and renal plasma flow are uniformly decreased compared to the increases in normal pregnancy. Blood urea nitrogen and serum creatinine often remain in the nonpregnant normal range, despite a significant decrease in GFR from the elevated levels of normal pregnancy. Simultaneous measurements of GFR and renal plasma flow indicate that the filtration fraction is lower during preeclampsia than in normal women during the last trimester of pregnancy.[18,25]

The urinary sediment is usually "bland" in preeclampsia, with few leukocytes, erythrocytes, or cellular casts. Hyaline casts may be present when proteinuria is heavy. The presence of many erythrocytes or erythrocyte casts suggests glomerulonephritis.

The proteinuria of preeclampsia is nonselective; that is, while most of the urinary protein is albumin, high molecular weight proteins are present as well.[25] After delivery, proteinuria usually disappears within 7 to 10 days, although in a few women, it may persist, although gradually diminishing, for 3 to 6 months.

Uric Acid

A disproportionate decrease in uric acid clearance is a key feature of preeclampsia. The serum uric acid concentration increases as preeclampsia progresses; a level >5.5 mg/dl (325 μmol/l) is a strong indicator of preeclampsia, and >7.8 mg/dl (460 μmol/l) is associated with significant maternal morbidity. The degree of uric acid elevation correlates with the severity of proteinuria and renal pathologic changes and with fetal demise.[10] Often, the elevation of uric acid precedes the onset of proteinuria and changes in GFR.

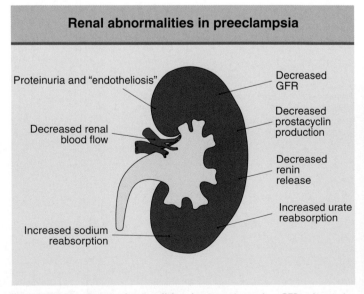

Renal abnormalities in preeclampsia

Proteinuria and "endotheliosis"
Decreased renal blood flow
Increased sodium reabsorption
Decreased GFR
Decreased prostacyclin production
Decreased renin release
Increased urate reabsorption

Figure 41.10 Renal abnormalities in preeclampsia. GFR, glomerular filtration rate.

Lowering serum uric acid by the administration of probenecid does not alter the hypertension and proteinuria of preeclampsia, so it is likely that hyperuricemia is a secondary rather than a primary phenomenon, analogous to the disproportionate decrease in urate clearance produced in normal human subjects by vasoconstrictors like angiotensin II and norepinephrine.[10] Nevertheless, recent rodent studies suggest that hyperuricemia may play a pathogenic role by contributing to the vascular damage and hypertension.[26]

Neurologic Abnormalities

The sudden development of seizures (eclampsia), together with headache, blurred vision, or temporary loss of vision, has been attributed to brain edema, thrombotic microangiopathy, and cerebral vasoconstriction. Sudden marked elevations of blood pressure usually contribute to the severe cerebral edema that is a hallmark at postmortem examination of women who die of eclampsia. Hyperactive tendon reflexes often precede convulsions. The cerebral edema of eclampsia involves predominantly the posterior portions of the white matter, is referred to as reversible posterior leukoencephalopathy syndrome, and is best visualized using magnetic resonance imaging.[27] Treatment with intravenous magnesium sulfate usually lowers blood pressure and reduces central nervous system irritability, but does not improve renal function. Occasionally, seizures occur postpartum, usually within 4 days but very rarely as long as 3 to 4 weeks after delivery in women in whom preeclampsia, although probably present, was not detected during the pregnancy.

HELLP Syndrome

This term is applied to patients with preeclampsia in whom the clinical picture is dominated by hemolysis, elevated liver enzymes and low platelets, all occurring as a result of the generalized maternal vascular dysfunction of preeclampsia.[28] Very occasionally subcapsular liver hemorrhage or liver rupture may develop. HELLP syndrome occurs in 10% to 20% of patients with preeclampsia and is one of its most severe forms. Symptoms and signs usually disappear promptly after delivery, although laboratory measures may transiently worsen in the first 24 hours, but improve within 7 days following delivery. Thrombocytopenia is a consequence of consumption coagulopathy, and usually disappears by 1 week postpartum.

Natural History

Following delivery, the hypertension and proteinuria of preeclampsia usually disappear within a few days to weeks, but complete resolution may occasionally take longer. In exceptional cases, proteinuria lingers up to 6 months after delivery. Renal biopsy is indicated if proteinuria persists >6 months or earlier if the proteinuria is accompanied by an active urine sediment or rapidly deteriorating renal function.

Considerable evidence suggests that preeclampsia predisposes women to late vascular disease.[29,30] Fifteen years after an episode of preeclampsia, the incidence of hypertension is five times that found in women with normal pregnancies who never had preeclampsia (37% versus 7%).[31] This tendency to later hypertension appears to be the result of preeclampsia rather than inherited factors since the same risk is not found in the siblings of preeclamptic patients.[31] Recent epidemiologic studies suggest that preeclampsia predicts remote cardiovascular deaths.[32]

Prevention

Because preeclampsia occurs more frequently in women with chronic hypertension, it is thought that if high blood pressure is controlled in such women, the risk of preeclampsia is lowered, but

this is not yet known with certainty. Low-dose aspirin (75 to 80 mg/day) is said to reduce the incidence of preeclampsia in those at high risk such as those with underlying renal disease or preexisting hypertension, but this has not been demonstrated in large prospective studies.[33] Oral calcium supplements may reduce the likelihood of preeclampsia in women whose calcium intake is extremely low.[34] Vitamins C and E do not protect against preeclampsia.[15]

Treatment

Figure 41.11 lists the key management options issues for patients with preeclampsia. The most reliable treatment of preeclampsia is delivery. Removal of the placenta usually produces prompt improvement, although in a few cases, in which the disease has been explosive, symptoms may progress for several days, even after delivery. Unexpected uterine hemorrhage may produce shock and cortical necrosis, and excessive saline infusions given to prevent that eventuality may trigger pulmonary edema or exacerbate hypertension.

The hypertension of preeclampsia usually responds to pharmacologic treatment. Prompt lowering of the blood pressure is important to reduce the risk of cerebral edema, cerebral hemorrhage, and eclampsia. Blood pressure should be maintained at <140/90 mm Hg; however, it is important not to lower the blood pressure to <120/80 mm Hg as relative hypotension may further compromise the fetoplacental blood flow. Figure 41.12 summarizes the recommended pharmacologic treatments for hypertension in pregnancy and preeclampsia. Angiotensin-converting enzyme inhibitors and angiotensin receptor blockers interfere with renal development in the fetus and should not be used in pregnancy. Although proteinuria may lessen as the blood pressure decreases, renal function usually does not improve, and the mother remains at risk of the development of HELLP syndrome and the fetus at risk of intrauterine death or placental abruption. Abrupt decreases in blood pressure produced by medication may produce renal cortical necrosis.

Management of preeclampsia	
Clinical Problem	Management
Assess indications for delivery	Always review whether an indication for delivery is present by clinical and laboratory monitoring
Control blood pressure (BP)	Acute treatment if BP ≥170/110 mm Hg Chronic treatment if BP ≥140/90 mm Hg
Eclampsia prophylaxis or treatment	Diazepam 10–20 mg IV to terminate convulsions Magnesium sulfate for persistent neurologic signs (also an indication for delivery): 4 g IV over 20 min, then 1.5 g/h for 48 h
Volume expander therapy	500–1000 ml colloid over 4–6 h for persistent oliguria 500 ml colloid in conjunction with parenteral antihypertensive therapy or before epidural anesthesia
Supportive therapies (sometimes required)	Platelet infusion if count <20–40 ×10⁹/l Fresh-frozen plasma for microangiopathy or for reduced clotting factors Dialysis for established acute renal failure
Progressive decline in renal, hepatic, or clotting function or of fetal growth	Delivery

Figure 41.11 Management of preeclampsia.

Common medications used in the treatment of hypertension in preeclampsia		
Type of Hypertension	Drug	Treatment Regimen
Acute	Hydralazine	5-mg IV bolus every 20–30 min to maximum of 20 mg, then infusion at 5–10 mg/h
	Labetalol	50 mg IV every 20 min to maximum 300 mg
	Nifedipine SR	20 mg oral
Chronic		
First-line choice	Methyldopa	500–2000 mg/day PO
	Clonidine	0.2–0.8 mg/day PO
	Oxprenolol	80–480 mg/day PO
	Labetalol	200–1200 mg/day PO
	Atenolol	50–100 mg/day PO
Second-line choice	Hydralazine	25–200 mg/day PO
	Prazosin	1–10 mg/day PO
	Nifedipine SR	40–100 mg/day PO

Figure 41.12 Common medications in the treatment of hypertension in preeclampsia. Diuretics and propranolol are not recommended. Angiotensin-converting enzyme inhibitors and angiotensin receptor blockers are contraindicated. SR, sustained release.

Infusions of magnesium sulfate are effective in preventing epileptic seizures and lowering blood pressure. At high concentrations, magnesium ions depress the respiratory center, and magnesium infusions should not be given if the deep tendon reflexes (e.g., patellar reflex) cannot be elicited. Intravenous dexamethasone is suggested to hasten recovery in HELLP syndrome, but this has not been confirmed by larger studies.[35] Platelet transfusions are indicated if there is significant maternal bleeding or if platelet counts are $<20 \times 10^9$ liters.

ACUTE RENAL FAILURE IN PREGNANCY

Acute Renal Failure and Renal Cortical Necrosis

The most common cause of acute renal failure during early pregnancy is dehydration owing to hyperemesis gravidarum. However, after 20 weeks of gestation, pregnancy-specific conditions such as preeclampsia may also lead to acute renal failure. Pregnancy has long been known to confer a peculiar susceptibility to the vascular effects of gram-negative endotoxin (Schwartzman phenomenon). Perhaps because of the physiologic increase in procoagulant factors that occurs in normal pregnancy, the thrombotic micro-angiopathy and renal cortical necrosis that characterize septic shock, especially with gram-negative organisms, are particularly pronounced during pregnancy. Renal cortical necrosis is a common complication, for example, of septic abortion.

Hemolytic Uremic Syndrome and Thrombotic Thrombocytopenic Purpura

Hemolytic uremic syndrome/thrombotic thrombocytopenic purpura (HUS/TTP) is a relatively rare complication that usually occurs toward the end of pregnancy or in the immediate postpartum period. The clinical features of HUS/TTP include thrombocytopenia, hemolysis, and variable organ dysfunction including acute renal failure. The distinction between HUS/TTP and HELLP syndrome of preeclampsia is often difficult, and occasionally there may be an overlap of both disorders. A history of proteinuria and hypertension and a predominant liver involvement are more suggestive of the HELLP syndrome, whereas renal failure and numerous schistocytes on the peripheral smears are more typical of HUS/TTP. The differentiation of HUS/TTP from HELLP syndrome is clinically important since plasma exchange is usually recommended for HUS/TTP and not for HELLP syndrome. The management is discussed further in Chapter 28.

Acute Fatty Liver of Pregnancy

Acute fatty liver of pregnancy is an extremely rare complication that is estimated to occur in about one in 10,000 pregnancies. The histologic abnormalities are swollen hepatocytes filled with microvesicular fat and minimal hepatocellular necrosis. A defect in mitochondrial fatty acid oxidation due to mutations in the long-chain 3-hydroxyacyl coenzyme A dehydrogenase deficiency has recently been hypothesized as a risk factor for the development of fatty liver of pregnancy.[36] Acute renal failure occurs in over half the patients, although the mechanisms of acute renal failure are unclear. Occasionally, there appears to be an overlap of this disorder with preeclampsia.

General Management of Acute Renal Failure in Pregnancy

The key issue in treatment of acute renal failure in pregnancy is restoration of fluid volume deficits and, in later pregnancy, delivery of the baby and placenta as quickly as possible. No specific therapy is effective in acute cortical necrosis. Both peritoneal dialysis and hemodialysis have been used during pregnancy, but peritoneal dialysis carries the risk of impairing uteroplacental blood flow.

REFERENCES

1. Packham D, Fairley KF: Renal biopsy: Indications and complications in pregnancy. Br J Obstet Gynaecol 1987;94:935–939.
2. Lindheimer MD, Davison JM: Renal disorders. In Barron WM, Lindheimer MD (eds): Medical Disorders During Pregnancy. Mosby Year Book, 1990, pp 42–72.
3. Smaill F: Antibiotics for asymptomatic bacteriuria in pregnancy. Cochrane Database Syst Rev 2001;2:D000490.
4. Rouse DJ, Andrews WW, Goldenberg RL, Owen J: Screening and treatment of asymptomatic bacteriuria of pregnancy to prevent pyelonephritis: A cost-effectiveness and cost-benefit analysis. Obstet Gynecol 1995;86: 119–123.
5. August P, Lindheimer MD: Chronic hypertension and pregnancy. In Laragh JH, Brenner BM (eds): Chesley's Hypertensive Disorders in Pregnancy, 2nd ed. Stamford, CT: Appleton & Lange, 1999.
6. Lindheimer MD, Richardson DA, Ehrlich EN, Katz AI: Potassium homeostasis in pregnancy. J Reprod Med 1987;32:517–522.
7. Strevens H, Wide-Swensson D, Hansen A, et al: Glomerular endotheliosis in normal pregnancy and pre-eclampsia. Br J Gynaecol 2003;110: 831–836.
8. Geller DS, Farhi A, Pinkerton N, et al. Activating mineralocorticoid receptor mutation in hypertension exacerbated by pregnancy. Science 2000;289:119–123.
9. ACOG Practice Bulletin. Diagnosis and management of preeclampsia and eclampsia. Number 33, January 2002. Obstet Gynecol 2002;99: 159–167.
10. Karumanchi SA, Maynard SE, Stillman IE, et al: Preeclampsia: A renal perspective. Kidney Int 2005;67:2101–2113.
11. Redman CW, Sargent IL: Latest advances in understanding preeclampsia. Science 2005;308:1592–1594.
12. Red-Horse K, Zhou Y, Genbacev O, et al: Trophoblast differentiation during embryo implantation and formation of the maternal-fetal interface. J Clin Invest 2004;114:744–754.

13. Podjarny E, Baylis C, Losonczy G: Animal models of preeclampsia. Semin Perinatol 1999;23:2–13.
14. Wallukat G, Homuth V, Fischer T, et al: Patients with preeclampsia develop agonistic autoantibodies against the angiotensin AT1 receptor. J Clin Invest 1999;103:945–952.
15. Poston L, Briley AJ, Seed PT, et al: Vitamin C and vitamin E in pregnant women at risk for pre-eclampsia (VIP trial): Randomized placebo-controlled trial. Lancet 2006;367:1145–1154.
16. Maynard SE, Min JY, Merchan J, et al: Excess placental soluble fms-like tyrosine kinase 1 (sFlt1) may contribute to endothelial dysfunction, hypertension, and proteinuria in preeclampsia. J Clin Invest 2003;111:649–658.
17. Levine RJ, Maynard SE, Qian C, et al: Circulating angiogenic factors and the risk of preeclampsia. N Engl J Med 2004;350:672–683.
18. Lafayette RA, Druzin M, Sibley R, et al: Nature of glomerular dysfunction in pre-eclampsia. Kidney Int 1998;54:1240–1249.
19. Eremina V, Sood M, Haigh J, et al: Glomerular-specific alterations of VEGF-A expression lead to distinct congenital and acquired renal diseases. J Clin Invest 2003;111:707–716.
20. Lam C, Lim KH, Karumanchi SA: Circulating angiogenic factors in the pathogenesis and prediction of preeclampsia. Hypertension 2005;46:1077–1085.
21. Levine RJ, Lam C, Qian C, et al: Soluble endoglin and other anti-angiogenic factors in pre-eclampsia. New Engl J Med 2006;355:992–1005.
22. Thadhani R, Ecker JL, Mutter WP, et al: Insulin resistance and alterations in angiogenesis: Additive insults that may lead to preeclampsia. Hypertension 2004;43:988–992.
23. Fisher KA, Luger A, Spargo BH, Lindheimer MD: Hypertension in pregnancy: Clinical-pathological correlations and remote prognosis. Medicine (Baltimore) 1981;60:267–276.
24. August P, Lenz T, Ales KL, et al: Longitudinal study of the renin-angiotensin-aldosterone system in hypertensive pregnant women: Deviations related to the development of superimposed preeclampsia. Am J Obstet Gynecol 1990;163:1612–1621.
25. Moran P, Baylis PH, Lindheimer MD, Davison JM: Glomerular ultrafiltration in normal and preeclamptic pregnancy. J Am Soc Nephrol 2003;14:648–652.
26. Kang DH, Finch J, Nakagawa T, et al: Uric acid, endothelial dysfunction and pre-eclampsia: Searching for a pathogenetic link. J Hypertens 2004;22:229–235.
27. Hinchey J, Chaves C, Appignani B, et al: A reversible posterior leukoencephalopathy syndrome. N Engl J Med 1996;334:494–500.
28. Sibai BM: Diagnosis, controversies, and management of the syndrome of hemolysis, elevated liver enzymes, and low platelet count. Obstet Gynecol 2004;103:981–991.
29. Sibai BM, el-Nazer A, Gonzalez-Ruiz A: Severe preeclampsia-eclampsia in young primigravid women: Subsequent pregnancy outcome and remote prognosis. Am J Obstet Gynecol 1986;155:1011–1016.
30. Irgens HU, Reisaeter L, Irgens LM, Lie RT: Long term mortality of mothers and fathers after pre-eclampsia: Population based cohort study. BMJ 2001;323:1213–1217.
31. Epstein FH: Late vascular effects of toxemia of pregnancy. N Engl J Med 1964;271:391–395.
32. Funai EF, Friedlander Y, Paltiel O, et al: Long-term mortality after preeclampsia. Epidemiology 2005;16:206–215.
33. Caritis S, Sibai B, Hauth J, et al: Low-dose aspirin to prevent preeclampsia in women at high risk. N Engl J Med 1998;338:701–705.
34. Villar J, Abdel-Aleem H, Merialdi M, et al: World Health Organization randomized trial of calcium supplementation among low calcium intake pregnant women. Am J Obstet Gynecol 2006;194:639–649.
35. Fonseca JE, Mendez F, Catano C, Arias F: Dexamethasone treatment does not improve the outcome of women with HELLP syndrome: A double-blind, placebo-controlled, randomized clinical trial. Am J Obstet Gynecol 2005;193:1591–1598.
36. Ibdah JA, Bennett MJ, Rinaldo P, et al: A fetal fatty-acid oxidation disorder as a cause of liver disease in pregnant women. N Engl J Med 1999;340:1723–1731.

Pregnancy with Pre-existing Kidney Disease

David Williams

INTRODUCTION

The kidneys undergo marked hemodynamic, renal tubular, and endocrine changes during pregnancy (see Chapter 40). A failure of these adaptations in women with chronic kidney disease (CKD) creates a suboptimal environment for fetal development and increases the risk for obstetric complications such as preeclampsia, preterm labor, and intrauterine growth restriction (IUGR). In turn, the diseased maternal kidneys are exposed to the damaging consequences of a prothrombotic state, ascending urinary infections, gestational hypertension, and altered hemodynamics that exacerbate proteinuria. Pre-existing hypertension, proteinuria, recurrent urinary tract infections, and, in women with diabetic nephropathy, poor glycemic control are all independently but cumulatively detrimental to maternal and fetal outcome. Advice to women with CKD regarding pregnancy must take into account all these parameters in an effort to answer the two most important questions:

1. What effect will the pregnancy have on the mother's kidney disease?
2. What effect will the mother's kidney disease have on the pregnancy?

IMPACT OF PREGNANCY ON PRE-EXISTING MATERNAL KIDNEY DISEASE

The effect of pregnancy-related changes on women with pre-existing CKD depends on the type of renal disease, the level of renal impairment, and the presence of hypertension, proteinuria, and infection (Fig. 42.1). Available data have not defined pre-existing renal disease using the now widely used classification of CKD originally proposed by the Kidney Disease Outcomes Quality Initiative (K/DOQI) but have mostly defined renal impairment on the basis of serum creatinine (SCr) values.

The normal gestational increment in glomerular filtration rate (GFR) is attenuated in women with moderate renal impairment and absent in those with SCr >2.3 mg/dl (202 μmol/l).[1–4] Similarly, the gestational increase in blood volume and erythropoiesis is inversely related to the preconception SCr.[3] At all levels of preconception CKD, the likelihood of renal damage as a consequence of pregnancy is increased by the coexistence of other factors, in particular hypertension, proteinuria, and infection.[1,3,5–7]

Pre-existing Proteinuria and Hypertension

Asymptomatic proteinuria (>500 mg/day) detected before 20 weeks' gestation usually indicates pre-existing renal disease.[8] These women have an increased risk for preeclampsia (30%), which increases further in those who also have chronic hypertension.[8] Limited postpartum follow-up of women with proteinuria

Features detrimental to long-term maternal renal function and pregnancy outcome	
Preconception impaired renal function	
Mild: (SCr <1.4 mg/dl, 123 μmol/l) or GFR >50 ml/min	Mild: Little or no decline in renal function[2,10]
Moderate: (SCr 1.5–1.9 mg/dl; 132–167 μmol/l) or GFR 25–50 ml/min	Moderate: 40% have a gestational decline in renal function, but 50% of these recover postpartum[9,11]
Severe: (SCr>2 mg/dl, 176 μmol/l) or GFR <25 ml/min	Severe: Two thirds of mothers have an accelerated decline in renal function, and one third develop ESRD in association with pregnancy[9]
	The worse the preconception renal function, the greater the risk for preterm labor, IUGR, and preeclampsia[1,3,9,15]
Preconception hypertension	Increased risk for preeclampsia, IUGR, and preterm labor[1,15]
	Accelerated decline in maternal renal function[1,3,5–7]
Proteinuria	Nephrotic range proteinuria associated with maternal thromboembolism[17,30]; variable reports of IUGR, preterm labor, and poorer long-term maternal renal prognosis[8,9,16]
Urinary tract infections	Increased maternal and fetal morbidity with acute pyelonephritis and preeclampsia
	Increased risk for preterm labor
Reduced plasma volume	IUGR
Hyperglycemia	Large-for-gestational-age babies
	But if microvascular disease: increased risk for IUGR[25]

Figure 42.1 **Features detrimental to long-term maternal renal function and pregnancy outcome.** ESRD, end-stage renal disease; GFR, glomerular filtration rate; IUGR, intrauterine growth restriction; SCr, serum creatinine.

identified in early pregnancy has shown that they have an increased risk for progressive renal impairment.[8] It is therefore important that women with proteinuria recognized during early pregnancy are investigated for previously occult renal disease and monitored serially throughout pregnancy for changes in renal function, level of proteinuria, blood pressure, and occult urinary infection. Chronic hypertension and preconception proteinuria usually worsen in the third trimester,[9] and in women with prepregnancy renal impairment, these parameters are associated with an increased risk for a further decline in renal function postpartum.[1,3,5–7]

Pre-existing Mild-to-Moderate Renal Impairment

Women who become pregnant with renal disease, but who have normal or near normal renal function at conception and SCr < 1.4 mg/dl (123 μmol/l), carry only a slightly increased risk for long-term damage to their kidneys from pregnancy compared with women with mild renal disease who had never become pregnant.[2,10] However, more accurate data using measurements or estimates of GFR as well as SCr are still needed.

In a large series, 40% of women with SCr 1.5 to 1.9 mg/dl (132–168 μmol/l) had a pregnancy-related deterioration in renal function, which persisted after delivery in about half.[9,11] Only 1 of 49 pregnancies (2%) in women with an initial SCr < 2 mg/dl (176 μmol/l) rapidly declined to end-stage renal disease (ESRD).[9]

Pre-existing Severe Renal Impairment

Two thirds of women with SCr > 2 mg/dl (176 μmol/l) have a gestational deterioration in renal function.[9] Unlike women who have mild to moderate renal impairment, this deterioration nearly always persists postpartum. One third of women with SCr > 2 mg/dl (176 μmol/l) will progress to ESRD during or after pregnancy.[9]

There is no guarantee that aborting the pregnancy will reverse a decline in renal function. Indeed, women with severe renal impairment who have a gestational decline in renal function requiring dialysis might consider continuing the pregnancy (in the absence of other complications) because, with modern management, there is an 80% chance of a live birth outcome when dialysis is started after conception.[12] Women who are established on dialysis with ESRD have no further renal function to lose, but they put themselves at high risk for morbidity from gestational syndromes such as preeclampsia.

IMPACT OF PRE-EXISTING RENAL IMPAIRMENT ON PREGNANCY OUTCOME

Women with preexisting CKD are more vulnerable to preeclampsia, preterm delivery, and fetal IUGR, especially when there is associated chronic hypertension.[2,13] Developments in neonatal and obstetric care during the past few decades are responsible for the impressive improvement in neonatal outcome from women with impaired renal function.[1,4,9] However, women with the most severe renal impairment still have the worst fetal outcomes.[1,3,9] Early pregnancy losses are often ignored in analyses of pregnancy outcome but are also more common in women with severe renal impairment.[1,14] Perinatal mortality rate is significantly higher with GFR < 70 ml/min.[15] A consistent observation is that SCr > 2.5 mg/dl (220 μmol/l) is associated with more preterm deliveries and lower birth weights than is lower SCr.[9] In one series, 73% of such women were delivered before 37 weeks, and 57% had IUGR, compared with 55% and 31%, respectively, for women with SCr < 2.5 mg/dl, although neonatal survival was 100%.[9]

A cesarean birth rate of about 60% is a consistent finding in most series of women who have markedly impaired renal function but relatively good perinatal outcome.[1,5,9] Therefore, when the fetus is put at risk by maternal disease, it seems inadvisable to prolong pregnancy beyond a point when neonatal survival is expected.

Clinical Parameters and Pregnancy Outcome

It is difficult to separate the independent contributions to poor fetal outcome of maternal hypertension, proteinuria, and renal impairment, but the balance of evidence suggests that each parameter is individually and cumulatively detrimental to fetal outcome.[1–3,14]

Pre-existing Hypertension

In one study, women with moderate to severe renal impairment (SCr 1.2–5.5 mg/dl [106–484 μmol/l]), who were hypertensive at conception or in early pregnancy had a 10 times higher relative risk for fetal loss compared with normotensive women with the same level of renal function.[1] Another study found that if the preconception blood pressure was > 140/90 mm Hg, perinatal mortality was 23% versus 4% for normotensive women with CKD.[15] Furthermore, treatment of chronic hypertension before conception reduces the incidence of fetal and maternal complications toward that of normotensive women.[14]

Pre-existing Proteinuria

Most studies indicate the negative impact of proteinuria in pregnancy outcome. In primary glomerulonephritis, there is a linear relationship between increasing proteinuria and decreasing infant weight.[16] Women with asymptomatic proteinuria (>500 mg/24 hours) in early pregnancy are reported to have > 95% live births, but 45% preterm deliveries, 23% complicated by IUGR and 62% with superimposed preeclampsia.[8] However, in another series of pregnancies affected by moderate to severe renal impairment, high-level proteinuria appeared to have no effect on pregnancy outcome.[9]

Glomerular Thrombosis

Women with renal disease typically have hyperfiltration through remaining glomeruli and associated microalbuminuria. During healthy pregnancy, women develop a prothrombotic and proinflammatory state, which even if preeclampsia does not occur, is often associated with a degree of glomerular endothelial swelling.[17] If preeclampsia does emerge, the glomerular capillary endothelial cells swell, and the narrowed lumen is filled with thrombus (Fig. 42.2). Thrombosis and infarction within glomerular capillaries lead to loss of functioning nephrons. Subclinical cortical necrosis due to glomerular capillary thrombosis is a possible explanation for the gestational loss of renal function associated with pregnancies complicated by moderate to severe renal impairment, especially in relation to sepsis due to recurrent urinary tract infections.[4] Prophylactic low-dose aspirin (50–150 mg/day) is given in an attempt to

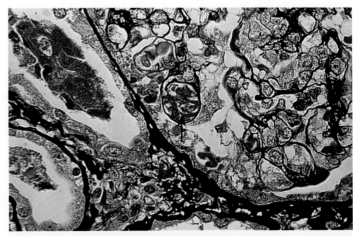

Figure 42.2 Glomerular fibrin deposition in pregnancy. Renal biopsy during pregnancy in a patient with reflux nephropathy showing fibrin thrombi in a glomerular capillary lumen (*arrow*).

prevent glomerular capillary thrombi, preserve maternal renal function, and reduce the risk for preeclampsia.[18] Pregnant women with proteinuria (>1–3 g/24 hours) are at high risk for systemic venous thrombosis and should receive thrombosis prophylaxis with low-molecular-weight (LMW) heparin until at least 6 weeks postpartum. Twice the nonpregnant thrombosis prophylaxis dose is required for clinical effectiveness owing to the gestational increase in renal clearance of heparin.

SPECIFIC RENAL DISEASES IN PREGNANCY

Primary Glomerulonephritis
The histologic type of primary glomerulonephritis does not affect pregnancy outcome as much as the clinical parameters of hypertension, proteinuria, level of renal impairment, and urinary tract infection (UTI).[15] The association of certain histopathologic diagnoses with a worse fetal or maternal outcome probably reflects the increased incidence of these clinical complications.[7,15] However, the presence of severe vascular lesions on renal biopsy specimens has been associated with increased perinatal mortality but surprisingly little effect on maternal complications.[14] On the rare occasion that sudden renal impairment (SCr > 1.4 mg/dl [123 μmol/l]), new-onset heavy proteinuria (>5 g/24 hours), or an active urinary sediment with red-cell casts occurs before 30 to 32 weeks' gestation in the absence of preeclampsia, a renal biopsy is indicated to exclude a steroid-responsive glomerular disease. In a heavily gravid woman, the plethoric kidney is less accessible and more prone to bleed, and renal biopsy should be undertaken by an experienced operator.[17] After 32 weeks, the option of waiting until an early delivery becomes possible. After delivery, gestationally induced proteinuria and renal impairment should improve, but if not, a renal biopsy becomes less difficult, and therapeutic options broaden.

IgA Nephropathy and Henoch-Schönlein Purpura
IgA nephropathy is the most common pattern of chronic primary glomerulonephritis in young people and is consequently highly represented in pregnant women. Pregnancy outcomes do not differ significantly from the general principles stated earlier. Women who have a preconception SCr > 1.4 mg/dl (120 μmol/l), GFR < 50 ml/min, with hypertension, heavy proteinuria, and the most severe histologic lesions on renal biopsy are most likely to have an accelerated deterioration in renal function and a pregnancy complicated by preeclampsia, IUGR, and preterm labor.[7,15]

Women who had Henoch-Schönlein nephritis as children are at increased risk for recurrent proteinuric hypertension during their pregnancies (70% in one series).[19] This may simply reflect the gestational changes of the kidney unmasking occult CKD; however, pregnancy has triggered recurrent Henoch-Schönlein purpura.

Autosomal Dominant Polycystic Kidney Disease
Women with autosomal dominant polycystic kidney disease (ADPKD) who have normal renal function and blood pressure usually have a successful, uncomplicated pregnancy.[20] However, preexisting hypertension in ADPKD is a significant risk factor for preeclampsia and fetal prematurity.[20]

Reflux Nephropathy
Reflux nephropathy is a common cause of CKD in young women, who frequently have reduced GFR, proteinuria, and hypertension. Pregnancy complications include superimposed preeclampsia (up to 75%), recurrent UTIs (28%–65%), deterioration of renal function (up to 13% have an irreversible decline in renal function), gestational ureteral obstruction requiring drainage (5%), and increased fetal morbidity and mortality influenced by maternal hypertension and SCr at conception.[4,21]

All women with reflux nephropathy, even those who have had vesicoureteral reflux (VUR) surgically treated by ureteral reimplantation during childhood, should be screened for asymptomatic bacteriuria every 4 to 6 weeks throughout pregnancy. Acute pyelonephritis is twice as common in women with persistent VUR as it is in those who have had spontaneous or surgical resolution of VUR.[4] After one urinary tract infection, low-dose prophylactic antibiotics, chosen according to the sensitivity of the most recent urine culture, reduce the risk for further UTIs and may therefore preserve renal function. Women with persistent VUR, especially those with a history of upper UTIs who are contemplating pregnancy, should consider prepregnancy correction of VUR to reduce maternal and fetal morbidity.

Upper Urinary Tract Obstruction
Women with congenital urologic defects, such as pelviureteral junction obstruction, are at increased risk for upper urinary tract obstruction requiring nephrostomy or stenting, even if they underwent urologic correction as children.[21] Throughout pregnancy, they should be monitored regularly with serial assessment of renal function, urine culture, and BP. Ultrasonography of the renal pelvis at the end of the first trimester will provide a useful baseline with which to compare future imaging. It is important to remember, however, that the pelvicalyceal systems and ureters dilate in normal pregnancy, particularly on the right side. The right pelvicalyceal system normally dilates by a maximum of 0.5 mm each week from 6 to 32 weeks, reaching a maximal diameter of about 20 mm (90th percentile), which is maintained until term.[22] The left pelvicalyceal system reaches a maximal diameter of 8 mm (90th percentile) at 20 weeks' gestation.[22] A repeat ultrasound scan is indicated if there is renal pain suggestive of obstruction, persistent infection, or a rise in SCr in a woman with a single kidney (Fig. 42.3).

Nephrolithiasis
The incidence of symptomatic renal stone disease during pregnancy is similar to that of the nongravid state. One large series has shown that symptomatic nephrolithiasis affects 1 in 244 pregnancies.[23] This is despite healthy pregnancy creating an ideal environment for renal stone formation that includes renal tract dilation, urinary stasis, and hypercalciuria. However, during pregnancy, there is also increased excretion of inhibitors of stone formation, such as magnesium, citrate, and nephrocalcin, an acidic glycoprotein. Symptomatic renal calculi are more common in Caucasians than Blacks and in multigravidas than primigravidas.[23] Renal colic is also more common in the second and third trimesters.[23]

UTIs associated with renal stones should be treated longer than isolated UTIs and followed up with antibiotic prophylaxis. The increased frequency of urinary infection with symptomatic renal stones is associated with an increased risk for preterm rupture of membranes.[23]

Pregnant women in the process of passing a renal calculus usually develop typical renal colic associated with fever, lower urinary tract infection, and hematuria. Ultrasound identifies a renal calculus in about half of these women. In those with a normal ultrasound, but suggestive symptoms, a plain abdominal radiograph and single-shot intravenous urogram can identify

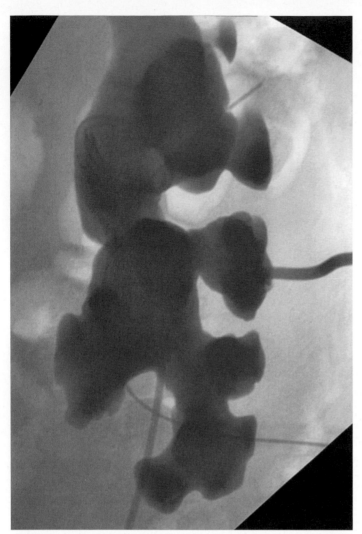

Figure 42.3 Upper urinary tract obstruction during pregnancy in a single kidney. Postpartum nephrostogram of a dilated collecting system in a solitary left kidney with crossed ectopia. The woman, a 28-year-old primigravida, presented at 22 weeks' gestation with severe hypertension (180/110 mm Hg), and her serum creatinine rose rapidly to 3.4 mg/dl (298 μmol/l) despite a urine output of 4 liters per 24 hr. Pelvicalyceal dilation (36 mm diameter) was noted, and within days of a nephrostomy, the patient's symptoms, hypertension, and serum creatinine had all returned to normal, and the pregnancy went to 37 weeks. The nephrostomy remained *in situ* until 6 weeks' postpartum, at which time a ureteral stent was inserted. Note the nephrostomy tube and ureteral stent.

most other renal calculi. In an effort to avoid even a small dose of radiation to the fetus, magnetic resonance urography has been used to differentiate between physiologic urinary tract dilation and obstruction due to calculi.

Up to 75% of pregnant women with renal colic pass the stones spontaneously with conservative management. Women must remain well hydrated and receive antibiotics and pain relief with either pethidine or, before the third trimester, a nonsteroidal anti-inflammatory drug. Continued symptoms may necessitate passage of a ureteral stent, but this is difficult to do without x-ray guidance. A percutaneous nephrostomy is another option, especially for an obstructed single kidney, but the nephrostomy must usually remain in place for the rest of the pregnancy. Recent advances in fiber-optics have allowed the development of holmium laser lithotripsy, which allows a ureteroscope to be passed into the upper renal tracts, delivering direct stone-crushing energy to within 0.5 mm of the laser fiber tip. This technique has been successfully and safely used in all stages of pregnancy.

Women who are recurrent stone formers with persistent gross hypercalciuria, despite increased fluid intake, can use thiazide diuretics in pregnancy to increase distal tubular reabsorption of calcium. Uric acid and cystine stones rarely form in pregnancy owing to gestational bicarbonaturia and consequent alkalinization of the urine. If problematic, both conditions may be controlled by increasing urine output and further alkalinizing the urine to pH > 6. During pregnancy, xanthine oxidase inhibitors for uric acid stones and D-penicillamine for cystine stones should be avoided if possible, especially during the first trimester.

Diabetic Nephropathy

The 80% gestational increase in renal blood flow in normal pregnancy is not associated with a rise in glomerular capillary pressure. Pregnancy does, however, further augment the hyperfiltration of early diabetic nephropathy, suggesting that diabetic and gestational hyperfiltration are working through separate, but synergistic, mechanisms. This partly explains the transient rise in microalbuminuria (30–300 mg/day) and preexisting proteinuria in women with diabetes during the third trimester.

Microalbuminuria in early pregnancy is associated with an increased prevalence of preeclampsia and as a consequence preterm delivery.[24] An elevated hemoglobin A1c in the first trimester,[24] prepregnancy duration of diabetes,[24] and maternal blood pressure[25] are all independently associated with an increased risk for preeclampsia. Improved perinatal care is now responsible for an almost 95% perinatal survival rate of babies born to women with diabetes.[25] Stillbirths are most common in women with diabetic nephropathy and suboptimal glycemic control, smoking, and low social status.

Pregnancy in women with diabetes does not precipitate the onset of diabetic nephropathy, and those who have established diabetic nephropathy with well-preserved renal function do not progress more rapidly to ESRD as a consequence of pregnancy. Conversely, women with diabetic nephropathy and moderate to severe renal impairment (SCr > 1.4 mg/dl; 125 μmol/l) have more than a 40% chance of an accelerated decline in renal function, usually associated with preeclampsia or an exacerbation of hypertension.[26] Good control of maternal blood glucose levels and hypertension before conception and during pregnancy improves both perinatal and maternal outcomes.[25]

Lupus Nephritis

Systemic lupus erythematosus (SLE) is a multisystem autoimmune disorder that predominantly affects young women and is characterized by a relapsing and remitting course. Renal involvement (lupus nephritis) is recognized by proteinuria, elevated SCr, hypertension, and often thrombocytopenia and hyperuricemia. Consequently, a relapse of lupus nephritis during the second half of pregnancy is difficult to distinguish from preeclampsia. Clinical features that may be discriminatory are the presence of an active urinary sediment with hematuria and red-cell casts in active lupus nephritis, as well as extrarenal manifestations affecting the skin and joints. The laboratory findings of active lupus include a rising titer of double-stranded DNA antibodies and low serum C3 and C4 complement. However, a gestational rise in complement levels may mask disease-induced consumption; complement is not consumed during active preeclampsia. In healthy pregnancy, the erythrocyte sedimentation rate (ESR) can rise as high as 80 mm/hour and is therefore not useful in identifying a flare of lupus nephritis during pregnancy. The C-reactive protein (CRP) level is unchanged in active lupus and is not influenced by pregnancy. If there is clinical doubt remote from term (before 30–32 weeks' gestation), a renal biopsy may help to differentiate between active lupus nephritis and preeclampsia.

Women with quiescent lupus nephritis, absent antiphospholipid (APL) antibodies, normal or near-normal renal function (SCr < 123 μmol/l), proteinuria (<500 mg/24 hours), and controlled hypertension for at least 6 months before conception can expect a good fetal and maternal outcome.[27] Relapses are more common in pregnant women who have had more than three flares before pregnancy and who have APL antibodies, C3 hypocomplementemia, and hypertension. Women with active lupus nephritis at conception, especially in association with proteinuria, hypertension, and APL antibodies, have an increased risk for early pregnancy loss, IUGR, preterm delivery, preeclampsia, and perinatal and maternal mortality.[27] The presence of maternal APL antibodies is specifically associated with an increased risk for early pregnancy loss. Those women with extractable nuclear antibodies (anti-Ro and anti-La) are at increased risk (about 1:20) for having an infant affected by congenital lupus. Neonatal lupus is associated with irreversible heart block or transient cutaneous lupus.

Management of Lupus Nephritis in Pregnancy

Prednisolone, azathioprine, and hydroxychloroquine have all been safely used to control SLE during pregnancy for many years. It is safe for a woman to remain on maintenance treatment with these agents with the goal of sustaining remission during pregnancy. A flare of lupus nephritis during pregnancy is usually treated with intravenous methylprednisolone, 500 mg daily for 3 days, and an increase of oral prednisolone to about 40 mg daily. Steroid-resistant and progressive lupus nephritis has been successfully treated during pregnancy with intravenous cyclophosphamide. However, when a severe flare of lupus nephritis occurs during pregnancy, the effects of this life-threatening condition on the mother, as well as the effects of toxic drugs on the fetus, need to be balanced against the likelihood of a successful fetal outcome. Sometimes, difficult decisions regarding continuation of the pregnancy need to be made. Additional treatment includes antihypertensive medication to keep blood pressures 140/90 mm Hg or lower and thrombosis prophylaxis with low-dose aspirin and LMW heparin, especially in the presence of APL antibodies and proteinuria > 1 g/24 hours. Lupus nephritis is slightly more likely to flare postpartum, but the consensus is not to use prophylactic steroids peripartum unless there are signs of disease activity.

DISTINCTION BETWEEN PRE-EXISTING RENAL DISEASE AND PREECLAMPSIA

Some women are not known to have CKD before pregnancy, and the distinction between preeclampsia, pre-existing CKD, and preeclampsia superimposed on CKD can be challenging when a woman is first seen for evaluation of proteinuria and hypertension in mid-pregnancy. The differential diagnosis is not always helped by the presence of hyperuricemia and IUGR, which are common features of both preeclampsia and CKD, but the presence of raised hepatic transaminases and thrombocytopenia support a diagnosis of preeclampsia (Fig. 42.4).[28]

This can be a crucial differential diagnosis because it will influence how the woman is advised. If a difficult first pregnancy with a threatened fetal outcome has occurred when there is underlying CKD, the woman must be advised of the high risk that subsequent pregnancies may have a similar course. Preeclampsia alone does not usually recur in a second pregnancy, and when it does, the condition is often milder and later in a subsequent pregnancy. The risk for recurrent preeclampsia is

Differential diagnosis of preeclampsia and primary renal disease		
During Pregnancy	Preeclampsia	Pre-existing Renal Disease
Proteinuria	After 20 weeks gestation	May occur before 20 weeks
Hematuria	—	May occur
Cast	Rarely seen	Often seen
Hypertension	After 20 weeks gestation	May occur before 20 weeks
Thrombocytopenia	Occurs in moderate and severe preeclampsia	Not usually seen
Elevated hepatic transaminases	Occur in moderate and severe pre-eclampsia	Not usually seen

Figure 42.4 Differential diagnosis of preeclampsia and primary renal disease in pregnancy. Although serum uric acid is often raised in preeclampsia (>4.5 mg/dl [270 μmol/l]), this is not reliable in distinguishing preeclampsia from preexisting renal disease.

related to the severity of and gestational week at which preeclampsia occurred in the first pregnancy; the earlier and more severe, the greater the risk for recurrence.

Among those diagnosed with preeclampsia, 2% to 5% of women are shown to have underlying renal disease when assessed more than 3 months postpartum.[29] Gestational hypertension usually resolves within 3 months of delivery, but heavy proteinuria due to preeclampsia can take up to 12 months to disappear.

GENERAL MANAGEMENT OF PREGNANCY IN CHRONIC KIDNEY DISEASE

The management of pregnancy in women with CKD is summarized in Figure 42.5.

Prepregnancy Counseling and Decision Making

Ideally, women with CKD have the opportunity for prepregnancy discussions to inform their decisions about pregnancy. Women should be informed of the risks to fetal and maternal outcomes based on the general information shown in Figure 42.1 along with any disease-specific advice. For some women, the decisions will be psychologically taxing. For example, a woman in her 30s with progressive severe CKD may be advised against pregnancy yet know that the slow rate of progression of her renal disease probably means that she will be beyond her reproductive years by the time she has a functioning renal transplant that would make successful pregnancy a realistic prospect.

If pregnancy is planned, medications may need to be changed: Angiotensin-converting enzyme (ACE) inhibitors and angiotensin receptor blockers (ARBs) should be discontinued once pregnancy has been confirmed. Statins should also be avoided in pregnancy, but there is evidence that pravastatin may not be associated with the same developmental problems as other statins. Folic acid, 400 μg daily, should be started in anticipation of conception until 12 weeks' gestation and aspirin, 50–150 mg daily, commenced once pregnancy has been confirmed until delivery.

Hypertension

Blood pressure should be maintained at about 140/90 mm Hg throughout pregnancy. Lower targets do not reduce maternal

---

Management of women with CKD during pregnancy

Prepregnancy

Advise—increased risk of pregnancy complications (IUGR, preeclampsia, preterm labor; see Fig 42.1)
Advise—increased risk of deteriorating maternal renal function (see Fig 42.1)

Discontinue inappropriate medication——statins, ACE inhibitors, ARB

Aspirin 75 mg/day
Folic acid 5 mg daily

Prenatal monitoring

Urine culture every 4–6 weeks—after one infection, keep urine sterile with prophylactic antibiotics

Proteinuria >3 g/24 hr—thrombosis prophylaxis with LMW heparin; 1–3 g/24 hr—prophylaxis if other risk factors

Hematuria—if red-cell casts suggesting active renal parenchymal disease, consider renal biopsy or delivery if >32 weeks

Blood pressure—maintain BP ≤140/90 mm Hg with antihypertensive medication

Serum creatinine, BUN—recognize acute or chronic renal impairment and need for dialysis

FBC and iron status—use iron and EPO if necessary to keep Hb 10–11 g/dl

Baseline renal ultrasound (pelvicalyceal dimensions)

Postnatal

Close monitoring of BP and fluid balance
Continue LMW heparin for 6 weeks
Return to nonpregnant medication regimen over 2 weeks

Figure 42.5   Management of women with chronic kidney disease (CKD) during pregnancy. ACE, angiotensin-converting enzyme; ARB, angiotensin receptor blocker; BUN, blood urea nitrogen; EPO, erythropoietin; FBC, full blood count; Hb, hemoglobin; IUGR, intrauterine growth restriction; LMW, low-molecular-weight. See text for further discussion.

morbidity and may be associated with further compromise of fetoplacental blood flow and IUGR.

Women can conceive on ACE inhibitors and ARBs, and these appear safe until the 6th week of pregnancy, but because of their effect on fetal renal development and other teratogenic effects, they should be stopped as soon as pregnancy is diagnosed. Some women have continued these drugs throughout the first trimester, without apparent harm to the neonate, but studies have lacked assessment of neonatal renal function. Under exceptional circumstances, for example, in association with severe peripartum preeclampsia or heart failure, the acute benefit of ACE inhibitors or ARBs to maternal health may exceed the potential harm to the developing fetus.

Antihypertensive medications that can be safely used to control hypertension in pregnant women with renal impairment include methyldopa, labetalol, nifedipine SR, and α-blockers (see Chapter 41, Fig. 41.12). There is no strong evidence to support the use of one drug over another with regard the management of CKD-related hypertension in pregnancy. Methyldopa has the most detailed and reassuring safety data for use in pregnancy, but it is not as well tolerated as nifedipine slow release (SR) or labetalol. When possible, the author prescribes those drugs that controlled a woman's hypertension outside of pregnancy, or nifedipine SR or labetalol for first-line new-onset gestational hypertension. Thiazide diuretics mildly attenuate gestational

plasma volume expansion and are associated with an increased risk for IUGR. These drugs are therefore best avoided in hypertensive pregnancies complicated by CKD.

Proteinuria

Other than appropriate blood pressure control, there are no specific strategies to reduce proteinuria during pregnancy. Nephrotic syndrome carries an increased risk for thromboembolism, and pregnant women are already in a prothrombotic state, with thromboembolism a major cause of maternal death.[30] Thrombosis prophylaxis with LMW heparin is therefore essential for all pregnant women with proteinuria >3 g/24 hours. In women with 1 to 3 g proteinuria per 24 hours, thrombosis prophylaxis should be considered, especially if additional risk factors exist, such as obesity (body mass index >30), maternal age >35 years, cigarette smoking, and immobility. If proteinuria persists postpartum, LMW heparin should be continued for at least 6 weeks. The prophylactic dose of heparin is usually doubled during pregnancy because the gestational rise in GFR leads to an increased renal clearance of heparin. For example, enoxaparin, 40 mg given subcutaneously once daily, and dalteparin, 5000 units given subcutaneously once daily, are standard prophylaxis during pregnancy and for 6 weeks postpartum. There is no evidence to support a reduction of LMW heparin dose in women with a reduced GFR. Because

LMW heparin is safe in pregnancy and the consequences of thromboembolism potentially devastating, it is the author's practice to maintain the same prophylactic dosing for women with impaired renal function. Increasing proteinuria alone is not an indication for delivery because, after correction for prematurity, massive proteinuria (>10 g/24 hours) has no significant effect on neonatal outcome.

Progressive Renal Impairment and Early Delivery

If, despite these management strategies, there is a gestational decline in GFR, a decision may need to be made to either institute dialysis in an attempt to prolong pregnancy and achieve fetal viability or to deliver the baby. Fetal viability and well-being are determined in conjunction with fetal medicine specialists and obstetricians. Fetal growth is often compromised in pregnancies complicated by renal impairment, but a small fetus may still benefit from continuing the pregnancy until there is evidence of fetal compromise from umbilical artery Doppler studies.

There are no absolute criteria for the initiation of dialysis. If this option is being considered, the mother should be given the option of ending the pregnancy. However, there is no guarantee that aborting the pregnancy will reverse a decline in renal function. Indeed, women with severe renal impairment who have a gestational decline to ESRD, might consider continuing the pregnancy (in the absence of other complications) because there is an 80% chance of a live birth outcome when dialysis is started after conception.[12] Usually, dialysis is instituted when GFR is about 20 ml/min. Hemodialysis (HD) using a tunneled central venous catheter is the typical modality.

RENAL REPLACEMENT THERAPY AND PREGNANCY

Maintenance Dialysis and Pregnancy

The management of pregnancy in women on maintenance dialysis is summarized in Figure 42.6. Women with ESRD have reduced fertility, but improvements in HD and the use of erythropoietin (EPO) to treat CKD-induced anemia have increased the likelihood of women conceiving and producing a surviving infant. The incidence of women conceiving while on HD has been variably reported between 0.4% and 7%, depending on the criteria that define the female dialysis population.[31] Up to 60% of reported pregnancies now result in a live infant,[31] but 80% of pregnancies end preterm at about 32 weeks.[31] Urea crosses the placenta to the fetus, and a high fetal urinary urea causes an osmotic diuresis, which probably explains the polyhydramnios associated with more than 50% of dialysis pregnancies. Premature rupture of membranes and maternal hypertension are other causes for preterm delivery.

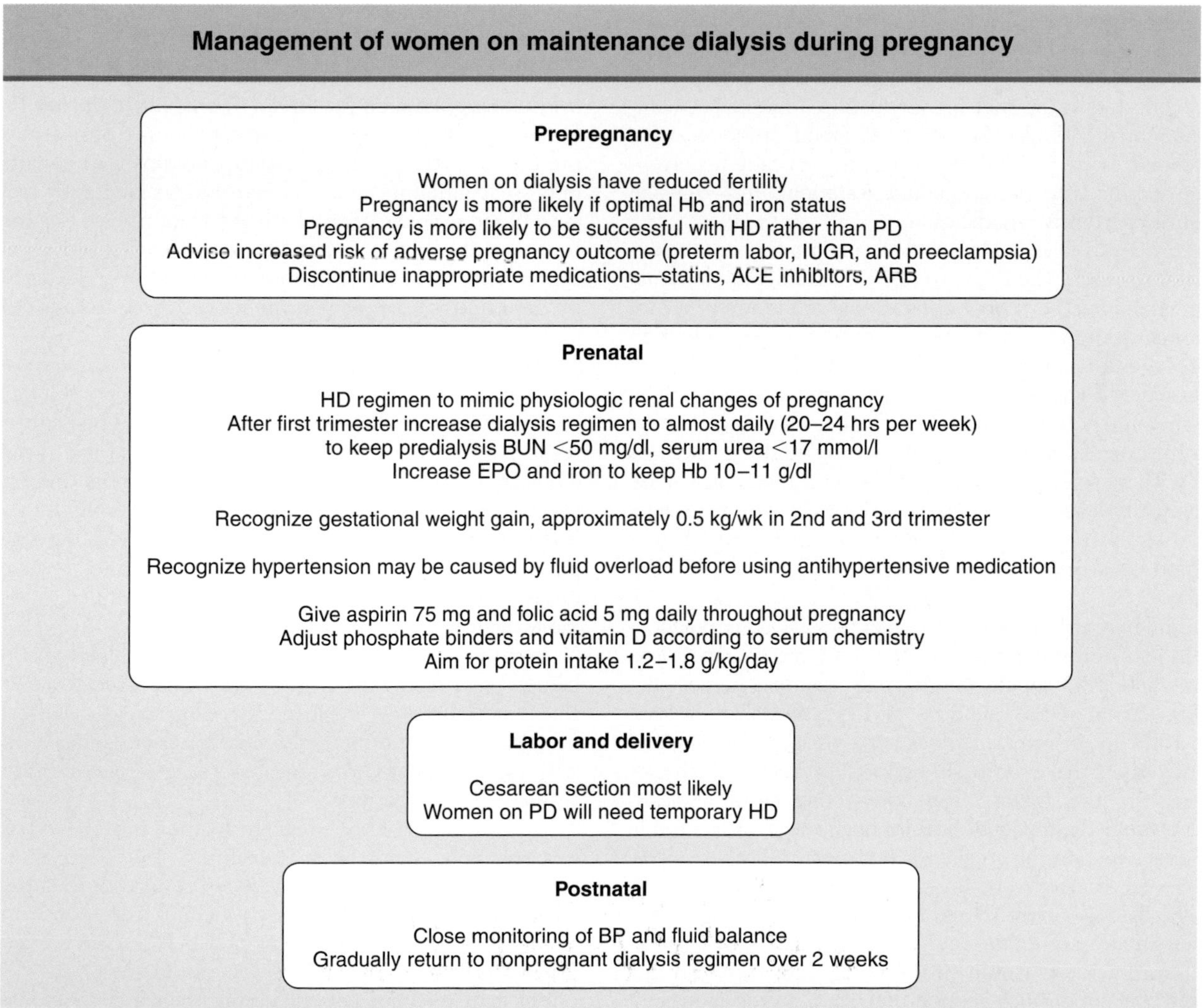

Management of women on maintenance dialysis during pregnancy

Prepregnancy

Women on dialysis have reduced fertility
Pregnancy is more likely if optimal Hb and iron status
Pregnancy is more likely to be successful with HD rather than PD
Advise increased risk of adverse pregnancy outcome (preterm labor, IUGR, and preeclampsia)
Discontinue inappropriate medications—statins, ACE inhibitors, ARB

Prenatal

HD regimen to mimic physiologic renal changes of pregnancy
After first trimester increase dialysis regimen to almost daily (20–24 hrs per week)
to keep predialysis BUN <50 mg/dl, serum urea <17 mmol/l
Increase EPO and iron to keep Hb 10–11 g/dl

Recognize gestational weight gain, approximately 0.5 kg/wk in 2nd and 3rd trimester

Recognize hypertension may be caused by fluid overload before using antihypertensive medication

Give aspirin 75 mg and folic acid 5 mg daily throughout pregnancy
Adjust phosphate binders and vitamin D according to serum chemistry
Aim for protein intake 1.2–1.8 g/kg/day

Labor and delivery

Cesarean section most likely
Women on PD will need temporary HD

Postnatal

Close monitoring of BP and fluid balance
Gradually return to nonpregnant dialysis regimen over 2 weeks

Figure 42.6   Management of maintenance dialysis patients during pregnancy. ACE, angiotensin-converting enzyme; ARB, angiotensin receptor blocker; BUN, blood urea nitrogen; EPO, erythropoietin; Hb, hemoglobin; HD, hemodialysis; IUGR, intrauterine growth restriction; PD, peritoneal dialysis. See text for further discussion.

Women on peritoneal dialysis (PD) are less likely to conceive than women on HD.[31] Furthermore, as pregnancy progresses, it is increasingly difficult to achieve PD adequacy to meet the physiologic demands of pregnancy, and a switch to HD may be necessary. There are, however, several case reports of successful pregnancies in women on PD. Complications include peritonitis, which should be treated in the same way as in nonpregnant patients, with intraperitoneal antibiotics. When it is necessary to initiate dialysis during pregnancy (see earlier discussion), HD is the preferred modality.

Management of Pregnancy on Dialysis

The key to a successful pregnancy on dialysis is to use renal replacement therapy to mimic as closely as possible the healthy gestational changes to kidney function. This requires knowledge of the timing and extent of these pregnancy-related changes and a willingness by the woman to accept almost daily HD in later pregnancy. Frequent dialysis should aim to keep the predialysis blood urea nitrogen <50 mg/dl (serum urea <17 mmol/l). There are no accepted criteria for adequacy using urea kinetic modelling in pregnancy. Frequent dialysis also reduces the need for large fluid shifts, which may compromise uteroplacental blood flow. In those women who have some residual renal function, fluid balance is easier to manage, which increases the likelihood of a successful pregnancy outcome.

Women who increase their HD regimen to more than 20 hours per week are more likely to have a successful pregnancy outcome. Further improvements are likely with more than 24 hours per week. Fluid balance and weight gain should recognize an average gestational weight gain of 1 lb (0.5 kg) per week during the second and third trimesters. Maternal blood pressure should be maintained at about 140/90 mm Hg. Rises in blood pressure might initially respond to extra fluid removal, but resistant hypertension in a euvolemic woman may herald gestational hypertension requiring antihypertensive medication.

Increased dialysis leads to hypokalemia and a higher concentration of potassium in the dialysate, or potassium supplements may be necessary. Furthermore, a gestational reduction in serum sodium concentration necessitates a concomitant reduction in dialysate sodium concentration to about 135 mmol/l, and the gestational reduction in serum bicarbonate concentration (18–22 mmol/l) should be matched with a low bicarbonate dialysate. In pregnancy, there is also a respiratory alkalosis associated with increased tidal volume, and this mixed acid-base disorder typically leaves serum pH within the reference range. Increased dialysis frequency will also allow a greater protein intake, which is variably recommended to be between 1.2 and 1.8 g/kg/day.[31]

Anemia and hemorrhage are common in the dialysis population. Hemoglobin and iron status need to be monitored monthly; iron supplements and EPO should be given to maintain hemoglobin between 10 and 11 g/dl. The dose of EPO needs to increase by 50% to 100% in pregnancy. It does not cross the placenta, and consequently, there have been no reports of teratogenicity or polycythemia in the infant. The long-acting erythropoiesis-stimulating protein, darbepoetin, has also been successfully used in a transplant recipient during pregnancy, but more information with regard to its safety is needed before widespread use can be recommended. The dialysis circuit should be heparinized as usual. Folic acid supplementation (2–5 mg/day) is recommended throughout pregnancy, and low-dose aspirin (50–150 mg/day) taken starting shortly after conception may reduce the risk for preeclampsia.[18] The requirement for calcium and vitamin D supplements is also likely to change as pregnancy progresses, and plasma levels of calcium, phosphate, and vitamin D need to be monitored and doses of phosphate binders and vitamin D analogues adjusted accordingly.

Cesarean birth is necessary in about 50% of pregnancies in women on dialysis. After cesarean birth, women on PD should discontinue this form of dialysis for up to 72 hours, after which time, 1-liter exchanges can be reintroduced, gradually building back up to a full regimen.

Renal Transplantation and Pregnancy

The management of pregnancy in women with a functioning renal transplant is summarized in Figure 42.7. Women with ESRD are far more likely to have a successful pregnancy outcome if they have a renal transplant compared with those on dialysis. After renal transplantation, a woman's fertility usually returns to normal after about 6 months.[32] Pregnancy should be delayed, however, until renal function and immunosuppressive therapy have stabilized.[32] Pregnancy is increasingly common among female transplant recipients. About 1 in 20 of all women of childbearing age who have a functioning kidney transplant will become pregnant. About 20% of pregnancies will end in spontaneous abortion in early pregnancy, but of those that go beyond the first trimester, at least 90% will end successfully. These pregnancies, however, are more likely to be complicated by preterm labor (30%–50%), preeclampsia (30%–37%), and IUGR (20%–33%). Despite these complications, most controlled studies have shown that pregnancy has no influence on long-term maternal renal function if SCr < 1.5 mg/dl (132 μmol/l).[32] However, as for all CKD, obstetric and maternal outcome is worse if there is hypertension, recurrent UTIs, proteinuria, and renal impairment (SCr > 132 μmol/l).

Immunosuppression for Renal Transplants during Pregnancy

Pregnancy does not appear to affect the rate of rejection.[32] Prednisolone (5–10 mg) rarely causes problems for neonates because only small amounts cross the placenta, as judged by maternal-to-cord blood ratios of about 10:1. Azathioprine passes easily across the placenta, but it is not converted to its active metabolite, 6-mercaptopurine, by the immature fetal liver. It has been taken by thousands of pregnant women over three to four decades and appears to be safe.

However, the gestational rise in plasma volume leads to a fall in plasma concentration of calcineurin inhibitors (CNIs). There is controversy as to whether CNI dosage should be adjusted according to plasma levels. Small studies suggest that it is unnecessary to increase the dose of cyclosporine to prevent rejection, and it is the author's practice to minimize increments in CNIs, aiming to keep levels at the lower end of the therapeutic range. Postpartum, the plasma volume rapidly returns to nonpregnancy levels, and CNI doses should be readjusted in a timely manner, otherwise the kidney can be exposed to toxic levels.

Women taking cyclosporine have small-for-gestational-age babies compared with women who take prednisolone and azathioprine. However, cyclosporine is otherwise well tolerated in pregnancy, with no increased risk for teratogenesis. Experience with tacrolimus has now revealed a side-effect and safety profile similar to cyclosporine.[32]

At present, very few pregnant women have been treated with mycophenolate mofetil and sirolimus, but successful pregnancies and healthy offspring have been reported. In anticipation of pregnancy, it seems prudent to switch from those drugs with an unknown safety profile to those for which experience in pregnancy is reassuring.

An acute rejection episode during pregnancy should be managed conventionally with pulse intravenous methylprednisolone. Too few women have received OKT3 or antithymocyte globulin to

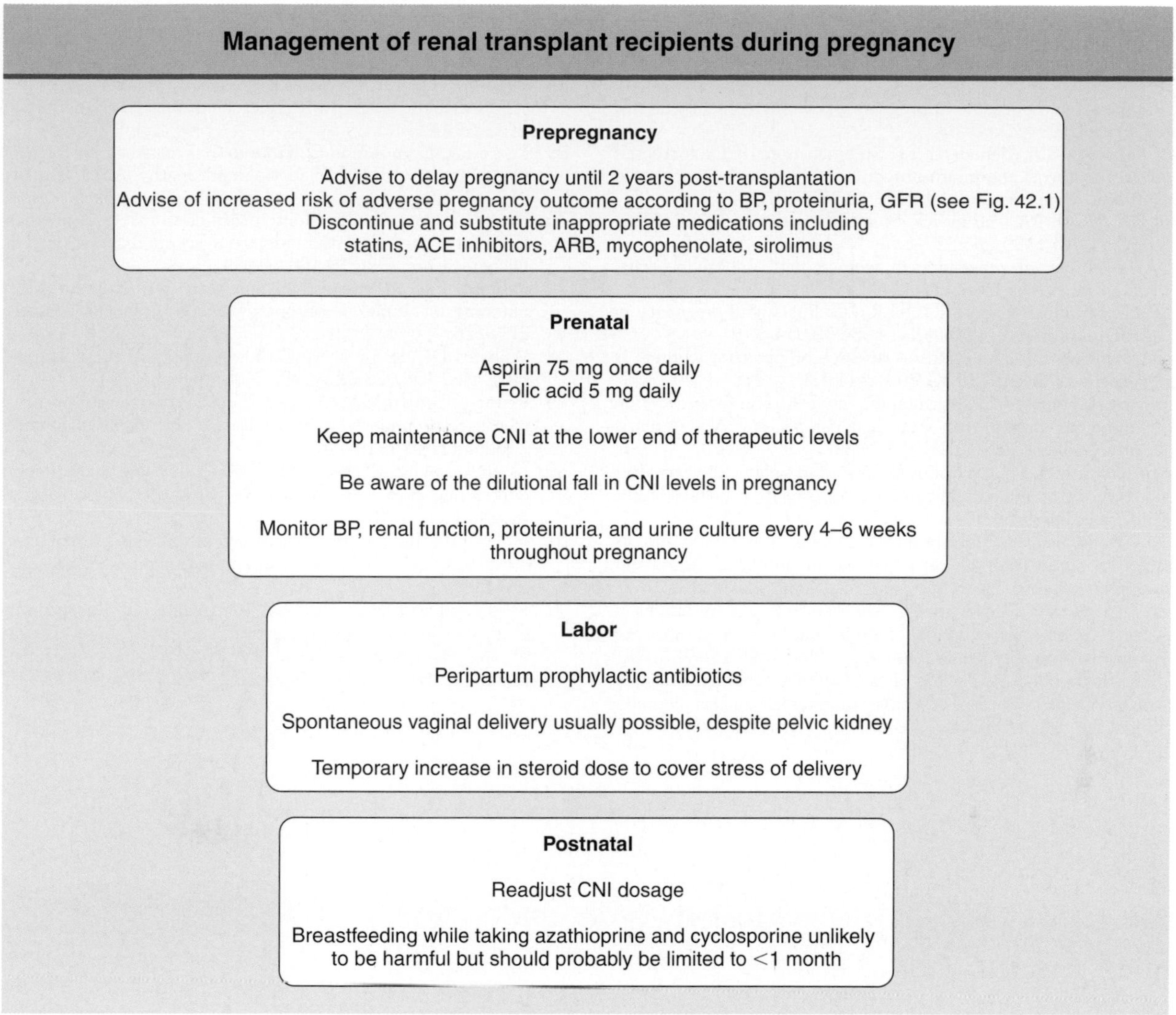

Management of renal transplant recipients during pregnancy

Prepregnancy

Advise to delay pregnancy until 2 years post-transplantation
Advise of increased risk of adverse pregnancy outcome according to BP, proteinuria, GFR (see Fig. 42.1)
Discontinue and substitute inappropriate medications including
statins, ACE inhibitors, ARB, mycophenolate, sirolimus

Prenatal

Aspirin 75 mg once daily
Folic acid 5 mg daily

Keep maintenance CNI at the lower end of therapeutic levels

Be aware of the dilutional fall in CNI levels in pregnancy

Monitor BP, renal function, proteinuria, and urine culture every 4–6 weeks
throughout pregnancy

Labor

Peripartum prophylactic antibiotics

Spontaneous vaginal delivery usually possible, despite pelvic kidney

Temporary increase in steroid dose to cover stress of delivery

Postnatal

Readjust CNI dosage

Breastfeeding while taking azathioprine and cyclosporine unlikely
to be harmful but should probably be limited to <1 month

Figure 42.7 Management of renal transplants during pregnancy. ACE, angiotensin-converting enzyme; ARB, angiotensin receptor blocker; CNI, calcineurin inhibitor; GFR, glomerular filtration rate.

recommend their use in pregnancy, but difficult decisions sometimes need to be made between treating steroid-resistant rejection and continuing the pregnancy.

Pregnant women on immunosuppression therapy should receive prophylactic antibiotics for all surgical interventions, including delivery. Furthermore, monthly urine cultures should be taken to screen for asymptomatic bacteriuria, and treated when isolated. Just one UTI during pregnancy in a transplant recipient is an indication for low-dose antibiotic prophylaxis for the duration of the pregnancy.

The transplanted pelvic kidney does not obstruct labor; therefore, a spontaneous vaginal delivery should be the aim if obstetric circumstances allow. Cesarean birth is necessary, however, in 50% of women with renal transplants.[32] The dose of corticosteroids should be temporarily increased in the perioperative period. Azathioprine does not appear in breast milk, but the presence of cyclosporine in breast milk suggests that breast-feeding should be limited, although additional exposure for a few weeks postpartum is unlikely to be harmful compared with *in utero* exposure over the previous 9 months.

REFERENCES

1. Jungers P, Chauveau G, Choukroun G, et al: Pregnancy in women with impaired renal function. Clin Nephrol 1997;47:281–288.
2. Katz AI, Davison JM, Hayslett JP, et al: Pregnancy in women with kidney disease. Kidney Int 1980;18:192–206.
3. Cunningham FG, Cox SM, Harstad TW, et al: Chronic renal disease and pregnancy outcome. Am J Obstet Gynecol 1990;163:453–459.
4. Jungers P, Houillier P, Chauveau D, et al: Pregnancy in women with reflux nephropathy. Kidney Int 1996;50:593–599.
5. Imbasciatti E, Pardi G, Capetta P, et al: Pregnancy in women with chronic renal failure. Am J Nephrol 1986;6:193–198.
6. Hemmelder MH, de Zeeuw D, Fidler V, de Jong PE: Proteinuria: A risk factor for pregnancy-related renal function decline in primary glomerular disease? Am J Kidney Dis 1995;26:187–192.
7. Jungers P, Houillier P, Forget D, Henry-Amar M: Specific controversies concerning the natural history of renal disease in pregnancy. Am J Kidney Dis 1991;17:116–112.
8. Stettler RW, Cunningham FG: Natural history of chronic proteinuria complicating pregnancy. Am J Obstet Gynecol 1992;167:1219–1224.
9. Jones DC, Hayslett JP: Outcome of pregnancy in women with moderate or severe renal insufficiency. N Engl J Med 1996;335:226–232.

10. Jungers P, Houillier P, Forget D, et al: Influence of pregnancy on the course of primary glomerulonephritis. Lancet 1995;346:1122–1124.

11. Epstein FH: Pregnancy and renal disease. N Engl J Med 1996;335:277–278.

12. Hou S: Frequency and outcome of pregnancy in women on dialysis. Am J Obstet Gynecol 1994;23:60–63.

13. Fink JC, Schwartz SM, Benedetti TJ, Stehman-Breen CO: Increased risk of adverse maternal and infant outcomes among women with renal disease. Paediatr Perinat Epidemiol 1998;12:277–287.

14. Packham DK, North RA, Fairley KF, et al: Primary glomerulonephritis and pregnancy. QJM 1989;266:537–553.

15. Abe S: An overview of pregnancy in women with underlying renal disease. Am J Kidney Dis 1991;17:112–115.

16. Barcelo P, Lopez-Lillo J, Cabero L, Del Rio G: Successful pregnancy in primary glomerular disease. Kidney Int 1986;30:914–919.

17. Lupton M, Williams DJ: The ethics of research on pregnant women: Is maternal consent sufficient? BJOG 2004;111:1307–1312.

18. Coomarasamy A, Honest H, Papaioannou S, et al: Aspirin for prevention of preeclampsia in women with historical risk factors: A systematic review. Obstet Gynecol 2003;101:1319–1332.

19. Ronkainen J, Nuutinen M, Koskimies O: The adult kidney 24 years after childhood Henoch-Schonlein purpura: A retrospective cohort study. Lancet 2002;360:666–679.

20. Chapman AB, Johnson AM, Gabow PA: Pregnancy outcome and its relationship to progression of renal failure in autosomal dominant polycystic kidney disease. J Am Soc Nephrol 1994;5:1178–1185.

21. Mansfield JT, Snow BW, Cartwright PC, Wadsworth K: Complications of pregnancy in women after childhood reimplantation for vesicoureteral reflux: An update with 25 years of follow-up. J Urol 1995;154:787–790.

22. Faundes A, Bricola-Filho M, Pinto e Silva LC: Dilatation of the urinary tract during pregnancy: Proposal of a curve of maximal caliceal diameter by gestational age. Am J Obstet Gynecol 1998;178:1082–1086.

23. Lewis DF, Robichaux AG 3rd, Jaekle RK, et al: Urolithiasis in pregnancy. Diagnosis, management and pregnancy outcome. J Reprod Med 2003;48:28–32.

24. Ekbom P, Damm P, Feldt-Rasmussen B, et al: Pregnancy outcome in type 1 diabetic women with microalbuminuria. Diabetes Care 2001;24:1739–1744.

25. Reece EA, Leguizamon G, Homko C: Pregnancy performance and outcomes associated with diabetic nephropathy. Am J Perinatol 1998;15:413–421.

26. Purdy LP, Hantsch CE, Molitch ME, et al: Effect of pregnancy on renal function in patients with moderate to severe diabetic renal insufficiency. Diabetes Care 1996;19:1067–1074.

27. Rahman FZ, Rahman J, Al-Suleiman SA, Rahman MS: Pregnancy outcome in lupus nephropathy. Arch Gynecol Obstet 2005;271:222–226.

28. Williams DJ, de Swiet M: Pathophysiology of pre-eclampsia. Intensive Care Med 1997;23:620–629.

29. Reiter L, Brown MA, Whitworth JA: Hypertension in pregnancy: The incidence of underlying renal disease and essential hypertension. Am J Kidney Dis 1994;24:883–887.

30. Lewis G: Why Mothers Die 2000–2002: The Sixth Report of Confidential Enquiries into Maternal Deaths in the United Kingdom. London, RCOG Press, 2004.

31. Holley JL, Reddy SS: Pregnancy in dialysis patients: A review of outcomes, complications and management. Semin Dial 2003;16:384–387.

32. EBPG Expert Group on Renal Transplantation. European best practice guidelines for renal transplantation. Section IV: Long-term management of the transplant recipient. IV 10. Pregnancy in renal transplant recipients. Nephrol Dial Transplant 2002;17(Suppl 4):50–55.

CHAPTER

43

Autosomal Dominant Polycystic Kidney Disease

Deirdre A. O'Sullivan and Vicente E. Torres

INTRODUCTION AND DEFINITION

Autosomal dominant polycystic kidney disease (ADPKD) is a multisystem disorder characterized by multiple, bilateral renal cysts associated with cysts in other organs such as liver, pancreas, and arachnoid membranes.[1,2] Noncystic, extrarenal manifestations of ADPKD include mitral valve prolapse, intracranial aneurysms, and hernias. It is a genetic disorder, expressed in an autosomal dominant pattern, with 100% penetrance but variable expression. ADPKD is a genetically heterogeneous disease. Because of the possibility of clinical presentation in infancy, the term autosomal dominant polycystic kidney disease is preferred to adult polycystic kidney disease, and the latter has been abandoned. Although benign renal cysts are common, multiple bilateral cysts are not. Therefore, an underlying inherited disease should be considered in patients with normal renal function and multiple bilateral renal cysts.

ETIOLOGY AND PATHOGENESIS

Genetics

PKD1 is the gene responsible for 85% to 90% of clinically detected cases. A second gene, in the long arm of chromosome 4, *PKD2*, has been identified. A third gene may exist, as evidenced by absence of linkage to *PKD1* and *PKD2* in certain families with ADPKD phenotype.[3–6] Autosomal dominant polycystic liver disease (ADPLD) also exists as an independent entity. Like ADPKD, ADPLD is genetically heterogeneous, with the first two genes identified (*PRKCSH* in chromosome 19 and *Sec63* in chromosome 6) accounting for about one third of isolated ADPLD cases.[7,8]

The intron-exon sequences of the *PKD1* and *PKD2* genes are illustrated in Figure 43.1.[9] Although *PKD2* is a larger gene, the open reading frame of *PKD1* is larger than *PKD2*. About 75% of the *PKD1* gene is duplicated at least three times on chromosome 16. These duplicated segments are designated homologous genes. The *PKD1* gene contains three long polypyrimidine tracts within introns 1, 21, and 22, which may predispose to triple helix formation, erroneous repair, and mutations during transcription. The mutations of both *PKD1* and *PKD2* are unique and dispersed over the entire gene.

Although ADPKD is caused by an inherited germline mutation, only a small percentage of nephrons develop cysts. These observations can be explained by a two-hit tumor suppressor model of cystogenesis.[10,11] Cysts arise from clonal expansion of a single cell. Loss of heterozygosity with deletion of a wild-type *PKD* allele can be demonstrated in about 30% of cysts. Mice with single *PKD1* or

PKD2 copies have a mild phenotype. Homozygous *Pkd1* or *Pkd2* null mouse embryos have severe cystic changes. *PKD2*(WS25/WS25) and *PKD2*(WS25/-) mice [*PKD2*(WS25) is an unstable allele that results in an increased rate of somatic mutations by intragenic homologous recombination] have an intermediate phenotype. These observations are consistent with a two-hit mechanism. On the other hand, transheterozygous *PKD1/PKD2* mutations (e.g., somatic mutations of *PKD2* in cells carrying a germline *PKD1* mutation) also occur in cyst-derived cells. *Pkd1* overexpression or *Pkd1* aberrant splicing (with transcript levels 13%–20% of controls) also induce a cystic phenotype. These observations suggest that other genetic mechanisms, in addition to two-hit inactivation of *PKD1* or *PKD2*, may contribute to cyst formation.[12–15]

Disease Mechanisms

The proteins encoded by *PKD1* and *PKD2* have been named polycystin 1 and polycystin 2. Their structures predicted by gene sequences have been determined by computer modeling[3–6] (see Fig. 43.1). Polycystin-1 and polycystin-2 play an important role in the regulation of intracellular Ca^{2+} homeostasis.[16–18] Polycystin-1 has a large extracellular region, 11 transmembrane domains, and a short cytoplasmic tail. The extracellular region has homology to domains usually involved in protein–protein or protein–carbohydrate interactions and to a family of sperm expressed sea urchin proteins involved in sperm–egg interactions and the acrosome reaction. The C-terminal tail of polycystin-1 physically interacts and regulates the function of polycystin-2 and may also activate a number of intracellular pathways (G protein, Wnt, and JAK/STAT signaling). Polycystin-2 is smaller than polycystin-1 and is predicted to have cytoplasmic N- and C-termini and six transmembrane domains. It acts as a Ca^{2+} permeable cation channel, and its transmembrane region has homology to transient receptor potential channel (TRPC) subunits.

Recent studies have focused on the localization of the polycystin complex in primary cilia and on its well-documented role in mediating calcium fluxes in response to mechanical stimulation.[19,20] The primary cilium is a single hair-like organelle arising from the centrosome, the microtubule-organizing center of the cell, and projecting from the surface of most mammalian cells. In tubular epithelial cells, the cilium projects into the lumen of the tubule and is thought to have a sensory role. The demonstration that the polycystins and most other proteins mutated in inherited renal cystic diseases are located in the primary cilia or centrosomes and that a targeted disruption of the primary cilia in the principal cells of the collecting ducts results in polycystic kidney disease

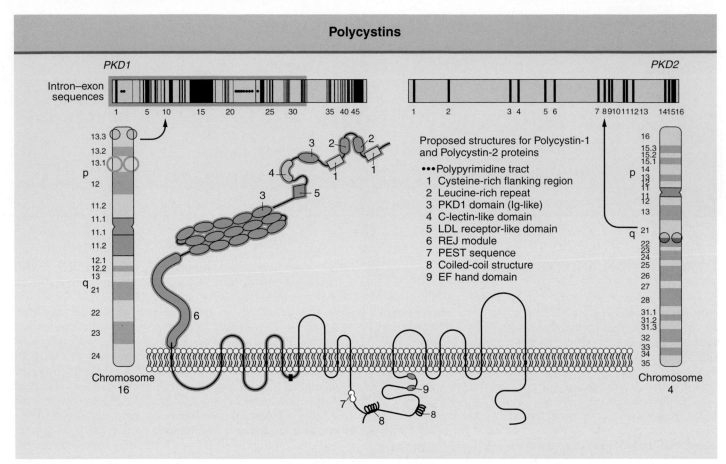

Figure 43.1   Polycystins: genes, mRNAs, and proteins. Diagrammatic representation of chromosome 16 (left) and chromosome 4 (right). Intron-exon sequences of *PKD1* (upper left) and *PKD2* (upper right). Diagram of proposed structural features of the polycystin-1 and polycystin-2 proteins (center).

provides strong support for a major role of primary cilia in the pathogenesis of this disease.

Polycystin-1 is also found in focal adhesions, desmosomes, adherens, and tight junctions, and polycystin-2 in the endoplasmic reticulum.[16–18] Polycystin-1 in the plasma membrane may interact with polycystin-2 in the adjacent endoplasmic reticulum. Polycystin-2 has also been shown to interact physically with TRPC1. Therefore, the role of the polycystins in the regulation of intracellular Ca^{2+} may go beyond the primary cilia. Overexpression of polycystin-2 in LLPCK cells amplifies the Ca^{2+} release from intracellular stores in response to agonist stimulation. In certain cells, such as vascular smooth muscle and B-lymphoblastoid cells, a haploinsufficient state (i.e., 50% reduction in polycystin-2 content) is sufficient to significantly alter intracellular Ca^{2+} homeostasis.[21,22]

In the past two decades, many studies have established that the development of polycystic kidney disease is characterized by a switch from a well-differentiated, nonproliferative, mainly reabsorptive cellular phenotype to a partially dedifferentiated, secretory phenotype characterized by polarization defects and high rates of proliferation and apoptosis. Evidence pointing to a major role for cyclic adenosine monophosphate (cAMP) in cystogenesis by promoting fluid secretion and cell proliferation[23] has accumulated. Fluid secretion by ADPKD epithelia, as well as by normal collecting ducts, is driven by chloride entering the cell through basolateral Na^+Cl^- or $Na^+K^+2Cl^-$ cotransporters and exiting through apical cAMP-dependent Cl^- channels (Fig. 43.2). Cyclic AMP has opposing effects on cell proliferation in wild-type and ADPKD epithelial cells. Although it exerts an inhibitory effect on wild-type human kidney cortex cells, it activates the ERK cascade and increases the proliferation of ADPKD cells. Treatment of collecting duct principal cells with calcium channel blockers or with a dominant negative polycystin-1 C-tail construct replicates the abnormal proliferative response of the ADPKD cells to cAMP, suggesting a link between the cystic phenotype and the alterations in intracellular Ca^{2+} that likely result from disrupting the polycystin pathway.[24]

EPIDEMIOLOGY

ADPKD affects between 1 in 400 and 1 in 1000 individuals, making it one of the most common hereditary diseases.[25] In the United States, about 400,000 people are affected, and about 1800 begin hemodialysis each year. Given its inheritance pattern, it has an equal gender distribution, but males appear to manifest slightly more severe disease. ADPKD occurs worldwide and in all races. The disease may be less common in Africa. In the United States, ADPKD may be less common in African Americans than Caucasians.

CLINICAL MANIFESTATIONS

ADPKD is a multisystem disorder. Multiple renal and extrarenal manifestations of ADPKD have been described that cause significant complications. Familiarity with these associated manifestations is essential so that they can be readily recognized and intervened with to limit morbidity and mortality to the ADPKD patient.

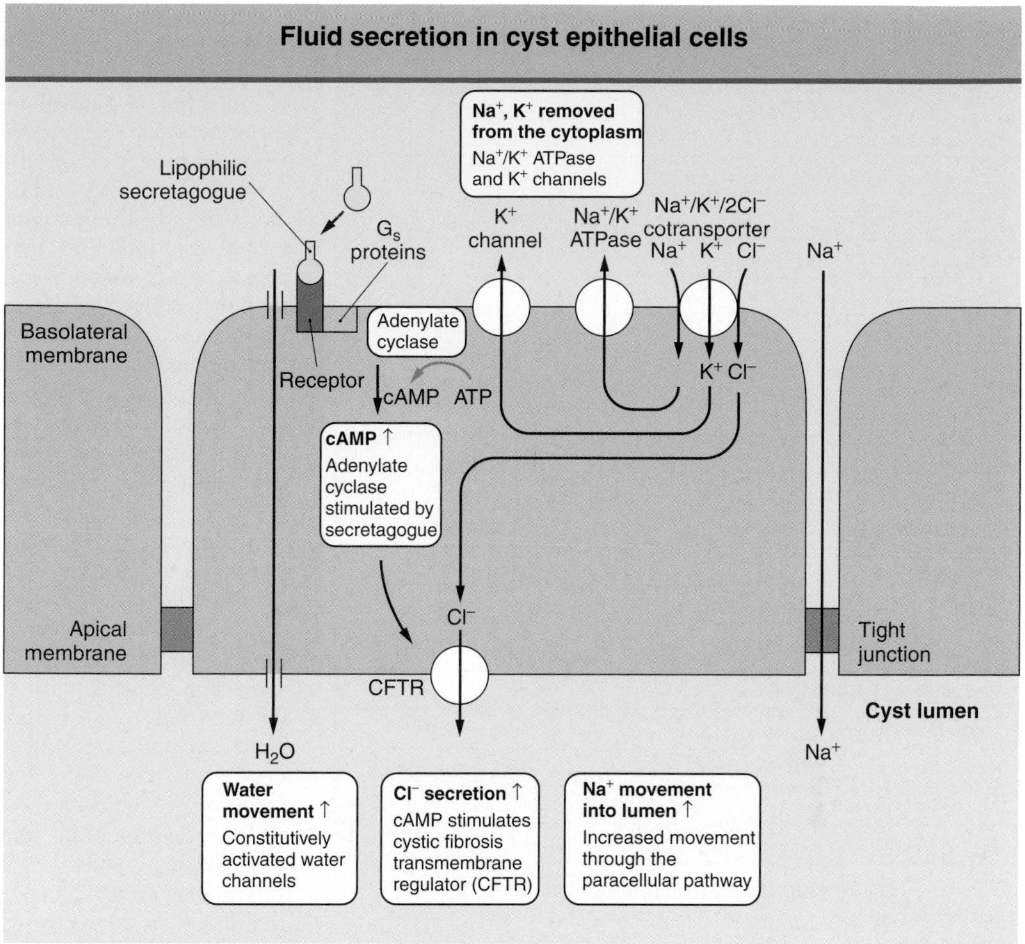

Figure 43.2 Mechanism of fluid secretion in cyst epithelial cells. Relative to normal tubular cells, cyst cells have decreased apical Na channels and increased apical Cl⁻ channels. The basolateral $Na^+K^+2Cl^-$ cotransporter is activated, creating a favorable electrochemical gradient for movement of Na^+ through paracellular channels into the cyst lumen. Intracellular cAMP stimulates Cl⁻ secretion by apical CFTR Cl⁻ channels. An endogenous lipophilic secretagogue present in polycystic kidneys is one of several agonists that may activate adenylate cyclase to form cAMP and thereby increase and activate Cl⁻ channels in the apical plasma membranes. This cAMP-dependent loss of Cl⁻ from the cytoplasm promotes entry of Cl⁻ from the interstitium via $Na^+K^+2Cl^-$ cotransporters. The accompanying Na^+ and K^+ are removed from the cell by the Na^+K^+ ATPase and K^+ channels on the basolateral membrane. Water moves via constitutively activated water channels and follows Cl⁻ transport rather than Na^+. (From Martinez JR, Grantham JJ: Polycystic kidney disease: Etiology, pathogenesis and treatment. Disease-a-Month 1995;41:697–765.)

Renal Manifestations

A number of clinical features that result from renal damage that can be identified (Fig. 43.3). Reduction in urinary concentrating capacity and glomerular hyperfiltration are early functional abnormalities that can be observed in some children and adolescents with ADPKD.

Pain and Renal Size

Renal size increases with age, and renal enlargement eventually occurs in 100% of patients with ADPKD. The severity of structural abnormality correlates with the manifestations of ADPKD, such as pain, hematuria, hypertension, and renal insufficiency.[25] Massive renal enlargement can lead to compression of local structures, resulting in such complications as inferior vena cava compression and digestive symptoms. Episodes of acute pain are seen frequently, but chronic, severe pain is rare. Potential causes of acute flank pain include cyst hemorrhage, infection, stone, and rarely tumor, and these must be investigated thoroughly. A small subset of ADPKD patients with renal enlargement and structural distortion develop chronic flank pain without specifically identifiable etiology.

Hematuria and Cyst Hemorrhage

Gross hematuria may be the initial presenting symptom of ADPKD. It occurs in up to 40% of ADPKD patients at some time during the course of the disease. Many have recurrent episodes. Differential diagnosis of hematuria in ADPKD patients includes cyst hemorrhage, stone, infection, or tumor. Cyst hemorrhage is a frequent complication. When the cyst communicates with the

collecting system, gross hematuria is observed. Frequently, the cyst does not communicate with the collecting system, and flank pain without hematuria occurs. It can present with fever, raising the possibility of cyst infection. Occasionally, a hemorrhagic cyst will rupture, resulting in a retroperitoneal bleed that can be significant, potentially requiring transfusion. In most patients, cyst hemorrhage is self-limited, resolving within 2 to 7 days. If symptoms of hematuria or flank pain last longer than 1 week or if the initial episode of hematuria occurs after the age of 50 years, a detailed investigation to exclude neoplasm should be undertaken.

Urinary Tract Infection and Cyst Infection

Urinary tract infection (UTI) is common in ADPKD, but its incidence may have been overestimated because of the occurrence of sterile pyuria in many of these patients. UTIs occur in the form of cystitis, pyelonephritis, cyst infection, and perinephric abscesses. As in the general population, females are affected more frequently than males. Most infections are caused by *Escherichia coli*, *Klebsiella* species, *Proteus* species, and other Enterobacteriaceae. The route of infection in pyelonephritis and cyst infection is usually retrograde from the bladder; therefore, cystitis should be promptly treated to prevent complicated infections.

The imaging modality of choice has not been defined in comparative studies. Computed tomography (CT) and magnetic resonance imaging (MRI) are sensitive to detect complicated cysts and provide anatomic definition, but the findings are not specific for infection. Nuclear imaging, especially indium-labeled white-cell scanning, is useful, but both false-negative and false-positive results are possible. In the appropriate clinical setting of fever and

Renal manifestations of ADPKD
Functional Manifestations
Concentrating defect
Reduced urine NH₄ relative to pH
Reduced renal blood flow
Hypertension → Target Organ Damage
Cardiac
Cerebrovascular
Arteriolosclerosis and glomerulosclerosis
Peripheral vascular disease
Pain, Caused by
Cyst hemorrhage
Gross hematuria
Nephrolithiasis
Infection
Renal enlargement
Renal Failure, Possibly Due to
Interstitial inflammation
Apoptosis of tubular epithelial cells
Nephroangiosclerosis
Compression atrophy

Figure 43.3 Renal manifestations of ADPKD.

flank pain and suggestive diagnostic imaging, if blood and urine cultures are negative, cyst aspiration under ultrasound or CT guidance should be undertaken to culture the organism and assist in selection of antimicrobial therapy.

Nephrolithiasis

The frequency of renal stone disease is increased, occurring in about 20% of patients. Most stones are uric acid, calcium oxalate, or both in composition. Uric acid stones are more common in stone formers with ADPKD than without ADPKD. Urinary stasis thought secondary to distorted renal anatomy possibly plays a role in the pathogenesis of nephrolithiasis. Predisposing metabolic factors include decreased ammonia excretion, low urinary pH, and low urinary citrate concentration.[26]

Stones can be difficult to diagnose in ADPKD by imaging studies because of the presence of cyst wall and parenchymal calcification. The distorted anatomy can cause difficulty localizing stones to the collecting system on plain films. Intravenous urography (IVU) has the advantage of specifically localizing stone material to the collecting system and can assist in the determination of stone composition. IVU can also detect pericaliceal tubular ectasia, found in 15% of ADPKD patients. CT scanning is more sensitive in detecting small or radiolucent stones and for differentiating stones from tumor, clot, and cyst wall or parenchymal calcification.

Hypertension

Hypertension is an important complication of ADPKD associated with significant morbidity and mortality. Hypertension is present in at least 75% of ADPKD patients before the onset of renal failure, and the prevalence increases with age. There is a statistical

correlation between renal size and prevalence of hypertension in ADPKD. The most widely accepted hypothesis involves reduced renal blood flow, increased intrarenal angiotensin effect, increased filtration fraction, and abnormal renal handling of sodium resulting in intravascular volume expansion with resultant hypertension. Evidence for activation of the intrarenal renin-angiotensin system in ADPKD includes (1) partial reversal of the reduced renal blood flow, of the increased renal vascular resistance, and of the increased filtration fraction by acute or chronic administration of angiotensin-converting enzyme (ACE) inhibitors; (2) a shift of immunoreactive renin from the juxtaglomerular apparatus to the walls of the arterioles and small arteries; (3) detection of renin in the epithelium of dilated tubules and cysts; and (4) the association in some studies of double deletion (DD) ACE gene polymorphism with worse renal outcome.

Recent studies have shown that nitric oxide (NO) endothelium-dependent vasorelaxation is impaired in small subcutaneous resistance vessels from ADPKD patients with normal- or near-normal renal function before the development of hypertension as compared with healthy control subjects. Furthermore, the decrease of renal plasma flow in response to the intravenous infusion of a competitive inhibitor of NO synthase has been found to be significantly reduced in ADPKD patients compared with normal controls or subjects with essential hypertension. The interactions between angiotensin II and NO at the level of endothelium are of key importance in determining whether end-organ damage develops in response to the hemodynamic stress of hypertension; an imbalance between the generation of angiotensin II and that of NO may be responsible for the severity of the renal vascular lesions observed in ADPKD.[27]

Unrecognized hypertension can lead to target-organ damage that has been shown to significantly affect the life expectancy of patients with ADPKD. Hypertension also accelerates loss of renal function (Fig. 43.4). Proteinuria and microalbuminuria correlate with elevated mean arterial pressure and are independent risk factors for accelerated decline in renal function. Hematuria, a risk factor for the progression of renal failure in ADPKD, is more common in hypertensive patients. Left ventricular hypertrophy (LVH) occurs early in the course of ADPKD and may be a consequence of higher nocturnal blood pressures reported in young ADPKD patients. Valvular heart disease is also common in

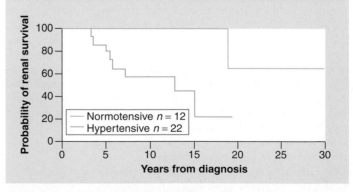

Effect of blood pressure on renal survival in autosomal dominant polycystic kidney disease

— Normotensive n = 12
— Hypertensive n = 22

Figure 43.4 Patients with polycystic kidney disease and hypertension at diagnosis have less probability of renal survival than those with normal blood pressure. (From Iglesias CG, Torres VE, Offord KP, et al: Epidemiology and ADPKD. Olmsted County, Minnesota: 1935–1980. Am J Kidney Dis 1983; 2:630–639.)

ADPKD and may be aggravated by hypertension. Hypertension may be a risk factor for intracranial aneurysm (ICA) rupture and may contribute to morbidity associated with rupture.

End-Stage Renal Disease

End-stage renal disease (ESRD) is not inevitable in ADPKD. Up to 77% of patients are alive with preserved renal function at age 50 years, and 52% at age 73 years. Fifty percent of ADPKD patients have reached ESRD by the ages of 57 to 73 years. *PKD1* is associated with a 15-year earlier onset of ESRD than *PKD2*. The influence of environmental factors and of genetic background is demonstrated by intrafamilial variability in the severity of disease. Once renal insufficiency has begun, the rate of decline in renal function is linear, with a loss of about 5.0 to 6.4 mL/min/year on average in patients with moderate renal failure. Males tend to progress to renal failure more rapidly and require renal replacement therapy at a younger age than females. Other risk factors for renal failure include Black race, diagnosis of ADPKD before the age of 30 years, first episode of hematuria before the age of 30 years, onset of hypertension before the age of 35 years, hyperlipidemia, low high-density lipoprotein (HDL) cholesterol, sickle cell trait, and in some studies, DD ACE polymorphism.[28] The location of the *PKD1* and *PKD2* mutations may also influence the clinical outcome. Patients with mutations in the 5′ region of *PKD1* were found to have significantly more severe disease than the patients with 3′ mutations (18.9% vs. 39.7% with adequate renal function at 60 years).[29]

The mechanism by which ADPKD causes renal failure is incompletely understood. An adverse association between renal volume and progression of renal failure has been recognized in younger patients, suggesting that compression of normal renal parenchyma by expanding cysts plays a role. However, cyst decompression does not improve renal function or delay the progression to renal failure. Hyperfiltration was also thought to play a role, although ADPKD patients who have undergone unilateral nephrectomy for urologic emergencies show no difference in the slope of decline in renal function than controls. Histologically, ADPKD is characterized by advanced vascular sclerosis of afferent and interlobular arteries, even in the absence of hypertension, and interstitial fibrosis.[30] Angiotensin II may play a role in the pathogenesis of interstitial inflammation and interstitial fibrosis. It potentiates the mitogenic effects of epidermal growth factor and stimulates the synthesis of osteopontin, a strong chemotactic factor for macrophages, and of transforming growth factor-β by tubular epithelial cells. Transforming growth factor-ß in turn stimulates the synthesis of collagen type IV and metalloproteinase inhibitors, which inhibit degradation of extracellular matrix.

Extrarenal Manifestations
Polycystic Liver Disease

Polycystic liver disease (PLD) is the most common extrarenal manifestation of ADPKD.[31] It is associated with both *PKD1* and non-*PKD1* genotypes. In addition, PLD also occurs as a genetically distinct disease in the absence of renal cysts. Developmentally, liver cysts arise from a ductal plate abnormality, with abnormal development and differentiation of the bile ducts.

PLD refers to any liver cysts in the presence of ADPKD. In the absence of renal cystic disease, PLD should be suspected when four or more cysts are present in the hepatic parenchyma. The number of cysts can help distinguish PLD from simple hepatic cysts. Most simple cysts are solitary, and no more than three cysts are present in those with multiple cysts. The liver in PLD contains multiple microscopic or macroscopic cysts that

result in hepatomegaly (Fig. 43.5) but typically there is preservation of normal hepatic parenchyma and liver function. Other pathologic findings in PLD include biliary hamartomas, biliary fibroadenomas, cystic dilation of peribiliary glands, and dilation of intrahepatic and extrahepatic bile ducts.

Hepatic cysts are exceedingly rare in children with ADPKD. Frequency increases with age; cysts are identified in 20% of patients in the third decade and in 75% by the seventh decade. Females develop more cysts, at an earlier age than men. Women who have multiple pregnancies or who have used oral contraceptive agents or estrogen replacement therapy postmenopausally have worse disease, suggesting a direct role of estrogen exposure in hepatic cyst growth.

Typically, PLD is asymptomatic. Reported symptoms have become more frequent as the lifespan of ADPKD patients is prolonged with dialysis and transplantation. Symptoms result from mass effect or from complications related to the cysts themselves. Symptoms typically caused by massive enlargement

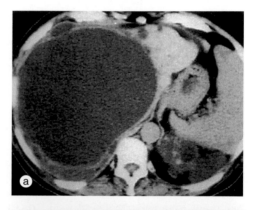

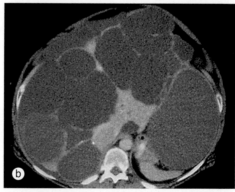

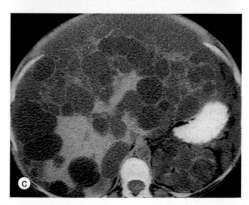

Figure 43.5   Variable presentation of symptomatic polycystic liver disease. *a,* Hepatomegaly caused by a very large, isolated, dominant cyst. *b,* Hepatomegaly caused by several large cysts. *c,* Hepatomegaly caused by multiple smaller cysts throughout the hepatic parenchyma.

of the liver or by mass effect from a single or a limited number of dominant cysts include dyspnea, orthopnea, early satiety, gastroesophageal reflux, mechanical low back pain, uterine prolapse, and even rib fracture. Other complications caused directly by mass effect include hepatic venous outflow obstruction, inferior vena cava compression, portal vein compression, and bile duct compression presenting as obstructive jaundice. Hepatic venous outflow obstruction is an uncommon condition caused by severe extrinsic compression of the intrahepatic inferior vena cava and hepatic veins by cysts, in rare cases with superimposed thrombosis. Cyst aspiration and alcohol sclerosis, laparoscopic fenestration, or combined hepatic resection and cyst fenestration can relieve the obstruction of the intrahepatic inferior vena cava and hepatic veins. In these cases, prognosis is good, unless there is superimposed hepatic vein thrombosis. Symptomatic cyst complications include cyst hemorrhage, which occurs less frequently than renal cyst hemorrhage; cyst infection; and the rare occurrence of torsion or rupture of cysts. Hepatic cyst infection can be a serious complication and typically presents with localized pain, fever, leukocytosis, an elevated sedimentation rate, and often an elevated alkaline phosphatase. Enterobacteriaceae are the most common microorganisms causing cyst infection. Localization of the infected cyst by imaging techniques may be difficult. MRI may be the most sensitive technique to differentiate a complicated from an uncomplicated hepatic cyst.

Intracranial Aneurysms

ICAs occur in about 8% of the ADPKD population. There appears to be familial clustering, occurring in 5% of patients with a negative family history and 22% of those with a positive family history. Most are asymptomatic. Focal findings such as cranial nerve palsy or seizure may result from compression of local structures by an enlarging aneurysm (Fig. 43.6). Yearly rupture rates increase with size, ranging from less than 0.5% for aneurysms less than 5 mm in diameter to 4% for aneurysms greater than 10 mm in diameter. Rupture carries a 35% to 55% risk for combined severe morbidity and mortality. The mean age at rupture is lower in the ADPKD

population than in the general population (39 vs. 51 years), with a range of 15 to 69 years. Most patients have normal renal function, and up to 29% have normal blood pressure at the time of rupture.

Widespread screening is not indicated because most ICAs found by presymptomatic screening are small, have a low risk for rupture, and require no treatment. Indications for screening in patients with a good life expectancy include family history of ICA or subarachnoid hemorrhage (SAH), previous aneurysmal rupture, preparation for elective surgery with potential hemodynamic instability, high-risk occupations (e.g., airline pilots), and significant anxiety on the part of the patient despite adequate information about the risks. Magnetic resonance angiography is the diagnostic imaging modality of choice for presymptomatic screening because it is noninvasive and does not require intravenous contrast material.[32] CT angiography is a satisfactory alternative in cases in which there is no contraindication to the administration of intravenous contrast.

Other Vascular Abnormalities

In addition to intracranial aneurysms, ADPKD has been associated with other vascular abnormalities such as thoracic aortic and cervicocephalic arterial dissections and coronary artery aneurysms (Fig. 43.7). Thoracic aortic dissection is seven times more common in the ADPKD population than in the general population by

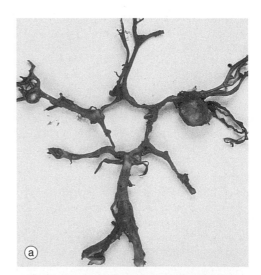

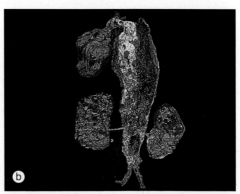

Figure 43.7 **Vascular manifestations of ADPKD.** *a,* Gross specimen demonstrating bilateral aneurysms of the middle cerebral arteries. *b,* Gross specimen demonstrating a thoracic aortic dissection extending into the abdominal aorta in a patient with ADPKD.

Clinical manifestations and classification of intracranial aneurysms

Intracranial aneurysm

Unruptured

Asymptomatic
Incidental
Concurrent

Symptomatic
Cranial nerve compression
Compression of other CNS structures
Distal embolization (TIAs)
Seizures
Headache

Ruptured
Thunderclap headache
Neck stiffness
Lower back pain
Loss of consciousness
Focal neurologic signs
Preretinal/subhyaloid hemorrhage

Figure 43.6 **Intracranial aneurysms.** Clinical manifestations and classification.

autopsy series, but actual case reports are rare. Rare patients with coronary aneurysms can present with cardiac ischemia and thrombus in the aneurysm in the absence of atherosclerotic disease. Several case reports describe abdominal aortic aneurysms in ADPKD patients. However, a prospective, sonographic study showed neither a wider aortic diameter nor a higher prevalence of abdominal aortic aneurysms in ADPKD patients compared with unaffected kindred in any age group. Pathologically, tissues from arterial aneurysms and dissections demonstrate disruption of elastic tissue. Recent immunohistochemical studies demonstrated both polycystin-1 and polycystin-2 expression in the myocytes of elastic and large distributive arteries, suggesting a direct pathogenetic role for ADPKD-related mutations in the arterial complications of this disease.[33,34]

Valvular Heart Disease

Mitral valve prolapse is the most common valvular abnormality and has been demonstrated in up to 25% of ADPKD patients by echocardiography. Mitral insufficiency, tricuspid insufficiency, and tricuspid prolapse also occur more frequently in ADPKD than in unaffected kindred. Aortic insufficiency has been reported in association with dilation of the aortic root. Histologically, valvular tissue shows myxoid degeneration with disruption of collagen, as seen in Marfan and Ehlers-Danlos syndromes. Overall, the risk for valvular abnormalities is unclear; although the lesions may progress with time, they rarely require valve replacement.

Screening echocardiography is not indicated unless a murmur is detected on physical examination.

Other Associated Conditions

Cyst formation has been described in such diverse organs as the pancreas, seminal vesicles, and arachnoid membrane (Fig. 43.8). Seminal vesicle cysts, usually multiple and bilateral, were found in 40% of ADPKD, as compared with 2% in nonaffected, males. In addition, spinal meningeal diverticula have been described in these patients and may present with intracranial hypotension, presumably due to cerebrospinal fluid leak. Ovarian cysts are not associated with ADPKD. An association between ADPKD and colonic diverticula has been described but is controversial. These associated conditions are typically asymptomatic and require no intervention. Male sterility due to low sperm motility has also been associated with ADPKD.

PATHOLOGY

Polycystic kidneys are diffusely cystic and enlarged (Fig. 43.9). Size varies from normal to weighing greater than 4000 g. The outer and cut surfaces show numerous spherical cysts of varying size, which are distributed evenly between cortex and medulla. The collecting system typically is distorted. The epithelium lining the cysts is characterized by hyperplastic changes, including flat nonpolypoid hyperplasia, polypoid hyperplasia and microscopic adenomas[35] (Fig. 43.10), and increased rates of cell proliferation and apoptosis.[36] Despite the frequency of hyperplastic lesions and microscopic adenomas, the incidence of renal cell carcinoma is not increased.

Cysts arise from focal dilation of existing renal tubules.[37] As they grow, they dissociate from the parent tubule and eventually become isolated, fluid-filled sacs. Early microdissection studies showed that cysts in ADPKD arise from all segments of the nephron and collecting ducts. Some also showed abnormal branching or diffuse enlargement of collecting ducts and larger size of cysts of collecting duct origin. Cysts with fluid sodium, chloride, potassium, and urea concentrations similar to those of plasma (nongradient cysts) have been thought to be derived from proximal tubules, whereas cysts with low sodium and chloride and high potassium and urea concentrations have been considered to be distally derived. Some histochemical studies have suggested an origin predominantly from collecting tubules. In a study of 10 ADPKD kidneys, in which cysts were defined

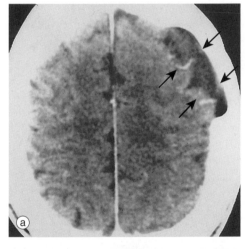

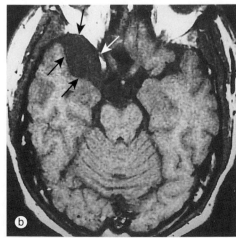

Figure 43.8 Extrarenal manifestations of ADPKD. Arachnoid cysts (*arrow*) demonstrated by CT (*a*) and MRI (*b*).

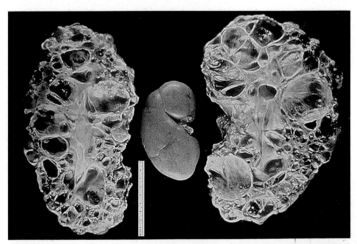

Figure 43.9 Markedly enlarged polycystic kidneys from a patient with ADPKD in comparison to a normal kidney in the middle.

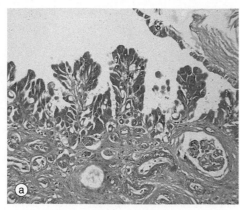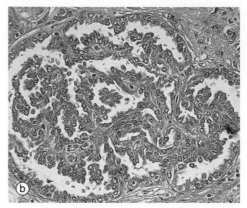

Figure 43.10 Renal cyst histology in ADPKD. *a*, Papillary hyperplasia of cyst epithelium. *b*, Papillary microscopic adenoma in an ADPKD kidney (original magnification ×200). (From Dunn MD, Portis AJ, Elbahnasy AM, et al: Laparoscopic nephrectomy in patients with end-stage renal disease and autosomal dominant polycystic kidney disease. Am J Kidney Dis 2000;35:720–725.)

as tubular dilations at least 1 mm in diameter, 70% of the cysts stained positively for collecting duct markers, whereas the remaining 30% were negative for all markers, possibly owing to cellular dedifferentiation. Another study using aquaporin (AQP) antibodies showed that 30% of ADPKD cysts, but only 11% of large cysts, were positive for AQP-1 (presumably from proximal tubular origin). A third study that did not take into account the size of the cysts showed that only a minority of the cysts stained positively for AQP-2 (a collecting duct marker). Because these observations were made mostly in kidneys with advanced or end-stage renal disease, it is possible that obstruction and acquired renal cystic disease could account for the observed proximal tubular dilations and small cysts. A predominant distal or collecting tubule origin of the cysts has been observed in the *Pkd2(-/WS25)* mouse model and a new *Pkd1(nl/nl)* model of ADPKD. Consistent with a predominant origin from collecting tubules is the observation that epithelial cells from human ADPKD cysts in primary culture exhibit a larger cAMP response to vasopressin than to parathyroid hormone.

Polycystic kidneys demonstrate advanced sclerosis of preglomerular vessels, interstitial fibrosis, and tubular epithelial hyperplasia, even in patients with normal renal function or early renal failure.[30] Sclerosis involves both afferent arterioles and interlobular arteries. This is more prominent in ADPKD than in patients with glomerular disease and comparable renal function and may be attributable to hypertension and the activation of the renin-angiotensin system demonstrated in ADPKD. Interstitial fibrosis is also prominent, even in early disease. It is associated with an interstitial infiltrate of macrophages and lymphocytes.

DIAGNOSIS AND DIFFERENTIAL DIAGNOSIS

Presymptomatic screening of patients at risk for ADPKD is by ultrasound or identification of a mutated *PKD* gene by linkage or direct mutational analysis. Diagnostic ultrasonographic criteria for individuals known to be at 50% risk by positive family history include two cysts, either unilateral or bilateral, in patients younger than 30 years; two cysts in both kidneys in patients 30 to 59 years of age; and at least four cysts in each kidney in patients older than 60 years.[1] Presymptomatic screening by ultrasound before age 20 years may not be conclusive and is not generally recommended. In addition, these criteria may not be sufficiently sensitive in *PKD2* patients younger than 30 years.[2] Genetic diagnosis by linkage analysis requires participation of other family members with and without the disease. It allows for prenatal diagnosis and

is important in the evaluation of young, living, related kidney donors with indeterminate diagnosis by imaging studies. Improvements in methodology now allow direct mutation analysis of the *PKD1* and *PKD2* genes with yields exceeding 90% and 70%, respectively.[38] Only individuals who have been properly informed about the advantages and disadvantages of screening should be offered presymptomatic screening. If ADPKD is diagnosed, the patient can receive appropriate genetic counseling, and risk factors such as hypertension can be identified and intervention instituted early. If ADPKD is absent, the patient is reassured. The disadvantages of presymptomatic screening relate to insurability and employability. Recommendations will change when more effective therapy for the disease becomes available.

Preimplantation genetic diagnosis (PGD) has been used for many inherited conditions causing severe morbidity and mortality. During PGD, genetic analysis is carried out on single blastomeres from preimplantation embryo biopsies obtained after *in vitro* fertilization, and only embryos unaffected by the disease under investigation are selected for transfer. PGD for ADPKD is complicated by the genetic heterogeneity of the disease and by the large size and complex structure of the *PKD1* gene. PGD for ADPKD has been performed in very few cases.[39]

Renal cystic disease can be a manifestation of many other systemic diseases. Important conditions to keep in mind when renal cystic disease is detected but the presentation is not typical of ADPKD include autosomal recessive PKD, tuberous sclerosis complex, von Hippel-Lindau disease, and orofaciodigital syndrome type 1, as well as medullary sponge kidney and simple renal cysts. These are discussed further, including differential diagnosis, in Chapter 44. If the patient has ESRD, acquired cystic disease should also be considered (see Chapter 79).

NATURAL HISTORY

ADPKD is a heterogeneous disease with significant variability in clinical presentation occurring between families. Even within the same family, significant variability in clinical presentation can occur. The natural history of renal insufficiency in ADPKD is as variable as the clinical presentation.[25] ESRD occurs in 50% of patients by the age of 57 to 73 years, depending on the clinical series. Risk factors for progressive renal failure include *PKD1* genotype, male gender, diagnosis before age 30 years, first episode of hematuria before age 30 years, and onset of hypertension before age 35 years.[28] Hyperlipidemia and low HDL cholesterol may also worsen patient outcomes. Even though the degree of structural abnormality and renal size correlates with worse renal function in ADPKD, surgical decompression of renal cysts does not have a beneficial effect on preserving renal function. Once renal failure begins, renal function tends to decline linearly with time.

TRANSPLANTATION

Transplantation has become the treatment of choice for ESRD in ADPKD. Several studies have demonstrated no difference in patient or graft survival between ADPKD patients and other ESRD populations. The 1997 U.S. Renal Data System (USRDS) data show a 1-year survival probability for cadaveric transplants in ADPKD of 87% versus 85% overall, and at 5 years, 68% in ADPKD versus 59% overall. Living donor transplants also have graft survival no different than non-ADPKD populations. Because of the genetic nature of the disease, living-related transplantation has only recently been widely practiced in the ADPKD population. The number of living related transplants for ADPKD increased from 12% in 1990 to 22% in 1995. In 1999, 30% of kidney transplants for ADPKD patients were from living donors.

Complications after transplantation are no greater in the ADPKD population than in the general population, and specific complications directly related to ADPKD are rare. One study showed a higher rate of cyst infection after transplantation relative to before transplantation, although the difference was not statistically significant. No significant increase in the incidence of symptomatic mitral valve prolapse, aortic aneurysm rupture, hepatic cyst infection, or native cancers was observed. Another study showed a higher rate of diverticulosis and perforation in ADPKD patients than in controls, but the association with colonic diverticulosis remains controversial.

Although practiced routinely in the past, pretransplantation nephrectomy has fallen out of favor. Nephrectomy is an extensive procedure often with prolonged convalescence. In addition, native kidneys contribute to the maintenance of hemoglobin levels and assist in fluid management in ESRD. Indications for nephrectomy include a history of infected cysts, frequent bleeding, severe hypertension, or massive renal enlargement with extension into the pelvis. There is no evidence for an increased risk for renal cell carcinoma developing in native ADPKD kidneys after transplantation; thus, pretransplantation nephrectomy is not indicated as cancer prophylaxis. More recently, hand-assisted laparoscopic nephrectomy has been used in ADPKD patients who require a nephrectomy. After devascularization of the kidneys, drainage of cyst fluid is usually necessary for size reduction. Laparoscopic nephrectomy may have less associated morbidity and mortality than open nephrectomy in these patients.

TREATMENT

Current therapy is directed toward the renal and extrarenal complications of the disease in an effort to limit morbidity and mortality. Advances in the understanding of the genetics of ADPKD and mechanisms of cyst development and growth have raised hopes for treatments specifically directed toward limiting the development and progression of the disease.

Flank Pain

Causes of flank pain that may require intervention, such as infection, stone, or tumor, should be excluded. Nonopioid agents are preferred, and care should be taken to avoid long-term administration of nephrotoxic agents such as combination analgesics and nonsteroidal anti-inflammatory drugs. Narcotic analgesics should be reserved for the management of acute episodes of pain. Patients with chronic flank pain are at risk for narcotic and analgesic dependence, and a psychological evaluation and an understanding and supportive attitude on the part of the physician are essential for avoiding this. Reassurance, lifestyle modification, and avoidance of aggravating activities may be helpful. Tricyclic antidepressants are helpful as in other chronic pain syndromes, with a generally well-tolerated side-effect profile. Splanchnic nerve blockade with local anesthesia or steroids has been shown to result in pain relief prolonged beyond the duration of the local anesthetic.

When distortion of the kidneys by large cysts is deemed responsible for the pain, and conservative measures fail, therapy can be directed toward cyst decompression with cyst aspiration and sclerosis, surgical cyst decompression, or laparoscopic cyst decompression. Cyst aspiration, under ultrasound or CT guidance, is a relatively simple procedure; to prevent the reaccumulation of cyst fluid, sclerosing agents such as 95% ethanol or acidic solutions of minocycline are commonly used. There is a success rate of greater than 90% in benign renal cysts using 95% ethanol. Minor complications include microhematuria, localized pain, transient fever, and systemic absorption of the alcohol. More serious complications such as pneumothorax, perirenal hematoma, arteriovenous fistula, urinoma, and infection are rare. Complications from aspiration of centrally located cysts are more common, and the morbidity of the procedure is proportional to the number of cysts treated.

If multiple cysts are contributing to pain, laparoscopic or surgical cyst fenestration through lumbotomy or flank incision may be of benefit. Surgical decompression is effective in 80% to 90% of patients at 1 year, and 62% to 77% have sustained pain relief for greater than 2 years (Fig. 43.11). Surgical intervention

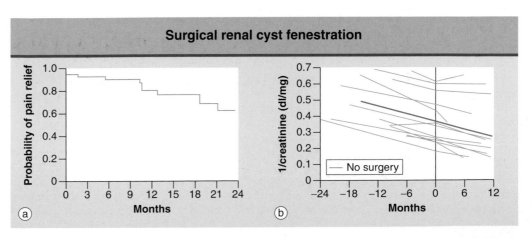

Figure 43.11 Surgical cyst fenestration for symptomatic ADPKD. *a*, Effects on relief of pain. *b*, Rate of decline of renal function. (From Elzinga LW, Barry JM, Torres VE, et al: Cyst decompression surgery for autosomal dominant polycystic kidney disease. J Am Soc Nephrol 1992;2: 1219–1226.)

does not accelerate the decline in renal function, as once thought, but does not appear to preserve declining renal function either (see Fig. 46.10). Laparoscopy is equally effective as open surgical fenestration in short-term follow-up in patients with limited disease, and there is a shorter, less complicated recovery period compared with open surgery. Previous abdominal surgery with possible adhesion formation is a relative contraindication to the procedure.[40]

There are a number of novel interventions for the management of pain in ADPKD whose roles have not yet been fully defined. Laparoscopic renal denervation has been used in combination with cyst fenestration and may be considered, particularly in polycystic kidneys without large cysts. Laparoscopic and retroperitoneoscopic nephrectomy and arterial embolization have been used to treat symptomatic polycystic kidneys in ADPKD patients with ESRD.[41–43]

Cyst Hemorrhage

Episodes of cyst hemorrhage are self-limited and respond well to conservative management with bedrest, analgesics, and adequate fluid intake to prevent obstructing clots. Rarely, bleeding is more severe, with extensive subcapsular or retroperitoneal hematoma causing significant decrease in hematocrit and hemodynamic instability. This requires hospitalization, transfusion, and investigation by CT or angiography. In cases of unusually severe or persistent hemorrhage, segmental arterial embolization can be successful. If not, surgery may be required to control bleeding.

Urinary Tract and Cyst Infection

Because most upper UTIs begin as cystitis, prompt treatment of symptomatic cystitis and asymptomatic bacteriuria is indicated to prevent retrograde seeding of the renal parenchyma. Antibiotics that require glomerular filtration, such as highly polar aminoglycosides, are not effective for upper UTI in advanced renal insufficiency. Cyst infection is often difficult to treat despite prolonged therapy with an antibiotic to which the organism is susceptible. Treatment failure occurs because certain antibiotics do not penetrate the cyst epithelium and achieve therapeutic concentrations within the cysts. With gradient cysts, the epithelium lining the cyst has functional and ultrastructural characteristics of the distal tubule epithelium. Penetration is through tight junctions, allowing only lipid-soluble agents access. Nongradient cysts, which are more common, allow solute access through diffusion, suggesting that water-soluble agents should gain entry to the cysts. However, kinetic studies indicate that these agents penetrate nongradient cysts slowly and irregularly, giving rise to unreliable drug concentrations within the cysts. Lipophilic agents have been shown to penetrate both gradient and nongradient cysts equally and reliably and have a pKa that allows for favorable electrochemical gradients into acidic cyst fluid. Therapeutic agents of choice include trimethoprim-sulfamethoxazole and fluoroquinolones, both of which have shown favorable intracystic therapeutic concentration gradients at physiologic pH in gradient and nongradient cysts, and chloramphenicol.

If fever persists after 1 to 2 weeks of appropriate antimicrobial therapy, percutaneous or surgical drainage of infected cysts should be undertaken. In the case of end-stage polycystic kidneys, nephrectomy should be considered. If fever recurs after stopping antibiotics, complicating features such as obstruction, perinephric abscess, or stone should be excluded. If no such complicating features are identified, the antibiotic course should be extended and may require several months to fully eradicate infection.

Nephrolithiasis

Treatment of nephrolithiasis in patients with ADPKD is not different from that in patients without ADPKD. Potassium citrate is the treatment of choice in the three conditions associated with ADPKD: uric acid lithiasis, hypocitraturic calcium oxalate nephrolithiasis, and distal acidification defects. Extracorporeal shock-wave lithotripsy and percutaneous nephrostolithotomy are reported to be 82% and 80% successful, respectively, without significant complication.[26]

Hypertension

Control of hypertension is essential because uncontrolled hypertension accelerates the decline in renal function and aggravates extrarenal complications. Antihypertensive agents of choice and optimal blood pressure targets in ADPKD have not been established. ACE inhibitors or angiotensin receptor blockers (ARBs) increase renal blood flow in ADPKD, have a low side-effect profile, and may have renoprotective properties that go beyond blood pressure control. Small numbers of patients, short duration of follow-up, inclusion of patients with widely different levels of renal function, and small doses of medication that might not have achieved the desired pharmacologic effect limit the validity of some studies that have failed to demonstrate a beneficial effect of ACE inhibitors on the progression of ADPKD.[44–47] An extended follow-up of the MDRD study showed a delayed onset of kidney failure and composite outcome of kidney failure and all-cause mortality in the low blood pressure group (51% of them taking ACE inhibitors) compared with those in the usual blood pressure group (32% of them taking ACE inhibitors).[48] This was also true in the ADPKD patients, who accounted for about one fourth of the patients in the study. An ongoing study (HALT-PKD) is designed to determine whether combined therapy with an ACE inhibitor and an ARB is superior to an ACE inhibitor alone in delaying the progression of the cystic disease in patients with preserved renal function or in slowing down the decline of renal function in patients with chronic kidney disease stage 3. HALT-PKD will also determine whether a low blood pressure target is superior to a standard blood pressure target in the group of patients with preserved function. Although these definitive studies are needed, on available evidence, we recommend tight blood pressure control to 125/75 mm Hg with a regimen that includes ACE inhibitors or ARBs to block the renin-angiotensin system.

Progressive Renal Failure

General strategies to delay progression of chronic kidney disease are discussed in Chapter 69. A subgroup analysis of the MDRD trial, however, showed no beneficial effect on renal function in ADPKD of strict compared with standard blood pressure control, and only a slight beneficial effect of borderline significance of a very-low-protein diet. Because these interventions were introduced at a late stage of the disease (glomerular filtration rate of 13–55 ml/min per 1.73 m^2), these results do not exclude a beneficial effect of earlier interventions.

Actuarial data indicate that ADPKD patients do better on dialysis than patients with ESRD from other causes, particularly for age over 47 years. Females also appear to do better than males. The good outcome in ADPKD may be due to higher endogenous erythropoietin production and better maintenance of hemoglobin or to lower comorbidity. Rarely, hemodialysis can be complicated by intradialytic hypotension if there is inferior vena cava compression by a medially located renal cyst. Despite renal size, peritoneal dialysis can usually be performed in ADPKD patients, although they are at increased risk for inguinal and umbilical hernias, which require surgical repair.

Polycystic Liver Disease

Most cases of PLD are asymptomatic and require no treatment. When symptomatic, therapy is directed toward reducing cyst volume and hepatic size. Noninvasive measures include avoiding ethanol, other hepatotoxins, and possibly, cAMP agonists (e.g., caffeine) because the latter have been shown to stimulate fluid secretion by the cysts *in vitro*. Histamine-2 blockers and somatostatin have been suggested to reduce secretion of secretin and secretory activity of cyst walls. Estrogens likely contribute to cyst growth, but the use of oral contraceptive agents and postmenopausal estrogen replacement therapy is contraindicated only if the liver is significantly enlarged and the risk for further hepatic cyst growth outweighs the benefits of estrogen therapy. Rarely, symptomatic PLD may require invasive measures to reduce cyst volume and hepatic size. Options include percutaneous cyst aspiration and sclerosis, laparoscopic fenestration, or open surgical fenestration.[31] Cyst aspiration is the procedure of choice if symptoms are caused by one or a few dominant cysts or by cysts that are easily accessible to percutaneous intervention. To prevent the reaccumulation of cyst fluid, sclerosis with minocycline or 95% ethanol is often successful. Laparoscopic fenestration can be considered for large cysts that are more likely to recur after ethanol sclerosis or if several cysts are present that would require multiple percutaneous passes to treat adequately. Partial hepatectomy with cyst fenestration is an option because PLD often spares a part of the liver with adequate preservation of hepatic parenchyma and liver function (Fig 43.12). In the rare case in which no segments are spared, liver transplantation may be necessary.

When a hepatic cyst infection is suspected, any cyst with unusual appearance on an imaging study should be aspirated for diagnostic purposes. The best management is percutaneous cyst drainage in combination with antibiotic therapy. Long-term oral antibiotic suppression or prophylaxis should be reserved for relapsing or recurrent cases. Antibiotics of choice are trimethoprim-sulfamethoxazole and the fluoroquinolones, which are effective against the typical infecting organisms and concentrate in the biliary tree and cysts.

Intracranial Aneurysm

Ruptured or symptomatic ICA requires surgical clipping of the neck of the aneurysm. Asymptomatic aneurysms measuring less than 5 mm, diagnosed by presymptomatic screening, can be observed initially and followed at yearly intervals. If the size increases, surgery is indicated. Definitive management of aneurysms between 6 and 9 mm remains controversial. Surgical intervention is usually indicated for all unruptured aneurysms 10 mm in diameter or greater. For patients with high surgical risk or with technically difficult lesions, endovascular treatment with detachable platinum coils may be indicated.

Novel Therapies

Advances in the understanding of the genetics of ADPKD and the mechanisms of cyst development and growth have led to testing of a number of potential therapies, mostly in animal models of polycystic kidney disease. Among them, epidermal growth factor receptor tyrosine kinase inhibitors[49] and rapamycin,[50] which are

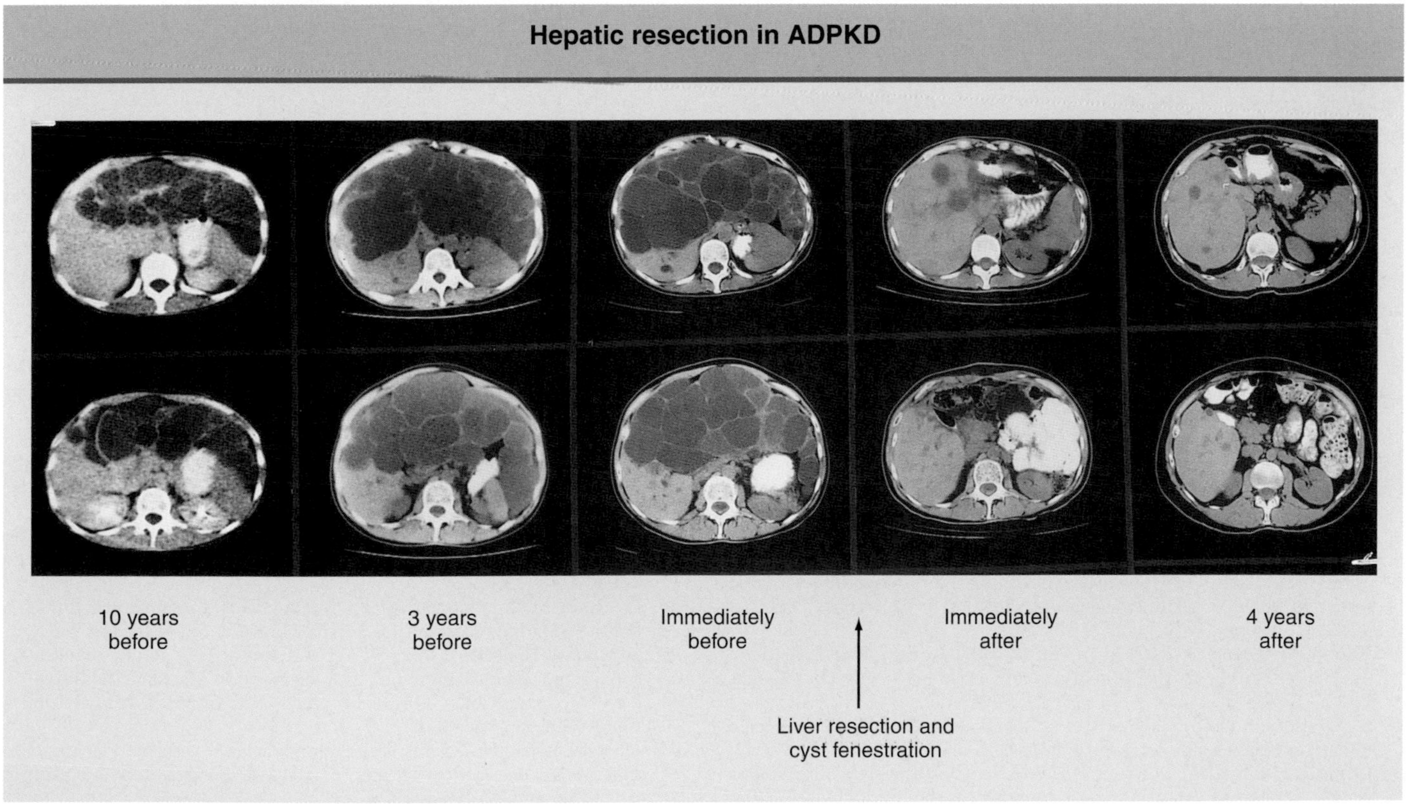

Hepatic resection in ADPKD

10 years before · 3 years before · Immediately before · Immediately after · 4 years after

Liver resection and cyst fenestration

Figure 43.12 Hepatic resection in ADPKD. CT scans of the abdomen. Ten years before (column 1), 3 years before (column 2), immediately before (column 3), immediately after (column 4), and 4 years after (column 5) liver resection and cyst fenestration demonstrating long-term, sustained reduction in liver size after the procedure. (From Que F, Nagorney DM, Gross JB, Torres VE: Liver resection and cyst fenestration in the treatment of severe polycystic liver disease. Gastroenterology 1995;108:487–494.)

both antiproliferative agents, may in the future be considered for clinical trial. A clinical trial of vasopressin-2 (V$_2$) receptor antagonist has been initiated.[51,52] The rationale for this trial includes the effect of vasopressin (through V$_2$ receptors) on adenyl cyclase in principal cells; the predominant origin of the cysts from collecting ducts; the cystogenic effect of cAMP; the favorable results of preclinical studies of V$_2$ receptor antagonists in animal models of polycystic kidney disease; and the safety of these drugs in clinical trials for water-retaining states.

Surrogate markers of disease progression will be essential for clinical trials in ADPKD. The Consortium for Radiologic Imaging Studies of Polycystic Kidney Disease (CRISP) study, a National Institutes of Health–funded prospective observational study, examined the potential of radiologically measured structural changes as indicators of progressive renal function decline in early ADPKD.[53] Preliminary results from this study indicate that sequential determinations of renal volume quantify the rate of disease progression and that higher rates of kidney enlargement are associated with a more rapid decrease in renal function.

A small, randomized, crossover, placebo-controlled trial has shown that long-acting somatostatin slows renal volume expansion, as measured by CT.[54] This study demonstrates for the first time that the course of ADPKD in humans can be modified by pharmacologic interventions.

REFERENCES

1. Ravine D, Gibson RN, Walker RG, et al: Evaluation of ultrasonographic diagnostic criteria for autosomal dominant polycystic kidney disease 1. Lancet 1994;343:824–827.
2. Nicolau C, Torra R, Badenas C, et al: Autosomal dominant polycystic kidney disease types 1 and 2: Assessment of US sensitivity for diagnosis. Radiology 1999;213:273–276.
3. Hughes J, Ward CJ, Peral B, et al: The polycystic kidney disease 1 (*PKD1*) gene encodes a novel protein with multiple cell recognition domains. Nat Genet 1995;10:151–160.
4. Consortium TIPKD: Polycystic kidney disease: The complete structure of the PKD1 gene and its protein. Cell 1995;81:289–298.
5. Consortium TAP: Analysis of the genomic sequence for the autosomal dominant polycystic kidney disease (*PKD1*) gene predicts the presence of a leucine-rich repeat. Hum Mol Genet 1995;4:575–582.
6. Mochizuki T, Wu G, Hayashi T, et al: PKD2, a gene for polycystic kidney disease that encodes an integral membrane protein. Science 1996;272:1339–1342.
7. Reynolds DM, Falk CT, Li AR, et al: Identification of a locus for autosomal dominant polycystic liver disease, on chromosome 19p13.2–13.1. Am J Hum Genet 2000;67:1598–1604.
8. Davila S, Furu L, Gharavi AG, et al: Mutations in SEC63 cause autosomal dominant polycystic liver disease. Nat Genet 2004;36:575–577.
9. Torres V: New insights into polycystic kidney disease and its treatment. Curr Opin Nephrol Hypertens 1998;7:159–169.
10. Qian F, Watnick TJ, Onuchic LF, Germino GG: The molecular basis of focal cyst formation in human autosomal dominant polycystic kidney disease type 1. Cell 1996;87:979–987.
11. Germino G: Autosomal dominant polycystic kidney disease: A two-hit model. Hosp Pract 1997;32:81–102.
12. Pritchard L, Sloane-Stanley JA, Sharpe J, et al: A human *PKD1* transgene generates functional polycystin-1 in mice and is associated with a cystic phenotype. Hum Mol Genet 2000;9:2617–2627.
13. Koptides M, Mean R, Demetriou K, et al: Genetic evidence of a transheterozygous model for cystogenesis in autosomal dominant polycystic kidney disease. Hum Mol Genet 2000;9:447–452.
14. Watnick T, He N, Wang K, et al: Mutations of *PKD1* in ADPKD2 cysts suggest a pathogenic effect of trans-heterozygous mutations. Nat Genet 2000;25:143–144.
15. Lantinga-van Leeuwen IS, Dauwerse JG, Baelde HJ, et al: Lowering of Pkd1 expression is sufficient to cause polycystic kidney disease. Hum Mol Genet 2004;13:3069–3077.
16. Delmas P, Padilla F, Osorio N, et al: Polycystins, calcium signaling, and human diseases. Biochem Biophys Res Commun 2004;322:1374–1383.
17. Wilson PD: Polycystic kidney disease. N Engl J Med 2004;350:151–164.
18. Torres VE, Harris PC: Mechanisms of disease: Autosomal dominant and recessive polycystic kidney disease. Nat Clin Pract Nephrol 2006;2:40–55.
19. Nauli SM, Alenghat FJ, Luo Y, et al: Polycystins 1 and 2 mediate mechanosensation in the primary cilium of kidney cells. Nat Genet 2003;33:129–137.
20. McGrath J, Somlo S, Makova S, et al: Two populations of node monocilia initiate left-right asymmetry in the mouse. Cell 2003;114:61–73.
21. Qian Q, Hunter LW, Li M, et al: *Pkd2* haploinsufficiency alters intracellular calcium in vascular smooth muscle cells. Hum Mol Genet 2003;12:1875–1880.
22. Aguiari G, Banzi M, Gessi S, et al: Deficiency of polycystin-2 reduces Ca^{2+} channel activity and cell proliferation in ADPKD lymphoblastoid cells. FASEB J 2004;18:884–886.
23. Grantham JJ: Lillian Jean Kaplan International Prize for advancement in the understanding of polycystic kidney disease. Understanding polycystic kidney disease: A systems biology approach. Kidney Int 2003;64:1157–1162.
24. Yamaguchi T, Wallace DP, Magenheimer BS, et al: Calcium restriction allows cAMP activation of the B-Raf/ERK pathway, switching cells to a cAMP-dependent growth-stimulated phenotype. J Biol Chem 2004:40419–40430.
25. Gabow P: Definition and natural history of autosomal dominant polycystic kidney disease. In Watson M, Torres V, eds: Polycystic Kidney Disease. Oxford, UK, Oxford University Press, 1996, pp 333–355.
26. Torres VE, Wilson DM, Hattery RR, Segura JW: Renal stone disease in autosomal dominant polycystic kidney disease. Am J Kidney Dis 1993;22:513–519.
27. Wang D, Iversen J, Strandgaard S: Endothelium-dependent relaxation of small resistance vessels is impaired in patients with autosomal dominant polycystic kidney disease. J Am Soc Nephrol 2000;11:1371–1376.
28. Johnson A, Gabow P: Identification of patients with autosomal dominant polycystic kidney disease at highest risk for end-stage renal disease. J Am Soc Nephrol 1997;8:1560–1567.
29. Rossetti S, Burton S, Strmecki L, et al: The position of the polycystic kidney disease 1 (PKD1) gene mutation correlates with the severity of renal disease. J Am Soc Nephrol 2002;13:1230–1237.
30. Zeier M, Fehrenbach P, Geberth S, et al: Renal histology in polycystic kidney disease with incipient and advanced renal failure. Kidney Int 1992;42:1259–1265.
31. Torres V: Polycystic liver disease. In Watson MT, VE, ed: Polycystic Kidney Disease. Oxford, UK, Oxford Medical Publications, 1996, pp 500–529.
32. Huston J, Torres V, Wiebers D, Schievink W: Follow-up of intracranial aneurysms in autosomal dominant polycystic kidney disease by magnetic resonance angiography. J Am Soc Nephrol 1996;7:2135–2141.
33. Griffin MD, Torres VE, Grande JP, Kumar R: Vascular expression of polycystin. J Am Soc Nephrol 1997;8:616–626.
34. Torres VE, Cai Y, Chen X, et al: Vascular expression of polycystin 2. J Am Soc Nephrol 2001;12:1–9.
35. Gregoire J, Torres V, Holley K, Farrow G: Renal epithelial hyperplastic and neoplastic proliferation in autosomal dominant polycystic kidney disease. Am J Kidney Dis 1987;9:27–38.
36. Woo D: Apoptosis and loss of renal tissue in polycystic kidney diseases. N Engl J Med 1995;333:18–25.
37. Torres VE: Vasopressin antagonists in polycystic kidney disease. Kidney Int 2005;68:2405–2418.
38. Rossetti S, Strmecki L, Gamble V, et al: Mutation analysis of the entire *PKD1* gene: Genetic and diagnostic implications. Am J Hum Genet 2001;68:46–63.
39. De Rycke M, Georgiou I, Sermon K, et al: PGD for autosomal dominant polycystic kidney disease type 1. Mol Hum Reprod 2005;11:65–71.
40. Segura JW, King BF, Jowsey SG, et al: Chronic pain and its medical and surgical management in renal cystic diseases. In Watson ML, Torres VE, eds: Polycystic Kidney Disease. Oxford, UK, Oxford Medical Publications, 1996, pp 462–480.
41. Ubara Y, Katori H, Tagami T, et al: Transcatheter renal arterial embolization therapy on a patient with polycystic kidney disease on hemodialysis. Am J Kidney Dis 1999;34:926–931.
42. Dunn MD, Portis AJ, Elbahnasy AM, et al: Laparoscopic nephrectomy in patients with end-stage renal disease and autosomal dominant polycystic kidney disease. (See comments). Am J Kidney Dis 2000;35:720–725.

43. Valente JF: Laparoscopic renal denervation for intractable ADPKD-related pain. Nephrol Dial Transplant 2001;16:160.
44. Ecder T, Chapman A, Brosnahan G, et al: Effect of antihypertensive therapy on renal function and urinary albumin excretion in hypertensive patients with autosomal dominant polycystic kidney disease. Am J Kid Dis 2000;35:427–432.
45. Jafar T, Schmid C, Landa M, et al: Angiotensin-converting enzyme inhibitors and progression of nondiabetic renal disease: A meta-analysis of patient-level data. Ann Intern Med 2001;135:73–87.
46. Schrier RW, McFann KK, Johnson AM: Epidemiological study of kidney survival in autosomal dominant polycystic kidney disease. Kidney Int 2003;63:678–685.
47. Schrier R, McFann K, Johnson A, et al: Cardiac and renal effects of standard versus rigorous blood pressure control in autosomal-dominant polycystic kidney disease: results of a seven-year prospective randomized study. J Am Soc Nephrol 2002;13:1733–1739.
48. Sarnak MJ, Greene T, Wang X, et al: The effect of a lower target blood pressure on the progression of kidney disease: Long-term follow-up of the modification of diet in renal disease study. Ann Intern Med 2005; 142:342–351.
49. Sweeney WE, Jr., Hamahira K, Sweeney J, et al: Combination treatment of PKD utilizing dual inhibition of EGF-receptor activity and ligand bioavailability. Kidney Int 2003;64:1310–1319.
50. Tao Y, Kim J, Schrier RW, Edelstein CL: Rapamycin markedly slows disease progression in a rat model of polycystic kidney disease. J Am Soc Nephrol 2005;16:46–51.
51. Torres VE, Wang X, Qian Q, et al: Effective treatment of an orthologous model of autosomal dominant polycystic kidney disease. Nat Med 2004;10:363–364.
52. Gattone VH, Wang X, Harris PC, Torres VE: Inhibition of renal cystic disease development and progression by a vasopressin V2 receptor antagonist. Nat Med 2003;9:1323–1326.
53. Grantham JJ, Torres VE, Chapman AB, et al: Volume progression in polycystic kidney disease. N Engl J Med 2006;354:2181–2183.
54. Ruggenenti P, Remuzzi A, Ondei P, et al: Safety and efficacy of long-acting somatostatin treatment in autosomal dominant polycystic kidney disease. Kidney Int 2005;68:206–216.

Other Cystic Kidney Diseases

Lisa Guay-Woodford

INTRODUCTION

In addition to autosomal dominant polycystic kidney disease (ADPKD), there are numerous other disorders that share renal cysts as a common feature[1,2] (Fig. 44.1). These disorders may be inherited or acquired, and their manifestations may be confined to the kidney or expressed systemically. They may present at a wide range of ages, from the perinatal period to old age (Fig. 44.2). The renal cysts may be single or multiple, and the associated renal morbidity may range from clinical insignificance to progressive parenchymal destruction with resultant renal insufficiency.

The clinical context often helps distinguish these renal cystic disorders from one another. Echogenic, enlarged kidneys in a

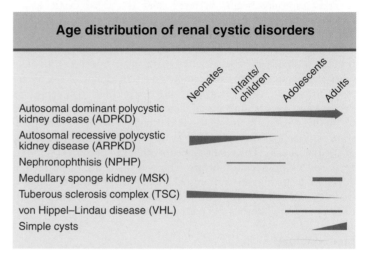

Figure 44.2   Age distribution of renal cystic disorders.

neonate or infant should raise suspicion about autosomal recessive polycystic kidney disease (ARPKD), ADPKD, tuberous sclerosis complex (TSC), or one of the many congenital syndromes associated with renal cystic disease. Renal insufficiency in an adolescent suggests juvenile nephronophthisis (NPHP)–medullary cystic disease complex or ARPKD as possible etiologies. The finding of a solitary cyst in a 5-year-old may indicate a calyceal diverticulum, whereas this finding in a 50-year-old is most compatible with a simple renal cyst. Renal stones occur in ADPKD and medullary sponge kidneys (MSKs). For those disorders with systemic manifestations, such as ADPKD, TSC, and von Hippel–Lindau disease (VHL), the associated extrarenal features may provide other important differential diagnostic clues.

For an increasing number of conditions, genetic testing is available in expert laboratories around the world. These are listed at www.genetests.org.

AUTOSOMAL RECESSIVE POLYCYSTIC KIDNEY DISEASE

Introduction and Definition

ARPKD is an inherited malformation complex with varying degrees of renal collecting duct dilation and biliary ductal ectasia.[3]

Etiology and Pathogenesis
Genetic Basis of Autosomal Recessive Polycystic Kidney Disease
ARPKD is associated with mutations in the very large gene, *PKHD1*, which encodes several alternatively spliced isoforms predicted to form both membrane-bound and secreted proteins.[4–6]

Renal cystic disorders	
Renal Cystic Disorder	Mendelian Inheritance*
Nongenetic	
Developmental	
Medullary sponge kidney	
Renal cystic dysplasia	
Multicystic dysplasia	
Cystic dysplasia associated with lower urinary tract obstruction	
Diffuse cystic dysplasia—syndromal and nonsyndromal	
Acquired	
Simple cysts	
Hypokalemic cystic disease	
Acquired cystic disease (in advanced renal failure)	
Genetic	
Autosomal dominant	
Autosomal dominant polycystic kidney disease	601313; 173910
von Hippel–Lindau syndrome	193300
Tuberous sclerosis	191100
Adult-onset medullary cystic disease	174000; 603860
Autosomal recessive	
Autosomal recessive polycystic kidney disease	263200
Juvenile nephronophthisis	256000; 602088; 6044387; 606966; 609254
Meckel-Gruber syndrome	24900; 607361
X-linked	
Orofaciodigital syndrome type I	311200

Figure 44.1   Renal cystic disorders. *Mendelian inheritance in man (www.ncbi.nlm.nih.gov).

The largest protein product of *PKHD1*, termed *fibrocystin* or *polyductin*, contains one membrane spanning domain and an intracellular C-terminal tail. Recent reports demonstrate that fibrocystin/polyductin localizes, at least in part, to the primary cilium and the centrosome in renal epithelial cells.[7] The basic defects observed in ARPKD suggest that fibrocystin/polyductin mediates the terminal differentiation of the collecting duct and biliary tract. However, the exact function of the numerous isoforms has not been defined, and the widely varying clinical spectrum of ARPKD may depend, in part, on the nature and number of splice variants that are disrupted by specific *PKHD1* mutations.

Pathogenesis

ARPKD typically begins *in utero*, and the renal cystic lesion appears to be superimposed on a normal developmental sequence. The tubular abnormality primarily involves fusiform dilation of the collecting ducts. Detailed microdissection studies have excluded tubular obstruction as a primary pathogenic mechanism.[8] The biliary lesion appears to involve defective remodeling of the ductal plate *in utero*. As a result, primitive bile duct configurations persist, and progressive portal fibrosis evolves.[9] The remainder of the liver parenchyma develops normally. The defect in ductal plate remodeling is accompanied by abnormalities in the branching of the portal vein. The resulting histopathologic pattern is referred to as congenital hepatic fibrosis. The weight of the experimental evidence from human and animal model studies suggests that a maturational arrest in both renal and biliary tubuloepithelial differentiation underlies the pathogenesis of ARPKD.

Epidemiology

The estimated incidence of ARPKD is 1 per 20,000 live births.[10] The disorder appears to occur more frequently in Caucasians than in other ethnic populations.[11,12]

Clinical Manifestations

The clinical spectrum of ARPKD is variable and depends on the age at presentation. Most cases are identified either *in utero* or at birth. The most severely affected fetuses have enlarged echogenic kidneys and oligohydramnios due to poor fetal renal output. These fetuses develop the Potter phenotype, with pulmonary hypoplasia, a characteristic facies, and deformities of the spine and limbs. At birth, these neonates often have a critical degree of pulmonary hypoplasia that is incompatible with survival. Renal function, although frequently compromised, is rarely a cause of neonatal death. For those infants who survive the perinatal period, morbidity and mortality result from severe systemic hypertension, renal insufficiency, and portal hypertension due to portal tract hyperplasia and fibrosis.

Hypertension usually develops in the first several months and ultimately affects 70% to 80% of patients.[13] ARPKD patients have defects in both urinary diluting capacity and concentrating capacity. Newborns can have hyponatremia, presumably resulting from defects in free water excretion. Although net acid excretion may be reduced, metabolic acidosis is not a significant clinical feature.

Abnormal urinalyses are common in both infants and older children.[13] Microscopic or gross hematuria, proteinuria, and sterile pyuria have all been reported. Two retrospective studies report an increased incidence of culture-confirmed urinary tract infections.

In the first 6 months of life, ARPKD infants may have a transient improvement in their glomerular filtration rate (GFR) due to renal maturation. Subsequently, a progressive but variable decline in renal function occurs, with some patients not progressing to end-stage renal disease (ESRD) until adolescence or early adulthood. With advances in effective therapy for ESRD, prolonged survival is common, and for many patients, the hepatic complications become the dominant clinical issue.

In children who present later in childhood or in adolescence, portal hypertension is frequently the predominant clinical abnormality, with hepatosplenomegaly and bleeding esophageal or gastric varices, as well as hypersplenism with consequent thrombocytopenia, anemia, and leukopenia. Hepatocellular function is usually preserved. Ascending suppurative cholangitis is a serious complication and can cause fulminant hepatic failure.[14]

Pathology
Kidney

The renal involvement is invariably bilateral and largely symmetric. The histopathology varies depending on the age of presentation and the extent of cystic involvement (Fig. 44.3a, b).

In the affected neonate, the kidneys can be 10 times normal size, but retain their reniform configuration. Dilated, fusiform collecting ducts extend radially through the cortex. In the medulla, the dilated collecting ducts are more often cut tangentially or transversely. Up to 90% of the collecting ducts are involved. Associated

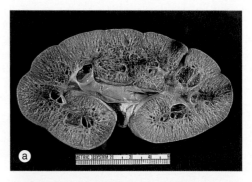

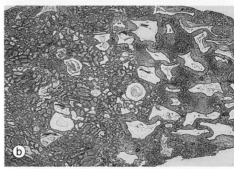

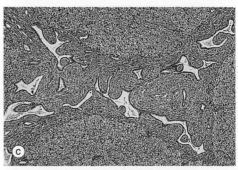

Figure 44.3 Pathologic features of ARPKD. *a*, Cut section: ARPKD kidney from 1-year-old child with discrete medullary cysts and dilated collecting ducts. *b*, Light microscopy: later-onset ARPKD kidney with prominent medullary ductal ectasia, H&E × 10. *c*, Light microscopy: congenital hepatic fibrosis. There is extensive fibrosis of the portal area with ectatic, tortuous bile ducts, and hypoplasia of the portal vein, H&E × 40.

interstitial fibrosis is minimal in neonates and infants, but increases with progressive disease.

In patients diagnosed later in childhood, the kidney size and extent of cystic involvement tend to be more limited. Cysts can expand up to 2 cm in diameter and assume a more spherical configuration. Progressive interstitial fibrosis is probably responsible for secondary tubular obstruction. In older children, medullary ductal ectasia is the predominant finding.

Cysts are lined with a single layer of nondescript cuboidal epithelium. The glomeruli and nephron segments proximal to the collecting ducts are initially structurally normal but are often crowded between ectatic collecting ducts or displaced into subcapsular wedges. The presence of cartilage or other dysplastic elements indicates a diagnosis other than ARPKD, such as cystic dysplasia.

Liver

The liver in ARPKD can be either normal in size or somewhat enlarged. The hepatic parenchyma may be intersected by delicate fibrous septa, which link the portal tracts. Bile ducts are dilated (biliary ectasia), and marked cystic dilation of the entire intra-hepatic biliary system (Caroli's disease) has been reported.[15] In neonatal ARPKD, the bile ducts are increased in number, rather tortuous in configuration, and often located around the periphery of the portal tract. In older children, the biliary ectasia is accompanied by increasing portal fibrosis and hypoplasia of the small portal vein branches (see Fig. 44.3c). The portal fibrosis may be quite extensive, but the hepatocytes are seldom affected.

DIAGNOSIS

Prenatal Diagnosis

The diagnosis of ARPKD can be suggested by fetal ultrasound scanning. Enlarged echogenic kidneys, oligohydramnios, and decreased urine in the bladder may become evident as early as the 16th week of gestation, but most often occur after the 20th week. However, these findings are not specific to ARPKD and may also be evident in ADPKD, glomerulocystic kidney disease, and Meckel's syndrome (Fig. 44.4).

Clinical and genetic features of pediatric renal cystic disease						
	ARPKD	NPHP	Meckel-Gruber	GCKD	ADPKD	TSC
Clinical onset (years)	Perinatal	NPHP2: 0–5 NPHP: 10–18	Perinatal	Infancy, older children	Infancy, older children	Infancy, older children
Enlarged kidneys	Yes	NPHP2: yes NPHP: no	Yes	—		Occurs
Renal pathology	Multiple cysts	NPHP2: multiple cysts NPHP: few cysts at cortico-medullary junction	Multiple cysts	Multiple cortical cysts	Multiple cysts	Few to multiple cysts; angiomyo-lipoma
Cyst infection	Uncommon	No	Uncommon	No	Occurs	Uncommon
Blood pressure	Normal increased	NPHP2: increased NPHP: normal	Normal	Normal increased	Normal increased	Normal
Renal function	Normal, impaired	Normal, impaired	Normal, impaired	Normal	Normal	Normal
Nephrocalcinosis/ nephrolithiasis	Nephrocalcinosis up to 25%	No	No	No	Nephrolithiases occur	No
Congestive heart failure	Yes	Rare	Yes	No	10%–15% infantile ADPKD	No
Pancreas lesions	No	No	No	MODY5	No	No
Central nervous system involvement	No	Joubert syndrome[4]	Encephalocele; mental retardation	No	No	Seizures, mental retardation
Disease gene	PKHD1	NPHP1-NPHP5	MSK1 MSK3	PKD1 HNF1-β	PKD1 PKD2	TSC1 TSC2
Genetic testing	Yes	Yes	No	Yes	Yes	Yes

Figure 44.4   Clinical and genetic features of pediatric renal cystic disease. Meckel-Gruber syndrome is a severe, often lethal, autosomal recessive disorder characterized by bilateral renal cystic dysplasia, biliary ductal dysgenesis, polydactyly, and variable central nervous system malformations. Glomerulocystic kidney disease (GCKD) can occur as the infantile manifestation of autosomal dominant polycystic kidney disease (ADPKD). Familial hypoplastic GCKD, due to mutations in the gene encoding hepatocyte nuclear factor (HNF)-1β, can be associated with maturity-onset diabetes of the young, type V (MODY5). A contiguous germline deletion of both the PKD1 and TSC2 genes (the PKDTS contiguous gene syndrome) occurs in a small group of patients with features of TSC as well as massive renal cystic disease reminiscent of ADPKD, severe hypertension, and a progressive decline in renal function with the onset of end-stage renal disease in the second or third decade of life. Joubert syndrome (JBTS) is an autosomal recessive disorder characterized by cerebellar vermis aplasia, coloboma, retinitis pigmentosa, congenital hypotonia, and either ocular motor apraxia or irregularities in breathing patterns during the neonatal period. The disease can be associated with nephronophthisis (NPHP), and mutations in *NPHP1* have been described in a small subset of patients (JBTS4). Mutations in the gene *AHI1* (Abelson helper integration site 1) were recently identified as the cause of JBTS3 in families with or without renal involvement.[27] ARPKD, autosomal recessive polycystic kidney disease.

In families known to be at risk for ARPKD, the genetic mapping data and the absence of genetic heterogeneity have allowed for haplotype-based prenatal diagnosis.[10] However, haplotype-based genotyping requires the accurate diagnosis of ARPKD in previous affected siblings and the availability of DNA from the index case. In cases with diagnostic uncertainties or families in which no DNA from the index case is available, direct analysis of the *PKHD1* gene would be required. Recent studies have refined the mutation detection strategies and improved the mutation detection rate to 80% to 85% in ARPKD patients.[16,17] Therefore, new algorithms that include gene-based analysis and haplotype-based genotyping (in informative families) can now provide reliable prenatal diagnosis testing for ARPKD. Genetic diagnosis is currently available for ARPKD and is particularly useful for prenatal testing (see www.genetests.org).

Postnatal Diagnosis

The renal ultrasound findings vary with patient age and the severity of renal involvement. Kidney size typically peaks at 1 to 2 years of age, then gradually declines relative to the child's body size and stabilizes by 4 to 5 years of age.[18,19] In affected neonates, the kidneys are typically symmetrically enlarged and diffusely echogenic with poor demarcation from surrounding tissues, as well as among the cortex, medulla, and renal sinus. With high-resolution ultrasound, the radial array of dilated collecting ducts may be imaged (Fig. 44.5a). As patients age, there is increased medullary echogenicity with scattered small cysts, measuring <2 cm in diameter. These cysts and progressive fibrosis can alter the reniform contour, causing ARPKD in some older children to be mistaken for ADPKD. Contrast-enhanced CT scanning can be useful in delineating the renal architecture in these children (see Fig. 44.5b). In several small studies, bilateral pelvicaliectasis and renal calcification have been reported in 25% and 50% of ARPKD patients, respectively.[19–21] In adults with medullary ectasia alone, the cystic lesion may be confused with MSK.

The liver may be either normal in size or enlarged. It is usually less echogenic than the kidneys. Prominent intrahepatic bile duct dilation suggests associated Caroli's disease. With age, the portal fibrosis tends to progress, and in older children, ultrasound typically reveals hepatosplenomegaly and a patchy increase in hepatic echogenicity.

Natural History

The estimated perinatal mortality rate is 30% to 50%. For those who survive the first month of life, the reported mean 5-year patient survival rate is 80% to 95%.[12,22] On average, those infants with serum creatinine values > 2.2 mg/dl (200 μmol/l) progress to ESRD within 5 years, but this is highly variable. In one longitudinal study, the probability of survival without ESRD was 85% at 1 year, 76% at 5 years, and 63% at 15 years.[22] Effective management of systemic and portal hypertension, coupled with successful renal replacement therapy, has allowed long-term patient survival. Therefore, the prognosis in ARPKD, particularly for those children who survive the first month of life, is far less bleak than popularly thought, and aggressive medical therapy is warranted. In patients with ESRD and severe portal hypertension, combined kidney and liver transplantation may be indicated.

Treatment

The survival of ARPKD neonates has improved significantly in the past decade because of advances in mechanical ventilation and other supportive measures. Aggressive interventions such as unilateral or bilateral nephrectomies and continuous hemofiltration have been advocated in neonatal management, but prospective, controlled studies have yet to be performed.

For children who survive the perinatal period, careful blood pressure monitoring is required. Angiotensin-converting enzyme (ACE) inhibitors, calcium channel blockers, β-blockers, and loop diuretics are effective antihypertensive agents. The management of ARPKD children with declining GFR should follow the standard guidelines established for chronic renal insufficiency in pediatric patients.[23,24]

Given the relative urinary concentrating defect, ARPKD children should be monitored for dehydration during intercurrent illnesses associated with fever, tachypnea, nausea, vomiting, or diarrhea. In infants with severe polyuria, thiazide diuretics may be used to decrease distal nephron solute and water delivery. Acid-base balance should be closely monitored and supplemental bicarbonate therapy initiated as needed.

Close monitoring for portal hypertension is warranted in all ARPKD patients. The severity of portal hypertension and its progression can be followed by serial ultrasound and Doppler flow studies. Hematemesis or melena suggests the presence of esophageal varices. Medical management may include sclerotherapy, variceal banding, or transjugular intrahepatic portosystemic shunt (TIPS). Surgical approaches such as portocaval or splenorenal shunting may be indicated in some patients. Although hypersplenism occurs fairly commonly, splenectomy is seldom warranted. Unexplained fever with or without elevated transaminase levels suggests bacterial cholangitis and requires meticulous evaluation, sometimes including a percutaneous liver biopsy, to make the diagnosis and guide aggressive antibiotic therapy.[25]

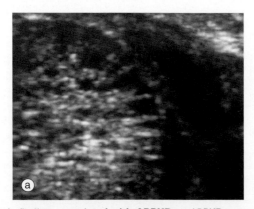 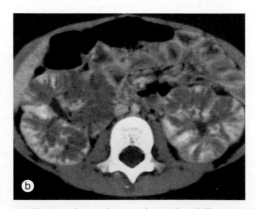

Figure 44.5 Radiologic findings associated with ARPKD. *a*, ARPKD in a neonate. High-resolution ultrasound reveals radially arrayed dilated collecting ducts. *b*, ARPKD in a symptomatic 4-year-old girl. Contrast-enhanced CT shows a striated nephrogram and persistent corticomedullary differentiation.

Transplantation

A prolonged period of dialysis in childhood has been associated with both cognitive and educational impairment.[26] Therefore, renal transplantation is the treatment of choice for ARPKD patients who develop ESRD. For children, renal allografts are more commonly obtained from living-related than cadaveric donors. Because ARPKD is a recessive disorder, either parent may be a suitable kidney donor. Native nephrectomies may be warranted in patients with massively enlarged kidneys to allow allograft placement.

In some patients, combined kidney-liver transplantation is appropriate. Indications include the combination of renal failure and either recurrent cholangitis or significant complications of portal hypertension, such as recurrent variceal bleeding, refractory ascites, and the hepatopulmonary syndrome. In addition, liver transplantation may be a reasonable option for patients with a single episode of cholangitis in the context of marked abnormalities in the biliary system (Caroli's syndrome).[27]

JUVENILE NEPHRONOPHTHISIS–MEDULLARY CYSTIC DISEASE COMPLEX

Introduction and Definitions

Juvenile NPHP and medullary cystic kidney disease share the same triad of histopathologic features: tubular basement membrane irregularities, tubular atrophy with cyst formation, and interstitial cell infiltration with fibrosis. These histopathologically similar disorders differ only in their mode of transmission and age of onset. Juvenile NPHP is an autosomal recessive disorder that presents in childhood, whereas medullary cystic disease is an autosomal dominant disorder that occurs in adults. The inclusive term juvenile NPHP–medullary cystic disease complex has been used to describe these disorders. However, juvenile NPHP is far more common than medullary cystic disease and has been reported both as an isolated renal disease and in association with retinitis pigmentosa, congenital hepatic fibrosis, oculomotor apraxia, and skeletal anomalies. Therefore, these entities will be considered separately.

AUTOSOMAL RECESSIVE JUVENILE NEPHRONOPHTHISIS

Etiology and Pathogenesis
Genetic Basis of Juvenile Nephronophthisis

Five genes (NPHP1–NPHP5) involved in juvenile NPHP have been identified.[28] About 60% of the cases of purely renal NPHP have defects in NPHP1, with large, homozygous deletions detected in 80% of affected family members and in 65% of sporadic cases.[29] The NPHP1 and NPHP3–5 genes encode cytosolic proteins that are collectively called the nephrocystins. The NPHP2 gene, involved in infantile NPHP, encodes inversin, a protein that is critical for normal left-to-right patterning in the vertebrate embryo. Inversin, nephrocystin-3, and nephrocystin-4 each bind to nephrocystin, and all these proteins are expressed in or at the base of primary cilia in renal epithelial cells, suggesting a common pathway in cilia function.[28] However, the subcellular localization of these proteins is not confined to the cilium. Nephrocystin and nephrocystin-4 have also been localized to cell junctions and shown to interact with components of cell-cell and cell-matrix interaction complexes. These observations suggest that NPHP proteins may have multiple functions depending on their localization in different cell compartments and their association with distinct protein complexes.

Clinical Manifestations
Renal Disease

NPHP accounts for 6% to 15% of ESRD in children and adolescents. Three distinct forms of the disease (infantile, juvenile, and adolescent) have been described, based on the age of onset of ESRD. However, further clinical, pathologic, and genetic analyses indicate that the adolescent and juvenile forms are virtually indistinguishable, so these two forms are described with the single designation, juvenile NPHP.[29] In juvenile NPHP (the most common form), ESRD occurs at a mean age of 13 years; whereas in the infantile form, the age of onset of ESRD consistently occurs before 5 years of age.

Decreased urinary concentrating capacity is an invariable finding in NPHP patients and usually precedes the decline in renal function, with onset in school-aged children. Polyuria and polydipsia are common symptoms. Salt wasting develops in most patients with renal insufficiency, and sodium supplementation is often required until the onset of ESRD. One third of patients become anemic before the onset of renal insufficiency, possibly due to a defect in the functional regulation of erythropoietin production by peritubular fibroblasts.[30] Growth retardation, out of proportion to the degree of renal insufficiency, is a common finding.

Slowly progressive decline in renal function is typical of juvenile NPHP. Although symptoms can be detected after the age of 2 years, they may progress insidiously, such that 15% of affected patients are recognized only after ESRD has developed. There is no specific treatment. The disease is not known to recur in renal allografts.

Children with the infantile variant develop symptoms in the first few months of life and rapidly progress to ESRD, usually before the age of 2 years, but invariably by 5 years of age. This disorder is a distinct genetic entity with a characteristic renal histopathology and has not been reported in sibships with classic juvenile NPHP.[31]

Unlike patients with polycystic kidney disease or MSK, NPHP patients rarely develop flank pain, hematuria, hypertension, urinary tract infections, or renal calculi.

Associated Extrarenal Abnormalities

Extrarenal abnormalities have been described in about 10% to 15% of juvenile NPHP patients.[29] The most frequently associated anomaly is retinal dystrophy due to tapetoretinal degeneration (Senior-Loken syndrome). Severely affected patients present with coarse nystagmus, early blindness, and a flat electroretinogram (Leber's amaurosis), whereas those with moderate retinal dystrophy typically have mild visual impairment and retinitis pigmentosa. Other extrarenal anomalies include oculomotor apraxia (Cogan's syndrome), mental retardation, and cone-shaped epiphyses of the bones. Congenital hepatic fibrosis occurs occasionally in NPHP patients, but the associated bile duct proliferation is mild and qualitatively different from that found in ARPKD.

Pathology

In juvenile NPHP, the kidneys are moderately contracted, with parenchymal atrophy causing a loss of corticomedullary demarcation.[32] Histopathologic findings include tubular atrophy with thickened tubular basement membrane, diffuse and severe interstitial fibrosis, and cysts of variable size distributed in an irregular pattern at the corticomedullary junction and in the outer medulla. However, up to 25% of NPHP kidneys have no grossly visible cysts.

In the typical NPHP renal lesion, clusters of atrophic tubules alternate with either groups of viable tubules showing dilation or marked compensatory hypertrophy or groups of collapsed tubules. Although this histopathologic pattern is not unique, the abrupt transition from one type of tubular profile to another is suggestive of NPHP. Moderate interstitial fibrosis, usually without a significant inflammatory cell infiltrate, is interspersed among the atrophic tubules. Spherical, thin-walled cysts lined with a simple cuboidal epithelium may be evident at the corticomedullary junction, in the medulla, and even in the papillae. Microdissection studies indicate that these cysts arise from the loop of Henle, distal convoluted tubules, and collecting ducts. Glomeruli may be normal, although some may be completely sclerosed, others show periglomerular fibrosis, and still others show dilation of Bowman's space (Fig. 44.6).

In comparison, the infantile form has features of both juvenile NPHP, such as tubular cell atrophy, interstitial fibrosis, and tubular cysts, and polycystic kidney disease, including enlarged kidneys and widespread cystic involvement.[32]

Diagnosis and Differential Diagnosis

In a child with NPHP and renal insufficiency, renal ultrasonography reveals normal-sized or small kidneys with loss of corticomedullary differentiation and increased echogenicity. Occasionally, cysts can be detected at the corticomedullary junction or in the medulla. Thin-section CT may be more sensitive than ultrasonography in detecting these cysts.

The pathologic findings in NPHP are not unique; hence, in the early stages of the disease, neither renal imaging nor histopathology can confirm the clinical diagnosis. As an alternative strategy, molecular testing may become increasingly useful in establishing the diagnosis of NPHP. An algorithm for gene-based diagnosis addresses four critical diagnostic issues: (1) detection of the classic homozygous deletion of *NPHP1*; (2) detection of rare, smaller homozygous deletions of *NPHP1*; (3) testing for a heterozygous deletion; and (4) potential exclusion of linkage to *NPHP1*.[33] Genetic testing is currently available for *NPHP1*-related disease (see www.genetests.org). As new genes are identified and their relative contribution to the NPHP disease spectrum determined, mutational algorithms will be expanded to include analyses of these NPHP genes.

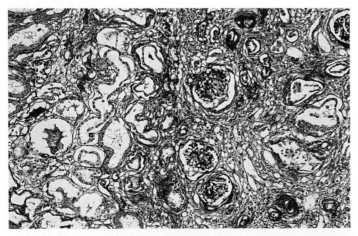

Figure 44.6 **Renal pathology in juvenile nephronophthisis.** Light microscopy: tubulointerstitial nephropathy. Atrophic tubules with irregularly thickened basement membranes are surrounded by interstitial fibrosis. Dilated tubules are evident at the corticomedullary junction, H&E × 40.

AUTOSOMAL DOMINANT MEDULLARY CYSTIC KIDNEY DISEASE

Medullary cystic kidney disease is histopathologically indistinguishable from recessive NPHP and occurs with male-to-male transmission in successive generations, suggesting an autosomal dominant mode of inheritance. Some patients have had phenotypically unaffected parents but an affected second- or third-degree relative, raising the possibility of variable penetrance. This disorder appears to be rare compared with recessive NPHP. Although the clinical manifestations of the two disorders are similar, medullary cystic kidney disease is distinguished by its dominant mode of inheritance, later age of onset, progression to ESRD in the third to fourth decade of life, and lack of associated growth retardation and extrarenal manifestations.

Genetic linkage analyses indicate that defects in at least two loci (*MCKD1*, *MCKD2*) can cause medullary cystic kidney disease. Uremia occurs after 60 years of age in type 1 disease, whereas in type 2, progression to ESRD occurs at about 30 years of age. Mutations in the gene *UMOD*, which encodes uromodulin or Tamm-Horsfall protein, were recently identified as the cause of medullary cystic kidney disease type 2.[34] Subsequently, *UMOD* mutations have also been identified in families with familial juvenile hyperuricemic nephropathy (Mendelian Inheritance of Man [MIM] 162000), a dominantly transmitted disorder characterized by medullary cystic kidney disease, hyperuricemia, and gout.[35] The diagnosis can usually be made based on the family history, the clinical associations of hyperuricemia and gout, and the sonographic finding of medullary cysts. Genetic testing is now available for *UMOD*-related disease (see www.genetests.org).

MEDULLARY SPONGE KIDNEY

Introduction and Definition

MSK is a relatively common disorder characterized by dilated medullary and papillary collecting ducts that give the renal medulla a spongy appearance.[36]

Etiology and Pathogenesis

MSK is likely the result of a developmental defect, as evidenced by the occasional presence of embryonal tissue in the affected papillae and coexistence of other urinary tract anomalies. In addition, MSK occurs more frequently in individuals with other congenital defects, including congenital hemihypertrophy, Beckwith-Wiedemann syndrome, Ehlers-Danlos syndrome, and Marfan syndrome.[36] Fewer than 5% of cases are familial, and a clear genetic basis for MSK has not been established.

Epidemiology

In the general population, the frequency of MSK may be underestimated because some affected individuals remain entirely asymptomatic. Up to 20% of patients with nephrolithiasis have at least a mild degree of MSK, but excretory urography in *unselected* patients indicates a disease frequency of about 1 in 5000 individuals.[37]

Clinical Manifestations

MSK disease is asymptomatic unless complicated by nephrolithiasis, hematuria, or infection. Symptoms typically begin between the fourth and fifth decades of life, but adolescent presentations have been reported.[37] In MSK patients, stones or granular debris are composed of either pure apatite (calcium phosphate) or a mixture of apatite and calcium oxalate. Several factors appear to contribute to stone formation, including urinary stasis within the ectatic ducts, hypercalciuria, and hyperoxaluria. Hyperparathyroidism has also been reported.

Hematuria, unrelated to either coexisting stones or infection, may be recurrent. The bleeding is usually asymptomatic, but with gross hematuria, clot formation may cause colic. Urinary tract infection may occur in association with nephrolithiasis or as an independent event. Of those patients with stones, infections are more likely to occur in females than in males.

About one third to one half of MSK patients have hypercalcemia,[36] but the mechanism has not been established. Decreased renal concentrating ability and impaired urinary acidification have been reported. In most patients, the acidification defect is not associated with systemic acidosis.

Pathology

The pathologic changes are confined to the renal medullary and intrapapillary collecting ducts. Multiple spherical or oval cysts measuring 1 to 8 mm may be detected in one or more papillae. These cysts may be isolated or may communicate with the collecting system. The cysts are frequently bilateral and often contain spherical concretions composed of apatite. The affected pyramids and associated calyces are usually enlarged, and nephromegaly can result when many pyramids are involved. The renal cortex, medullary rays, calyces, and pelvis appear normal, unless complications such as pyelonephritis or urinary tract obstruction become superimposed.

Diagnosis

Plain films of the abdomen often reveal radiopaque concretions in the medulla (Fig. 44.7a). The diagnosis is established by intravenous urography (see Fig. 44.7b). Retention of contrast media by the ectatic collecting ducts appears either as spherical cysts or, more commonly, as diffuse linear striations. The latter imparts a characteristic blushlike pattern to the papillae, the so-called bouquet of flowers or paintbrush appearance. CT is usually not necessary, but nonenhanced CT may help distinguish MSK from papillary necrosis or even ADPKD (see Fig. 44.7c).

Natural History

With proper management of the clinical complications, the long-term prognosis is excellent. Progression to renal insufficiency is distinctly unusual.

Treatment

Asymptomatic patients in whom MSK is detected as an incidental finding require no therapy. Hematuria in the absence of stones or infection requires no intervention. If the tubular ectasia is unilateral and segmental, partial nephrectomy may alleviate recurrent nephrolithiasis and urinary tract infection. However, for most patients who have bilateral disease, medical management is sufficient.

Hypercalciuria is the predominant cause of nephrolithiasis in MSK. The mainstay of treatment is high fluid intake, in order to increase urine output and reduce the precipitation of calcium salts in ectatic ducts. Patients with documented hypercalciuria may benefit from thiazide diuretics.[36] If thiazides are poorly tolerated or contraindicated, inorganic phosphate therapy may be useful. To avoid struvite stone formation, oral phosphates should *not* be used in patients with previous urinary tract infections caused by urease-producing organisms. Patients who form and pass stones recurrently may benefit from periodic lithotripsy. Urinary tract obstruction must be considered during acute episodes of renal colic, and surgical intervention may be indicated.

Urinary tract infection should be treated with standard antibiotic regimens, and for some patients, prolonged therapy may be warranted. Urease-producing organisms, such as coagulase-negative staphylococci, are particularly problematic as urinary pathogens in MSK. Positive urine cultures, even with relatively insignificant colony counts, must be vigorously pursued.

TUBEROUS SCLEROSIS COMPLEX

Introduction and Definition

TSC is an autosomal dominant, tumor suppressor gene syndrome in which tumor-like malformations, called hamartomas, develop in multiple organ systems, including the kidneys, brain, heart, lungs, and skin.

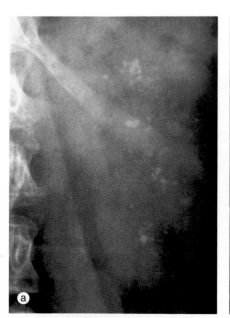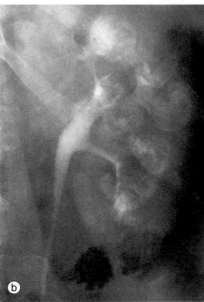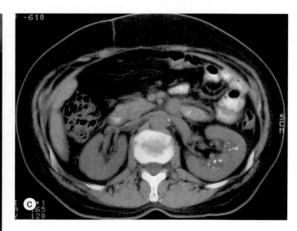

Figure 44.7   Radiologic findings associated with medullary sponge kidney (MSK). MSK in a 52-year-old, symptomatic woman. *a,* Plain film shows medullary nephrolithiases in the left kidney. *b,* Ten-minute film from an intravenous urography shows clusters of rounded densities in the papillae amidst discrete linear opacities (paintbrush appearance). *c,* Nonenhanced CT reveals densely echogenic foci in the medulla.

Etiology and Pathogenesis
Genetic Basis of Tuberous Sclerosis Complex

TSC results from inactivating mutations in one of two genes, *TSC1* on chromosome 9q32-q34[38] and *TSC2* on chromosome 16p13, adjacent to the *PKD1* gene.[39]

The molecular defect in TSC appears to disrupt cell migration and differentiation in neural crest derivatives. The focal nature of TSC-associated disease and the variability of disease expression even within families have suggested that *TSC1* and *TSC2* function as tumor suppressor genes.[40] The tumor suppressor gene paradigm was first proposed by Knudson, who hypothesized that two successive mutations are necessary to inactivate a tumor suppressor gene and cause tumor formation. The first mutation, inherited and therefore present in all cells, is necessary but not sufficient to produce tumors. A second mutation is required after fertilization to induce tumor transformation. The inactivating germline mutations identified in *TSC1* and *TSC2*, as well as the loss of heterozygosity detected in 50% of *TSC2*-associated hamartomas and about 10% of *TSC1*-associated hamartomas, support the hypothesis that both *TSC1* and *TSC2* function as tumor suppressor genes.

The past 5 years have seen remarkable progress in understanding the normal cellular functions of the TSC1/TSC2 protein complex. The *TSC2* gene product, tuberin, interacts with hamartin, the product of the *TSC1* gene. As described in Figure 44.8, the hamartin/tuberin (TSC1/TSC2) complex functions in multiple cellular pathways,[41] primarily by inhibiting mammalian target of rapamycin (mTOR) kinase activity. The mTOR pathway regulates nutrient uptake, cell growth, and protein translation.[42]

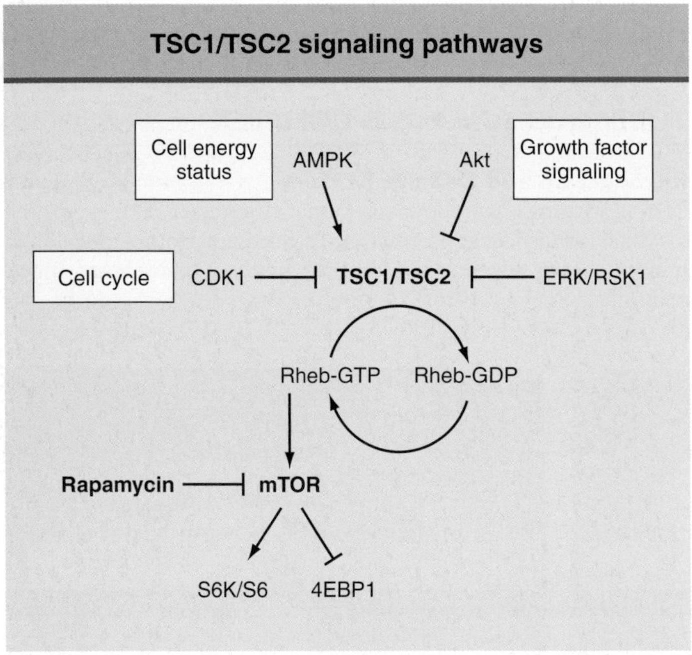

Epidemiology

TSC affects 1 in 6000 individuals. The disease penetrance is quite variable. About two thirds of TSC patients are sporadic cases with no family history, and the disease apparently results from new mutational events. Among patients with sporadic disease, mutations in *TSC2* are about five times more common than mutations in *TSC1*, whereas the ratio is 1:1 in familial cases. *TSC1*-related disease is milder, apparently because of a reduced rate of second hits.[42]

Clinicopathologic Manifestations

The clinical features of *TSC1*- and *TSC2*-linked disease are similar, although *TSC2*-linked disease tends to be more severe. The most common clinical manifestations include seizures, mental retardation or autism, skin lesions, and tumors in the brain, retina, kidney, and heart. In affected individuals older than 5 years of age, the most common skin lesions are facial angiofibromas (Fig. 44.9), hypomelanotic macules, and ungual fibromas.[43]

Kidney involvement occurs frequently in TSC. The principal manifestations include angiomyolipomas, cysts, and renal malignancies. Some of the malignant tumors originally thought to be renal cell carcinoma are now regarded as malignant epithelioid angiomyolipomas.[44] Other renal neoplasms, interstitial fibrosis with focal segmental glomerulosclerosis (FSGS), glomerular microhamartomas, and peripelvic and perirenal lymphangiomatous cysts have also been observed in TSC patients.

Renal Angiomyolipomas

Angiomyolipomas are hamartomatous structures composed of abnormal, thick-walled vessels, varying amounts of smooth muscle–like cells, and adipose tissue (Fig. 44.10a, b) These are the most common renal lesion in TSC patients and are evident in about 80% of TSC patients by age 10 years.[40] Although solitary angiomyolipomas are found in the general population, particularly among older women, TSC-associated angiomyolipomas are distinguished by the young age of onset, the multiple number, and the bilateral distribution. Angiomyolipomas rarely occur before 5 years of age but increase in frequency and size with age.[45] These tumors

TSC1/TSC2 signaling pathways

Cell energy status — AMPK — Akt — Growth factor signaling

Cell cycle — CDK1 ⊣ **TSC1/TSC2** ⊣ ERK/RSK1

Rheb-GTP → Rheb-GDP

Rapamycin ⊣ mTOR

S6K/S6   4EBP1

Figure 44.8 The TSC1/TSC2 signaling pathways. Hamartin (TSC1) and tuberin (TSC2) integrate cues from extracellular growth factor binding (via Akt and ERK/RSK1), the intracellular energy status (via AMPK), and the cell cycle (via CDK1) to direct signaling pathways that regulate cellular proliferation, differentiation, and migration. Tuberin contains a GTPase-activating protein (GAP) domain in its carboxy terminus, and when it forms a complex with hamartin (TSC1/TSC2 complex), the small GTPase Rheb is converted from its active GTP-bound state to an inactive GDP-bound state. Rheb is an activator of the mTOR kinase, which regulates a number of processes linked to protein synthesis and cell growth (via the ribosomal S6 kinases and the eukaryotic initiation factor 4E-binding protein (4E-BP1). mTOR is activated physiologically in response to growth factor signaling, which causes phosphorylation of tuberin, dissociation of the TSC1/TSC2 complex, and increased levels of Rheb-GTP. Inactivation of the TSC1/TSC2 complex through mutations in *TSC1* or *TSC2* leads to inappropriate activation of mTOR. Rapamycin is an mTOR inhibitor. (Adapted from Henske E: Tuberous sclerosis and the kidney: From mesenchyme to epithelium and beyond. Pediatr Nephrol 2005;20:854–857.)

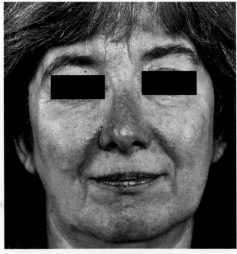

Figure 44.9 Facial angiofibromas. This 49-year-old patient has tuberous sclerosis complex.

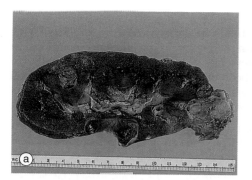 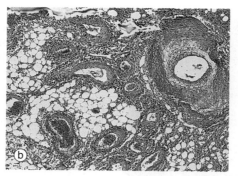 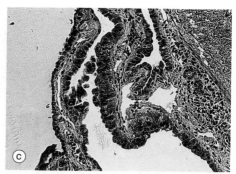

Figure 44.10 **Renal pathology in tuberous sclerosis complex (TSC).** *a,* Cut section: multiple angiomyolipomas in the kidney of a 60-year-old symptomatic woman. *b,* Light microscopy: angiomyolipoma containing adipose tissue and spindle smooth muscle–like cells interspersed between abnormal vessels with thickened walls, H&E × 16. *c,* Light microscopy: TSC cysts lined with a distinctive epithelia consisting of large, acidophilic cells with hyperchromatic nuclei, H&E × 65.

can be locally invasive, extending into the perirenal fat or, more rarely, the collecting system, renal vein, and even the inferior vena cava and right atrium. Lymph node and splenic involvement likely represent multifocal origin rather than metastases.

The clinical manifestations relate to the potential for hemorrhage (gross hematuria, intratumoral or retroperitoneal hemorrhage) and to mass effects (abdominal or flank masses and tenderness, hypertension, renal insufficiency). Women tend to have more numerous and larger angiomyolipomas than men. Pregnancy appears to increase the risk for rupture and hemorrhage.

Renal Cystic Disease

Renal cysts occur less frequently than angiomyolipomas in TSC patients (47% vs. 80% in one recent study).[45] However, like angiomyolipomas, renal cysts tend to increase in size and number over time. The concurrence of cysts and angiomyolipomas, easily detected by CT, is strongly suggestive of TSC.

The cysts in TSC can develop from any nephron segment. When their number is limited and the size is small, they are predominantly cortical. In some cases, glomerular cysts predominate. The epithelial lining of the cysts is distinctive and appears to be unique to TSC, with large and acidophilic epithelia containing large hyperchromatic nuclei with occasional mitotic figures (see Fig. 44.10c). Associated papillary hyperplasia and adenomas are common.

A small subset of affected infants can present with massive renal cystic disease reminiscent of ADPKD, severe hypertension, and a progressive decline in renal function with the onset of ESRD in the second or third decade of life. Most of these patients have a contiguous germline deletion of both the *TSC2* and *PKD1* genes, the PKDTS contiguous gene syndrome (MIM 600273).[46] Early detection, strict blood pressure control, and prompt therapy for the associated infantile spasms may favorably affect the overall prognosis.

Renal Neoplasms

Both benign and malignant epithelial tumors of the kidney, such as papillary adenomas and oncocytomas and renal cell carcinomas, as well as leiomyosarcomas, have been identified in TSC patients. However, despite the multiplicity of benign tumors, neoplastic transformation is rare, and malignancies occur primarily in the kidney, with a lifetime risk of 2% to 3%.[42]

TSC-associated renal carcinomas are characterized by pathologic heterogeneity, with clear cell, papillary, and chromophobe carcinomas reported.[44] These carcinomas are often bilateral and occur with a higher frequency and earlier age of onset than in the general population. The median age at diagnosis is 28 years. The prognosis of TSC-associated renal carcinomas compared with

sporadic renal carcinomas in the general population is unknown. Malignant transformation of angiomyolipomas has been reported and appears to portend a poor prognosis.[44]

Diagnosis

TSC is a pleiotropic disease in which the size, number, and location of the lesions can be variable, even among members of the same family. Specific clinical criteria have been defined to assist in the diagnosis of TSC (Fig. 44.11). Imaging is the mainstay for diagnosis of TSC-associated renal lesions. The presence of small cysts and fat-containing angiomyolipomas is strongly suggestive of TSC. Although the median age at presentation for both renal cysts and angiomyolipomas is 9 years, these lesions have been detected in patients as young as 16 days of age and 4 months of age, respectively.[45]

Ultrasound may be more sensitive than CT for detecting small angiomyolipomas because fatty tissue is highly echogenic. Conversely, CT may be superior for detecting small angiomyolipomas

Clinical diagnostic criteria for tuberous sclerosis complex

Neurologic (definite diagnosis: single lesion with histologic confirmation; multiple lesions with imaging studies or ophthalmoscopy)
    Cortical tuber
    Subependymal glial nodule/giant cell astrocytoma
    Retinal hamartoma

Dermatologic (definite diagnosis)
    Facial angiofibromas
    Fibrous forehead plaque
    Ungual fibroma
    Shagreen patch* (histologic confirmation)

Visceral (presumptive diagnosis)†
    Multiple renal angiomyolipomas
    Multiple cardiac rhabdomyomas
    Multiple renal cysts and an angiomyolipoma
    Pulmonary lymphangioleiomyomatosis and a renal angiomyolipoma

Suggestive
    Hypomelanotic skin macules, enamel pits
    Hamartomatous rectal polyps
    Radiographic sclerotic bone patches and cysts
    Angiomyolipoma of kidney, liver, adrenal, or gonads
    Thyroid adenoma (papillary or fetal type)
    Infantile spasms

Figure 44.11 **Clinical diagnostic criteria for tuberous sclerosis complex (TSC).** *Shagreen patch is a raised skin lesion in the lumbosacral region. †Individuals with only these findings have borne children with TSC. (Adapted from Kwiatkowski D, Manning B: Tuberous sclerosis: A GAP at the crossroads of multiple signaling pathways. Hum Mol Genet 2005;14:R1–R8.)

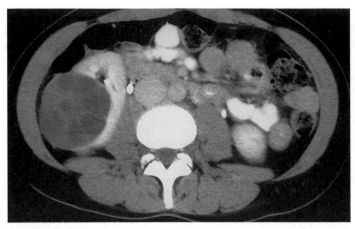

Figure 44.16 Solitary multilocular cyst. Contrast-enhanced CT shows a solitary, septated, well-circumscribed renal cystic lesion in the right kidney.

The cystic phenotype is widely variable, and the underlying pathogenesis is unclear. The dilation may involve a single lymphatic channel or multiple channels. The lymphangiectasis may be unilateral or bilateral or limited to the hilar region, or it may extend into the renal parenchyma to the corticomedullary junction. Occasionally, renal lymphangiomatosis may be very extensive and simulate ADPKD. The thin-walled cysts are lined by lymphatic endothelium, and the cyst fluid is quite distinct from that in ADPKD cysts because it contains lymphatic constituents such as albumin and lipid. The characteristic ultrasound or CT findings include multiple, bilateral small peripelvic cysts that splay the renal hilum, as well as capsular cysts in the perirenal space, both separated by thin septations. Treatment is usually not required because renal lymphangiomas are most often asymptomatic. However, the condition may be exacerbated by pregnancy, resulting in large perinephric lymph collections and ascites that may require percutaneous drainage.

GLOMERULOCYSTIC KIDNEY DISEASE

Cystic glomeruli are evident in three different clinical contexts: (1) isolated glomerulocystic kidney disease (GCKD); (2) glomerulocystic kidneys associated with inherited malformation syndromes, such as tuberous sclerosis, orofaciodigital syndrome type I, trisomy 13, Jeune's asphyxiating thoracic dystrophy syndrome, and Zellweger's cerebrohepatorenal syndrome; and (3) glomerular cysts present in dysplastic kidneys.[62]

GCKD can occur as a sporadic condition, a familial disorder, or the infantile manifestation of ADPKD. Pathologically, the kidney architecture is normal, with no dysplastic elements in the cortex and no evidence of urinary tract obstruction. Cystic dilation predominantly involves Bowman's space and the initial proximal tubule. The glomerular cysts are <1 cm in size and distributed from the subcapsular zone to the inner cortex. Because of this pathologic lesion, the typical sonographic pattern in GCKD involves echogenicity of the renal cortex with minute

cysts, smaller than those evident in ADPKD.[56] Young infants with either familial or sporadic forms of GCKD may also have renal medullary dysplasia and biliary dysgenesis.[62]

In most cases, GCKD is transmitted as an autosomal dominant trait. Autosomal dominant GCKD is usually discovered in infants with a familial history of ADPKD. In these infants, the kidneys are bilaterally enlarged and diffusely cystic. In addition, familial GCKD has been observed in infants, older children, and adults in whom the disease locus is not linked to *PKD1* or *PKD2*, but the specific causative gene has yet to be identified. In these non–ADPKD-associated GCKD families, the kidneys are typically normal in size, although occasionally enlarged kidneys are observed. Finally, several sporadic cases of nonsyndromal GCKD have been described, suggesting either new spontaneous mutations or a recessively transmitted disorder.[56]

Familial hypoplastic GCKD (MIM 137920) is probably a different type of GCKD. The kidneys are smaller than normal and often associated with medullocalyceal abnormalities. The disease is pleiotropic among affected family members with variable associations of hypoplastic GCKD, gynecologic abnormalities, and maturity-onset diabetes of the young, type V (MODY5). MODY5 results from mutations in the gene encoding hepatocyte nuclear factor-1β.[63]

OTHER ACQUIRED CYSTIC DISEASES

Hypokalemic Cystic Disease

Renal cysts are often seen in association with chronic hypokalemia due to primary hyperaldosteronism or other renal potassium wasting disorders. Nearly 50% of patients with idiopathic adrenal hyperplasia and 60% of patients with adrenal tumors have been found to have renal cysts, which are distributed primarily in the renal medulla. These cysts typically regress after adrenalectomy.[64]

Hilar Cysts

Hilar cysts are spherical accumulations of clear, fat droplet–containing fluid within the renal sinus. These cystic structures are not lined by epithelia. They are most commonly seen in debilitated patients and may represent atrophy of the renal sinus fat.

Perinephric Pseudocysts

Perinephric pseudocysts are also unlined cavities. They typically occur under the renal capsule or in the perirenal fascia as a result of urine extravasation from a renal cyst following traumatic or spontaneous rupture[65] or as the posterior extension of a pancreatic pseudocyst.[66] Surgical intervention is indicated for associated urinary tract obstruction. Otherwise, treatment is directed to the underlying cause.

Acquired Cystic Disease In Renal Failure

Acquired cystic disease (ACD) is a significant complication of prolonged renal failure. It should be considered in the differential diagnosis of cystic disease presenting with renal failure (see Fig. 44.14). ACD is discussed further in Chapter 79.

REFERENCES

1. Fick G, Gabow P: Hereditary and acquired cystic disease of the kidney. Kidney Int 1994;46:951–964.
2. D'Agata I, Jonas M, Perez-Atayde A, Guay-Woodford L: Combined cystic disease of the liver and kidney. Semin Liver Dis 1994;14: 215–228.
3. Guay-Woodford LM, Desmond RA: Autosomal recessive polycystic kidney disease: The clinical experience in North America. Pediatrics 2003;111: 1072–1080.
4. Ward C, Hogan M, Rossetti S, et al: The gene mutated in autosomal recessive polycystic kidney disease encodes a large, receptor-like protein. Nat Genet 2002;30:259–269.
5. Onuchic L, Furu L, Nagasawa Y, et al: *PKHD1*, the polycystic kidney and hepatic disease 1 gene, encodes a novel large protein containing multiple IPT domains and PbH1 repeats. Am J Hum Genet 2002;70: 1305–1317.

6. Xiong H, Chen Y, Yi Y, et al: A novel gene encoding a TID multiple domain protein is a positional candidate for autosomal recessive polycystic kidney disease. Genomics 2002;80:96–104.
7. Menezes F, Cai Y, Nagasawa Y, et al: Polyductin, the PKHD1 gene product, comprises isoforms expressed in plasma membrane, primary cilium and cytoplasm. Kidney Int 2004;66:1345–1355.
8. Osathanondh V, Potter E: Pathogenesis of polycystic kidneys. Type 1 due to hyperplasia of interstitial portions of the collecting tubules. Arch Pathol 1964;77:466–473.
9. Desmet V: Pathogenesis of ductal plate abnormalities. Mayo Clin Proc 1998;73:80–89.
10. Zerres K, Becker J, Muecher G, et al: Haplotype-based prenatal diagnosis in autosomal recessive polycystic kidney disease (ARPKD). Am J Med Genet 1998;76:137–144.
11. Guay-Woodford L: Autosomal recessive disease: Clinical and genetic profiles. In Watson M, Torres V, eds: Polycystic Kidney Disease. Oxford, UK, Oxford University Press, 1996, pp 237–267.
12. Bergmann C, Senderek J, Windelen E, et al: Clinical consequences of PKHD1 mutations in 164 patients with autosomal recessive polycystic kidney disease (ARPKD). Kidney Int 2005;67:829–848.
13. Guay-Woodford L, Desmond R: Autosomal recessive polycystic kidney disease (ARPKD): The clinical experience in North America. Pediatrics 2003;111:1072–1080.
14. Davis ID, Ho M, Hupertz V, Avner ED: Survival of childhood polycystic kidney disease following renal transplantation: The impact of advanced hepatobiliary disease. Pediatr Transplant 2003;7:364–369.
15. Jung G, Benz-Bohm G, Kugel H, et al: MR cholangiography in children with autosomal recessive polycystic kidney disease. Pediatr Radiol 1999;29:463–466.
16. Sharp A, Messiaen L, Page G, et al: Comprehensive genomic analysis for PKHD1 mutations in ARPKD cohorts. J Med Genet 2005;42:336–349.
17. Bergmann C, Senderek J, Schneider F, et al: PKHD1 mutations in families requesting prenatal diagnosis for autosomal recessive polycystic kidney disease (ARPKD). Hum Mutat 2004;23:453–463.
18. Lieberman E, Salinas-Madrigal L, Gwinn J, et al: Infantile polycystic disease of the kidneys and liver: Clinical, pathological and radiological correlations and comparison with congenital hepatic fibrosis. Medicine (Baltimore) 1971;50:277–318.
19. Melson G, Shackelford G, Cole B, McClennan B: The spectrum of sonographic findings in infantile polycystic kidney disease with urographic and clinical correlations. J Clin Ultrasound 1985;13:113–119.
20. Capisonda R, Phan V, Traubuci J, et al: Autosomal recessive polycystic kidney disease: Clinical course and outcome, a single center experience. Pediatr Nephrol 2003;18:119–126.
21. Lucaya J, Enriquez G, Nieto J, et al: Renal calcifications in patients with autosomal recessive polycystic kidney disease: Prevalance and cause. Am J Radiol 1993;160:359–362.
22. Roy S, Dillon M, Trompeter R, Barratt T: Autosomal recessive polycystic kidney disease: Long-term outcome of neonatal survivors. Pediatr Nephrol 1997;11:302–306.
23. Warady B, Alexander S, Watkins S, et al: Optimal care of the pediatric end-stage renal disease patient on dialysis. Am J Kidney Dis 1999;33:567–583.
24. Seikaly M, Ho P, Emmett L, et al: Chronic renal insufficiency in children: The 2001 Annual Report of the NAPRTCS. Pediatr Nephrol 2003;18:796–804.
25. Kashtan C, Primack W, Kainer G, et al: Recurrent bacteremia with enteric pathogens in recessive polycystic kidney disease. Pediatr Nephrol 1999;13:678–682.
26. Groothoff J: Long-term outcomes of children with end-stage renal disease. Pediatr Nephrol 2005;20:849–853.
27. Shneider B, Magid M: Liver disease in autosomal recessive polycystic kidney disease. Pediatr Transplant 2005;9:634–649.
28. Hildebrandt F, Otto E: Cilia and centrosomes: A unifying pathogenic concept for cystic kidney disease? Nat Rev Genet 2005;6:928–940.
29. Saunier S, Salomon R, Antignac C: Nephronophthisis. Curr Opin Genet Dev 2005;15:324–331.
30. Ala-Mello S, Kivivuori S, Ronnholm K, et al: Mechanism underlying early anemia in children with familial juvenile nephronophthisis. Pediatr Nephrol 1996;10:578–581.
31. Otto E, Schermer B, Obara T, et al: Mutations in INVS encoding inversin cause nephronophthisis type 2, linking renal cystic disease to the function of primary cilia and left-right axis determination. Nat Genet 2003;l34:413–420.
32. Salomon R, Gubler M, Antignac C: Nephronophthisis. In Davidson A, Cameron J, Grunfeld J, et al, eds: Oxford Text Book of Clinical Nephrology. Oxford, UK, Oxford University Press, 2005, pp 2325–2334.
33. Heninger E, Otto E, Imm A, et al: Improved strategy for molecular genetic diagnostics in juvenile nephronophthisis. Am J Kidney Dis 2001;37:1131–1139.
34. Wolf MT, Mucha BE, Attanasio M, et al: Mutations of the uromodulin gene in MCKD type 2 patients cluster in exon 4, which encodes three EGF-like domains. Kidney Int 2003;64:1580–1587.
35. Scolari F, Caridi G, Rampoldi L, et al: Uromodulin storage diseases: Clinical aspects and mechanisms. Am J Kidney Dis 2004;44:987–999.
36. Yendt E: Medullary sponge kidney. In Gardner K, Bernstein J, eds: The Cystic Kidney. Dordrecht, Netherlands, Kluwer, 1990, pp 379–391.
37. Glassberg K: Renal dysgenesis and cystic disease of the kidney. In Walsh P, Retik E, Vaughan E, Wein AJ, eds: Campbell's Urology, 8th ed. Philadelphia, WB Saunders, 2002, pp 1925–1994.
38. The European Chromosome 16 Tuberous Sclerosis Consortium: Identification and characterization of the tuberous sclerosis gene on chromosome 16. Cell 193;75:1305–1315.
39. van Slegtenhorst M, Hoogt RD, Hermans C, et al: Identification of the tuberous sclerosis gene TSC1 on chromosome 9q34. Science 1997;277:805–808.
40. Henske E: Tuberous sclerosis and the kidney: From mesenchyme to epithelium and beyond. Pediatr Nephrol 2005;20:854–857.
41. Karbowniczek M, Henske E: The role of tuberin in cellular differentiation: Are B-Raf and MAPK involved? Ann N Y Acad Sci 2005;1059:168–173.
42. Kwiatkowski D, Manning B: Tuberous sclerosis: A GAP at the crossroads of multiple signaling pathways. Hum Mol Genet 2005;14:R1–R8.
43. Torres V: Tuberous sclerosis complex. In Torres V, Watson M, eds: Polycystic Kidney Disease. Oxford, UK, Oxford University Press, 1996, pp 283–308.
44. Pea M, Bonetti F, Martignoni G, et al: Apparent renal cell carcinomas in tuberous sclerosis are heterogeneous: The identification of malignant epithelioid angiomyolipoma. Am J Surg Pathol 1998;22:180–187.
45. Casper K, Donnelly L, Chen B, Bissler JJ: Tuberous sclerosis complex: renal imaging findings. Radiology 225:451–456.
46. Sampson J, Maheshwar M, Aspinwall R, et al: Renal cystic disease in tuberous sclerosis: role of the polycystic kidney disease 1 gene. Am J Hum Genet 1997;61:843–851.
47. Lee L, Sudentas P, Donohue B, et al: Efficacy of a rapamycin analog (CCI-779) and IFN-gamma in tuberous sclerosis mouse models. Genes Chromosomes Cancer 2005;42:213–227.
48. Schillinger F, Montagnac R: Chronic renal failure and its treatment in tuberous sclerosis. Nephrol Dial Transplant 1996;11:481–485.
49. Joerger M, Koeberle D, Neumann H, Gillessen S: Von Hippel-Lindau disease: A rare disease important to recognize. Onkologie 2005;28:159–163.
50. Kaelin WG Jr: The von Hippel-Lindau tumor suppressor gene and kidney cancer. Clin Cancer Res 2004;10:6290S–6295S.
51. Friedrich C: Genotype-phenotype correlations in von Hippel-Lindau syndrome. Hum Mol Genet 2002;10:763–767.
52. Couch V, Lindor N, Karnes P, Michels V: Von Hippel-Lindau disease. Mayo Clin Proc 2000;75:265–272.
53. Grubb RR, Choyke P, Pinto P, et al: Management of von Hippel-Lindau-associated kidney cancer. Nat Clin Pract Urol 2005;2:248–255.
54. Ravine D, Gibson R, Donlan J, Sheffield L: An ultrasound renal cyst prevalence survey: Specificity data for inherited renal cystic diseases. Am J Kidney Dis 1993;22:803–807.
55. Nascimento A, Mitchell D, Zhang X, et al: Rapid MR imaging detection of renal cysts: Age-based standards. Radiology 2001;221:628–632.
56. Bisceglia M, Galliani C, Senger C, et al: Renal cystic diseases: A review. Adv Anat Pathol 2006;13:26–56.
57. Pedersen J, Emanian S, Nielsen M: Significant association between simple renal cysts and arterial blood pressure. Br J Urol 1997;79:688–692.
58. Isreal G, Bosniak M. An update of the Bosniak renal cyst classification system. Urology 2005;86:484–488.
59. Novick A, Campbell S: Renal tumors. In Walsh P, Retik A, Vaughan E, Wein AJ, eds: Campbell's Urology, 8th ed. Philadelphia, WB Saunders, 2002, pp 2672–2731.
60. Castillo O, Boyle EJ, Kramer S: Multilocular cysts of kidney: A study of 29 patients and review of literature. Urology 1991;37:156–162.
61. Androulakakis P, Kirayianis B, Deliveliotis A: The parapelvic renal cyst: A report of 8 cases with particular emphasis on diagnosis and management. Br J Urol 1980;52:342–344.
62. Bernstein J: Glomerulocystic kidney disease: Nosological considerations. Pediatr Nephrol 1993;7:464–470.
63. Bingham C, Hattersley A: Renal cysts and diabetes syndrome resulting from mutations in hepatocyte nuclear factor-1b. Nephrol Dial Transplant 2004;19:2703–2708.
64. Torres V, Young W, Offord K, Hattery R: Association of hypokalemia, aldosteronism, and renal cysts N Engl J Med 1990;322:345–351.
65. Meyers M: Uriniferous perirenal pseudocyst: New observations. Radiology 1975;117:539–545.
66. Lilienfeld R, Lande A: Pancreatic pseudocysts presenting as thick-walled renal and perinephric cysts. J Urol 1976;115:123–125.

Alport's and Other Familial Glomerular Syndromes

Clifford E. Kashtan

ALPORT'S SYNDROME

Introduction and Definition

Alport's syndrome (AS) is a generalized, inherited disorder of basement membranes due to mutations affecting specific proteins of the type IV (basement membrane) collagen family. The major features of AS are hematuria, progressive nephritis with proteinuria and declining renal function, sensorineural deafness, and ocular abnormalities. The course of AS is gender dependent: affected males typically have severe disease, whereas the manifestations of AS in women are usually mild. In 1902, Guthrie provided the first description of familial hematuria.[1] Later studies of Guthrie's family by Hurst[2] and Alport[3] revealed the progressive nature of the nephropathy, its association with deafness, and the poorer prognosis in affected males. In the 1970s, the glomerular basement membrane (GBM) was recognized as the site of the primary abnormality in AS.[4–6] Indirect evidence of abnormalities in type IV collagen[7,8] was followed by mapping of the major Alport locus to the X chromosome,[9] cloning of a new type IV collagen gene (COL4A5) and its assignment to the same X-chromosomal region,[10] and identification of the first COL4A5 mutations in patients with X-linked AS (XLAS).[11]

Etiology and Pathogenesis
Type IV Collagen
Genes and Proteins   Type IV collagen is a major constituent of basement membranes. The type IV collagen family of proteins comprises six isomeric chains, designated $\alpha 1(IV)$ to $\alpha 6(IV)$.[12] These chains show extensive sequence homology and share basic structural features, including a major collagenous domain of about 1400 residues containing the repetitive triplet sequence glycine (Gly)-X-Y, in which X and Y represent a variety of other amino acids; a C-terminal noncollagenous (NC1) domain of about 230 residues; and a noncollagenous N-terminal sequence of 15 to 20 residues. The collagenous domain of each chain contains about 20 interruptions of the collagenous triplet sequence, whereas each NC1 domain contains 12 completely conserved cysteine residues that participate in critical disulfide bonds.

Each type IV collagen molecule is a heterotrimer composed of three α chains. Formation of these heterotrimers is initiated by C-terminal NC1 domain interactions, accompanied by folding of the collagenous domains into triple helices. There is evidence for at least three types of type IV collagen heterotrimer: $\alpha 1(IV)_2–\alpha 2(IV)$, $\alpha 3(IV)–\alpha 4(IV)–\alpha(IV)$, and $\alpha 5(IV)_2–\alpha 6(IV)$. Type IV collagen triple helices form open, nonfibrillar networks

that associate with laminin assemblies through interactions mediated by nidogen to form basement membranes.

The six type IV collagen genes are arranged in pairs on three chromosomes (Fig. 45.1). The 5′ ends of each gene pair are adjacent to each other, separated by sequences of varying length that contain motifs involved in the regulation of transcriptional activity.

Tissue Distribution   Several distinct type IV collagen networks appear to exist in basement membranes: a ubiquitous network comprising the $\alpha 1(IV)$ and $\alpha 2(IV)$ chains, and other networks, restricted in distribution, composed of $\alpha 3(IV)$, $\alpha 4(IV)$, and $\alpha 5(IV)$ chains, or $\alpha 5(IV)$ and $\alpha 6(IV)$ chains. GBM contains separate $\alpha 1/\alpha 2(IV)$ and $\alpha 3/\alpha 4/\alpha 5(IV)$ networks, whereas epidermal basement membranes contain separate networks of $\alpha 1/\alpha 2(IV)$ chains and $\alpha 5/\alpha 6(IV)$ chains. It is likely that these networks have different functional characteristics and interact differently with other matrix components and with adjacent cells.

Genetics
Three forms of AS have been established on a molecular genetic basis: an X-linked dominant form resulting from mutations at the COL4A5 locus, primarily affecting the $\alpha 5(IV)$ chain; an autosomal recessive form arising from mutations at the COL4A3 locus or the COL4A4 locus, affecting the $\alpha 3(IV)$ and $\alpha 4(IV)$ chains, respectively; and an autosomal dominant form due to heterozygous mutations in COL4A3 or COL4A4 (Fig. 45.2).

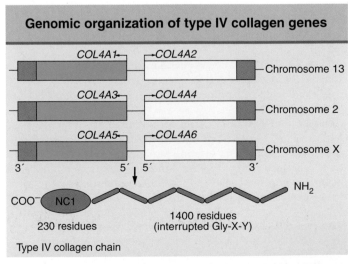

Figure 45.1   Genomic organization of type IV collagen genes.

Molecular genetics of Alport's syndrome		
Inheritance	Affected Locus	Gene Product
X-linked (XLAS)	COL4A5	α5(IV)
X-linked + leiomyomatosis	COL4A5 + COL4A6	α5(IV) + α6(IV)
Autosomal recessive (ARAS)	COL4A3 COL4A4	α3(IV) α4(IV)
Autosomal dominant	COL4A3 COL4A4	α3(IV) α4(IV)

Figure 45.2   Molecular genetics of Alport's syndrome.

X-linked Alport's Syndrome   XLAS is the predominant form of the disease, accounting for about 80% of patients. Several hundred COL4A5 mutations have been described.[13,14]

Missense mutations, splice-site mutations, and deletions of fewer than 10 base pairs account for most COL4A5 mutations. A common missense mutation involves replacement of a glycine residue in the collagenous domain of the α5(IV) chain by another amino acid. Such mutations are thought to interfere with the normal folding of the α5(IV) chain into triple helices with other α(IV) chains.

Male patients with COL4A5 deletions consistently progress to end-stage renal disease (ESRD) during the second or third decade of life and have deafness.[15] Most of the missense, nonsense, and splicing mutations of COL4A5 described so far are also associated with early progression to ESRD and deafness. Several missense mutations of COL4A5 have been associated with late-onset (after the third decade) ESRD and with late development of deafness or normal hearing. The severity of disease in a female heterozygous for a COL4A5 mutation probably depends primarily on the relative activities of the mutant and normal X chromosomes in renal, cochlear, and ocular tissues.

Autosomal Recessive Alport's Syndrome   Autosomal recessive Alport's syndrome (ARAS) arises from mutations affecting both alleles of COL4A3 or COL4A4.[16,17] ARAS should be suspected when an individual exhibits the typical clinical and pathologic features of the disease but lacks a positive family history, especially when a young female has findings indicative of severe disease such as deafness, renal insufficiency, and nephrotic syndrome. However, sporadic cases of AS may represent *de novo* mutations at the COL4A5 locus or a germline COL4A5 mutation in the proband's mother.

Phenotypic information in ARAS is somewhat sparse. Based on available data, it appears that most patients with ARAS develop ESRD and deafness before age 30 years, regardless of gender.

Autosomal Dominant Alport's Syndrome   Heterozygous mutations in COL4A3 or COL4A4 typically result in asymptomatic hematuria[16,17] but in some families may also be associated with progressive nephropathy, that is, autosomal dominant Alport's syndrome (ADAS).[18,19] ADAS patients tend to have a slower course to ESRD than those with XLAS or ARAS.[20]

Type IV Collagen in Alport's Basement Membranes
The GBMs and tubular basement membranes (TBMs) of males with XLAS usually fail to stain for the α3(IV), α4(IV), and α5(IV) chains but do express the α1(IV) and α2(IV) chains (Fig. 45.3).[21]

Women with XLAS frequently exhibit mosaicism of GBM expression of the α3(IV), α4(IV), and α5(IV) chains, whereas expression of the α1(IV) and α2(IV) chains is preserved (see Fig. 45.3). Most males with XLAS show no epidermal basement membrane (EBM) expression of α5(IV), whereas female heterozygotes frequently display mosaicism (Fig. 45.4). Lens capsules of some males with XLAS do not express the α3(IV), α4(IV), or α5(IV) chains, whereas expression of these chains appears normal in other patients.[22]

In most patients with ARAS, GBM shows no expression of the α3(IV), α4(IV), or α5(IV) chains, but α5(IV) and α6(IV) are expressed in Bowman's capsule, distal TBM, and EBM (Fig. 45.5).[21] Therefore, XLAS and ARAS may be differentiated by immunohistochemical analysis. Basement membrane expression of type IV collagen α chains appears to be normal in patients with ADAS.

These observations indicate that a mutation affecting one of the chains involved in the α3–α4–α5(IV) network can prevent GBM expression not only of that chain, but also of the other two chains. At this time, the bulk of observational and experimental evidence supports the hypothesis that these effects reflect post-translational events. Some mutant chains are unable to participate in the formation of trimers; as a result, the normal chains that are prevented from forming trimers undergo degradation. Other mutations may allow formation of abnormal trimers that are degraded before deposition in basement membranes can occur.

Clinical Manifestations
Renal Defects
Hematuria is the cardinal finding of AS. Affected males have persistent microscopic hematuria. Many also have episodic gross hematuria, precipitated by upper respiratory infections, during the first two decades of life. Hematuria has been discovered in the first year of life in affected boys, in whom it is probably present from birth. Boys who are free of hematuria during the first 10 years of life are unlikely to be affected.

More than 90% of females with XLAS have persistent or intermittent microscopic hematuria, but about 7% of obligate heterozygotes never manifest hematuria.[23] Hematuria appears to be persistent in both males and females with ARAS. About 50% of carriers of COL4A3 or COL4A4 mutations have hematuria.[16,17]

Proteinuria is usually absent early in life but develops eventually in all males with XLAS and in both males and females with ARAS. Proteinuria increases progressively with age and may result in the nephrotic syndrome. Proteinuria develops eventually in most heterozygous females.[23] Hypertension also increases in incidence and severity with age. Similar to proteinuria, hypertension is more likely to occur in affected males than in affected females with XLAS, but there are no gender differences in the hypertension frequency in ARAS.

ESRD develops in all affected males with XLAS. The rate of progression to ESRD in affected males is determined primarily by the nature of the underlying COL4A5 mutation.[15] Thus, the rate of progression is fairly constant among affected males within a particular family, but there is significant interkindred variability. Significant intrakindred variability in the rate of progression to ESRD has been reported in some families with missense COL4A5 mutations.

Progression to ESRD in females with XLAS was, until recently, considered an unusual event. However, a recent study of several hundred XLAS females found that 12% developed ESRD before

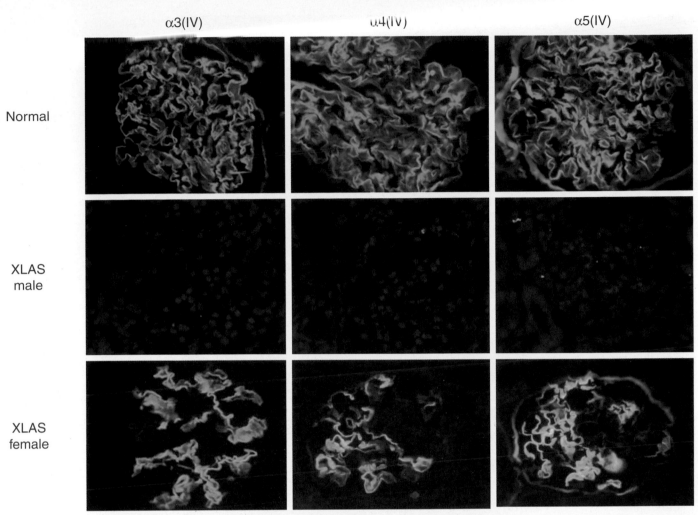

Figure 45.3   Immunohistochemistry of glomerular basement membrane (GBM) in X-linked Alport's syndrome. In a normal individual, GBM stains strongly for the α3(IV), α4(IV), and α5(IV) chains of type IV collagen. Staining of GBM of an affected male is negative for each of these chains, whereas an affected female shows mosaic immunoreactivity.

age 40 (compared with 90% of XLAS males), increasing to 30% by age 60 and 40% by age 80.[23] The risk for ESRD was significantly increased in heterozygotes with proteinuria. The outcome of XLAS in females is presumed to be dependent on the relative activities of the normal and mutant X chromosomes, but this has yet to be proved. Previous work had shown that gross hematuria in childhood, nephrotic syndrome, and the finding of diffuse GBM thickening by electron microscopy are risk factors for chronic renal failure in affected females.[21,24] Sensorineural deafness and anterior lenticonus are also indicative of an unfavorable outcome in affected women. Both males and females with ARAS appear likely to progress to ESRD during the second or third decade of life.

Cochlear Defects

Deafness is frequently but not universally associated with the Alport's renal lesion, occurring in about 80% of males and 25% to 30% of females with the disease.[15,23] In some families with Alport's nephropathy and apparently normal hearing, deafness may be a late and very slowly progressive phenomenon.

Hearing loss in AS is never congenital and usually becomes apparent by late childhood to early adolescence in boys with XLAS and in both boys and girls with ARAS. Hearing impairment in members of families with AS is always accompanied by evidence of renal involvement. There is no convincing evidence

that deaf males lacking renal disease can transmit AS to their offspring. In its early stages, the hearing deficit is detectable only by audiometry, with bilateral reduction in sensitivity to tones in the 2000 to 8000 Hz range. In affected males, the deficit extends progressively to other frequencies, including those of conversational speech.

Ocular Defects

Ocular defects occur in 30% to 40% of XLAS males and in about 15% of XLAS females.[15,23] The spectrum and frequencies of ocular lesions appear to be similar in XLAS and ARAS.[25] Anterior lenticonus, which is virtually pathognomonic of AS, occurs in about 15% of XLAS males and is almost entirely restricted to AS families with progression to ESRD before age 30 years and deafness.[15] Anterior lenticonus is absent at birth, usually appearing during the second to third decade of life, and is bilateral in 75% of patients (Fig. 45.6a).

Another common ocular manifestation of AS is a maculopathy, which consists of whitish or yellowish flecks or granulations in a perimacular distribution (see Fig. 45.6b), and occurs in 15% to 30% of patients. The maculopathy does not appear to be associated with any visual abnormalities.

Corneal endothelial vesicles (posterior polymorphous dystrophy) have been observed in Alport's patients and may indicate

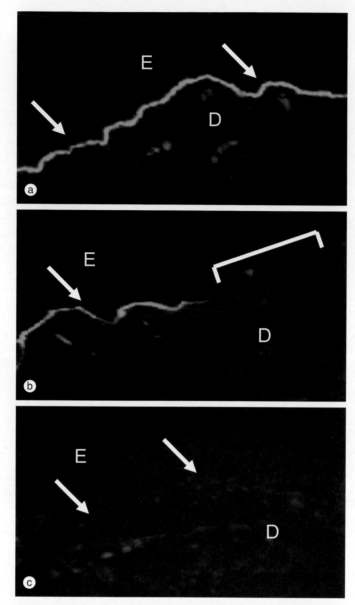

Figure 45.4   Immunohistochemistry of epidermal basement membrane (EBM) in X-linked Alport's syndrome. *a,* In a normal male, EBM shows strong staining for α5(IV) at the dermoepidermal junction *(arrows)* between dermis (D) and epidermis (E). *b,* In an affected female, EBM shows mosaic staining *(arrow)*; the bracket identifies a length of EBM negative for α5(IV). *c,* In affected males, staining of EBM *(arrows)* for α5(IV) is absent.

defects in Descemet's membrane, the basement membrane underlying the corneal endothelium. Recurrent corneal erosion in Alport's patients has been attributed to alterations of the corneal epithelial basement membrane.

Leiomyomatosis

The association of AS with leiomyomatosis of the esophagus and tracheobronchial tree has been reported in about 20 to 30 families.[14] Affected females typically exhibit genital leiomyomas as well, with clitoral hypertrophy and variable involvement of the labia majora and uterus. Bilateral posterior subcapsular cataracts also occur frequently in affected individuals. Symptoms usually appear in late childhood and include dysphagia, postprandial vomiting, retrosternal or epigastric pain, recurrent bronchitis, dyspnea, cough, and stridor. All patients with AS–diffuse leiomyomatosis complex have been found to have deletions that encompass the 5' ends of *COL4A5* and *COL4A6*.

Hematologic Defects

An autosomal dominant syndrome of hereditary nephritis, deafness, and megathrombocytopenia, Epstein's syndrome, has been described in a handful of families. Families with Fechtner's syndrome exhibit these features as well as leukocyte inclusions (May-Hegglin anomaly). Both Epstein's and Fechtner's syndromes arise from mutations in nonmuscle myosin heavy-chain IIA.[26] Basement membranes of these patients do not exhibit abnormalities in expression of type IV collagen α chains. Therefore, Epstein's and Fechtner's syndromes are best considered as distinct forms of hereditary nephritis, rather than as variants of AS.

Pathology

There are no pathognomonic lesions by light microscopy or direct immunofluorescence in AS. Indirect immunofluorescence of type IV collagen α-chain expression in renal or skin basement membranes can be diagnostic (see earlier discussion) and is increasingly available in specialized laboratories around the world.

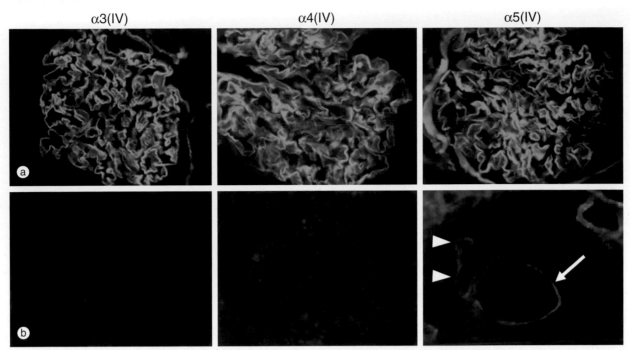

α3(IV) α4(IV) α5(IV)

Figure 45.5 Immunohistochemistry of the kidney in a patient with autosomal recessive Alport's syndrome (ARAS). *a,* Normal glomerular basement membranes (GBMs) and Bowman's capsule staining for α3(IV), α4(IV), and α5(IV). *b,* Patient shows no GBM staining, but it is present in Bowman's capsule *(arrow)* and distal tubular basement membranes *(arrowheads)*.

Electron microscopy frequently reveals diagnostic abnormalities. The cardinal fine structural feature of the kidney in AS is the variable thickening, thinning, basket-weaving, and lamellation of the GBM (Fig. 45.7). This lesion occurs in most patients with AS. The thick segments measure up to 1200 nm in depth, usually have irregular outer and inner contours, and are found more commonly in males than in females. The lamina densa is transformed into a heterogeneous network of membranous strands, which enclose clear electron-lucent areas that may contain round granules of variable density measuring 20 to 90 nm in diameter. The altered capillary walls typically demonstrate variable degrees of epithelial foot process fusion.

Not all Alport's kindred demonstrate these characteristic ultrastructural features. Thick, thin, normal, and nonspecifically altered GBM have all been described. Affected young males, heterozygous females at any age, and, on occasion, affected adult

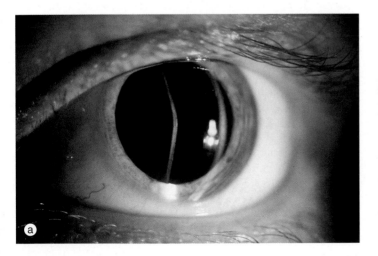

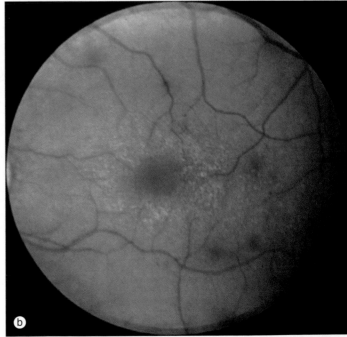

Figure 45.6 Ocular abnormalities in Alport's syndrome. *a,* Anterior lenticonus shown by slit-lamp ophthalmoscopy. *b,* Perimacular flecks. (From Flinter FA: Disorders of the basement membrane: Hereditary nephritis. In Morgan SH, Grunfeld J-P [eds]: Inherited Disorders of the Kidney. Oxford, UK, Oxford University Press, 1998).

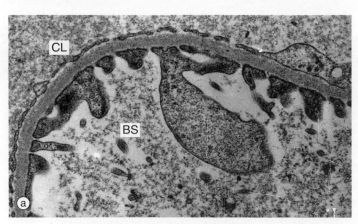
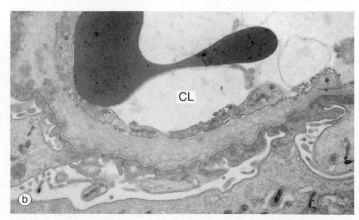

Figure 45.7   Renal biopsy in Alport's syndrome. *a*, A normal glomerular capillary wall is shown. *b*, Glomerular capillary wall from a patient with Alport's syndrome, at the same magnification. Note the thickening of the glomerular basement membrane (GBM), the splitting of the lamina densa into multiple strands, and the marked irregularity of the epithelial aspect of the GBM in the patient with Alport's syndrome. BS, Bowman's lumen; CL, capillary space.

males may have diffusely attenuated GBM measuring as little as 100 nm or less in thickness, rather than the pathognomonic lesion. Although diffuse attenuation of GBM has been considered the hallmark of thin basement membrane nephropathy (as discussed elsewhere in this chapter), some patients with this abnormality are members of kindred with a history of progression to renal failure. Therefore, the significance of an ultrastructural finding of thin GBM must be considered in the context of the family history, basement membrane expression of type IV collagen α chains, and, if available, molecular genetic information.

Diagnosis and Differential Diagnosis

A summary of the evaluation of patients with hematuria and a positive family history is given in Figure 45.8. AS should be included in the initial differential diagnosis of patients with persistent microscopic hematuria, once structural abnormalities of the kidneys or urinary tract have been excluded. The presence of diffuse thickening and multilamellation of the GBM, as demonstrated by electron microscopy, predicts a progressive nephropathy, regardless of family history. However, in a patient with a negative family history, electron microscopy cannot differentiate *de novo* XLAS from ARAS. In some patients, the biopsy findings may be ambiguous, particularly females and young patients of either sex. Furthermore, families with progressive nephritis and *COL4A5* mutations in association with GBM thinning have been described, indicating that the classic Alport's GBM lesion is not present in all Alport's kindred.

It is not unusual to see a patient with hematuria and discover that multiple relatives also have hematuria, although none has ever undergone kidney biopsy. Who should undergo biopsy in such instances? The natural history of the Alport's renal lesion suggests that older, male subjects are more likely to exhibit diagnostic ultrastructural GBM abnormalities. In families in which a firm diagnosis of AS has been established, evaluation of individuals with newly recognized hematuria can be limited to ultrasound of the kidneys and urinary tract to exclude coincidental tumor or structural anomalies of the urinary tract.

Absence of the α3, α4, and α5 chains of type IV collagen from GBM and distal TBM has not been described in any condition other than AS, making this a diagnostic finding on kidney biopsy (Fig. 45.9). Examination of skin biopsies by immunofluorescence for expression of α5(IV) in the epidermal basement membrane is an additional tool for diagnosing AS. However, apparently normal expression of type IV collagen α chains in basement membranes does not exclude the diagnosis of AS. Heterozygous females frequently express α5(IV) mosaically. Although mosaic expression of α5(IV) is diagnostic of the carrier state, a normal result does not exclude heterozygosity. A female member of an Alport's kindred who does not have hematuria may still be a carrier but is less likely to exhibit detectable mosaicism than a female with hematuria.

A firm histologic diagnosis of AS cannot always be established, or it may not be possible to determine the mode of transmission, despite careful evaluation of the pedigree and application of the full range of histologic methods. In these situations, genetic analysis has the potential to provide information essential for determining prognosis and guiding genetic counseling. The inheritance of AS in a family can be determined by linkage analysis, which does not require identification of a particular mutation. However, genetic analysis for AS is not yet widely available.

Glomerular diseases that typically occur sporadically may on occasion be heritable and should be considered in the differential diagnosis. These include focal segmental glomerulosclerosis, membranous nephropathy, membranoproliferative glomerulonephritis, and IgA nephropathy.

Natural History

The tissue pathology of AS arises from underexpression of the α3, α4, and α5 chains of type IV collagen. As a result, the networks formed by these chains are absent or are defective in structure and function. Microhematuria, the first and invariable renal manifestation of AS, probably reflects GBM thinning and a tendency to develop focal ruptures because of defective expression of the α3–α4–α5(IV) network. Anterior lenticonus most likely results from the inability of the abnormal lens capsule to maintain the normal conformation of the lens. A recent description of the ultrastructural pathology of the Alport's cochlea suggested that the hearing deficit may be attributable to a specific defect in adherence of the organ of Corti to the basilar membrane.[27]

AS in its early stages is clinically and often histologically indistinguishable from thin basement membrane nephropathy (TBMN), which typically has a benign outcome. GBM attenuation is therefore an insufficient explanation for the divergent natural histories of the two conditions. What factors initiate and drive the progression of Alport's nephropathy to ESRD? Reduction in the quantity of α3(IV), α4(IV), and α5(IV) chains

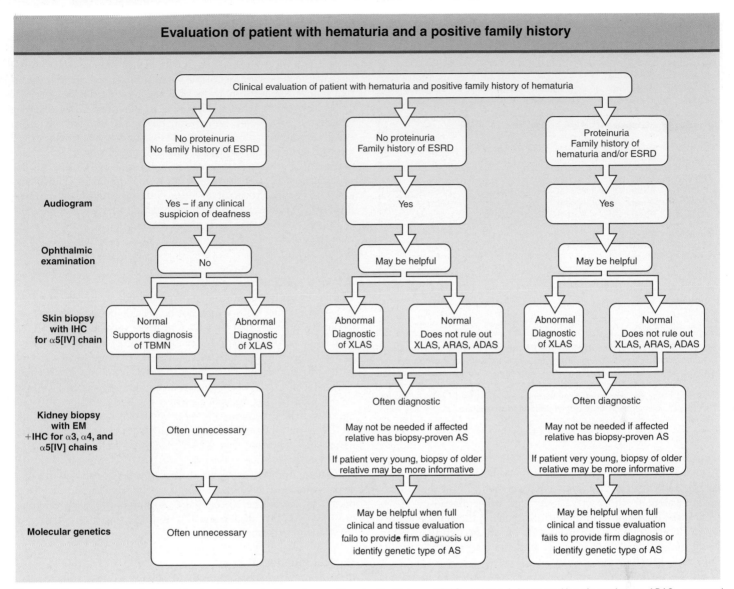

Figure 45.8 Evaluation of the patient with hematuria and a positive family history. ADAS, autosomal dominant Alport's syndrome; ARAS, autosomal recessive Alport's syndrome; AS, Alport's syndrome; EM, electron microscopy; ESRD, end-stage renal disease; IHC, immunohistochemistry; TBMN, thin basement membrane nephropathy; XLAS, X-linked Alport's syndrome.

in GBM, as likely occurs in TBMN, probably has different consequences than complete loss of these chains, as occurs in most males with XLAS and most patients with ARAS. There is increasing information about the molecular events that occur consequent to the loss of the α3(IV)–α4(IV)–α5(IV) network. In the GBM, the normal transition from the $\alpha1(IV)_2–\alpha2(IV)_1$ network of nascent glomeruli to the α3(IV)–α4(IV)–α5(IV) network of mature glomeruli fails to occur, and α1(IV) and α2(IV) chains accumulate in Alport's glomeruli as the disease progresses.[28,29] Alport's GBM has overexpression of other matrix proteins that are normally absent from GBM or present in scant quantities, including type V collagen, type VI collagen, laminin α2 chain, and fibronectin. These alterations in GBM composition are unique to AS.[30] Both glomerular endothelial cells and podocytes appear to contribute to the accumulation of these proteins in Alport's GBM. Alterations in glomerular extracellular matrix are accompanied by changes in glomerular cell behavior, including expression of transforming growth factor-β1, integrins, and matrix metalloproteinases.[31] Activation

of fibrogenic pathways in the renal interstitium presumably represents a downstream consequence of glomerular pathology.

Treatment

Clinical trials of therapy for the Alport's nephropathy have not been conducted. The availability of canine and murine models of AS should allow the testing of genetic or pharmacologic therapies, in order to select promising treatments for human trials.[32,33] AS resembles other chronic glomerulopathies in that deterioration of glomerular filtration rate is closely correlated with fibrosis of the renal interstitium.[34] It is possible that therapies that interfere with interstitial fibrosis may be of benefit to AS patients, without correcting the primary abnormalities of type IV collagen expression. Cyclosporine appeared to stabilize renal function in a small, uncontrolled study of Alport's males[35]; confirmatory studies will need to be published before this therapeutic approach can be recommended. Results of studies of angiotensin blockade in animals with AS suggest that this approach could be beneficial in human AS, although clinical trials have not been organized.[36]

Immunostaining for type IV collagen in Alport's syndrome

Type IV Collagen Group	Glomerular Basement Membranes	Bowman's Capsules	Distal Tubular Basement Membrane	Epidermal Basement Membrane
Normal (males and females)				
α3(IV)	Present	Present	Present	Absent
α4(IV)	Present	Present	Present	Absent
α5(IV)	Present	Present	Present	Present
X-linked (males)*				
α3(IV)	Absent	Absent	Absent	Absent
α4(IV)	Absent	Absent	Absent	Absent
α5(IV)	Absent	Absent	Absent	Absent
X-linked (females)†				
α3(IV)	Mosaic			Absent
α4(IV)	Mosaic			Absent
α5(IV)	Mosaic			Mosaic
Autosomal recessive (males and females)*				
α3(IV)	Absent	Absent	Absent	Absent
α4(IV)	Absent	Absent	Absent	Absent
α5(IV)	Absent	Present	Present	Present

Figure 45.9 Immunostaining for type IV collagen in Alport's syndrome. *In some Alport's syndrome kindreds, staining of basement membranes for type IV collagen chains is entirely normal. Therefore, a normal result does not exclude a diagnosis of X-linked Alport's syndrome. †Some heterozygous females have normal basement membrane immunoreactivity for type IV collagen chains. Therefore, a normal result does not exclude the carrier state.

Transplantation

At present, renal transplantation is the only available treatment for AS. Allograft survival rates in patients with familial nephritis are equivalent to those in patients with other diagnoses. However, anti-GBM glomerulonephritis involving the renal allograft is a rare, but dramatic, manifestation of AS, occurring in 2% to 3% of male Alport's patients who undergo transplantation. This is discussed further in Chapter 22.

Should women who are heterozygous for COL4A5 mutations be allowed to serve as kidney donors? Clearly, those with proteinuria, hypertension, or renal insufficiency will not be allowed to donate, and the same should apply if any hearing loss is present. What about heterozygotes with hematuria but normal renal function and hearing? There is no long-term follow-up information on the impact of uninephrectomy in such women. Given the recent finding that 30% to 40% of heterozygous women may eventually develop ESRD, it seems prudent to discourage kidney donation. The wishes of a heterozygous woman with asymptomatic microhematuria should be thoughtfully considered, but it must be assumed at this time that the risk to such an individual of ultimately developing significant renal insufficiency is substantially higher than it is for the usual kidney donor.

THIN BASEMENT MEMBRANE NEPHROPATHY: FAMILIAL AND SPORADIC

Introduction and Definition

Isolated glomerular hematuria may occur as a familial or sporadic condition and is often associated with a renal biopsy finding of excessively thin GBM. The term *benign familial hematuria* has been used to describe the disease kindred in which multiple individuals in several generations have isolated hematuria without progression to ESRD. More recently, *thin basement membrane nephropathy* (TBMN) has been used to identify both familial and sporadic isolated hematuria associated with attenuated GBM. It is likely that several disorders that differ at the molecular level can be associated with GBM thinning, and in some instances, it is probably a normal variant. In general, the discussion that follows applies to both familial and sporadic TBMN.

Similar to AS, familial TBMN is an inherited GBM disorder manifested by chronic hematuria, but it differs clinically from AS in several important respects: (1) extrarenal abnormalities are rare; (2) proteinuria, hypertension, and progression to ESRD are unusual; (3) gender differences in expression of TBMN are not apparent; and (4) transmission is autosomal dominant. TBMN and early AS may be difficult to differentiate histologically because diffuse GBM attenuation is characteristic of both. However, the GBM of TBMN patients remains attenuated over time, rather than undergoing the progressive thickening and multilamellation that occurs in AS.

Etiology and Pathogenesis

TBMN is usually transmitted as an autosomal dominant condition. A negative family history may not be reliable because patients are frequently unaware that they have relatives with hematuria. In one Dutch kindred with isolated hematuria,[37] affected individuals were found to be heterozygous for a missense mutation in COL4A4. After this initial report, familial TBMN has been localized to COL4A3 or COL4A4 in numerous additional kindreds.[38] About 50% or more of heterozygous carriers of a COL4A3 or COL4A4 mutation exhibit hematuria.[16,17] However, linkage to COL4A3 and COL4A4 has been excluded in other families with isolated hematuria, indicating that TBMN is a genetically heterogeneous condition.

To date, immunohistologic studies of type IV collagen in GBM of patients with TBMN have found no abnormalities in the distribution of any of the six α chains. Immunohistologic evaluation of GBM type IV collagen may be useful in the differentiation of TBMN from AS (see later discussion).

Clinical Manifestations

It has been estimated that 20% to 25% of patients referred to a nephrologist for evaluation of persistent hematuria will prove to have thin GBM on renal biopsy. Individuals with TBMN typically exhibit persistent microhematuria that is first detected in childhood. In some patients, microhematuria is intermittent and may not be detected until adulthood. Episodic gross hematuria, often in association with upper respiratory infections, is not unusual. The hematuria of TBMN appears to be lifelong.

Overt proteinuria and hypertension are unusual in TBMN but have been reported. Some of these patients may have actually had AS, in which the predominant abnormality of GBM was attenuation rather than thickening and multilamellation. Other glomerular disorders, such as IgA nephropathy and focal or global glomerulosclerosis, may occur concurrently with TBMN, altering the expected natural history and histopathology of the condition.

Pathology

Light and immunofluorescence microscopy are unremarkable in typical cases of TBMN. Most patients exhibit diffuse thinning of the whole GBM and of the lamina densa (Fig. 45.10). GBM width is age and gender dependent in normal individuals. Both the lamina densa and the GBM increase rapidly in thickness between birth and age 2 years, followed by gradual thickening into adulthood. GBM thickness in adult men (373 ± 42 nm) exceeds that in adult women (326 ± 45 nm).[31] Each electron

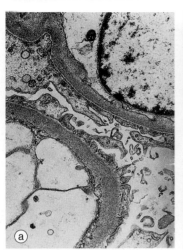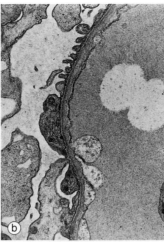

Figure 45.10 Thin basement membrane nephropathy. Electron micrographs of renal biopsies. *a*, Normal glomerular capillary wall. *b*, Thin basement membrane nephropathy at the same magnification. Note the diffuse and uniform attenuation of the glomerular basement membrane and the lamina densa. (From Warrell DA, Cox TM, Firth JD, Benz EJ Jr [eds]: Oxford Textbook of Medicine. Oxford, UK, Oxford University Press, 2003, p 322.)

microscopy laboratory should establish a consistent technique for measuring GBM thickness and determine its own reference range for GBM width to make comparisons with published data meaningful. Typically, a cutoff value of 250 nm will accurately separate adults with normal GBM from those with TBMN.[39] For children, the cutoff is in the range of 200 to 250 nm. Intraglomerular variability in GBM width is small in individuals with TBMN.

Diagnosis and Differential Diagnosis

If the patient's family history indicates autosomal dominant transmission of hematuria, if there is no history of chronic renal failure, and if kidney and urinary tract imaging are normal, a presumptive diagnosis of TBMN can often be made without kidney biopsy (see Fig. 45.7). When family history is negative or unknown, or there are atypical coexisting features such as proteinuria or deafness, renal biopsy may be very informative. A finding of thin GBM may be further characterized by examining the distribution of type IV collagen α chains in the kidney. Normal distribution of these chains provides supportive, although not conclusive, evidence for a diagnosis of TBMN. Marked variability in GBM width within a glomerulus in a patient with persistent microhematuria should raise suspicion of AS, although focal lamina densa splitting has been described in TBMN.

Treatment

Patients who are given a diagnosis of TBMN should be reassured but not lost to follow-up examination. The risk for chronic renal insufficiency appears to be small but real. Urinalysis and measurement of blood pressure and renal function are recommended every 1 to 2 years.

FABRY'S DISEASE (ANDERSON-FABRY DISEASE)

Introduction and Definition

Fabry's disease comprises the clinical and pathologic manifestations of hereditary deficiency of the enzyme α-galactosidase A (α-Gal A), resulting in the intracellular accumulation of neutral

glycosphingolipids with terminal α-linked galactosyl moieties (globotriaosylceramide, Gb3; Fig. 45.11). Anderson[40] and Fabry[41] each described the characteristic skin lesions of this condition in 1898 and noted the association of proteinuria with the skin lesion, for which Fabry coined the term *angiokeratoma corporis diffusum.*

Etiology and Pathogenesis

More than 100 mutations causing Fabry's disease have been identified in the gene for α-Gal A, which is located on the X chromosome. Most of the described mutations are associated with the classic Fabry's phenotype, in which there is multisystem involvement. Certain missense mutations have been identified in patients with a mild phenotype limited to cardiac abnormalities (see later discussion).[42]

Deficiency of α-Gal A leads to progressive intracellular accumulation of neutral glycosphingolipids, particularly those with α-galactosyl moieties, the most abundant of which is globotriaosylceramide (Gb3). Glycosphingolipids are normal constituents of the plasma membrane, the membranes of intracellular organelles, and circulate in association with apolipoproteins. The glycosphingolipids that accumulate in Fabry's disease are identical to those found in normal tissue. All tissues except red blood cells accumulate Gb3, with the highest concentrations found in the diseased kidney.

Clinical Manifestations and Pathology

Classic Fabry's disease is a multisystem disorder, with prominent and potentially devastating involvement of the kidneys, heart, and peripheral and central nervous system. As expected for an X-linked disorder, severe clinical manifestations occur in hemizygous males, whereas heterozygous females exhibit a variable but typically less severe course. In affected males, the initial features of the disease are seen in childhood and early adolescence and consist of paresthesias and pain in the hands and feet with episodic pain crises. The course of the disease is variable but usually leads to ESRD in the third to sixth decade. Myocardial or cerebral infarctions are typical terminal events. Severe Fabry's disease in a female reflects extensive inactivation of the X chromosome carrying the normal α-Gal A allele.

Renal Defects

Although the earliest manifestation of renal involvement is a concentrating defect, the nephropathy of Fabry's disease typically manifests as mild to moderate proteinuria, sometimes with

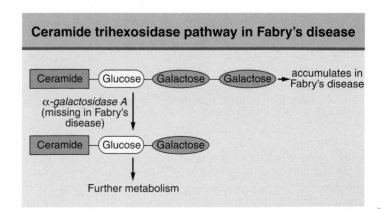

Figure 45.11 The ceramide trihexosidase pathway in Fabry's disease. α-Galactosidase A deficiency leads to tissue accumulation of trihexosylceramide.

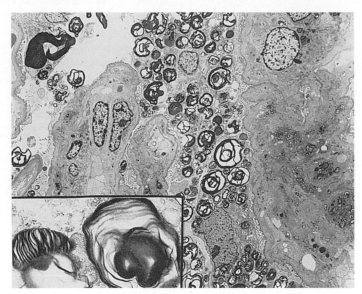

Figure 45.12 Electron micrograph of a renal biopsy in Fabry's disease. Glycosphingolipid is deposited in cytoplasmic vacuoles in glomerular visceral epithelial cells. *Insert:* Cytoplasmic vacuoles contain electron-dense material in parallel arrays (zebra bodies) and in concentric whorls (myelin figures). (Courtesy of J. Carlos Manivel, MD.)

microhematuria, beginning in the third decade of life. Nephrotic syndrome is unusual. Urinary oval fat bodies, exhibiting a Maltese cross configuration when viewed with a polarizing microscope, may be seen as a result of the large amounts of glycosphingolipid in the urine (see Chapter 4, Fig. 4.4b). Deterioration of renal function is gradual, with hypertension and ESRD developing by the fourth or fifth decade of life. Heterozygous women typically display mild renal involvement but may develop ESRD.

Light microscopy shows striking glomerular changes, with additional abnormalities of tubular epithelium and vessels. Glomerular visceral epithelial cells are enlarged and packed with small, clear vacuoles, which represent glycosphingolipid material that has been extracted during processing. Vacuoles may also be seen in parietal epithelial cells and the epithelial cells of the distal convoluted tubule and loop of Henle, but only rarely in mesangial cells, glomerular endothelial cells, or proximal tubular epithelial cells. With time, glomeruli exhibit segmental and global sclerosis. Vacuoles are also observed in endothelial cells and smooth muscle cells of arterioles and arteries.

Ultrastructural examination reveals abundant inclusions within lysosomes, particularly within visceral epithelial cells (Fig. 45.12). The inclusions ("myelin figures") are typically round, comprising concentric layers of dense material separated by clear spaces. The layers may be arranged in parallel ("zebra bodies").

Detachment of visceral epithelial cells from the underlying basement membrane may be observed. Inclusions are also observed in heterozygous females, although usually in smaller numbers than in affected males. Typical inclusions may be noted in excreted renal tubular cells.

The progression of the Fabry's nephropathy to ESRD probably reflects two parallel processes. Visceral epithelial cell dysfunction, which results in proteinuria, is followed by visceral epithelial cell detachment and necrosis leading to capillary loop collapse and segmental sclerosis. Simultaneously, progressive impairment of arterial flow may develop, as enlarging endothelial cells impinge on vascular lumina, resulting in ischemic glomerular damage.

Heart Defects

Glycosphingolipid accumulation in coronary arterial endothelial cells and in the myocardium results in coronary artery narrowing, which may lead to angina, myocardial infarction, or congestive heart failure. Arrhythmias and valvular lesions have been identified. Certain missense mutations affecting α-Gal A may present as isolated left ventricular hypertrophy.[42]

Nervous System

Autonomic dysfunction is a prominent feature of Fabry's disease, commonly manifested by hypohidrosis, acral paresthesias, and altered intestinal motility. Cerebrovascular symptoms tend to appear during the fourth decade of life and include hemiparesis, vertigo, diplopia, dysarthria, nystagmus, nausea and vomiting, headache, ataxia, and memory loss. The vertebrobasilar circulation is preferentially involved. Symptoms are often recurrent. Life-threatening intracerebral hemorrhage and infarction are not unusual. Dementia arising from glycosphingolipid accumulation in small cerebral blood vessels has also been described.

Skin

Angiokeratomas usually appear during the second decade of life, presenting as dark red macules or papules of variable size (Fig. 45.13). Typical locations include the lower trunk, buttocks, hips, genitalia, and upper thighs. The number of lesions varies from none to 20 to 40. Histologically, angiokeratomas consist of dilated small veins in the upper dermis, covered by hyperkeratotic epidermis. Telangiectasias may be noted, especially behind the ears.

Eyes

Characteristic corneal opacities are common in both men and women with Fabry's disease. These lesions, termed *verticillata*, are identified by slit-lamp examination and are whorls of whitish discoloration that radiate from the center of the cornea. Cataracts and dilated conjunctival or retinal vessels may be observed.

Lungs

Dyspnea and cough are common in men with Fabry's disease, often with airflow limitation on spirometry. This may be a consequence of fixed narrowing of the airways owing to glycosphingolipid accumulation.

Diagnosis

Diagnosis of affected males can usually be made on clinical grounds with the additional information from slit-lamp examination of

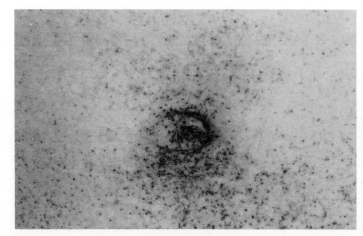

Figure 45.13 Angiokeratoma in Fabry's disease. Note the multiple periumbilical angiokeratomas. (Courtesy of Dr. S. Waldek.)

the eye. The diagnosis should be confirmed by demonstrating decreased or absent α-Gal A activity in serum, leukocytes, cultured skin fibroblasts, or tissue. Atypical variants may have enzyme activity up to 35% of normal. Heterozygous females have intermediate levels of α-Gal A activity, but values may be in the low-normal range, making measurement of enzyme activity an insensitive way of diagnosing carriers. Alternatives include careful slit-lamp eye examination, measuring urinary ceramide digalactoside and trihexoside, or molecular techniques using restriction fragment-length polymorphisms of either the α-Gal A gene or closely linked markers on the X-chromosome. Identification of carriers is particularly relevant when family members are being considered as living kidney donors.

Fabry's disease should be considered in patients with unexplained ESRD,[43] especially if left ventricular hypertrophy is present or there is a history of stroke.[44]

Treatment

Until recently, clinicians could offer little beyond palliative, symptomatic care to patients with Fabry's disease, including carbamazepine and gabapentin, or narcotics, for neuropathic pain, supplemented by antihypertensive therapy and platelet antagonists. However, the introduction of enzyme replacement therapy using recombinant human α-Gal A (agalsidase) has transformed the treatment of Fabry's disease. In 2001, preclinical studies in α-Gal A–deficient mice showing that agalsidase, lowered tissue and plasma Gb3, providing the rationale for human treatment trials.[45] Randomized clinical trials showed that agalsidase administration over 5 to 6 months resulted in reduced plasma and urine Gb3; amelioration of neuropathic pain; enhanced quality of life; clearing of Gb3 deposits from kidney, heart, and skin; and improved cerebral blood flow.[46,47] A multicenter longitudinal study showed that agalsidase stabilized renal function in patients with mild to moderate renal impairment at baseline and reduced left ventricular mass in those with left ventricular hypertrophy at baseline, over 1 to 2 years of treatment.[48] In patients with ESRD, agalsidase infusion may be combined with hemodialysis because there is little clearance of the enzyme by dialysis.[49] Agalsidase therapy has been recommended for all affected males and symptomatic carrier females.[50] The clinical significance of the development of neutralizing antibodies to agalsidase remains to be determined.[51]

Renal transplantation is an effective treatment for advanced Fabry's nephropathy but does not ameliorate the extrarenal manifestations. Transplanted kidneys from cadaveric donors or unaffected living donors may exhibit glycosphingolipid inclusions, but these are generally infrequent and clinically insignificant. The use of Fabry's heterozygotes as kidney donors should be avoided. Coronary artery and cerebrovascular disease are the major causes of death in patients with Fabry's disease who have undergone renal transplantation. Renal allograft recipients with Fabry's disease are candidates for agalsidase treatment.[50]

Fabry's Disease in Childhood

Because it is often not appreciated that the signs and symptoms of Fabry's disease, particularly pain crises, acroparesthesias, angiokeratomas, and corneal opacities, typically have their onset in childhood, a specific diagnosis is frequently delayed until well into adulthood.[51,52] Symptomatic children with Fabry's disease are potential candidates for agalsidase therapy, and treatment

trials in children are now under way in the United States and Europe.[51]

NAIL-PATELLA SYNDROME

Definition

Nail-patella syndrome (NPS) is an autosomal dominant condition characterized by hypoplasia or absence of the patellae, dystrophic nails, dysplasia of the elbows and iliac horns, and renal disease.

Etiology and Pathogenesis

The NPS locus was identified in 1998 as the LIM homeodomain transcription factor *LMX1B*.[53,54] Targeted disruption of the murine homologue resulted in skeletal defects (hypoplastic nails and absent patellae) as well as renal dysplasia in transgenic mice.[53] *LMX1B* and the NPS locus were mapped to chromosome 9q34, leading to the discovery of *LMX1B* mutations in patients with NPS.[54] A variety of mutations in *LMX1B* have been found in NPS patients, including missense, splicing, insertion or deletion, and nonsense alterations. The results of *in vitro* studies of the transcriptional effects of mixing wild-type and mutant *LMX1B* suggest that NPS results from haploinsufficiency of *LMX1B*, rather than a dominant-negative effect.[55] Although *LMX1B* appears to be important for normal limb and kidney development, the precise mechanisms for the renal effects of *LMX1B* mutations remain under investigation.

Clinical Manifestations
Renal Defects

Clinically apparent renal disease occurs in less than half of NPS patients. The nephropathy is usually benign, with about a 10% risk for progression to ESRD. The clinical signs of NPS nephropathy appear in adolescence or young adulthood and typically include microhematuria and mild proteinuria, although some patients develop nephrotic syndrome and mild hypertension. The severity of the renal manifestations may differ substantially in related individuals.

Skeletal Defects

The patellae are absent or hypoplastic in more than 90% of patients with NPS (Fig. 45.14) and may be associated with effusions and osteoarthritis of the knees. In about 80% of patients, there are osseous processes projecting posteriorly from the iliac wings (iliac horns), which are pathognomonic (Fig. 45.15). Anomalies of the elbows include aplasia, hypoplasia, and posterior processes at the distal ends of the humeri.

Nails

Nail abnormalities occur in about 90% of patients and are typically bilateral and symmetric. Fingernails are more commonly affected than toenails. The nails may be absent or dystrophic with discoloration, koilonychia, longitudinal ridges, or triangular lunulae.

Pathology

Although there are no specific light or immunofluorescence microscopic features of the NPS renal lesion, by electron microscopy, the GBM exhibits multiple irregular lucencies, giving it a moth-eaten appearance (Fig. 45.16). Such lucencies may also be observed in the mesangium. These lucent areas sometimes appear to contain cross-banded collagen fibrils, which are more easily

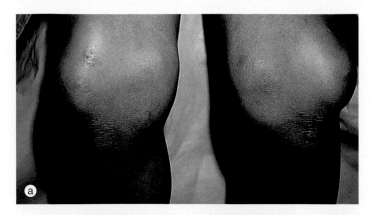

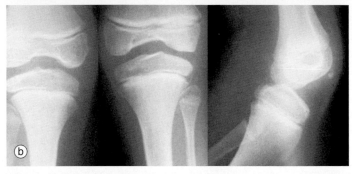

Figure 45.14 Nail-patella syndrome. Clinical *(a)* and radiologic *(b)* appearance of absence of the patellae. (Courtesy of Dr. R. Vernier)

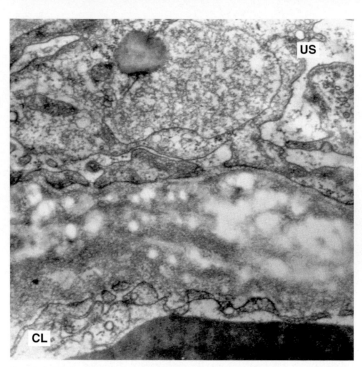

Figure 45.16 Electron micrograph of renal biopsy in nail-patella syndrome. The glomerular basement membrane appears moth-eaten on routine staining. CL, capillary lumen; US, urinary space. (Courtesy of Dr. R. Vernier)

observed after staining with phosphotungstic acid (Fig. 45.17). The fibrils tend to be arranged in clusters, and the surrounding GBM is often thickened. These fibrils may be observed in the kidneys in the absence of clinically evident renal disease, but they have not been found in extraglomerular basement membranes. These fibrils were recently identified as type III collagen.[56] Cross-banded fibrils of type III collagen have been seen in GBM of patients with glomerular disease who lack nail or skeletal abnormalities, sometimes as a familial condition with autosomal recessive inheritance (collagen type III glomerulopathy, see Chapter 27). Whether a pathogenetic relationship between collagen type III glomerulopathy and NPS exists remains to be determined.

Treatment

There is no specific therapy for the nephropathy of NPS. Renal transplantation has been performed successfully, without apparent recurrence of the disease in the transplanted kidney. Because NPS is an autosomal dominant disorder, careful evaluation of potential living-related kidney donors for features of the disease is essential.

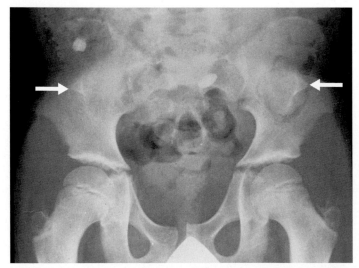

Figure 45.15 Nail-patella syndrome. Iliac horns *(arrows)*. (Courtesy of Dr. R. Vernier)

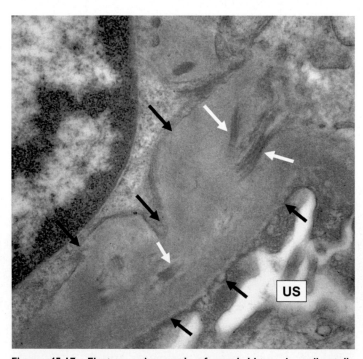

Figure 45.17 Electron micrograph of renal biopsy in nail-patella syndrome stained with phosphotungstic acid. *Black arrows* show margins of irregular glomerular basement membrane. Staining with phosphotungstic acid reveals fibrillar collagen *(white arrows)*. US, urinary space.

REFERENCES

1. Guthrie LG: "Idiopathic," or congenital, hereditary and familial hematuria. Lancet 1902;1:1243–1246.
2. Hurst AF: Hereditary familial congenital haemorrhagic nephritis occurring in sixteen individuals in three generations. Guy's Hosp Rec 1923;3:368–370.
3. Alport AC: Hereditary familial congenital haemorrhagic nephritis. BMJ 1927;1:504–506.
4. Spear GS, Slusser RJ: Alport's syndrome: Emphasizing electron microscopic studies of the glomerulus. Am J Pathol 1972;69:213–222.
5. Hinglais N, Grunfeld J-P, Bois LE: Characteristic ultrastructural lesion of the glomerular basement membrane in progressive hereditary nephritis (Alport's syndrome). Lab Invest 1972;27:473–487.
6. Churg J, Sherman RL: Pathologic characteristics of hereditary nephritis. Arch Pathol 1973;95:374–379.
7. McCoy RC, Johnson HK, Stone WJ, Wilson CB: Absence of nephritogenic GBM antigen(s) in some patients with hereditary nephritis. Kidney Int 1982;21:642–652.
8. Kashtan C, Fish AJ, Kleppel M, et al: Nephritogenic antigen determinants in epidermal and renal basement membranes of kindreds with Alport-type familial nephritis. J Clin Invest 1986;78:1035–1044.
9. Atkin CL, Hasstedt SJ, Menlove L, et al: Mapping of Alport syndrome to the long arm of the X chromosome. Am J Hum Genet 1988;42:249–255.
10. Hostikka SL, Eddy RL, Byers MG, et al: Identification of a distinct type IV collagen α chain with restricted kidney distribution and assignment of its gene to the locus of X chromosome-linked Alport syndrome. Proc Natl Acad Sci U S A 1990;87:1606–1610.
11. Barker DF, Hostikka SL, Zhou J, et al: Identification of mutations in the COL4A5 collagen gene in Alport syndrome. Science 1990;248:1224–1227.
12. Zhou J, Reeders ST: The α chains of type IV collagen. Contrib Nephrol 1996;117:80–105.
13. Lemmink HH, Schröder CH, Monnens LAH, Smeets HJM: The clinical spectrum of type IV collagen mutations. Hum Mutat 1997;9:477–499.
14. Antignac C, Heidet L: Mutations in Alport syndrome associated with diffuse esophageal leiomyomatosis. Contrib Nephrol 1996;117:172–182.
15. Jais JP, Knebelmann B, Giatras I, et al: X-linked Alport syndrome: Natural history in 195 families and genotype-phenotype correlations in males. J Am Soc Nephrol. 2000;11:649–657.
16. Boye E, Mollet G, Forestier L, et al: Determination of the genomic structure of the COL4A4 gene and of novel mutations causing autosomal recessive Alport syndrome. Am J Hum Genet 1998;63:1329–1340.
17. Heidet L, Arrondel C, Forestier L, et al: Structure of the human type IV collagen gene COL4A3 and mutations in autosomal Alport syndrome. J Am Soc Nephrol 2001;12:97–106.
18. van der Loop FTL, Heidet L, Timmer EDJ, et al: Autosomal dominant Alport syndrome caused by a COL4A3 splice site mutation. Kidney Int 2000;58:1870–1875.
19. Ciccarese M, Casu D, Wong FK, et al: Identification of a new mutation in the α4(IV) collagen gene in a family with autosomal dominant Alport syndrome and hypercholesterolaemia. Nephrol Dial Transplant 2001;16:2008–2012.
20. Pochet JM, Bobrie G, Landais P, et al: Renal prognosis in Alport's and related syndromes: Influence of the mode of inheritance. Nephrol Dial Transpl 1989;4:1016–1021.
21. Kashtan CE, Kleppel MM, Gubler MC: Immunohistologic findings in Alport syndrome. Contrib Nephrol 1996;117:142–153.
22. Cheong HI, Kashtan CE, Kim Y, et al. Immunohistologic studies of type IV collagen in anterior lens capsules of patients with Alport syndrome. Lab Invest 1994;70:553–557.
23. Jais JP, Knebelmann B, Giatras I, et al: X-linked Alport syndrome: Natural history and genotype-phenotype correlations in girls and women belonging to 195 families: A "European Community Alport Syndrome Concerted Action" study. J Am Soc Nephrol 2003;14:2603–2610.
24. Grunfeld J-P, Noel LH, Hafez S, Droz D: Renal prognosis in women with hereditary nephritis. Clin Nephrol 1985;23:267–271.
25. Colville D, Savige J, Morfis M, et al: Ocular manifestations of autosomal recessive Alport syndrome. Ophthalmic Genet 1997;18:119–128.
26. Heath KE, Campos-Barros A, Toren A, et al: Nonmuscle myosin heavy chain IIA mutations define a spectrum of autosomal dominant macrothrombocytopenias: May-Hegglin anomaly and Fechtner, Sebastian, Epstein and Alport-like syndromes. Am J Hum Genet 2001;69:1033–1045.
27. Merchant SN, Burgess BJ, Adams JC, et al: Temporal bone histopathology in Alport syndrome. Laryngoscope 2004;114:1609–1618.
28. Kashtan CE, Kim Y: Distribution of the α1 and α2 chains of collagen IV and of collagens V and VI in Alport syndrome. Kidney Int 1992;42:115–126.
29. Kalluri R, Shield CF, Todd P, et al: Isoform switching of type IV collagen is developmentally arrested in X-linked Alport syndrome leading to increased susceptibility of renal basement membranes to endoproteolysis. J Clin Invest 1997;99:2470–2478.
30. Kashtan CE, Kim Y, Lees GE, et al: Abnormal glomerular basement membrane laminins in murine, canine, and human Alport syndrome: Aberrant laminin alpha2 deposition is species independent. J Am Soc Nephrol 2001;12:252–260.
31. Rao VH, Lees GE, Kashtan CE, et al: Increased expression of MMP-2, MMP-9 (type IV collagenases/gelatinases), and MT1-MMP in canine X-linked Alport syndrome (XLAS). Kidney Int 2003;63:1736–1748.
32. Kashtan CE: Animal models of Alport syndrome. Nephrol Dial Transpl 2002;17:1359–1362.
33. Rheault MN, Kren SM, Thielen BK, et al: Mouse model of X-linked Alport syndrome. J Am Soc Nephrol 2004;15:1466–1474.
34. Kashtan CE, Gubler MC, Sisson-Ross S, Mauer M: Chronology of renal scarring in males with Alport syndrome. Pediatr Nephrol 1998;12:269–274.
35. Callis L, Vila A, Carrera M, Nieto J: Long-term effects of cyclosporine A in Alport's syndrome. Kidney Int 1999;55:1051–1056.
36. Gross O, Schulze-Lohoff E, Koepke ML, et al: Antifibrotic, nephroprotective potential of ACE inhibitor vs AT1 antagonist in a murine model of renal fibrosis. Nephrol Dial Transplant 2004;19:1716–1723.
37. Lemmink HH, Nillesen WN, Mochizuki T, et al: Benign familial hematuria due to mutation of the type IV collagen α4 gene. J Clin Invest 1996;98:1114–1118.
38. Savige J, Rana K, Tonna S, et al: Thin basement membrane nephropathy. Kidney Int 2003;64:1169–1178.
39. Steffes MW, Barbosa J, Basgen JM, et al: Quantitative glomerular morphology of the normal human kidney. Lab Invest 1983;49:82–86.
40. Anderson W: A case of "angio-keratoma." Br J Dermatol 1898;10:113–117.
41. Fabry J: Ein Beitrag zur Kenntniss der Purpura haemorrhagica nodularis (Purpura papulosa haemorrhagica Hebrae). Arch Dermatol Syph 1898;43:187–200.
42. Nakao S, Takenaka T, Maeda M, et al: An atypical variant of Fabry's disease in men with left ventricular hypertrophy. N Engl J Med 1995;333:288–293.
43. Ichinose M, Nakayama M, Ohashi T, et al: Significance of screening for Fabry disease among male dialysis patients. Clin Exp Nephrol 2005;9:228–232.
44. Rolfs A, Bottcher T, Zschiesche M, et al: Prevalence of Fabry disease in patients with cryptogenic stroke. Lancet 2005;366:1794–1796.
45. Ioannou YA, Zeidner KM, Gordon RE, et al: Fabry disease: Preclinical studies demonstrate the effectiveness of alpha-galactosidase A replacement in enzyme-deficient mice. Am J Hum Genet 2001;68:14–25.
46. Eng CM, Banikazemi M, Gordon RE, et al: A phase 1/2 clinical trial of enzyme replacement in Fabry disease: Pharmacokinetic, substrate clearance, and safety studies. Am J Hum Genet 2001;68:711–722.
47. Schiffmann R, Kopp JB, Austin HA, et al: Enzyme replacement therapy in Fabry disease: A randomized controlled trial. JAMA 2001;285:2743–2749.
48. Beck M, Ricci R, Widmer U, et al: Fabry disease: Overall effects of agalsidase alpha treatment. Eur J Clin Invest 2004;34:838–844.
49. Kosch M, Koch HG, Oliveira JP, et al: Enzyme replacement therapy administered during hemodialysis in patients with Fabry disease. Kidney Int 2004;66:1279–1282.
50. Desnick RJ, Brady R, Barranger J, et al: Fabry disease, an under-recognized multisystemic disorder: Expert recommendations for diagnosis, management, and enzyme replacement therapy. Ann Intern Med 2003;138:338–346.
51. Linthorst GE, Hollak CE, Donker-Koopman WE, et al: Enzyme therapy for Fabry disease: Neutralizing antibodies toward agalsidase alpha and beta. Kidney Int 2004;66:1589–1595.
52. Desnick RJ, Brady RO. Fabry disease in childhood. J Pediatr 2004;144:S20–26.

53. Chen H, Lun Y, Ovchinnikov D, et al: Limb and kidney defects in Lmx1b mutant mice suggest an involvement of LMX1B in human nail patella syndrome. Nat Genet 1998;19:51–55.

54. Dreyer SD, Zhou G, Baldini A, et al: Mutations in LMX1B cause abnormal skeletal patterning and renal dysplasia in nail patella syndrome. Nat Genet 1998;19:47–50.

55. Dreyer SD, Morello R, German MS, et al: LMX1B transactivation and expression in nail-patella syndrome. Hum Mol Genet 2000;9: 1067–1074.

56. Heidet L, Bongers EM, Sich M, et al: In vivo expression of putative LMX1B targets in nail-patella syndrome kidneys. Am J Pathol 2003; 163:145–155.

Inherited Disorders of Sodium and Water Handling

Peter Gross and Peter Heduschka

INTRODUCTION

Glomerular filtration yields about 150 L of water, 21,000 mmol of Na^+, and 750 mmol of K^+ in a healthy individual in 24 hours, yet only minute fractions of these quantities are excreted eventually as urine. This remarkable volume reduction is accomplished by highly active tubular transport. Inherited defects of tubular transport proteins may thus lead to major fluid and electrolyte derangements. This chapter describes disorders arising in the thick ascending limb of Henle's loop and thereafter; proximal tubular disorders are described in Chapter 47 and disturbances of acidification in Chapter 12.

Genetic studies of the past decade have been able to unravel the molecular basis of most of the inherited tubular disorders. The new information has helped to establish specific diagnoses more clearly and to explain the corresponding pathogenesis more reliably than was possible before. It is hoped that improved therapies will be developed in time. Diagnostic genetic testing is available for a number of the disorders discussed in this chapter (see www.genetests.org).

PHYSIOLOGY OF SODIUM AND WATER REABSORPTION

Sodium Reabsorption

The cellular machinery of tubular sodium reabsorption follows a certain basic pattern: in all tubular epithelial cells, a basolateral energy requiring Na^+K^+-ATPase will ensure that intracellular Na^+ is kept at low levels while K^+ is high. The resulting concentration gradients of Na^+ across the apical cell membrane drive passive Na^+ reabsorption from the tubular lumen to the cell interior. Apical Na^+ channels and transport proteins serve to regulate the Na^+ reabsorption, and the proteins involved differ from one tubular segment to the next.

In the proximal tubule, an apical Na^+H^+ exchange protein (NHE-3) facilitates most of the Na^+ reabsorbed. It is inhibitable by acetazolamide. The thick ascending limb has an apical $Na^+K^+Cl^-$ cotransporter (NKCC2; Fig. 46.1), which can be blocked by furosemide and bumetanide. For an efficient Na^+ reabsorption by NKCC2, this segment requires that K^+ is returned through a K^+ channel called ROMK from the cell to the low K^+ tubular fluid (see Fig. 46.1). It is also important that salt transport by this segment is dependent on a basolateral Cl^-

channel (ClC-Kb) and an accessory protein of ClC-Kb called *barttin* (see Fig. 46.1).

The distal convoluted tubule reabsorbs Na^+ by a unique apical Na^+Cl^- cotransporter (NCCT). The protein is specifically inhibited by thiazides (Fig. 46.2). A basolateral ClC-Kb chloride channel is also necessary for efficient sodium reabsorption.

In the collecting duct, an apical Na^+ channel called ENaC regulates Na^+ reabsorption. Amiloride and triamterene block ENaC specifically. On the other hand, the mineralocorticoid aldosterone upregulates ENaC (Fig. 46.3). An overview of segmental proteins of Na^+ reabsorption and of their corresponding inheritable disorders is provided in Figure 46.4.

Water Reabsorption

In most nephron segments, water follows NaCl passively through aquaporins, constitutively open water transport proteins in apical and basolateral tubular cell membranes. However, the collecting duct is different. It is equipped with apical aquaporin-2, which is

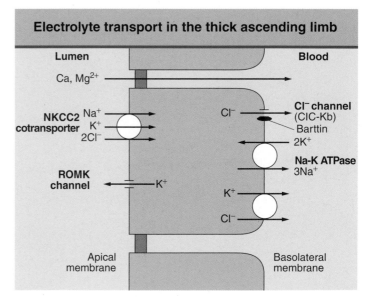

Figure 46.1 Electrolyte transport in the thick ascending limb of the loop of Henle. The furosemide-sensitive $Na^+K^+2Cl^-$ (NKCC2) cotransporter is driven by low intracellular Na^+ and Cl^- concentrations produced by the Na^+-K^+ ATPase pump, K^+Cl^- cotransporter, and the basolateral Cl^- channel (ClC-Kb). The ß-subunit (barttin) is crucial for normal functioning of the ClC-Kb channels. Apical K^+ recycling via the low-conductance, ATP-sensitive renal medullary K^+ (ROMK) channel ensures the efficient functioning of the NKCC2 cotransporter.

Electrolyte transport in the distal convoluted tubule

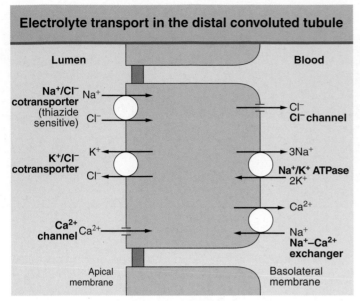

Figure 46.2 Electrolyte transport in the distal convoluted tubule. Reabsorption of Na$^+$ and Cl$^-$ occurs across the apical membrane by the thiazide-sensitive Na$^+$Cl$^-$ cotransporter (NCCT), and these ions leave the cell through the Cl$^-$ channels and via the Na$^+$-K$^+$ ATPase pump. Calcium ions enter the cell through the Ca^{2+} channels and exit via the Na$^+$Ca^{2+} exchanger.

the sole water channel in the kidney that can be regulated on a short-term basis by vasopressin. In this way, the collecting duct provides for eventual fine-tuning of water reabsorption or excretion (Fig. 46.5).

DISORDERS OF SODIUM HANDLING

An overview of inherited disorders of Na$^+$ transport is shown in Figure 46.6.

Electrolyte transport in the collecting tubule

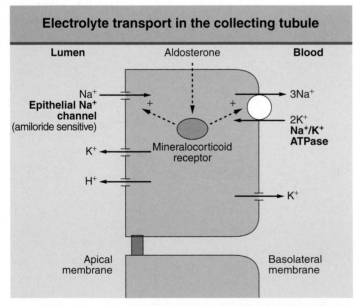

Figure 46.3 Electrolyte transport in the principal cell of the collecting tubule. Reabsorption of Na$^+$ occurs via the amiloride-sensitive epithelial Na$^+$ channel (ENaC). Its uptake is coupled to K$^+$ and H$^+$ secretion. Aldosterone increases the activity of ENaC and Na$^+$-K$^+$ ATPase, which increases Na$^+$ reabsorption and K$^+$ and H$^+$ secretion, resulting in hypokalemic alkalosis. Cortisol is also a ligand for the mineralocorticoid receptor but is normally removed by oxidation by 11β-hydroxysteroid dehydrogenase to cortisone.

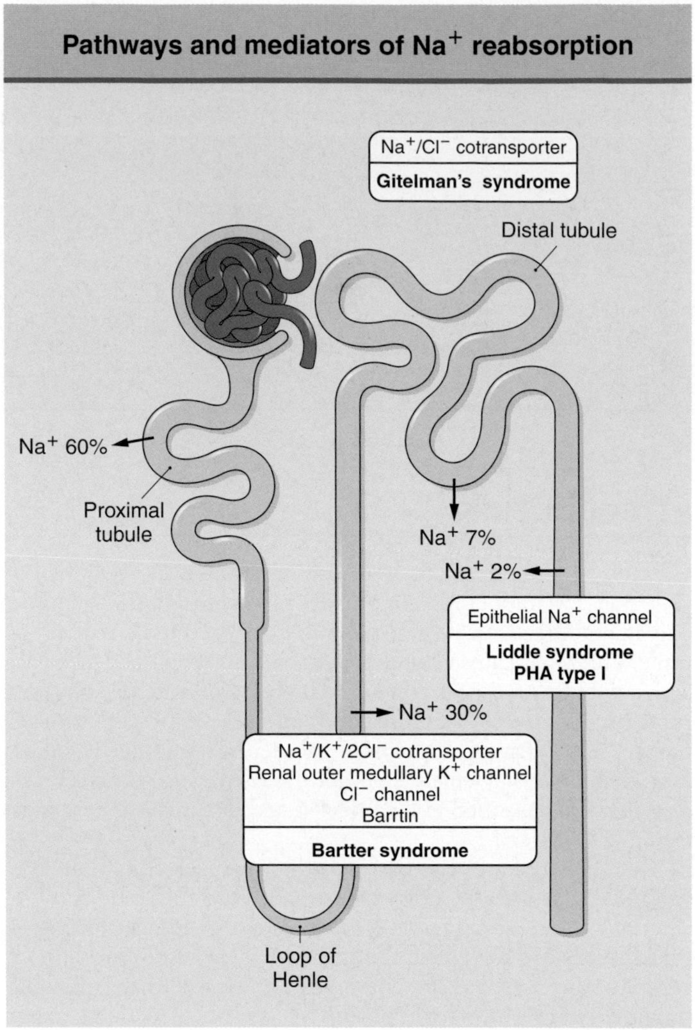

Pathways and mediators of Na$^+$ reabsorption

Figure 46.4 Pathways and mediators involved in Na$^+$ reabsorption. Almost 60% of the filtered Na$^+$ is reabsorbed in the proximal tubule. The distal portions of the nephron reabsorb the remainder. The chief mediators involved in Na$^+$ reabsorption and disorders resulting from their mutations are shown in boxes. PHA, pseudohypoaldosteronism.

On clinical grounds, it is possible to broadly distinguish four different phenotypes:

1. Hypokalemia and normal blood pressure (Bartter syndrome, Gitelman's syndrome)
2. Hypokalemia and high blood pressure (Liddle syndrome, apparent mineralocorticoid excess [AME], glucocorticoid remediable hyperaldosteronism, adrenal 17α-hydroxylase deficiency, adrenal 11-β hydroxylase deficiency
3. Hyperkalemia and normal blood pressure (pseudohypoaldosteronism [PHA], adrenal 21-hydroxylase deficiency, adrenal aldosterone synthase deficiency)
4. Hyperkalemia and high blood pressure (Gordon's syndrome)

Some of the disorders are caused by mutated renal transport proteins (e.g., Gitelman's syndrome), whereas in others, the genetic defect resides in the adrenals, and the changes of adrenal mineralocorticoids and glucocorticoids bring about the renal phenotype.

Water reabsorption in the distal tubule

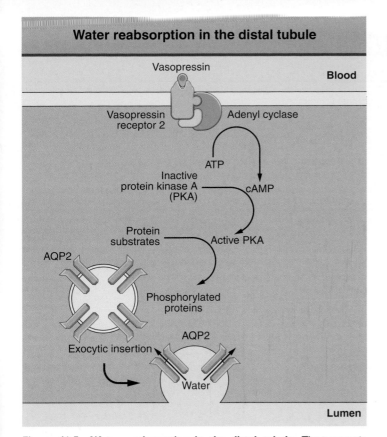

Figure 46.5 Water reabsorption in the distal tubule. The aquaporin AQP2, which is exclusively present in the principal cells of the collecting tubules and ducts, is the chief vasopressin-regulated water channel. Activation of cAMP-dependent protein kinase A mediates protein phosphorylation that triggers exocytic insertion of AQP2 channels into the apical membrane. These channels increase the water permeability of the apical membrane, facilitating water transport. PKA, protein kinase A.

Features of inherited defects of sodium handling

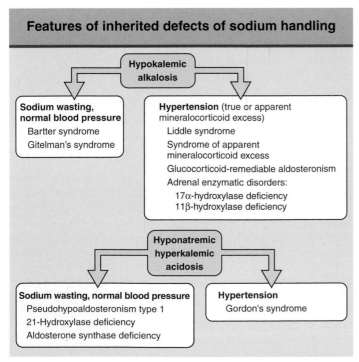

Figure 46.6 Features of inherited defects of sodium handling.

CONDITIONS WITH HYPOKALEMIA, METABOLIC ALKALOSIS, AND NORMAL BLOOD PRESSURE

Bartter Syndrome

Bartter syndrome is a rare abnormality. It manifests in childhood or in the perinatal period with severe hypokalemia, metabolic alkalosis, and low normal blood pressure, all of which are caused by tubular wasting of Na^+ and Cl^-.[1] In contrast, Gitelman's syndrome is mostly a disorder of adults, and hypomagnesemia is a defining feature.[2]

Pathogenesis

Bartter syndrome is due to dysfunction of the thick ascending limb and is caused by inactivating mutations of each of its major transport proteins[3-6] (NKCC2, Bartter syndrome type I; ROMK, type II; ClC-Kb, type III; barttin, type IV; Figs. 46.1 and 46.7). The pathogenic consequences of these mutations are broadly similar in all four varieties except that the more severe phenotypes (type I, II and IV) manifest earlier in life.

Loss of function of any single one of the four transport proteins will impair NaCl reabsorption by the thick ascending limb. Consequently, the delivery of salt to the distal nephron will increase, and it will stimulate NaCl reabsorption in those segments. Although this activity will provide only partial compensation of the salt wasting, it is associated with distal secretion of K^+ and $H.^+$ On balance, the loss of NaCl from the nephron will cause plasma volume contraction, low normal blood pressure, and secondary hyperaldosteronism. The loss of K^+ and H^+ will be followed by severe hypokalemia and metabolic alkalosis. Hypokalemia and increased angiotensin II will also serve to stimulate prostaglandin E_2 (PGE_2) production.

Reduced Cl^- absorption in the loop of Henle inhibits voltage-driven paracellular absorption of Ca^{2+} causing hypercalciuria. The latter is an important feature of Bartter syndrome. It may be associated with the development of nephrocalcinosis.

Inactivating mutations of barttin, in addition to the pathogenesis described so far, cause deafness because barttin-dependent chloride transport is crucial to endolymph production in the inner ear.[6] In some individuals with mutation of ClC-Kb (type III), there is a mixed Bartter and Gitelman's syndrome.[7] In these patients, the features of Bartter syndrome are associated with hypomagnesemia and hypocalciuria. Age at presentation is 1 month to 29 years. Because the ClC-Kb chloride channel is normally also expressed in the distal tubule, the site affected in Gitelman's syndrome, the mixed syndrome is tentatively explained by the overlapping distribution of ClC-Kb.[7] Finally, gain of function mutations in the extracellular calcium ion–sensing receptor also cause a Bartter-like syndrome.[8] The receptor is normally expressed in the thick ascending limb, and its activation inhibits salt reabsorption similarly to furosemide; in addition, this syndrome is associated with hypocalcemia.[8]

Clinical Manifestations

Bartter syndrome from mutations in NKCC2, ROMK, or barttin has a more severe phenotype than is observed in that caused by mutations of ClC-Kb. The more severe phenotype typically presents in the perinatal period and is called *antenatal* Bartter syndrome. The milder variety is called *classic* Bartter syndrome.

The clinical features of antenatal Bartter syndrome include hypokalemia and metabolic alkalosis in a newborn with vomiting and failure to thrive. There may also be a history of polyhydramnios and premature delivery. Polyuria, hypercalciuria, and high

Inherited single gene defects of sodium and water handling			
Syndrome	Inheritance	Gene Localization	Gene Product
Neonatal Bartter syndrome	AR	15q	Na-K-2Cl cotransporter *NKCC2*
Neonatal Bartter syndrome	AR	11q	Renal potassium channel *ROMK*
Classic Bartter syndrome	AR	1p	Renal chloride channel *ClC-Kb*
Bartter syndrome with deafness	AR	1p	β-Subunit of ClC-Kb *Barttin*
Gitelman's syndrome	AR	16q	Na-Cl cotransporter *NCCT*
Liddle syndrome	AD	16p	Epithelial sodium channel *ENaC*
Syndrome of apparent mineralocorticoid excess	AR	16q	11β-hydroxysteroid dehydrogenase type II
Glucocorticoid-remediable aldosteronism	AD	8q	Aldosterone synthase *CYP11B2*
Pseudohypoaldosteronism type I	AD AR	4p 12p, 16p	Mineralocorticoid receptor ENaC
Gordon's syndrome	AD	12p 17q 1q	WNK1 WNK4 Not identified
Congenital adrenal hyperplasia	AR AR AR	6p 8q 10q	21 hydroxylase 11β-hydroxylase 17α-hydroxylase
Nephrogenic diabetes insipidus	X-linked AR	Xq 12q	AVP receptor 2 Aquaporin 2

Figure 46.7 Inherited single gene defects of sodium and water handling. AD, autosomal dominant; AR, autosomal recessive; AVP, arginine vasopressin.

urinary chloride concentrations are regularly present. Nephrocalcinosis may manifest later in life. A prenatal diagnosis of Bartter syndrome may be made by demonstrating high Cl⁻ concentrations in amniotic fluid.

Patients with classic Bartter syndrome develop normally during the first 2 to 5 years of life. Thereafter, vomiting, polyuria, recurrent episodes of dehydration, and fever may become apparent. Carpopedal spasms and fatigue have been seen frequently. Many children show developmental delay. The blood pressure is low normal. The laboratory features are comparable to those described previously, but nephrocalcinosis is usually absent.

Diagnosis

A newborn or a young child with vomiting, dehydration, low-normal blood pressure, severe hypokalemia, and metabolic alkalosis is likely to have Bartter syndrome if it shows high urinary excretion rates of Cl⁻ and K⁺. The suspected diagnosis will receive further support when it is found that supplements of K⁺ and Cl⁻ are inefficient in correcting the severe hypokalemia and the blood pressure. Diuretics in the urine will not be found. Hypomagnesemia and hypocalciuria are absent. Secondary hyperaldosteronism is a regular feature. In questionable cases, genotyping should be used to confirm the diagnosis.

Differential Diagnosis

In syndromes of chronic severe hypokalemia with metabolic alkalosis, the differential diagnosis may be facilitated greatly by taking into consideration the associated blood pressure and the urinary chloride concentration (Fig. 46.8).

If the syndrome occurs in the setting of hypertension, this observation alone puts it into the category of hyperaldosteronism-related disorders.

If, however, the syndrome is associated with a normal or low-normal blood pressure, extrarenal or renal Cl⁻ and Na⁺ losses are the culprits. Extrarenal loss of sodium occurs in diarrhea,

vomiting, or burns. It is characterized by very low Cl⁻ concentrations in the urine, often as low as 1 mmol/l. By contrast, renal loss of salt with high urinary Cl⁻ and Na⁺ is typical of Bartter syndrome, Gitelman's syndrome, and diuretic use. The absence of hypomagnesemia and hypocalciuria will then argue against Gitelman's syndrome (Fig. 46.9). Genotyping is recommended to diagnose overlap of Bartter and Gitelman's syndromes.

Treatment

Patients with the neonatal form of Bartter syndrome have marked fluid and electrolyte disturbances that need to be corrected carefully. Saline infusion may be required in the neonatal period. Potassium chloride supplementation is always necessary.[9] Addition of spironolactone or triamterene may be useful in correcting hypokalemia, but the effect of these drugs is usually transient. Angiotensin-converting enzyme (ACE) inhibitors have been used for correction of hypokalemia, with conflicting results. Magnesium deficiency may aggravate renal K⁺ wasting and, if present, should be corrected.

The efficacy of long-term treatment with prostaglandin synthase inhibitors, such as indomethacin (1–3 mg/kg per 24 hours) or ibuprofen, is well established.[9] They act by reducing cortical perfusion and decreasing delivery of Na⁺ and Cl⁻ to the distal nephron, ameliorating many of the features of the disease. The amplifying effect of prostaglandins on the renal tubules is also neutralized. Treatment results in reduction of polyuria and polydipsia, restitution of normal growth and activity, and correction of hypokalemia; serum K⁺, however, rarely exceeds 3.5 mmol/l. Plasma levels of renin and aldosterone reduce to the normal range.

Outcome

If not treated, patients may succumb to episodes of dehydration, electrolyte disturbance, or intercurrent infection. With appropriate therapy, most children improve clinically and show catch-up growth; pubertal and mental developments are usually

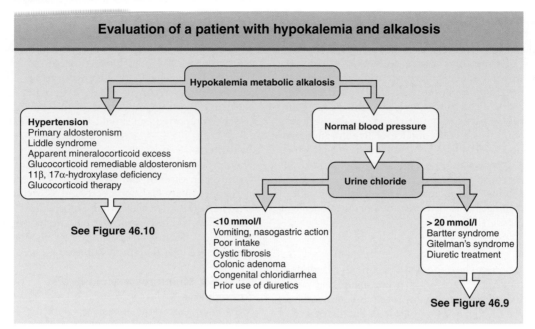

Figure 46.8 Evaluation of a patient with hypokalemia and metabolic alkalosis.

normal. Lifelong therapy is needed. Chronic tubulointerstitial nephropathy owing to persistent hypokalemia, hypercalciuria, and nephrocalcinosis may lead to progressive decline in renal function. There are anecdotal reports of renal transplantation in patients with end-stage renal disease (ESRD). The biochemical parameters return to normal after transplantation.

Gitelman's Syndrome
Gitelman's syndrome is an autosomal recessive condition also characterized by hypokalemic metabolic alkalosis, but with hypocalciuria and hypomagnesemia.

Pathogenesis
The similarity between the features of Gitelman's syndrome and those caused by thiazide administration originally suggested the defect might be in the distal convoluted tubule. The condition has now been linked to inactivating mutations in the gene for NCCT (see Figs 46.2 and 46.4).[10] Loss of NCCT function results in Na^+ and Cl^- wasting from this segment, leading to hypovolemia with secondary activation of the renin-aldosterone system. The resulting increase in collecting tubule Na^+ reabsorption is, however, counterbalanced by K^+ and H^+ excretion, causing hypokalemic alkalosis. The distal convoluted tubule normally reabsorbs only 7% to 8% of the filtered Na^+ and Cl^- load. The degree of volume contraction, stimulation of the renin-angiotensin system, and the amount of K^+ loss are, therefore, not substantial enough to stimulate PGE_2 production.

The hypocalciuria is due to the associated plasma volume contraction. The renal magnesium wasting is caused by downregulation of the epithelial Mg^{2+} channel Trpm6 in distal convoluted tubules.

Features differentiating Bartter and Gitelman's syndromes			
Features	Neonatal Bartter Syndrome	Classic Bartter Syndrome	Gitelman's Syndrome
Age at onset	Neonatal period	Infancy/childhood	Childhood/later
Maternal hydramnios	Common	Rare	Absent
Polyuria, polydipsia	Marked	Present	Rare
Dehydration	Present	Often present	Absent
Tetany	Absent	Rare	Present
Growth retardation	Present	Present	Absent
Urinary calcium	Very high	Normal or high	Low
Nephrocalcinosis	Present	Rare	Absent
Serum magnesium	Normal	Occasionally low	Low
Urine prostaglandins (PGE_2)	Very high	High or normal	Normal
Response to indomethacin (improvement of hypokalemia and renal salt wasting)	Good	Good	Rare

Figure 46.9 Features differentiating Bartter and Gitelman's syndromes. In addition to these clinical and laboratory features, molecular diagnosis is now possible (see text).

Clinical Manifestations and Diagnosis

Most adults believed to have Bartter syndrome will turn out to suffer from Gitelman's syndrome, and this diagnosis is not very rare. The severity of symptoms varies widely. More severely affected patients complain of generalized and muscular weakness, inability to work for extended periods, salt craving, and a preference for licorice. Cardiac disturbances, muscle cramps, and tetany are only exceptionally present. Chondrocalcinosis of the knees does occur later in life; it is a consequence of hypomagnesemia. Laboratory evaluation will show moderate hypomagnesemia, severe hypokalemia, hypocalciuria, a high urinary chloride concentration, and an absence of thiazides from the urine. The blood pressure will be in the low-normal range. These findings establish the diagnosis. Genotyping should be performed in questionable or incomplete syndromes.

Treatment

There is no consensus on the best mode of treatment. Magnesium aspartate (5–15 mmol Mg^{2+}/day), magnesium oxide, and potassium supplements are usually given to improve muscular weakness or cramps. However, dosing may be limited by diarrhea and abdominal discomfort. In exceptional cases, parenteral Mg^{2+} has been infused. Indomethacin, cyclooxygenase-2 inhibitors, and spironolactone are usually not helpful. The long-term prognosis for cardiac and renal function, as well as for general health, is good.

CONDITIONS WITH HYPOKALEMIA, METABOLIC ALKALOSIS, AND HYPERTENSION

Conditions with hypokalemia, metabolic alkalosis, and hypertension all have true or apparent mineralocorticoid excess (AME).

Liddle Syndrome (Pseudohyperaldosteronism)

Liddle syndrome is an autosomal dominant syndrome of hypertension and variable degrees of hypokalemic metabolic alkalosis. The patients resemble those with primary hyperaldosteronism, but levels of mineralocorticoid hormones are not increased. Renin and aldosterone are suppressed, and there is no response to spironolactone.[11] However, triamterene and amiloride, aldosterone-independent inhibitors of distal Na^+ transport, correct hypertension, renal K^+ loss, and hypokalemia.[12]

Pathogenesis

Liddle syndrome is related to mutations of the β or γ subunits of the collecting duct sodium channel, ENaC.[13] The mutations result in truncations of the cytoplasmic C-terminal tail of the affected subunits. Collecting duct sodium reabsorption is dependent on the channel density present in the apical cell membrane. Channel density is regulated by removal of ENaC from the cell membrane, ubiquitination, and degradation. In Liddle syndrome, the mutated ENaC protein cannot be recognized by NEDD4, a ubiquitin ligase protein; hence, the channels remain in the cell membrane for prolonged periods.[12] This action results in enhanced sodium reabsorption, hypertension, and hypokalemic alkalosis (see Fig. 46.3).

Clinical Manifestations and Diagnosis

Liddle syndrome is a rare disorder of hypertension in teenage children[12] that is associated with hypokalemic metabolic alkalosis and low blood levels of renin and aldosterone. The original patient developed renal failure from an unknown cause and eventually underwent transplantation.[14] Thereafter her blood pressure normalized, and renin and aldosterone responded normally to provocative measures.

This condition should be differentiated from primary hyperaldosteronism, AME, and glucocorticoid-remediable aldosteronism (Fig. 46.10), as well as 11β-hydroxylase (steroid 11β-mono-oxygenase) or 17α-hydroxylase (steroid 17α-mono-oxygenase) deficiency. Activating mutations of the mineralocorticoid receptor have been reported and should also be differentiated.[15]

Treatment

Therapy consists of sodium restriction and K^+ supplements. Triamterene directly inhibits apical Na^+ channels, resulting in increased urinary Na^+ and decreased K^+ excretion and resolution of hypertension. Amiloride also normalizes the blood pressure and K^+ levels. However, most patients continue to have growth retardation. Because the pathogenetic disorder is not correctable with age, lifelong therapy is required.

Apparent Mineralocorticoid Excess
Pathogenesis

AME is an autosomal recessive condition resulting from deficiency of the type II (renal and placental) isoform of the enzyme 11β-hydroxysteroid dehydrogenase. Clinical features of this condition closely mimic those of Liddle syndrome.[16]

In normal conditions, aldosterone is the chief mineralocorticoid regulating electrolyte and water balance, through its effects on distal renal tubules and cortical collecting ducts. After its binding to the mineralocorticoid receptor (MR), aldosterone increases synthesis of various proteins, chiefly Na^+K^+-ATPase on the basolateral surface and ENaC on the apical surface. These proteins increase Na^+ reabsorption and K^+ secretion in the distal tubules (see Fig. 46.3). Cortisol is also a ligand for MR and shows potent sodium-retaining activity. Cortisol is, however, normally metabolized by 11β-hydroxysteroid dehydrogenase to cortisone, which lacks such an action.

Loss of function mutations in the gene encoding 11β-hydroxysteroid dehydrogenase have been detected in patients with the inherited form of AME.[17,18] As a consequence, in the kidney, intracellular metabolic clearance of cortisol is severely impaired. The accumulation of cortisol causes nonspecific stimulation of the MR. This will be followed by increased sodium reabsorption together with K^+ and H^+ secretion.

The 11β-hydroxysteroid dehydrogenase is also expressed in the placenta. In AME-reduced placental 11β-hydroxysteroid dehydrogenase, activity might be related to the low birth weight that is characteristic of AME patients.

Carbenoxolone and glycyrrhizic acid (found in licorice compounds) are potent inhibitors of this enzyme. Consumption of these agents may be associated with features similar to AME.

Clinical Manifestations and Diagnosis

Apparent mineralocorticoid excess is characterized by an onset of hypertension in childhood, hypokalemia, metabolic alkalosis, very low plasma levels of renin and aldosterone, and increased metabolites of cortisol in the urine. There may be a history of low birth weight and subsequent failure to thrive.

The diagnosis of AME is made by finding, on gas chromatography or mass spectroscopy, elevated urinary levels of hydrogenated metabolites of cortisol (tetrahydrocortisol plus allotetrahydrocortisol) compared with cortisone (tetrahydrocortisone). The ratio of urinary free cortisol to cortisone is also increased.[19] Heterozygotes may occasionally show hypertension, normal serum K^+, suppressed plasma renin and aldosterone, and moderately elevated urinary

Features of Liddle syndrome, apparent mineralocorticoid excess, and glucocorticoid-remediable aldosteronism

Features	Syndromes with Hypokalemia, Metabolic Alkalosis, and Hypertension		
	Liddle Syndrome	AME	GRA
Inheritance	Autosomal dominant	Autosomal recessive	Autosomal dominant
Chief features	Significant hypertension, polyuria, growth retardation	Low birth weight, early-onset hypertension, polyuria, growth retardation	Significant hypertension, hemorrhagic stroke
Plasma aldosterone	Reduced	Reduced	Elevated
Plasma renin activity	Reduced	Reduced	Reduced
Urinary mineralocorticoid metabolites	Normal	Elevated ratios of THF + alloTHF to THE; free cortisol to cortisone	Elevated cortisol C-18 oxidation products
Response of the hypertension to			
Glucocorticoids	No	Satisfactory	Satisfactory
Triamterene	Satisfactory	Satisfactory	Satisfactory
Spironolactone	No	Satisfactory	Satisfactory

Figure 46.10 Features of Liddle syndrome, apparent mineralocorticoid excess (AME), and glucocorticoid-remediable aldosteronism (GRA). THE, tetrahydrocortisone; THF, tetrahydrocortisol.

cortisol-to-cortisone metabolite ratio. A variant of AME, called AME type II, has similar clinical features but a milder urinary steroid profile.[20]

Treatment

Treatment with oral dexamethasone (0.75–5 mg/day) suppresses cortisol secretion, resulting in reduced Na^+ reabsorption and amelioration of hypertension and hypokalemia. Urinary concentrations of metabolites of cortisol and cortisone are only moderately affected. As in Liddle syndrome, patients respond to treatment with K^+ supplements combined with triamterene or amiloride. Spironolactone is effective in AME, although not in Liddle syndrome. Renal transplantation is followed by normalization of cortisol metabolism, biochemical abnormalities, and hypertension.[21]

Glucocorticoid-Remediable Aldosteronism

Glucocorticoid-remediable aldosteronism (GRA) appears to be the most common monogenic form of human hypertension. Genetic analysis has revealed that the disease is transmitted in an autosomal dominant fashion. Patients present typical features of primary hyperaldosteronism: hypertension, suppressed plasma renin activity, and hypokalemia. As the most striking difference to primary hyperaldosteronism (i.e., due to aldosterone-producing adrenal adenoma), hypersecretion of aldosterone in GRA can be reversed by the administration of glucocorticoids. Affected individuals have early-onset hypertension. The prevalence of hemorrhagic stroke, largely as a result of ruptured intracranial aneurysms, seems to be high.

Hypokalemia is typically mild but becomes more pronounced when patients are treated with diuretics. Potassium levels may occasionally be normal.

Pathogenesis

Patients with GRA have adrenocorticotropic hormone (ACTH)-sensitive aldosterone production occurring in the zona fasciculata of the adrenal gland, which is usually only responsible for cortisol synthesis. Normal subjects synthesize aldosterone in the zona glomerulosa. Two isoenzymes of 11β-hydroxylase are involved in the biosynthesis of aldosterone and cortisol: steroid 11β-hydroxylase (CYP11B1) and aldosterone synthase (CYP11B2), respectively (Fig. 46.11). The genes for these isoenzymes are located close to each other on the long arm of chromosome 8. Unequal meiotic crossovers may produce hybrid genes by fusion of the promoter end of CYP11B1 with the coding sequence of CYP11B2.[16] CYP11B2 encoding aldosterone synthase will now be inappropriately regulated by ACTH, as is CYP11B1. Abnormal expression of this chimeric gene in the adrenal zona fasciculata has been shown by *in situ* hybridization.

Diagnosis

Patients are often misdiagnosed as having essential hypertension. Hypertensive subjects with early-onset hypertension, early cerebral hemorrhage, hypokalemia after treatment with diuretics, and refractoriness to standard antihypertensive medication are candidates for GRA testing. Similar to other genetic forms of hypertension (Liddle syndrome, AME, Gordon's syndrome), plasma renin activity is low. Although the mean aldosterone levels are high, determination of serum aldosterone has poor sensitivity as a screening test. In GRA, the aldosterone-to-renin ratio is elevated (>300), whereas in essential hypertension, AME, and Liddle syndrome, it is not.

The biochemical hallmark of GRA is overproduction and excretion of cortisol C-18 oxidation products. These characteristics reflect the action of aldosterone synthase on cortisol in the zona fasciculata. Large amounts of the so-called hybrid steroids (18-hydroxycortisol and 18-oxocortisol) can be found in the urine by specialized steroid laboratories.

Dexamethasone leads to suppression of blood aldosterone levels. When 0.5 mg of dexamethasone is given every 6 hours for 2 days, it suppresses aldosterone to undetectable levels (<4 ng/dl).

Direct screening for the hybrid gene *CYP11B1/CYP11B2* can also be performed and confirms the diagnosis[22] (test can be obtained via www.bwh.partners.org).

Treatment

Treatment with low-dose corticosteroid is effective. Typically, 0.125 to 0.25 mg of dexamethasone or 2.5 to 5 mg of prednisolone is administered at bedtime. Therapeutic goals are normotension and normalization of biochemical markers (urinary

Biosynthesis of aldosterone and cortisol

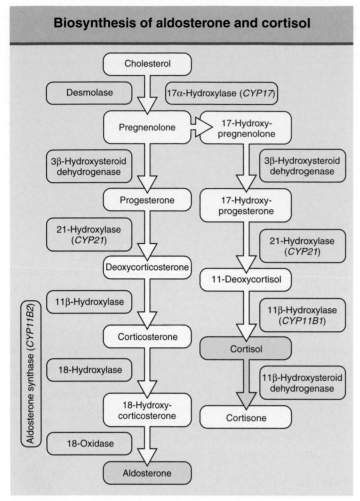

Figure 46.11 Biosynthesis of aldosterone and cortisol. Although cortisol and aldosterone both require 11β-hydroxylation of precursors, these steps are catalyzed by different isoenzymes: steroid 11β-hydroxylase (*CYP11B1*) and aldosterone synthase (*CYP11B2*), respectively. Aldosterone synthase also mediates two further conversions. Common enzyme deficiencies leading to derangement in sodium and water balance are shown in boxes. Cortisol is converted peripherally by 11β-hydroxysteroid dehydrogenase to cortisone.

18-oxosteroid, serum aldosterone). Mineralocorticoid receptor antagonists (spironolactone, eplerenone) and ENaC antagonists such as amiloride and triamterene may be used as useful treatments. Antihypertensive therapy with ß-blockers and ACE inhibitors is less likely to be effective.

Incomplete Phenotypes

Occasional patients with Liddle syndrome, AME, or GRA either do not express the complete phenotype or have mild clinical or biochemical features and are considered to have essential hypertension. Poor blood pressure control with conventional therapy should raise suspicion of an alternative diagnosis. Hypokalemia may not be present at the onset but develops after institution of diuretic treatment. These conditions should be considered in patients with early-onset hypertension, failure to thrive, or an impressive family history. The response to specific treatment with potassium-sparing diuretics or corticosteroids may suggest the diagnosis.

Adrenal Enzymatic Disorders

Inherited deficiency of 11β- or 17α-hydroxylase also causes mineralocorticoid excess with hypertension and hypokalemic metabolic alkalosis (see Fig. 46.11).

Deficiency of 17α-hydroxylase (*CYP17*) impairs normal production of cortisol and adrenal androgens, resulting in pseudohermaphroditism in genetic males and primary amenorrhea in females. Cortisol deficiency results in increased ACTH secretion, low levels of renin and aldosterone, hypokalemia, metabolic alkalosis, and hypertension. Diagnosis is confirmed by finding excessive levels of deoxycorticosterone and corticosterone in the urine. Glucocorticoid replacement corrects the mineralocorticoid excess state.

Deficiency of 11β-hydroxylase (*CYP11B1*) also impairs cortisol production but results in excessive androgens. Genetic females show pseudohermaphroditism, whereas males have virilization. The cortisol deficiency results in high blood levels of ACTH, deoxycortisol, and deoxycorticosterone; corticosterone levels are normal. Hypokalemia is variable. Diagnosis is confirmed by measuring high levels of tetrahydro-11-deoxycortisol in the urine. Hypokalemia is variable. Treatment with glucocorticoids corrects hypertension and hypokalemia; renin levels increase, but aldosterone remains low because of the biosynthetic defect.

CONDITIONS WITH HYPONATREMIA, HYPERKALEMIA, METABOLIC ACIDOSIS, AND NORMAL BLOOD PRESSURE

Conditions with hyponatremia, hyperkalemia, metabolic acidosis, and normal blood pressure have features of mineralocorticoid deficiency, either because of a synthetic defect or because of end-organ resistance.

Pseudohypoaldosteronism

PHA is a state of renal tubular (and other tissue) unresponsiveness to the action of aldosterone.[23] Symptoms start in early infancy with marked salt wasting and failure to thrive. PHA type 1 includes at least two major entities, with either renal or multiple target-organ defects; the former is more common.

The inheritance of renal PHA type 1 is autosomal dominant but may be sporadic. Loss of function mutations of the gene for MR (located on 4p) have been identified.[24]

Multiple end-organ PHA type 1 is a severe autosomal recessive disorder with multiple target-organ resistance to the action of mineralocorticoids and is associated with inactivating mutations of α, β, or γ subunits of ENaC.[25] Differences between the two major types are shown in Figure 46.12.

Aldosterone Biosynthetic Defects

Patients with defects in aldosterone biosynthesis show salt wasting with hyponatremia, hyperkalemia, hypovolemia, and elevated plasma renin activity.[26]

The enzymes cholesterol desmolase, 3β-hydroxysteroid dehydrogenase, and 21-hydroxylase are required for synthesis of cholesterol and aldosterone, whereas aldosterone synthase is selectively responsible for aldosterone production in the adrenal cortex (see Fig. 46.11). Characteristics of diseases with aldosterone biosynthetic defects are shown in Figure 46.13.

Deficiency of 21-Hydroxylase

Mutations in the gene encoding 21-hydroxylase (*CYP21*) result in two major forms of the disease: a virilizing form and the more common salt-wasting type.[27] Patients with signs only of androgen excess are said to have the virilizing form. Female infants show varying degrees of pseudohermaphroditism, whereas affected males have normal or precocious sexual development. The salt-wasting type presents with hyponatremia, hyperkalemia, and moderate to severe volume depletion.

Differential features of renal-limited and multisystem forms of pseudohypoaldosteronism type 1

Feature	Renal-Limited Form	Multisystem Form
Underlying defect	Mineralocorticoid receptor	Epithelial sodium channel
Affected organs	Kidney only	Kidney, sweat, salivary glands, distal colon
Inheritance	Autosomal dominant	Autosomal recessive
Salt wasting	Variable	Severe
Blood renin, aldosterone	Very high	Very high aldosterone
Sweat, salivary Na$^+$	Normal	High
Clinical features	Salt wasting variable, during stress	Severe salt wasting, often life-threatening (e.g., hyperkalemia, infections of the skin), often respiratory tract (mimics cystic fibrosis) destabilization
Treatment	Sodium chloride supplements for 1–3 years Carbenoloxone is effective in some patients (creates situation akin to AME)	Lifelong sodium chloride supplements, strict potassium restriction, prophylactic antibiotics to prevent skin sepsis, no response to carbenoloxone
Prognosis	Improvement usually by 6–8 years, need for salt supplement diminishes	Improvement rare with age

Figure 46.12 Features of renal-limited and multisystem forms of pseudohypoaldosteronism type 1. AME, apparent mineralocorticoid excess.

The diagnosis of 21-hydroxylase deficiency should be suspected in any newborn with genital ambiguity, salt wasting, or hypotension. Blood levels of progesterone, 17-hydroxyprogesterone, and dehydroepiandrosterone are raised several fold above normal.

Patients with electrolyte imbalance and shock require resuscitation with intravenous fluids and salt supplements. Replacement therapy with oral hydrocortisone and 9α-fludrocortisone is required long term. Some amelioration of the tendency to salt wasting may be seen with age, because of the ability of children to regulate their dietary salt intake and maturation of proximal tubular function.

Reconstructive genital surgery may be required in females with genital ambiguity. Fetal DNA analysis and demonstration of elevated 17-hydroxyprogesterone in amniotic fluid allows prenatal detection of affected female infants. Treatment of the mother with dexamethasone from early in gestation reduces virilization of genitalia of the affected female fetus.

CONDITIONS WITH HYPERKALEMIA, METABOLIC ACIDOSIS, AND HYPERTENSION

Pseudohypoaldosteronism Type 2 (Gordon's Syndrome)

Gordon's syndrome is the clinical inverse of Gitelman's syndrome. It is characterized by hypertension, hyperkalemia, and slight hyperchloremic metabolic acidosis. Defects in PHA type 2 are inherited as an autosomal dominant trait.

Pathogenesis

Two responsible genes have been identified.[28] They encode two members of the with-no-lysine kinase family: *WNK1* and *WNK4*. The WNK kinases are both expressed in the kidney within the convoluted tubule and the collecting ducts.

WNK4 acts as a negative regulator of thiazide-sensitive Na$^+$Cl$^-$ cotransporter (NCCT) function (see Fig 46.2). The kinase reduces the number of NCCT on the cell surface. In addition, *WNK4* downregulates the potassium channel ROMK and epithelial chloride flux.

Mutations in *WNK4* are missense mutations and cause a loss of function. As a result, *WNK4* loses its ability to suppress NCCT and ROMK. Transporter overactivity consequently leads to sodium and potassium retention.

WNK1 prevents *WNK4* from interacting with NCCT. Mutations in *WNK1* are intronic deletions that increase *WNK1* expression. WNKs are intriguing targets for novel antihypertensive agents.

Aldosterone biosynthesis defects

Defective enzyme	21-hydroxylase	3β-hydroxysteroid dehydrogenase	Cholesterol desmolase	Aldosterone synthase
Incidence	Most common (1:11,000–23,000)	Rare	Rare	Rare
Aldosterone	Deficient	Deficient	Deficient	Deficient
Cortisol production	Deficient	Deficient	Deficient	Normal cortisol
ACTH	Loss of feedback inhibition	Loss of feedback inhibition	Loss of feedback inhibition	Normal feedback inhibition
Adrenal hyperplasia	Yes	Yes	Yes	No
Genital ambiguity	In females	In females	In females	No
Clinical features	Children with failure to thrive; hyponatremia, hyperkalemia, acidosis, and hypotension			
Elevated metabolites	17-Hydroxyprogesterone	Dehydroepiandrosterone	Dehydroepiandrosterone	Corticosterone
Therapy	Oral hydrocortisone and 9α-fludrocortisone			9α-fludrocortisone

Figure 46.13 Characteristics of diseases with aldosterone biosynthetic defects. ACTH, adrenocorticotropic hormone.

Clinical Manifestations and Diagnosis

Hyperkalemia may be present from birth, but as in GRA, hypertension may not present until later in life. Patients show hyperchloremic metabolic acidosis with a normal glomerular filtration rate (GFR); plasma renin and aldosterone are reduced to variable degrees.

Treatment

As a specific inhibitor of the NCCT, hydrochlorothiazide is able to correct clinical features of Gordon's syndrome. Treatment with drugs results in complete reversal of clinical and biochemical abnormalities.

NEPHROGENIC DIABETES INSIPIDUS

Congenital nephrogenic diabetes insipidus (NDI) is a rare polyuric disorder identified by the failure to concentrate urine despite normal or elevated levels of vasopressin. GFR and solute excretion rate are normal. Acquired diabetes insipidus is much more common, and its diagnosis and management are discussed in Chapter 8.

Pathogenesis

More than 90% of patients have X-linked recessive NDI with mutations in *AVPR2*, the gene at Xq28 coding for the arginine vasopressin receptor (AVPR). Mutant proteins are conformationally different from the wild-type protein. As a result, mutations usually cause intracellular trapping of the receptor, which is retained in the endoplasmic reticulum (ER). Occasionally, the receptor may be expressed on the cell surface but is unable to bind vasopressin or to trigger an appropriate cyclic adenosine monophosphate (cAMP) response.[29] In less than 10% of the families, congenital NDI has an autosomal recessive inheritance, and mutations have been identified in the gene for aquaporin-2 located on chromosome 12q13. Similarly to X-linked NDI, most autosomal recessive *AQP2* mutations were found to be held back in the ER.

An autosomal dominant form of NDI, also caused by mutation in *AQP2*, has been reported. These mutations lead to mistransporting of *AQP2* mutant proteins to the basolateral membrane instead of the apical membrane.[30] Reduced expression of *AQP2* may result in acquired NDI secondary to lithium or demeclocycline therapy.

Clinical Features

Manifestations of congenital NDI appear within the first weeks of life. Males with *AVPR2* mutations show marked polyuria and excessive thirst; these features are often not recognized in early infancy. Unless the condition is suspected early, children have recurrent episodes of severe hypernatremic dehydration, occasionally complicated by convulsions.[31] Delayed development and mental retardation are possible consequences of these episodes. Cranial computed tomography may occasionally show dystrophic calcification in the basal ganglia and the cerebral cortex.

A reduced intake of calories because of the large quantities of water that are ingested leads to growth failure beginning in early childhood. Increased urine volumes may result in dilation of the lower urinary tract. Renal cortical damage, because of recurrent episodes of severe dehydration, may result in impairment of renal function. Heterozygous females may show variable degrees of polyuria and polydipsia. The onset and severity of clinical features of autosomal recessive NDI are similar to those of the X-linked form.

Diagnosis

Episodes of dehydration are marked by hypernatremia, hyperchloremia, and occasionally, elevated levels of urea and creatinine. Polyuria with low urine osmolality (<200 mOsm/kg) and hypernatremia with plasma Na^+ >150 mmol/l and plasma osmolality >300 mOsm/kg is highly suggestive of either vasopressin deficiency (central diabetes insipidus) or resistance to its action (NDI). Central diabetes insipidus is more common than NDI. Primary polydipsia resembles true diabetes insipidus in that compulsive water drinking results in polyuria with low urine osmolality; however, the plasma osmolality in primary polydipsia is normal or borderline low.

To confirm the lack of renal concentrating ability and distinguish NDI from central diabetes insipidus and primary polydipsia, a vasopressin test is performed. Desamino-8-D-arginine vasopressin (DDAVP) is administered nasally (5–10 μg in neonates and infants, 20 μg in children) or by an intramuscular injection (0.4–1.0 μg in infants and young children, 2 μg in older children). Hourly urine collection is done over the next 6 hours. After administration of DDAVP, patients with NDI fail to show a rise of urine osmolality, which remains below 200 to 300 mOsm/kg (normal, >800 mOsm/kg). Those with central diabetes insipidus and primary polydipsia concentrate urine appropriately.

Persistence of polyuria for years may result in a washout of the medullary countercurrent concentration mechanism. Several days of treatment with DDAVP may be required to elicit an appropriate response in these patients. In patients in whom the diagnosis of primary polydipsia is strongly suspected, supervised reduction of fluid intake over several days may restore normal sensitivity to DDAVP.

Differential Diagnosis

Patients with central diabetes insipidus show hypernatremia with inappropriately dilute urine, no primary renal disease, and a rise in urine osmolality after administration of vasopressin or its analogues. Central diabetes insipidus usually results from posterior pituitary neuronal damage, which may be secondary to tumors (craniopharyngioma, optic glioma, metastasis), Langerhans cell histiocytosis, trauma (e.g., fracture of base of skull), or infections (meningitis, encephalitis). Deficiency of vasopressin may also be familial, with an autosomal dominant inheritance. Mutations of *AVP-NPII*, the gene for vasopressin–neurophysin II, located on chromosome 20p, have been reported.[32] The onset of vasopressin deficiency, in the familial form, is usually delayed and may not be apparent until after the first few years of life. Central diabetes insipidus may also occur with the syndrome of diabetes insipidus, diabetes mellitus, optic atrophy, and deafness (DIDMOAD, or Wolfram syndrome), which is autosomal recessive. A Wolfram gene has recently been mapped to chromosome 4p16.1, but there is evidence for locus heterogeneity.

Many patients with central diabetes insipidus or NDI have a partial defect in vasopressin secretion or action. They are, therefore, able to concentrate urine to varying degrees after DDAVP administration, making precise diagnosis difficult. Measurement of levels of plasma vasopressin in relation to plasma osmolality following an osmotic stimulus, such as fluid restriction, allows differentiation in these patients. Patients with severe or partial central diabetes insipidus always show subnormal vasopressin levels relative to plasma osmolality. In contrast, the values from patients with NDI or psychogenic polydipsia are always within or above the normal range.

Magnetic resonance imaging of the brain produces a bright spot on T1-weighted images of the posterior pituitary in normal individuals and also those with NDI or primary polydipsia. This signal is absent in most patients with central diabetes insipidus.

The differential response of clotting factors and urine osmolality to DDAVP is useful in differentiating X-linked (*AVPR2* abnormalities) from autosomal recessive (*AQP2* mutations) NDI. Patients with *AQP2* abnormalities show normal increases in factor VIII and von Willebrand factor after DDAVP infusion; this response is absent in those with an *AVPR2* defect.[31,33] Sequencing of *AVPR2* and *AQP2* is useful in identification of the molecular defect underlying NDI. Congenital NDI should also be differentiated from acquired forms of NDI (see Chapter 8).

Treatment

Appropriate management of patients with NDI prevents episodes of dehydration, allowing normal physical growth and development. Patients must have adequate water intake to prevent dehydration. The renal solute load is minimized by restriction of dietary protein and salt intake. Adequate energy and nutrients, depending on the age, should be provided to promote normal growth and development.

Thiazide diuretics, such as hydrochlorothiazide (1–2 mg/kg every 12 hours), when combined with reduction of salt intake, are effective in reducing urine output. Thiazides inhibit salt reabsorption in distal convoluted tubules, which leads to mild volume depletion. Hypovolemia stimulates fluid reabsorption in the proximal tubules, thereby diminishing water delivery to vasopressin sensitive sites in the collecting ducts. The antipolyuric effect can be enhanced by combination therapy with amiloride (0.1–0.2 mg/kg every 8–12 hours).

Because prostaglandins normally antagonize the action of vasopressin, prostaglandin synthase inhibitors are also effective in reducing urine volume and free water clearance. Not all non-steroidal anti-inflammatory drugs are equally potent in inhibiting renal prostaglandin synthesis. The agent most commonly used is indomethacin (1 mg/kg every 12 hours). Indomethacin may, however, reduce GFR and cause gastrointestinal side effects.

REFERENCES

1. Bartter FC, Pronove P, Gill J, MacCardle R: Hyperplasia of the juxtaglomerular complex with hyperaldosteronism and hypokalemic alkalosis. Am J Med 1962;33:811–828.
2. Gitelman HJ, Graham JB, Welt LG: A new familial disorder characterized by hypokalemia and hypomagnesemia. Trans Assoc Am Physic 1966;79:221–235.
3. Shaer AJ: Inherited primary renal tubular hypokalemic alkalosis: A review of Gitelman and Bartter syndromes. Am J Med Sci 2001;322:316–332.
4. Simon DB, Karet FE, Hamblan JM, et al: Bartter syndrome, hypokalemic alkalosis with hypercalciuria, is caused by mutations in the $Na^+K^+2Cl^-$ co-transporter NKCC2. Nat Genet 1996;13:183–188.
5. International Collaborative Study Group for Bartter-like Syndromes: Mutations in the gene encoding the inwardly-rectifying renal potassium channel, ROMK, cause the antenatal variant of Bartter syndrome: Evidence for genetic heterogeneity. Hum Mol Genet 1997;6:17–26.
6. Birkenhager R, Otto E, Schurmann MJ, et al: Mutations of BSND cause Bartter syndrome with sensorineural deafness and kidney failure. Nat Genet 2001;29:310–314.
7. Zelikovic I, Szargel R, Hawash A, et al: A novel mutation in the chloride channel gene, ClCKB, as a cause of Gitelman and Bartter syndromes. Kidney Int 2003;63:24–32.
8. Vargas-Poussou R, Huang C, Hulin P, et al: Functional characterisation of a calcium-sensing receptor mutation in severe autosomal dominant hypocalcemia with a Bartter like syndrome. J Am Soc Nephrol 2002;13:2259–2266.
9. Dillon MJ, Shah V, Mitchell MD: Bartter syndrome: 10 cases in childhood. Results of long term indomethacin therapy. Q J Med 1979;48:429–446.
10. Simon DB, Nelson-Williams C, Bia MJ, et al: Gitelman variant of Bartter syndrome, inherited hypokalemic alkalosis, is caused by mutations in the thiazide-sensitive Na^+Cl^- co-transporter. Nat Genet 1996;12:24–30.
11. Liddle GW, Bledsoe T, Coppage WS: A familial renal disorder simulating primary aldosteronism but with negligible aldosterone secretion. Trans Assoc Am Physic 1963;76:199–213.
12. Palmer BF, Alpern RJ: Liddle's syndrome. Am J Med 1998;104:310–319.
13. Rossier BC, Pradervand S, Schild L, Hummler E: Epithelial sodium channel and the control of sodium balance: Interaction between genetic and environmental factors. Annu Rev Physiol 2002;64:877–897.
14. Botero-Velez M, Curtis JJ, Warnock DG: Liddle's syndrome revisited: A disorder of sodium reabsorption in the distal tubule. N Engl J Med 1994;330:178–181.
15. Geller DS, Farhi A, Pinkerton N, et al: Activating mineralocorticoid receptor mutation in hypertension exacerbated by pregnancy. Science 2000;289:119–123.
16. White PC: Abnormalities of aldosterone synthesis and action in children. Curr Opin Pediatr 1997;9:424–430.
17. Stewart PM, Krozowski Z, Gupta A, et al: Hypertension in the syndrome of apparent mineralocorticoid excess due to mutations of the 11β-hydroxysteroid dehydrogenase type 2 gene. Lancet 1996;347:88–91.
18. White PC: 11β-hydroxysteroid dehydrogenase and its role in the syndrome of apparent mineralocorticoid excess. Am J Med Sci 2001;322:308–315.
19. Palermo M, Delitala G, Mantero F, et al: Congenital deficiency of 11β-hydroxysteroid dehydrogenase (apparent mineralocorticoid excess syndrome): Diagnostic value of urinary free cortisol and cortisone. J Endocrinol Invest 2001;24:17–23.
20. Li A, Tedde R, Krozowski ZS, et al: Molecular basis for hypertension in the "type II variant" of apparent mineralocorticoid excess. Am J Hum Genet 1998;63:370–379.
21. Palermo M, Delitala G, Sorba G, et al: Does kidney transplantation normalise cortisol metabolism in apparent mineralocorticoid excess syndrome? J Endocrinol Invest 2000;23:457–462.
22. McMahon GT, Dluhy RG: Glucocorticoid-remediable aldosteronism. Cardiol Rev 2004;12:44–48.
23. Dillon MJ, Leonard JV, Buckler JM, et al: Pseudohypoaldosteronism. Arch Dis Child 1980;55:427–434.
24. Geller DS, Rodriaguez Soriano J, Boado AV, et al: Mutations in the mineralocorticoid receptor gene causes autosomal dominant pseudohypoaldosteronism type 1. Nat Genet 1998;19:279–281.
25. Chang SS, Grunder S, Hanukoglu A, et al: Mutations in subunits of the epithelial sodium channel cause salt wasting with hyperkalemic acidosis, pseudohypoaldosteronism type 1. Nat Genet 1996;12:248–253.
26. White PC: Aldosterone synthase deficiency and related disorders. Mol Cell Endocrinol 2004;217:81–87.
27. Speiser PW: Congenital adrenal hyperplasia owing to 21-hydroxylase deficiency. Endocrinol Metab Clin North Am 2001;30:31–59.
28. Mein CA, Caulfield MJ, Dobson RJ, et al: Genetics of essential hypertension. Hum Mol Genet 2004;13:169–175.
29. Fujiwara MT, Bichet DG: Molecular biology of hereditary diabetes insipidus. Am Soc Nephrol 2005;16:2836–2846.
30. Sasaki S: Nephrogenic diabetes insipidus: update of genetic and clinical aspects. Nephrol Dial Transplant 2004;19:1351–1353.
31. Bichet DG, Oksche A, Rosenthal W: Congenital nephrogenic diabetes insipidus. J Am Soc Nephrol 1997;8:1951–1958.
32. Heppner C, Kotzka J, Bullmann C, et al: Identification of mutations of the arginine vasopressin-neurophysin II gene in two kindreds with familial central diabetes insipidus. J Clin Endocrinol Metab 1998;83:693–696.
33. Nguyen MK, Nielsen S, Kurtz I: Molecular pathogenesis of nephrogenic diabetes insipidus. Clin Exp Nephrol 2003;7:9–17.

Fanconi Syndrome and Other Proximal Tubule Disorders

John W. Foreman

INTRODUCTION

The proximal tubule is responsible for the reabsorption of the bulk of a number of solutes, including glucose, amino acids, bicarbonate, and phosphate. A number of disorders, mainly heritable, that affect proximal tubule reabsorption are described in this chapter, but renal tubular acidosis and familial forms of hyperphosphaturia are discussed in Chapters 12 and 10, respectively.

Most nonelectrolyte solutes are reabsorbed in the proximal tubule through specific transport proteins that cotransport them in conjunction with sodium (Fig. 47.1). The driving force for this solute transport is the electrochemical gradient for sodium entry maintained by the enzyme, Na^+K^+-ATPase. Most disorders of isolated solute reabsorption are related to defects in specific transport proteins, whereas disorders affecting multiple solutes, such as Fanconi syndrome, are probably secondary to defects in

energy generation, Na^+K^+-ATPase activity, or dysfunction of cellular organelles involved with membrane protein recycling.

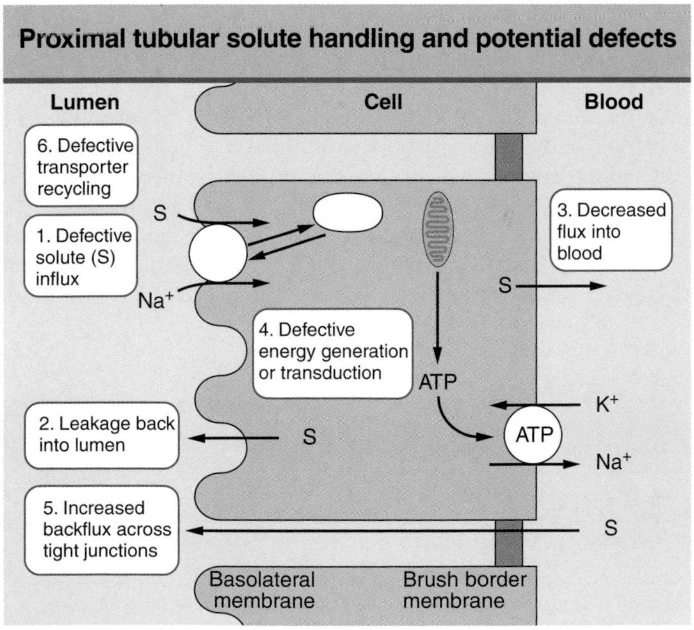

FAMILIAL GLUCOSE-GALACTOSE MALABSORPTION AND HEREDITARY RENAL GLYCOSURIA

Definition
Renal glycosuria refers to the appearance of readily detectable glucose in the urine when the plasma glucose is in a normal range. When the plasma glucose is in a physiologic range, virtually all the filtered glucose is reabsorbed in the proximal tubule. Filtered glucose enters the proximal tubule through two specific carriers (SGLT1 and SGLT2) coupled to sodium and exits the cell through the sugar transporters, GLUT1 and GLUT2 (Fig. 47.2). However, when the plasma level exceeds the physiologic range, the filtered load exceeds the capacity of these carriers, and glucose begins to appear in the urine; this is termed the *renal threshold*.

Etiology and Pathogenesis
Familial glucose-galactose malabsorption is a rare autosomal disorder that is due to mutations in the gene coding for the brush border sodium-glucose cotransporter SGLT1, which is found in the intestinal cell and the S3 segment of the proximal renal tubule cell. The disorder is characterized by the neonatal onset of life-threatening diarrhea from the intestinal malabsorption of glucose and galactose that resolves rapidly with the removal of the offending sugars and their dipeptide, lactose, from the diet. These patients frequently also have a mild renal glycosuria.

Hereditary renal glycosuria occurs with an incidence of 1 in 20,000 and appears to be inherited as an autosomal recessive trait. This disorder is due to mutations in SGLT2 glucose transporter found in the early portion of the proximal tubule. The gene (SLC5A2) for this has been mapped to chromosome 16p11.2. Renal glycosuria has been divided into three types based on the reabsorption patterns observed during glucose infusion studies (Fig. 47.3), although this separation has been called into question.[1] In type A, there is lowering of both the threshold and the maximal rate of tubular reabsorption of glucose. In type B, the maximal rate of glucose reabsorption is normal, but the threshold is low, and there is exaggerated splay in the tubular reabsorption versus filtered load curve. In type O, described by Brodehl and colleagues, there is virtually no reabsorption of filtered glucose, with the clearance of glucose nearly the same as that of inulin.[1] These authors call into question this typing system because their data and those

Figure 47.1   Defects and potential defects in proximal tubular solute handling. Solute uptake by the brush border membrane from the lumen is coupled to Na^+ influx. The favorable electrochemical driving force for luminal Na^+ is maintained by the Na^+K^+-ATPase pump. Transported solute is then either used by the cell or returned to the blood across the basolateral membrane. Fanconi syndrome could arise because of a defect in one of six areas, shown. ATP, adenosine triphosphate.

Within figure 47.1:

Proximal tubular solute handling and potential defects

Lumen | Cell | Blood

6. Defective transporter recycling

1. Defective solute (S) influx

3. Decreased flux into blood

4. Defective energy generation or transduction

2. Leakage back into lumen

5. Increased backflux across tight junctions

Basolateral membrane | Brush border membrane

Proximal tubule glucose reabsorption

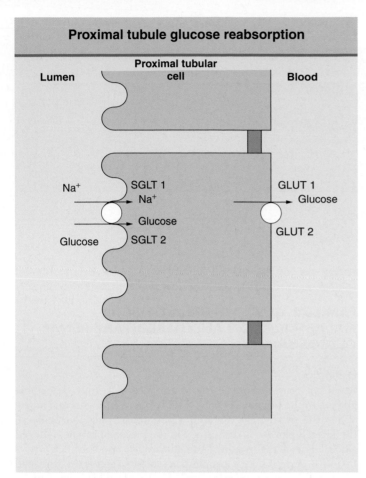

Figure 47.2 Proximal tubule glucose reabsorption. Glucose enters the proximal tubule cell coupled to Na+ reabsorption from the lumen through a high-capacity, low-affinity transporter (SGLT2) in the early proximal tubule and a low-capacity, high-affinity transporter (SGLT1) in the late proximal tubule. Glucose exits the cell through the transporters GLUT1 and GLUT2 located in the late and early proximal tubule, respectively.

Renal tubular glucose reabsorption

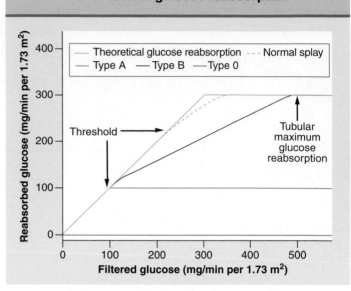

Figure 47.3 Renal glucose titration curves. The observed normal reabsorption curve follows the theoretical renal tubular glucose reabsorption until near the maximal reabsorption rate when the observed rate deviates from the theoretical rate (splay). The point of deviation is the threshold. Stylized titration curves for types A, B, and O renal glycosuria are shown. (Adapted from Brodehl J, Oemer BS, Hoyer PF: Renal glucosuria. Pediatr Nephrol 1987;1:502–508.)

of others suggest that patients with renal glycosuria have rates of glucose reabsorption that vary from virtually no reabsorption to nearly normal rates, rather than three distinct types, probably reflecting different mutations in the *SLC5A2* gene.

Natural History

Patients with familial glucose-galactose malabsorption appear to grow and develop normally with removal of the offending sugars from the diet. The clinical course of hereditary renal glycosuria is benign, except for a few patients with polyuria, and is not a precursor to diabetes mellitus.

AMINOACIDURIAS

Like glucose, amino acids are nearly completely reabsorbed in the proximal tubule by a series of specific carriers. A number of inherited disorders resulting in the incomplete reabsorption of a specific amino acid or a group of amino acids have been described[2] (Fig. 47.4).

Cystinuria
Definition

Cystinuria is characterized by the excessive urinary excretion of cystine and the dibasic amino acids ornithine, lysine, and arginine.[3]

Etiology and Pathogenesis

These four amino acids share a transport system on the brush border membrane of the proximal tubule. Because of the relative insolubility of cystine when its urine concentration exceeds 250 mg/l (1 mmol/l), patients with cystinuria have recurrent renal calculi.

Cystinuria is an autosomal recessive trait with a disease incidence of 1 in 20,000.[4] Initially, there appeared to be three genetic types, based on *in vitro* studies of intestinal transport and amino acid excretion in heterozygotes. More recently, two genes have been identified that are defective in cystinuria. The gene *SLC3A1* is carried on the short arm of chromosome 2; heterozygotes for this defect have normal excretion rates for cystine. The second gene, *SLC7A9*, is carried on the long arm of chromosome 19; heterozygotes for this gene defect have cystine excretion rates that range from normal to nearly that of homozygous patients. Based on these data, a new classification has been proposed. Type A involves

Inherited aminoacidurias

Disease	Clinical Findings	Urine Amino Acids
Cystinuria	Urolithiasis	Cystine, lysine, ornithine, arginine
Hartnup disease	Rash, neurologic disease	Neutral amino acids
Iminoglycinuria	None	Proline, hydroxyproline glycine
Lysinuric protein intolerance	Hyperammonemia, vomiting, diarrhea	Dibasic amino acids

Figure 47.4 Inherited aminoacidurias.

mutations in both *SCLC3A1* genes and type B mutations in *SLC7A9.*[4] Type AB is compound heterozygote.

Clinical Manifestations
Cystine stones are typically yellow-brown (Fig. 47.5a) and are radio-opaque (see Fig. 47.5b). Cystine crystals appear as microscopic, flat hexagons in the urine (see Fig. 47.5c), and this is a clue to the diagnosis.

Diagnosis
Patients can be screened for cystinuria with the cyanide-nitroprusside test, but type B heterozygotes may also give a positive result. The definitive test is to quantify cystine and dibasic amino acid excretion in a 24-hour urine specimen. Homozygotes excrete more than 118 mmol cystine/mmol creatinine (250 mg/g).

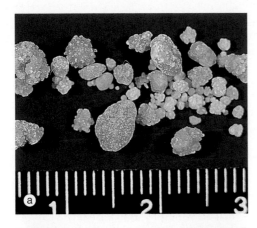

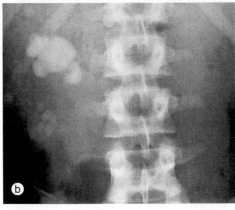

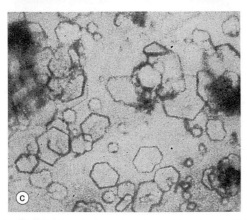

Figure 47.5 Cystinuria. *a,* Both rough and smooth cystine calculi. *b,* Plain radiograph of a cystine calculus in the right renal pelvis and further multiple parenchymal calculi. *c,* Urine microscopy showing characteristic flat hexagonal crystals.

Treatment
The aim of therapy in cystinuria is to lower the urine cystine concentration to below 300 mg/l (1.25 mmol/l). The first step is to increase the fluid intake. However, because most patients with cystinuria excrete 0.5 to 1 g/day of cystine, a urine output of 2 to 4 liters/day is needed to achieve this goal. Cystine solubility increases in alkaline urine, but the urine pH must be above 7.5 to be effective. In patients with recurrent stone disease, thiols, such as penicillamine, are extremely useful through the formation of a more soluble mixed disulfide of the thiol and cysteine from cystine. The thiols also reduce the overall excretion of cystine through an unknown mechanism. Penicillamine should be started at 250 mg/day and gradually increased (maximum, 2 g/day) over 3 months to achieve a urine cystine concentration below 300 mg/l in conjunction with a high fluid intake. Thiola is equally effective and is better tolerated than penicillamine. It should also be started at a low dose and slowly increased (maximum, 2 g/day). Captopril can be useful (an effect resulting from its thiol structure not its angiotensin-converting enzyme [ACE] inhibitor effect), but the dose range (75–150 mg/day) may be limited by its hypotensive effects.

Hartnup Disease
Hartnup disease is an autosomal recessive trait characterized by a neutral aminoaciduria that arises from a defect in a specific carrier for neutral amino acid transport present in both the intestine and the proximal renal tubule. The gene responsible for Hartnup disease is *SLC6A19,* residing on chromosome 5, and codes for the neutral amino acid transporter, B^0T^1. From newborn screening programs, the genetic defect is more common than originally thought because most individuals with the aminoaciduria never manifest any symptoms. Individuals who become symptomatic with Hartnup disease have pellagra-like clinical features, including a photosensitive dermatitis, ataxia, and psychotic behavior. These symptoms appear to be secondary to niacin deficiency that is in part due to inadequate intestinal absorption of tryptophan, the precursor for niacin synthesis. However, most individuals who inherit the Hartnup transport defect do not have symptoms, so there must be other environmental or genetic factors that lead to disease. Nicotinamide supplementation leads to clearing of the skin disease and, on occasion, some of the neurologic problems. The renal loss of neutral amino acids appears to have little clinical importance.

Iminoglycinuria
Iminoglycinuria is a benign heritable defect in the proximal tubule transporter PAT1, leading to incomplete reabsorption of proline, hydroxyproline, and glycine.

Lysinuric Protein Intolerance
Lysinuric protein intolerance is associated with recurrent bouts of hyperammonemia after a protein load, resulting from the decreased renal and intestinal dibasic amino acid transport.

Other Aminoacidurias
Rare individuals have been described with abnormalities in the excretion of other amino acids. These usually occur in association with mental retardation.

HEREDITARY DEFECTS IN URIC ACID HANDLING

Hereditary Renal Hypouricemia

Hereditary renal hypouricemia is a rare autosomal recessive disorder characterized by very low serum uric acid levels (<2.5 mg/dl [<150 μmol/l] in adult males and <2.1 mg/dl [<124 μmol/l] in adult women) and increased uric acid clearance, ranging from 30% to 150% of the filtered load.[5] In the normal kidney, uric acid is both reabsorbed and secreted in the proximal tubule by two different uric acid–anion exchange transporters and a voltage-sensitive pathway. In some patients, the defect is in the gene *SLC22A12* that codes for the protein URAT1. Most patients do not have symptoms and are found incidentally when a low serum uric acid is noted during routine serum chemistry evaluation. About one fourth of patients with renal hypouricemia have had renal stones, but only one third of these were uric acid stones. A few patients have also had hypercalciuria, and a few patients have had exercise-induced acute renal failure. Most patients require no treatment, but if they are forming uric acid stones, they should maintain a high fluid intake. Urine alkalinization and allopurinol can be used for patients with persistent uric acid stones.

Familial Juvenile Hyperuricemic Nephropathy and Medullary Cystic Kidney Disease Type 2

Familial juvenile hyperuricemic nephropathy (FJHN) is a rare autosomal dominant condition characterized by hyperuricemia associated with a tubular defect in uric acid excretion.[6] Children develop progressive renal insufficiency with interstitial fibrosis and glomerulosclerosis. The hyperuricemia is due to renal underexcretion of uric acid. Diagnosis is suggested by a fractional excretion of uric acid of <5% (normal, 10% to 15%). Controversy exists as to whether lowering serum uric acid slows the progression of renal failure; the studies reporting benefit have usually involved starting a xanthine oxidase inhibitor early in the course of the disease. Isosthenuria and hypertension are common, and some patients have renal salt wasting. Many of the features of FJHN are also seen in medullary cystic kidney disease type 2 (MCKD 2). Most of these patients have a defect in the gene *UMOD*, located on chromosome 16p12, coding for the Tamm-Horsfall/uromodulin protein. There is some evidence that this mutation may interfere with the function of the Na-K-2Cl transporter, leading to a secondary increase in proximal sodium and urate reabsorption.

FANCONI SYNDROME

Introduction and Definition

In the 1930s, de Toni, Debre, and coworkers and Fanconi independently described several children with the combination of renal rickets, glycosuria, and hypophosphatemia. This clinical entity is now called Fanconi syndrome and refers to a global dysfunction of the proximal tubule leading to excessive urinary excretion of amino acids, glucose, phosphate, bicarbonate, and other solutes handled by this nephron segment. These losses lead to the clinical problems of acidosis, dehydration, electrolyte imbalance, rickets, osteomalacia, and growth failure. Numerous disorders, ranging from inborn errors of metabolism to exogenous toxins, are associated with Fanconi syndrome (Fig. 47.6).

Etiology and Pathogenesis

The sequence of events leading to Fanconi syndrome is incompletely defined and probably varies with each cause. Possible

Causes of Fanconi syndrome
Inherited Causes
Cystinosis
Hereditary fructose intolerance
Tyrosinemia
Wilson's disease
Lowe syndrome
Glycogenosis
Mitochondrial cytopathies
Idiopathic
Acquired Causes
Drugs: *cisplatin, ifosfamide,* gentamicin, azathioprine, valproic acid (sodium valproate), suramin, streptozocin (streptozotocin), ranitidine
Dysproteinemias: multiple myeloma, Sjögren syndrome, light-chain proteinuria, amyloidosis
Heavy metal poisoning: lead, cadmium
Other poisonings: glue sniffing, diachrome, Chinese herbal medicine
Other: nephrotic syndrome, renal transplantation, mesenchymal tumors

Figure 47.6   Causes of Fanconi syndrome. More common causes are shown in *italics*.

mechanisms include widespread abnormality of most or all the proximal tubule carriers, for example, a defect in sodium binding to the carrier or insertion of the carrier into the brush border membrane; "leaky" brush border membrane or tight junctions; inhibited or abnormal Na$^+$K$^+$-ATPase pump; or impaired mitochondrial energy generation (see Fig. 47.1). An abnormality in energy generation has been implicated in a number of disorders, including hereditary fructose intolerance, galactosemia, mitochondrial cytopathies, and heavy metal poisoning, as well as in a number of experimental models of Fanconi syndrome. Abnormal subcellular organelle function, such as the lysosome in cystinosis or the megalin-cubulin-endocytic pathway in Dent disease, is also a cause of Fanconi syndrome (Fig. 47.7).

Fanconi syndrome can be inherited or acquired (see Fig. 47.6). In adults, the most common causes of persistent Fanconi syndrome are an endogenous or exogenous toxin, such as a heavy metal or a dysproteinemia; in children, the most common persistent cause is an inborn error of metabolism, such as cystinosis. Specific causes of Fanconi syndrome are discussed after a general description of the clinical manifestations and treatment of the syndrome.

Clinical Manifestations of Fanconi Syndrome

Fanconi syndrome gives rise to a number of abnormalities (Fig. 47.8).

Aminoaciduria

Aminoaciduria is a cardinal feature of Fanconi syndrome. Virtually every amino acid is found in excess in the urine, hence the term *generalized aminoaciduria*. There are, however, no clinical consequences because the losses are trivial in relation to the dietary intake.

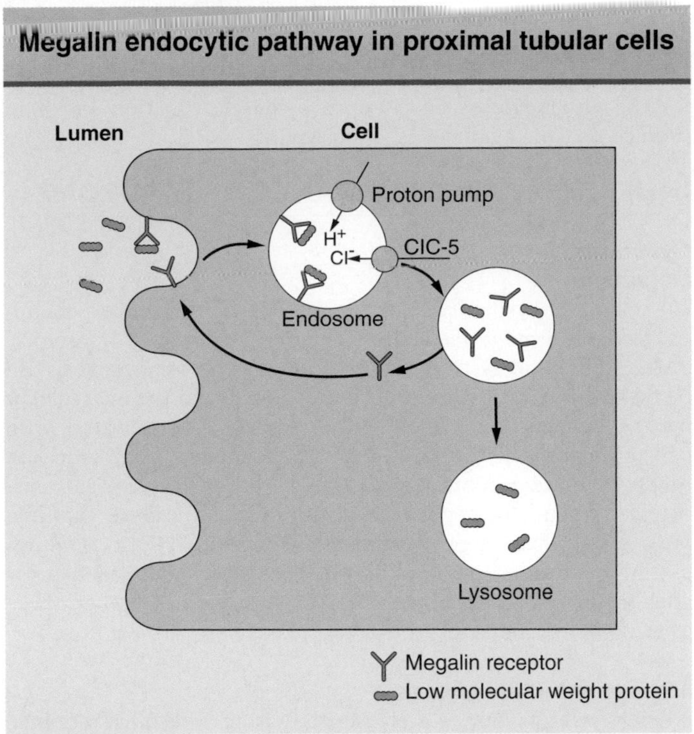

Megalin endocytic pathway in proximal tubular cells

Figure 47.7 **Megalin-cubulin-endocytic pathway in proximal tubular cells.** Low-molecular-weight proteins in the luminal fluid bind to the megalin-cubulin complex and are endocytosed. The recycling of megalin and further catabolism of these proteins are dependent on acidification of the vesicle by a proton pump. The ClC-5 chloride channel provides an electrical shunt for efficient functioning of the proton pump. This endocytosis pathway may also play a role in membrane transporter recycling, and disruption of this pathway could interfere with absorption of other luminal solutes.

Glycosuria

Glycosuria secondary to proximal tubule dysfunction is another of the cardinal features of Fanconi syndrome and occurs because of impaired tubular reabsorption of glucose. It is often one of the first diagnostic clues. Like aminoaciduria, it rarely causes symptoms.

Hypophosphatemia

Hypophosphatemia, secondary to impairment in phosphate reabsorption, is a common finding in Fanconi syndrome. Assessment of tubular phosphate handling can be made by measuring the maximum phosphate reabsorption in relation to the glomerular filtration rate (T_mP/GFR) on fasting urine and blood samples. Elevated parathyroid hormone (PTH) and low vitamin D levels also may play a role in the phosphaturia of Fanconi syndrome, although these hormonal abnormalities are not always present. A few patients have impaired conversion of 25-hydroxyvitamin D to 1,25-hydroxyvitamin D; metabolic acidosis, another feature of Fanconi syndrome, may also impair this conversion. Another possible mechanism for the hypophosphatemia is impairment of the megalin-dependent reabsorption and degradation of filtered PTH. Unabsorbed PTH could then bind to receptors in more distal portions of the proximal tubule. This would lead to increased endocytosis of apical phosphate transporters and increased phosphaturia. The hypophosphatemia, especially if accompanied by hyperparathyroidism and low 1,25-hydroxyvitamin D levels, often leads to significant bone disease, presenting with pain, fractures, rickets, or growth failure.

Features of Fanconi syndrome

Metabolic Abnormalities
Hyperaminoaciduria
Glucosuria
Hypophosphatemia
Hypokalemia
Hypouricemia
Hypocarnitinemia
Clinical Features
Rickets, osteomalacia
Growth retardation
Polyuria
Dehydration
Proteinuria
Acidosis

Figure 47.8 **Features of Fanconi syndrome.**

Hyperchloremic Metabolic Acidosis

Hyperchloremic metabolic acidosis, another feature of Fanconi syndrome, is a result of impaired bicarbonate reabsorption by the proximal tubule (proximal, or type II renal tubular acidosis [RTA], see Chapter 12). This impaired reabsorption can lead to the loss of more than 30% of the normal filtered load. As the serum bicarbonate falls, the filtered load falls, and excretion drops such that the serum bicarbonate usually remains between 12 and 18 mmol/l. Occasionally, there is an associated defect in distal acidification, usually in association with long-standing hypokalemia or nephrocalcinosis. Ammoniagenesis is usually normal or increased, because of the hypokalemia and acidosis, unless there is an associated impairment in GFR.

Natriuresis and Kaliuresis

Natriuresis and kaliuresis are common in Fanconi syndrome and can give rise to significant, even life-threatening, problems. These electrolyte losses are, in part, related to impaired bicarbonate reabsorption, with the subsequent urinary excretion of sodium and potassium ions with the bicarbonate. In some cases, sodium and potassium losses are so great that metabolic alkalosis and hyperaldosteronism result, simulating Bartter syndrome despite the lowered bicarbonate threshold. The clearance of potassium may be twice that of the GFR, and the resulting hypokalemia can cause sudden death.

Polyuria and Polydipsia

Polyuria, polydipsia, and frequent bouts of severe dehydration are common symptoms in young patients with Fanconi syndrome. The polyuria is mainly related to the osmotic diuresis from the excessive urinary solute losses, but in some patients, there is an associated concentrating defect, especially in patients with prolonged hypokalemia.

Growth Retardation

Growth retardation in children with Fanconi syndrome is multifactorial. Hypophosphatemia, disordered vitamin D metabolism, and acidosis contribute to growth failure, as do chronic hypokalemia and extracellular volume contraction. Glycosuria and aminoaciduria probably do not play a role. However, even with correction of all these metabolic abnormalities, most patients fail to grow, especially those with cystinosis.

Hypouricemia

Hypouricemia, caused by impairment in renal handling of uric acid, is often present in Fanconi syndrome, especially in adults. Urolithiasis from the uricosuria has only rarely been reported, probably because the urine flow and pH are increased, inhibiting uric acid crystallization.

Proteinuria

Proteinuria, another feature of Fanconi syndrome, is usually minimal, except when Fanconi syndrome develops in association with the nephrotic syndrome. Typically, only low-molecular-weight proteins (<30,000 daltons) are excreted, for example, enzymes, immunoglobulins, light chains, and hormones.

Treatment of Fanconi Syndrome

Therapy, whenever possible, should be directed at the underlying causes (see later discussion), for example, avoidance of the offending nutrient in galactosemia, hereditary fructose intolerance, or tyrosinemia; treatment of Wilson's disease with penicillamine and other copper chelators; or treatment of heavy metal intoxication by chelation therapy. In these cases, resolution of Fanconi syndrome usually is complete.

In other instances, therapy is directed at the biochemical abnormalities secondary to the renal solute losses and at the bone disease that is often present in these patients. The proximal RTA usually requires large doses of alkali for correction. Some patients benefit from hydrochlorothiazide to minimize the volume expansion associated with these large doses of alkali. Potassium supplementation is also commonly needed, especially if there is a significant RTA. The use of potassium citrate, lactate, or acetate will correct not only the hypokalemia but also the acidosis. A few patients will require sodium supplementation along with potassium. Again, the use of a metabolizable anion will aid in the correction of the acidosis. Rarely, patients may need sodium chloride supplementation. Usually, these patients have alkalosis when untreated as a result of large urinary sodium chloride losses, which lead to volume contraction that overrides the RTA. Magnesium supplementation may be required. Adequate fluid intake is essential. Correction of hypokalemia and its effect on the concentrating ability of the distal tubule may lessen the polyuria.

Bone disease is multifactorial, including hypophosphatemia, decreased synthesis of calcitriol in some patients, hypercalciuria, and chronic acidosis. Hypophosphatemia should be treated with 1 to 3 g/day of oral phosphate with the goal of normalizing serum phosphate levels. Many patients will require supplemental vitamin D for adequate treatment of the rickets and osteomalacia. It is unclear whether standard vitamin D (calciferol [ergocalciferol]) or a vitamin D metabolite is better for supplementation. Currently, most clinicians use a vitamin D metabolite, such as 1.25-dihydroxycholecalciferol (calcitriol). These metabolites obviate the concern of inadequate vitamin D hydroxylation by the proximal tubule mitochondria and reduce the risk for prolonged hypercalcemia because of their shorter half-life. Vitamin D therapy will also improve the hypophosphatemia and lessen the risk for hyperparathyroidism. Supplemental calcium is indicated in those with hypocalcemia after starting supplemental vitamin D.

Hyperaminoaciduria, glycosuria, proteinuria, and hyperuricosuria usually do not lead to clinical difficulties and do not require specific treatment. Carnitine supplementation, to compensate for the urinary losses, may improve muscle function and lipid profiles, but the evidence is inconsistent.

INHERITED CAUSES OF FANCONI SYNDROME

Cystinosis
Definition
Cystinosis, or cystine storage disease, is characterized biochemically by excessive intracellular storage, particularly in lysosomes, of the amino acid cystine.[7] Three different types of cystinosis can be distinguished, based on the clinical course and the intracellular cystine content. Benign or adult cystinosis is associated with cystine crystals in the cornea and bone marrow only and the mildest elevation in intracellular cystine levels; there is no renal disease. Infantile or nephropathic cystinosis is the most common form and is associated with the highest intracellular levels of cystine and the earliest onset of renal disease. The intermediate or adolescent form has intracellular cystine levels in between those of the infantile and adult forms and later onset of renal disease.

Etiology and Pathogenesis
Nephropathic cystinosis is transmitted as an autosomal recessive trait localized to the short arm of chromosome 17, with an estimated incidence of 1 in 200,000 live births. *CTNS*, a gene mapped to chromosome 17p13, codes for a lysosomal membrane protein, cystinosin, which mediates the transport of cystine from the lysosome.[8] A number of mutations have been described in this gene in children with nephropathic cystinosis, the most common being a large 57-kb deletion. Both the benign and intermediate forms of cystinosis are also associated with mutations in this gene. However, in these patients, the mutations still result in some functional transport protein leading to lower intracellular cystine levels and slower onset of renal disease in the intermediate form and no renal disease in the benign form.

Clinical Manifestations
The first clinical symptoms and signs in nephropathic cystinosis are those of Fanconi syndrome and usually appear in the latter half of the first year of life. Subtle abnormalities of tubular function can be demonstrated earlier in families with index cases, but there always is a delay between birth and the first symptoms. Rickets is common after the first year of life, along with growth failure. The growth failure occurs before the GFR declines and despite correction of electrolyte and mineral deficiencies. The GFR invariably declines, and end-stage renal disease (ESRD) occurs by late childhood. Nephrocalcinosis is relatively common, and a few patients have developed renal calculi. Photophobia is another common symptom that occurs by 3 years of age and is progressive. Older patients with cystinosis may develop visual impairment and blindness. Children with cystinosis usually have fair complexions and blond hair, but dark hair has been observed in some. Cystinosis has been observed in other ethnic groups but is less common than in Caucasians. The diagnosis is based on the demonstration of elevated intracellular levels of cystine, usually in white blood cells or skin fibroblasts. Patients with nephropathic and intermediate cystinosis have intracellular cystine levels that exceed 2 nmol half cystine/mg protein. Normal patients have levels that are less than 0.2 nmol half-cystine/mg protein. Heterozygotes for cystinosis will have levels that range from 0.2 to 1 nmol half-cystine/mg protein. A slit-lamp demonstration of corneal crystals is strongly suggestive

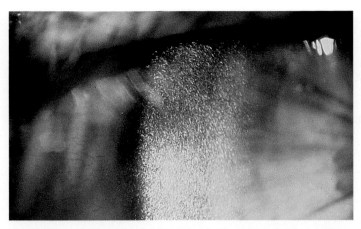

Figure 47.9   Corneal opacities in cystinosis. Tinsel-like refractile opacities in the cornea of a patient with cystinosis under slit-lamp examination. (From Foreman JW: Cystinosis and the Fanconi syndrome. In Avner ED, Harmon WE, Niaudet P [eds]: Pediatric Nephrology, 5th ed. Philadelphia, Lippincott Williams & Wilkins, 2004, p 789.)

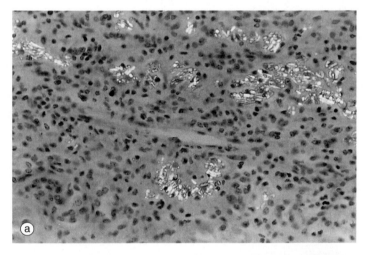

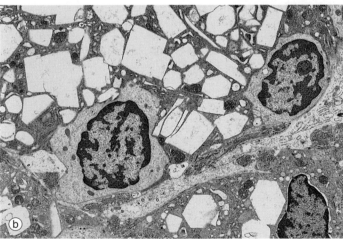

Figure 47.10   Cystine crystals in the kidney in cystinosis. *a*, Crystals are seen in a photomicrograph of an alcohol-fixed nephrectomy specimen, taken through incompletely crossed polarizing filters. Birefringent crystals are evident in tubular epithelial cells and free in the interstitium. *b*, Electron micrograph of a renal biopsy showing hexagonal, rectangular, and needle-shaped crystals in macrophages within the interstitium (original magnification × 3000). (*a*, From Schnaper HW, Cottel J, Merrill S, et al: Early occurrence of end-stage renal disease in a patient with infantile nephropathic cystinosis. J Pediatr 1992;120:576; *b*, from van't Hoff WG, Ledermann SE, Waldron M, Trompter RS: Early-onset chronic renal failure as a presentation of infantile cystinosis. Pediatr Nephrol 1995;9:483–484.)

of the diagnosis[9] (Fig. 47.9). A prenatal diagnosis can be made with amniocytes or chorionic villi.

Common late complications of cystinosis include hypothyroidism, splenomegaly and hepatomegaly, decreased visual acuity, swallowing difficulties, and corneal ulcerations. Less commonly, older patients have developed insulin-dependent diabetes mellitus, myopathy, and progressive neurologic disorders. Decreased brain cortex has also been noted in some patients.

Pathology

The morphologic features of the kidney in cystinosis vary with the stage of the disease. Early in the disease, cystine crystals are present in tubular epithelial cells, interstitial cells, and rarely, glomerular epithelial cells[10,11] (Fig. 47.10a). A swan-neck deformity or thinning of the first part of the proximal tubule is an early finding, but is not unique to cystinosis. Later, there is pronounced tubular atrophy, interstitial fibrosis, and abundant crystal deposition with giant cell formation of the glomerular visceral epithelium, segmental sclerosis, and eventual glomerular obsolescence. Electron microscopy studies have demonstrated intracellular crystalline inclusions consistent with cystine (see Fig. 47.10b). Peculiar "dark cells," unique to the cystinotic kidney, have also been observed.

Treatment

Until recently, treatment of infantile cystinosis has been limited to vitamin D therapy and replacement of the urinary electrolyte losses, followed, in due course, by the management of the progressive renal failure. (Fig. 47.11) Cysteamine has now been shown to lower tissue cystine and to slow the decline in GFR, especially in children with a normal serum creatinine treated before 2 years of age[12] (Fig. 47.12). Cysteamine therapy also improves linear growth but not Fanconi syndrome. The most common problems associated with cysteamine therapy are

Treatment of cystinosis	
Problem	**Therapy**
Removal of lysosomal cystine	Cysteamine, 0.325 g/m²q 6hr to maintain leukocyte cystine level <1 nmol half-cystine*/mg protein
Correction of Tubulopathy	
Dehydration	2–6 l/d fluid
Acidosis	2–15 mg/kg/d K⁺ citrate
Hypophosphatemia	1–4 g/d K⁺ phosphate
Rickets	0.25–1 μg/d calcitriol
Adjunct therapies	NaCl, carnitine, indomethacin, hydrochlorothiazide
Later Therapies	
Growth failure	Growth hormone
Hypothyroidism	Thyroxine
Renal failure	Renal replacement therapy, ideally renal transplantation

Figure 47.11   Treatment of cystinosis. *By convention, units are half-cystine because the cystine originally was converted to two cystine molecules, or "broken in half," before measurement.

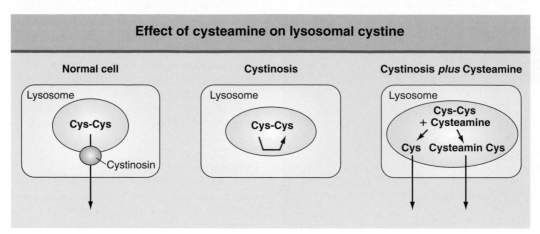

Figure 47.12   Effect of cysteamine on lysosomal cystine. In cystinosis, the transporter (cystinosin) for cystine (Cys-Cys) egress from the lysosome is defective. Cysteamine can easily enter the lysosome and combine with cystine, forming cysteine (Cys) and the mixed disulfide cysteamine-cysteine. Both of these compounds can exit the lysosome through a transporter other than the cystine carrier.

nausea, vomiting, and a foul odor and taste. Treatment should begin with a low dose of cysteamine soon after the diagnosis is made, increased over 4 to 6 weeks to 1.3 g/m² daily in four divided doses as close to every 6 hours as possible. Slowly increasing the dose minimizes the risk for a serum sickness–like reaction. Leukocyte cystine levels should be checked every 3 to 4 months to monitor effectiveness and compliance, with the goal of achieving and maintaining a cystine level of below 2.0 and preferably below 1.0 nmol half cystine/mg protein. A 50 mM solution of cysteamine applied topically onto the eye has proved useful in depleting the cornea of cystine crystals but requires administration 6 to 12 times a day to be effective.

Treatment of ESRD in these children poses no greater problems than with other children. Successful renal transplantation reverses the renal failure and Fanconi syndrome but does not appear to improve the extrarenal manifestations of cystinosis. Cystine does not accumulate in the transplanted kidney, except in infiltrating immunocytes.

Galactosemia
Etiology and Pathogenesis
Galactosemia is an autosomal recessively inherited disorder of galactose metabolism. It is most commonly the result of deficient activity of the enzyme galactose 1-phosphate uridyl transferase; this occurs with an incidence of 1 in 62,000 live births.[13] The gene for this enzyme is found on the short arm of chromosome 9. Deficiency of this enzyme leads to the intracellular accumulation of galactose 1-phosphate, with damage to the liver, proximal renal tubule, ovary, brain, and lens. A less frequent cause of galactosemia is a deficiency of galactose kinase, which forms galactose 1-phosphate from galactose. Cataracts are the only manifestation of this form of galactosemia. The pathogenesis of the symptoms of galactosemia is not clear. Accumulation of galactose 1-phosphate subsequent to the ingestion of galactose can inhibit a number of pathways for carbohydrate metabolism, and there is some correlation of its level with clinical symptoms. Defective galactosylation of proteins has also been postulated. Formation of galactitol from galactose by aldose reductase has been proposed as a pathogenetic mechanism, and this is probably responsible for the cataract formation.

Clinical Manifestations
Affected infants ingesting milk containing lactose, the most common source of galactose in the diet, rapidly develop vomiting,

diarrhea, and failure to thrive. Jaundice from unconjugated hyperbilirubinemia is common, along with severe hemolysis. Continued intake of galactose leads to hepatomegaly and cirrhosis. Cataracts appear within days after birth, although they often are detectable only with a slit lamp. Mental retardation may develop within a few months. Fulminant *Escherichia coli* sepsis has been described in a number of infants, which may be a consequence of inhibited leukocyte bactericidal activity.

In addition to these clinical findings, galactose intake leads within days to hyperaminoaciduria and albuminuria. Raised urine sugar excretion is principally a result of galactosuria and not glucosuria. There seems to be little or no impairment in glucose handling by the renal tubule. Galactosemia should be suspected whenever there is a urinary reducing substance that does not react in a glucose oxidase test. The diagnosis can be confirmed by demonstrating deficient transferase activity in red blood cells, fibroblasts, leukocytes, or hepatocytes.

Treatment
Galactosemia is treated by eliminating galactose from the diet. Acute symptoms and signs resolve in a few days. Cataracts will also regress to some extent. However, even with early elimination of galactose, developmental delay, speech impairment, ovarian dysfunction, and growth retardation are a common outcome in galactosemia. Profound intellectual deficits are rare even in infants treated late.

Hereditary Fructose Intolerance
Etiology and Pathogenesis
Hereditary fructose intolerance is another disorder of carbohydrate metabolism associated with Fanconi syndrome.[14] It is inherited as an autosomal recessive trait with an incidence estimated to be 1 in 20,000. It is caused by a deficiency of the B isoform of the enzyme fructose 1-phosphate aldolase, which cleaves fructose 1-phosphate into D-glyceraldehyde and dihydroxyacetone phosphate. Deficient activity of aldolase B leads to tissue accumulation of fructose 1-phosphate and reduced levels of adenosine triphosphate (ATP). The gene for aldolase B resides on the long arm of chromosome 9.

Clinical Manifestations
Symptoms of hereditary fructose intolerance appear at weaning when fruit, vegetables, and sweetened cereals that contain fructose

or sucrose are introduced. Children with this disorder experience nausea, vomiting, and symptoms of hypoglycemia shortly after ingesting fructose, sucrose, or sorbitol. These symptoms may progress to convulsions, coma, and even death, depending on the amount consumed. Young infants, when exposed to fructose, may have a catastrophic illness, with severe dehydration, shock, acute liver impairment, bleeding, or acute renal failure. Concomitant serum biochemical findings after fructose ingestion are a fall in glucose, phosphate, and bicarbonate with a rise in uric acid and lactic acid. Chronic exposure to fructose leads to failure to thrive, hepatomegaly, jaundice, hepatic cirrhosis, and nephrocalcinosis. Children with hereditary fructose intolerance learn to avoid sweets and as a result have few dental caries.

Diagnosis

The diagnosis should be suspected when symptoms develop after the ingestion of fructose. Confirmation can be made either by a carefully applied fructose tolerance test or by assaying the activity of fructose 1-phosphate aldolase in a liver biopsy specimen.

Treatment

Treatment involves strict avoidance of foods containing fructose and sucrose. Most patients develop a strong aversion to such foods, making this interdiction easy. The greatest risk occurs during infancy before affected individuals learn to avoid fructose.

Glycogenosis

Most patients with glycogen storage disease and Fanconi syndrome have an autosomal recessive disorder characterized by heavy glycosuria and glycogen storage in the liver and kidney, known as the Fanconi-Bickel syndrome, or a renal glucose-losing syndrome because the glucose losses can be massive.[15] The defect is deficient activity of the sugar transporter, GLUT2 (see Fig. 47.2). GLUT2 facilitates sugar exit from the basolateral side of the proximal tubule and intestinal cell and sugar entry and exit from the hepatocyte and pancreatic β-cell. A few patients with type I glycogen storage disease have mild Fanconi syndrome, but not Fanconi-Bickel syndrome. The therapy of this disorder is directed at the renal solute losses, treatment of rickets, which can be quite severe and frequent feeding to prevent ketosis. Uncooked cornstarch has been shown to lessen the hypoglycemia and improve growth.

Tyrosinemia
Definition

Hereditary tyrosinemia type I, also known as hepatorenal tyrosinemia, is a defect of tyrosine metabolism affecting the liver, kidneys, and peripheral nerves.[16]

Etiology and Pathogenesis

The cause of hereditary tyrosinemia type I is a deficiency of fumarylacetoacetate hydrolase (FAH) activity. It is an autosomal recessive disorder carried on the long arm of chromosome 15. Decreased or absent FAH activity leads to accumulation of maleylacetoacetate (MAA) and fumarylacetoacetate (FAA) in affected tissues. These compounds can react with free sulfydryl groups, reduce intracellular levels of glutathione, and act as alkylating agents. MAA and FAA are not detectable in plasma or urine but are converted to succinylacetoacetate and succinylacetone. The latter is structurally similar to maleic acid, a compound that causes

Fanconi syndrome experimentally in rats and may be the cause of Fanconi syndrome in humans affected with tyrosinemia.

Clinical Manifestations

The liver is the major organ affected, and this may be evident as early as the first month of life. Such infants usually have severe disease and die in the first year of life. All children will eventually develop macronodular cirrhosis, and many develop hepatocellular carcinoma. Acute, painful peripheral neuropathy and autonomic dysfunction can also occur in tyrosinemia. Proximal renal tubular dysfunction is evident in all patients with tyrosinemia, especially those presenting after infancy. Nephromegaly is very common, and nephrocalcinosis may be seen. Glomerulosclerosis and impaired GFR may be seen with time.

Diagnosis

The diagnosis should be suspected with elevated plasma tyrosine and methionine levels together with their p-hydroxy metabolites. The presence of succinylacetone in blood or urine is diagnostic of hereditary tyrosinemia type I.

Treatment

The institution of a diet low in phenylalanine and tyrosine dramatically improves the renal tubular dysfunction. Nitrotrifluorobenzoylcyclohexadione, which inhibits the formation of MAA and FAA, dramatically improves the renal and hepatic dysfunction.[16] Liver transplantation has been successfully used to treat patients with severe liver failure and to prevent the development of hepatoma. Liver transplantation leads to rapid correction of Fanconi syndrome.

Wilson's Disease
Definition

Wilson's disease is an inherited disorder of copper metabolism that affects numerous organ systems.[17] It has an overall incidence of 1 in 30,000. About 40% of patients present with liver disease, 40% with extrapyramidal symptoms, and 20% with psychiatric or behavioral abnormalities.

Etiology and Pathogenesis

Wilson's disease is a defect in a P-type copper-transporting ATPase in the liver. It impairs biliary copper excretion and the incorporation of copper into ceruloplasmin. These abnormalities cause excessive intracellular accumulation of copper in the liver, with subsequent overflow into other tissues such as brain, cornea, and renal proximal tubule. The gene for this enzyme has been localized to chromosome 13q14.3.

Clinical Manifestations

Excessive storage of copper in the kidney leads to renal tubular dysfunction in most patients and full-blown Fanconi syndrome in some. Hematuria also has been noted. Renal plasma flow and GFR decrease as the disease progresses, but death from extrarenal causes occurs before the onset of renal failure. Fanconi syndrome usually appears before the onset of hepatic failure. Hypercalciuria with the development of renal stones and nephrocalcinosis also has been reported. Besides proximal tubular dysfunction, abnormalities in distal tubular function, decreased concentrating ability, and distal RTA have also been observed.

Pathology

Histologically, the kidney in untreated Wilson's disease shows either no alteration on light microscopy or only some flattened proximal tubular cells without recognizable brush borders. Electron microscopy shows loss of the brush border, disruption of the apical tubular network, electron-dense bodies probably representing metalloproteins in the subapical region of tubule cell cytoplasm, and cavitation of the mitochondria with disruption of the normal cristae pattern. Rubeanic acid staining shows intracytoplasmic copper granules. The copper content of kidney tissue is markedly elevated.

Diagnosis

The diagnosis of Wilson's disease should be suspected in children and young adults with unexplained neurologic disease, chronic active hepatitis, acute hemolytic crisis, behavioral or psychiatric disturbances, or the appearance of Fanconi syndrome. In such patients, the presence of Kayser-Fleischer rings is an important clue in making the diagnosis. Serum ceruloplasmin levels are decreased in 96% of patients with Wilson's disease. A markedly increased urinary copper level is also useful in making the diagnosis, especially if it increases significantly with D-penicillamine. Liver copper levels are increased in untreated patients.

Treatment

Treatment with D-penicillamine reverses the renal dysfunction and may reverse the hepatic and neurologic disease, depending on the degree of damage before the onset of therapy. Recovery, however, is quite slow. Trientine can also chelate copper and is indicated in patients who cannot tolerate D-penicillamine. Tetrathiomolybdate is a very potent agent in removing copper from the body and has been used in some patients with neurologic disease to prevent the immediate worsening of symptoms that can occur with penicillamine. Zinc salts, which induce intestinal metallothionein and blockade of intestinal absorption of copper, are useful in maintenance therapy. Liver transplantation has been successful in some patients but should be reserved for those with liver failure.

Lowe Syndrome

Lowe syndrome (oculocerebrorenal syndrome) is characterized by congenital cataracts and glaucoma, severe mental retardation, hypotonia with diminished-to-absent reflexes, and renal abnormalities.[18] Fanconi syndrome is followed by progressive renal insufficiency. ESRD usually does not occur until the third to fourth decade of life.

Lowe syndrome is transmitted as an X-linked recessive trait mapped to Xp24-26. Despite this inheritance pattern, Lowe syndrome has occurred in a few females. This gene codes for a phosphatidylinositol bisphosphate phosphatase localized in the Golgi complex.

Light microscopy of the kidney is normal early in the disorder, with endothelial cell swelling and thickening and splitting of the glomerular basement membrane seen by electron microscopy. In the proximal tubule cells, there is shortening of the brush border and enlargement of the mitochondria, with distortion and loss of the cristae. Only symptomatic treatment is available.

Dent Disease
Definition

Dent disease is an X-linked recessive disorder characterized by low-molecular-weight proteinuria, hypercalciuria, nephrolithiasis, nephrocalcinosis, and rickets.[19] In addition, affected males often have aminoaciduria, phosphaturia, and glucosuria. Renal failure is common and may occur by late childhood. Hemizygous females usually have only proteinuria and mild hypercalciuria. X-linked recessive nephrolithiasis, X-linked recessive hypophosphatemic rickets, and Japanese idiopathic low-molecular-weight proteinuria have similar features and all are now known to be part of the clinical spectrum of a defect in the renal ClC-5 chloride channel.

Etiology and Pathogenesis

All these disorders are caused by a mutation in the *CLCN5* gene located on chromosome Xp11.22 leading to inactive ClC-5 chloride channel function. The ClC-5 chloride channel spans the membrane of pre-endocytic vesicles just below the brush border of the proximal tubule. There it facilitates the entry of Cl⁻ that is necessary for the active acidification of the vesicles by a proton pump. Lack of this Cl⁻ channel interferes with protein reabsorption from the tubule through the megalin-cubilin receptor system and cell surface receptor recycling, which may explain the phosphaturia, glucosuria, and aminoaciduria.

Filtered parathyroid hormone (PTH) is also reabsorbed by the megalin-cubilin system for degradation in the lysosome. Decreased PTH reabsorption allows increased binding to luminal PTH receptors and increased endocytosis of luminal phosphate transporters, leading to increased phosphaturia.

Mitochondrial Cytopathies
Definition

Mitochondrial cytopathies are a diverse group of diseases with abnormalities in mitochondrial DNA that lead to mitochondrial dysfunction in various tissues.[20]

Clinical Manifestations

Most of the mitochondrial cytopathies present with neurologic disorders such as myopathy, myoclonus, ataxia, seizures, external ophthalmoplegia, strokelike episodes, and optic neuropathy. Other manifestations include pigmentary retinitis, diabetes mellitus, exocrine pancreatic insufficiency, sideroblastic anemia, sensorineural hearing loss, pseudo-obstruction of the colon, hepatic disease, cardiac conduction disorders, and cardiomyopathy. These various manifestations tend to group together in specific syndromes and reflect specific mutations in mitochondrial DNA (Fig. 47.13).

The most common renal manifestation associated with mitochondrial cytopathies is Fanconi syndrome, although a number of patients have been described with focal segmental glomerulosclerosis and steroid-resistant nephrotic syndrome. All the patients

Mitochondrial cytopathies
MERRF: myoclonic epilepsy with ragged red fibers
NARP: neuropathy, ataxia, and retinitis pigmentosa
MELAS: mitochondrial encephalopathy, lactic acidosis, and strokelike episodes
LHON: Leber's hereditary optic neuropathy
Leigh disease: maternally inherited Leigh disease (somnolence, blindness, deafness, peripheral neuropathy, degeneration of brainstem)
Pearson's syndrome: pancytopenia, exocrine pancreatic deficiency, hepatic dysfunction
Kearns-Sayre syndrome: ophthalmoplegia, pigmentary retinopathy, heart block, ataxia
Alpers' disease: intractable epilepsy, liver disease, neuronal degeneration

Figure 47.13 Mitochondrial cytopathies.

with renal abnormalities have had extrarenal disorders, mainly neurologic disease. Most patients present in the first months of life and die soon afterward.

Diagnosis

A clue to these disorders is elevated serum or cerebrospinal fluid lactate levels, especially if associated with an altered lactate-to-pyruvate ratio, suggesting a defect in mitochondrial respiration. The presence of "ragged red fibers," a manifestation of abnormal mitochondria, in a muscle biopsy is another clue, especially with large abnormal mitochondria on electron microscopy of muscle tissue.

Treatment

There is little to offer these patients in terms of definitive therapy. Low complex III activity can be treated with menadione or ubidecarenone. Deficient complex I activity may be treated with riboflavin and ubidecarenone. Ascorbic acid has been used to minimize oxygen free radical injury. High-lipid, low-carbohydrate diet has been tried in cytochrome *c* oxidase deficiency.

Idiopathic Fanconi Syndrome

A number of patients develop the complete Fanconi syndrome in the absence of any known cause. Traditionally, these cases have been called *adult Fanconi syndrome* because it was thought that only adults were affected. However, it is clear that children may be affected, and a more proper designation is idiopathic Fanconi syndrome. All the features of Fanconi syndrome may not be present when the patients are first seen but do appear with time. Idiopathic Fanconi syndrome can be inherited in an autosomal dominant, autosomal recessive, or even X-linked pattern. However, most cases occur sporadically, without any evidence of genetic transmission. The prognosis is quite variable, and some develop chronic renal failure 10 to 30 years after the onset of symptoms. A few patients have undergone renal transplantation, and in some of these, Fanconi syndrome has recurred in the allograft without evidence of rejection, suggesting an extrarenal cause for the idiopathic Fanconi syndrome.

Renal morphologic descriptions of such cases are scanty. In some reports, no abnormalities were found, and in others, tubular atrophy with interstitial fibrosis was interspersed with areas of tubular dilation. Markedly dilated proximal tubules with swollen epithelium and grossly enlarged mitochondria with displaced cristae have also been noted.

ACQUIRED CAUSES OF FANCONI SYNDROME

Numerous substances can injure the proximal renal tubule (see Fig. 47.6), and this injury can range from an incomplete Fanconi syndrome to acute tubular necrosis and renal failure. The extent of the tubular damage is quite variable and is dependent on the type of toxin, the amount ingested, and the host. A careful history of possible toxin exposure is therefore important in patients with tubular dysfunction.

Heavy Metal Intoxication

A major cause of proximal tubular dysfunction is heavy metal intoxication, principally lead and cadmium. In lead poisoning, the renal tubular dysfunction, mainly aminoaciduria and mild glycosuria and phosphaturia, is usually overshadowed by the involvement of other organs, especially the central nervous system. Fanconi syndrome associated with cadmium poisoning is associated with severe bone pain, giving rise to the name *itai-itai* ("ouch-ouch") *disease* for its occurrence in Japanese patients affected by industrial contamination of the soil.

Tetracycline

Outdated tetracycline causes a reversible Fanconi syndrome even in therapeutic doses. Recovery is rapid when the degraded drug is stopped. The compound responsible for the tubule dysfunction is anhydro-4-tetracycline formed from tetracycline by heat, moisture, and a low pH.

Cancer Chemotherapy Agents

A number of cancer chemotherapy agents have been associated with Fanconi syndrome and renal tubule dysfunction, especially cisplatin and ifosfamide. Carboplatin has been associated with reduced GFR and magnesium wasting but not Fanconi syndrome. The nephrotoxicity of both is dose dependent and often irreversible. Besides the usual manifestations of Fanconi syndrome, cisplatin toxicity is characterized by hypomagnesemia, caused by hypermagnesuria, which can be extremely severe, persistent, and difficult to treat. Ifosfamide is more commonly associated with hypophosphatemic rickets. Chloroacetaldehyde, a metabolite of ifosfamide, appears experimentally to cause Fanconi syndrome. Both ifosfamide and cisplatin can cause an irreversible reduction in GFR.

Other Drugs and Toxins

Exposure to a wide range of toxins may give rise to Fanconi syndrome, often in association with a reduced GFR, including methyl 3-chromone (diachrome), 6-mercaptopurine, toluene (glue sniffing), and Chinese herbal medicines containing an *Aristolochia* species. There have also been anecdotal reports associating Fanconi syndrome with valproic acid (valproate), suramin, Lysol (a cresol-based antiseptic), gentamicin, and ranitidine.

Dysproteinemias

Dysproteinemia from multiple myeloma, light-chain proteinuria, Sjögren syndrome, and amyloidosis is sometimes associated with Fanconi syndrome, which appears to be correlated with specific light chains or light-chain fragments (Bence-Jones proteins) that crystallize within the tubular cells.

Glomerular Disease

Nephrotic syndrome has rarely been associated with Fanconi syndrome. Most of these patients have focal segmental glomerulosclerosis, and the occurrence of Fanconi syndrome heralds a poor prognosis.

After Acute Tubular Necrosis

Tubular dysfunction during recovery from acute renal failure from any cause can occur, whether or not a known tubular toxin was originally implicated.

After Renal Transplantation

Fanconi syndrome has appeared rarely after renal transplantation. The pathogenesis probably is multifactorial, for example, sequelae of acute tubular necrosis, rejection, nephrotoxic drugs, ischemia from renal artery stenosis, and residual hyperparathyroidism.

REFERENCES

1. Brodehl J, Oemer BS, Hoyer PF: Renal glucosuria. Pediatr Nephrol 1987;1:502–508.
2. Chillaron J, Roca R, Valencia A, et al: Heteromeric aminoacid transporters: Biochemistry, genetics, and physiology. Am J Physiol Renal Physiol 2001; 281:F995–1018.
3. Reynolds TM: Best Clinical Practice No 181. Chemical pathology, clinical investigation, and management of nephrolithiasis. J Clin Pathol 2005:58:134–140.
4. Strologo LD, Pras E, Pontesilli C, et al: Comparison between SLC3A1 and SLC7A9 cystinuria patients and carriers: A need for a new classification. J Am Soc Nephrol 2002;13:2547–2523.
5. Sperling O: Hereditary renal hypouricemia. In: Scriver CR, Beaudet AL, et al (eds): Metabolic and Molecular Bases of Inherited Disease, 8th ed. New York, McGraw-Hill, 2001, pp 5069–5085.
6. Dahan K, Devuyst O, Smaers M, et al: Cluster of mutations in the UMOD gene causes familial juvenile hyperuricemic nephropathy with abnormal excretion of uromodulin. J Am Soc Nephrol 2003;14: 2883–2893.
7. Gahl WA, Thoene JG, Schneider JA: Cystinosis. N Engl J Med 2002; 347:111–121.
8. Town M, Jean G, Cherqui S, et al: A novel gene encoding an integral membrane protein is mutated in nephropathic cystinosis. Nat Genet 1998;18:319–324.
9. Foreman JW: Cystinosis and the Fanconi syndrome. In Avner ED, Harmon WE, Niaudet P (eds): Pediatric Nephrology, 5th ed. Philadelphia, Lippincott Williams & Wilkins, 2004, p 789.
10. Schnaper HW, Cottel J, Merrill S, et al: Early occurrence of end-stage renal disease in a patient with infantile nephropathic cystinosis. J Pediatr 1992;120:576.
11. van't Hoff WG, Ledermann SE, Waldron M, Trompter RS: Early-onset chronic renal failure as a presentation of infantile cystinosis. Pediatr Nephrol 1995;9:483–484.
12. Kleta R, Gahl WA: Pharmacological treatment of nephropathic cystinosis with cysteamine. Expert Opin Pharmacother 2004;5:2255–2262.
13. Tyfield LA: Galactosemia and allelic variation at the galactose-1-phophate uridyltransferase gene: A complex relationship between genotype and phenotype. Eur J Pediatr 2000;159:S204–207.
14. Wong D: Hereditary fructose intolerance. Mol Genet Metab 2005;85: 165–167.
15. Santer S, Steinmenn B, Schaub J: Fanconi-Bickel syndrome: A congenital defect of facilitative glucose transport. Curr Mol Med 2002;2:213–227.
16. Grompe M: The pathophysiology and treatment of hereditary tyrosinemia type I. Semin Liver Dis 2001;21:563–571.
17. Riordan SM, Williams R: The Wilson's gene and phenotypic diversity. J Hepatol 2001;34:165–171.
18. Charnas LR, Bernadini I, Radar D, et al: Clinical and laboratory finding in the oculocerebrorenal syndrome of Lowe, with special reference to growth and renal function. N Engl J Med 1991;324:1318–1325.
19. Thakker RV: Pathogenesis of Dent's disease and related syndromes of X-linked nephrolithiasis. Kidney Int 2000;57:787–793.
20. Niaudet P, Roetig A: Renal involvement in mitochondrial cytopathies. Pediatr Nephrol 1996;10:368–373.

Jan C. ter Maaten, Rijk O. B. Gans, and Paul E. de Jong

INTRODUCTION AND DEFINITIONS

Sickle cell disease is an autosomal recessive inherited disorder, predominantly of the African American race. The gene for sickle hemoglobin (hemoglobin S, or HbS) results in the replacement of the normal glutamine by valine in the β-globin subunit, thereby changing the configuration of the hemoglobin molecule and enhancing the aggregation of hemoglobin molecules. This aggregation decreases the pliability of the red cells and may distort their shape to a characteristic crescentic or sickle shape. This event results in premature destruction of red cells (hemolysis) and frequent, widespread vaso-occlusive episodes with subsequent organ damage. Sickle cell anemia occurs in those homozygous for HbS. Sickle cell trait occurs in those heterozygous for HbS. Sickle cell nephropathy describes the structural and functional abnormalities of the kidney in sickle cell disease.

SICKLE CELL DISEASE

Epidemiology

Sickle cell disease was first recognized in West Africa. The high prevalence of HbS in this region probably represents a survival benefit because the presence of sickle cell trait protects against malaria. Nowadays, sickle cell disease is a worldwide health problem because HbS has spread throughout Africa, around the Mediterranean, to the Middle East and India, as well as to the Caribbean, North America, and Northern Europe. The prevalence of the sickle cell gene is about 8% in African Americans; about 25% in some areas in equatorial Africa, Greece, Saudi Arabia, and India; and up to 50% in local West African areas.

Restriction enzyme techniques have identified several hemoglobin S haplotypes, mutations of the HbS molecule, which have probably arisen independently of each other. There are four major types in Africa—the Benin, Senegal, Cameroon, and Bantu (or Central African Republic)—and one Asian haplotype.

Pathogenesis
Genetics

Sickle cell disease comprises a group of heterogenous disorders that share the presence of the gene for HbS, either homozygous (i.e., sickle cell anemia, HbSS) or double heterozygous (i.e., the combination of HbS with another abnormal hemoglobin).[1,2] Sickle cell anemia is the most common form. The most common double heterozygous disorders are the combinations of hemoglobin S with hemoglobin C (HbSC) or β-thalassemia (HbS-thal). Subjects with the latter may also produce reduced amounts of normal β-chains (HbS-β+-thal), but not always (HbS-β0-thal). Subjects with a sickle cell trait or carrier state are heterozygous for HbS only.

Pathophysiology

The characteristic pathophysiologic feature in sickle cell disease is the episodic vaso-occlusive episodes, which can be triggered by several factors, including infection, hypoxia, volume depletion, hypothermia, acidosis, and hyperosmolality. The common denominator is the occurrence of inflammation or cellular stress. The two key processes in the pathophysiology of vaso-occlusion are adhesive interactions between the sickle red cells and the endothelium and the subsequent polymerization of HbS.

Sickle Cell Adherence Sickle cells have enhanced adherence to the endothelium compared with that of normal red cells. This is further increased by endothelial cell activation, which may occur through stimulation by many infective and inflammatory agents, including proinflammatory cytokines such as tumor necrosis factor-α (TNF-α), interleukin-1β (IL-1β), and interferon-γ (IFN-γ). These induce the expression of cellular adhesion molecules on endothelial cells. In addition, inflammatory stress may induce a procoagulant state by increasing the release of von Willebrand factor, thrombospondin, and other proteins that contribute to the adhesion process (Fig. 48.1). The adhesive interaction between sickle red cells and endothelium delays the capillary transit time, which allows polymerization of HbS and the sickling of red cells to occur.

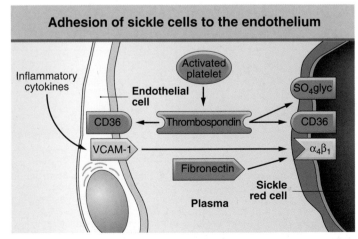

Adhesion of sickle cells to the endothelium

Figure 48.1 **Principal interactions responsible for the adhesion of a sickle red cell to the microvascular endothelium.** Thrombospondin acts as a bridging molecule by binding to CD36 on the surface of an endothelial cell and to CD36 or sulfated glycans (SO₄glyc) on a sickle reticulocyte. Vascular cell adhesion molecule 1 (VCAM-1) on endothelial cells can bind directly to the α₄β₁-integrin on the sickle reticulocyte. (Modified from Bunn HF: Pathogenesis and treatment of sickle cell disease. N Engl J Med 1997;337:762–769. Copyright ©1997 Massachusetts Medical Society. All rights reserved.)

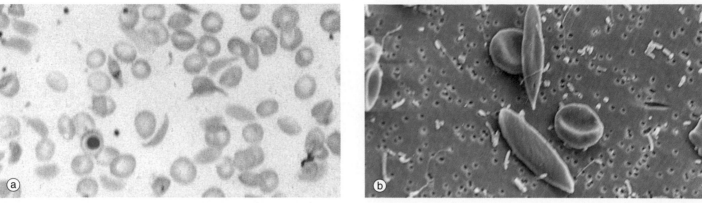

Figure 48.2 Sickle cells. *a*, Characteristic sickle cell erythrocytes in peripheral blood film of a patient with homozygous sickle cell anemia. *b*, Electron micrograph showing two normal and two sickle-shaped erythrocytes. (Courtesy of Professor Sally C. Davies.)

Polymerization of Hemoglobin S When HbS polymerizes, the hemoglobin molecules adhere to each other and aggregate into chain-like formations.[3] Polymerization changes the shape of the red cell, increases its rigidity, and thus causes sickling of red cells. (Fig 48.2) Polymerization is a dynamic event and depends primarily on three independent variables: the degree of cellular hypoxia, the intracellular hemoglobin concentration, and the presence or absence of hemoglobin F (fetal hemoglobin, or HbF).[3] Deoxygenation of HbS causes a change in the conformation of the β-globin subunits, which promotes the interaction of HbS molecules. The intracellular hemoglobin concentration in red cells can increase through cellular dehydration caused by membrane transport lesions, especially activated potassium-chloride cotransport and calcium-activated potassium efflux. The presence of

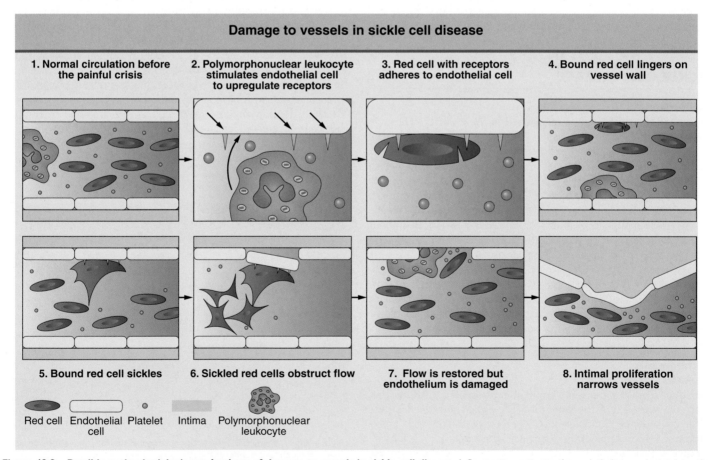

Figure 48.3 Possible pathophysiologic mechanisms of damage to vessels in sickle cell disease. Inflammation activates the endothelium and stimulates the upregulation of adhesion molecules and adherence of sickle cells to the endothelium. This promotes the sickling of red cells, increases the blood viscosity, and causes sludging in the microcirculation (eventually with microvascular thrombosis and infarction). After restoration of blood flow, vascular remodeling may contribute to persistent impairment of tissue blood flow. (Modified from Platt OS: Easing the suffering caused by sickle cell disease. N Engl J Med 1994;330:783–784. Copyright ©1997 Massachusetts Medical Society. All rights reserved.)

HbF decreases the polymerization tendency by reducing the concentration of HbS. Possible mechanisms of vaso-occlusion and ensuing vessel damage are shown in Figure 48.3.[4]

Clinical Manifestations

The clinical manifestations of sickle cell disease show an individual and age-dependent variation (Fig. 48.4). A chronic low-grade hemolytic anemia always occurs and predisposes to gallstones. The most prevalent clinical problem is periodic crises of bone pain. During the first years of life, it presents as the hand-foot syndrome, and in the course of life, it can result in avascular necrosis of the heads of the femur and humerus. Other important disabling problems are stroke resulting from occlusion of major cerebral vessels, the acute chest syndrome, priapism, chronic leg ulceration, and chronic pulmonary disease with pulmonary hypertension.[5,6]

Patients with sickle cell disease are prone to infections because of functional asplenia early in life as a result of splenic sequestration, recurrent splenic infarction, and consequent autosplenectomy. Ordinary bacterial infections can be fatal in these patients. Bacterial isolates during invasive bacterial infections show *Streptococcus pneumoniae* (38%), *Salmonella* species (33%), *Haemophilus influenzae* (14%), *Escherichia coli* (11%) and *Klebsiella* species (4%).[7] *S. pneumoniae* and *H. influenzae* occur predominantly before 5 years of age, *Salmonella* increases almost linearly with age, and *Klebsiella* and *E. coli* predominate in patients older than 10 years. Pneumococcal infections carry high morbidity and mortality rates in the early years of life, necessitating vaccination or prophylaxis.[1]

Fever is a cause of concern in patients with sickle cell disease. Common complications accompanying fever are painful crisis and acute chest syndrome.[8] Bacteremia is not always confirmed. The cause of fever often remains unclear and is presumed to be of viral origin or related to infections due to atypical organisms. Nevertheless, early antibiotic treatment is recommended pending microbiologic information.

There are remarkable differences in clinical severity and outcome of disease. Sickle cell trait is a rather benign condition. Patients with HbSS tend to have a more severe disease than those with HbSC. Likewise, subjects with HbS-β^+-thal do better than those with HbS-β^0-thal. The Bantu haplotype is associated with the highest frequency of organ damage. However, the severity of disease may also differ among subjects with an identical genotype. In part, these differences can be explained by the amount of HbF present because HbF may protect against clinical severity. In addition, endothelial factors probably play an important role. It has been shown that the degree of adherence between sickle red cells and endothelial cells correlates with the clinical severity of disease. Also, a relation has been found between circulating activated endothelial cells of microvascular origin and the onset of painful sickle cell crises.[9]

Natural History

Life expectancy is reduced in sickle cell disease, especially in subjects with symptomatic disease. An increased risk for early death is associated with low levels of HbF, renal failure, the acute chest syndrome, and seizures.[10] Childhood survival to age 20 years has improved during the past decades. In the course of life, irreversible organ damage due to arterial and capillary microcirculation obstructive vasculopathy gradually becomes more prevalent. The diagnosis of a clinically evident form of organ damage such as leg ulcer, osteonecrosis, or retinopathy predicts the development of a more lethal form of organ damage such as chronic lung disease, renal failure, or stroke.[11] Overall, the primary causes of death in patients with sickle cell anemia are chronic lung disease in 20%, chronic renal failure in 14%, and stroke in 10%. In younger patients, the primary cause of death is infection; in older patients, the primary cause of death is irreversible organ damage (Fig. 48.5).

Treatment

Management of sickle cell disease is primarily directed at the relief of symptoms and prevention of complications, whereas newer treatments are being devised that target the pathophysiology of the disease.[5,12] Daily oral penicillin for children 2 to 5 years of age is effective in reducing both the infection rate and the mortality related to pneumococcal infection.[13] Immunization against pneumococcus is recommended for children at 2 years of age, with booster doses at 5 years of age,[12] although protection from current vaccines is imperfect. Immunization against influenza in children is also important.[14] The empiric antibiotic treatment of choice in adults with fever is amoxicillin.

Sickle cell crises are managed with oxygen therapy, red cell transfusions, and analgesia. Hydroxyurea treatment in subjects with sickle cell anemia and recurrent vaso-occlusive events decreases the incidence of painful crises and acute chest syndrome, and overall mortality.[5,14,15] Hematopoietic stem cell transplantation is a potentially curative for sickle cell disease; it is associated with an 80% to 85% disease-free survival rate in several series.[16]

Age distribution of clinical problems in sickle cell disease

Symptom	Age (years)
	0　5　10　15　20　25　30
Pain	
Digits	
Long bones	
Trunk	
Sequestration	
Splenic	
Hepatic	
Chest syndrome	
Mesenteric syndrome	
Infection	
Pneumococcus	
Parvovirus	
Salmonella	
Priapism	
Upper airways obstruction	
Stroke	
Subarachnoid hemorrhage	
Retinopathy	
Gallstones	
Avascular necrosis	
Hyposthenuria	
Delayed growth and development	
Leg ulcers	
Chronic renal failure	
Chronic sickle lung	

Figure 48.4　Age distribution of clinical problems in sickle cell disease. (Modified from Davies SC, Oni L: Management of patients with sickle cell disease. BMJ 1997;315:656–660.)

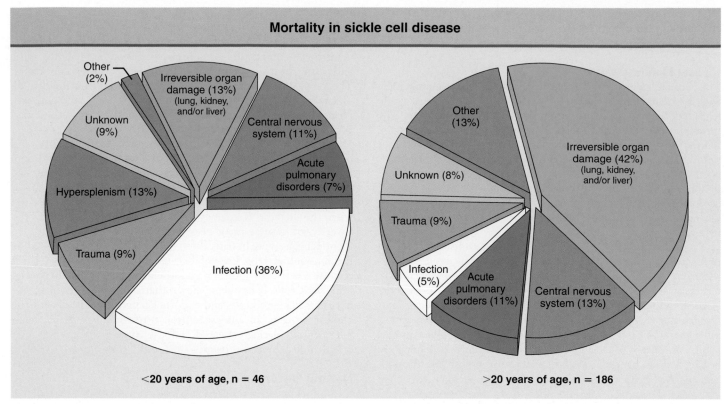

Figure 48.5 Mortality in sickle cell disease. Causes of death among 232 HbSS patients, comparing patients <20 years old (46 died) with patients >29 years old (186 died). The "infection" category includes both bacterial and viral diseases. (Modified from Powars DR, Chan LS, Hiti A, et al: Outcome of sickle cell anemia: A 4-decade observational study of 1056 patients. Medicine 2005;84:363–376.)

Young and presymptomatic patients with high-risk features of severe disease benefit the most from hematopoietic stem cell transplantation.

SICKLE CELL NEPHROPATHY

Pathogenesis
The hallmark of sickle cell nephropathy is the combination of an impaired renal concentrating capacity and a normal diluting capacity.[17,18]

Concentrating Capacity
The defect in concentrating capacity results from loss of the countercurrent exchange mechanism in the inner renal medulla through loss of the vasa recta and long loops of Henle of the juxtamedullary nephrons (Fig. 48.6). The vasa recta of the juxtamedullary nephrons presents an ideal setting for the sickling of red cells. The renal medulla is relatively hypoxic and hyperosmotic, the blood viscosity is increased in the medullary circulation, and medullary blood flow is slow. Studies in transgenic sickle cell mice have demonstrated distension and congestion of the vasa recta under hypoxic conditions. This environment facilitates the sickling of erythrocytes, formation of intravascular microthrombi, and obstruction of blood flow through the vasa recta. The loss of vasa recta has been confirmed by microradioangiographic studies[19] (Fig. 48.7). Histologic examination of the medulla shows edema, focal scarring, and interstitial fibrosis resulting in tubular atrophy. Ischemic infarction in the vasa recta sometimes causes papillary necrosis. The concentration defect is found to be reversible in

young children when sickling is prevented after multiple transfusions of normal blood, but it becomes irreversible thereafter. Adults with sickle cell anemia cannot concentrate the urine above 450 mOsm/kg H_2O. This relates to the interstitial osmolality at the transition of the outer and inner medulla, at the tips of the short loops of Henle of the cortical nephrons. Subjects with sickle cell trait or hybrid sickling disorders show intermediate concentrating defects. Maximal osmolality varies from 400 to 900 mOsm/kg H_2O in sickle cell trait and from 400 to 700 mOsm/kg H_2O in HbSC and declines further with aging.

Diluting Capacity
The diluting capacity is normal as a result of the intact reabsorptive function of the superficial loops of Henle of the cortical nephrons. These are supplied by peritubular capillaries, which present a less ideal setting for the sickling of red cells than the vasa recta. In contrast to the diluting capacity, the free water reabsorption, or capacity to generate negative free water balance, is impaired by defective trapping of solute in the inner medulla.

Other Tubular Abnormalities
Defects in urinary acidification and potassium excretion are other distal nephron function abnormalities.[20] These may become overt only when there is an increased supply of acid and potassium, for example, during rhabdomyolysis. The exact causes of these defects are unknown, but they likely reflect failure to maintain the necessary energy-requiring hydrogen ion and electrochemical gradients along the collecting ducts owing to the impaired medullary blood flow and hypoxia. The impaired potassium excretion is aldosterone independent.

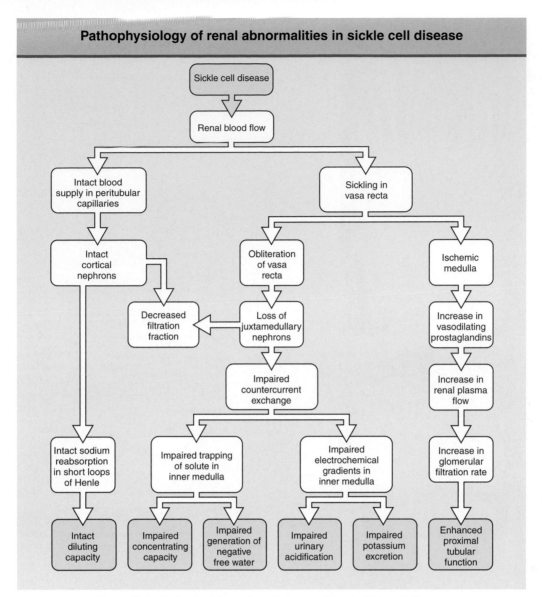

Figure 48.6   Pathophysiology of renal abnormalities in sickle cell disease.

In contrast to the functional abnormalities of the distal nephron, proximal tubular function is enhanced. Reabsorption of phosphate and β_2-microglobin and secretion of uric acid and creatinine in the proximal tubule are increased. Therefore, creatinine clearance overestimates glomerular filtration rate (GFR) considerably. The cause of the enhanced proximal function is not clear, but it probably represents a secondary compensatory mechanism to correct for defects in medullary function.

Renal Hemodynamics

Renal hemodynamics show remarkable changes in the course of the disease (Fig. 48.8). Young subjects with sickle cell disease have increases in renal plasma flow (RPF) and renal blood flow and, to a lesser extent, in GFR. The increased RPF is ascribed to increased release of vasodilator prostaglandins as a result of medullary ischemia because prostaglandin inhibition significantly reduces RPF and GFR. Studies in transgenic sickle cell mice suggest that increased nitric oxide production also contributes to renal vasodilation. The decrease in filtration fraction may be

caused by selective damage of juxtamedullary nephrons, which have the highest filtration fractions.

Glomerular Injury

Glomerular hypertrophy is an early manifestation of sickle cell nephropathy. Histologic examination of the kidneys of young children shows glomerular enlargement and congestion, especially in the juxtamedullary glomeruli. Both afferent and efferent arterioles of these glomeruli may be dilated. In young adult patients with sickle cell anemia, there is a distinct pattern of glomerular dysfunction, with impaired glomerular permselectivity, increased ultrafiltration coefficient, glomerular hyperfiltration, and proteinuria.[21,22] Prolonged glomerular hyperfiltration may cause further glomerular injury. This is supported by the common histologic finding of focal segmental glomerulosclerosis (FSGS) in adult patients with sickle cell disease[23] (Fig. 48.9). Two consecutive patterns of FSGS have been described: a "collapsing" and an "expansive" pattern.[24] The initial collapsing pattern has been attributed to progressive obliteration of glomerular capillaries by red blood cell sickling in maximally

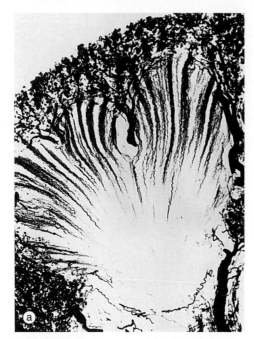

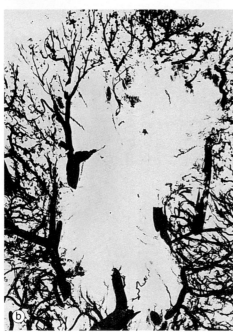

Figure 48.7   Microradioangiography showing loss of vasa recta in sickle cell nephropathy. *a,* Kidney from a control subject, showing normal vasa recta. *b,* A patient with sickle cell anemia, with the absence of the vasa recta. (Modified from Statius Eps LW van, Pinedo-Veels C, Vries CH de, Koning J de: Nature of concentrating defect in sickle cell nephropathy, microradioangiographic studies. Lancet 1970;1:450–452.)

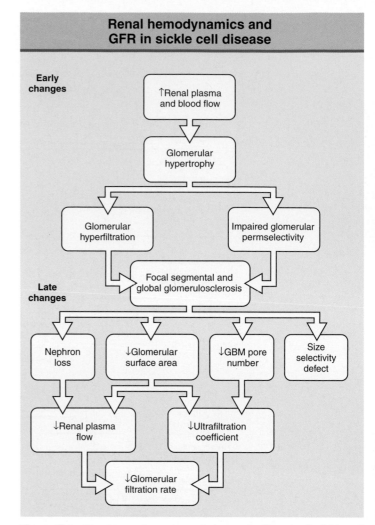

Renal hemodynamics and GFR in sickle cell disease

Figure 48.8   Renal hemodynamics and glomerular filtration in sickle cell nephropathy. GBM, glomerular basement membrane; GFR, glomerular filtration rate.

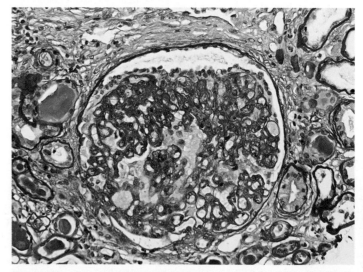

Figure 48.9   Focal segmental glomerulosclerosis in sickle cell nephropathy. Segmental sclerosis involving the upper half of the glomerulus. (Courtesy of Professor J. Weening.)

hypertrophied glomeruli. The expansive pattern is characterized by an expansive sclerosis with increased mesangial matrix and further capillary obliteration; it is ascribed to sustained or increasing hyperfiltration.[24]

In older subjects, progressive ischemia and fibrosis with obliteration of glomeruli can be found. Glomerular function studies show a decrease in glomerular basement membrane pore number and a size selectivity defect in subjects with renal insufficiency.[25] Ultimately, a combined decrease in ultrafiltration capacity and RPF can result in end-stage renal disease (ESRD).[21]

Hormones in Sickle Cell Nephropathy

There is relative *erythropoietin* deficiency in sickle cell disease; that is, erythropoietin levels do not increase to the expected level for the degree of anemia, perhaps due to the right-shifted hemoglobin-oxygen dissociation curve. In addition, erythropoietin levels fall with the decline in renal function, probably as a result of renal damage due to the sickling process.

Elevated values of *renin* and *aldosterone* have been reported in some studies, both under standard and volume-depleted conditions, although in general normal values are found in sickle cell anemia.[17]

Hormone infusion studies have helped to localize sites of action in the kidney. Failure of low-dose infusion of *atrial natriuretic peptide* (ANP) to increase natriuresis in sickle cell anemia[26] suggests that ANP at this dosage exerts its natriuretic effect in the long loops of Henle of the juxtamedullary nephrons, whereas *insulin* induces a similar sodium retention in patients with sickle cell anemia and normal subjects,[26] suggesting its antinatriuretic effect is probably localized at a distal tubular site other than the long loops of Henle.

Urinary endothelin-1 is elevated in asymptomatic sickle cell disease patients. It correlates with a urine-concentrating defect and microalbuminuria.[27]

CLINICAL MANIFESTATIONS OF SICKLE CELL NEPHROPATHY

The presentation of the clinical manifestations of sickle cell nephropathy shows an age-dependent pattern. The frequency and etiology of the renal abnormalities associated with sickle cell anemia, sickle cell trait, and the most common double heterozygous disorders (HbSC and HbS-thal) are listed in Figure 48.10.

Hematuria

Hematuria is a common clinical manifestation in sickle cell anemia and the hybrid sickling disorders and occurs in 3% to 4% of subjects with sickle cell trait at some time. There is often persistent microscopic hematuria with episodic gross hematuria. The hematuria may follow relatively minor trauma. Hematuria occurs more often in males and is usually unilateral, originating from the left kidney in 80% of patients.

Pathogenesis

Sickling The main mechanism of hematuria probably relates to the sickling of erythrocytes in the vasa recta and microthrombotic infarction and extravasation of blood in the renal medulla. Histologic examination typically shows severe stasis in peritubular capillaries of the cortex and, especially, the medulla, and extravasation of blood into the collecting system.

Papillary Necrosis Papillary necrosis is a frequent cause of hematuria in sickle cell anemia, hybrid sickling disorders, and sickle cell trait (Fig. 48.11). The incidence of papillary necrosis varied from 23% to 67% in several studies of selected patients with sickle cell disease.[28] This complication results from obliteration of the vasa recta, with medullary necrosis and fibrosis. The

Frequencies and etiology of renal abnormalities associated with sickle cell disease

Type of Renal Disease	Etiology	Frequencies in Subsets of Sickle Cell Disease		
		Sickle Cell Anemia	Sickle Cell Trait	HbSC and HbS-thal
Impaired concentrating capacity	Loss of vasa recta of juxtamedullary	Irreversible defects in all adults	Intermediate defects in all adults' nephrons	Intermediate defects in all adults
Impaired urinary acidification	Incomplete form of distal renal tubular acidosis	Almost all, during acid loading	Rare	At least 30%, during acid loading
Impaired potassium excretion	Aldosterone independent	Almost all, during potassium loading	Rare	Unknown; probably at least 30%
Hematuria	Infarction, extravasation of blood in renal medulla	Common	3%–4%	Common
Proteinuria	Glomerular hyperfiltration plus impaired permselectivity	Up to 50%–60% with increasing age	Rare	20%–25%
Nephrotic syndrome	FSGS most common	About 4%	Rare	0%–4%
Chronic renal failure	See Figure 48.8	4.2%–4.6%	Rare	About 2.4%
Renal carcinoma	Possible genetic predisposition	Rare	Absolutely rare, relatively frequent	Rare

Figure 48.10 Frequencies and etiology of renal abnormalities associated with sickle cell disease.

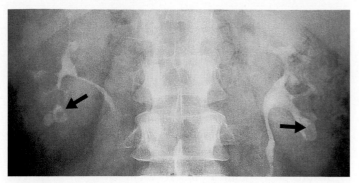

Figure 48.11 Papillary necrosis in sickle cell disease. Intravenous urography shows abnormal calyces with filling defects *(arrows)*.

large analgesic consumption by these patients because of their bone pain may also contribute to papillary necrosis. The most common presenting symptom is painless macroscopic hematuria. Other presentations are renal colic caused by the passage of blood clots or necrotic papillae, microscopic hematuria, symptoms of urinary tract infection, and, rarely, acute renal failure. Papillary necrosis may also be asymptomatic and is frequently an incidental finding during radiography.

Nutcracker Phenomenon The left-sided predominance of hematuria has been attributed to the so-called nutcracker phenomenon, compression of the left renal vein between the aorta and the superior mesenteric artery, thereby increasing the pressure in the renal vein. This may especially contribute to the development of hematuria in sickle cell patients because the increased renal vein pressure could lead to a relatively increased anoxia in the renal medulla, thereby increasing the likelihood of sickling in the left kidney.

Clinical Manifestations

Painless macroscopic hematuria often presents after physical activity or minor renal trauma or is associated with hypoxic challenges, for example, airplane flights. It usually is accompanied by a substantial fall in hematocrit. Bleeding typically remits spontaneously within a few days.

Diagnosis and Differential Diagnosis

Urinalysis can exclude the presence of myoglobinuria and rhabdomyolysis, which can mimic hematuria. Rhabdomyolysis can be provoked during strenuous exercise and dehydration and may also occur during severe sickle cell crises. The coexistence of hematuria with leukocyturia or pyuria is not unusual and does not necessarily indicate a urinary tract infection, even in combination with flank pain. Infection must be confirmed by examination of the urinary sediment and urine cultures.

Sickle cell trait has been reported in 50% of African Americans with ESRD caused by autosomal dominant polycystic kidney disease (ADPKD) but in only 7.5% of African American patients with other causes of ESRD. In addition, patients with ADPKD and sickle cell trait had an earlier onset of ESRD.[29]

Recently, renal medullary carcinoma has been recognized as a specific entity in sickle cell nephropathy.[30–32] It is a very aggressive form of renal cell carcinoma that appears uniquely to affect patients with sickle cell trait or HbSC, especially occurring in teenagers and young adults. The relationship between renal medullary carcinoma and sickle hemoglobinopathy has been explained by chronic medullary hypoxia secondary to hemoglobinopathy.[32] The tumors tend to be metastatic at the time of diagnosis, with a reported mean survival from the time of surgery of only 15 weeks. The tumors are resistant to chemotherapy. Possibly, only early recognition may improve prognosis. One should consider hematuria as a potentially ominous harbinger of malignancy, particularly in young patients with sickle cell trait.

Further evaluation is indicated for patients with severe or prolonged hematuria, which is resistant to conservative therapeutic measures. Ultrasound examination will be normal unless there is papillary necrosis or a coincidental cause of hematuria such as polycystic kidney disease, renal calculus, or tumor. Intravenous urography used to be the method of choice to diagnose papillary necrosis but may provide confounding information because blood clots in the renal pelvis may cause radiocontrast translucencies resembling neoplasm, calculus, or hemangioma. Ultrasound is, therefore, preferred. The role of magnetic resonance imaging in this setting has not yet been sufficiently evaluated. The presence of von Willebrand's disease has occasionally been described in subjects with sickle cell trait and gross hematuria.

Cystoscopy is not routinely required but is indicated if the episode of hematuria is atypical, for example, a first episode of macroscopic hematuria in a patient over the age of 40 years or an episode that persists for more than 2 weeks. Cystoscopy may also be required to lateralize the source of the bleeding if surgical intervention is considered (see later discussion).

Renal angiography only rarely identifies the bleeding source, but when it does so, it can be followed by embolization. However, the optimal approach in any institution depends on local experience with specific investigations.

Treatment

The therapeutic strategy for hematuria depends on the severity and duration of a specific bleeding episode. Bleeding will stop in most patients spontaneously or after a period of bed rest, although it may occasionally last for weeks or months. About half of patients will have recurrent episodes.

Initial therapeutic measures include bed rest and interventions aimed at retardation of the sickling process in the anoxic renal medulla. A high urine flow rate should be induced by intravenous fluid administration and diuretics to further reduce medullary tonicity and the urine alkalinized by administration of sodium bicarbonate by mouth or by vein, with a target of urine pH 8. Blood transfusion with normal HbA is indicated if anemia becomes severe; this may also decrease the sickling process. If necessary, bladder irrigation is performed for removal of blood clots.

Hyperbaric oxygen therapy may be helpful but has not been formally evaluated. Irrigation of the pelvicalyceal system with silver nitrate has also been described. The antifibrinolytic agent, ε-aminocaproic acid, may be effective, but unfortunately sometimes leads to the formation of large blood clots and obstruction in the urinary collecting system. Therefore, this therapy should be used with care, starting at a low dose, 1 g/1.73 m^2 body surface area orally, 3 times daily, increasing cautiously until the bleeding subsides.

Unilateral nephrectomy has occasionally been necessary in patients with persistent, life-threatening hematuria refractory to a conservative approach. Full evaluation for another cause of hematuria, including cystoscopy to exclude a bladder lesion and to establish which kidney is the source of bleeding, is required before proceeding with nephrectomy.

Urinary Tract Infection

Subjects with sickle cell disease have an increased susceptibility to bacterial infections; even low-grade bacteremia with a common organism may be fatal. In addition to the impaired immunity that is a consequence of autosplenectomy, there is opsonic antibody deficiency, which predisposes to bacterial infections. The relative incidence of urinary tract infections is not exactly known. However, the incidence of asymptomatic bacteriuria during pregnancy and the puerperium appears to be twice as high in women with sickle cell disease or trait than in women without sickle cell disease and requires appropriate therapy (see Chapter 44).

Pyelonephritis and urosepsis, like any other infection, may precipitate a sickle cell crisis. One should especially be aware of this possibility in young children, who often do not complain of urinary tract symptoms. Most common organisms isolated include *E. coli*, *Klebsiella* species, and other gram-negative Enterobacteriaceae. Invasive bacterial infections with *E. coli* occur especially in females after the age of 15 years, suggesting a greater chance of urinary tract infections in relation to sexual activity.[7]

Acute Renal Failure

Acute renal failure (ARF), defined as a doubling of serum creatinine, has been reported in 10% of patients hospitalized with sickle cell anemia.[33]

Etiology

A prerenal cause of ARF will be found in more than half of patients, especially volume depletion in the setting of sickle cell crisis. Patients with sickle cell disease are prone to ARF caused by volume depletion because of impaired urine-concentrating capacity; it is therefore typically nonoliguric. A less frequent prerenal cause is congestive heart failure.

Typical intrinsic renal causes of ARF are rhabdomyolysis, sepsis, and drug nephrotoxicity. Less common are renal vein thrombosis and hepatorenal syndrome (caused by hemosiderosis-induced hepatic failure). Both exertional and nontraumatic rhabdomyolysis have been reported in patients with sickle cell disease. The latter especially occurs during a sickle cell crisis and has been ascribed to intravascular sickling and muscle ischemia. Rhabdomyolysis is a common finding in patients who develop multiorgan failure during severe sickle cell crises, in addition to the acute chest syndrome, which further contributes to ARF.

The most typical postrenal cause of ARF is urinary tract obstruction by necrotic papillae or blood clots.

Treatment

Treatment and recovery of renal function depends on the specific underlying pathology. Metabolic acidosis may be prominent and should be actively corrected with sodium bicarbonate. Patients with volume depletion have a favorable outcome after fluid replacement.[33] Renal function may recover in patients with sepsis and rhabdomyolysis, although temporary renal function replacement therapy may be necessary. ARF as a part of multiorgan failure during a severe sickle cell crisis may show a dramatic improvement with aggressive red cell transfusion therapy, although some renal function loss may persist.

Proteinuria and Nephrotic Syndrome

Microalbuminuria has been reported in 19% to 26% of children with sickle cell anemia.[34,35] The presence of microalbuminuria is directly related to age and inversely related to hemoglobin levels. Proteinuria has been reported in 17% to 33% of subjects with sickle cell disease in several studies using semiquantitative or dipstick measurements. The prevalence of proteinuria is lower in subjects with coinheritance of sickle cell anemia and α-thalassemia than in those with sickle cell anemia and intact α-globin genes (13% versus 40%).[36] The "renoprotective" effect of α-globin gene microdeletions could be related to a lower mean corpuscular volume or lower erythrocyte hemoglobin concentration in sickle erythrocytes. The frequency of proteinuria increases with age (56% in subjects ≥40 years[37]) and its presence is associated with renal impairment.

The nephrotic syndrome has been estimated to occur in 4% of patients with sickle cell anemia.[38] The eventual development of renal failure appears virtually inevitable once the patient has nephrotic syndrome.

Pathology

The most common pathologic lesion is FSGS,[23,24] which is also the major lesion in patients who develop renal failure. Another specific pathologic lesion is a form of membranoproliferative glomerulonephritis (MPGN) with mesangial expansion and basement membrane duplication.[2] The general absence of immune complexes and electron-dense deposits discriminates this entity from idiopathic MPGN. It has been proposed that this form of MPGN is caused by intracapillary red cell fragmentation. Fragments of red cells become lodged in isolated capillary loops and are continuously phagocytosed by mesangial cells. As a result, the mesangium expands and lays down new basement membrane material.[20,38]

Patients may become hepatitis C positive from multiple blood transfusions, which may also be associated with MPGN. Occasionally, other causes have been reported, such as poststreptococcal glomerulonephritis, minimal change disease, and immune complex–mediated glomerulonephritis. Glomerulonephritis has also been described in association with aplastic crises in parvovirus infection.[39] Renal vein thrombosis should be considered when nephrotic syndrome develops in sickle cell disease, but its incidence is not exactly known.

Treatment

Theoretically, dietary protein restriction may reduce hyperfiltration and retard the development of renal failure in those with FSGS, but this has not been evaluated specifically in sickle cell disease.

Short-term treatment with angiotensin-converting enzyme (ACE) inhibitors significantly reduces the degree of proteinuria without affecting blood pressure or renal hemodynamics.[23] More prolonged ACE inhibition reduces proteinuria with a slight decrease in blood pressure.[40] However, it remains to be established whether long-term treatment with ACE inhibitors or angiotensin receptor blockers (ARBs) delays the development of progressive renal failure.

Prevention of hyperfiltration can, theoretically, also be obtained with nonsteroidal anti-inflammatory drugs (NSAIDs), but these drugs reduce RPF and GFR in sickle cell anemia[17] and are not recommended.

Sodium and Acid-Base Disturbances
Distal Tubular Function

Distal tubular function abnormalities are impaired potassium excretion and impaired urinary acidification caused by an incomplete form of distal tubular acidosis. However, hyperkalemia and metabolic acidosis are not present under normal circumstances and may only become manifest during potassium or acid loading, with mild renal insufficiency or volume depletion, and during rhabdomyolysis.[17,18] Hyperkalemia may also develop more readily during treatment with NSAIDs, ACE inhibitors, β-blockers, potassium-sparing diuretics, or heparin.

Urine pH does not fall below 5 during acid-loading tests unless maximal acidifying stimuli are used. The titratable acid and hydrogen ion excretion is reduced, whereas the ammonium excretion is either normal or decreased. Metabolic acidosis developing during renal insufficiency or intercurrent diseases in sickle cell disease requires active treatment with sodium bicarbonate because acidosis stimulates the sickling process. Plasma bicarbonate should be monitored routinely and oral sodium bicarbonate supplements given to keep it within the reference range.

Proximal Tubular Function

Proximal tubular function abnormalities modify solute handling, producing increased reabsorption of phosphate and increased secretion of uric acid. Hyperphosphatemia may develop easily when renal function declines, necessitating dietary phosphate restriction and the use of phosphate binders early in renal insufficiency. The increased uric acid secretion protects patients with sickle cell disease against elevated uric acid production resulting from hemolysis. However, the incidence of hyperuricemia and risk for gout increase with age as renal function declines.

Hypertension
Epidemiology

The prevalence of hypertension in patients with sickle cell anemia is about 2% to 6%, which is significantly lower than in age- and sex-matched control subjects.[17,41] However, blood pressure levels in patients with sickle cell anemia are higher than in matched subjects with β-thalassemia and similar levels of anemia. Hypertension in sickle cell anemia especially occurs in the presence of advanced renal failure.

Pathogenesis

It is not yet clear whether the relative hypotension compared with control subjects relates to the pathologic renal medullary condition in sickle cell disease or to other mechanisms. The kidney in sickle cell disease has a normal overall capacity for sodium conservation, despite a tendency to lose sodium and water through the medullary defect.[17,41] This sodium conservation in sickle cell disease may follow stimulation of the renin-angiotensin-aldosterone system, which has been described in some but not all studies. The relative hypotension may be related to general vasodilation because skeletal vascular resistance is reduced in sickle cell patients. Increased production of vasodilatory prostaglandins or nitric oxide may be involved. Systemic vasodilation and increased flow is a compensatory mechanism for microcirculatory flow disturbances and intermittent microvascular occlusion.[42] Finally, reduced vascular reactivity has been demonstrated in sickle cell patients and may protect against blood pressure elevation.[41]

Treatment

The antihypertensive treatment of choice is ACE inhibitors or ARB, because of the potential beneficial effects on the progression of proteinuria and renal failure, and because of the reported increments in plasma renin activity. However, the risk for hyperkalemia is increased.

An alternative therapeutic option is a calcium channel blocker, but it is not yet known whether these drugs reduce proteinuria in sickle cell disease. Loop diuretics are less effective in patients with sickle cell disease because of the specific medullary defect.

Chronic Renal Failure
Epidemiology

In a prospective, 25-year longitudinal study, chronic renal failure (CRF) developed in 4.2% of 725 patients with sickle cell anemia and in 2.4% of 209 patients with HbSC.[43] The patients with sickle cell anemia were much younger at the time of the diagnosis of renal failure than those with HbSC (median age, 23.1 and 49.9 years, respectively). However, in another study in 368 patients with sickle cell anemia with an overall prevalence of CRF of 4.6%, the prevalence of CRF clearly increased with age.[37] Probably, the prevalence of CRF will increase even more in the future with further improved medical care and longer life expectancy.

Predictors of CRF are hypertension, proteinuria, hematuria, increasingly severe anemia, the nephrotic syndrome, and inheritance of the Bantu, or Central African Republic, β-globin gene cluster haplotype.[43] Apart from an apparent genetic predisposition, the presence of glomerular capillary hypertension and prolonged glomerular hyperfiltration seem to be very important in the development of renal failure.

Natural History

Patients with sickle cell anemia and CRF have an increased mortality rate compared with patients without renal failure (Fig. 48.12). Patients with renal failure are also prone to other manifestations of sickle-induced vasculopathy and nonrenal organ failure, such as cerebrovascular accidents, chronic restrictive lung disease, and leg ulcers.[43] In the United States Renal Data System, patients with sickle cell nephropathy and ESRD had an independently increased risk for mortality (hazard ratio, 1.52; 95% confidence interval, 1.27–1.82) compared with other patients with ESRD. However, patients with sickle cell nephropathy were less likely to be listed for or receive renal transplantation, and the increased mortality risk did not persist after adjustment for receipt of renal transplantation.[44]

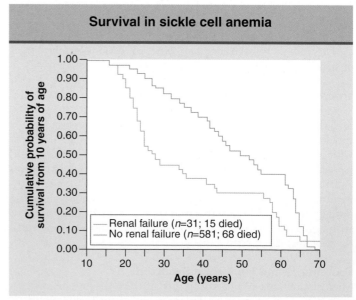

Figure 48.12 Survival in sickle cell anemia in the presence and absence of renal failure. (Modified from Powars DR, Elliott-Mills DD, Chan L, et al: Chronic renal failure in sickle cell disease: Risk factors, clinical course, and mortality. Ann Intern Med 1991;115:614–620.)

Treatment

To delay the development of progressive renal failure, it is important to control hypertension and to avoid the use of nephrotoxic drugs, especially NSAIDs. Although plausible, it remains to be established whether the reduction of the degree of proteinuria with either ACE inhibitors or a low-protein diet retards the progression of renal failure.

The response to erythropoietin therapy is poor, even when high doses are used over long treatment periods.[45] Erythropoietin treatment predominantly results in the release of HbS-containing reticulocytes, with only a modest increase in the more stable HbF. A marked increase in hemoglobin levels, although unexpected, may precipitate sickle cell crisis. Routine use of erythropoietin is therefore not recommended, but it can be tried on an individual basis with higher doses than needed in other forms of ESRD. As an alternative, supportive red cell transfusion may be given regularly to these subjects. Excessive iron accumulation should be prevented in patients undergoing regular transfusions, who are at risk for hemochromatosis, although organ dysfunction caused by tissue iron overload seems less predictable in sickle cell disease than in thalassemia major. Metabolic acidosis is also prominent and requires correction with sodium bicarbonate supplements.

ESRD in sickle cell disease has been treated successfully with hemodialysis, peritoneal dialysis, and transplantation. So far, hemodialysis has been used relatively more frequently than peritoneal dialysis in patients with sickle cell disease. Sickle cell crises are not common despite the potential for hypotension, hypoxemia, and cytokine release during hemodialysis. The 30-month survival rate of a group of 77 patients who were predominantly treated with hemodialysis was 59%, a figure comparable to the survival rates in other groups of patients with multisystem disorders receiving dialysis.

TRANSPLANTATION

Transplantation is an appropriate form of renal replacement therapy for those with sickle cell nephropathy who develop ESRD. After kidney transplantation, 1- and 3-year patient survivals rates are 90% and 75%, respectively; 1- and 3-year graft survival rates are 82% and 54%, respectively.[46] These outcomes compare unfavorably to kidney transplantation for most other patient groups. Compared with other transplant recipients, the adjusted mortality risk in sickle cell patients undergoing transplantation is higher at 1 year (relative risk, 2.95) and at 3 years (relative risk, 2.82).[36] Nevertheless, transplantation probably confers a survival advantage in patients with sickle cell disease; there is a trend toward improved survival in transplant recipients compared with dialysis-treated patients with sickle cell disease on the transplant waiting list.[47]

In sickle cell disease, perioperative risks such as severe crisis and massive sickling can be reduced by preoperative transfusions of normal blood, thereby reducing the proportion of HbS. After transplantation, hematocrit values increase and are even higher than in patients with sickle cell disease and normal renal function. Sickle cell crisis may occur after transplantation, but it is not yet clear whether the increase in hematocrit values enhances the risk for a crisis. Standard immunosuppressive therapy does not increase the risk for sickle cell crisis. However, caution is warranted with the use of antilymphocyte antibodies because the onset of a crisis has been related to this therapy in a few patients, perhaps as a consequence of increased cytokine release. Occasionally, the recurrence of hyposthenuria and sickle cell nephropathy after transplantation has been described.

REFERENCES

1. Davies SC, Oni L: Management of patients with sickle cell disease. BMJ 1997;315:656–660.
2. Serjeant GR: Sickle-cell disease. Lancet 1997;350:725–730.
3. Bunn HF: Pathogenesis and treatment of sickle cell disease. N Engl J Med 1997;337:762–769.
4. Platt OS: Easing the suffering caused by sickle cell disease. N Engl J Med 1994;330:783–784.
5. Stuart MJ, Nagel RL: Sickle-cell disease. Lancet 2004;364:1343–1360.
6. Gladwin MT, Sachdev V, Jison ML, et al: Pulmonary hypertension as a risk factor for death in patients with sickle cell disease. N Engl J Med 2004;350:886–895.
7. Magnus SA, Hambleton IR, Moosdeen F, Serjeant GR: Recurrent infections in homozygous sickle cell disease. Arch Dis Child 1999;80:537–541.
8. Wierenga KJJ, Hambleton IR, Wilson RM, et al: Significance of fever in Jamaican patients with homozygous sickle cell disease. Arch Dis Child 2001;84:156–159.
9. Solovey A, Lin Y, Browne P, et al: Circulating activated endothelial cells in sickle cell disease. N Engl J Med 1997;337:1584–1590.
10. Platt OS, Brambilla DJ, Rosse WF, et al: Mortality in sickle cell disease. Life expectancy and risk factors for early death. N Engl J Med 1994;330:1639–1644.
11. Powars DR, Chan LS, Hiti A, et al: Outcome of sickle cell anemia: A 4-decade observational study of 1056 patients. Medicine 2005;84:363–376.
12. Steinberg MH: Management of sickle cell disease. N Engl J Med 1999;340:1021–1030.
13. Hord J, Byrd R, Stowe L, et al: Streptococcus pneumoniae sepsis and meningitis during penicillin prophylaxis era in children with sickle cell disease. J Pediatr Hematol Oncol 2002;24:470–472.
14. Claster S, Vichinsky EP: Managing sickle cell disease. BMJ 2003;327:1151–1155.
15. Steinberg MH, Barton F, Castro O, et al: Effect of hydroxyurea on mortality and morbidity in sickle cell anemia: Risks and benefits up to 9 years of treatment. JAMA 2003;289:1645–1651.
16. Vermylen C: Hematopoietic stem cell transplantation in sickle cell disease. Blood Rev 2003;17:163–166.
17. Jong PE de, Statius Eps LW van: Sickle cell nephropathy: New insights into pathophysiology. Kidney Int 1985;27:711–717.
18. Allon M: Renal abnormalities in sickle cell disease. Arch Intern Med 1990;150:501–504.
19. Statius Eps LW van, Pinedo-Veels C, Vries CH de, Koning J de: Nature of concentrating defect in sickle cell nephropathy, microradioangiographic studies. Lancet 1970;1:450–452.
20. Pham PT, Pham PT, Wilkinson AH, Lew SQ: Renal abnormalities in sickle cell disease. Kidney Int 2000;57:1–8.
21. Guasch A, Cua M, Mitch WE: Early detection and the course of glomerular injury in patients with sickle cell anemia. Kidney Int 1996;49:786–791.
22. Schmitt F, Martinez F, Brillet G, et al: Early glomerular dysfunction in patients with sickle cell anemia. Am J Kidney Dis 1998;32:208–214.
23. Falk RJ, Scheinman J, Phillips G, et al: Prevalence and pathologic features of sickle cell nephropathy and response to inhibition of angiotensin-converting enzyme. N Engl J Med 1992;326:910–915.
24. Bhathena DB, Sondheimer JH: The glomerulopathy of homozygous sickle hemoglobin (SS) disease: Morphology and pathogenesis. J Am Soc Nephrol 1991;1:1241–1252.
25. Guasch A, Cua M, You W, Mitch WE: Sickle cell anemia causes a distinct pattern of glomerular dysfunction. Kidney Int 1997;51:826–833.
26. Maaten JC ter, Serné EH, Statius Eps LW van, et al: Effects of insulin and atrial natriuretic peptide on renal tubular sodium handling in sickle cell disease. Am J Physiol 2000;278:F499–F505.

27. Tharaux PL, Hagege I, Placier S, et al: Urinary endothelin-1 as a marker of renal damage in sickle cell disease. Nephrol Dial Transplant 2005;20:2408–2413.

28. Vaamonde CA: Renal papillary necrosis in sickle cell haemoglobinopathies. Semin Nephrol 1984;4:48–64.

29. Yium J, Gabow P, Johnson A, et al: Autosomal dominant polycystic kidney disease in blacks: Clinical course and effects of sickle-cell hemoglobin. J Am Soc Nephrol 1994;4:1670–1674.

30. Saborio P, Scheinman JI: Sickle cell nephropathy. J Am Soc Nephrol 1999;10:187–192.

31. Bruno D, Wigfall DR, Zimmerman SA, et al: Genitourinary complications of sickle cell disease. J Urol 2001;166:803–811.

32. Swartz MA, Karth J, Schneider DT, et al: Renal medullary carcinoma: Clinical, pathologic, immunohistochemical, and genetic analysis with pathogenetic implications. Urology 2002;60:1083–1089.

33. Sklar AH, Perez JC, Harp RJ, Caruana RJ: Acute renal failure in sickle cell anemia. Int J Artif Organs 1990;13:347–351.

34. McBurney PG, Hanevold CD, Hernandez CM, et al: Risk factors for microalbuminuria in children with sickle cell anemia. J Pediatr Hematol Oncol 2002;24:473–477.

35. Dharnidharka VR, Dabbagh S, Atiyeh B, et al: Prevalence of microalbuminuria in children with sickle cell disease. Pediatr Nephrol 1998;12:475–478.

36. Guasch A, Zayas CF, Eckman JR, et al: Evidence that microdeletions in the a globin gene protect against the development of sickle cell glomerulopathy in humans. J Am Soc Nephrol 1999;10:1014–1019.

37. Sklar AH, Campbell H, Caruana RJ, et al: Population study of renal function in sickle cell anemia. Int J Artif Organs 1990;13:231–236.

38. Bakir AA, Hathiwala SC, Ainis H, et al: Prognosis of the nephrotic syndrome in sickle glomerulopathy: A retrospective study. Am J Nephrol 1987;7:110–115.

39. Wierenga KJJ, Pattison JR, Brink N, et al: Glomerulonephritis after human parvovirus infection in homozygous sickle-cell disease. Lancet 1995;346:475–476.

40. Foucan L, Bourhis V, Bangou J, et al: A randomized trail of captopril for microalbuminuria in normotensive adults with sickle cell anemia. Am J Med 1998;104:339–402.

41. Hatch FE, Crowe LR, Miles DE, et al: Altered vascular reactivity in sickle hemoglobinopathy. A possible protective factor from hypertension. Am J Hypertens 1989;2:2–8.

42. Maaten JC ter, Serné EH, Bakker SJL, et al: Effects of insulin on glucose uptake and leg blood flow in patients with sickle cell disease and normal subjects. Metabolism 2001;50:387–392.

43. Powars DR, Elliott-Mills DD, Chan L, et al: Chronic renal failure in sickle cell disease: Risk factors, clinical course, and mortality. Ann Intern Med 1991;115:614–620.

44. Abbott KC, Hypolite IO, Agodoa LY: Sickle cell nephropathy at end-stage renal disease in the United States: Patient characteristics and survival. Clin Nephrol 2002;58:9–15.

45. Ataga KI, Orringer EP: Renal abnormalities in sickle cell disease. Am J Hematol 2000;63:205–211.

46. Bleyer AJ, Donaldson LA, McIntosch M, Adams PL: Relationship between underlying renal disease and renal transplantation outcome. Am J Kidney Dis 2001;37:1152–1161.

47. Ojo AO, Govaerts TC, Schmouder RL, et al. Renal transplantation in end-stage sickle cell nephropathy. Transplantation 1999;67:291–295.

CHAPTER 49

Congenital Abnormalities of the Renal Tract

Guy H. Neild and John O. Connolly

INTRODUCTION

This chapter discusses malformations of the urinary tract that can result in renal problems and renal failure. Nearly half the children and young adults who develop end-stage renal disease (ESRD) have asymmetric irregularly shaped kidneys.[1] This appearance, often referred to as *bilateral renal scarring*, is frequently associated with vesicoureteral reflux (VUR). It is generally a consequence of congenital malformations of the kidneys and urinary tract and is variously described as reflux nephropathy or formerly as chronic pyelonephritis.

The most serious conditions involve bladder outflow obstruction, and many can now be detected antenatally.[2] With the advances of molecular medicine, there has been rapid progress in genetics and developmental biology of these conditions. What is becoming clearer is that malformations of the ureter, bladder, and urethra can be associated with primary renal malformations (renal dysplasia). This is a change from the view that renal scarring and damage are secondary to the outflow problem and ureteral reflux. The concept of acquired scarring is often wrong.

CLINICAL PRINCIPLES

Congenital renal tract abnormalities may present in one of five settings:
1. Antenatal diagnosis by fetal ultrasound screening[2]
2. Failure to thrive in an infant or young child
3. Investigation of urinary tract infection (UTI)
4. An incidental finding in a child or adult
5. An adult with abnormal urinalysis, stones, hypertension, or renal insufficiency

The identification of these problems always poses the following questions:
- What is the cause?
- What is the natural history?
- Is surgical intervention required?

Such patients fall into two broad groups. First, there is a group who appear to have normal bladders without outflow obstruction and normal-caliber ureters when not micturating, described as having either primary VUR or primary renal dysplasia. Second, there is a group with some form of bladder outflow dysfunction that causes a secondary VUR and dilated upper urinary tracts, of which posterior urethral valves (PUV) in males is the most common cause.

As predicted by the Brenner hypothesis,[3] small asymmetric kidneys with reduced glomerular filtration rate (GFR) develop all the features of glomerular hyperfiltration, with the onset of progressive renal failure signaled by increasing proteinuria. This can now be significantly modified by treatment with renin-angiotensin

blockade.[4] The details of antenatal and pediatric management of these patients are beyond the scope of this chapter, which focuses on their management in adolescence and adult life.

DEVELOPMENT OF THE URINARY TRACT

The urinary tract develops from the cloaca and intermediate mesoderm in parallel with the early differentiation of the metanephric blastema (future kidney)[5–7] (Fig. 49.1). At the 5th week of fetal life, the mesonephric (Wolffian) duct connects to the allantois and the cloaca. By the 6th week, the urorectal fold appears and divides this cavity, which separates the urinary system (urogenital sinus) from the rectum. Growth of the anterior abdominal wall between the allantois and the urogenital membrane is accompanied by an increase in size and capacity of this bladder precursor. The allantois remains attached to the apex of the fetal bladder and extends into the umbilical root, although it loses its patency and persists as the urachal remnant, the median umbilical ligament, which connects the bladder to the umbilicus. By the 7th week, there is a separate opening of the mesonephric duct into the bladder at what will become the vesicoureteral opening and the area known as the *trigone*. The distal part of the primitive urogenital sinus will form the definitive urogenital sinus. In females, this gives rise to the entire urethra and the vestibule of the vagina. In males, it gives rise to the posterior urethra, whereas the anterior urethra is formed from the closure of the urethral folds.

In the 6-week embryo, the mesonephric and paramesonephric (Müllerian) ducts run in parallel. By 7 weeks, in the male, the latter starts to regress, and the Wolffian duct will eventually develop into the epididymis and the caudal part of the vas deferens. In the female, the Müllerian ducts fuse to become the uterovaginal cord, which opens into the urogenital sinus and will develop into the vagina.

As the urogenital tract develops, there is simultaneous development of the fetal kidney (see Fig. 49.1). In the absence of the ureteral bud, the metanephric kidney does not form. Fetal urine makes a significant contribution to the amniotic fluid by 16 weeks.

Pathogenesis of Maldevelopment

Renal development is orchestrated by the expression of transcription factors, growth and survival factors, and adhesion molecules.[6,8,9] Mutations of genes encoding all classes of these molecules cause urinary tract malformations in mice.[8–10] One family of transcription factor proteins contains the paired DNA-binding domain and is encoded by the *PAX* group of genes. Studies in mice show these *PAX* genes regulate the development of brain, eyes, lymphoid system, musculature, neural crest, and vertebrae.[11,12] *PAX-2* is expressed in the metanephros and in cell lineages that are forming nephrons and also in those that are destined to differentiate into

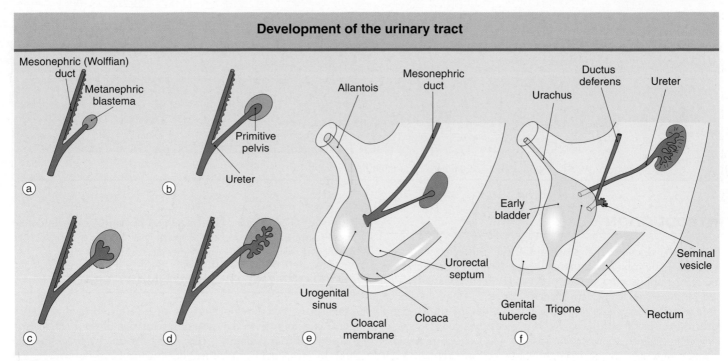

Development of the urinary tract

Figure 49.1   Development of the urinary tract. Growth and development of the ureter, pelvis, and calyces are shown in *a–d*. *a*, The metanephric kidneys first become detectable as small areas in the mesoderm close to the aorta. The primitive epithelial ureter buds off from the mesonephric duct and makes contact with the metanephric mesenchyme. *b*, Under the influence of signals from the ureter, the mesenchyme condenses and proliferates around the ureteral tip, while there is simultaneous elongation and branching of the ureteral tip. *c* and *d*, A primitive pelvis appears, which then branches to form the divisions of the calyces. The branching process continues with the epithelial system eventually differentiating into the nephrons of the renal parenchyma. As the fetus grows, there is ascent of the kidney owing to the continuous rostral growth. *e*, Growth and development of the cloaca during weeks 5–6. *f*, Growth and development of the urogenital sinus into bladder and outflow tract during weeks 8–9.

the ureter, renal pelvis, and branching collecting duct system. The ablation of a single *PAX-2* allele in knock-out mice causes impaired metanephric growth and fewer nephrons than normal, as well as megaureter, a finding consistent with gross VUR.[12] *WT1*, which is mutated in a proportion of Wilms' tumors, is another transcription factor whose mutation is associated with abnormal urinary tract development. Primary VUR, the most common of all malformations leading to renal failure, maps to a locus on chromosome 1[13] and is not associated with *PAX-2* or *WT1*.

Angiotensin type 2 receptor gene null mutant mice display congenital anomalies of the kidney and urinary tract. These include unilateral agenesis, unilateral megaureter and hydronephrosis, and pelvic–ureteral junction (PUJ) obstruction and mimic a range of abnormalities found in humans.[14] Administration of angiotensin-converting enzyme (ACE) inhibitors throughout pregnancy can cause hypotension and anuria in the baby with histologic features of renal tubular dysplasia. This phenotype is also caused by mutations in genes encoding renin, angiotensinogen, ACE, and angiotensin II receptor type 1.

Other syndromes associated with dysplasia and agenesis in which the mutation is now known include branchio-oto-renal syndrome (*EYA1* mutation, transcription factor–like protein); Fraser syndrome (*FRAS1* mutation, putative cell adhesion molecule); Kallmann syndrome (X-linked form, *KAL1* mutation, cell adhesion molecule; autosomal form, *FGFR1* mutation, growth factor receptor); renal cysts and diabetes syndrome (*HNF1* mutation, transcription factor).[8]

RENAL MALFORMATIONS

Congenitally abnormal kidneys may be large or small, cystic or irregular in outline, and absent or misplaced.

We have traditionally discussed these conditions on the basis of findings on intravenous urography (IVU), but we are entering a transition period in which the findings on computed tomography (CT) and magnetic resonance imaging (MRI) are increasingly being emphasized.

Large Kidneys
Enlarged kidneys resulting from congenital problems are usually hydronephrotic or cystic. Wilms' tumor must also be considered. The differential diagnosis in adults of enlarged kidneys, both congenital and acquired, is shown in Chapter 5, Figure 5.2, and the differential diagnosis of cystic kidney disease is discussed further in Chapters 43 and 44.

Irregular Kidneys
Irregularity of the renal outline may result from fetal lobulation or a "dromedary hump", neither of which have any functional implications. Much more important is the diagnosis of renal dysplasia.

Renal Dysplasia
The range of dysplastic and other malformations of the kidney is presented in Figure 49.2. It is clear that abnormalities of the ureter, bladder, and urethra are often associated with renal dysplasia.[15,16] All types of renal dysplasia can also occur as isolated developmental anomalies. Renal dysplasia, although typically producing small, irregular kidneys, may sometimes be cystic or multicystic renal dysplasia.

Renal Hypoplasia (Oligomeganephronia)
Hypoplasia is defined as a congenitally small kidney (2 standard deviations below the expected mean) that lacks evidence of parenchymal maldifferentiation (renal dysplasia) or of acquired

Definitions of renal dysplasia and malformation

Term	Characteristics
Renal agenesis	Absence of the kidney or an identifiable metanephric structure
Renal aplasia	Severe dysplasia with an extremely small kidney, sometimes identifiable only by histologic examination
Renal dysplasia	Abnormal differentiation of the renal parenchyma with the development of abnormal structures, including primitive ducts surrounded by collars of connective tissue, metaplastic cartilage, a variety of nonspecific malformations such as preglomeruli of the fetal type, and reduced branching of the collecting ducts with cystic dilations and primitive tubules
Renal hypoplasia	Significantly reduced renal mass and nephron number without evidence of maldevelopment of the parenchyma
Renal multicystic dysplasia	Severe cystic dysplasia with extremely enlarged kidney full of cystic structures. It occurs as an isolated renal lesion in response to ureteral atresia and urethral obstruction. Ten percent of patients have a family history.

Figure 49.2   Definitions of renal dysplasia and malformation.

disease sufficient to explain the reduced size. The term, however, is often used very loosely, and most patients with a small kidney and other malformations will have oligomeganephronia. This is a type of renal hypoplasia resulting from a congenital reduction in the number of nephrons. It results from arrested development of the metanephric blastema at 14 to 20 weeks' gestation with subsequent hypertrophy of glomeruli and tubules in the kidney. The hypertrophy and hyperfiltration result later in life in progressive nephron injury and sclerosis. Oligomeganephronia is recognized on renal biopsy by the large size of the glomeruli and tubules and the small number of glomeruli seen in a good core of renal cortex. It is reported in congenital syndromes caused by mutations in *PAX-2* and hepatocyte nuclear factor-1β (*HNF-1β*).

Differential Diagnosis of Scarred Kidneys: Dysplasia Versus Reflux

Progressive scarring and renal failure were once considered chronic parenchymal infection (so-called chronic pyelonephritis) and as such were a consequence of VUR. However, in the 1980s, there was retreat from the paradigm of the primary role of infection, and emphasis was placed on scarring as a result of reflux and the progressive nature of the glomerular lesion associated with glomerular hypertension (or hyperfiltration), so-called reflux nephropathy.[3,17–19] The emphasis is changing again to the concept that scarring is often a consequence of renal dysplasia and that the reflux is a secondary feature (Fig. 49.3). Thus, irregular kidneys with normal-caliber ureters are more likely caused by primary dysplasia, and there may be no evidence of VUR.

Disease in Adults

A practical clinical problem is the differential diagnosis of scarred, asymmetric kidneys. With older patients, the differential diagnosis of scarred or "lumpy bumpy" kidneys widens. Whereas in the 1970s, this appearance was often attributed to analgesic nephropathy, today it is often designated as reflux nephropathy. In older patients, multiple scarring from atheromatous arterial disease and

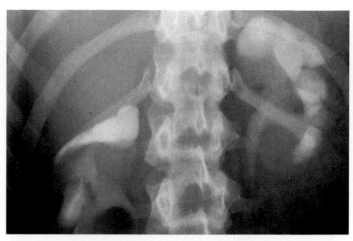

Figure 49.3   Renal dysplasia. Gross bilateral scarring in a 20-year-old woman who has been assessed since the age of 2 years. Progressive scarring has been observed in the absence of urinary tract infections and obstruction. This probably represents primary renal dysplasia.

embolization of the kidney is an increasingly important cause of renal failure. The diagnosis is, in theory, made by the radiologic features of an IVU, but in practice, patients often have advanced renal insufficiency and are unable to excrete enough radiocontrast to delineate the anatomy of the calyces and pelvis and their relationship to the scarring. With urologic conditions, there will be distortion and clubbing of calyces, whereas with other conditions, the calyceal pattern should be normal (except for examples of papillary necrosis; Fig. 49.4). Scarring is best demonstrated by a ^{99m}Tc-labeled dimercaptosuccinic acid (DMSA) scintigram.

Absent Kidneys
Unilateral Renal Agenesis

Complete absence of one kidney occurs in 1 in 500 to 1000 births. It can be familial, and the term *hereditary renal aplasia* is used by pediatricians. It is an autosomal dominant trait with incomplete penetrance and variable expression and can be associated with bilateral renal agenesis or severe dysplasia. In some families, mutations in uroplakin IIIa are found.[20]

Typically, there is no ureter, and the ipsilateral half of the bladder trigone is missing. The remaining kidney is usually hypertrophic, but it may be ectopic, malrotated, or hydronephrotic with a megaureter (Fig. 49.5). The more severe the dysplasia of the remaining kidney, the earlier the presentation. The ipsilateral testis and seminal tract are usually absent, and in 10% of cases, the adrenal gland is also missing. Girls can have an absent fallopian tube, ovary, or malformation of the vagina or uterus. Other associations include imperforate anus and malformations of the vertebrae and cardiovascular system. Agenesis could result from failure in formation of either the metanephros or the ureteral bud; however, when it is associated with cloacal abnormalities, the latter is more likely.

Normality of the single kidney should be confirmed by a ^{99m}Tc-DMSA scintigram, a normal isotopic GFR, and the absence of proteinuria. If the remaining kidney is not normal, lifelong follow-up is necessary. Ultrasound study of the kidneys of first-degree relatives is recommended in all families in which there is an individual with unilateral or bilateral renal agenesis.

Bilateral Renal Agenesis

Bilateral renal agenesis is lethal. It is associated with pulmonary hypoplasia and a characteristic facial appearance (Potter's facies) caused by intrauterine compression, which is a consequence of

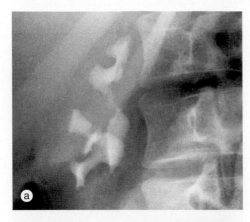

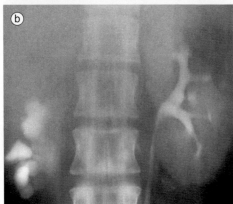

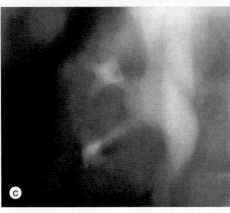

Figure 49.4   Differential diagnosis of "lumpy bumpy" kidneys from the intravenous urogram appearance. *a,* Sickle cell disease: papillary necrosis. Missing papillae leave a round hole in the medulla and give a clubbed appearance. Otherwise, the calyceal architecture is relatively well preserved. *b,* Reflux nephropathy. There is gross scarring and distortion of the calyceal pattern of the right kidney, giving rise to clubbed appearance of the dilated calyces. With reflux, there is a predilection for scarring of the upper and lower poles, whereas with papillary necrosis or analgesic nephropathy, changes are less predictable. *c,* Analgesic nephropathy: the uniformly small shrunken kidney has relative preservation of the calyceal pattern. A plain film showed areas of calcification in both kidneys.

oligohydramnios. The prevalence is about 1 in 10,000, with risk for occurrence in siblings of about 3%; unless there is a family history of agenesis, when risk rises to 15% to 20%.

Misplaced Kidneys
Renal Ectopia, Malrotation, and Crossed Fused Kidneys
The starting position of the fetal kidney is deep in the pelvis. Kidneys that fail to ascend properly and, therefore, remain lower than usual occur in 1 in 800 births. During development and ascent

of the kidney, the renal pelvis comes to face more medially. The most common anomaly is for the pelvis to face forward. The more ectopic the kidney, the more severe the rotation and abnormal the appearance (Fig. 49.6). This is best visualized on an IVU, except when the kidney overlies the pelvic bone and may be impossible to see. In this case, or if one is simply looking for the kidney, a DMSA renogram is best. Symptoms and complications are caused by associated reflux or PUJ obstruction.

Horseshoe Kidney
If both kidneys are low, they may join at the lower pole and are usually drained by two ureters (Fig. 49.7). They lie lower than normal, and further ascent is prevented by the root of the inferior mesenteric artery. This occurs in 1 in 400 to 1800 births and is more common in males (2:1). Patients present, if at all, with complications of reflux, obstruction, or stone formation.

Calyceal Abnormalities
Hydrocalyx and Hydrocalycosis
Dilated calyces are usually caused by obstruction. Focal dilation can also be caused by congenital infundibular stenosis, extrinsic compression from vessel or tumor, stones, or tuberculosis. If

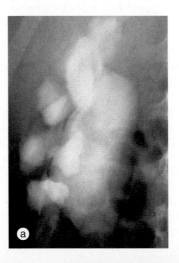

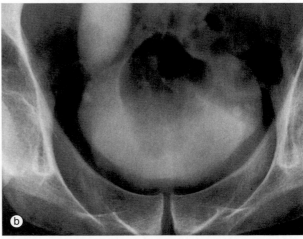

Figure 49.5   Megaureter and hydronephrosis. Intravenous urogram in a 50-year-old man showing a right megaureter and hydronephrosis. There was left renal agenesis. His glomerular filtration rate was 70 ml/min, and he had never had a urine infection or urinary tract symptoms. *a,* Despite the grossly dilated appearance of the calyces, there was no evidence of obstruction on dynamic scans. *b,* There is a single dilated megaureter. A micturating cystogram showed no evidence of reflux.

obstruction is excluded, the appearance is likely to be a congenital abnormality and can be an incidental finding. Moreover, if the GFR is normal and the divided function of the kidneys is 50:50, surgery to "improve" the anatomy should not be attempted.

Megacalycosis

In megacalycosis, there is bizarre dysplasia of the calyceal system with an increase in the number of calyces. There is no obstruction, and it results from malformation of renal papillae. Megacalycosis is congenital, usually unilateral, and an incidental finding. It is much more common in males (6:1) and occurs only in Caucasians.

Bilateral disease is confined to males, and segmental, unilateral disease to females, which suggests an X-linked partially recessive gene with reduced penetrance in females. There may be an associated ipsilateral segmental megaureter, usually affecting the distal third.

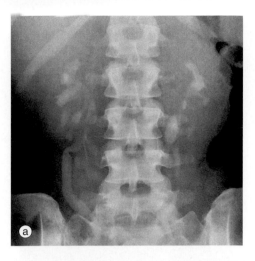

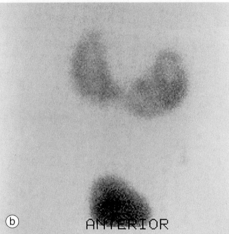

Figure 49.7 Horseshoe kidney. *a,* Intravenous urogram soon after pregnancy in a 25-year-old woman shows not only the horseshoe kidney joining in the midline but also dilated ureters following her pregnancy. *b,* Dimercaptosuccinate scan showing a horseshoe kidney.

Calyceal Diverticulum (Calyceal Cyst)

Calyceal diverticulum is a cavity, peripheral to a minor calyx that is not a closed cyst but is connected to the calyx by a narrow channel. It is usually an incidental finding in 5 per 1000 IVUs and is best seen on a delayed film (Fig. 49.8). If present, symptoms relate to stones or infection within the cavity.

Bardet-Biedl Syndrome

Multiple calyceal clubbing and calyceal diverticula are the characteristic features of the renal dysplasia seen in Bardet-Biedl syndrome (formerly known as Laurence-Moon-Biedl syndrome).[21] This autosomal recessive condition is characterized by retinitis pigmentosa, dysmorphic extremities (sometimes with polydactyly), obesity, and hypogonadism. Calyceal malformation is associated with parenchymal dysplasia; renal failure in early adult life is common.

Bardet-Biedl syndrome is probably the result of a lack of cilia formation or function caused by a defect of the basal body of ciliated cells. The *TTC8* gene mutation encodes a protein with a prokaryotic domain, pilF, involved in pilus formation and twitching mobility.[22]

Pelvic-Ureteral Junction Obstruction

PUJ obstruction is one of the most frequent causes of obstructive uropathy in children. The condition is usually congenital but

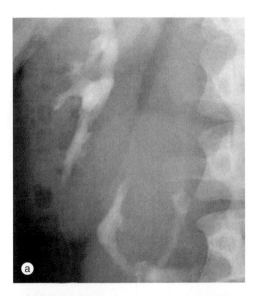

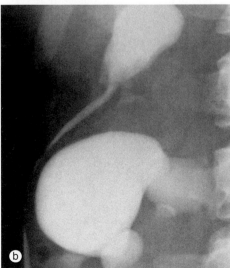

Figure 49.6 Crossed ectopia visualized by intravenous urography. *a,* A relatively normal right kidney and below it a crossed ectopic left kidney. *b,* A crossed left kidney with pelvic-ureteral junction obstruction. After furosemide (frusemide), the upper kidney washed out completely, whereas the appearance in the lower kidney did not change. It is often impossible to tell from the intravenous urogram whether the kidneys are fused, and this may require an isotopic dimercaptosuccinate renogram.

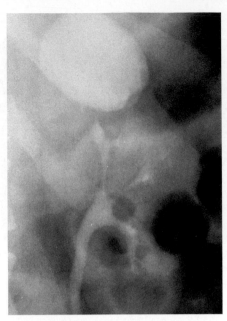

Figure 49.8 Calyceal cyst. Intravenous urogram showing an upper pole calyceal cyst. The plain abdominal film showed a group of stones in the floor of the cyst.

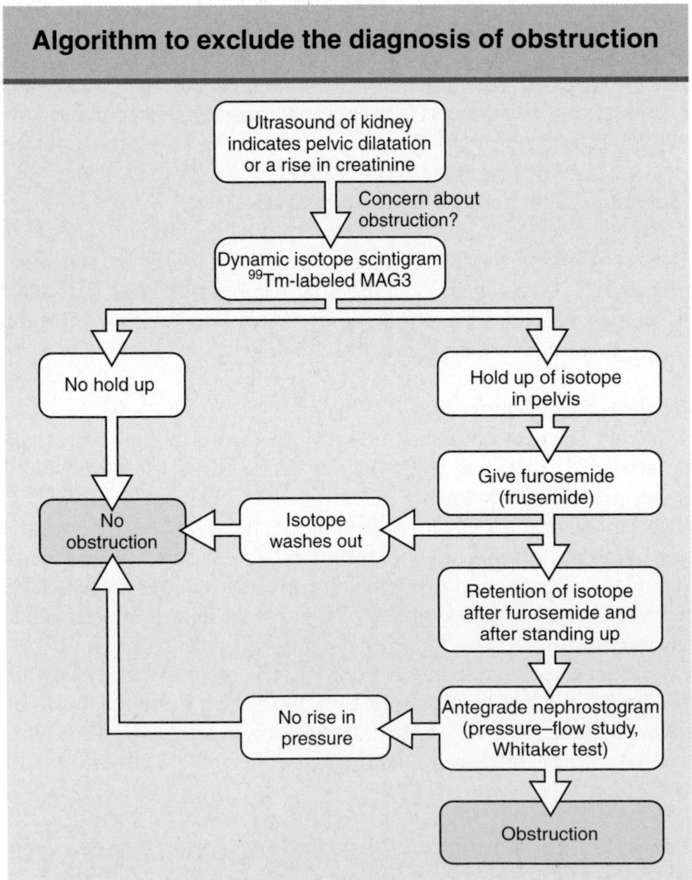

Algorithm to exclude the diagnosis of obstruction

Ultrasound of kidney indicates pelvic dilatation or a rise in creatinine

Concern about obstruction?

Dynamic isotope scintigram ^{99}Tm-labeled MAG3

No hold up

Hold up of isotope in pelvis

Give furosemide (frusemide)

No obstruction

Isotope washes out

Retention of isotope after furosemide and after standing up

No rise in pressure

Antegrade nephrostogram (pressure–flow study, Whitaker test)

Obstruction

Figure 49.9 Algorithm to exclude the diagnosis of obstruction.

can have an acquired mechanical basis caused by stenosis or external compression from adhesions, aberrant lower pole vessels, or kinking of the most proximal ureter. Associated abnormalities are common, and up to 50% of infants have another urologic abnormality, such as contralateral PUJ, a contralateral renal dysplastic and multicystic kidney, minor degrees of VUR, and contralateral renal agenesis.

Older children can present with an abdominal mass or with pain in the flank, hematuria secondary to mild trauma, or UTI. Hypertension is unusual but can occur temporarily after surgical correction.

Diagnostic procedures have to differentiate between significant obstruction (Fig. 49.9) that requires surgical correction and congenital ectasia of the renal pelvis, in which case surgery is not indicated. Indications for surgical intervention include impairment of renal function, pyelonephritis, renal stones, and pain. Kidneys with good function can generally be left alone, and surgery is only indicated when function is clearly shown to deteriorate.[23]

Gonadal Dysgenesis

The problems of intersex, gender identity, and micropenis are beyond the scope of this chapter and rarely encountered in adult practice. Patients will be met, however, with ESRD who are phenotypically female but are genotype XY and have mutations of *WT1* (Denys-Drash and Frasier syndromes). They have gonadal dysgenesis and must have their streak ovaries removed; otherwise, they will develop gonadoblastomas.

URETERAL ABNORMALITIES

Duplex Ureters

Duplication of the ureter and the renal pelvis is a common anomaly, with an incidence of about 1 in 150 births; unilateral duplication is six times more frequent than bilateral. It is more common in girls. If duplication has been detected in a patient, the likelihood of another sibling with duplication rises to 1 in 8.

Pathogenesis

If the ureteral bud bifurcates after its origin from the mesonephric duct but arises at a normal site, an incomplete ureteral duplication with a Y-ureter will develop.[7] Complete ureteral duplication occurs if there are two ureteral buds, one in the normal location and the other in a low position. The normal bud ends in a correct site on the trigone in the bladder and is nonrefluxing. The lower bud, representing the ureter of the lower pole of the kidney, ends in the bladder as a lateral orifice with a short submucosal tunnel. The lower pole ureter is, therefore, often associated with VUR, and scarring of the lower pole can result.

If there are two ureteral buds, one with a normal location and one with a high position, the upper ureter is incorporated into the developing bladder, ending more distally and medial to the normal one. Thus, the upper pole ureter ends ectopically and as a consequence of either obstruction or dysplasia, and there is often severe scarring of the upper pole moiety.

Clinical Manifestations

In most adult patients, ureteral reduplication is asymptomatic and causes no long-term problems. Children with ureteral duplication often have VUR. The spontaneous disappearance of reflux is less common in duplex ureters than in patients with a single ureter.[24] Duplex ureters are best diagnosed by IVU and cystoscopy. PUJ obstruction of the ureter draining the lower pole of the kidney can occur.

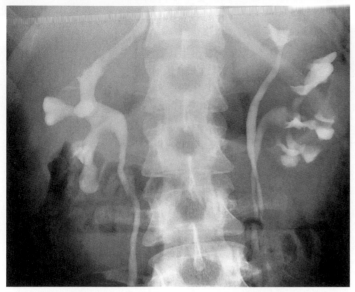

Figure 49.10 **Duplex kidney.** Intravenous urogram shows a duplex left kidney. The lower pole is scarred and shows evidence of reflux damage. The two ureters entered the bladder separately, with the lower pole ureter in the abnormal location. The right kidney also shows features of reflux, with clubbing of the calyces and some scarring.

Associated conditions such as ectopic ureters or ureterocele (see later discussion) usually cause problems in early life and, therefore, have been dealt with by adolescence. Upper pole scarring is associated with an ectopic ureter, lower pole scarring with VUR (Fig. 49.10).

Ectopic Ureters

Ectopic ureters are almost always associated with ureteral reduplication, and 10% are bilateral. There is a female-to-male ratio of 7:1. The ectopic ureter comes from the upper pole and inserts into the bladder more distally and toward the bladder neck, or it opens into the upper urethra. In females, the ureter may end in the urethra, vagina, or vulva, and patients present with incontinence, UTIs, or a persistent vaginal discharge, particularly if the external sphincter is damaged, for example, during labor.

Ectopic ureters are rare in males and present as UTI. Usually, there is a single ureter associated with a dysplastic kidney, which ends in the posterior urethra, ejaculatory duct, seminal vesicle, or vas. Males are usually continent because the ureter is proximal to the external sphincter.

Ectopic ureters are best visualized by an IVU, although a small dysplastic kidney may be missed. A micturating cystourethrogram shows reflux into the lower pole of the kidney in 50% of patients.

Ureterocele

Ureteroceles are cystic dilations of the terminal segments of the ureter and are caused by maldevelopment of the caudal ureter. They occur more commonly in females (4:1) and almost exclusively in Caucasians, and 10% are bilateral.

Ectopic ureters and those with ureteroceles frequently (80%) drain the upper pole and are often associated with dysplastic or nonfunctional renal tissue. They usually present in childhood with infection; when large, they can obstruct the bladder neck or even the contralateral ureter. In adults, they commonly present with stones in the lower ureter. The treatment of simple ureteroceles is surgical excision with reimplantation of the ureter, or simple incision if they subtend a well-functioning moiety. There are usually no medical sequelae.

Megaureter

Isolated dilation of the ureter does not necessarily imply obstruction. There are three broad groups of conditions with widely dilated ureters:

1. *Obstruction of the ureter itself.* This may be intrinsic (e.g., stone) or extrinsic (e.g., retroperitoneal fibrosis); it is not associated with reflux.
2. *Bladder outflow obstruction, with secondary ureteral obstruction.* Examples would include a neuropathic bladder or posterior urethral valves; it may or may not be associated with reflux.
3. *A dilated but nonobstructed ureter for which there is no apparent cause.* This often occurs without reflux, and there can be normal renal function; sometimes, this is caused by an adynamic segment of the lower ureter (see Fig. 49.5).

Pathogenesis

In the normal ureter, there is a characteristic helical orientation of muscle fibers. When the megaureter is secondary to bladder outflow obstruction, there is muscular hyperplasia and hypertrophy of the ureteral wall. In megaureters for which there is no apparent cause, a variety of abnormalities of muscle orientation are described, or there may even be absence of muscle fibers at the proximal end of the undilated segment. By electron microscopy, there is an increase in collagen between the muscle bundles at the level of the obstructing segment.[25] Obstruction appears to be caused by a failure of peristalsis through the distal ureteral segment.

Clinical Manifestations

Most cases of megaureter associated with obstruction present in childhood with severe infections, often complicated by septicemia. In such cases, there is a high incidence of other congenital abnormalities. In less severe cases or when there is no obstruction, patients can present with abdominal pain, loin pain, hematuria, and UTI. Renal stones can form easily in the dilated systems. The exclusion of obstruction is often only established by an antegrade pressure–flow study (Whitaker test), in which a nephrostomy is placed in the renal pelvis and contrast infused at 10 ml/min.[26]

Treatment

A definite diagnosis (is there obstruction or not?) must be made (see Fig. 49.9). The current view is that patients with nonobstructed asymptomatic disease should be managed conservatively, and most do very well with this approach.

BLADDER AND OUTFLOW DISORDERS

Prune Belly Syndrome

The prune belly syndrome occurs in males and consists of absence of the muscles of the anterior abdominal wall, bizarre malformations of the urinary tract with gross dilatation of the bladder and ureters, and bilateral undescended testes.[27–29] When diagnosed early, renal outcome is related to the degree of renal dysplasia. There are incomplete forms of the syndrome (pseudo-prune). Rarely, a similar megacystis or megaureter may be seen in either sex.

Pathogenesis

No gene defect or unifying hypothesis has emerged to explain these features. The incidence varies from 1 in 30,000 to 50,000. There are a few familial cases, and the condition has been reported in twins, but there is 100% discordance reported in identical twins, which is a powerful argument against a genetic basis. There is evidence for a primary, localized arrest of mesenchymal development. This is supported by the lack of prostatic differentiation: the epithelial element in the prostate is absent or hypoplastic. Ultrastructure studies of the ureter show massive replacement of smooth muscle with fibrous and collagen tissue and the absence of nerve plexuses. A nearly identical syndrome can occur as a consequence of fetal urethral obstruction, including urethral atresia.

Clinical Manifestations

The prognosis is dependent on the degree of renal dysplasia and injury. Three groups can be distinguished. In group I, complete urethral obstruction causes stillbirth or neonatal death (20%); in group II, acute, early presentation requires diversion and reconstruction (20%); in group III, good health and renal function exist despite urologic appearances (60%).

There is complete absence or incomplete formation of the rectus abdominis and other muscles, which leads to the wrinkled abdominal wall of the prune infant. This gives way to a fairly smooth "pot belly" in later life (Fig. 49.11). Reconstructive surgery is not normally required. The patients grow up physically active and strong but cannot sit up directly from a supine position. Abnormalities of the thoracic cage, such as pectus excavatum, are common.

Although true outflow obstruction is sometimes present, the gross and irregular dilation of the urinary tract that is characteristic of this syndrome is primarily caused by a developmental defect with a variable degree of smooth muscle aplasia leading to aperistaltic ureters (Fig. 49.12). Urodynamics are often difficult to interpret because of gross VUR, but typically there is a low-pressure bladder. With late presentation, some patients have detrusor instability.

Differential Diagnosis

In severe cases of megacystis or megaureter with gross impairment of renal function (often with dysplastic kidneys), the differential diagnosis includes posterior urethral valves, renal dysplasia with

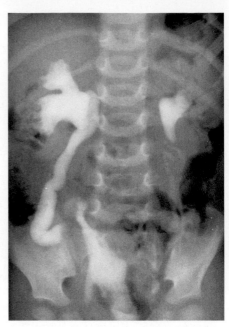

Figure 49.12 Prune belly syndrome. Typical intravenous urogram appearance of a patient with prune belly syndrome and good renal function. Often, the ureters are extremely dilated and tortuous.

or without multiple congenital defects, neuropathic bladder, and nephrogenic diabetes insipidus.

Natural History

Once any outflow obstruction is dealt with, usually in infancy, the renal function should remain stable despite the frightening radiologic appearances. In those patients followed in our unit for up to 40 years, renal deterioration and hypertension have been rare. In the small number who have progressed, recurrent infection, hypertension, and proteinuria have been warning signs of impending trouble.

Renal scarring should be assessed by isotopic DMSA scintigrams, and renal function followed by serial isotopic GFR measurements. Lifelong attention to blood pressure, UTIs, and stones is necessary.

Treatment

In all children, even with good renal function, there should be a careful search for obstruction, beginning with the urethra and working up to the PUJ, but often no obstruction is found and no surgery is required. In many others, the floppy bladder is not anatomically obstructed, but bladder emptying is improved by urethrotomy ("functional obstruction"). In infancy, there is debate about the need for reconstructive surgery. There is certainly a group of patients born with severely compromised renal function who do require reconstruction after stabilization by early diversion.[30]

The current view is that the testes should be brought down to the scrotum in infancy. It is hoped that earlier surgery will produce proper germ cell development and thus preserve fertility. So far, however, no prune patient has been shown to be fertile.

Bladder Exstrophy (Ectopia Vesicae)

Classic exstrophy is the failure of the anterior abdominal wall and bladder to close, but there are a range of defects from epispadias of an otherwise normal penis to major cloacal abnormalities (Fig. 49.13).

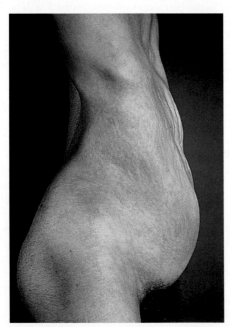

Figure 49.11 Prune belly syndrome. Note the lax abdominal musculature leading to a pot-bellied appearance. There is also marked thoracic cage deformity. (Courtesy of Mr. C. R. J. Woodhouse.)

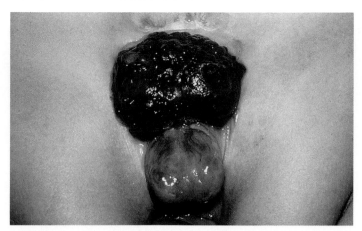

Figure 49.13   Bladder exstrophy. The entire length of the penis is also open (epispadias). (Courtesy of Mr. C. R. J. Woodhouse.)

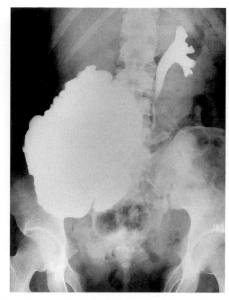

Figure 49.14   Cystography in bladder exstrophy. A 26-year-old woman with bladder exstrophy who has a continent Mitrofanoff system using the colon to create a reservoir. There is reflux into the left kidney. There is also reflux into the right kidney, but the kidney is obscured by the full reservoir. Her glomerular filtration rate is 130 ml/min.

Pathogenesis

Failure of growth of the lower abdominal wall between the allantois and the urogenital membrane, coupled with breakdown of the urogenital membrane, leaves a small, open bladder plate, a low-placed umbilical root, and diastasis of the pubic bones. The genital tubercle is probably placed lower in these patients, and the cloacal membrane ruptures above it, leading to a penis with an open dorsal surface that is continuous with the bladder plate. A midline closure defect causes a failure of fusion of the lower anterior abdominal wall, including the symphysis pubis, lower urinary tract, and external genitalia. There are rare reports of a familial incidence. The condition occurs in 1 in 10,000 to 50,000 births. The male-to-female ratio is 2:1.

Clinical Manifestations

In severe cases, the bladder mucosa lies exposed on the lower abdominal wall, with the bladder neck and urethra laid open. The prostate and testes are normal. Most patients have normal kidneys at birth (although many reports do not record the state of the kidneys at birth). In one series, 33% had dilated ureters at presentation, but an IVU was usually normal after diversion. However, in another series, one third of patients were said to have unilateral renal agenesis.[31] Renal function may be preserved after the diversion, although reflux is common (Fig. 49.14).

Other congenital abnormalities are only rarely present. More severe cloacal abnormalities are associated with imperforate anus and either high or low rectal atresia.

Natural History

Long-term renal outcome depends on the bladder. In the long term (up to 25 years), the kidneys survive much better with a well-functioning bladder: 13% of those with a good bladder had significant renal damage, compared with 82% with ileal conduits, 22% with nonrefluxing colonic conduits, and 33% with ureterosigmoidostomy.[32] Today, the bladder is augmented (enterocystoplasty, ileocystoplasty, cecocystoplasty) or replaced by bowel (intestinal reservoir). In a study of 53 such patients, who were followed for more than 10 years, renal function deteriorated (fall in GFR of 20% or more) in only 10 (20%).[33]

Treatment

When the infant is born, the three urologic treatment goals are to close the abdominal wall, to establish urinary continence and preserve renal function, and to reconstruct cosmetically acceptable genitalia.

The aim of initial surgery is to convert the patient's defect to a complete epispadias (Fig. 49.15). At 4 years of age, reconstruction of the bladder neck and correction of the epispadias can be performed. If the bladder is small, intestinal augmentation is required. Patients may be able to void, but many have to use catheters. Incontinence may be a long-term problem.

Neuropathic Bladder

In childhood, the most common cause of a neuropathic bladder is myelomeningocele. A neuropathic bladder may also be seen without associated neurologic or other obvious causes (Fig. 49.16). The principal consequences are incontinence, infection, and reflux with upper tract dilation and subsequently renal failure. Early urodynamic assessment is essential (Fig. 49.17).

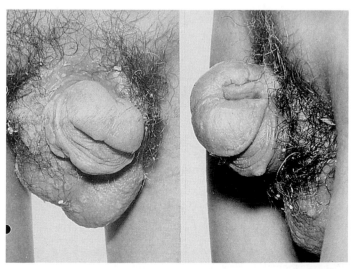

Figure 49.15   Epispadias. Result of multiple surgery to close the epispadias and lengthen the penis. (Courtesy of Mr. C. R. J. Woodhouse.)

Causes of neuropathic bladder	
Area Affected	Causes
Cerebral	Cerebrovascular accident/cerebral palsy, encephalopathy, trauma, Parkinson's disease, dementia
Spinal	Isolated (no other neurologic features), trauma, multiple sclerosis, compression, spina bifida, spinal dysraphism, tethered cord, sacral agenesis, sacral teratoma
Peripheral nerve	Pelvic surgery, diabetes

Figure 49.16   Causes of neuropathic bladder.

Three different patterns of bladder behavior are seen: contractile, intermediate, and acontractile.

Contractile Behavior

An overactive detrusor (hyperreflexia) can produce some bladder emptying (incontinence). Unfortunately, 95% of patients have sphincter dyssynergia (inability to relax urethral sphincter), which results in no relaxation and incomplete emptying of the bladder. Patients with incomplete lesions may have some control of the distal sphincter and normal anal and sacral reflexes. Ironically, although this latter group has the least neurologic deficit, they have the worst bladder situation, generating high pressures and great risk for renal injury. The bladder becomes progressively hypertrophic, fibrotic, and poorly compliant.

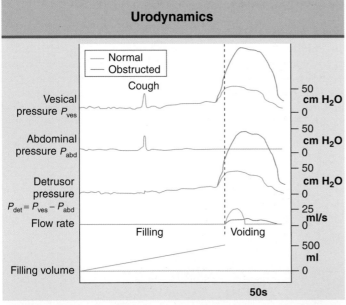

Figure 49.17   Urodynamic assessment by a cystometrogram (CMG). The vesical pressure is measured simultaneously with the abdominal pressure through the rectum; the detrusor pressure is the difference. A cough is used as a marker to show that the system is working. Normally during filling, the first desire to void is at a detrusor pressure of <10 cm H_2O. This point is noted. Normally, the voiding pressure should be <40 cm H_2O (and is lower in women). Detrusor instability is an unstable (spontaneous) contraction occurring with a detrusor pressure >15 cm H_2O. Higher pressure can cause incontinence. When combined with radiologic imaging (VCMG), the following are all recorded: bladder neck, closed/open; bladder pressure, end-filling; voiding detrusor pressure; bladder stability; compliance; flow rate, maximum; sensation, first; volume, voided/residual. (Courtesy of Professor M. Craggs.)

Intermediate Behavior

These patients have some detrusor activity, but not sufficient to empty the bladder. Their bladders are poorly compliant, and they have no voluntary control of their sphincters, so any rise in bladder pressure tends to cause incontinence, or the high intravesical pressures lead to renal injury.

Acontractile Behavior

In about 25% of patients, there is no detrusor activity, and the bladder overflows when it is sufficiently full. This is not usually associated with renal failure.

Myelodysplasia

Myelodysplasia refers to a group of neural tube anomalies that primarily affect the lumbar and sacral segment of the spinal cord and are the most common cause of neurogenic bladder dysfunction in children. Spina bifida means the defective fusion of the posterior vertebral arches. Meningocele implies that the meninges extend beyond the confines of the vertebral canal with no neural elements contained inside. A myelomeningocele has neural tissue protruding with the meningocele. Spinal dysraphism (symptomatic spina bifida occulta) defines a group of structural anomalies of the caudal end of the spinal cord that do not result in an open vertebral canal but are associated with incomplete fusion of the posterior vertebral arches. Sacral agenesis is a rare anomaly in which part or all of two or more vertebral bodies are absent. It occurs early in fetal development when there is failure of ossification of the lowest vertebral segments. The only known teratogen is insulin. Sacral agenesis occurs in 1% of children born to insulin-dependent mothers. Partial sacral agenesis can be associated with an anterior meningocele.

Pathogenesis

Normally, the neural tube forms as the neural folds close over and fuse, starting in the cervical region and progressing caudally. It is believed that the embryologic defect is an incomplete tubularization of the neural tube, with inadequate mesodermal invagination and subsequent arrest of vertebral arch formation.

The incidence of myelodysplasia varies from 1 to 5 in 1000 live births, but there are wide geographic variations. Monozygotic twins are often discordant for spina bifida, but siblings are at increased risk (1:10–20), and children of affected parents have a 4% chance of having a similarly affected child. Myelomeningocele accounts for more than 90% of myelodysplastic infants. Folic acid supplements taken during the last trimester reduce the incidence of myelodysplasia by 50%.

Clinical Manifestations

All causes of tethered cord can produce a variable neurologic deficit. During development, some children develop progressive neurologic disturbance with bladder dysfunction, bowel dysfunction, scoliosis, and a syndrome of pes cavus and limb growth failure.

Bladder Dysfunction   Neuropathic bladder can be an isolated problem with abnormal urodynamic studies but a normal neurologic examination.[34]

Bowel Dysfunction   Bowel dysfunction is often present and needs to be treated accordingly. There may be severe constipation and overflow incontinence. The antegrade continent enterostomy procedure has been developed to improve the management. The appendix is brought out to the abdominal surface, and thus the colon can be irrigated antegradely with saline.

Intelligence Patients with myelomeningocele may have some intellectual impairment, especially those who have required ventriculoperitoneal shunting for associated hydrocephalus. Manual dexterity may also be affected. These are very important issues in long-term management.

Natural History

About 14% of patients have renal complications at birth and are at high risk in the next few years. Ultimately, about 50% will develop upper tract problems, although these can take up to 30 years to occur (Fig. 49.18). In one prospective study, renal outcome could be predicted by the urodynamic findings, with worst outcomes related to increased bladder wall thickness, the degree of reflux, urethral pressures above 70 cm H_2O, and reduced bladder capacity. VUR occurs in 3% to 5% of newborns with detrusor hypertonicity or dyssynergia. Without treatment, this figure increases to 30% to 40% by the age of 5 years.[35]

Treatment

The management of the bladder depends on the urodynamic findings. In the 1970s, clean intermittent self-catheterization (CISC) was introduced,[36] but before that time, urinary diversion was the usual treatment. Today, when reflux and hydroureter are present, the management is principally with CISC and anticholinergic drugs that increase bladder compliance.[37]

Bladder Neck Obstruction

Congenital bladder neck obstruction is rare and is usually caused by a neuropathic bladder, posterior urethral valves, or an ectopic ureterocele.

Posterior Urethral Valves

Posterior urethral valves are the most common cause of severe subvesical obstruction in the male infant (although in the newborn,

they account for only 10% of cases of hydronephrosis). As a consequence, bilateral hydronephrosis and megaureter occur. Obstruction is caused by a diaphragm that extends from the floor to the roof of the urethra at the apex of the prostate. Valves appear as mucosal folds in the posterior urethra below the verumontanum. There is dilation of the proximal urethra and bladder wall hypertrophy and trabeculation. Above the valves, there is dilation of the prostatic urethra, which undermines the bladder neck. The valves only obstruct flow in one direction, and therefore a catheter can be passed without difficulty.

Pathogenesis

The urethra develops in two parts: differentiation of the urogenital sinus part (posterior urethra) and tubularization of the urethral plate (anterior urethra). Early obstruction during renal development can result in severe renal dysplasia.

Clinical Manifestations

Most cases of posterior urethral valves are now detected antenatally by ultrasound. Half of all patients present before the age of 1 year. Infants present with a palpably distended bladder and enlarged kidneys, abnormal urine stream, or failure to thrive owing to renal failure. At diagnosis, 30% to 50% of children have VUR. Children with less severe disease present with poor stream, hematuria, incontinence, acute UTI, or renal failure; however, late presentation is also associated with worse outcome.[38]

There are three abnormal features that can help to protect the kidney. These all act to reduce the high pressures generated during voiding. They are massive unilateral reflux, usually with ipsilateral renal dysplasia (thereby protecting the other kidney); large bladder diverticulum; and urinary extravasation, often with urinary ascites. These protective mechanisms are referred to as "pop-off" mechanisms[39] (see Fig. 49.18). Ultrasound can show the bladder thickening, dilated system, and dilation of the

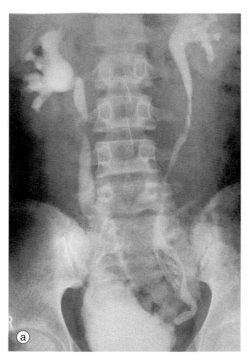
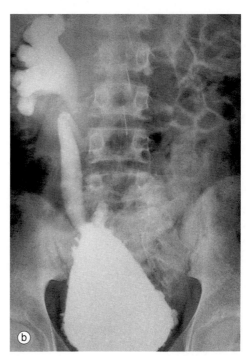

Figure 49.18 Sacral spina bifida with neuropathic bladder. a, Intravenous urogram shows evidence of a previous hydronephrosis and subsequent scarring of the right kidney. The architecture of the left kidney is well preserved. b, Micturating cystogram. The typical tapering, hypertrophied, trabeculated bladder giving the characteristic fir cone appearance. Note the gross reflux on the right side. This is probably helping to protect the left kidney by acting as a pop-off mechanism. This is analogous to the protection that can occur in boys with posterior urethral valves.

posterior urethra. A specific diagnosis should be documented by videocystometrogram (VCMG; see later discussion).

Natural History

In the 1960s, 25% of children died within the first 12 months, and 25% died later in childhood, including "renal death" (i.e., ESRD). By the late 1990s, the early mortality rate was less than 5%, and after 15 years of follow-up, only 15% to 20% of patients had reached ESRD.[40]

The bladder may become stretched, resulting in poor emptying, or unstable, leading to poor compliance, unsuppressed detrusor contractions, and high storage pressure. Both these situations are exaggerated by progressive polyuria. It is not uncommon for such patients to have a daily urine volume of 5 liters. Urodynamic follow-up studies suggest that instability decreases with time; bladder capacity increases, but there are unsustained voiding contractions. The prognosis correlates with the nadir creatinine value. Despite adequate early treatment, many children develop chronic renal insufficiency owing to renal dysplasia.[38,41]

Treatment

All children have had transurethral resection of their valves in infancy. Bladder diversion should be avoided. The question of "undiversion" of ileal conduits (created in earlier times) is discussed later. Bladder instability and poor bladder compliance must be treated, irrespective of whether they are causing symptoms. Boys with substantial residual volumes can be managed by CISC, but there is often poor compliance with this either because of urethral discomfort or because previous urethral surgery has made the passage of catheters difficult. Compliance is a particular problem with adolescents who are continent and for whom renal failure is too abstract a concept. Continence often improves spontaneously at puberty but can be helped by imipramine. Deterioration in renal function will require further examination of urine flow rate and exclusion of urethral stricture.

Urethral Diverticulum

Urethral diverticulum usually occurs in boys and is rare. It may present with UTI, obstruction, or stones. There are two types: anterior or posterior. The former can be associated with anterior urethral valves and obstruction.

GENERAL MANAGEMENT OF CONGENITAL TRACT ABNORMALITIES

The principles of management of congenital tract abnormalities are shown in Figure 49.19. The most important part of the management is ensuring that the patient, family, and primary care physician know what can and must be done. The first thing to make clear is the necessity of long-term follow-up at no more than annual intervals. ESRD commonly occurs when a patient is lost to follow-up, often presenting later with accelerated hypertension and rapid loss of renal function.

Clinical Evaluation

By the time the adolescent is passed on to an adult physician, it is assumed that the urinary tract is not obstructed and further surgery is not required. Nevertheless, it is the responsibility of the nephrologists and urologists who care for these children to review this aspect from time to time.

Symptomatic UTI is common and must be treated promptly. Increase in frequency or severity of infections must lead to

Management of congenital renal tract abnormalities
Educate and explain to encourage compliance
Review urologic status
Find cause of urinary tract obstruction and treat
Control blood pressure
Monitor renal function and proteinuria
Treat acidosis
Prevent bone disease
Check for stones
Clean intermittent self-catheterization for chronic retention
Maintain bladder storage pressure below 40 cm H_2O
Maintain bladder volume below 400 ml

Figure 49.19 General principles of management of congenital renal tract abnormalities.

investigations to find the cause.[42] The blood pressure must be monitored regularly and kept normal. Finally, renal function must be monitored, proteinuria assessed, and the cause of any deterioration identified. As in any other renal condition, the remnant kidney function may decline inexorably, and this is associated with increasing proteinuria and hypertension. As with other renal conditions, function is usually stable when there is little or no proteinuria. Deterioration in the absence of proteinuria must alert the physician to the likelihood of obstruction or some other cause of acute-on-chronic renal failure, such as a nephrotoxic drug.

A number of routine investigations should be performed to document the current situation and to act as a reference point for the future (Fig. 49.20). If the bladder empties completely with an adequate flow rate (15 ml/sec), no problems should arise. If there is any doubt about the condition of the bladder, urodynamic investigations are necessary. If the clinical situation changes, further investigations are required. An increase in UTIs

Monitoring patients with congenital renal tract abnormalities	
Baseline Measurements	Reason for Test
Radiology	
Abdominal x-ray	Exclude stones
Ultrasound of kidneys	Baseline
Ultrasound of bladder postmicturition	Assess residual volume
Urine flow rate	Ensure adequacy
Scintigraphy	
Glomerular filtration rate: ^{51}Cr-labeled EDTA	Baseline
Dynamic isotope scan with ^{99}Tc-labeled MAG3 or DTPA	Assess outflow obstruction/holdup
Static isotope scan with ^{99}Tc-labeled DMSA	Assess scarring and divided function
Biochemistry	
Urine-protein creatinine ratio	Baseline

Figure 49.20 Monitoring patients with congenital renal tract abnormalities. Routine investigations for assessment of clinical status.

might suggest a stone or increase in residual urine. With an unexpected decline in renal function, obstruction has to be excluded all over again.

It is helpful and important for the patient to keep a 24-hour urine-volume diary every 6 to 12 months. Patients are asked to write down the time that they voided and measure and record the volume passed. It is best to ask them to do this on 2 consecutive days, so that one can determine the maximum bladder capacity and the total 24-hour urine volume. This should be done before urodynamic investigations because results can be misleading if bladder is not filled to capacity.

Exclude Obstruction

Obstruction must always be excluded if there is a change in renal function. The possibility of obstruction may be raised by a routine ultrasound (see Fig. 49.9) and should be pursued with an MAG3 scintigram to exclude obstruction (Fig. 49.21).

In patients with conduits, obstruction can be excluded by infusing contrast into the loop (loopogram) and demonstrating reflux up the ureter.

Rarely, in patients with large bladders or in transplant recipients, the kidney may become obstructed when the bladder reaches a certain volume. This can be investigated by filling the bladder by a catheter and performing a ^{99m}Tc-labeled MAG3 scintigram, initially with the bladder full. If there is no excretion, the bladder

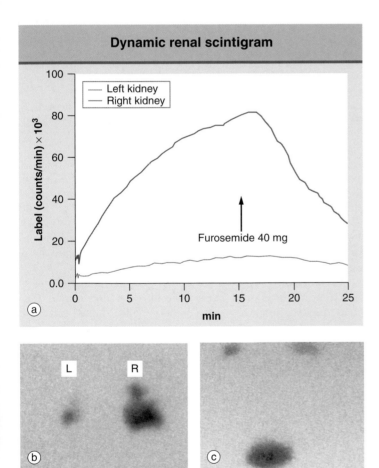

Figure 49.21   Dynamic ^{99}Tc-labeled MAG3 renal scintigram. *a*, Time-activity curve showing accumulation of isotope in right kidney, which washes out after furosemide, thus excluding significant obstruction. Images from the same study, showing holdup of isotope in dilated right renal pelvis (*b*), which washes out into the bladder after furosemide (*c*), excluding significant obstruction.

volume can be reduced in 100-ml increments until there is flow down the ureter (Fig. 49.22).

Urodynamics

Any urodynamic investigation should start with a free urine flow rate. Provided that the flow rate is normal and the bladder empties completely (leaving no residual volume on postmicturition ultrasound), it can be assumed that there is no significant bladder outflow obstruction.

Complete investigation of abnormalities of bladder and urethral function requires synchronous recordings of intravesical and intrarectal pressures taken during bladder filling and emptying (see Fig. 49.18). Combined with radiologic imaging, the study is known as a VCMG.

Surgical Correction of the Urinary Tract

A normal bladder acts as a low-pressure, good-volume urine reservoir that is continent, is sterile, and empties freely and completely. Any other form of urine reservoir aims to recreate such an environment. When this is not achieved in either a natural or a reconstructed bladder, complications such as sepsis and renal dysfunction can occur.

A variety of conduits and continent reservoirs have been developed to replace unusable bladders. Ileal conduit diversion has been most widely used for native kidneys, although deterioration in renal function commonly occurs secondary to long-term complications including urosepsis, renal calculi, and, most commonly, stenosis leading either to obstruction or to reflux with ureteral dilation. There is an overall complication rate of 45%, but with a high index of suspicion and an aggressive diagnostic and therapeutic approach, many of these problems can be detected and treated early, with resultant good long-term function of native kidneys. Similar results may be obtained when renal transplantation is performed in these patients.[43] Other forms of urinary diversion that are continent and, therefore, more socially acceptable to patients are now widely used in general urologic practice and are being encountered in renal transplantation (Fig. 49.23; see also Fig. 49.14). These forms include augmented bladders draining through the urethra and augmented or intestinal bladders draining through continent stomas.

Undiversion of Conduits

The only certain improvement with undiversion is cosmetic. Initially, undiversion was undertaken because of poor results or complications from conduits. Short-term results of undiversion are very promising, and the major indications today would be convenience and cosmetic appearance (see Fig. 49.23). Long-term results, however, are not available.

Before considering undiversion, four factors must be considered:
1. Is there residual obstruction?
2. What is the function of the bladder?
3. What is the function of the sphincters?
4. What is the normal 24-hour urine output?

In particular, the bladder storage pressure must be considered because one must achieve a low-pressure reservoir. This is a particular problem when patients are polyuric. The potential capacity of the bladder will often have to be reassessed after a period of bladder cycling, when the bladder is repeatedly filled through a suprapubic catheter and the volume, voiding capacity, and residual volume are determined. If the native bladder is not of sufficient volume and compliance, some form of augmentation will be required.

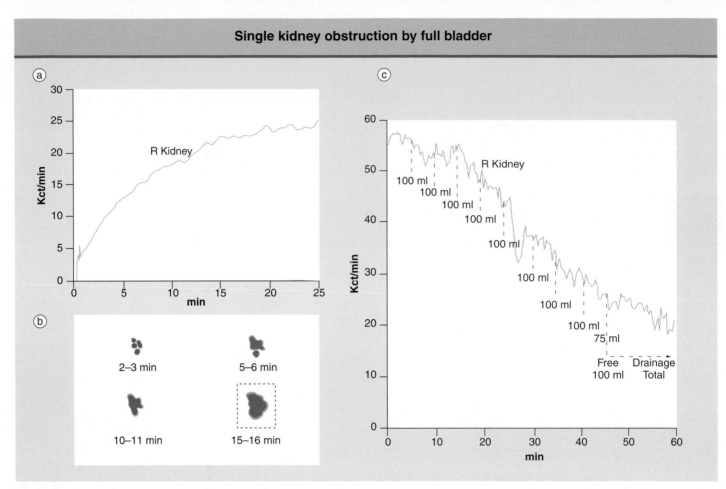

Figure 49.22 **Dynamic isotope scan (MAG3) starting with bladder full in a patient with solitary right kidney.** *a*, Rising curve of tracer accumulating in kidney and showing no excretion. *b*, Accumulation of isotope in hydronephrotic pelvis without excretion to bladder. *c*, 100-ml increments of fluid removed from bladder result in eventual free drainage of the kidney.

COMPLICATIONS

Urinary Tract Infections (To Treat or Not To Treat)
Symptomatic UTIs are common.[42] Risk factors include stagnation of urine, stones, foreign bodies (stents, catheters), previous infections, and renal scarring. UTIs must be treated promptly after a urine culture (midstream or catheter specimen) has been taken.

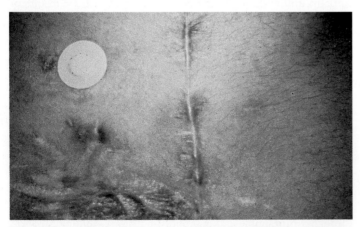

Figure 49.23 **Mitrofanoff stoma.** A patient born with bladder exstrophy who has had a successful renal transplant for the past 11 years. Her kidney is plumbed into a colonic reservoir, and she catheterizes herself through a continent Mitrofanoff stoma, which in the picture is covered by a small piece of bandage.

Recurrent UTIs, particularly after a period of stability, must lead to further investigations to exclude stones or obstruction, including abdominal x-ray, renal ultrasound, and postmicturition bladder ultrasound.

Asymptomatic UTIs often do not require treatment (except during pregnancy). For patients with urinary diversions, it is important to get a catheter specimen of urine because urine taken from a bag is invariably infected.

Sometimes it is appropriate to give prophylactic antibiotics, such as trimethoprim or nitrofurantoin, to eradicate infection. Many patients believe that cranberry juice helps them; it reduces the incidence of *Escherichia coli* infection, but will not treat a symptomatic infection. Tetracycline and oxytetracycline are contraindicated because they are toxic to damaged tubules and cause acute-on-chronic renal failure. Doxycycline, however, can be used. Nitrofurantoin and nalidixic acid are avoided if GFR is reduced below 50 ml/min because they are both renally excreted and toxic in renal failure. Quinolones should not be used for prophylaxis, if possible, because of the risk for inducing resistance. Attempts to sterilize the urinary tract, when foreign bodies such as stones remain, are unlikely to be successful.

If prophylactic antibiotics are no longer effective at preventing infection, it is advisable to stop all antibiotics and to give the patient a supply of antibiotics to treat symptoms at home as they occur.

Hypertension and Glomerular Hyperfiltration

If renal function is declining and proteinuria and hypertension are present, glomerular hyperfiltration is likely, although all other causes of renal dysfunction must be excluded. Patients should be treated with angiotensin antagonists (ACE inhibitors and angiotensin receptor blockers [ARBs]).[4]

Proteinuria and Progressive Renal Failure

Can progression to ESRD be predicted, and does treatment with ACE inhibitors delay or prevent this?[4] We investigated this in a retrospective review of patients with scarred irregular kidneys as a consequence of either primary renal dysplasia or abnormal bladder function. All patients had at least 5 years of follow-up, and when ACE inhibitors were started, estimated GFR (eGFR) was <60 ml/min/1.73 m^2 (mean, 41 ml/min), with mean proteinuria of 1.7 g/24 hours. ESRD developed in 46% of the patients, but in none with proteinuria less than 0.5 g/24 hours and in only 2 of 18 patients with eGFR >50 ml/min. The renal outcome of the two groups was similar whether there was primary renal dysplasia or abnormal bladder function. There was a watershed GFR of 40 to 50 ml/min above which ACE inhibitor treatment improved renal outcome.[4] The similar outcome of the two groups indicates that progressive renal failure in young men born with abnormal bladders is due to intrinsic renal pathophysiology, in contrast to the view that it is a consequence of poor bladder function.

Hypertension

Hypertension is common in the presence of scarred kidneys, but it is usually controlled easily with one or two drugs. Patients in whom chronic renal failure is secondary to obstruction tend to have volume contraction and, therefore, often have normal blood pressure or only mild hypertension. ACE inhibitors or ARBs are preferred for patients with proteinuria and progressive renal failure. Diuretics are likely to cause unacceptable side effects if the patient is volume contracted.

Stones

Stones that form in the presence of infected urine are typically made of magnesium ammonium phosphate (struvite) and calcium phosphate stones (hydroxyl-apatite, carbonate-apatite, calcium hydrogen phosphate [Brushite], tri-calcium phosphate [Whitlockite]). These salts are poorly soluble in alkaline urine. In 90% of patients, the infecting organism is *Proteus* species,[44] but other urea-splitting organisms (including some staphylococci and *Pseudomonas* species) also generate ammonia.[42]

Stones, usually calcium phosphate, are common in conduits because of the alkaline environment and occur in 5% to 30% of ileal conduits. Stones must be suspected if UTIs recur or become more frequent, if renal function suddenly deteriorates, or if there is an unexplained sterile pyuria.

Tubular Dysfunction

In patients whose renal failure is secondary to obstruction, there is significant tubular injury. This may cause problems, in particular with urinary concentration, acidification, and sodium reabsorption.

Polyuria

Nocturia is one of the most significant symptoms in the assessment of patients in whom obstruction or tubular dysfunction is suspected. Overfilling of the bladder or reservoir is an important cause of intermittent upper tract obstruction and deteriorating function. The 24-hour urine-volume diary is a simple way to assess this.

Salt Depletion

Patients with tubular damage may have a salt-losing tendency. Patients typically have a cool periphery and constricted hand veins with no peripheral edema. Increasing salt intake can relieve cramps, improve renal function, and reduce hyperuricemia, but at the cost of increasing blood pressure. With patients who are salt depleted, it is important to give sodium chloride because it is the chloride anion that is deficient and responsible for the reduction in circulating volume.

Acidosis

There is often a metabolic acidosis disproportionate to the degree of renal impairment. This is secondary both to a proximal tubular failure of bicarbonate reabsorption and a distal tubular failure to secrete hydrogen ions. It is our practice to give sufficient sodium bicarbonate to correct the plasma bicarbonate into the normal range.

Bone Disease

In addition to the typical bone disease of progressive renal failure, acidosis contributes significantly to osteomalacia. Growing children are particularly vulnerable to osteomalacia, and great care must be taken to correct acidosis and manage bone disease carefully.

Urinary Diversions
Ureterosigmoidostomy

Fortunately, it is now rare to meet a patient who still has a ureterosigmoidostomy, which was widely used as a technique for urinary diversion until the 1970s. The ureters were anastomosed directly into the sigmoid colon with no disruption of bowel continuity. This technique was most commonly used in patients with bladder exstrophy. Although patients start with normal renal function, there is frequently deterioration in function. In one series of 25 patients, significant renal damage occurred in 50%. Stones, infection, and ureteral strictures are common, and patients remain at risk for colonic carcinoma, with a 10% incidence of carcinoma at 20-year follow-up. However, this diversion is probably best known for the hyperchloremic, hypokalemic acidosis that occurs. Once the urine is in contact with the colonic mucosa, the urinary sodium exchanges for potassium and the chloride for bicarbonate, and large quantities of ammonium ions are produced by the action of the fecal bacteria on urinary ammonia. Ammonium ions are absorbed both with chloride and in exchange for sodium. The severe acidosis is a consequence of the ammonium ion retention and stool loss of bicarbonate. Patients are managed with large doses of oral sodium bicarbonate, which is titrated to keep the plasma bicarbonate in the normal range (>22 mmol/l).

Ileal Conduits

Unlike the sigmoidostomy in which urine enters a reservoir, the ileal conduit is free flowing, with rapid urinary transit and no reservoir. Therefore, metabolic complications are much less common, although again the bowel can exchange sodium and chloride for potassium and bicarbonate.[45,46] There are a number of other complications of ileal and colonic conduits that can lead to progressive loss of renal function (Fig. 49.24).

Enterocystoplasty and Intestinal Urinary Reservoirs

In a study of 53 patients with bladder exstrophy, who were followed for more than 10 years and had serial isotopic GFRs, renal function deteriorated (decrease in GFR of 20% or more) in only 10 (20%).[33] Loss of function was caused principally by chronic retention with or without infection in poorly compliant patients who did not catheterize regularly. Patients must also be

Long-term complications of urinary diversion
Pyelonephritis and scarring
Calculi
Obstruction
Strictures
Bladder mucus causing obstruction
Cancer at intestinal–ureteral anastomosis
Hyperchloremic acidosis
Delayed linear growth in children
Effects of intestinal loss from gastrointestinal tract, e.g., vitamin B_{12} deficiency
Complications related to abnormal pelvic anatomy, e.g., in pregnancy
Psychological and body image problems

Figure 49.24   Long-term complications of urinary diversion.

checked regularly to ensure that anastomotic stenoses and high-pressure reservoirs do not occur. Stones are very common and occur in up to 50% of patients.[47]

END-STAGE RENAL DISEASE AND TRANSPLANTATION

This group of patients presents two important problems at ESRD. First, because of multiple abdominal operations, continuous ambulatory peritoneal dialysis (CAPD) is often impossible, although if there is any doubt, CAPD should be attempted. Second, the bladder and urinary reservoir must be suitable for renal transplantation. If a bladder has just destroyed two perfectly good native kidneys, it is likely to do the same to a transplant kidney. Most patients will be maintained on hemodialysis, but it is frequently difficult to establish a good arteriovenous fistula because of chronic hypovolemia and venoconstriction. Patients on dialysis often continue to pass 1 liter or more of urine per 24 hours, and they also remain at risk for serious UTI and pyelonephritis.

Transplantation
Pretransplantation Assessment
Transplantation into the abnormal lower urinary tract requires careful evaluation and follow-up. Thorough preoperative assessment of bladder function is essential. Patients considered to have normal bladders require at least a postmicturition bladder ultrasound examination and urinary flow rate.

All patients with abnormal bladders or reservoir must have a full VCMG to ensure that the bladder reservoir is large and adequately compliant. If the bladder is small or has not been used for some time, bladder cycling, which involves periodically filling and distending the bladder through a suprapubic catheter, may be required. A study of urodynamics before transplantation indicated that poor bladder function as shown by small bladder volumes was a predictor of graft loss even in patients with previously normal bladder function.[48]

Intermittent self-catheterization is safe and effective for a patient with a poor flow rate who fails to empty the bladder. This, however, is only possible with a normal urethra and a cooperative patient. When this is not practical, we attempt to establish suprapubic drainage through a continent stoma, for example, a Mitrofanoff stoma (see Fig. 49.23). If a conduit is to be used, then a loopogram and endoscopy must ensure that it is

in good condition. We do not remove native kidneys unless they are causing recurrent UTI.

Transplant Outcome
In an 18-year experience, we transplanted 65 patients with abnormal bladders, with a total of 72 renal transplants.[49] In 52 cases, the ureters were transplanted into unaugmented bladder; in 20 cases, there was some form of augmentation or diversion. Results were compared with 59 transplants in 55 patients who had renal failure from renal dysplasia and whose bladder function was considered to be normal. There was no difference in actuarial graft survival in the two groups at 10 years (abnormal bladders, 66%; normal bladders, 61%), although longer follow-up showed an advantage for normal bladders, with a kidney half-life of 29 to 33 years, compared with 15 years for the abnormal bladders.[49] UTIs were relatively common in all patients but only produced problems in patients with abnormal bladders.

Management
We routinely use double-J ureteral stents at the time of transplant surgery. Adequacy of urinary drainage must be assessed frequently, even when graft function seems to be good. Two months after transplantation, when the ureteral stent has been removed, we perform as a baseline the following tests:
- ^{51}Cr-EDTA GFR
- Postmicturition ultrasound of kidney and bladder
- Dynamic ^{99}Tc-MAG3 scintigram
- Static ^{99}Tc-DMSA scintigram, as a baseline for renal scarring

The GFR is repeated at 6 months and then annually. Ultrasound and ^{99}Tc-MAG3 scintigraphy are repeated at 1 year, and then when indicated. The protein-to-creatinine ratio is measured on a random urine sample at every outpatient visit. If there is renal dysfunction, imaging tests are repeated, and if there is a change from baseline, renal biopsy is performed to exclude an immunologic cause of graft dysfunction. If there is a documented deterioration in renal function in the absence of rejection or calcineurin inhibitor toxicity, the DMSA scan is repeated (to see whether there has been new scarring) and the bladder reassessed urodynamically.[50]

Complications
UTIs must be detected and treated early, and recurrent infections may require long courses of antibiotics or even removal of the native tracts.

In our experience, symptomatic UTIs are common in the first 3 months after transplantation (63%); fever and systemic symptoms occur in 39% with normal bladders and 59% with abnormal bladders. UTI directly contributes to graft loss in patients with abnormal bladders, but causes no consequences in those with normal bladders.[43] In our practice, prophylactic antibiotics for the first 6 months has halved the subsequent incidence of UTI.

When UTIs recur, a cause must be sought with ultrasound of kidney and bladder. A plain abdominal x-ray is essential to look for stones in native or transplant kidneys and the bladder, or for urinary diversion. If there is a residual volume after double micturition, the patient must be instructed to perform clean intermittent self-catheterization. With these measures, good results are obtained.

ACKNOWLEDGMENTS

We would like to thank all our colleagues who have helped in the preparation of this chapter and contributed material from their clinical practice, in particular Drs. M. J. Kellett and J. Bomanji, Professors M. Craggs and C. R. J. Woodhouse, and Mr. P. J. R. Shah.

REFERENCES

1. British Association for Paediatric Nephrology: Report from the Paediatric Renal Registry. In Ansell D, Feest TG, Byrne C (eds): The UK Renal Registry 5th Annual Report. 2002, pp 253–273. www.renalreg.com

2. James CA, Watson AR, Twining P, Rance CH: Antenatally detected urinary tract abnormalities: Changing incidence and management. Eur J Pediatr 1998;157:508–511.

3. Brenner BM, Meyer TW, Hostetter TH: Dietary protein intake and the progressive nature of kidney disease: The role of hemodynamically mediated glomerular injury in the pathogenesis of progressive glomerular sclerosis in aging, renal ablation, and intrinsic renal disease. N Engl J Med 1982;307:652–659.

4. Neild GH, Thomson G, Nitsch D, et al: Renal outcome in adults with renal insufficiency and irregular asymmetric kidneys. BMC Nephrol 2004;5:12–22.

5. Woolf AS, Winyard PJ, Hermanns MM, Welham SJM: Maldevelopment of the human kidney and lower urinary tract. In Vize PD, Woolf AS, Bard JBL (eds): The Kidney: From Normal Development to Congenital Disease. London, Academic Press, 2003, pp 377–394.

6. Woolf AS, Jenkins D: Development of the kidney. In Jennette JC, Olson JL, Schwartz MM, Silva FG (eds): Heptinstall's Pathology of the Kidney, 6th ed. Philadelphia: Lippincott Williams & Wilkins, 2006.

7. Rascher W, Roesch WH: Congenital abnormalities of the urinary tract. In Davison AM, Cameron JS, Grunfeld J-P, et al (eds): Oxford Textbook of Clinical Nephrology, 3rd ed. Oxford, UK, Oxford University Press, 2005, pp 2471–2494.

8. Woolf AS, Price KL, Scambler PJ, Winyard PJ: Evolving concepts in human renal dysplasia. J Am Soc Nephrol 2004;15:998–1007.

9. Miyazaki Y, Ichikawa I: Ontogeny of congenital anomalies of the kidney and urinary tract, CAKUT. Pediatr Int 2003;45:598–604.

10. Bassuk JA, Grady R, Mitchell M: Review article: The molecular era of bladder research. Transgenic mice as experimental tools in the study of outlet obstruction. J Urol 2000;164:170–179.

11. Dressler GR, Wilkinson JE, Rothenpieler UW, et al: Deregulation of Pax-2 expression in transgenic mice generates severe kidney abnormalities. Nature 1993;362:65–67.

12. Torres M, Gomez PE, Dressler GR, Gruss P: Pax-2 controls multiple steps of urogenital development. Development 1995;121:4057–4065.

13. Feather SA, Malcolm S, Woolf AS, et al: Primary, nonsyndromic vesicoureteric reflux and its nephropathy is genetically heterogeneous, with a locus on chromosome 1. Am J Hum Genet 2000;66:1420–1425.

14. Ichikawa I, Kuwayama F, Pope JC, et al: Paradigm shift from classic anatomic theories to contemporary cell biological views of CAKUT. Kidney Int 2002;61:889–898.

15. Risdon RA, Yeung CK, Ransley PG: Reflux nephropathy in children submitted to unilateral nephrectomy: a clinicopathological study. Clin Nephrol 1993;40:308–314.

16. Hiraoka M, Hori C, Tsukahara H, et al: Congenitally small kidneys with reflux as a common cause of nephropathy in boys. Kidney Int 1997;52:811–816.

17. Cotran RS: Glomerulosclerosis in reflux nephropathy. Kidney Int 1982;21:528–534.

18. Kincaid-Smith P, Becker G: Reflux nephropathy and chronic atrophic pyelonephritis: A review. J Infect Dis 1978;138:774–780.

19. Bhathena DB, Weiss JH, Holland NH, et al: Focal and segmental glomerular sclerosis in reflux nephropathy. Am J Med 1980;68:886–892.

20. Jenkins D, Bitner-Glindzicz M, Malcolm S, et al: De novo uroplakin IIIa heterozygous mutations cause human renal adysplasia leading to severe kidney failure. J Am Soc Nephrol 2005;16:2141–2149.

21. O'Dea D, Parfrey PS, Harnett JD, et al: The importance of renal impairment in the natural history of Bardet-Biedl syndrome. Am J Kidney Dis 1996;27:776–783.

22. Ansley SJ, Badano JL, Blacque OE, et al: Basal body dysfunction is a likely cause of pleiotropic Bardet-Biedl syndrome. Nature 2003;425:628–633.

23. Koff SA, Campbell KD: The nonoperative management of unilateral neonatal hydronephrosis: Natural history of poorly functioning kidneys. J Urol 1994;152:593–595.

24. Lee PH, Diamond DA, Duffy PG, Ransley PG: Duplex reflux: A study of 105 children. J Urol 1991;146:657–659.

25. Ehrlich RM, Brown WJ: Ultrastructural anatomic observations of the ureter in the prune belly syndrome. Birth Defects Orig Artic Ser 1977;13:101–103.

26. Whitaker RH, Johnston JH: A simple classification of wide ureters. Br J Urol 1975;47:781–787.

27. Woodhouse CRJ: Long-Term Paediatric Urology. Oxford, UK, Blackwell Scientific Publications, 1991.

28. Woodhouse CR, Ransley PG, Innes WD: Prune belly syndrome: Report of 47 cases. Arch Dis Child 1982;57:856–859.

29. Burbige KA, Amodio J, Berdon WE, et al: Prune belly syndrome: 35 Years of experience. J Urol 1987;137:86–90.

30. Woodard JR, Parrott TS: Reconstruction of the urinary tract in prune belly uropathy. J Urol 1978;119:824–828.

31. Hurwitz RS, Manzoni GA, Ransley PG, Stephens FD: Cloacal exstrophy: A report of 34 cases. J Urol 1987;138:1060–1064.

32. Husmann DA, McLorie GA, Churchill BM: A comparison of renal function in the exstrophy patient treated with staged reconstruction versus urinary diversion. J Urol 1988;140:1204–1206.

33. Fontaine E, Leaver R, Woodhouse CR: The effect of intestinal urinary reservoirs on renal function: A 10-year follow-up. BJU Int 2000; 86:195–198.

34. Johnston LB, Borzyskowski M: Bladder dysfunction and neurological disability at presentation in closed spina bifida. Arch Dis Child 1998;79:33–38.

35. McLorie GA, Perez MR, Csima A, Churchill BM: Determinants of hydronephrosis and renal injury in patients with myelomeningocele. J Urol 1988;140:1289–1292.

36. Lapides J, Diokno AC, Silber SJ, Lowe BS: Clean, intermittent self-catheterization in the treatment of urinary tract disease. J Urol 1972;107:458–461.

37. Edelstein RA, Bauer SB, Kelly MD, et al: The long-term urological response of neonates with myelodysplasia treated proactively with intermittent catheterization and anticholinergic therapy. J Urol 1995;154:1500–1504.

38. Tejani A, Butt K, Glassberg K, et al: Predictors of eventual end stage renal disease in children with posterior urethral valves. J Urol 1986;136:857–860.

39. Rittenberg MH, Hulbert WC, Snyder HM, Duckett JW: Protective factors in posterior urethral valves. J Urol 1988;140:993–996.

40. Smith GH, Canning DA, Schulman SL, et al: The long-term outcome of posterior urethral valves treated with primary valve ablation and observation. J Urol 1996;155:1730–1734.

41. Parkhouse HF, Barratt TM, Dillon MJ, et al: Long-term outcome of boys with posterior urethral valves. Br J Urol 1988;62:59–62.

42. Neild GH: Urinary tract infection. Medicine 2003;31:85–90.

43. Crowe A, Cairns HS, Wood S, et al: Renal transplantation following renal failure due to urological disorders. Nephrol Dial Transplant 1998;13:2065–2069.

44. Dretler SP: The pathogenesis of urinary tract calculi occurring after ileal conduit diversion. I. Clinical study. II. Conduit study. 3. Prevention. J Urol 1973;109:204–209.

45. McDougal WS: Metabolic complications of urinary intestinal diversion. J Urol 1992;147:1199–208.

46. Silverman SH, Woodhouse CR, Strachan JR, et al: Long-term management of patients who have had urinary diversions into colon. Br J Urol 1986;58:634–639.

47. Woodhouse CR, Robertson WG: Urolithiasis in enterocystoplasties. World J Urol 2004;22:215–221.

48. Kashi SH, Wynne KS, Sadek SA, Lodge JP: An evaluation of vesical urodynamics before renal transplantation and its effect on renal allograft function and survival. Transplantation 1994;57:1455–1457.

49. Neild GH, Dakmish A, Wood S, et al: Renal transplantation in adults with abnormal bladders. Transplantation 2004;77:1123–1127.

50. Cairns HS, Spencer S, Hilson AJ, et al: 99mTc-DMSA imaging with tomography in renal transplant recipients with abnormal lower urinary tracts. Nephrol Dial Transplant 1994;9:1157–1161.

Urinary Tract Infections in Adults

Thomas Hooton

DEFINITION

Urinary tract infection (UTI) in adults can be categorized into six groups: young women with acute uncomplicated cystitis, young women with recurrent cystitis, young women with acute uncomplicated pyelonephritis, adults with acute cystitis and conditions that suggest occult renal or prostatic involvement, complicated UTI, and asymptomatic bacteriuria (Fig. 50.1).[1] A discussion of UTI in pregnancy is provided in Chapter 41 and of vesicoureteral reflux in children in Chapter 58.

A complicated UTI is one that is associated with a condition that increases the risk for serious complications or treatment failure. Distinction between uncomplicated and complicated UTIs is important mainly because of implications regarding pretreatment and post-treatment evaluation, type and duration of antimicrobial treatment, and the extent of evaluation of the urinary tract that is required. It is not always possible, however, to classify patients definitively as having complicated or uncomplicated infections when they first present, and the distinction is sometimes made only when a patient has a poor response to treatment. Patients with certain complicating conditions, such as those presented in Figure 50.1, are at greatly increased risk

for serious complications of UTI and warrant special concern. These conditions only serve as guidelines for the clinician who must decide, based on limited clinical information, whether to embark on a more extensive evaluation and treatment course when confronted with a patient with UTI.

EPIDEMIOLOGY

Acute uncomplicated UTIs are among the most common medical conditions, with several million episodes of acute cystitis and at least 250,000 episodes of acute pyelonephritis occurring annually in the United States. One recent survey estimated that as many as 11 million women in the United States had at least one treated UTI in 1995, and that the cost of evaluating and managing UTIs was $1.6 billion U.S.[2] In a prospective study of young sexually active women, the incidence of cystitis was about 0.5 per 1 person-year.[3] Acute uncomplicated cystitis may recur in 27% to 44% of healthy women, even though they have a normal urinary tract.[4] The incidence of pyelonephritis in young women is about 3 per 1000 person-years.[5] The self-reported incidence of symptomatic UTI in postmenopausal women is about 10% per year.[6] The incidence of symptomatic UTI in adult men younger

Categories of urinary tract infection in adults
Acute uncomplicated cystitis in young women
Recurrent acute uncomplicated cystitis in young women
Acute uncomplicated pyelonephritis in young women

Acute uncomplicated cystitis in adults with a following condition suggesting possible occult renal or prostatic involvement but without other known complicating factors:
    Male sex
    Elderly
    Pregnancy
    Recent urinary tract instrumentation
    Childhood urinary tract infection
    Recent antimicrobial use
    Symptoms for more than 7 days at presentation
    Diabetes mellitus

Complicated urinary tract infection*
    Obstruction or other structural factor: urolithiasis, malignancies, ureteral and urethral strictures, bladder diverticula, renal cysts, fistulas, ileal conduits, and other urinary diversions
    Functional abnormality: neurogenic bladder, vesicoureteral reflux
    Foreign bodies: indwelling catheter, ureteral stent, nephrostomy tube
    Other conditions: renal failure, renal transplantation, immunosuppression, multidrug-resistant uropathogens, hospital-acquired (nosocomial) infection, prostatitis-related infection, upper tract infection in an adult other than a young healthy woman, other functional or anatomic abnormality of the urinary tract

Asymptomatic bacteriuria

Figure 50.1   Categories of urinary tract infection in adults. *This is a selected list of complicating factors. Some factors complicate urinary tract infections through several mechanisms. (Data for complicating factors from Nicolle LE: A practical guide to the management of complicated urinary tract infection. Drugs 1997;53:583–592.)

than 50 years is much lower than in women, ranging from 5 to 8 per 10,000 men annually.

Complicated UTIs encompass an extraordinarily broad range of infectious entities (see Fig. 50.1). The incidence of nosocomial UTI, one of the most common types of complicated UTI, is about 5 per 100 admissions in a university tertiary care hospital, with catheter-associated infections accounting for 88% of the infections. More than 1 million nosocomial UTIs occur each year in the United States, and catheter-associated bacteriuria is the most common source of gram-negative bacteremia in hospitalized patients.[7]

Asymptomatic bacteriuria is defined as the presence of two separate consecutive clean-voided urine specimens both with $\geq 10^5$ colony-forming units (cfu)/ml of the same uropathogen in the absence of symptoms.[8,9] Asymptomatic bacteriuria is found in about 5% of young adult women,[10] but rarely in men aged younger than 50 years. The prevalence increases to 21% of ambulatory women and 12% of ambulatory men older than 65 years, and to 53% of elderly women and 37% of elderly men who are institutionalized. Asymptomatic bacteriuria may be persistent or transient and recurrent, and many patients have had previous symptomatic infection or develop symptomatic UTI soon after having asymptomatic bacteriuria. Asymptomatic bacteriuria is generally assumed to be a benign condition, although as discussed later, it may lead to serious complications in some clinical settings.

PATHOGENESIS

Uncomplicated Infection

Most uncomplicated UTIs in healthy women result when uropathogens (typically *Escherichia coli*) present in the rectal flora enter the bladder through the urethra after an interim phase of periurethral and distal urethral colonization. In the male, colonizing uropathogens may also come from a sex partner's vagina or rectum. Hematogenous seeding of the urinary tract by potential uropathogens such as *Staphylococcus aureus* is the source of some UTIs, but this is more likely to occur in the setting of persistent bloodstream infection or urinary tract obstruction.

Many host genetic, biologic, and behavioral factors predispose young healthy women to uncomplicated UTI[11] (Fig. 50.2).

Factors modulating risk for acute uncomplicated urinary tract infections in women	
Host Determinants	Uropathogen Determinants
Behavioral: sexual intercourse, use of spermicidal products, recent antimicrobial use, suboptimal voiding habits	*Escherichia coli* virulence determinants: P, S, Dr, and type I fimbriae; hemolysin; aerobactin; serum resistance
Genetic: enhanced epithelial cell adherence, antibacterial factors in urine and bladder mucosa, nonsecretor of ABO blood group antigens, P₁ blood group phenotype, previous history of recurrent cystitis	
Biologic: estrogen deficiency in postmenopausal, inflammatory, and immunologic response	

Figure 50.2 Factors modulating risk for acute uncomplicated urinary tract infections in women.

Important risk factors include sexual intercourse, use of spermicide products, and a history of previous recurrent UTI.[3,12] Nonsecretors of ABO blood group antigens have an increased risk for recurrent cystitis, and women with the P₁ blood group phenotype have an increased risk for recurrent pyelonephritis. The host's inflammatory and immunologic responses also help determine the clinical consequences of UTI.

In addition to these and other host factors that modulate UTI risk, certain strains of *E. coli* have a selective advantage for colonization and infection[13] (see Fig. 50.2). P-fimbriated strains of *E. coli* are associated with acute uncomplicated pyelonephritis, and their adherence properties may stimulate epithelial and other cells to produce cytokines and other proinflammatory factors that are responsible for some of the inflammatory response.[13] Other virulence determinants include adherence factors (types 1, S, and Dr fimbriae), toxins (hemolysin), aerobactin, and serum resistance.[13] Bacterial virulence determinants associated with cystitis and asymptomatic bacteriuria have been less well characterized.[10,13]

Factors affecting the large difference in UTI prevalence between men and women include the greater distance between the usual source of uropathogens (the anus and the urethral meatus), the drier environment surrounding the male urethra, the greater length of the male urethra, and the antibacterial activity of prostatic fluid. Risk factors associated with UTIs in healthy men include intercourse with an infected female partner, anal intercourse, and lack of circumcision, although these factors are often not present in men with UTI. Most uropathogenic strains infecting young men are highly virulent, suggesting that the urinary tract in healthy men is relatively resistant to infection.

Complicated Infection

The initial steps leading to uncomplicated UTI discussed earlier probably also occur in most individuals who develop a complicated UTI. Factors that predispose individuals to complicated UTI generally do so by causing obstruction or stasis of urine flow, facilitating entry of uropathogens into the urinary tract by bypassing normal host defense mechanisms, providing a nidus for infection that is not readily treatable with antimicrobials, or compromising the host immune system[1] (see Fig. 50.1). UTIs are more likely to become complicated in the setting of impaired host defense, as occurs with indwelling catheter use, vesicoureteral reflux, obstruction, neutropenia, and immune deficiencies. Diabetes mellitus, in particular, is associated with several syndromes of complicated UTI, including renal and perirenal abscess, emphysematous pyelonephritis and cystitis, papillary necrosis, and xanthogranulomatous pyelonephritis.[14] Uropathogen virulence determinants appear to be of much less importance in the pathogenesis of complicated UTIs compared with uncomplicated UTIs. However, infection with multidrug-resistant uropathogens is more likely with complicated UTI.

ETIOLOGIC AGENTS

The spectrum of etiologic agents is similar in uncomplicated upper and lower UTI, with *E. coli* the causative pathogen in 70% to 95% and *Staphylococcus saprophyticus* in 5% to more than 20% (Fig. 50.3). *S. saprophyticus* may be a less common cause of acute pyelonephritis.[15] Occasionally, other Enterobacteriaceae such as *Proteus mirabilis*, *Klebsiella* species, or enterococci are isolated from such patients. Group B streptococcci also appear to cause occasional episodes and, rarely, *Pseudomonas aeruginosa*, *Citrobacter* species, or other uropathogens cause uncomplicated UTI.

Bacterial etiology of urinary tract infections		
	Urinary Tract Infection (%)	
Organisms	Uncomplicated	Complicated
Gram-negative organisms		
Escherichia coli	70–95	21–54
Proteus mirabilis	1–2	1–10
Klebsiella species	1–2	2–17
Citrobacter species	<1	5
Enterobacter species	<1	2–10
Pseudomonas aeruginosa	<1	2–19
Other	<1	6–20
Gram-positive organisms		
Coagulase-negative staphylococci (S. saprophyticus)	5–20 or more	1–4
Enterococci	1–2	1–23
Group B streptococci	<1	1–4
Staphylococcus aureus	<1	1–2
Other	<1	2

Figure 50.3 Bacterial etiology of urinary tract infections. (Data for complicated infections from Nicolle LE: A practical guide to the management of complicated urinary tract infection. Drugs 1997;53:583–592.)

Unlike the narrow and predictable spectrum of causative agents in uncomplicated infection, a broad range of bacteria can cause complicated infections, and many are resistant to multiple antimicrobial agents. Although E. coli is the predominant uropathogen in complicated UTI, uropathogens other than E. coli, including Citrobacter species, Enterobacter species, P. aeruginosa, enterococci, and S. aureus, account for a relatively higher proportion of cases compared with uncomplicated UTIs[1] (see Fig. 50.3). The proportion of infections caused by fungi, especially Candida species, is increasing (see Chapter 52). Patients with chronic conditions, such as spinal cord injury and neurogenic bladder, are relatively more likely to have polymicrobic and multidrug-resistant infections.

CLINICAL SYNDROMES

Acute Uncomplicated Cystitis in Young Women

Women with acute uncomplicated cystitis generally present with acute onset of symptoms including dysuria, frequency, urgency, or suprapubic pain. Acute dysuria in a young sexually active woman is usually caused by acute cystitis; acute urethritis from Chlamydia trachomatis, Neisseria gonorrhoeae, or herpes simplex virus infections or vaginitis caused by Candida species or Trichomonas vaginalis.[7] A distinction among these three entities can usually, but not always, be made with a high degree of certainty with data from the history and physical examination and simple laboratory tests. Pyuria is present in almost all women with acute cystitis, as well as in most women with urethritis caused by N. gonorrhoeae or C. trachomatis, and its absence strongly suggests an alternative diagnosis. Hematuria is common in women with UTI but not in women with urethritis or vaginitis.

The definitive diagnosis of UTI is the presence of significant bacteriuria, the traditional standard for which is $\geq 10^5$ uropathogen/ml of voided midstream urine. Recent studies, however, have shown that up to one third of patients with cystitis have lower colony counts, which are missed using the traditional definition. The Infectious Disease Society of America consensus definition of cystitis is $\geq 10^3$ cfu/ml (sensitivity, 80%; specificity, 90%).[16] Urine cultures are generally not necessary in women

with uncomplicated cystitis because the causative organisms are predictable and the culture results become available only after therapeutic decisions have been made.

E. coli in patients with uncomplicated UTI are often resistant to sulfonamides and amoxicillin. Moreover, there has been an increase in resistance to trimethoprim and trimethoprim-sulfamethoxazole (cotrimoxazole) among outpatient urinary strains in the United States and Europe, which is cause for concern.[17] Recent data showing that a high proportion of drug-resistant strains found in different parts of the country are clonal have led to speculation that resistant strains may enter new environments by contaminated products ingested by community residents.[18] The prevalence of E. coli resistance to nitrofurantoin is generally <5%, although nitrofurantoin is inactive against Proteus species and some Enterobacter and Klebsiella strains. Fluoroquinolones remain active against almost all E. coli strains causing uncomplicated cystitis, although resistance is increasing in certain areas of the world.

Three-day regimens are recommended for the treatment of acute uncomplicated cystitis because of comparable efficacy, better compliance, lower cost, and lower frequency of adverse reactions than with longer regimens. Single-dose regimens, although highly effective in most women (especially trimethoprim-sulfamethoxazole and fluoroquinolones), are somewhat less effective than longer regimens.[19] Higher cure rates generally have been observed with trimethoprim-sulfamethoxazole and fluoroquinolones than with ß-lactams regardless of the site of infection and duration of treatment. Fosfomycin tromethamine, a single-dose regimen for uncomplicated cystitis, is less effective than 7- to 10-day regimens of ciprofloxacin or trimethoprim-sulfamethoxazole.

Optimal management of acute uncomplicated cystitis is summarized in Figures 50.4 and 50.5. Trimethoprim or trimethoprim-sulfamethoxazole in a 3-day oral regimen should be considered the first-line agent for uncomplicated cystitis in women who can tolerate this agent and in areas where resistance is infrequent.[20] Fluoroquinolones are reasonable first-line agents in women who are known or suspected to have antimicrobial-resistant organisms, who are allergic or otherwise do not tolerate more conventional regimens, or who live in areas where resistance to trimethoprim-sulfamethoxazole is more than 20%. A recent large trial comparing a 5-day regimen of nitrofurantoin to a 3-day regimen of trimethoprim-sulfamethoxazole for the treatment of acute cystitis in young women showed that the two regimens were comparable in clinical outcomes and adverse events (Hooton TM, unpublished data, 2005). However, nitrofurantoin should be used in regimens of 5 days or longer because there are no convincing data that 3-day regimens are as effective as trimethoprim-sulfamethoxazole or fluoroquinolones. Broad-spectrum oral cephalosporins (such as cefixime, cefpodoxime, cefprozil, and cefaclor) demonstrate in vitro activity against most uropathogens causing uncomplicated cystitis, but clinical data are sparse. Amoxicillin-clavulanate (co-amoxiclav) is approved for treatment of UTI but has a high rate of gastrointestinal side effects, and a recent trial demonstrated that a 3-day regimen of amoxicillin-clavulanate was significantly inferior to a 3-day regimen of ciprofloxacin, even in women infected with uropathogens susceptible to the drugs with which they were treated.[21]

Routine post-treatment cultures in asymptomatic women are not indicated because of the considerable costs necessary to detect a single case of asymptomatic bacteriuria, and because the benefit of detecting and treating asymptomatic bacteriuria in healthy women has been demonstrated only in pregnancy and before urologic instrumentation or surgery.[8] In women whose symptomatic infection persists or recurs within 2 weeks, a urine culture and antimicrobial susceptibility testing should be

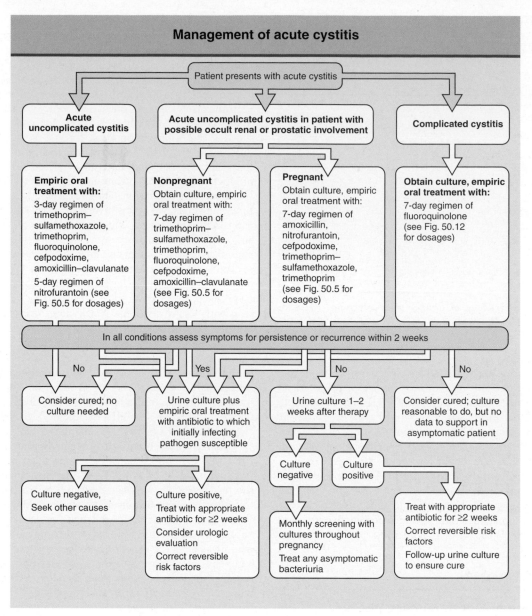

Figure 50. 4   Algorithm for management of acute cystitis.

performed, and a longer course of therapy, usually with a fluoro-quinolone, should be used. In those women whose infection resolves but recurs after 2 weeks, the approach should be the same as with sporadic infections.

Recurrent Acute Uncomplicated Cystitis in Women

Most episodes of recurrent cystitis in healthy women are reinfections, which, in many cases, are caused by the initially infecting strain persisting in the fecal flora.[22] Recent research in mice has led to the alternative hypothesis that some same-strain recurrent UTIs may be caused by a latent reservoir of uropathogens in the bladder wall that persist after the initial UTI.[23] Such a phenomenon has yet to be demonstrated in humans. Women with recurrent cystitis may benefit from modification of certain behavioral factors (Fig. 50.6), such as increasing fluid intake and ensuring postcoital micturition, although this has not been proved. Several small studies suggest that ingestion of cranberry products has preventive properties, and *in vitro* studies have shown that cranberry juice blocks adherence of *E. coli* to epithelial cells. More definitive

clinical trials are currently in progress, but it is reasonable to recommend daily cranberry juice (or other cranberry products) to women with frequent recurrences of UTI. Women who do not wish to try or who get no benefit from the preceding approaches should be offered antimicrobial management.

Antimicrobial prophylaxis is highly effective in preventing recurrent UTI in women (Fig. 50.7; see also Fig. 50.6). Prophylaxis should be considered for women who experience three or more infections over a 12-month period, or whenever the woman feels her life is being adversely affected by frequent recurrences. Several approaches have been shown to be effective in the management of recurrent uncomplicated UTIs, including continuous prophylaxis, postcoital prophylaxis, or intermittent self-treatment (which is not really a prophylaxis method). In postmenopausal women with recurrent UTI, intravaginal estriol has been demonstrated to be effective, presumably by normalizing the vaginal flora, which reduces the risk for coliform colonization of the vagina.[22] This offers an alternative for such women to the antimicrobial strategies discussed earlier (see Fig. 50.6).

Oral regimens for acute uncomplicated cystitis			
Drug	Dose (mg)	Interval	Comment
Trimethoprim-sulfamethoxazole	160/800	q 12 hr	Widely used in pregnancy, although not an approved use. Avoid in first trimester.
Trimethoprim	100	q 12 hr	Widely used in pregnancy, although not an approved use. Avoid in first trimester.
Fluoroquinolones			Avoid fluoroquinolones if possible in pregnancy, nursing mothers, or persons <18 years old
Ciprofloxacin	100–250	q 12 hr	
Ciprofloxacin extended release	500	q 24 hr	
Levofloxacin	250	q 24 hr	
Ofloxacin	200	q 12 hr	
Cefpodoxime proxetil	100	q 12 hr	Data are sparse
Nitrofurantoin			Less active against *Proteus* species
Monohydrate/macrocrystals	100	q 12 hr	An effective and safe alternative to fluoroquinolones for acute uncomplicated cystitis. Avoid in conditions with possible occult renal involvement except for pregnancy.
Macrocrystals	50	q 6 hr	
Amoxicillin	250	q 8 hr	Used only when causative pathogen is known to be susceptible or for empiric treatment of mild cystitis in pregnancy
Amoxicillin-clavulanate	500/125	q 12 hr	Inferior to ciprofloxacin in 3-day regimen

Figure 50.5 **Oral antimicrobial agents for acute uncomplicated cystitis or cystitis in patient with possible occult renal or prostatic involvement.** Duration of therapy depends on the clinical setting (see text and Fig. 50.4).

Acute Uncomplicated Pyelonephritis in Women

Acute pyelonephritis is suggested by fever (temperature ≥38.5° C), chills, flank pain, nausea and vomiting, and costovertebral angle tenderness. Cystitis symptoms are variably present. Symptoms may vary from a mild illness to a sepsis syndrome with or without shock and renal failure. Pyuria is almost always present, but leukocyte casts, specific for UTI, are infrequently seen. Gram stain of the urine sediment may aid in differentiating gram-positive and gram-negative infections, which can influence empiric therapy. A urine culture, which should be performed in all women with acute pyelonephritis, will have ≥10^4 cfu/ml uropathogens in up to 95% of patients.[16]

Pathologically, the kidney shows a focal inflammatory reaction with neutrophil and monocyte infiltrates, tubular damage, and interstitial edema (Fig. 50.8). Although imaging studies are generally not performed, the infected kidney is often enlarged, and contrast computed tomography (CT) shows decreased opacification of the affected parenchyma, typically in patchy, wedge-shaped, or linear patterns (Fig. 50.9).

The availability of effective oral antimicrobials, especially the fluoroquinolones, allows for initial oral therapy in appropriate patients or, in those requiring parenteral therapy, the timely conversion from intravenous to oral therapy and reduced need for hospitalization. Indications for admission to the hospital include inability to maintain oral hydration or take medications, uncertain social situation or concern about compliance, uncertainty about the diagnosis, and severe illness with high fevers, severe pain, and marked debility. Outpatient therapy has been shown to be safe and effective for selected patients, who can be stabilized with parenteral fluids and antibiotics in an urgent care facility and sent home on oral antibiotics under close supervision.

The management strategy for acute uncomplicated pyelonephritis is shown in Figure 50.10. There are many effective parenteral (Fig. 50.11) and oral (Fig. 50.12) regimens for use in patients with acute uncomplicated pyelonephritis. For those patients who can be managed in the outpatient setting, an oral fluoroquinolone should be used for initial empiric treatment

of infection caused by gram-negative bacilli.[20] Trimethoprim-sulfamethoxazole or other agents can be used if the infecting strain is known to be susceptible. If enterococci are suspected from the Gram stain, amoxicillin should be added to the treatment regimen until the causative organism is identified. Cefixime, cefpodoxime proxetil, cefaclor, or cefprozil also appear to be effective for the treatment of acute uncomplicated pyelonephritis, although published data are sparse. Nitrofurantoin should not be used for the treatment of pyelonephritis because it does not achieve reliable tissue levels.

For hospitalized patients, ceftriaxone is an effective and inexpensive agent if the Gram stain is not suggestive of infection caused by gram-positive pathogens. If enterococci are suspected based on the Gram stain, ampicillin plus gentamicin, ampicillin-sulbactam, and piperacillin-tazobactam are reasonable broad-spectrum empiric choices. Trimethoprim-sulfamethoxazole should not be used alone for empiric therapy for pyelonephritis in areas with a high prevalence of resistance to this combination. Patients with acute uncomplicated pyelonephritis can often be switched to oral therapy after 24 to 48 hours, although longer intervals of parenteral therapy are occasionally indicated in patients whose symptoms and signs do not improve rapidly (such as those with continued high fever, severe flank pain, or persistent nausea and vomiting).

Six-week regimens are no more effective than 14-day regimens for uncomplicated pyelonephritis and cause more side effects.[24] Although there are few published data demonstrating that regimens shorter than 14 days are as effective as longer regimens, one recent study demonstrated superiority of a 7-day ciprofloxacin regimen over a 14-day trimethoprim-sulfamethoxazole regimen. The difference was accounted for entirely by the higher rate of resistance to trimethoprim-sulfamethoxazole compared with ciprofloxacin among the uropathogens.[15] In general, for those mild to moderately ill patients who have a rapid response with resolution of fever and symptoms soon after initiating treatment, treatment can be discontinued after 7 to 10 days. Of note, however, ß-lactam regimens shorter than 14 days have been associated with unacceptably high failure rates. Routine post-treatment urine cultures in

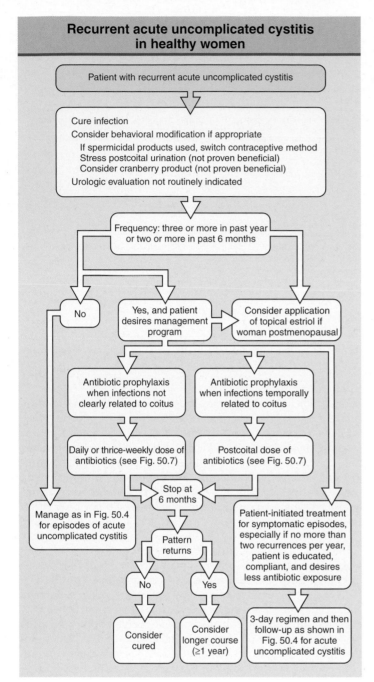

Recurrent acute uncomplicated cystitis in healthy women

Patient with recurrent acute uncomplicated cystitis

↓

Cure infection
Consider behavioral modification if appropriate
   If spermicidal products used, switch contraceptive method
   Stress postcoital urination (not proven beneficial)
   Consider cranberry product (not proven beneficial)
Urologic evaluation not routinely indicated

↓

Frequency: three or more in past year or two or more in past 6 months

→ No

→ Yes, and patient desires management program

→ Consider application of topical estriol if woman postmenopausal

Antibiotic prophylaxis when infections not clearly related to coitus
→ Daily or thrice-weekly dose of antibiotics (see Fig. 50.7)

Antibiotic prophylaxis when infections temporally related to coitus
→ Postcoital dose of antibiotics (see Fig. 50.7)

→ Stop at 6 months

Manage as in Fig. 50.4 for episodes of acute uncomplicated cystitis

Pattern returns → No / Yes

Patient-initiated treatment for symptomatic episodes, especially if no more than two recurrences per year, patient is educated, compliant, and desires less antibiotic exposure

No → Consider cured
Yes → Consider longer course (≥1 year)

3-day regimen and then follow-up as shown in Fig. 50.4 for acute uncomplicated cystitis

Figure 50.6 **Management strategies for recurrent acute uncomplicated cystitis.**

Prophylaxis for recurrent acute uncomplicated cystitis

Drug	Dose (mg)	Frequency
Continuous prophylaxis		
Trimethoprim-sulfamethoxazole	40/200	Daily
Trimethoprim-sulfamethoxazole	40/200	Thrice weekly
Trimethoprim	100	Daily
Nitrofurantoin	50 or 100	Daily
Cefaclor	250	Daily
Cefalexin (cephalexin)	125 or 250	Daily
Norfloxacin	200	Other fluoro-quinolones are likely to be as effective*
Postcoital prophylaxis		
Trimethoprim-sulfamethoxazole	40/200	Single dose
Trimethoprim-sulfamethoxazole	80/400	Single dose
Nitrofurantoin	50 or 100	Single dose
Cefalexin	250	Single dose
Ciprofloxacin*	125	Single dose
Norfloxacin*	200	Single dose
Ofloxacin*	100	Single dose

Figure 50.7 **Antimicrobial prophylaxis regimens for women with recurrent acute uncomplicated cystitis.** See text and Fig. 50.6 for management strategy. *Women should be cautioned about pregnancy when fluoroquinolones are being used.

laboratory findings in this group are the same as in uncomplicated cystitis. Urethritis must be excluded in dysuric sexually active men with a urethral Gram stain or a first-voided urine specimen wet mount evaluation for urethral leukocytosis.

The management approach to patients in this category is shown in Figure 50.4. Empiric use of the agents discussed previously for uncomplicated cystitis in women is suitable for the treatment of UTIs in these patients. Nitrofurantoin generally should be avoided because of poor tissue penetration, except for the treatment of mild cystitis in pregnancy. The recommended duration of treatment is at least 7 days, but studies of shorter-course regimens are lacking. A pretreatment urine culture should be obtained routinely in patients in this category, whereas the need for a post-treatment culture is less certain, except in pregnant women (see Fig. 50.4). In men, early recurrence of UTI with the same species suggests

asymptomatic patients are not cost effective, but cultures should be performed if symptoms recur. Recurrent infections are treated with a second 2-week course, but in patients whose infection persists with the same strain as the initial infecting strain, complicating factors should be looked for and corrected if found.

Acute Cystitis in Healthy Adults with Possible Occult Renal or Prostatic Involvement

Episodes of acute cystitis in healthy individuals other than young women are more likely to involve occult renal or prostatic infection (see Fig. 50.1) and may respond poorly to short-course therapy. Some patients, such as those with diabetes or pregnancy, warrant special attention because of the serious complications that can occur if treatment is inadequate. Symptoms, signs, and

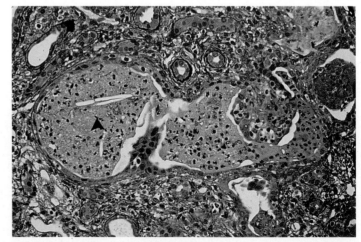

Figure 50.8 **Acute pyelonephritis.** Renal tissue shows a dilated tubule with neutrophils enmeshed in proteinaceous debris ("pus casts"; *arrowhead*) with adjacent interstitial inflammation. (Courtesy of C. Alpers.)

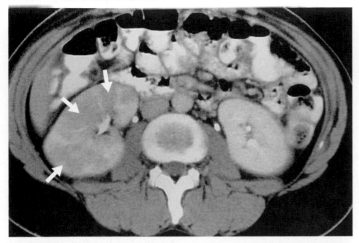

Figure 50.9 Acute pyelonephritis. Contrast computed tomography scan shows areas of lower density owing to infection and edema (*arrows*). (Courtesy of W. Bush.)

a prostatic source of infection and warrants a 4- to 6-week regimen of either a fluoroquinolone (preferable) or trimethoprim-sulfamethoxazole.

Complicated Infections

In addition to the classic signs of cystitis and pyelonephritis, complicated UTIs may also be associated with nonspecific symptoms such as fatigue, irritability, nausea, headache, abdominal or back pain, or other vague symptoms, especially in patients at the extremes of age and patients with neurologic disease. Signs and symptoms may occasionally be insidious and exist for weeks to months before diagnosis. Complicated UTI, like uncomplicated UTI, is generally associated with pyuria and bacteriuria, although these may be absent if the infection does not communicate with the collecting system. Because of the diverse spectrum of causative uropathogens and their unpredictable susceptibility profile, a urine culture should always be performed in patients with suspected complicated UTI. As with uncomplicated UTI, a colony count threshold of $\geq 10^3$ cfu/ml should be used to diagnose complicated UTI except when urine cultures are obtained through a catheter, in which case a level of $\geq 10^2$ cfu/ml is evidence of infection.[16]

The wide variety of underlying conditions (see Fig. 50.1), diverse spectrum of possible etiologic agents (see Fig. 50.3), and paucity of controlled clinical trials with stratification according to specific complicating factors make generalizing about antimicrobial therapy difficult. The management strategy for complicated cystitis is shown in Figure 50.4 and that for complicated infections other than cystitis in Figure 50.10. Attempts must be made to correct any underlying anatomic, functional, or metabolic defect because otherwise antibiotics alone will often not be successful.[1] For empiric therapy in patients with mild to moderate illness who can be treated with oral medication, the fluoroquinolones provide the broadest spectrum of antimicrobial activity, cover most expected pathogens, and achieve high levels in the urine and urinary tract tissue. Exceptions are sparfloxacin, grepafloxacin, trovafloxacin, and moxifloxacin, which, in contrast to other fluoroquinolones, may not achieve sufficient concentration in urine to be effective for complicated UTI. If the infecting pathogen is known to be susceptible, trimethoprim-sulfamethoxazole or other agents are reasonable therapeutic choices. For initial treatment in more seriously ill, hospitalized patients, several parenteral antimicrobial agents are available (see Fig. 50.11). In contrast to uncomplicated UTI, *S. aureus* is relatively more likely to be found in complicated

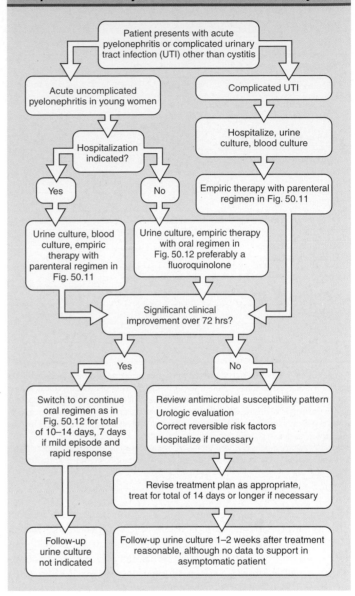

Figure 50.10 Management algorithm for acute uncomplicated pyelonephritis and complicated urinary tract infection other than cystitis.

UTIs, and if suspected, the therapeutic regimen should have activity against this pathogen.

The antimicrobial regimen can be modified when the infecting strain has been identified and antimicrobial susceptibilities are known. Patients who are given parenteral therapy can be switched to oral treatment after clinical improvement. At least 10 to 14 days of therapy is generally recommended, but longer therapy may be indicated in patients in whom an underlying complicating factor delays clinical response. By comparison, many patients in this category who have mild cystitis can be successfully treated with a 7-day regimen.

Catheter-Associated Infections

The incidence of bacteriuria associated with indwelling catheterization is 3% to 10% per day of catheterization, and the duration of catheterization is the most important risk factor for the development of catheter-associated bacteriuria. Catheter-associated

Parenteral regimens for acute uncomplicated pyelonephritis and complicated urinary tract infection

Drug	Dose (mg)	Interval
Ceftriaxone	1000–2000	q 24 hr
Cefepime*	1000–2000	q 12 hr
Fluoroquinolones[†]		
Ciprofloxacin	200–400	q 12 hr
Levofloxacin	250–500	q 24 hr
Ofloxacin	200–400	q 12 hr
Gentamicin (± ampicillin)	3–5 mg/kg body weight	q 24 hr
	1 mg/kg body weight	q 8 hr
Ampicillin (+ gentamicin)	1000	q 6 hr
Trimethoprim-sulfamethoxazole[‡]	160/800	q 12 hr
Aztreonam	1000	q 8–12 hr
Ampicillin-sulbactam*	1500	q 6 hr
Ticarcillin-clavulanate*	3200	q 8 hr
Piperacillin-tazobactam*	3375	q 6–8 hr
Imipenem-cilastatin*	250–500	q 6–8 hr
Ertapenem*	1000	q 24 hr
Vancomycin[§]	1000	q 12 hr

Figure 50.11 **Parenteral regimens for acute uncomplicated pyelonephritis and complicated urinary tract infection.** Duration depends on clinical setting (see text and Fig. 50.10). *Recommended if methicillin-susceptible *Staphylococcus aureus* coverage is desirable, as for treatment of a renal or perirenal abscess or when the Gram stain suggests *S. aureus* infection and no risk factors for methicillin-resistant *S. aureus* (e.g., injection drug use, recently in health care setting or jail, HIV-positive). [†]Avoid, if possible, in pregnancy. [‡]Widely used in pregnancy, although not an approved use. [§]Recommended if methicillin-resistant *S. aureus* is suspected or known.

Oral regimens for acute uncomplicated pyelonephritis and complicated urinary tract infection

Drug	Dose (mg)	Interval	Comment
Fluoroquinolones			Preferred for empiric treatment, avoid if possible in pregnancy, nursing mothers, or persons <18 years old.
Ciprofloxacin	500	q 12 hr	
Ciprofloxacin extended release	1000	q 24 hr	
Levofloxacin	250–500	q 24 hr	
Ofloxacin	200–300	q 12 hr	
Trimethoprim-sulfamethoxazole	160/800	q 12 hr	Widely used in pregnancy, although not an approved use. Avoid in first trimester.
Cefpodoxime proxetil	200	q 12 hr	Data are sparse.
Amoxicillin	500	q 8 hr	Used only when the causative pathogen is known to be susceptible or in addition to a broad-spectrum agent when empiric coverage against enterococci is desirable.

Figure 50.12 **Oral regimens for acute uncomplicated pyelonephritis and complicated urinary tract infection.** Duration depends on clinical setting (see text and Fig. 50.10).

bacteriuria is the most common source of gram-negative bacteremia in hospitalized patients. Complications of long-term catheterization (>30 days) include almost universal bacteriuria, often with polymicrobic and antibiotic-resistant flora, and (in addition to cystitis, pyelonephritis, and bacteremia as seen with short-term catheterization) frequent febrile episodes, catheter obstruction, stone formation associated with urease-producing uropathogens, local genitourinary infections, fistula formation, and bladder cancer. An increase in mortality risk has been reported with catheter-associated bacteriuria, but it is difficult to distinguish the role of the catheter because most deaths occur in patients who have severe underlying disease.

Most episodes of catheter-associated bacteriuria are asymptomatic and do not require routine screening or treatment because treatment does not reduce the complications of bacteriuria and can lead to antimicrobial resistance.[25] Symptomatic infections, often polymicrobial and caused by multidrug-resistant uropathogens, warrant broad-spectrum therapy as described previously. Because bacteria may be sequestered and protected from antibiotics in a biofilm on the catheter surface, it is reasonable to replace the catheter during antibiotic therapy, although there are few data to support this recommendation.[7]

Preventive measures are indicated to reduce the morbidity, mortality, and costs of catheter-associated infection. Effective strategies include avoidance of a catheter when possible and, when the catheter is necessary, sterile insertion, prompt removal,

and strict adherence to a closed collecting system.[7,26] Although randomized trials have not been performed, intermittent catheterization appears to result in lower rates of bacteriuria compared with long-term indwelling catheterization. Prophylactic systemic antimicrobial agents are generally not recommended but may be useful in patients at high risk for serious complications if UTI occurs, such as pregnant women or patients undergoing urologic surgery who are undergoing short-term catheterization. Prophylaxis has also been demonstrated to be beneficial in patients undergoing renal transplantation and requiring indwelling catheterization.

Spinal Cord Injury

Spinal cord injury alters the dynamics of voiding and often requires the use of bladder drainage with catheters. The diagnosis of UTI in patients with spinal cord injuries is often problematic and is based on the combination of symptoms and signs, which are often nonspecific, pyuria, and significant bacteriuria, with uropathogens often present in quantities >10^5 cfu/ml. Fluoroquinolones are the empiric oral agents of choice in patients with mild to moderate infection, although many uropathogens, even in the outpatient setting, are resistant to this class of antibiotic, and parenteral antibiotics may be needed.

Treatment of asymptomatic bacteriuria in patients with spinal cord injuries has not been shown to be beneficial and increases the risk for infection with antimicrobial-resistant uropathogens.[25,27] Likewise, antibiotic prophylaxis is generally not recommended except for selected outpatients with frequent symptomatic UTIs for whom there are no correctable risk factors.

Prostatitis

Prostatitis occurs in about 2% to 10% of men during their lifetime, but it is caused by acute or chronic bacterial infection in a minority.[28] The current National Institutes of Health classification system categorizes prostatitis within a complex series of syndromes that vary widely in clinical presentation and response to treatment. The most common organisms causing bacterial prostatitis are gram-negative bacilli, including *E. coli*, *Proteus* species, *Klebsiella* species, *P. aeruginosa*, and, less commonly, enterococci and *S. aureus*. The pathogenesis of prostatitis is believed to be related to reflux of infected urine from the urethra into the prostatic ducts. Prostatic calculi, commonly found in adult men, may provide a nidus for bacteria and protection from antibacterial agents.

Acute bacterial prostatitis is rare. Patients present with dysuria, frequency, urgency, obstructive voiding symptoms, fever, chills, and myalgias. The prostate is tender and swollen. Prostatic massage is contraindicated in men in whom the diagnosis of acute prostatitis is being considered, because of the risk for precipitating bacteremia. The patient will usually have pyuria and a positive urine culture. Patients who are severely ill require hospitalization and parenteral antibiotics, but many patients can be treated in the outpatient setting with oral fluoroquinolones. The duration of treatment is recommended to be at least 30 days to help to prevent the development of chronic bacterial prostatitis.[29] Abscess formation may rarely occur.

Chronic bacterial prostatitis is characterized by recurrent UTIs with the same uropathogen with intervening asymptomatic periods. The prostate typically is normal to palpation during asymptomatic periods. Chronic bacterial prostatitis is characterized microscopically by the presence of ≥10 leukocytes/high-power field in expressed prostatic secretions or postmassage voided urine in the absence of significant pyuria in first-voided and midstream urine specimens, and a uropathogen colony count that is at least 10-fold higher in the expressed prostatic secretions or postmassage voided urine compared with the first-voided midstream urine. In addition, macrophage-laden fat droplets (oval fat bodies) are usually prominent in the prostatic secretions. These tests, however, are infrequently performed by urologists. Cure rates, which historically have been low, are now up to 60% to 80% with the fluoroquinolones, which are the antibiotics of choice. The optimal duration of treatment is unknown, but most authorities recommend at least 1 to 3 months. Some patients require long-term, low-dose suppressive therapy to prevent symptomatic UTIs. Surgical intervention is only rarely considered and is associated with high morbidity.

Renal Abscess

Renal cortical and corticomedullary abscesses and perirenal abscesses occur in 1 to 10 per 10,000 hospital admissions.[30] Patients usually present with fever, chills, back or abdominal pain, and costovertebral angle tenderness but may have no urinary symptoms or findings if the abscess does not communicate with the collecting system, as is often the case with a cortical abscess. Bacteremia at the time of diagnosis is more common with corticomedullary and perirenal abscesses. The clinical presentation may be very insidious and nonspecific, especially with perirenal abscess, and the diagnosis may not be made until admission to a hospital or at autopsy. CT is recommended to establish the diagnosis and location of a renal or perirenal abscess (Fig. 50.13). Empiric antibiotic therapy should be broad and cover *S. aureus* and other uropathogens causing complicated UTI (see Figs. 50.10 and 50.11) and modified once urine culture results are known.

A renal cortical abscess (renal carbuncle) is usually caused by *S. aureus*, which reaches the kidney through the hematogenous route. Treatment with antibiotics is usually effective, and drainage is not required unless the patient is slow to respond. A renal corticomedullary abscess, in contrast, usually results from ascending

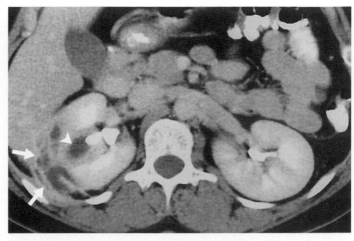

Figure 50.13 Renal abscess. Contrast computed tomography shows an abscess in the medulla of the kidney *(arrowhead)* with penetration and extension into the perinephric space *(arrows)*. (Courtesy of L. Towner.)

UTI in association with an underlying urinary tract abnormality, such as obstructive uropathy or vesicoureteral reflux, and is usually caused by common uropathogenic species such as *E. coli* and other coliforms. Such abscesses may extend deep into the renal parenchyma, perforate the renal capsule, and form a perirenal abscess. Treatment with antimicrobial agents without drainage is usually effective if the abscess is not very large and if the underlying urinary tract abnormality can be corrected. Aspiration of the abscess may be necessary in some patients, and nephrectomy may occasionally be required in patients with diffuse renal involvement or with severe sepsis. Perirenal abscesses usually occur in the setting of obstruction or other complicating factors (see Fig. 50.1) and result from ruptured intrarenal abscesses, hematogenous spread, or spread from a contiguous infection. Causative uropathogens are those commonly found in complicated UTIs (see Fig. 50.3), including *S. aureus* and enterococci; polymicrobic infections are common. Anaerobes or *Mycobacterium tuberculosis* may be causative. A previously high mortality rate has been lowered with earlier diagnosis and therapy. In contrast to the other types of abscess, drainage of pus is the cornerstone of therapy, and nephrectomy is sometimes indicated.

Papillary Necrosis

More than half of those who develop papillary necrosis have diabetes, almost always in conjunction with a UTI, but the condition also complicates sickle cell disease, analgesic abuse, and obstruction. Renal papillae are vulnerable to ischemia because of the sluggish blood flow in the vasa recta, and relatively modest ischemic insults may cause papillary necrosis. The clinical features are those typical of pyelonephritis. In addition, passage of sloughed papillae into the ureter may cause renal colic, renal insufficiency or failure, or obstruction with severe urosepsis. Papillary necrosis in the setting of pyelonephritis is associated with pyuria and a positive urine culture. Causative uropathogens are those typical of complicated UTI. The retrograde pyelogram is the preferred diagnostic procedure. Radiologic findings include an irregular papillary tip, dilated calyceal fornix, extension of contrast material into the parenchyma, and a separated crescent-shaped papilla surrounded by contrast, called the *ring sign*. Broad-spectrum antibiotics are indicated. Papillae obstructing the ureter may require removal with a cystoscopic ureteral basket or relief of obstruction by insertion of a ureteral stent.

Emphysematous Pyelonephritis

Emphysematous pyelonephritis is a fulminant, necrotizing, life-threatening variant of acute pyelonephritis caused by gas-forming organisms, including *E. coli*, *K. pneumoniae*, *P. aeruginosa*, and *P. mirabilis*.[31] Up to 90% of cases occur in diabetic patients, and obstruction may be present. Symptoms are suggestive of pyelonephritis, and a flank mass may be present. Dehydration and ketoacidosis are common. Pyuria and a positive urine culture are usually present. Gas is usually detected by a plain abdominal radiograph or ultrasound (Fig. 50.14). CT is the diagnostic modality of choice, however, because it can better localize the gas than ultrasonography. Accurate localization of gas is important because gas may also form in an infected obstructed collecting system or renal abscess; although serious, these conditions do not carry the same grave prognosis and are managed differently. Emergency nephrectomy in conjunction with broad-spectrum antibiotics is the treatment of choice. Medical treatment is associated with a mortality rate of 60% to 80%, which is lowered to 20% or less with surgical intervention.

Renal Malacoplakia

Malacoplakia is a chronic granulomatous disorder of unknown etiology involving the genitourinary, gastrointestinal, skin, and pulmonary systems.[32] It is characterized by an unusual inflammatory reaction to a variety of infections and is manifested by the accumulation of macrophages containing calcified bacterial debris called *Michaelis-Gutmann bodies* (Fig. 50.15). The underlying disorder appears to be a monocyte-macrophage bactericidal defect. The diagnosis is made by histologic examination of involved tissue. Genitourinary malacoplakia, most commonly involving the bladder, is usually associated with gram-negative UTI. Patients with renal malacoplakia generally have fever, flank pain, pyuria and hematuria, bacteriuria, and if both kidneys are involved, renal insufficiency. CT scanning usually shows enlarged kidneys with areas of poor enhancement, and the condition may be indistinguishable from other infectious or neoplastic lesions. Occasionally, the malacoplakia may extend through the renal capsule into the perinephric space, simulating a renal carcinoma (see Fig. 50.15). Treatment consists of therapy with a fluoroquinolone, correction of any underlying complicating conditions if possible, and improvement of renal function. Nephrectomy is recommended for

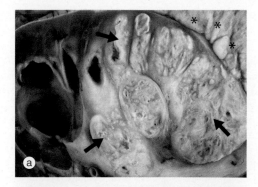

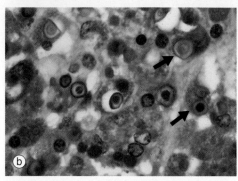

Figure 50.15   Renal malacoplakia. *a,* Malacoplakia involving most of the kidney *(arrows)* with extension through the capsule *(asterisks).* A small portion of normal kidney is present that is associated with hydronephrosis secondary to obstruction by the malacoplakia. *b,* The kidney tissue shows many macrophages containing intracytoplasmic inclusions *(arrows identify two particularly well-demarcated macrophages with Michaelis-Gutmann bodies).* (Courtesy of Luan Truong and Neil Sheerin.)

advanced unilateral disease. When the disease is bilateral or occurs in a transplanted kidney, the prognosis is very poor.

Xanthogranulomatous Pyelonephritis

Xanthogranulomatous pyelonephritis is a poorly understood, uncommon, but severe chronic renal infection associated with obstruction of the urinary tract.[30] It is characterized by replacement of renal parenchyma with a diffuse or segmental cellular infiltrate of lipid-laden macrophages called *foam cells*. The process may also extend beyond the renal capsule to the retroperitoneum. Its pathogenesis appears to be multifactorial, with infection complicating obstruction and leading to ischemia, tissue destruction, and accumulation of lipid deposits. Patients with xanthogranulomatous pyelonephritis are characteristically middle-aged women and have chronic symptoms such as flank pain, fever, chills, and malaise. Flank tenderness, a palpable mass, and irritative voiding symptoms are often present. The urine culture is usually positive with *E. coli*, other gram-negative bacilli, or *S. aureus*. CT generally shows an enlarged nonfunctioning kidney, a large calculus, low-density masses (xanthomatous tissue), and in some cases, involvement of adjacent structures (Fig. 50.16). It may be difficult to distinguish from neoplastic disease. Broad-spectrum antimicrobials are indicated, but total or partial nephrectomy is usually necessary for cure.

ASYMPTOMATIC BACTERIURIA

Asymptomatic bacteriuria, as noted previously, is a common and generally benign infection.[8,25] Pyuria is often present, especially in elderly people, and is a predictor for subsequent symptomatic UTI in some groups.[9] Causative uropathogens are the same as

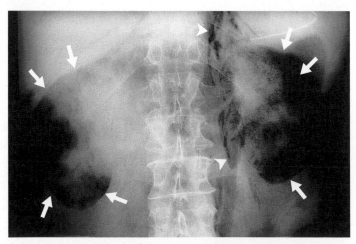

Figure 50.14   Emphysematous pyelonephritis. A plain radiograph in this febrile diabetic subject revealed diffuse gas formation throughout both kidneys (outlined by *arrows*) and gas dissecting in the left retroperitoneal space *(arrowheads).* (Courtesy of W. Bush.)

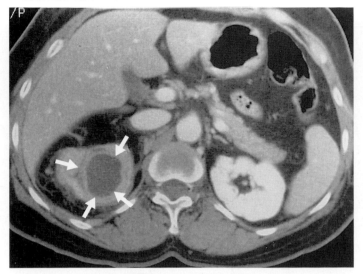

Figure 50.16 Xanthogranulomatous pyelonephritis. Contrast computed tomography scan with the inflammatory mass outlined by *arrows*. Pathologic diagnosis confirmed xanthogranulomatous pyelonephritis. (Courtesy of W. Bush.)

UROLOGIC EVALUATION

Urologic consultation and evaluation of the urinary tract should be considered in patients who present with symptoms or signs of obstruction, urolithiasis, flank mass, or urosepsis. Similarly, such an evaluation should be considered for those patients with presumptive uncomplicated or complicated UTI who have not had a satisfactory clinical response after 72 hours of treatment to exclude the presence of a complicating factor. Contrast-enhanced CT scanning of the kidneys is the most effective imaging modality in adult patients with renal infection because of its superior resolution and sensitivity in detecting renal abnormalities and perirenal fluid collections.[33] Spiral (helical) CT may be superior to conventional CT.[34] Noncontrast spiral CT appears to be a rapid, safe, and sensitive method for evaluating patients with suspected renal stones. Renal ultrasound is useful for detection of stones and abscesses and is often more readily accessible than CT. However, it is less sensitive than CT for detection of many of the conditions present in patients with complicated UTI. The role of magnetic resonance imaging remains to be determined. Radionuclide imaging procedures have no role in the evaluation of adults with UTI, although they are very useful in children with pyelonephritis (see Chapter 58). A plain abdominal radiograph may be used to detect gas in the urinary tracts of diabetic patients with suspected pyelonephritis, but it is not as sensitive or specific as CT.

Studies of the value of excretory urography and of cystoscopy in women with recurrent cystitis have demonstrated that significant abnormalities that influence subsequent management of UTIs are very uncommon.[4] Therefore, routine urologic evaluation of patients with recurrent cystitis results in unnecessary expense and potential toxicity. Likewise, routine urologic investigation of young women with acute pyelonephritis is generally not cost effective and has a low diagnostic yield, although it is reasonable to obtain such an evaluation after two episodes of pyelonephritis or if any complicating factor (see Fig. 50.1) is identified with any of the recurrences. A urologic evaluation is probably not necessary in a man who has had a single UTI with no obvious complicating factors and whose infection responds promptly to treatment.

those causing UTIs in the same population. Treatment of asymptomatic bacteriuria is generally not warranted.[25] However, patients at high risk for serious complications may warrant a more aggressive approach to diagnosis and treatment, including pregnant women and patients undergoing urologic surgery.[25] Current management strategies in patients with a renal transplant, including long-term antimicrobial prophylaxis, help prevent both asymptomatic bacteriuria and symptomatic urinary infection. It is not clear whether screening for or treatment of asymptomatic bacteriuria in such patients is worthwhile.[25] Some authorities advise treatment of asymptomatic bacteriuria found in patients with anatomic or functional abnormalities of the urinary tract, diabetic patients, and patients with urea-splitting bacteria, such as *P. mirabilis*, *Klebsiella* species, and others.[8] Evidence-based guidelines for screening and treatment of asymptomatic bacteriuria in these populations are needed.

REFERENCES

1. Nicolle LE: A practical guide to the management of complicated urinary tract infection. Drugs 1997;53:583–592.
2. Foxman B, Barlow R, D'Arcy H, et al: Urinary tract infection: Self-reported incidence and associated costs. Ann Epidemiol 2000;10:509–515.
3. Hooton TM, Scholes D, Hughes JP, et al: A prospective study of risk factors for symptomatic urinary tract infection in young women. N Engl J Med 1996;335:468–474.
4. Hooton TM, Stamm WE: Diagnosis and treatment of uncomplicated urinary tract infection. Infect Dis Clin North Am 1997;11:551–581.
5. Scholes D, Hooton TM, Roberts PL, et al: Risk factors associated with acute pyelonephritis in healthy women. Ann Intern Med 2005;142:20–27.
6. Foxman B, Barlow R, D'Arcy H, et al: Urinary tract infection: Self-reported incidence and associated costs. Ann Epidemiol 2000;10:509–515.
7. Stamm WE, Hooton TM: Management of urinary tract infections in adults. N Engl J Med 1993;329:1328–1334.
8. Zhanel GG, Harding GKM, Guay DRP: Asymptomatic bacteriuria: Which patients should be treated? Arch Intern Med 1990;150:1389–1396.
9. Nicolle LE: Asymptomatic bacteriuria: When to screen and when to treat. Infect Dis Clin North Am 2003;17:367–394.
10. Hooton TM, Scholes D, Stapleton AE, et al: A prospective study of asymptomatic bacteriuria in young sexually active women. N Engl J Med 2000;343:992–997.
11. Sobel JD: Pathogenesis of urinary tract infection: Role of host defenses. Infect Dis Clin North Am 1997;11:531–549.
12. Scholes D, Hooton TM, Roberts PL, et al: Risk factors for recurrent urinary tract infection in young women. J Infect Dis 2000;182:1177–1182.
13. Svanborg C, Godaly G: Bacterial virulence in urinary tract infection. Infect Dis Clin North Am 1997;11:513–529.
14. Patterson JE, Andriole VT: Bacterial urinary tract infections in diabetes. Infect Dis Clin North Am 1997;11:735–750.
15. Talan DA, Stamm WE, Hooton TM, et al: Comparison of ciprofloxacin (7 days) and trimethoprim-sulfamethoxazole (14 days) for acute uncomplicated pyelonephritis in women: A randomized trial. JAMA 2000;283:1583–590.
16. Rubin UH, Shapiro ED, Andriole VT, et al: Evaluation of new anti-infective drugs for the treatment of urinary tract infection. Clin Infect Dis 1992;15:S216–227.
17. Gupta K, Hooton TM, Stamm WE: Increasing antimicrobial resistance and the management of uncomplicated community-acquired urinary tract infections. Ann Intern Med 2001;135:41–50.
18. Manges AR, Jonson JR, Foxman B, et al: Widespread distribution of urinary tract infection caused by a multi-drug-resistant *Escherichia coli* clonal group. N Engl J Med 2001;345:1055–1057.
19. Norrby SR: Short-term treatment of uncomplicated lower urinary tract infections in women. Rev Infect Dis 1990;12:458–467.

20. Warren JW, Abrutyn E, Hebel JR, et al: Guidelines for antimicrobial treatment of uncomplicated acute bacterial cystitis and acute pyelonephritis in women. Clin Infect Dis 1999;29:745–758.

21. Hooton TM, Scholes D, Gupta K, et al. Amoxicillin-clavulanate vs ciprofloxacin for the treatment of uncomplicated cystitis in women: A randomized trial. JAMA 2005;293:949–955.

22. Stapleton A, Stamm WE: Prevention of urinary tract infection. Infect Dis Clin North Am 1997;11:719–733.

23. Anderson GG, Dodson KW, Hooton TM, et al: Intracellular bacterial communities of uropathogenic *Escherichia coli* in urinary tract pathogenesis. Trends Microbiol 2004;12:424–430.

24. Stamm WE, McKevitt M, Counts GW: Acute renal infection in women: Treatment with trimethoprim-sulfamethoxazole or ampicillin for two or six weeks. A randomized trial. Ann Intern Med 1987;106:341–345.

25. Nicolle LE, Bradley S, Colgan R, et al: Infectious Diseases Society of America guidelines for the diagnosis and treatment of asymptomatic bacteriuria in adults (IDSA GUIDELINES). Clin Infect Dis 2005;40:643.

26. Warren JW: Catheter-associated urinary tract infections. Infect Dis Clin North Am 1997;11:609–622.

27. Cardenas DD, Hooton TM: Urinary tract infection in persons with spinal cord injury. Arch Phys Med Rehabil 1995;76:272–280.

28. Habermacher GM, Chason JT, Schaeffer AJ: Prostatitis/chronic pelvic pain syndrome. Annu Rev Med 2006;57:195–206.

29. Brannigan RE, Schaeffer AJ: Prostatitis syndromes. Curr Opin Infect Dis 1996;9:37–41.

30. Dembry LM, Andriole VT: Renal and perirenal abscesses. Infect Dis Clin North Am 1997;11:663–680.

31. McHugh TP, Albanna SE, Stewart NJ: Bilateral emphysematous pyelonephritis. Am J Emerg Med 1998;16:166–169.

32. Dobyan DC, Truong LD, Eknoyan G: Renal malacoplakia reappraised. Am J Kidney Dis 1993;22:243–252.

33. Kaplan DM, Rosenfield AT, Smith RC: Advances in the imaging of renal infection. Infect Dis Clin North Am 1997;11:681–705.

34. Wyatt SH, Urban BA, Fishman EK: Spiral CT of the kidneys: role in characterization of renal disease. Part I: Nonneoplastic disease. Crit Rev Diagn Imag 1995;36:1–37.

CHAPTER 51

Tuberculosis of the Urinary Tract

R. Kasi Visweswaran and Suresh Bhat

INTRODUCTION AND DEFINITION

Tuberculosis (TB), caused by *Mycobacterium tuberculosis*, affects 15 to 20 million people worldwide, of which 8 to 10 million are infectious. About 8 million people develop active disease annually from the stage of asymptomatic infection.[1] According to an estimate by the World Health Organization (WHO), between 1999 and 2020, nearly 1 billion more people will be newly infected, 200 million will get sick, and 70 million will die from TB if control measures are not improved. In developed countries, TB commonly affects older individuals and ethnic migrants. In recent years, the incidence is increasing owing to the prevalence of human immunodeficiency virus (HIV) infection. The incidence of TB in HIV-infected patients is 100 times greater than that observed in the general population. When a tuberculin-positive individual develops HIV, active disease is estimated to occur in 7% to 10% annually, which contrasts with the 5% to 10% per lifetime in the immunocompetent host.[2]

Extrapulmonary TB occurs in about 15% of active cases in the non–HIV-infected population.[3] Genitourinary TB is one of the more common forms of extrapulmonary TB and constitutes 30% of the extrapulmonary cases. It is almost always secondary to a symptomatic or asymptomatic primary lesion, most often in the lung. Renal involvement may also occur as a part of miliary TB.

ETIOLOGY

The tubercle bacillus, which was first identified by Robert Koch in 1882, is a nonmotile, nonsporing, strictly aerobic straight or slightly curved rodlike bacillus that is weakly gram positive and acid and alcohol fast. Mycobacteria possess several unique features that help in their intracellular existence, including a cell wall that contains a lipid shell ("lipid barrier"), mycolic acid derivatives that allow the organism to resist proteolysis and uptake into phagolysosomes, muramyl dipeptide that stimulates a T cell response that elicits the characteristic granuloma, and cell wall glycolipids (lipoarabinomannan) that inhibit macrophage function. This surrounding coat of inert lipids and surface proteins allows mycobacteria to survive inside phagocytes, where they may remain dormant for years.[4]

Other pathogenic mycobacteria may rarely cause clinical disease, usually in immunocompromised hosts; these include *M. avium-intracellulare*, and rarely *M. kansasii*, *M. bovis*, *M. fortuitum*, and *M. szulgai*. However, most cases of genitourinary TB are due to *M. tuberculosis*.[4]

PATHOGENESIS

The clinical and pathologic manifestations of TB vary depending on the virulence of the organism and the effectiveness of the host response. The host response may lead to complete containment of infection or result in an illness of varying severity. Evidence is accumulating that there are strain-to-strain differences that may determine whether an infected person develops primary TB, reactivation TB, or a chronic asymptomatic infection. The clinical manifestations of TB represent not only the consequence of bacterial proliferation but also host destructive and reparative processes.

When an infected droplet with the size of 1 to 5 μm is deposited in the respiratory tract, tonsillar fossa, or gastrointestinal tract, a primary focus develops in which there is formation of a nonspecific asymptomatic granuloma. The organisms from the primary focus drain to the regional lymph gland causing its enlargement, resulting in the *primary complex*. This is often asymptomatic and self-limited.

However, the bacilli from the regional lymph node may reach the systemic circulation through the thoracic duct, where they undergo silent hematogenous dissemination (Fig. 51.1). The bacilli are initially disseminated throughout the cortices of both kidneys and are deposited in the glomeruli. The high blood flow to the renal cortex, oxygen saturation in the glomeruli, and increased viscosity of blood toward the efferent arteriolar end of the glomerular capillary tuft favor the localization of bacteria in this location. Here they stimulate an inflammatory response, leading to the formation of granulomas in the cortex that may heal and form a scar, remain dormant for many years, or rupture into the proximal tubule of the nephron as a result of proliferation of mycobacteria. The bacilli in the nephron are trapped at the level of the loop of Henle, where they multiply. The relatively poor blood flow, hypertonicity, and high ammonia concentration in the renal medullary region may lead to weakening of immune responses locally and favor the formation of medullary granulomas. These granulomas (tuberculomas), which contain macrophages, may undergo coagulative necrosis (driven by macrophage production of cytokines), forming cheeselike caseous material (Fig. 51.2) and occasionally rupturing into the calyx.[5]

The renal medulla is the most common site of involvement of clinical renal TB[6] and is usually unilateral (Fig. 51.3). When this caseous focus ruptures into the collecting system, cavities and ulcers are formed, and involvement of renal papillae may lead to sloughing and papillary necrosis. Healing in the kidney occurs by fibrosis and scarring, resulting in strictures and obstruction. Dystrophic calcification of damaged structures may result in a nonfunctioning kidney called "putty" or "cement" kidney. Spread of TB to contiguous structures may occur; ureteritis is common and may result in long segment strictures or multiple strictures and obstructive uropathy (Fig. 51.4). The bladder may develop hyperemia near the ureteral orifice followed by superficial ulcers and granulomatous changes involving all layers (pancystitis).

Pathogenesis of urinary tuberculosis

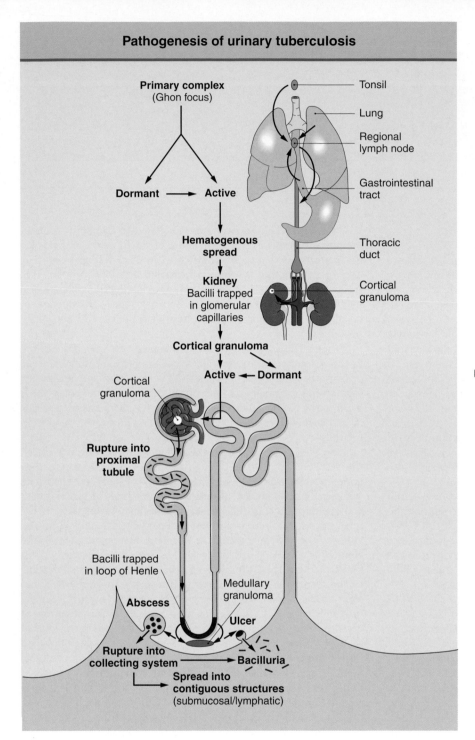

Figure 51.1   Pathogenesis of urinary tuberculosis.

Healing by fibrosis at the ureteral orifice results in a refluxing "golf-hole" ureter. Extensive fibrosis of the bladder wall results in a thick, small-capacity bladder ("thimble" bladder). Involvement of the genital tract is also common. As many as 70% to 80% of males with TB of the urinary tract have epididymitis, prostatitis, seminal vesiculitis, orchitis, or cold abscesses. In females, genital tract involvement is uncommon, but if present, usually presents as salpingitis that is often diagnosed during investigation for infertility.

Although genitourinary TB usually results from hematogenous dissemination from a primary lung site, the urinary tract may also be primarily involved following instillation of bacille Calmette-Guérin (BCG) in the bladder as part of treatment of superficial bladder carcinomas. Transplanted kidneys may also transmit TB to their recipients.[7]

CLINICAL MANIFESTATIONS

Urinary tract TB may be asymptomatic or mimic other disorders. It may present with constitutional symptoms or symptoms related to the lower urinary tract, abdomen, or genitalia (Fig. 51.5). A high index of suspicion enables early diagnosis. Most patients are between 20 and 40 years of age, with a male-to-female ratio of 2:1. Increased risk factors for TB include close contact with sputum

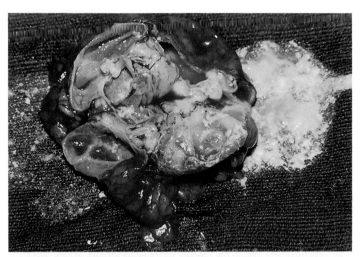

Figure 51.2 Renal tuberculosis. A cut section of kidney showing areas of cavitation and caseation necrosis (white chalky material).

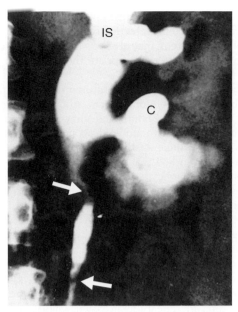

Figure 51.4 Multiple ureteral strictures. Strictures *(arrows)* associated with dilated lower ureter, infundibular stenosis (IS), and caliectasis (C) are seen in this intravenous urogram. (Courtesy of Professor K. Sasidharan, Kasthurba Medical College, Manipal, India.)

smear–positive individuals, vagrancy, social deprivation, neglect, immunosuppression, HIV infection or AIDS, diabetes mellitus, renal failure, and other debilitating illness.

Nearly 25% of patients are asymptomatic, and the diagnosis is made while investigating for other diseases, during surgery, or even at autopsy. Another 25% may have asymptomatic urinary abnormalities, usually persistent asymptomatic pyuria or hematuria. In patients with persistent pyuria, conventional urine cultures do not yield any growth, and the urine is usually acidic, hence the term *acid-sterile pyuria*. Of the patients who are symptomatic, lower urinary tract symptoms such as frequency, urgency, dysuria, nocturia, frank pyuria, or hematuria occur in more than 75%. Increased frequency of micturition is one of the early symptoms and results from inflammation of the bladder and the acidic nature of the urine. The defect in the urinary-concentrating mechanism explains the occurrence of nocturia.

Recurrent bouts of painless macroscopic hematuria should alert the clinician to the possible diagnosis of urinary TB, although diseases such as IgA nephropathy should also be considered. Macroscopic hematuria in urinary TB occurs as a result of bleeding from the ulcerating lesions, inflammation of the urothelium, or rupture of blood vessel in the vicinity of

a cavity. Colicky pain may occur as a presenting manifestation of urinary TB when associated with stone, clot, or acute obstruction.

In advanced diseases, frequency and urgency related to reduced bladder capacity (thimble bladder) occur. Incomplete emptying, increased susceptibility to infection, and secondary vesicoureteral reflux may also occur. In chronic ureteral obstruction, enlargement of the kidney, infection, or perinephric collection leads to a dull aching loin pain. Severe suprapubic pain with backache and dysuria

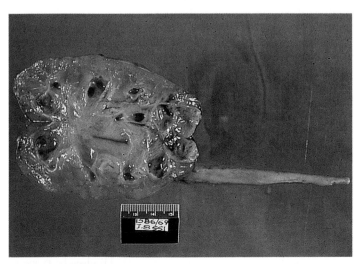

Figure 51.3 Renal tuberculosis. Ulcerocavernous lesions. A cut section of kidney showing areas of destruction in medulla and renal cortex. (Courtesy of Professor K. Sasidhara, Kasthurba Medical College, Manipal, India.)

Clinical features of urinary tuberculosis		
Features	Frequency (%)	Symptoms
Asymptomatic	25	Detected during autopsy, surgery, or investigations for other diseases
Asymptomatic urinary	25	Persistent pyuria, microscopic abnormalities, hematuria
Lower urinary tract symptoms (most common)	40	Frequency, urgency, dysuria, incontinence, nocturia, suprapubic pain, perineal pain
Male genital tract involvement	75	Epididymitis, hemospermia, infertility, reduced semen volume
Female genital tract involvement	<5	Amenorrhea, infertility, vaginal bleeding, pelvic pain
Constitutional symptoms	<20	Fever, reduced appetite, anorexia, weight loss, night sweats
Miscellaneous	—	Urolithiasis, hypertension, acute renal failure, chronic renal failure, abdominal colic, abdominal mass

Figure 51.5 Clinical features of urinary tuberculosis.

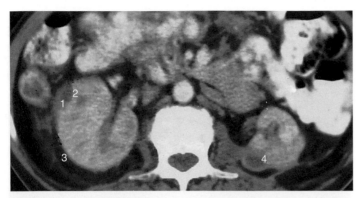

Figure 51.9   Renal tuberculosis. Computed tomography shows an enlarged left kidney with multiple cavities present bilaterally (marked 1, 2, 3, and 4). (Courtesy of Professor K. Sasidharan, Kasthurba Medical College, Manipal, India.)

is the most sensitive investigation for identifying renal calcification and cavitary lesions, which occur in more than half of cases of renal TB (Fig.51.9). Cortical thinning is a common CT finding and may be either focal or global. These imaging modalities are helpful in the follow-up of patients with cavities or mass lesions in the kidney. Cystoscopy under general anesthesia with adequate muscle relaxation helps to visualize the mucosal lesions, the golf-hole ureteral orifice, or the efflux of toothpaste-like caseous material. Biopsy during the acute stage is avoided for fear of dissemination of TB.

TB mimics numerous diseases both clinically and radiologically. Chronic nonspecific urinary infections may be confused with renal TB. This is confounded by the finding that in about 20% of patients with renal TB, secondary bacterial infection may occur. Absence of response to usual antibiotics should arouse suspicion of urinary TB. Conditions causing recurrent painless hematuria, such as IgA nephropathy and bilharziasis (schistosomiasis, see Chapter 53), are often misdiagnosed as TB in endemic areas. In interstitial cystitis, lower urinary symptoms similar to tuberculous cystitis may occur, but the urinalysis does not show gross pyuria, and cultures for acid-fast bacilli are negative. Radiologically, chronic pyelonephritis, renal papillary necrosis, medullary sponge kidney, calyceal diverticulum, renal carcinoma, xanthogranulomatous pyelonephritis, and multiple small renal calculi have to be differentiated from TB. Of late, a few cases of pseudotuberculous pyelonephritis have been reported in which caseating granulomas resembling TB were observed in the renal parenchyma but no mycobacteria or other microorganisms were detected in the renal tissue or urine culture.[15,16]

NATURAL HISTORY

The overall prognosis of TB of the urinary tract depends on the host resistance and the load and virulence of the organism. In many cases, foci in the urinary tract remain dormant indefinitely. Progression occurs through formation of tuberculous granuloma, caseation, ulceration, and dystrophic calcification. Most manifestations result from the complications, which can be prevented by timely chemotherapy and appropriate surgical intervention when indicated. With the advent of effective chemotherapeutic measures, the long-term complications and sequelae of TB have decreased significantly.

TREATMENT

Patients are managed mainly by medical treatment. Surgery is reserved for correction of anatomic abnormalities and removal

of infected or dead tissues and pus. Chemotherapy of TB can be planned adequately only after considering certain peculiarities of the mycobacteria. The tendency of the organism to remain dormant in many parts of the body poses a special problem, which is often not seen in other chronic infections. Three populations of organisms are believed to survive in the body in different environments (Fig. 51.10).

Curative therapy requires a combination of bactericidal drugs that will eradicate all three groups of mycobacteria. In addition to streptomycin, isoniazid, rifampin (rifampicin), and pyrazinamide, which are bactericidal, other bacteriostatic antituberculous drugs are also used (Fig. 51.11). Fixed-dose combinations of anti-TB drugs incorporating two or more drugs in the same tablet have advantages, including increased compliance, administration of adequate dose, minimization of inadvertent medication errors, and avoidance of drug resistance. Genitourinary TB is more amenable to medical treatment because of the presence of significantly fewer organisms in the lesion compared with lesions in the lungs. Many of the drugs reach the kidneys, urinary tract, urine, and cavitary lesions in high concentration.

A short-course regimen is usually recommended. Treatment is started with daily rifampin, 600 mg, isoniazid, 300 mg, and pyrazinamide, 1500 mg, in the morning. Unless the culture sensitivity indicates otherwise, pyrazinamide is discontinued after 2 months, and isoniazid and rifampin (rifampicin) are continued for another 4 months. In instances in which the patient is very sick with irritative bladder symptoms, streptomycin in daily doses of 1 g may be added during the first 2 months. However, if the patient

Subpopulations of *M. tuberculosis*		
Type of *M. tuberculosis*	Type of lesion	Ideal bactericidal drug

Group I
Extracellular
  Neutral/alkaline pH
  Rapid multiplication
	Cavitating lesions in medulla	Streptomycin
		Isoniazid
		Rifampin (Rifampicin)

Group II
Intracellular
  Acidic pH
  Slow or intermittent multiplication
	Macrophage	Pyrazinamide
		Rifampin (Rifampicin)
		Isoniazid

Group III
Closed caseous lesion
  Neutral pH
  Slow or intermittent multiplication
	Closed caseous lesions
	Cold abscess
		Rifampin (Rifampicin)

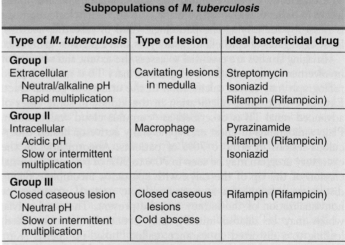

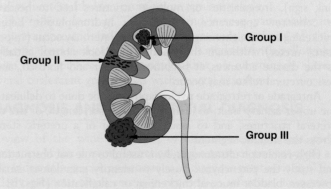

Figure 51.10   Subpopulations of mycobacteria in the kidney. The localization of three populations of *Mycobacterium tuberculosis* and their drug susceptibility are shown.

Antituberculous drugs

Drug	Dose Form	Dosage	Side Effects	Mode of Action	Remarks
Isoniazid	Tablet: 100 mg, 300 mg	5 mg/kg daily (oral) (maximum, 300 mg/day)	Peripheral neuritis, hepatitis, hyper-sensitivity reactions	Bactericidal for groups I and II	Pyridoxine (50 mg) prophylaxis necessary
Rifampin (Rifampicin)	Capsule or tablet: 150, 300, 450 mg	10 mg/kg daily (oral) (maximum, 600 mg/day)	Hepatitis, febrile reactions, acute interstitial nephritis	Bactericidal for groups I, II, and III	
Pyrazinamide	Tablet: 400, 500 mg	25 mg/kg daily (oral) (maximum, 2 g/day)	Hepatotoxicity, hyperuricemia	Bactericidal for group II	Combination with aminoglycoside useful
Streptomycin	Powder for injection: 1 g	15 mg/kg daily IM (maximum dose, 1 g; dose reduced in those >40 years of age)	Ototoxicity, nephrotoxicity	Bactericidal for group I	
Ethambutol	Tablet: 100, 400 mg	15–25 mg/kg daily (oral) (maximum, 2.5 g/day)	Optic neuritis (reversible), skin rash	Bacteriostatic for groups I and II	Used to inhibit development of resistant mutants; use with caution in renal failure
Thiacetazone	Tablet: 150 mg	150 mg (oral) (not for intermittent therapy)	Skin rashes, exfoliative dermatitis, hepatic failure	Bacteriostatic and inhibits emergence of INH resistance	Not used in renal failure
Ciprofloxacin	Tablet: 250, 500 mg	500–1000 mg (oral)	Hypersensitivity, drug interaction		Not used in children
Ofloxacin	Tablet: 200, 400 mg	400–500 mg (oral)			Not approved by FDA for tuberculosis
Capreomycin Kanamycin		15–30 mg/kg daily IM	Ototoxicity, nephrotoxicity	Bactericidal for group I	Avoided in older patients and those with renal failure

Figure 51.11 Antituberculous drugs. The main drugs are listed with dosage form, dosage, side effects, and mode of action.

is older than 40 years, the daily dose of streptomycin may be reduced to 0.75 g with periodic monitoring for ototoxicity and vestibular toxicity.

In situations in which the probability of drug resistance is high, ethambutol in daily doses of 800 to 1200 mg may also be used in the first 2 months. Longer courses of antituberculous treatment ranging from 9 months to 2 years are useful in patients who do not tolerate pyrazinamide, those responding slowly to a standard regimen, those with miliary or central nervous system disease, and children with multiple-site involvement.

During treatment, healing by fibrosis may lead to obstruction of one or both ureters, with hydronephrosis, parenchymal damage, and renal failure. Dehydration or salt depletion may occur as a result of tubulointerstitial damage, resulting in altered tubular function. Adrenal involvement may contribute to salt wasting. Oliguric acute renal failure caused by allergic interstitial nephritis may occur in patients receiving intermittent rifampin therapy.

Surgical Treatment

The role of surgical treatment in urinary TB is limited. For ureteral strictures, timely introduction of stents across the narrow segment may help to avoid the need for major surgical procedures. Two broad types of surgical treatments are considered.

Reconstructive surgery involves the correction of obstruction to the ureter by pyeloplasty, ureteroureterostomy, correction of reflux by ureteral reimplantation, and increasing the bladder capacity by augmentation cystoplasty, which involves anastomosing an isolated segment of bowel to the contracted bladder.

Ablative surgery involves removal of the diseased parts together with the infected material containing the dormant organisms. The need for removal of a unilateral nonfunctioning kidney is controversial. Because prolonged antituberculous treatment for 18 to 24 months effectively sterilizes caseous and calcified masses of the tuberculous cement kidney, nephrectomy is advocated only in cases of secondary sepsis, pain, bleeding, uncontrollable hypertension, or continued positive urinary cultures. Tuberculous abscesses can be aspirated under ultrasound or CT guidance and antituberculous drugs directly instilled into the cavity.

Treatment Regimens in Special Situations

Standardized treatment regimens have been devised for a number of special situations.[17]

Women during Pregnancy and Lactation

Most antituberculous drugs are safe for use during pregnancy. However, streptomycin, which is ototoxic to the fetus, is avoided. If a four-drug schedule is indicated, streptomycin is replaced by ethambutol. There is no contraindication to the use of these drugs during breast-feeding, and it is not necessary to isolate the baby from the mother. The baby should receive BCG immunization and isoniazid prophylaxis. Because rifampin interacts with the efficacy of oral contraceptive pills, women taking these agents together should be advised to take a higher dose of estrogen or use alternative methods of contraception.

Treatment of Patients with Liver Disorders

The usual short-term chemotherapy regimen can be used in patients with liver disorders if there is no evidence of chronic liver disease, hepatitis virus carrier state, past history of acute hepatitis, or excessive alcohol consumption. In chronic liver disease, isoniazid, rifampin and one or two nonhepatotoxic drugs (streptomycin and ethambutol) can be used for 8 to 12 months. Pyrazinamide is contraindicated. In those with acute hepatitis unrelated to TB or its therapy, it would be safer to defer the chemotherapy until the acute hepatitis has resolved. If immediate treatment of TB during acute hepatitis is mandatory, streptomycin plus ethambutol for a period of 3 months followed by isoniazid and rifampin for 6 months may be advised.

Treatment of Patients with Renal Failure

In patients with renal failure, isoniazid, rifampin, and pyrazinamide, which are eliminated by the biliary route, can be given in normal dosages. Those receiving isoniazid should also be given pyridoxine (50 mg/day) to prevent peripheral neuropathy. Because streptomycin and ethambutol are excreted by the kidney, dosage modification of these drugs is necessary in renal failure. Streptomycin (15 mg/kg) is administered every 24 to 72 hours for a creatinine clearance between 10 and 50 ml/min, and every 72 to 96 hours for a creatinine clearance less than 10 ml/min to maintain a therapeutic peak level of 20 to 30 μg/ml. Monitoring

for high-pitched tinnitus, sense of fullness in the ears, and audiography may be useful. For ethambutol, the dose is administered every 24 to 36 hours if the creatinine clearance is between 10 and 50 ml/min and every 48 hours if the creatinine clearance is below 10 ml/min. Monthly questioning for symptoms of visual dysfunction (alterations in visual fields, acuity, and blue-green color vision) with early referral for ophthalmic examination may identify ethambutol toxicity early with potential reversibility.

Treatment in AIDS

Even in patients with AIDS, short-term chemotherapy is sufficient. If the follow-up cultures are positive, prolonged therapy for up to 2 years may be needed based on the antibiotic sensitivity.

Monitoring of Patients

After 2 months of intensive chemotherapy, urine is cultured for *M. tuberculosis* for 3 consecutive days. If cultures are still positive, sensitivity is done and treatment modified accordingly. After completion of treatment, all patients should have three consecutive early-morning samples of urine for *M. tuberculosis* culture, and this is repeated after 3 months and 1 year. Intravenous urography is repeated at the end of 2 months and at the completion of treatment to detect any evidence of obstruction. In cases of renal calcification, the patient should be evaluated yearly by three early-morning samples of urine for culture for mycobacteria and plain x-ray abdomen for up to 10 years because calcification may harbor *M. tuberculosis* and may progress to destruction of the kidney.[18]

REFERENCES

1. Raviglione MC, Srider DE, Kochi A: Global epidemiology of tuberculosis. JAMA 1995;273:220–226.
2. Selwyn PA, Hartel D, Lewis VA, et al: A prospective study of the risk of tuberculosis among intravenous drug users with human immunodeficiency virus infection. N Engl J Med 1989;370:546–547.
3. Schafer M, Kim D, Weiss J, et al: Extrapulmonary tuberculosis in patients with HIV infection. Medicine 1991;70:384–396.
4. Ho JL, Rilay LW: Defenses against tuberculosis. In Crystal RG, West JB, Weibel ER, Barnes PJ (eds): The Lung: Scientific Foundations, 2nd ed. Philadelphia, Lippincott-Raven, 1997, pp 2381–2391.
5. Turk JL: Granulomatous diseases. In McGee JOD, Isacson PG, Wright NA (eds): Oxford Textbook of Pathology. Oxford, UK, Oxford University Press, 1992, pp 394–404.
6. Simon HB, Weinstein AJ, Pasternak MS, et al: Genitourinary tuberculosis: Clinical features in a general hospital population. Am J Med 1977;63: 410–414.
7. Mourad G, Soullilon JP, Chong G, et al: Transmission of mycobacterium TB with renal allografts. Nephron 1985;41:82–85.
8. Wismia LG, Jukol S, Lopez de SM, et al: Renal function damage in 131 cases of urogenital tuberculosis. Urology 1978;11:457–461.
9. De Frongs RA: Hyperkalemia and hyporenenemic hypoaldosteronism. Kidney Int 1980;17;118–134.
10. Mallinson WJW, Fuller RW, Levison DA, et al: Diffuse interstitial renal tuberculosis: An unusual cause of renal failure. Q J Med 1981;50: 137–148.
11. Marks LS, Poutasse EF: Hypertension from renal tuberculosis: Operative cure predicted by renal vein renin. J Urol 1973;109:149–152.
12. Shankar MS, Aravindan AN, Sohal PM, et al: The prevalence of tuberculin sensitivity and anergy in chronic renal failure in an endemic area: Tuberculin test and the risk of post-transplant tuberculosis. Nephrol Dial Transplant 2005;20:2720–2724.
13. Baniel J, Maunia A, Liamen G: Fine needle cytodiagnosis of renal tuberculosis. J Urol 1999;146:689–691.
14. Vijayaraghavan SB, Kandasamy SV, Arul M, et al: Spectrum of high-resolution sonographic features of urinary tuberculosis. J Ultrasound Med 2004;23:585–594.
15. Casasole SV, Muntaner LP, Alonso UJ: Pseudo tuberculous pyelonephritis. Arch Esp Urol 1994;47:172–174.
16. Hoorens AV, Niepen PV, Kauppens F, et al: Pseudotuberculous pyelonephritis: Associated with urolithiasis. Am J Surg Pathol 1993;17: 314–316.
17. Maher D, Chaulet P, Spinaci S, Harries A (eds): Standardised treatment regimens. In Treatment of Tuberculosis: Guidelines for National Programmes, 2nd ed. Geneva, WHO, 1997, pp 25–31.
18. Gow GJ, Barbosa S: Genitourinary tuberculosis: A study of 1117 cases over a period of 34 years. Br J Urol 1984;56:449–455.

Fungal Infection of the Urinary Tract

Jack D. Sobel

INTRODUCTION

Since the 1980s, there has been a marked increase in opportunistic fungal pathogens involving the urinary tract, of which *Candida* species are the most prevalent.[1,2] The kidney and urinary tract become infected as a result of hematogenous spread or from an ascending infection, usually in the presence of urinary obstruction. *Candida* species are common causes of ascending infection in catheterized and obstructed urinary tracts, particularly in patients with diabetes. Patients receiving immunosuppressive therapy for renal transplantation are at risk of invasive fungal urinary tract infections (UTIs) caused by *Candida*, *Aspergillus*, and *Cryptococcus* species. Acquired immunodeficiency syndrome (AIDS) is associated with mucosal *Candida* infections but not candiduria; however, disseminated histoplasmosis and cryptococcosis, both common complications of AIDS, frequently involve the urinary tract (Fig. 52.1).

Candida species are the main fungal species commonly associated with urethritis, cystitis, and pyelonephritis. Nevertheless, many species of fungi can cause prostatitis, epididymitis, chronic bladder inflammation or ulceration, and ureteral obstruction (see Fig. 52.1). In the absence of obstruction, fungal infections rarely cause renal insufficiency. Fungal infection should always be considered in the differential diagnosis of filling defects in the collecting system.

URINARY CANDIDIASIS

Epidemiology

Candida frequently exists as saprophytes on the external genitalia or urethra; however, yeast in measurable quantities is found in less than 1% of clean voided urine specimens. *Candida* infections currently account for 5% of urine isolates in the general hospital and 10% of positive urinary cultures in tertiary care centers.[3] Candiduria is especially common in the intensive care unit (ICU) and may represent the most common urinary infection in surgical ICUs.[4] At present, 10% to 15% of nosocomial UTIs are caused by *Candida* species.[5–11] Nosocomial candidiasis is also common in neonatal and pediatric ICUs.[6] Most positive cultures are isolated or transient and represent colonization rather than true infection; however, candiduria may lead to symptomatic UTI and/or fungemia.[12]

Microbiology

Candida albicans tends to be the most common fungal species isolated from the urine and in one large study was found in 446 (52%) of 861 patients with funguria.[4] *Candida glabrata* accounts for 25% to 35% of infections, whereas 8% to 28% of infections are due to *Candida tropicalis*, *Candida krusei*, and *Candida parapsilosis*.[4,7,13] Nevertheless, many recent epidemiologic microbiologic studies have reported a marked increase in infections caused by non–*C. albicans* species, especially *C. glabrata* and *C. tropicalis*.[14] Unusual species are common in hospitalized patients, especially those with diabetes, with chronic indwelling bladder catheters. Mixed infections caused by more than one *Candida* species are not infrequent, as is concomitant bacteriuria.

Pathogenesis

Candida UTIs generally occur in the presence of predisposing factors or in immunocompromised hosts (Fig. 52.2). Most infections are associated with the use of indwelling urinary devices including Foley catheters, internal stents, and percutaneous

Urinary tract involvement by invasive mycoses				
Infection	Prostate	Bladder	Kidney	Penis/Cutaneous
Blastomycosis	+++	±	+	+
Histoplasmosis	++	+	++	++
Coccidioidomycosis	+	+	++	+
Aspergillosis	+	+	+++	+
Cryptococcosis	+++	+	+++	+
Candidiasis	+++	++++	++++	++

Figure 52.1 Urinary tract involvement by invasive mycoses.

Risk factors for candidal urinary tract infections	
Route	Risk Factors
Renal hematogenous candidiasis (anterograde)	Neutropenia (prolonged), intravascular drug use, burns, recent surgery (abdominal, thoracic), systemic infection
Lower urinary ascending tract infection (retrograde) (UTI)	Foley catheter, female gender, extremes of age, instrumentation, diabetes mellitus, obstruction/stasis, recent antibacterial therapy, recent bacterial UTI, ureteral stent, nephrostomy tube, renal transplantation
Pyelonephritis ascending	Diabetes, obstruction/stasis, instrumentation, postoperative, nephrostomy tube, ureteral stent, nephrolithiasis

Figure 52.2 Risk factors for candidal urinary tract infections. UTI, urinary tract infection.

Infectious sources for candiduria

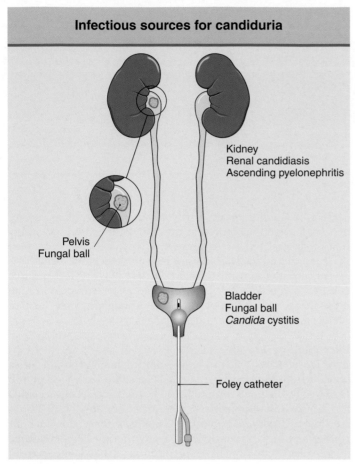

Kidney
Renal candidiasis
Ascending pyelonephritis

Pelvis
Fungal ball

Bladder
Fungal ball
Candida cystitis

Foley catheter

Figure 52.3 Infectious sources for candiduria. Candiduria may originate in the upper or lower urinary tract. Most infections occur by the ascending route, but not infrequently Candiduria may be the result of hematogenous seeding of the kidneys.

nephrostomy tubes (Fig. 52.3). Individuals with diabetes have an increased overall risk of UTI for both bacterial and fungal infection.[2,4] *Candida* growth in urine is enhanced when urinary levels of glucose exceed 150 mg/dl (8.3 mmol/l). Women with diabetes have higher perineal and periurethral *Candida* colonization rates. Patients with diabetes also have impaired phagocytic and fungicidal activity of neutrophils; however, the dominant predisposing factor to candiduria is increased instrumentation, urinary stasis, and obstruction secondary to autonomic neuropathy.

Antibiotic therapy has a major role in predisposing to candiduria.[15] No antibiotic appears exempt from this complication, although there is a higher risk with either prolonged use or with broad-spectrum agents. By suppressing susceptible endogenous bacterial flora in the gastrointestinal and lower genital tracts, antibiotic use results in the emergence of fungi colonizing these epithelial surfaces with ready access to the urinary tract, especially in the presence of indwelling bladder catheters.

Most lower UTIs are caused by genital or perineal colonization with retrograde infection from an indwelling catheter. The upper urinary tract may rarely become involved via ascending infection and then usually only in the presence of urinary obstruction, reflux, or diabetes.[11]

The majority of cases of renal candidiasis occur not as a result of ascending spread from the lower urinary tract but as a consequence of hematogenous seeding of the renal parenchyma. *Candida* species express a tropism for the kidney. An autopsy

study performed by Lehner[16] documented that 90% of the patients dying of disseminated candidiasis had renal involvement, although renal infection (candidiasis) may occur as an isolated site of metastatic spread, especially after transient candidemia. Autopsy studies demonstrated multiple abscesses in the renal interstitium, glomeruli, and peritubular vessels, with not infrequent papillary necrosis and, rarely, complicating emphysematous pyelonephritis.

Clinical Features

Most patients with candiduria are asymptomatic. Patients who have an indwelling bladder catheter most often are colonized rather than infected with a *Candida* species. Hospitalized patients with candiduria with constitutional or systemic symptoms usually have another cause of their symptoms. However, patients with *Candida* cystitis may present with frequency, dysuria, urgency, hematuria, and pyuria. Cystoscopy reveals soft, pearly white, slightly elevated patches that resemble oral thrush, as well as hyperemia and inflammation of the bladder mucosa (Fig 52.4). Most symptomatic patients with *Candida* cystitis are not catheterized and the converse also applies.

Ascending infection, although rare, may result in *Candida* pyelonephritis characterized by fever, leukocytosis, rigors, and costovertebral angle tenderness. Ultrasonography and computed tomography scanning are useful in diagnosing an intrarenal and perinephric abscess. Excretory urography may reveal ureteropelvic fungal balls with or without accompanying papillary necrosis. Ascending infection with *Candida* species uncommonly causes candidemia, with 3% to 10% of episodes of candidemia being secondary to candiduria.[17] When candidemia occurs, it invariably complicates anatomic obstruction, manipulation, or a urologic procedure.

Fungal bezoars may develop anywhere in the urinary drainage system but most commonly are found in the pelvis or upper ureters (Fig. 52.5). Fungal balls are rare, and their presence is suggested by signs of ureteral obstruction associated with candiduria. When bilateral, they may induce obstruction sufficient to cause azotemia. Obstruction may be intermittent or passage of the fungal balls may result in renal colic or the passage of "soft" stones. Excretory urography or retrograde pyelography reveals a filling defect in the collecting system. Fungal balls in the urinary tract have also been described with *Aspergillus* and *Penicillium* species and *Zygomycetes*.

Renal candidiasis secondary to hematogenous spread represents a systemic infection usually accompanied by fever and other constitutional manifestations of sepsis (Fig. 52.6). Positive blood cultures may be obtained; however, often when the

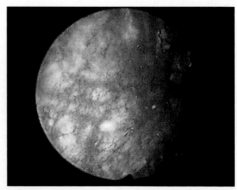

Figure 52.4 Macroscopic appearances of extensive cystitis caused by *Candida krusei* as visualized on cystoscopy. Note the extensive hyperemic, exudative reaction resembling a "snowstorm."

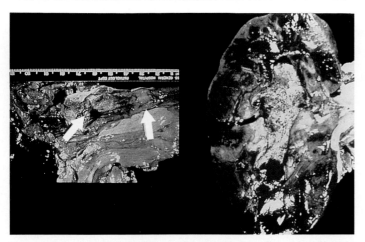

Figure 52.5 Fungal bezoars. Autopsy specimens showing large fungal bezoars in dilated renal pelvices (*arrows*).

diagnosis of renal candidiasis is considered, blood cultures are no longer positive, causing difficulty in diagnosis. Manifestations of disseminated candidiasis may include maculopapular skin rash and endophthalmitis. Most patients with candiduria secondary to renal candidiasis are febrile but lack other clinical manifestations that indicate renal involvement other than variable reduction in renal function. Accordingly, finding candiduria may be the only clue to the diagnosis of invasive and disseminated candidiasis.[18]

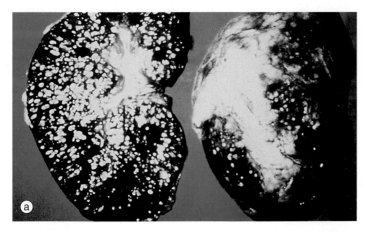

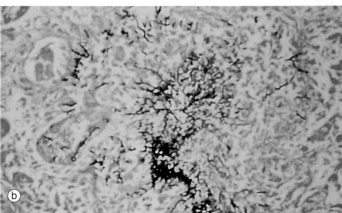

Figure 52.6 Hematogenous renal candidiasis. *a*, Autopsy shows macroscopic seeding of the kidneys. *b*, On microscopic examination, multiple small abscesses caused by *Candida* are evident.

Diagnosis

Isolation of *Candida* species from a urine sample may represent contamination, vulvovestibular or catheter colonization, or a superficial/deep infection of the lower or upper urinary tract. Contamination of the sample is common in women with vulvovaginal colonization. Contamination can usually be excluded by repeating the urine culture with special attention to proper collection techniques. Two consecutive positive isolates of *Candida* are essential before initiating antifungal therapy. Rarely, in hospitalized female patients, a bladder urine sample obtained with a straight catheter is necessary to determine the source.

Differentiating infection from colonization of the urinary tract is difficult, if not impossible, especially in patients with catheters. Clinical features are not specific, and in critically ill patients in ICUs, fever and leukocytosis may have other sources. The presence of pyuria in catheterized patients does not differentiate infection from colonization, as an indwelling catheter may itself lead to pyuria from mechanical irritation of bladder mucosa and because of concomitant bacteriuria. Quantitative urine colony counts are also not of value in the patient with an indwelling catheter. Fungal morphology (such as the presence of hyphae) is only helpful if hyphae or pseudohyphae are found within hyaline or granular casts (Fig. 52.7).

In patients without catheters, there is greater likelihood of true infection in the presence of candiduria, particularly if urinary counts are greater than 10,000 to 15,000 colony-forming units/ml urine. However, renal candidiasis has rarely been reported with a colony count of greater than 10^3 colony-forming units/ml. Therefore, considerable overlap occurs and quantitative cultures are not the final determinant in therapeutic decision making; similarly, negative urine cultures cannot be used to exclude renal candidiasis.

After candiduria is determined to represent infection, the challenge to the clinician is to localize the anatomic level of infection. Localization is critical in the management of candiduria. No useful test to differentiate *Candida* invasion of kidneys from the frequent lower tract *Candida* infection exists, other than the rare detection of *Candida* hyphae or pseudohyphae within

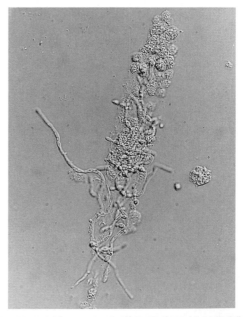

Figure 52.7 Photomicrograph of renal tubular cast containing *Candida* organisms forming hyphae, indicating renal involvement.

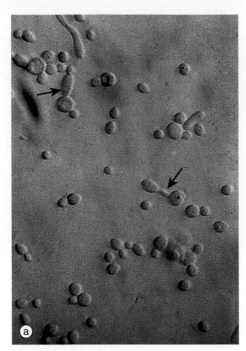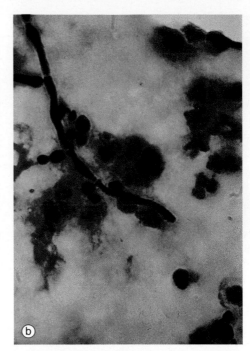

Figure 52.8 Photomicrograph of urine specimens containing *Candida*. *a*, A high-power (×100) examination of urine demonstrates singlets and yeast (blastospores), budding yeast (*arrows*), and pseudohyphae in a patient with *Candida albicans* infection. *b*, A Gram stain of urine obtained from the same patient, showing pseudohyphae.

casts (see Fig. 52.7). Quantitative cultures, fungal morphology on microscopy, and pyuria also have little value in localizing infection (Fig. 52.8). Nonspecific evidence of upper UTI is suggested by declining renal function, constitutional features, and radiographic findings on computed tomography scans and ultrasonography. Serologic tests for *Candida* enolase as a marker for parenchymal invasion remain insensitive. A 5-day bladder irrigation with amphotericin solution (50–100 mg/l 5% dextrose in water) may be effective in establishing the source of candiduria, in that persistent postirrigation candiduria is indicative of fungal infection originating above the bladder. This implies the need for further investigation and raises the suspicion of renal candidiasis. Unfortunately, the lengthy nature of the conventional amphotericin irrigation test excludes its utility in febrile, critically ill patients with candiduria. A 3-hour rapid bladder irrigation test using amphotericin at 200 mg/l has been recommended based on *in vitro* studies but has yet to be shown to be reliable in patients.[19]

Significance of Candiduria

Several epidemiologic studies dealing with the diverse populations of patients with candiduria have concluded that candiduria is associated with a reduced long-term survival rate when compared to matched controls. This is particularly evident in critically ill populations[20] and postrenal transplantation.[21] It is thought that the candiduria reflects the greater severity of illness and the increased use of invasive devices and is therefore a surrogate marker for these comorbidities that directly affect the mortality rate.[22] It is likely that candiduria in asymptomatic, catheterized patients also reflects opportunistic colonization of the urinary tract in severely ill patients whose mortality is predicated on comorbidities, organ failure, and severity of illness rather than on candiduria.[21]

In contrast, in the febrile, critically ill patient, candiduria must be evaluated for possible acute pyelonephritis and as the sole indicator of disseminated or systemic candidiasis. These possibilities are more likely in patients with urinary tract obstruction.

Treatment of Candiduria
Asymptomatic Candiduria

Asymptomatic colonization with *Candida* is the most common syndrome associated with candiduria and requires no therapy. The candiduria is often transient and, even if persistent, uncommonly results in serious morbidity. The risk of invasive complications is small and almost invariably associated with urinary obstruction.[4,17]

In a prospective, multicenter, placebo-controlled study, Sobel and colleagues[23] found that asymptomatic candiduria resolved with urinary catheter elimination in approximately 41% of hospitalized, catheterized patients. After the catheter was changed, untreated candiduria resolved in 20% of patients. Storfer and associates[24] reported a similar rate of resolution of untreated candiduria.

While antifungal therapy, either with systemic amphotericin or fluconazole or with local amphotericin irrigation, can eliminate candiduria in catheterized patients,[5,25,26] there is no evidence that patients benefit from therapy. Furthermore, relapse is frequent. For example, Sobel and coworkers[23] reported that fluconazole treatment resulted in high short-term rates of eradication of *Candida* from the urine, but 2 weeks after therapy was discontinued, the frequency of candiduria was similar in the fluconazole and placebo groups. Interestingly, C. *glabrata* responded equally well to fluconazole as C. *albicans* despite having higher minimal inhibitory concentrations (MICs) to fluconazole. This may be due to the high concentrations (10-fold that of serum) that fluconazole achieves in the urine.

Persistent asymptomatic candiduria in patients without catheters should be investigated for upper tract disease since the likelihood of obstruction or stasis is relatively high. Persistent asymptomatic candiduria in catheterized low birth weight infants or in the afebrile neutropenic patient may also require antifungal therapy and investigation to exclude the possibility of renal or systemic involvement. Candiduria in these patients should be considered a complicated UTI; hence, when treatment is indicated as described in the following, therapy should generally be for at least 14 days (Fig. 52.9).

Treatment recommendations for urinary tract infections with *Candida*		
1. Asymptomatic candiduria	No treatment indicated (especially in catheterized patients) **Exceptions**	
	1. Afebrile neutropenia	Systemic amphotericin 0.6 mg/kg/day or fluconazole 6 mg/kg/day for 14 days (IV/PO)
	2. After renal transplantation	Systemic fluconazole 6 mg/kg/day for 14 days (IV/PO) (controversial)
	3. Prior to elective urologic surgery	Systemic antifungal or amphotericin bladder irrigation (50 mg/l) for 7 days if catheterized
	4. Catheterized low birth weight infant	Systemic antifungal (see text)
2. *Candida* cystitis		**Options**
		1. Systemic fluconazole 6 mg/kg/day for 14 days
		2. Systemic amphotericin
		a. Single dose 0.3 mg/kg
		b. Multidose 0.6 mg/kg/day for 10–14 days
		3. Flucytosine for non–*Candida albicans* (e.g., *Candida glabrata*) 150 mg/kg/day for 14 days
		4. If catheterized, amphotericin irrigation (50 mg/l) for 5–7 days
3. Ascending pyelonephritis		1. Amphotericin 0.6 mg/kg/day for at least 14 days
		2. Fluconazole 6–12 mg/kg/day (based on species)
4. Disseminated/renal candidiasis		Amphotericin 0.6 mg/kg/day for 4–6 weeks (based on species)

Figure 52.9   Treatment recommendations for urinary tract infections with *Candida*.

The management of asymptomatic candiduria in the renal transplant patient is particularly perplexing. Many of the patients are diabetic, are receiving perioperative antibiotics and immunosuppressive agents, and have Foley catheters and intraoperative ureterocystic stent placement. The risk of ascending infection is high given the frequent presence of a stent, glycosuria, short ureter, and frequent reflux. Nevertheless, parenchymal invasion of the graft and candidemia is rare in the absence of obstruction.[17] Safdar and colleagues[21] performed a large nested case-control study involving 1738 renal transplant patients seen over an 8-year period, 192 of whom had 276 episodes of candiduria (11%). *C. glabrata*, recovered from 98 (51%), was the most common *Candida* species. Most case patients were asymptomatic. Risk factors for candiduria were similar to those for hospitalized patients who had not received a transplant and included female sex (odds ratio = 12.5), ICU admission, antibiotic use during the month before candiduria, the presence of an indwelling bladder catheter, diabetes, a neurogenic bladder, and malnutrition. Most importantly, candiduria was associated with reduced survival rate, possibly a proxy for severity of illness (see previous discussion). A variety of treatment regimens were used, including removal of the catheter within 1 week after diagnosis in 119 patients (62%). Overall, candiduria cleared in 148 case patients (77%). Of note, treatment of candiduria was not associated with an improved survival rate.[21] Accordingly, many experts prefer to observe these patients with candiduria until all foreign bodies are removed. When fever and sepsis due to invasive candidiasis supervene, antifungal therapy is justified.

Patients with asymptomatic candiduria in whom urologic instrumentation or surgery is planned should have the candiduria eliminated or suppressed before and during the procedure in order to avoid the risk of invasive candidiasis and candidemia. Successful elimination can be achieved with amphotericin or miconazole bladder irrigation or with systemic therapy using amphotericin, flucytosine, or fluconazole.

Candida Cystitis

Symptomatic cystitis requires treatment with either amphotericin bladder instillation (50 mg/l) or systemic therapy, using intravenous amphotericin, flucytosine, or fluconazole.[5–7,23,25–27] In

contrast to fluconazole, in which 80% of the drug is excreted unchanged in the urine, both ketoconazole and itraconazole are poorly excreted in the urine and should not be used. Similarly, the latest generation of azoles such as voriconazole and posaconazole are not excreted in the urine. The echinocandin class includes several new agents, including caspofungin, micafungin, and anidulafungin, but these agents similarly achieve low concentrations in the urine and should not be used to treat funguria. The advanced generation azoles (voriconazole and posaconazole) and, to a lesser extent, the echinocandin class of drugs also interact with immunosuppressive drugs used in the transplant setting, adding a further complexity to their use in patients with candiduria.

Although lipid formulations of amphotericin are safer and less toxic than conventional amphotericin, reduced renal excretion occurs when using these combinations and therefore they should not be used to treat lower urinary tract infection secondary to *Candida*. In contrast, single-dose intravenous amphotericin 0.3 mg/kg has been shown to be highly efficacious in the treatment of lower urinary tract candidiasis, with therapeutic urine concentrations continuing for a considerable time after administration. This regimen may be preferable for resistant fungal species. Most patients without indwelling catheters are more conveniently managed with oral fluconazole (see Fig. 52.9).

After being used for four decades as the principal and often only modality of treatment of fungemia, amphotericin irrigation has been considered obsolete by several experts.[28] Certainly, its use as a diagnostic modality has largely failed and the 5-day irrigation regimen is time-consuming, labor-intensive, and expensive. Critics suggest that antifungal therapy should be systemic rather than local. Drew[28] concluded that amphotericin irrigation is rarely needed today and therapy for candiduria can be achieved by urinary catheter removal and, if necessary, administration of fluconazole. What is abundantly clear is that all forms of therapy, topical or systemic, are currently expensive and frequently unnecessarily undertaken. The first response to this argument is that most candiduria patients require no treatment at all. Nevertheless, local irrigation with amphotericin remains useful in a subset of patients (often elderly or with renal failure) in which antifungal drug delivery to the urinary tract may be impaired or in which the *Candida* species are resistant to fluconazole (such as C. *glabrata* and C. *krusei*), especially when the Foley catheter cannot be removed.[29]

Ascending Pyelonephritis and *Candida* Urosepsis

Invasive upper tract infections require systemic antifungal therapy and immediate investigation and visualization of the urinary drainage system to exclude urinary obstruction, papillary necrosis, and fungal ball formation.[30] Previously, the most widely accepted therapy was intravenous amphotericin 0.6 mg/kg/day. Duration of therapy depends on the severity of infection, presence of candidemia, and response to therapy and usually requires a total of 1–2 g. Unfortunately the less nephrotoxic lipid formulations of amphotericin do not achieve adequate urinary levels.[31]

As an alternative to amphotericin, systemic therapy with fluconazole 5–10 mg/kg/day (intravenous or oral) is effective and less toxic. Since fluconazole is excreted unchanged into the urine, coexistent severe renal failure may frequently result in subtherapeutic urinary concentrations of fluconazole. Accordingly, systemic doses of fluconazole should not be reduced in renal failure and candiduria associated with urinary tract obstruction.[25]

The echinocandin class, for example, caspofungin 50 mg/day IV, offers a safe, broad-spectrum alternative to amphotericin. Caspofungin is not nephrotoxic and requires no dose adjustments even with advanced renal failure achieving therapeutic renal parenchymal concentrations. However, in the presence of a fungal bezoar or urinary tract obstruction, poor urinary excretion of echinocandins would preclude their use.

Infection refractory to medical management should be treated surgically with drainage or, in cases of a nonviable kidney, nephrectomy. An obstructed kidney with hydronephrosis requires a percutaneous nephrostomy. The management of ureteral fungal balls depends on the extent, site, and severity of infection. In some patients, bezoars spontaneously lyse or become dislodged during placement of ureteral stents.[30] In many patients, upper tract external drainage via a nephrostomy tube must be combined with local amphotericin or fluconazole irrigation. Occasionally, the fungal bezoars must be removed surgically.

Renal and Disseminated Candidiasis

Management of renal candidiasis secondary to hematogenous spread is essentially that of systemic candidiasis. Various treatments include intravenous amphotericin 0.6 mg/kg/day, intravenous fluconazole 400 mg/day, caspofungin 50 mg/day, or intravenous voriconazole 3 mg/kg twice daily.[32] Dose modifications may be necessary in the presence of severe azotemia. Prognosis depends on correction of the underlying factors, such as resolution of neutropenia or removal of infected intravascular catheters. Systemic candidiasis requires prolonged therapy over 4–6 weeks. Lipid formulations of amphotericin, although less nephrotoxic than the standard desoxycholate form, have not been shown to be superior but are less toxic and also regarded as first-line therapy for disseminated candidiasis.

CRYPTOCOCCAL URINARY TRACT INFECTIONS

Both symptomatic and asymptomatic UTI secondary to *Cryptococcus neoformans* infection can occur in AIDS patients as well as in patients with other immunocompromised conditions. In systemic cryptococcosis, cryptococcuria may occur as an early event preceding meningitis.[33] It may coexist with meningitis (30% to 40%) and, in this case, is a poor prognostic factor indicative of widely disseminated disease. It may occur after apparent successful antifungal therapy and may be a source of systemic infection relapse. Finally, isolated cryptococcal UTI can exist in the absence of systemic infection. However, the fact that systemic recurrence, meningitis, and death have occurred after relapse from a urinary source indicates that even in the absence of pulmonary or meningeal cryptococcosis, cryptococcuria is not benign. Hence, patients presenting with cryptococcuria should be evaluated for systemic and meningeal infection and their genitourinary tracts should also be investigated.

Clinical infection of the genitourinary tract may take three forms. Pyelonephritis is usually asymptomatic or may rarely present as a clinical pyelonephritis, particularly in immunosuppressed or diabetic patients. These patients are often found at autopsy to have disseminated infection, cryptococcal prostatitis is the most common presentation (see later discussion), and occult cryptococcal UTI can occur, in which no localizing signs are observed. Most occult involvement occurs without an increase in serum cryptococcal antigen titer. Nevertheless, occult infection with isolated cryptococcuria and no localizing signs may represent disseminated disease, as autopsy studies have shown that disseminated cryptococcal infection is associated with renal foci of infection in 26% to 57% of patients. Treatment of symptomatic or asymptomatic cryptococcuria requires systemic antifungal agents, including intravenous amphotericin 0.7 mg/kg/day or fluconazole 5 to 10 mg/kg/day. Duration of antifungal therapy is controversial and depends on whether associated immunosuppression or immunodeficiency exists. In the absence of defective cell-mediated immunity, all therapy should continue for 6 weeks. In the presence of impaired cell-mediated immunity, lifetime therapy may be indicated. The serum cryptococcal antigen should be used as a guide to therapy.

FUNGAL PROSTATITIS

Fungal prostatitis may result from local inoculation (*Candida* and *Trichosporon* species) by contaminated or infected urine, or from hematogenous spread (blastomycosis, histoplasmosis, coccidioidomycosis, aspergillosis, cryptococcosis, candidiasis, and zygomycosis). Frequently, prostatic involvement by fungi is chronic and asymptomatic and is discovered at the time of prostatectomy or autopsy.[1,33,34]

Candida species are the most common fungi that infect the urinary tract and hence the most common cause of prostatitis, followed by blastomycosis and cryptococcosis. Risk factors for candidal prostatitis are similar to those for UTI and include diabetes mellitus, antibiotic administration, indwelling catheters, and anatomic abnormalities. Considering the high prevalence of candiduria, especially in catheterized patients, *Candida* abscesses of the prostate gland are rare.

Acute prostatitis caused by *Candida* species presents with fever, constitutional findings, perineal pain, discomfort, urinary bladder irritative symptoms, and, possibly, urinary obstruction. The last is more likely in the presence of a *Candida* prostatic abscess. In most patients, urine cultures for *Candida* are positive, although rare instances of sterile urine have been reported. The presence of an abscess is confirmed by transrectal ultrasonography or computed tomography. In addition to systemic antifungal therapy, focal suppuration requires drainage, either by the percutaneous route or, occasionally, by performing a transurethral prostatectomy.

Most prostatic fungal infections other than those due to *Candida* result from hematogenous dissemination, especially *Blastomyces dermatitidis*. Clinical features are identical for all the invasive mycoses. The diagnosis of chronic fungal prostatitis is usually considered when symptomatic patients have laboratory signs of urinary inflammation (pyuria) but negative bacterial cultures. A negative fungal culture of urine or prostatic secretions should not, however, exclude the diagnosis of chronic fungal prostatitis, given the pathology of granulomatous fungal prostatitis.

Cryptococcal infection of the prostate occurs secondary to hematogenous seeding in immunocompromised patients (especially patients with AIDS) and may accompany pulmonary infection or meningitis. Most cases of prostatic infection are asymptomatic and are only diagnosed at autopsy. Patients with AIDS are more likely to develop a prostatic abscess, which may be symptomatic and present with dysuria, frequency, nausea, and fever. Physical examination may only reveal variable prostatic enlargement. Although the mainstay of treatment remains intravenous amphotericin, often in combination with flucytosine, fluconazole by virtue of its oral convenience, relative lack of toxicity, penetration, and efficacy in UTI has become the long-term treatment of choice. Nevertheless, treatment failures with fluconazole have been reported. Importantly, prostatic infection is an important site of relapse of cryptococcosis after seemingly successful treatment in patients with AIDS.[34,35]

REFERENCES

1. Wise GJ, Silver DA: Fungal infections of the genitourinary system. J Urol 1993;149:1377–1388.
2. Platt R, Polk BT, Murdock B, et al: Risk factors for nosocomial urinary tract infection. Am J Epidemiol 1986;124:977.
3. Rivett AG, Perry JA, Cohen J: Urinary candidiasis: A prospective study in hospitalized patients. Urol Res 1986;14:183–186.
4. Kauffman CA, Vazquez JA, Sobel JD, et al: Prospective multicenter surveillance study of funguria in hospitalized patients. Clin Infect Dis 2000;30:14–18.
5. Jacobs LG, Skidmore EA, Freeman K, et al: Oral fluconazole compared with amphotericin B bladder irrigation for fungal urinary tract infections in the elderly. Clin Infect Dis 1996;22:30–35.
6. Phillips JR, Karlowicz MG: Prevalence of *Candida* species in hospital-acquired urinary tract infections in a neonatal intensive care unit. Pediatr Infect Dis J 1997;16:190–194.
7. Febre N, Silva V, Medeiros EA, et al: Microbiological characteristics of yeasts isolated from urinary tracts of intensive care unit patients undergoing urinary catheterization. J Clin Microbiol 1999;37:1584–1586.
8. Kobayashi CC, de Fernandes OF, Miranda KC, et al: Candiduria in hospital patients: A study prospective. Mycopathologia 2004;158:49–52.
9. Shay AC, Miller LG: An estimate of the incidence of candiduria among hospitalized patients in the United States. Infect Control Hosp Epidemiol 2004;25:894–895.
10. Carvalho M, Guimaraes CM, Mayer JR Jr, et al: Hospital-associated funguria: Analysis of risk factors, clinical presentation and outcome. Braz J Infect Dis 2001;5:313–318.
11. Occhipinti DJ, Gubbins PO, Schreckenberger P, Danziger LH: Frequency, pathogenicity and microbiologic outcome of non-*Candida albicans* candiduria. Eur J Clin Microbiol Infect Dis 1994;13:459–467.
12. Kauffman CA: Candiduria. Clin Infect Dis 2005;41(Suppl 6):S371–S376.
13. Kozinn PJ, Taschdjian CL, Goldberg PK, et al: Advances in the diagnosis of renal candidiasis. J Urol 1978;119:184–187.
14. de Oliveira RD, Maffei CM, Martinez R: Nosocomial urinary tract infections by *Candida* species. Rev Assoc Med Bras 2001;47:231–235.
15. Harris AD, Castro J, Sheppard DC, et al: Risk factors for nosocomial candiduria due to *Candida glabrata* and *Candida albicans*. Clin Infect Dis 1999;29:926–928.
16. Lehner T: Systemic candidiasis and renal involvement. Lancet 1964;1:1414–1416.
17. Ang BSP, Telenti A, King B, et al: Candidemia from a urinary tract source: Microbiological aspects and clinical significance. Clin Infect Dis 1993;17:622–626.
18. Nassoura Z, Ivatury RR, Simon RJ, et al: Candiduria as an early marker of disseminated infection in critically ill surgical patients: The role of fluconazole therapy. J Trauma 1995;35:290–295.
19. Fong LW, Cheng PC, Hinton NA: Fungicidal effects of amphotericin B in urine: In vitro study to assess feasibility of bladder washout for localization of site of candiduria. Antimicrob Agents Chemother 1991;35:1856–1859.
20. Alvarez-Lerma F, Nolla-Salas J, Leon C, et al. and the EPCAN Study Group: Candiduria in critically ill patients admitted to intensive care medical units. Intensive Care Med 2003;29:1069–1076.
21. Safdar N, Slattery WR, Knasinski V, et al: Predictors and outcomes of candiduria in renal transplant recipients. Clin Infect Dis 2005;40:1413–1421.
22. Abbott KC, Hypolite I, Poropatich RK, et al: Hospitalizations for fungal infections after renal transplantation in the United States. Transpl Infect Dis 2001;3:203–211.
23. Sobel JD, Kauffman CA, McKinsey D, et al: Candiduria—a randomized double-blind study of treatment with fluconazole and placebo. Clin Infect Dis 2000;30:19–24.
24. Storfer SP, Medoff G, Fraser VJ, et al: Candiduria: Retrospective review in hospitalized patients. Infect Dis Clin Pract 1994;3:23–29.
25. Fan-Havard P, O'Donovan C, Smith SM, et al: Oral fluconazole versus amphotericin B bladder irrigation for treatment of candidal funguria. Clin Infect Dis 1995;21:960–965.
26. Leu HS, Huancy CT: Clearance of funguria with short course antifungal regimens: A prospective randomized controlled study. Clin Infect Dis 1995;20:1152–1157.
27. Wong-Beringer A, Jacobs RA, Guglielma BJ: Treatment of funguria: A critical review. JAMA 1992;267:2780–2785.
28. Drew RH, Arthur RR, Perfect JR: Is it time to abandon the use of amphotericin B bladder irrigation? Clin Infect Dis 2005;40:1465–1470.
29. Wise GJ: Do not abandon amphotericin B as an antifungal bladder irrigant. Clin Infect Dis 2005;41:1073–1074.
30. Irby PB, Stoller MI, McAninch JW: Fungal bezoars of the upper urinary tract. J Urol 1990;143:447–451.
31. Agustin J, Lacson S, Raffalli J, et al: Failure of a lipid amphotericin B preparation to eradicate candiduria: Preliminary findings based on three cases. Clin Infect Dis 1999;29:686–687.
32. Pappas PG, Rex JH, Sobel JD, et al., Infectious Diseases Society of America: Guidelines for treatment of candidiasis. Clin Infect Dis 2004;38:161–189.
33. Byrne R, Hammil RJ, Rodriguez-Barradas MC: Cryptococcuria: Case reports and literature review. Infect Dis Clin Pract 1997;6:573–576.
34. Bailly MP, Boibieux A, Biron F, et al: Persistence of *Cryptococcus neoformans* in the prostate: Failure of fluconazole despite high doses. J Infect Dis 1991;164:435–438.
35. Larsen RA, Bozzette S, McCutchan JA, et al: Persistent *Cryptococcus neoformans* infection of the prostate after successful treatment of meningitis: California Collaborative Treatment Group. Ann Intern Med 1989;111:125–128.

The Kidney in Schistosomiasis

Rashad S. Barsoum

INTRODUCTION

Schistosomiasis is a parasitic disease usually acquired by teenagers, often leading to complications that may extend into the fourth or fifth decades of life. It was known to the Ancient Egyptians as "the bloody urine disease"[1] and is also known as *bilharziasis* in honor of its discoverer, Theodore Bilharz, the German physician who practiced in Egypt in the 1850s.

The life cycle of the parasite is shown in Figure 53.1. Infection is acquired through contact with contaminated waters in the ponds and slow-flowing canals originating from certain rivers such as the Nile. Cercariae enter through the skin or mucous membranes and migrate through the lymphatics and blood circulation into the portal or perivesical venous system, where they mature into sexually differentiated adult worms and live in almost continuous copulation. Females leave the males only to lay eggs, traveling against the blood flow aiming at the rectal or bladder mucosa. The ova are driven out by visceral contraction during defecation or urination in the respective excreta. Contact with fresh water within a

couple of days allows the eggs to hatch, releasing *miracidia*, which infect specific snails. In this "intermediate" host, they mature asexually into *cercariae*, which are eventually released, searching for their "definitive" host, usually humans and occasionally apes and cattle. The snail demography defines the endemicity and intensity of schistosomiasis in different geographic regions. Because this is largely influenced by climatic factors such as temperature and humidity, it is possible to accurately monitor the global epidemiology of schistosomiasis by satellite remote sensing.[2]

About 200 million inhabitants of 76 countries on five continents are infected, and an additional 400 million are at risk. Of the infected subjects, 60% are symptomatic, 10% have serious sequelae, and 1% die of the disease each year, mainly in China, the Philippines, Egypt, Brazil, northern Senegal, and Uganda.

Only three species are responsible for almost all the morbidity from the disease: *Schistosoma haematobium*, throughout Africa and adjacent regions; *Schistosoma mansoni*, in Africa, South America, and the Caribbean islands; and *Schistosoma japonicum*, in the Far East (Fig. 53.2). *S. haematobium* affects the urinary

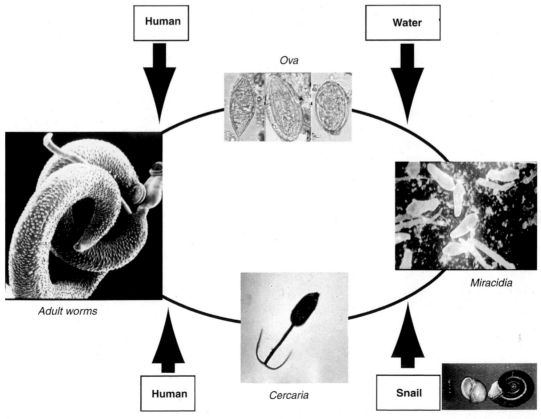

Figure 53.1   Life cycle of schistosomes.

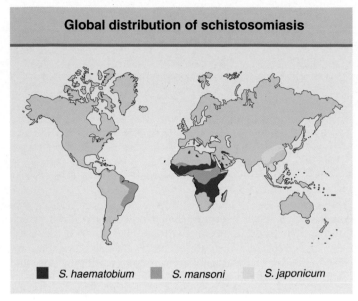

Figure 53.2 World map showing the geographic distribution of the main pathogenic schistosomes.

tract, whereas *S. mansoni* and *S. japonicum* affect the colon and rectum, ultimately reaching the liver and inducing periportal fibrosis. Sporadically, all three species cause "metastatic lesions" when ova are driven by the bloodstream to the lungs, brain, spinal cord, heart muscle, eyes, and other sites.[3]

Morbidity from infection is variable and depends on the virulence of the infective strains, host resistance, environmental factors, and standards of primary medical care. For example, chronic lower urinary tract pathology among infected subjects is reported to vary from 2% in Nigeria in the West of Africa to 52% in Tanzania in the East.[4]

PATHOGENESIS

Schistosomes causes morbidity through two major mechanisms (Fig. 53.3): (1) local reactions around the ova deposited in different tissues, and (2) systemic effects attributed to the host's response to circulating antigens released from the worms or the ova.[4,5]

The local reaction is a cell-mediated immune response to soluble egg antigens (SEAs) diffusing out of trapped ova through micropores in the eggshell. The initial response is innate, being driven by tissue macrophages, and involves natural killer (NK) cells, neutrophils, and complement. This is followed by a specific immune response orchestrated by the helper CD4+ T lymphocytes.

The schistosomal granuloma (Fig.53.4) is composed of mononuclear cells, eosinophils, neutrophils, basophils, and fibroblasts, which are recruited and activated by a variety of T helper (Th) lymphokines as well as specific chemoattractants of parasitic origin. These cells are involved in the elimination of the parasite by direct phagocytosis (monocytes), lymphocytotoxicity (T lymphocytes), antibody-dependent cytotoxicity (eosinophils), and antibody- and complement-dependent cytotoxicity (neutrophils). Later, the granuloma tends to be modulated through gradual switching from Th1 to Th2 activation, largely mediated by a critical change in the monokine profile that favors the release of interleukin-4 (IL-4), which is associated with a phenotypic change of the committed tissue macrophages. At this stage, the intensity of the inflammatory reaction is reduced, and progressive fibrosis is induced largely through the release of IL-4, IL-5, IL-10, somatostatin, and transforming growth factor-β (TGF-β). Finally, fibrotic granulomas in the bladder, lower ureters, and seminal vessels tend to become calcified.[6]

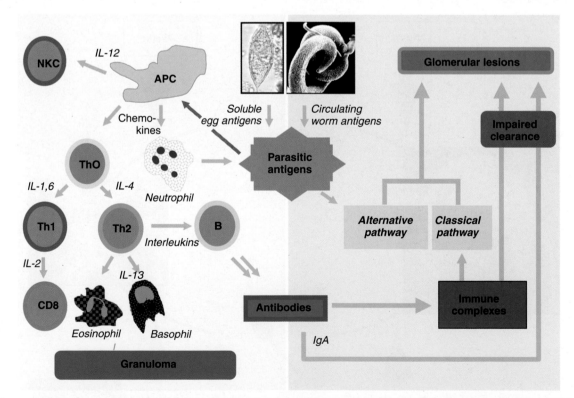

Figure 53.3 Immune response to schistosomal infection. The local immune response to deposited ova leading to granuloma formation is shown on the *left*; all cells shown in the diagram, in conjunction with antibodies or complement, participate in eventual parasite elimination (see text). The systemic immune response is shown on the *right*; note the important role of impaired clearance of schistosomal antigens and immunoglobulin A (IgA) in the development of glomerular lesions. APC, antigen-presenting cell; IL, interleukin; NKC, natural killer cell.

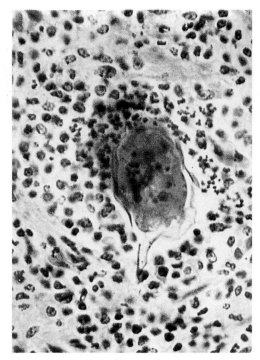

Figure 53.4 *Schistosoma haematobium* **granuloma.** Note the egg's terminal spike, which identifies *S. haematobium*, and the distortion of shell from proteases and oxidants released by the local neutrophil infiltration. (Hematoxylin and eosin, ×500.)

The systemic immune response is primarily a humoral reaction to *circulating* schistosomal antigens. The latter originate mainly from the worm's digestive enzymes (gut antigens), with a minor contribution from the tegument and ova. The gut antigens consist of a positively charged glycoprotein and a negatively charged proteoglycan (circulating cathodal antigens [CCAs] and circulating anodal antigens [CAAs]), respectively). These antigens are present in most of the schistosomal immune complex–mediated lesions, particularly in glomeruli.[7] The antibody response is biphasic, reflecting the successive Th1 and Th2 stages of lymphocyte activation. In the former, B cells tend to synthesize immunoglobulin M (IgM), IgG1, and IgG3 under the influence of IL-2. During the Th2 phase, IgG2, IgG4, and IgA predominate. The latter have a limited ability to fix complement and may even block its deposition, hence their importance in modulating the granulomas.[4,6]

CLINICAL MANIFESTATIONS

The renal tract lesions in schistosomiasis mirror the two major pathogenetic mechanisms. On one hand, there are local lesions, mostly affecting the lower urinary tract, caused by the local granulomatous response to *S. haematobium* ova.[8] On the other hand are those lesions caused by immune complex deposition in the glomeruli, usually associated with *S. mansoni* infections of the intestine and less commonly with *S. haematobium* infections.[9]

Lower Urinary Schistosomiasis
The lower urinary tract is the site of *S. haematobium* infection. Clinical disease starts by the coalescence of multiple granulomas that form small "pseudotubercles" in the bladder mucosa (Fig. 53.5). These may consolidate to form sessile, occasionally

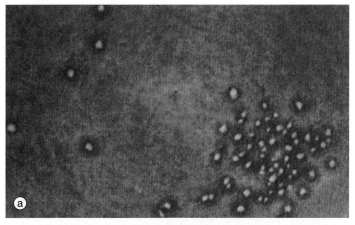

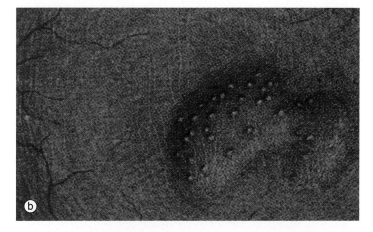

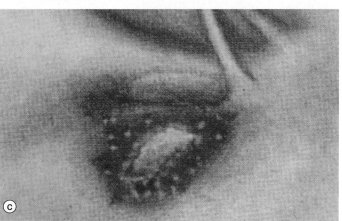

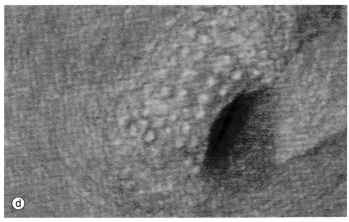

Figure 53.5 Cystoscopic appearances in urinary schistosomiasis. *a,* Pseudotubercles. *b,* Sessile mass covered by pseudotubercles. *c,* Ulcer surrounded by pseudotubercles. *d,* Sandy patches. (Courtesy of Professor Naguib Makar.)

Most patients are 20- to 40 year-old men, with evidence of hepatosplenic schistosomiasis. Renal involvement is asymptomatic in up to 40% of those, being identified by accidental or surveillance urinalysis, which may display microalbuminuria, various grades of proteinuria, or abnormal sediment. Some 15% of those with hepatosplenic schistosomiasis have overt disease, presenting with proteinuria and microhematuria, with or without the nephrotic syndrome, hypertension, and impaired renal function. Liver function tests are often normal. A polyclonal gammopathy is seen in most cases, whereas a monoclonal IgM response is seen in those with associated hepatitis C virus (HCV) and cryoglobulinemia. Rheumatoid factor activity and anti-DNA antibodies are detected in 5% to 10% of cases, particularly when associated with salmonella infection (see later discussion), but they do not correlate with clinical severity. Rheumatoid seropositivity is detected in much higher titers when HCV infection is associated.[13]

There are six histologic classes of schistosomal GN (Figs. 53.10 and 53.11).[4,6,9,13] Classes I (mesangial proliferative), III (membranoproliferative), and IV (focal segmental glomerulosclerosis) result from the deposition of immune complexes representing different stages in the evolution of "pure schistosomal" hepatosplenic disease. The main deposits in class I are schistosomal antigens, IgM and C3; and in classes III and IV, IgG and IgA, usually without schistosomal antigens. The IgA deposits parallel the severity of proteinuria and mesangial proliferation. Impaired hepatic clearance and increased mucosal synthesis of IgA have been documented in those patients.[14] Whereas class I lesions are seen in most asymptomatic cases, classes III and IV are usually symptomatic and progressive, even with eradication of the parasitic infection.

Class II (diffuse proliferative and exudative) is associated with coinfection with salmonella strains, usually *Salmonella paratyphi* A in Africa and *Salmonella typhimurium* in Brazil, which are attached to specific receptors in the tissues of adult schistosomes. C3 and salmonella antigens were detected in the glomerular capillary walls and the mesangium. In these patients, the clinical presentation is typical of acute postinfectious glomerulonephritis, associated with manifestations of salmonella-related toxemia (fever, exanthema, and severe anemia).

Amyloid A protein deposits are detected by special stains or electron microscopy in up to 15% of biopsy samples from patients with classes III and IV, whereas amyloidosis may be the predominant lesion (class V) in less than 5% of patients with clinically overt schistosomal glomerulopathy. It occurs with heavy, often mixed, infection regardless of the anatomic site. Minimal amyloid deposits do not seem to alter the clinical presentation or prognosis, but typical class V cases are grossly nephrotic and relentlessly progressive.

A class VI lesion was recently described in patients with hepatosplenic schistosomiasis and hepatitis C viral infection.[13] This association is common, particularly in Egypt, where it is believed that the virus was acquired many decades earlier, along with contemporary intravenous injections used for mass treatment of schistosomiasis. Some evidence also suggests that the virus may be transmitted with the infected cercariae. Regardless of the mode of infection, those patients appear to have created a critical pool in

Class	Histology	Immunofluorescence	Etiologic Agent	Prevalence	Clinical Findings	Treatment of Renal Disease
	Classification of schistosomal glomerulonephritis					
I	Mesangioproliferative (GN)	IgM, C3 Schistosomal gut antigens	*S. haematobium* *S. mansoni* *S. japonicum*	27%–60% of asymptomatic patients, 10%–40% of patients with renal disease	Microhematuria Proteinuria	No
II	Diffuse proliferative exudative (GN)	C3, *Salmonella* antigens	*S. haemotabium* *S. mansoni* + *Salmonella* species	*Salmonella* infections Reduced serum C3	Acute nephritic syndrome, toxemia	Treatment of *Salmonella* infection
III	Membranoproliferative (GN)	IgG, IgA, C3, schistosomal antigens	*S. mansoni* (*S. haematobium*?)	7%–20% of asymptomatic patients and in 80% of patients with overt renal disease	Hepatosplenomegaly, nephrotic syndrome, hypertension, renal failure	No
IV	Focal segmental glomerulosclerosis	IgM, IgG (occasionally IgA)	*S. mansoni*	11%–38%	Hepatosplenomegaly, nephrotic syndrome, hypertension, renal failure	No
V	Amyloid	AA protein	*S. mansoni* *S. haematobium*	16%–39%	Hepatosplenomegaly, nephrotic syndrome, hypertension, renal failure	No
VI	Cryoglobulinemic (GN)	IgM, C3	*S. mansoni* + hepatitis C virus	Unknown	Hepatosplenomegaly, nephrotic syndrome, purpura, vasculitis, arthritis, hypertension, renal failure	? Interferon + ribavirin, corticosteroids, immunosuppression, plasmapheresis

Figure 53.10 Classification of schistosomal glomerulonephritis.

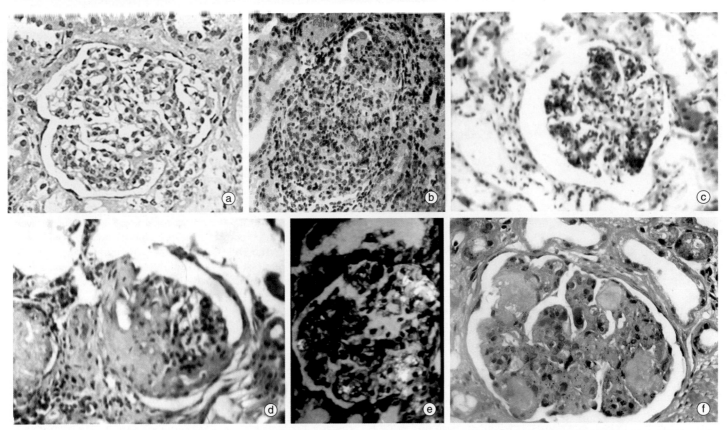

Figure 53.11   Schistosomal glomerulopathy. *a,* Mesangial proliferative glomerulonephritis, hematoxylin and eosin (H&E) stain (class I). *b, Schistosoma-* and *Salmonella-* associated exudative glomerulonephritis, H&E stain (class II). *c,* Membranoproliferative (mesangiocapillary) glomerulonephritis type I, H&E stain (class III). *d,* Focal and segmental glomerulosclerosis, Masson trichrome stain (class IV). *e,* Green birefringence under polarized light in a glomerulus with mesangial proliferation in a patient with mixed *S. haematobium* and *S. mansoni* infection, Congo Red stain (class V). *f,* Amyloid deposits and cryoglobulin capillary thrombi (red stain) in a glomerulus displaying focal mesangial proliferation in a patient with schistosomal hepatic fibrosis and associated hepatitis C virus infection (class VI).

the community that became a reservoir for the spread of infection by other means. The lesion consists of a mixture of mesangial proliferation, amyloid deposition, fibrinoid necrosis, and cryoglobulinemic thrombi in the glomerular capillaries with tubular casts. Patients present with chronic hepatitis, cirrhosis, nephrotic syndrome, cryoglobulinemic skin vasculitis, polyarthritis, and rapidly progressive renal failure associated with severe protein-calorie malnutrition.

DIAGNOSIS

Schistosoma haematobium Urinary Tract Disease

The bedside diagnosis of lower urinary schistosomiasis is easily made, particularly if patients present with the typical pattern of painful terminal hematuria following exposure to fresh river waters in an endemic area. Diagnosis is more difficult when the history of exposure is less convincing (e.g., swimming pools), or when the clinical presentation is atypical (such as bacterial pyelonephritis, typhoid, or amyloidosis).

The diagnosis is made by finding ova in a fresh urine sample, which is easy owing to their abundance, large size, and typical appearance. Live ova, containing mobile miracidia, indicate active infection, whereas dead, calcified ova may continue to be shed from fibrotic lesions for many months or even years.

Serologic diagnosis is based on finding circulating schistosomal antigens or antibodies by gel diffusion, precipitation, complement fixation, chromatography, immunoelectrophoresis, indirect hemagglutination, microfluorometry, radioimmunoassay, or various forms of enzyme-linked immunosorbent assay (ELISA) techniques. The circumoval precipitin is most frequently used in clinical laboratories. These techniques are useful in confirming the diagnosis in the absence of ova, which occurs with old infections when the worms are sterile but continue to release their antigens. Serologic tests are also useful in assessing the response to treatment because titers usually become negative within 3 to 6 months of complete eradication of infection.

The radiologic appearances of bladder and seminal vesicle calcification are so typical that no further confirmatory tests are needed. Cystoscopic findings are equally pathognomonic although seldom required. Early pseudotubercles are easily distinguished from mycobacterial infection by their size and the surrounding mucosal pathology. The presence of sandy patches with associated masses, polyps, and even neoplasms makes the diagnosis. Tissue biopsy confirms the parasitic nature of the lesions. Different imaging techniques (e.g., ultrasonography, intravenous urography [IVU], ascending cystograms) are useful in the diagnosis of upstream complications (see Chapter 55).

The main differential diagnosis for urinary schistosomiasis is tuberculosis, which also causes hematuria, strictures, back pressure, and chronic renal failure that can be resolved with appropriate parasitologic and bacteriologic techniques (see Chapter 51).

Schistosoma mansoni Glomerular Disease

Overt glomerular disease in patients with hepatosplenic schistosomiasis is suspected in those who develop new hypertension, nephrotic or nephritic syndrome, or renal insufficiency. Occult

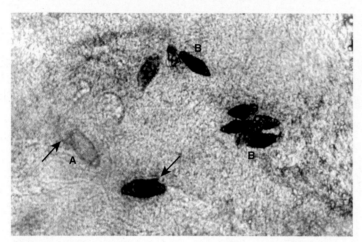

Figure 53.12   Stool smears showing living (A) and dead (B) *Schistosoma mansoni* ova. Species are identified by the lateral spike (*arrows*).

glomerular disease is detected by the presence of abnormal urinary sediment or renal function. Although renal biopsy is essential for the diagnosis and classification, none of the lesions is pathognomonic unless schistosomal antigens are detected by immunofluorescence, which is unusual in clinically overt cases. Identifying *S. mansoni* eggs in the stools (Fig. 53.12) or submucosal rectal snips supports the diagnosis. Concomitant salmonella or HCV infection can be detected by appropriate microbiologic tests. The various serologic abnormalities described are of limited diagnostic value, except the high rheumatoid factor, monoclonal IgM expansion, and low C4 that are typical of class VI.

Other glomerular disorders associated with hepatic fibrosis, such as secondary IgA nephropathy and hepatic glomerulosclerosis, may be considered in the differential diagnosis. However, in both these conditions, the renal lesions are relatively mild, presenting mainly with microhematuria but rarely with significant proteinuria or impaired renal function. The glomerular deposits are mostly mesangial, in contrast to those seen in schistosomiasis, in which subendothelial and intramembranous deposits may also be present.

TREATMENT

Schistosoma haematobium Urinary Tract Disease

S. haematobium is susceptible to antimony compounds, organophosphates (Metrifonate), and niridazole, but the current drug of choice is praziquantel, being the most effective and least toxic. It is administered as a single oral dose of 40 mg/kg body weight. Antiparasitic treatment cures the early bladder pathology, yet it has no effect on sandy patches or other fibrotic lesions. Interestingly, ureteral distention with radiologic evidence of hydronephrosis may be reversed a few weeks after successful treatment.

Antibacterial therapy usually controls acute episodes of cystitis and pyelonephritis. However, it must be combined with simultaneous eradication of parasitic infection if the latter is still active, especially if the urinary bacterial infection is due to typhoid (*Salmonella typhi*).

Chronic fibrotic lesions are difficult to treat. Surgery or the placement of stents may be necessary for the relief of an obstructive lesion. However, particular caution is required while dealing with the ureterovesical junction to avoid induction of reflux. Several plastic procedures are available to restore the distorted ureteral, bladder, or urethral anatomy. Associated bacterial infections may require long-term low-dose antibiotics.

Regular dialysis in such patients can be difficult, owing to the negative effects of chronic infection; associated schistosomal lesions in the liver, lungs, and other organs; and the comorbid impact of undernutrition, viral infection, or malignancy. The same factors reflect on the outcome of renal transplantation, with the additional risk for urinary leakage, which is many folds higher than usual, owing to the presence of fibrotic granulomas and anatomic distortion in the bladder wall. Reinfection with *S. haematobium* has also been described in patients living in an endemic area.[15]

Schistosoma mansoni Glomerular Disease

S. mansoni is more resistant to treatment but does respond to single-dose treatment with either praziquantel (40–50 mg/kg body weight) or oxamniquine (15 mg/kg body weight in South America or 30 mg/kg body weight in Africa). However, eradication of the parasite can be curative only in classes I and II. In the latter, it must be combined with antibiotics for the control of salmonella infection (usually ampicillin and cotrimoxazole) Antischistosomal therapy (praziquantel or oxamniquine) and immunosuppressive therapy are ineffective in all other classes.[9]

Dialysis may be difficult in those who reach end-stage renal disease because of the frequent presence of esophageal or gastric varices that carry the risk for bleeding with anticoagulation for hemodialysis. Endoscopy is essential before starting regular hemodialysis, with prophylactic sclerotherapy if necessary. Although peritoneal dialysis is a viable option in some cases, it is impossible in those with significant ascites, owing to the risk for excessive protein loss in the effluent.

The overall results of renal transplantation are not different from those with other renal disorders. Uncomplicated residual hepatic fibrosis in the recipient does not seem to significantly modify the pharmacokinetics of the immunosuppressive agents used in transplant recipients. However, variations in cyclosporine blood levels have been noticed by certain groups[15] and attributed to altered absorption of the drug. Associated viral hepatitis may have a considerable impact on the protocols of donor selection and prophylactic immunosuppression, and on the eventual outcome (see Chapters 91–94).

Recurrence of schistosomal GN has been described in a few patients,[16] suggesting the persistent release of antigens from living worms. Prophylactic antischistosomal chemotherapy (i.e., praziquantel) is therefore recommended before renal transplantation for recipients known to have been previously infected with the parasite.

REFERENCES

1. Ghalioungui P: Magic and Medical Science in Ancient Egypt. London, Hodder and Stoughton, 1963.
2. Yang GJ, Vounatsou P, Zhou XN, et al: A review of geographic information system and remote sensing with applications to the epidemiology and control of schistosomiasis in China. Acta Trop 2005;96:17–29.
3. Abdel-Wahab MF: Schistosomiasis in Egypt. Boca Raton, Fla, CRC Press, 1982.
4. Barsoum RS: Schistosomiasis. In Davison AM, Cameron JS, Grunfeld JP, et al (eds): Oxford Textbook of Clinical Nephrology, 3rd ed. Oxford, UK, Oxford University Press, 2005, pp 1173–1184.
5. Wahl SM, Frazier-Jessen M, Jin WW, et al: Cytokine regulation of schistosome-induced granuloma and fibrosis. Kidney Int 1997;51:1370–1375.
6. Barsoum RS: Schistosomiasis and the kidney. Semin Nephrol 2003; 23:4–41.

7. de Water R, Van Marck EA, Fransen JA, Deelder AM: *Schistosoma mansoni*: Ultrastructural localization of the circulating anodic antigen and the circulating cathodic antigen in the mouse kidney glomerulus. Am J Trop Med Hyg 1988;38:118–124.

8. Badr MM: Surgical management of urinary bilharziasis. In Dudley H, Pories WJ, Carter DC, McDougal WS (eds): Rob Smith's Operative Surgery. London, Butterworth, 1986.

9. Barsoum RS: Schistosomal glomerulopathies. Kidney Int 1993;44:1–12.

10. Mostafa MH, Sheweita SA, O'Connor PJ: Relationship between schistosomiasis and bladder cancer. Clin Microbiol Rev 1999;12:97–111.

11. Houba V: Experimental renal disease due to schistosomiasis. Kidney Int 1979;16:30–43.

12. Ezzat E, Osman R, Ahmed KY, Soothill JF: The association between *Schistosoma haematobium* infection and heavy proteinuria. Trans R Soc Trop Med Hyg 1974;68:315–317.

13. Barsoum R: The changing face of schistosomal glomerulopathy. Kidney Int 2004;66:2472–2484.

14. Barsoum R, Nabil M, Saady G, et al: Immunoglobulin A and the pathogenesis of schistosomal glomerulopathy. Kidney Int 1996;50:920–928.

15. Mahmoud KM, Sobh MA, El-Agroudy AE, et al: Impact of schistosomiasis on patient and graft outcome after renal transplantation: 10 years' follow-up. Nephrol Dial Transplant 2001;16:2214–2221.

16. Azevedo LS, de Paula FJ, Ianhez LE, et al: Renal transplantation and schistosomiasis *mansoni*. Transplantation 1987;44:795–798.

CHAPTER

54 Nephrolithiasis and Nephrocalcinosis

Rebeca D. Monk and David A. Bushinsky

INTRODUCTION

Nephrolithiasis refers to stone formation within the renal tubules or collecting system, although calculi are often found within the ureters or in the bladder. The principal types of renal calculi are calcium oxalate, calcium phosphate, struvite, urate, and cystine. Kidney stones vary in clinical presentation from asymptomatic small stones to large, obstructing staghorn calculi that can severely impair renal function and lead to chronic kidney disease. The severity of stone disease depends on the pathogenetic factors contributing to the rate of stone formation, in addition to the stone type, size, and location. In its most classic form, nephrolithiasis presents as renal colic, but it may also commonly present with hematuria or urinary tract infection. Certain disorders can lead to small diffuse renal parenchymal calcifications termed *nephrocalcinosis*. The calcifications, usually calcium phosphate or calcium oxalate, may deposit in the renal cortex or medulla, depending on etiology. Among the most common causes of nephrocalcinosis are primary hyperoxaluria and medullary sponge kidney.

NEPHROLITHIASIS

A discussion of the general aspects of nephrolithiasis is followed by specific features of the pathogenesis and management of the common types of renal stones.

Epidemiology

Kidney stones are common in industrialized nations, with an annual incidence of more than 1 per 1000 persons and a lifetime risk for forming stones of 5% to 13%.[1-5] In the United States, the prevalence of nephrolithiasis has increased from 3.2% in the late 1970s to 5.2% in the 1990s.[6] Incidence peaks in the third and fourth decades, and prevalence increases with age until about 70 years in men and 60 years in women.[4,7] Factors that determine renal stone prevalence include age, sex, race, and geographic distribution. In the United States, Caucasians are much more likely to develop renal stones than African Americans, Hispanics, or Asian Americans. Men are more prone to stone formation than women, at a ratio of 2:1 to 4:1. In the United States, the tendency for the development of stones also depends on geographic location, with an increasing prevalence from North to South and, to a lesser degree, from West to East. Some have postulated that the increase in nephrolithiasis rates in the American Southeast may be linked to the greater sunlight exposure in this area, leading to an increase in insensible losses through sweating, resulting in more concentrated urine. The sun exposure may also enhance vitamin D production, with a subsequent increase in intestinal calcium absorption and subsequent urine calcium excretion.[1,8] The augmented urine calcium excretion in a smaller urine volume

will markedly increase the concentration of urinary calcium and consequent urine supersaturation promoting stone formation.

Stone type also varies with worldwide geography and genetic predisposition. In the Mediterranean and Middle Eastern countries, the percentage of stones composed of uric acid may be as high as 75%, whereas in the United States, most stones are composed primarily of calcium with oxalate or phosphate (>70%), with less than 10% formed purely of uric acid. Magnesium ammonium phosphate (struvite) stones account for roughly 10% to 25% of stones formed (with a higher incidence in the United Kingdom), and cystine stones constitute about 2% of all stones formed[4,9,10] (Fig. 54.1).

Pathogenesis

Stones form through a complex series of events that can only occur in urine that is supersaturated with respect to the ionic constituents of the specific stone. Supersaturation is dependent on the product of the free ion activities of stone components rather than on their molar concentrations. Although an increasing concentration of crystal components increases their free ion activity, other factors may serve to diminish it. If one were to dissolve calcium and oxalate in pure water, for example, the solution would become saturated when the addition of any more calcium or oxalate would not result in further dissolution. However, urine, unlike pure water, contains numerous other ions and molecules that can form soluble complexes with the ionic components of a stone. The interactions with these other solutes (e.g., citrate) may result in a decrease in free ion activity, which allows the stone constituents to increase in total concentration to levels that would normally cause stone formation. Urinary pH

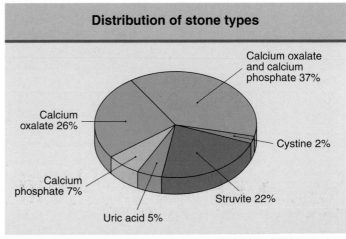

Distribution of stone types

Calcium oxalate and calcium phosphate 37%

Calcium oxalate 26%

Cystine 2%

Calcium phosphate 7%

Struvite 22%

Uric acid 5%

Figure 54.1   Proportion of stone types in a typical U.S. population.

can also influence free ion activity. The level of chemical free ion activity in which stones will neither grow nor dissolve is referred to as the *equilibrium solubility product*, or the *upper limit of metastability*. Above this level, the urine will be supersaturated, and any stone present will grow in size.

When the solution becomes supersaturated with respect to a solid phase, ions can join together to form the more stable, solid phase. This process, termed *nucleation*, can be homogeneous or heterogeneous. Homogeneous nucleation refers to the joining of similar ions into crystals. The more common and thermodynamically favored heterogeneous nucleation results when crystals grow around dissimilar crystals or other substances in the urine such as sloughed epithelial cells. Calcium oxalate crystals, for example, can nucleate around uric acid crystals. In order for stones to grow sufficiently large in size to obstruct before being excreted in the urine, several small crystals generally bond together rapidly in a process termed *aggregation*.

A next essential step in stone formation that allows crystal growth into a clinically significant calculus is *anchoring* of crystals to the renal epithelium. Calcium oxalate crystals have been shown to anchor on areas of calcium phosphate deposits termed *Randall's plaques*. These plaques are located in the renal papillae and are composed of apatite crystals. The apatite appears to originate around the thin loop of Henle in the tubular basement membrane and extends into the interstitium without filling the tubular lumen or damaging the tubular cells. In addition to the apatite crystals, organic material also extends from the same tubular basement membrane area to the uroepithelial surface of the renal papillae. Calcium oxalate crystals attach to these plaques, allowing significant stone growth.[7,11,12]

Clinical Manifestations

The two most characteristic symptoms of nephrolithiasis are pain and hematuria. Other presentations include urinary tract infection and acute renal failure owing to obstructive uropathy if stones cause bilateral renal tract obstruction or unilateral obstruction in a single functioning kidney (Fig. 54.2).

Pain

The classic presentation of pain in patients with nephrolithiasis is ureteral colic. This discomfort of abrupt onset intensifies over time into an excruciating, severe flank pain that only resolves with stone passage or removal. The pain may migrate anteriorly along the abdomen and inferiorly to the groin, testicles, or labia majora as the stone moves toward the vesicoureteral junction. Gross hematuria, urinary urgency, frequency, nausea, and vomiting may

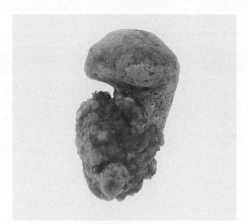

Figure 54.3 Ureteral calculus. This 1-cm wide calcium oxalate stone provoked ureteral colic and required surgical removal.

be also present. Stones smaller than 5 mm are likely to pass spontaneously with hydration, whereas larger stones often require urologic intervention[7,13] (Fig. 54.3). Ureteral colic is not exclusive to stone disease and may also occur with the passage of clots from hematuria of many causes ("clot colic") or with papillary necrosis. As well as colic, nephrolithiasis may provoke less-specific loin pain that may be poorly localized to the kidney and, therefore, has a wide differential diagnosis, particularly if not associated with other urinary symptoms. The finding of a stone on radiologic examination does not preclude the concurrent presence of other pathology.

Hematuria

Stone disease is a common cause of hematuria, both microscopic and macroscopic. Macroscopic hematuria occurs most commonly with large calculi and during urinary infection and colic. Although typically associated with loin pain or ureteral colic, the hematuria of nephrolithiasis may also be painless. The clinical differential of hematuria is therefore wide and includes tumor, infection, and stones, as well as glomerular and interstitial renal parenchymal disease (Fig. 54.4). Painless microscopic hematuria in children may occur with hypercalciuria in the absence of demonstrable stones.

Loin Pain Hematuria Syndrome

Loin pain hematuria syndrome is a poorly understood condition that must always be considered in the differential diagnosis of nephrolithiasis. It is diagnosed by exclusion when patients (most typically young and middle-aged females) present with loin pain and persistent microscopic or intermittent macroscopic hematuria.[14] Careful evaluation is required to exclude small stones, tumor, urinary infection, and glomerular disease. Angiographic abnormalities implying intrarenal vasospasm or occlusion have been reported, as have renal biopsy abnormalities typified by deposition of complement C3 in arteriolar walls. However, these findings are not consistent, nor do they provide a coherent framework to explain the pathogenesis of this condition.

In a recent study, 43 consecutive patients with clinical manifestations of loin pain hematuria syndrome were evaluated by renal biopsy after other causes of their symptoms were excluded with at least two imaging studies.[15] Thirty-four subjects were considered to have idiopathic loin pain hematuria syndrome after 9 with histologic evidence of IgA nephropathy were excluded. Of these, 66.5% had glomerular basement membranes that were either unusually thick or thin on electron microscopy, and 47% had a history of kidney stones, although none had

Clinical presentations of nephrolithiasis	
Presentation	Characteristics
Pain	Ureteral colic, loin pain, dysuria
Hematuria	—
Urinary tract infection	Recurrent, chronic infection; pyelonephritis
Asymptomatic urine abnormality	Microscopic hematuria, proteinuria, sterile pyuria
Interruption of urinary stream	—
Calculus anuria	—

Figure 54.2 Clinical presentations of nephrolithiasis.

Causes of hematuria
Nephrolithiasis
Infection: cystitis, prostatitis, urethritis, acute pyelonephritis, tuberculosis, schistosomiasis
Malignancy: renal cell carcinoma, transitional cell carcinoma, prostatic carcinoma, Wilms' tumor
Trauma
Glomerular disease
Interstitial nephritis
Polycystic kidney disease
Papillary necrosis
Medullary sponge kidney
Coagulopathy: bleeding disorders, anticoagulation therapy
Miscellaneous: loin pain hematuria syndrome, arteriovenous malformation, chemical cystitis, caruncle, factitious

Figure 54.4   Causes of hematuria.

obstructing stones at the time of assessment. Glomerular hematuria was evident in a significantly greater percentage of the biopsy specimens of patients with loin pain hematuria syndrome compared with those of healthy living kidney donors (controls) who also underwent renal biopsy. The investigators postulate that the structurally abnormal glomerular basement membranes in most of these patients may lead to rupture of the glomerular capillary walls, with consequent hemorrhage into the renal tubules. Tubular obstruction by red blood cells and also, potentially, by microcrystals, ensues. Local and global renal parenchymal edema follow, ultimately resulting in stretching of the renal capsule and in severe flank pain.

Loin pain hematuria syndrome is a chronic condition requiring reassurance, careful management of analgesia, and ongoing psychological support. The condition usually remits after several years. Denervation of the kidney by autotransplantation is rarely successful.[16] The extreme measure of nephrectomy has been used but pain often recurs promptly in the contralateral kidney. Bilateral nephrectomy and renal replacement therapy have been reported as an approach of very last resort.

Asymptomatic Stone Disease
Even large staghorn calculi that have been present for a number of years may remain entirely asymptomatic, being a coincidental finding during the investigation of unrelated abdominal or musculoskeletal disease. Obstructive uropathy caused by calculi may be painless; therefore, nephrolithiasis should always be considered in the differential diagnosis of unexplained renal failure. Ultrasound is a poor imaging technique for ureteral stones and may not identify such stones in a patient with hydronephrosis (see Chapter 55, and the later section on Radiologic Evaluation).

Clinical Evaluation of Stone Formers
All patients with recurrent nephrolithiasis merit evaluation with the goal of determining the cause of their kidney stones. However, evaluation of patients with a single stone is somewhat controversial because of the undetermined cost-to-benefit ratio of stone evaluation and therapy. A National Institutes of Health Consensus Development Conference on the Prevention and Treatment of Kidney Stones determined that all patients, even those with a single stone, should undergo a basic evaluation, which need not

include a 24-hour urine collection. Those with metabolically active stones (stones growing in size or number within 1 year), all children, noncalcium stone formers, and patients in demographic groups not typically prone to stone formation (non-Caucasians), warrant a more complete evaluation, which includes a 24-hour urine collection on the patient's typical diet.[17]

Basic Evaluation
The clinical evaluation of stone formers includes a general history and physical examination and requires specific data gathering on stone formation as well as specific laboratory studies (Fig. 54.5). In addition to the basic medical history, family history, medications, a stone history, as well as careful review of diet, fluid intake, occupation, and lifestyle, should be included.

History   The medical history serves to uncover a systemic etiology for nephrolithiasis. Any disease that can lead to hypercalcemia (including malignancy, hyperparathyroidism, and sarcoidosis) can result in hypercalciuria and increase the risk for calcium stone formation. A number of malabsorptive gastrointestinal disorders (including Crohn's disease and sprue [celiac disease]) can result in calcium oxalate stone formation as a result of volume depletion and hyperoxaluria. Uric acid stones often occur in patients with a history of gout and increasingly in patients with insulin resistance.[10]

The stone history (see Fig. 54.5) includes the number and frequency of stones formed, patient age at incidence of first stone, size of stones, stone type (if known), and whether the patient

Basic evaluation of nephrolithiasis

Stone history
    Number of stones formed
    Frequency of stone formation
    Age at first onset
    Size of stones passed or still present
    Kidney involved (left, right, or both)
    Stone type, if known
    Need for urologic intervention, e.g., extracorporeal shock-wave
        lithotripsy, percutaneous nephrolithotomy
    Response to surgical procedure
    Are stones associated with urinary tract infections?

Medical history
Medications
Family history
Occupation, lifestyle
Fluid intake, diet
Physical examination   Evidence of systemic causes of stones, e.g., tophi

Laboratory data
    Urinalysis
    Urine culture
    Stone analysis

Blood chemistry
    Sodium, potassium, chloride, bicarbonate
    Creatinine, calcium, phosphorus, uric acid
    Parathyroid hormone level if calcium elevated

Radiologic evaluation
    Plain abdominal radiography
    Spiral computed tomography
    Intravenous urography
    Ultrasound

Figure 54.5   The basic evaluation of nephrolithiasis.

required surgical removal of the calculi. This information indicates the severity of the stone disease and provides clues to the possible etiology of the stone formation. For example, large staghorn calculi that do not pass spontaneously and recur despite frequent surgical intervention are more consistent with struvite than calcium oxalate stones. Stones that develop at a young age may be caused by cystinuria or primary hyperoxaluria. Stone response to surgical intervention is also significant. Cystine stones, for example, do not fragment well with lithotripsy. If stones recur frequently in a single kidney, a congenital abnormality in that kidney, such as megacalyx or medullary sponge kidney, should be explored.

Family history is important because a number of stone types have a genetic basis. Idiopathic hypercalciuria is most likely a polygenic disorder; cystinuria is autosomal recessive; and, in some patients, hyperuricosuria has been associated with rare inherited metabolic disorders. In addition, nephrolithiasis and nephrocalcinosis can result from a variety of monogenic disorders, including X-linked diseases.[1,7,12,18,19]

Review of all medications is essential. A number of medications are known to potentiate calcium stone formation (e.g., loop diuretics promote calcium excretion), and several have been implicated in uric acid lithiasis (salicylates, probenecid; Fig. 54.6). Certain drugs can precipitate into stones themselves, such as rapidly infused intravenous acyclovir, triamterene, and the antiretroviral agents, indinavir and nelfinavir.[20]

The social history in these patients should include details regarding their occupation and lifestyle. Cardiothoracic surgeons and real estate agents, for example, may minimize fluid intake to avoid bathroom breaks during the workday. People who engage in vigorous outdoor activities, such as running, may not rehydrate adequately to keep up with insensible losses. In patients already

Medications associated with nephrolithiasis and nephrocalcinosis
Calcium Stone Formation
Loop diuretics
Vitamin D
Glucocorticoids
Calcium supplements
Antacids (calcium and noncalcium antacids)
Theophylline
Acetazolamide*
Amphotericin B*
Uric Acid Stone Formation
Salicylates
Probenecid
Allopurinol (usually associated with xanthine stones)
Medications That May Precipitate into Stones
Triamterene
Acyclovir (if infused rapidly intravenously)
Indinavir
Nelfinavir

Figure 54.6   Medications associated with nephrolithiasis and nephrocalcinosis. *Associated with nephrocalcinosis.

Foods high in oxalate and purine
High Oxalate Foods (avoid in setting of hyperoxaluria)
Green beans
Beets
Celery
Green onions
Leeks
Leafy greens: collard greens, dandelion greens, Swiss chard, spinach, escarole, mustard greens, sorrel, kale, rhubarb
Cocoa
Chocolate
Black tea
Berries: blackberries, blueberries, strawberries, raspberries, currants, gooseberries
Orange peel
Lemon peel
Dried figs
Summer squash
Nuts, peanut butter
Tofu (bean curd)
High Purine Foods (avoid in setting of hyperuricosuria)
Organ meats: sweetbreads, liver, kidney, brains, heart
Shellfish
Meat: beef, pork, lamb, poultry
Fish: anchovies, sardines (canned), herring, mackerel, cod, halibut, tuna, carp
Meat extracts: bouillon, broth, consommé, stock
Gravies
Certain vegetables: asparagus, cauliflower, peas, spinach, mushrooms, lima and kidney beans, lentils

Figure 54.7   Foods high in oxalate and purine.

prone to nephrolithiasis, this may lead to production of excessively concentrated urine and precipitation of stone crystals.

A complete dietary history and review of fluid intake is essential in determining potential causes or contributors to stone formation. It is important to have the patient cite commonly consumed foods with each meal, with particular attention paid to sodium-containing foods, as well as quantities of calcium, animal protein, purine, and oxalate (Fig. 54.7). It is particularly important to review dietary calcium because many patients with nephrolithiasis are erroneously instructed to eliminate all calcium from their diet, a suggestion that can result not only in bone demineralization, particularly in women and children, but also in an increase in stone formation.[21-24]

Physical Examination   The physical examination may be helpful in uncovering systemic disorders that predispose patients to nephrolithiasis. Although most patients with idiopathic hypercalciuria are healthy and have a normal physical examination, the presence of tophi in others may provide evidence for hyperuricosuria and uric acid stone formation. Similarly, a patient with paraplegia and a chronic indwelling bladder catheter may be predisposed to chronic urinary tract infections and struvite stone production.

Laboratory Findings The basic evaluation includes several urine and blood tests that help to determine metabolic factors that may lead to stone formation. The urinalysis is particularly useful: the urine pH is generally high in patients with struvite and calcium phosphate stones but low in patients with uric acid and calcium oxalate stones. The specific gravity, if high, will confirm inadequate fluid intake. Hematuria may imply active stone disease with crystal or stone passage. Examination of the urine may reveal red blood cells along with characteristic crystals (Fig. 54.8; see also Fig. 4.7g). The presence of bacteria in urine with a pH greater than 6 to 6.5 may be indicative of struvite stone disease. In this case, a urine culture should be obtained. Because many bacteria can produce urease even when urine bacterial colony counts are low, the microbiology laboratory should be instructed to type the organism even if there are fewer than 100,000 colony-forming units (cfu)/ml.

Blood tests required in the basic evaluation are electrolytes (sodium, potassium, chloride, and bicarbonate), creatinine, calcium, uric acid, and phosphorus. If the serum calcium is elevated or at the upper limit of normal, especially if the serum phosphorus is low, a serum parathyroid hormone level should also be measured. A low potassium or bicarbonate level may indicate a cause for hypocitraturia, such as occurs in distal renal tubular acidosis.

Stone Analysis Patients should be encouraged, whenever possible, to retrieve any stone they excrete for chemical analysis. This stone analysis may be most helpful in defining an underlying metabolic abnormality and indicating a direction for treatment.

Radiologic Evaluation Patients with no contraindication to radiographic evaluation should have a plain film of the abdomen performed that includes views of the kidneys, ureters, and bladder (KUB). This will reveal any opacifications in the areas of the kidneys and ureters that could be attributed to calcium, cystine, or struvite stones (Fig. 54.9). Uric acid and xanthine calculi are radiolucent, however, and will not be visible on plain films. The unenhanced helical computed tomography (CT) scan, also known as spiral CT, multidetector CT, or computed tomography–intravenous urography (CT-IVU), has replaced intravenous urography (IVU) as the test of choice for the diagnosis of acute renal colic (Fig. 54.10). This test has a higher sensitivity and specificity than IVU for detecting ureteral stones and ureteral obstruction.[13] Another advantage of spiral CT over standard IVU is that it can, and virtually always should, be performed without radiographic contrast. This test is more likely to reveal other etiologies of symptoms that may not be stone related. It is also a more rapid test, with results being available in minutes rather than hours, making it a more practical test in the emergency room setting, although an experienced radiologist, generally required for optimal interpretation of the images, may not be available at all times in urgent care facilities. Disadvantages of the spiral CT include the radiation dose, which is about three times that of a conventional IVU, and the greater cost of the procedure. Both tests should be avoided or limited in patients at risk for radiation exposure, such as children and pregnant women.[25-29]

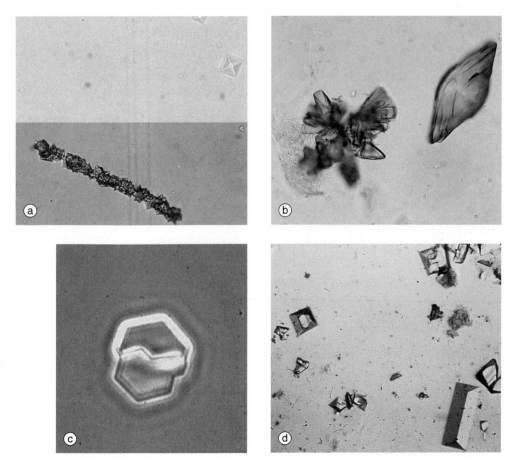

Figure 54.8 **Urine crystals.** *a,* Oxalate crystals: a pseudocast of calcium oxalate crystals accompanied by crystals of calcium oxalate dihydrate. *b,* Uric acid crystals: complex crystals suggestive of acute uric acid nephropathy or uric acid nephrolithiasis. *c,* A typical hexagonal cystine crystal; a single crystal provides a definitive diagnosis of cystinuria. *d,* Coffin-lid crystals of magnesium ammonium phosphate (struvite). (Courtesy of Dr. Patrick Fleet.)

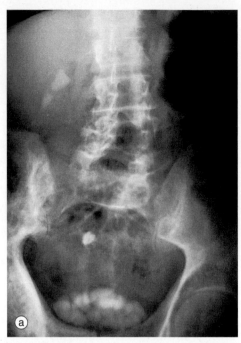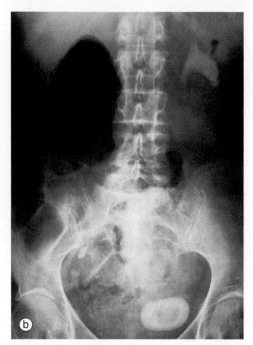

Figure 54.9   Radiopaque renal calculi on plain abdominal radiography. *a,* Multiple cystine stones in the right kidney, right ureter, and bladder. *b,* Struvite stones: left staghorn calculus and a single bladder stone.

The standard IVU has largely been supplanted by spiral CT and should be avoided in patients with renal insufficiency or other contraindications to the use of contrast. The IVU generally demonstrates urinary tract obstruction caused by calculi (Fig. 54.11). In addition, the IVU can demonstrate abnormalities of the genitourinary tract that may predispose the patient to stone formation, such as medullary sponge kidney (see Chapter 44) or calyceal anomalies (see Chapter 49). During acute episodes of colic, the radiographic contrast used in the IVU, by creating a strong osmotic diuresis, may assist in moving the stone along the ureter.

Renal ultrasound provides great specificity in the evaluation of stones, but is not a sensitive screening test. Both radiolucent and radiopaque stones within the kidneys should be detectable on ultrasound, but ureteral stones are often missed. Nonetheless,

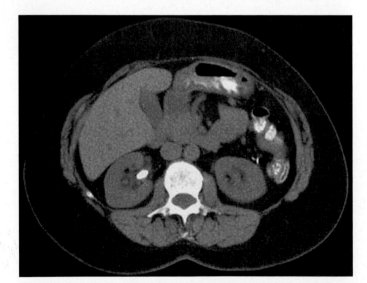

Figure 54.10   Stone in the right renal pelvis. Spiral CT scan showing a single stone in the right renal pelvis. (From http://www. gehealthcare.com/usen/ct/products/urologyimagegallery.html.)

this is the test of choice for those patients who must avoid radiation exposure.

If a KUB demonstrates radiopaque stones, subsequent radiographs can be obtained if a patient develops new symptoms suggestive of recurrent stone disease. Periodic monitoring, if deemed necessary, should be obtained with a KUB rather than spiral CT, whenever possible, to minimize radiation exposure.

Complete Evaluation

A complete evaluation should be undertaken in patients with multiple or metabolically active stones (i.e., stones that grow in size or increase in number within a year). All children, non-Caucasians (demographic groups not typically prone to stone formation), and patients who form stones other than calcium-containing calculi should also undergo a complete evaluation. In addition to the basic evaluation, the complete evaluation includes a 24-hour urine collection for quantification of supersaturation for calcium oxalate, brushite (calcium phosphate), and uric acid (Fig. 54.12). Urine for supersaturation analysis has been shown to correlate well with stone composition.[30] Patients can bring their specimens to a local laboratory or may directly mail them to specialized laboratories that measure calcium, oxalate, citrate, uric acid, creatinine, sodium, potassium, magnesium, sulfate, phosphorus, chloride, urine urea nitrogen, and pH. The levels can be used to calculate supersaturation for calcium oxalate, calcium phosphate, and uric acid using a software program such as EQUIL2.[31] Desirable levels of supersaturation are noted in the results, as well as dietary and pharmacologic recommendations that may assist in achieving them.[32] Calculation of supersaturation from a 24-hour urine will provide an average prevailing supersaturation that will certainly be lower than the peak supersaturation that may dictate stone formation. Postprandial spikes in ion excretion may result in supersaturation that initiates stone formation. Only an undersaturated urine ensures that stones will not recur; the risk for stone formation rises with increasing supersaturation.

In the absence of urine for supersaturation analysis, most laboratories assess urine volume and the quantity of calcium, oxalate,

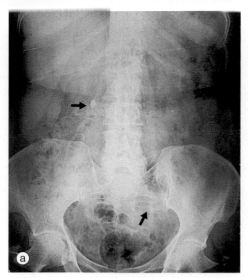 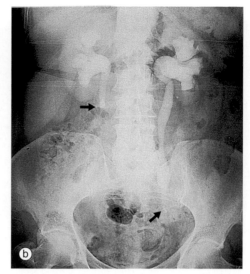

Figure 54.11 Obstructive uropathy resulting from nephrolithiasis in a patient with acute renal impairment. *a,* Plain abdominal radiograph showing a stone in the right upper ureter and a very small stone in the lower left ureter *(arrows)*. *b,* Intravenous urography at the same time showing bilateral hydronephrosis caused by ureteral obstruction.

phosphorus, uric acid, sodium, citrate, and creatinine excreted in a 24-hour urine collection (see Fig. 54.12). Urine creatinine is useful in assessing adequacy of the collection. In an adequate collection, men should excrete greater than 15 mg/kg (132 μmol/kg) daily, and women should excrete greater than 10 mg/kg (88 μmol/kg) daily. A disadvantage of the standard 24-hour urine collection is that laboratories vary in the preservatives required to process the various constituents. Many require more than one collection to measure all the urinary constituents, limiting compliance with the collection and therefore the accuracy of the results. Additionally, determination of supersaturation is far more informative than evaluation of the individual urinary constituents.

Patients should be encouraged to perform the collection on a typical day while eating a typical diet, although many patients prefer to collect the urine at weekends when their diet and habits may differ from usual workdays. Specialized testing, such as the use of high- or low-calcium diets, is not recommended.[17] When collecting the 24-hour urine, the first morning urine should be discarded, then all urine should be collected for the next 24 hours, including the next first morning urine. This procedure must be explicitly reviewed with the patient, or an overcollection or undercollection may result.

General Treatment

Intervention for stone removal may be required when pain, obstruction, or infection due to nephrolithiasis does not respond to conservative management. These aspects of stone management, including extracorporeal shock-wave lithotripsy (ESWL) and both endoscopic and percutaneous surgical techniques, are discussed in Chapter 56. The risk for developing renal insufficiency varies with different types of stone, and this must also be taken into account in planning the management of nephrolithiasis.[33] Here, we discuss medical management strategies to minimize stone recurrence.

Patients who are seen by stone specialists often have a decrease in stone recurrence even without pharmacologic intervention.[34] This phenomenon, termed the *stone clinic effect*, has been ascribed to modifications in diet and fluid intake. These nonpharmacologic measures include an increase in fluid intake, which will concomitantly increase urine volume; restriction of dietary sodium, which leads to a reduction of urine calcium excretion; restriction of animal protein, which also leads to a reduction of urine calcium excretion and an increase in excretion of the calcification inhibitor citrate; and ingestion of an age- and gender-appropriate amount of dietary calcium. Although dietary calcium restriction continues to be prescribed by many physicians, increasing evidence indicates that this is not beneficial and can actually increase the rate of stone formation (see later discussion, Calcium Stones).[3,22]

Fluid Intake

An increase in urine volume to greater than 2 to 2.5 liters daily is of proven efficacy in reducing the incidence of stone formation.[34-36] Larger urine volumes are known to reduce calcium oxalate supersaturation, as well as precipitation of other crystals.

Optimal 24-hour urine values in recurrent nephrolithiasis	
Urine Values in 24 Hours	
Volume	>2–2.5 l
Calcium	<4 mg/kg (0.1 mmol/kg), ~300 mg (7.5 mmol) in men, ~250 mg (6.3 mmol) in women
Oxalate	<40 mg (0.36 mmol)
Uric acid	<750 mg (4.5 mmol) in women, <800 mg (4.7 mmol) in men (can be pH dependent)
Citrate	>320 mg (17 mmol)
Sodium	<3000 mg (<130 mmol)
Phosphorus	<1100 mg (35 mmol)
Creatinine >10 mg/kg (88 μmol/kg) in women and >15 mg/kg (132 μmol/kg) in men, if specimen is a complete collection	
Urine Supersaturation Values*	
Calcium oxalate supersaturation	<5
Calcium phosphate supersaturation	0.5–2
Uric acid supersaturation	0–1

Figure 54.12 Evaluation of nephrolithiasis: optimal 24-hour urine values.
*The ratio between the actual ion-activity product and its solubility product.

Increased fluid intake to augment urine volume has also been the mainstay of therapy for patients with uric acid and cystine stones. The period of maximum risk for stone formation is at night, when urine concentration is physiologically increased. Patients should be encouraged to drink enough fluid in the evening to provoke nocturia and then drink further fluid before returning to bed.

Salt Intake

Sodium excretion by the renal tubules augments urine calcium excretion.[37] Conversely, dietary salt restriction, which diminishes sodium excretion, is associated with a decrease in calcium excretion. Patients should be instructed to limit daily sodium intake to 2 g (about 87 mmol sodium).

Dietary Protein

Animal protein ingestion increases the frequency of renal stone formation by a number of mechanisms. Metabolism of certain amino acids leads to generation of sulfate ions, which render urinary calcium ions less soluble.[38,39] In addition, the metabolic acidosis that results from protein ingestion leads to calcium release from bone and a consequent increase in the filtered load of calcium.[38,39] Acidosis also decreases renal tubule calcium reabsorption, which leads to hypercalciuria. Urinary citrate excretion is also pH dependent, with acidosis leading to a decrease in citrate excretion. The result of increased animal protein intake is an increase in urinary calcium ions that are rendered less soluble because of concomitant sulfate excretion and hypocitraturia. The low urine pH during acidosis, coupled with increased uric acid excretion from the metabolism of animal protein, can result in uric acid lithiasis. For these reasons, stone formers should consume only a moderate protein diet (0.8–1.0 g/kg daily).[4]

Dietary Calcium

Despite conventional wisdom, recent studies have demonstrated a decrease in stone incidence when people consume diets adequate in calcium.[36,40-42] The beneficial effect of dietary calcium on reducing stone formation has been attributed to the binding of ingested oxalate by the additional calcium. Given the high lithogenic potential of oxalate, a decrease in absorbed and excreted oxalate would diminish calcium oxalate crystal formation. Women also appear to have reduced stone formation on a higher calcium diet but may be prone to forming stones when taking calcium supplements, especially with supplemental vitamin D.[43] Some have postulated that this increase may be due to timing the supplemental calcium ingestion apart from meals, which would enhance calcium absorption without reducing oxalate absorption.

Previously, there were attempts to divide hypercalciuric patients into distinct pathophysiologic groups: those with excessive renal calcium excretion ("renal leak"), and those who absorbed excessive amounts of calcium through the gastrointestinal tract ("absorptive hypercalciuria"). For the latter group, a low-calcium diet was suggested. However, studies have shown that hypercalciuric patients generally do not have a transport defect limited to a single site. In both hypercalciuric rats and humans placed on a low-calcium diet, there is a continuous, wide spectrum of calcium excretion, with many subjects excreting more calcium than they consume. This negative calcium balance must be derived from demineralization of bone, by far the largest repository of calcium in the body.[21,23,44]

Clinical support for the use of an age- and gender-appropriate amount of dietary calcium to prevent recurrent calcium oxalate stone formation in hypercalciuric men was recently provided by a randomized prospective study comparing the rate of stone formation in men assigned to a low calcium diet with that of those assigned to a normal-calcium, low-sodium, and low–animal protein diet.[22] The 60 men assigned to the low-calcium diet were twice as likely to have recurrent stones over 5 years, compared with those on the normal-calcium, low-sodium, and low–animal protein diet. Urinary calcium oxalate supersaturation also diminished more rapidly in those on the higher-calcium diet and remained lower than that of men on the low-calcium diet for most of the 5-year study. This reduction in supersaturation was due to a greater fall in urinary oxalate in the men eating the normal-calcium, low-sodium, and low–animal protein diet.[22,45]

Others have shown that patients prescribed low-calcium diets can avoid excessive hyperoxaluria when adequately instructed on a low-oxalate diet.[46] They contend that patients who demonstrate excessive intestinal absorption of calcium associated with severe hypercalciuria may benefit from calcium restriction without risk for significant osteopenia.

We believe, however, that although "excessive" dietary calcium intake and calcium supplements should be avoided in patients with calcium nephrolithiasis, an age- and gender-appropriate calcium diet is highly recommended. The benefits of reducing stone formation with normal calcium intake, in addition to the risk for bone demineralization with calcium restriction, have rendered the low-calcium diet obsolete.[22,23,45]

SPECIFIC FORMS OF STONE DISEASE

Calcium Stones

Calcium-containing kidney stones are most common, constituting about 70% of all stones formed. Most calcium stones are composed of calcium oxalate, either alone or in combination with calcium phosphate or urate. A small percentage of stones are composed entirely of calcium phosphate.[4] Most calcium stones do not exceed 1 to 2 cm in width, although surgical intervention is often required when they grow larger than 5 mm.

Calcium stones may develop as a result of excessive excretion of calcium (hypercalciuria), oxalate (hyperoxaluria), and uric acid (hyperuricosuria); insufficient citrate excretion (hypocitraturia); renal tubular acidosis; certain medications; and congenital abnormalities of the genitourinary tract (Fig. 54.13). Specific therapy for patients with calcium stones depends on the underlying metabolic abnormalities detected on evaluation. Nonspecific or general therapy as outlined earlier should always be instituted; however, more often, more definitive treatment is required.

Hypercalciuria

Etiology Hypercalciuria with no other demonstrable metabolic abnormality is termed *idiopathic hypercalciuria*. These patients generally exhibit excessive intestinal calcium absorption and may also have decreased renal tubular calcium reabsorption and decreased bone mineralization. The etiology of this systemic disorder in calcium transport has, in hypercalciuric stone-forming rats and in humans, been linked to an excessive number of receptors for vitamin D.[47] Metabolic disorders leading to an elevation in serum calcium, parathyroid hormone, or $1,25(OH)_2$ vitamin D_3 also may result in hypercalciuria.

Treatment For hypercalciuria, the usual first-line therapy is a thiazide diuretic. Chlorthalidone, 25 to 50 mg, is the drug of choice because it requires only once daily administration. Indapamide, 1.25 to 2.5 mg daily, does not tend to raise serum lipids as much as other thiazides and is often preferred for patients with cardiac risk factors or elevated serum lipids. On commencing

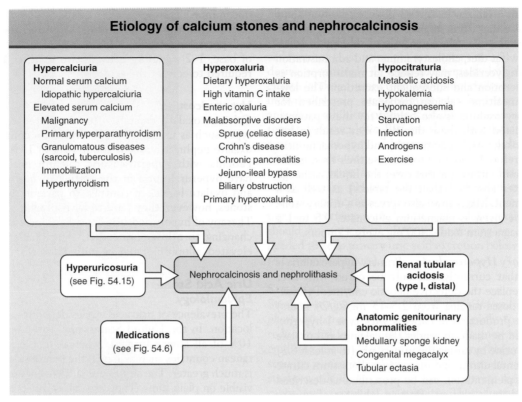

Figure 54.13 Etiology of calcium stones and nephrocalcinosis.

these medications, patients should be instructed to increase their dietary potassium intake, and a serum potassium level should be checked 7 to 10 days later. If the level is low, oral potassium supplementation should be initiated. Potassium citrate is preferred over potassium chloride because citrate complexes urinary calcium, further lowering supersaturation. However, most patients find potassium citrate liquid preparations unpalatable, and a wax matrix tablet (Urocit-K) that is well tolerated is available in some countries. Generally, patients are able to maintain a normal serum potassium level with potassium citrate, 20 to 40 mmol daily. Serum potassium and bicarbonate levels should be rechecked 7 to 10 days later for further dose adjustment. Because citrate is a base, potassium citrate may excessively raise the serum bicarbonate level, and a change to potassium chloride may be required. The 24-hour urine calcium, sodium, and citrate should be rechecked after several weeks. If the calcium excretion remains elevated, the thiazide dose should be increased. If the sodium excretion also remains high, patients should be encouraged to limit their sodium intake further because they will not have adequate response to the diuretic on a high-sodium diet. If the potassium remains low despite supplementation or the calcium excretion remains high despite increased thiazide dosing, addition of a potassium-sparing diuretic may be advantageous. Triamterene can precipitate into stones; therefore, amiloride (starting dose 5 mg daily) should be used, or a combination tablet that includes both a thiazide and amiloride.[4,48,49]

For dietary recommendations see the earlier section on General Treatment.

Hyperoxaluria

Etiology Elevated urinary oxalate levels can result from excessive dietary intake (dietary oxaluria), gastrointestinal disorders that can lead to malabsorption (enteric oxaluria), or an inherited enzyme deficiency that results in excessive metabolism of oxalate (primary hyperoxaluria)[50] (see Fig. 54.13).

Dietary excess of oxalate generally does not raise urinary oxalate values to levels exceeding 60 mg/24 hours (0.54 mmol/24 hours). Enteric oxaluria may occur in a number of disorders in which malabsorption results in excessive colonic absorption of oxalate. These include sprue (celiac disease), Crohn's disease, chronic pancreatitis, and short bowel syndrome. Urinary oxalate values are generally greater than 60 mg/24 hours and can exceed 100 mg/24 hours (0.54 and 0.9 mmol/24 hours).[51] In primary hyperoxaluria, the tremendous oxalate production results in widespread calcium oxalate deposition throughout the body at an early age. This infiltration of calcium oxalate into organs can result in cardiomyopathy, bone marrow suppression, and renal failure. Urinary oxalate values may range from 80 to 300 mg/24 hours (0.72–2.70 mmol/24 hours).

There are two types of primary hyperoxaluria with unique enzymatic defects in the liver glyoxylate pathway.[52] In type I, the defective enzyme is alanine-glyoxylate aminotransferase, encoded by the gene *AGXT* on chromosome 2. Type II tends to be a milder disorder and is caused by mutations in the *GRHPR* gene on chromosome 9, which result in failure of glyoxylate reduction to glycolate.[7,50,53]

Treatment of Dietary and Enteric Hyperoxaluria Treatment of dietary oxaluria consists of dietary oxalate restriction. Patients should be given a list of foods that have high oxalate content and told to either avoid them or eat them in moderation (see Fig. 54.7). In addition, calcium carbonate (500–650 mg/tablet, two to three tablets with each meal) may be added at meals and snacks to bind intestinal oxalate and prevent its absorption.

Specific therapy of the malabsorptive disorder, such as a gluten-free diet for patients with sprue, is the first line of

Factors associated with struvite stone formation
Urease-producing bacteria*
Proteus
Haemophilus
Yersinia
Staphylococcus epidermidis
Pseudomonas
Klebsiella
Serratia
Citrobacter
Ureaplasma
Elevated urinary pH

Figure 54.16 Factors associated with struvite stone formation. *Escherichia coli* is *not* a urease producer.

maintained or the calculi are completely eradicated. Given the need for complete stone removal in order to effect a cure, early urologic intervention is advised. Stones smaller than 2 cm may respond well to ESWL; however, larger stones will likely require percutaneous nephrolithotomy (PCNL) or a combination of both ESWL and PCNL (see Chapter 56). Any stone fragments retrieved should be cultured and culture-specific antibiotics continued. Once the urine is sterile, usually about 2 weeks after initiation of therapy, the dose is halved. Monthly urine cultures should be obtained, and if they remain sterile for 3 consecutive months, antibiotics may be discontinued, although surveillance urine cultures should continue monthly for a full year.[60]

Adjunct medical therapies include urease inhibitors and chemolysis. The most commonly used urease inhibitor is acetohydroxamic acid. By inhibiting urease, these agents retard stone growth and prevent new stone formation. Unfortunately, they have numerous side effects that limit their use, although adverse effects resolve on discontinuation of the drug. In addition, they require adequate renal clearance to be effective and therefore are not useful in patients with renal insufficiency (creatinine >2 mg/dl [176 μmol/l]).[59,61] Chemolysis refers to irrigation of the kidney through a nephrostomy tube or the ureter with a solution designed to dissolve the stones. The most common solution is 10% hemiacidrin, which contains carbonic acid, citric acid, D-gluconic acid, and magnesium at pH 3.9. Use of lavage chemolysis is controversial because it has been associated with a high mortality rate in the past. However, it is thought to be relatively safe with appropriate monitoring for urinary tract infections, obstruction to flow, intrapelvic pressures, and magnesium levels. Although not a treatment of choice for large stones, it may be useful when surgical techniques have been effective but have left residual stone fragments.

Cystine Stones
Cystinuria is an autosomal disorder in which there is a tubular defect in dibasic amino acid transport, resulting in increased cystine, ornithine, lysine, and arginine excretion (see Chapter 47). More than 100 mutations of the *SL3A1* gene on chromosome 2 and more than 60 mutations of the *SCLC7A9* gene on chromosome 19 have been identified.[62] The pattern of inheritance may be autosomal recessive as well as autosomal dominant with incomplete penetrance. The stone disease is usually clinically manifest by the second and third decades of life. Because of the high sulfur content of the cystine molecule, the stones are apparent on plain radiographs (see Fig. 54.9a) and will often present as staghorn calculi or multiple bilateral stones. Cystinuria, in which cystine accumulates only in the lumen of the renal tubules, is distinct from cystinosis, in which there is widespread intracellular cystine accumulation. Cystinosis and cystinuria are discussed further in Chapter 47.

Cystine is poorly soluble, with a solubility of only about 300 mg/l (1.25 mmol/l) at a neutral pH. Normal cystine excretion of about 30 to 50 mg (0.12–0.21 mmol) per day is readily soluble in the usual daily urine output of about 1 liter. However, homozygote cystinuric patients often excrete 250 to 1000 mg (1.04–4.20 mmol) of cystine per day, with heterozygotes excreting an intermediate amount. Treatment must be directed at decreasing the urinary cystine concentration below the limits of solubility. The dietary precursor of cystine, methionine, is an essential amino acid; therefore, it is impractical to reduce intake. Increasing urine volume so that cystine remains below the limits of solubility is often practical; however, sometimes 4 l of urine per day is necessary. A low sodium diet may help reduce cystine excretion. Increasing urine pH above 7.5 will increase cystine solubility, but this is often difficult to achieve on a long-term basis. D-Penicillamine (starting dose, 250 mg daily; maximum dose, 2 g daily) or tiopronin will both bind cystine and reduce urinary supersaturation; however, side effects may limit their use. The angiotensin-converting enzyme inhibitor captopril may be effective by forming a thiol-cysteine disulfide bond that is more soluble than cystine.[63]

NEPHROCALCINOSIS

Introduction
Nephrocalcinosis refers to augmented calcium content within the kidney.[12,64] The disorder may be symmetric, or in anatomic disorders such as medullary sponge kidney, it may involve only a single kidney.

Etiology and Pathogenesis
Medullary Nephrocalcinosis
Medullary nephrocalcinosis, in which the calcification tends to occur in the area of the renal pyramids, accounts for most cases of nephrocalcinosis. It is typically associated with elevated urinary levels of constituents that can precipitate, most commonly calcium, phosphate, and oxalate; or it can occur in the setting of alkaline urine (Fig. 54.17). Any disorder that can lead to hypercalcemia or hypercalciuria may be implicated. Instead of stone formation, smaller parenchymal calcifications deposit in the medulla that are usually bilateral and relatively symmetric (Fig. 54.18). Some metabolic disorders, particularly oxalosis due to primary hyperoxaluria, can result in both medullary and cortical nephrocalcinosis[64] (Fig. 54.19).

The common etiologies for nephrocalcinosis vary considerably with age. In adults, the most common causes of medullary nephrocalcinosis are primary hyperparathyroidism, renal tubular acidosis, and medullary sponge kidney, as well as medications such as acetazolamide, amphotericin B, and triamterene (see Fig. 54.6).

Although a similar range of disorders can be seen in children, the most common associations are with furosemide therapy and the hereditary disorders associated with hypercalciuria.[12,18] Furosemide, when used in premature neonates and older infants with congestive heart failure, can result in nephrocalcinosis with or without hypercalciuria. The lesions often resolve with discontinuation of therapy. A normal calcium-to-creatinine ratio

Causes of nephrocalcinosis
Medullary

Disturbed calcium metabolism
  Hyperparathyroidism
  Sarcoidosis
  Milk-alkali syndrome
  Rapidly progressive osteoporosis
  Idiopathic hypercalciuria

Other tubular disease
  Distal (type I) renal tubular acidosis
  Oxalosis*
  Dent disease (X-linked hypercalciuric nephrolithiasis)
  X-linked hypophosphatemic rickets
  Bartter syndrome
  Hypomagnesemia-hypercalciuria syndrome

Anatomic disease
  Medullary sponge kidney
  Papillary necrosis

Medications
  Acetazolamide
  Amphotericin B
  Triamterene

Cortical
Cortical necrosis
Transplant rejection
Chronic glomerulonephritis
Trauma
Tuberculosis
Oxalosis*

Figure 54.17 Causes of nephrocalcinosis. *Oxalosis typically causes both medullary and cortical nephrocalcinosis.

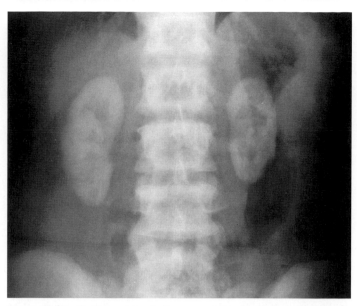

Figure 54.19 Nephrocalcinosis. Dense cortical and medullary calcification in the shrunken kidneys of a patient with oxalosis and long-standing renal failure.

at the time of diagnosis of nephrocalcinosis (about 0.40 [mg:mg] in premature infants) appears to be a good predictor of resolution.

There are many hereditary disorders associated with nephrocalcinosis, including X-linked hypercalciuric nephrolithiasis, X-linked hypophosphatemic rickets, hypomagnesemia-hypercalciuria syndrome, and Bartter syndrome.

X-linked hypercalciuric nephrolithiasis has also been termed *Dent disease* in the United Kingdom, *low-molecular-weight proteinuria*

with hypercalciuria and nephrocalcinosis in Japan, and *X-linked recessive hypophosphatemic rickets* in Italy.[65] A number of mutations affecting the *CLCN5* gene on the X-chromosome have been identified that lead to inactivation of CLC-5 voltage-gated chloride channels. The result is a clinical syndrome typically affecting young boys and usually including hypercalciuria, nephrocalcinosis, nephrolithiasis, and hematuria, as well as low-molecular-weight proteinuria, glycosuria, aminoaciduria, hypophosphatemia, renal failure, and rickets.[65,66]

In X-linked hypophosphatemic rickets, the recommended treatment, with phosphate repletion and vitamin D, may itself result in hypercalcemia, hypercalciuria, and nephrocalcinosis.

Another cause of medullary nephrocalcinosis in children is primary hypomagnesemia-hypercalciuria syndrome.[7,12,67] This rare autosomal recessive condition results from defective production of the cellular tight-junction protein, paracellin-1. This claudin family protein is necessary for adequate calcium and magnesium reabsorption in the thick ascending limb (TAL) of the loop of Henle. Children typically present with symptoms of urinary tract infection (most likely due to nephrolithiasis), polyuria, tetanic seizures (due to hypomagnesemia), and muscle cramps and weakness. Hypercalciuria, hypermagnesuria, and a urinary-concentrating defect also occur. Patients often have renal insufficiency and may require renal replacement therapy by the third decade of life. Sensorineural hearing disorders and ocular impairment may accompany the renal manifestations in a subset of patients. Several predominantly autosomal recessive genetic mutations result in Bartter syndrome.[7,12] In this disorder, defects in the sodium potassium chloride cotransporter (NKCC2), the renal outer medullary potassium channel (ROMK), or the basolateral chloride channel (CLC-Kb) lead to sodium chloride wasting at the TAL. Defective sodium transport results in diminished calcium reabsorption, as well as intravascular volume depletion and aldosterone-mediated metabolic alkalosis. The consequences are clinically similar to excessive furosemide intake; hypercalciuria, nephrocalcinosis and nephrolithiasis are often present as well. These inherited tubular disorders are discussed further in Chapter 46.

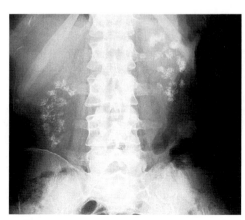

Figure 54.18 Medullary nephrocalcinosis. Plain radiograph showing bilateral metastatic medullary nephrocalcinosis in a patient with distal renal tubular acidosis.

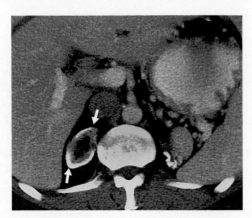

Figure 54.20 Cortical nephrocalcinosis. Noncontrast computed tomography scan showing cortical nephrocalcinosis (arrows) in the right kidney following cortical necrosis.

Cortical Nephrocalcinosis

Cortical nephrocalcinosis is usually the result of dystrophic calcification, which follows parenchymal tissue destruction rather than the precipitation of excessive urinary constituents. It is secondary to infarction, neoplasm, and infection. It is typically asymmetric and is usually localized to the renal cortex (Fig. 54.20). Causes of cortical nephrocalcinosis include transplant rejection, cortical necrosis, tuberculosis, ethylene glycol toxicity, and chronic glomerulonephritis.

Clinical Manifestations

Patients who do not have nephrolithiasis associated with nephrocalcinosis are often asymptomatic. Ultrasonography and CT scanning are sensitive diagnostic tests for both cortical and medullary nephrocalcinosis, demonstrating the parenchymal calcifications before they can be visualized on plain radiographs. The extent of calcification correlates poorly with renal function. Patients with extensive calcification may have minimal renal impairment.

Treatment

Similar to nephrolithiasis, treatment of nephrocalcinosis relies on therapy of the underlying disease, as well as measures to reduce hypercalcemia, hyperphosphatemia, and oxalosis, if possible.[68] The goal of treatment is usually to prevent further deposits because therapy cannot eradicate existing calcium deposits.

REFERENCES

1. Moe OW: Kidney stones: Pathophysiology and medical management. Lancet 2006;367:333–344.
2. Monk RD, Bushinsky DA: Kidney stones. In Larsen PR, Kronenberg HM, Melmed S, Polonsky KS (eds): Williams Textbook of Endocrinology, 11th ed. Philadelphia, WB Saunders, in press.
3. Bushinsky DA: Renal lithiasis. In Humes HD (ed): Kelly's Textbook of Medicine. New York, Lippincott Williams & Wilkins, 2000, pp 1243–1248.
4. Monk RD: Clinical approach to adults. Semin Nephrol 1996;16:375–388.
5. Bushinsky DA: Kidney stones. Adv Intern Med 2001;47:219–238.
6. Stamatelou KK, Francis ME, Jones CA, et al: Time trends in reported prevalence of kidney stones in the United States: 1976–1994. Kidney Int 2003;63:1817–1823.
7. Coe FL, Evan A, Worcester E: Kidney stone disease. J Clin Invest 2005;115:2598–2608.
8. Soucie JM, Thun MJ, Coates RJ, et al: Demographic and geographic variability of kidney stones in the United States. Kidney Int 1994;893–899.
9. Mandel N: Mechanism of stone formation. Semin Nephrol 1996;16:364–374.
10. Maalouf NM, Cameron MA, Moe OW, Sakhaee K: Novel insights into the pathogenesis of uric acid nephrolithiasis. Curr Opin Nephrol Hypertens 2004;13:181–189.
11. Evan AP, Lingeman JE, Coe FL, et al: Randall plaque of patients with nephrolithiasis begins in basement membranes of thin loops of Henle. J Clin Invest 2003;111:607–616.
12. Sayer JA, Carr G, Simmons NL: Nephrocalcinosis: Molecular insights into calcium precipitation within the kidney. Clin Sci 2004;106:549–561.
13. Teichman JMH: Acute renal colic from ureteral calculus. N Engl J Med 2004;350:684–693.
14. Weisberg LS, Bloom PB, Simmons RL, Viner ED: Loin pain hematuria syndrome. Am J Nephrol 1993;13:229–237.
15. Spetie DN, Nadasdy T, Nadasdy G, et al: Proposed pathogenesis of idiopathic loin pain–hematuria syndrome. Am J Kidney Dis 2006;47:419–427.
16. Sheil AG, Chui AK, Verran DJ, et al: Evaluation of the loin pain/hematuria syndrome treated by renal autotransplantation or radical renal neurectomy. Am J Kidney Dis 1998;32:215–220.
17. Consensus Conference: Prevention and treatment of kidney stones. JAMA 1988;260:977–981.
18. Moe OW, Bonny O: Genetic hypercalciuria. J Am Soc Nephrol 2005;16:729–745.
19. Gambaro G, Vezzoli G, Casari G, et al: Genetics of hypercalciuria and calcium nephrolithiasis: From the rare monogenic to the common polygenic forms. Am J Kidney Dis 2004;44:963–986.
20. Daudon M, Jungers P: Drug-induced renal calculi: Epidemiology, prevention and management. Drugs 2004;64:245–275.
21. Coe FL, Favus MJ, Crockett T, et al: Effects of low-calcium diet on urine calcium excretion, parathyroid function and serum $1,25(OH)_2D_3$ levels in patients with idiopathic hypercalciuria and in normal subjects. Am J Med 1982;72:25–32.
22. Borghi L, Schianchi T, Meschi T, et al: Comparison of two diets for the prevention of stone recurrences in idiopathic hypercalciuria. N Engl J Med 2002;346:77–84.
23. Asplin JR, Bauer KA, Kinder J, et al: Bone mineral density and urine calcium excretion among subjects with and without nephrolithiasis. Kidney Int 2003;63:662–669.
24. Freundlich M, Alonzo E, Bellorin-Font E, Weisinger JR: Reduced bone mass in children with idiopathic hypercalciuria and in their asymptomatic mothers. Nephrol Dial Transplant 2002;17:1396–1401.
25. Denton ER, Mackenzie A, Greenwell T, et al: Unenhanced helical CT for renal colic: Is the radiation dose justifiable? Clin Radiol 1999;54:444–447.
26. Smith RC, Coll DM: Helical computed tomography in the diagnosis of ureteric colic. BJU Int 2000;86:33–41.
27. Nakada SY, Hoff DG, Attai S, et al: Determination of stone composition by noncontrast spiral computed tomography in the clinical setting. Urology 2000;55:816–819.
28. Smith RC, Verga M, McCarthy S, Rosenfield AT: Diagnosis of acute flank pain: Value of unenhanced helical CT. AJR Am J Roentgenol 1996;166:97–101.
29. Smith RC, Rosenfield AT, Choe KA, et al: Acute flank pain: Comparison of non-contrast-enhanced CT and intravenous urography. Radiology 1995;159:735–740.
30. Parks JH, Coward M, Coe FL: Correspondence between stone composition and urine supersaturation in nephrolithiasis. Kidney Int 1997;51:894–900.
31. Werness PG, Brown CM, Smith LH, et al: A BASIC computer program for the calculation of urinary saturation. J Urol 1985;134:1242–1244.
32. Asplin J, Parks J, Lingeman J, et al: Supersaturation and stone composition in a network of dispersed treatment sites. J Urol 1998;159:1821–1825.
33. Gambaro G, Favaro S, D'Angelo A: Risk of renal failure in nephrolithiasis. Am J Kidney Dis 2001;37:233–243.
34. Hosking DH, Erickson SB, Van Den Berg CJ, et al: The stone clinic effect in patients with idiopathic calcium urolithiasis. J Urol 1983;130:1115–1118.
35. Borghi L, Meschi T, Amato F, et al: Urinary volume, water, and recurrences in idiopathic calcium nephrolithiasis: A 5-year randomized prospective study. J Urol 1996;155:839–843.

36. Lemann J Jr, Pleuss JA, Worcester EM, et al: Urinary oxalate excretion increases with body size and decreases with increasing dietary calcium intake among healthy adults. Kidney Int 1996;49:200–208 (Erratum: Kidney Int 1996;50:341).

37. Muldowney FP, Freaney R, Moloney MF: Importance of dietary sodium in the hypercalciuria syndrome. Kidney Int 1972;22:292–296.

38. Frassetto L, Morris RC Jr, Sebastian A: Long-term persistence of the urine calcium-lowering effect of potassium bicarbonate in postmenopausal women. J Clin Endocrinol Metab 2005;90:831–834.

39. Lemann J Jr, Bushinsky DA, Hamm LL: Bone buffering of acid and base in humans. Am J Physiol Renal Physiol 2003;285:F811–F832.

40. Curhan GC, Willett WC, Rimm EB, Stampfer MJ: A prospective study of dietary calcium and other nutrients and the risk of symptomatic kidney stones. N Engl J Med 1993;328:833–838.

41. Stauffer JQ: Hyperoxaluria and intestinal disease: The role of steatorrhea and dietary calcium in regulating intestinal oxalate absorption. Digest Dis 1977;22:921–928.

42. Curhan GC, Willett WC, Speizer FE, et al: Comparison of dietary calcium with supplemental calcium and other nutrients as factors affecting the risk for kidney stones in women. Ann Intern Med 1997;126:497–504.

43. Jackson RD, LaCroix AZ, Gass M, et al, for the Women's Health Initiative Investigators: Calcium plus vitamin D supplementation and the risk of fractures. N Engl J Med 2006;354:669–683.

44. Monk RD, Bushinsky DA: Pathogenesis of idiopathic hypercalciuria. In Coe F, Favus M, Pak C, Parks J, Preminger G (eds): Kidney Stones: Medical and Surgical Management. Philadelphia, Lippincott-Raven, 1996, pp 759–772.

45. Bushinsky DA: Recurrent hypercalciuric nephrolithiasis: Does diet help? N Engl J Med 2002;346:124–125.

46. Pak CYC, Odvina CV, Pearle MS, et al: Effect of dietary modification on urinary stone risk factors. Kidney Int 2005;68:2264–2273.

47. Bushinsky DA, Frick KK, Nehrke K: Genetic hypercalciuric stone-forming rats. Curr Opin Nephrol Hypertens 2006;15:403–418.

48. Coe FL, Parks JH, Asplin JR: The pathogenesis and treatment of kidney stones. N Engl J Med 1992;327:1141–1152.

49. Coe FL, Parks JH, Bushinsky DA, et al: Chlorthalidone promotes mineral retention in patients with idiopathic hypercalciuria. Kidney Int 1988;33:1140–1146.

50. Asplin JR: Hyperoxaluric calcium nephrolithiasis. Endocrinol Metab Clin North Am 2002;31:927–949.

51. Worcester EM: Stones from bowel disease. Endocrinol Metab Clin North Am 2002;31: 979–999.

52. Milliner DS: The primary hyperoxalurias: An algorithm for diagnosis. Am J Nephrol 2005;25:154–160.

53. Danpure CJ: Molecular etiology of primary hyperoxaluria type 1: New direction for treatment. Am J Nephrol 2005;25:303–310.

54. Smith LH: Hyperoxaluric states. In Coe FL, Favus MJ (eds): Disorders of Bone and Mineral Metabolism. New York, Raven, 2000, pp 707–727.

55. Pak CYC, Fuller C: Idiopathic hypocitraturic calcium oxalate nephrolithiasis successfully treated with potassium citrate. Ann Intern Med 1986;104:33–37.

56. Millman S, Strauss AL, Parks JH, et al: Pathogenesis and clinical course of mixed calcium oxalate and uric acid nephrolithiasis. Kidney Int 1982;366–370.

57. Ettinger B, Tang A, Citron JT, et al: Randomized trial of allopurinol in the prevention of calcium oxalate calculi. N Engl J Med 1986;315:1386–1389.

58. Asplin JR: Uric acid stones. Semin Nephrol 1996;16:412–424.

59. Rodman JS: Struvite stones. Nephron 1999;81:50–59.

60. Wong HY, Riedl CR, Griffith DP: Medical management and prevention of struvite stones. In Coe FL, Favus MJ, Pak CYC, et al (eds): Kidney Stones: Medical and Surgical Management. Philadelphia, Lippincott-Raven, 1996, pp 941–950.

61. Rodman JS: Struvite stones. In Pak CYC (ed): Renal Stone Disease: Pathogenesis, Prevention, and Treatment. Boston, Martinus-Nijhoff, 1987, pp 225–251.

62. Font-Llitjos M, Jimenez-Vidal M, Bisceglia L, et al: New insights into cystinuria: 40 New mutations, genotype-phenotype correlation, and digenic inheritance causing partial phenotype. J Med Genet 2005;42:58–68.

63. Sakhaee K: Pathogenesis and medical management of cystinuria. Semin Nephrol 1996;16:435–447.

64. Ramchandani P, Pollack HM: Radiologic evaluation of patients with urolithiasis. In Coe FL, Favus MJ, Pak CYC, et al (eds): Kidney Stones: Medical and Surgical Management. Philadelphia, Lippincott-Raven, 1996, pp 369–435.

65. Scheinman SJ: X-linked hypercalciuric nephrolithiasis: Clinical syndromes and chloride channel mutations. Kidney Int 1998;53:3–17.

66. Scheinman SJ, Guay-Woodford LM, Thakker RV, Warnock DG: Genetic disorders of renal electrolyte transport. N Engl J Med 1999;340:1177–1187.

67. Benigno V, Canonica CS, Bettinelli A, et al: Hypomagnesaemia-hypercalciuria-nephrocalcinosis: A report of nine cases and a review. Nephrol Dial Transplant 2000;15:605–610.

68. Alon US: Nephrocalcinosis. Curr Opin Pediatr 1997;9:160–165.

Urinary Tract Obstruction

Kevin P. G. Harris

INTRODUCTION AND DEFINITIONS

Obstructive uropathy refers to the structural or functional changes in the urinary tract that impede the normal flow of urine, whereas *obstructive nephropathy* refers to the renal disease caused by impaired flow of urine or tubular fluid. *Hydronephrosis* refers to dilation of the urinary tract; it can occur without functional obstruction to the urinary tract and can be absent in established obstruction and is therefore not necessarily synonymous with obstructive uropathy.

Obstructive uropathy and nephropathy frequently coexist, and their management requires close collaboration between nephrologists and urologists. Some surgical aspects of obstruction to the urinary tract are discussed in Chapter 56.

Obstructive uropathy is classified according to the site, the degree, and the duration of the obstruction. Acute or chronic obstruction can occur anywhere in the urinary tract, including intrarenal causes (casts, crystals) as well as extrarenal causes, which can be further subdivided into upper urinary tract obstruction (usually unilateral obstruction occurring above the vesicoureteral junction [VUJ]) and lower urinary tract obstruction (bilateral obstruction located below the VUJ). Complete obstruction of the urinary tract is termed *high grade*, whereas partial or incomplete obstruction is termed *low grade*.

Unilateral obstruction in a patient with two normal kidneys will not result in significant renal impairment because the contralateral kidney is able to compensate. However, if the obstruction is bilateral (or unilateral in a single functioning kidney), renal failure will result. In acute urinary tract obstruction, changes are mainly functional, whereas with more chronic obstruction, structural damage to the kidney commonly results. The acute functional changes may recover after the effective release of the obstruction, but any structural changes will be permanent, leading to chronic impairment of renal function. Obstruction of the urinary tract remains a major cause of renal impairment worldwide.

ETIOLOGY AND PATHOGENESIS

The etiology of renal obstruction is quite varied, but this leads to common functional and structural events in the kidney. The causes of obstructive uropathy affecting the upper and lower urinary tracts are summarized in Figures 55.1 and 55.2.

Congenital Urinary Tract Obstruction

Congenital urinary tract obstruction occurs most frequently in males, most commonly as a result of either posterior urethral valves or pelvic-ureteral junction (PUJ) obstruction. If obstruction occurs early during development, the kidney fails to develop and becomes dysplastic. If the obstruction is bilateral, there is a

Causes of upper urinary tract obstruction	
Intrinsic Causes	Extrinsic Causes

Intraluminal
  Intratubular deposition of crystals
    (uric acid, drugs)
  Stones
  Papillary tissue
  Blood clots
  Fungal ball
	Originating in the reproductive
	    system
	  Cervix: *carcinoma*
	  Uterus: *pregnancy, tumors,*
	    prolapse, endometriosis, pelvic
	    inflammatory disease
	  Ovary: abscess, tumor, cysts
	  Prostate: *carcinoma*

Intramural
  Functional: pelvic-ureteral or
    vesicoureteral junction dysfunction
  Anatomic: tumors (benign or
    malignant)
  Infections, granulomas, strictures
	Originating in the vascular system
	  Aneurysms: aorta, iliac vessels
	  Aberrant arteries: pelviureteral
	    junction
	  Venous: ovarian veins, retrocaval
	    ureter

	Originating in the gastrointestinal
	    tract
	  Crohn's disease
	  Pancreatitis
	  Appendicitis
	  Diverticulitis
	  Tumors

	Originating in the retroperitoneal
	    space
	  Lymph nodes
	  Fibrosis: idiopathic, drugs, or
	    inflammatory
	  Tumors: primary or metastatic
	  Hematomas
	  Radiation therapy

	Surgical disruption or ureteral ligation

Figure 55.1 Causes of upper urinary tract obstruction. The most common causes are in *italics*.

high mortality rate as a result of severe renal failure. If the obstruction occurs later in gestation and is low grade or unilateral, hydronephrosis and nephron loss will still occur, but renal function may be sufficient to allow survival, and such patients may not present until later in childhood. PUJ obstruction, if mild, may not present until adulthood and in some patients may be an incidental finding (Fig. 55.3). However, with increased use and improved sensitivity of antenatal scanning, congenital abnormalities of the urinary tract are now frequently identified early, allowing prompt postnatal (and in some cases antenatal) intervention to relieve the obstruction and hence preserve renal function. Congenital causes of obstruction are discussed further in Chapter 49.

About 2 to 5 hours after obstruction, renal blood flow begins to decline, whereas intratubular pressure continues to increase. Within 5 hours, proximal tubular pressure begins to decline toward control values. From this time, the main determinant of the decrease in GFR is the fall in intraglomerular capillary pressure as a result of an increase in resistance of afferent arterioles. This results in a progressive fall in renal plasma flow, which reaches 30% to 50% of control values by 24 hours. Preferential constriction of the preglomerular blood vessels lowers both plasma flow and glomerular capillary pressure, resulting in a greater decrement in GFR than in plasma flow and a fall in filtration fraction. A falling filtration fraction also occurs as a result of diversion of blood to nonfiltering areas of the kidney or a reduction in the ultrafiltration coefficient. The relative changes in ureteral pressure, renal plasma flow, and GFR are summarized in Figure 55.5.

The intrarenal vasoconstriction results from the generation of angiotensin II and thromboxane A_2, the release of vasopressin (antidiuretic hormone), and a decrease in the production of nitric oxide. Angiotensin II and thromboxane A_2 may also reduce the ultrafiltration coefficient.[2,3] The central role of these two vasoconstrictors has been demonstrated by studies in rats, in which pretreatment with angiotensin-converting enzyme (ACE) inhibitors and thromboxane synthase inhibitors virtually normalized renal function after the relief of short-term ureteral obstruction.[4]

Intrarenal angiotensin II generation occurs secondary to an increase in renin release either through reduced delivery of sodium and chloride to the distal nephron (macula densa mechanism) or through a reduction in transmural pressure at the baroreceptor as a consequence of the prostaglandin-dependent dilation of the afferent arteriole. Generation of thromboxane A_2 after ureteral obstruction occurs both in glomeruli and in interstitial infiltrating cells.

An interstitial infiltrate, predominantly macrophages, develops in response to chemoattractants such as monocyte chemoattractant protein 1 and osteopontin, which are presumably released in response to the increase in tubular pressure. This infiltrate plays a key role in the acute functional changes after ureteral obstruction[5] and has also been implicated in the pathogenesis of the late structural changes that occur after obstruction.

The extent to which glomerular function recovers after the release of ureteral obstruction depends on the duration of the obstruction. Whole kidney GFR may return to normal after short-term obstruction (days); however, recovery may be incomplete after prolonged obstruction. Evidence from studies in rats now suggests that even with shorter periods of obstruction (72 hours), there may be a permanent loss of nephrons, and whole kidney GFR returns to normal only at the expense of hyperfiltration (increase in single nephron GFR) in the remaining functional nephrons.[6]

Changes in Tubular Function

Abnormalities in tubular function are common in urinary tract obstruction and manifest as altered renal handling of electrolytes as well as changes in the regulation of water excretion.[2] The degree and nature of the tubular defects after obstruction depend in part on whether the obstruction is bilateral or unilateral. These differences could result from the dissimilar hemodynamic responses, different intrinsic changes within the nephron, or differences in extrinsic factors (e.g., volume expansion and accumulation of natriuretic substances in bilateral obstruction) between the two states, or a combination of all three.

After ureteral obstruction, the ability to concentrate the urine is markedly impaired, with maximum values of 350 to 400 mOsm/kg reported in the rat. Causative factors include a loss of medullary

tonicity and an overall decrease in GFR in deep nephrons. The collecting duct is also unresponsive to vasopressin, which appears to result from a cyclooxygenase-2 (COX-2)–dependent loss of expression of renal aquaporins.[7] It is possible that the interstitial macrophage infiltrate contributes to both functional and structural tubular changes.[8]

Patients with urinary tract obstruction often have urinary acidification defects. This may only be detected by exogenous acid loading, but hyperchloremic acidosis caused by impaired distal acid secretion, hyporeninemic hypoaldosteronism (type IV renal tubular acidosis), and a combination of these findings have been described. This acidifying defect results from a marked increase in bicarbonate excretion or from a distal acidification defect, possibly as a result of abnormalities of the H^+ ATPase activity of intercalated cells of the collecting duct after ureteral obstruction.

Obstruction alters renal potassium handling. In the presence of a normal functioning contralateral kidney, potassium excretion is reduced after relief of obstruction, either in proportion to or perhaps even greater than the fall in GFR (i.e., fractional excretion of potassium is unaltered or slightly reduced). There is a defect in the distal potassium secretory mechanism after unilateral obstruction that may possibly be secondary to an unresponsiveness of that segment of the nephron to aldosterone. By contrast, after release of bilateral ureteral obstruction, there is a marked increase in the net and fractional excretion of potassium. The major mechanism by which potassium losses occur in this setting is an increased delivery of sodium to the distal tubule, resulting in an accelerated sodium-potassium exchange.

Recovery of tubular function after release of obstruction is slow and may remain abnormal even after whole kidney GFR has returned to normal. In rats, acidification and potassium-handling abnormalities persist for at least 14 days and urinary concentrating ability is abnormal for up to 60 days after the release of 24 hours of unilateral ureteral obstruction. These observations are consistent with persistent alterations in distal tubular and collecting duct function or a loss in functioning juxtaglomerular nephrons after the release of the obstruction.

PATHOLOGY

The morphologic alterations in renal architecture are similar irrespective of the cause of the obstruction. Initially, there is renal enlargement and edema with pelvicalyceal dilation (Fig. 55.6). Microscopically, the cortex may initially appear normal. Subsequently, there is tubular dilation predominantly of the collecting duct and distal tubular segments; cellular flattening and atrophy of the cells lining the proximal tubule can also occur. In most instances, glomerular structures are initially preserved, although Bowman's space may be dilated and contain Tamm-Horsfall protein; ultimately, some periglomerular fibrosis may develop.

Inadequately treated obstruction to the urinary tract eventually causes irreversible structural changes to the renal tract. The renal pelvis becomes widely dilated, with the renal papillae either flattened or hollowed out. The cortex and medulla become markedly thinned such that the kidney becomes a thin rim of renal tissue surrounding a large saccular pelvis (Fig. 55.7). Histologic examination demonstrates tubulointerstitial fibrosis and obliteration of nephrons. There is tubular proliferation and apoptosis, epithelial-mesenchymal transition, (myo)fibroblast accumulation, increased extracellular matrix deposition, and tubular atrophy and apoptosis. Ischemia as a result of the decreased renal blood flow

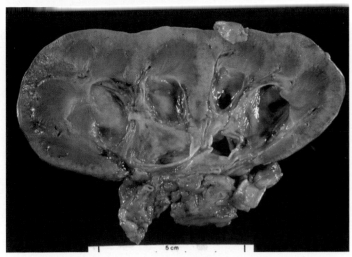

Figure 55.6 Autopsy specimen of a kidney showing the early effects of ureteral obstruction. The kidney is enlarged and edematous with pelvicalyceal dilation. There is good preservation of the renal parenchyma.

contributes to the parenchymal damage after obstruction. In both genetic and interventional studies, an important pathologic role for angiotensin II and transforming growth factor-β (TGF-β) has been established.[9,10] Infiltrating macrophages and T cells also play a pivotal role not only in the acute functional changes that occur after obstruction but also in the chronic structural damage that results[11] (Fig. 55.8). These biologically active cells release a number of profibrogenic cytokines, such as TGF-β, that promote the progressive fibrosis characteristic of prolonged ureteral obstruction. Local angiotensin II generation may also stimulate the production of TGF-β by tubular cells.

Obstruction to venous drainage and bacterial infection (pyelonephritis) may also play a role in the development of parenchymal fibrosis.

EPIDEMIOLOGY

Obstructive uropathy is a common entity and can occur at all ages. The prevalence of hydronephrosis at autopsy is 3.5% to 3.8%, with about equal distribution between males and females.[12] This is an

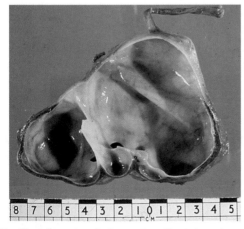

Figure 55.7 Chronic ureteral obstruction. Surgical specimen of a kidney showing gross dilation of the pelvicalyceal system and the reduction of the renal cortex to a thin fibrotic rim of tissue. There would have been no prospect for any significant functional recovery in this kidney after the relief of the obstruction.

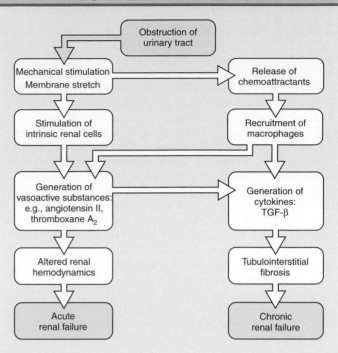

Impairment of function and structural damage in obstructive nephropathy

Figure 55.8 Events leading to acute impairment of renal function and chronic structural damage in obstructive nephropathy. TGF-β, transforming growth factor-β.

underestimate of the true incidence because these figures exclude temporary obstruction (i.e., from renal calculi). The frequency and etiology of obstruction vary in both sexes with age. Antenatal ultrasonography has significantly increased the detection rate of urinary tract anomalies as an incidental finding in the fetus, although the exact long-term significance of many of such observations remains to be determined. In children younger than 10 years, obstruction is more common in males, with congenital anomalies of the urinary tract (urethral valves, PUJ obstruction) accounting for most cases. The overall prevalence of hydronephrosis found at autopsy in this age group is about 2%.[13] In North America, obstructive uropathy remains the most common cause of end-stage renal disease (ESRD) in pediatric patients registered for renal transplantation, accounting for 16% of cases.[14] In addition, congenital obstructive uropathy accounts for 0.7% of all patients maintained on renal replacement therapy; these patients have a median age of 31 years, demonstrating the continued impact of this disease into adult life.[15] In young adults (<20 years of age), the frequency of urinary tract obstruction is similar in males and females. Beyond 20 years of age, obstruction becomes more common in females, mainly as a result of pregnancy and gynecologic malignancies. The peak incidence of renal calculi occurs in the second and third decades of life, with three times more males than females being affected. After the age of 60 years, obstructive uropathy occurs more frequently in males than in females because of the increased incidence of benign prostatic hypertrophy and carcinoma of the prostate. About 80% of men older than 60 years have some symptoms of bladder outflow obstruction, and up to 10% have hydronephrosis. In Europe, acquired urinary tract obstruction accounts for 3% to 5% of the cases of ESRD in patients older than 65 years, most as a result of prostatic disease.[16] In the United States, the number of patients on renal replacement therapy as a result of acquired obstruction continues to increase, accounting for 1.4% of prevalent patients, although the rise is not as rapid as with other causes of ESRD.[15]

CLINICAL MANIFESTATIONS

Obstruction of the urinary tract can present with a wide range of clinical symptoms, depending on the site, degree, and duration of obstruction.[2] The clinical manifestations of upper and lower urinary tract obstruction differ. Symptoms can be caused by mechanical obstruction of the urinary tract (usually pain) or can result from the complex alterations in glomerular and tubular function that occur subsequent to obstruction (obstructive nephropathy). The latter commonly present as alterations in urine volume and as renal failure, which can be acute or chronic. For example, patients with complete obstruction present with anuria and ARF, whereas those with partial obstruction may present with polyuria and polydipsia as a result of acquired vasopressin resistance in the distal nephron. Alternatively, there may be a fluctuating urine output, alternating from oliguria to polyuria. However, it is important to note that obstructive uropathy and hence obstructive nephropathy can occur without symptoms and with minimal clinical manifestations. Thus, obstruction of the urinary tract should always be considered in the differential diagnosis of any patient with renal impairment.

Pain

Pain is a frequent complaint in patients with obstructive uropathy, particularly in those with ureteral calculi. The pain is thought to be caused by stretching of the collecting system or the renal capsule. Its severity correlates with the degree of distention and not with the degree of dilation of the urinary tract. Occasionally, the location of the pain helps to determine the site of obstruction. With upper ureteral or pelvic obstruction, flank pain and tenderness typically occur, whereas lower ureteral obstruction causes pain that radiates to the groin, the ipsilateral testicle, or the labia. Acute high-grade ureteral obstruction may be manifested by a steady and severe crescendo flank pain radiating to the labia, the testicles, or the groin ("classic" renal colic). The acute attack may last less than half an hour, or as long as a day. In contrast, pain radiating into the flank during micturition is said to be pathognomonic of VUR. By comparison, patients with chronic slowly progressive obstruction, such as those with retroperitoneal fibrosis, may have no pain or minimal pain during the course of their disease. In such patients, any pain that does occur is rarely colicky in nature. In PUJ obstruction, pain may only be present after fluid loading to promote a high urine flow rate.

Lower Urinary Tract Symptoms

Obstructive lesions of the bladder neck or bladder pathology may cause difficulties in micturition: decrease in the force or caliber of the urine stream, intermittency, postvoid dribbling, hesitancy, or nocturia. Urgency, frequency, and urinary incontinence can result from incomplete bladder emptying. Such symptoms commonly result from prostatic hypertrophy and are frequently referred to as *prostatism*, but they are not pathognomonic of this condition.

Urinary Tract Infections

Urinary stasis as a result of obstruction predisposes to the development of urinary tract infection. As a result, the patient may develop cystitis with dysuria and frequency or pyelonephritis with loin pain and systemic symptoms. Infection occurs more often in patients with lower urinary tract obstruction than in those with upper urinary tract obstruction.

Urinary tract infection in men or young children of either sex, recurrent or persistent infections in women, infections with unusual organisms such as *Pseudomonas* species, and a single attack of ascending infection (acute pyelonephritis) require further investigation to exclude obstruction. When obstruction is present, eradication of the infection is usually difficult. Infections of the urinary tract with a urease-producing organism such as *Proteus mirabilis* predispose to stone formation. These organisms generate ammonia, which results in urine alkalinization and favors the development of magnesium ammonium phosphate (struvite) stones. This calculus can expand to fill the entire renal pelvis, forming a staghorn calculus that can eventually lead to loss of the kidney if untreated. Thus, stone formation and papillary necrosis can also be a consequence of urinary tract obstruction as well as a cause of obstruction.

Hematuria

Calculi may cause trauma to the uroepithelium of the urinary tract and result in either macroscopic or microscopic hematuria. Any neoplastic lesion that obstructs the urinary tract and, in particular, uroepithelial malignancies may bleed, resulting in macroscopic hematuria. In addition, bleeding into the urinary tract may result in obstruction, giving rise to clot colic when in the ureter or clot retention when in the bladder.

Changes in Urine Output

Complete bilateral obstruction or unilateral obstruction in patients with a single functioning kidney (such as a renal transplant) will result in anuria. However, when the obstructive lesion is partial, urine output may be normal or increased (polyuria). A pattern of alternating oliguria and polyuria or the presence of anuria strongly suggests obstructive uropathy.

Abnormal Physical Findings

Physical examination can be completely normal. Some patients with upper urinary tract obstruction may have flank tenderness; long-standing obstructive uropathy may result in an enlarged kidney, resulting in an increased abdominal girth or a palpable flank mass. Hydronephrosis is a common cause of a palpable abdominal mass in children. Lower urinary tract obstruction causes a distended, palpable, and occasionally painful bladder. A rectal examination and, in women, a pelvic examination should be performed because they may reveal a local malignancy or the presence of prostatic enlargement.

Acute or chronic hydronephrosis, either unilateral or bilateral, may cause hypertension as a result of impaired sodium excretion with expansion of extracellular fluid volume or from abnormal release of renin (renin-dependent hypertension). Occasionally, in patients with partial urinary tract obstruction, hypotension occurs as a result of polyuria and volume depletion.

Abnormal Laboratory Findings

Urinalysis may show hematuria, bacteriuria, pyuria, crystal deposition, and low-grade proteinuria, depending on the cause of obstruction. However, urinalysis may be completely negative despite advanced obstructive nephropathy.

In the acute phase of obstruction, urinary electrolytes are similar to those seen in a "prerenal" state, with a low urinary sodium (<20 mmol/l), a low fractional excretion of sodium (<1%), and a high urinary osmolality (>500 mOsm/kg). However, with more prolonged obstruction, there is a decreased ability to concentrate the urine and an inability to reabsorb sodium and other solutes. These changes are particularly marked after the release of chronic obstruction and give rise to the syndrome commonly referred to as *postobstructive diuresis.*

Polycythemia, which may subside after relief of the obstruction, has been described in obstructive uropathy. It probably results from increased erythropoietin production by the obstructed kidney.

Increases in serum urea and creatinine are the most significant laboratory abnormalities in patients with obstructive uropathy. Electrolyte abnormalities may also occur, including a hyperchloremic hyperkalemic (type IV) metabolic acidosis, and hypernatremia as a result of acquired nephrogenic diabetes insipidus.

If obstruction develops in patients with underlying chronic kidney disease, it may cause acceleration in the rate of progression. Occasionally, ESRD may be caused by chronic obstructive uropathy that had been asymptomatic.

Symptoms of Obstruction in Neonates or Infants

Although with the advent of routine antenatal scanning, the diagnosis of hydronephrosis and genitourinary abnormalities is now frequently made antenatally, obstructive uropathy may not be suspected until failure to thrive, voiding difficulties, fever, hematuria, or symptoms of renal failure appear. Oligohydramnios at the time of delivery should raise the suspicion of obstructive uropathy, as should the presence of congenital anomalies of the external genitalia. Nonurologic anomalies such as ear deformities, a single umbilical artery, imperforate anus, or a rectourethral or rectovaginal fistula should prompt investigation for urinary tract obstruction. Any infant with neurologic abnormalities may have a neurogenic bladder with associated obstructive uropathy.

DIAGNOSIS

Prompt diagnosis of urinary tract obstruction is essential to allow treatment to limit any long-term adverse consequences. Symptoms such as "renal colic" may suggest the diagnosis and prompt appropriate investigation. However, obstruction to the urinary tract should be considered in any patient with unexplained acute or chronic kidney impairment and appropriate investigations performed. The diagnostic approach has to be tailored to the clinical presentation (Fig. 55.9), but a careful

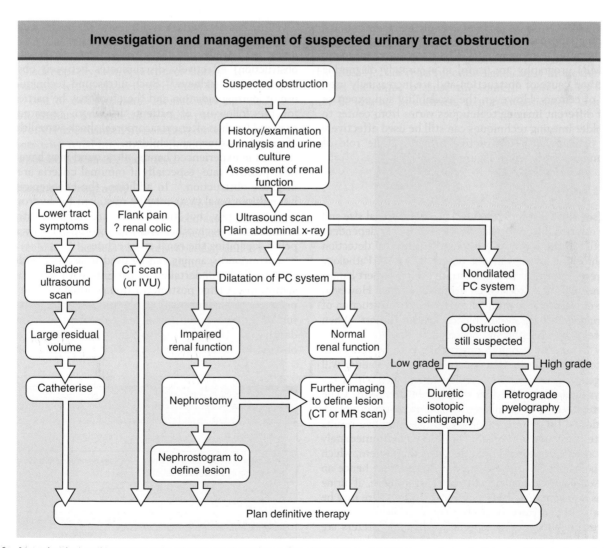

Figure 55.9 Investigation and management of suspected urinary tract obstruction. A full history and examination should be performed, together with urinalysis, urine microscopy and culture, and measurement of renal function and serum electrolytes. Ultrasound is a useful first-line investigation for any patient with suspected urinary tract obstruction. Computed tomography (CT) is now the preferred imaging technique when renal calculi are suspected. Either CT or magnetic resonance (MR) urography can accurately diagnose both the site and cause of obstruction in most cases. If there is renal impairment, insertion of a nephrostomy allows the effective relief of the obstruction and time for renal function to recover while definitive therapy is planned. IVU, intravenous urography.

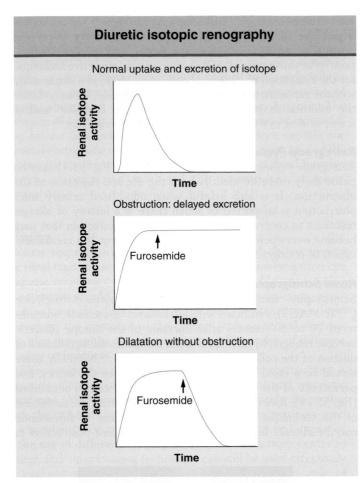

Figure 55.14   Diuretic isotopic renography. Idealized tracings for normal, obstructed, and dilated kidneys without obstruction of the upper urinary tract. In obstruction, there is delayed excretion of ^{99m}Tc-MAG3 despite administration of furosemide. When there is dilation of the upper urinary tract without obstruction, the isotope is retained but is rapidly excreted after the administration of furosemide.

children younger than 2 years because the renal pelvis normally expands during diuresis in this age group.

Pressure Flow Studies

The cause and functional significance of obstruction to the renal tract can usually be defined using modern imaging techniques including diuretic isotopic renography. A pressure flow study (Whitaker test),[25] in which the collecting system is punctured with a fine-gauge needle and, after catheterization of the bladder, fluid is perfused at a rate of 10 ml/min, is now rarely required. The differential pressure between the bladder and the collecting system should not exceed 15 cm H_2O, and a pressure greater than 20 cm H_2O indicates obstruction. An antegrade pyeloureterograms can be obtained at the same time to define the site of the obstruction.

Other Evaluations

Lower urinary tract obstruction may be evaluated by cystoscopy, which allows a visual inspection of the entire urethra and the bladder. Urodynamic studies (see Chapter 49, Fig. 49.7) may be useful in assessing bladder outlet obstruction, allow the measurement of residual urine volume after voiding, and can detect functional abnormalities of the bladder. An IVU with oblique films of the bladder and urethra during voiding (excretory cystogram)

and postvoiding can also help evaluate the site of lower urinary tract obstruction and the amount of residual urine, but this has now largely been superseded by the use of ultrasound, CT, and MR urography. A retrograde cystourethrogram will give better definition of the bladder and urethra, but bladder catheterization is required, which may be difficult if the infravesical obstruction is caused by urethral stricture or prostatic cancer.

DIFFERENTIAL DIAGNOSIS

Diagnostic uncertainty arises with nonobstructive dilation of the upper urinary tract. This condition may be seen with VUR, diuretic administration, diabetes insipidus, congenital megacalyces, chronic pyelonephritis, and postobstructive atrophy. Diuresis renography or retrograde pyelography may be required to exclude obstruction. A voiding cystogram may demonstrate the presence of VUR as a cause of the dilation of the urinary tract.

NATURAL HISTORY

Obstructive uropathy is one of the few potentially curable renal diseases, but left untreated, it will result in the progressive irreversible loss of nephrons, with renal parenchyma being replaced by extracellular matrix (Fig. 55.15). If both kidneys are affected or if there is only a solitary kidney, ESRD will result. The exact prognosis will depend on the pathology responsible for the obstruction, the duration of the obstruction, and the presence or absence of urosepsis. Relief of short-term obstruction (<1–2 weeks) usually results in an adequate return of renal function (both glomerular and tubular). With chronic progressive obstruction (>12 weeks), there is often irreversible destruction of renal parenchyma, and renal functional recovery may be minimal even after relief of the obstruction. However, the degree of functional recovery after relief of obstruction is difficult to predict, and some patients recover independent renal function after relief of months of chronic obstruction. In general, however, the earlier obstruction is

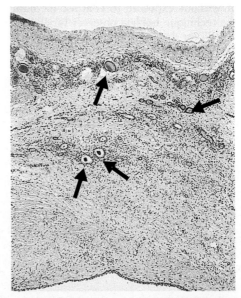

Figure 55.15   Pathology of chronic ureteral obstruction. This is a section of the rim of renal tissue from the kidney shown in Figure 55.7. The renal capsule is at the top, the urinary space at the bottom. The cortex is considerably thinned, and only a few atrophic tubules remain (arrows) within an interstitium comprising dense fibrous tissue and a mononuclear cell infiltrate (blue staining nuclei). No glomeruli can be seen. This demonstrates why there would be no prospect for any significant functional recovery in this kidney even after the relief of the obstruction.

diagnosed and hence relieved, the better the prognosis for renal functional recovery.

TREATMENT

General Considerations

The treatment of obstructive uropathy is dictated by the location of the obstruction, the underlying cause, and the degree (if any) of renal impairment. If renal impairment is present, the treatment of obstruction requires close collaboration between nephrologists and urologists in order to reduce the risks associated with the metabolic and electrolyte consequences of renal failure and to optimize the chances for long-term recovery of renal function. For example, complete bilateral ureteral obstruction presenting as ARF is a medical emergency and requires rapid intervention to salvage renal function. Prompt intervention to relieve the obstruction should result in a rapid improvement in renal function. With modern techniques, dialysis should rarely be required in patients with ARF secondary to obstruction except to get the patient fit for intervention, for example, when there is life-threatening hyperkalemia or fluid overload. The rapid relief of obstruction minimizes permanent renal damage by reducing the stimulus for renal atrophy and fibrosis. However, if acute tubular necrosis has occurred as a result of obstruction, renal function may not recover immediately.

Some surgical aspects of the management of obstructive uropathy are discussed in Chapter 56. The site of obstruction frequently determines the approach. If the obstruction is distal to the bladder, a urethral catheter or, if this cannot be passed, a suprapubic cystostomy will effectively decompress the kidneys. Placement of nephrostomy tubes or cystoscopy and passage of a retrograde ureteral catheter will relieve upper urinary tract obstruction. Insertion of nephrostomy tubes is generally the appropriate emergency treatment for upper urinary tract obstruction, especially in the setting of ARF. They can be inserted under local anesthetic and should allow rapid recovery of renal function in most patients (>70%), avoiding the need for dialysis. Once the obstruction is relieved by a nephrostomy, the specific site and nature of the obstructing lesion can be determined by infusing x-ray contrast media down the nephrostomy tube (nephrostogram, Fig. 55.16), and time can be taken to plan definitive therapy. Major complications of nephrostomy (abscess, infection, and hematoma) occur in less than 5% of patients. If both kidneys are obstructed, the nephrostomy should initially be placed in the kidney with the best-preserved parenchyma, but in time, bilateral nephrostomies may be required to maximize the potential for the recovery of renal function.

Infection may occur above a ureteral obstruction (pyonephrosis). In such patients, drainage of the kidney with nephrostomy tubes can play an important therapeutic role with appropriate antibiotics and supportive therapy.

A nephrostomy can be used to gauge the potential for functional recovery in patients with chronic obstruction. Failure of the kidney to recover after several weeks of drainage through a nephrostomy suggests that it has sustained irreversible structural damage and that there will be no benefit from performing a more definitive surgical correction of the obstructing lesion.

Long-term nephrostomy is increasingly used as a definitive therapy for patients who are unsuitable for major surgical intervention and for those with a limited life expectancy because of incurable malignancy.

Specific Therapies

Calculi are the most common cause of ureteral obstruction, and their treatment includes relief of pain, elimination of obstruction, and treatment of infection (see Chapter 56). Ureteral obstruction by papillary tissue, blood clots, or a fungus ball is treated by procedures similar to those used for calculi. When obstruction is caused by neoplastic, inflammatory, or neurologic disease, there is unlikely to be spontaneous remission of the

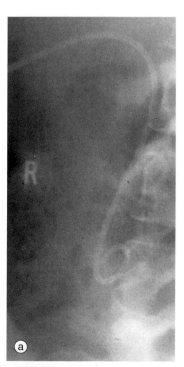 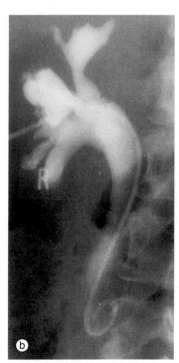 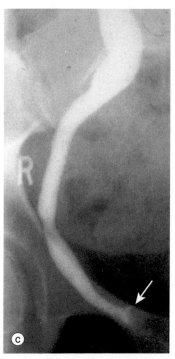

Figure 55.16 **Nephrostogram.** *a*, A nephrostomy has been placed percutaneously into the dilated collecting system of the kidney under ultrasound control. Following infusion of contrast down the nephrostomy, the dilated pelvicalyceal system and upper ureter (*b*) and the lower ureter (*c*) are outlined. The ureter is dilated along its length but tapers abruptly at the vesicoureteral junction (*arrow*). In this case, the obstruction was caused by a radiolucent stone.

obstruction, and some form of urinary diversion such as an ileal conduit should be considered. Some obstructing neoplastic lesions, such as lymphadenopathy from lymphoma, may respond to appropriate aggressive chemotherapy. Management of malignant urinary tract obstruction is discussed further in Chapter 56.

In idiopathic retroperitoneal fibrosis, ureterolysis (in which the ureters are surgically freed from their fibrous encasement) may be beneficial, especially if combined with steroid therapy to prevent recurrence.

Functionally significant PUJ obstruction should be corrected surgically. Either an open (Anderson-Hynes pyeloplasty) or a laparoscopic approach can be used. The latter results in significantly less morbidity and has good long-term outcomes that are identical to those of the open procedure. Balloon dilation of the abnormal segment of ureter is also possible, but the recurrence rate is high.

Benign prostatic hypertrophy is the most common cause of lower urinary tract obstruction in men. It may be mild and does not always progress. A patient with minimal symptoms, no infection, and a normal upper urinary tract can continue with assessment until he and his physician agree that further treatment is desirable. Medical therapy with either α-adrenergic blockers or 5α-reductase inhibitors may be used in patients with moderate symptoms. α-Blockers relax the smooth muscle of the bladder neck and prostate and, thus, decrease urethral pressure and outflow obstruction. 5α-Reductase inhibitors inhibit the conversion of testosterone to the active metabolite dihydrotestosterone and, thus, reduce prostatic hypertrophy. These agents may act synergistically when given in combination. If medical treatment fails or if prostatic hypertrophy results in debilitating symptoms and urinary retention, or if there is recurrent infection or evidence of renal parenchymal damage, surgical intervention with transurethral resection of the prostate (TURP) is generally required. Laser prostatectomy is a less invasive alternative to TURP, although long-term outcomes remain to be determined.

Urethral strictures in men can be treated by dilation or direct-vision internal urethrotomy. The incidence of bladder neck and urethral obstruction in women is low, and urethral dilation, internal urethrotomy, meatotomy, and revision of the bladder neck in females are seldom indicated. Suprapubic cystostomy may be necessary for bladder drainage in patients who cannot void after injury to the urethra or in those who have an impassable urethral stricture.

When obstruction is the result of neuropathic bladder function, dynamic studies are essential to determine therapy. The goals of therapy are to establish the bladder as a urine storage organ without causing renal parenchymal injury and to provide a mechanism for bladder emptying that is acceptable to the patient. Patients may either have an atonic bladder secondary to lower motor neuron injury or unstable bladder function resulting from upper motor neuron dysfunction. In both cases, ureteral reflux and parenchymal damage may develop, although this is more common in patients with a hypertonic bladder. Asking the patient to void at regular intervals may be sufficient to achieve satisfactory emptying of the bladder. The best treatment for patients with an atonic bladder and significant residual urine retention associated with recurrent bouts of urosepsis is the establishment of clean intermittent self-catheterization. The aim should be to catheterize four or five times per day to ensure that the amount of urine drained from the bladder on each occasion is less than 400 mL. External sphincterotomy has also been used in men with an atonic bladder and may relieve outlet obstruction and promote bladder emptying, but it may cause

urinary incontinence and the need to wear an external collection device. In patients with a hypertonic bladder, improvement in the storage function of the bladder may be obtained with anticholinergic agents. Occasionally, chronic clean intermittent self-catheterization is necessary.

Whenever possible, chronic indwelling catheters should be avoided in patients with a neurogenic bladder because they may lead to the formation of bladder stones, urosepsis, and urethral erosion, and they predispose to squamous cell carcinoma of the bladder. Patients who have chronic indwelling catheters for more than 5 years should have yearly cystoscopic examinations.

If deterioration in renal function occurs despite conservative measures, or there is intractable incontinence or a small contracted bladder, then an upper urinary tract diversion procedure such as an ileal conduit may be used to treat lower urinary tract obstruction.

Management of Postobstructive Diuresis

Marked polyuria (postobstructive diuresis) is frequently seen after the release of bilateral obstruction or obstruction in a single functioning kidney. Release of unilateral obstruction rarely results in a postobstructive diuresis,[26] despite the presence of tubular dysfunction and a concentrating defect. This may result from intrinsic differences in the tubular response to unilateral and bilateral obstruction. Probably more importantly, in bilateral obstruction, salt and water retention and renal impairment will have occurred (this is not seen in unilateral obstruction because of the presence of a contralateral normal kidney). As a result, there is an increase in natriuretic factors (including atrial natriuretic peptide) and substances able to promote an osmotic diuresis such as urea.[27] Thus, the postobstructive diuresis may be in part appropriate and result from the excretion of water and electrolytes that were retained during the period of obstruction and in part inappropriate as a result of tubular dysfunction. If the latter condition is not managed correctly, there is potential for severe volume depletion (suggested by orthostatic hypotension and tachycardia) and electrolyte imbalance, and renal function may fail to recover. Intravenous fluid, as well as oral fluid, replacement is usually required. Careful and regular assessment of the patient's fluid balance and serum electrolytes is essential to tailor the fluid replacement regime appropriately. Once the patient is euvolemic, urine losses plus an allowance for insensible losses should be replaced. Urine volume should be measured regularly (hourly) to determine the rate of fluid administration, and serum electrolytes should be measured at least daily and as frequently as every 6 hours when there is a massive diuresis. Weighing the patient daily is also helpful. Commercially available intravenous fluid preparations vary from country to country, but replacement regimens should include sodium chloride, a source of bicarbonate, and potassium. Calcium, phosphate, and magnesium replacement may also be necessary.

If fluid administration is overzealous, the kidney will not recover its concentrating ability and a continued "driven" diuresis will result.[28] On occasion, it may be necessary to decrease fluid replacement to levels below those of the urine output and observe the patient carefully for signs of volume depletion.

Future Prospects

Understanding the pathophysiologic changes that follow ureteral obstruction has allowed the development of rational therapies to hasten the recovery of renal function and limit any permanent damage to renal tissue. A number of approaches have been shown to prevent chronic interstitial damage in experimental models of obstructive uropathy. These include angiotensin receptor blockers (which decrease the degree of tubulointerstitial fibrosis), pentoxifylline (which attenuates tubulointerstitial fibrosis, e.g., by blocking Smad3/4-activated transcription and profibrogenic effects of connective tissue growth factor), simvastatin (which reduces renal interstitial inflammation and prevents tubular activation and transdifferentiation), and dietary arginine supplementation (which significantly reduces fibrosis, apoptosis, and macrophage infiltration presumably by increasing NO availability). Bone morphogenetic protein-7 (which preserves the epithelial cell phenotype and inhibits epithelial–mesenchymal transdifferentiation and epithelial cell apoptosis) and hepatocyte growth factor have also been shown to be beneficial.

However, to date, such therapies have only been shown to be effective in animal models of obstruction, and their value in human disease remains speculative. Thus, the best treatment option in humans remains the prompt and effective relief of the obstruction.

REFERENCES

1. Harris KPG: Models of obstructive nephropathy. In Gretz N, Strauch M (eds): Experimental and Genetic Rat Models of Chronic Renal Failure. Basel, Switzerland, Karger, 1993, pp 156–168.
2. Klahr S, Harris KPG: Obstructive uropathy. In Seldin D, Giebisch G (eds): The Kidney: Physiology and Pathophysiology, 2nd ed. New York, Raven Press, 1992, pp 3327–3369.
3. Klahr S, Harris KPG: Effects of obstruction on renal function. Pediatr Nephrol 1988;2:34–42.
4. Purkerson ML, Klahr S: Prior inhibition of vasoconstrictors normalizes GFR in postobstructed kidneys. Kidney Int 1989;35:1305–1314.
5. Harris KPG, Schreiner GF, Klahr S: Effect of leukocyte depletion on the function of the postobstructed kidney in the rat. Kidney Int 1989;36:210–211.
6. Bander SJ, Buerkert JE, Martin D, Klahr S: Long-term effects of 24-hour unilateral ureteral obstruction on renal function in the rat. Kidney Int 1985;28:614–620.
7. Norregaard R, Jensen BL, Li C, et al: Cox-2 inhibition prevents down-regulation of key renal water and sodium transport proteins in response to bilateral ureteral obstruction. Am J Physiol Renal Physiol 2005;289:322–333.
8. Schreiner GF, Kohan DE: Regulation of renal transport processes and hemodynamics by macrophages and lymphocytes. Am J Physiol 1990;258:F761–767.
9. Misseri R. Meldrum KK: Mediators of fibrosis and apoptosis in obstructive uropathies. Curr Urol Rep 2005;6:40–45.
10. Bascands JL, Schanstra JP: Obstructive nephropathy: Insights from genetically engineered animals. Kidney Int 2005;68:25–37.
11. Ricardo SD, Diamond JR: The role of macrophages and reactive oxygen species in experimental hydronephrosis. Semin Nephrol 1998;18:12–21.
12. Bell ET: Renal Diseases. Philadelphia, Lea & Febiger, 1946, pp 113–139.
13. Campbell MF: Urinary obstruction. In Campbell MF, Harrison JH (eds): Urology, 3rd ed. Philadelphia, WB Saunders, 1970, pp 1772–1193.
14. Talley L, Stablein MD, et al: The 2005 Annual Report of the North American Pediatric Renal Transplant Cooperative Study (NAPRTCS). Available at: http://spitfire.emmes.com.
15. U.S. Renal Data System, USRDS 2005 Annual Data Report: Atlas of End-Stage Renal Disease in the United States. Bethesda, Md, National Institutes of Health, National Institute of Diabetes and Digestive and Kidney Diseases, 2005.
16. Sacks SH, Aparicio SA, Bevan A, et al: Late renal failure due to prostatic outflow obstruction: A preventable disease. BMJ 1989;298:156–159.
17. Webb JA: Ultrasonography in the diagnosis of urinary tract obstruction. BMJ 1990;301:944–946.
18. Rascoff JH, Golden RA, Spinowitz BS, Charytan C: Nondilated obstructive nephropathy. Arch Intern Med 1983;143:696–698.
19. Mostbeck GH, Zontsich T, Turetschek K: Ultrasound of the kidney: Obstruction and medical diseases. Eur Radiol 2001:11:1878–1889.
20. Dorio PJ, Pozniak MA, Lee FT Jr, Kuhlman JE: Non-contrast-enhanced helical computed tomography for the evaluation of patients with acute flank pain. Wisc Med J 1999;98:30–34.
21. Regan F, Kuszyk B, Bohlman ME, Jackman S: Acute ureteric calculus obstruction: Unenhanced spiral CT versus HASTE MR urography and abdominal radiograph. Br J Radiol 2005;78:6–11.
22. Blandino A, Gaeta M, Minutoli F, et al: MR pyelography in 115 patients with a dilated renal collecting system. Acta Radiol 2001;42:532–536.
23. Rodriguez LV, Spielman D, Herfkens RJ, Shortliffe LD: Magnetic resonance imaging for the evaluation of hydronephrosis, reflux and renal scarring in children. J Urol 2001;166:1023–1027.
24. O'Reilly P: Diuresis renography 8 years later: An update. J Urol 1986;136:993–999.
25. Whitaker RH, Buxton-Thomas MS: A comparison of pressure flow studies and renography in equivocal upper urinary tract obstruction. J Urol 1984;131:446–449.
26. Gillenwater JY, Westervelt FB Jr, Vaughan ED Jr, Howards SS: Renal function after release of chronic unilateral hydronephrosis in man. Kidney Int 1975;7:179–186.
27. Harris RH, Yarger WE: The pathogenesis of postobstructive diuresis: The role of circulating natriuretic and diuretic factors including urea. J Clin Invest 1975;56:880–887.
28. Bishop MC: Diuresis and renal functional recovery in chronic retention. Br J Urol 1985;57:1–5.

Urologic Issues for the Nephrologist

Sunjay Jain and J. Kilian Mellon

INTRODUCTION

Close interaction between nephrologists and urologists is crucial to the optimal management of a number of common clinical problems. A proper understanding of urologic strategies helps the nephrologist to ensure that patients presenting with these problems are given clear information and are optimally managed.

Areas where such coordinated work is most important are discussed in this chapter. They include the management of stone disease, the surgical approach to urinary tract obstruction, the investigation of hematuria, and the management of renal tract malignancy.

SURGICAL MANAGEMENT OF STONE DISEASE

In the past 20 years, the management of urinary tract stones has been irrevocably changed by the introduction of extracorporeal shock-wave lithotripsy (ESWL), percutaneous nephrolithotomy (PCNL), and ureteroscopy. Because of the effectiveness of ESWL, many endoscopic procedures for stones are now more complex than previously. Open stone surgical techniques are a second- or third-line treatment in most cases. Figure 56.1 indicates the changing use of different modalities of stone treatment since the introduction of the newer techniques.[1]

Advances in Imaging for Urinary Tract Stones

In the past few years, the standard imaging modality for stone diagnosis has become plain abdominal computed tomography (CT) scanning (Fig. 56.2). This has been brought about with the

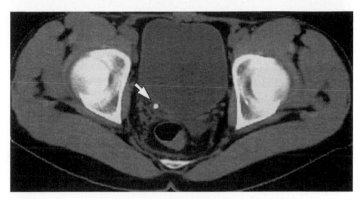

Figure 56.2 Computed tomography (CT) scan demonstrating ureteral calculus. Noncontrast CT showing a calculus (*arrow*) at the right vesicoureteral junction.

development of modern spiral scanners, which can acquire images in only a few minutes. CT offers increased sensitivity compared with intravenous urography (IVU) (99% vs. 70%) without the need for intravenous contrast. CT does require an increased radiation dose, but this is lessening with modern machines. Comparative doses are 1 millisievert (mSv) for a plain x-ray of kidneys, ureters, and bladder (KUB), 2.5 mSv for an IVU, and 4 mSv for noncontrast CT.

Indications for Surgical Intervention

Spontaneous stone passage can be expected in up to 80% of patients with a stone size <4 mm. Conversely, for stones with a diameter >7 mm, the chance of spontaneous stone passage is very low. As well as size, other factors influencing the decision for active stone removal relate to stone shape, stone composition (if known), presence of infection, and stone position. Some 70% of distal ureteral stones pass spontaneously, but only 45% of midureteral stones and 25% of proximal ureteral stones do so. Active stone removal is strongly recommended when there is persistent pain (>72 hours) despite adequate analgesia, persistent obstruction with risk for impaired renal function (for example, with pre-existing renal impairment or in a single kidney), bilateral obstruction, or associated urinary tract sepsis.

Acute Surgical Intervention

The main goal of acute surgical intervention is to relieve obstruction, and in the setting of possible infection, percutaneous nephrostomy (PCN) is the preferred option because it can be done under local anesthesia and has less chance of causing septicemia than endoscopic surgery (Fig. 56.3). If the patient is considered well enough for general anesthesia, ureteroscopic stone destruction can be attempted in most cases. If this is unsuccessful, a double J stent (a uretreal stent with two coiled ends) can be inserted, which will relieve obstruction until subsequent

Changing use of techniques for stone removal			
	1984	1990	1999
Location (%)			
Calyceal stones	35	43	46
Pelvic stones	42	20	13
Staghorn stones	8	3	1
Ureteral stones	15	34	40
Treatment modality (%)			
ESWL	64	79	78
PCNL	20	5	2
Ureteroscopy	11	15	20
Open surgery	9	1	0.1

Figure 56.1 Changing use of techniques for stone removal. The changes in the application of surgical techniques for stone removal since the introduction of extracorporeal shock-wave lithotripsy (ESWL) and percutaneous nephrolithotomy (PCNL). (Data from Rassweiler JJ, Renner C, Eisenberger F: The management of complex renal stones. BJU Int 2000;86:919–928.)

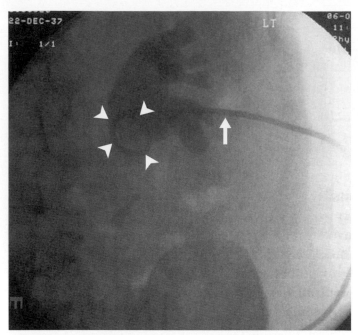

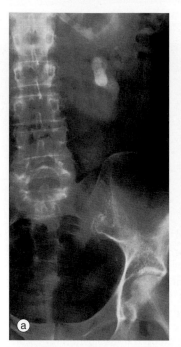

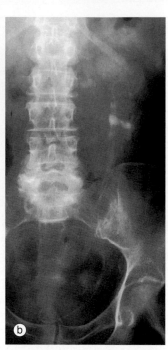

Figure 56.3 Nephrostogram in ureteral obstruction due to a stone. Contrast is injected through a percutaneous nephrostomy tube placed in the lower pole calyx *(arrow)*. The contrast outlines a single large calculus *(arrowheads)* producing complete obstruction at the pelviureteral junction.

Figure 56.5 Extracorporeal shock-wave lithotripsy (ESWL) complicated by Steinstrasse. *a,* Preoperative plain radiograph showing stones in the left renal pelvis. *b,* After ESWL, note the disappearance of the pelvic stone, the string of stone fragments throughout the length of the ureter, and the double J ureteral stent placed to facilitate their passage. (From Weiss R, George N, O'Reilly P: Comprehensive Urology. Philadelphia, Elsevier, 2001.)

stone treatment (Fig. 56.4). Rarely, when neither of these options is feasible, it may be necessary to perform an urgent open surgical procedure to remove a stone.

Elective Surgical Intervention
Extracorporeal Shock-Wave Lithotripsy

ESWL achieves stone destruction by targeting on the stone (using ultrasound or fluoroscopy) acoustic shock-wave energy, which is generated by the lithotripter using electrohydraulic, electromagnetic, or piezoelectric energy.[2] Most patients have lithotripsy on an

outpatient basis under intravenous sedation and analgesia. Treatment sessions are usually of the order of 30 minutes, during which typically 1500 to 2500 shock waves are delivered. The number of treatments required depends on stone number, size, and composition.

Stone fragments may collect in the distal ureter after ESWL, giving rise to a condition referred to as *Steinstrasse* (literally, *stone street*; Fig. 56.5). Sometimes, a double J ureteral stent is placed endoscopically before ESWL treatment if the risk for obstruction by stone fragments is high. Other acute complications of ESWL include hemorrhage or hematoma, infection, injury to adjacent organs, and arrhythmias. The major late complication is stone recurrence; the risks for hypertension or renal impairment late after ESWL remain controversial.

ESWL is the first line treatment for >75% of stone patients. Figure 56.6 shows circumstances when ESWL is less effective and PCNL becomes the preferred surgical approach, or a combination of the two modalities is used. Lower pole stones are a particular situation in which ESWL may not provide optimal clearance because of problems with the drainage of residual fragments. A randomized controlled trial has shown that for lower pole stones larger than 10 mm, PCNL has much better clearance rates than ESWL (92% vs. 23%).[3]

Percutaneous Nephrolithotomy

Preoperatively, an IVU is used to plan access, and an ultrasound scan helps to determine the optimal site of puncture and the position of the stone in the kidney (ventral or dorsal) and to ensure that neighboring organs (e.g., spleen, liver, large bowel, pleura, or lungs) are not in the planned access path. Three-dimensional CT scan stone reconstruction to improve localization has recently been used in morbidly obese patients and those with malrotation and renal hypermobility when ultrasound and fluoroscopy are compromised.[4] The percutaneous puncture may be facilitated by

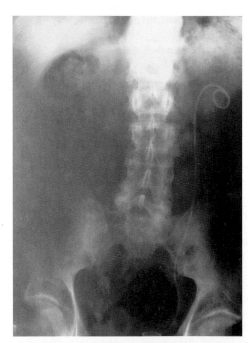

Figure 56.4 Ureteral stenting. Plain radiograph showing a double J ureteral stent in the left ureter. Note that the curled ends of the stent remain in the pelvis and the bladder despite ureteral peristalsis.

Indications for percutaneous nephrolithotomy		
Large Stones	Stone >3 cm or Staghorn	
Composition*	Struvite stones	Complete removal necessary to eliminate infection and minimize stone recurrence
	Calcium oxalate monohydrate stones	Difficult to pulverize by ESWL
	Cystine stones	Difficult to pulverize by ESWL
Stone position	Lower pole stones	Fragments less easily evacuated from dependent lower pole calyces, especially if collecting system dilated
Anatomic abnormalities	PUJ obstruction Calyceal diverticula	Prevent passage of fragments after ESWL
Patient characteristics	Morbid obesity Ureteral obstruction	Stone cannot be placed in focal point of ESWL machine

Figure 56.6 Indications for percutaneous nephrolithotomy (PCNL). ESWL is the first choice of treatment for stone intervention except in those circumstances, that may favor PCNL. *Stone composition can only be defined with certainty by direct stone analysis, but advances in imaging may ultimately provide a means to accurately assess stone composition *in situ* before treatment, thus allowing the urologist to select the treatment most likely to be successful.

the preliminary placement of a retrograde ureteral catheter to dilate and opacify the collecting system, which is then punctured using fluoroscopy. The most frequently used access site is the dorsal calyx of the lower pole. After tract dilation, the nephroscope is inserted, and stone fragmentation is undertaken by ultrasonic, electrohydraulic, or laser lithotripsy using a probe passed through the nephroscope and placed on the surface of the stone. After completion of PCNL, a self-retaining balloon nephrostomy tube is used to tamponade the tract and provide further access if needed. Complications of PCNL include hemorrhage (from renal or, rarely, intercostal arteries), which can usually be treated by selective angio-embolization. Other complications include sepsis; injury to spleen, pleura, or colon; extravasation; retained fragments; and stone granuloma due to migration of stone fragments into the ureteral wall. Perinephric scarring after PCNL may also make subsequent open surgery more difficult. PCNL usually results in minimal parenchymal injury, and the amount of renal damage averages only 0.15% of the total renal cortex.[5] *Mini-perc*, establishing a smaller-than-normal tract during the nephrostomy, has recently been advocated to reduce parenchymal damage even further; high stone-free rates are reported, and the procedure can be converted to a bigger tract if necessary.[6]

The PCNL technique is modified for special circumstances, usually by altering the site of puncture—for example, directly into a calyceal diverticulum—or if there are ureteral stones, using a higher-placed puncture to permit antegrade ureteroscopy. In a transplanted kidney, ureteral catheterization may be difficult, and ultrasound-guided puncture is an alternative approach.

Indications for PCNL are shown in Figure 56.6; these continue to evolve and are being challenged by developments in ureteroscopic techniques, which are allowing more upper ureteral and renal pelvis stones to be dealt with using a retrograde approach.

Ureteroscopy

Recent advances in the design of endoscopes for ureteronephroscopy have rendered the entire urinary tract accessible to endo-

scopic examination and manipulation. Ureteroscopes may be semirigid or flexible. Semirigid instrument channels vary in size and number and in whether the channel is straight or curved. Ultrasound probes require straight channels, but the lithoclast will pass through a gentle curvature. Flexible instruments are the only true ureteronephroscopes. They have poorer resolution and smaller working channels than rigid instruments. As well as stone fragmentation, ureteroscopy allows ureteral dilation by bougie or balloon techniques. The main energy source used for ureteroscopic stone destruction is the Holmium laser, and this has advantages of a flexible fiber (allowing intrarenal stone fragmentation), low tissue penetration, and minimal stone displacement during use. Success rates for laser fragmentation of ureteral stones are high, 70% to 80% overall. Graspers can be used to remove small fragments, but the use of baskets to remove stones whole is not now recommended because of the risk for ureteral detachment. Other complications of ureteroscopic techniques include perforation, extravasation, mucosal damage, hematuria, infection, and stricture.

Management of Staghorn Calculus

Staghorn calculus should usually be managed by intervention because reports of conservative therapy show a high rate of nephrectomy (up to 50%) and an increase in associated morbidity (mainly renal failure) and mortality (up to 28%).[7] Surgical options are ESWL monotherapy, complete endoscopic stone removal, or a combined approach using PCNL for debulking followed by ESWL. The advantage of the combined approach is the reduced need for additional renal access and secondary endourologic procedures. The choice of treatment depends on many factors, including the age and renal function of the patient. ESWL will not usually render the patient entirely stone free (the ideal goal of treatment), especially when treating large staghorns; nevertheless, achieving <40% of a staghorn persisting as fragments can still be considered successful.

SURGICAL MANAGEMENT OF URINARY TRACT OBSTRUCTION

Upper Tract Obstruction

The causes of upper tract obstruction are listed in Chapter 55, Figure 55.1, and a summary of the treatment of urinary tract obstruction is found toward the end of Chapter 55. Common surgical problems are the correction of pelvic-ureteral junction (PUJ) obstruction and the management of patients with upper tract malignancy due to an underlying malignancy.

Pelvic-Ureteral Junction Obstruction

Until recently, the standard approach to PUJ obstruction was the open surgical pyeloplasty. In recent years, minimally invasive surgery has offered alternatives, including percutaneous antegrade endopyelotomy, ureteroscopic endopyelotomy, and laparoscopic pyeloplasty. Of these, laparoscopic pyeloplasty appears to be emerging as the new gold standard because it is the only procedure with success rates equal to those of open pyeloplasty (95%).[8]

Upper Tract Obstruction Due to Malignancy

Upper tract obstruction due to malignancy can be a result of direct tumor invasion or external compression due to metastatic lymph node involvement or, rarely, due to true metastasis to the ureter. Some 70% of tumors causing ureteral obstruction are genitourinary (cervical, bladder, prostate) in origin, with breast and gastrointestinal carcinomas and lymphoma constituting the majority of the remainder.[9] Ureteral obstruction may also be secondary to retroperitoneal fibrosis following combinations of surgery, systemic chemotherapy, and pelvic irradiation. Upper tract obstruction due to malignancy rarely presents with classic acute ureteral colic, which is typically seen with ureteral obstruction due to a benign cause such as a stone. When obstruction is due to malignancy, progressive upper tract obstruction develops, often insidiously. Progressive obstruction of one upper tract remains unrecognized until the patient presents with anuria and uremia due to subsequent compromise of the contralateral ureter.

Techniques for Ureteral Decompression

When possible, a satisfactorily functioning double J ureteral stent is preferable. The most straightforward approach is to place the stent retrogradely through a cystoscope. Bilateral stents should be placed if technically possible. However, trigonal anatomy can be distorted owing to tumor infiltration, making identification of ureteral orifices for double J stent insertion impossible at the time of cystoscopy. Complications of ureteral stents include migration, obstruction with proteinaceous material, infection, and fragmentation. They may cause uncomfortable vesicoureteral reflux and erode through the urinary tract.[10] Patients may also experience bladder spasm from irritation of the trigone, which generally subsides within several weeks of stent placement.

If stents cannot be inserted, PCN is required. PCN may also be a safer initial approach in the acute situation, particularly if a uremic patient is hyperkalemic or septic. PCN can then be followed after an interval with antegrade ureteral stenting, and the success rate of this combined approach is high (>90%).[11] In patients with bilateral ureteral obstruction, it is not always necessary to insert bilateral PCN tubes. Significant palliation and return to near-normal renal function can be accomplished by the insertion of a single stent, targeted at the side with the better preserved renal parenchyma as determined by CT scan or ultrasound.

Once placed, PCN tubes or double J stents need to be replaced every 4 to 6 months. If left longer, they become increasingly brittle and encrusted and are liable to crack or break when manipulated.

Morbidity after stenting or PCN is similar.[12] The main problems with indwelling stents are the increased risk for recurrent obstruction (11% vs. 1%). PCN may have an increased infection rate, and there may be psychological issues relating to the need for an external drainage bag.

Extra-anatomic stents are an alternative for patients in whom conventional stent insertion has failed or for whom permanent nephrostomy drainage is unacceptable. An extra-anatomic stent is placed by an initial percutaneous puncture and insertion of the upper end of a long (50-cm double J stent) into the kidney. A subcutaneous tunnel is then created to bring the stent to the level of the iliac crest. A further tunnel is fashioned to bring the lower end of the stent out suprapubically, followed, finally, by suprapubic puncture of a full bladder and insertion of the lower end[13] (Fig. 56.7). Extra-anatomic stents are usually changed at intervals of 6 months.

Preliminary experience with metallic, self-expanding stents, used alone or in conjunction with double J stents for malignant ureteral obstruction, confirms their value in maintaining ureteral patency and avoiding PCN.[14]

Open Surgical Techniques

Today, open nephrostomy, cutaneous ureterostomy, and formal urinary diversion are rarely performed and would only be considered when endourologic procedures are unsuccessful. Major operative reconstruction (revision of ileal ureteral anastomoses,

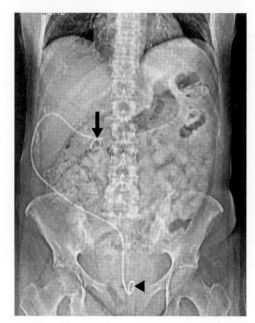

Figure 56.7 Extra-anatomic stenting for malignant ureteral obstruction. Magnetic resonance imaging study showing placement of an extra-anatomic stent for malignant obstruction of the right ureter. The upper end of the double J stent has been placed in the right renal pelvis (arrow). The stent then runs through a subcutaneous tunnel before the lower end enters the bladder (arrowhead).

ureteral reimplantation, ileal ureter interposition) is only considered when the patient is free of disease and has a relatively good prognosis.

When Is Ureteral Decompression Justified?

The diagnosis of upper tract obstruction due to cancer can pose significant ethical issues for those involved in the patient's care. The decision to offer ureteral decompression is not straightforward and requires input not only from the urologist but also from colleagues in radiation and medical oncology and the palliative care team, as well as careful discussion of the options with the patient and family. In addition, to reach an accurate diagnosis, the assistance of colleagues in radiology and pathology is often required, emphasizing the multidisciplinary approach that is mandatory in the management of this group of patients.

Ureteral decompression is justified when radiotherapy or systemic chemotherapy remain therapeutic options after improvement in renal function (discussed earlier) but may also be justified for palliation of pain or ongoing renal tract sepsis.

A review of patients undergoing PCN for obstructive uropathy secondary to pelvic malignant disease identified a group of patients with very poor survival in whom ureteral decompression is usually not justified[15] (Fig. 56.8). Patients with gastric or pancreatic cancer survive a median of only 1.4 months after ureteral decompression, questioning the benefit of such a procedure in this setting.[16] In another report, the average survival of patients with advanced malignancies undergoing endourologic diversion was only 5 months, half of which time was spent in the hospital.[17]

Lower Tract Obstruction

A list of causes of lower tract obstruction is given in Chapter 55, Figure 55.2. The most common causes relate to either benign or malignant disease of the prostate. Obstructive uropathy due to prostatic disease can be on the basis of bladder outlet obstruction (in benign prostatic hyperplasia or prostate cancer) or can

Percutaneous nephrostomy for malignant obstructive uropathy

	Median Survival (wk)	5-yr Survival Rate (%)
Group I: primary untreated malignancy	27	10
Group II: recurrent malignancy with further treatment	20	20
Group III: recurrent malignancy with no further treatment	6.5	None survived >1 yr
Group IV: benign disease as a result of previous treatment	Not stated	64
Overall	26	22

Figure 56.8 Percutaneous nephrostomy for malignant obstructive uropathy. Outcome in 77 patients undergoing percutaneous nephrostomy for obstructive uropathy secondary to pelvic malignant disease. (Data from Lau MW, Temperley DE, Mehta S, et al: Urinary tract obstruction and nephrostomy drainage in pelvic malignant disease. Br J Urol 1995;76:565–569.)

be due to obstruction at the level of the vesicoureteral junctions (in prostate cancer). This distinction is easily made by the volume of residual urine in the bladder after urethral catheterization. The immediate management of bladder outlet obstruction, regardless of the prostatic pathology, is usually by the passage of a urethral catheter, although suprapubic catheterization may be required if the urethral anatomy is distorted. Obstructive uropathy due to tumor invasion of the vesicoureteral junctions requires insertion of either a PCN or double J stents.

INVESTIGATION OF HEMATURIA

Macroscopic (visible) hematuria is perhaps the most important symptom in urologic practice and, quite apart from being alarming to the patient, can be the first presenting sign of an underlying malignant condition of the urinary tract (often a transitional cell tumor of the bladder). Studies show that 15% to 22% of patients with visible hematuria have an underlying genitourinary tract malignancy.

Patients with *macroscopic* hematuria must be distinguished from those who have been found to have *dipstick* hematuria or *microscopic* hematuria, in whom the risk for malignancy is significantly lower (malignancy rate, 2% to 11%).

The outcome of full evaluation of a large group of patients (with both macroscopic and microscopic hematuria) attending a hematuria clinic is shown in Figure 56.9.[18] As well as the small but important group of patients in whom malignancy was identified, there was a significant pickup rate of parenchymal renal disease (about 10%) in both macroscopic and microscopic hematuria. It is also important to note the sizable proportion of patients in whom a definitive diagnosis could not be reached.

Evaluation of Macroscopic Hematuria

All adults with a single episode of macroscopic hematuria require full urologic evaluation, including renal imaging and cystoscopy. The only exception to this rule occurs when an adult aged <40 years gives a history characteristic of glomerular hematuria such as is typically seen in immunoglobulin A (IgA) nephropathy, in which dark brown hematuria lasting 24 to 48 hours coincides with

intercurrent mucosal infection, usually of the upper respiratory tract. This hematuria may be painless, or there may be bilateral loin ache. These young adults should be referred first for nephrologic assessment.

Evaluation of Asymptomatic Microscopic Hematuria

The precise definition of microscopic hematuria remains contentious, and it has also been controversial whether these patients should be investigated by a urologist or nephrologist, and how patients should be followed if investigations are negative.[19]

In 2001, the recommendations of the American Urological Association (AUA) Best Practice Policy Panel on the management of asymptomatic microscopic hematuria in adults were published, providing an evidence-based set of guidelines for family physicians, urologists, and nephrologists in dealing with this condition.[20] Interpretation of the evidence continues to produce controversy about the likelihood of identifying a cause for hematuria.

Microscopic hematuria is very common—the prevalence is at least 2% of the population. It is more common in women and with increasing age (see Chapter 16, Fig. 16.7). There is no evidence to justify screening for microscopic hematuria except in specific high-risk groups, for example, those with occupational exposure to oncogenic chemicals or dyes (including benzene and aromatic amines).

The recommended definition of microscopic hematuria is three or more red blood cells per high-power field on microscopic evaluation of urinary sediment from two of three properly collected urinalysis specimens. It is important to appreciate that dipstick-positive hematuria may still herald significant disease in

Outcome of evaluation in a hematuria clinic

Diagnoses Found	All(%)	Microscopic Hematuria (%)	Macroscopic Hematuria (%)
No diagnosis	1168 (60.5)	670 (68.2)	498 (52.5)
Renal cancer	12 (0.6)	3 (0.3)	9 (0.9)
Upper tract transitional cell carcinoma	2 (0.1)	1 (0.1)	1 (0.1)
Bladder cancer	230 (11.9)	47 (4.8)	183 (19.3)
Prostate cancer	8 (0.4)	2 (0.2)	6 (0.6)
Stone disease	69 (3.6)	39 (4.0)	30 (3.2)
Urinary tract infection	251 (13.0)	128 (13.0)	123 (13.0)
Renal parenchymal disease	190 (9.8)	92 (9.4)	98 (10.3)

Likelihood of Finding Malignancy*	Microscopic Hematuria	Macroscopic Hematuria
Male, age > 40 yr	8	24
Male, age < 40 yr	1.7 (1 case)	6.5
Female, age > 40 yr	5.2	19
Female, age <40 yr	none	none

Figure 56.9 Outcome of evaluation in a hematuria clinic. *Percentage of cases investigated, according to age. (Data from Khadra MH, Pickard RS, Charlton M, et al: A prospective analysis of 1,930 patients with haematuria to evaluate current diagnostic practice. J Urol 2000;163:524–527.)

the absence of red cells on microscopy because red cells may lyse in alkaline or hypotonic urine before reaching the laboratory for analysis. Urine microscopy is discussed further in Chapter 4. If a careful history suggests a benign cause for the hematuria, the patient should undergo repeat urinalysis 48 hours after cessation of the implicated activity (i.e., menstruation, vigorous exercise, sexual activity, or trauma). No additional evaluation is warranted if the hematuria has resolved.

Two of three positive tests are sufficient to justify evaluation because intermittent hematuria still carries a significant risk for malignancy. Full evaluation should still be considered if there is only a single positive test or if there are only one or two red blood cells per high-power field, when there are risk factors for significant disease (Fig. 56.10).

Complete evaluation of microscopic hematuria includes a history and physical examination, laboratory analysis, and radiologic imaging of the upper urinary tract, followed by cystoscopic examination of the bladder (see Fig. 56.10). In women, urethral and vaginal examinations should be performed to exclude local causes of microscopic hematuria. In uncircumcised men, the foreskin should be retracted to expose the glans penis, if possible. If a phimosis is present, a catheter specimen of urine may be required. Patients with urinary tract infection should be treated appropriately, and urinalysis should be repeated 6 weeks after treatment. If the hematuria resolves with treatment, no additional evaluation is necessary. Serum creatinine should be measured. The remaining laboratory investigations are guided by specific findings of the history, physical examination, and urinalysis. In some instances, cytologic evaluation of exfoliated cells in the voided urine may also be performed. These AUA guidelines are likely to undergo continuing review. Voided urine cytology is becoming controversial as part of the urologic evaluation of hematuria because most urothelial tumors are detected by other modalities. The role of cystoscopy in the evaluation of low-risk patients is also increasingly debated. There is now evidence to justify avoiding cystoscopy in females <40 years. However, many authorities still recommend cystoscopy in males <40 years because the risk for bladder cancer, although very small, is higher than in young women. A number of urine tests are now available that claim to be more sensitive than urine cytology.[21] The ultimate aim is to avoid cystoscopy, but as yet none of the tests is sufficiently reliable. Virtual cystoscopy using three-dimensional reconstructions of cross-sectional imaging is also advancing to a level at which it may be an alternative to cystoscopy.[22]

The presence of significant proteinuria (>0.3 g/24 hours), red-cell casts, predominance of dysmorphic red blood cells in the urine (see Chapter 4), or renal insufficiency should prompt referral to a nephrologist and evaluation for parenchymal renal disease. When present, red-cell casts are virtually pathognomonic of glomerular bleeding, but they are often absent in low-grade glomerular disease. Accurate determination of red blood cell morphology requires inverted phase-contrast microscopy. In general, glomerular bleeding is associated with more than 80% dysmorphic red blood cells, and lower urinary tract bleeding is associated with more than 80% normal red blood cells.[23] This assessment is operator dependent. An alternative is to assess urinary red-cell size by Coulter counter analysis[19] because dysmorphic red cells are smaller than normal red cells, but this method is not useful when red-cell numbers in the urine are small. Even in the absence of features of glomerular bleeding, many patients with isolated microscopic hematuria have glomerular disease, most commonly IgA nephropathy or thin basement membrane nephropathy.[24] Because they have a low risk for progressive renal disease, renal biopsy in this setting is not usually recommended. Nevertheless, one study showed that microscopic hematuria unexplained by urologic evaluation carries a two-fold risk for eventual development of ESRD,[25] so these patients should be followed for the development of hypertension, renal insufficiency, or proteinuria.

INVESTIGATION OF A RENAL MASS

The widespread use of abdominal ultrasound and CT scanning has resulted in the increased detection of incidental renal masses. The primary goal in investigating a renal mass is to exclude an underlying malignancy. Ultrasound has been reported to be 79% sensitive for the detection of renal parenchymal masses but does not detect lesions <5 mm. Until recently, the gold standard method of assessing renal masses was CT scanning with contrast using no more than 5-mm slices. Magnetic resonance imaging (MRI), especially with T2-weighted turbo-spin echo images, may be superior to CT in the correct characterization of benign lesions.[26] Choice of imaging techniques and their interpretation is discussed further in Chapter 5.

The management of a solid mass is straightforward. Any solid mass >3 cm should be regarded as malignant and, unless there are exceptional circumstances (such as high operative risk because of comorbid conditions), requires surgical resection. An exception is when the radiologist can be confident the mass is an angiolipoma based on the presence of fat on CT images. Preoperative CT-guided biopsy is required if there is any suspicion that the histopathologic diagnosis is not renal cell carcinoma (RCC) because this may alter first-line treatment, for instance, if the diagnosis is lymphoma or metastasis from another site. Biopsy, however, is unhelpful in trying to distinguish benign from malignant lesions.

The management of mixed cystic and solid masses is more problematic. Figure 56.11 shows the Bosniak classification[27] of cystic renal masses, which has recently been updated. This classification, based on CT appearances, provides the basis for correct management according to risk for malignancy. The evaluation of multiple cystic lesions in the kidney is discussed further in Chapter 44.

NEPHRON-SPARING SURGERY FOR RENAL CELL CARCINOMA

Radical nephrectomy was for many years the standard surgical approach for RCC, and this is increasingly performed laparoscopically. With increasing detection of incidental low-stage RCC, there is great interest in nephron-sparing surgery, which appears to give satisfactory long-term survival, with careful patient selection and recent advances in renal imaging, as well as improved methods of preventing ischemia. In addition, in the past few years, minimally invasive ablative techniques such as cryotherapy and radiofrequency ablation (RFA) are being offered to patients with small renal tumors.

Indications for Partial Nephrectomy
Partial nephrectomy is indicated when preservation of functional renal mass has important benefits for the patient. A renal remnant of at least 20% is required to obviate the need for renal replacement therapy. When the residual renal mass is small, there is also significant risk for late sequelae, including proteinuria, glomerulosclerosis, and progressive renal failure.

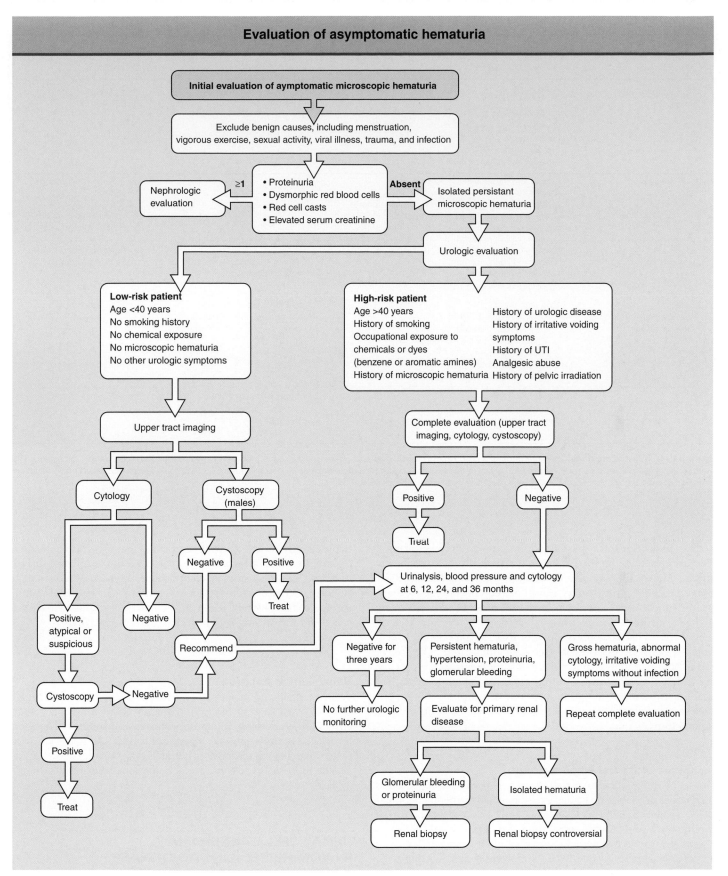

Figure 56.10 Evaluation of asymptomatic microscopic hematuria. UTI, urinary tract infection.

Classification and management of cystic renal masses			
Bosniak Class	Features on Imaging	Comment	Management
Class I: simple benign cyst	Round/oval Uniform density <20 H Unilocular No perceptible wall No contrast enhancement	Majority of asymptomatic cystic lesions	No further intervention required
Class II: benign cyst	One or two nonenhancing septa Calcifications in the wall or septum Hyperdense contents (50–90 H) resulting from the presence of blood, protein, or colloid <3 cm No contrast enhancement		No further intervention required
Class II F: probable benign cyst	Multiple hairline septa "Perceived" enhancement Nodular calcification Hyperdense lesions >3 cm	"Perceived" enhancement due to contrast within capillaries of septa	Surveillance with CT scans every 6–12 months

Class III: indeterminate exploration cystic lesions	One or more of
	  Thick, irregular borders
	  Irregular calcifications
	  Thickened or enhancing septa
	  Multilocular form
	  Uniform wall thickening
	  Small nonenhancing nodules
		About 40% are neoplastic
		Magnetic resonance imaging may improve characterization
			Surgical exploration

Class IV: presumed malignant cystic masses	Appear malignant Heterogeneous cysts Shaggy, thickened walls or enhancing nodules	Appearances result from necrosis and liquefaction of a solid tumor or a tumor growing in the wall	Surgical exploration

Figure 56.11 Classification and management of cystic renal masses. Approach to renal mass found incidentally by ultrasound or CT scanning. All patients with symptomatic renal masses should be referred for urologic assessment. Classification after Bosniak. H, Hounsfield units. (Data from Curry NS, Bissada NK: Radiologic evaluation of small and indeterminant renal masses. Urol Clin North Am 1997;24:493–505.)

The indications for partial nephrectomy include bilateral synchronous RCC and RCC in an anatomically or functionally solitary kidney. It may also be appropriate for unilateral RCC in patients with a functioning but impaired contralateral kidney, or any concomitant condition with the potential for adversely affecting future renal function.

The role of partial nephrectomy for RCC in von Hippel–Lindau disease (VHL) is controversial (see later discussion). The role of partial nephrectomy for unilateral RCC (including RCC, which is an incidental finding) with a normal contralateral kidney is not yet established. It is a valid option for those with tumors <4 cm but does have increased morbidity compared with laparoscopic radical nephrectomy.

Technique of Partial Nephrectomy
The technique of excision depends on size and location of tumor. Techniques used include wedge excision, polar segmental nephrectomy, major transverse resection, and extracorporeal partial nephrectomy and autotransplantation (for large central tumors).

Enucleation is problematic and should be reserved for cases of VHL in which multiple RCCs are often located within cysts.

Bilateral Renal Cell Carcinoma
Bilateral RCC is managed by staged bilateral partial nephrectomies or a partial nephrectomy on one side followed by a radical nephrectomy on the contralateral side. The less involved side is operated on first, which obviates the need for temporary dialysis if partial nephrectomy is complicated by postoperative acute tubular necrosis. Predisposing factors for acute renal failure include solitary kidney, tumor >7 cm, >50% parenchymal excision, >60 minutes of ischemia time, and *ex vivo* surgery.

Renal Tumor Ablation
As more small and incidental tumors are found, there has been a move to avoid surgery and perform tissue ablation, with cryotherapy and RFA appearing the most promising modalities.[28] These can be applied laparoscopically or percutaneously. The main disadvantage is that a tissue diagnosis is not always obtained. Follow-up can also be difficult because of artefact, and long-term results are not available.

RENAL CELL CARCINOMA IN VON HIPPEL–LINDAU DISEASE

VHL is a rare autosomal dominant condition with a predisposition to the development of RCC as well as retinal angiomas, hemangioblastomas of the brain and spinal cord, pheochromocytomas, cystadenomas of the pancreas and epididymis, and islet cell carcinomas of the pancreas. Individuals who inherit the associated gene may remain free of such manifestations or may develop tumors in one or more systems.[29] There is further discussion of the genetics, clinical manifestations, and general management of VHL in Chapter 44.

von Hippel–Lindau Disease and Renal Cell Carcinoma

RCC occurs in about 45% of patients with VHL. Histologically, the tumors are of the clear cell type and are often multifocal and bilateral. The mean age at diagnosis is 39 years, and there is a 30% to 35% risk for tumor progression and death.

A serial CT study identified 228 renal lesions (average, 8 per patient) in patients with VHL.[28] On CT appearance, 74% were classified as cysts, 8% as cysts with solid components, and 18% as solid masses. The solid components of cysts and the solid lesions almost always contained RCC. Over a mean 2.4-year follow-up (range, 1–12 years), most cysts remained the same size (71%) or enlarged (20%); 9% became smaller. Although it is generally thought that cysts are precursors of cancers, the transformation of a simple cyst to a solid lesion was observed in only two patients.

Some 95% of solid lesions enlarged. Surgery is recommended when the renal tumors approach 3 cm in size because below that size, the chance of metastasis is low.

Surgical Management

The results of nephron-sparing surgery for VHL appear less satisfactory than for sporadic RCC, with a high risk for local tumor recurrence. It is still unclear whether renal tumors in VHL are best managed by partial nephrectomy to preserve renal function or by immediate bilateral nephrectomy with subsequent renal replacement therapy. Bilateral nephrectomy is certainly favored in patients with multiple fast-growing tumors. In one report of surgery in 65 patients with VHL, 54 patients had bilateral and 11 unilateral surgery.[30] Sixteen patients underwent radical and 49 patients partial nephrectomy. Of the latter, 51% developed recurrent tumor, but only two developed metastases at a mean follow-up of 68 months. Five- and 10-year survival rates for the group undergoing partial nephrectomy were 100% and 81%, respectively. ESRD occurred in 23%. The evolving role of laparoscopic partial nephrectomy may affect the surgical management of these patients in the near future.

REFERENCES

1. Rassweiler JJ, Renner C, Eisenberger F: The management of complex renal stones. BJU Int 2000;86:919–928.
2. Rassweiler JJ, Renner C, Chaussy C, Thuroff S: Treatment of renal stones by extracorporeal shockwave lithotripsy: An update. Eur Urol 2001;39:187–199.
3. Buchholz NP: Three-dimensional CT scan stone reconstruction for the planning of percutaneous surgery in a morbidly obese patient. Urol Int 2000;65:46–48.
4. Albala DM, Assimos DG, Clayman RV, et al: Lower pole I: A prospective randomized trial of extracorporeal shock wave lithotripsy and percutaneous nephrostolithotomy for lower pole nephrolithiasis: Initial results. J Urol 2001;166:72–80.
5. Webb DR, Fitzpatrick JM: Percutaneous nephrolithotripsy: A functional and morphological study. J Urol 1985;134:587–591.
6. Chan DY, Jarrett TW: Techniques in endourology: Mini-percutaneous nephrolithotomy. J Endourol 2000;14:269–272.
7. Blandy JP, Singh M: The case for a more aggressive approach to staghorn calculi. J Urol 1976;115:505–506.
8. Adeyoju AB, Hrouda D, Gill IS: Laparoscopic pyeloplasty: The first decade. BJU Int 2004;94:64–67.
9. Zadra JA, Jewett MA, Keresteci AG, et al: Nonoperative urinary diversion for malignant ureteral obstruction. Cancer 1987;60:1353–1357.
10. Saltzman B: Ureteral stents: Indications, variations, and complications. Urol Clin North Am 1988;15:481–491.
11. Chitale SV, Scott-Barrett S, Ho ET, Burgess NA: The management of ureteric obstruction secondary to malignant pelvic disease. Clin Radiol 2002;57:118–121.
12. Ku JH, Lee SW, Jeon HG, et al: Percutaneous nephrostomy versus indwelling ureteral stents in the management of extrinsic ureteral obstruction in advanced malignancies: Are there differences? Urology 2004;64:95–99.
13. Minhas S, Irving HC, Lloyd SN, et al: Extra-anatomic stents in ureteric obstruction: Experience and complications. BJU Int 1999;84:762–764.
14. Sonnenberg E van, D'Agostino HB, O'Laoide R, et al: Malignant ureteral obstruction: Treatment with metal stents—technique, results, and observations with percutaneous intraluminal ureteral stents. Radiology 1994;191:765–768.
15. Lau MW, Temperley DE, Mehta S, et al: Urinary tract obstruction and nephrostomy drainage in pelvic malignant disease. Br J Urol 1995;76:565–569.
16. Donat SM, Russo P: Ureteral decompression in advanced non-urologic malignancies. Ann Surg Oncol 1996;3:393–399.
17. Shekarriz B, Shekarriz H, Upadhyay J, et al: Outcome of palliative urinary diversion in the treatment of advanced malignancies. Cancer 1999;85:998–1003.
18. Khadra MH, Pickard RS, Charlton M, et al: A prospective analysis of 1,930 patients with haematuria to evaluate current diagnostic practice. J Urol 2000;163:524–527.
19. Tomson C, Porter T: Asymptomatic microscopic or dipstick haematuria in adults: Which investigations for which patients? A review of the evidence. BJU Int 2002;90:185–198.
20. Grossfeld GD, Wolf JS Jr, Litwin MS, et al: Asymptomatic microscopic hematuria in adults: Summary of the AUA best practice policy recommendations. Am Fam Physician. 2001;63:1145–1154.
21. van Rhijn BW, van der Poel HG, van der Kwast TH: Urine markers for bladder cancer surveillance: A systematic review. Eur Urol 2005;47:36–48.
22. Nambirajan T, Sohaib SA, Muller-Pollard C, et al: Virtual cystoscopy from computed tomography: A pilot study. BJU Int 2004;94:28–31.
23. Santo NG De, Nuzzi F, Capodicasa G, et al: Phase contrast microscopy of the urine sediment for the diagnosis of glomerular and non-glomerular bleeding: Data in children and adults with normal creatinine clearance. Nephron 1987;45:35–39.
24. Topham PS, Harper SJ, Harris KPG, et al: Glomerular disease as a cause of isolated microscopic haematuria. Q J Med 1994;87:329–336.
25. Iseki K, Iseki C, Ikemiya Y, Fukiyama K: Risk of developing end-stage renal disease in a cohort of mass screening. Kidney Int 1996;49:800–805.
26. Curry NS, Bissada NK: Radiologic evaluation of small and indeterminant renal masses. Urol Clin North Am 1997;24:493–505.
27. Israel GM, Bosniak MA: An update of the Bosniak renal cyst classification system. Urology 2005;66:84–88.
28. Weld KJ, Landman J: Comparison of cryoablation, radiofrequency ablation and high-intensity focused ultrasound for treating small renal tumours. BJU Int 2005;96:224–229.
29. Choyke PL, Glenn GM, Walther MM, et al: The natural history of renal lesions in von Hippel-Lindau Disease: A serial CT study in 28 patients. AJR Am J Roentgenol 1992;159:1229–1234.
30. Steinbach F, Novick AC, Zincke H, et al: Treatment of renal cell carcinoma in von Hippel-Lindau disease: A multicenter study. J Urol 1995;15:1812–1816.

CHAPTER

57 Acute Interstitial Nephritis

Jérôme A. Rossert and Evelyne A. Fischer

DEFINITION

Acute interstitial nephritis (AIN) is an acute, often reversible disease characterized by the presence of inflammatory infiltrates within the interstitium. It is only a rare cause of acute renal failure, but this nephropathy should not be overlooked because it usually requires specific therapeutic interventions.

PATHOGENESIS

Most studies suggest AIN is an immunologically induced hypersensitivity reaction to an antigen that is classically a drug or an infectious agent. Evidence for a hypersensitivity reaction in drug-induced AIN includes the following: it only occurs in a small percentage of individuals; it is not dose dependent; it is often associated with extrarenal manifestations of hypersensitivity; it recurs after accidental re-exposure to the same drug or to a closely related one; and it is sometimes associated with evidence for delayed-type hypersensitivity reaction (renal granulomas). Similarly, AIN secondary to infections can be differentiated from pyelonephritis by the relative absence of neutrophils in the interstitial infiltrates and the failure to isolate the infective agent from the renal parenchyma, again suggesting an immunologic basis for the disease.

Studies of experimental models of AIN have shown that three major categories of antigens can induce an AIN.[1,2] Antigens may be tubular basement membrane (TBM) components (such as the glycoproteins 3M-1 or TIN-Ag/TIN1), secreted tubular proteins (such as Tamm-Horsfall protein), or nonrenal proteins (such as from immune complexes).

Although some types of human AIN may be secondary to an immune reaction directed against a renal antigen, most cases of AIN are probably induced by extrarenal antigens, being produced in particular by drugs or infectious agents. These antigens may be able to induce AIN by a variety of mechanisms, including binding to kidney structures ("planted antigen"); acting as haptens that modify the immunogenicity of native renal proteins; mimicking renal antigens, resulting in a cross-reactive immune reaction; or precipitating within the interstitium as circulating immune complexes.

Studies of experimental models of AIN show that their pathogenesis involves either cell-mediated immunity or antibody-mediated immunity[1,2] (Fig. 57.1). In humans, most forms of AIN are not associated with antibody deposition, which suggests that cell-mediated immunity plays a major role. This hypothesis is reinforced by the fact that interstitial infiltrates usually contain numerous T cells and that these infiltrates sometimes form granulomas. Nevertheless, deposition of anti-TBM antibodies or of immune complexes can be observed occasionally in renal biopsy specimens, and in these cases, antibody-mediated immunity may play a role in the pathogenesis of the disease.

Formation of immune complexes within the interstitium, or interstitial infiltration with T cells, will result in an inflammatory reaction. This reaction is triggered by many events, including activation of the complement cascade by antibodies and release of inflammatory cytokines by T lymphocytes and phagocytes[2,3] (see Fig. 57.1). Although the interstitial inflammatory reaction may resolve without sequelae, it sometimes induces interstitial fibroblast proliferation and extracellular matrix synthesis, leading to interstitial fibrosis and chronic renal failure.[4] Cytokines such as transforming growth factor-β (TGF-β) appear to play a key role in this latter process.

EPIDEMIOLOGY

AIN is an uncommon cause of acute renal failure and is identified in only about 2% to 3% of all renal biopsy specimens.[5–7] However, it may account for up to 10% of patients undergoing renal biopsy for unexplained acute renal failure and for up to 25% of patients undergoing biopsy for drug-induced acute renal failure.[7,8] Although AIN can occur at any age, it appears to be rare in children.

Before antibiotics were available, AIN was most commonly associated with infections, such as scarlet fever or diphtheria. Currently, AIN is most often induced by drugs, particularly antimicrobial agents, proton pump inhibitors, and nonsteroidal anti-inflammatory drugs (NSAIDs).

DRUG-INDUCED ACUTE INTERSTITIAL NEPHRITIS

Clinical Manifestations

In the 1960s and 1970s, most cases of drug-induced AIN were caused by methicillin, and the clinical manifestations of methicillin-induced AIN were considered the prototypical presentation of AIN. Since then, many other drugs have been implicated in the induction of AIN (Fig. 57.2), of which antimicrobial agents (in particular, β-lactam antibiotics, sulfonamides, fluoroquinolones, and rifampin) and NSAIDs (especially fenoprofen), as well as cyclooxygenase-2 (COX-2) inhibitors, have been most commonly involved. Antiulcer agents, diuretics, phenindione, phenytoin, and allopurinol have also been reported to cause AIN, and the increasing number of AIN cases induced by proton pump inhibitors should be emphasized.[9] Most other drugs have only rarely been linked with AIN (see Fig. 57.2). The clinical characteristics of drug-induced AIN are now recognized as much more varied and nonspecific than the spectrum seen in classic methicillin-induced AIN[4,10] (Fig. 57.3).

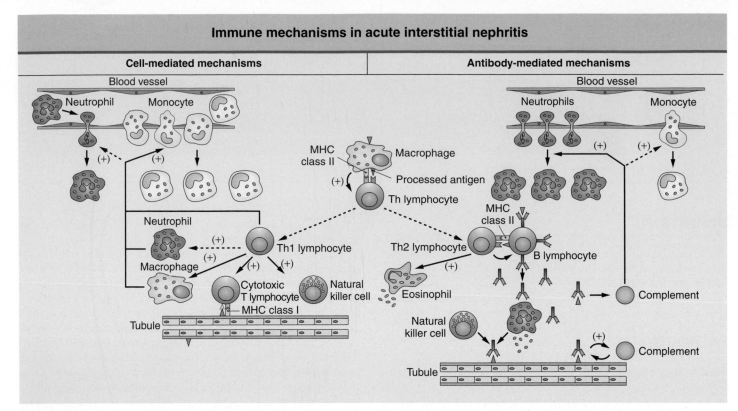

Figure 57.1 Immune mechanisms that can be involved in acute interstitial nephritis. Both cell-mediated and antibody-mediated mechanisms occur. The cell-mediated mechanism is primarily associated with macrophages and T cells; the antibody-mediated mechanism is frequently associated with neutrophil or eosinophil infiltration, as well as local complement activation. MHC, major histocompatibility complex. (Data from references [1-3].)

Renal Manifestations

Symptoms of AIN develop within 3 weeks after starting the inciting drug in about 80% of patients, although this can range from 1 day to more than 2 months after the beginning of the treatment. The typical presentation is that of a sudden impairment in renal function, associated with mild proteinuria (<1 g/day) and abnormal urinalysis, in a patient with flank pain, normal blood pressure, and no edema. In patients with AIN not caused by methicillin, the clinical presentation is often incomplete (see Fig. 57.3), and AIN should be considered in any patient with unexplained acute renal failure.[4,10] The renal dysfunction may be mild or severe, with dialysis being required in about one third of patients. Hematuria and pyuria are present in about half of patients, and although leukocyte casts are common, hematuria is almost never associated with red blood cell casts. Flank pain, reflecting distention of the renal capsule, is observed in about one third of patients and can be the main complaint upon hospital admission. Occasional patients have a low fractional excretion of sodium.

Standard imaging procedures show kidneys normal in size or slightly enlarged, and ultrasonography usually discloses an increased cortical echogenicity (comparable to or higher than that of the liver).

Extrarenal Manifestations

Extrarenal symptoms consistent with a hypersensitivity reaction are occasionally observed, including low-grade fever, maculopapular rash (Fig. 57.4), mild arthralgias, and eosinophilia. If patients with methicillin-induced AIN are not considered, each of these symptoms is present in less than half of patients (see Fig. 57.3), and all these symptoms are present together in less than 10% of patients.[4,7,10] With some drugs, other manifestations of hypersensitivity, such as hemolysis or hepatitis, can be present. Serum IgE levels may also be elevated.

The association of acute renal failure either with a clinical sign suggestive of hypersensitivity or with an eosinophilia should lead to consideration of a diagnosis of AIN, but signs of hypersensitivity can also be observed in patients with acute renal failure not related to AIN. In a study of 81 patients with acute renal failure who had a renal biopsy, signs of hypersensitivity were found in 14% of patients with drug-induced acute tubular necrosis.[8]

Other Specific Drug Associations

The clinical and biologic manifestations of AIN may have some specificity, depending on the drug involved.

As outlined earlier, methicillin-induced AIN was characterized by a high frequency of abnormal urinalysis and extrarenal symptoms and by a good preservation of renal function: renal failure has been reported in only about 50% of patients[11-13] (see Fig. 57.3).

More than 200 cases of rifampin-induced acute renal failure have been reported.[14-16] Most have been observed either after readministration of rifampin or several months after intermittent administration of the drug. Renal failure is usually associated with the sudden onset of fever, gastrointestinal symptoms (nausea, vomiting, diarrhea, abdominal pain), and myalgias. It may also be associated with hemolysis, thrombocytopenia, and less frequently, hepatitis. Renal biopsy typically discloses important tubular lesions, in addition to interstitial inflammatory infiltrates. Although circulating antirifampin antibodies are usually found in these patients, immunofluorescence staining of renal biopsies has been negative in most cases, suggesting that cell-mediated immunity plays a key role in the induction of the nephropathy. In a few cases, AIN developed after continuous treatment with rifampin for 1 to 10 weeks. It was

Drugs responsible for acute interstitial nephritis			
Antimicrobial Agents	Rifampin* (rifampicin*) Ethambutol Isoniazid	**Antalgics**	**Others**
Penicillin G* (benzylpenicillin*)	Nitrofurantoin* Sulfonamides*	Aminopyrine Antipyrine	Allopurinol* Alpha methyldopa
Ampicillin* Amoxicillin	Cotrimoxazole* Acyclovir	Dipyrone (nor- amidopyrine,	Amlodipine Azathioprine
Methicillin* Oxacillin*	(aciclovir) Foscarnet	metamizole) Clometacin*	Bethanidine* Bismuth salts
Cloxacillin Carbenicillin	Atanavir Indinavir	Antrafenine Floctafenine*	Captopril* Carbimazole
Mezlocillin Piperacillin	Interferon Quinine	Glafenine*	Chlorpropa- mide*
Nafcillin Aztreonam			Cyclosporine (cyclosporin A)
Cefaclor Cefamandole	**NSAIDs Including Salicylates**	**Anticonvulsants**	Clofibrate Clozapine
Cefazolin Cephalexin	Aspirin (acetyl sali-	Carbamazepine*	Cyamemazine* Cytosine
Cephaloridine Cephalothin	cylic acid Mesalamine	Diazepam Phenobarbital	arabinoside Diltiazem
Cephapirin Cephradine	(mesalazine, 5-ASA) Sulfasalazine	(phenobarbitone) Phenytoin*	D-penicillamine Fenofibrate*
Cefixime Cefoperazone	Diflunisal* Fenoprofen*	Valproic acid (valproate sodium)	Gold salts Griseofulvin
Cefoxitin Cefotetan	Ibuprofen* Naproxen		Interleukin-2 Lamotrigine*
Cefotaxime Latamoxef	Benoxaprofen Fenbufen	**Diuretics**	Nicergoline Phenindione*
Ciprofloxacin* Levofloxacin*	Flurbiprofen Ketoprofen	Chlorthalidone	Phenothiazine Phentermine/
Moxifloxacin Norfloxacin	Pirprofen Suprofen	Ethacrynic acid Furosemide*	Phendimetrazine Phenylpropa-
Piromidic acid Azithromycin	Indomethacin* Tolmetin	Hydrochlorothiazide* Indapamide	nolamine Probenecid
Erythromycin* Flurithromycin	Zomepirac Sulindac	Ticnilic acid* Triamterene*	Propranolol Propylthiouracil
Lincomycin Tetracycline	Alclofenac Diclofenac		Streptokinase Sulphinpyrazone
Minocycline Spiramycine*	Fenclofenac Mefenamic acid	**Antiulcer Agents**	Warfarin Zopiclone
Gentamicin Colistin	Niflumic acid Piroxicam*	Cimetidine* Famotidine	
Polymixin B* Vancomycin	Meloxicam Azapropazone	Ranitidine Esomeprazole	
Teicoplamin	Phenylbutazone Phenazone	Lansoprazole Omeprazole	
	Rofecoxib Celecoxib	Pantoprazole Rabeprazole	

Figure 57.2 Drugs responsible for acute interstitial nephritis. NSAID, nonsteroidal anti-inflammatory drug. *Causes granulomatous interstitial nephritis.

almost never associated with extrarenal symptoms or with antirif-ampin antibodies, and renal biopsies disclosed severe interstitial infiltrates but few tubular lesions.

Phenindione-induced AIN is generally associated with the development of hepatitis, which can be fatal. Allopurinol-induced AIN appears to occur more often in patients with chronic reduction in renal function and is usually seen in association with rash

and liver dysfunction. It has been suggested that the decreased excretion of oxypurinol, a metabolite of allopurinol, might favor the occurrence of AIN. A reduced dose (100 mg/day) is generally recommended in patients with chronic renal disease to decrease the risk for this complication.

AIN occurring secondary to NSAIDs is associated with nephrotic syndrome in about three fourths of cases.[17,18] This

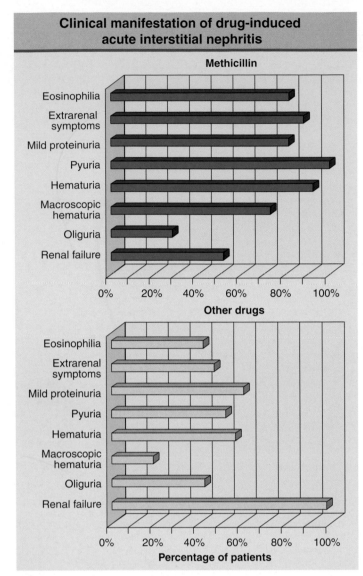

Figure 57.3 Clinical manifestations of drug-induced acute interstitial nephritis (AIN). Data were pooled from different case reports, including 95 patients with methicillin-induced AIN and 175 patients with other drug–induced AIN. Patients with AIN associated with a nephrotic syndrome were not considered.

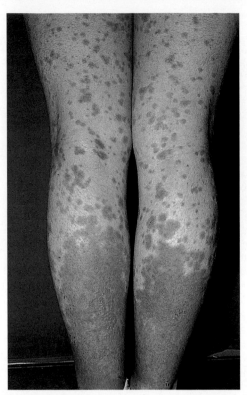

Figure 57.4 Maculopapular rash in a patient with drug-induced acute interstitial nephritis (AIN). Such cutaneous lesions occur in about 40% of patients with drug-induced AIN, but they can also be seen in patients with drug-induced acute tubular necrosis.

Pathology

The hallmark of AIN is the presence of inflammatory infiltrates within the interstitium (Fig. 57.6). These infiltrative lesions are often patchy, predominating in the deep cortex and in the outer medulla, but they can be diffuse in most severe diseases. They are composed mostly of T cells and monocyte-macrophages, but

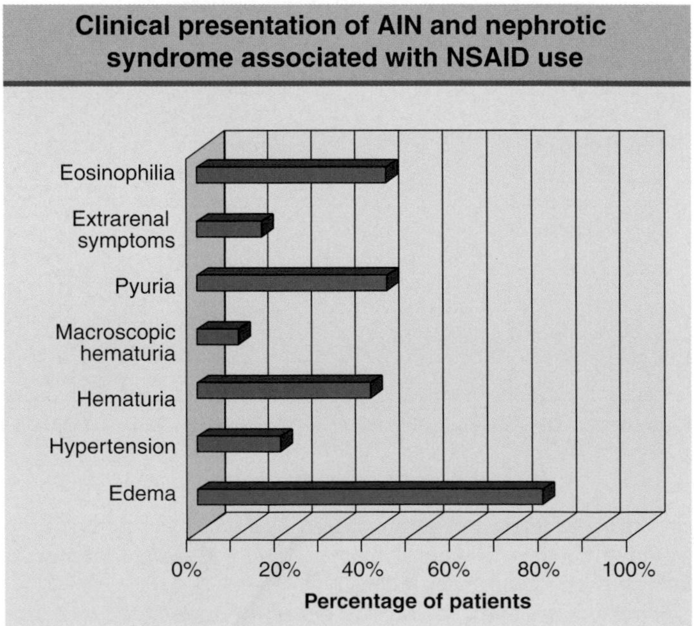

nephropathy usually occurs in patients older than 50 years, and although it has been observed with all NSAIDs, including COX-2 selective inhibitors, half of the incidents have been reported with fenoprofen. Most occurrences develop after the patient has taken NSAIDs for a few months (mean, 6 months), but AIN can occur within days or after more than a year. With the exception of the heavy proteinuria and associated edema, the presentation of these patients is quite similar to that of patients with other drug-induced AIN (Fig. 57.5). The main difference is that extrarenal symptoms are present in only about 10% of patients. Renal disease caused by NSAIDs must be differentiated from other NSAID-induced nephropathies, including hemodynamically mediated acute renal failure, papillary necrosis, and NSAID-induced membranous nephropathy.[17] Drugs other than NSAIDs can, rarely, induce an AIN associated with a nephrotic syndrome; a few cases have been reported after administration of ampicillin, rifampin, lithium, interferon, phenytoin, and D-penicillamine.

Clinical presentation of AIN and nephrotic syndrome associated with NSAID use

(bar chart: Eosinophilia, Extrarenal symptoms, Pyuria, Macroscopic hematuria, Hematuria, Hypertension, Edema; Percentage of patients 0%–100%)

Figure 57.5 Clinical presentation of acute interstitial nephritis and nephrotic syndrome associated with nonsteroidal anti-inflammatory drug use. Data were pooled from different case reports of 65 patients.

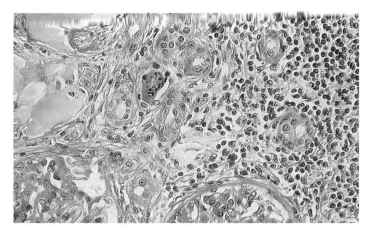

Figure 57.6   Drug-induced acute interstitial nephritis. On light microscopy, the characteristic feature is of an interstitial infiltration with mononuclear cells and normal glomeruli. It is usually associated with interstitial edema and with tubular lesions. (Courtesy of Dr. B. Mougenot.)

plasma cells, eosinophils, and a few neutrophilic granulocytes may also be present. The relative number of CD4+ T cells and CD8+ T cells appears to be quite variable from one patient to another and to be influenced by various factors, including the drug. In some cases, T lymphocytes infiltrate across the TBM and between tubular cells, mainly in distal tubules, and the resulting lesion is referred to as *tubulitis*.

In some cases of drug-induced AIN, renal biopsy discloses interstitial granulomas (Fig. 57.7). These granulomas are usually sparse and non-necrotic, with few giant cells, and are associated with nongranulomatous interstitial infiltrates. Granulomas are also found in AIN related to infection, sarcoidosis, Sjögren's syndrome, and Wegener's granulomatosis.

Interstitial infiltrates are always associated with an interstitial edema, which is responsible for separating the tubules (see Fig. 57.6). They can also be associated with focal tubular lesions, which range from mild cellular alterations to extensive necrosis of epithelial cells, and which are sometimes associated with a disruption of the TBM. These tubular lesions usually predominate where the inflammatory infiltrates are most extensive.

Tubulointerstitial lesions are not associated with vascular or glomerular lesions. Even in AIN associated with a nephrotic syndrome, glomeruli appear normal on light microscopy, glomerular lesions being similar to those seen in minimal change disease (see Chapter 17).

In most patients with AIN, renal biopsies do not show immune deposits, and both immunofluorescence and electron microscopy are negative. Nevertheless, staining of the tubular or capsular basement membrane for IgG or complement may occasionally be seen by immunofluorescence, the staining pattern being either granular or linear (Fig. 57.8). Linear fixation of IgG along the TBM indicates the presence of antibodies directed against membrane antigens, or against drug metabolites bound to the TBM, and in some cases, circulating anti-TBM antibodies have been detected. These linear deposits are seen mostly in patients taking methicillin, NSAIDs, phenytoin, or allopurinol.

Diagnosis of Acute Interstitial Nephritis

The most accurate way to diagnose AIN is by renal biopsy. However, both eosinophiluria and gallium scanning have been suggested as helpful in making the diagnosis.

Eosinophils can be detected in urine using either Wright's stain or Hansel's stain, which are both eosin-methylene blue combinations, but the latter appears to be much more sensitive.[19,20] This test is usually considered positive if more that 1% of urinary white blood cells are eosinophils. However, although eosinophiluria is frequently used to corroborate the diagnosis of drug-induced AIN, review of four large series shows that this test has rather low sensitivity (67%) and also a low positive predictive value, even when only patients with acute renal failure are considered (50%)[19–22] (Fig. 57.9). In these series, the specificity of the test was 87%, and eosinophiluria was also observed in patients with acute tubular necrosis, postinfectious or crescentic glomerulonephritis, atheroembolic renal disease, urinary tract infection, urinary schistosomiasis, and even prerenal azotemia. In particular, 28% of patients with urinary tract infection had eosinophiluria.

An increased renal uptake of gallium-67 has been reported in AIN.[23] Analysis of available series shows that in 45 patients with AIN, 88% had a positive renal scan (maximum after 48 hours), whereas it was negative in 17 of 18 patients with acute tubular necrosis. However, one should recognize that these studies were small and retrospective and also that gallium-67 renal scanning is not specific for AIN and may be positive in patients with pyelonephritis, cancer, or glomerular disease.

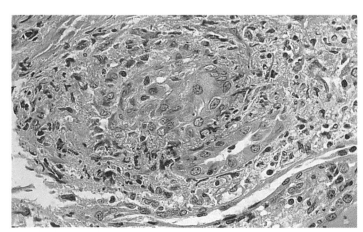

Figure 57.7   Drug-induced granulomatous acute interstitial nephritis. Some drugs can induce the formation of interstitial granulomas, which reflect a delayed-type hypersensitivity reaction. (Courtesy of Dr. B. Mougenot.)

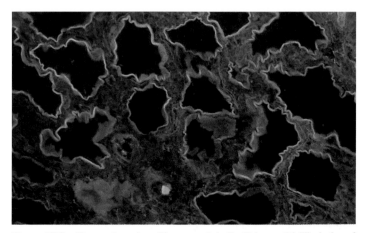

Figure 57.8   Linear deposits of immunoglobulin G in methicillin-induced acute interstitial nephritis. Deposits along the tubular basement membrane (TBM) are shown on immunofluorescence microscopy. These antibodies recognize either a component of the TBM or a methicillin metabolite (dimethoxyphenyl penicilloyl) bound to the TBM. (Courtesy of Dr. B. Mougenot.)

Vesicoureteral Reflux and Reflux Nephropathy

Kelvin Lynn

DEFINITION

Primary vesicoureteral reflux (VUR) is a common congenital abnormality of the urinary tract that may be inherited. The most common presentations are fetal renal dilation (dilation of the renal pelvis *in utero*) or a urinary tract infection in early childhood. Repeated infections in infants and children with congenital or hereditary VUR may lead to renal scarring. The small, contracted, irregularly scarred kidney that occurs in association with VUR is termed *reflux nephropathy*[1] (Fig. 58.1). Reflux nephropathy may present with urinary tract infections, hypertension, proteinuria, or renal failure; and its presentation may not occur until adulthood.[2] Although reflux nephropathy usually refers to a tubulointerstitial lesion with grossly scarred kidneys, some cases may also be associated with a glomerular lesion (focal and segmental glomerulosclerosis and hyalinosis), proteinuria, and progressive deterioration of renal function.[3]

Most cases of chronic interstitial inflammation associated with leukocytes (lymphocytes and polymorphonuclear cells) and macroscopic scars are caused by reflux nephropathy, although similar histologic lesions (previously referred to as *chronic pyelonephritis*) may occur with obstructive uropathy or analgesic nephropathy[4] (see Chapter 59).

There is scanty evidence in humans that urinary tract infection, without VUR, leads to the development or progression of renal scarring. Urinary tract infection in adults with VUR is also only rarely associated with the formation of new renal scars or progressive renal disease.

EPIDEMIOLOGY

VUR is the most common disorder affecting the urinary tract, with a prevalence of 0.4% to 1.8%.[5] The most widely used classification is that developed by the International Reflux Study in Children and includes five grades, with two grades to describe gross VUR[6] (Figs. 58.2 and 58.3). VUR may be detected *in utero* by fetal ultrasound from 16 weeks' gestation. A dilated renal pelvis (>5 mm anteroposterior diameter) suggests the diagnosis. VUR, in varying degrees of severity, has been detected as a result of ultrasonography in up to 1.0% of healthy neonates, 60% of whom are boys. Premature infants have an increased incidence of VUR that disappears spontaneously by the time of expected maturity.[7] In babies born at term, VUR demonstrated in the first few days of life may also disappear by 4 weeks of age and will resolve spontaneously in 80% of patients with grades I to III disease by 1 year of age; grade V VUR usually persists.[8] Only a small number of children with VUR subsequently develop reflux nephropathy.

Fetal renal dilation is a common fetal urinary tract abnormality. VUR is subsequently demonstrated during the neonatal period in 13% to 22% of such cases, depending on the fetal renal pelvic diameter chosen to initiate postnatal investigation.[9,10] Low-grade VUR (international grades I and II) is found in about 40% and high-grade VUR (international grades III–V) in about 60% of cases. Obstruction (pelviureteral and vesicoureteral) is found in 3% to 4% of children with antenatal renal dilation.

Severe VUR and renal damage in early life are more common in boys. Urinary tract infections in neonates are associated with equal frequency of VUR in both males and females. After the first year of life, urinary tract infections are rare in boys, even if they have VUR.[11,12]

Reflux nephropathy is responsible for about 10% of all cases of treated end-stage renal disease (ESRD)[13] and is the most common cause of ESRD in children.[2] ESRD from reflux nephropathy in children younger than 16 years at the time of starting renal replacement therapy is about equal for both sexes, and for older patients, there is only a small female preponderance.[14]

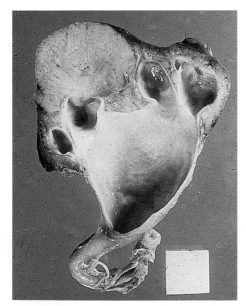

Figure 58.1   Renal pathology in reflux nephropathy. Small kidney damaged by gross vesicoureteral reflux shows focal cortical scarring and a preserved renal lobe. (From Bailey RR: Vesicoureteric reflux and reflux nephropathy. In Schrier RW, Gottschalk GW (eds): Diseases of the Kidney. Boston, Little, Brown, 1988, pp 747–783.)

Factors contributing to progression of renal impairment in reflux nephropathy
Extensive renal damage in childhood
Hypertension
Secondary focal segmental glomerulosclerosis
Altered intrarenal glomerular hemodynamics
? Angiotensin-converting enzyme DD genotype
Immunologic injury (e.g., immunologic response to intrarenal Tamm-Horsfall glycoprotein)

Figure 58.8   Factors contributing to progression of renal impairment in reflux nephropathy.

with age and growth. Ongoing high-grade VUR may slow or arrest overall renal growth.

Primary, Congenital Renal Scarring

Risdon reported a less common, but more severe, form of reflux nephropathy that is observed primarily in boys with congenital renal maldevelopment and gross VUR in the absence of urinary infection.[4] The kidneys in such children are small and smooth without gross focal scarring and have histologic evidence of dysplasia. This form of reflux nephropathy is often associated with fetal pelvic dilation and renal impairment. Although the pathogenetic relationship between VUR and this type of renal dysplasia is controversial (see Chapter 49), the degree of renal damage appears to be primarily the consequence of the severity of the VUR.[10] In one third of cases, there is renal impairment without a previous history of urinary tract infection. Half of the boys with gross VUR have a hypercontractile, small-volume bladder.[8]

Progression to End-Stage Renal Disease

Progression to ESRD occurs in patients with gross VUR whose kidneys have sustained severe, bilateral renal scarring (Fig. 58.8). Most of the initiating injury occurs during the first 5 years of life.[2] Less often, patients with lesser degrees of renal scarring, and sometimes only one kidney apparently involved, progress to ESRD. These patients often have proteinuria and focal segmental glomerulosclerosis in the unscarred areas of a reflux-damaged kidney or in the contralateral, macroscopically normal kidney

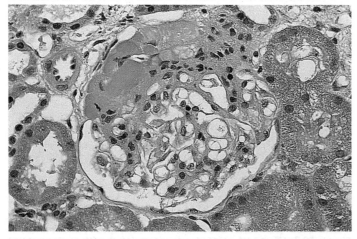

Figure 58.9   Renal pathology of reflux nephropathy. Light microscopy of a glomerulus showing segmental glomerulosclerosis and hyalinosis. (Hematoxylin and eosin stain; original magnification ×400.)

Clinical presentations of VUR
Complicated urinary infection—usually acute pyelonephritis in infants and children
Loin pain

Asymptomatic
    Detected in the workup of members of an affected family
    Detected by fetal ultrasonography
    Detected during assessment of other urologic congenital abnormalities

Figure 58.10   Clinical presentations of vesicoureteral reflux.

(Fig. 58.9). It is suggested that the renal progression occurring in these patients is independent of VUR and urinary tract infection but rather is due to loss of renal mass that leads to maladaptive hemodynamic changes in the remaining glomeruli, resulting in progressive segmental focal and global glomerulosclerosis.

CLINICAL MANIFESTATIONS

The most common presentation of both VUR and reflux nephropathy is a complicated urinary tract infection. The presentations of VUR and reflux nephropathy are summarized in Figures 58.10 and 58.11.

Urinary Tract Infections

It is not fully understood why patients with VUR are prone to urinary infections. With severe VUR, stasis owing to the large volumes of refluxing urine probably plays a role. In 15% to 60% of infants and children with urinary tract infection, there will be some form of VUR,[5] and 8% to 13% of these will have radiologic evidence of reflux nephropathy[1] (Fig. 58.12).

In neonates, urinary infection usually presents as fever, jaundice, or failure to thrive. Therefore, the diagnosis of urinary tract infection may be difficult. Suprapubic aspiration of urine is a safe and effective method for obtaining uncontaminated urine.

About 1% of all neonates, usually boys, have bacteriuria, and about half of these have VUR of varying severity. Bacteriuria can be found on suprapubic aspiration of urine in 10% of sick infants, again mostly males. In one study of 100 infants (68 boys and 32 girls), who presented consecutively with urinary tract infection, 36 infants had VUR, mostly grade III or IV.[7] These studies show that, in neonates and infants, urinary infections are more common in boys, and that with both sexes there is a high incidence of

Clinical presentations of reflux nephropathy
Complicated urinary infection—usually acute pyelonephritis in infants and children
Hypertension: benign or accelerated
During pregnancy: urinary infection, hypertension, preeclampsia
Proteinuria
Chronic renal failure
Urinary calculi

Asymptomatic
    Detected in the workup of members of an affected family
    Detected by fetal ultrasonography
    Detected during assessment of other urologic congenital abnormalities

Figure 58.11   Clinical presentations of reflux nephropathy.

Prevalence of VUR in patients with urinary tract infection, according to age	
Age	Percentage with VUR
2–3 days	57
3–6 days	51
2–6 months	60
7–12 months	35
1–4 years	50
5–9 years	35
10–14 years	14
14 years	10
Adult	5

Figure 58.12   Prevalence of vesicoureteral reflux (VUR) in patients with urinary tract infection, according to age. (Data from Bailey RR: The relationship of vesico-ureteric reflux to urinary tract infection and chronic pyelonephritis-reflux nephropathy. Clin Nephrol 1973;1:132–141.)

associated VUR. Studies of infants and young children with acute pyelonephritis, as defined by an abnormal scintigram using technetium-99m (^{99m}Tc)-labeled dimercaptosuccinic acid (DMSA) as the tracer, have shown that 30% to 60% have VUR. In another study of preschool children, the risk factors for recurrent urinary tract infections were age less than 6 months and VUR of grades III to V.[25]

After the first year of life, the prevalence of asymptomatic bacteriuria is very low in boys but is about 1% in girls. VUR is seen in one third of preschool children with urinary infection.[1,26]

Most authorities still recommend that every infant or child undergo urinary tract investigation after the first bacteriologically proven urinary tract infection,[2,11] although doubts have been

raised as to the usefulness of this practice.[27] There are a number of options for the appropriate investigation in such children.[11,28] A logical application of currently available techniques should take into account that (1) renal scarring is unusual after the age of 5 years, (2) VUR tends to resolve spontaneously with time, and (3) VCUG is perceived as an invasive and unpleasant procedure. In children younger than 2 years, the first investigation remains VCUG, together with imaging of the upper urinary tract (Fig. 58.13). If gross VUR has been present from birth, renal scarring should be apparent by this age. If VUR is demonstrated, further renal imaging with a DMSA scan is indicated (see Chapter 5). VCUG can be reliably carried out as soon as any symptomatic urinary tract infection has been controlled. Delaying this investigation because of concerns of false-positive findings is unfounded.

With increasing age, other presentations of VUR become more common. Young women with urinary tract infections associated with onset of sexual activity may be shown to have reflux nephropathy not detected in infancy or early childhood. These patients may present with bacterial cystitis or acute pyelonephritis, often recurrent. About 5% of sexually active women with urinary tract infection have reflux nephropathy. The diagnosis of VUR or reflux nephropathy may also be made after detection of asymptomatic bacteriuria in pregnancy.

Hypertension

Reflux nephropathy often causes hypertension, and 60% of adults with reflux nephropathy are hypertensive at presentation. About 15% of adults with reflux nephropathy present with hypertension or its complications and no history of urinary tract infection. Hypertension affects 10% of children with reflux nephropathy and is the most common cause of severe hypertension in children.[28] In adults, the hypertension is usually benign but may follow an accelerated course with deteriorating renal function. Hypertension may become apparent in women if they take the combined oral contraceptive or become pregnant. The risk for

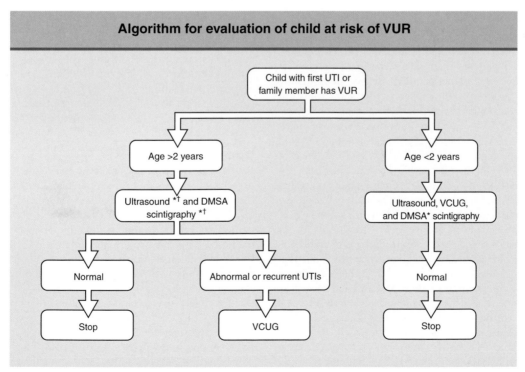

Figure 58.13   Algorithm for the evaluation of the child at risk for vesicoureteral reflux (VUR). *MAG3 renogram if evidence of obstruction. †Older than 5 years only with acute pyelonephritis. DMSA, dimercaptosuccinic acid; UTI, urinary tract infection; VCUG, voiding cystourethrography.

hypertension appears to be greater in males and increases with the degree of VUR and the extent of renal damage.[29–31] Any role of the renin-angiotensin system remains unproved. The role of nephrectomy of a small contracted kidney, when the contralateral kidney is normal or hypertrophied, in hypertensive patients for cure, or in normotensive patients for prevention of hypertension, is unclear. Hypertension accelerates the progression of reflux nephropathy; thus, meticulous control of blood pressure is one of the most important aspects of its management.

Proteinuria

Proteinuria suggests that the patient is likely to have focal segmental glomerulosclerosis (see Fig. 58.9) and a poor prognosis.[4] Proteinuria may not be detected for many years after the renal scarring has occurred, although it may be present in childhood in patients with bilateral renal scarring. Proteinuria is more common in patients with renal impairment and severe bilateral reflux nephropathy and is one of the most serious complications of reflux nephropathy.[30,31] It is uncommon for the nephrotic syndrome to complicate reflux nephropathy.

Presentation During Pregnancy

A pregnant woman with previously unrecognized reflux nephropathy may present during pregnancy with asymptomatic or symptomatic urinary tract infection, hypertension in early pregnancy, or severe preeclampsia.

About 5% of women have asymptomatic bacteriuria in the first trimester of pregnancy, and 5% to 33% of these women have a urinary tract abnormality, most commonly reflux nephropathy. About 4% of women with severe or atypical preeclampsia have reflux nephropathy. The dilation of the ureter seen with normal pregnancy can be distinguished from that seen with VUR. In pregnancy, the midportion of the ureter, more commonly the right, is dilated, and the renal parenchymal morphology is normal.

Renal Failure

Reflux nephropathy is an important cause of chronic renal failure usually presenting with renal impairment, proteinuria, or hypertension. Only a small proportion of patients with renal failure have a history of urinary tract infection.[14] The urinary sediment findings are nonspecific. Older patients may have accompanying type IV renal tubular acidosis and hyperkalemia. Reflux nephropathy should be excluded in any patient presenting with renal insufficiency and proteinuria, with or without hypertension or urinary tract infections. About 10% of patients entering dialysis or transplant programs have reflux nephropathy. These patients develop ESRD at a mean age of 30 years (Fig. 58.14). The incidence of renal failure caused by reflux nephropathy is about equal between the sexes, in contrast to the female preponderance of reflux nephropathy in adults. This discrepancy is probably explained by the higher incidence of symptomatic urinary tract infection in girls, leading to the discovery of underlying reflux nephropathy. In patients younger than 16 years, reflux nephropathy is probably the most common cause of treated ESRD. Pretransplantation bilateral nephrectomy may occasionally be necessary when there is ongoing VUR with infection that cannot be eradicated. Craig and colleagues analyzed the incidence of ESRD in patients aged 5 to 44 years who were reported to the Australian and New Zealand Dialysis and Transplantation Registry (ANZDATA) between 1971 and 1998.[32] They concluded that the treatment of VUR with ureteric reimplantation or prophylactic antibiotic therapy had not achieved a significant reduction in the incidence of renal failure due to reflux nephropathy. ESRD from reflux nephropathy is relatively rare

Incidence of end-stage reflux nephropathy in Australia and New Zealand, 1971–2000						
	1971–1980		**1981–1990**		**1991–2000**	
Patient Group	Male	Female	Male	Female	Male	Female
No of patients starting renal replacement therapy	2651	2147	4689	3844	9700	7202
No. of patients with reflux nephropathy (%)	173 (6.5)	203 (9.5)	293 (6.2)	368 (9.6)	360 (3.7)	492 (6.8)
No. of patients <16 years of age	110	87	162	133	202	152
No.of patients <16 years old with reflux nephropathy (%)	27 (24.5)	29 (33.3)	31 (19.1)	28 (21.1)	35 (17.3)	18 (11.8)

Figure 58.14   Incidence of end-stage reflux nephropathy in Australia and New Zealand, 1971–2000.

in Swedish children. Radionuclide GFR changed little over two decades in children with renal scarring detected after their first urinary tract infection.[33] Swedish practice guidelines for the management of urinary tract infection and VUR emphasize the importance of early recognition and treatment of symptomatic urinary tract infections.[11]

Familial Vesicoureteral Reflux

Primary VUR is inherited in many patients (see Fig. 58.5). In some patients, it may be accompanied by renal dysplasia.[15] There is a high degree of concordance in identical twins and support for autosomal dominant inheritance from fraternal twin and family studies. It is estimated that the gene frequency is 1 in 600, making VUR among the most common autosomal dominant defects in humans. VUR is found in about half of asymptomatic siblings and offspring of affected patients.[16,29] If a genetic marker for VUR could be identified, it would provide an excellent tool for screening populations at risk for VUR.

Other Clinical Features

Patients with reflux nephropathy may develop renal calculi and present with loin pain or ureteral colic. Calculi usually develop in the medullary cavities or clubbed calyces of the scarred regions of the kidney. Most renal calculi are radiopaque and can be demonstrated on plain radiograph if they are >4 mm in diameter. There is usually no evidence of a metabolic cause for the renal calculi. Patients with uncontrolled or recurrent infections, particularly those caused by *Proteus mirabilis*, may develop staghorn calculi.

Loin pain may pose a significant management problem in patients with VUR or reflux nephropathy. In the absence of urinary tract obstruction, continuing gross VUR, or acute pyelonephritis, reflux nephropathy does not cause pain. However, gross VUR in older children and adults may cause loin pain, particularly when the bladder is full or on the initiation of voiding. These patients may benefit from antireflux surgery.

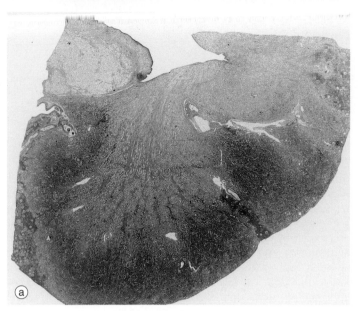
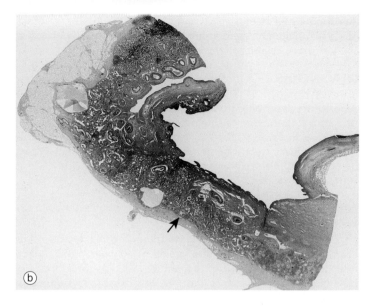

Figure 58.15   Renal pathology of reflux nephropathy. Light microscopy of a small kidney removed from an adult with advanced reflux nephropathy. *a*, Preserved renal lobe. *b*, Full-thickness scar *(arrow)*. (Hematoxylin and eosin stain.)

Nocturnal enuresis and lower urinary tract dysfunction are common in children with VUR. A number of urologic abnormalities, including hypospadias, undescended testes, a bifid collecting system, and pelviureteral junction obstruction, may be associated with primary VUR.

PATHOLOGY

Reflux nephropathy is only one of several causes of chronic tubulointerstitial nephritis, and its histologic features are nonspecific. The presence of urinary infection is insufficient to confirm the diagnosis. The recognition of the pivotal role that VUR plays in the pathogenesis of reflux nephropathy has improved the understanding of chronic pyelonephritis.[2] The pathologic diagnosis of reflux nephropathy requires, in addition to the demonstration of a chronic tubulointerstitial nephritis, assessment of clinical features, particularly by radiology, and macroscopic examination of the kidney.[3]

The gross changes and cardinal features of reflux nephropathy are coarse, segmental scars, most commonly at the renal poles, involving the medulla and cortex and overlying a clubbed calyx (Fig. 58.15; see also Fig. 58.1). Depending on the degree of scarring, the kidneys may be reduced in size. One or both kidneys may be involved. The degree of atrophy varies from lobe to lobe. Commonly, there is at least one normal or hypertrophied renal lobe. If gross VUR has persisted, the ureter will be tortuous, dilated, and hypertrophied. There may be generalized dilation of the pelvicalyceal system with atrophy of pyramids and hypertrophy of the pelvicalyceal smooth muscle. The capsule may be thickened and adherent, particularly when urinary infections have been frequent and severe. The relationship of the full-thickness scar to the underlying dilated calyx is the critical feature that differentiates reflux nephropathy from other causes of renal scarring or small kidneys[4] (see Figs. 58.15 and 59.5).

In the scarred areas of the kidney, the major microscopic changes are tubular atrophy or complete loss. There are variable degrees of interstitial fibrosis and chronic inflammation, with a cellular infiltrate composed mostly of lymphocytes and plasma cells

(Fig. 58.16). The severity of interstitial nephritis is usually correlated with the presence of urinary infection. Lymphoid follicles may be present. Collections of dilated atrophic tubules lined by atrophic epithelium and filled with homogeneous eosinophilic casts may give a thyroid-like appearance. These changes are not specific for reflux nephropathy. Rounded masses of pale-staining material that include Tamm-Horsfall glycoprotein, which has apparently extravasated from ruptured tubules, can be seen in the outer medullary and cortical interstitium. Glomeruli within scarred areas are crowded together and may appear normal, collapsed, or completely hyalinized. Collagenous thickening of Bowman's capsule may lead to periglomerular fibrosis. Vascular changes are frequent within scars, with medial hypertrophy and concentric fibroelastic intimal hyperplasia and luminal narrowing.

In patients without severe bilateral renal scarring, ongoing VUR, hypertension, or recurrent urinary infection, renal failure may develop. These patients are characterized clinically by the

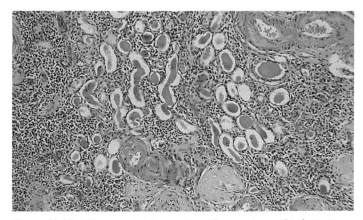

Figure 58.16   Microscopic changes in reflux nephropathy. Low-power view of renal cortex showing sclerosed glomeruli, chronic cellular infiltrate, and dilated, atrophic tubules, with eosinophilic casts and thick-walled blood vessels. (Hematoxylin and eosin stain; original magnification ×40.)

development of hypertension and histologically by the presence of focal segmental glomerulosclerosis and hyalinosis affecting the unscarred regions of the kidney[4] (see Fig. 58.9).

DIAGNOSIS

Algorithms describing the investigation of a child after the first urinary tract infection or the finding of fetal renal pelvic dilation are shown in Figures 58.13 and 58.17. Screening of individuals without urinary tract infection or clinical renal disease may also be warranted in the siblings and offspring of those with VUR or reflux nephropathy.

Diagnosis of Vesicoureteral Reflux
Voiding Cystourethrography

VCUG remains the most accurate method for detecting VUR (Figs. 58.18 and 58.19; see also Fig. 58.6). Radiographs are taken after bladder filling and during voiding. Bladder pressures and flow rates may also be measured. VUR is classified according to the extent and degree of ureteral filling and dilation and the degree of dilation of the collecting system, particularly the minor calyces. The bladder volume at which reflux is first seen and any intrarenal reflux should be recorded. The most widely used classification is that developed by the International Reflux Study in Children[6] (see Figs. 58.2 and 58.3).

VCUG is not usually indicated in adults. However, it may rarely be considered when surgical correction of anticipated VUR (to manage recurrent acute pyelonephritis or flank pain with voiding) is a possibility.

Radionuclide Micturating Cystography

Substituting a radionuclide for contrast medium is an effective and sensitive means of demonstrating VUR but is less useful for demonstrating anatomic or voiding abnormalities. The estimated dose of gonadal radiation is similar to that of conventional VCUG. Radionuclide micturating cystography is a useful technique for follow-up of patients whose VUR is managed conservatively.

Ultrasonography

Ultrasonography demonstrates the normal renal parenchyma, collecting system, and bladder. By utilizing color Doppler and contrast enhancement, dynamic information on ureteric function and the position of the ureteric orifices can be obtained, and VUR may be demonstrated.

Diagnosis of Reflux Nephropathy
Radionuclide Scanning

Radionuclide scanning with DMSA is now the preferred technique for imaging reflux nephropathy.[34] Focal defects seen with radionuclide scanning represent areas of underperfusion that are shown by reduced proximal tubular uptake of radionuclide and indicate areas of scarring (see Figs. 58.18 and 58.19). In addition, the DMSA scan provides information on individual kidney function. The DMSA scan is capable of detecting scars not apparent on ultrasound. DMSA scanning is also the preferred imaging technique for adults with suspected reflux nephropathy; intravenous urography is no longer used in this context.

Ultrasonography

Ultrasonography can demonstrate many of the features of reflux nephropathy and is now used as the first renal imaging technique in the workup of children with a urinary tract infection (see Figs. 58.13 and 58.18). Ultrasonography is noninvasive, does not use ionizing radiation, and gives a rapid overview of renal anatomy and the dimensions of the pelvicalyceal collecting system.

Other Techniques

^{99m}Tc-labeled mercaptoacetyl triglycine (MAG3) scintigraphy is a dynamic study that provides information on both the renal parenchymal uptake and the urine flow through the renal pelvis and ureters. It is particularly useful in infants in the first months of life and for the quantification of urinary tract obstruction.

Computed tomography will readily demonstrate focal renal scarring but is not used routinely because of the need for intravenous contrast medium, the radiation dose, and cost.

Magnetic resonance imaging (MRI) will demonstrate focal scarring, and dynamic studies of renal function and voiding can be performed. At this point, these studies can only be done in cooperative patients because of the scan times involved. If rapid sequences can be developed, MRI may become more widely used in children.

Antenatal Detection of Vesicoureteral Reflux

VUR is found in 13% to 22% of neonates or infants with antenatally detected renal dilation or other renal abnormalities using a cut-off point of 5 mm anteroposterior fetal renal pelvic diameter. Postnatal urinary tract investigations should include urinary tract ultrasonography and VCUG (see Fig. 58.17). The degree of fetal renal pelvic dilation does not predict the presence of postnatal dilation, nor does the severity of VUR demonstrated by VCUG, but when a cut-off point of 10 mm is used, most high-grade VUR and most obstructive lesions are identified.[9,35]

DIFFERENTIAL DIAGNOSIS

Reflux nephropathy should be considered in any patient, particularly a child, with unexplained renal impairment or hypertension.

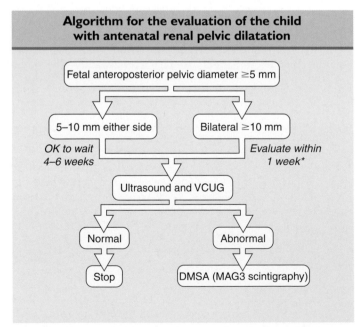

Figure 58.17 Algorithm for the evaluation of the child with antenatal renal pelvic dilation. DMSA, dimercaptosuccinic acid; VCUG, voiding cystourethrography. *Immediately after birth in boys if urethral valves are suspected.

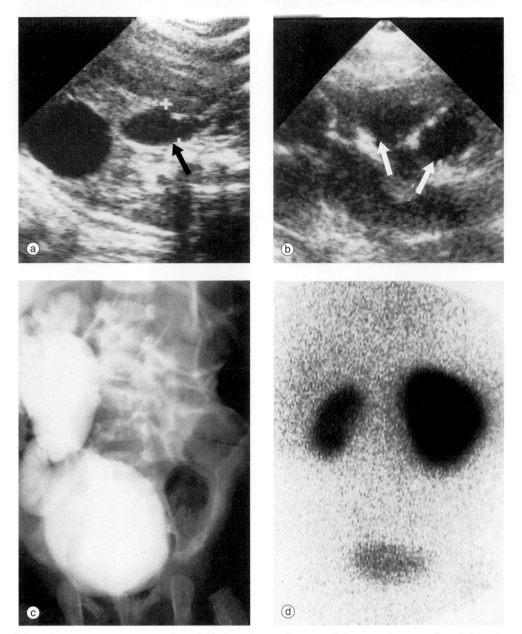

Figure 58.18 Infant with moderate to severe antenatal renal dilation, abnormal postnatal ultrasound scan, and grade V vesicoureteral reflux (VUR). *a,* Antenatal ultrasound scan at 25 weeks' gestation showing longitudinal view of markedly dilated right upper urinary tract (anteroposterior diameter of renal pelvis, 17 mm) *(arrow)*. *b,* Postnatal sonogram of right kidney showing pelvicalyceal dilation *(arrows)* and thinning of renal parenchyma. *c,* Voiding cystourethrogram showing grade V VUR on the right and grade II VUR on the left. *d,* Dimercaptosuccinic acid scan *(anterior view)* showing globally scarred right kidney with 12% uptake. (From Anderson NG, Abbott GD, Mogridge N, et al: Vesicoureteric reflux in the newborn: Relationship to fetal renal pelvic diameter. Pediatr Nephrol 1997;11:610–616.)

The absence of a history of urinary tract infection does not exclude the diagnosis. The urinary sediment findings are unremarkable, but most patients have low-grade pyuria. Nephrotic-range proteinuria is rare. In children, the differential diagnosis of a small kidney will include obstructive uropathy from a pelviureteral junction obstruction or achalasia of the ureter and congenital renal dysplasia.

Appropriate radiologic investigations should enable confident differentiation in most cases. In the adult, the differential diagnoses include obstructive uropathy, analgesic nephropathy, and ischemic nephropathy. The radiologic changes in these conditions are usually distinct from reflux nephropathy. Patients with analgesic nephropathy have a lengthy history of consumption of compound analgesics, or nonsteroidal anti-inflammatory agents, and papillary necrosis. Obstructive uropathy results in global, not focal, changes to the kidney. Patients with ischemic nephropathy usually have evidence of atheromatous vascular disease affecting heart, brain, or limbs; although focal scars may occur, the usual morphologic change is a global regular reduction in renal size.

NATURAL HISTORY

It is well recognized that some kidneys subjected to VUR become progressively damaged, whereas others remain unaffected. The severity of VUR is the single most important factor predicting renal scarring.[24] Bailey reported on the long-term follow-up of 31 infants (16 boys) with gross VUR identified during the first year of life—24 with urinary tract infection.[36] None of the children underwent ureteral reimplantation. Twelve of the 26 children who

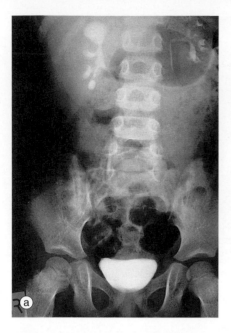 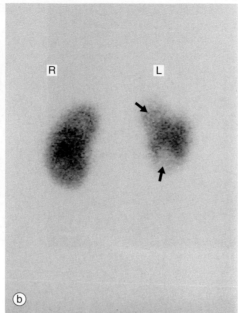 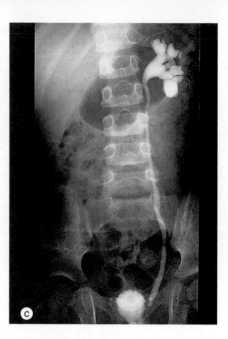

Figure 58.19 **Investigation of reflux nephropathy.** Investigation of a 3-year-old child with urinary tract infection. *a*, Intravenous urogram showing calyceal diverticulum in the upper pole of the right kidney and renal scarring in upper pole and, probably, the lower pole of the left kidney. *b*, DMSA scintigraphy (*anterior view*), demonstrating upper and lower pole scarring (*arrows*) in the left kidney. *c*, Voiding cystourethrogram showing grade IV vesicoureteral reflux on the left.

developed reflux nephropathy had renal scarring at the time of diagnosis of VUR. The remaining 14 patients who subsequently developed reflux nephropathy did so by the age of 5 years and mostly by the age of 3 years. A group of 20 patients were followed for up to 34 years. None developed new scars, and 2 of the 5 with bilateral renal scarring had renal impairment.

Two hundred twenty-six children with VUR, 85 of whom had renal scarring, who presented at a median age of 5 years were followed for up to 41 years.[13] One hundred and ninety-three were managed conservatively, and 33 were treated surgically. VUR resolved in 69%, and no renal scars developed after puberty. Hypertension, renal impairment, or both developed in 17 (7.5%) in adulthood.

Kidneys subjected to gross reflux usually undergo a steady decline in function, probably mediated by hemodynamic and non-immunologic mechanisms[29] (see Fig. 58.8). Kidneys with lesser degrees of VUR, or no continuing reflux, are less likely to suffer a decline in individual function. Assessment of individual kidney glomerular filtration rate by radionuclide techniques has shown that only the kidneys suffering gross VUR have reduced function.

TREATMENT

The most important aim in the treatment of the patient with VUR is the prevention of renal scarring and subsequent renal failure. There is no place for antireflux surgery to prevent renal scarring in adults with ongoing VUR, but such surgery may be indicated in a few adults with VUR to prevent recurrent acute pyelonephritis or flank pain with voiding. The question of the best treatment for children is much more contentious. It is unclear whether medical treatment with continuous antimicrobial therapy or surgical repair is the best treatment for VUR. Surgery corrects VUR in more than 95% of cases but does not decrease the incidence of urinary infections, with the possible exception of recurrent acute pyelonephritis. Few surgeons now operate on grades I to III VUR (see Fig. 58.2), which tend to resolve spontaneously.

Surgical versus Medical Treatment

There have been five controlled trials comparing medical and surgical therapy for grades II to IV VUR[27] and one for grade V VUR.[37] Unfortunately, they have not resolved the controversy regarding the best treatment for VUR, nor have they provided reassurance that either form of therapy reduces the incidence of ESRD from reflux nephropathy.[32] A meta-analysis of 10 trials involving 964 children compared the benefits and harms of the different treatment options for primary VUR. The reviewers concluded that it was uncertain whether any of the interventions benefited children with VUR. Up to 5 years after intervention, there was no difference in the risk for urinary tract infection between those treated with surgery and those treated with prophylactic antibiotic therapy. None of the interventions significantly reduced the risk for new or progressive renal damage.[27]

Surgery is of no benefit if proteinuria, renal impairment, or hypertension is present.[38] Prospective studies in girls older than 4 years have shown that reflux nephropathy rarely develops in kidneys that are normal even when there is ongoing VUR and urinary infections.[39]

Surgery and medical treatment can be seen as equally effective, or ineffective. Each treatment has its advantages and disadvantages. Consideration of the best treatment for any child should be determined by the preferences of the parents, expected compliance with long-term medical therapy, and the knowledge that spontaneous resolution of the severe grades of VUR is uncommon. Infancy and early childhood are the critical times for the formation of scars in children with gross VUR. With this in mind, it is advisable that those at most risk for VUR and reflux nephropathy (siblings and the offspring of those with VUR) undergo screening, including renal imaging with ultrasonography or DMSA scintigraphy and VCUG, early in life (see Fig. 58.13).

Urinary Tract Infections

The management of urinary tract infections in patients with VUR is the same as for any complicated urinary infection (see Chapter 50). The aim of therapy is to alleviate symptoms and to prevent bacterial invasion of the kidney. Bacteriologically confirmed urinary infections should be treated with a curative course of antibiotic therapy, usually over 5 days.[2] Combined or single-dose therapy is not indicated for infants and children with VUR and cystitis or acute pyelonephritis.

There is no evidence from randomized studies to guide the choice or duration of therapy. Some authorities recommend that infants with VUR of grade II or more should be given prophylactic antibiotics until puberty or the spontaneous or surgical correction of VUR, but the benefit of this is unproved.[27] Antibiotics that have proved effective and safe are nitrofurantoin, trimethoprim, and cotrimoxazole.

Children and adults may experience recurrent urinary infections. In addition to the treatment of symptomatic episodes, management includes maintenance of an adequate fluid intake, postcoital voiding for sexually active women, and consideration for prophylactic antimicrobial therapy (see Chapter 50). Antimicrobial prophylaxis should be for 3 to 6 months initially, and then according to patient and physician choice. If there is no urinary obstruction or calculus, there is no risk for further renal scarring in adults with VUR and asymptomatic or symptomatic urinary tract infection.

Blood Pressure

Hypertension in patients with reflux nephropathy, whether benign or accelerated, is usually easily controlled with standard drug therapy. Excellent control of blood pressure is the most important aspect of the long-term management of the patient with reflux nephropathy. Patients with reflux nephropathy who are hypertensive are about four times more likely to develop renal failure than normotensive patients.[40] Many physicians prefer to use an ACE inhibitor, particularly in patients with proteinuria and renal impairment. Currently, there are no data to indicate that any group of antihypertensive drugs is to be preferred for patients with reflux nephropathy. There is a small amount of evidence that removal of a small scarred kidney in hypertensive patients with unilateral reflux nephropathy may improve or cure hypertension.[2]

Pregnancy

During pregnancy, women with reflux nephropathy should be screened for bacteriuria at the time of diagnosis and then in each trimester. If bacteriuria is detected, it should be eradicated to reduce the risk for acute pyelonephritis. If bacteriuria recurs, antimicrobial prophylaxis (e.g., nitrofurantoin 50 mg at night) should be given throughout the remainder of the pregnancy. Chapter 41 discusses antibiotics and antihypertensives that are safe in pregnancy. Pregnant women with reflux nephropathy, normal blood pressure, no proteinuria, and normal renal function should be carefully supervised but are at low risk for developing problems during pregnancy. Urinary tract infection in the mother does not usually affect fetal outcome. There is increased risk for fetal death in pregnant women with hypertension, proteinuria, and renal impairment, although long-term observations have shown recent improvement in fetal outcomes. Women with reflux nephropathy and a plasma creatinine concentration >1.8 mg/dl (159 μmol/l) may experience an irreversible deterioration in renal function during pregnancy.[41] A prospective study of 54 pregnancies in 46 women with reflux nephropathy found preeclampsia in 24% with an increased risk associated with pre-existing hypertension. Deterioration in renal function occurred in 18% of pregnancies, and women with mild or moderate renal impairment were at greatest risk.[42] The offspring of patients with known VUR or who have a first-degree relative with VUR should be investigated as soon after birth as possible (see Fig. 58.5).

REFERENCES

1. Bailey RR: The relationship of vesico-ureteric reflux to urinary tract infection and chronic pyelonephritis-reflux nephropathy. Clin Nephrol 1973;1:132–141.
2. Bailey RR: Vesicoureteric reflux and reflux nephropathy. In Schrier RW, Gottschalk GW (eds): Diseases of the Kidney. Boston, Little, Brown, 1988, pp 747–783.
3. Becker GJ, Kincaid-Smith P: Reflux nephropathy: The glomerular lesion and progression of renal failure. Pediatr Nephrol 1993;7:365–369.
4. Risdon RA: Pyelonephritis and reflux nephropathy. In Tisher CG, Brenner BM (eds): Renal pathology with clinical and functional correlations. Philadelphia, JB Lippincott, 1994, pp 832–862.
5. Sargent MA: What is the normal prevalence of vesicoureteral reflux? Pediatr Radiol 2000;30:587–593.
6. International Reflux Study Committee: Medical versus surgical treatment of primary vesicoureteral reflux: A prospective international reflux study in children. J Urol 1981;125:277–283.
7. Bourchier D, Abbott GD, Maling TM: Radiological abnormalities in infants with urinary tract infections. Arch Dis Child 1984;59:620–624.
8. Sillen U: Vesicoureteral reflux in infants. Pediatr Nephrol 1999;13:355–361.
9. Acton C, Pahuja M, Opie G, Woodward A: A 5-year audit of 778 neonatal renal scans. Part 1: Perplexing pyelectasis and suggested protocol for investigation. Australas Radiol 2003;47:349–353.
10. McIlroy PJ, Abbott GD, Anderson NG, et al: Outcome of primary vesicoureteric reflux detected following fetal renal pelvic dilatation. J Paediatr Child Health 2000;36:569–573.
11. Jodal U, Lindberg U: Guidelines for management of children with urinary tract infection and vesico-ureteric reflux. Recommendations from a Swedish state-of-the-art conference. Swedish Medical Research Council. Acta Paediatr Suppl 1999;88:87–89.
12. Wennerstrom M, Hansson S, Jodal U, Stokland E: Primary and acquired renal scarring in boys and girls with urinary tract infection. J Pediatr 2000;136:30–34.
13. Smellie JM, Prescod NP, Shaw PJ, et al: Childhood reflux and urinary infection: A follow-up of 10–41 years in 226 adults. Pediatr Nephrol 1998;12:727–736.
14. Bailey RR, Lynn KL, Robson RA: End-stage reflux nephropathy. Ren Fail 1994;16:27–35.
15. Woolf AS: A molecular and genetic view of human renal and urinary tract malformations. Kidney Int 2000;58:500–512.
16. Feather SA, Malcolm S, Woolf AS, et al: Primary, nonsyndromic vesicoureteric reflux and its nephropathy is genetically heterogeneous, with a locus on chromosome 1. Am J Hum Genet 2000;66:1420–1425.
17. Mak RH, Kuo HJ: Primary ureteral reflux: Emerging insights from molecular and genetic studies. Curr Opin Pediatr 2003;15:181–185.
18. Hohenfellner K, Wingen AM, Nauroth O, et al: Impact of ACE I/D gene polymorphism on congenital renal malformations. Pediatr Nephrol 2001;16:356–361.
19. Ozen S, Alikasifoglu M, Saatci U, et al: Implications of certain genetic polymorphisms in scarring in vesicoureteric reflux: Importance of ACE polymorphism. Am J Kidney Dis 1999;34:140–145.
20. Greenfield SP, Wan J: The relationship between dysfunctional voiding and congenital vesicoureteral reflux. Curr Opin Urol 2000;10:607–610.
21. Maling TM, Rolleston GL: Intra-renal reflux in children demonstrated by micturating cystography. Clin Radiol 1974;25:81–85.
22. Ransley PG, Risdon RA: Renal papillary morphology in infants and young children. Urol Res 1975;3:111–113.
23. Fanos V, Cataldi L: Antibiotics or surgery for vesicoureteric reflux in children. Lancet 2004;364:1720–1722.
24. Rolleston GL, Shannon FT, Utley WL: Relationship of infantile vesicoureteric reflux to renal damage. BMJ 1970;1:460–463.
25. Panaretto K, Craig J, Knight J, et al: Risk factors for recurrent urinary tract infection in preschool children. J Paediatr Child Health 1999;35:454–459.
26. Craig JC, Irwig LM, Knight JF, et al: Symptomatic urinary tract infection in preschool Australian children. J Paediatr Child Health 1998;34:154–159.

27. Wheeler DM, Vimalachandra D, Hodson EM, et al: Interventions for primary vesicoureteric reflux. Cochrane Database of Systematic Reviews 2004, Issue3. Art. No.:CD001532.pub2. DOI: 10.1002/14651858. CD001532.pub2.

28. Agarwal S: Vesicoureteral reflux and urinary tract infections. Curr Opin Urol 2000;10:587–592.

29. Dillon MJ, Goonasekera CD: Reflux nephropathy. J Am Soc Nephrol 1998;9:2377–2383.

30. Kohler JR, Tencer J, Thysell H, et al: Long-term effects of reflux nephropathy on blood pressure and renal function in adults. Nephron 2003;93:C35–C46.

31. Zhang Y, Bailey RR: A long term follow up of adults with reflux nephropathy. N Z Med J 1995;108:142–144.

32. Craig JC, Irwig LM, Knight JF, Roy LP: Does treatment of vesicoureteric reflux in childhood prevent end-stage renal disease attributable to reflux nephropathy? Pediatrics 2000;105:1236–1241.

33. Wennerstrom M, Hansson S, Jodal U, et al: Renal function 16 to 26 years after the first urinary tract infection in childhood. Arch Pediatr Adolesc Med 2000;154:339–345.

34. Stokland E, Hellstrom M, Jakobsson B, Sixt R: Imaging of renal scarring. Acta Paediatr Suppl 1999;88:13–21.

35. Anderson NG, Abbott GD, Mogridge N, et al: Vesicoureteric reflux in the newborn: Relationship to fetal renal pelvic diameter. Pediatr Nephrol 1997;11:610–616.

36. Bailey RR: Long-term follow-up of infants with gross vesicoureteric reflux. In Hodson CJ, Heptinstall RH, Winberg J (eds): Reflux Nephropathy Update. Basel, Karger, 1983, pp 146–151.

37. Smellie JM, Barratt TM, Chantler C, et al: Medical versus surgical treatment in children with severe bilateral vesicoureteric reflux and bilateral nephropathy: A randomised trial. Lancet 2001;357:1329–1333.

38. Kohler J, Thysell H, Tencer J, et al: Long-term follow-up of reflux nephropathy in adults with vesicoureteral reflux: Radiological and pathoanatomical analysis. Acta Radiol 2001;42:355–364.

39. Cardiff-Oxford Bacteriuria Study Group: Long-term effects of bacteriuria on the urinary tract in schoolgirls. Radiology 1979;132:343–350.

40. El Khatib MT, Becker GJ, Kincaid-Smith PS: Reflux nephropathy and primary vesicoureteric reflux in adults. Q J Med 1990;77:1241–1253.

41. El-Khatib M, Packham DK, Becker GJ, Kincaid-Smith P: Pregnancy-related complications in women with reflux nephropathy. Clin Nephrol 1994;41:50–55.

42. North RA, Taylor RS, Gunn TR: Pregnancy outcome in women with reflux nephropathy and the inheritance of vesico-ureteric reflux. Aust N Z J Obstet Gynaecol 2000;40 :280–285.

Chronic Interstitial Nephritis

Masaomi Nangaku, Toshiro Fujita

DEFINITIONS

Chronic interstitial nephritis is a histologic entity characterized by progressive scarring of the tubulointerstitium, with tubular atrophy, macrophage and lymphocytic infiltration, and interstitial fibrosis. Because the degree of tubular damage accompanying interstitial nephritis is variable, the term *tubulointerstitial nephritis* is used interchangeably with *interstitial nephritis*. *Tubulitis* refers to infiltration of the tubular epithelium by leukocytes, usually lymphocytes.

There are many primary as well as secondary causes of chronic interstitial nephritis (Fig. 59.1). Tubulointerstitial injury is clinically important because it is a better predictor of present and future renal function than the degree of glomerular injury. Although any glomerular disease can injure the tubulointerstitium secondarily through mechanisms including the direct effects of proteinuria and ischemia, we will restrict our discussion to primary chronic interstitial nephritis.

PATHOGENESIS

The tubulointerstitium can be injured by toxins (e.g., heavy metals), drugs (e.g., analgesics), crystals (e.g., calcium phosphate, uric acid), infections, obstruction, immunologic mechanisms, and ischemia. Regardless of initiating mechanism, however, the tubulointerstitial response shows little variation.[1] Tubular injury results in the release of chemotactic substances and the expression of leukocyte adhesion molecules that attract inflammatory cells into the interstitium. Tubular cells express human leukocyte antigens (HLAs), serve as antigen-presenting cells, and secrete complement components and vasoactive mediators, all of which may further stimulate or attract macrophages and T cells. Growth factors released by tubular cells and macrophages, such as platelet-derived growth factor (PDGF) and transforming growth factor-β (TGF-β), may stimulate fibroblast proliferation and activation, leading to matrix accumulation. The source of fibroblasts in renal interstitial fibrosis remains controversial; however, candidates

Major etiologies of chronic interstitial nephritis	
Diseases in Which the Kidneys Are Macroscopically Normal	Diseases in Which the Kidneys Are Macroscopically Abnormal
Drugs and toxins (e.g., aristolochic acid, lithium, cyclosporine, tacrolimus, indinavir, cisplatin)	Analgesic nephropathy
Metabolic (hyperuricemia, hypokalemia, hypercalcemia, hyperoxaluria, cystinosis)	Chronic obstruction (see Chapters 55 and 58)
Heavy metals (lead, cadmium, arsenic, mercury, gold, uranium)	Hereditary (nephronophtisis, medullary cystic kidney disease, familial juvenile hyperuricemic nephropathy, autosomal dominant polycystic kidney disease, autosomal recessive polycystic kidney disease)
Radiation	Infection (chronic pyelonephritis, malacoplakia, xanthogranulomatous pyelonephritis; see Chapter 50)
Balkan nephropathy	
Immune-mediated systemic lupus erythematosus, Sjögren's syndrome, sarcoidosis, Wegener's granulomatosis, other vasculitides	
Vascular diseases (atherosclerotic kidney disease) (see Chapter 61)	
Transplantation (chronic transplant rejection)	
Hematologic disturbances (multiple myeloma, light-chain deposition disease, lymphoma, sickle cell disease, paroxysmal nocturnal hemoglobinuria) (see Chapters 26, 48, and 60)	
Progressive glomerular disease of all etiologies (e.g., glomerulonephritides, diabetes, hypertension)	
Idiopathic	

Figure 59.1 Major etiologies of chronic interstitial nephritis. Note that kidneys of any clinical entity can be shrunken at the end stage. Some diseases categorized as "macroscopically normal" can show macroscopically abnormal kidneys. For example, kidneys of sickle cell nephropathy are macroscopically normal unless there is papillary necrosis.

include an intrinsic fibroblast population, migration of circulating fibrocytes from perivascular areas, or transdifferentiation of tubular cells into fibroblasts.[2,3] Fibrocytes are circulating cells with the unique characteristic of expressing the hemopoietic stem cell antigen CD34. They rapidly enter sites of tissue injury and synthesize connective tissue matrix molecules. Tubular epithelial-to-mesenchymal transdifferentiation (EMT) is a complex process involving disruption of polarized tubular epithelial cell morphology into cells with spindle-shaped mesenchymal morphology, loss of cell-to-cell adhesions, destruction of basement membrane, and increased cell migration and invasion. An important regulator in this context is the composition of the extracellular matrix. Type IV collagen maintains the epithelial phenotype of proximal tubular epithelial cells, whereas type I collagen promotes EMT.[4]

Chronic interstitial nephritis eventually results in a focal loss of peritubular capillaries, which occurs in association with expansion of the interstitium. The tubular basement membrane (TBM) is thickened with increased matrix, especially collagen type IV. Loss of peritubular capillaries and decreased oxygen diffusion due to expansion of the interstitium renders the kidney hypoxic and leads to the progression of kidney failure.[5] Progressive apoptosis of the cell populations results in a densely fibrotic and hypocellular lesion. Renal function by this stage is severely decreased, and renal replacement therapies are required.

EPIDEMIOLOGY

The changes in chronic interstitial nephritis described earlier characterize progressive renal disease of all etiologies. Despite this, relatively few patients with primary forms of chronic interstitial nephritis reach end-stage renal disease (ESRD). Reports from different regions of the world have indicated a variable incidence in patients with ESRD, ranging from 42% in Scotland to 3% in the United States.[6] The variability in incidence may relate to differences in how diagnoses are made, etiologies and toxin or drug exposure, and treatment modalities.

PATHOLOGY

The identification of specific histologic features in chronic interstitial nephritis is problematic. Virtually all are nonspecific, and it is rather the absence of specific glomerular features that points to the tubulointerstitium as the primary area of insult.

The pathologic features of chronic interstitial nephritis include tubular cell atrophy with flattened epithelial cells and tubular dilation, interstitial fibrosis, and areas of mononuclear cell infiltration within the interstitial compartment and between tubules. The TBM is thickened, and tubules are often separated from each other by dense interstitial fibrosis. Tubular lumina vary in diameter but may occasionally show marked dilation, with homogeneous casts producing a thyroid-like appearance, hence the term *thyroidization*. Casts may contain desquamated tubuloepithelial cells embedded in Tamm-Horsfall protein; occasionally, they take on a homogenous waxy appearance in dilated tubules, suggesting long-standing disease.

Interstitial cell infiltration is not an invariable finding. The pattern of infiltration is usually patchy (focal) but may be more diffuse. Cells in the infiltrate include lymphocytes and monocyte-macrophages, but most infiltrating mononuclear cells are T lymphocytes. Depending on the etiology, other cells, such as neutrophils, eosinophils, or plasma cells, may accumulate.

The cardinal features for a diagnosis of chronic interstitial nephritis are interstitial fibrosis and tubular atrophy. Fibrosis is

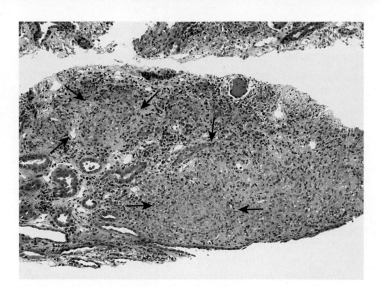

Figure 59.2 Renal tuberculosis. Noncaseating granuloma of epithelioid cells in miliary tuberculosis (*arrows*). Although the typical pathologic change is granuloma with caseous necrosis and Langhans-type giant cells, these nontypical granulomas can be observed in tuberculosis and should be differentiated from sarcoidosis. (Hematoxylin and eosin staining.) (Courtesy of Noriko Uesugi.)

characterized by expansion of the interstitial space with increased interstitial collagens, of varying patterns (focal or diffuse) dependent on the nature of the original insult. The deposited extracellular matrix is a combination of types I, III, and V collagen derived from interstitial fibroblasts and type IV collagen derived from endothelial and tubular epithelial cells. Although small arteries and arterioles typically show fibrointimal thickening of variable severity, vasculitis is not a feature.

Whereas a noncaseating granulomatous pattern is observed in sarcoidosis, interstitial granulomatous reactions also occur in response to infection of the kidney by mycobacteria (Fig. 59.2), fungi, or bacteria; to drugs (sulfonamides and narcotics); and to oxalate or urate crystal deposition. Interstitial granulomatous reactions also have been noted in renal malakoplakia, Wegener's granulomatosis, and heroin abuse and after jejunoileal bypass surgery.

CLINICAL MANIFESTATIONS

Renal insufficiency is slow to develop, and the early manifestations of the disease are those of tubular dysfunction, which may go undetected (Fig. 59.3). Because of its insidious nature, chronic interstitial nephritis is often diagnosed incidentally on routine laboratory screening or evaluation of hypertension, which occurs after significant decrements in glomerular filtration rate (GFR). In one series of biopsy-documented chronic interstitial nephritis, creatinine clearance at presentation was below 50 ml/min in 75% of cases and below 15 ml/min in roughly 33%.[7]

Most patients with primary chronic interstitial nephritis have mild proteinuria, often less than 1 g/day. Urinary sediment usually demonstrates occasional white blood cells and, rarely, white blood cell casts. Hematuria is uncommon. Anemia occurs relatively early in the course of certain forms of chronic interstitial nephritis, presumably because of early destruction of erythropoietin-producing interstitial cells.

Some causes of chronic interstitial nephritis display characteristic patterns that reflect the main site of injury. Proximal tubular defects present as aminoaciduria, phosphaturia, proximal

Functional manifestations of chronic interstitial nephritis
Deterioration of glomerular filtration rate with insidious onset
Tubular proteinuria mainly composed of low-molecular-weight protein (generally <1 g/day)
Inactive urinary sediment
Renal anemia at a relatively early stage
Proximal tubular dysfunction (aminoaciduria, phosphaturia, proximal renal tubular acidosis, Fanconi syndrome)
Distal tubular dysfunction (type IV renal tubular acidosis)
Medullary dysfunction (concentrating defects)
Salt-wasting syndrome
Salt-sensitive hypertension

Figure 59.3 **Functional manifestations of chronic interstitial nephritis.**

renal tubular acidosis (RTA), or, rarely, Fanconi syndrome. Distal tubular defects can be associated with type IV RTA (see Chapter 12). Concentrating defects can be a sign of medullary dysfunction and may be severe enough to result in nephrogenic diabetes insipidus.

More often, however, the pattern of tubular dysfunction is generalized. Although many diseases are associated with the inability to conserve salt on a low-salt diet and subsequent salt-wasting syndrome, certain tubulointerstitial diseases, particularly if accompanied by microvascular disease, may also be associated with a relative inability to excrete salt and resultant salt-sensitive hypertension.[8]

TREATMENT

Treatment should be focused on the primary disease. In many cases, the identification and elimination of any exogenous agents (drugs, heavy metals) or conditions (obstruction, infection) associated with the chronic interstitial lesion is crucial. Good control of blood pressure is important, and most clinicians favor the use of angiotensin-converting enzyme (ACE) inhibitors or angiotensin receptor blockers (ARBs), which reduce glomerular and systemic pressures, decrease proteinuria, and increase renal blood flow. Other strategies include a low-protein diet to reduce glomerular hyperfiltration and subsequent work load on tubular epithelial cells, and consequent decreases in ammoniagenesis, complement activation, and production of various oxygen radicals. Corticosteroids may be a good choice in some conditions in which there is evidence of ongoing inflammation in the tubulointerstitium, or in which the renal lesion is secondary to a systemic condition such as systemic lupus erythematosus or sarcoidosis. More specific therapies against each clinical entity are discussed later.

DRUG-INDUCED CHRONIC INTERSTITIAL NEPHRITIS

Analgesic Nephropathy
Definition and Epidemiology
The clinical syndrome analgesic nephropathy results from the abuse of compound analgesics containing aspirin or antipyrine, in combination with phenacetin, acetaminophen or salicylamide, and caffeine or codeine. It is likely that a similar lesion can be induced by the chronic use of nonsteroidal anti-inflammatory

drugs (NSAIDs). Variations in the incidence of analgesic nephropathy parallel patterns of analgesic use: various estimates have suggested that analgesic nephropathy is responsible for 1% to 3% of cases of ESRD in the United States as a whole, up to 10% in areas of North Carolina, and 10% to 20% in Australia and some countries in Europe (such as Belgium and Scotland).

Epidemiologic studies have shown that the risk for analgesic nephropathy with compound analgesics is generally dose dependent. The amount of phenacetin-acetaminophen combination required to produce chronic interstitial nephritis has been estimated to be at least 2 to 3 kg over many years. Not surprisingly, restrictions in compound analgesic sales over the past 10 to 15 years have been followed by marked reductions in the number of new cases of analgesic nephropathy.

Pathogenesis
The site of renal injury in chronic analgesic abuse is the medulla, likely for two reasons: the buildup in toxic metabolite concentrations that occur here through the countercurrent mechanism and the relative hypoxia in this site under physiologic conditions.

The injury itself may relate to the net effects of several metabolites. For example, phenacetin is converted to acetaminophen, which can deplete cells of glutathione with subsequent generation of oxidative and alkylating metabolites. The inhibition of vasodilatory prostaglandin synthesis can exacerbate medullary damage from ischemia. Collectively, these substances may lead to oxidant and ischemic injury to the medulla, an effect that is exacerbated in the setting of volume depletion.

Pathology
The major pathologic change in analgesic nephropathy is renal papillary necrosis. Necrotic tissues may then slough into the urine, or remain *in situ*, where they atrophy and become calcified. Papillary necrosis is induced by thrombosis and infarction that involves the medulla. The cortical changes of chronic interstitial nephritis overlying the necrotic papilla are secondary and include tubular atrophy, interstitial fibrosis, and a mononuclear cellular infiltrate (Fig. 59.4). The medullary rays traversing the cortex are usually spared and become hypertrophic, imparting a characteristic cortical nodularity to the now shrunken kidneys. The presence of a golden-brown lipofuscin-like pigment in tubular cells and characteristic capillary sclerosis is highly indicative of an analgesic etiology.

Clinical Manifestations
Analgesic nephropathy is five to seven times more common in women than men. Patients typically have a history of chronic pain syndrome. Although flank pain or hematuria from a sloughed papilla may be present, these symptoms are often obscured by nonspecific complaints of headache, malaise, weight loss, and dyspepsia.

The renal manifestations of analgesic nephropathy are nonspecific. They consist of slowly progressive chronic renal failure with impaired urine-concentrating ability, urinary acidification defects, impaired sodium conservation, and urinalysis that may be normal or may reveal sterile pyuria, mild proteinuria, or both. Hypertension and anemia are commonly seen with moderate to advanced disease. Anemia is attributable to both the renal failure and chronic blood loss from peptic ulcer disease. Hyperkalemia may follow NSAID administration in patients with normal and abnormal renal function owing to hyporeninemic hypoaldosteronism created by the use of the NSAID. The natural history depends on the severity of the renal damage at the time of

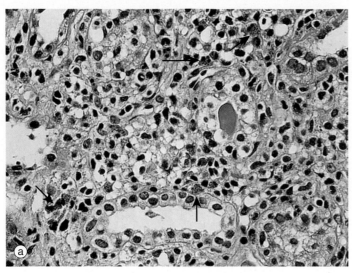
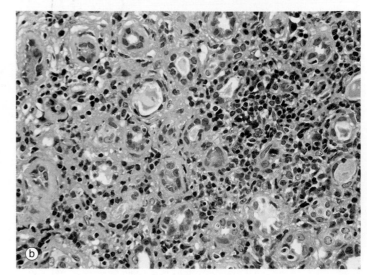

Figure 59.4   Histologic changes in analgesic nephropathy. *a*, Interstitial nephritis in a patient with analgesic nephropathy associated with marked mononuclear cellular infiltrate including eosinophils (*arrows*). (Hematoxylin and eosin stain; original magnification ×600.) *b*, Analgesic nephropathy with interstitial fibrosis and inflammatory cell infiltration. (Masson-Trichrome stain; original magnification ×400.) (Courtesy of Drs. Akira Shimizu and Hideki Takano.)

presentation and whether the drug therapy is discontinued. Patients with analgesic nephropathy are at increased risk for transitional cell carcinoma of the uroepithelium (renal pelvis, ureter, bladder, and proximal urethra).

Diagnosis

Early diagnosis is important because discontinuation of drug use can often halt renal progression. Although papillary necrosis is present histologically in almost all patients, this can be detected radiologically only if part or all of the papilla has sloughed. Of note, papillary necrosis is not pathognomonic of analgesic nephropathy because similar changes can occur in other disorders, including diabetic nephropathy (particularly during an episode of acute pyelonephritis), urinary tract obstruction, sickle cell nephropathy, renal tuberculosis, and, very rarely, obstructive uropathy and reflux nephropathy. The differential diagnosis of analgesic nephropathy from reflux nephropathy is clinically important and is summarized in Figure 59.5.

Because intravenous urography has low sensitivity and potential nephrotoxicity, noncontrast CT scanning serves as an important diagnostic tool, with the major findings being papillary calcifications, decreased renal size, and "bumpy" renal contours (Fig. 59.6). The diagnostic criteria of the renal imaging investigations of analgesic nephropathy (decrease in renal mass plus either bumpy contours or papillary calcifications) established by the Analgesic Nephropathy Network of Europe (ANNE) was shown to be highly sensitive and specific in a population with a daily consumption of analgesic mixtures for a minimum of 5 years.[9]

Treatment

Management consists of stopping or at least reducing the intake of analgesic medications. No specific treatment is available, and management is similar to that for all patients with chronic renal insufficiency (see Chapter 69). Because of the increased incidence of uroepithelial tumors, close follow-up is necessary. New hematuria should be evaluated with urinary cytology with early referral for urologic evaluation. It may also be prudent to obtain yearly urine cytology for the first several years if analgesics are discontinued or indefinitely if drug intake persists.

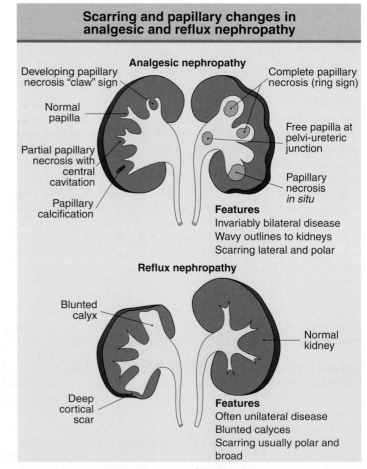

Scarring and papillary changes in analgesic and reflux nephropathy

Analgesic nephropathy

Developing papillary necrosis "claw" sign

Complete papillary necrosis (ring sign)

Normal papilla

Free papilla at pelvi-ureteric junction

Partial papillary necrosis with central cavitation

Papillary necrosis *in situ*

Papillary calcification

Features
Invariably bilateral disease
Wavy outlines to kidneys
Scarring lateral and polar

Reflux nephropathy

Blunted calyx

Normal kidney

Deep cortical scar

Features
Often unilateral disease
Blunted calyces
Scarring usually polar and broad

Figure 59.5   Pattern of scarring and range of papillary changes in analgesic nephropathy compared with reflux nephropathy.

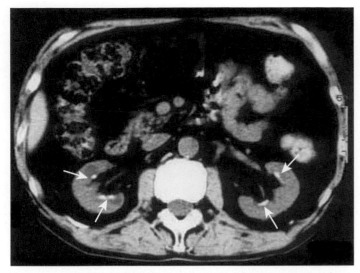

Figure 59.6 Papillary calcifications in analgesic nephropathy. Noncontrast computed tomography scanning of a patient with long-time analgesic abuse showed thinning of the renal parendyma and typical papillary calcifications (*arrows*). (Courtesy of Dr. Yoshifumi Ubara.)

Aristolochic Acid–associated Nephropathy (Chinese Herbs Nephropathy)
Definition and Epidemiology
In 1992, nine women in Brussels, Belgium presented with a rapidly progressive renal failure associated with extensive tubulointerstitial fibrosis.[10] All had followed the same "slimming" regimen, which included Chinese herbs, in the same medical clinic. It was found that one of the herbs (*Stephania tetranda*) had been inadvertently replaced with *Aristolochia fangchi.* Similar cases have now been reported all around the world (reviewed in refs. 11 and 12).

Pathogenesis
Aristolochic acid is the causative agent because its administration to experimental animals reproduced the tubulointerstitial disease and uroepithelial atypia.[13,14] This entity is now called *aristolochic acid–associated nephropathy* or *Chinese herbs nephropathy.*

Pathology
The major lesion is extensive hypocellular interstitial fibrosis with tubular loss, predominantly in the cortex. There may be thickening of the interlobular and afferent arterioles. Glomeruli may show mild collapse of capillaries and wrinkling of the basement membrane consistent with ischemia. The clinical and histologic features of the interstitial disease are similar to those observed in Balkan nephropathy (see later discussion).

Clinical Manifestations
Affected patients typically present with progressive renal insufficiency over several months with other findings that are typical of chronic interstitial nephritis (see earlier discussion). Fanconi syndrome is often present. The risk for renal progression increases with the duration of exposure and, in those with severe disease, may continue to ESRD even if further exposure to the causative herb is prevented.

Treatment
Although one study with 12 patients showed a potential benefit of corticosteroid therapy, most patients are managed conservatively.

Patients with aristolochic acid–associated nephropathy treated by dialysis or renal grafting are now systematically offered bilateral removal of their native kidneys and ureters. Without this precaution, multifocal high-grade transitional cell carcinomas, mainly in the upper urinary tract, will develop in about half of these patients.[15,16]

LITHIUM NEPHROPATHY

Definition and Epidemiology
Lithium is commonly used in the treatment of bipolar disorder. Complications of lithium treatment include nephrogenic diabetes insipidus, acute lithium intoxication, and chronic lithium nephrotoxicity. A meta-analysis of 14 studies involving 1172 patients receiving chronic lithium therapy showed that the prevalence of reduced GFR was 15%.[17]

Pathogenesis
Diabetes insipidus results from accumulation of lithium in the collecting tubular cells after entry into these cells through sodium channels in the luminal membrane. Lithium interferes with the ability of vasopressin to increase water reabsorption by two mechanisms, first by inhibiting adenylate cyclase activity, and hence cyclic adenosine monophosphate production, and second by decreasing the apical membrane expression of aquaporin-2, the collecting tubule water channel.[18]

The mechanism of chronic lithium-induced interstitial nephritis is poorly understood. *In vivo*, lithium induces inositol depletion[19] and inhibits cell cycle progression, probably by induction of p21.[20] The potential role of these molecular events in lithium nephrotoxicity remains to be investigated.

Pathology
Biopsies in patients reveal a focal chronic interstitial nephritis with interstitial fibrosis, tubular atrophy, and glomerular sclerosis. Interstitial inflammation ranges from scant to absent. The specificity of chronic interstitial nephritis attributed to lithium was questioned after the finding of similar changes in a group of psychiatric patients without a history of lithium therapy, but the presence of microcystic changes in the distal tubule clearly differentiated lithium nephropathy from that in psychiatric patients who did not receive lithium.[21] A recent report on 24 patients with biopsy-proven chronic lithium nephrotoxicity revealed interstitial nephritis with disproportionately severe tubular atrophy and interstitial fibrosis, and lesser degrees of glomerulosclerosis and vascular disease.[22] The degree of interstitial fibrosis is related to the duration of administration and cumulative dose.[23]

Clinical Manifestations
Lithium-Associated Diabetes Insipidus   The most common of the three patterns of lithium-induced nephrotoxicity is nephrogenic diabetes insipidus, characterized by resistance to vasopressin, polyuria, and polydipsia. Impaired renal concentrating ability is found in about 50% of patients, and polyuria due to nephrogenic diabetes insipidus occurs in about 20% of patients chronically treated with lithium.[17]

Lithium is also (unusually) a cause of hypercalcemia, which could potentially exaggerate the tubular concentrating defect and contribute to the development of chronic interstitial nephritis in lithium-treated patients. Further, nephrogenic diabetes insipidus in lithium treatment is sometimes associated with distal RTA, although this partial functional defect is virtually never of clinical importance.

Chronic Lithium Nephropathy The side effect of nephrogenic diabetes insipidus by lithium may persist despite the cessation of treatment, indicating the presence of irreversible renal damage. A large number of studies have shown a correlation between the duration of lithium therapy and persistent impairment of urine-concentrating ability.

In one study, the mean serum creatinine of patients with biopsy-proven chronic lithium nephrotoxicity was 2.8 mg/dl (247 μmol/l), and 42% of patients had proteinuria of greater than 1 g/day at the time of biopsy.[22] After renal biopsy, all but one patient discontinued treatment with lithium, but seven patients nevertheless progressed to ESRD. A study of 74 lithium-treated patients in France showed that lithium-induced nephropathy developed slowly over several decades, with an average latency between the start of therapy and ESRD of 20 years.[23]

Treatment

After other potential causes of polyuria and polydipsia have been excluded, particularly psychogenic polydipsia, the first step to consider is a reduction in lithium dosage. Thiazide diuretics are effective against lithium-induced polyuria but should be avoided because they pose a risk for acute lithium intoxication owing to the resultant volume contraction causing an increase in sodium and lithium reabsorption in the proximal tubule. The potassium-sparing diuretic amiloride also reduces urine output by up to 50% and has the added advantage of blocking lithium uptake through sodium channels in the collecting duct.[24]

A practical approach to patients receiving long-term lithium treatment should include the annual estimation of renal function, measured as serum creatinine, estimated GFR, and 24-hour urine volume. Monitoring of lithium levels with dose adjustments is essential because lithium has a narrow therapeutic index. Effective and safe concentrations are between 0.6 and 1.25 mmol/l. The severity of chronic lithium intoxication correlates directly to the serum lithium concentrations and may be categorized as mild (1.5–2.0 mmol/l), moderate (2.0–2.5 mmol/l), or severe (>2.5 mmol/l).

Because progressive renal injury with a reduced GFR in patients without prior acute lithium intoxication is unusual, raised serum creatinine should initially be treated by a dose reduction. For persistently elevated serum creatinine levels, a renal biopsy should be considered, although the result will seldom lead to a recommendation to cease lithium entirely; at all times, the risk for discontinuation in a patient with a severe unipolar or bipolar affective disorder needs to be considered against the relatively low risk for progressive renal injury.

Cyclosporine-induced and Tacrolimus-induced Nephropathy

Definition and Epidemiology

These agents can cause acute and chronic nephrotoxicity by their potent vasoconstrictive effects. Although chronic interstitial nephritis induced by cyclosporine or tacrolimus is common among patients receiving kidney, heart, liver, and pancreas transplants, it is rare in bone marrow transplant recipients because they receive the drugs for a short time and generally at lower doses. In renal transplant recipients, the clinical presentation of cyclosporine agents or tacrolimus-induced interstitial nephritis is similar to chronic rejection. From a clinicopathologic point of view, the effects of these two reagents on the kidney can be considered essentially the same.

Pathogenesis

There is evidence of systemic and intrarenal renin-angiotensin system activation by cyclosporine, which may play a pathogenic role in cyclosporine nephropathy. Cyclosporine also stimulates renal and systemic overproduction of TGF-β. It is likely that chronic cyclosporine nephropathy is the result of a combination of events inducing persistent preglomerular vasoconstriction and of mechanisms directly operating on tubulointerstitial cells, ultimately leading to the development of arteriolopathy and interstitial fibrosis.

Pathology

Long-term use of cyclosporine is associated with patchy interstitial fibrosis, usually in a striped pattern reminiscent of ischemic injury. This injury is classically associated with degenerative hyaline changes in the afferent arteriole walls, consisting of endothelial swelling, nodular hyaline protein deposition, and areas of smooth muscle cell lesions and necrosis (Fig. 59.7). Morphologic changes associated with tacrolimus and cyclosporine are quite similar.

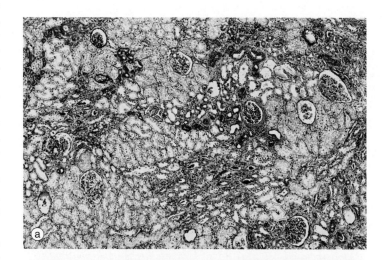

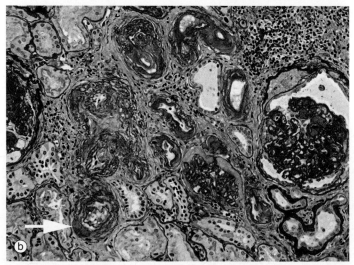

Figure 59.7 Cyclosporine nephropathy. *a,* Long-term cyclosporine toxicity is associated with interstitial fibrosis and tubular atrophy. (Periodic acid–Schiff stain; original magnification ×40.) *b,* Obstructive arteriolopathy with ischemic glomerulosclerosis is observed in cyclosporine nephropathy. The arterioles and small arteries show hyalinization (*arrow*). (Periodic acid–Schiff stain; original magnification ×400.) (Courtesy of Dr. Yutaka Yamaguchi.)

Clinical Manifestations

Both cyclosporine and tacrolimus frequently cause hypertension, hyperuricemia, and hyperkalemia. Hypomagnesemia caused by renal magnesium wasting is also common. Thrombotic microangiopathy may also result from either cyclosporine or tacrolimus, especially in the setting of elevated drug blood levels.

Treatment

Cyclosporine-induced adverse events are usually dose related and can be minimized to some extent by careful titration of dosage and drug blood levels. Regular monitoring of cyclosporine trough blood levels in order to maintain drug concentration within its narrow therapeutic window is an appropriate means of preventing this nephrotoxicity. Concomitant use of calcium channel blockers to induce afferent arteriole vasodilation may be protective, and in experimental studies, ACE inhibitors and ARBs have been shown to be protective.

CHRONIC INTERSTITIAL NEPHRITIS DUE TO METABOLIC DISORDERS

Chronic Urate Nephropathy
Definition and Epidemiology

Although extreme hyperuricemia (especially in the treatment of myeloproliferative disease) can cause acute renal failure, the nature of chronic urate or chronic "gouty" nephropathy—or even its existence as such—has been the subject of much debate.

In the early 1980s, the concept of "gouty nephropathy" as a disease was challenged because of the report that the association of hyperuricemia with chronic interstitial nephritis might be attributed to coexistent hypertension, vascular disease, or aging.[25] Furthermore, an increase in serum uric acid levels in patients with renal insufficiency could also be attributed to the effect of a low GFR to result in urate retention. Recently, the possibility that uric acid may have a role in kidney disease has been readdressed based on experimental studies that implicate a pathogenic role for urate in the progression of tubulointerstitial injury.[26-28]

Pathogenesis

It has been suggested that chronic hyperuricemia and uricosuria result in intratubular sodium urate crystal deposition, with local obstruction, rupture into the interstitium, and a subsequent granulomatous response and interstitial fibrosis. The determinants of uric acid solubility are its concentration and the pH of the tubular fluid, and the major sites of urate deposition are the renal medulla. If deposition occurs in an acid medium, as in the tubular fluid, birefringent uric acid crystals are formed, whereas in an alkaline medium, as in the interstitium, amorphous urate salts are deposited.

Although it is difficult to ascribe diffuse renal disease to the presence of focal crystalline deposits, recent experimental studies have suggested that hyperuricemia may induce chronic renal injury independent of crystal formation.[26,27] The mechanism of this was shown to involve three steps, namely activation of the renin-angiotensin system, stimulation of cyclooxygenase-2, and inhibition of local nitric oxide synthases with a reduction in endothelial nitric oxide.[25,26]

Pathology

Renal functional abnormalities are observed in 30% to 50% of patients who have had gout for many years, and histologic changes are observed in more than 90%.[28] Histologically, the lesion is characterized by tubulointerstitial fibrosis, often with arteriolosclerosis and glomerulosclerosis. Within the kidney, one can often find precipitated uric acid crystals in the tubules and in the interstitium (particularly in the medulla; Fig. 59.8).

Clinical Manifestations

Patients present with hypertension with mild azotemia, mild proteinuria, an unremarkable urinary sediment, and minimal tubular dysfunction (usually impairment of urine-concentrating ability manifest as isosthenuria). Uric acid nephropathy should be particularly considered if there is a disproportionate elevation in serum uric acid in relation to the degree of renal insufficiency (Fig. 59.9).

Diagnosis

The most important differential diagnosis for gouty nephropathy is chronic lead nephropathy. Familial juvenile hyperuricemic

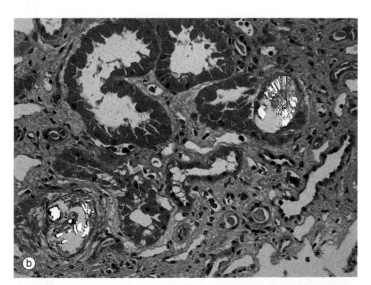

Figure 59.8 Chronic urate nephropathy. *a,* Large collections of elongated or fragmented urate crystals are present in association with atrophic tubules. (Hematoxylin and eosin stain; original magnification ×400.) *b,* The crystalline masses are refractile under polarized light. (Courtesy of Drs. Akira Shimizu and Hideki Takano.)

Expected relationship of serum creatinine and uric acid levels			
Serum Creatinine		**Corresponding Serum Uric Acid Level**	
mg/dl	μmol/l	mg/dl	μmol/l
<1.5	132	9	536
1.5–2.0	132–176	10	595
>2.0	176	12	714

Figure 59.9 Expected relationship of serum creatinine and uric acid levels. Serum uric acid disproportionately elevated above the expected values for the serum creatinine suggests a diagnosis of chronic uric acid nephropathy. (Adapted from Murray T, Goldberg M: Chronic interstitial nephritis: Etiologic factors. Ann Intern Med 1975;82:453–459.)

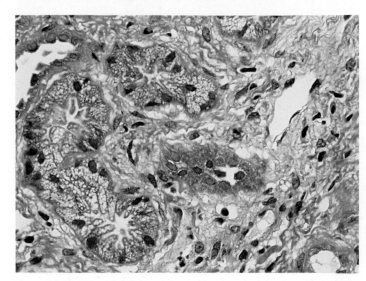

Figure 59.10 Hypokalemic nephropathy. Vacuolization of the renal tubules is observed in association with interstitial fibrosis in a patient with hypokalemic nephropathy. (Masson-trichrome stain; original magnification ×400.) (Courtesy of Drs. Akira Shimizu and Hideki Takano.)

nephropathy is a rare autosomal dominant disease that mimics chronic urate nephropathy but that presents in adolescence or during early childhood (see Chapter 47).

Treatment
Treatment consists of lowering uric acid with xanthine oxidase inhibitors (allopurinol). As allopurinol is excreted by the kidneys, it is prudent to initiate treatment at a dose of 50 to 100 mg per day, increasing to 200 or 300 mg/day if tolerated. A small percentage of patients develop a hypersensitivity syndrome (0.1%) that can be fatal, and this risk is increased in patients with renal dysfunction. One recent prospective, randomized, controlled trial demonstrated that allopurinol therapy was associated with preservation of the renal function in mild to moderate chronic kidney disease,[29] emphasizing a pathogenic role of chronic hyperuricemia and justifying its treatment in patients with kidney diseases.

Hypokalemic Nephropathy
Definition and Epidemiology
Hypokalemia, if persistent for prolonged periods, can induce the development of renal cysts, chronic interstitial nephritis, and progressive loss of renal function, so-called hypokalemic nephropathy. Both inherited and acquired forms of hypokalemic nephropathy have been identified.[30,31]

Pathology
The characteristic finding is vacuolation of the renal tubules due to dilation of cisternae of the endoplasmic reticulum and basal folding, which is generally limited to the proximal tubule segments (Fig. 59.10). This abnormality requires at least 1 month to develop and is reversible with potassium supplementation. More prolonged hypokalemia can lead to more severe changes, predominantly in the renal medulla, including interstitial fibrosis, tubular atrophy, and cyst formation. There is experimental evidence that hypokalemic injury may be due to hypokalemia-induced renal vasoconstriction with ischemia. Local ammonia production stimulated by hypokalemia may also lead to intrarenal complement activation that may contribute to the renal injury. Furthermore, the associated intracellular acidosis can stimulate cell proliferation, which may account for the occasional development of cysts in hypokalemic subjects.[32]

Clinical Manifestations
Impaired urine-concentrating ability, symptomatically characterized by nocturia, polyuria, and polydipsia, may occur, particularly when plasma potassium concentration is consistently <3.0 mmol/l for months or years. The average duration of hypokalemia reported in patients with chronic hypokalemic nephropathy is between 3.5 and 9 years. The renal defect is associated with decreased collecting tubule responsiveness to vasopressin, possibly due to decreased expression of aquaporin-2.

Diagnosis
Although degenerative changes in proximal tubular cells are a consistent but nonspecific finding in hypokalemic nephropathy, vacuolar degeneration in the proximal tubules is characteristic and diagnostic. Similar vacuolization of the convoluted tubules is observed in diethylene glycol poisoning.

Treatment
Usually, hypokalemia can be treated with oral potassium supplements. Details about treatment of hypokalemia are described in Chapter 9. Coarse cytoplasmic vacuoles may persist for some time after normalization of serum potassium values.

Hypercalcemic Nephropathy
Definition and Epidemiology
Hypercalcemia of any cause may produce chronic interstitial nephritis secondary to tubular cell necrosis and intratubular obstruction. Even transient hypercalcemia can lead to chronic renal insufficiency.

Pathology
Focal degeneration and necrosis of the tubular epithelium, primarily in the medulla where calcium is concentrated, occur shortly after persistent hypercalcemia. Although focal degenerative and

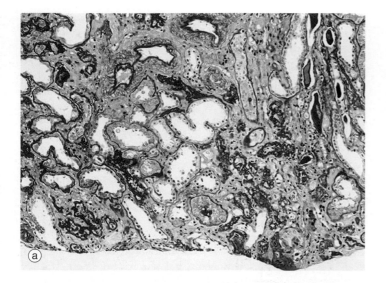

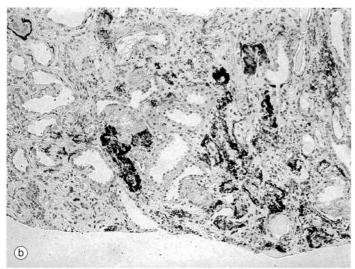

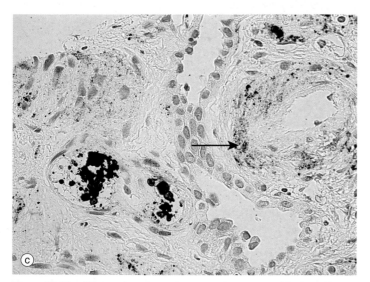

Figure 59.11 Hypercalcemic nephropathy due to sarcoidosis. *a*, Marked tubular atrophy and interstitial fibrosis with mild lymphocytic infiltrate. *b*, Dense calcium deposits are seen in the thickened basement membrane of the atrophic tubules and in the fibrotic area of interstitium (serial section of *a*). *c*, Intraluminal calcium plaque in the atrophic tubules. Granular calcium deposits are observed in the arterial wall *(arrow)*. (*a*, Period acid–Schiff staining; *b* and *c*, von Kossa staining.) (Courtesy of Noriko Uesugi.)

necrotic lesions of the tubular epithelium can be observed in acute hypercalcemic patients, the most distinctive histologic feature of long-standing hypercalcemia is the occurrence of calcific deposits in the interstitium ("nephrocalcinosis"; Fig. 59.11). Deposition begins in the medullary tubules, followed by the cortical proximal and distal tubules and within the interstitial space, and secondarily leads to mononuclear cell infiltration and tubular necrosis.

Clinical Manifestations
Macroscopic nephrocalcinosis is often detected on x-ray or ultrasound. A defect in urinary concentration is the most notable tubular dysfunction and manifests as polyuria and polydipsia. The mechanism is incompletely understood, but the impairment relates both to a reduction in medullary solute content and to interference with the cellular response to vasopressin. Reversible impairment of renal function can result from either acute or chronic hypercalcemia as a result of decreased renal blood flow and GFR. Irreversible renal failure is a rare consequence of long-standing hypercalcemia and is almost invariably associated with calcium crystal deposition in the interstitium of the kidney.

Hyperoxaluria
Hyperoxaluria is described in detail in Chapter 54.

Cystinosis
Cystinosis is described in detail in Chapter 47.

CHRONIC INTERSTITIAL NEPHRITIS DUE TO HEREDITARY DISEASES OF THE KIDNEY

Nephronophthisis (NPHP) and medullary cystic kidney disease (MCKD) (or the NPHP-MCKD complex) are hereditary diseases associated with renal cysts at the corticomedullary junction. These disorders are described in detail in Chapters 44 and 47.

CHRONIC INTERSTITIAL NEPHRITIS ASSOCIATED WITH HEAVY METAL EXPOSURE

Lead Nephropathy
Definition and Epidemiology
Acute lead intoxication is rare but may present with abdominal pain, encephalopathy, hemolytic anemia, peripheral neuropathy, and proximal tubular dysfunction. Because lead has a biologic half-life of several decades, both intermittent acute poisoning and low-level environmental exposure result in chronic cumulative lead poisoning. An epidemic of childhood lead poisoning in Queensland, Australia established chronic lead nephropathy as a recognized clinical and pathologic entity.[33] The pathogenesis of the renal disease may be related to the accumulation of reabsorbed lead in the proximal tubule cells.

Epidemiologic studies have suggested that low-level exposure may be associated with chronic renal insufficiency or hypertension in the general population.[34,35] Accelerated deterioration of renal insufficiency by low-level environmental lead exposure was recently confirmed in a prospective study of 121 patients with chronic renal insufficiency.[36]

Pathology

The kidneys are reduced in size.[33] The characteristic morphology is relatively acellular, interstitial nephritis. The earliest histologic findings show proximal tubular injury, with intranuclear inclusion bodies composed of a lead–protein complex. Glomeruli are normal, and arteries and arterioles demonstrate medial thickening and luminal narrowing, probably related to hypertension. Immunofluorescence studies are noncontributory.

Clinical Manifestations

Chronic lead nephropathy is usually identified when a source of high exposure is known (occupational hazard, or consumption of illicitly distilled spirits [moonshine]). The earliest renal manifestations are primarily limited to impaired proximal tubular function, which gives rise to hyperuricemia ("saturnine gout" resulting from diminished uric acid secretion) and, occasionally, aminoaciduria or renal glycosuria. Urine sediment is benign, and urinary protein excretion is less than 2 g/day. Hypertension is almost always present, and in the absence of appropriate testing or a careful exposure history, lead nephropathy is often misdiagnosed as hypertensive kidney disease. Gouty arthritis affects about half of patients. Patients with chronic lead intoxication may occasionally manifest other signs, including peripheral motor neuropathies, anemia with "basophilic" stippling, and perivascular cerebellar calcifications.

Diagnosis

Lead nephropathy is underdiagnosed because no simple diagnostic blood test is available. Lead nephropathy is easily confused with chronic urate nephropathy, in which urate deposits (tophi) may form in the renal interstitium. All patients with hyperuricemia and renal insufficiency should have a history of occupational lead exposure excluded. The blood lead concentration is an insensitive measure of cumulative body stores. A clinical diagnosis of lead nephropathy is based on a history of exposure, evidence of renal dysfunction, and a positive calcium disodium edentate (CaNa$_2$ EDTA) lead chelation test.[37] The association between gout and chronic renal failure is strong enough to merit lead chelation screening in patients with chronic renal failure who have gout. CaNa$_2$ EDTA is administered (two doses of 0.5 g in 250 ml, 5% dextrose given 12 hours apart), and urine is collected for 3 days because urinary excretion is slowed in the setting of renal failure. Normal urinary lead levels are less than 650 mg per 3 days. X-ray fluorescence, which provokes the emission of fluorescent photons from the target area, is an alternative method that detects increased bone lead levels, which are also a reflection of cumulative lead exposure.

Treatment

Treatment involves the infusions of CaNa$_2$ EDTA together with removal of the source of lead. The likelihood of a satisfactory response to CaNa$_2$ EDTA is influenced by the degree of interstitial fibrosis that has already occurred.

In industrial and occupational settings, such as in foundry workers and individuals working with lead-based paints and glazes, preventative measures to minimize exposure and low-level absorption are essential. Although the oral chelating agent succimer (Chemet) has proved highly successful in treating children, it has not been widely used in adults. Chelation therapy may slow progressive renal insufficiency, even in patients with mild lead intoxication.[38]

Other Heavy Metal–Induced Nephropathies

Cadmium is a metal with a wide variety of industrial uses, including the manufacture of glass, metal alloys, and electrical equipment. Cadmium is preferentially concentrated in the kidney, principally in the proximal tubule, in the form of a cadmium–metallothionein complex that has a biologic half-life of about 10 years. A major outbreak of cadmium toxicity occurred in Japan as a result of industrial contamination. The disease was called *itai-itai*, or "ouch-ouch," because of the presence of significant bone pain as the major clinical manifestation. Other manifestations included proximal tubular dysfunction, renal stones caused by hypercalciuria, anemia, and rarely, progressive chronic interstitial nephritis. The mechanism by which cadmium elicits chronic inflammation and fibrosis in the kidney is relatively unstudied. The diagnosis is suggested by a history of occupation exposure, increased urinary β_2-microglobulin, and increased urinary cadmium levels (>7 μg/g creatinine). Once manifested, renal injury tends to be progressive, even if exposure is discontinued. Chelation has not been effective in humans, and prevention is the only effective treatment.

Arsenic, used as a poison gas in the First World War, is present in insecticides, weed killers, wallpaper, and paints. Chronic arsenic toxicity most commonly manifests as sensory and motor neuropathies, distal extremity hyperkeratosis, palmar desquamation, diarrhea and nausea, Aldrich-Mees lines (white bands on the nails), and anemia. In rare cases, it may cause renal disease, manifested by both proximal renal tubular acidosis and chronic interstitial fibrosis. Diagnosis is made by demonstrating an elevated urinary arsenic level.

Mercury is found in alloy plants, mirror plants, and in batteries, and mercury intoxication usually occurs as a result of accidental exposure to mercury vapor. Although mercury has been shown to induce membranous nephropathy in experimental animals, the nephrotic syndrome is so uncommon in humans exposed to mercury that its etiologic role has been doubted. Whereas neither elemental mercury nor the mercurous salt (Hg_2Cl_2) produces sustained renal tubular injury, mercury dichloride ($HgCl_2$) may produce acute tubular necrosis and subsequent chronic interstitial nephritis. However, a report of endemic methyl mercury poisoning in Japan revealed a clinical picture dominated by neurologic sequelae; renal disease in these patients was surprisingly benign, consisting only of tubular proteinuria without changes in serum creatinine.

RADIATION NEPHRITIS

Definition and Epidemiology

Although radiation nephritis was relatively common decades ago, the incidence has decreased considerably because recognition of radiation-induced renal damage has altered protocols for the administration of therapeutic radiation. In general, direct exposure of the kidney to 20 to 30 Gy (1 Gy = 100 rad) over 5 weeks or less will produce radiation nephritis.

Pathology

The initial target of ionizing radiation within the kidney appears to be endothelial cells, leading to endothelial cell swelling. Subsequent vascular occlusion develops with resultant tubular atrophy. Electron microscopy reveals a split appearance of the capillary wall due to the interposition of mesangial matrix between the glomerular basement membrane and endothelial cells. In addition, the subendothelial space is markedly widened by a nondescript fluffy material. These features are shared by hemolytic-uremic syndrome and thrombotic thrombocytopenic purpura, suggesting a common pathogenic mechanism originating from endothelial injury. Severe disease is characterized by progressive interstitial fibrosis and the presence of interstitial inflammatory cells.

Clinical Manifestations

In general, vascular and glomerular lesions of the thrombotic microangiopathy may predominate. However, tubulointerstitial changes of varying severity are also usually present. Hypertension is commonly observed. Progression to a "chronic" form of radiation nephritis may result from the failure of the acute radiation nephritis to improve. These patients present with proteinuria, progressive azotemia, and eventual development of ESRD several years after irradiation in the absence of an acute phase.

Treatment

Prevention is the best approach. The risk for developing radiation nephritis can be minimized by shielding of the kidneys or fractioning the total-body irradiation into several small doses over several days. No specific treatment is available for established radiation nephritis; consequently, control of hypertension and supportive treatment for renal insufficiency is the general approach.

ENDEMIC DISEASES

Balkan Nephropathy
Definition and Epidemiology

This is an endemic kidney disease confined to discrete, well-defined settlements in the Balkans (i.e., Albania, Bosnia, Croatia, Serbia, Macedonia, Romania, Bulgaria) [39] (Fig. 59.12). The etiology of Balkan nephropathy has never been precisely established. The disease occurs in indigenous or immigrant individuals who have resided in an endemic area for at least 15 to 20 years and does not occur among residents who move to nonendemic areas.

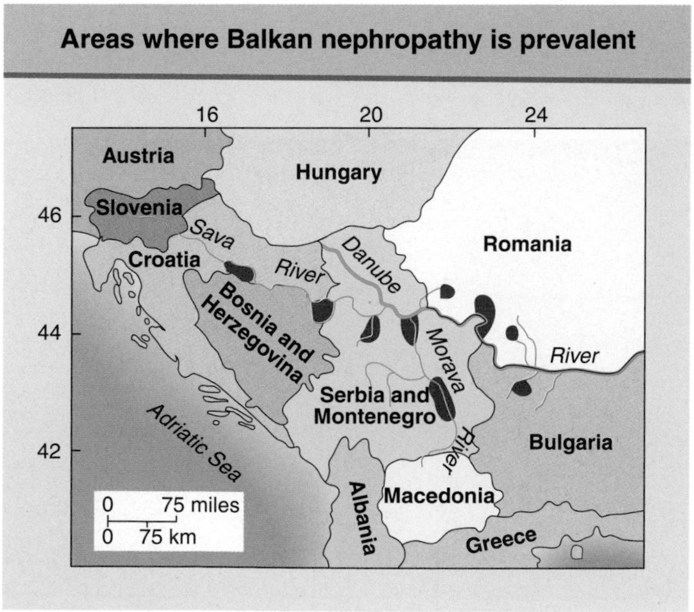

Figure 59.12 Balkan endemic nephropathy. Geographic regions where Balkan nephropathy is prevalent. The endemic areas are in *red*.

Pathogenesis

The familial nature of Balkan nephropathy has led some to suggest that it is a polygenic disorder in which the phenotype might be influenced by the environment. Bulgarian genetic studies favor an autosomal dominant form of inheritance with linkage to 3q25 on chromosome 3.[40] Various trace elements and fungal and plant toxins have also been investigated as possible pathogens. Some studies have implicated a fungal toxin, ochratoxin, which grows in moist grains in storage. The most interesting association has been with the contamination of wheat flour with aristolochic acids, which are derived from the seeds of *Aristolochia clematis*, because the clinical features of Balkan nephropathy are essentially identical to those of aristolochic acid–associated nephropathy. Thus, the disease most likely occurs in genetically predisposed individuals who are chronically exposed to a causative (but as yet unidentified) factor in the environment within endemic areas.

Pathology

The kidneys are usually of normal size early in the course of the disease. A symmetric, smooth reduction in size is observed in late-stage disease. Renal biopsy findings are characterized by proximal tubular lesions in the early stage of disease, with predominantly focal tubular atrophy, interstitial edema and sclerosis, and sometimes mononuclear cell infiltrates. Disease progression is associated with marked tubular atrophy, peritubular capillary damage, and interstitial fibrosis. Early glomerular changes are mild and focal, whereas most glomeruli are hyalinized or sclerotic in advanced stages of the disease.

Clinical Manifestations

Balkan nephropathy typically manifests clinically in the fourth or fifth decade of life and is only rarely seen in individuals younger than 20 years. One of the first signs, detected only when prospective monitoring is performed, is tubular proteinuria. Proteinuria is usually mild or intermittent but may increase in the advanced stages. An unremarkable urinary sediment is characteristic. Other manifestations of abnormal renal tubular dysfunction include impaired acidification, decreased ammonia and increased uric acid excretion, and urine-concentrating defects with renal salt wasting, which may precede the decrease in GFR. The disease slowly progresses to ESRD.

An early feature is normochromic normocytic anemia disproportionate to the degree of renal impairment, whereas patients are usually without edema and are normotensive; hypertension only develops with end-stage disease.

The increased incidence of uroepithelial carcinomas is similar to that observed in both analgesic nephropathy and aristolochic acid–associated nephropathy. Patients with macroscopic hematuria need attention and should be investigated for the presence of uroepithelial tumors.

Treatment

Because the etiology of Balkan nephropathy remains unknown, there are no effective preventive measures, probably apart from moving out of an endemic area. Treatment is primarily supportive. For advancing disease with proteinuria or hypertension, ACE inhibitors or ARBs are recommended.

INTERSTITIAL NEPHRITIS MEDIATED BY IMMUNOLOGIC MECHANISMS

Sjögren's Syndrome
Definition and Epidemiology
Sjögren's syndrome may be associated with chronic interstitial nephritis. The reported prevalence of renal involvement in Sjögren's syndrome has varied widely, ranging from 2% to 67%, principally owing to different definitions of kidney involvement or disease.[41,42]

Pathology
Histologically, the lesion is characterized by infiltration of lymphocytic and plasmacytic cells in the interstitium with tubular cell injury and, rarely, granuloma formation. This progresses to tubular atrophy and interstitial fibrosis over time. Immunofluorescence reveals granular deposits of IgG and C3 along the TBM.

Clinical Manifestations
The clinical and biochemical manifestations of interstitial nephritis may be the presenting or only features of Sjögren's syndrome. Plasma creatinine concentration is generally only mildly elevated and is associated with a relatively benign urinalysis and abnormalities in tubular function, including Fanconi syndrome, type 1 RTA (25% of patients), hypokalemia, and nephrogenic diabetes insipidus. Sjögren's syndrome is one of the most common causes of acquired distal (type 1) RTA in adults and the hypokalemia may be marked, resulting in a clinical presentation of severe weakness. Hypokalemia may occur in the absence of RTA, resulting from salt wasting and secondary hyperaldosteronism.

Treatment
Treatment with corticosteroids at the stage of cellular infiltration is frequently beneficial for protecting renal function. Although the renal disease has a slow and protracted course and renal insufficiency develops over time, progression to ESRD is rare.

Sarcoidosis
Definition and Epidemiology
Histologic evidence of interstitial nephritis with noncaseating granulomas is common in patients with sarcoidosis, but the frequency of clinically significant disease is low. It may present as either an acute interstitial nephritis (see Chapter 57) or a chronic interstitial nephritis.

Pathology
Renal biopsy reveals normal glomeruli; interstitial infiltration, mostly with mononuclear cells; noncaseating granulomas in the interstitium; tubular injury; and with more chronic disease, interstitial fibrosis. Immunofluorescence and electron microscopic studies typically show no immune deposits.

Clinical Manifestations
Most affected patients have clear evidence of diffuse active sarcoidosis, although some present with an isolated elevation in plasma creatinine concentration and no or only minimal extrarenal manifestations.[43–45] The urine analysis, if not normal, shows only sterile pyuria or mild proteinuria.

In addition, hypercalcemia induced by increased production of calcitriol (1,25-dihydroxyvitamin D) by activated mononuclear cells (particularly macrophages) in the lung and lymph nodes[45] occasionally results in renal problems (see the previous discussion of Hypercalcemic Nephropathy).

Treatment
Corticosteroid therapy tends to improve renal function, although recovery is often incomplete. Rapid tapering of steroid can result in relapse.

Systemic Lupus Erythematosus
Definition and Epidemiology
Interstitial nephritis with immune complexes implies the presence of granular deposits of immunoglobulins and complement in the TBM, interstitium, or both. Systemic lupus erythematosus is the most common reason for this type of interstitial nephritis (Fig. 59.13), and interstitial involvement is present in half of kidney biopsy specimens from patients. Rarely, tubulointerstitial immune complex disease may be the only manifestation of lupus nephritis.[46] The presentation is often of an acute interstitial nephritis (see Chapters 24 and 57) but may present as a chronic interstitial nephritis.

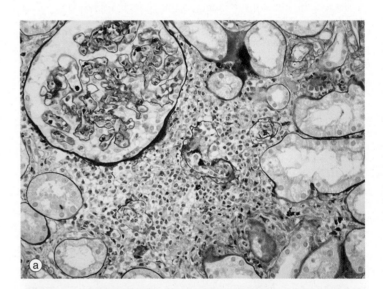

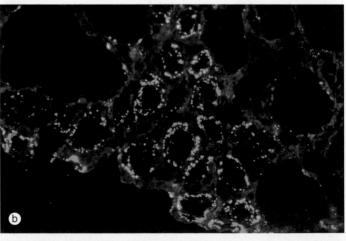

Figure 59.13 **Chronic interstitial nephritis in lupus.** *a*, Interstitial nephritis observed in patients with systemic lupus erythematosus. (Period acid–Schiff staining; original magnification ×400.) *b*, Immunofluorescence study of the same patient revealed deposition of IgG in the interstitium tubular cells and along the fubular basement membrane. (Courtesy of Drs. Akira Shimizu and Hideki Takano.)

Clinical Manifestations

The possibility of interstitial involvement (without glomerular disease) is suggested by a rising plasma creatinine concentration and urinalysis showing relatively benign or normal urine sediment. Interstitial involvement may be accompanied by signs of tubular dysfunction such as type I or type IV RTA, by isolated hyperkalemia resulting from impaired distal potassium secretion, or by hypokalemia resulting from salt wasting. The potentiating effects of sodium wasting on potassium secretion include an increase in sodium delivery to the potassium secretory site in the collecting tubules and associated volume depletion with subsequent stimulation of aldosterone secretion.

Treatment

Corticosteroid therapy is usually effective in subsiding tubular dysfunction and preserving renal function.

RARER FORMS OF IMMUNE-MEDIATED INTERSTITIAL NEPHRITIS

Primary anti-TBM nephritis is an extremely rare form of interstitial nephritis that usually is acute and is characterized by linear deposits of immunoglobulins and complement in the TBM together with tubular interstitial inflammation and anti-TBM antibodies in the serum.[47] Anti-TBM antibodies may also be found in 50% to 70% of patients with anti-GBM nephritis, and occasionally in patients with membranous nephropathy, lupus, IgA nephropathy, minimal change disease, and malignant hypertension.

Although the most frequent renal complications of Crohn's disease are calcium oxalate stones and renal amyloidosis, several cases of interstitial nephritis were recently reported in patients treated for chronic inflammatory bowel disease. Whereas mesalazine was responsible for the development of chronic nephropathy in most cases, some patients were reported to have biopsy-proven interstitial nephritis before the diagnosis of Crohn's disease.[48]

An acute interstitial nephritis with anterior uveitis (TINU syndrome) has been occasionally reported, primarily in young women, and is usually responsive to steroid therapy (see Chapter 57). However, some cases will progress to chronic interstitial disease.

Obstructive Uropathy

Complete or partial urinary tract obstruction is accompanied by pathologic changes in both the tubulointerstitium and glomeruli consisting of interstitial fibrosis, tubular atrophy, and occasionally focal glomerular sclerosis. Details are discussed in Chapters 55 and 58.

Vascular Diseases

Kidney disease in this category is variably termed *ischemic nephropathy*, *renovascular disease*, and *nephrosclerosis*. Ischemia due to intrarenal vascular involvement causes tubular atrophy, interstitial fibrosis, and cellular infiltration. Of note, chronic ischemia in the tubulointerstitial compartment also plays a crucial role in the progression of a variety of glomerular and tubulointerstitial diseases.[5] For details, refer to Chapter 61.

Virus-associated Chronic Interstitial Nephritis

Although a variety of bacteria and viral infections can be associated with acute interstitial nephritis (see Chapters 25 and 57), chronic interstitial nephritis secondary to infectious agents appears to be rare. Chronic bacterial infections can result in xanthogranulomatous pyelonephritis or renal malakoplakia (see Chapter 50). In addition, there have been reports that some cases of idiopathic chronic interstitial nephritis may represent chronic infection with Epstein-Barr virus (EBV).[49] EBV DNA has been demonstrated to be present in the proximal tubular cells by *in situ* hybridization in these patients.

REFERENCES

1. Eddy AA: Molecular basis of renal fibrosis. Pediatr Nephrol 2000;15:290–301.
2. Liu Y: Epithelial to mesenchymal transition in renal fibrogenesis: Pathologic significance, molecular mechanism, and therapeutic intervention. J Am Soc Nephrol 2004;15:1–12.
3. Kalluri R, Neilson EG: Epithelial-mesenchymal transition and its implications for fibrosis. J Clin Invest 2003;112:1776–1784.
4. Zeisberg M, Bonner G, Maeshima Y, et al: Renal fibrosis: Collagen composition and assembly regulates epithelial-mesenchymal transdifferentiation. Am J Pathol 2001;159:1313–1321.
5. Nangaku M: Chronic hypoxia and tubulointerstitial injury: A final common pathway to end-stage renal failure. J Am Soc Nephrol 2006;17:17–25.
6. Rastegar A, Kashgarian M: The clinical spectrum of tubulointerstitial nephritis. Kidney Int 1998;54:313–327.
7. Eknoyan G, McDonald MA, Appel D, Truong LD: Chronic tubulointerstitial nephritis: Correlation between structural and functional findings. Kidney Int 1990;38:736–743.
8. Johnson RJ, Herrera-Acosta J, Schreiner GF, Rodriguez-Iturbe B: Subtle acquired renal injury as a mechanism of salt-sensitive hypertension. N Engl J Med 2002;346:913–923.
9. Elseviers MM, Waller I, Nenoy D, et al: Evaluation of diagnostic criteria for analgesic nephropathy in patients with end-stage renal failure: Results of the ANNE study. Analgesic Nephropathy Network of Europe. Nephrol Dial Transplant 1995;10:808–814.
10. Vanherweghem JL, Depierreux M, Tielemans C, et al: Rapidly progressive interstitial renal fibrosis in young women: Association with slimming regimen including Chinese herbs. Lancet 1993;341:387–391.
11. Cosyns JP: Aristolochic acid and "Chinese herbs nephropathy": A review of the evidence to date. Drug Saf 2003;26:33–48.
12. Isnard Bagnis C, Deray G, Baumelou A, et al: Herbs and the kidney. Am J Kidney Dis 2004;44:1–11.
13. Debelle FD, Nortier JL, De Prez EG, et al: Aristolochic acids induce chronic renal failure with interstitial fibrosis in salt-depleted rats. J Am Soc Nephrol 2002;13:431–436.
14. Cosyns JP, Dehoux JP, Guiot Y, et al: Chronic aristolochic acid toxicity in rabbits: A model of Chinese herbs nephropathy? Kidney Int 2001;59:2164–2173.
15. Nortier JL, Martinez MC, Schmeiser HH, et al: Urothelial carcinoma associated with the use of a Chinese herb (Aristolochia fangchi). N Engl J Med 2000.342:1686–1692.
16. Cosyns JP, Martinez MC, Squifflet JP, et al: Urothelial lesions in Chinese-herb nephropathy. Am J Kidney Dis 1999;33:1011–1017.
17. Boton R, Gaviria M, Batlle DC: Prevalence, pathogenesis, and treatment of renal dysfunction associated with chronic lithium therapy. Am J Kidney Dis 1987;10:329–345.
18. Marples D, Christensen S, Christensen EI, et al: Lithium-induced downregulation of aquaporin-2 water channel expression in rat kidney medulla. J Clin Invest 1995;95:1838–1845.
19. Williams RS, Cheng L, Mudge AW, Harwood AJ: A common mechanism of action for three mood-stabilizing drugs. Nature 2002;417:292–295.
20. Mao CD, Hoang P, DiCorleto PE: Lithium inhibits cell cycle progression and induces stabilization of p53 in bovine aortic endothelial cells. J Biol Chem 2001;276:26180–26188.
21. Hestbech J, Hansen HE, Amdisen A, Olsen S: Chronic renal lesions following long-term treatment with lithium. Kidney Int 1977;12:205–213.
22. Markowitz GS, Radhakrishnan J, Kambham N, et al: Lithium nephrotoxicity: A progressive combined glomerular and tubulointerstitial nephropathy. J Am Soc Nephrol 2000;11:1439–1448.

23. Presne C, Fakhouri F, Noel LH, et al: Lithium-induced nephropathy: Rate of progression and prognostic factors. Kidney Int 2003;64:585–592.
24. Timmer RT, Sands JM: Lithium intoxication. J Am Soc Nephrol 1999; 10:666–674.
25. Yu TF, Berger L: Impaired renal function gout: Its association with hypertensive vascular disease and intrinsic renal disease. Am J Med 1982;72:95–100.
26. Mazzali M, Hughes J, Kim YG, et al: Elevated uric acid increases blood pressure in the rat by a novel crystal-independent mechanism. Hypertension 2001;38:1101–1106.
27. Kang D-H, Nakagawa T, Feng L, et al: A role for uric acid in the progression of renal disease. J Am Soc Nephrol 2002;13:2888–2897.
28. Johnson RJ, Kivlighn SD, Kim YG, et al: Reappraisal of the pathogenesis and consequences of hyperuricemia in hypertension, cardiovascular disease, and renal disease. Am J Kidney Dis 1999;33:225–234.
29. Siu Y-P, Leung K-T, Tong MK-H, Kwan T-H: Use of allopurinol in slowing the progression of renal disease through its ability in lowering serum uric acid level. Am J Kidney Dis 2006;47:51–59.
30. Wallace MR, Bruton D, North A, Wild DJ: End-stage renal failure due to familial hypokalaemic interstitial nephritis with identical HLA tissue types. N Z Med J 1985;98:5–7.
31. Kraikitpanitch S, Lindeman RD, Mandal AK: Case report: Severe hyperuricemia, hypokalemic alkalosis and tubulointerstitial nephritis. Am J Med Sci 1976;271:77–83.
32. Alpern RJ, Toto RD: Hypokalemic nephropathy: A clue to cystogenesis? N Engl J Med 1990;322:398–399.
33. Inglis JA, Henderson DA, Emmerson BT: The pathology and pathogenesis of chronic lead nephropathy occurring in Queensland. J Pathol 1978;124:65–76.
34. Kim R, Rotnitsky A, Sparrow D, et al: A longitudinal study of low-level lead exposure and impairment of renal function. The Normative Aging Study. JAMA 1996;275:1177–1181.
35. Muntner P, He J, Vupputuri S, et al: Blood lead and chronic kidney disease in the general United States population: Results from NHANES III. Kidney Int 2003;63:1044–1050.
36. Yu CC, Lin JL, Lin-Tan DT: Environmental exposure to lead and progression of chronic renal diseases: A four-year prospective longitudinal study. J Am Soc Nephrol 2004;15:1016–1022.
37. Wedeen RP, Malik DK, Batuman V: Detection and treatment of occupational lead nephropathy. Arch Intern Med 1979;139:53–57.
38. Lin JL, Lin-Tan DT, Hsu KH, Yu CC: Environmental lead exposure and progression of chronic renal diseases in patients without diabetes. N Engl J Med 2003;348:277–286.
39. Feder GL, Radovanovic Z, Finkelman RB: Relationship between weathered coal deposits and the etiology of Balkan endemic nephropathy. Kidney Int 1991;34:S9–11.
40. Stefanovic V: Balkan endemic nephropathy: A need for novel aetiological approaches. Q J Med 1998;91:457–463.
41. Pertovaara M, Korpela M, Pasternack A: Factors predictive of renal involvement in patients with primary Sjogren's syndrome. Clin Nephrol 2001;56:10–18.
42. Bossini N, Savoldi S, Franceschini F, et al: Clinical and morphological features of kidney involvement in primary Sjogren's syndrome. Nephrol Dial Transplant 2001;16:2328–2336.
43. Brause M, Magnusson K, Degenhardt S, et al: Renal involvement in sarcoidosis: A report of 6 cases. Clin Nephrol 2002;57:142–148.
44. Robson MG, Banerjee D, Hopster D, Cairns HS: Seven cases of granulomatous interstitial nephritis in the absence of extrarenal sarcoid. Nephrol Dial Transplant 2003;18:280–284.
45. Gobel U, Kettritz R, Schneider W, Luft F: The protean face of renal sarcoidosis. J Am Soc Nephrol 2001;12:616–623.
46. Berden JH: Lupus nephritis. Kidney Int 1997;52:538–558.
47. Bergstein J, Litman N: Interstitial nephritis with anti-tubular-basement-membrane antibody. N Engl J Med 1975;292:875–878.
48. Izzedine H, Simon J, Piette AM, et al: Primary chronic interstitial nephritis in Crohn's disease. Gastroenterology 2002;123:1436–1440.
49. Becker JL, Miller F, Nuovo GJ, et al: Epstein-Barr virus infection of renal proximal tubule cells: possible role in chronic interstitial nephritis. J Clin Invest 1999;104:1673–1681.

Myeloma and the Kidney

Ashley B. Irish

INTRODUCTION

Multiple myeloma (MM) is an uncommon hematologic malignancy, accounting for about 1% of all malignancies and 10% of all hematologic malignancies. Although all common ethnic groups are affected, African Americans have about twice the incidence of Caucasians, and males predominate over females. It is a disease of the elderly, with the median age of diagnosis older than 65 years. Whereas MM is a hematologic malignancy, the dysregulated overproduction of immunoglobulin (Ig), and especially the light-chain (LC) component, provides particular hazards for the kidney. (see Chapter 26). Myeloma with acute renal failure (ARF) is a medical emergency that requires prompt diagnosis and intervention to avoid irreversible renal failure.

ETIOLOGY AND PATHOGENESIS OF MYELOMA

MM is an incurable B cell–derived malignancy of incompletely differentiated plasma cells that have two prominent features: increased production of monoclonal Ig and bone destruction. Normally, plasma cells derive from mature uncommitted B cells and, after antigen stimulus, undergo heavy-chain class switching from μ (IgM) expression to α, δ, ε, and γ. Whole Ig production requires the intracellular assembly of two heavy chains and two LC, κ or λ chains to derive whole IgG, IgA, IgD, and IgE. Normally, LCs are excreted in slight excess, with a κ:λ ratio of about 2:1. In MM, a clone of cells secretes excessive quantities of a specific Ig or LC (the paraprotein or M protein). The genetic and somatic abnormalities underlying this malignant clone are complex and remain incompletely understood but have important implications for prognosis and treatment.[1] Both deregulation of cell cycling and impaired apoptosis account for their progressive and dysfunctional accumulation within the bone marrow, and occasionally other organs. Plasma cells express little surface Ig and are recognized by surface expression of CD38 and CD138, and they normally reside only in the bone marrow. In MM, unrestrained plasma cell growth is supported by a complex milieu of autocrine and paracrine cytokines, especially interleukin-6 (IL-6), preventing apoptosis. These cytokines are secreted from stromal cells, endothelial cells, or osteoclasts and maintain MM cell growth, survival, and migration, and they also contribute to local organ dysfunction (e.g., bone resorption, fracture, and anemia).[2]

ETIOLOGY AND PATHOGENESIS OF RENAL DISEASE

Free light chains (FLCs) circulate as monomers and dimers with a very short half-life (hours) owing to free glomerular filtration (molecular weight, 22,000), whereas the much larger whole Ig circulates intact for several weeks. The filtered FLC is reabsorbed in the proximal tubule cell (PTC) by receptor-mediated endocytosis after binding with the glycoprotein receptor cubilin[3] (Fig. 60.1). LC in excess can induce an inhibitory effect on endocytosis *in vitro* and are associated with lysosomal overload and rupture, releasing enzymatic contents into the cytosol, manifesting histologically by evidence of crystallization, vacuolation, and desquamation of the PTC. Endocytosis of light chains induces the release of the proinflammatory cytokines IL-6, IL-8, and monocyte chemoattractant protein-1 (MCP-1) through the activation of NF-κB in the PTC.[4] This mechanism suggests that LC overload induces factors promoting interstitial injury and fibrosis, a model noted in other proteinuric states. LC may also be cytotoxic to the PTC, possibly through direct DNA injury and the induction of apoptosis.[5,6] Less common manifestations of PTC injury include Fanconi syndrome, which is invariably associated[7,8] with specific variant κ light chains and, pathologically, often crystalline inclusions.[9]

Injury to the PTC allows escape or overflow of LCs to the distal nephron, where it can interact with the Tamm-Horsfall protein (THP) secreted by the cells of the thick ascending loop of Henle (TAL). Variations in the specificity of the binding region of different LCs modifies the affinity of the LC for binding with THP, which could in part explain the variability in risk for nephrotoxicity of LC.[10] This specificity of the individual LC for THP was illustrated by the finding that the same renal injury can be induced in animals, by the intraperitoneal installation of LC isolated from humans with specific renal LC-associated disease.[11]

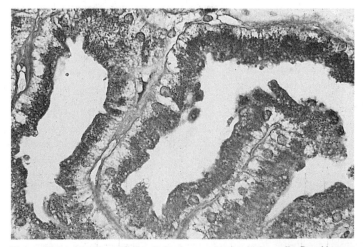

Figure 60.1 Uptake of light chains by proximal tubular cells. Renal biopsy from a patient excreting κ light chains. Immunoperoxidase staining showing κ light chains along the brush border and in the cytoplasm of proximal tubular cells.

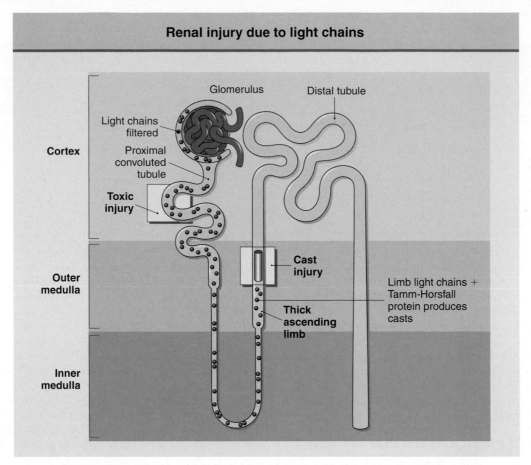

Figure 60.2   Renal injury caused by light chains. Sites *(white boxes)* where light chains injure the tubule. In the proximal tubule, there is direct tubular cytotoxicity. In the distal tubule, there is cast injury.

Although renal injury occurs only in the presence of urinary LCs, not all LCs are associated with injury, and neither the amount nor type of LC correlates with the severity of cast formation. Nevertheless, in general, the higher the urinary excretion of LCs, the more likely is a presentation with renal failure.[12,13] In addition to LC-specific factors, environmental factors affecting tubular solute composition and tubular flow rates modulate the tendency to cast formation. In animals, urinary acidification, furosemide, sodium, and calcium concentration may affect the tendency to increased binding or aggregation of LCs with THP, whereas colchicine may reduce this tendency in animals but not in humans.[14,15] The formation and passage of casts distally can occlude the tubule and allow intratubular obstruction, with rupture and even backflow of contents (Fig. 60.2).

EPIDEMIOLOGY

Most cases of MM present *de novo*, although a small number evolve from patients with monoclonal gammopathy of undetermined significance (MGUS) each year. In Europe, about 50 cases per million occur annually, with a median age at presentation of about 70 years. In patients with newly diagnosed MM, the prevalence rates of IgG, IgA, IgD, and FLC-only MM were 52%, 21%, 2%, and 16%, respectively.[12] IgM and IgE MM are extremely uncommon. Nonsecretory MM (in which no whole Ig or LCs are detectable by serum or urine protein electrophoresis) is not associated with renal disease. About 70% of patients with MM also have a urinary M protein. At the time of diagnosis of myeloma, up to 50% of patients have evidence of renal functional impairment judged by increased

serum creatinine levels, with about 25% presenting with serum creatinine >2 mg/dl (177 μmol/l).[12,13] In unselected series, 2% to 10% of patients present with severe renal failure requiring dialysis; this figure is higher in series reported from renal units. In contrast to the general distribution of M-protein types in MM, LC and IgD myeloma are particularly associated with the risk for renal disease, being present in nearly half of patients with severe renal disease requiring dialysis.[16]

CLINICAL PRESENTATION

Most patients present with constitutional symptoms (fatigue, weight loss) and skeletal pain, especially back pain. Renal impairment is common, and the causes are shown in Figure 60.3. A smaller proportion of patients may present with severe renal failure, and the diagnosis is made or suggested by renal biopsy. In general, these patients have more advanced disease with high morbidity and mortality.[16] Clinical features of renal disease are nonspecific; patients usually present with normal-sized kidneys and bland urine. Urinary protein excretion may be marked owing to the presence of LCs, whereas urinary dipstick analysis may reveal only small amounts of protein because this measures albumin. Normal or elevated albumin-corrected calcium, lytic bone lesions on x-ray, hypogammaglobulinemia, or reductions in levels of other Ig classes and significant cytopenia are clues to the possibility of myeloma. Clinical and laboratory findings that may distinguish myeloma kidney (MK) from other monoclonal immunoglobulin deposition diseases (MIDDs) are listed in Figure 60.4 and discussed in Chapter 26.

Etiology of renal injury and clinical manifestations

Type	Cause	Manifestation
Prerenal	Volume depletion secondary to hypercalcemia, GI losses (nausea and vomiting)	Polyuria and polydipsia Hypotension
	Hemodynamic secondary to sepsis, NSAIDs or hyperviscosity (IgA, IgG3)	Fever Oliguria/hyperkalaemia Mental state alterations
Renal	Proximal tubular injury from light chains, urate, hypercalcemia, and radiocontrast dye Distal tubular injury from casts and crystals	Fanconi syndrome Tubular proteinuria Crystalluria Tumor lysis
	Glomerular disease (LCDD, amyloid)	Nephrotic proteinuria Hematuria/active sediment
Postrenal	Calculi	Colic

Figure 60.3 **Etiology of renal injury and clinical manifestations.** GI, gastrointestinal; Ig, immunoglobulin; LCDD, light-chain deposition disease; NSAIDs, nonsteroidal anti-inflammatory drugs.

PATHOLOGY

Histologic examination of the kidney in MM has diagnostic and prognostic benefits, although this is not uniformly required. Biopsy may be required for the initial diagnosis of acute renal failure or

Differentiating features of myeloma kidney and other monoclonal immune deposition diseases

	Myeloma Kidney	Other MIDDs
Proteinuria	<3 g/l	>3 g/l
Hematuria	Rare	LCDD, occasional Amyloidosis, rare
Hypercalcemia (or normal corrected calcium)	Common	Absent
Hypertension	Uncommon	LCDD common Amyloidosis uncommon
Cytopenias	Anemia very common Leukopenia and thrombocytopenia, occasional	Uncommon
Immune paresis*	Very common	Uncommon
Lytic bone lesions	Very common	Absent
Renal impairment	Common	Common
Heavy chain	IgA, IgD, IgG	None
Type of light chain	Either	Amyloid $\lambda > \kappa$ LCDD $\kappa > \lambda$
Urinary light-chain excretion	Higher	Lower

Figure 60.4 **Clinical features of myeloma kidney compared with monoclonal immunoglobulin deposition diseases (MIDDs; amyloidosis and light-chain deposition disease).** *Defined as a reduction in the nonparaprotein globulin fractions.

Patterns of pathologic involvement of the kidney in multiple myeloma

Histologic Finding	Approximate Prevalence (%)
Myeloma kidney (myeloma cast nephropathy)	30–50
Interstitial nephritis nephritis/fibrosis without cast nephropathy	20–30
Amyloidosis	10
Light-chain deposition disease	5
Acute tubular necrosis	10
Other (urate nephropathy, tubular crystals, hypercalcemia, focal segmental glomerulosclerosis)	5

Figure 60.5 **Pathologic involvement of the kidney in multiple myeloma.** (Data from refs. 17, 30, and Touchard G: Renal biopsy in multiple myeloma and in other monoclonal immunoglobulin-producing diseases. Ann Med Interne [Paris] 1992;143[Suppl 1]:80–83; Sanders PW, Herrera GA, Kirk KA, et al: Spectrum of glomerular and tubulointerstitial renal lesions associated with monotypical immunoglobulin light chain deposition. Lab Invest 1991;64:527–537; Ivanyi B: Frequency of light chain deposition nephropathy relative to renal amyloidosis and Bence Jones cast nephropathy in a necropsy study of patients with myeloma. Arch Pathol Lab Med 1990;114:986–987.)

clarification of the type of renal involvement and reversibility, especially in elderly patients who may not be eligible for aggressive therapies.[17] Figure 60.5 lists the likely findings and prevalence of renal injury noted at histological or autopsy sampling. MK (or *myeloma cast nephropathy*) is the most common histologic finding, occurring in 30% to 50% of patients (Figs. 60.6 and 60.7a). MK is characterized by many distal tubular casts, which are strongly eosinophilic and consist of the monoclonal LC and laminated THP, which often appear fractured after fixation. Similar casts can occasionally be seen in other disease states, such as Waldenström's macroglobulinemia, lymphoma, and rarely pancreatic adenocarcinoma and thyroid carcinoma.[18] Casts are associated with the infiltration of polymorphonuclear leukocytes and monocyte-macrophages and the development of giant cells, which appear to be recruited from both resident and hematopoietic-derived cells and engulf the casts, usually when rupture of the basement membrane occurs.[18,19] In 30% of cases of renal impairment, renal biopsy does not reveal extensive cast formation despite the development of interstitial tubular injury and fibrosis. Prolonged exposure to nephrotoxic LCs can therefore be associated with intense interstitial inflammation, fibrosis, and tubular atrophy as the hallmark of renal injury[20] (see Fig. 60.7b and c). Involvement of the glomerulus is not a usual feature of myeloma but is associated with additional injury and pathologic response related to

Histologic features of myeloma kidney

Many eosinophilic, often fractured casts (medullary portion of the distal nephron predominantly)
Intratubular and interstitial macrophages and giant cells in response to casts
Interstitial inflammation, fibrosis, tubular atrophy, crystalline inclusions
Minimal glomerular abnormality
Minimal or no vascular changes

Figure 60.6 **Histologic features of myeloma cast nephropathy.**

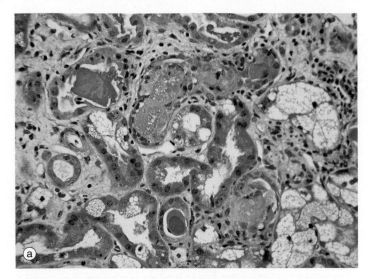

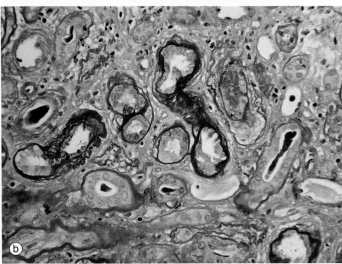

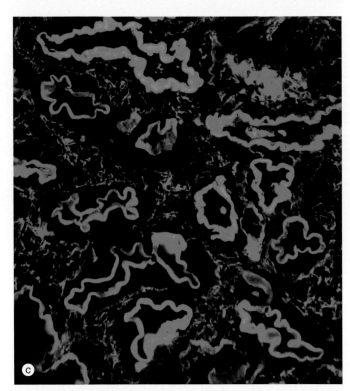

Figure 60.7   Myeloma cast nephropathy. *a,* Myeloma kidney. Many dilated tubules are obstructed by densely eosinophilic hard casts, with giant cell reaction and inflammatory cell infiltrates. There is also vacuolation and degeneration of tubules. (Hematoxylin and eosin stain; ×160). *b,* Light-chain deposition along tubular basement membrane in myeloma kidney without casts. There is marked thickening of the tubular basement membrane by PAS–positive deposits and interstitial fibrosis and mild chronic inflammation. (Periodic acid–Schiff stain; ×160). *c,* Light-chain deposition along tubular basement membrane. Strong linear deposition of κ light chain in the thickened tubular basement membrane (direct immunofluorescence anti-κ light chain; ×160). (Courtesy of Professor R. Sinniah, Perth, Australia.)

specific, often polymeric-forming LC components, which may or may not be associated or overlap with myeloma, such as light-chain deposition disease (LCDD) and amyloidosis[21] (see Chapter 26).

DIAGNOSIS AND DIFFERENTIAL DIAGNOSIS

Patients with acute MM may present to either hematologists or nephrologists, and the diagnosis is usually straightforward when all of the required diagnostic components are met. The International Myeloma Working Group (2003) diagnostic criteria for symptomatic MM require (1) the detection and quantification of a monoclonal protein by serum electrophoresis (SEP) and characterization by immunofixation (IFE), (2) bone marrow (clonal) plasma cells or biopsy-proven plasmacytoma, and (3) the demonstration of any end-organ damage not otherwise explained by other pathology (including hypercalcemia, renal failure, anemia, and lytic bone disease).[22] The monoclonal M protein is the key abnormality required for diagnosis, and 97% of patients have either an intact Ig or a free LC by SEP and IFE. The quantity of the M protein is estimated from the SEP and may be used both for diagnosis and to monitor response to therapy. Urinary LC (Bence Jones protein) is determined from a concentrated sample, but despite this, LC may still be below the level of detection by IFE. The use of a new specific quantitative FLC assay (which measures only LC not bound to whole Ig) for both urine and serum is

significantly more sensitive for diagnosis and management than SEP and IFE alone and increases the detection of FLC when IFE is negative.[23,24] Synthesis of serum FLC is independent of whole Ig, and serum FLC has a short half-life compared with whole Ig. FLC increases with renal failure and age, but the ratio is maintained. An abnormal monoclonal FLC alters the normal ratio of FLC (0.26–1.65 κ:λ) to reflect the oversecretion of the abnormal LC band (<0.26 for λ FLC, >1.65 for κ). This ratio remains diagnostic even in patients with reduced glomerular filtration rate (GFR) or on hemodialysis because both LCs are equally retained and the ratio preserved unless an abnormal LC is present and alters the ratio.[25] Monitoring of serum FLC for diagnosis and therapy therefore has significant advantages in nonsecretory MM (by detecting FLC in 70% of cases in which both SEP and IFE are negative), LC-only MM, and potentially MM and renal failure.[26,27]

Diagnostic difficulties can arise in elderly patients who are evaluated for newly diagnosed renal impairment and in whom a routine SEP reveals an M protein. About 3% of the population older than 70 years will have a serum M protein, most consistent with MGUS. Because diabetes, vascular disease, and hypertension are also highly prevalent in this age group, the chance association of these diseases with serum and urinary paraproteins will commonly arise, raising the question of which condition is responsible for the renal dysfunction. Distinguishing MGUS from MM is a clinical decision based on the level of M protein (<3 g/dl), absent or very low urinary LC (<1 g/24 hours), and the absence of end-organ injury (no lytic lesions, <10% plasma cells on bone marrow aspirate).[22] This distinction is important because most patients with MGUS die from an unrelated disease, and only 1% a year progress to MM.[28] Most renal disease in patients with MGUS is unrelated to the M protein,[29] although rare cases of focal segmental glomerulosclerosis have been associated with the dysproteinemia.[30] Evidence supportive of alternative disease processes and their duration (diabetes and albuminuria, vascular disease), along with a period of observation, may clarify the significance of the M protein, although renal biopsy and occasionally even a bone marrow biopsy may be required when diagnostic uncertainty persists.

NATURAL HISTORY

Most patients with renal impairment at presentation will show resolution of these predominantly functional changes with therapeutic measures that include withdrawal of nephrotoxins, rehydration, treatment of hypercalcemia, treatment of sepsis, and reduction in LC load with chemotherapy. Indeed, response to treatment by improvement in renal function is associated with improved clinical outcomes.[31] Reversibility occurs more frequently with lesser degrees of initial renal impairment, lower LC excretion, and hypercalcemia. Although most patients demonstrate improvement in renal function, about 10% present with, or progress to, end-stage renal disease (ESRD) requiring dialysis. Patients receiving dialysis have reported rates of recovery as low as 5% to 15% or, most recently, up to 30%.[32] Sometimes this recovery occurs many months after presentation.

TREATMENT

The key issue in the management of MK is to rapidly identify and manage possible contributing factors to renal impairment, which are present in about half of patients, to prevent or reverse oliguria. Hypercalcemia, sepsis, and nonsteroidal anti-inflammatory drugs (NSAIDs) are the most common precipitants.[16] The solubility of urinary LC is adversely affected by reductions in glomerular filtration, which increases the relative tubular LC concentration, overwhelms the capacity of the PTC reabsorptive capacity, and delivers a high concentration of LC distally. In states of circulating volume reduction (e.g., hypercalcemia or sepsis), higher LC concentration per nephron and altered composition of tubular solute with higher calcium and a more acidic urine favor cast formation in the distal tubule. Hence, volume expansion to increase glomerular filtration can reduce single-nephron LC concentration and increase tubular flow. Excessive delivery of distal tubular sodium and especially the use of furosemide to promote diuresis should be avoided because these may favor cast formation. There is no clinical evidence of the superiority of volume expansion with sodium bicarbonate over sodium chloride, although prevention of urinary acidification is in theory desirable and in severe renal failure may be necessary for management of metabolic acidosis. The maintenance of a high fluid intake (3 liters per day) with water after initial volume correction and restoration of urine output with crystalloid to maintain high urine flow rates are suggested. The sudden deterioration of patients previously stable in whom abrupt declines in GFR may occur with the use of NSAIDs, sepsis, or radiocontrast agents, however, suggests incipient vulnerability to rapid cast formation and acute distal tubular obstruction.[33-36] Avoidance of fasting coupled with adequate hydration before the use of contrast agents for radiologic or other procedures is essential.

Along with increasing tubular flow, efforts to rapidly reduce the circulating LC load should be initiated promptly once the diagnosis is suspected or proven. The immediate commencement of high-dose dexamethasone, 40 mg daily, is recommended because plasma cells are highly responsive to steroids, which induce rapid apoptosis and lowering of LC concentration. Despite some previous enthusiasm, the routine addition of plasma exchange to conventional treatment did not improve either recovery from renal failure or patient survival.[32] The large volume of distribution of LC (which freely crosses cell membranes) is not well suited to plasma exchange, and the use of continuous convective therapies with enhanced clearance of small molecules may offer greater benefits but is untested. A suggested algorithm for management of MM and acute renal failure is shown in Figure 60.8.

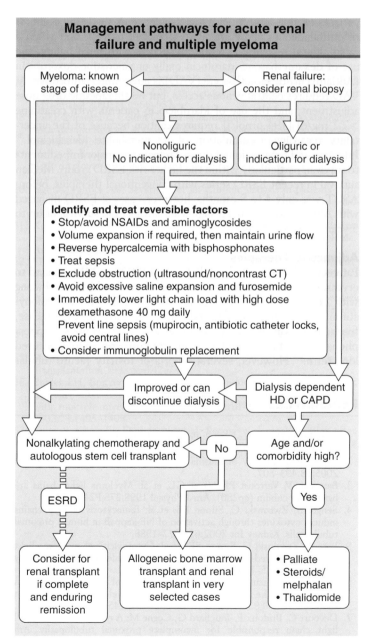

Management pathways for acute renal failure and multiple myeloma

Myeloma: known stage of disease ⟷ Renal failure: consider renal biopsy

Nonoliguric No indication for dialysis | Oliguric or indication for dialysis

Identify and treat reversible factors
- Stop/avoid NSAIDs and aminoglycosides
- Volume expansion if required, then maintain urine flow
- Reverse hypercalcemia with bisphosphonates
- Treat sepsis
- Exclude obstruction (ultrasound/noncontrast CT)
- Avoid excessive saline expansion and furosemide
- Immediately lower light chain load with high dose dexamethasone 40 mg daily
  Prevent line sepsis (mupirocin, antibiotic catheter locks, avoid central lines)
- Consider immunoglobulin replacement

Improved or can discontinue dialysis ← Dialysis dependent HD or CAPD

Nonalkylating chemotherapy and autologous stem cell transplant ← No — Age and/or comorbidity high? — Yes

ESRD

Consider for renal transplant if complete and enduring remission | Allogeneic bone marrow transplant and renal transplant in very selected cases | • Palliate • Steroids/ melphalan • Thalidomide

Figure 60.8 Algorithm for the management of myeloma and acute renal failure. CAPD, continuous ambulatory peritoneal dialysis; CT, computed tomography; ESRD, end-stage renal disease; HD, hemodialysis; NSAIDs, nonsteroidal anti-inflammatory drugs.

Atheromatous and Thromboembolic Renovascular Disease

Julia Lewis and Barbara Greco

INTRODUCTION

Renal arterial and venous occlusive disease presents as a wide variety of clinical syndromes, ranging from vascular catastrophe with acute renal infarction to progressive decline in renal function due to chronic renal ischemia. Improved sensitivity of screening tests allows easy identification of renal artery stenosis, renal infarction, and vascular abnormalities. Advances in pharmacologic management of hypertension and technical advances in endovascular and surgical revascularization have led to more frequent referrals for intervention. This chapter provides an overview of the causes and clinical presentations of atherosclerotic renovascular disease and thromboembolic processes involving the renal arterial and venous circulation, along with approaches to diagnosis and treatment in both native kidney and renal transplant settings. Thrombotic microangiopathies are discussed in Chapter 28, and renovascular hypertension is covered in Chapter 35.

RENAL ARTERY ANATOMY

The anatomic considerations that affect the clinical outcome of renal arterial thromboembolic events include the size of the vessel involved, from the main renal artery to the branch vessels to the arterioles or glomerular capillaries, and the condition of the collateral blood supply. In most individuals, the kidney has a single artery ranging in diameter from 3 to 7 mm. The incidence of multiple renal arteries is about 30%.

Acute occlusion of the renal artery may result in sudden and irreversible renal infarction, particularly if there is a single vessel with inadequate collateral circulation. In the setting of chronic ischemia, such as might exist on a background of atheromatous renovascular disease, the collateral circulation may be more extensively developed and able to maintain renal viability in the face of acute main renal artery occlusion.

The main collateral vessels to the kidney include the suprarenal, the lumbar, and the ureteral vessel complexes, which can maintain renal parenchymal viability in the face of main renal arterial occlusion. The collateral circulation to the kidney is depicted in Figure 61.1. In a study examining 301 aortograms, the adrenal arteries supplied collateral circulation to the kidney in 60% of cases, the lumbar arteries in 55%, the ureteric in 15%, and the gonadal in 13%.[1] The factors determining the development and caliber of these vessels are poorly understood but likely relate to individual anatomic peculiarities, the state of the aorta, the rate of progression of main renal artery narrowing, and the condition of the intrarenal perforating arteries.

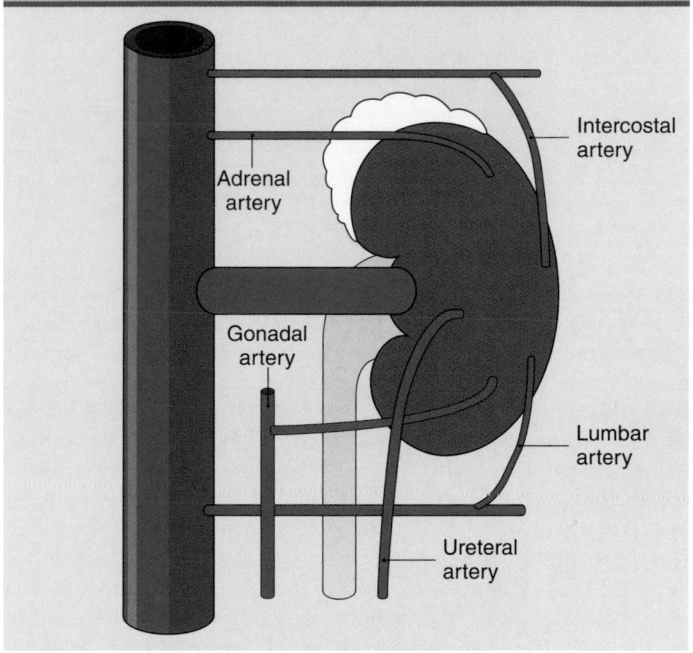

Figure 61.1 Renal collateral circulation. Diagrammatic representation of the potential collateral arterial vessels to the kidney.

CLINICAL SYNDROMES SECONDARY TO ATHEROMATOUS AND RENAL THROMBOEMBOLIC DISEASE

Irrespective of etiology, renal vascular occlusive disease results in renal ischemia, which may present as one of several clinical syndromes, with some overlap (Fig. 61.2). The extent of renal ischemia and the acuteness of the event determine whether the patient presents with predominantly hypertension, renal insufficiency, or overt renal infarction.

There are several major syndromes involving renal vascular disease. First, nonhemodynamically significant renal artery stenosis (RA stenosis; stenosis <60%) may have no clinical signs or symptoms. Because these lesions may progress to more significant stenosis with hypertension or renal ischemia, or lead to distal cholesterol embolization, close follow-up is necessary. Second, hemodynamically significant RA stenosis, fibromuscular dysplasia,

Clinical syndromes associated with atheromatous and thromboembolic renovascular disease
Nonhemodynamically significant atheromatous involvement of the renal vessels in a patient with extrarenal atherosclerosis: requires close follow-up to detect progression to significant disease
Renovascular hypertension (see Chapter 35)
Ischemic renal disease Angiotensin-converting enzyme inhibitor–induced acute renal failure Azotemia in a patient with renovascular hypertension Flash pulmonary edema Unexplained azotemia in the elderly Acute renal failure superimposed on chronic hypertension and renal insufficiency
Chronic kidney disease and unilateral renal artery stenosis
Acute renal infarction Dissection of the aorta and/or renal artery Aneurysm of the renal artery Thrombosis of the renal artery Embolism to the renal artery Acute renal vein thrombosis
Atheroembolic renal disease (cholesterol embolization)
Transplant renal artery stenosis
Chronic renal vein thrombosis

Figure 61.2 Clinical syndromes associated with atheromatous and thromboembolic renovascular disease.

and renal artery aneurysms may present as renovascular hypertension (RVH) without significant detectable renal insufficiency (see Chapter 35). Third, hemodynamically significant RA stenosis may present as renal insufficiency usually, but not always, associated with some degree of hypertension. When RA stenosis affects all functioning renal parenchyma, this clinical entity is termed *ischemic renal disease* (IRD), *ischemic nephropathy*, or *renovascular renal insufficiency*. Fourth, unilateral RA stenosis often presents in association with renal dysfunction of the contralateral kidney due to long-standing hypertension and associated nephrosclerosis or other primary renal disease, such as diabetic nephropathy. In this situation, the renal insufficiency is multifactorial, with injury related to both the primary intrinsic renal disease and the unilateral renal ischemia. Fifth, atheroembolism (cholesterol embolization) may result from proximal aortorenal atherosclerosis and has a clinical course distinct from the other clinical syndromes. Finally, acute renal infarction may result from other causes, including renal artery thrombosis in the setting of inadequate collateral vascular supply or secondary to embolism, dissection, or aneurysm of the renal vessel. Transplant RA stenosis and thrombosis are discussed separately in this section, as is renal vein thrombosis (RVT).

ATHEROSCLEROTIC RENOVASCULAR DISEASE

Epidemiology

Atherosclerotic renovascular disease affects older patients (generally >50 years of age) with evidence of generalized atherosclerosis. When atherosclerotic RA stenosis is present, extrarenal atherosclerotic disease is present 85% of the time. Conversely, many angiographic studies have confirmed the presence of RA stenosis in 11% to 42%[2–3] of patients undergoing angiography of the peripheral or coronary circulation. Predictors of the presence of RA stenosis include a history of hypertension, presence of renal insufficiency, coexisting peripheral, carotid, or coronary artery disease, the presence of abdominal bruits, and a history of smoking.[4]

The true prevalence of RA stenosis is dependent on the population screened. One population-based study of a cohort of 870 patients older than 65 years found a 6.8% prevalence of RA stenosis by renal artery duplex sonography (RDS) screening.[5] Autopsy series report an overall prevalence of 4% to 20%, with higher rates for those older than 60 years (25%–30%) and 75 years (40%–60%).[6] Although Caucasians were historically considered to be more prone to renovascular disease, a recent elderly population-based study detected RA stenosis by RDS with equal prevalence in blacks and whites, suggesting that screening should not be limited by race.[7]

Natural History

Both serial angiographic studies and evaluations using RDS have documented progression of renal artery stenosis in 40% to 50% of patients with atherosclerotic renovascular disease over a 1- to 2-year period[8] (Fig. 61.3). Progression is usually defined as a greater than 25% luminal diameter narrowing or progression from severe stenosis to vascular occlusion. In addition to progression of the arterial lesions, progression is likely if there is a 1-cm or more decrease in renal size.[9]

The factors predicting progression have been somewhat elusive, but one consistent finding has been the close correlation between the degree of initial stenosis and progression on follow-up examination, with high-grade stenoses more likely to progress. Interestingly, progression of renovascular disease often occurs without significant change in blood pressure control, reflecting the effectiveness of current antihypertensive agents. Similarly, hyperlipidemia, a known risk factor for atherosclerosis, has not been shown to be an independent predictor of progression.

ISCHEMIC RENAL DISEASE

Definition

Critical reduction in renal blood flow to the functioning renal parenchyma as a result of atheromatous RA stenosis can reduce glomerular filtration rate (GFR). Over time, progressive renal injury and atrophy develop, and this can lead to permanent loss of renal structural and functional integrity. Generally, the term IRD refers to the hemodynamic and, therefore, potentially reversible component of this chronic ischemic state, although it is important for the clinician to recognize the irreversible consequences of untreated chronic renal ischemia.

Anatomy

IRD is associated with three anatomic variations: (1) unilateral stenosis or occlusion in a single kidney, (2) bilateral critical RA stenosis or occlusion, or (3) unilateral critical RA stenosis or occlusion with contralateral renal nonfunction (Fig. 61.4). Atherosclerotic RA stenosis most often involves the proximal or ostial portion of the vessel. The degree of luminal diameter narrowing requires careful, calibrated measurements. A standard approach to determining the hemodynamic significance of a stenotic lesion involves measurement of the pressure gradient across the stenosis during angiography. A gradient of 20 mm Hg is considered unequivocally hemodynamically significant.

Epidemiology

The incidence of IRD as a cause of renal failure has been estimated from data derived from end-stage renal disease (ESRD) programs. The ESRD population worldwide is aging, and in the United States, the median age of patients entering renal replacement therapy is

Natural history of renal artery stenosis						
Authors	Modality	Year	No. of Patients	Length of Follow-up (mo)	Progression (%)	Occlusion (%)
Meaney et.al.	Angiography	1968	39	6–120	36	8
Wollenweber et al.	Angiography	1968	30	12–88	63	—
Dean et al.	Angiography	1981	35	6–102	29	11
Schreiber et al.	Angiography	1984	85	12–60	44	16
Tollefson and Ernst	Angiography	1991	48	15–180	71	15
Zierler et al.	Renal duplex sonography	1994	80	6–24	42	11

Figure 61.3 Natural history of renal artery stenosis. (Adapted from Greco, BA, Breyer JB: Atherosclerotic ischemic renal disease. Am J Kidney Dis 1997; 29:167–187.)

between 60 and 65 years. Several centers have screened their populations entering ESRD therapy for the existence of significant renal artery stenosis, either by clinical criteria or using angiography or RDS. These data suggest IRD may have a contributory role in between 11% and 22% of all patients with ESRD on dialysis.[10]

Etiology and Pathogenesis

IRD develops when atheromatous disease compromises blood flow to the functioning renal parenchyma. This usually requires a stenosis of 60% or higher that results in a reduction in renal perfusion pressure below the limits of autoregulation, resulting in a reduction in glomerular capillary pressure and GFR. Chronic ischemia may cause variable progressive renal atrophy and fibrosis. Because the kidney receives a large percentage of the cardiac output, it is unclear whether the renal scarring is actually due to diminished oxygen delivery to the renal parenchyma.

Chronic ischemia leads to renal scarring and atrophy, as well as to the production of vasoactive mediators, which can increase blood pressure and promote renal fibrosis. The kidney decreases in size, with preferential thinning of the renal cortex. Histologic correlates consist of tubular simplification, glomerular involution, and wrinkling of the glomerular capillary wall (Fig. 61.5).

Renal atrophy may occasionally be reversed by restoration of renal perfusion, with recovery of renal function and an increase in

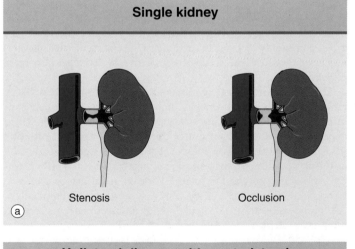

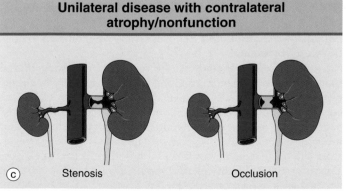

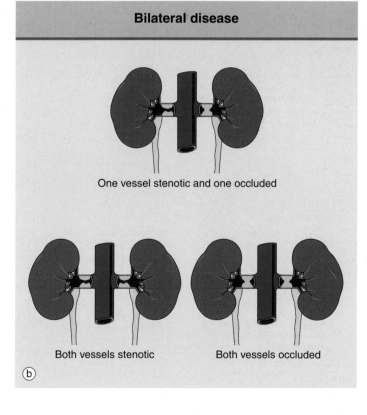

Figure 61.4 Anatomic variations of ischemic renal disease. The renal artery can be partially or totally occluded in situations of single functioning kidney (*a*), bilateral disease (*b*), or unilateral disease with contralateral nonfunction (*c*).

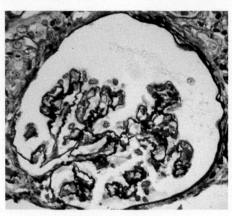

Figure 61,5 Ischemic glomerular changes. This Jones silver stain of a glomerulus demonstrates the glomerular collapse associated with wrinkling of the basement membrane characteristic of ischemia. (Courtesy of Dr. R. Horn.)

renal size after revascularization. More commonly, renal atrophy is associated with irreversible patchy areas of cortical scarring, sclerotic glomeruli, and interstitial fibrosis. The mechanisms responsible for these changes are unclear and may include occult atheroembolic events and microinfarctions due to repeated acute hypoperfusion events (Fig. 61.6). These considerations complicate decisions regarding the optimal approach to a poststenotic or postocclusion atrophic kidney, even when distal vessel reconstitution is visible angiographically. The ultimate renal functional response to aggressive intervention depends on the relative contributions of the hemodynamic and structural effects of diminished perfusion to the overall reduction in GFR.

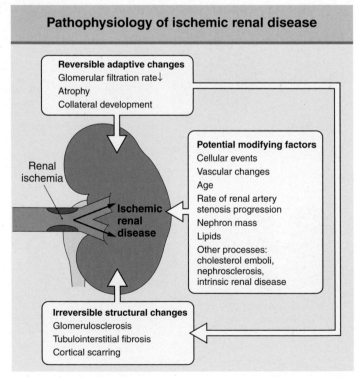

Pathophysiology of ischemic renal disease

Reversible adaptive changes
Glomerular filtration rate↓
Atrophy
Collateral development

Renal ischemia

Ischemic renal disease

Potential modifying factors
Cellular events
Vascular changes
Age
Rate of renal artery stenosis progression
Nephron mass
Lipids
Other processes: cholesterol emboli, nephrosclerosis, intrinsic renal disease

Irreversible structural changes
Glomerulosclerosis
Tubulointerstitial fibrosis
Cortical scarring

Figure 61.6 Pathophysiology of ischemic renal disease. Chronic ischemia of the kidney is associated with reversible functional involution and atrophy as well as irreversible structural changes. A number of external factors influence the renal response to chronic ischemia. (Adapted from Greco, BA, Breyer JB: Atherosclerotic ischemic renal disease. Am J Kidney Dis 1997;29:167–187.)

Clinical Manifestations

IRD should be considered in several clinical settings.

Acute Renal Failure Precipitated by Treatment of Hypertension

Acute renal failure may be precipitated in IRD by the treatment of hypertension, particularly with angiotensin-converting enzyme (ACE) inhibitors or angiotensin receptor blockers (ARBs). The sudden reduction in systemic blood pressure, in the setting of critical RA stenosis, may lead to renal hypoperfusion. With ACE inhibitors and ARBs, there may also be alterations in glomerular hemodynamics independent of any effect on systemic blood pressure. ACE inhibitors and ARBs decrease efferent arteriolar resistance and, hence, decrease glomerular capillary filtration pressure. In the setting of renal arterial disease, the GFR may be critically dependent on angiotensin-mediated increased efferent arteriolar resistance. Acute renal failure in this setting typically occurs 1 to 14 days after the start of antihypertensive therapy and is usually, but not always, reversible.

Most patients with renal vascular disease who are treated with ACE inhibitors or ARBs will not develop acute renal failure;[11] this is likely because those with unilateral stenosis often have preserved function in the nonstenosed kidney and because those with bilateral renovascular disease often have sodium retention, and the GFR is no longer angiotensin II dependent. However, ACE inhibitors and ARBs are more likely to precipitate renal failure in patients with bilateral renal vascular disease if the patients are taking diuretics that will reduce the blood volume and unmask the angiotensin II dependence of the GFR.

Because most patients with renovascular disease treated with ACE inhibitors or ARBs do not develop acute renal failure, it cannot be assumed that these patients do not have IRD. Conversely, acute renal failure can occur with the use of ACE inhibitors in hypertensive patients in the absence of IRD. This most commonly occurs in patients with intravascular volume depletion because, in this setting, GFR is also angiotensin II dependent.[12]

Despite widespread awareness of the potential for ACE inhibitor–induced acute renal failure, surveys in England of primary care physicians have revealed that only about one third of physicians routinely monitor renal function after initiating ACE inhibitor therapy.[13] However, in a prospective study, the criterion of a 20% increase in serum creatinine was 100% sensitive and 70% specific for bilateral severe renal artery stenosis. No case of acute renal failure was encountered in that study.[14] After the resolution of acute renal failure, patients should undergo evaluation for the presence of IRD. ARF can also be precipitated in a patient with IRD in the setting of hypovolemia, intrarenal cholesterol emboli, or sudden renal arterial occlusion.

Patients with Established Renovascular Hypertension Who Develop Azotemia

Patients with RVH should also be suspected of having IRD if they develop azotemia or are found to have a decrease in kidney size (by ultrasound). An atrophic kidney has a 70% chance of being associated with ipsilateral significant RA stenosis. Most patients who present with hypertensive azotemia have either primary renal disease or hypertensive nephrosclerosis. However, given the high frequency of bilateral RA stenosis (between 30% and 50%), the possibility of IRD should always be considered in patients with known prior RVH.

Clinical factors that help distinguish RVH from essential hypertension were identified in the Cooperative Study of Renovascular

Hypertension and include older age, a shorter duration of hypertension, difficult to control blood pressure, recent worsening of blood pressure, or accelerated hypertension.[15] In addition, histories of peripheral vascular disease, coronary artery disease, or cerebral vascular disease were more common in patients with RVH. Patients with RVH also have an increased prevalence of moderate or severe hypertensive retinopathy and abdominal or flank bruits. A decrease in renal function or small or asymmetric kidneys by ultrasound in the presence of these clinical clues suggests the presence of RVH and IRD. By far the most common presentation of atherosclerotic RA stenosis is the setting of unilateral involvement in a patient with chronic kidney disease associated with longstanding hypertension. Here, the cause of renal insufficiency cannot be defined as IRD because the RA stenosis affects only one of the kidneys. The kidney supplied by the stenotic vessel may be ischemic, resulting in diminished GFR, renovascular hypertension, and atrophy. The contralateral kidney with the patent renal vessel often hypertrophies and compensates with hyperfiltration. However, over time, this kidney develops significant parenchymal injury. Much of the time, the kidney with the patent renal artery has worse renal function than the ischemic kidney. The optimal approach to patients with this clinical picture is unclear, particularly given the availability of agents to block the renin-angiotensin system.

Patients with "Flash" Pulmonary Edema

IRD may present as recurrent episodes of "flash" pulmonary edema. These episodes can be unpredictable, sudden, and life threatening and may be associated with normal or low blood pressure at the time of presentation. In one series of patients undergoing renal revascularization, 9% had a clinical picture of recurrent pulmonary edema and poorly controlled hypertension.[16] Renal revascularization aborted the cyclical flash pulmonary edema and improved pulmonary function even in those patients with a very poor preoperative pulmonary status. In another series, 41% of subjects with bilateral RA stenosis had a history of pulmonary edema, compared with 12% with unilateral renovascular disease. Seventy-seven percent of the patients with bilateral RAS had no further pulmonary edema after renal artery stent placement in one or both arteries. The patients who did have recurrent pulmonary edema all had evidence of stent thrombosis or restenosis.[17] Although the mechanism of the pulmonary edema is unclear, it is likely that the severe hypertension associated with IRD leads to hypertensive heart disease. As renal insufficiency progresses, the ability of the kidney to excrete salt and water becomes limited. Severe episodic increases in blood pressure in these chronically volume-overloaded patients with hypertensive heart disease may explain the episodes of flash pulmonary edema. Therefore, patients who present with recurrent episodes of acute pulmonary edema associated with severe hypertension and renal insufficiency should be evaluated for the presence of IRD.

Unexplained Azotemia in Elderly Patients

Diagnosis of IRD should also be considered in unexplained azotemia in elderly patients, particularly in those with diffuse atherosclerotic disease. Elderly patients who have documented peripheral vascular, cerebral vascular, or coronary artery atherosclerosis are at higher risk for occult IRD. The diagnosis of IRD should also be considered in elderly patients with unexplained azotemia who have recent onset of hypertension or in whom there is a recent difficulty controlling hypertension. It is important to remember that essential hypertension typically presents before the age of 60. Therefore, IRD should be considered if the patient has new-onset hypertension after age 60 years, especially if the patient is azotemic.

Acute Renal Failure Superimposed on Chronic Renal Insufficiency

Patients with RA stenosis are at risk for renal artery occlusion. When RA stenosis is bilateral or unilateral in the setting of a single functioning kidney, progression to total occlusion presents as anuric acute renal failure often associated with a hypertensive emergency. The clinical clue to this diagnosis is anuria. In this setting, the kidney parenchyma may be viable despite lack of function. Although renal arterial disease may lead to ischemia and renal atrophy, in some patients collateral vessels may maintain renal viability in the face of proximal renal artery occlusion. Clues to this situation include preserved renal length and evidence of renal contrast enhancement ("renal blush") seen on delayed or venous phase images during renal angiography. The kidney is viable despite nonfunction in this setting. When these factors are present and the clinical course is consistent with recent occlusion, there is a good chance of retrieval of renal function if revascularization is feasible clinically and anatomically. In this setting, urgent vascular surgical consultation should be sought, and it should be assumed that the kidneys may be viable for up to 6 weeks.

Diagnosis
Screening Tests

The diagnosis of IRD involves both the identification of critical renovascular disease in patients with renal insufficiency and an assessment of the role that diminished renal perfusion is playing in the decrement in GFR.

The three best noninvasive screening tests for RAS are magnetic resonance angiography (MRA), renal duplex sonography (RDS), and computed tomography angiography (CTA; Fig. 61.7). A recent meta-analysis evaluated studies using CTA, MRA, RDS, captopril renal scintigraphy, and the captopril test for identifying RA stenosis in patients suspected of having RVH. MRA and CTA proved to have better diagnostic accuracy than ultrasonography in this population.[18]

If the clinician has a moderate index of suspicion for the presence of renovascular disease and there are no contraindications, MRA is probably the best screen for the presence of significant RA stenosis in patients with renal insufficiency. Studies have shown gadolinium-enhanced three-dimensional MRA to be highly sensitive (92%–100%) and specific (69%–95%) for accurately identifying high-grade RAS, with negative predictive values as high as 100%. The MRA may overestimate the degree of stenosis, particularly in the mid to distal renal vessels, and segmental renal branches are not reliably seen. Accessory renal arteries may also be missed by MRA, and there is some interobserver variability regarding the judgment of degree of stenosis. MRA is also associated with a significant number of false-positive results, with low positive-predictive values in some series.[19] Subtle forms of fibromuscular dysplasia may be missed by MRA.[20] It is important to note that smaller hospitals may not be able to report the same rates of specificity and sensitivity that are achieved in large specialist centers. CTA has similar sensitivity and specificity as MRA but has the disadvantage of requiring intravenous radiocontrast administration (usually 100–150 ml) with its attendant risk for contrast-induced acute renal failure. It may prove useful in following stented renal arteries for restenosis.

Noninvasive testing for ischemic renal disease

Test	Comment
Intravenous urogram and/or renal ultrasound	Not directly helpful: can define renal anatomy (kidney size, one or two kidneys) and rule out obstruction
Plasma renin activity and captopril-stimulated plasma renin activity	Reduced specificity with renal insufficiency
Renal vein renins	Not directly helpful when bilateral disease is present
Isotopic renal blood flow and functional scans	Not directly helpful because of bilateral renal artery disease and because it is difficult to differentiate from intrinsic disease
Captopril renography	Excellent for renovascular hypertension but not accurate in severe renal insufficiency and requires great care for accuracy with moderate renal insufficiency
Doppler ultrasonography	Can be technically difficult if bowel gas or obesity interferes
Magnetic resonance angiography	Blood flow turbulence can exaggerate measured stenosis

Figure 61.7 Noninvasive testing for ischemic renal disease. (Adapted from Greco BA, Breyer JB: Atherosclerotic ischemic renal disease. Am J Kidney Dis 1997;29:167–187.)

An in-depth discussion of RDS is provided in Chapter 5. Direct examination of the main renal artery, as well as indirect duplex evaluation of the distal arterial tree, can detect lesions with ≥60% RA stenosis. A peak systolic velocity in the main renal artery of more than 200 cm/second and a renal-to-aortic ratio of >3.5 detects stenosis in more than 60%. This technique has been reported to be highly sensitive and specific, but caveats to technical success include operator dependency and patient factors, including habitus, echogenicity of fascia, depth or angle of arteries, and bowel gas interference. Hence, not all centers have been able to reproduce the high accuracy rates of RDS. Indeed, one prospective study comparing RDS to MRA found MRA to have greater sensitivity and negative predictive value in predicting RA stenosis.[21] However, RDS is useful for following renal vessels with stents for the development of restenosis. Finally, determination of resistive index values (defined as [1 – end-diastolic velocity/maximal systolic velocity] × 100) using RDS has been shown to predict the renal function and blood pressure response to renal revascularization, with indices greater than 80 having a poor chance of improvement.[22]

There are no good screening tests to determine the functional significance of RA stenosis. Isotopic renal blood flow and functional scan studies are not directly helpful in diagnosing IRD because they depend on a comparison of an involved and an uninvolved side, whereas IRD often involves both kidneys. Captopril renography, an accurate, noninvasive screen for RVH, can be helpful in assessing the significance of renovascular disease, but its specificity is diminished with advancing renal insufficiency. Both plasma renin activity and renal vein renin measurements also have reduced specificity in the setting of renal insufficiency.[23]

Diagnostic Tests

The diagnosis of IRD depends on the detection of critical RA stenosis in the setting of clinical criteria for IRD as opposed to other causes of acute or chronic kidney disease. For patients with renal insufficiency, MRA has become the imaging modality of choice because of its sensitivity and lack of risk. Because MRA will miss some accessory vessels and tends to overestimate luminal diameter narrowing, renal angiography remains the most accurate diagnostic study.

Renal arteriography can be performed by conventional aortography, intravenous subtraction angiography, intra-arterial subtraction angiography, or angiography using alternative non-nephrotoxic contrast agents (Fig. 61.8). Figure 61.9a shows an aortogram of a patient with bilateral atherosclerotic reno-occlusive disease with total occlusion of the right renal artery. Initially, the right kidney was not visualized, but the delayed view (see Fig. 61.9b) demonstrates a right renal blush and distal reconstitution of the ipsilateral artery.

In very-high-risk patients such as those with IRD, arteriography can be performed using either carbon dioxide or gadolinium. Carbon dioxide digital subtraction imaging provides images of the proximal renal vessels comparable to those obtained with traditional iodinated contrast agents. However, visualization of mid, distal, and segmental renal vessels requires the use of a small amount (usually <20 ml) of supplemental radiocontrast because of rapid dissipation of carbon dioxide and inadequate filling of distal vessels. More recently, gadolinium, the traditional contrast agent used in MRA, has been used as an alternative to iodinated contrast in conventional angiography of high-risk patients.

Three-dimensional, volume-rendered CTA provides as much detailed anatomic information, including location of accessory vessels and venous anatomy as conventional aortography. However, the contrast volume required (120–150 ml) for CTA poses a higher risk for contrast-induced acute renal failure than selective digital subtraction arteriography, and subsequent endovascular intervention for IRD would require additional contrast.[24] Hence, renal arteriography is preferable in patients with IRD.[25]

Differential Diagnosis

The differential diagnosis of IRD includes hypertensive nephrosclerosis, atheroembolic renal disease, diabetic nephropathy, and other unsuspected interstitial processes, such as drug-induced interstitial nephritis, urate nephropathy, autoimmune processes, and even

Angiography in the diagnosis of ischemic renal disease

Test	Volume of Contrast	Arterial Puncture	Risk of Emboli (Catheterization)	Quality of Images
Conventional aortography	++	Yes	+++	+++
Intravenous subtraction angiography	+++	No	No	+
Intra-arterial subtraction angiography	+	Yes	++	++
Carbon dioxide angiography	None	Yes	+++	+

Figure 61.8 Angiography in the diagnosis of ischemic renal disease. Comparative features of available angiographic techniques. The symbols + to ++++ indicate increasing effect. (Adapted from Greco BA, Breyer JB: Atherosclerotic ischemic renal disease. Am J Kidney Dis 1997;29:167–187.)

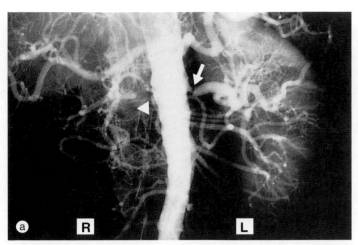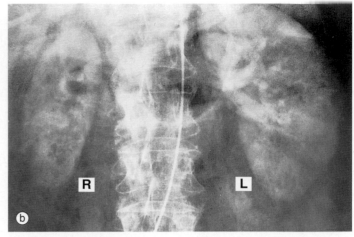

Figure 61.9 Aortogram demonstrating bilateral reno-occlusive disease. *a,* This aortogram demonstrates one of the anatomic variations of ischemic renal disease: the left renal artery has a tight proximal stenosis *(arrow),* and the right renal artery is totally occluded *(arrowhead).* Collateral vessels are visualized on the right. A contrast blush clearly shows the left kidney, but the right kidney is not visible on this early film. *b,* Delayed nephrogram, at a later time during the same aortogram, shows a viable right kidney, which appears as a delayed contrast blush. The right kidney is viable because of the collateral blood supply, but in the setting of chronic proximal renovascular disease, the kidney has atrophied.

occult glomerular diseases (e.g., focal segmental glomerulosclerosis). In patients with coexistent congestive heart failure, RA stenosis is often present, but the predominant insult to renal function is the poor cardiac output owing to myocardial failure rather than the hemodynamic influence of the main renovascular disease. These factors make it difficult for the clinician to predict *a priori* those patients who will benefit from renal revascularization. Several investigators have commented that the only proof of the diagnosis of IRD is in the renal functional response to reperfusion. Even this is unreliable in cases in which chronic ischemia has resulted in severe irreversible renal injury, often accompanied by significant atrophy. Renal biopsy has not been helpful in terms of predicting reversibility because pathologic ischemic changes are often patchy. Thus, the clinician must carefully weigh all the factors in the individual patient before assigning the diagnosis of clinically significant IRD.

Proteinuria >2 g/day is rare and should lead to consideration of other diagnoses. Although most patients (52% in one study) have minimal proteinuria (<0.5 g/24 hours), proteinuria does increase with worsening renal function in patients with IRD, and this suggests that the proteinuria may be a marker for worse parenchymal disease due to atherosclerotic or hypertensive parenchymal disease (including cholesterol emboli, glomerulosclerosis with ischemic changes).[26] In addition to the absence of significant proteinuria, clues to the diagnosis of potentially reversible (hemodynamic) IRD as the cause of renal insufficiency include recent decline in renal function, as opposed to slow, steady deterioration over years; preserved renal length; and a bland urinary sediment.

Natural History

IRD is associated with poor long-term survival. A recent retrospective analysis reported a mortality rate of 34% over 2.5 years in patients with RA stenosis,[27] which is largely due to cardiovascular events or stroke. Five- and 10-year survival rates for patients reaching ESRD due to IRD are as low as 18% and 5%, respectively.[28] In a retrospective analysis of patients with unilateral RA stenosis followed for a mean of 31 months, the mortality rate correlated with GFR at study entry. Patients with severe renal dysfunction requiring renal replacement therapy had the greatest mortality, with median survival <1 month. In a different study of

angiographically defined RA stenosis and RVH, age, reduced renal function, bilateral renal artery stenosis, ischemic heart disease, and congestive heart failure were associated with greater risk for death. Patients who underwent renal artery interventions did not have a higher survival rate.[29] Others have reported that severe carotid disease, ACE DD genotype, smoking, duration (>12 years) of hypertension, and uncontrolled hypertension are risk factors for mortality.[30] However, other studies suggest that intervention to improve renal function may improve survival in this group of patients with diffuse atherosclerotic disease. Watson and colleagues reported 2-year survival rates of 80% among patients with ischemic nephropathy who underwent endovascular stenting.[31] Clearly, the presence of RA stenosis is a marker for more diffuse atherosclerotic vascular disease. More information is needed to determine whether renovascular interventions alter mortality in these patients and which subgroups are most likely to benefit.

Treatment

The clinician treating patients with RA stenosis causing IRD or unilateral RA stenosis in patients with RVH or chronic kidney disease is faced with the dilemma that there are no evidenced-based standards directing the optimal treatment. Six treatment options have been used to manage RA stenosis causing IRD. These include medical management alone, percutaneous transluminal renal angioplasty (PTRA), PTRA with endovascular stenting, primary renal artery stent placement, and surgical revascularization (Fig. 61.10). Regardless of whether medical or surgical intervention is performed, all patients with RAS should be considered at high risk for cardiovascular events.[32]

Medical Management

Studies from the 1980s of patients (ages 45–65 years) with RA stenosis and IRD randomized to medical therapy documented deterioration of renal function over 1 to 2 years in 35% to 50% of patients.[33] However, this was before the availability of a number of therapeutic agents, such as statins. Current medical treatment addresses all risk factors for atherosclerosis, including optimizing blood pressure, based on the Seventh Joint National Committee on Prevention, Detection, Evaluation, and Treatment of High Blood Pressure (JNC 7) guidelines; treatment of hyperlipidemia; encouraging cessation of smoking; optimizing control

---

Therapeutic strategies in ischemic renal disease

Surgical renal artery revascularization
   Aortorenal bypass: vein, Dacron, or polytetrafluoroethylene
   Extra-anatomic repair: splenorenal, hepatorenal, ileorenal, superior
     mesenterorenal arteries
   Autotransplantation
   Ex vivo branch vessel repair
   Transaortic transrenal endarterectomy
   Concomitant aortic replacement and renal revascularization

Percutaneous transluminal renal angioplasty
Endovascular renal artery stenting
Medical or supportive therapy

Figure 61.10 Therapeutic strategies in ischemic renal disease.

of diabetes when present; and managing chronic kidney disease according to the National Kidney Foundation's Kidney Disease Outcomes Quality Initiative (KDOQI) guidelines. All treatments known to benefit cardiovascular and renal outcomes should be applied to this group of patients, including the use of ACE inhibitors and ARBs. Whether modern medical management will result in better outcomes than other options is unclear. A number of ongoing studies trials are comparing optimal medical therapy with endovascular interventions.

Because IRD can progress, it is important that patients with renovascular hypertension and stable mild renal insufficiency whose blood pressure is controlled with medical therapy be followed carefully at 4- to 6-month intervals for changes in renal size and function.[34–36] Indeed, a recent retrospective study of 68 patients with RA stenosis treated without revascularization reported worsening creatinine in 14% of patients followed for an average of 38 months, with an overall rise in the serum creatinine in the entire cohort of 1 to 2 mg/dl (88–176 μmol/l).[37]

Percutaneous Transluminal Renal Angioplasty

Since its introduction in 1978, PTRA has proved successful in treating renal artery fibromuscular dysplasia as well as atherosclerotic renovascular disease. Immediate technical success rates of 75% to 80% with complication rates of 3% to 10% have been reported.[38] However, PTRA alone is limited by high early restenosis rates (up to 30% at 6 to 12 months) and inferior results in the common setting when ostial disease is present. PTRA also has a lower technical success rate when the lesions are longer or more diffuse or when the vessel is totally occluded.

Successful dilation of the vessel can be associated with good renal functional outcomes. However, most PTRA data derive from studies with short follow-up periods. In a study undertaken in the era before the use of endovascular stents, 56% of patients who underwent PTRA eventually required surgical revascularization, with an actuarial renal artery patency of 81% in the surgical group and only 17% in the PTRA group.[39] Although PTRA can be repeated, this approach is undesirable in IRD because repeated contrast studies and endovascular procedures in patients with renal insufficiency pose significant risks to renal function and may offset the benefit gained by improving proximal renal blood flow.

Renal complications of PTRA include hematoma, hemorrhage, pseudoaneurysm, or dissection of the access vessel; rupture, dissection, or thrombosis of the renal artery; cholesterol embolization; and acute renal failure. In addition, cardiac morbidity and mortality have been reported. PTRA should not be undertaken lightly in this patient population.

Endovascular Stents

Endovascular renal artery stent placement has largely replaced PTRA alone as the preferred renal artery revascularization procedure in most centers. Comparisons of PTRA alone versus PTRA with stent placement show superior immediate and long-term results with stents. After initial studies with high complication rates, the past decade has seen renal artery stenting achieve excellent technical success with more acceptable morbidity rates and better long-term patency rates.

Renal artery stenting carries morbidity and rarely mortality with similar complications as seen with angioplasty and with a higher risk for renal artery intimal dissection, thrombosis, or rupture.[40] Patients are typically placed on antiplatelet therapy for several weeks after stenting to prevent thrombosis. A 2-week postprocedure visit followed by visits every 3 months is recommended to adjust antihypertensives and screen for complications and restenosis. Most restenoses occur in the first 6 months after intervention and are more common for smaller vessels. The frequency of restenosis ranges between 17% and 30% at 1 year, depending on the intensity of surveillance. Indicators of restenosis include worsening of blood pressure control or renal function after initial response, or silent renal atrophy as measured by renal ultrasound. In many centers, RDS of the stented vessel is useful in screening for restenosis, whereas artifact produced by the stent makes MRA a poor screening test in stented vessels. Confirmation of restenosis and retreatment requires angiography.

Figure 61.11 summarizes the data from studies of more than 1000 patients undergoing renal artery stent placement for either hypertension or renal function preservation. The overall rate of improvement in blood pressure control approached 50%, with 68% of patients experiencing stabilization or improvement in renal function over a mean of 17 months.[38] However, these studies are largely single-center experiences, not randomized trials.

The effects of renal artery stenting on the course of renal insufficiency in patients with RA stenosis remain controversial. In nearly all studies reporting renal function outcome after stenting, the percentage of patients experiencing improvement in renal function essentially matches that with worsening renal function, about 20% to 30%. Those whose renal function improves the most tend to be those whose renal function was actively deteriorating over the preceding year.[41,42] Patients who show deterioration of renal function after stenting presumably suffer from complications such as thrombosis, distal cholesterol embolization, or contrast acute renal failure. Newer techniques using distal embolic protection devices to guard against cholesterol embolization–associated renal microinfarcts are under investigation.

There are several problems with retrospective reports of renal stents. First, most studies report data on patients with unilateral and bilateral reno-occlusive disease, which represent two different subgroups of renal disease, one with potential IRD and one with a combination of unilateral RA stenosis and contralateral nephrosclerosis. Furthermore, most studies fail to document clinical and angiographic indicators of hemodynamic significance of the renal lesions. Second, many studies report changes in renal function as changes in serum creatinine, which is a poor surrogate for changes in individual kidney GFR. Finally, long-term follow-up data regarding outcome and the durability of patency are scarce, and the few randomized studies comparing renal intervention to medical therapy alone fail to demonstrate a clear benefit of intervention.

Surgical Revascularization

Although renal artery stenting has supplanted surgical revascularization for RA stenosis in many centers, there have been no

Renal function outcomes after endovascular stenting

Year	Author	No. of Patients	Follow-up	Renal Function Outcome (%)			Restenosis (%)
				Improved	Stable	Worse	
1991	Rees	100*	7 mo	36	36	28	25
1994	Hennequin	100*	32 mo	17	50	33	20
1995	van de Ven	92*	6 mo	36	64	0	13
1996	Iannone	86*	10 mo	36	45	19	14
1997	Boisclair	100*	13 mo	41	35	24	ND
1997	Harden	100*	6 mo	34	34	32	13
1998	Shannon	100*	9 mo	43	29	28	0
1998	Dorros	163*	6–48 mo	66–75§ 25–33			
2000	Baumgartner	107†	12 mo	33	42	25	21
2000	Watson	25	8 mo	72	28	0	ND
2000	Burket	37†/127*	15 mo	43	24	33	ND
2001	Bush	69	20 mo	22	48	25	ND
2001	Beutler	63	23 mo	12	68	19	17–19

Figure 61.11 Renal function outcomes after endovascular stenting. ND, not done. *Includes patients with and without renal insufficiency. †Patients with renal insufficiency. §Includes those with stable or improved renal function at last follow-up; the 75% and 25% values represent those stented for bilateral renal artery stenosis. (Adapted from Leertouwer TC, Gussenhoven EJ, Bosch J: Stent placement for renal arterial stenosis: Where do we stand? A meta-analysis. Radiology 2000;216:78–85.)

prospective studies comparing efficacy in preservation or reversal of renal function and long-term vessel patency. Certainly, in situations of occluded renal arteries, a surgical approach is optimal. Despite a population with diffuse atherosclerotic disease, many studies report good renal function outcomes in 70% to 80% of patients undergoing surgical revascularization with low mortality rates and with excellent long-term patency rates up to 93% at 5 years (Fig. 61.12). In surgical series, predictors of good renal function outcome include lower preoperative serum creatinine (<2.0 mg/dl), the presence of bilateral renovascular disease, and recent rapid decline in renal function. These predictors are consistent with the concept that improvement is most likely when the IRD is the cause of the decrement in renal function and there is minimal intrinsic renal parenchymal disease.[43]

Diabetic patients form a significant subgroup of those with IRD. Surgical revascularization in this group is associated with similar renal functional responses but an inferior rate of blood pressure responses and a higher postoperative risk for death or eventual dialysis dependence.[44]

In patients with IRD who are dialysis dependent, recovery of renal function has also been reported after surgical revascularization.[45] The best predictor of successful and sustained

Renal outcomes and mortality of surgical renal revascularization in ischemic renal disease

Source	Year	No. of Patients	Renal Function Outcome (%)			Mortality Rate (%)
			Improved	Stable	Worse	
Luft et al.	1983	12	67	17	17	17
Jamieson et al.	1984	23	65	0	35	17
Novick et al.	1987	161	58	31	11	11
Hallett et al.	1987	91	22	53	25	7.1
Nally et al.	1992	55	58	31	11	2.1
Hansen et al.	1992	70	49	36	15	2.5
Messina et al.	1992	17	77	12	11	0
Bredenberg et al.	1992	40	55	25	20	3
Chaikof et al.	1994	50	42	54	44	2.0
Libertino et al.	1992	91	49	35	16	6
Cambria et al.	1996	139	54	19	27	8

Figure 61.12 Renal outcomes and mortality of surgical renal revascularization in ischemic renal disease. (Adapted from Greco BA, Breyer JB: Atherosclerotic ischemic renal disease. Am J Kidney Dis 1997;29:167–187.)

withdrawal from dialysis is a rapid and recent preoperative decline in GFR, often associated with occlusion of a critically stenotic main renal artery and a kidney with preserved size and extensive collateral supply. The demonstration of postocclusion reconstitution of the renal artery by angiography is also a good predictor of successful revascularization in this setting.

When renal arterial disease accompanies an abdominal aortic aneurysm, the issue arises as to whether to perform combined aortic and renal artery repair, carry out staged surgical procedures, or use endovascular stenting to address the renal lesion and simplify the surgical procedure. There are no data to define an optimal approach in this setting. Although early reports of combined surgical procedures reported high mortality rates, these have dropped to between 2% and 13% depending on the population and the center. However, in most centers, the mortality rate of combined procedures still exceeds that for aortic or renal artery repair alone, although the margin is closing.[46,47]

In addition to mortality rates and renal functional outcomes, the long-term survival of patients undergoing renal revascularization is improving. A study from the Cleveland Clinic reported a 2.2% mortality rate in a predominantly Caucasian population with a mean age of 59 years with documented diffuse atherosclerosis. The actuarial 5- and 10-year survival data were 81% and 53%, respectively.[48] More elderly patients in whom this disease is common would likely have worse outcomes. Cardiovascular death and stroke remain the leading causes of mortality in these patients. Improved outcomes appear to result from improved screening of patients for occult cardiovascular and cerebrovascular disease, better patient selection for surgical revascularization, and optimal postoperative care. Whether the results of centers with experienced, designated renovascular surgeons can be generalized to other surgical settings is unclear.

In many centers, transaortic renal endarterectomy is the preferred operative approach to ostial renovascular disease. Aortorenal bypass with autogenous or synthetic grafts can also address the totally occluded artery or vessels with smaller luminal diameter in many cases. When severe aortic atherosclerosis is present, extra-anatomic approaches, such as hepatorenal, splenorenal, and iliorenal bypasses, are often used to avoid transecting a severely diseased aorta. Subdiaphragmatic supraceliac and thoracic aortorenal bypass techniques are also gaining popularity because of the relative sparing of these aortic segments by the atherosclerotic process.

Treatment Recommendations

Figure 61.13 presents an algorithm for the management of suspected IRD. All patients should receive optimal medical therapy for atherosclerosis, hypertension, and cardiovascular risk, as well as careful management of chronic kidney disease. Nephrologic evaluation should include a careful assessment to determine the likelihood that the renal insufficiency is due to IRD. For any given patient, the overall risk profile must include assessment of cardiovascular status, cerebrovascular and peripheral vascular disease, age, the condition of the aorta, other comorbid conditions affecting longevity, and quality-of-life issues.

If the patient is likely to reach ESRD due to IRD in his or her lifetime, and if that patient would be considered a candidate for dialysis therapy, then revascularization should be considered. Revascularization should be particularly considered in IRD associated with recent worsening renal function, bouts of pulmonary edema with normal cardiac function, and inability to tolerate blockade of the renin angiotensin system (RAS) owing to side effects or development of acute renal failure. Although controversial, in elderly patients with IRD, the data demonstrating the high mortality rate

in this subgroup, once dialysis dependent, supports an aggressive approach to preventing ESRD. The initial screening test should likely be the MRA. The final decision on the type of intervention should take into account the local endovascular interventional and renal vascular surgical expertise, the patient's renal artery and aortic anatomy, and cardiovascular risk factors (see Fig. 61.13).

RENAL INFARCTION

Acute Renal Artery Occlusion

Unlike thrombotic occlusion of a long-standing stenotic atherosclerotic RA stenosis, acute renal arterial occlusion is almost always symptomatic, presenting with loin or flank pain, low back pain or abdominal pain, microscopic hematuria, and proteinuria. Nausea, vomiting, and renal colic are also common. When infarction leads to release of renin, hypertension occurs. When occlusion to a single functioning kidney occurs, the patient presents with oliguria, anuria, and uremic symptoms. Systemic signs of renal infarction associated with renal artery occlusion include leukocytosis, fever, and elevations of lactate dehydrogenase (LDH), transaminases, creatine phosphokinase (CPK), and alkaline phosphatase. Studies in experimental animals with acute renal artery occlusion have shown that the collateral circulation can maintain renal viability for up to 3 hours after occlusion.[49] Whether revascularization beyond this time results in renal salvage is unclear and may depend on the state of the renal vessels before occlusion.

Etiology

Causes of acute renal arterial occlusion leading to renal infarction are presented in Figure 61.14.

Embolism

Because of the relatively high renal blood flow, the kidneys are frequently the target for emboli from thrombus originating in the heart, with the left renal artery more often involved because of the more acute angle at which it comes off the aorta. Atrial fibrillation, cardiac thrombus after myocardial infarction, atrial myxoma or other cardiac tumors, endocarditis, paradoxical emboli, and aortic thrombus represent most of the conditions associated with renal embolism. Atrial fibrillation is one of the most common causes, with a rate of embolism four times higher than that of the general population, and with the highest risk during the first year after the diagnosis of atrial fibrillation. In addition to cardiac thrombi, numerous other causes of renal emboli have been reported in the literature, including fiber or foam related to cardiac bypass procedures and materials, calcium from valve annuli, and even "bullet emboli" in the setting of trauma.

Clinical presentation of renal artery embolism includes abrupt onset of pain (flank or abdominal) often associated with nausea, vomiting, fever, leukocytosis, and hematuria. Many cases may be asymptomatic but noted as enhancing or functional defects on renal imaging. Based on one large autopsy series, renal emboli have an estimated frequency of 1.4% in the general population, of which only 1% were diagnosed clinically. The diagnosis can be made definitively by renal angiography in 100% of cases, but contrast-enhanced computed tomography (CT) is positive in most cases as well. Isotope scans are less sensitive and specific.[50]

Paradoxical Embolism

Renal artery embolism may occur in patients with right-to-left cardiac shunts. The most common cardiac shunt is due to atrial septal defect and is present in up to 9% to 35% of the general population. The diagnosis of paradoxical embolism requires the

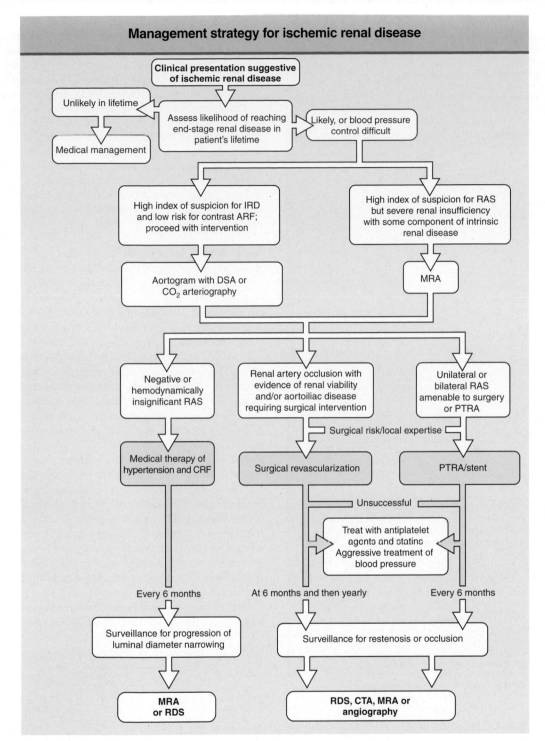

Figure 61.13 Management strategy for ischemic renal disease. ARF, acute renal failure; CO_2, carbon dioxide; CRF, chronic renal failure; CTA, computed tomographic angiography; DSA, digital subtraction angiography; IRD, ischemic renal disease; MRA, magnetic resonance angiography; PTRA, percutaneous transluminal renal angioplasty; RAS, renal artery stenosis; RDS, renal artery duplex sonography.

presence of venous thrombus; an abnormal communication between the right and left circulations; clinical, angiographic, or pathologic evidence of systemic embolism; and favorable pressure gradient within the cardiac cycle for the passage of clot from the right to left side of the heart.

Thrombosis Due to Hypercoagulable Disorders

Several clotting disorders predispose to arterial thrombosis that may involve the renal artery and cause renal infarction. Some are

more commonly associated with renal vein thrombosis (RVT) and are discussed later. Cases of renal artery thrombosis have been reported in patients with protein S and protein C deficiency, antithrombin III deficiency, and rarely factor V Leiden mutations. Dehydration, polycythemia, and the use of oral contraceptive agents can increase chances of thrombosis when these underlying disorders are present.

Antiphospholipid antibody syndrome is associated with both arterial and venous thrombotic events, which can involve the

Causes of renal infarction

Thrombosis: spontaneous
  Atherosclerotic disease of aorta and renal artery
  Fibromuscular dysplasia of renal artery
  Aneurysms of aorta or renal artery
  Dissection of aorta or renal artery
    Marfan syndrome
    Ehlers-Danlos syndrome
  Vasculitis involving the renal artery
    Polyarteritis nodosa
    Takayasu's arteritis
    Kawasaki disease
    Thromboangiitis obliterans
    Other necrotizing vasculitides
  Inflammatory disease of the aorta or renal artery
    Syphilis
    Tuberculosis
    Mycoses
  Hypercoagulable states
    Nephrotic syndrome
    Antiphospholipid syndrome
    Antithrombin III deficiency
    Homocystinuria
  Thrombotic microangiopathies
    Hemolytic-uremic syndrome
    Thrombotic thrombocytopenic purpura
    Antiphospholipid syndrome
    Malignant hypertension
    Scleroderma
    Sickle cell nephropathy
    Polycythemia vera
    Postpartum hemolytic-uremic syndrome
    Hyperacute vascular allograft rejection

Thrombosis: induced
  Traumatic
  Following endovascular intervention
  Post renal transplantation

Embolism
  Cardiac source
    Atrial fibrillation or other arrhythmias
    Native and prosthetic valvular heart disease
    Infective endocarditis
    Marantic endocarditis
  Myocardial infarction with mural thrombi
    Left atrial myxoma or other tumor
  Noncardiac sources
    Atheromatous embolic disease
    Paradoxical emboli
    Fat emboli
    Tumor emboli
  Therapeutic renal embolization

Figure 61.14   Causes of renal infarction.

renal circulation at almost every level. In patients younger than 50 years, the antiphospholipid syndrome can account for 15% to 20% of all deep vein thromboses and 30% of strokes. It is the most common cause of spontaneous arterial thrombosis. In one report of 16 cases of renal involvement with this syndrome, 15 of 16 subjects had either arterial or venous thrombosis, 10 had intrarenal microangiopathy, 1 patient had suprarenal aortic occlusion, and 1 had main renal artery thrombosis.[51] Concomitant thromboses in the mesenteric and cerebral circulation have been reported.

Traumatic Renal Infarction
Traumatic injuries to the renal arteries make up 1% to 4% of all nonpenetrating abdominal trauma.[52] Classically, trauma to the kidney results from a deceleration injury such as a fall from a great height with the patient landing upright on impact. This results in

stretching of the renal arteries as the kidneys continue downward after the rest of the body has stopped. The subsequent stretching and recoiling of the renal arteries can result in acute thrombosis, which is typically bilateral. Direct blunt trauma to the loin or flank regions associated with motor vehicle crashes, street fights, and sports injuries can also result in renal artery thrombosis.

Evidence of lumbar vertebral injury should raise suspicion in the emergency room for renal vascular trauma. Even when diagnosed early, the success rate for renal revascularization after trauma to the renal blood vessels remains low, between 0% and 29%.[52] Injuries to the renal pedicle that result in diminished perfusion to a single functioning kidney or to both kidneys require rapid intervention, and endovascular stabilization of renal blood flow may be helpful as a bridge to more definitive renal revascularization.[52]

Renal Artery Aneurysms
Renal artery aneurysms are rare and associated with atheromatous, fibromuscular, and vasculitic disease involving the renal circulation (Fig. 61.15). Other causes include syphilis, tuberculosis, pyelonephritis, and trauma. They can be a cause of renovascular hypertension, which is the presenting feature in 55% to 75% of cases. Aneurysm rupture is a concern for those greater than 1.5 cm, with the greatest risk during the third trimester of pregnancy. Elective repair of renal aneurysms should be considered in women of childbearing age and in hypertensive patients with single kidneys as well as when aneurysms are causing renovascular hypertension. Other complications of renal artery aneurysms include distal embolization, thrombosis, and arteriovenous fistula formation.

Aortic and Renal Artery Dissection
Aortic dissection can involve the origin of either renal artery, with the false lumen occluding the vessel and impairing renal perfusion. In this setting, the predictors of renal salvage are the same as those for occlusion due to atherosclerotic RA stenosis and include preserved renal size, renal resistive index less than 0.8, collateral circulation permitting renal viability, and blush on imaging studies. In a recent report, despite renal atrophy, aortic stent graft placement allowed for renal reperfusion and restoration of renal size and function.[53]

Aortic dissection occurs most commonly associated with atheromatous vascular disease but can occur in collagen disorders such as

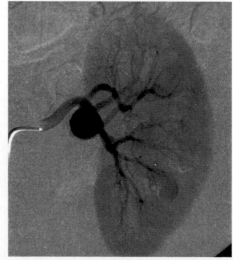

Figure 61.15   Renal artery aneurysm. Angiogram showing large renal artery aneurysm. The aneurysm is patent but is a risk factor for renal artery thrombosis.

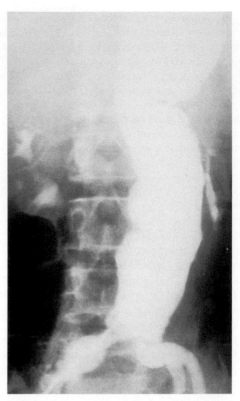

Figure 61.16 Aortogram in a patient with Takayasu's disease. Note the ragged appearance of the aorta. (Courtesy of Dr. J. Reidy.)

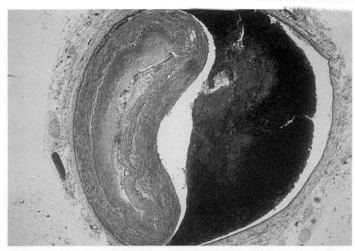

Figure 61.17 Cross-section of a renal artery with dissection after renal angioplasty. Shown is the dissection with thrombosis. The kidney could not be salvaged at subsequent surgery.

Ehlers-Danlos type IV or Marfan syndrome, or associated with arteritis such as Takayasu's disease (Fig. 61.16). Spontaneous renal artery dissection in otherwise healthy individuals has also been reported. Risk factors for dissection include age, hypertension, connective tissue disorders, pregnancy, bicuspid aortic valve, and coarctation of the aorta. A high index of suspicion and rapid imaging confirmation are critical to improve chances of survival. Although MRA is nearly 100% sensitive for diagnosing aortic dissection, CTA has a sensitivity of 93% and is more readily available and practical, providing a more rapid turn-around time; is less dependent on patient factors; and is usually the imaging modality of choice.

Complications of Endovascular Interventions

Renal artery thrombosis, dissection, laceration, or embolism can occur secondary to vascular interventions of any kind, but especially those associated with placement of endovascular stents (Fig. 61.17). Over the past decade, endovascular aortic stents have been used to treat infrarenal abdominal aortic aneurysms. When the stent crosses the orifice of the renal artery, renal perfusion is impaired, and there is a significant risk for renal artery thrombosis. Renal artery stent placement has also been reported to cause intimal dissection and thrombosis of the renal artery and even aortic dissection.

Middle Aortic Syndrome

A rare entity, middle aortic syndrome is a diffuse narrowing of the aorta, considered a form of coarctation, causing renovascular hypertension. The cause is unknown, but associations with fibromuscular dysplasia, congenital anomalies, neurofibromatosis, Williams syndrome, and Takayasu's arteritis have been hypothesized. It can present as aortic thrombosis involving the renal arteries.

Repair of middle aortic syndrome before thrombosis is the goal, with angioplasty or surgical repair or autotransplantation of

ischemic organs. Figure 61.18 demonstrates an aortogram of a patient with this disorder, and Figure 61.19 shows an occluded aorta due to atherosclerosis.

Rare Causes of Renal Infarction

Rare causes of renal infarction include autoimmune diseases such as Behçet's syndrome, systemic lupus and other autoimmune diseases, Henoch-Schönlein purpura, chronic Chagas' disease, and drug abuse, such as intravenous injection or nasal insufflation of cocaine, or even smoking marijuana. The exact mechanisms involved in the pathogenesis of renal infarction in some of these situations are unclear.

Treatment of Acute Renal Vascular Catastrophe

Unlike acute or chronic atherosclerotic renovascular disease, the management of renal artery occlusion due to thrombosis associated with hypercoagulable state or embolism from a central source almost always involves systemic anticoagulation. In patients with renal artery thrombosis secondary to antiphospholipid syndrome or antiphospholipid antibody-mediated hypercoagulability, antithrombin III deficiency, or nephrotic syndrome lifelong anticoagulation is indicated. Salvage of the kidney by acute thrombolytic therapy has been attempted with limited success.

When embolism from a central source results in renal infarction or renal artery occlusion, a search for the source should include evaluation for atrial fibrillation, cardiac mural or atrial thrombus,

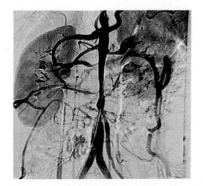

Figure 61.18 Middle aortic syndrome. Angiogram showing typical smooth narrowing of the aorta. There is bilateral stenosis of paired renal arteries. (From Panayiotopoulos YP, Tyrrell MR, Koffman G, et al: Mid-aortic syndrome presenting in childhood. Br J Surg 1996;83:235–240.)

737

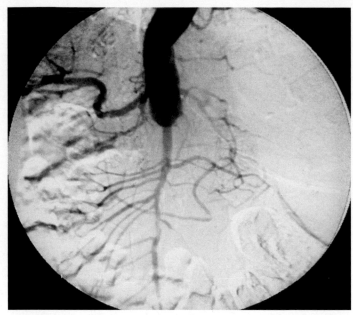

Figure 61.19 Atherosclerotic aorta. (From Streather C, Wlodarczyk ZC, Sneddon F, et al: Progression of occlusive renal vascular disease and axillofemoral bypass grafts. Nephrol Dial Transplant 1993;8:1186–1187.)

and mass and search for valvular lesions. Except in the situation of septic emboli, anticoagulation is indicated to prevent recurrent embolic events.

There is no evidence that thrombolytic therapy can limit infarct size if administered in the acute setting. When no cardiac source is found, echocardiographic "bubble" study should be considered to rule out right-to-left shunts as a route for paradoxical embolism.

ATHEROEMBOLIC RENAL DISEASE

Atheroembolic renal disease is a common clinical syndrome and an important clinical presentation of atheromatous renovascular disease, accounting for up to 10% of unexplained renal failure in the elderly. Indeed, ipsilateral RA stenosis has been reported in up to 80% of patients with renal cholesterol embolization. Conversely, in one study in which 44 patients underwent surgical revascularization and simultaneous renal biopsy, cholesterol emboli were found in the kidneys of 36% of the cases.[54] These findings support the concept that cholesterol embolization may be one factor contributing to the loss of renal function in patients with atherosclerotic IRD. Autopsy studies have identified renal cholesterol embolization in 15% to 30% of all patients with autopsy evidence of significant atherosclerosis or abdominal aortic aneurysms.

Cholesterol embolization most commonly occurs after arterial manipulation: arteriography, vascular surgery, angioplasty, and stent placement. In patients with extensive atherosclerosis with unstable plaques, this same process can occur spontaneously, independent of any vascular intervention, or after the administration of oral or intravenous anticoagulants or thrombolytic agents. The incidence of atheroembolic disease following vascular interventions is unclear, but recent data suggest that it is common.[55] Three large series of cardiac catheterization cited incidences <0.2%. In selected patient groups, the incidence is clearly much higher. A recent study evaluated the frequency of renal perfusion defects in patients after endovascular stent repair of abdominal aortic aneurysms. Eighteen percent of the cases had identifiable renal perfusion defects, and the occurrence of these infarcts was significantly associated with atherosclerotic burden as quantified by three-dimensional volume-rendered CTA.[56] Atheroembolism may therefore be expected to occur in up to 30% of patients with extensive aortic atherosclerosis.

Typically, patients are older than 50 years with generalized atherosclerosis. They often have a history of recent vascular surgery or signs or symptoms of atherosclerotic vascular disease, such as claudication, abdominal pain, angina, myocardial infarction, transient ischemic attacks, retinal artery emboli, amaurosis fugax, stroke, abdominal aortic aneurysm, renovascular hypertension, or IRD. Many have a history of risk factors for atherosclerosis, including hypertension, hypercholesterolemia, and smoking.

Clinical Presentation

Acute or subacute renal insufficiency due to renal microinfarctions is the most common clinical problem leading to the diagnosis of cholesterol embolization (see Chapter 63). The clinical picture is multisystemic in nature and involves the kidneys in about 75% of patients. At autopsy, renal involvement is observed in 92% to 100%.

If a large shower of atheroemboli causes significant tubular damage, the acute renal failure may have an oliguric phase characterized by a high fractional excretion of sodium. More often, the renal failure is nonoliguric and progressive because of ongoing embolization from a nidus of unstable ulcerative plaque. Some patients develop only a moderate impairment in renal function, and others progress to ESRD. Atheroembolic renal disease can also present as a more slowly progressive chronic renal insufficiency. Urinalysis findings are nondiagnostic but may include mild proteinuria, microhematuria, pyuria, and eosinophiluria. Renin release by ischemic tissue in areas of embolization can lead to labile, even malignant, hypertension early in the course, sometimes associated with transient marked proteinuria. Fever, often low-grade, is characteristic.

Although the kidneys are the most common organs involved, extrarenal cholesterol embolization will provide clues for diagnosis. Cutaneous findings present in up to 60% of patients at initial presentation include purple toes, mottled skin or livedo reticularis, petechiae, and purpura or necrotic ulceration in areas of skin embolization, such as the lower back, buttocks, lower abdomen, legs, feet, or digits (Fig. 61.20).

Other organs often involved include spleen (in 55% of cases), pancreas (52%), gastrointestinal tract (31%), liver (17%), and brain (14%). This involvement can result in a number of clinical symptoms, including abdominal or muscle pain, nausea, vomiting, ileus, gastrointestinal bleeding, ischemic bowel, hepatitis, angina, or neurologic deficits. When retinal cholesterol embolization occurs, refractile yellow deposits known as *Hollenhorst plaques* may be seen at the bifurcation of retinal vessels on funduscopic examination (Fig. 61.21).

Diagnosis

The diagnosis of atheroembolic renal disease is strongly suspected when subacute renal failure develops after a vascular intervention in the presence of livedo reticularis. A myriad of laboratory abnormalities indicative of tissue injury are associated with cholesterol embolization, including elevated sedimentation rate (in 97% of cases), elevated serum amylase (60%), leukocytosis (57%), anemia (46%), hypocomplementemia (25%–70%), and elevated LDH and CPK (38%–60%). Eosinophilia, which may be transient, is seen in up to 57% of patients. Serum lactate is usually not elevated unless concomitant ischemic bowel is present.

Although associated laboratory findings can be supportive, definitive diagnosis is made by biopsy of an involved organ or

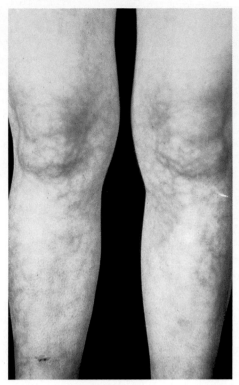

Figure 61.20 Livedo reticularis. The mottled skin changes associated with peripheral cholesterol embolization may be seen over the legs, buttocks, back, or flank and may be transient.

system showing the cholesterol clefts within the vascular lumina, representing atherosclerotic debris that has embolized, with adjacent ischemic or infarcted segments of tissue (Fig. 61.22). A cutaneous or muscle biopsy in an involved area can preclude the need for renal biopsy.

Differential Diagnosis

The systemic nature of this syndrome may mimic infection or vasculitis that may lead to delayed or missed diagnosis. Contrast nephropathy with nonoliguric acute tubular necrosis may also occur after angiography, angioplasty, or an aortic vascular surgical procedure but is often more rapid as opposed to the subacute presentation of atheroemboli. Clinical presentation with eosinophilia and eosinophiluria, rash, fever, and renal

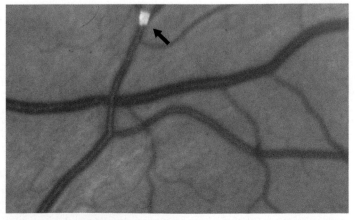

Figure 61.21 Cholesterol embolus of a retinal arteriole (arrow). (Courtesy of Mr. Richard Mills.)

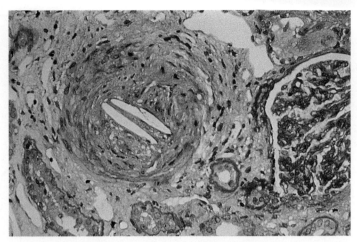

Figure 61.22 Cholesterol emboli in a kidney biopsy. Light microscopic section demonstrating cholesterol clefts with giant cell reaction and recanalization in the lumen of a medium-sized renal vessel. (Periodic acid–Schiff stain.) (Courtesy of Dr. R. Horn.)

dysfunction may also be misdiagnosed as acute interstitial nephritis (see Chapter 57).

Pathology and Pathophysiology

If clinical or other pathologic evidence has not secured the diagnosis, renal biopsy may be helpful. The diagnostic finding on biopsy is the presence of birefringent, biconvex, elongated cholesterol crystals or biconcave clefts within the lumina of small vessels left behind in formalin-fixed tissue (see Fig. 61.22). Because of the patchy nature of this disorder, open-wedge renal biopsy guided by visualization of areas of ischemic infarction of the cortex has a higher likelihood of successfully finding diagnostic pathologic changes than percutaneous needle biopsy. The pathologist should be alerted by the clinician that cholesterol embolization is in the differential diagnosis before the biopsy specimen is processed. In frozen sections of tissue, the cholesterol material can be identified using polarized light microscopy. The pathologic findings may also include intimal thickening and concentric fibrosis of vessels, giant cell reaction to the cholesterol particles, vascular recanalization, endothelial proliferation, tubulointerstitial fibrosis with both eosinophil and mononuclear cell infiltrates, glomerular ischemia, and even a collapsing glomerulopathy, a subtype of focal segmental glomerulosclerosis.[57] In the kidney, the most commonly affected vessels are the arcuate and interlobular arterioles, leading to patchy ischemic changes in glomeruli distal to these vessels.

Natural History

The natural history of atheroembolic renal disease is variable and is determined by the extent of organ involvement and the degree of the embolization. In one series of cases diagnosed by renal biopsy, renal function declined rapidly in 29%, with a more slowly progressive course seen in 79%.[58] Among the latter group, the decline in renal function was thought to result from a combination of cholesterol embolization and IRD. In another series, the peak serum creatinine occurred within 8 weeks after an angiographic procedure.[59] Patients may also manifest acute or subacute renal insufficiency followed by partial recovery of renal function. Conversely, the outcome can be dismal, particularly when cerebral embolization occurs or when there is a large unstable atheromatous burden. Some patients with cholesterol embolization may develop ESRD. These patients have a mortality rate of 35% to 40% over 5 years, even when dialysis is offered.[59]

Treatment

The risk for cholesterol embolization should be considered before undertaking angiographic and vascular surgical procedures in patients with diffuse, extensive atherosclerotic disease. Because prevention is the most effective management strategy, patients with extensive aortic atherosclerosis should be considered for alternative approaches to cardiac catheterization, such as through the brachial artery. If vascular intervention is performed, signs of embolization should be sought in both the immediate postoperative period and for several months thereafter. When feasible, distal embolic protection devices should be used to trap embolic material and remove it from the circulation to avoid end-organ damage by embolic debris.

After the diagnosis of cholesterol embolization is established, further endovascular interventions should be avoided. Poor outcomes have been reported in patients with cholesterol emboli that subsequently undergo coronary artery bypass surgery. When clinical factors dictate the need for aortic, renal, or peripheral arterial surgery, optimal timing and surgical approach are critical. Conversely, there is a growing surgical experience with segmental aortic replacement to remove the source of emboli, particularly when atheroembolic disease occurs spontaneously. Transesophageal echocardiography is often used to identify mobile ulcerative plaque in the aorta.

ACE inhibitors are effective in managing the labile hypertension seen early in the course of cholesterol embolization. Corticosteroids have been used with some success in patients with systemic cholesterol embolization and associated inflammatory symptoms.[60] There have also been several reports documenting improvement or stabilization of skin signs of cholesterol embolization after administration of statins,[61] which should be part of the treatment of the generalized atherosclerosis in these patients. Cholesterol embolization has also occurred after treatment with anticoagulants. Although direct causality between anticoagulants and cholesterol embolization has not been established, the proposed mechanism is that anticoagulants prevent thrombus organization over the ulcerative plaques. Therefore, anticoagulation should be avoided in the acute setting of cholesterol embolization unless a strong life-threatening indication for anticoagulation is present.

TRANSPLANT RENAL ARTERY STENOSIS AND THROMBOSIS

Epidemiology

Transplant RA stenosis is a relatively common post-transplantation complication occurring most often in the period between 3 months and 2 years after transplantation (see Chapter 92). The highest reported incidence is 23% in a patient cohort screened angiographically, compared with reported incidences of between 1.3% and 12% when other screening tests are used.[62] In many reports, the hemodynamic significance of the stenosis is poorly documented, and recent data suggest that often anastomotic stenoses are not hemodynamically significant.[62] The use of pediatric kidneys in adult recipients is associated with a higher rate of stenosis owing to smaller donor vessel size, leading to greater turbulences and mismatch between donor and recipient vessels. As the transplant population ages, there has been increasing recognition of another subset of patients with "pseudotransplant" RA stenosis, in which vascular disease proximal to the allograft artery, particularly involving the iliac vessel, results in renal ischemia.

Pathogenesis

The pathophysiologic basis for transplant RA stenosis is multifactorial and may include atheromatous disease in the donor artery, intimal scarring and hyperplasia in response to trauma to the vessel during harvesting, and anastomotic stenosis, which is most commonly associated with end-to-end anastomoses and may be related to suture technique. In end-to-side anastomoses, stenosis tends to develop in the postanastomotic site, suggesting that turbulence or other hemodynamic factors play a role. Immunologic causes of transplant RA stenosis have also been proposed based on histologic similarities with chronic vascular rejection and reports that it is associated with prior rejection. Other proposed candidates include calcineurin inhibitor toxicity and cytomegalovirus infection.

Clinical Presentation

Patients typically present with new-onset hypertension or difficult-to-control blood pressure with or without graft dysfunction occurring 3 to 24 months after transplantation. Patients may also present with acute renal failure or hypotension after placement on ACE inhibitors or ARBs. Systolic bruits over the transplant are not diagnostic because they may represent turbulent flow in the main vessels in the absence of stenosis or biopsy-related arteriovenous fistulas. Risk factors for the development of RA stenosis include male gender, hyperlipidemia, and elevated serum creatinine at discharge from transplantation.

Diagnosis

RDS is the screening test of choice for transplant RA stenosis because the vessel is superficial and easy to interrogate. The ratio of velocity in the renal and iliac vessels and the resistive index in the kidney have been shown to predict the hemodynamic response to PTRA. Phase-contrast MRA has advantage over arteriography in viewing tortuous renal arteries and may provide additional information over Doppler ultrasound regarding the aorta and iliac vessels. However, with MRA, the surgical clip artifact may obscure the proximal renal artery and often cannot resolve peripheral renal vessels. High false-positive rates are associated with sharp anastomotic angles. Spiral CT has advantage over MRA from an imaging standpoint but requires a large amount of contrast. The gold standard is selective digital subtraction angiography of the transplant artery. In situations in which the risk for contrast-induced acute renal failure is high, carbon dioxide angiography can be performed safely.

Treatment

Long-term observation of untreated transplant RA stenosis suggests progressive loss of renal function.[63] PTRA is the preferred initial approach to RA stenosis in the transplant setting, with initial success rates of up to 75% and patency for follow-up periods of up to 30 months. The average complication rate for PTRA of the allograft artery is 10%. It is often unsuccessful when there is arterial kinking and is associated with a high complication rate in this setting. The reported rates of late restenosis are between 10% and 33%, necessitating repeated procedures. Recent reports document the safety and efficacy of endovascular stenting in treating transplant RA stenosis, with fewer complications than with earlier reports for both PTRA and stenting.[64]

Surgical revascularization is reserved for patients in whom PTRA has been unsuccessful or complicated, or in whom stenoses are distal. Although there are some data supporting the superiority of surgical repair over PTRA in terms of long-term patency, blood pressure control, and allograft function, surgical repair is fraught with difficulty and is associated with significant mortality in the transplantation setting. Extensive fibrosis develops around the allograft and often involves the renal vessels, making surgical access difficult and risky. Complications include graft loss (in 15% to 30% of cases), ureteral injury (14%), and death (5%).

RENAL VEIN THROMBOSIS

RVT is a rare event primarily observed in children with severe dehydration (with an incidence in neonates of 0.26% to 0.7%) or in adults with nephrotic syndrome, renal cancer, hypercoagulable states, or following surgery or trauma to the renal vessels.[65] When it occurs in adults, the diagnosis is often never considered. Thrombosis of the longer left (7.5 cm) renal vein may also involve the ureteric, gonadal, adrenal, and phrenic branches that drain into the left vein, whereas on the shorter right renal vein (2.5 cm), the adrenal and gonadal veins drain directly into the inferior vena cava. The renal veins also communicate with perirenal veins outside of Gerota's fascia as part of the retroperitoneal collateral venous network: tributaries of the portal system, lumbar, azygos, and hemiazygos. Because of this network of venous complexes, occlusion of the left renal vein results in enlargement of the systemic collateral vessels and provides some protection against infarction.

Experimentally, acute RVT is associated with immediate enlargement of the kidney with marked increase in renal vein pressure (from 6 to 135 mm Hg in a study in dogs), leading to a marked decrease in renal arterial flow. Complications include hemorrhagic infarction, kidney rupture, or retroperitoneal hemorrhage. In the dog, the kidney enlarges over the course of 1 week, then proceeds to atrophy as a result of progressive fibrosis. In contrast, slow, progressive ("chronic") thrombosis may allow collateral formation, resulting in minimal symptoms.

Clinical Presentation

Acute RVT is usually symptomatic and associated with loin, testicular, or flank pain, low-grade temperature, and in the setting of single kidney or renal transplant, symptoms of renal failure. Often, nausea and vomiting accompany acute RVT, and symptoms might be confused with acute pyelonephritis. Leukocytosis can accompany acute thrombosis. Clinical signs include renal enlargement, which in infants manifests as a palpable abdominal mass. Hematuria is nearly universal and most often is microscopic. The high venous pressures result in a marked increase in proteinuria. Oliguric renal failure occurs when RVT results in renal infarction of both kidneys or in subjects with a single kidney. In some cases, RVT is diagnosed only after the patient develops an acute pulmonary embolus and the source of the embolus is investigated.

Chronic RVT may be asymptomatic and is associated with extensive venous collaterals and minimal impairment of renal function and structure. Often, however, microhematuria, an increase in proteinuria, and some renal dysfunction is present, particularly when indices of differential renal function are sought, such as with nuclear studies.

Causes of Renal Vein Thrombosis

Causes of RVT are listed in Figure 61.23. In the neonate, the most common cause is dehydration. In both infants and adults, all hypercoagulable states can lead to RVT, including nephrotic syndrome, pregnancy, and abnormalities of the clotting cascade, such as factor V Leiden mutations.

Nephrotic Syndrome

RVT is the most common thromboembolic event in nephrotic syndrome. The prevalence of RVT in nephrotic syndrome is unclear because it is largely undiagnosed; studies report frequencies between 5% and 62%.[65] Numerous abnormalities promoting a prothrombotic state occur secondary to heavy proteinuria (see Chapter 16). Interestingly, RVT appears more common in membranous nephropathy and lupus nephritis, but RVT can complicate any cause of proteinuric renal disease. When it presents in this setting, RVT can lead to an increase in baseline proteinuria and present with acute renal failure superimposed on chronic renal insufficiency.

Diagnosis of RVT requires imaging. Conventional ultrasonography may demonstrate alterations in size and echogenicity. RDS may show increases in resistive indices, and ultrasound can directly visualize the filling defect, but this may depend on the angle of the vein, the body habitus of the patient, and operator experience. Both CT and magnetic resonance venography can demonstrate RVT (Fig. 61.24), avoiding the need for direct renal venography. Magnetic resonance venography has the advantage of avoiding nephrotoxic contrast agents.

Renal Vein Thrombosis in Renal Transplantation

RVT after transplantation is rare and occurs in less than 0.1% of transplants, usually within the first week after transplantation. It usually leads to graft infarction. Causes include volume depletion

Causes of renal vein thrombosis
Thrombosis of the inferior vena cava

Rheologic abnormalities
   Neonatal or (rarely) adult dehydration
      Maternal diabetes, diarrhea, sepsis, adrenal hemorrhage,
         hypoglycemia, seizure disorder, hypoxia
   Infants with sickle cell disease
   Neonatal polycythemia
   Hyperleukocytosis associated with leukemia
   Thrombophilia, thrombocytosis
   Hyperhomocystinemia

Nephropathies
   Membranous glomerulonephritis
   Lupus nephritis
   Nephrotic syndrome associated with other glomerulopathies
   Amyloidosis

Tumor
   Renal cell carcinoma
   Leiomyosarcoma of the inferior vena cava
   Extrinsic compression by retroperitoneal tumor, lymphoma, or fibrosis

Acute pancreatitis
Acute pyelonephritis
Venous hypertensive states   Tricuspid insufficiency, constrictive pericarditis

Hypercoagulable states
   Oral contraceptives
   Antiphospholipid syndrome
   Trousseau's syndrome
   Factor V Leiden mutation
   Protein S and C deficiency
   Antithrombin III deficiency
   Prothrombin G20210A mutation
   Postpartum state of pregnancy

Inferior vena cava filter in the renal vein
Surgical dissection or division of the renal vein
Blunt trauma
Renal transplantation

Figure 61.23 Causes of renal vein thrombosis.

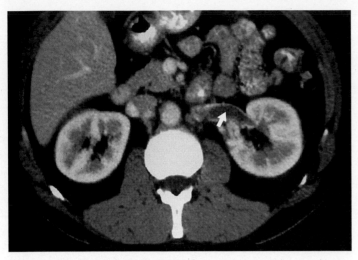

Figure 61.24 **Renal vein thrombosis.** Computed tomography scan showing left renal vein thrombosis *(arrow)*. (Courtesy of Dr. S. Rankin.)

or a hypercoagulable state. Factor V Leiden mutation, which occurs in 2% to 5% of the population is a risk factor for transplant RVT and should be sought when it occurs. There is some data supporting the protective effects of low dose aspirin in this population.

Renal Vein Thrombosis in Pregnancy
Pregnancy and the postpartum state are hypercoagulable states. There have been reports of spontaneous RVT in the postpartum period associated with renal infarction. RVT complicating pregnancy should be suspected when clinical clues such as flank pain or hematuria are present.

Renal Vein Thrombosis in Malignancy
RVT can result from invasion of tumor of renal origin into the renal vein. About half of renal cell carcinomas are associated with RVT at autopsy. In addition, neoplasia originating in the renal vein or inferior vena cava, such as leiomyosarcoma, can cause RVT. Extrinsic compression of the renal vein by tumor or retroperitoneal fibrosis may also cause this syndrome.

Treatment
Treatment is controversial and depends on the acuteness and renal consequences. Surgical interventions include nephrectomy, thrombectomy, and retroperitoneal surgery for non–renal-associated abnormalities such as tumor, retroperitoneal fibrosis, aortic aneurysm, or acute pancreatitis. Surgery tends to be reserved for situations in which the RVT results in hemorrhage due to capsular rupture or for long-term consequences of RVT such as hypertension or infection of a nonfunctioning kidney. Over the past decade, there has been a shift from surgical intervention to medical or conservative therapy. In neonatal RVT, which often results in renal nonfunction, thrombolytic therapy and anticoagulation have been used with variable results. In two recent reports of neonatal RVT, supportive care was recommended for unilateral RVT without extension into the inferior vena cava while thrombolytics were used for bilateral cases with impending renal failure.

In adults with acute RVT secondary to hypercoagulable state, catheter-directed thrombolytic therapy with urokinase or tissue plasminogen activator with or without percutaneous mechanical thrombectomy can be successful in regaining patency of the vessel and restoring renal function. There are even reports of successful thrombolytic therapy used in pregnancy-associated RVT. The long-term benefit of this approach is unclear, and it is less successful when the thrombotic process initiates in the small intrarenal venules rather than the major veins as is often the case when primary renal disease or hypercoagulable state initiates the process. In addition, a conservative approach may be favored when left RVT occurs because of the extensive collateral venous supply on that side, ultimately allowing venous drainage and improvement in renal function. Systemic anticoagulation is indicated acutely to prevent extension of thrombus into the inferior vena cava and for prevention of pulmonary emboli. Anticoagulation should be continued indefinitely in patients with persistent hypercoagulable state following RVT. In addition, eventual recanalization of the venous system can result in delayed improvement in renal function as measured by nuclear medicine studies.

REFERENCES

1. Yune Hy, Klatte EC: Collateral circulation to an ischemic kidney. Radiology 1976;119:539–546.
2. Conlon PJ, O'Riordan EO, Kalra PA: New insights into the epidemiologic and clinical manifestations of atherosclerotic renovascular disease. Am J Kidney Dis 2000;35:573–587.
3. Olin JW, Melia M, Young JR, et al: Prevalence of atherosclerotic RAS in patients with atherosclerosis elsewhere. Am J Med 1990;88(Suppl 1):56N–61N.
4. Harding MB, Smith LR, Himmelstein SI, et al: Renal artery stenosis: Prevalence and associated risk factors in patients undergoing cardiac catheterization. J Am Soc Nephrol 1992;2:1608–1614.
5. Hansen KJ, Edwards MS, Craven TE, et al: Prevalence of renovascular disease in the elderly: A population-based study. J Vasc Surg 2002;36:43–51.
6. Kuroda S, Nishida N, Uzu T, et al: Prevalence of renal artery stenosis in autopsy patients with stroke. Stroke 2000;31:64–65.
7. Sica DA, Hansen KJ, Deitch JS, et al: Renovascular disease in blacks: Prevalence and result of operative management. Am J Med Sci 1998;315:37–342.
8. Greco, BA, Breyer JB: Atherosclerotic ischemic renal disease. Am J Kidney Dis 1997;29:167–187.
9. Caps MT, Perissinotto C, Zierler RE, et al: Prospective study of atherosclerotic disease progression in the renal artery. Circulation 1998;98:2866–2872.
10. van Ampting JM, Penne EL, Beek FJ, et al: Prevalence of atherosclerotic renal artery stenosis in patients starting dialysis. Nephrol Dial Transpl 2003;18:147–151.
11. Hricik DE, Browning PJ, Kopelman R: Captopril induced functional renal insufficiency in patients with bilateral renal-artery stenosis or renal-artery stenosis in a solitary kidney. N Engl J Med 1983;308:373–376.
12. Toto RD, Mitchell HC, Lee HC: Reversible renal insufficiency due to angiotensin converting enzyme inhibitions in hypertensive nephrosclerosis. Ann Intern Med 1991;15:513–519.
13. Kulra PA, Kumwenda M, MacDowell P, Roland MO: ACE inhibitor usage and monitoring in general practice: The need for guidelines to prevent renal failure. BMG 1999;318:234–237.
14. Hollenberg GG, Clarkson AB, Woodroffe AJ: Medical therapy of renovascular hypertension: Efficacy and safety of captopril in 269 patients. Cardiovasc Res 1983;4:852–876.
15. Maxwell MH, Bleifer KH, Franklin SS: Cooperative study of renovascular hypertension: Demographic analysis of the study. JAMA 1972;220:1195–204.
16. Messina LM, Zelenock GB, Yao KA: Renal revascularization for recurrent pulmonary edema in patients with poorly controlled hypertension and renal insufficiency: A distinct subgroup of patients with arterosclerotic renal artery occlusive disease. J Vasc Surg 1992;15:73–82.

17. Bloch MJ, Trost DW, Pickering TG, et al: Prevention of recurrent pulmonary edema in patients with bilateral renovascular disease through renal artery stent placement. Am J Hypertens 1999;12:1–7.

18. Vasbinder GB, Nelemans PJ, Kessels AG, et al: Diagnostic tests for renal artery stenosis in patients suspected of having renovascular hypertension: A meta-analysis. Ann Intern Med 2001;135:401–411.

19. Patel ST, Mill JL: The limitations of magnetic resonance angiography in the diagnosis of renal artery stenosis: Comparative analysis with conventional angiography. J Vasc Surg 2005;41:462–468.

20. De Cobelli F, Venturini M, Vanzulli A, et al: Renal artery stenosis: Prospective comparison of color Doppler US and breath-hold, three-dimensional, dynamic, gadolinium-enhanced MR angiography. Radiology 2000;214:373–380.

21. Vasbinder GB, Nelemens PJ: Accuracy of computed tomography angiography and magnetic resonance angiography for diagnosing renal artery stenosis. J Vasc Interv Radiol 2005;16:432.

22. Radermacher J, Chavan A, Bleck J, et al: Use of Doppler ultrasonography to predict the outcome of therapy for renal artery stenosis. N Engl J Med 2001;344:410–417.

23. Vaughn BFR Jr, Laragh JH: Renovascular hypertension: Renin measurements to indicate hypersecretion and contralateral suppression, estimate renal plasma flow, and score for surgical curability. Am J Med 1973;55:402–414.

24. Urban BA, Ratner LF, Fishman EK: Three-dimensional volume-rendered CT angiography of the renal arteries and veins: Normal anatomy, variants and clinical applications. Radiographics 2001;21:373–386.

25. Martin LG, Rundback JH, Sacks D, et al: Society of Interventional Radiology Standards of Practice Committee. Quality improvement guidelines for angiography, angioplasty, and stent placement in the diagnosis and treatment of renal artery stenosis in adults. J Vasc Interv Radiol 2003;14(Pt 2):S297–S310.

26. Makanjuola AD, Suresh M, Laboi P, et al: Proteinuria in atherosclerotic renovascular disease. Q J Med 1999;92:515–518.

27. Siddiqui S, MacGregor MS, Glynn C, et al: Factors predicting outcome in a cohort of patients with atherosclerotic renal artery stenosis diagnosed by magnetic resonance angiography. Am J Kidney Dis 2005;46:1068–1073.

28. Mailloux LU, Bellucci AG, Mossey RG, et al: Predictors of survival in patients undergoing dialysis. Am J Med 1988,84:855–862.

29. Johannson M, Herlitz H, Jensen G, et al: Increased cardiovascular mortality in hypertensive patients with renal artery stenosis: Relation to sympathetic activation, renal function and treatment regimens. J Hypertens 1999;17:1743–1750.

30. Losito A, Parente B, Cao PG, et al: ACE gene polymorphism and survival in atherosclerotic renovascular disease. Am J Kidney Dis 2000,35:211–215.

31. Watson PS, Hudjipetrou P, Cox SV, et al: Effect of renal artery stenting on renal function and size in patients with atherosclerotic renovascular disease. Circulation 2000;102:1671–1677.

32. Edwards MS, Craven TE, Burke GL, et al: Renovascular disease and the risk of adverse coronary events in the elderly: A prospective, population-based study. Arch Intern Med 2005;165:207–213.

33. Dean RH, Kieffer RW, Smith BM, et al: Renovascular hypertension: Anatomic and renal function changes during drug therapy, Arch Surg 1981;116:1408–1415.

34. Scarpioni R, Michieletti E, Cristinelli L, et al: Atherosclerotic renovascular disease: Medical therapy versus medical therapy plus renal artery stenting in preventing renal failure progression: The rationale and study of a prospective multicenter and randomized trial. J Hypertens 2005;Oct 23:S5–S13.

35. Murphy TP, Cooper CJ, Dworkin LD, et al: The Cardiovascular Outcomes with Renal Atherosclerotic Lesions (CORAL) study: Rationale and methods. J Vasc Interv Radiol 2005;16:1295–1300.

36. Bax L, Mali WP, Buskens E, et al: The benefit of stent placement and blood pressure and lipid-lowering for the prevention of progression of renal dysfunction caused by atherosclerotic ostial stenosis of the renal artery. The STAR study: Rationale and study design. J Nephrol 2003;16:807–812.

37. Chabova V, Schirger A, Stanson AW, et al: Outcomes of atherosclerotic renal artery stenosis managed without revascularization. Mayo Clin Proc 2000;75:37–44.

38. Leertouwer TC, Gussenhoven EJ, Bosch J: Stent placement for renal arterial stenosis: Where do we stand? A meta-analysis. Radiology 2000;216:78–85.

39. Erdoes LS, Berman SS, Hunter GC, Mills JL: Comparative analysis of percutaneous transluminal angioplasty and operation for renal revascularization. Am J Kidney Dis 1996;27:496–503.

40. Ivanovic V, McKusick MA, Johnson CM, et al: Renal artery stent placement: Complications at a single tertiary care center. J Vasc Interv Radiol 2003;14(Pt 1):217–225.

41. Korsakas S, Mohaupt M, Dinkel H, et al: Delay of dialysis in end-stage renal failure: Prospective study on percutaneous renal artery interventions. Kidney Int 2004;65:251–258.

42. Beutler JJ, Van Ampting JM, van de Ven PJ, et al: Long-term effects of arterial stenting on kidney function for patients with ostial atherosclerotic renal artery stenosis and renal insufficiency. J Am Soc Nephrol 2001;12:1475–1481.

43. Novick AC: Surgical revascularization for renal artery disease: current status. BJU Int 2005;95(Suppl 2):75–77.

44. Hansen KJ, Lundbert AH, Benjamin ME, et al: Is renal revascularization in diabetic patients worthwhile? J Vasc Surg 1996;24:383–393.

45. Hansen KJ, Cherr GS, Craven TE, et al: Management of ischemic nephropathy: Dialysis-free survival after surgical repair. J Vasc Surg 2000;32:472–482.

46. Cambria RP, Brewster DC, L'Italien GJ, et al: Renal artery reconstruction for the preservation of renal function. J Vasc Surg 1996;24:371–382.

47. Marone LK, Clouse WD, Dorer DJ, et al: Preservation of renal function with surgical revascularization in patients with atherosclerotic renovascular disease. J Vasc Surg 2004;39:22–29.

48. Steinbach F, Novick AC, Campbell S, Dykstra D: Long-term survival after surgical revascularization for atherosclerotic renal artery disease. J Urol 1997;158:388–341.

49. Lohse Jr, Shore RM, Belzer FO: Acute renal artery occlusion. Arch Surg 1982;117:801–804.

50. Hazanov N, Somin M, Attali M, et al: Acute renal embolism: Forty-four cases of renal infarction in patients with atrial fibrillation. Medicine 2004;83:92–99.

51. Nochy DE, Daugas E, Droz D, et al: The intrarenal vascular lesions associated with primary antiphospholipid syndrome. J Am Soc Nephrol 1999;10:506–518.

52. van der Wal MA, Wisselink W, Rauwerda JA: Traumatic bilateral renal artery thrombosis: Case report and review of the literature. Cardiovasc Surg 2003;11:27–29.

53. Verhoye J, De Latour B, Heautot J: Return of renal function after endovascular treatment of aortic dissection. N Engl J Med 2005;352:824–1825.

54. Krishnamurthi V, Novick AC, Myles JL: Atheroembolic renal disease: Effect on morbidity and survival after revascularization for atherosclerotic renal artery stenosis. J Urol 1999;161:93–96.

55. Polu KR, Wolf M: Needle in a haystack. N Engl J Med 2006;354:68–73.

56. Harris JR, Fan CM, Geller SC, et al: Renal perfusion defects after endovascular repair of abdominal aortic aneurysms. J Vasc Interv Radiol 2003;14:329–333.

57. Greenberg A, Bastacky SI, Iqbal A, et al: Focal segmental glomerulosclerosis associated with nephrotic syndrome in cholesterol atheroembolism: clinicopathologic correlations. Am J Kidney Dis 1997;29:334–344.

58. Blenfant X, Meyrier A, Jacquot C: Supportive treatment improves survival in multivisceral cholesterol crystal embolism. Am J Kidney Dis 1999;33:840–850.

59. Scolari F, Ravani P, Pola A, et al: Predictors of renal and patient outcomes in atheroembolic renal disease: A prospective study. J Am Soc Nephrol 2003;14:1584–1590.

60. Graziani G, Sanostasi S, Angelini C, et al: Corticosteroids in cholesterol emboli syndrome. Nephron 2001;87:371–373.

61. Finch TM, Ryatt KS: Livedo reticularis caused by cholesterol embolization may improve with simvastatin. Br J Dermatol 2000;143:1319–1320.

62. Fervenza FC, Lafayette RA, Alfrey EJ, et al: Renal artery stenosis in kidney transplants. Am J Kidney Dis 1998;31:142–148.

63. Deglise-Favre A, Hiesse C, Lantz O, et al: Long-term follow-up of 40 untreated cadaveric kidney transplant renal artery stenoses. Transplant Proc 1991;23:1342–1343.

64. Bertoni E, Zanazzi M, Rosat A, et al: Efficacy and safety of Palmaz stent insertion in the treatment of renal artery stenosis in kidney transplantation. Transplant Int 2000;13:S425–430.

65. Harris R, Ismail N: Extrarenal complications of nephrotic syndrome. Am J Kidney Dis 1994;23:477–497.

CHAPTER
62 Geriatric Nephrology

Edgar V. Lerma, Leon Ferder, and Richard J. Johnson

INTRODUCTION

Aging is a slow, inflammatory biologic process that affects many organs, of which the kidney is one of the main targets. Aging is associated with a decline in renal function coincident with a progressive loss of nephrons, with glomerular and tubulointerstitial scarring. These changes begin in the fourth decade of life and accelerate between the fifth and sixth decades, resulting in alterations in glomerular and tubular function, systemic hemodynamics, and body homeostasis. Although aging-related changes begin in midlife, most of the discussion in this chapter revolves around the management of the older population, defined as >65 years of age.

It is important to realize that aging-associated renal disease may not be an inevitable consequence of life. Some subjects do not show age-related decline in GFR, and in some populations, hypertension does not increase with aging, the latter occurring primarily in non-Westernized groups habitually on low sodium diets. This has led some to hypothesize that aging-associated renal disease may be an active process that is potentially preventable.

ANATOMIC CHANGES

The human kidney reaches a maximum size of about 400 g (corresponding to 12 cm in length) in the fourth decade of life. After this, there is a natural decline in renal size, amounting to about a 10% decrease in renal mass per decade, with a tendency for decrease to be greater in males than females. This decrease is associated with progressive cortical thinning and loss in the number of functional nephrons. Renal biopsies show progressive focal and segmental glomerulosclerosis, tubulointerstitial fibrosis, and arteriolar hyalinosis (Fig. 62.1).

GLOMERULAR CHANGES

Several structural changes occur in the glomerulus with aging. Preserved glomeruli often show an increase in overall tuft cross-sectional area, consistent with glomerular hypertrophy.[1] The glomerular basement membrane also thickens with age. Most evident is the development of focal and segmental or, rarely, global, glomerulosclerosis. Whereas the prevalence of glomerulosclerosis is <5% of glomeruli at birth, this increases to 10% to 30% of glomeruli by the eighth decade[2] (Fig. 62.2). In aging mice and rats, which show similar histologic changes, a strong relationship between the glomerular hypertrophy and glomerulosclerosis has been shown,[3] consistent with the hypothesis that glomerular hypertrophy may predispose to the development of glomerulosclerosis.[4] The glomerulosclerosis is associated with mesangial matrix expansion and a progressive loss of capillary loops. Periglomerular

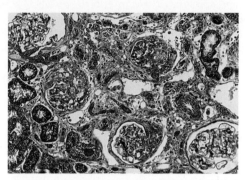

Figure 62.1 Glomerulosclerosis and tubulointerstitial fibrosis in an aging rat. Similar changes, consisting of focal segmental glomerulosclerosis, tubular atrophy, and interstitial fibrosis, occur in humans. (Trichrome stain, original magnification ×400).

fibrosis is often prominent, and there may be "atubular glomeruli," in which the exit from Bowman's capsule to the proximal tubular lumen is blocked by fibrosis.

TUBULAR AND INTERSTITIAL CHANGES

Tubulointerstitial injury is greatest in the outer medulla and medullary rays, with tubular dilatation and atrophy, mononuclear cell infiltration, and interstitial fibrosis. Many tubules express osteopontin, which is a marker of tubular injury and a chemotactic protein. The infiltrating interstitial cells consist of macrophages and myofibroblasts, and the fibrosis is due in part to the deposition of types I and III collagen,[5] which appears to be mediated by the local expression of transforming growth

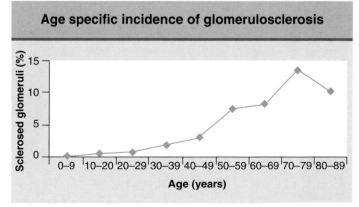

Figure 62.2 Glomerulosclerosis increases with aging. (Adapted from Kaplan C, Pasternack B, Shah H, Gallo G: Age-related incidence of sclerotic glomeruli in human kidneys. Am J Pathol 1975;80:227–234.)

factor-β (TGF-β).[6] Some tubules (especially of the distal tubule and collecting duct) may develop small diverticula; it has been suggested that these diverticula play a role in the development of upper urinary tract infections (pyelonephritis) by harboring bacteria, thereby predisposing to recurrent infection.[7]

VASCULAR CHANGES

Arterioles often develop hyalinosis with aging. Thickening of the arterioles with an increase in the medial thickness–to–lumen diameter ratio is common with aging but is observed almost exclusively in hypertensive individuals.[7] The arcuate arteries become more angulated and irregular with aging, and there is increased tortuosity and spiraling of the interlobar vessels. These changes occur independently of hypertension but are augmented in its presence. With aging, some afferent arterioles, particularly of juxtamedullary glomeruli, develop vascular shunts to the efferent arterioles, thereby bypassing glomeruli, leading to "aglomerular arterioles."[8] Studies in rats have also demonstrated focal losses of glomerular capillary loops and peritubular capillaries consistent with a state of impaired angiogenesis.[9]

FUNCTIONAL CHANGES

Glomerular Filtration Rate

Serum creatinine is a relatively unreliable indicator of renal function in the aging population. This is because creatinine generation reflects muscle mass, and muscle mass decreases with aging. Normally, males excrete 20 to 25 mg/kg body weight of creatinine in the urine each day, and women excrete 15 to 20 mg/kg body weight of creatinine. However, after the age of 60 years, there is a progressive decrease in urinary creatinine excretion, resulting in excretion rates lower than these ranges[10] (Fig. 62.3).

When accurate creatinine clearances are performed, there is clear evidence for a reduction in renal function with age. In one study, the mean creatinine clearance fell from 140 ml/min/1.73 m² at age 30 years to 97 ml/min/1.73 m² at age 80 years.[11] Interestingly, serum creatinine was not different between these groups because of the loss of muscle mass that occurs with aging. The decrease in renal function has been corroborated by

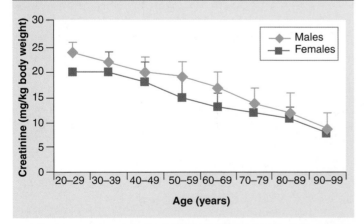

Figure 62.3 Urinary creatinine excretion (factored for body weight) decreases with age. (Adapted from Epstein M: Aging and the kidney. J Am Soc Nephrol 1996;7:1106–1122.)

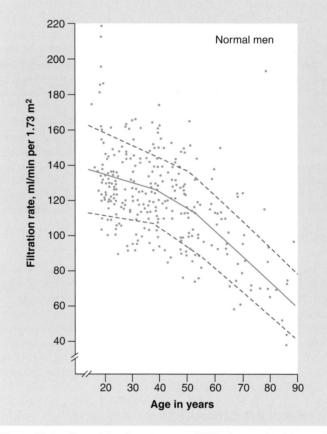

Figure 62.4 Glomerular filtration rate (GFR) decreases with age. GFR (inulin clearance) begins to fall at age 40 years, and the rate of decline is more rapid in men than women. (Adapted from Wesson LG Jr: Renal hemodynamics in physiological states. In Physiology of the Human Kidney. New York, Grune and Stratton, 1969, pp 96–108.)

inulin clearance studies, which show a progressive fall in GFR after the age of 40 years, with a relatively greater decline in men[12] (Fig. 62.4).

Formulas such as the MDRD (Modification of Diet in Renal Disease) equation or the Cockcroft-Gault formula (see Chapter 3) take into account changes with age. Both have a tendency to underestimate true GFR in the aging (>65 years) population when compared with standard techniques such as technetium-99m diethylenetriaminepenta-acetic acid (^{99m}Tc-DTPA). However, the MDRD appears to be more accurate than the Cockcroft-Gault formula.[13,14]

In addition to the decrease in GFR with aging, there may be a reduction in renal "reserve." Usually, GFR increases with a protein load or with feeding. Some studies suggest that aging humans show a normal increase in GFR after amino acid infusion. However, a more profound challenge was performed in aging rats; in this study, aging rats showed a markedly blunted increase in GFR with feeding.[15]

Not all individuals show a decrease in GFR with aging. In particular, in as many as one third of subjects who remain normotensive, there is no decrease in creatinine clearance with age.[7]

Renal Plasma Flow

There is also a decrease in renal plasma flow (RPF) with aging. RPF measured by para-amino hippurate (PAH) clearance decreases from a mean of 650 ml/min in the fourth decade to 290 ml/min by the ninth decade, and this is associated with increasing renal vascular resistance[12] (Fig. 62. 5). The fall in RPF tends to be greater in males than in females and is also greater in elderly subjects who are hypertensive.[16] Because RPF decreases relatively more than GFR, filtration fraction (defined as GFR/RPF) increases with age.

The decrease in RPF does not simply reflect a decrease in renal mass. Studies using a Xenon washout technique demonstrated there is a true reduction in renal blood flow when factored for renal mass.[17] The decrease in renal blood flow especially involves the cortex, and blood flow to the medulla is relatively preserved.

Capillary Permeability and Proteinuria

The prevalence of both microalbuminuria (urinary albumin levels of 30–300 mg/day) and albuminuria increases progressively in the U.S. population after the age of 40 years. The increased prevalence is most marked in diabetic and hypertensive subjects but is also observed in patients lacking these risk factors[18] (Fig. 62.6). The prevalence of microalbuminuria and albuminuria is higher in African Americans, Mexican Americans, and those with elevated serum creatinine.[18] This is clinically relevant because microalbuminuria is an independent risk factor for cardiovascular disease (such as carotid disease and left ventricular hypertrophy) and cardiovascular mortality.

Sodium Balance and Hypertension

Sodium balance is also altered in aging. There is evidence for both impaired sodium excretion of a salt load[19] and defective conservation in the setting of sodium restriction.[20] Proximal sodium reabsorption (reflected by lithium clearance) is increased in aging, whereas distal sodium reabsorption may be reduced.[21] Studies in rats suggest that pressure natriuresis is impaired in aging.[22] Because the diet of most individuals in developed countries contains excess sodium (8–10 g salt/day), there is a tendency in the elderly population for total body sodium excess.

The relative defect in sodium excretion and increased total body sodium may be a predisposing factor for the development of hypertension. Blood pressure increases with age. After the age of 60 years, most of the population is hypertensive[23] (Fig. 62.7). Most cases of hypertension (>85%) in the aging population are sodium sensitive, in that restricting sodium will result in a significant fall (>10 mm Hg) in mean arterial pressure.[24] Populations that ingest low-sodium diets, such as the Yanomamo Indians of Southern Venezuela, do not show an increase in blood pressure with age.[25] Other mechanisms may also be involved in aging-associated hypertension, including loss of vascular compliance due

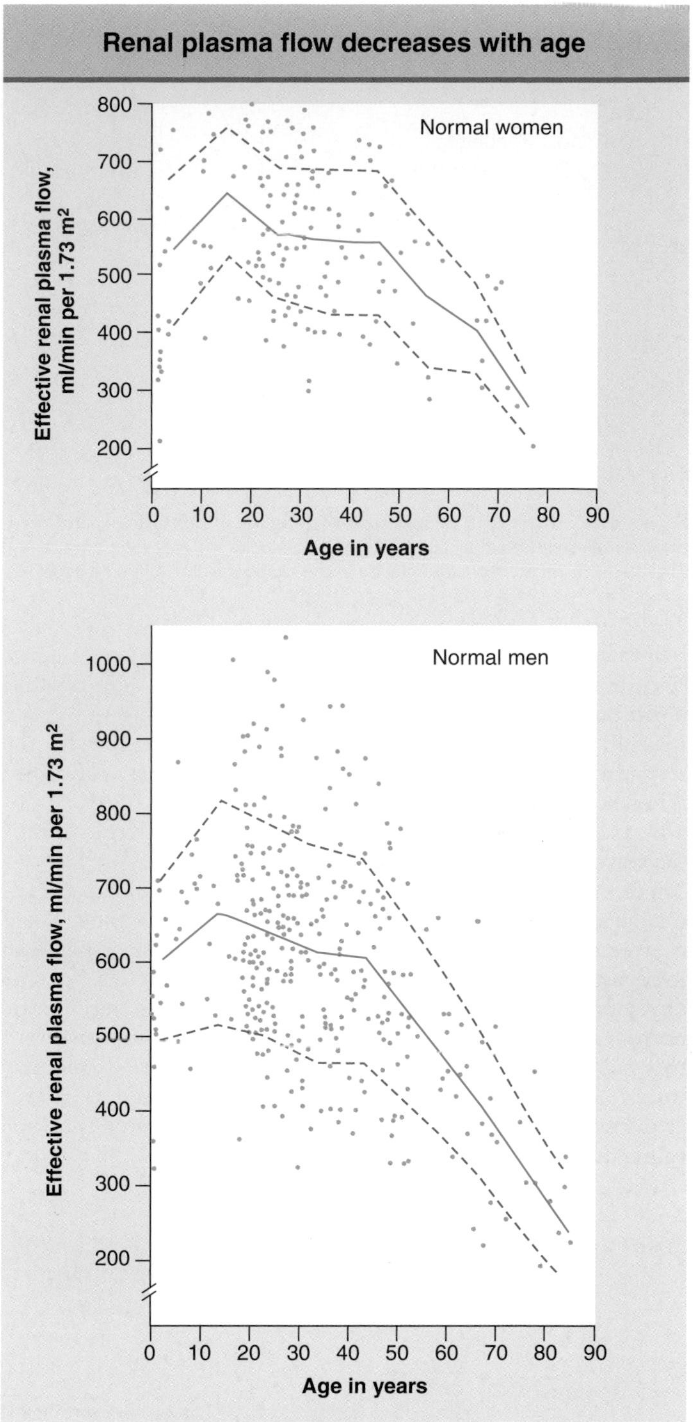

Renal plasma flow decreases with age

Figure 62.5 **Renal plasma flow (RPF) decreases with age.** RPF (PAH clearance) begins to fall rapidly after the age of 50 years, and the rate of decline is more rapid in men than women. (Adapted from Wesson LG Jr: Renal hemodynamics in physiological states. In Physiology of the Human Kidney. New York, Grune & Stratton, 1969, pp 96–108.)

to collagen deposition in the larger arterial vessels. Endothelial dysfunction, perhaps mediated by oxidative stress, has been shown to be increased in the aging population and may contribute to the development of increased blood pressure.

The observation that aging-associated renal and vascular changes may be responsible for the high frequency of hypertension in the population likely explains why correction of secondary forms of hypertension (such as primary aldosteronism, Cushing's syndrome,

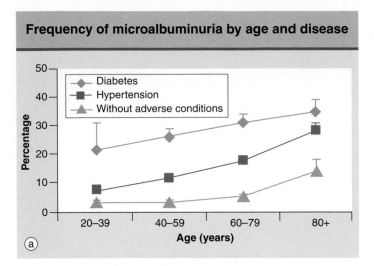

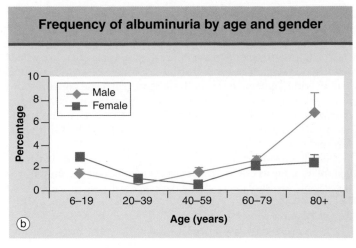

Figure 62.6   Increased proteinuria with aging. *a,* Microalbuminuria increases with age, with the greatest prevalence in diabetes, followed by hypertension and then the absence of either condition. *b,* Albuminuria increases with age, and the prevalence is greater in men than women. (Adapted from Jones CA, Francis ME, Eberhardt MS, et al: Microalbuminuria in the US population: Third National Health and Nutrition Examination Survey. Am J Kidney Dis 2002;39:445–449.)

renovascular hypertension, and hypothyroidism) is more effective at curing hypertension in younger patients. In one study, diastolic blood pressure fell to <90 mm Hg in 24 of 25 subjects younger than 40 years after treating the mechanism responsible for the secondary hypertension but in only 38 of 61 subjects older than 40 years.[26]

Osmoregulation and Water Handling

There is also impaired water handling with aging. Both concentration and dilution are affected, and nocturia is common. There is a reduced maximal urinary osmolality and thirst response to hyperosmolality, which may be predisposing factors for the development of dehydration. Subjects respond to antidiuretic hormone (vasopressin) with an increase in urine osmolarity, but this is blunted compared with younger subjects. Total body water also decreases with age. Conversely, there is slower excretion of a water load, leading to an increased predisposition to hyponatremia.

Other Tubular Defects and Electrolyte Problems

Potassium excretion is impaired and is likely due to decreased tubular mass. Hyperkalemia occurs more frequently in elderly subjects treated with drugs that interfere with potassium excretion (such as potassium-sparing diuretics) than in younger people. Other predispositions to hyperkalemia in the elderly include decreased GFR and lower basal levels of aldosterone. Hypokalemia is also common because of renal or extrarenal losses. Acid-base disturbances may result from the impaired distal tubular acidification that occurs with aging; aging subjects do not excrete an acid load as effectively as younger subjects.

Hypercalcemia occurs in 2% to 3% of institutionalized elderly patients. Causes are multifactorial and include malignant tumors, hyperparathyroidism, immobilization, and thiazide diuretic use. Hypocalcemia is less common and is observed mainly in patients with chronic renal failure, chronic malabsorption, and severe malnutrition. Aging is associated with increased parathyroid hormone levels (which correlate inversely with GFR) and a

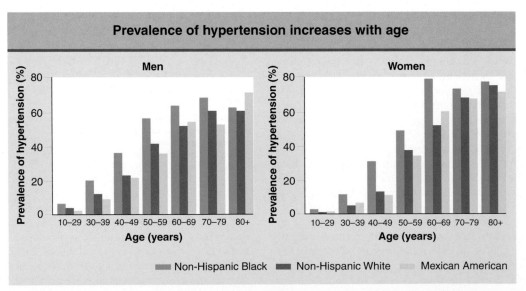

Figure 62.7   Prevalence of hypertension based on age, gender, and race. (Adapted from Burt VL, Whelton P, Roccella EJ, et al: Prevalence of hypertension in the US adult population. Results from the Third National Health and Nutrition Examination Survey, 1988–1991. Hypertension 1995;25:305–313.)

decrease in serum calcitriol and phosphate.[21] Hypomagnesemia may be present in as many as 7% to 10% of elderly patients admitted to the hospital; most commonly, this is the result of malnutrition, laxatives, or diuretic use. Hypermagnesemia is less common and is found primarily in patients with chronic renal failure or who are taking large doses of magnesium-containing antacids. Gout (as well as an elevation in serum uric acid levels) is also more common in the aging population.

RISK FACTORS FOR AGING-RELATED DISEASE

Variability in the severity of aging-related renal disease in humans and experimental animals has suggested that there may be specific risk factors for its development. For example, it is known that a percentage of normal subjects who remain normotensive will not show age-related decreases in GFR (measured as creatinine clearance).[7] In experimental models, aging-related histologic changes vary according to the genetic strain, gender, body mass index, and diet. Specifically, disease is worse in male and obese animals, and aging changes can be retarded with protein or caloric restriction.[22]

PATHOGENESIS OF PROGRESSIVE RENAL DISEASE IN AGING

A variety of mechanisms have been proposed for aging-related renal changes (Fig. 62.8). Senescence is associated with progressive telomere shortening of chromosomal DNA that may limit replicative capacity. In particular, a loss of mitochondrial DNA and total mitochondria occurs with aging.[27] A favored hypothesis is that it is due to the production of oxygen-derived free radicals that cause cumulative oxidative injury to tissues over time.[28] A loss of mitochondria interferes with mitochondrial respiration and cellular energetics and may predispose to cell injury or death. Senescence is associated with accelerated apoptosis, and increased numbers of apoptotic tubular and interstitial cells have been shown in the aging rat.[5]

Glomerular number also decreases from about 1 million per kidney to 600,000 or less by the eighth decade. A loss of nephrons results in hyperfiltration with increased glomerular hydrostatic pressure and glomerular hypertrophy, which are known risk factors for glomerular scarring.[29] However, studies in aging rats have shown that the initiation of renal damage with aging may occur independently of glomerular hypertension. Depending on the strain, glomerular hydrostatic pressures may be either elevated

Proposed mechanisms for aging-associated renal disease
Oxidative stress
Senescence (with telomere shortening and loss of mitochondria)
Glomerular hypertension and hyperfiltration
Intrarenal activation of the renin angiotensin system
Endothelial dysfunction (loss of nitric oxide)
Renal ischemia
Renal TGF-β expression
Accumulation of advanced glycation end products (AGEs)
Chronic effects of uric acid

Figure 62.8 Proposed mechanisms for aging-associated renal disease. TGF-β, transforming growth factor-β.

or normal with aging.[22] It is thus likely that glomerular hypertension, when it occurs with a decrease in nephron mass, is a contributor, rather than an initiator, of the aging-associated decline in renal function.

The renin angiotensin system also has a role in the renal changes of aging. Although aging is associated with extracellular volume expansion and a reduction in plasma renin activity, there is evidence in aging rats that renal angiotensin II levels are elevated. Furthermore, rats or mice treated with angiotensin-converting enzyme (ACE) inhibitors or angiotensin receptor blockers (ARBs) from shortly after birth have less glomerulosclerosis, less glomerular hypertrophy, and less tubulointerstitial fibrosis with aging.[30] The renoprotection may be mediated by both hemodynamic (decreasing glomerular hydrostatic pressure and increasing renal blood flow) and nonhemodynamic (direct effect to block angiotensin II–mediated cell growth or cytokine (TGF-β) generation) mechanisms.[31] Blockade of the renin angiotensin system also reduces aging-associated oxidative stress and preserves mitochondria in renal proximal tubules in association with upregulation of cellular antioxidant enzymes as rats age.[32,33] In addition, lifelong blockade of the renin angiotensin system in rats results in less left ventricular hypertrophy and myocardial fibrosis, improvement in learning capacity, increased sexual activity, and decreased liver fibrosis.[31–33]

Endothelial function also declines with aging, and this is greater in men than women. The decline in endothelial function is associated with a progressive reduction in nitric oxide (NO) production by endothelial cells and is reflected clinically by a reduction in brachial artery reactivity.[34] The loss of nitric oxide may be due to the accumulation of asymmetric dimethyl arginine (ADMA, an inhibitor of NO synthesis), to biologic effects of serum uric acid (which reduces endothelial NO bioavailability), or to the local generation of oxidants (which scavenge NO). There is also a loss of neuronal NO synthase in the aging kidney, which is associated with renal progression. The loss of normal endothelial vasodilatory substances may account for the increased renal vasoconstrictive response observed in aging rats to agents such as angiotensin II and endothelin-1. In addition, the endothelial changes may predispose to preglomerular vascular disease, resulting in impaired renal autoregulation (and glomerular hypertension), as well as inhibit renal angiogenesis with progressive capillary loss and ischemia.

Other potential mediators of aging-associated renal disease include TGF-β (an important profibrotic growth factor with increased expression in aging kidneys). Advanced glycation end products (AGEs), although classically associated with diabetes, also accumulate in aging. Chronic administration of aminoguanidine (an inhibitor of AGE synthesis) reduces glomerulosclerosis in the aging rat. Chronic hyperuricemia is also associated with renal functional and histologic changes similar to those observed with aging. It is thus of interest that experimental hyperuricemia induces arteriolar hyalinosis and thickening, glomerular hypertrophy, glomerulosclerosis, and interstitial fibrosis, likely through an effect of uric acid to inhibit endothelial NO bioavailability, block neuronal NO synthase, and activate the renin angiotensin system.[35] Thus, it is possible that chronic effects of uric acid may have a role in the pathogenesis of aging-associated renal disease.

CLINICAL MANIFESTATIONS

General Considerations
The practical implications of these limitations of glomerular and tubular function in elderly people are considerable. Fluid and electrolyte management need constant vigilance to minimize

morbidity. Although fluid and electrolyte homeostasis is well maintained in everyday settings, older people are easily destabilized by intercurrent challenges that are well tolerated by younger patients. Moderate fluid loss (e.g., episode of diarrhea) or moderate fluid loading (e.g., inappropriate perioperative intravenous fluids) are both poorly tolerated and may lead to hypovolemia and fluid overload, respectively. Overzealous administration of water as 5% dextrose or 0.45% saline may result in hyponatremia. The acid load provoked by ischemic tissue injury or hypoxemia will be more severe in the elderly owing to inadequate renal compensation. Potassium homeostasis is easily altered by inaccurate estimation of intravenous or potassium requirements. Subjects are also more prone to complications from various drugs. For example, the use of nonsteroidal anti-inflammatory drugs (NSAIDs) in the elderly is associated with increased risk for hyponatremia, hyperkalemia, hypertension, and renal insufficiency.

Glomerular Diseases

In general, the types of glomerular disease seen in elderly people are similar to those seen in the general population, although certain disorders may have an increased prevalence. For instance, renal complications of type 2 diabetes mellitus are seen with increasing frequency in the aging population. Also seen with increased frequency are amyloidosis, membranous nephropathy, poststreptococcal glomerulonephritis, Wegener's granulomatosis, and membranoproliferative glomerulonephritis[36,37] (Fig. 62.9). In contrast, certain glomerular disorders are uncommon in elderly people, such as lupus nephritis and immunoglobulin A (IgA) nephropathy. Only 2% of patients with systemic lupus erythematosus present after the age of 60 years.[36] In particular, most positive fluorescent antinuclear antibody tests performed in elderly patients are false-positive tests. Other diseases may be less typical in the elderly. For example, minimal change disease may have superimposed renal changes of aging or hypertension, and elderly patients respond more slowly to steroids than children with the disease (see Chapter 17).

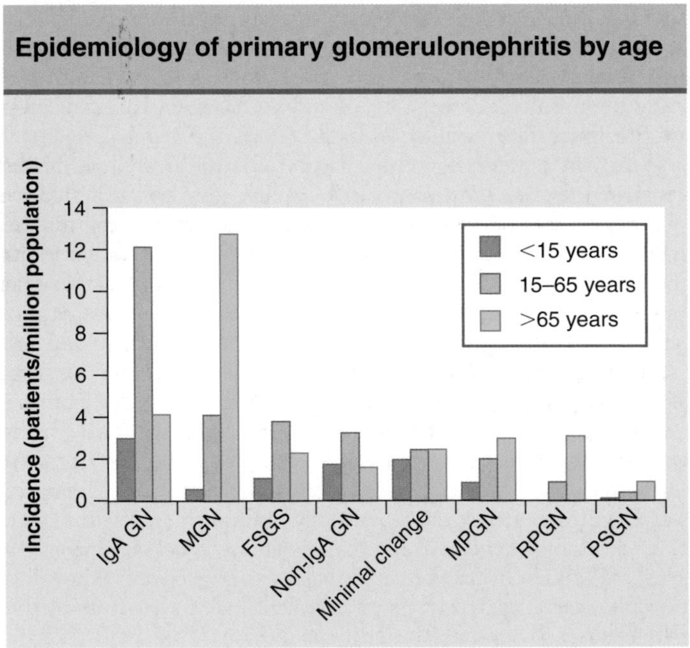

Renovascular and Atheroembolic Disease

There is also an increased frequency of renovascular and atheroembolic disease with aging. The observation of hypertension and an elevated serum creatinine, especially in an individual with a history of vascular disease, should prompt a screening test for renovascular disease, such as by magnetic resonance angiography (MRA) or by renal artery duplex scanning (see Chapter 61).

Acute Renal Failure

Elderly subjects are at marked increased risk for acute renal failure, particularly after cardiovascular surgery. In some studies, the increased risk for acute renal failure approaches a twofold to threefold increase compared with younger subjects. It is likely that several mechanisms account for this finding in aging subjects, including the reduction in functional renal reserve and the impaired renal autoregulation. Indeed, the functional (relative loss of NO) and structural (arteriolar disease) changes in the preglomerular vasculature likely play a role in the impaired ability of the kidney to regulate glomerular filtration and renal blood flow despite only modest changes in systemic hemodynamics.

Urinary Tract Infections

There is an increased risk for asymptomatic bacteriuria with aging (see Chapter 50). The prevalence in women increases from 5% (<50 years) to 21% (ambulatory, >65 years) to 53% (institutionalized, >65 years). In men, the prevalence increases from 0% (<50 years) to 12% (ambulatory, >65 years) to 37% (institutionalized, >65 years). In men, this may relate to the increased risk for prostatic hypertrophy and urinary calculi with age. Chronic use of indwelling catheters in elderly subjects is also associated with increased bacterial colonization rates; treatment of these urinary tract infections should generally be based on the presence of symptoms or signs (fever, elevated white blood cell count, or dysuria). Exceptions would include high-risk subjects such as those with frequent or recurrent urinary tract infections, or structural defects of the urinary tract; patients scheduled to undergo urologic surgery; neutropenic patients; and renal transplant recipients. The treatment of catheter-associated infections is discussed in Chapter 50.

Obstructive Uropathy

Obstructive disease involving the urinary tract is common in elderly men, primarily because of the propensity of the prostate gland to enlarge and block urine flow, as well as the greater length of the male urethra. The most common causes of obstructive uropathy are benign prostatic hypertrophy, prostate cancer, and urethral strictures. The incidence of obstructive uropathy in females is about one third to one half that in males and is primarily due to malignancies of the genitourinary tract. Diagnosis of lower urinary tract obstruction should be excluded by measuring the postvoid residual bladder volume, either by a bedside ultrasound bladder scan or by placement of a straight catheter. Ultrasonography is the

Epidemiology of primary glomerulonephritis by age

Figure 62.9 **Epidemiology of primary glomerulonephritis by age.** FSGS, focal segmental glomerulosclerosis; IgA GN, IgA, nephropathy; MGN, membranous nephropathy; MPGN, membranoproliferative glomerulonephritis; non-IgA GN, other mesangial proliferative GN; PSGN, poststreptococcal glomerulonephritis; RPGN, rapidly progressive glomerulonephritis. (Adapted from Vendemia F, Gesualdo L, Schena FP, D'Amico G: Epidemiology of primary glomerulonephritis in the elderly. Report from the Italian Registry of Renal Biopsy. J Nephrol 2001;14:340–352.)

most appropriate imaging study to diagnose upper urinary tract obstruction (see Chapter 55).

Urinary Incontinence

The lower urinary tract also undergoes significant changes with aging. Decreased bladder contractility occurs secondary to weakening and thinning of the detrusor smooth muscle. This leads to a dysfunctional pattern, eventually culminating in involuntary detrusor contractions. Bladder capacity decreases, whereas postvoid residual bladder volume increases by about 50 to 100 ml. Because of a decrease in renal concentrating capability (see earlier discussion), elderly people also have a higher frequency of nocturia, which may be associated with an increased incidence of sleep disorders.

Transient urinary incontinence accounts for about 50% of incontinence cases in the elderly and has multiple potentially treatable causes, which may be elucidated by the DIAPPERS mnemonic[38] (Fig. 62.10). In males, overflow incontinence from prostatic obstruction is common, whereas in women, a prolapsed uterus is frequently the cause. In the absence of identification of a rapidly reversible mechanism, referral to a neurologist (to rule out conditions such as normal pressure hydrocephalus) and to a urologist is recommended.

Treatment of urinary incontinence in elderly patients is tailored to the individual. The first line of therapy usually consists of nonsurgical options, such as behavioral therapy and biofeedback, pelvic floor exercises, catheterization, and pharmacologic therapy (e.g., α-adrenergic antagonists to reduce prostatic hypertrophy). Surgical therapy may be required for conditions such as large cystoceles, vaginal-vault prolapse, and postprostatectomy stress incontinence.[38]

Evaluation of Hematuria

Malignancies of the urinary tract are more common in older subjects. Bladder carcinoma is rarely observed before the age of 40 years in men and is even more uncommon in women younger than 40 years; it increases progressively after the fourth decade. Renal cell carcinomas are most commonly observed in the seventh decade, with a median age of diagnosis of 66 years

and a median age of death of 70 years. As a consequence, the development of microhematuria or macrohematuria generally requires an investigation of both the lower (cystoscopy and in men, a prostate examination) and upper (imaging studies) tract. A search for other diagnoses (including glomerular lesions, stones, idiopathic hypercalciuria, etc.) may also be indicated in the evaluation of hematuria, as discussed in Chapters 16 and 56.

Nephrotoxicity and Drug Dosing

Elderly subjects are prone to increased nephrotoxicity both as a consequence of their decreased renal mass and because they are often administered medicines on the assumption that a normal or near-normal serum creatinine is consistent with normal renal function. As a result, elderly subjects are prone to nephrotoxicity from nonsteroidal agents, cyclooxygenase-2 inhibitors, aminoglycosides, radiocontrast, and chemotherapy (e.g., cisplatin).

Drug dosing needs to be carefully adjusted in the aging patient. Certain common drugs frequently need adjusting for renal function; these include aminoglycosides, digoxin, procainamide, tetracycline, and vancomycin. Other drugs may be commonly associated with the development of hyponatremia; these include thiazides and chlorpropamide. Other drugs commonly prescribed in elderly subjects are rarely associated with the development of nephrotic syndrome. These include nonsteroidal agents, pamidronate, gold, and penicillamine.

End-Stage Renal Disease, Dialysis, and Transplantation

Given the normal decrease in GFR with aging, it is not surprising that end-stage renal disease (ESRD) is common in the elderly. Both the incidence and prevalence of ESRD are higher in older subjects[39] (Fig. 62.11). Indeed, the mean age for a patient to initiate renal replacement therapy is currently 63 years in the United States. Most cases of ESRD in older subjects are due to either diabetes or hypertension. Glomerulonephritis and polycystic kidney disease are less common.

The clinical presentation of ESRD in the elderly may differ from that in younger patients. Patients may present with uremic symptoms (anorexia, nausea, and pruritus), with only modest elevations in serum creatinine. Occasional subjects may present with unexplained dementia or change in personality or behavior, unexplained exacerbation of congestive heart failure, or simply a change in sense of well-being. To complicate diagnosis further, such uremic manifestations may have been attributed to the "aging process" or other diseases associated with aging.

The decision to offer renal replacement therapy is no longer based on the age of the individual. Patients often do very well with either hemodialysis or peritoneal dialysis unless there are comorbid conditions such as cardiovascular disease. Unfortunately, cardiac disease is common in elderly subjects with ESRD[40] (Fig. 62.12).

As with younger subjects, vascular access remains the Achilles heel of hemodialysis. It must be emphasized, however, that even in this population the survival of arteriovenous fistulas is significantly greater than that of arteriovenous grafts. Some surgeons tend to justify constructing more vascular grafts in the elderly on the grounds that their blood vessels tend to be fragile and significantly atherosclerotic. However, in those subjects in whom arteriovenous fistulas successfully mature, not only are longevities and patencies more prolonged, but also

Transient causes of urinary incontinence (DIAPPERS)	
D	Delirium/confusional state
I	Infection—urinary (symptomatic)
A	Atrophic urethritis/vaginitis
P	Pharmaceuticals (diuretics, etc.)
P	Psychological, especially depression
E	Endocrine (hypercalcemia, hypokalemia, glycosuria)
R	Restricted mobility
S	Stool impaction

Figure 62.10 Transient causes of urinary incontinence in the elderly (DIAPPERS). (Adapted from Sirls LT, Rashid T: Urinary incontinence in the elderly. In Oreopoulos DG, Hazzard WR, Luke R [eds]: Nephrology and Geriatrics Integrated, 1st ed. Dordrecht, The Netherlands, Kluwer Academic Publishers, 2000, pp 179–198.)

Incidence and prevalence of ESRD in the United States, by age

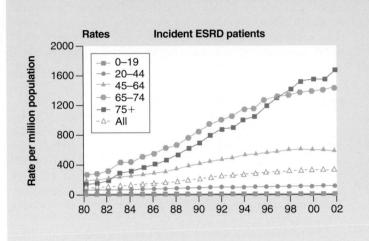
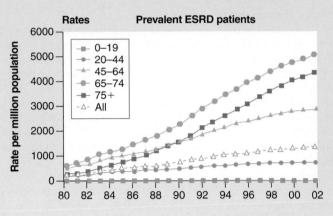

Figure 62.11 **Incidence and prevalence of end-stage renal disease (ESRD) in the United States, by age.** Subjects older than 65 years have a higher incidence and prevalence of ESRD. Factored for gender and race. (Adapted from U.S. Renal Data System (USRDS): 2005 Annual Data Report. Am J Kid Dis 2006; 47[Suppl 1]:S65–S81.)

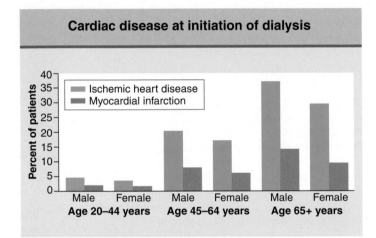

Figure 62.12 **Prevalence of cardiac disease in patients with end-stage renal disease being initiated on dialysis in the United States.** (Adapted from U.S. Renal Data System (USRDS): 2005 Annual Data Report. Am J Kid Dis 2001;38[Suppl 3]:S37–S195.)

the incidence of infections, thromboses, and complications is decreased.

Transplantation should be considered in the management of elderly subjects, although only a minority of elderly patients with ESRD is suitable for transplantation because of comorbid conditions, particularly cardiovascular disease and malignancy. The proportion of patients with ESRD who are older than 65 years and on the transplant waiting list has tripled in the past 10 years and currently exceeds 12%.[41] Transplantation of subjects between the ages of 65 and 74 years is associated with superior survival compared with patients of the same age who remain on a transplant waiting list, although this benefit becomes less apparent the longer the patient waits before transplantation.[42] Elderly subjects also have a lower rate of graft rejection than younger patients. However, because they have a higher rate of death with functioning grafts, overall graft survival is similar to that in younger subjects.[42] This result may provide an argument for lower doses of immunosuppression in elderly subjects.[43]

REFERENCES

1. McLachlan MS: The aging kidney. Lancet 1978;2:143–145.
2. Kaplan C, Pasternack B, Shah H, Gallo G: Age-related incidence of sclerotic glomeruli in human kidneys. Am J Pathol 1975;80: 227–234.
3. Ferder L, Inserra F, Romano L, et al: Decreased glomerulosclerosis in aging by angiotensin-concerting enzyme inhibitors. J Am Soc Nephrol 1994;5: 1147–1152.
4. Fogo AB: Glomerular hypertension, abnormal glomerular growth, and progression of renal diseases. Kidney Int 2000;57:S15–21.
5. Thomas SE, Anderson S, Gordon KL, et al: Tubulointerstitial disease in aging: Evidence for underlying peritubular capillary damage. A potential role for renal ischemia. J Am Soc Nephrol 1998;9:231–242.
6. Ruiz-Torres MP, Bosch RJ, O'Valle F, et al: Age-related increase in expression of TGF-β1 in the rat kidney: Relationship to morphologic changes. J Am Soc Nephrol 1998;9;782–791, 485–508.
7. Lindeman, RD, Goldman R: Anatomic and physiologic age changes in the kidney. Exp Gerontol 1986;21:379–406.
8. Takazakura E, Sawabu N, Handa A, et al: Intrarenal vascular changes with age and disease. Kidney Int 1972;2:224–230.
9. Kang DH, Anderson S, Kim Y-G, et al: Impaired angiogenesis in the aging kidney: Vascular endothelial growth factor and thrombospondin-1 renal disease. Am J Kidney Dis 2001:37;601–611.
10. Epstein M: Aging and the kidney. J Am Soc Nephrol 1996;7:1106–1122.
11. Rowe JW, Andres R, Tobin J, et al: The effect of age on creatinine clearance in man: A cross-sectional and longitudinal study. J Gerontol 1976;31:155–163.
12. Wesson LG Jr: Renal hemodynamics in physiological states. In Physiology of the Human Kidney. New York, Grune & Stratton, 1969, pp 96–108.
13. Harmoinen A, Lehtimaki T, Korpela M, et al: Diagnostic accuracies of plasma creatinine, cystatin C, and glomerular filtration rate calculated by the Cockroft-Gault and Levey (MDRD) formulas. Clin Chem 2003; 49:1223–1225.
14. Verhave JC, Fesler P, Ribstein J, et al: Estimation of renal subjects with normal serum creatinine levels: Influence of age and body mass index. Am J Kidney Dis 2005;46:233–241.
15. Corman B, Chami-Khazraji J, Schaeverbeke J, Michel JB: Effect of feeding on glomerular filtration rate and proteinuria in conscious aging rats. Am J Physiol Renal Physiol 1988; 255:F250–F256.

16. Baylis C: Changes in renal hemodynamics and structure in the aging kidney: Sexual dimorphism and the nitric oxide system. Exp Gerontol 2005;40:271–278.
17. Hollenberg NK, Adams DF, Solomon HS, et al: Senescence and the renal vasculature in normal man. J Lab Clin Med 1976;87:411–417.
18. Jones CA, Francis ME, Eberhardt MS, et al: Microalbuminuria in the US population: Third National Health and Nutrition Examination Survey. Am J Kidney Dis 2002;39:445–449.
19. Luft, FC, Grim CE, Gineberg N, Weinberger MC: Effects of volume expansion and contraction in normotensive whites, blacks, and subjects of different ages. Circulation 1979;59:643–650.
20. Epstein M, Hollenberg NK: Age as a determinant of renal sodium conservation in normal man. J Lab Clin Med 1976;87:411–417.
21. Filser D, Franek E, Joest M, et al: Renal function in the elderly: Impact of hypertension and cardiac function. Kidney Int 1997;51:1196–1204.
22. Baylis C, Corma B: The aging kidney: Insights from experimental studies. J Am Soc Nephrol 1998;9:699–799.
23. Burt VL, Whelton P, Roccella EJ, et al: Prevalence of hypertension in the US adult population. Results from the Third National Health and Nutrition Examination Survey, 1988–1991. Hypertension 1995;25:305–313.
24. Weinberger MH, Fineberg NS: Sodium and volume sensitivity of blood pressure: Age and pressure change over time. Hypertension 1991;18:67–71.
25. Oliver WB, Cohen EL, Neel JV: Blood pressure, sodium intake, and sodium related hormones in the Yanomamo Indians, a "no-salt" culture. Circulation 1975;52:146–151.
26. Streeten DHP, Anderson GP, Wagner S: Effect of age on response of secondary hypertension to specific treatment. Am J Hypertens 1990;3:360–365.
27. Polson CD, Webster JC: Loss of mitochondrial DNA in mouse tissues with age. Age 1982;5:5–133.
28. Beckman KB, Ames BN: The free radical theory of aging matures. Physiol Rev 1998;78:547–581.
29. Anderson S, Brenner BM: Progressive renal disease: A disorder of adaptation. Q J Med 1989;70:185–189.
30. Anderson S, Rennke HG, Zatz R: Glomerular adaptations with normal aging and with long-term converting enzyme inhibition in rats. Am J Physiol Renal Physiol 1994;36:F35–43.
31. Basso N, Paglia N, Stella I, et al: Protective effect of the inhibition of the rennin-angiotensin system on aging. Regul Pept 2005;128:247–252.
32. Ferder LF, Inserra F, Romano L, et al: Effects of angiotensin-converting enzyme inhibition on mitochondrial number in the aging mouse. Am J Physiol Cell Physiol 1993;34:C15–18.
33. de Cavanagh EM, Piotrkowski B, Basso N, et al: Enalapril and losartan attenuate mitochondrial dysfunction in aged rats. FASEB J 2003;17:1096–1098.
34. Campo C, Lahera V, Garcia-Robles R, et al: Aging abolishes the renal response to L-arginine infusion in essential hypertension. Kidney Int 1996;49:S126–S128.
35. Nakagawa T, Mazzali M, Kang D-H, et al: Hyperuricemia causes glomerular hypertrophy in the rat. Am J Nephrol 2003;23:2–7.
36. Glassock RJ: Glomerular disease in the elderly population. In Oreopoulos DG, Hazzard WR, Luke R (eds): Nephrology and Geriatrics Integrated. Dordrecht, The Netherlands, Kluwer Academic Publishers, 2000, pp 57–66.
37. Vendemia F, Gesualdo L, Schena FP, D'Amico G: Epidemiology of primary glomerulonephritis in the elderly. Report from the Italian Registry of Renal Biopsy. J Nephrol 2001;14:340–352.
38. Sirls LT, Rashid T: Urinary incontinence in the elderly. In Oreopoulos DG, Hazzard WR, Luke R (eds): Nephrology and Geriatrics Integrated. Dordrecht, The Netherlands, Kluwer Academic Publishers, 2000, pp 179–198.
39. U.S. Renal Data System (USRDS): 2005 Annual Data Report. Am J Kid Dis 2006;47(Suppl 1):S65–S81.
40. U.S. Renal Data System (USRDS): 2005 Annual Data Report. Am J Kid Dis 2001;38(Suppl 3):S37–S195.
41. Gaston RS, Alveranga DY, Becker BN, et al: Kidney and pancreas transplantation. Am J Transplantation 2003;3:S64–S67.
42. Tesi RJ, Elkhammas EA, Davis EA, et al: Renal transplantation in older people. Lancet 1994;343:461–464.
43. Meier-Kriesche H, Ojo A, Hanson J, et al: Increased immunosuppressive vulnerability in elderly renal transplant recipients. Transplantation 2000;69:885–889

CHAPTER

63

Pathophysiology and Etiology of Acute Renal Failure

J. Ashley Jefferson and Robert W. Schrier

DEFINITION

Acute renal failure (ARF) is a clinical syndrome denoted by an abrupt decline (over days to a few weeks) in glomerular filtration rate (GFR) sufficient to decrease the elimination of nitrogenous waste products (urea and creatinine) and other uremic toxins. The urine volume in ARF is variable and is determined not only by GFR but also by tubular reabsorption. Although ARF is defined by a reduced *glomerular* filtration rate, the underlying etiology of the renal impairment is typically due to tubular and vascular factors.

The etiology of ARF is broad and must be considered in a systematic fashion to avoid missing multiple factors that may be contributing to the condition. The traditional paradigm divides ARF into prerenal, renal, and postrenal causes. Prerenal azotemia may be due to hypovolemia or a decreased effective arterial volume (see Chapter 66). Postrenal obstructive renal failure is usually diagnosed by urinary tract dilation on renal ultrasound or computed tomography (CT) scanning. Renal causes of ARF should be considered under the different anatomic components of the kidney (vascular supply, glomerular, tubular, and interstitial disease; Fig. 63.1). Major extra renal artery or venous occlusion must also be considered in the differential diagnosis (see Chapter 61). Similarly, disorders of the small intrarenal vasculature can result in ARF (e.g., vasculitis, thrombotic microangiopathy, malignant hypertension, eclampsia, postpartum states, disseminated intravascular coagulation [DIC], scleroderma; see Chapters 23, 28, 32, 41, and 61). All

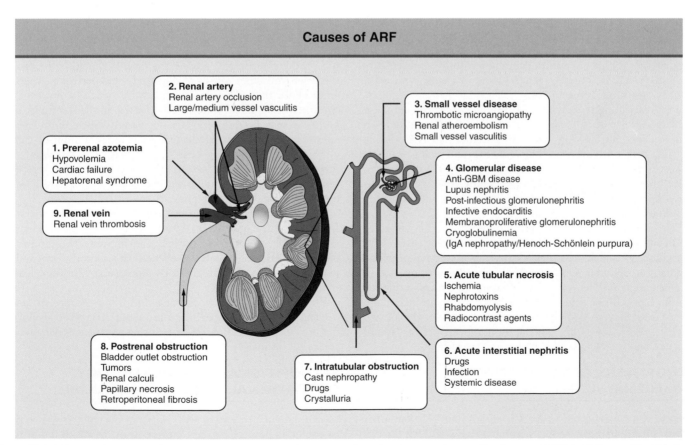

Causes of ARF

2. Renal artery
Renal artery occlusion
Large/medium vessel vasculitis

3. Small vessel disease
Thrombotic microangiopathy
Renal atheroembolism
Small vessel vasculitis

1. Prerenal azotemia
Hypovolemia
Cardiac failure
Hepatorenal syndrome

9. Renal vein
Renal vein thrombosis

4. Glomerular disease
Anti-GBM disease
Lupus nephritis
Post-infectious glomerulonephritis
Infective endocarditis
Membranoproliferative glomerulonephritis
Cryoglobulinemia
(IgA nephropathy/Henoch-Schönlein purpura)

5. Acute tubular necrosis
Ischemia
Nephrotoxins
Rhabdomyolysis
Radiocontrast agents

8. Postrenal obstruction
Bladder outlet obstruction
Tumors
Renal calculi
Papillary necrosis
Retroperitoneal fibrosis

7. Intratubular obstruction
Cast nephropathy
Drugs
Crystalluria

6. Acute interstitial nephritis
Drugs
Infection
Systemic disease

Figure 63.1 Causes of acute renal failure (ARF). ARF is classified into prerenal, renal, and postrenal causes. Renal causes of ARF should be considered under the different anatomic components of the kidney (vascular supply, glomerular, tubular, and interstitial disease). GBM, glomerular basement membrane.

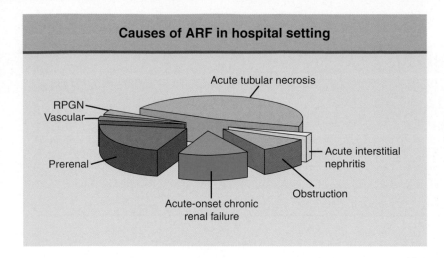

Figure 63.2 Causes of acute renal failure (ARF) in the hospital setting. RPGN, rapidly progressive glomerulonephritis.

forms of acute glomerulonephritis can present as ARF, as can acute inflammation and space-occupying processes of the renal interstitium (e.g., drug-induced, infectious, and autoimmune disorders, leukemia, lymphoma, sarcoidosis).

In the hospital setting, prerenal uremia and acute tubular necrosis (ATN) account for the majority of ARF cases[1] (Fig. 63.2). The term "tubular necrosis" is a misnomer because the alterations are not limited to the tubular structures and true cellular necrosis in human ATN is often minimal. However, the term ATN is commonly employed in the clinical setting. To make things even more confusing, the terms ATN and ARF are frequently used interchangeably in the literature. The term ATN should be reserved for cases of ARF in which a renal biopsy (if performed) would show the characteristic changes of tubular cell injury (Fig 63.3).

The typical course of *uncomplicated* ATN is recovery over 2 to 3 weeks; however, superimposed renal insults often alter this pattern. For example, episodes of hypotension induced by hemodialysis may lead to additional ischemic lesions, potentially prolonging renal functional recovery, and patients with ARF often have multiple comorbidities.

In critically ill patients with ARF, the outcomes remain poor. In a large multinational study of nearly 30,000 patients in intensive care units (ICUs), 5.7% of patients had ARF during their ICU stay, with an overall hospital mortality rate of 60%.[2] Of those who survived to leave the intensive care unit, often despite prolonged renal replacement therapy, 86% were able to achieve independent renal function, albeit often with a degree of residual chronic renal impairment.[2]

There are significant geographic differences in the causes of ARF. In tropical countries, ATN is also the dominant cause, with hypovolemia caused by diarrheal disease an important problem, particularly in children. Obstetric ARF remains more common in emerging countries. There are also different patterns of accidental and deliberate self-poisoning. In Africa, herbal toxins are a common cause of ARF. Severe hemolysis may also occur in malaria, with drugs in association with glucose-6-phosphate dehydrogenase deficiency, and following spider, snake, and insect bites.

PATHOPHYSIOLOGY AND ETIOLOGY OF PRERENAL AZOTEMIA

Impaired renal perfusion with a resultant fall in glomerular capillary filtration pressure is a common cause of ARF. In this setting, tubular function is typically normal, renal reabsorption of sodium and water is increased, and consequently, urine chemistries

reveal a low urine sodium (<10 mmol/l) and a concentrated urine (urine osmolality >500 mOsm/kg).

A marked reduction in renal perfusion may overwhelm autoregulation (see Chapter 2) and precipitate an acute fall in GFR. With lesser degrees of renal hypoperfusion, glomerular filtration pressures and GFR are maintained by afferent arteriolar vasodilation (mediated by vasodilatory eicosanoids) and efferent arteriolar vasoconstriction (mediated by angiotensin II). In this setting, ARF may be precipitated by agents that impair afferent arteriolar dilation (nonsteroidal anti-inflammatory drugs [NSAIDs]) or efferent vasoconstriction (angiotensin-converting enzyme [ACE] inhibitors and angiotensin receptor blockers [ARB]).

Prerenal azotemia is commonly secondary to extracellular fluid volume depletion due to gastrointestinal losses (diarrhea, vomiting, prolonged nasogastric drainage), renal losses (diuretics, osmotic diuresis in hyperglycemia), dermal losses (burns, extensive sweating), or possibly sequestration of fluid, so-called third spacing (e.g., acute pancreatitis, muscle trauma). It should be recognized that there are other causes of impaired renal perfusion when the extracellular fluid volume may actually be increased; however, the *effective arterial* blood volume is decreased. In these settings, renal perfusion may be reduced by a decreased cardiac output (heart failure) or by arterial vasodilation with redistribution of cardiac output to other vascular beds (e.g., sepsis, liver cirrhosis). The presence of ARF in the setting of severe heart failure has been termed the *cardiorenal syndrome* and is often exacerbated by the use of ACE inhibitors and diuretics.

An unusual cause of prerenal ARF is the hyperoncotic state. Infusion of large quantities of osmotically active substances such as mannitol, dextran, or protein can increase the glomerular oncotic pressure enough to exceed the glomerular capillary hydrostatic pressure, which stops glomerular filtration, leading to an anuric form of ARF.

Prerenal azotemia can be corrected if the extrarenal factors causing the renal hypoperfusion are rapidly reversed. Failure to restore renal blood flow (RBF) during the functional prerenal stage will ultimately lead to ischemic ATN.

PATHOPHYSIOLOGY AND ETIOLOGY OF POSTRENAL ACUTE RENAL FAILURE

In any patient presenting with ARF, an obstructive cause must be excluded because prompt intervention can result in improvement or complete recovery of renal function (see Chapter 55). Postrenal forms of ARF are divided into intrarenal (tubular) and

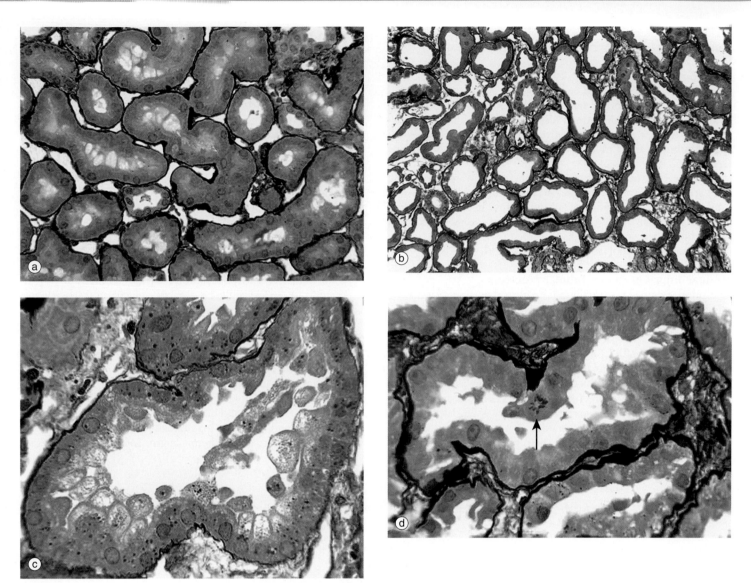

Figure 63.3 Renal pathology in acute tubular necrosis (ATN). *a,* Normal cortical renal tubules. *b* and *c,* ATN: note the flattened epithelium, bare basement membranes, and intraluminal cellular debris. *d,* Recovering ATN showing a tubular epithelial cell mitotic figure *(arrow).* (Courtesy of Erika Bracamonte, MD, University of Washington.)

extrarenal. Tubular precipitation of insoluble crystals (methotrexate, acyclovir, sulfonamides, indinavir, uric acid, triamterene, oxalic acid) or protein (hemoglobin, myoglobin, paraprotein) can increase intratubular pressure. If sufficiently high, this opposes glomerular filtration pressure and can decrease GFR. Similarly, obstruction of the extrarenal collecting system at any level (renal pelvis, ureters, bladder, or urethra) can lead to postrenal ARF. Obstructive uropathy is common in older men with prostatic disease and in patients with a single kidney or intra-abdominal, particularly pelvic, cancer. Severe ureteral obstruction is also seen with small inflammatory aortic aneurysms. Most causes of obstructive uropathy are amenable to therapy, and the prognosis is generally good, depending on the underlying disease.

Important clinical sequelae of postrenal ARF are the postobstructive diuresis and the presence of hyperkalemic renal tubular acidosis. Profuse diuresis, ranging from 4 to 20 l/day, can occur after the release of the obstruction, and some patients may become volume depleted, necessitating careful monitoring and adjustment of the volume and electrolyte status during the diuretic phase.

PATHOPHYSIOLOGY OF ACUTE TUBULAR NECROSIS

ATN commonly occurs in high-risk settings, which include postvascular and postcardiac surgery, severe burns, pancreatitis, sepsis, and chronic liver disease. ATN is responsible for most cases of hospital-acquired ARF and is usually considered to be due to ischemic or nephrotoxic injury.[3,4] In the intensive care unit, two thirds of cases of ARF are due to the combination of impaired renal perfusion, sepsis, and nephrotoxic agents.[5]

The importance of combined injurious mechanisms is also emphasized by experimental data. In animal studies, severe and prolonged hypotension (<50 mm Hg for 2–3 hours in the rat) does not cause ATN. Similarly, animal models require very high doses of single nephrotoxic agents to induce ARF. These features may reflect an inherent resistance to ATN in animal models, but also illustrate the fact that a single insult alone is rarely sufficient to induce ATN. Fever may exacerbate ATN by increasing the renal tubular metabolic rate, thereby increasing adenosine triphosphate (ATP) consumption. In an experimental model (renal artery occlusion in the rat), renal ischemia for 40 minutes resulted in minimal renal injury at 32°C but marked ARF at 39.4°C.

Histology

The typical features of ATN on renal biopsy include vacuolization and loss of brush border in proximal tubular cells. Sloughing of tubular cells into the lumen leads to cast obstruction, manifested by tubular dilation. Interstitial edema can produce widely spaced tubules, and a mild leukocyte infiltration may be present (see Fig. 63.3).

Despite the term acute tubular "necrosis," frankly necrotic cells are not a common finding on renal biopsy, and often only limited histologic evidence of injury is present despite marked functional impairment. This implies that factors other than just tubular cell injury (such as vasoconstriction and tubular obstruction) are important in the loss of GFR.

Tubular Injury in Acute Tubular Necrosis

The tubular damage is usually due to a combination of ischemic injury resulting in depletion of cellular ATP and direct tubular epithelial cell injury by nephrotoxins. Most accept that the S3 segment of the proximal tubule and the medullary thick ascending limb (mTAL) are particularly vulnerable (Fig. 63.4). There are several reasons for this vulnerability:

1. Blood supply—The blood flow to the kidney is not uniform, and most of it is directed to the renal cortex for glomerular filtration where the cortical tissue Po_2 is 50–100 mm Hg. By contrast, the outer medulla and medullary rays are watershed areas receiving their blood supply from vasa rectae. Countercurrent oxygen exchange occurs, leading to a progressive fall in Po_2 from cortex to medulla, which results in medullary cells living on the "brink of hypoxia" (medullary Po_2 as low as 10–15 mm Hg). The S3 segments of proximal tubule cells and distal medullary thick ascending limbs are thus exposed to borderline chronic oxygen deprivation.

2. High tubular energy requirements—The cells of the S3 region and mTAL have high metabolic activity, principally owing to sodium reabsorption driven by basolateral membrane Na^+-K^+-ATPase. Indeed, blocking sodium reabsorption in the mTAL with loop diuretics raises the medullary tissue Po_2 from about 15 to 35 mm Hg. Of note, the reduction of GFR in the setting of ARF may be renoprotective by diminishing sodium filtration and hence limiting ATP-dependent sodium reabsorption.

3. Glycolytic ability of tubular cells—Proximal tubular cells have minimal glycolytic machinery and rely almost solely on oxidative phosphorylation for the generation of ATP. In contrast, mTAL cells have a large glycolytic capacity and are more resistant to hypoxic or ischemic insults.

Hemodynamic Factors in the Development of Acute Tubular Necrosis
Impaired Renal Autoregulation

Autoregulation normally occurs between systolic blood pressures of 80 and 150 mm Hg, and between these ranges, RBF, glomerular pressures, and GFR are maintained. Below 80 mm Hg, this autoregulation fails, and ischemic injury may result. In certain

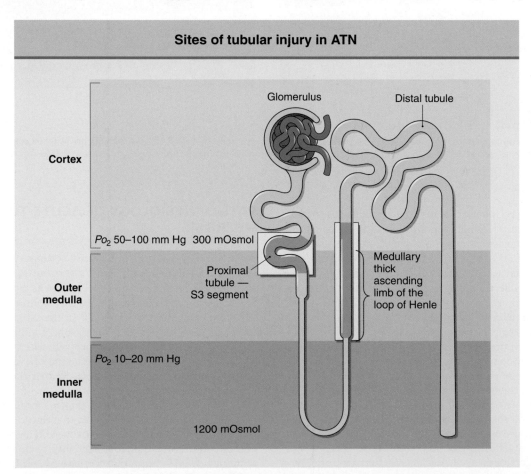

Figure 63.4 Sites of tubular injury in acute tubular necrosis (ATN). The S3 segment of the proximal tubule and the medullary thick ascending limb are particularly vulnerable to ischemic injury because of the combination of borderline oxygen supply and high metabolic demands.

conditions, such as aging or chronic renal disease, autoregulation is abnormal, and ischemic injury may occur more easily with reductions in perfusion pressure. In addition, experimental studies demonstrate impaired autoregulation in ischemic ATN. In settings of low renal perfusion (e.g., volume depletion, left ventricular failure, edematous states, renal artery stenosis), GFR may be dependent on autoregulation mediated by vasodilatory prostaglandins acting on the afferent arteriole and angiotensin II–mediated efferent arteriolar vasoconstriction to maintain glomerular pressure. Any interference with these mechanisms (e.g., administration of ACE inhibitors or acute inhibition of cyclooxygenase-1 or -2 [COX-1 or -2] by NSAIDs) may produce a precipitous fall in GFR (see Chapter 64).

Intrarenal Vasoconstriction

In established ATN, RBF is decreased by 30% to 50%. Indeed in ARF, rather than the normal autoregulatory renal vasodilation that occurs in response to decreased perfusion pressure, there is evidence of renal vasoconstriction. A number of vasoconstrictors have been implicated in this vasoconstrictive response, including angiotensin II, endothelin-1, adenosine, thromboxane A_2, prostaglandin H_2, leukotrienes C_4 and D_4, and sympathetic nerve stimulation. Tubuloglomerular feedback contributes to this vasoconstriction. Some of these vascular abnormalities may be mediated by increased cytosolic calcium content in afferent arterioles as a result of ischemia.

Tubuloglomerular Feedback

The role of tubuloglomerular feedback (TGF; see Chapter 2) in the setting of ARF may be partly beneficial because the resultant decrease in GFR limits sodium delivery to damaged tubules and decreases ATP-dependent tubular reabsorption, protecting against intracellular ATP depletion augmenting renal injury. In this respect, adenosine A1 receptor knockout mice with absent TGF have augmented acute renal injury after ischemia reperfusion.

Endothelial Cell Injury and the Development of Acute Tubular Necrosis

Renal cell injury is not limited to the tubular cell, and endothelial cell injury occurs partly as a result of acute renal ischemia and oxidant injury.[4] Endothelial injury is characterized by cell swelling, upregulation of adhesion molecules (with enhanced leukocyte–endothelial cell interactions), and impaired vasodilation (decreased endothelial nitric oxide synthase and vasodilatory prostaglandins) and may mediate some of the impaired autoregulation and intrarenal vasoconstriction described earlier. Endothelial injury within the peritubular capillaries (vasa rectae) may produce congestion in the outer medulla, exacerbating hypoxic injury to the S3 segment of the proximal tubule and the thick ascending loop of Henle.

Tubular Factors in the Development of Acute Tubular Necrosis

The tubular cell may be injured because of ischemia, with resulting depletion of cellular energy stores (ATP), or from direct cytotoxic injury. After acute renal ischemia, tubular cell injury may also result from the restoration of RBF (reperfusion injury). Mediators of tubular cell injury include reactive oxygen species (ROS), intracellular calcium influx, nitric oxide, phospholipase A_2, complement, and cell-mediated cytotoxicity. ROS may be derived from local sources (including xanthine oxidase and cyclooxygenases, and secondary to mitochondrial injury) or from infiltrating leukocytes. In models of ischemic ATN, a variety of methods that inhibit ROS protect against renal injury (reviewed in ref. 6).

Factors that affect the integrity and function of the renal tubular epithelial cells and contribute to the reduction in GFR include the following (Fig. 63.5):

1. *Cell death*—Despite the term acute tubular necrosis, only a small percentage of tubular cells undergo cell death, and of these, many actually die by apoptosis rather than necrosis. Indeed, recent studies in animal models have shown amelioration of renal injury using caspase inhibitors that inhibit apoptosis.

2. *Disruption of actin cytoskeleton*—A characteristic feature of sublethally injured cells is the disruption of the actin cytoskeleton. Activation of the cysteine protease calpain (partly due to increased intracellular calcium) can degrade actin-binding proteins such as spectrin and ankyrin. This leads to abnormal translocation of Na^+-K^+-ATPase and other proteins from the basolateral membrane to the cytoplasm or apical membranes. In the proximal tubular cell, this loss of polarity results in impaired proximal reabsorption of filtrate with resultant increased distal NaCl delivery and activation of tubuloglomerular feedback.

3. *Cast obstruction*—Tubular cells are attached to the tubular basement membrane by $\alpha_3\beta_1$ integrins, which recognize RGD (arginine-glycine-aspartate) sequences in matrix proteins. Disruption of the actin cytoskeleton results in movement of integrins from basolateral positions to the apical membrane leading to impaired cell matrix adhesion and cell detachment. Many of these detached cells are still viable and can be cultured from urine of patients with ATN. Sloughed proximal tubular cells can bind to RGD sequences in Tamm-Horsfall protein, resulting in cast formation and intratubular obstruction. In models of ischemic ARF, the elevation in tubular pressures may be inhibited by synthetic RGD peptides mitigating the obstructive process.

4. *Backleak*—The loss of adhesion molecules (E-cadherin) and tight junction proteins (ZO-1, occludin) results in the weakening of junctions between cells, allowing filtrate to leak back into the renal interstitium. Although this does not alter the actual GFR at the level of the glomerulus, the net effect is a reduction in the measured GFR. Earlier dextran sieving experiments suggest only a modest effect of backleak on the decrement of GFR in ARF (about 10%); however, in the renal allograft with delayed graft function due to severe ATN, backleak has been calculated to account for up to 50% of the reduction in inulin clearance.

Inflammatory Factors in the Development of Acute Tubular Necrosis

The inflammatory response plays an important role in ATN.[7] Inflammatory mediators may be derived from local cell populations or from infiltrating leukocytes. Renal tubular epithelial cells may produce proinflammatory cytokines (such as tumor necrosis factor-α [TNF-α], interleukin-6 [IL-6], IL-1β) and chemokines (such as MCP-1, IL-8, RANTES) promoting infiltration of leukocytes. Neutrophils and mononuclear cells may be seen in peritubular capillaries on renal biopsy.

Experimental studies have helped to elucidate the role of the inflammatory cells in ATN. Neutrophil activation with the release of proteases and ROS can exacerbate injury. By contrast, neutrophil depletion with antibody, or inhibiting neutrophil adhesion molecules (ICAM-1) with antibody or antisense oligonucleotides, ameliorates injury in ischemic ATN. ICAM-1 knockout mice are similarly protected.

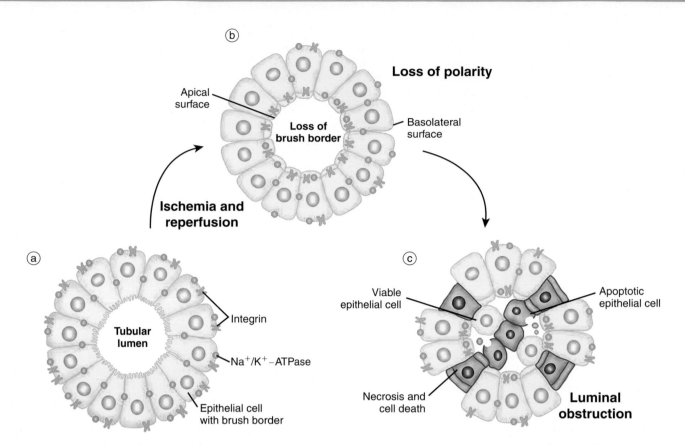

Figure 63.5 **Tubular factors in the development of acute tubular necrosis.** Loss of cell polarity results in weakening of cell-to-cell and cell matrix adhesion, resulting in cast obstruction and backleak of tubular fluid. (Adapted from Schrier RW, Wang W, Poole B, Mitra A: Acute renal failure: Definitions, diagnosis, pathogenesis, and therapy. J Clin Invest 2004;114:5–14.)

More recently, the role of T lymphocytes has emerged. Experimental ischemic reperfusion injury may be ameliorated by T cell depletion or blockade of T cell costimulatory pathways. In addition, CD4-deficient mice (helper T cells) or mice that are unable to mount a Th1 response are protected against ischemia reperfusion injury.

Recovery Phase
Recovery from ATN requires the restoration of tubular cell number and coverage of denuded tubular basement membrane. A marked increase in cell proliferation occurs in recovering human ATN, and mitotic figures may be seen by light microscopy (see Fig. 63.3). There has been some debate about the origin of the restored tubular cells. Some studies have suggested that mesenchymal stem cells may locate to areas of tubular injury and transform into proximal tubular cells. Indeed, experimental models of ischemic reperfusion injury may be ameliorated by infusions of mesenchymal stem cells. More recent evidence, however, suggests that the restoration of tubular cell number is due to the dedifferentiation and proliferation of surviving tubular cells.[8] A number of growth factors have been implicated in the proliferative response, including insulin-like growth factor-1 (IGF-1) and hepatocyte growth factor (HGF); however, a therapeutic trial of subcutaneous recombinant IGF-1 in critically ill patients failed to show an acceleration in renal functional recovery[9] (see Chapter 64). After tubular epithelial cell proliferation, the dedifferentiated cells must migrate to areas of denuded tubular basement membrane, attach to the basement membrane, and differentiate into mature polar tubular epithelial cells.

SPECIFIC ETIOLOGIES OF ACUTE RENAL FAILURE

Nephrotoxic Agents and Mechanisms of Toxicity
The identification and avoidance of nephrotoxic agents in ARF is critical in the management of this condition because ARF may be rapidly reversible upon removal of the offending agent. The mechanisms of nephrotoxicity are very broad and include alterations in renal hemodynamics, induction of direct tubular injury, generation of allergic reactions resulting in interstitial nephritis, and intratubular obstruction. The list is extensive, but the more common agents are presented in Figure 63.6.

Nonsteroidal Anti-Inflammatory Drugs
The NSAIDs are a common cause of ARF in the community because of the large amounts of these drugs either prescribed or bought over the counter.[10] The newer COX-2–specific NSAIDs do not appear to be significantly less nephrotoxic.

ARF may be due to a hemodynamically mediated reduction in GFR in particular clinical situations, such as atherosclerotic cardiovascular disease in elderly patients, pre-existing chronic renal insufficiency, states of renal hypoperfusion including sodium depletion, diuretic use, hypotension, and sodium-avid states such as cirrhosis, nephrotic syndrome, and congestive heart failure. There is little evidence that NSAIDs impair renal function in otherwise healthy individuals. However, a recent population study found that NSAID users had a threefold greater risk for developing a first-ever diagnosis of clinical ARF compared with nonusers. This risk increased with concomitant use of NSAIDs

Nephrotoxic agents leading to acute renal failure

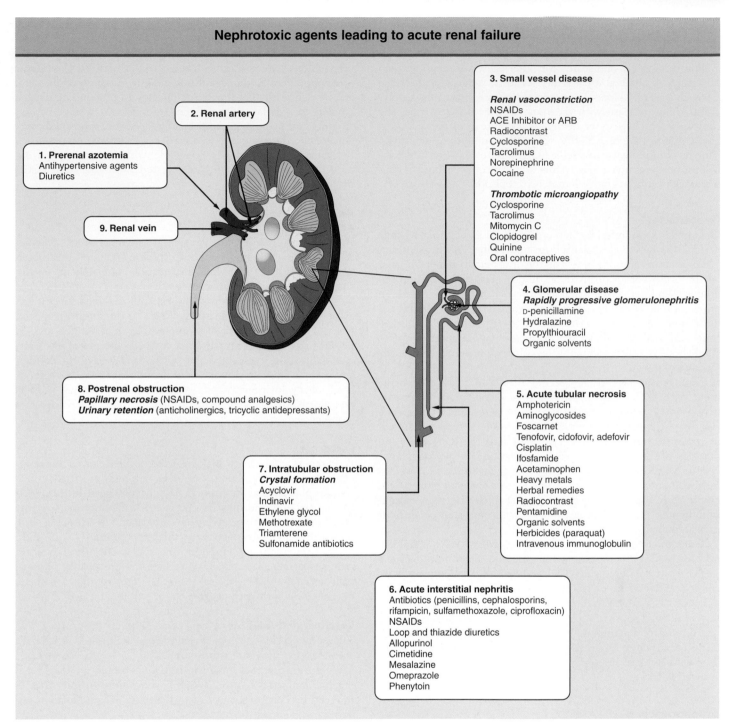

3. Small vessel disease

Renal vasoconstriction
NSAIDs
ACE Inhibitor or ARB
Radiocontrast
Cyclosporine
Tacrolimus
Norepinephrine
Cocaine

Thrombotic microangiopathy
Cyclosporine
Tacrolimus
Mitomycin C
Clopidogrel
Quinine
Oral contraceptives

2. Renal artery

1. Prerenal azotemia
Antihypertensive agents
Diuretics

9. Renal vein

4. Glomerular disease
Rapidly progressive glomerulonephritis
D-penicillamine
Hydralazine
Propylthiouracil
Organic solvents

8. Postrenal obstruction
Papillary necrosis (NSAIDs, compound analgesics)
Urinary retention (anticholinergics, tricyclic antidepressants)

5. Acute tubular necrosis
Amphotericin
Aminoglycosides
Foscarnet
Tenofovir, cidofovir, adefovir
Cisplatin
Ifosfamide
Acetaminophen
Heavy metals
Herbal remedies
Radiocontrast
Pentamidine
Organic solvents
Herbicides (paraquat)
Intravenous immunoglobulin

7. Intratubular obstruction
Crystal formation
Acyclovir
Indinavir
Ethylene glycol
Methotrexate
Triamterene
Sulfonamide antibiotics

6. Acute interstitial nephritis
Antibiotics (penicillins, cephalosporins,
rifampicin, sulfamethoxazole, ciprofloxacin)
NSAIDs
Loop and thiazide diuretics
Allopurinol
Cimetidine
Mesalazine
Omeprazole
Phenytoin

Figure 63.6 Common nephrotoxic agents leading to acute tubular necrosis. ACE, angiotensin-converting enzyme; ARB, angiotensin receptor blocker; NSAIDs, nonsteroidal anti-inflammatory drugs.

and diuretics and calcium channel blockers.[11] This form of ARF is usually reversible in 2 to 7 days upon discontinuation of the drug. Less frequently, NSAIDs induce ATN or, even more rarely, papillary necrosis.[10]

NSAIDs may also cause an acute interstitial nephritis, often with a subacute presentation, associated with white cells and white-cell casts in the urine. About 85% of these patients also have heavy proteinuria due to a concomitant minimal change type injury. Possibly as a result of the anti-inflammatory effects of these drugs, the signs of rash, fever, and eosinophilia are often absent.

Other renal side effects of NSAIDs include fluid and electrolyte disturbances such as sodium retention exacerbating hypertension and congestive heart failure, hyponatremia, and hyperkalemia.

Angiotensin-Converting Enzyme Inhibitors and Angiotensin Receptor Blockers
ACE inhibitors and ARBs may also cause a hemodynamically induced ARF in the setting of reduced renal perfusion due to impaired vasoconstriction of the efferent arteriole. They may also directly impair renal perfusion by their antihypertensive effects.

In situations in which the initial increase in serum creatinine is greater than 30% or repeated measurements show a progressive increase, the appropriate response is to discontinue the ACE inhibitors and ARB and search for other causes of renal dysfunction, such as bilateral renal artery stenosis, stenosis of the renal artery in a solitary kidney, intrarenal diffuse nephrosclerosis, polycystic kidney disease with the renal arteries being extrinsically compressed by large cysts, decreased absolute or effective arterial blood volume, use of NSAIDs, calcineurin inhibitors, and sepsis. Patients chronically treated with ACE inhibitors have an increased risk for postoperative renal dysfunction,[12] most probably as a consequence of intraoperative hypotensive episodes.

Gentamicin

Gentamicin is excreted by glomerular filtration, and toxicity may occur if the dose is not adjusted for underlying renal impairment. Cationic amino groups (NH_3^+) on the drug bind to anionic megalin on the brush border of proximal tubular epithelial cells, and the drug is then internalized by endocytosis. The drug accumulates in proximal tubular cell lysosomes and can reach 100 to 1000 times its serum concentration. The drug interferes with cellular energetics, impairs intracellular phospholipases, and induces oxidative stress; however, the exact pathways culminating in tubular necrosis remain unknown.[13]

Nonoliguric ARF usually occurs after 5 to 10 days of treatment with gentamicin. Involvement of distal tubular segments may produce polyuria, potassium, and magnesium wasting. The risk for ARF correlates with the accumulation of gentamicin in proximal tubular cells and is related to the daily dose and duration of therapy. Prolonged accumulation in proximal tubular cells may allow development of ARF even after the drug has been discontinued. Additional risk factors for gentamicin toxicity include increasing age, pre-existing renal disease, hypotension, concurrent liver disease, sepsis syndrome, and concurrent nephrotoxins.

Gentamicin serum levels should be followed to minimize nephrotoxicity. When possible, the drug may be administered in a single daily total dose, which leads to lower renal proximal tubular cell accumulation. Gentamicin, tobramycin, and netilmicin appear to have similar nephrotoxic effects. However, amikacin, which has fewer amino groups per molecule, may be less nephrotoxic.

The macrolide antibiotic vancomycin is rarely associated with acute renal failure when used as monotherapy. However, when used with gentamicin, it may increase the risk for aminoglycoside-induced ARF.

Amphotericin B

This polyene macrolide antibiotic binds to sterols in the cell membranes of both fungal walls (ergosterol) and mammalian (cholesterol) cell membranes, resulting in the formation of aqueous pores, which increase membrane permeability. The increased sodium influx leads to increased Na^+-K^+-ATPase activity and depletion of cellular energy stores. Additionally, the standard amphotericin B formulation is suspended in the bile salt deoxycholate, which has a detergent effect on cell membranes.[14] Nephrotoxicity relates to cumulative dosage, usually occurring after administration of 2 to 3 g.

Early signs of nephrotoxicity include a loss of urine-concentrating ability, followed by a decrease in GFR. Hypokalemia and hypomagnesemia due to distal tubular toxicity are common. A distal renal tubular acidosis may be present due to proton backleak in the cortical collecting duct.

Prevention of nephrotoxicity requires the maintenance of high urine flow rates by saline loading during amphotericin administration. The much more expensive liposomal amphotericin B preparations reduce the incidence of ARF by 50%. The binding of amphotericin B to ergosterol is more avid than to cholesterol, and by delivering the drug as a cholesterol liposome, diminished binding to tubular epithelial cell membranes results without altering fungal binding. Additionally, liposomal preparations do not contain deoxycholate (see earlier discussion). Amphotericin B–induced ARF is usually reversible with discontinuing treatment, although distal injury manifested by magnesium wasting may persist.

Antiviral Therapy

Acyclovir

Nephrotoxicity is typically seen after intravenous acyclovir administration and may be due to the formation of intratubular acyclovir crystals. The latter appear as birefringent needle-shaped crystals on urine microscopy. However, crystals may also be seen in non-ARF patients, and renal biopsy data suggest that an acute interstitial nephritis may be the predominant mechanism of toxicity. Ceftriaxone appears to increase the risk for nephrotoxicity. By contrast, ganciclovir has little nephrotoxicity.

Oliguric ARF typically occurs within a few days of treatment and may be associated with abdominal or loin pain. High serum levels of acyclovir due to decreased renal clearance may produce neurologic toxicity. The ARF is usually mild and recovers on stopping the drug.

Foscarnet

Foscarnet is a phosphate analogue used in the treatment of severe cytomegalovirus infection but also inhibits proximal tubule sodium-phosphate cotransport. ARF occurs in 10% to 20% of treated patients and may be due to ATN or intratubular crystal obstruction and acute interstitial nephritis. The ARF is usually nonoliguric and associated with mild proteinuria (<1 g) and a benign urine sediment. Hypocalcemia due to chelation of calcium may be present. The renal failure is usually reversible, although recovery may take several months. Prehydration markedly decreases the incidence of ARF.

Cidofovir and Adefovir

These nucleotide analogues have been associated with ARF secondary to proximal tubular injury in 12% to 24% of cases. They are transported into the proximal tubule by the human organic anion transporter (hOAT), and nephrotoxicity may be reduced by concurrent use of probenecid, which blocks hOAT and volume expansion.

Other Antiviral Agents

Most other antiviral agents are not nephrotoxic. In the treatment of hepatitis C virus (HCV), there have been rare reports of ATN secondary to interferon-α.

Immunosuppressive Agents

See also Chapter 90.

Calcineurin Inhibitors

Cyclosporine and tacrolimus may cause acute renal impairment due to afferent arteriolar vasoconstriction partly mediated by endothelin. This is usually reversible upon dose reduction. Persistent injury may lead to chronic interstitial fibrosis in a striped pattern along medullary rays reflecting the ischemic nature of the insult as well as the development of arteriolar hyalinosis. Associated clinical features may include hypertension, hyperkalemia, hyperuricemia, and wasting of phosphate and magnesium from tubular injury. Calcineurin inhibitors may also cause endothelial injury, leading to thrombotic microangiopathy (see Chapter 28).

Other Immunosuppressive Agents

The monoclonal anti-CD3 antibody (OKT3) or polyclonal anti-lymphocyte and antithymocyte preparations (ALG, ATG) may cause a first-dose cytokine release syndrome and prerenal azotemia secondary to capillary leak. OKT3 has rarely been associated with a hemolytic uremic syndrome. Intravenous immunoglobulin (IVIG) can cause ARF, which may be partly mediated by the high sucrose concentration in these products. Tubular uptake of sucrose may result in osmotic cell swelling and injury. Methotrexate is toxic to proximal tubular epithelial cells and rarely may cause intratubular crystal obstruction.

Acetaminophen (Paracetamol)

Isolated ATN may occur in rare cases, but renal injury is more typically associated with an acute hepatitis. Renal and liver toxicity usually occur when >15 g have been taken, but in alcoholics, normal doses may be toxic. Acetaminophen is conjugated in the liver and undergoes renal excretion. Less than 5% undergoes metabolism by P-450 (CYP2E1) enzymes to form a toxic metabolite, *N*-acetylimidoquinone, which is inactivated by the thiol group of glutathione. With high levels of acetaminophen, glutathione becomes depleted, and *N*-acetylimidoquinone can bind to thiol groups on intracellular proteins, resulting in cell injury. Because glutathione is a major intracellular antioxidant, its loss may predispose to oxidative injury to the tubular cells.

Clinically, acute hepatitis and ATN only begin once glutathione levels are depleted, and clinical manifestations usually present 3 to 4 days after ingestion. *N*-acetyl cysteine can be protective, if administered early, because it provides a free thiol group, substituting for glutathione.

Ethylene Glycol

Ethylene glycol, found in antifreeze, remains a cause of both deliberate and accidental injury. It is rapidly metabolized by alcohol dehydrogenase to glycoaldehyde and glyoxylate, which are toxic to tubular cells. Further metabolism generates oxalic acid, which can precipitate in renal tubules, leading to intratubular obstruction.

The diagnosis is suggested by the presence of a severe anion gap metabolic acidosis and the presence of a serum osmolal gap. Oxalate crystals are typically, but not always, seen on the urine microscopy (see Chapter 4, Fig. 4.7). Management includes inhibition of alcohol dehydrogenase with intravenous ethanol (aiming for blood levels of 100–200 mg/dl) or the specific alcohol dehydrogenase inhibitor fomepizole. Hemodialysis should be performed to remove the ethylene glycol and metabolites when the level is >20 mg/dl and continued until it is <5 mg/dl. Methanol intoxication may present with similar metabolic abnormalities, but rarely causes ARF (see Chapter 12).

Illicit Drug Use

ARF is a common condition in those who abuse drugs and may be due to nephrotoxicity of the drug, coexistent viral infection (HIV, HCV), sepsis, infective endocarditis, rhabdomyolysis, or alcohol abuse.

Cocaine

Cocaine induces intense vasoconstriction, which may lead to severe hypertension and rhabdomyolysis.[15] Mechanisms for rhabdomyolysis include coma and pressure necrosis; vasospasm leading to ischemic muscle injury; adrenergic stimulation and hyperpyrexia leading to increased cellular metabolism. It typically occurs in those who inject cocaine, and the patient often presents with fever, hypertension, tachycardia, and a decreased mental state.

Other illicit drugs associated with acute renal failure include opiates (coma-associated, pressure-induced rhabdomyolysis); phencyclidine (PCP; rhabdomyolysis secondary to hyperpyrexia and vasoconstriction); and amphetamines (ARF secondary to rhabdomyolysis, acute interstitial nephritis, or acute necrotizing angiitis).

Bisphosphonates

ARF due to tubular injury has been described with both intravenous zoledronate and intravenous pamidronate. This typically occurs after several months of treatment.

Occupational Toxins
Heavy Metals

Lead intoxication usually causes a chronic nephropathy (see Chapter 59). Rarely, acute tubular injury occurs that may be associated with Fanconi syndrome. ATN may also occur in cadmium and mercury poisoning.

Organic Solvents

Organic solvents may cause acute tubular injury due to peroxidation of membrane lipids. A subacute renal failure due to anti–glomerular basement membrane (anti-GBM) antibody disease has also been reported with exposure to halogenated hydrocarbons.

Herbal Remedies

Specific herbs used in traditional African medicine (e.g., Cape aloes, *Callilepis laureola*) are common causes of ARF in parts of Africa. A subacute form of renal failure due to aristolochic acid found in certain herbs used in traditional Chinese medicine is also described (see Chapter 59).

Heme Pigment Nephropathy

Heme pigment nephropathy is a common cause of ARF and usually secondary to the breakdown of muscle fibers (rhabdomyolysis), which release potentially nephrotoxic intracellular contents (particularly myoglobin) into the systemic circulation. Less commonly, heme pigment nephropathy may occur due to massive intravascular hemolysis. Prevention and therapy of heme pigment nephropathy are discussed in Chapter 64.

Causes of Rhabdomyolysis

Muscle trauma is the most common cause of rhabdomyolysis. The initial description was by Bywaters and Beall during the bombing of London in World War II.[16] Other common causes of muscle injury include marked exercise, seizures, pressure necrosis secondary to coma, alcohol abuse, and limb ischemia (Fig. 63.7). In the patient with alcohol abuse, rhabdomyolysis is often multifactorial due to pressure necrosis from coma ("found down"), direct myotoxicity from ethanol seizures, and electrolyte abnormalities (hypokalemia and hypophosphatemia). Therapy with statins may be associated with rhabdomyolysis. The risk is increased by concomitant therapy with fibrates, cyclosporine, or erythromycin.

Causes of rhabdomyolysis	
Muscle injury/ischemia	Trauma, pressure necrosis, electric shock, burns, acute vascular disease
Myofiber exhaustion	Seizures, excessive exercise, heat exhaustion
Toxins	Alcohol, cocaine, heroin, amphetamines, Ecstasy, phencyclidine, snakebite
Drugs	Statins, fibrates, zidovudine, neuroleptic malignant syndrome, azathioprine, theophylline, lithium, diuretics
Electrolyte disorders	Hypophosphatemia, hypokalemia, excess water shifts (hyperosmolality)
Infections	Viral (influenza, HIV, coxsackievirus, Epstein-Barr virus), bacterial (*Legionella*, *Francisella*, *Streptococcus pneumoniae*, *Salmonella*, *Staphylococcus aureus*)
Familial	McArdle's disease, carnitine palmitoyl transferase deficiency, malignant hyperthermia
Other	Hypothyroidism, polymyositis, dermatomyositis

Figure 63.7   Causes of rhabdomyolysis.

Familial myopathies such as McArdle's syndrome and carnitine palmitoyl transferase deficiency should be suspected in patients with a history of recurrent episodes of rhabdomyolysis associated with muscle pain, positive family history, onset in childhood, and the absence of other identifiable causes (reviewed in ref. 17).

Causes of Hemoglobinuria

Intravascular hemolysis results in circulating free hemoglobin. If the hemolysis is mild, the released hemoglobin is bound by circulating haptoglobin. However, with massive hemolysis, haptoglobin becomes exhausted, and hemoglobin (69 kd) dissociates into α-β dimers (34 kd), which are small enough to be filtered, resulting in hemoglobinuria, hemoglobin cast formation, and heme uptake by proximal tubular cells. Like myoglobin, these processes can result in ATN and filtration failure. Causes of hemoglobinuric ARF include incompatible blood transfusion, autoimmune hemolytic anemia, malaria (blackwater fever), glucose-6-phosphate dehydrogenase deficiency, paroxysmal nocturnal hemoglobinuria, and toxins (dapsone, venoms).

Pathogenesis of Heme Pigment Nephropathy
Muscle Injury

A variety of environmental, metabolic, and infective insults may produce muscle injury, but the final common pathway is often ATP depletion from tissue ischemia or metabolic abnormalities, and mitochondrial injury leading to the generation of oxygen free radicals. Muscle hyperthermia may potentiate injury by increasing the metabolic rate. Pronounced hypophosphatemia (i.e., serum levels <0.5 mmol/l [>1.56 mg/dl]) may impair ATP production, and hypokalemia may inhibit glycogen synthesis. Additionally, potassium is an important vasodilator in the muscle microcirculation. Hypokalemia reduces endothelial nitric oxide and thereby may inhibit the hyperemia of exercising muscle and exacerbate ischemia.

During the period of tissue ischemia, cell viability may be maintained by limited calcium delivery, decreased production of oxidative radicals by mitochondria due to oxygen lack, and the

protective effect of local acidosis. Reperfusion removes these protective mechanisms, and much of the myocyte damage occurs not during the ischemic period but after the restoration of blood flow (reperfusion injury). It is also during this time that myoglobin gains access to the systemic circulation and fluid sequestration in injured muscle occurs that can lead to intravascular volume contraction. Furthermore, the release of potassium and phosphate from damaged cells may obscure electrolyte abnormalities underlying rhabdomyolysis.

Renal Injury

The renal injury is due to a combination of factors, including volume depletion, renal vasoconstriction, direct heme-protein–mediated cytotoxicity, and intraluminal cast formation (Fig. 63.8). Volume depletion is often prominent in this condition owing to the sequestration of large amounts of fluid (up to 15–20 liters) in injured muscle. Volume depletion activates the sympathetic nervous system and renin angiotensin system, resulting in renal vasoconstriction, which may be exacerbated by the scavenging of nitric oxide by circulating heme proteins. Myoglobin (17 kd) is freely filtered at the glomerulus and is toxic to tubular epithelial cells. The heme center of myoglobin may directly induce lipid peroxidation and renal injury,[18] and liberated free iron catalyzes the formation of hydroxyl radical through the Fenton reaction inducing free radical–mediated injury. Renoprotection has been demonstrated in animal models with free iron scavengers and various antioxidants. Finally, the precipitation of myoglobin with Tamm-Horsfall protein and sloughed proximal tubular cells may result in obstructing casts in the distal nephron. This is enhanced by increased concentrations of tubular heme protein due to volume depletion with low tubular fluid flow rates. The binding of myoglobin to Tamm-Horsfall protein is enhanced in acid urine.

Clinical Features of Heme Pigment (Hemoglobin, Myoglobin) Acute Renal Failure

Heme pigment nephropathy typically presents with oliguric ARF; however, both rhabdomyolysis and hemolysis may occur without ARF. In rhabdomyolysis, large amounts of fluid may be sequestered in injured muscle, and volume depletion is prominent. Blood pressure may be preserved despite marked volume depletion due to the scavenging effect of myoglobin on nitric oxide. The injured muscle may not be clinically apparent on examination and muscle pain may be absent. In limb muscles confined to rigid compartments, cell swelling after injury may result in increased intracompartmental pressures impairing local microvascular circulation leading to compartment syndrome (Fig. 63.9).

Myoglobin causes a red-brown discoloration of the urine and a positive dipstick urinalysis for heme. Urine microscopy reveals multiple pigmented casts. The absence of red cells with a positive urinalysis for heme implies the presence of myoglobinuria or hemoglobinuria. The finding of urine myoglobin is nonspecific because this test may be positive with only minor muscle injury. Urine electrolytes may show a low fractional excretion of sodium due to volume depletion and renal vasoconstriction. The level of serum creatinine kinase (CK) is usually greater than 10,000 U/liter, although levels correspond poorly with the degree of renal failure. The release of other cellular constituents may produce life-threatening hyperkalemia, hyperphosphatemia, and hyperuricemia. A lactic acidosis may be present from increased muscle anaerobic metabolism. Calcium levels are typically low in the acute stage owing to calcium phosphate deposition in injured muscle tissue and an inhibition of renal 1,25-dihydroxyvitamin D synthesis within the

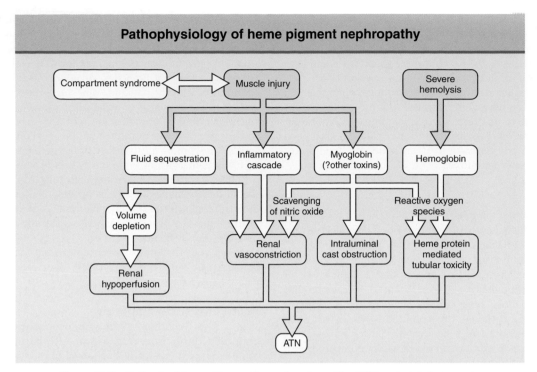

Figure 63.8   Pathophysiology of heme pigment nephropathy. ATN, acute tubular necrosis.

damaged kidney. Hypercalcemia occurs in 25% of subjects during the recovery phase and results from the mobilization of deposited calcium from muscle, a rebound in 1,25-dihydroxyvitamin D levels, and elevated parathyroid hormone levels (the latter stimulated by the previous hypocalcemia).

Radiocontrast-induced Nephropathy

ARF secondary to contrast nephrotoxicity (reviewed in ref. 19) typically occurs in patients with underlying renal impairment and is rarely seen in patients with normal renal function. It may occur with both intravenous and intra-arterial contrast, but not with oral contrast (assuming an intact bowel). The incidence of contrast nephrotoxicity is about 20% and 50% in patients with serum

creatinine levels >2 mg/dl and 5 mg/dl (176 and 440 μmol/l), respectively. Other risk factors for the development of this condition include diabetic nephropathy, advanced age (>75 years) congestive heart failure, volume depletion, and high or repetitive doses of radiocontrast agent. High osmolar contrast is more nephrotoxic than low or iso-osmolar contrast agents. Concurrent use of potentially nephrotoxic agents such as NSAIDs or ACE inhibitors may increase the risk (see also Chapters 5 and 64).

Pathogenesis

Medullary hypoxia and direct tubular epithelial cell toxicity are the main factors in the pathogenesis of contrast nephrotoxicity. Typically, a biphasic hemodynamic response is seen. An initial

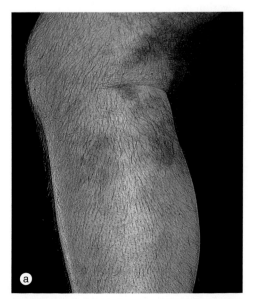
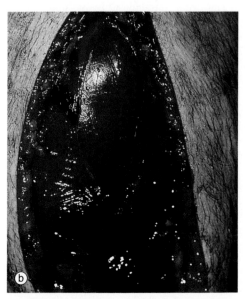

Figure 63.9   Compartment syndrome. a, Severe calf swelling due to anterior and posterior compartment syndromes after ischemia-reperfusion. b, Appearance following emergency fasciotomy: note edematous muscle and hematoma. (Courtesy of Mr. M. J. Allen, FRCS.)

vasodilation (lasting a few seconds to minutes) is followed by a more prolonged renal vasoconstriction. The consequent medullary hypoxia may be exacerbated by the osmotic diuresis, leading to increased sodium delivery to the medullary thick ascending loop and requiring greater oxygen consumption for reabsorption.

Radiocontrast agents also cause direct tubular epithelial cell injury. Human studies have demonstrated low-molecular-weight proteinuria, suggestive of proximal tubular injury, partly mediated by ROS. Increased markers of lipid peroxidation have been described, and the administration of antioxidants ameliorates contrast nephrotoxicity in animals.

Clinical Features

Typically, the serum creatinine begins to rise within 24 to 48 hours of radiocontrast administration, peaks after 4 to 5 days, and returns to baseline over 7 to 10 days. The patient is usually nonoliguric, and examination of the urine sediment reveals granular casts and some tubular epithelial cells. In some, contrast nephrotoxicity may lead to treatment delays, prolong hospital stay, or require short-term hemodialysis (particularly patients with diabetes who may be oliguric). Although this condition typically recovers, several studies have confirmed a significantly increased mortality in patients who develop contrast nephrotoxicity compared with matched controls.[20] Failure to return to baseline renal function suggests the presence of additional renal insults such as renal atheroembolism (see later discussion). Prevention and therapy of contrast nephrotoxicity is discussed in Chapter 64.

Atheroembolic Renal Disease (Syndrome of Multiple Cholesterol Emboli)

This condition is more frequent than previously suspected, and large series of patients suffering from this condition have been described.[21] It occurs predominantly in older patients with atherosclerotic vascular disease either spontaneously or, more frequently, precipitated by arteriography, vascular surgery, thrombolysis (streptokinase and tissue plasminogen activator), and anticoagulation. Destabilization of atherosclerotic plaques primarily in the aorta results in showers of cholesterol that lodge in small arteries in the kidneys (see Fig. 61.22) and typically the lower extremities (see Fig. 61.20). At times, significant embolization of extrarenal intra-abdominal vessels can occur, inducing ischemic injury (e.g., bowel and pancreas). Needle-shaped clefts may be seen on renal or skin biopsy, denoting the localization of cholesterol plaques before dissolution with tissue fixation. The cholesterol emboli produce a marked and progressive inflammatory reaction, resulting in occlusion of the involved vasculature. Flank pain, with or without moderate fever and leukocytosis, is the initial symptom. Typically, a subacute renal failure occurs that is progressive and is usually associated with systemic embolic phenomena of digital infarcts, livedo reticularis, and distal cyanosis ("purple toes"). Eosinophilia and hypocomplementemia may be found, mimicking a systemic vasculitis.

The condition is an important differential diagnosis in older patients undergoing vascular interventions. When ARF due to cholesterol emboli appears after an angiographic procedure, it usually presents after 2 to 4 weeks, in contrast to radiographic contrast ATN, which usually develops in a few days. In cases of cholesterol emboli, renal recovery is not observed in 30% to 40% of cases. There is currently no effective treatment for this condition, although ACE inhibitors have been suggested to slow progressive renal damage. Atheroembolic renal disease is discussed further in Chapter 61.

Other Vascular Causes of Acute Renal Failure

ARF caused by complete renal artery thrombosis occurs when the occlusion is bilateral or, in the case of unilateral acute occlusion, with a single nonfunctioning kidney. Thrombosis of the renal artery, its intrarenal branches, or noncholesterol emboli is more common in elderly patients. One important risk for intrarenal emboli is the presence of atrial fibrillation, in which the relative risk for peripheral embolization (aorta, renal and pelvic arteries, and arteries of the extremities) has been calculated to be 4 in men and 5.7 in women compared with the general population.

Flank pain, with or without low-grade fever and leukocytosis, is the most common presenting symptom. Macroscopic or microscopic hematuria is not always present. Whereas total occlusion of both renal arteries usually manifests as anuria, minimal output of urine may be observed, and the differential diagnosis of ARF may become difficult.

Renal vein thrombosis most commonly occurs in the setting of nephrotic syndrome and rarely may cause ARF if bilateral (see Chapter 61).

Acute Interstitial Nephritis

This is most commonly a drug-induced phenomenon and is an important differential diagnosis in ARF because removal of the offending agent can result in reversal of the condition. Less commonly, it may be due to infection or immune-mediated diseases. Acute interstitial nephritis is discussed further in Chapter 57.

Hemorrhagic Fever with Renal Syndrome

Hemorrhagic fever with renal syndrome (HFRS) is caused by a rodent-transmitted hantavirus (see also Chapter 57). Humans may become infected through inhalation of aerosols of dried excreta, inoculation through the conjunctiva, or entry through broken skin or rodent bites. Depending in part on the causative virus, HFRS can manifest as mild, moderate, or severe disease: severe HFRS is usually attributed to Dobrava and Hantaan viruses, moderate HFRS (Korean hemorrhagic fever) to Seoul virus, and mild HFRS (nephropathia epidemica or benign epidemic nephropathy) to Puumala virus.

The diagnosis of hantavirus infection can be made from the clinical manifestations plus high level of IgG antibody titers. Laboratory findings reveal leukocytosis, thrombocytopenia, and elevation of lactate dehydrogenase.

Most cases occur in Central and Eastern Europe and Central and East Asia. Incubation time is estimated to be 2 to 3 weeks, followed by a febrile phase (prodrome) associated with head, often severe abdominal, and back pain and ending with appearance of proteinuria that lasts for 3 to 7 days. A hypotensive phase follows, lasting several hours to 2 days, and hemorrhage and lethal shock syndrome in the most severe cases. About 50% of deaths occur during the subsequent oliguric phase with duration of 3 to 7 days. ARF presents as a reversible acute hemorrhagic interstitial nephritis but can progress to a chronic form. Treatment consists of supportive measures.

Specific Clinical Situations

Determining the etiology of ARF is often aided by recognizing common patterns of presentation and determining the likely causes arising in each of these situations.

Acute Renal Failure in the Patient with Multiorgan Failure

About 20% of patients with sepsis syndrome and 50% of those with septic shock develop ARF. Sepsis is classically associated with infection. A similar condition, termed the *systemic inflammatory response syndrome* (SIRS), may occur secondary to noninfectious insults (such as acute pancreatitis, major trauma, or ischemia reperfusion). The causes of the ARF in this setting are typically multifactorial, due to a combination of hypotension, impaired renal perfusion, inflammatory mediators, and nephrotoxic agents.[22–25]

Initial activation of the innate immune system may occur after the interaction of a number of bacterial products (lipopolysaccharide, flagellin, lipoteichoic acid, others) with pattern recognition receptors (such as toll-like receptors) on immune cells. This leads to the activation of a wide range of cellular and humoral mediator systems, including the cytokine cascade (TNF-α, IL-1β, IL-6); the complement, coagulation, and fibrinolytic systems; and the release of mediators such as eicosanoids, platelet-activating factor, endothelin-1, and nitric oxide. Widespread endothelial injury results, leading to peripheral vasodilation, increased vascular permeability, and leukocyte infiltration. Peripheral vasodilation causes hypotension, with consequent activation of the renin angiotensin system, increased vasopressin, and increased cardiac output to maintain organ perfusion.

Clinical Features

Diagnostic criteria for sepsis or SIRS include tachypnea, tachycardia, and fever or hypothermia and leukocytosis (Fig. 63.10). Systemic vasodilation produces a hyperdynamic circulation with warm extremities. The blood pressure is initially maintained by a markedly increased cardiac output, but at later stages, sepsis has depressant effects on myocardial function, and hypotension develops. Organ dysfunction is manifested by ARF, acute respiratory distress syndrome, liver dysfunction, and hypoperfusion with lactic acidosis. This combination has been described as the multiorgan dysfunction syndrome (MODS). Renal dysfunction is an early feature of sepsis syndrome. Initially, there is a prominent prerenal aspect from systemic hypotension and intrarenal vasoconstriction, which often progresses to ATN.

There is no specific therapy for ARF in this condition other than management of the associated SIRS.[26] Prevention of ARF in sepsis is discussed in Chapter 64.

Acute Renal Failure in the Postoperative Patient

ARF in the postoperative period is commonly due to problems with fluid balance, perioperative hemodynamic instability, or nephrotoxic agents. The critically ill postoperative patient may develop SIRS. ARF may be particularly common after vascular, cardiac, and hepatobiliary surgery (see Chapter 64).

There is evidence that anesthetic agents may impair renal function. This may be partly due to their hypotensive effects, but the metabolism of fluorinated agents can lead to the production of potentially nephrotoxic fluoride ions. Modern inhaled agents (e.g., isoflurane, halothane, enflurane) all cause a transient decrease in GFR, and methoxyflurane had to be discontinued because of nephrotoxicity.

After Vascular Surgery

In patients with peripheral vascular disease, prior ischemic renal disease is often present, and preoperative renal function is the strongest predictor of the risk for postoperative ARF. In aortic aneurysm surgery, most aneurysms are infrarenal; however, surgery that directly involves the renal arteries or aortic cross-clamping above the renal arteries can result in severe renal ischemia. Furthermore, aortic manipulation may dislodge atherosclerotic plaque, resulting in renal atheroembolism. Peripheral limb surgery may be complicated by rhabdomyolysis, and radiocontrast is frequently used for diagnostic purposes.

After Cardiac Surgery

Risk factors for postoperative ARF include duration of cardiac bypass, preoperative renal function, age, diabetes, valvular surgery, blood transfusions, and poor cardiac function.[27] ARF after cardiac surgery is independently associated with an increased mortality and cost. The surgery is often performed with the patient cooled to less than 30°C to protect cells against ischemic injury; however, systemic hypothermia may cause intravascular coagulation. Aortic instrumentation and clamping may lead to renal atheroembolism. Cardiac bypass causes exposure of blood to a nonendothelialized surface, resulting in activation of neutrophils, platelets, complement, and fibrinolytic systems. Significant hemolysis may also occur, potentially resulting in hemoglobinuria. Perioperative myocardial infarction or left ventricular dysfunction may impair renal perfusion postoperatively, although the low cardiac output is often transient and recovers within 24 to 48 hours. Atrial fibrillation is a common complication and may be associated with peripheral embolization.

After Hepatobiliary Surgery

Surgery to relieve obstructive jaundice is more commonly associated with ARF than other forms of abdominal surgery. This may be due to the absence of bile salts in the gut lumen, which normally break down lipopolysaccharide endotoxin, preventing absorption. One study suggested a decreased incidence of postoperative endotoxemia when treated with oral bile salts. Other factors may include direct nephrotoxic effects of bilirubin or bile salts on renal tubular cells and an increased incidence of biliary sepsis.

Abdominal Compartment Syndrome

Markedly raised intra-abdominal pressures (>20 mm Hg) may occur after trauma, after abdominal surgery, or secondary to massive fluid resuscitation resulting in ARF.[28] The mechanism remains unclear, but may be due to increased renal venous pressure and vascular resistance. Ureteral compression is not considered a factor. Efforts to reduce intra-abdominal pressures, including paracentesis, nasogastric suction, ultrafiltration, or surgical decompression, may occasionally improve renal function.

Pulmonary-Renal Syndromes

The term *pulmonary-renal syndrome* describes the presence of pulmonary hemorrhage in a patient with ARF and is most commonly due to anti-GBM disease (Goodpasture's syndrome), systemic vasculitis, or systemic lupus erythematosus (Fig. 63.11; see Chapters 22–24).

Clinical definitions of sepsis	
Moderate sepsis	Temperature >38°C or <36°C Heart rate >90 beats/min Respiratory rate >20 breaths/min (or partial pressure of arterial CO_2 <32 mm Hg) White cell count >12,000/mm³ (or >10% immature neutrophils [band forms]) Evidence of infection
Severe sepsis	Sepsis associated with organ dysfunction (lactic acidosis, oliguria, or acute alteration of mental status)
Septic shock	Sepsis-associated hypotension (systolic blood pressure <90 mm Hg) despite adequate fluid resuscitation

Figure 63.10   Clinical definitions of sepsis.

Causes of pulmonary-renal syndrome	
Systemic vasculitis	Anti-GBM disease, Wegener's granulomatosis, microscopic polyarteritis, lupus erythematosus, Churg-Strauss syndrome, Henoch-Schönlein purpura, Behçet's disease, essential mixed cryoglobulinemia, rheumatoid vasculitis, rarely, drugs (penicillamine, hydralazine, propylthiouracil)
Infection	Severe bacterial pneumonia, post-infectious glomerulonephritis, *Legionella*, hantavirus, opportunistic infection in immunocompromised patients, infective endocarditis
Pulmonary edema and ARF	Volume overload, severe left ventricular failure
Multiorgan failure	Adult respiratory distress syndrome and ARF
Other	Paraquat poisoning, renal vein or inferior vena cava thrombosis with pulmonary emboli

Figure 63.11 Causes of pulmonary-renal syndrome. ARF, acute renal failure; GBM, glomerular basement membrane.

A similar clinical presentation may occur due to pulmonary edema secondary to volume overload in ARF. Other conditions that may masquerade as a pulmonary renal syndrome include upper respiratory infection triggering a flair of IgA nephropathy; severe bacterial pneumonia complicated by ATN or postinfectious glomerulonephritis; *Legionella* species infection causing a severe atypical pneumonia, and acute interstitial nephritis or rhabdomyolysis.

Thrombotic Microangiopathy

Thrombotic microangiopathy (TMA) constitutes a wide range of conditions that should be considered when a patient presents with ARF and thrombocytopenia, although it should be recognized that the condition may occur in the absence of a low platelet count (see Figs. 28.10 and 28.12). Endothelial activation is followed by the formation of platelet thrombi which occlude small vessels and lead to downstream ischemic injury. Renal biopsy may be required to confirm the diagnosis, although it should be recognized that histology is unable to differentiate among the different causes of TMA. TMA is discussed further in Chapter 28.

Acute Renal Failure and Liver Disease

The patient with liver cirrhosis is predisposed to the development of ARF, and the differential diagnosis typically falls between prerenal azotemia, hepatorenal syndrome, and ATN. Assessment of intravascular volume status can be difficult, and a therapeutic trial of volume replacement is typically undertaken. Impaired renal perfusion and hyperbilirubinemia are predisposing risk factors. Alternatively, the same etiologic agent may be responsible for both the liver and renal injury. This occurs with certain infections (e.g., leptospirosis, hantavirus) and nephrotoxic agents (Fig. 63.12). Rarely, hyperbilirubinemia from hemolysis may cause jaundice in the absence of liver disease. ARF and liver disease is discussed further in Chapter 67.

Acute Renal Failure in Patients with HIV Infection

ARF is common in patients with HIV infection and may be related to the disease itself (e.g., HIV nephropathy; see Chapter 25), the therapy, opportunistic infections, or coexistent infections (HCV) and intravenous drug abuse[29] (Fig. 63.13). A hemolytic-uremic syndrome has also been described in HIV infection. In view of the wide differential diagnosis, renal biopsy should be considered when ARF does not respond to supportive measures. In the HIV-infected intravenous drug user, ARF may be due to concomitant HCV infection associated with membranoproliferative glomerulonephritis or to complications related to intravenous drug use (most notably endocarditis-associated renal disease or rhabdomyolysis).

Drug Therapy

Protease inhibitors may cause ARF in patients with HIV infection. This occurs most commonly with indinavir, which can cause intratubular crystal obstruction or obstructing renal calculi, but has also been reported with ritonavir. Reverse transcriptase inhibitors may also produce ARF (e.g., tenofovir, nevirapine).

Treatment of opportunistic infections often requires the use of potentially nephrotoxic drugs such as aminoglycosides or amphotericin B. *Pneumocystis* species infection may be treated with high dose cotrimoxazole (acute interstitial nephritis or intratubular crystal obstruction) or pentamidine (ATN in 25% of cases). Resistant cytomegalovirus infection may require foscarnet therapy (acute interstitial nephritis or intratubular crystal obstruction).

Causes of acute renal failure and liver disease	
Prerenal uremia	Diuretic use, gastrointestinal loss, peritoneal aspiration, hypoalbuminemia
Hepatorenal syndrome	
Acute tubular necrosis	Hyperbilirubinemia, sepsis, toxic shock syndrome
Drugs	Acetaminophen (paracetamol), NSAIDs, tetracycline, rifampicin, isoniazid, anesthetic agents, sulfonamides, allopurinol, methotrexate
Infections	Hepatitis C and cryoglobulinemia, hepatitis B and polyarteritis nodosa, leptospirosis, hantavirus, Epstein-Barr virus, gram-negative sepsis, spontaneous bacterial peritonitis
Other	Papillary necrosis and obstruction, inhalation of chlorinated hydrocarbons, mushroom poisoning (*Amanita phalloides*)

Figure 63.12 Causes of acute renal failure (ARF) and liver disease. NSAIDs, nonsteroidal anti-inflammatory drugs.

Causes of acute renal failure in patients with HIV infection	
Prerenal	Diarrhea, nausea and vomiting, cirrhosis and hepatorenal syndrome, sepsis
Vascular	Thrombotic microangiopathy
Glomerular	Immune complex glomerulonephritis (MPGN secondary to hepatitis C virus, postinfectious glomerulonephritis), HIVAN
Acute tubular necrosis	Sepsis, hypotension, nephrotoxins (aminoglycosides, amphotericin, acyclovir, cidofovir, tenofovir, pentamidine), rhabdomyolysis
Acute interstitial nephritis	Drug induced (cotrimoxazole, rifampicin, foscarnet, nevirapine), CMV infection, DILS
Drug-induced intratubular obstruction	Sulfadiazine, indinavir, foscarnet, acyclovir
Postrenal obstruction	Stones, tuberculosis, fungal ball, tumor
Associated with IV drug use	Sepsis, endocarditis, heroin-associated nephropathy (FSGS), rhabdomyolysis

Figure 63.13 Causes of acute renal failure (ARF) in patients with HIV infection. CMV, cytomegalovirus; DILS, diffuse infiltrative lymphocytosis syndrome; FSGS, focal segmental glomerulosclerosis; HIVAN, HIV-associated nephropathy; MPGN, membranoproliferative glomerulonephritis.

Acute Renal Failure in the Cancer Patient

Patients with cancer are prone to ARF as a consequence of both their underlying disease and its treatment.[30] Also, there is a high incidence of prerenal azotemia in this patient group due to the high frequency of nausea, vomiting, and diarrhea (Fig. 63.14). More specific causes of ARF are noted in the following sections.

Tumor Lysis Syndrome

Necrosis of large numbers of tumor cells, typically following chemotherapy, may release large amounts of nephrotoxic intracellular contents (uric acid, phosphate, xanthine) into the circulation.[31] It usually occurs with lymphomas (particularly Burkitt's) and leukemias, but may be seen with solid tumors. Rarely, a spontaneous form of tumor lysis syndrome occurs in rapidly growing tumors that outstrip their blood supply.

In earlier days, hyperuricemia resulted in acute urate nephropathy due to intratubular crystal obstruction and interstitial nephritis, but this is now uncommon owing to the prophylactic use of allopurinol before chemotherapy. Other intracellular components are now more commonly involved, such as phosphate release with the precipitation of calcium phosphate in the tubules.

The ARF is typically oligoanuric, and the condition should be suspected in patients with high lactate dehydrogenase levels suggestive of massive cell lysis. Markedly elevated phosphate and urate levels may also be found. Hyperkalemia may be prominent and life threatening.

Preventive measures include the use of high-dose allopurinol (600–900 mg/day) started 2 to 3 days before chemotherapy, and either oral or intravenous fluid loading to ensure a urine output >2.5 l/day. Urine alkalinization is controversial because it may promote tubular calcium phosphate deposition; however, it should be considered when serum uric acid levels are elevated (>12 mg/dl [714 μmol/l]) or urinary uric acid crystals are present. Recombinant uricase (rasburicase) is very effective in

Causes of acute renal failure in patients with cancer	
Prerenal	Nausea and vomiting, hypercalcemia, cardiomyopathy secondary to chemotherapy
Vascular	Thrombotic microangiopathy (adenocarcinoma of stomach, pancreas, prostate; radiation nephropathy), renal vein thrombosis secondary to hypercoagulability, disseminated intravascular coagulation (acute promyelocytic leukemia)
Glomerular	Rapidly progressive glomerulonephritis
Acute tubular necrosis	Sepsis and antibiotic nephrotoxicity, hypercalcemia
Malignant infiltration	Lymphoma, acute lymphoblastic leukemia
Intraluminal obstruction	Tumor lysis syndrome, cast nephropathy
Postrenal obstruction	Transitional cell carcinoma of the ureters/bladder, extrinsic ureteral compression (tumor, nodes, retroperitoneal fibrosis)
Chemotherapeutic agents Tubular toxicity	Cisplatin, ifosfamide, plicamycin (mithramycin); 5-fluorouracil, thioguanine (6-thioguanine), cytarabine
Thrombotic microangiopathy	Mitomycin C, bleomycin, cisplatin, calcineurin inhibitors
Other mechanisms	Capillary leak syndrome (IL-2 therapy), acute interstitial nephritis (interferon-α), intraluminal obstruction (methotrexate)

Figure 63.14 Causes of acute renal failure (ARF) in patients with cancer. IL-2, interleukin-2.

lowering serum uric acid levels (to <1 mg/dl in 24 hours) and should be considered for prophylaxis in high-risk patients.

Once the patient develops ARF with hyperuricemia, rasburicase, which lowers uric acid much more effectively than dialysis, should be considered. If this is not available or the patient is markedly hyperphosphatemic, early dialysis should be considered to remove these potential causes of further renal damage. Because phosphate is less well removed by dialysis than urate, frequent (every 12–24 hours) or prolonged treatments should be considered.

Hypercalcemia

Volume depletion secondary to hypercalcemia-induced nausea and vomiting may cause ARF, which may be exacerbated by hypercalcemia-induced nephrogenic diabetes insipidus. Other hypercalcemia-associated factors that may contribute to ARF include direct intrarenal vasoconstriction, acute interstitial nephritis, and intratubular obstruction.

Renal Infiltration

Direct infiltration of the kidneys by tumor is not uncommon; however, this rarely results in renal failure. ARF may be seen with slow-growing lymphomas or leukemias, when the patient presents with nonoliguric ARF, a benign urine sediment and enlarged kidneys on ultrasound scan. Renal function may improve depending on the responsiveness of the tumor to treatment.

Chemotherapeutic Agents

Cisplatin is commonly associated with a nonoliguric renal impairment.[32] Nephrotoxic injury affects both the proximal and distal nephron and clinically may be associated with magnesium wasting, impaired urinary concentration, and rarely salt wasting with volume depletion. Chloride ions in the *cis* position on the molecule may be replaced by water, releasing toxic hydroxyl radicals. Prophylaxis against nephrotoxicity includes volume loading, possibly with hypertonic saline, and the use of the antioxidant amifostine as a thiol donor. The alternative agent carboplatin appears to be less nephrotoxic. Once renal impairment is present, recovery may be poor, and magnesium wasting may persist.

Ifosfamide is a cyclophosphamide analogue with a nephrotoxic metabolite, chloroacetaldehyde. Cyclophosphamide itself has no significant nephrotoxicity. ARF is usually mild, although proximal tubular dysfunction (Fanconi syndrome) and hypokalemia may be prominent.

REFERENCES

1. Liano F, Pascual J: Epidemiology of acute renal failure: A prospective, multicenter, community-based study. Madrid Acute Renal Failure Study Group. Kidney Int 1996;50:811–818.
2. Uchino S, Kellum JA, Bellomo R, et al: Acute renal failure in critically ill patients: A multinational, multicenter study. JAMA 2005;294:813–818.
3. Schrier RW, Wang W, Poole B, Mitra A: Acute renal failure: Definitions, diagnosis, pathogenesis, and therapy. J Clin Invest 2004;114:5–14.
4. Bonventre JV, Weinberg JM: Recent advances in the pathophysiology of ischemic acute renal failure. J Am Soc Nephrol 2003;14:2199–2210.
5. Brivet FG, Kleinknecht DJ, Loirat P, Landais PJ: Acute renal failure in intensive care units: Causes, outcome, and prognostic factors of hospital mortality. A prospective, multicenter study. French Study Group on Acute Renal Failure. Crit Care Med 1996;24:192–198.
6. Nath KA, Norby SM: Reactive oxygen species and acute renal failure. Am J Med 2000;109:665–678.
7. Bonventre JV, Zuk A: Ischemic acute renal failure: an inflammatory disease? Kidney Int 2004;66:480–485.
8. Duffield JS, Park KM, Hsiao LL, et al: Restoration of tubular epithelial cells during repair of the postischemic kidney occurs independently of bone marrow-derived stem cells. J Clin Invest 2005;115:1743–1755.
9. Hirschberg R, Kopple J, Lipsett P, et al: Multicenter clinical trial of recombinant human insulin-like growth factor I in patients with acute renal failure. Kidney Int 1999;55:2423–2432.
10. Cheng HF, Harris RC: Renal effects of non-steroidal anti-inflammatory drugs and selective cyclooxygenase-2 inhibitors. Curr Pharm Des 2005;11:1795–1804.
11. Huerta C, Castellsague J, Varas-Lorenzo C, Garcia Rodriguez LA: Nonsteroidal anti-inflammatory drugs and risk of ARF in the general population. Am J Kidney Dis 2005;45:531–539.
12. Evenepoel P: Acute toxic renal failure. Best Pract Res Clin Anaesthesiol 2004;18:37–52.
13. Rougier F, Claude D, Maurin M, Maire P: Aminoglycoside nephrotoxicity. Curr Drug Targets Infect Disord 2004;4:153–162.
14. Deray G: Amphotericin B nephrotoxicity. J Antimicrob Chemother 2002;49(Suppl 1):37–41.
15. Nzerue CM, Hewan-Lowe K, Riley LJ Jr: Cocaine and the kidney: A synthesis of pathophysiologic and clinical perspectives. Am J Kidney Dis 2000;35:783–795.
16. Bywaters EGL, Beall D: Crush injuries with impairment of renal function. BMJ 1941;1:427–432.
17. Lofberg M, Jankala H, Paetau A, et al: Metabolic causes of recurrent rhabdomyolysis. Acta Neurol Scand 1998;98:268–275.
18. Holt S, Moore K: Pathogenesis of renal failure in rhabdomyolysis: The role of myoglobin. Exp Nephrol 2000;8:72–76.
19. Lin J, Bonventre JV: Prevention of radiocontrast nephropathy. Curr Opin Nephrol Hypertens 2005;14:105–110.
20. Levy EM, Viscoli CM, Horwitz RI: The effect of acute renal failure on mortality: A cohort analysis. JAMA 1996;275:1489–1494.
21. Belenfant X, Meyrier A, Jacquot C: Supportive treatment improves survival in multivisceral cholesterol crystal embolism. Am J Kidney Dis 1999;33:840–850.
22. Schrier RW, Wang W: Acute renal failure and sepsis. N Engl J Med 2004;351:159–169.
23. Riedemann NC, Guo RF, Ward PA: The enigma of sepsis. J Clin Invest 2003;112:460–467.
24. De Vriese AS: Prevention and treatment of acute renal failure in sepsis. J Am Soc Nephrol 2003;14:792–805.
25. Hotchkiss RS, Karl IE: The pathophysiology and treatment of sepsis. N Engl J Med 2003;348:138–150.
26. Dellinger RP, Carlet JM, Masur H, et al: Surviving Sepsis Campaign guidelines for management of severe sepsis and septic shock. Crit Care Med 2004;32:858–873.
27. Bove T, Calabro MG, Landoni G, et al: The incidence and risk of acute renal failure after cardiac surgery. J Cardiothorac Vasc Anesth 2004;18:442–445.
28. Sugrue M: Abdominal compartment syndrome. Curr Opin Crit Care 2005;11:333–338.
29. Franceschini N, Napravnik S, Eron JJ Jr, et al: Incidence and etiology of acute renal failure among ambulatory HIV-infected patients. Kidney Int 2005;67:1526–1531.
30. Lameire NH, Flombaum CD, Moreau D, Ronco C: Acute renal failure in cancer patients. Ann Med 2005;37:13–25.
31. Davidson MB, Thakkar S, Hix JK, et al: Pathophysiology, clinical consequences, and treatment of tumor lysis syndrome. Am J Med 2004;116:546–554.
32. Kintzel PE: Anticancer drug-induced kidney disorders. Drug Saf 2001;24:19–38.

Epidemiology, Clinical Evaluation, and Prevention of Acute Renal Failure

Norbert Lameire, Wim Van Biesen, and Raymond Vanholder

CLASSIFICATION OF ACUTE RENAL FAILURE

Acute renal failure (ARF) is defined as a rapid (over hours to weeks) and usually at least partially reversible decline in glomerular filtration rate (GFR) that may occur either in the setting of pre-existing normal renal function (classic ARF) or in someone with pre-existing renal disease (acute-on-chronic renal failure).[1] Clinically, it is often further divided into oliguric (<500 ml/day) or nonoliguric (>500 ml/day) ARF, and whether it is dialysis dependent. The International Acute Dialysis Quality Initiative Group has provided definitions for ARF and acute-on-chronic renal failure for research purposes.[2] This classification (Fig. 64.1) uses GFR and urine output criteria, whichever is worse, to define three increasing levels of renal dysfunction. Patients are classified according to *r*isk of renal dysfunction, type of kidney *i*njury, and degree of

kidney *f*ailure with two clinical outcomes: *l*oss and *e*nd-stage kidney disease (RIFLE). ARF (loss) is defined as the need for renal replacement therapy (RRT) for >4 weeks, whereas end-stage renal disease is defined as the need for dialysis for >3 months.

In patients presenting with acute renal dysfunction without any baseline measure of renal function, one should evaluate for the presence of pre-existing chronic kidney disease (CKD; see later discussion). In the event that no evidence of pre-existing chronic renal disease is present, one can use the Modification of Diet in Renal Disease formula (see Chapter 3) to calculate the GFR that the patient would normally have been predicted to have. This should help in the assessment of the severity of the ARF episode.

Small increases in serum creatinine, which often correspond to important declines in GFR but no need for RRT, may have a dramatic negative impact on the outcome of critically ill patients

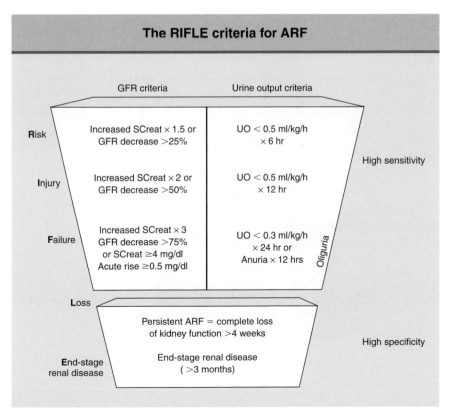

Figure 64.1 **The RIFLE (risk, injury, failure, loss, end-stage renal disease) criteria for acute renal failure (ARF).** GFR, glomerular filtration rate; SCreat, serum creatine; UO, urine output. (Redrawn from Bellomo R: Defining, quantifying, and classifying acute renal failure. Crit Care Clin 2005;21:223–237.)

(see later discussion). In such cases, the term *acute kidney injury* will probably be used in the future and the term *acute renal failure* will be reserved for cases requiring RRT.

EPIDEMIOLOGY OF ACUTE RENAL FAILURE

The epidemiology of ARF is difficult to ascertain due to the differences in definitions and classifications and the patient populations studied. The epidemiology of ARF is different whether it occurs in the general population, the hospitalized population, or in critically ill patients admitted to the intensive care unit (ICU).

Community-Acquired Acute Renal Failure

ARF, defined as an acute elevation in serum creatinine occurring outside the hospital, is noted in about 1% of all hospital admissions. In a Spanish study, the incidence of community-acquired ARF was 209 cases per million population (Fig. 64.2).[3] *De novo* ARF in African Americans occurred in 0.7% of all admissions over a 1-year period; community-acquired ARF was 3.5 times more frequent than hospital-acquired ARF.[4]

Community-acquired ARF may also occur in comatous patients due to rhabdomyolysis in massive disasters, after earthquakes, or other causes of crush syndromes (see Chapter 63). In children, postinfectious glomerulonephritis and in particular diarrhea-associated hemolytic uremic syndrome are common causes of ARF. The latter occurred in 0.7 cases per 100,000 population per year in the United Kingdom.[5] In the developing world, herbs and infections remain the most common etiologic factors in the medical subgroup of ARF in Africa. In India, infectious diarrheal diseases, malaria, leptospirosis, intravascular hemolysis due to glucose-6-phosphate dehydrogenase deficiency, snake bites, and insect stings constitute >60% of ARF, while in Nigeria, edible plants (djenkol beans, *Amanita* mushrooms) and medicinal herbs (impila, cat's claw) are involved in 50% of ARF cases. In contrast, in these countries, obstetric causes have decreased over the years.[6] Nephrotoxicity caused by chemicals can be secondary to accidental occupational exposure in industrial work places (e.g., chromic acid), or after suicidal or homicidal attempts (e.g., copper sulfate, ethylene dibromide, ethylene glycol).

Hospital-Acquired Acute Renal Failure

The incidence of ARF in hospitalized patients increases and now varies between 0.15% and 7.2% of all hospitalizations.[4,7] The major causes of hospital-acquired ARF are ischemic and/or toxin-induced acute tubular necrosis (ATN), but often the cause is multifactorial and iatrogenic (see Chapter 63).

Acute Renal Failure in the Critically Ill

Severe ARF requiring admission to an ICU occurs in 11 patients per 100,000 population per year, and in these critically ill patients, ARF occurs in up to 30% of all ICU admissions and is usually a manifestation of a multiorgan failure syndrome.[8] When the more liberal RIFLE definition is applied, approximately two thirds of ICU patients develop an episode of acute renal dysfunction. Of concern is the finding that increasing RIFLE severity grades correspond with increasing mortality in these patients.[9] Furthermore, this high incidence is likely an underestimate due to the underreporting of terminal patients who are not considered for treatment for ARF.

In the ICU patient, severe sepsis and septic shock are increasingly common and the leading cause of ARF. ARF occurs in ~20% of patients with bacteremia but increases to 50% of patients with concurrent septic shock.[10] Mortality in patients with sepsis-associated ARF (~70%) is greater than in patients with ARF unrelated to sepsis (~45%).

The Changing Spectrum of Acute Renal Failure

The spectrum of particularly hospital-acquired ARF has changed over the past 20 years in view of the increasing acuity and severity of illnesses in people now admitted to hospitals.[11] In present

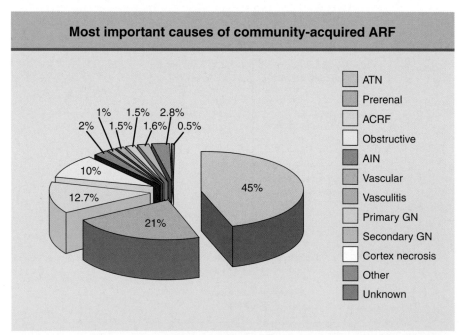

Most important causes of community-acquired ARF

1%   1.5%   2.8%
2%   1.5%   1.6%   0.5%
10%
12.7%
21%
45%

- ATN
- Prerenal
- ACRF
- Obstructive
- AIN
- Vascular
- Vasculitis
- Primary GN
- Secondary GN
- Cortex necrosis
- Other
- Unknown

Figure 64.2 Most important causes of community-acquired acute renal failure (ARF). ACRF, acute-on-chronic renal failure; AIN, acute interstitial nephritis; ATN, acute tubular necrosis; GN, glomerulonephritis. (Redrawn from Liano F, Pascual J: Epidemiology of acute renal failure: A prospective, multicenter, community-based study. Madrid Acute Renal Failure Study Group. Kidney Int 1996; 50:811–818.)

Risk factors for the development of acute renal failure in common clinical situations

Postoperative (general)	Cardiac Surgery	Critically Ill	Sepsis	Contrast Nephropathy	Nephrotoxic Antibiotics
Cardiac	Female gender	Active cancer	Serum bilirubin	Systolic BP<80 mm Hg	Amphotericin
Hemodynamic instability	Congestive heart failure	Low serum albumin	>1.5 mg mg/dl at	for >1 hr and need for	Volume depletion
Congestive heart failure	LV ejection fraction	A-a gradient*	diagnosis of sepsis	inotropic support or IABP	Concurrent
Aortic cross clamping	<35%		Age	24 hr after procedure	administration of
Major vascular surgery	Preoperative intra-aortic		SCreat >1.3 mg/dl at	Use of IABP pump	other nephrotoxins
Hypertension	balloon pump (IABP)		diagnosis of sepsis	Heart failure (NYHA class	Aminoglycosides
Infection	Chronic obstructive		Elevated CVP>8 cm	3 or 4), history of	Duration of >7 days
Sepsis	pulmonary disease		H_2O under colloid	pulmonary edema, or	Volume depletion
Multiorgan failure	Insulin-requiring diabetes		substitution for	both	Divided-dose regimens
Gastrointestinal	Previous cardiac surgery		hemodynamic	Age >75 yrs	Sepsis
and endocrine	Emergency surgery		instability	Hematocrit <39% for men	Liver disease
Liver cirrhosis	Valve surgery only		Systolic BP <80 mm	or <36% for women	Old age
Biliary surgery	Combination of		Hg for >1 hr	Diabetes mellitus	Pre-existing CKD
Diabetes mellitus	CABG + valve surgery			Volume of contrast >100 ml	
Obstructive jaundice	Other cardiac surgery			SCreat >1.5 mg/dl or	
Renal	Preoperative			eGFR <60 ml/min/1.73m²	
Transplantation	SCreat >2.1 mg/dl				
Oliguria <400 ml/day					
SCreat >2 mg/dl					
Miscellaneous					
Age >70 yrs					
Trauma					
Massive blood transfusion					

Figure 64.3 Risk factors for the development of acute renal failure (ARF) in common clinical situations. *A-a gradient: alveolar-arterial oxygen gradient calculated using the sea level standard formula $[(713 \times (FiO_2) - (PCO_2/0.8) - PaO_2]$ where FiO_2 is the fractional inspired oxygen concentration, PaO_2 is the arterial partial oxygen pressure, PCO_2 is the partial CO_2 pressure. The normal A-a gradient varies with age and ranges from 7 to 14 mm Hg when breathing room air. BP, blood pressure; CABG, coronary artery bypass graft; CKD, chronic kidney disease; CVP, central venous pressure; eGFR, estimated glomerular filtration rate; LV, left ventricular; NYHA, New York Heart Association; SCreat, serum creatine.

hospitalized patient populations, those with ARF are characterized by older age, male gender, much higher frequency of comorbidities, diagnostic and therapeutic interventions, and nonrenal organ dysfunction. In addition, human immunodeficiency virus (HIV) and related treatment as well as more frequent nonrenal organ transplantations contribute to the changing spectrum. Figure 64.3 summarizes the most important common and specific risk factors for the development of ARF in six common clinical conditions.

Patient Age

The percentage of ARF patients older than 80 years of age in one unit in Paris increased to about 40% in 1995 to 1996, while in the United States, average ARF rates during a 10-year study period were 19 and 29 cases per 1000 discharges for the age groups younger than 64 and older than 85 years, respectively.[12]

Pre-existent Chronic Kidney Disease

Patients with underlying chronic kidney disease (CKD) were approximately three times more likely to develop hospital-acquired ARF than patients with normal renal function. Underlying CKD is a particular risk factor for perioperative and nephrotoxic, especially radiocontrast-induced ARF.[13]

Irreversible Acute Renal Failure

Mainly due to the older age and pre-existent CKD (Fig. 64.4), there is a growing frequency of irreversible ARF, defined as need for RRT for >3 months. Many of these patients become permanently dialysis dependent. However, not only elderly patients but also children with ARF have a significant risk of residual renal injury, end-stage renal disease, and mortality, irrespective of the ARF cause.[14] In particular, those with primary renal/urologic conditions leading to ARF had lower renal survival rate than others (69% versus 96% after 3 to 5 years).

Postoperative Acute Renal Failure

Postoperative ARF continues to be a major cause of ARF, particularly after complicated surgeries such as cardiothoracic, aortic, or liver and cardiac transplantation accounting for 14% of all episodes of hospital-acquired ARF occurring in 1996.[7] A recent series described ARF occurring in 3.4% of patients undergoing cardiac surgery with cardiopulmonary bypass, with 1.9% of them requiring RRT. Sex, age, emergency surgery, low ejection fraction, need for intra-aortic balloon pumping, repetitive surgery, diabetes, mitral valve surgery, cardiopulmonary bypass duration, and preoperative CKD were

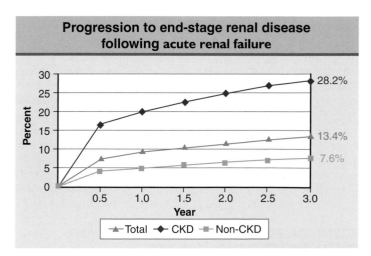

Figure 64.4 Progression to end-stage renal disease (ESRD) after acute renal failure depending on chronic kidney disease (CKD) status at onset of acute renal failure. "CKD" refers to patients who developed ARF following a diagnosis code of any CKD. (Courtesy of P. Eggers, presented at the 2004 American Society of Nephrology Congress).

independently associated with ARF.[15] In aortic aneurysm surgery, ARF occurs in ~5% of elective cases and ~25% of emergent cases.

Hematologic and Oncologic Diseases

ARF can result directly from these diseases and, when RRT is required, is associated with a poor prognosis. ARF in patients with acute leukemia and treated with chemotherapy is observed in ~30%. ARF frequencies in patients receiving a hematopoietic progenitor cell transplant range from a low of 6.5% in some hematopoietic progenitor cell transplant series using an autologous transplant to a mean of 26% to 64% in most series and to an extreme of 81% with allogenic transplantation.[16]

Solid Organ Transplantation and Acute Renal Failure

The frequency of delayed graft function (DGF) of kidneys from cadaveric donors varies from 2% to 50% between countries.[11] These large differences in reported DGF mainly may be due to differences in logistical and allocation strategies since DGF increases rapidly when cold ischemia time is >24 hours. In orthotopic liver transplantations, the incidence of RRT requiring ARF increased from 8% between 1985 and 1995 to 12% between the years 1996 and 1999, along with increased median waiting times. In heart transplantations, this incidence was 4.5%. In both latter situations, perioperative ARF is associated with increased mortality and morbidity.[11]

Infection-Associated Acute Renal Failure

In HIV-infected patients, the risk and causes of ARF have changed in view of improved survival and lower hospitalization rates due to highly active antiretroviral therapy (HAART), a variety of potential nephrotoxic drugs for the treatment of HIV (e.g., tenofovir, indanavir), co-infections (e.g., hepatitis C virus), and comorbidities (e.g., diabetes, hypertension). ARF occurred in nearly 10% of ambulatory HIV patients with an incidence rate of 5.9 episodes of ARF per 100 person-years.[17] Many of these events are community acquired due to prerenal causes or ATN associated with opportunistic infections and drugs.

ARF also complicates *Plasmodium falciparum* malaria infection. Nonimmune Europeans are more frequently (25% to 30%) affected than native patients (1% to 4.8%) in endemic areas. In India, 6% of patients with ARF presented with malaria (*P. falciparum* or *P. vivax*) between 1990 and 1999; 80% of them required RRT. Imported malaria in nontropical countries may be complicated by ARF in 31% of patients.

Toxin- and Drug-Induced Acute Renal Failure

Despite the widespread appreciation of the role of nephrotoxins and drugs in ARF (see Chapter 63, Fig. 63.6), in a recent series they were still causally implicated in about 25% of cases of ARF, little different from incidences reported 17 years ago.[7] Radiocontrast nephropathy is still one of the most frequent causes of hospital-acquired ARF and ranges between 1% and 45%, depending largely on the comorbidities of the study population and the parameters that are used to define it. Heme pigment nephropathy (caused by myoglobin or hemoglobin) has been implicated in 10% to 15% of hospitalized patients with ARF in the United States.

CLINICAL EVALUATION OF THE PATIENT WITH ACUTE RENAL FAILURE

The clinical evaluation of ARF should aim to answer the following five questions:

1. Is the renal failure acute, acute-on-chronic, or chronic?
2. Is there evidence of true hypovolemia or reduced effective arterial blood volume, that is, prerenal ARF?
3. Has there been a major vascular occlusion?
4. Is there evidence of parenchymal renal disease other than ATN?
5. Is there renal tract obstruction, that is, postrenal ARF?

An algorithm summarizing the approach to a patient with presumed ARF is provided in Figure 64.5. This approach will reveal the likely cause of ARF in most patients. This enables the clinician to develop a rational therapeutic plan that will facilitate the rapid restoration of renal function in patients with pre- or postrenal ARF and will provide a logical basis for the treatment of patients with intrinsic parenchymal renal diseases.

Acute versus Chronic Renal Failure

A semilogarithmic plot, or even a simple flow sheet, of remote and recent serum creatinine values versus time and incorporating changes in drug therapy and other interventions (e.g., radiocontrast investigations) is invaluable for differentiation of ARF and chronic renal failure and the identification of the cause of ARF. When previous measurements of serum creatinine are not available, the findings of anemia, hyperphosphatemia, hypocalcemia, hyperparathyroidism, neuropathy, band keratopathy on presentation, and radiographic evidence of renal osteodystrophy or small scarred kidneys are useful pointers to a chronic process. However, it should be noted that anemia, hyperphosphatemia, and hypocalcemia, if prolonged, may also complicate ARF, and renal size can be normal or increased in a variety of chronic renal diseases (e.g., diabetic nephropathy, amyloidosis, polycystic kidney disease). Once a diagnosis of ARF is established, the patient's history, physical findings, laboratory tests, and imaging procedures usually answer the remainder of the preceding questions and identify a specific etiology of ARF.

History and Record Review

The medical history should include previous urea, creatinine and electrolyte results, health checks, systemic conditions (e.g., diabetes, hypertension, ischemic heart or peripheral artery disease, jaundice), urinary symptoms (pyelonephritis, urinary tract infection), recent procedures (surgery, angiography, other radiographic procedures), known infections (e.g., HIV, hepatitis), and known immunosuppressive therapy (transplant recipients, patients with malignancies). Drug history should include over-the-counter formulations and herbal remedies or recreational drugs. The social history should include foreign travel (malaria, schistosomiasis), exposure to waterways or sewage systems (leptospirosis), and exposure to rodents (Hantavirus).

With respect to the setting in which ARF has developed, community-acquired ARF can usually be attributed to a single cause, whereas ARF acquired on a hospital ward mostly occurs in the setting of comorbidity and is often multifactorial. ARF acquired in the ICU is almost always multifactorial and associated with sepsis and multiorgan failure. Unique causes of ARF can be seen in the setting of malignancy, HIV infection, pregnancy, and the postoperative state (see Chapter 63). Patients with liver disease are susceptible to prerenal and intrarenal ARF as well as the hepatorenal syndrome (see Chapter 67).

The clinical history with regard to events associated with intravascular volume loss or volume sequestration and impaired cardiac function is important in determining the cause of ARF. A history of thirst, orthostatic lightheadedness or hypotension, and symptoms of congestive heart failure support a prerenal etiology of ARF.

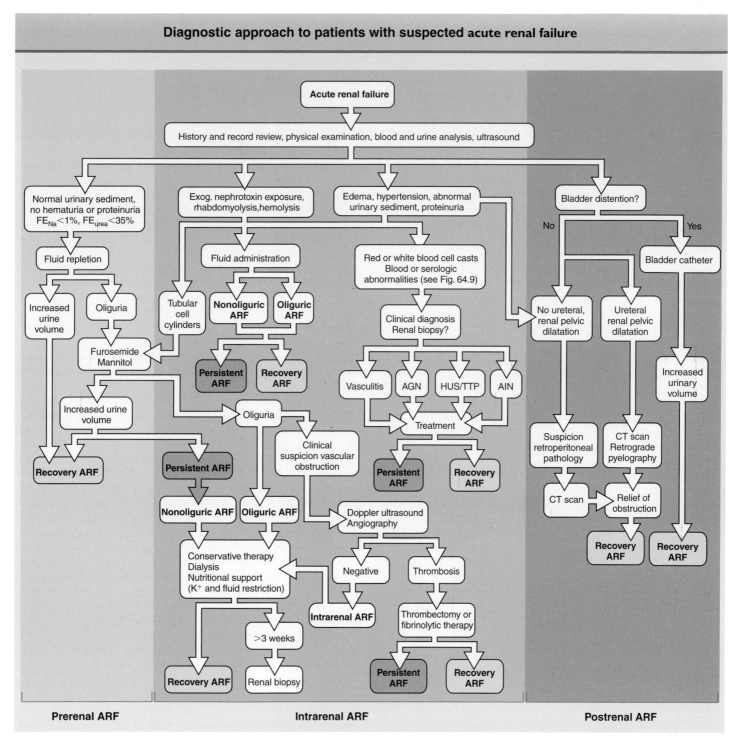

Figure 64.5 Algorithm for the diagnostic approach to patients with suspected acute renal failure (ARF). AGN, acute glomerulonephritis; AIN, acute interstitial nephritis; CT, computed tomography; Exog., exogenous; HUS/TTP, hemolytic uremic syndrome/thrombotic thrombocytopenic purpura.

A history of factors that predispose to vascular disease or pre-existent cardiovascular morbidity, arterial catheterization involving the aorta, and atrial fibrillation are compatible with vascular embolic events leading to ARF. A history of systemic infection or the presence of systemic symptoms may support a glomerular cause of ARF. Medication exposure or a history of acute pyelonephritis may point to acute interstitial nephritis as the cause of ARF. The presence of disorders associated with either rhabdomyolysis or intravascular hemolysis suggests the possibility of heme pigment nephropathy (see Chapter 63).

Postrenal causes of ARF are common at the extremes of age, with a history of changes in the size and force of urine stream; the presence of bladder, prostate, or pelvic cancer; the use of anti-cholinergic and α-adrenergic medications; the presence of anuria, suprapubic pain, or urolithiasis; or exposure to medications known to cause hyperuricemia or crystalluria. Patients with either a single kidney or a significant baseline decrease in the function of one kidney should make the clinician even more concerned about the possibility of postrenal ARF because a single lesion may obstruct the normal kidney. In this case, anuria is frequent.

Physical Examination

Assessing the volume status of patients with ARF is critical but sometimes difficult (Fig. 64.6). Orthostatic tachycardia and hypotension have diagnostic value in detecting hypovolemia. Decreased skin turgor or impaired capillary refill time have limited sensitivity and specificity. Assessment of the jugular venous pressure (JVP) with the patient reclining at 45 degrees is mandatory. The normal JVP is between 0 and 3 cm above the sternal angle, which corresponds to a right atrial pressure of ~8 cm of water. If the JVP is difficult to visualize, gentle pressure over the liver to increase venous return can be helpful (the hepatojugular reflux). Recording the patient's daily body weight in conjunction with fluid balance charts and clinical examination can aid to estimate the evolution of the fluid balance. Although clinical assessment provides a satisfactory index of cardiac output and tissue perfusion in most patients, invasive hemodynamic monitoring (central venous and/or Swan-Ganz catheterization) is often necessary in critically ill patients.

Ophthalmic examination may reveal plaques suggestive of atheroemboli (Hollenhorst plaques, i.e., intraluminal retinal cholesterol/fibrin deposits) or findings compatible with bacterial endocarditis, vasculitis, or malignant hypertension. Neck examination for jugular venous pressure and carotid pulses and sounds may be helpful in detecting heart failure, aortic valve disease, or vascular disease. Cardiovascular examination for rate, rhythm, murmurs, gallops, and rubs may be helpful in detecting the presence of heart failure and possible sources of emboli. Lung examination can assist in determining the presence of either heart failure or a pulmonary-renal syndrome associated with ARF. Abdominal examination can reveal findings compatible with vascular disease (e.g., bruits, palpable abdominal aortic aneurysm), masses that could be malignant, a distended bladder, possible sources of bacteremia, or evidence of liver disease. Examination of the extremities for symmetry and strength of pulses and edema can be helpful. Skin examination may reveal palpable purpura (vasculitis), a fine maculopapular rash (drug-induced interstitial nephritis), livedo recticularis, purple toes, and other embolic stigmata (atheroemboli). If neurologic signs are present, systemic disorders such as vasculitis, thrombotic microangiopathy, subacute bacterial endocarditis, and malignant hypertension warrant consideration. Peripheral neuropathy in the presence of ARF raises the possibility of nerve compression caused by rhabdomyolysis,

heavy metal intoxication, or plasma cell dyscrasia. Pelvic examination in females and rectal examination in both females and males may detect an obstructive cause of ARF.

Laboratory Tests
Urine Volume

Urine volume in ARF can vary from oliguria (i.e., <500 ml/24 hr or <20 ml/hr) to anuria (i.e., <100 ml/24 hr) to extreme polyuria. In most patients with ARF in the ICU, an indwelling urinary catheter allows accurate measurement of hourly urine output, a parameter useful in monitoring the initial response to fluid resuscitation until the intravascular fluid volume of the patient is adequately restored. Once this state is reached, hourly urine volumes are less useful in guiding management and increased urine flow should not be regarded as a primary treatment goal. Once patients are established to be oligoanuric, the urinary catheter should be removed to reduce the risk of infection. Severe ARF can exist despite normal urine output (i.e., nonoliguria), but changes in urine output can occur long before biochemical changes are apparent. Nonoliguric ARF is more common than oliguric ARF, particularly in ICU patients, because of the more frequent monitoring via daily serum creatinine changes and/or earlier intervention with fluid loading and diuretics. The spontaneous nonoliguric forms usually have a better prognosis compared to the oliguric forms. This may well relate to a less severe renal insult or a higher incidence of nephrotoxin-induced ARF in the nonoliguric group.

Anuria is seen with cessation of glomerular filtration (e.g., rapidly progressive glomerulonephritis, acute cortical necrosis, total renal arterial or venous occlusion) or complete urinary tract obstruction. Brief (<24 to 48 hours) episodes of oligoanuria occur in some cases of ATN. Prerenal forms of ARF nearly always present with oliguria, although nonoliguric forms have been reported. Postrenal and renal forms of ARF can present with any pattern of urine flow. The presence of alternating anuria and polyuria is an uncommon but classic manifestation of urinary tract obstruction, for example, due to a stone that changes its position. In rare cases, unilateral obstruction can lead to anuria and ARF; vascular or ureteral spasm, mediated by autonomic activation, is thought to be responsible for the loss of function in the nonobstructed kidney.

Urine Dipstick and Microscopic Examination

Routine dipstick and microscopic analysis of urine (see also Chapter 4) are often helpful in determining the cause of ARF. Generally, a normal urinalysis in the setting of ARF suggests a pre- or postrenal cause and an abnormal urinalysis a renal cause. However, patients with prerenal ARF can have a significant number of casts (due to the precipitation of Tamm-Horsfall protein in concentrated, acidic urine) and cellular elements in their urine in addition to small urine volumes, high specific gravity, and acidic urine.

Urinary protein measurement by dipstick is specific for albumin. Small amounts of protein found by dipstick, with larger amounts found by laboratory urinary protein tests (such as sulfosalicylic acid) suggest the presence of light chains (see Chapter 4). If the dipstick reaction for protein is moderately or strongly positive in the setting of ARF, quantification is indicated. The presence of >1 to 2 g/day of urine protein suggests a glomerular cause of ARF.

Examination of the urine sediment is of great value in ARF (Figs. 64.7 and 64.8). Gross or microscopic hematuria suggests a glomerular, vascular, interstitial, or other structural renal cause (e.g., stone, tumor, infection, trauma) of ARF and is rarely seen with ATN (see also Chapter 56). Red blood cell casts in the urine

Clinical evaluation of volume status		
	Intravascular Volume Depletion	Volume Overload (CHF)
History and chart review	Thirst, dry mucosae, oliguria Excessive fluid losses Fluid balance (intake/output, daily body weight)	Ankle swelling, weight gain Orthopnea, paroxysmal nocturnal dyspnea
Physical examination	Reduced skin turgor Dry mucosae, absent axillary sweat Reduced jugular venous pressure Postural tachyardia or hypotension Supine tachycardia or hypotension	Pitting edema Jugular venous distention Third heart sound Pulmonary crackles Pleural effusion

Figure 64.6 Clinical evaluation of volume status. CHF, congestive heart failure.

sediment strongly suggest a glomerular or vascular cause of ARF but have also been observed with acute interstitial nephritis. Studies of the urinary red blood cell morphology in ARF of different causes are lacking. Lack of urinary red cells despite a positive dipstick reaction for blood is typical of ARF induced by myoglobinuria or hemoglobinuria.

Large numbers of white blood cells (WBCs) and in particular of leukocyte casts on urinalysis suggest either pyelonephritis or interstitial nephritis. Eosinophiluria (>1% urine WBCs) is nonspecific. However, this finding is diagnostically valuable when ARF occurs in a setting compatible with either allergic interstitial nephritis (drug exposure, fever, rash, peripheral eosinophiluria) or cholesterol embolism.

Collecting duct cells and total casts in urine detected by cytodiagnostic quantitative assessment are increased in ARF but lack sufficient sensitivity, specificity, and predictive power for routine clinical use.

Crystals in the urine sediment should be assessed using fresh warm urine, polarizing microscopy, knowledge of the urine pH, and an experienced microscopist (see Chapter 4). A large number

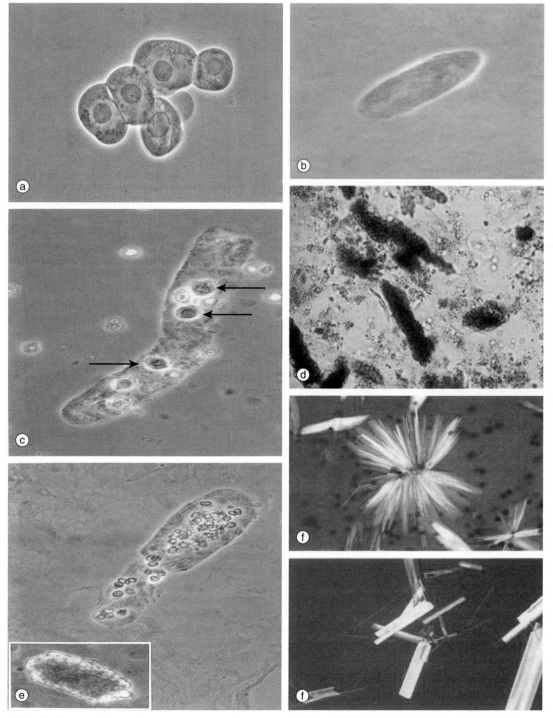

Figure 64.7 Examples of urinary sediments in common cases of acute renal failure (ARF). *a*, Epithelial cell aggregate. *b*, Hyaline cast as can be seen in prerenal ARF. *c*, Epithelial cast as can be seen in early acute tubular necrosis (ATN; *arrows* indicate epithelial cells.). *d*, Muddy brown cast, typical for established ATN. *e*, Erythrocyte cast as seen in glomerulonephritis and vasculitis. *Inset*: Hemoglobin cast. *f*, Two forms of indinavir crystals.

Blood and serum findings pointing to specific causes of acute renal failure	
Laboratory Finding	Cause of ARF
Anemia	Pre-existent chronic renal failure, hemorrhage, hemolysis
Anemia with rouleaux formation	Plasma cell dyscrasia
Eosinophilia	Atheroemboli, acute interstitial nephritis, or polyarteritis nodosa
Leukopenia	SLE (see Chapter 24)
Thrombocytopenia	SLE, Hantavirus infection, DIC, rhabdomyolysis, advanced liver disease with hypersplenism, heparin-induced thrombocytopenia (HIT) syndrome
Thrombocytopenia, reticulocytosis, elevated LDH, schistocytes on peripheral smear	Thrombotic microangiopathy (see Chapter 28)
Coagulopathy	Liver disease, DIC, antiphospholipid antibody syndrome
Hyperkalemia >5.5 mmol/l	Various causes, tumor lysis syndrome, hemolysis, use of NSAIDs, ACE inhibitors or ARB
Marked hyperkalemia, hyperphosphatemia, hypocalcemia, elevated serum uric acid and CK, AST, and LDH	Rhabdomyolysis (crush syndrome, heat stroke, seizures, immobilization, influenza, etc.)
Marked hyperkalemia, hyperphosphatemia, hypocalcemia, very high serum uric acid, normal or marginally elevated CK	Acute uric acid nephropathy, tumor lysis syndrome
Hypercalcemia	Malignancy, sarcoidosis, vitamin D intoxication, etc. (see Chapter 10)
Widening of serum anion and osmolal gap*	Ethylene glycol or methanol intoxication
Marked acidosis, anion gap* >5–10 mmol/l	Ethylene glycol poisoning, rhabdomyolysis, lactic acidosis from sepsis (see Chapter 12)
Hypergammaglobulinemia	SLE, bacterial endocarditis, and other chronic infections
Paraprotein (M-gradient), hypergammaglobulinemia	Myeloma (see Chapter 26)
Urine electrophoresis showing free light chains	Myeloma, low-grade plasma cell dyscrasias (even in the absence of serum abnormalities)
Elevated serum IgA	IgA nephropathy (see Chapter 21)
Elevated antinuclear antibodies	Autoimmune diseases including SLE, scleroderma, mixed connective tissue disease, Sjögren's syndrome etc.
Elevated anti–double-strand DNA antibodies	SLE
Elevated anti-C1q antibodies	SLE, MPGN, some cases of IgA nephropathy
Elevated ANCA titer	Wegener's granulomatosis, microscopic polyangiitis
Antiglomerular basement membrane antibodies	Anti-GBM nephritis, Goodpasture's syndrome (see Chapter 22)
Cryoglobulins	Hepatitis C, lymphoproliferative disorder (see Chapter 20)

Figure 64.12 Blood and serum findings pointing to specific causes of ARF. ACE, angiotensin-converting enzyme; ARB, angiotensin receptor blocker; AST, asparagine aminotransferase; CK, creatinine kinase; DIC, disseminated intravascular coagulation; GBM, glomerular basement membrane; LDH, lactate dehydrogenase; MPGN, membranoproliferative glomerulonephritis; NSAIDs, nonsteroidal anti-inflammatory drugs; SLE, systemic lupus erythematosus. *Mild metabolic acidosis occurs frequently as a consequence of ARF and is often associated with a modest (5 to 10 mEq/l) increase in the anion gap.

fibrosis, encased the retroperitoneal ureters and renal pelvis, preventing their dilatation. In the elderly, partial obstruction may be obscured by volume depletion. When there is a strong suspicion of obstruction, the ultrasonographic examination should be repeated after volume repletion.

Increased ultrasonographic renal size without hydronephrosis may occur with acute glomerulonephritis, with infiltration by amyloid or malignancy, in diabetes, and in renal vein thrombosis. The finding of reduced renal size and increased echogenicity points to chronic renal failure. Even if the kidneys are reduced in size, the possibility of prerenal ARF or acute-on-chronic renal failure must always be considered.

Ultrasound contrast media can improve the diagnostic capabilities in ARF by allowing the visualization of altered renal blood flow (RBF) and renal perfusion defects.

Doppler Ultrasonography

Doppler studies have been suggested to differentiate prerenal cause from renal cause ARF. Partly as a result of intrarenal

Value of renal ultrasonography in differential diagnosis of acute renal failure	
Observation	Clue to Diagnosis Of
Shrunken kidneys	Chronic intrinsic renal disease
Normal-sized kidneys Echogenic	Acute glomerulonephritis, acute tubular necrosis
Normal echo pattern	Prerenal acute renal failure, acute renal artery occlusion
Enlarged kidneys	Malignant infiltration, renal vein thrombosis, amyloid, human immunodeficiency virus (HIV)–associated nephropathy
Pelvicalyceal dilatation*	Obstructive nephropathy

Figure 64.13 Value of renal ultrasonography in differential diagnosis of acute renal failure. *Pelvicalyceal dilatation is usual but not universal in presence of obstruction.

vasoconstriction, ATN usually produces a reduction in RBF. Increases of the resistance index (RI; see Chapter 5) to >0.75 have been described in 91% of kidneys with ATN, compared with <0.75 in kidneys with acute prerenal failure. However, the RI results overlap between these two major causes and high RIs are also observed in acute obstruction, which markedly reduces its usefulness to obtain a specific diagnosis.

Other Radiographic Investigations

Intravenous urography nowadays is largely abandoned in patients with ARF, particularly given the need for potentially nephrotoxic radiocontrast agents.

A plain radiograph of the abdomen (sometimes called KUB [kidney, ureter, and bladder]) is a mandatory investigation in any patient in whom an obstructive cause of ARF is suspected since it can detect even small radio-opaque stones and ureteral stones not found by ultrasonography.

The presence and site of obstruction are accurately diagnosed by antegrade or retrograde pyelography (see Chapter 5). If obstruction is present, a ureteral stent or percutaneous nephrostomy can be placed in the same session.

A computed tomography (CT) scan performed without contrast is of comparable diagnostic value to the renal ultrasonography but more costly and less convenient. However, CT is superior in the evaluation of ureteral obstruction since it can delineate the level of obstruction and define retroperitoneal inflammatory tissue (in retroperitoneal fibrosis) or a retroperitoneal malignant mass.

Magnetic resonance imaging (MRI) is not usually used for evaluation of ARF, but if imaging is necessary, it should be preferred to contrast-enhanced CT and other radiocontrast-requiring radiographic techniques. An altered corticomedullary relationship is frequently recognized in patients with ARF but also in other acute renal diseases on T-weighted images. When postrenal ARF is suspected, MRI is valuable in assessing hydronephrosis and detecting the cause and site of obstruction. MR angiography can be useful for detecting abnormalities in the renal artery and vein. The diagnosis of acute renal cortical necrosis, in particular, becomes more reliable with gadolinium-enhanced MRI (Fig. 64.14). The rim sign is characteristic for this infrequent cause of ARF.

Renal angiography can be indicated when renal artery occlusion (by embolization, thrombosis, or a dissecting aneurysm) is suspected based on the clinical history (e.g., in a patient with atrial fibrillation and acute flank pain) or on duplex scanning, to confirm the exact anatomy of the occlusion and to assess the

potential for intervention. However, in this setting, MR angiography or helical CT is superior. Hepatic or renal angiography may also be useful in diagnosing classic polyarteritis nodosa.

Doppler ultrasonography, MRI, MR angiography, and CT are used frequently in the evaluation of thromboembolic disease and acute cortical necrosis, and have also largely replaced renal venography to confirm a clinical suspicion of renal vein thrombosis (see Chapter 5). When a diagnosis of acute renal artery occlusion is considered, renal angiography should be obtained urgently, as early surgical or thrombolytic therapy may be necessary to salvage the kidney. However, where the complete occlusion occurs in a background of chronic occlusive disease, sufficient collateral blood supply may be provided and even delayed intervention can result in recovery of renal function.

Renal Biopsy

Renal biopsy is reserved for patients in whom prerenal and postrenal failure have been excluded and the cause of intrinsic renal ARF is unclear. Renal biopsy is particularly useful when clinical assessment, urinalysis, and laboratory investigation suggest diagnoses other than ischemic or nephrotoxic injury that may respond to specific therapy, for example, rapidly progressive glomerulonephritis (see Chapters 22 and 23), and allergic interstitial nephritis (see Chapter 57). Renal biopsy should also be considered in ARF when there are symptoms or signs of a systemic illness, such as persistent fever or unexplained anemia. Unexpected causes of ARF, such as myeloma, interstitial nephritis, endocarditis (associated glomerular disease), and cryoglobulinemia, may be revealed by renal biopsy in these situations. In patients diagnosed with ATN and normal-sized kidneys who do not recover renal function after 3 to 4 weeks, a renal biopsy may be indicated to confirm the cause of ARF, exclude other treatable causes, and determine the prognosis. Finally, renal biopsy is a routine diagnostic procedure in patients with ARF after transplantation when it is often essential for distinguishing between ischemic ATN, acute rejection, and calcineurin inhibitor toxicity.

PREVENTION OF ACUTE RENAL FAILURE[22]

General Measures

Until recently, the evolution of ATN was divided somewhat arbitrarily into an initiation, maintenance, and recovery phase. Given the important role of the outer medullary ischemia and of endothelium-leukocyte interactions, a fourth extension phase has been described that connects the initiation and maintenance phases.[23] It has been suggested that most of the preventive interventions in human ATN should be active during this extension phase.

In any critically ill patient, appropriate intensive care and stabilization of the general hemodynamics with optimization of the cardiac output and blood pressure can prevent ARF. Potential causes of acute prerenal failure should be avoided, and careful attention should always be given to the volume status of the patient, which is one of the key interventions with proven benefit for patients prone to ARF or with established ARF.

Figure 64.15 summarizes the most important potential clinical strategies that have been proposed to prevent ARF in general and more specifically in surgery (Fig. 64.16). In sepsis, few interventions have led to a reduction in total mortality and none has reduced the incidence of septic ARF, except administration of activated protein C. However, early fluid resuscitation of critically ill patients with sepsis, initiated already in the emergency department, may reduce not only the mortality but also renal failure in these patients.

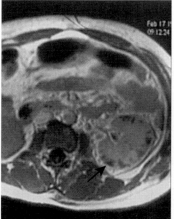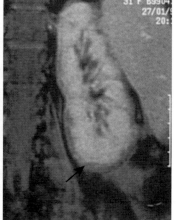

Figure 64.14 **Magnetic resonance image of cortex necrosis (gadolinium contrast).** Irregularly shaped hypointense areas (*arrows*) are present in the renal cortes.

Strategies to decrease acute renal failure

Proven Efficacy

Avoidance of nephrotoxins
Single daily dosing of aminoglycosides
Drug modifications
    Liposomal amphotericin
    Nonionic, low or iso-osmolar radiocontrast agents
Hydration
    Radiocontrast
    Cisplatin
    Rhabdomyolysis
    Tumor lysis syndrome
Activated protein C in sepsis

Possibly Effective

Monitoring drug levels
Adequate renal perfusion
Low-dose fenoldopam
N-acetylcysteine (in contrast nephropathy)
Atrial and B natriuretic peptides
Alkalinization of the urine
    Rhabdomyolysis
    Methotrexate
    Tumor lysis syndrome
Mannitol (in kidney transplantation, aorta surgery, rhabdomyolysis)
Tight glycemia control in the critically ill

Ineffective

Low-dose dopamine
Loop diuretics (furosemide, bumetanide, torasemide)
Aminophylline

Figure 64.15 Strategies to decrease acute renal failure.

Adverse effects of hyperglycemia have been described in critically ill postsurgical patients, and a controlled trial showed a reduction in ARF incidence and mortality with strict control of blood glucose concentration.[24] However, a follow-up study in patients in a medical ICU showed that intensive insulin therapy reduced blood glucose levels but did not significantly reduce

Measures for minimizing surgical acute renal failure

Optimizing volume status with correction of hypovolemia by appropriate fluid administration guided by CVP line, aiming for a CVP > 10 cm of water and a urine output of >40 ml/min

Pulmonary catheter monitoring in high-risk patients, such as those undergoing cardiac surgery or those with impaired cardiac function; aim for a PCWP 10–12 mm Hg or higher depending on cardiac function and response to fluid challenge

Mean arterial pressure >80 mm Hg, achieved and maintained by adequate volume replacement with or without inotropic support

Strategies to reduce the incidence of nosocomial infections, such as the conservative use and rapid removal of intravascular and bladder catheters

Cautious use of antibiotics

Sepsis needs to be aggressively investigated and treated

Restricted use and, where possible, total avoidance of potentially nephrotoxic agents

Figure 64.16 Measures for minimizing surgical acute renal failure. CVP, central venous pressure; PCWP, pulmonary capillary wedge pressure.

in-hospital mortality in patients who stayed in the ICU for <3 days, By contrast, in patients who stayed in the ICU for ≥3 days and received intensive insulin therapy, in-hospital mortality was significantly reduced, in part by the prevention of newly acquired kidney injury.[25]

Prevention of ARF also includes the avoidance of risk factors such as nephrotoxic drugs or agents (e.g., by replacing hyperosmolar with iso-osmolar radiocontrast agents in patients at risk of contrast-induced nephropathy; see Chapter 5), stopping particular drugs in high-risk situations (e.g., nonsteroidal anti-inflammatory drugs and/or ACE inhibitors or angiotensin receptor blockers prior to surgery) and the guidance of drug dosing based on plasma concentrations (e.g., aminoglycoside antibiotics, calcineurin inhibitors). In the case of amphotericin B, the use of lipid formulations and changes in the rate of drug infusion may prevent renal dysfunction.

Allopurinol and the recently introduced rasburicase, a recombinant urate oxidase preparation, decrease levels of uric acid in patients with leukemia and lymphoma who are prone to uric acid nephropathy and tumor lysis syndrome.[16]

Volume Expansion

Both animal and human studies suggest that intravascular fluid expansion decreases the risk of ARF from radiocontrast agents and various nephrotoxic insults, from surgery of the aorta or of obstructive jaundice, and following renal transplantation.[22] However, what role it plays in preventing ARF in patients in the ICU with multiple risk factors who may also have capillary leak syndrome and impaired pulmonary function is speculative.

The superiority of colloid over crystalloid fluids in the resuscitation of critically ill patients is controversial and the recent Saline versus Albumin Fluid Evaluation (SAFE) trial found that fluid resuscitation with saline or albumin gave similar results in critically ill patients. In randomized trials of trauma or postoperative patients with sepsis or patients after cardiac surgery, mortality and ARF incidences were similar in patients resuscitated with hydroxyethyl starch or albumin, and since hydroxyethyl starch is cheaper than albumin, this should at present be the preferred fluid when colloids are required.

In the prevention of radiocontrast medium–associated nephropathy, lower risk patients should increase oral fluid intake and high-risk patients should receive intravenous hydration. In the latter, it has been found that hydration with isotonic saline starting on the morning of the procedure or immediately before in cases of emergency intervention is superior to the routinely recommended half-isotonic saline. It was also reported that hydration with isotonic sodium bicarbonate (154 mmol/l NaHCO$_3$ in 5% dextrose at 3 ml/kg/hr for 6 hours starting 1 hour preprocedure) is more effective than hydration with isotonic NaCl for prophylaxis of ARF. The initial infusion was followed by the same fluid at a rate of 1 ml/kg/h during the contrast exposure and for 6 hours after the procedure.

In the prevention of myoglobin-induced nephropathy following crush syndrome, intravenous hydration should be initiated before the crush is relieved to prevent precipitation of the pigment in the tubular lumen. As much as 1 to 1.5 L of 0.9% saline can be given within the first hour; within the first 24 hours, up to 10 liters or more of total intravenous fluid may be given in monitored patients in whom there is adequate urine output, aiming for a urine volume of 300 ml/hr. Alkalinization of the urine (achieving a urinary pH >6.5) may also reduce the risk of pigment nephropathy. When the urine output is sufficient to prevent bicarbonate and mannitol accumulation in serum, one commonly used regimen for coadministering them uses isotonic fluid prepared by adding sodium bicarbonate (100 ml of 100 mmol/l $NaHCO_3$) and mannitol (100 ml of 25% mannitol) to 800 ml of 5% dextrose. One liter of this solution can be infused over 4 hours. Care must be taken to avoid a $NaHCO_3$-induced decrease in ionized calcium (due to metabolic alkalosis), which can trigger seizures, worsening already existent muscle damage. An alkaline diuresis is ineffective if the patient already has established ARF and accumulation of mannitol in this setting may actually exacerbate renal injury. Swelling of injured muscle may produce a compartment syndrome with impaired local tissue perfusion. Urgent fasciotomy may be required when intracompartment pressures exceed 40 mm Hg.

A difficult problem may arise in the ICU patient with decreased renal perfusion resulting from cardiac failure. Vigorous fluid challenge may result in pulmonary edema. Likewise in septic patients, volume restitution, even under Swan-Ganz monitoring, may result in fluid redistribution, with preferential sequestration into a third-space compartment (i.e., into the bowel lumen, abdominal cavity, pleural space). Intervention with early ultrafiltration or dialysis to rescue the patient should fluids be pushed too far is necessary to avoid the major risk factor of volume overload in these patients (the so-called renal support concept). The primary therapeutic approach with ultrafiltration, if needed, is here to prevent or cure pulmonary edema.

Pharmacologic Approaches

A variety of drugs are effective in altering the course of experimental models of ATN. However, only a few have consistently been shown to be of benefit in clinical ATN (see Fig. 64.15).

Vasopressors

Vasopressors and inotropes are generally used to improve vascular tone and cardiac output, respectively, when volume expansion alone is not able to restore adequate hemodynamic function or during fluid resuscitation in the setting of life-threatening hypotension.

Norepinephrine reduces RBF in healthy animals and humans, but its ultimate effect on renal perfusion depends on a complex interplay of its actions on different vascular beds and the underlying condition of the patient. The net effect on renal vascular resistance hinges on the increase in systemic blood pressure with a decreased renal sympathetic tone through a baroreceptor response, resulting in vasodilatation; an autoregulatory vasoconstriction resulting from an increase in renal perfusion pressure; and a direct α_1-mediated renal vasoconstriction. It was mainly in noncontrolled studies in sepsis that norepinephrine infusion was associated with an augmented urine output and GFR.

Dobutamine has no effect on the kidney and primarily acts on the heart, where it stimulates β_1 receptors. It also stimulates β_2 vascular receptors, provoking a peripheral vasodilation. The major beneficial effects of dobutamine in ARF are thus the result of an increase in cardiac output and consequently an augmentation of RBF. In stable, critically ill patients, it improved creatinine clearance without a significant change in urine output.

Dopexamine, a synthetic dopamine analogue, is a dopamine 1 and less potent dopamine 2 receptor agonist. It is also a β-agonist, primarily at β_2-adrenoreceptors, and it inhibits neuronal reuptake of norepinephrine. Studies performed in critically ill or in patients undergoing surgery have revealed contradictory results.

In view of the recognition of relative vasopressin deficiency, enhanced arteriolar sensitivity to vasopressin (despite reduced sensitivity to norepinephrine) after endotoxin exposure, and the potent vasopressor effect of arginine vasopressin, vasopressin infusions should be considered in refractory shock in doses of 0.01 to 0.04 U/min.[10]

The long-acting vasopressin analogue terlipressin may also increase mean arterial pressure despite lower norepinephrine doses and increase urine output and creatinine clearance.

Therefore, vasopressors can be used safely to restore blood pressure without compromising renal function, particularly in patients with distributive shock. At present, norepinephrine is preferable to dopamine, and in patients refractory to norepinephrine, early use of arginine vasopressin is recommended.

Renal Vasodilating Agents

Dopamine, when infused in so-called renal doses, is a renal vasodilator and increases sodium excretion in normal individuals. Low-dose dopamine (1 to 2 μg kg^{-1}·min^{-1} intravenously) has frequently been used alone or in combination with furosemide, particularly in ICU patients with oliguria. Prospective, controlled trials and a careful meta-analysis have concluded that dopamine does not reduce mortality or promote the recovery of renal function; moreover, potential risks, such as arrhythmias, are associated with low-dose dopamine regimens.

Fenoldopam is a highly selective dopamine type 1 agonist that preferentially dilates the renal and splanchnic vasculature. Fenoldopam mesylate has been tested in some high-risk patients for radiocontrast nephropathy and in patients undergoing aorta surgery or elective repair of a thoracoabdominal aortic aneurysm; it showed reductions in mortality, dialysis requirements, and length of hospital and ICU stay in these patients. However, two recent prospective, randomized trials in septic patients[26] and critically ill patients[27] found no difference in patient survival or the need for RRT.

Atrial natriuretic peptide (ANP) is reported to dilate the glomerular afferent arteriole but to constrict the efferent arteriole and to inhibit almost all vasoconstrictors that affect glomerular blood flow. Despite many controversial results with ANP in the past, a recent large and rigidly controlled clinical trial with a long-term infusion of ANP compared to placebo in patients with established ischemic or nephrotoxic ATN[28] showed a decrease in the incidence of dialysis and an increase in the dialysis-free survivorship in the subgroup of oliguric ARF patients and long-term infusion (>48 hours) of ANP-improved RBF and GFR in patients with acute renal impairment after cardiac surgery. In a randomized, placebo-controlled, double-blind study of 20 patients undergoing upper abdominal surgery, patients who received ANP had increased urinary electrolyte excretion and urine output compared to the control group.[29] This renal vasodilatory effect was maintained during the infusion and seemed to be hemodynamically safe.

B-natriuretic peptide was tested in patients undergoing orthotopic heart transplantation, not responding to inotropes and escalating doses of diuretics, and with elevated filling pressures with a serum creatinine >2.5 mg/dl.[30] B-natriuretic peptide was started 48 hours after transplantation and continued for 48 to 72 hours. Most intravascular hemodynamics improved, and the mean urine output increased significantly in the first 24 hours of therapy with no increase in diuretics and a decrease in serum creatinine was observed.

Several natriuretic peptides have been discovered, including urodilatin, with an equal or even greater natriuretic potency compared to human ANP. However, urodilatin did not improve renal function or reduce the need for RRT in critically ill ARF patients.

At present more data are needed to recommend these vasodilating drugs because, in most of the randomized, placebo-controlled studies, they have been shown to be ineffective.

Diuretics

Assessments of loop diuretics (e.g., furosemide, bumetanide, torasemide) and mannitol in the prevention or reversal of ATN have given inconsistent results. Prophylactic mannitol has been promoted in patients considered to be at high risk of ATN, in particular, those with rhabdomyolysis (see previous discussion) and patients undergoing surgery. While in most of these instances, mannitol increases urine flow, it is highly probable that mannitol does not convey additional beneficial effects beyond adequate hydration on the incidence of ATN. In radiocontrast-induced nephropathy, loop diuretics and mannitol in one study were shown to exacerbate ARF. More convincing are the results obtained with the preventive administration of mannitol, just before clamp release, during renal transplantation.

With adequate circulating volume, loop diuretics may convert oliguric to nonoliguric ATN in humans, but they have no effect on the duration of ATN, need for dialysis, or survival. A retrospective review of a recent trial of diuretics in critically ill patients with ATN raised concerns because their administration was associated with a higher mortality and delayed recovery from ARF. Most of the increased risk was seen in patients unresponsive to high doses of diuretics, implying they had more severe disease.[31] These adverse effects were recently not confirmed in a large multicenter database analysis.[32]

Loop diuretics in the setting of ARF are not without hazards. Transient episodes of tinnitus and/or vertigo and very rarely deafness may be present if high doses are administered intravenously in <6 hours. Furosemide dose should not exceed 1000 mg/day. Coprescription of aminoglycosides with diuretics increases the risk of ototoxicity and should be avoided. As loop diuretics have not shown real benefits for either patient or renal prognosis, their use cannot be recommended.

Acetylcysteine

Several meta-analyses over the past 2 to 3 years have concluded that, compared to periprocedural hydration alone, oral acetylcysteine, together with hydration, significantly lowers the risk of radiocontrast nephropathy in patients with chronic renal insufficiency. However, acetylcysteine without adequate hydration is not sufficient and in some studies the individual contribution of acetylcysteine is difficult to delineate. Every meta-analysis also found studies showing no benefit.[28] Furthermore, acetylcysteine seems to affect the tubular handling of creatinine directly, so a decrease in serum creatinine concentration with this drug does not necessarily imply protection of the GFR.[33] More data are needed before acetylcysteine can be strongly recommended for the prevention of radiocontrast-induced nephropathy.

Calcium Channel Blockers

If administered prophylactically, calcium blockers protected against post-transplantation delayed graft failure in some studies. However, a meta-analysis found no definitive benefit of calcium entry blockers in the prevention of post-transplantation ATN. In other settings of ARF and after cardiac surgery, the preventive role of calcium channel blockers was more promising.

Endothelin Receptor Blockers or Adenosine Antagonists

Studies with endothelin receptor blockers or adenosine antagonists were either negative or inconclusive.

Drugs to Promote Recovery from Acute Renal Failure

These drugs include growth factors (e.g., insulin-like growth factor I) and thyroxine. None of these drugs were associated with a positive effect on patient survival or on GFR in either critically ill patients or in preventing post–kidney transplantation DGF.[22] In contrast with animal data, a recent retrospective, propensity-adjusted analysis showed that erythropoietin did not influence the renal recovery in critically ill patients with ARF.[34] Thyroxine even had a negative effect on outcome through prolonged suppression of thyroid-stimulating hormone and should not be administered in critically ill patients.

REFERENCES

1. Lameire N, Van BW, Vanholder R: Acute renal failure. Lancet 2005;365: 417–430.
2. Bellomo R: Defining, quantifying, and classifying acute renal failure. Crit Care Clin 2005;21:223–237.
3. Liano F, Pascual J: Epidemiology of acute renal failure: A prospective, multicenter, community-based study. Madrid Acute Renal Failure Study Group. Kidney Int 1996;50:811–818.
4. Obialo CI, Okonofua EC, Tayade AS, Riley LJ: Epidemiology of de novo acute renal failure in hospitalized African Americans: Comparing community-acquired vs hospital-acquired disease. Arch Intern Med 2000;160:1309–1313.
5. Lynn RM, O'Brien SJ, Taylor CM, et al: Childhood hemolytic uremic syndrome, United Kingdom and Ireland. Emerg Infect Dis 2005;11: 590–596.
6. Barsoum RS: Tropical acute renal failure. Contrib Nephrol 2004;144: 44–52.
7. Nash K, Hafeez A, Hou S: Hospital-acquired renal insufficiency. Am J Kidney Dis 2002;39:930–936.
8. Joannidis M, Metnitz PG: Epidemiology and natural history of acute renal failure in the ICU. Crit Care Clin 2005;21:239–249.
9. Abosaif NY, Tolba YA, Heap M, et al: The outcome of acute renal failure in the intensive care unit according to RIFLE: Model application, sensitivity, and predictability. Am J Kidney Dis 2005;46: 1038–1048.
10. Schrier RW, Wang W: Acute renal failure and sepsis. N Engl J Med 2004; 351:159–169.
11. Lameire N, Van Biesen W, Vanholder R: The changing epidemiology of acute renal failure. Nat Clin Pract Nephrol 2006;2:364–377.
12. Xue JL, Daniels F, Star RA, et al: Incidence and mortality of acute renal failure in Medicare beneficiaries, 1992 to 2001. J Am Soc Nephrol 2006; 17:1135–1142.
13. Evenepoel P: Acute toxic renal failure. Best Pract Res Clin Anesthesiol 2004;18:37–52.
14. Askenazi DJ, Feig DI, Graham NM, et al: 3-5 year longitudinal follow-up of pediatric patients after acute renal failure. Kidney Int 2006;69:184–189.
15. Rosner MH, Okusa MD: Acute kidney injury associated with cardiac surgery. Clin J Am Soc Nephrol 2006;1:19–32.
16. Lameire NH, Flombaum CD, Moreau D, Ronco C: Acute renal failure in cancer patients. Ann Med 2005;37:13–25.
17. Franceschini N, Napravnik S, Eron JJ Jr, et al: Incidence and etiology of acute renal failure among ambulatory HIV-infected patients. Kidney Int 2005;67:1526–1531.
18. Carvounis CP, Nisar S, Guro-Razuman S: Significance of the fractional excretion of urea in the differential diagnosis of acute renal failure. Kidney Int 2002;62:2223–2229.
19. Lassnigg A, Schmidlin D, Mouhieddine M, et al: Minimal changes of serum creatinine predict prognosis in patients after cardiothoracic surgery: A prospective cohort study. J Am Soc Nephrol 2004;15:1597–1605.
20. Herget-Rosenthal S, Marggraf G, Husing J, et al: Early detection of acute renal failure by serum cystatin C. Kidney Int 2004;66:1115–1122.
21. Han WK, Bonventre JV: Biologic markers for the early detection of acute kidney injury. Curr Opin Crit Care 2004;10:476–482.

22. Lameire NH, Vanholder RC: Acute renal failure: Pathophysiology and prevention. In Davison AM, Cameron JS, Grünfeld J-P, et al. (eds): Oxford Textbook of Clinical Nephrology, 3rd ed. Oxford, UK: Oxford University Press, 2005, pp 1445–1464.
23. Molitoris BA, Sutton TA: Endothelial injury and dysfunction: Role in the extension phase of acute renal failure. Kidney Int 2004;66:496–499.
24. Van den Berghe G, Wouters P, Weekers F, et al: Intensive insulin therapy in the critically ill patients. N Engl J Med 2001;345:1359–1367.
25. Van den Berghe G, Wilmer A, Hermans G, et al: Intensive insulin therapy in the medical ICU. N Engl J Med 2006;354:449–461.
26. Morelli A, Ricci Z, Bellomo R, et al: Prophylactic fenoldopam for renal protection in sepsis: A randomized, double-blind, placebo-controlled pilot trial. Crit Care Med 2005;33:2451–2456.
27. Tumlin JA, Finkel KW, Murray PT, et al: Fenoldopam mesylate in early acute tubular necrosis: A randomized, double-blind, placebo-controlled clinical trial. Am J Kidney Dis 2005;46:26-34.
28. Venkataraman R: Prevention of acute renal failure. Crit Care Clin 2005;21:281–289.
29. Koda M, Sakamoto A, Ogawa R: Effects of atrial natriuretic peptide at a low dose on water and electrolyte metabolism during general anesthesia. J Clin Anesth 2005;17:3–7.
30. Feldman DS, Ikonomidis JS, Uber WE, et al: Human B-natriuretic peptide improves hemodynamics and renal function in hear transplant patients immediately after surgery. J Cardiac Failure 2004;10:292–296.
31. Mehta RL, Pascual MT, Soroko S, Chertow GM: Diuretics, mortality, and nonrecovery of renal function in acute renal failure. JAMA 2002; 288: 2547–2553.
32. Uchino S, Doig GS, Bellomo R, et al: Diuretics and mortality in acute renal failure. Crit Care Med 2004;32:1669–1677.
33. Hoffmann U, Banas B, Fischereder M, Kramer BK: N-acetylcysteine in the prevention of radiocontrast-induced nephropathy: Clinical trials and end points. Kidney Blood Press Res 2004;27:161–166.
34. Park J, Gage BF, Vijayan A: Use of EPO in critically ill patients with acute renal failure requiring renal replacement therapy. Am J Kidney Dis 2005; 46:791–798.

Nondialytic Management of Acute Renal Failure

A. Ahsan Ejaz and Emil P. Paganini

INTRODUCTION

Once measures to prevent acute renal failure (ARF; see Chapter 64) have not succeeded, the central question is whether ARF can be treated with nondialytic therapy alone or whether renal replacement therapy (RRT) is necessary. This chapter covers nondialytic aspects, whereas the question of when to initiate RRT in ARF and which type of RRT to choose is covered in Chapters 66 and 87. Key issues in the nondialytic management of such patients relate to fluid and electrolyte disturbances as well as the metabolic state (Fig. 65.1).

GENERAL MANAGEMENT

The patient with dysfunctional kidneys requires attention to a variety of details that may have been less important with good renal function. Beyond the volume, electrolyte, and acid/base aspects of care (see later discussion), drug dosages and invasive procedures need to be considered.

Patients with ARF are prone to infection. Common sources of infection include the operative site, intravascular lines, lungs, and urinary tract. This relationship underlines the need to restrict the use of invasive monitors or additional blood access devices. Indeed, aggressive fluid control in an attempt to reduce intubation time is rewarded with a reduction of ventilator-associated pneumonia.

Avoiding any potentially nephrotoxic agents should also be a strong consideration. Anti-infective agents such as aminoglycosides, amphotericin, acyclovir, and pentamidine should be restricted or the dose significantly altered to avoid further insult. Any other medications associated with ARF (i.e., hemodynamic, toxic, immune mediated) such as allopurinol, phenytoin, and nonsteroidal anti-inflammatory drugs (NSAIDs) should also be avoided when possible. A review of radiographic diagnostic investigations should be undertaken with a focus on avoiding iodine-containing dyes. Alternative contrast measures such as CO_2 may serve the same purpose and not carry potential renal injury.

Whether the use of erythropoietin supplementation can help with treatment of anemia, which is commonly associated with ARF, and reduce blood transfusions is debated. The economic aspects of using an expensive medication in a situation of increased inflammation and decreased drug responsiveness is balanced against the physiologic aspects of decreased endogenous production. While there have been situations where erythropoietin has been used successfully, its routine use in ARF should currently be discouraged.

FLUID AND ELECTROLYTE MANAGEMENT

Perhaps the largest area of controversy is in the type of fluid to use when challenging a "dry" patient or in correcting a specific

Supportive management of acute renal failure	
Complication	**Treatment**
Intravascular volume excess	Restrict salt (1–2 g/day) and water (usually <1 l/day) intake Diuretics (usually loop diuretics ± thiazides) Ultrafiltration or dialysis
Hyponatremia	Restrict free water intake (<1 l/day) Avoid hypotonic intravenous solutions (including dextrose solutions)
Hyperkalemia	Restrict dietary K^+ intake (usually <50 mmol/day) Eliminate K^+ supplements and K^+-sparing diuretics Potassium-binding ion exchange resins Glucose (50 ml of 50% dextrose) and insulin (10 units) Sodium bicarbonate (usually 50–100 mmol) β_2 agonist inhaled (e.g., albuterol [salbutamol] 10–20 mg inhaled or 0.5–1 mg IV) Calcium gluconate (10 ml of 10% solution over 2–5 minutes)
Metabolic acidosis	Restrict dietary protein (usually 0.8–1.0 g/kg/day of high biologic value) Sodium bicarbonate (maintain serum bicarbonate >15 mmol/l and arterial pH >7.2)
Hyperphosphatemia	Restrict dietary phosphate intake (usually <800 mg/day) Phosphate-binding agents (calcium acetate, calcium carbonate, aluminum hydroxide, and sevelamer)
Hypocalcemia	If symptomatic: IV calcium gluconate (10–20 ml of 10% solution) or IV calcium chloride (10–20 ml of 10% solution via central line) If aysmptomatic: calcium carbonate 500 mg orally three times daily
Hypermagnesemia	Discontinue magnesium-containing antacids
Hyperuricemia	Treatment usually not necessary if uric acid <15 mg/dl (<900 µmol/l)
Nutrition	Restrict dietary protein (0.8–1.0 g/kg/day) if not catabolic Carbohydrate (>100 g/day, adjust according to non–protein calorie requirement) Enteral or parenteral nutrition (if prolonged course or very catabolic)

Figure 65.1 Supportive management of acute renal failure (ARF).

electrolyte abnormality. Figure 65.2 gives an approximation of the compartment distribution of various types of fluid used. Water will distribute across all compartments, while colloid will remain intravascular. Thus, when offering a fluid challenge, using normal saline with or without colloid would be the most efficacious, while combination solutions may be more appropriate for the correction of electrolytes. An algorithm of how to approach an oliguric patient is shown in Figure 65.3.

Intravenous fluids are commonly administered in the intensive care unit (see also Chapter 66) to achieve and maintain normovolemia and hemodynamic stability, optimize oxygen delivery and consumption, and ensure adequate plasma colloid osmotic pressure. Prerenal ARF can be rapidly reversed with restoration of renal perfusion by replacement fluids. The composition of replacement fluid varies depending on the source of fluid loss: packed red blood cells are favored in hypovolemia due to hemorrhage, whereas isotonic saline is preferred in patients with hemodynamic instability. A liberal transfusion policy, however, is to be avoided because excess packed red blood cell transfusion has been associated with an increase in in-hospital mortality. Optimal strategies remain uncertain, but recommendations are that critically ill patients receive red cell transfusions when their hemoglobin concentrations decrease to <7 g/dl and that hemoglobin concentrations should be maintained between 7 and 9 g/dl. Higher hemoglobin levels may not necessarily provide more benefit.[1] Recently, colloids and crystalloids have been demonstrated to be clinically equivalent treatments for intravascular volume resuscitation in critically ill patients. Fluid losses are initially replaced by fluids of equal tonicity (e.g., 0.45% saline for urinary losses); subsequent therapy is based on the volume and osmolar content of excreted or drained fluids (Fig. 65.4).

The clinical effect of the administration of resuscitation fluid can be time and rate dependent. Early and vigorous replacement of the enormous insensible and isotonic fluid losses with a judicious mixture of water and crystalloid solutions and aggressive infection control can reduce the incidence of ARF (1% to 30%) and mortality (73% to 100%) in burn injury victims. ARF immediately after burn injury is mostly due to the decrease in renal perfusion from hypovolemia and occasionally from pigment-induced renal tubular damage from rhabdomyolysis. Later, excessive fluid and protein losses from the burn wound may lead to hypoalbuminemia and a shift of fluid into the interstitial space, further depleting the circulating volume and increasing the risk of ARF.[2] In catastrophic crush injury patients, a similar prompt, massive, and alkaline fluid resuscitation (to maintain urine output more than 300 ml/h) is the key to the prevention of renal failure (see Chapter 64).[3]

The role of fluid resuscitation in established ARF is less clear. Fluid resuscitation is targeted to a specific preload, stroke volume, or cardiac output rather than to a specific mean arterial pressure. However, the lack of correlation between surrogate markers of preload (such as filling pressure, central venous pressure, and pulmonary capillary wedge pressure) and ventricular end-diastolic volume in the sickest of patients often leads to the administration of fluid challenges to assess volume status. The choice of fluids is controversial; there are no studies of fluid resuscitation regimens in patients with ARF that show clear evidence of the superiority of any fluid type.[4,5]

In postobstructive diuresis, the urine is hypotonic; therefore, hypotonic solutions (0.45% saline) are initially preferred for the replacement of urine and insensible fluid losses. In the case of pigment (myoglobin)-related or protein deposition (myeloma)–related postrenal ARF, alkalinization of the urine is achieved by adding sodium bicarbonate to a solution of glucose, water, or hypotonic saline.

Acute renal failure superimposed on chronic kidney disease is an increasingly recognized form of ARF.[6] Intravascular volume deficiency is a common feature in this entity, and its correction may improve renal function.

Diuretic Therapy

Diuretics are frequently used in the critical care setting to minimize fluid overload (Fig. 65.5) and prevent ARF due to their theoretical benefit of flushing casts through the tubular lumen and reducing tubular oxygen consumption. They do not appear to protect against ARF but rather increase mortality and nonrecovery of renal function in an intensive care unit setting (see Chapter 64). The mechanisms by which diuretics may exacerbate ARF are not well understood, but could relate to effects on renal perfusion. Indeed, their utilization is greatest in the sickest patients with sepsis, elevated extracellular volume with third-spacing, respiratory distress, and after cardiovascular surgery, a time where renal vasoconstriction and reduced renal blood flow are marked.

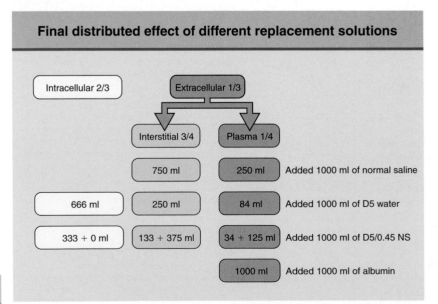

Final distributed effect of different replacement solutions

Intracellular 2/3	Extracellular 1/3	
	Interstitial 3/4	Plasma 1/4
	750 ml	250 ml	Added 1000 ml of normal saline
666 ml	250 ml	84 ml	Added 1000 ml of D5 water
333 + 0 ml	133 + 375 ml	34 + 125 ml	Added 1000 ml of D5/0.45 NS
		1000 ml	Added 1000 ml of albumin

Figure 65.2 Final distributed effect of different replacement solutions. D5, 5% dextrose; NS, normal saline.

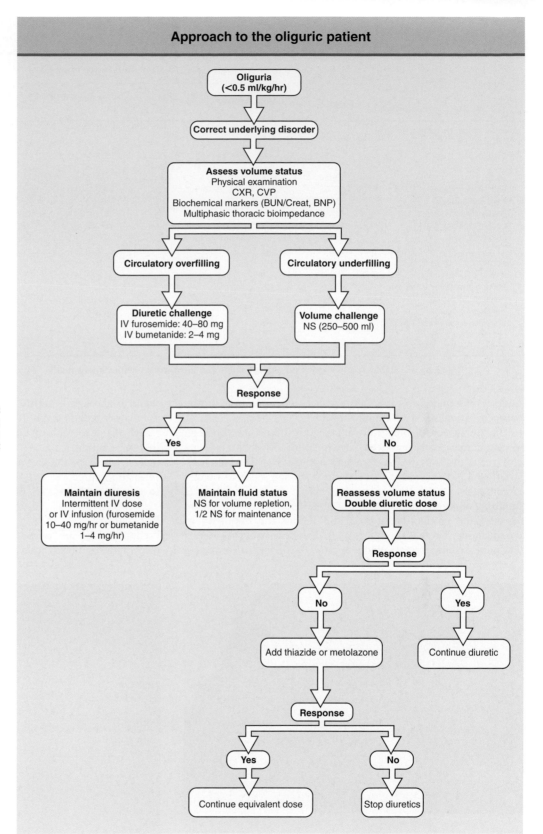

Figure 65.3 Approach to the oliguric patient. BNP, brain natriuretic peptide; BUN, blood urea nitrogen; Creat, creatine; CVP, central venous pressure; CXR, chest radiograph; NS, normal saline

Diuretics may worsen the relative underfilling of the arterial circulation and intravascular blood volume and reduce renal perfusion, resulting in either prerenal azotemia or ARF. There are insufficient data to support the routine administration of mannitol or natriuretic peptides to oliguric patients. Furthermore, mannitol may cause pulmonary edema and severe hyponatremia due to expansion of intravascular volume. The administration of anaritide (atrial natriuretic peptide) did not improve the overall rate of dialysis-free survival or reduction in dialysis in critically ill patients with acute tubular necrosis in a multicenter clinical trial.[7] These

	Electrolyte composition of body fluids and intravenous replacement fluids							
	Electrolyte (mmol/l)							
Fluids	Na⁺	K⁺	H⁺	Cl⁻	HCO₃⁻	Ca²⁺	Glucose (mmol/l [mg/dl])
Plasma, sweat, or gastrointestinal secretion							
Plasma	136–145	3.5–5.0	4 ×10⁻⁶ (40 mmol/l)	98–106	21–30	2.20–2.63	4.2–6.4 (75–115)
Sweat	30–50	5	—	45–55	—	—	—
Gastric secretions	40–65	10	90*	100–140	—	—	—
Pancreatic fistula	135–155	5	—	55–75	70–90	—	—
Biliary fistula	135–155	5	—	80–110	35–50	—	—
Ileostomy fluid	120–130	10	—	50–60	50–70	—	—
Diarrhea fluid	25–50	30–60	—	20–40	30–45	—	—
Common replacement fluids							
Isotonic saline (0.9%)	150	—	—	150	—	—	—
Half normal saline (0.45%)	75	—	—	75	—	—	—
Solution 18 (0.18%)	30	—	—	30	—	—	22.2 (400)
Ringer's solution	147	4	—	156	—	2.2	—
Hartman's solution/Ringer's lactate solution	131	5	—	111	29	2	—
5% dextrose	—	—	—	—	—	—	27.7 (500)

Figure 65.4 Electrolyte composition of body fluids and intravenous replacement fluids. *Variable (e.g., lower in achlorhydria).

results again underscore the importance of prevention in the management of ARF (see Chapter 64).

The conversion of oliguric to nonoliguric status has also been one of the universally practiced early measures offered to patients with renal dysfunction. A standard approach to this situation is outlined (see Fig. 65.3), but there does not seem to be any outcome advantage to this conversion.[8] What does seem helpful is the lifting of severe fluid restrictions in patients who can maintain a good urine production; it may also reduce the frequency of hyperkalemia. There is often a delay in dialytic support in patients with increased interstitial volume because of the fear of converting them to an oliguric status. Whether the oliguria is secondary to the dialysis technique *per se* (e.g., membrane interaction, dialysate reactivity) or a result of intravascular volume changes during the therapy continues to be elusive. The delay in dialytic support may result in pulmonary edema and tissue hypoxia, mechanical ventilation, infection, and acute respiratory dysfunction and lead to a worse outcome.[9]

Potassium
Predominantly an intracellular cation, its movement across membranes and into the extracellular space is quite variable. Thus,

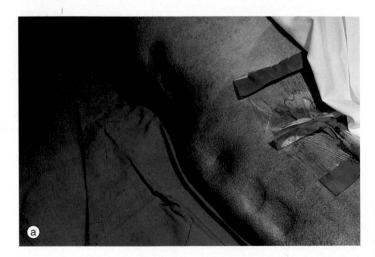

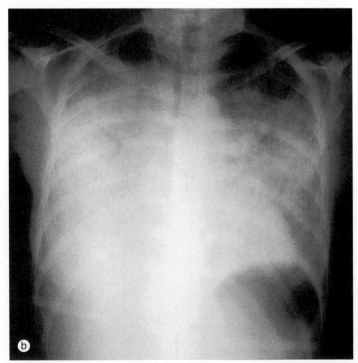

Figure 65.5   Fluid overload in acute renal failure (ARF). *a*, Gross pitting edema in a patient with ARF in whom femoral venous access has been established to initiate hemodialysis. *b*, Severe pulmonary edema.

small variations in serum levels may have less significance than larger and sustained serum concentrations or rapid concentration swings. Changes in serum pH contribute to this movement, with low pH (acidemia) inducing a higher serum potassium and alkalemia associated with a lower plasma concentration. Thus, when evaluating a control strategy, one must consider the anticipated concomitant acid-base change.

Hyperkalemia is defined as a serum potassium >5.5 mmol/l and may occur from an intracellular to extracellular shift (due to acidosis, insulin deficiency, β-adrenergic blockade, or hyperosmolarity), tissue release (tumor lysis, rhabdomyolysis), increased intake, or decreased urinary excretion (see Chapter 9). While hyperkalemia may cause symptoms such as muscle weakness, its primary risk is on cardiac conduction where it may cause bradycardia or asystole. Electrocardiographic changes begin with peaked T waves in the precordial leads (K$^+$ 5.5 to 6.0 mmol/l), followed by widening of the PR and QRS intervals, progression to a nodal rhythm, and eventually a sinus wave pattern and ventricular asystole (Fig. 65.6; see Chapter 9). It is often said that patients with chronic kidney disease (CKD) or end-stage renal disease may tolerate a higher serum level, although there is little solid evidence of this. The symptoms associated with hyperkalemia include muscle weakness and respiratory failure. An electrocardiogram can reveal a variety of abnormalities, from peaked T waves (tenting) to prolonged QRS complexes to asystolic arrest (see Fig. 65.6). The lack of electrocardiographic abnormalities should not lessen the urgency of treatment, especially in the higher ranges of hyperkalemia.

Initial treatment will depend on urgency. Removing the source of continued delivery is obvious (antibiotics, nutritional substitutes, fluids) as is discontinuing potentially offending medication (aldosterone blockade, angiotensin-converting enzyme [ACE] inhibition, NSAIDs, and β-blockers). If more aggressive therapy is required, depending on the absolute level, loop diuretics (furosemide 40 to 80 mg IV) or binder therapy with oral resins (sodium polystyrene sulfonate 15 to 30 g with 30% sorbitol) may be adequate. Resin enemas should be avoided due to the risk of colonic necrosis (see Chapter 77). Other rapidly acting measures, including correction of acidosis, nebulized β$_2$-adrenergic receptor

agonists, insulin, and glucose infusions as well as calcium gluconate injection are discussed in Chapter 9. It is important to watch for potassium rebound as the effects of these maneuvers wear off. For definitive control, administration of a loop diuretic or, for patients on RRT, aggressive high-flow dialytic intervention (diffusive rather than convective) is effective.

Hypokalemia (see also Chapter 9) is defined as serum levels <3.5 mmol/l. Cardiac arrhythmias are frequently encountered, especially in patients with underlying myocardial disease receiving digitalis therapy. The source is usually gastrointestinal losses from diarrhea, intracellular shifts from alkalosis, or renal losses from diuretics. Not infrequently, medications such as carbenicillin and amphotericin B may promote exaggerated renal losses as well.

Therapy should be gentle. Oral supplements or low-dose IV infusions can be delivered slowly (10 to 20 mmol/l over 1 hour). Care should be taken when using a central line, as the position of the catheter tip may create problems if situated in the right atrium. A more rapid infusion (administration of 5 to 10 mmol of KCl intravenously over 15 to 20 minutes with close, continuous monitoring of the serum potassium concentration and the electrocardiogram) may be warranted if treating severe hypokalemia in a patient requiring emergent surgery or a patient with an acute myocardial infarction and malignant ventricular arrhythmia. If on dialytic support, a change in either the potassium concentration of the dialysate (replacement solution) or in the dialysate flow rate will resolve the imbalance.

Sodium

Serum osmolality is determined predominantly by serum sodium levels. With the free flow of water among the various compartments (see Fig. 65.2) any acute change in the concentration of sodium will result in a fluid shift to maintain osmolality across the compartments. Thus, rapid correction of either hyper- or hyponatremia will result in volume changes within compartments. Exaggerated drops in serum sodium concentrations may result in cerebral edema or cell swelling, while rapid increases in

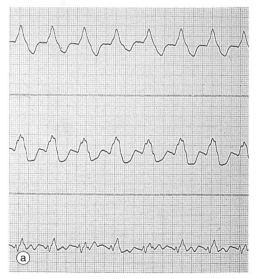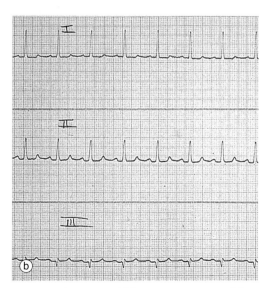

Figure 65.6 Electrocardiography (ECG) in hyperkalemia. *a*, ECG recorded in a patient with acute renal failure, serum potassium 6.8 mmol/l. Note the bizarre broad complex recording with no P waves, which is typical of hyperkalemia. *b*, ECG in the same patient, 15 minutes later, following administration of 10 ml 10% calcium gluconate. Serum potassium is unchanged, but the ECG has recovered.

concentration may result in pontine myelinolysis and potential cerebral hemorrhage.

Hypernatremia (see also Chapter 8), defined as serum sodium concentrations of >145 mmol/l, is usually the result of either an exaggerated loss of water or the addition of an excessive amount of sodium. Water loss can either be primarily from losses through the gastrointestinal tract or, more frequently, with the use of osmotic diuretics, from unrecognized insensible losses, or from nephrogenic diabetes insipidus (CKD, hypokalemia, hypercalcemia, medications, decreased protein intake). Excessive hypertonic saline, sodium bicarbonate administration as well as aggressive steroid therapy are the usual causes of intake-induced hypernatremia.

Serum sodium <135 mmol/l, and certainly below 130 mmol/l, is considered hyponatremia. In the absence of pseudohyponatremia, such as due to a hyperglycemic state, hyponatremia reflects a state of hypo-osmoality. The condition may be associated with hypovalemia (e.g., from vomiting or diarrhea), euvolemia (e.g., the syndrome of inappropriate ADH [SIADH] release), or with hypervolemia (such as with edematous states, e.g., cirrhosis). Treatment depends on the condition (see Chapter 8). For SIADH the classic treatment consists of free water restriction, followed by more aggressive therapies (e.g., normal saline and furosemide, hypertonic saline, or treatment with the new V2 receptor antagonists for vasopressin (see Chapter 8).

Once again, especially in patients with cardiorenal syndrome, the use of extracorporeal therapeutic interventions may help correct both the renal dysfunction and the electrolyte abnormality. Indeed, a clear advantage here is the ability to accurately calculate the speed at which the correction will occur by controlling the sodium concentration of the bath (replacement solution). Conversely, great care should be taken in hyponatremic patients to adjust the dialysate sodium to low values.

Calcium, Phosphorus, and Magnesium Disorders

Hyperphosphatemia and hypocalemia are common in ARF. A reduction of renal phosphorus loss with ARF and its continued release from tissues will create an increase in serum levels. If the tissue injury is great (as in rhabdomyolysis) or acute tissue death is induced (as in tumor lysis), the level of hyperphosphatemia may be quite high (>12 mg/dl; >3.9 mmol/l). As phosphorus increases, calcium will decrease, resulting in hypocalcemia. The levels of reduction are usually mild to moderate with total calcium levels dropping to 7 to 8 mg/dl (1.75 to 2.0 mmol/l). Because of the frequent presence of metabolic acidosis, the ionized calcium is usually adequate, but may become problematic with correction of acidosis. One issue of concern, however, is a high calcium phosphorus product (>60 mg^2/dl^2; >4.84 $mmol^2/l^2$) and the associated tissue deposition of calcium. Calcium deposition can cause both skin irritation and cardiac arrhythmia.

Other reasons for low calcium in ARF beyond tissue deposition are (1) skeletal resistance to parathyroid hormone and (2) low levels of calcitriol production from the dysfunctional kidney. The combination may be the reason for a lack of calcium release from bone despite the hypocalcemic state. The most effective nondialytic treatment for the high phosphorus is phosphate binding (see Chapter 74). Control of the phosphorus

level will usually be enough to normalize the level of calcium as well. If, however, there are symptoms associated with the low calcium, a calcium gluconate infusion may be indicated.

Hypercalcemia is a rare occurrence in ARF and is usually seen in the recovery phase of rhabdomyolysis. The calcium is released from calcium-containing complexes in muscle. Also, with the reestablished production of calcitriol by the recovering kidney, enhanced responsiveness to parathyroid hormone is seen. These calcium levels are rarely problematic and can be easily treated with dialytic maneuvers or a loop diuretic.

Mild hypermagnesemia is a frequent state in ARF. Clinical consequences of these levels are usually absent unless very high levels are provoked by using a magnesium-containing medication.

Acid-Base Disorders

The approach to acid/base disturbances in early ARF needs to be balanced against the background status of the patient. Review of the pH, $PaCO_2$, and HCO_3^- will guide the physician toward establishing the predominant disorder. The approach to defining metabolic acidosis is listed in Figure 12.1.

While metabolic acidosis is the most frequently encountered abnormality, triple acid-base disturbances are not infrequent. The situation involves metabolic acidosis and metabolic alkalosis with one primary respiratory disorder. In high anion gap acidosis, the relative change in serum bicarbonate (ΔHCO_3^-) is informative. If the excess anion gap is greater than ΔHCO_3^-, there is a superimposed metabolic alkalosis. If the anion gap is less than ΔHCO_3^-, a combined high gap and normal gap acidosis must be considered. In a patient with metabolic acidosis, if the anion gap plus the measured HCO_3^- is >30, there is underlying metabolic alkalosis, while if this number is <23, there is an associated nongap acidosis. Although this may seem academic, its clinical value becomes apparent during treatment.

There is controversy surrounding the treatment of acute metabolic acidosis. Normal gap metabolic acidosis is associated with a greater impairment of immune response, a greater stimulation of cytokine release, and a higher state of inflammation than the high gap acidemia. While it seems reasonable to treat the acute acidosis with sodium bicarbonate, application of this approach in high-gap acidemia has not been associated with improved outcome. This may be explained by other effects of the bicarbonate beyond correcting the serum pH: significant increase in CO_2 generation, potential worsening of the respiratory component of the acidemia, and worsening of intracellular acidosis have been described. Rapid improvement in the acidemic state may also lead to hypocalcemia, which may result in a depression of cardiac output. Alternative forms of base treatment are not of proven benefit in patients with ARF. Tris(hydroxymethyl)aminomethane (THAM) depends on renal excretion for efficacy. Other approaches have not been studied adequately in ARF.

Restriction of protein intake has been recommended as another method of acidosis control. Protein breakdown has been associated with worsening acidosis, and thus restricting intake is thought to be beneficial. The addition of sodium acetate or sodium lactate to parenteral nutrition has also been practiced. While acetate at rates delivered via total parenteral nutrition is usually well tolerated, lactate may still create problems, especially in subjects with severe lactic acidosis.

Nutritional Considerations

Not all patients with ARF require the addition of nutritional therapy and may actually be able to maintain their requirements through feeding. It is the underlying cause of ARF and the status of the patient beyond renal dysfunction that usually dictate this requirement. One important issue, however, is the baseline nutritional status of the premorbid patient. Those individuals who are deficient will have a higher risk of a poor outcome than those patients with good nutritional status. This is frequently judged by their entry level of serum albumin (half-life of approximately 20 days), level of serum creatinine either at baseline or during renal dysfunction, and other markers that are much less accurate (serum cholesterol, transferrin, prealbumin) in ARF.

Monitoring of nitrogen balance to assess the effectiveness of supplemental nutritional therapy is determined by measuring protein intake over 12 or 24 hours and urinary excretion of urea nitrogen over the same time interval. A positive or negative protein balance is used to determine the adequacy of protein intake of the patient. It is calculated as follows:

Nitrogen balance = (protein intake/6.25) – (UUN + 4),

where protein intake and urinary urea nitrogen (UUN) are each expressed in grams.

Establishing a nitrogen balance may be difficult, particularly in the patient with rapidly declining renal function, and impossible in the oligoanuric patient. Grouping patients according to their measured nitrogen balance may, however, provide some direction in supplemental therapy decisions.

The goal of nutritional support is to preserve lean body mass, maintain immunocompetence, offer substrate for the acute inflammatory state, and help promote wound healing. The conservative levels of protein usually recommended in chronic renal failure are not appropriate in ARF. Indeed, underdelivery of protein in these patients is one of the most frequently found problems. Timing is also problematic. Initiation of support should be considered early in the course of ARF in patients already compromised or undernourished.

As we have already seen, both fluid and electrolyte considerations are important in the choice of appropriate nutritional supplement. When possible, enteral feeding should be the primary supplemental mode. The primary issues with enteral feeding in ARF are osmolality and subsequent episodes of diarrhea balanced with the content of sodium, potassium, and chloride; caloric load and how that is handled; and protein delivery and its solute balance with urea appearance. Basic energy requirements (calories per 24 hours) may be estimated from the Harris-Benedict equation to obtain a corrected resting energy requirement when factored by a patient-specific stress factor (Fig. 65.7).

In general, 25 to 35 kcal/kg/day is the energy required by patients with ARF. The best source of energy is still debated, but most prefer to use a combination of carbohydrates and lipids again depending more on the underlying patient condition than the level of renal function.

Tight glucose control (90–120 mg/dl [5–6.7 mmol/l]) has recently been suggested to improve patient outcome. While there continues to be debate around the published trial, early glucose control and continued close attention to serum potassium levels make this more difficult in patients with ARF. Variations in renal catabolism of insulin may pose problems with hypoglycemia.

Estimation of basic energy requirement (calories per 24 hours) using the Harris-Benedict equation		
Men:	BER = 66 + (13.7 × weight) + (5 × height) – (6.8 × age)	
Women:	BER = 655 + (9.6 × weight) + (1.8 × height) – (4.7 × age)	
where weight* is expressed in kg, height in cm, and age in years		
BER is multiplied with a stress factor		
Postoperative, no complications:		1.0
Patient with peritonitis/sepsis:		1.2–1.3
Patient with severe infection:		1.2–1.4
Patient with polytrauma:		1.3
Burns (factor for percentage burned):		1.2–1.4

Figure 65.7 Estimation of basic energy requirement (BER) (calories per 24 hours) using the Harris-Benedict equation. *The weight in these equations should be the usual (baseline) weight of the patient for those without significant weight loss, current weight for those with significant weight loss, and ideal body weight for obese patients.

Protein delivery needs to be higher in severe ARF with poor general status than those stated for patients with CKD. Since renal preservation is not an issue here, but rather supplying the needed protein to serve in catabolic states, a rate of 1.2 to 1.8 g/kg/day is usually employed. Protein restriction should be considered only in the simple ARF patient. However, in those with multiorgan failure or in highly catabolic states, higher protein delivery and perhaps early dialytic support is usually preferable.

TREATMENT FOR SPECIFIC CAUSES OF ACUTE RENAL FAILURE

The management of ARF must be modified to the underlying disorder. In addition to the general measures discussed previously, treatment may include immunosuppressive agents (glomerulonephritis, vasculitis), plasma exchange (hemolytic uremic syndrome/thrombotic thrombocytopenic purpura, Goodpasture's syndrome), systemic anticoagulation (renal artery or vein thrombosis), angiotensin-converting enzyme inhibitors (scleroderma), and aggressive control of systemic blood pressure (preeclampsia). Recombinant urate oxidase (rasburicase) can effectively lower serum urate levels in acute urate nephropathy. However, it is contraindicated in patients with glucose-6-phosphate dehydrogenase deficiency as it may cause hemolytic anemia and methemoglobinemia.[10]

Detailed description of treatment strategies for various entities is discussed throughout the book, but ARF in patients with congestive heart failure is mentioned here due to the prevalence and challenge of managing these patients in clinical practice. The majority of these patients have decreased glomerular filtration rate, are at increased risk of cardiovascular mortality, and have acute-onset CKD. ARF is mostly the result of either overdiuresis or decreased cardiac output from poor pump function that causes decreased renal blood flow. Discontinuation of diuretics and cautious fluid replacement may improve ARF in some, but inotropes and vasodilators may be required in those with severe cardiac pump failure. Nesiritide (brain natriuretic peptide) is used because of its beneficial hemodynamic effects in acute congestive heart failure and causes a small increase in the urine volume; however, there is lack of evidence of its use in the management of ARF.

REFERENCES

1. Hebert PC, Wells G, Blajchman MA, et al: A multicenter, randomized, controlled clinical trial of transfusion requirements in critical care. Transfusion Requirements in Critical Care Investigators, Canadian Critical Care Trials Group. N Engl J Med 1999;340:409–417.
2. Chrysopoulo MT, Jeschke MG, Dziewulski P, et al: Acute renal dysfunction in severely burned adults. J Trauma 1999;46:141–144.
3. Sever MS, Erek E, Vanholder R, et al: Marmara Earthquake Study Group: Treatment modalities and outcome of the renal victims of the Marmara earthquake. Nephron 2002;92:64–71.
4. Mehta RL, Clark WC, Schetz M: Techniques for assessing and achieving fluid balance in acute renal failure. Curr Opin Crit Care 2002;8: 535–543.
5. The SAFE Study Investigators: A comparison of albumin and saline for fluid resuscitation in the intensive care unit. N Engl J Med 2004;350: 2247–2256.
6. Liano F, Pascual J: Epidemiology of acute renal failure: A prospective, multicenter, community-based study. Madrid Acute Renal Failure Study Group. Kidney Int 1996;50:811–818.
7. Lewis J, Salem MM, Chertow GM, et al: Atrial natriuretic factor in oliguric acute renal failure. Anaritide Acute Renal Failure Study Group. Am J Kidney Dis 2000;36:767–774.
8. Cantarovich F, Rangoonwala B, Lorenz H, et al.; High-Dose Furosemide in Acute Renal Failure Study Group. High-dose furosemide for established ARF: A prospective, randomized, double-blind, placebo-controlled, multicenter trial. Am J Kidney Dis 2004;44:402–409.
9. Schrier RW, Wang W: Acute renal failure and sepsis. N Engl J Med 2004;351:159–169.
10. Browning LA, Kruse JA: Hemolysis and methemoglobinemia secondary to rasburicase administration. Ann Pharmacother 2005;39:1932–1935.

Intensive Care Unit Nephrology

Sevag Demirjian and Emil P. Paganini

INTRODUCTION

Acute renal failure (ARF), increasingly referred to as *acute kidney injury* (AKI), occurs in up to 30% of all intensive care unit (ICU) patients. Advances in the technology of organ support have led to extremely ill patients being aggressively supported and cared for by several specialists and subjected to more frequent and invasive interventions. In a closed ICU model, in which patient care is transferred to the intensivist, typically other specialists cannot directly prescribe therapy and can only recommend a course of treatment to the primary caregiver. Potential advantages of an intensivist-based management of ARF include immediate availability of service, cost containment, and decreased fragmentation of care.[1] Although the basic dialytic technologic expertise is easily acquired by the non-nephrologic staff, the nephrologist remains the specialist with the most experience and training pertaining to dialysis dosing, kidney design, dialysis mode, and membranes and their influence on drug kinetics. Moreover, ICU nephrology entails providing advice on fluid, acid-base, and electrolyte abnormalities. Overuse of extracorporeal techniques to achieve a goal that can be accomplished by the natural kidney has been the single most quoted point of contention between the nephrologist and other specialists. Overuse of extracorporeal techniques may compromise outcomes by exposing an unnecessary risk of procedures or may add to the cost of support where it was not needed. Therefore, timing or the appropriateness of initiation of renal replacement therapy (RRT) should be a joint decision with other members of the critical care team (multidisciplinary approach), led by a nephrologist. The latter is relevant in planning the continuity of care and dialytic support upon discharge of patients from the ICU.[2,3]

Complementary Training

Critical care specialists in the United States are brought through a broad and all-encompassing fellowship (Fig. 66.1). However, additional nephrology training gives a deeper understanding of the processes underlying renal dysfunction and their implications. Early consultation to nephrology has indeed been shown to improve patient outcome, principally owing to the added renal expertise brought earlier in the course of renal dysfunction.[4]

On the other hand, the presence of critical care physicians in the ICU offers distinct advantages to patient outcome and care. Their presence is continuous in many ICU situations and they are therefore able to respond immediately to a patient's need. They have a broader picture of the situation and can better correlate a variety of issues into a more coordinated approach. Ideally, a cooperative approach to patient care enhances the team concept in patients who frequently have multispecialty needs.

Critical care training core curriculum	
Physiology, pathology, pathophysiology, and therapy 　Respiratory 　Renal 　Central nervous system 　Infectious disease 　Hematology, oncology 　Gastrointestinal 　Genitourinary 　Obstetrics-gynecology	Procedural competence 　Airway, ventilation 　Circulation 　Central nervous system 　Renal 　Gastrointestinal 　Hematology 　Infection 　Metabolic, nutrition 　Trauma
Environmental hazards	Monitoring, bioengineering, statistics
Immunology, transplantation	Administration
Trauma	Pharmacokinetics

Figure 66.1　Critical care training core curriculum.

ACUTE RENAL INJURY IN THE INTENSIVE CARE UNIT PATIENT

Definition

Because of a lack of broadly accepted biomarkers of acute renal failure (ARF), renal dysfunction means different things to different groups. Volume control and renal clearance, but not renal cell injury, are frequently cited parameters of ARF. To successfully carry out and compare studies in patients with ARF, the RIFLE (risk, injury, loss, and end stage) criteria have been developed[5] (see Chapter 64, Fig. 64.1).

Treatment of Acute Renal Failure in the Intensive Care Unit Patient

Because of lack of prospective trials comparing alternative thresholds for initiation of dialysis, there can be wide variations between clinicians in different centers and even within the same center.

Initiation of RRT at lower levels of blood urea nitrogen (BUN; ≤80 vs. >80 mg/dl) suggested a survival benefit in a multicenter observational cohort of ICU patients, where BUN at time of therapy initiation was used as a proxy for the timing of dialysis initiation. However, BUN concentration is also a proxy for the degree of kidney injury, elevated catabolic state, bleeding, and parenteral nutrition. We advocate initiation of RRT when progressive azotemia is accompanied by inability to control electrolyte and acid-base balance, with less emphasis on absolute values of BUN or creatinine (Fig. 66.2). Moreover,

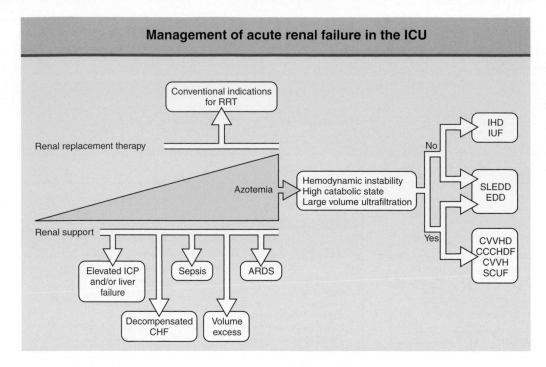

Management of acute renal failure in the ICU

Figure 66.2 Algorithm for acute renal failure management in the intensive care unit. Initiation of renal replacement therapy (RRT) may be based on azotemia (see text) or on the existence of comorbid conditions, which may necessitate earlier initiation in the form of renal support. ARDS, acute respiratory distress syndrome; CHF, congestive heart failure; CVVH(D, DF), continuous venovenous hemofiltration (hemodialysis, hemodiafiltration); EDD, extended daily dialysis; ICP, intracranial pressure; IHD, intermittent hemodialysis; IUF, isolated ultrafiltration; SCUF, slow continuous ultrafiltration; SLEDD, sustained low-efficiency daily dialysis.

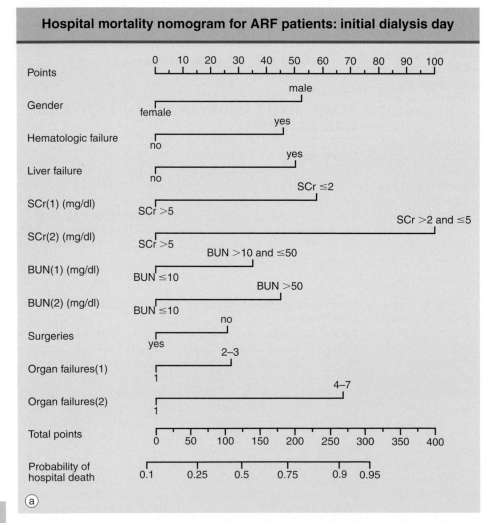

Hospital mortality nomogram for ARF patients: initial dialysis day

Figure 66.3 Mortality predictive scores at time of dialysis initiation and at day 5 of dialytic support.
1. Mark the value of each clinical predictor on its horizontal scale. (Note that the scale for the platelets begins on the bottom right and wraps over the top on the left as values increase.
2. At top is a line labeled "Points"; going directly above the locations marked on the individual variable scales to this topmost line gives the scores associated with each measure.
3. Mark the total of these scores on the "Total points" line (second from bottom).
4. The position directly below the bottom line gives the average probability of hospital mortality according to the model.
a, Liver failure: "yes" if bilirubin >2 mg/dl and SGOT >25 IU/l; hematologic failure: "yes" if platelets <50,000, leukocytes <2500, or bleeding diathesis; cardiac failure: "yes" if SBP <100 mm Hg requiring volume or pressors; respiratory failure: "yes" if requiring intubation/mechanical ventilation; gastrointestinal failure: "yes" if cholecystitis with perforation, bleeding requiring >2 units of blood in 24 hours, necrotizing enterocolitis, or necrotizing pancreatitis; neurologic failure: "yes" if severely disturbed consciousness (not induced by sedatives); vascular failure: "yes" if abdominal or thoracic aortic aneurysm, hypertension, or peripheral vascular disease.

there are instances in which extracorporeal support for other failing organs may be the driving force to initiate renal therapy, in the absence of traditional indications (see later discussion of Common Intensive Care Unit Conditions; see Fig. 66.2).

Survival benefit has not been demonstrated in several underpowered randomized clinical trials between intermittent hemodialysis (IHD) and continuous forms of renal replacement therapy (CRRT; see Chapter 87). An inherent difficulty of direct comparison of these modalities is the more prevalent use of continuous forms of therapy in patients with marked hemodynamic instability.

Continuous forms of RRT may be superior to IHD in solute clearance, hemodynamic stability, and ultrafiltration capacity. Continuous therapy is often feasible in patients requiring multiple and high doses of pressors (see Fig. 66.2). A distinct advantage of CRRT over IHD in the ICU setting is the capacity for ultrafiltration in patients with marginal systemic pressures, who often suffer from excess volume burden due to increased obligatory fluid intake resulting from nutritional demands, and liberal volume resuscitation resulting from sepsis or major surgery (see later discussion of Patients with Hypervolemia and Respiratory Failure). Solute clearance in CRRT (also to a certain extent in hybrid modalities) is more efficient than IHD due to better clearance when discrepancies in regional blood flow due to pressor use alter their single pool distribution.

Hybrid therapies (see Chapter 87), which combine the advantages of CRRT with the practicality of conventional IHD, have been increasingly popular in the recent years; however, data comparing outcomes with either CRRT or IHD are not available.

There are not yet sufficient data to develop evidence-based treatment guidelines for dialysis dose in ARF. An ongoing trial in the United States, the Acute Renal Failure Trial Network Study, examines survival in critically ill patients with ARF comparing usual to intensive dose dialysis, integrating IHD, sustained low-efficiency dialysis (SLED), and continuous venovenous hemodiafiltration.

Severity Scoring and Predictive Modeling

As discussed in Chapter 64, the presence of ARF in an ICU patient markedly worsens the outcome. Severity of illness indices are useful risk-stratifying tools for designing clinical trials and helpful prognostic indicators at the bedside in the detection of futile care. Generic severity score systems, such as the Acute Physiology and Chronic Health Evaluation III (APACHE III) and Simplified Acute Physiology Score (SAPS), do not accurately predict outcome in subjects with ARF. During the past decade, several ARF-specific scoring systems have been developed, but recent multicenter, multinational trial, the Beginning and Ending Supportive Therapy for the Kidney (BEST kidney), independently evaluated four ARF-specific and two generic scores with disappointing results.[6] Of note, a single lactate measurement at the time of enrollment had equivalent predictive power to the more sophisticated scoring systems.

Despite their limitations, we find severity scores clinically useful in two situations. First, they help in identifying patients undergoing fruitless renal support by objectively assessing the evolution of their clinical status overtime. We have used a series of predictive indicators that have been generated specifically at initiation of dialysis, day 5 of dialytic support, and day 10 of dialytic support (Fig. 66.3). This allows us to have frank

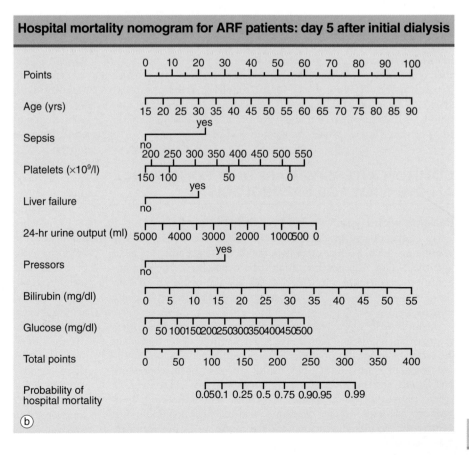

Figure 66.3, cont'd *b*, Liver failure: "yes" if either of the following:
1. Bilirubin >2 mg/dl and SGOT >25 IU/l
2. Bilirubin >1.5 mg/dl and/or [SGOT (2–3 × bl), SGPT (2–3 × normal)] (measured during current hospitalization up to time of consult)

Sepsis: "yes" if any of the following (measured at hospital admission and during ICU, except part 3, which is up to the time of consult):
1. Sepsis with presence of (+) blood culture and septic foci
2. Septic syndrome—fever or hypothermia, tachypnea, tachycardia, impaired organ system function or perfusion (i.e., altered mentation, hypoxemia, elevated lactate, oliguria, or clinical evidence of infection)
3. Sepsis (positive blood cultures and/or hemodynamic picture of sepsis, measured during current hospitalization up to time of consult)

Cleveland Clinic acute renal failure predictive score	
Risk Factor	**Points**
Female gender	1
Congestive heart failure	1
Left ventricular ejection fraction <35%	1
Preoperative use of IABP	2
COPD	1
Insulin-requiring diabetes	1
Previous cardiac surgery	1
Emergency surgery	2
Valve surgery only (reference to CABG)	1
CABG + valve (reference to CABG)	2
Other cardiac surgeries	2
Preoperative creatinine <1.2 mg/dl	0
Preoperative creatinine 1.2 to <2.1 mg/dl	2
Preoperative creatinine ≥2.1	5

Figure 66.4 Cleveland Clinic acute renal failure predictive score. Minimum score, 0; maximum score, 17. CABG, coronary artery bypass graft; COPD, chronic obstructive pulmonary disease; IABP, intra-aortic balloon pump.

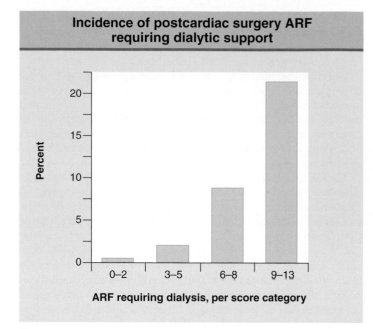

Figure 66.5 Incidence of postcardiac surgery acute renal failure (ARF) requiring dialytic support per Cleveland Clinic preoperative score. (See Fig. 66.4.)

discussions with family members and referring services regarding the continuation or cessation of dialytic support. (For further information, see www.bio.ri.ccf.org/arf.)

Second, in a more defined patient population, namely cardiac surgery, in which the timing of ARF is known, predictive modeling scores are extremely useful in the decision-making process. The Cleveland Clinic ARF predictive score, which has been validated in other cardiac surgery programs, utilizes preoperative indicators that characterize a patient in a population with a specific risk for postoperative acute renal injury requiring dialytic support (Figs. 66.4 and 66.5). Having this knowledge preoperatively may help to initiate protective maneuvers and avoid additional conditions or medications usually associated with ARF.

COMMON INTENSIVE CARE UNIT CONDITIONS: AN OVERVIEW FOR NEPHROLOGISTS

Patients with Hypervolemia and Respiratory Failure

Early in the course of ARF, salt and water retention results in volume overload. Moreover, depending on the definition of oliguria and the timing of assessment (at time of diagnosis, nephrology consultation, or initiation of RRT), and also the definition of ARF used, between 30% and 70% of patients with ARF in the ICU are oliguric.[7]

Intravascular volume assessment by physical examination is less informative in critically ill patients. Jugular-venous distention is not an accurate predictor of right ventricular filling pressures in the mechanically ventilated patient, in the setting of positive-pressure ventilation and positive end-expiratory pressure.[8] Moreover, in septic patients, baseline values of central venous pressure, pulmonary capillary wedge pressure, and echocardiographic left ventricular diastolic dimensions are inaccurate surrogates for intravascular volume status, particularly when they indicate that the

patient is well filled. A more reliable approach is to assess the effect of therapeutic maneuvers, such as fluid challenge, on filling pressures and stroke volume, and further adjust therapy accordingly. Respiratory changes in arterial pulse are good predictors of fluid responsiveness in septic patients on mechanical ventilation, provided they do not exhibit spontaneous breathing.[9,10] Perhaps the most accurate modality to assess fluid responsiveness in septic patients is measuring superior vena cava collapsibility obtained by routine bedside echocardiography.[10] Chest radiographic films provide invaluable information, such as enlarged heart or pulmonary interstitial edema.

Patients with extracellular fluid excess in the absence of intravascular hypervolemia may benefit from fluid removal if they develop abdominal compartment syndrome in which acute tense ascites may affect venous return, impairment of lung compliance and oxygenation, wound healing in postsurgical patients, prolonged ICU stay, and delay of ambulation. Traditionally, diuretics have been used in the early phases of oliguria to establish urine flow in order to better regulate volume status. However, diuretics improve neither survival nor renal recovery despite increased urine output (see Chapter 64).

Even when patients with moderate renal dysfunction and varying degrees of cardiac dysfunction are not oliguric, it still may be difficult to achieve a diuresis. In the event of diuretic resistance or intolerance due to worsening renal function, slow continuous ultrafiltration (SCUF) should be considered as an efficient alternative for nearly isotonic fluid removal. The latter could be achieved in patients with volume excess, in the setting of increased or even normal intravascular volume if the rate of removal is matched to that of vascular refill, with minimal effect on GFR.

Tissue edema has been known to decrease local blood flow and thus retard wound healing, as well as prevent adequate perfusion. Organ edema under these circumstances may also compromise function. Promoting fluid removal is a goal-directed use of aggressive diuretic administration or ultrafiltration either with or without a solute component to the therapy. Although the use of colloid to enhance the osmotic pull into the vascular system has been advocated by some, this approach has been a double-edged sword because it will also hold the fluid more tightly when presented to either membrane. Combination albumin-diuretics have met some success in the nephrotic syndrome patient, but have not been as successful in either the cirrhotic or the extravascular expanded subject with a serum albumin above 2.0 g/dl. Ongoing plasma volume analysis combined with slow yet continuous ultrafiltration has been the most effective approach.

Acute respiratory distress syndrome (ARDS) is defined as low arterial oxygen relative to high inspired oxygen, diffuse pulmonary infiltrates, and pulmonary capillary wedge pressure (PCWP) of less than 18 mm Hg. A recent randomized trial in patients with ARDS that compared liberal and conservative fluid management guided by central filling pressures (central venous pressure of 15–18 mm Hg vs. 9–13 mm Hg) mainly through diuresis, showed shorter duration of ventilatory support and ICU stay in the conservative group.[11] Ultrafiltration may reduce the accumulation of extravascular water by decreasing hydrostatic pressure in the lung, and by further reduction of the PCWP. However, the benefit of fluid removal in ARDS by means of CRRT or SCUF remains controversial.

Patients with Congestive Heart Failure

Congestive heart failure patients often present with low cardiac output, hypotension, sodium and water retention, diuretic resistance, and deterioration of renal function. Moreover, declining renal function precludes optimal management of heart failure and adversely influences the outcome of these patients. Diuretics, in conjunction with inotropes and afterload reducers, are the mainstay of therapy, often guided by filling pressures measured by pulmonary catheters. However, a significant proportion of patients do not diurese effectively despite optimization of cardiac function, persistent elevation of filling pressures, and volume overload over several days of ICU stay; continuous elevation in creatinine and BUN in this setting defines the "cardiorenal syndrome." SCUF, if maintained at a rate equal to the capillary refill rate, is an effective alternative to conventional therapy, with the added benefits of maintaining hemodynamic stability, and arguably is less nephrotoxic when compared with diuretics.[12] In recent years, there has been increasing use of ultrafiltration not only for patients who are refractory to diuresis but also as the first line of therapy (Fig. 66.6). Ultrafiltration, unlike diuretic use, achieves sustained decreases in various components of the neurohormonal axis, that is, norepinephrine, plasma renin activity, and aldosterone concentrations.[13,14] A recent randomized clinical trial showed that ultrafiltration was beneficial compared with intravenous diuretics for fluid removal in patients hospitalized for acute decompensated heart failure; decreased hospitalization in subjects receiving ultrafiltration became evident by a month after acute therapy without causing hypokalemia or untoward renal effects. Nevertheless, until further confirmation of these results, accompanied ideally with evidence of survival benefit, we reserve ultrafiltration for patients with large volume excess who prove refractory to diuresis or are at high risk for complications.

Patients with Lactic Acidosis

Lactic acid produced daily is buffered by HCO_3 to form sodium lactate. Subsequently, the liver restores the HCO_3 by oxidizing lactate, and achieving normal plasma lactate concentrations. Refractory causes of lactic acidosis in the ICU are typically due to

tissue hypoxia induced by circulatory failure, pulmonary failure, or restoration of ischemic areas. However, in patients with sepsis, the main source of lactate production is reported to be through exaggerated aerobic glycolysis rather than tissue hypoxia.[15]

In patients with critical circulatory compromise, the hypercapnia and acidemia at the level of the tissues are detected better in central venous blood rather than arterial blood gases due to large arteriovenous differences; arterial blood gases reflect pulmonary gas exchange.[16] The buildup of carbon dioxide is partly due to the buffering of the excess hydrogen ions by the bicarbonate administration in patients with compromised pulmonary blood flow. It has been suggested that acidosis will adversely affect cardiac contractility by reducing intracellular pH. On the other hand, bicarbonate administration has been proposed to worsen the intracellular acidosis due to the rise of P_{CO_2} and to compromise myocardial contractility due to lowering plasma ionized calcium.[17]

Therefore, the only effective treatment for lactic acidosis is improving tissue oxygenation to prevent acid production. Bicarbonate supplementation in patients with lactic acidosis and renal failure can result in volume overload, hypernatremia, and rebound metabolic alkalosis. Various means of bicarbonate supplementation, including tromethamine (tris-hydroxymethyl aminomethane [THAM]; trometanol), $NaHCO_3$, and dichloroacetate, have been used as temporizing measures, with disappointing results in clinical outcomes.[18,19]

CRRT is an attractive alternative in patients who would not tolerate the obligatory volume needed for bicarbonate administration. Bicarbonate-based hemofiltration has been suggested for the combination of ARF and lactic acidosis; however, lactate clearance compared with plasma clearance is <3% (at dialysate flow rate of 1 l/hour).[20] Lactate clearance through hemofiltration is about equal to the ultrafiltrate quantity (see Chapter 83). Subsequently, lactate clearance through hemofiltration will be in the range of 40 ml/min (at higher doses of hemofiltration—35 ml/kg/hour), much lower than the total plasma clearance and lactate production rate.[20] On the other hand, the controlled volume status and tonicity achieved with hemofiltration may allow a separate infusion of sodium bicarbonate.

Patients with Liver Failure

Patients with advanced hepatic failure frequently suffer from renal dysfunction, most commonly due to hepatorenal syndrome, ischemic injury, or nephrotoxic drugs (see Chapter 67). These patients have increased cardiac output, with low systemic vascular resistance, compounded by tissue hypoxia due to shunting of blood that results in further compromise in end-organ function.[21] Typically, they are cardiovascularly unstable. In addition, patients with advanced chronic hepatic failure and acute hepatic failure develop cerebral edema due to intracellular edema (excess circulating ammonia is converted to glutamine in astrocytes that exerts osmotic potential) and cerebrovascular vasodilation, which results in increased cerebral blood volume.[22] Other challenges in patients with decompensated liver failure include issues related to vascular access due to their bleeding diathesis, and susceptibility to infections (see Chapter 87).

Although CRRT is not a substitute for a failing liver, it remains the best support available as a bridge to urgent liver transplantation by allowing for the correction of hyponatremia, controlling volume, allowing space for nutrition, and reducing cerebral edema by means of solute control and ultrafiltration. Continuous therapy is preferred to achieve cardiovascular and intracranial stability in these critically ill patients[23] (see Chapter 87).

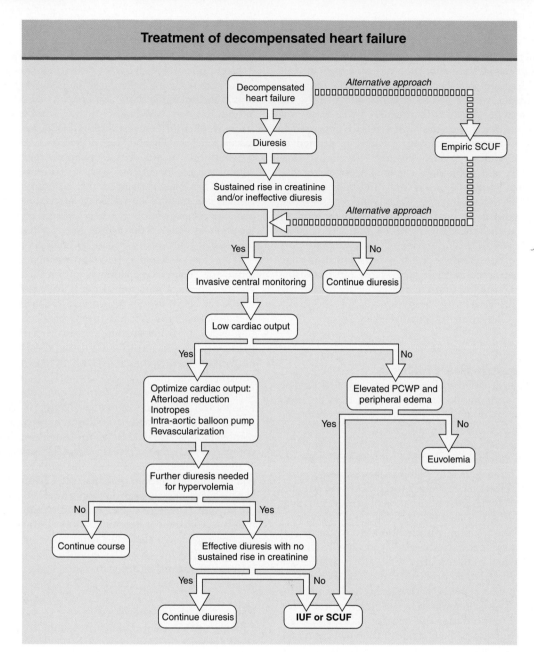

Figure 66.6 **Algorithm for the treatment of decompensated heart failure.** IUF, isolated ultrafiltration; PCWP, pulmonary capillary wedge pressure; SCUF, slow continuous ultrafiltration.

Patients with Cerebral Edema

Compromised renal function in the setting of elevated intracranial pressure (ICP) may hamper induction of a diuresis. The use of mannitol, in intermittent boluses to reduce ICP, can be problematic in oliguric patients (see Chapter 64). Circulating mannitol eventually diffuses to the brain tissue and exacerbates interstitial edema. Plasma osmolality should be closely monitored during CRRT, which does not readily clear mannitol. CRRT by virtue of its efficiency in fluid removal, without causing large variations in ICP and osmolality, is a useful modality in the volume overloaded and oliguric patient.

Patients Receiving Multiple Pressors

Vasopressin when titrated to the same mean arterial pressure (MAP) compared with norepinephrine is associated with higher GFR and urine output due to its preferential efferent arteriolar vasoconstriction. Despite its promising renal effects, the routine use of vasopressin in patients with septic shock needs further evaluation because of adverse events in other vascular beds (see Chapter 64). In critically ill patients with obligatory fluid intake and relative oliguria who are supported by multiple pressors, volume overload often precedes significant azotemia by several days (see Fig. 66.2).

NONUREMIC EXTRACORPOREAL THERAPY

Application of renal extracorporeal therapies to support nonrenal organ dysfunctions has been popular during the past decade.[24,25] These include sepsis and other inflammatory syndromes, such as acute respiratory distress syndrome, and refractory congestive heart failure.

Ultrafiltration techniques for fluid removal were outlined earlier. Some ultrafilters require a central access and blood flow rates above 100 ml/min, whereas others have been designed to work off peripheral access sites and at lower blood flow rates (10–40 ml/min). The lower the blood flow rate, the more porous the membrane to allow for fluid loss. As the membrane becomes more porous, the character of the fluid will also change. The "tighter" the membrane, the closer to plasma water; whereas the more porous, the more of the larger elements will cross into the ultrafiltrate. Over a short period, this may not have major consequences. Applied over a longer period, more substantial losses of albumin and amino acids may become problematic. Avoiding a central catheter altogether, or utilizing a peripherally inserted central line, has the advantage of lower complications and potential for use on regular hospital wards. Thus, ultrafiltration techniques that can be applied earlier and outside of specialized units may actually avoid the need for ICU transfer and thus lower both hospital costs and ICU bed utilization.

Overly aggressive fluid removal will also have significant negative effects. Intravascular depletion can compromise blood flow to other organs and thus create dysfunction based purely on hemodynamic factors. The use of intravascular monitoring can be accomplished either through central monitoring or by using measures of changes in the relative volume of plasma by measuring the hematocrit difference during ultrafiltration. This latter technique also avoids central catheter placement and uses the already exposed blood flow through the circuit to constantly measure the changing hematocrit, with the reciprocal change being used as the relative plasma volume status.

Another area of intense study for the application of dialytic techniques is in patients with sepsis. Originally observed to have a beneficial effect on the hemodynamics of patients in septic shock, continuous hemofiltration was quickly used with the theoretical advantage of cytokine removal. For example, work with a highly charged membrane (i.e., modified acrylonitrile) was thought to have absorption properties that might be used in cytokine control. A use of polymyxin B as an embedded substance in noncuprophane membranes has also shown promise in controlling endotoxin levels. This technique is currently in use in Japan and under clinical investigation in the United States for therapy in early sepsis and acute lung injury.

Another evolving technique is high-volume hemofiltration in septic shock. The observation of improved patient outcome with higher doses of hemofiltration (45 ml/kg/hour) among septic patients with ARF over the already high dose of 35 ml/kg/hour delivered to nonseptic patients with ARF stimulated several attempts at ultra-high-dose delivery with continuous hemofiltration techniques in nonrenal septic patients. Applied either as a "pulse" maneuver (100 ml/kg/hour × 8 hours) from a basis of 45 ml/kg/hour continuous venovenous hemofiltration (CVVH) or as a continuous ultra-high dose (60–100 ml/kg/hour), early results appear to show improved hemodynamic stability, but outcome data are still not well established.

The idea of cytokine removal either by adsorption or clearance has not been universally accepted. Until a reported dramatic decrease in patient mortality or a positive result from a prospective, adequately powered randomized study is established, this approach should be considered experimental.

In the United States and some other countries, the resistance of nephrology to become involved in these and other types of investigational maneuvers has widened the divide between intensivists and nephrologists. Nephrology expertise is not utilized by critical care practitioners, and the advances of nonrenal applications of dialytic techniques are resisted by the nephrology community.

Other Special Situations

Renal replacement therapy faces a particular dilemma in bleeding ICU patients, early postoperative patients, and patients with heparin-induced thrombocytopenia (HIT). In the former, regional anticoagulation of the extracorporeal circuit should be considered (see Chapter 87). Measures to counteract the uremic bleeding tendency, as well as alternatives to heparin, in chronic kidney disease patients with HIT type II are discussed in Chapter 73.

REFERENCES

1. Bellomo R, Cole L, Reeves J, Silvester W: Who should manage CRRT in the ICU? The intensivist's viewpoint. Am J Kidney Dis 1997;30(Suppl 4):S109–111.
2. Paganini EP: Continuous renal replacement therapy: A nephrological technique, managed by nephrology. Semin Dial 1996;9:200–203.
3. Yagi N, Paganini EP: Acute dialysis and continuous renal replacement: The emergence of new technology involving the nephrologist in the intensive care setting. Semin Nephrol 1997;17:406–420.
4. Mehta RL, McDonald B, Gabbai F, et al: Nephrology consultation in acute renal failure: Does timing matter? Am J Med 2002;113:56–61.
5. Bellomo R, Ronco C, Kellum JA, et al: Acute renal failure—definition, outcome measures, animal models, fluid therapy and information technology needs: The second international consensus conference of the acute dialysis quality initiative (ADQI) group. Crit Care 2004;8:204–212.
6. Uchino S, Kellum JA, Bellomo R, et al: Acute renal failure in critically ill patients: A multinational, multicenter study. JAMA 2005;294:13–18.
7. Mehta RL, Pascual MT, Soroko S, et al: Spectrum of acute renal failure in the intensive care unit: The PICARD experience. Kidney Int 2004; 66:613–621.
8. McGee SR: Physical examination of venous pressure: A critical review. Am Heart J 1998;136:10–18.
9. Michard F, Boussat S, Chemla D, et al: Relation between respiratory changes in arterial pulse pressure and fluid responsiveness in septic patients with acute circulatory failure. Am J Respir Crit Care Med 2000;162:34–38.
10. Vieillard-Baron A, Chergui K, Rabiller A, et al: Superior vena caval collapsibility as a gauge of volume status in ventilated septic patients. Intens Care Med 2004;30:734–739.
11. National Heart, Lung, and Blood Institute Acute Respiratory Distress Syndrome (ARDS) Clinical Trials Network: Pulmonary-artery versus central venous catheter to guide treatment of acute lung injury. N Engl J Med 2006;354:2213–2224.

12. Marenzi G, Lauri G, Guazzi M, et al: Cardiac and renal dysfunction in chronic heart failure: Relation to neurohumoral activation and prognosis. Am J Med Sci 2001;321:59–66.

13. Agostoni PG, Marenzi GC: Sustained benefit from ultrafiltration in moderate congestive heart failure. Cardiology 2001;96:83–89.

14. Clark WR, Paganini E, Weinstein D, et al: Extracorporeal ultrafiltration for acute exacerbations of chronic heart failure: Report from the acute dialysis quality initiative. Int J Artif Organs 2005;28:66–76.

15. Levy B, Gibot S, Franck P, et al: Relation between muscle Na$^+$K$^+$ ATPase activity and raised lactate concentrations in septic shock: A prospective study. Lancet 2005;365:871–875.

16. Mathias DW, Clifford PS, Klopfenstein HS: Mixed venous blood gases are superior to arterial blood gases in assessing acid-base status and oxygenation during acute cardiac tamponade in dogs. J Clin Invest 1988;82:33–38.

17. Lang RM, Fellner SK, Neumann A, et al: Left ventricular contractility varies directly with blood ionized calcium. Ann Intern Med 1988;108:24–29.

18. Cooper DJ, Walley KR, Wiggs BR, Russell JA: Bicarbonate does not improve hemodynamics in critically ill patients who have lactic acidosis: A prospective, controlled clinical study. Ann Intern Med 1990;112:92–98.

19. Stacpoole PW, Wright EC, Baumgartner TG, et al: A controlled clinical trial of dichloroacetate for treatment of lactic acidosis in adults: The dichloroacetate-lactic acidosis study group. N Engl J Med 1992;327:564–569.

20. Levraut JMD, Ciebiera J-MD, Jambou PMD, et al: Effect of continuous venovenous hemofiltration with dialysis on lactate clearance in critically ill patients. Crit Care Med 1997;25:58–62.

21. Wendon JA, Harrison PM, Keays R, et al: Effects of vasopressor agents and epoprostenol on systemic hemodynamics and oxygen transport in fulminant hepatic failure. Hepatology 1992;15:67–71.

22. Blei AT, Larsen FS: Pathophysiology of cerebral edema in fulminant hepatic failure. J Hepatol 1999;31:71–76.

23. Davenport A, Will EJ, Davidson AM: Improved cardiovascular stability during continuous modes of renal replacement therapy in critically ill patients with acute hepatic and renal failure. Crit Care Med 1993;21:28–38.

24. Schetz MR: Classical and alternative indications for continuous renal replacement therapy. Kidney Int Suppl 1998;66:S129–S132.

25. Schetz M: Non-renal indications for continuous renal replacement therapy. Kidney Int Suppl 1999;72:88–94.

Hepatorenal Syndrome

Ignatius K. P. Cheng and Felix F. K. Li

INTRODUCTION AND DEFINITION

Hepatorenal syndrome (HRS) is a reversible and functional renal failure that occurs in patients with acute or chronic liver disease, advanced hepatic failure, and portal hypertension. It is characterized by impaired renal function and marked abnormalities in the arterial circulation and endogenous vasoactive systems. In the kidney, there is pronounced vasoconstriction resulting in low glomerular filtration rate (GFR). In the splanchnic circulation, there is a predominance of arteriolar vasodilation, resulting in reduction of systemic vascular resistance and arterial hypotension.[1] Two forms of HRS can be identified based on the progression of the disease (Fig. 67.1). An acute form (type 1) is characterized by a rapid deterioration in renal function, whereas a chronic form (type 2) is marked by an insidious onset and a slowly progressive course.

Oliguric renal failure in advanced liver disease in the absence of significant histologic renal changes was first described by Austin Flint in 1863. However, the existence of HRS was not generally accepted until the detailed description by Hecker and Sherlock in the 1950s. The functional nature of the renal failure was established by studies that showed that such kidneys function normally after being transplanted into patients with chronic renal failure and that renal failure is rapidly reversed after successful orthotopic liver transplantation (OLT).

Pseudohepatorenal Syndrome

Pseudohepatorenal syndrome describes concurrent hepatic and renal dysfunction secondary to a wide variety of infectious, systemic, circulatory, genetic, and other diseases and after exposure to a variety of drugs and toxins. In these conditions, the liver does not play an etiologic role in the pathogenesis of renal failure, and they must be excluded before the diagnosis of HRS can be established.

ETIOLOGY AND PATHOGENESIS

The renal and systemic hemodynamic changes that occur in HRS result from complex interactions of multiple neurohumoral disturbances. HRS most likely represents one end of the spectrum of homeostatic abnormalities that accompany liver failure and portal hypertension.[2]

Renal and Systemic Hemodynamic Changes

In HRS, reduction in GFR occurs mainly as a result of renal cortical hypoperfusion following intense cortical renal vasoconstriction. The latter can be demonstrated angiographically as marked beading and tortuosity of the interlobular and proximal arcuate arteries and the absence of a distinct cortical nephrogram and vascular filling of the cortical vessels[3] (Fig. 67.2). The vasomotor abnormality in HRS is variable with time. Intense renal vasoconstriction occurs in the presence of splanchnic vasodilation. The latter gives rise to a low peripheral vascular resistance and a low systemic mean arterial blood pressure (MAP). This further compromises renal perfusion because intense renal vasoconstriction results in blunting of the autoregulation of renal blood flow, so that renal perfusion becomes more pressure dependent. In HRS, filtration fraction is also reduced, reflecting a dominant increase in afferent arteriolar tone and a decrease in the ultrafiltration coefficient. Serial systemic hemodynamic studies showed that HRS occurs in the setting of reduced MAP, cardiac output, wedge pulmonary pressure, and hepatic venous pressure. These findings suggest that the inability of the heart to increase its output to compensate for a decrease in cardiac preload also significantly contributes to the pathogenesis of HRS.[4]

Neurohumoral Abnormalities

A multitude of neurohumoral abnormalities characterize HRS. The sympathetic nervous system (SNS) is activated, and the sympathetic discharges through the renal nerves are markedly increased. Abnormalities in the plasma and urinary levels of a number of endogenous vasoactive substances are also observed (Figs. 67.3 and 67.4). Most of the neurohumoral abnormalities found in HRS are also detected, albeit to a lesser extent, in decompensated cirrhosis (with ascites) with normal renal function and in compensated cirrhosis (without ascites). This supports the hypothesis that HRS represents one end of the spectrum of homeostatic abnormalities that occur in liver failure and portal hypertension.

Definition of hepatorenal syndrome type 1 and type 2
Type 1 Hepatorenal Syndrome
Doubling of serum creatinine >2.5 mg/dl (220 μmol/l) or a 50% reduction in 24-hr creatinine clearance to <20 ml/min <2 wk
Frequently follows a precipitating event such as infection
Survival without treatment in the order of weeks
Type 2 Hepatorenal Syndrome
Less rapid renal functional deterioration than type 1
Mainly presents with refractory ascites
Survival without treatment in order of months

Figure 67.1   Definition of hepatorenal syndrome type 1 and 2.

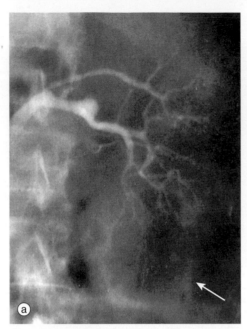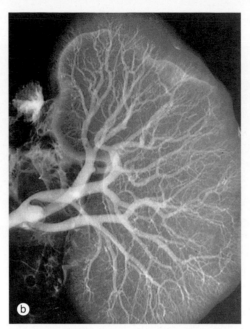

Figure 67.2 Hepatorenal syndrome (HRS). *a*, Renal angiogram (the *arrow* marks the edge of the kidney). *b*, The angiogram carried out in the same kidney at autopsy. Note complete filling of the renal arterial system throughout the vascular bed to the periphery of the cortex. The vascular attenuation and tortuosity seen previously (*a*) is no longer present. The vessels are also histologically normal. This indicates the functional nature of the vascular abnormality in HRS. (From Epstein M, Berk DP, Hollenberg NK, et al: Renal failure in the patient with cirrhosis: The role of active vasoconstriction. Am J Med 1970;49:175–185.)

Summary of Pathogenetic Events

Figure 67.5 is a simplified diagram of the pathogenetic events that lead to HRS.[5,6] Liver failure and portal hypertension increase vascular production of vasodilators in the splanchnic circulation, leading to the initiating event of splanchnic arteriolar vasodilation (the *peripheral arterial vasodilation hypothesis*). The vasodilators involved include nitric oxide, glucagons and other gut hormones, prostacyclin, and possibly false neurotransmitters (e.g., octopamine). Splanchnic vasodilation decreases arterial filling and reduces the effective arterial blood volume. The subsequent

stimulation of the central volume receptors leads to compensatory increases in arginine-vasopressin, in hormones of the renin angiotensin aldosterone system (RAAS), and in SNS activities, including increase in hormones of the SNS (norepinephrine and neuropeptide Y), which help to restore effective arterial blood volume. This restoration is achieved in patients with compensated cirrhosis but not in patients with decompensated cirrhosis. In the latter group of patients, progressive splanchnic arteriolar

Endogenous vasomotor substances in plasma in cirrhosis and hepatorenal syndrome			
Vasomotor Substances	Compensated Cirrhosis	Cirrhosis with Ascites	Hepatorenal Syndrome
Vasodilators			
Endotoxin	↔	↑	↑↑
Nitrite, nitrate	↑	↑↑	↑↑
Glucagon	↑	↑	↑↑
Vasoconstrictors			
Renin activity	↔↓	↑	↑↑
Norepinephrine	↔↓	↑	↑↑
Neuropeptide Y	↔	↔	↑
Vasopressin	↔	↑	↑↑
Platelet-activating factor	↔	↑	↑
Endothelin	↔	↑	↑↑
Isoprostanes (F_2)	↔	↔	↑

Figure 67.3 Endogenous vasomotor substances in plasma in cirrhosis and hepatorenal syndrome. (From Badalamenti S, Graziani G, Salerno F, et al: Hepatorenal syndrome: New perspectives in pathogenesis and treatment. Arch Intern Med 1993;153:1957–1967.)

Endogenous vasoactive substances in the urine in cirrhosis and hepatorenal syndrome			
Vasomotor Substances	Compensated Cirrhosis	Cirrhosis with Ascites	Hepatorenal Syndrome
Vasodilators			
Kallikrein	↔	↑	↓
Prostaglandin E_2	↔	↑	↓
6-Keto-$PGF_{1\alpha}$, a stable metabolite of renal prostacyclin	↔	↑	↓
2,3-Dinor-6-keto-$PGF_{1\alpha}$ (PG_1-M), a stable metabolite of systemic prostacyclin	↑	↑	↑
Vasoconstrictors			
Thromboxane β_2, a stable metabolite of thromboxane A_2	↔	↑	?
Leukotrienes	↔	↑	↑

Figure 67.4 Endogenous vasoactive substances in the urine in cirrhosis and hepatorenal syndrome. (From Badalamenti S, Graziani G, Salerno F, et al: Hepatorenal syndrome: New perspectives in pathogenesis and treatment. Arch Intern Med 1993;153:1957–1967.)

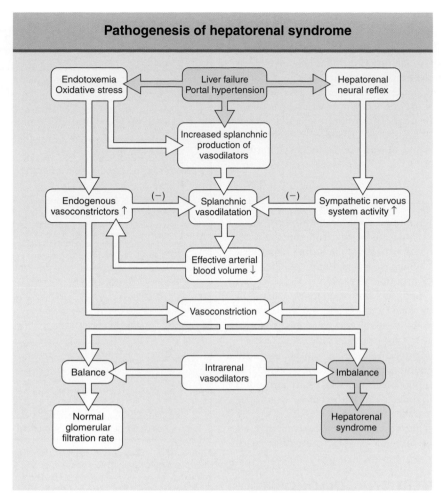

Pathogenesis of hepatorenal syndrome

Figure 67.5 The pathogenesis of hepatorenal syndrome.

vasodilation leads to increased splanchnic capillary pressure resulting in an increase in lymph formation, which exceeds reabsorption capacity. In parallel, contraction of the effective arterial blood volume leads to a reduction in systemic MAP and further stimulation of arginine-vasopressin, RAAS, and SNS, resulting in sodium and water retention. The net result of these combined effects is continuous ascites formation (the *forward theory of ascites formation*). The renal SNS activity is further enhanced by stimulation of the hepatorenal neural reflex arc as portal hypertension progresses. Progressive liver failure and portal hypertension through endotoxemia and oxidant stress also increase circulating or locally produced renal vasoconstrictors. These are thought to lead to the progressive renal vasoconstriction that characterizes HRS. Normally, the effect of renal vaso-constrictors is counterbalanced by the reactive production of intrarenal vasodilators. It is postulated that HRS develops when the balance of activities between the renal vasoconstrictors and intrarenal vasodilators finally breaks down. The likelihood that this will occur increases with progressive or acute deterioration in liver function or increasing severity of portal hypertension (e.g., following acute alcoholic hepatitis) and is precipitated by events that lead to further volume contraction and reduction of the effective arterial blood volume (see later discussion). The inability of the cirrhotic heart to respond to a reduction in cardiac preload after some of these acute effects also predisposes to the development of HRS.

EPIDEMIOLOGY

The possibility of developing HRS in the cirrhotic patient is estimated at 18% at 1 year and 39% at 5 years.[7] Neither the etiology nor the Child-Pugh score (http://homepage.mac.com/sholland/contrivances/childpugh.html) predict the incidence of HRS. Rather, independent predictors of HRS include low serum sodium concentration, high serum renin activity, absence of hepatomegaly,[7] abnormal renal duplex Doppler ultrasonography (resistive index >0.7),[8] and low cardiac output.[4]

CLINICAL MANIFESTATIONS

Type 1 HRS is characterized by a rapid decline in renal function and is most often observed in patients suffering from acute liver failure, acute alcoholic hepatitis, or acute decompensation on a back-ground of cirrhosis[1] (see Fig. 67.1). This group of patients tends to have severe hyperbilirubinemia, prolongation of prothrombin time, hyponatremia, and clinical evidence of portal hypertension and hepatic encephalopathy. Arterial blood pressure is usually low. Acute decompensation in type 1 HRS may be precipitated by bacterial infections (including spontaneous bacterial peritonitis), gastrointestinal bleeding, vigorous diuretic therapy, abdominal paracentesis, or the administration of substances such as non-steroidal anti-inflammatory drugs (NSAIDs) that further suppress intrarenal generation of vasodilators (e.g., prostaglandins). Left untreated, it tends to run a rapid and progressive downhill course resulting in death of the patient within weeks.

Type 2 HRS is characterized by insidious onset and slowly progressive deterioration of renal function. This is most often observed in patients with decompensated cirrhosis and portal hypertension. This group of patients tends to be less severely jaundiced and has refractory ascites. Low-normal arterial blood pressure, modest prolongation of prothrombin time, and hyponatremia are usually present. It tends to run a slowly progressive downhill course over months and most likely reflects the natural course of the disease.[2,6]

PATHOLOGY

HRS is by definition a functional renal disorder, and the presence of significant glomerular and tubular pathology excludes the diagnosis. However, glomerular abnormalities, including mesangial expansion, capillary wall thickening, mesangial and capillary wall electron-dense deposits, and immune deposits of C3 and the immunoglobulins IgA, IgM, and IgG are frequently found in cirrhotic patients with normal renal function and minimal urinary abnormalities. The presence of such glomerular abnormalities in a cirrhotic patient, therefore, does not exclude the diagnosis of HRS. Protrusion of the proximal tubular epithelium into Bowman's space (glomerulotubular reflux) is not specific for HRS, and is found in other conditions associated with profound renal ischemia and terminal hypotension. Although early autopsy studies demonstrate normal tubular morphology in patients dying from HRS, recent detailed light and electron microscopic studies have documented proximal tubular lesions consistent with ischemic injury.

DIAGNOSIS AND DIFFERENTIAL DIAGNOSIS

The diagnostic criteria for HRS were established by the International Ascites Club in 1996[1] and are now widely used (Fig. 67.6). The diagnosis of HRS is mainly one of exclusion (see major criteria, Fig. 67.6) although measurement of urinary electrolytes and osmolarity and plasma sodium may provide supportive evidence for the diagnosis.

HRS should be suspected in any patient with acute or chronic liver disease with advanced liver failure and portal hypertension who develops progressive renal insufficiency. Significant renal insufficiency may be present despite a normal serum creatinine or blood urea nitrogen (BUN) because these patients are frequently malnourished, with reduced lean body mass, and often have a low urea generation rate because of liver failure and low protein intake. Severe hyperbilirubinemia, which is often present in patients with HRS, interferes with the Jaffe reaction for creatinine quantification and may cause falsely low results. Creatinine assays employing creatininase or creatinine deaminase in the presence of bilirubin oxidase are less susceptible to high bilirubin levels. In cases of uncertainty, GFR may be assessed using serum cystatin C, ^{125}I-iothalamate, ^{51}Cr-labeled EDTA, or inulin clearance.[9]

Pseudohepatorenal syndrome (Fig. 67.7)[10] is usually easy to exclude because the etiologic agent is frequently known and both renal and liver functional abnormalities are often found at first clinical presentation, when evidence of advanced liver failure and portal hypertension is usually not initially present. In contrast, HRS invariably occurs after liver failure and portal hypertension are fully established and frequently develops when the patient is undergoing treatment for these conditions or their complications.

Diagnostic criteria for hepatorenal syndrome
Major Criteria
Chronic or acute liver disease with advanced hepatic failure and portal hypertension
Low glomerular filtration rate, as indicated by serum creatinine >1.5 mg/dl (133 μmol/l) or 24-hr creatinine clearance <40 ml/min
Absence of shock, ongoing bacterial infection, and current or recent treatment with nephrotoxic drugs
Absence of gastrointestinal fluid losses (repeated vomiting or intense diarrhea)
Absence of renal fluid losses in response to diuretic therapy (weight loss >500 g/day for several days in patients with ascites without peripheral edema or 1000 g/day in patients with peripheral edema)
No sustained improvement in renal function (decrease in serum creatinine to ≤1.5 mg/dl [133 μmol/l] or increase in creatinine clearance to >40 ml/min) after diuretic withdrawal and expansion of plasma volume with 1.5 liters of isotonic saline
Proteinuria <500 mg/day and no ultrasonographic evidence of obstructive uropathy or parenchymal renal disease
Additional Criteria
Urine volume <500 ml/day
Urine sodium <10 mmol/l
Urine osmolality greater than plasma osmolality
Urine red blood cells <50 per high-power field
Serum sodium concentration <130 mmol/l

Figure 67.6 Diagnostic criteria for hepatorenal syndrome. (Modified from Arroyo V, Gines P, Gerbes AL, et al: Definition and diagnostic criteria of refractory ascites and hepatorenal syndrome in cirrhosis. International Ascites Club. Hepatology 1996;23:164–176.)

In patients with pre-existing liver failure and portal hypertension, nephrotoxic agents (e.g., NSAIDs or aminoglycosides) must be stopped, and conditions leading to renal failure must be excluded by careful history, physical examination, urine examination, and ultrasonography before the diagnosis of HRS can be considered. The absence of shock, gastrointestinal bleeding, bacterial infection (especially spontaneous bacterial peritonitis), and excess gastrointestinal, peritoneal, or renal fluid loss must also be documented. Prerenal azotemia must be excluded by withdrawal of diuretics and fluid challenge (1.5 liters of isotonic saline or 100 g of albumin in 500 ml saline). The presence of oliguria <500 ml, urine sodium <10 mmol/l, urine osmolarity greater than plasma osmolarity, urinary red blood cells <50 per high-power field, and urinary protein <500 mg/l helps to exclude significant coexisting glomerular or tubulointerstitial disease leading to renal failure and supports the diagnosis of HRS. A low plasma sodium is often present in patients with HRS. The absence of debris or casts in the urine sediment is not a diagnostic criterion because they may appear late in the course of HRS owing to ischemic tubular injury.

NATURAL HISTORY

The prognosis of HRS is extremely poor. Without OLT, the median survival rate for type 1 HRS is only about 2 weeks, whereas that of type 2 HRS is about 6 months.[7] Recovery of renal function coincides with recovery of liver function and liver regeneration and follows therapeutic intervention. Renal failure

Causes of pseudohepatorenal syndrome		
Potential Causes	Predominantly Tubulointerstitial Involvement	Predominantly Glomerular Involvement
Infections	Sepsis, leptospirosis, brucellosis, tuberculosis, Epstein-Barr virus, hepatitis B virus	Hepatitis B and C viruses, HIV infection, *Schistosoma mansoni*, liver abscess
Drugs	Tetracycline, rifampin (rifampicin), sulfonamide, phenytoin, allopurinol, fluroxene, methotrexate (high dose), acetaminophen (overdose)	
Toxins	Carbon tetrachloride, trichloroethylene, chloroform, elemental phosphorus, arsenic, copper, chromium, barium, amatoxins,* raw carp bile toxins†	
Systemic disease	Sarcoidosis, Sjögren's syndrome	Systemic lupus erythematosus, vasculitis, cryoglobulinemia, amyloidosis
Circulatory failure	Hypovolemic or cardiogenic shock	
Malignancy	Lymphoma, leukemia	
Congenital and genetic disorders	Polycystic liver and kidney disease, nephronophthisis, and congenital hepatic fibrosis	
Miscellaneous	Fatty liver of pregnancy, Reye's syndrome	Eclampsia, HELLP syndrome, cirrhotic glomerulopathy

Figure 67.7 Causes of pseudohepatorenal syndrome. *Accidental poisoning after ingestion of mushroom of the *Amanita* genus. †Accidental poisoning after ingestion of the raw gallbladder or bile of the grass carp (a common practice in rural East Asia). (Adapted from Levenson D, Korecki KL: Acute renal failure associated with hepatobiliary disease. In Brenner BM, Lazarus JM [eds]: Acute Renal Failure. New York, Churchill Livingstone, 1988, pp 535–580.)

is infrequently an immediate cause of death, and most patients succumb to the other complications of liver failure and portal hypertension, such as hepatic encephalopathy, gastrointestinal bleeding, and sepsis. Despite this, renal failure refractory to therapy is an important determinant of outcome.[11,12]

TREATMENT

Preventive Measures

If one accepts the hypothesis that HRS represents one end of the spectrum of the homeostatic abnormalities in liver failure and portal hypertension and is precipitated by such events as volume contraction, sepsis, or the administration of potential nephrotoxic agents, it follows that a major focus of treatment must be to avoid the occurrence of such events, to have high awareness of their existence, and to treat them promptly when they occur. In patients with decompensated liver disease, the common

events that lead to volume contraction include gastrointestinal bleeding, injudicious use of lactulose (for treatment of hepatic encephalopathy) resulting in profuse diarrhea, and excessive diuretic therapy or paracentesis for the treatment of ascites. To avoid the last, a stepwise approach for the treatment of ascites is recommended.[2] All patients are advised to have bed rest and to follow a low-sodium diet (60–90 mmol/day, equivalent to about 1.5–2 g of salt per day). Following this, spironolactone is prescribed at increasing doses (100 mg/day as initial dosages; if there is no response within 4 days, 200 mg/day; if no further response, 400 mg/day). When there is no response to the highest dose of spironolactone, furosemide is added at increasing dosages every 2 days (40–160 mg/day). In diuretic resistance cases, therapeutic paracentesis, when combined with plasma volume expansion using albumin (8 g/l of ascites removed), is helpful and is associated with a low incidence of circulatory dysfunction after treatment. The threshold for antibiotic therapy for suspected sepsis should be low. Spontaneous bacterial peritonitis must be excluded by regular examination of ascites fluid and treated not only with broad-spectrum antibiotics but also with albumin infusion (1.5 g/kg initially and 1 g/kg 2 days later) because the latter has been shown to prevent the subsequent development of HRS.[13] The use of potentially nephrotoxic agents, including angiotensin-converting enzyme (ACE) inhibitors, NSAIDs, aminoglycosides, and radiologic contrast media, should be avoided as far as possible. Therapeutic agents (e.g., β-blockers and somatostatin) that are employed for the treatment of bleeding esophageal and gastric varices reduce GFR, and their use must be monitored carefully. Finally, there is evidence to suggest that prophylactic use of pentoxifylline (400 mg orally three times per day) prevents the development of HRS in patients suffering from acute alcoholic hepatitis, probably by inhibiting the synthesis of tumor necrosis factor-α (TNF-α).[14]

General Approach to Treatment

Once the diagnosis of HRS is made, patients should be assessed for OLT. Suitable candidates should be put on the urgent waiting list for cadaveric or living donor liver transplantation. In patients who are transplantation candidates, treatments that have been shown to be useful for HRS should be instituted as a bridge to OLT. These include pharmacotherapy, mechanical shunt, extracorporeal liver support therapy, and, in patients with advanced uremia, renal replacement therapy. Recent studies have shown that in some patients who are not transplantation candidates, prolonged survival in terms of months may still be achievable with some of these therapies.

Pharmacotherapy

At present, the most promising pharmacotherapies appear to be those targeted at reversing splanchnic arteriolar vasodilation (Fig. 67.8).

Vasopressin analogues have attracted the most attention as therapeutic agents in HRS. Vasopressin has a preferential vasoconstrictor action on the splanchnic versus the renal vascular bed. Ornipressin (8-ornithine vasopressin) is a synthetic polypeptide analogue of arginine-vasopressin that has equipotent vasoconstrictor activity but has markedly reduced antidiuretic properties. Prolonged intravenous administration of ornipressin for 15 days with daily albumin infusion or dopamine at a subpressor dose reversed HRS in about 50% of patients.[15,16] The longest patient survival following treatment without OLT was 8 months. The main limitations of the treatment were ischemic complications in one third of patients and included intestinal ischemia, tongue

Pharmacotherapies for hepatorenal syndrome
*Terlipressin, IV 0.5–2 mg q 4–12 hr (see Fig. 67.9)
*Midodrine, oral 7.5–12.5 mg tid + octreotide, SC 100–200 μg tid[25] or midodrine, oral 2.5 mg qd + octreotide, IV 25-μg bolus followed by IV 25 μg/hr[26]
Noradrenaline, IV 0.5–3 mg/hr[24]

Figure 67.8 Pharmacotherapies for hepatorenal syndrome. All are given with intravenous albumin, 20–40 g/day. *Preferred treatment.

necrosis, and ventricular arrhythmia. Terlipressin (triglycyllysine-vasopressin) is a newer synthetic analogue of vasopressin that, apart from having a greater effect on the vascular vasopressin receptors (V1) than the renal vasopressin receptors (V2), is a prodrug requiring transformation to the biologically active form, lysine-vasopressin. Because of this, terlipressin has a prolonged half-life and can be given as an intravenous bolus instead of a continuous intravenous infusion. This significantly reduces the incidence of systemic ischemic complications. Intravenous terlipressin given at 1 mg every 12 hours for 48 hours significantly increased mean blood pressure, creatinine clearance, and urine output and significantly decreased plasma renin and aldosterone levels in 10 patients with HRS.[17] A number of subsequent long-term retrospective and prospective studies in type 1 and 2 HRS utilizing different terlipressin treatment regimens showed an improvement in renal function in about two thirds of the treated patients[18–23] (Fig. 67.9). Most patients responded to a dose between 2 and 6 mg per day. Concomitant albumin infusion (20–40 g/day) appeared to be required for a favorable response in some studies. Improvement in renal function was not observed in untreated controls[18] or in patients suffering from renal failure secondary to organic renal

disease.[19] The probability of survival in treated patients was estimated to be 61% on day 15, 40% after 1 month, 28% after 2 months, 22% after 3 months, and 19% after 1 year.[12] Reversal of HRS was associated with improved survival.[11,12,20] Recurrence of HRS following successful treatment was variable, tended to increase with time, and appeared to be more common in type 2 than type 1 HRS.[11,19–22] Retreatment with terlipressin was successful in most patients.[11,20–22] Younger age, a Child-Pugh score of no greater than 13,[12] and administration of albumin[11] were independent predictors for a successful response to treatment. Ischemic side effects were uncommon and were reported in up to 5% of patients,[11,12] but patients with cardiovascular and peripheral vascular disease were excluded in all these studies.

Vasoconstrictors, apart from vasopressin analogues, have also been used in the treatment of HRS. Intravenous noradrenaline given at a mean dose of 0.8 ± 0.3 (range, 0.5 to 3) mg/hour for a mean of 10 ± 3 days, combined with intravenous albumin and furosemide, increased MAP, reduced plasma renin and aldosterone levels, and reversed type 1 HRS in 10 of 12 patients, with 3 surviving with OLT and 4 surviving for a median of 332 days (range, 180–450 days) without OLT.[24] Documented myocardial ischemia occurred in only 1 patient. Administration of midodrine, an orally active α-mimetic drug (7.5–12.5 mg given three times a day, titrated to achieve an increase in MAP of 15 mm Hg), subcutaneous octreotide (100–200 μg three times a day), and albumin infusion (20–40 g/day) was successful in reverting type 1 HRS in all of 5 treated patients, compared with only 1 of 8 patients treated with subpressor dose of dopamine and albumin.[25] Four of 5 treated patients survived longer than 1 month, 2 with OLT and 2 without OLT. Treatment could be maintained for up to 2 months, with 3 patients receiving treatment at home. Side effects were self-limiting, including tingling, goosebumps, and diarrhea. In another recent study, oral midodrine (2.5 mg daily) given in combination with intravenous octreotide (25-μg bolus

Long-term clinical studies on terlipressin in patients with HRS						
Investigators	No. of Patients*	Dose of Treatment	Albumin Infusion (yes/no)	Duration of Treatment (days)	Reversal of HRS (Complete/partial)[†]	Patients Surviving >1 m	Patients Undergoing OLT
Uriz et al., 2000[21‡]	9 (3)	0.5–1mg/4 hr	9/0	5–15	7 (7/0)	5	3
Mulkay et al., 2001[22]	12	2 mg/8–12 hr	12/0	8–68	11 (5/6)	9	3
Moreau et al., 2002[12‡]	91	3.2 ± 1.3 mg/day	68/23	11.4 ± 12.3	58 (NA)	36	13
Colle et al., 2002[20‡]	18	2.83 ± 0.07 mg/day	13/5	9.1 ± 1.3	11 (NA)	8	2
Halimi et al., 2002[23‡]	18 (2)	4 (1.5–12) mg/day	0/18	7 (2–16)	13 (8/5)	2	1
Alessandria et al., 2002[19‡]	11 (11)	1 mg/4 hr	11/0	>7[§]	8 (7/1)	8	NA
Ortega et al., 2002[11]	21 (5)	0.5–1 mg/4 hr	13/8	<15	14 (12/12)	11	5
Solanki et al., 2003[18]	12	1 mg/12 hr	12/0	<15	5 (NA)	0	0

Figure 67.9 Long-term clinical studies on terlipressin in patients with hepatorenal syndrome (HRS). *No. of patients with type 2 hepatorenal syndrome (in parentheses). [†]Complete reversal: serum creatinine ≤1.5 mg/dl; partial reversal: serum creatinine <20%–50% baseline level but >1.5 mg/dl. [‡]Retrospective study. [§]Transjugular intrahepatic portosystemic stent-shunt was performed in 9 patients subsequently. OLT, orthotopic liver transplantation; NA, information not available.

followed by 25 µg/hr) and albumin (50 g per day) for 14 ± 3 days (range, 5–47 days) reversed type 1 HRS in 10 of 14 patients.[26]

Specific inhibitors or antagonists of endogenous vasoactive substances thought to be important in inducing splanchnic vasodilation have also been studied in HRS. However, octreotide, an inhibitor of glucagon release with no adverse effect on renal hemodynamics and function, was ineffective in a randomized prospective double-blind placebo crossover trial.[27] As previously mentioned, the combination of midodrine or octreotide appears to be effective.[25,26] Octreotide may contribute to normalizing the response of the vasodilated splanchnic arterial vessels to midodrine, thereby avoiding the extrasplanchnic side effects of vasoconstrictor therapy.

A number of alternative approaches have been evaluated in patients with HRS, but none has produced sufficient clinical benefit or has been independently verified to be recommended for treatment. These approaches include nonspecific vasodilators (e.g., acetylcholine and papaverine) and α-adrenergic blockers (e.g., phentolamine) infused intra-arterially at low dose; oral misoprostol (a prostaglandin E_2 analogue); intravenous or intra-arterial infusion of prostaglandin E_1; intravenous and intra-arterial dopamine given at a subpressor dose (1–3 µg/kg per minute); combinations of intravenous prostacyclin and norepinephrine as well as low-dose dopamine and norepinephrine; inhibition of thromboxane A_2 generation using dazoxiben, a specific thromboxane synthetase inhibitor; specific endothelin A receptor antagonist; and intravenous infusion of N-acetylcysteine.

Transjugular Intrahepatic Portosystemic Stent-Shunt

Portal hypertension plays a central role in the pathogenesis of the homeostatic abnormalities in cirrhosis and hepatic failure and in HRS. The high operative mortality precludes side-to-side portacaval shunts in HRS patients. Transjugular intrahepatic portosystemic stent-shunting (TIPS) uses a metallic stent to reinforce a parenchymal track created by balloon dilation between a branch of the hepatic vein and a branch of the portal vein (Fig. 67.10). In experienced hands, this technique is associated with an operative mortality rate of 1% to 2% and a morbidity rate of 10%. Procedure-related complications include intra-abdominal bleeding, cardiac arrhythmia, shunt migration and thrombosis, hemolytic anemia, fever, infection, and reactions to radiocontrast media (including nephrotoxicity). The resultant diversion of portal blood flow from the liver to the systemic circulation may result in transient deterioration of liver function and development of encephalopathy. In a recent long-term study,[28] improvement of renal function was observed in 31 nontransplantable cirrhotic patients with HRS but without severe liver failure (bilirubin <15 mg/dl, Child-Pugh score <12, and absence of spontaneous severe encephalopathy) in whom limited portal decompression was achieved using 8- to 10-mm stents. For the whole group, the survival rates were 81%, 71%, 48%, and 35% at 3, 6, 12, and 18 months, respectively, and for 14 patients with type 1 HRS, they were 64%, 50%, and 20% at 3, 6, and 12 months, respectively. Shunt stenosis and occlusion in 7 patients could be treated in 6 by balloon dilation or stent prolongation.

The combined use of TIPS and pharmacotherapies in the treatment of HRS has been reported in two studies. In one, TIPS was performed in 9 patients with type 2 HRS after treatment with intravenous terlipressin.[19] All 7 patients who responded to terlipressin and relapsed after treatment cessation responded to TIPS, whereas 1 of 2 patients who did not respond to terlipressin showed a mild improvement in renal function. In another study, TIPS was performed in 5 patients with type 1 HRS after

successful treatment with midodrine, octreotide, and albumin.[26] Complete normalization of renal function, urinary sodium excretion, and plasma renin and aldosterone levels and elimination of ascites were observed in all patients 12 months after TIPS. In both studies, improvement or elimination of ascites was an added benefit.

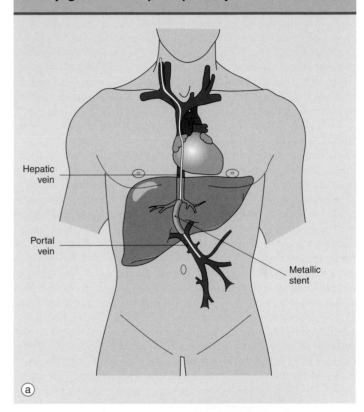

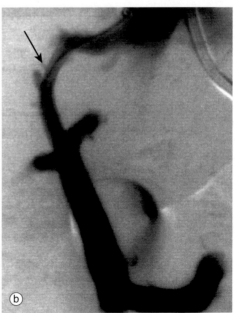

Figure 67.10 **Transjugular intrahepatic portosystemic stent-shunt.** *a,* An intrahepatic tract has been created between the right hepatic vein and the right portal vein. *b,* The tract is dilated (*arrow*) and stented, creating a shunt as demonstrated on shuntogram. (Courtesy of Dr. W. K. Tso.)

Extracorporeal Liver Support Therapy

Extracorporeal liver support therapy, as a bridge to OLT, relies on biologic (hepatocytes or whole liver organ from human or animal source in an *ex vivo* perfusion system) or nonbiologic methods, including hemodialysis, hemofiltration, plasma exchange, and hemoperfusion through charcoal or other adsorbent. The molecular adsorbents recirculating system (MARS) has emerged as a promising form of extracorporeal liver support therapy (see Chapter 100). In a prospective randomized controlled trial, MARS effectively removed strongly albumin-bound toxic metabolites (i.e., bilirubin and bile acids), improved renal function, and prolonged survival in 8 patients (mean survival, 25 ± 5 days) with type 1 HRS and severe liver failure (bilirubin >15 mg/dl, Child-Pugh score 12.5 ± 1.2) compared with 5 untreated control patients (mean survival, 4.6 ± 1.8 days).[29] Mild thrombocytopenia that did not lead to bleeding complications was observed. In addition to improvement in renal function, MARS has been shown to improve ascites and hepatic encephalopathy in these patients.[30]

Renal Replacement Therapy

Hemodialysis and peritoneal dialysis have been used for the treatment of advancing uremia in patients suffering from HRS, but both are fraught with difficulties. Systemic hypotension, which is invariably present, often means that conventional hemodialysis is not feasible or can only be carried out with difficulty. The presence of large amounts of ascites creates a huge "dead space" that reduces the efficiency of peritoneal dialysis. This could be overcome by complete drainage of the abdominal fluid between cycle exchanges, but this would result in substantial derangement of body fluid distribution, with resultant hypotension. Continuous venovenous hemofiltration (CVVH) has been advocated for the treatment of advancing uremia in HRS.[31] CVVH allows the administration of nutritional support, which is often vital to the survival of these patients and would optimize their condition before OLT. Furthermore, CVVH is associated with a fall in intracranial pressure in patients with HRS, an important consideration, especially in patients suffering from hepatic encephalopathy; whereas an increase is observed with intermittent hemofiltration or hemodialysis. It is, therefore, also safer to use in patients who suffer from severe hepatic encephalopathy. Anticoagulation should be minimized or may be avoided totally especially in patients with pre-existing coagulopathy, by giving the replacement fluid in the predilutional mode. When anticoagulation is needed, conventional or low-molecular-weight heparin is generally recommended. Because the liver plays a significant role in citrate metabolism,[32] dose adaptation and close metabolic monitoring would be required for regional citrate anticoagulation, especially after prolonged usage. Bicarbonate should be used instead of lactate as the buffer for the replacement solution to minimize metabolic acidosis. MARS may be combined with either CVVH or hemodialysis for the treatment of HRS. This approach may be most desirable in patients who also suffer from severe hepatic encephalopathy. For both MARS and CVVH, the site of dialysis catheter placement should be carefully chosen in a potential liver transplant recipient so that the right jugular and right femoral vein may be preserved for cannulation when going into bypass at the time of liver transplantation.

Orthotopic Liver Transplantation

OLT is the only definitive treatment for patients suffering from HRS. The clinical outcome of OLT in 56 patients with HRS has been compared with that of 513 patients without HRS.[33] The 5-year patient and graft survival rates were about 10% lower in the HRS group compared with the non-HRS group. Although renal function improved after transplantation in HRS patients, it never reached a level of function demonstrable in non-HRS patients. The HRS group required a longer stay in an intensive care unit, longer hospitalization, and more dialysis treatment after transplantation; however, pretransplantation or post-transplantation dialysis did not affect the clinical outcome. The incidence of end-stage renal disease in the HRS group was 7%, compared with 2% in the non-HRS group. Retransplantation rates and long-term liver function were similar in the two groups. Thus, OLT is associated with comparable liver outcome but inferior renal outcome in patients with HRS compared with those without HRS. This problem cannot be overcome by performing combined kidney and liver transplantation in HRS because the result was no better than that of OLT alone.[34] However, a recent study showed that pretransplantation reversal of HRS allows this group of patients to achieve renal and liver outcome comparable to that in patients without HRS after OLT.[35] These results suggest that HRS should be treated before OLT, and this strategy may improve the renal outcome in these patients.

THERAPEUTIC STRATEGY AND CHOICE OF TREATMENT MODALITIES

Figure 67.11 is an algorithm for the management of HRS. Although OLT is undoubtedly the treatment of choice for patients suffering from HRS, other treatments described earlier may be used as a bridge to OLT, and they may improve the renal outcome after successful OLT. In patients who are not transplantation candidates, these treatments are their only chance for increased survival and, in some cases, may improve their condition to an extent that may allow them to be reconsidered for transplantation. The choice of therapeutic modalities depends on the availability of resources and expertise on the one hand and on the severity of underlying renal and liver failure and the general condition of the patient on the other. In patients with relatively well-preserved liver function (bilirubin <15 mg/dl and Child-Pugh score <12 for TIPS and no greater than 13 for pharmacotherapy) with no or mild hepatic encephalopathy (grade <2), pharmacotherapy or TIPS would be the therapy of choice. In patients with severe liver failure and hepatic encephalopathy, MARS should be considered. In patients with advancing renal failure, CVVH is the treatment of choice and may be combined with other therapeutic modalities, especially MARS. Among the pharmacotherapies, intravenous terlipressin, combined with daily albumin infusion, is most established, but oral midodrine combined with subcutaneous octreotide or intravenous norepinephrine (both with daily albumin infusion) also appears promising. TIPS appears to be able to achieve complete normalization of renal function in selective patients following an initial successful response to pharmacotherapy and may be combined with the latter in the treatment of HRS. Because TIPS can eliminate or greatly reduce ascites formation, it would be particularly useful in patients with refractory ascites.

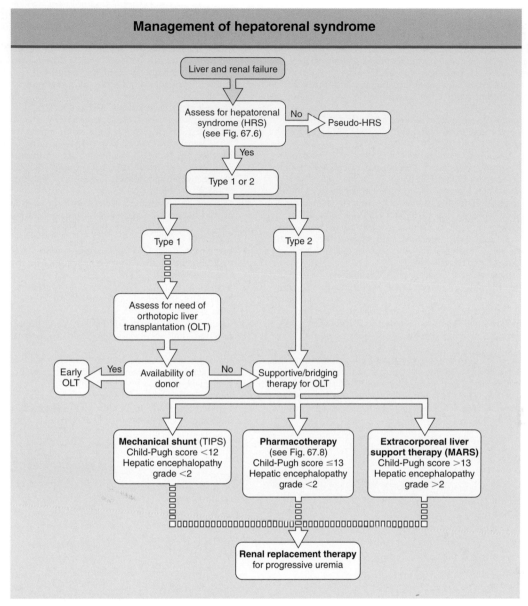

Figure 67.11   Algorithm for the management of hepatorenal syndrome. MARS, molecular adsorbents recirculating system.

REFERENCES

1. Arroyo V, Gines P, Gerbes AL, et al: Definition and diagnostic criteria of refractory ascites and hepatorenal syndrome in cirrhosis. International Ascites Club. Hepatology 1996;23:164–176.
2. Arroyo V, Colmenero J. Ascites and hepatorenal syndrome in cirrhosis: Pathophysiological basis of therapy and current management. J Hepatol 2003;38(Suppl 1):S69–89.
3. Epstein M, Berk DP, Hollenberg NK, et al: Renal failure in the patient with cirrhosis: The role of active vasoconstriction. Am J Med 1970;49:175–185.
4. Ruiz-Del-Arbol L, Monescillo A, Arocena C, et al: Circulatory function and hepatorenal syndrome in cirrhosis. Hepatology 2005;42:439–447.
5. Badalamenti S, Graziani G, Salerno F, et al: Hepatorenal syndrome: New perspectives in pathogenesis and treatment. Arch Intern Med 1993;153:1957–1967.
6. Gines P, Guevara M, Arroyo V, et al: Hepatorenal syndrome Lancet 2003;362:1819–1827.
7. Gines A, Escorsell A, Gines P, et al: Incidence, predictive factors, and prognosis of the hepatorenal syndrome in cirrhosis with ascites. Gastroenterology 1993;105:229–236.
8. Platt JF, Ellis JH, Rubin JM, et al: Renal duplex Doppler ultrasonography: A noninvasive predictor of kidney dysfunction and hepatorenal failure in liver disease. Hepatology 1994;20:362–369.
9. Demirtas S, Bozbas A, Akbay A, et al: Diagnostic value of serum cystatin C for evaluation of hepatorenal syndrome. Clin Chim Acta 2001;311:81–89.
10. Levenson D, Korecki KL: Acute renal failure associated with hepatobiliary disease. In Brenner BM, Lazarus JM (eds): Acute Renal Failure. New York, Churchill Livingstone, 1988, pp 535–580.
11. Ortega R, Gines P, Uriz J, et al: Terlipressin therapy with and without albumin for patients with hepatorenal syndrome: Results of a prospective, nonrandomized study. Hepatology 2002;36:941–948.
12. Moreau R, Durand F, Poynard T, et al: Terlipressin in patients with cirrhosis and type 1 hepatorenal syndrome: A retrospective multicenter study. Gastroenterology 2002;122:923–930.
13. Sort P, Navasa M, Arroyo V, et al: Effect of intravenous albumin on renal impairment and mortality in patients with cirrhosis and spontaneous bacterial peritonitis. N Engl J Med 1999;341:403–409.

14. Akriviadis E, Botla R, Briggs W, et al: Pentoxifylline improves short-term survival in severe acute alcoholic hepatitis: a double-blind, placebo-controlled trial. Gastroenterology 2000;119:1637–1648.

15. Guevara M, Gines P, Fernandez-Esparrach G, et al: Reversibility of hepatorenal syndrome by prolonged administration of ornipressin and plasma volume expansion. Hepatology 1998;27:35–41.

16. Gulberg V, Bilzer M, Gerbes AL: Long-term therapy and retreatment of hepatorenal syndrome type 1 with ornipressin and dopamine. Hepatology 1999;30:870–875.

17. Hadengue A, Gadano A, Moreau R, et al: Beneficial effects of the 2-day administration of terlipressin in patients with cirrhosis and hepatorenal syndrome. J Hepatol 1998;29:565–570.

18. Solanki P, Chawla A, Garg R, et al: Beneficial effects of terlipressin in hepatorenal syndrome: A prospective, randomized placebo-controlled clinical trial. J Gastroenterol Hepatol 2003;18:152–156.

19. Alessandria C, Venon WD, Marzano A, et al: Renal failure in cirrhotic patients: Role of terlipressin in clinical approach to hepatorenal syndrome type 2. Eur J Gastroenterol Hepatol 2002;14:1363–1368.

20. Colle I, Durand F, Pessione F, et al: Clinical course, predictive factors and prognosis in patients with cirrhosis and type 1 hepatorenal syndrome treated with terlipressin: A retrospective analysis. J Gastroenterol Hepatol 2002;17:882–888.

21. Uriz J, Gines P, Cardenas A, et al: Terlipressin plus albumin infusion: An effective and safe therapy of hepatorenal syndrome. J Hepatol 2000;33:43–48.

22. Mulkay JP, Louis H, Donckier V, et al: Long-term terlipressin administration improves renal function in cirrhotic patients with type 1 hepatorenal syndrome: A pilot study. Acta Gastroenterol Belg 2001;64:15–19.

23. Halimi C, Bonnard P, Bernard B, et al: Effect of terlipressin (Glypressin) on hepatorenal syndrome in cirrhotic patients: Results of a multicentre pilot study. Eur J Gastroenterol Hepatol 2002;14:153–158.

24. Duvoux C, Zanditenas D, Hezode C, et al: Effects of noradrenalin and albumin in patients with type I hepatorenal syndrome: A pilot study. Hepatology 2002;36:374–380.

25. Angeli P, Volpin R, Gerunda G, et al: Reversal of type 1 hepatorenal syndrome with the administration of midodrine and octreotide. Hepatology 1999;29:1690–1697.

26. Wong F, Pantea L, Sniderman K: Midodrine, octreotide, albumin, and TIPS in selected patients with cirrhosis and type 1 hepatorenal syndrome. Hepatology 2004;40:55–64.

27. Pomier-Layrargues G, Paquin SC, Hassoun Z, et al: Octreotide in hepatorenal syndrome: A randomized, double-blind, placebo-controlled, crossover study. Hepatology 2003;38:238–243.

28. Brensing KA, Textor J, Perz J, et al: Long term outcome after transjugular intrahepatic portosystemic stent-shunt in non-transplant cirrhotics with hepatorenal syndrome: A phase II study. Gut 2000;47:288–295.

29. Mitzner SR, Stange J, Klammt S, et al: Improvement of hepatorenal syndrome with extracorporeal albumin dialysis MARS: Results of a prospective, randomized, controlled clinical trial. Liver Transpl 2000;6:277–286.

30. Mitzner SR, Klammt S, Peszynski P, et al: Improvement of multiple organ functions in hepatorenal syndrome during albumin dialysis with the molecular adsorbent recirculating system. Therap Apher Dial 2001;5:417–422.

31. Epstein M, Perez GO: Continuous arterio-venous ultrafiltration in the management of the renal complications of liver disease. Int J Artif Organs 1986;9:217–218.

32. Kramer L, Bauer E, Joukhadar C, et al: Citrate pharmacokinetics and metabolism in cirrhotic and noncirrhotic critically ill patients. Crit Care Med 2003;31:2450–2455.

33. Gonwa TA, Klintmalm GB, Levy M, et al: Impact of pretransplant renal function on survival after liver transplantation. Transplantation 1995;59:361–365.

34. Jeyarajah DR, Gonwa TA, McBride M, et al: Hepatorenal syndrome: Combined liver kidney transplants versus isolated liver transplant. Transplantation 1997;64:1760–1765.

35. Restuccia T, Ortega R, Guevara M, et al: Effects of treatment of hepatorenal syndrome before transplantation on posttransplantation outcome: A case-control study. J Hepatol 2004;40:140–146.

CHAPTER

68

Epidemiology and Pathophysiology of Chronic Kidney Disease: Natural History, Risk Factors, and Management

Mohsen El Kossi and Meguid El Nahas

CHRONIC KIDNEY DISEASE: DEFINITION AND EPIDEMIOLOGY

Chronic kidney disease (CKD) is defined as kidney damage or glomerular filtration rate (GFR) <60 ml/min/1.73 m^2 for 3 months or more, irrespective of the cause. The Kidney Disease Outcomes Quality Initiative (K/DOQI) guidelines have classified CKD into five stages[1] (Fig. 68.1). Issues with these guidelines include labeling patients with mild and stable kidney damage as CKD and not differentiating between progressors and nonprogressors or between failure of native kidneys or a transplanted kidney and patients with advanced CKD not yet or already on dialysis. This prompted the Kidney Disease: Improving Global Outcomes (KDIGO) group to undergo reviews of this classification and suggest clarifications, including the addition of the suffixes T for patients with renal allografts and D to identify CKD stage 5 patients on dialysis.[2]

The true incidence and prevalence of CKD within a community are difficult to ascertain because early to moderate CKD is usually asymptomatic. However, various epidemiologic studies have made relatively similar observations:

- *United States*: In the third National Health and Nutrition Examination Survey (NHANES III, 1988–1994) an estimated 11% of the population (19 million individuals) had some degree of CKD.[3] Three percent of the population had an elevated serum creatinine (>1.4–1.6 mg/dl), 70% of whom were hypertensive. Albuminuria prevalence was about 12%.
- *Japan*: Proteinuria and hematuria increased with age, with 10% of subjects older than 65 years having one or the other[4]; less than 2% of those reached end-stage renal disease (ESRD) in 10 years.
- *United Kingdom*: In the EPIC-Norfolk Study, among 23,964 individuals aged 40–79 years, the prevalences of microalbuminuria and macroalbuminuria were 11.8% and 0.9%, respectively. Age, female gender, systolic blood pressure, and current smoking were independent predictors of albuminuria.
- *Germany*: The Monitoring of Trends and Determinants in Cardiovascular disease–Augsburg (MONICA) study showed the prevalence of albuminuria to be significantly higher in elderly and obese individuals.
- *The Netherlands*: In the city of Groningen, the Prevention of Renal and Vascular End Stage Disease (PREVEND) study detected albuminuria in about 7% of adults.[5]
- *Australia*: Among 11,247 Australians aged 25 years or older, the Australian Diabetes, Obesity, and Lifestyle (AusDiab) study found proteinuria in 0.6%, albuminuria in 6%, hematuria in 3.7%, and reduced GFR (<60 ml/min/1.73 m^2) in 9.7%[6]; about 16% had at least one indicator of kidney damage. Age, diabetes mellitus, and hypertension were independently associated with proteinuria. Age, gender, and hypertension were associated with hematuria and reduced GFR.[6]

In developing countries, renal replacement therapy (RRT) is less widely available, and ESRD often equates with death. The International Society of Nephrology, therefore, made the detection and prevention of CKD one of its top health care priorities.

	Classification of CKD based on GFR as proposed by the Kidney Disease Outcomes Quality Initiative (K/DOQI) guidelines	
CKD Stage	Description
1	Normal or increased GFR; some evidence of kidney damage reflected by microalbuminuria/proteinuria, hematuria, or histologic changes
2	Mild decrease in GFR (89–60 ml/min/1.73 m^2)
3	Moderate decrease in GFR (59–30 ml/min/1.73 m^2)
4	Severe decrease in GFR (29–15 ml/min/1.73 m^2)
5	GFR <15 ml/min/1.73 m^2; when renal replacement therapy in the form of dialysis or transplantation has to be considered to sustain life

Figure 68.1 Classification of chronic kidney disease (CKD) based on glomerular filtration rate (GFR) as proposed by the Kidney Disease Outcomes Quality Initiative (K/DOQI) guidelines. (Data from National Kidney Foundation: K/DOQI kidney disease outcome quality initiative. Am J Kidney Dis 2002;39:(Suppl I):S1–S266.)

Incidence and prevalence of RRT per million population in different parts of the world in 2002		
Continent or Country	Incidence	Prevalence
United States		
Total population	333	1446
Caucasians	255	1060
African Americans	982	4467
Native Americans	514	2569
Asians	344	1571
Hispanics	481	1991
Australia	94	658
Aboriginal, Torres Strait Islanders	393	1904
Europe	129	770
United Kingdom	101	626
France	123	898
Germany	174	918
Italy	142	864
Spain	126	950
Japan	262	1726

Figure 68.2   Incidence and prevalence of renal replacement therapy (RRT) per 1 million population in different parts of the world in 2002.

EPIDEMIOLOGY OF END-STAGE RENAL DISEASE

In the United Kingdom, the incidence of ESRD treated by RRT is about 100 new patients per 1 million population (pmp) per year[7] (Fig. 68.2); this has doubled over the past decade and is expected to continue to rise by 5% to 8% annually but remains well below the European average (about 129 pmp/year) and that of the United States (333 pmp/year).[8] Disparities in the incidence of ESRD within and between developed countries reflect racial and ethnic diversity as well as the prevalence of diabetes and hypertension.

The rise in ESRD patients worldwide most likely reflects aging of the population (annual incidence of ESRD in the population older than 65 years in the United Kingdom >350 pmp, United States >1200 pmp) and the global epidemic of type 2 diabetes mellitus. It is predicted that the number of diabetic people worldwide (currently about 154 million) will double within the next 20 years, with the highest increase in the developing world. In addition, increasing access to RRT worldwide has encouraged the referral and treatment of patients who, in the past, were denied RRT.

The cost of treating patients with ESRD is substantial and affects provision of care. By 2010, more than 2 million individuals worldwide will be treated by RRT at a cost of $1 trillion.[9] More than 100 countries have no provision for RRT,[10] and consequently, more than 1 million individuals will die each year from ESRD.

SCREENING FOR CHRONIC KIDNEY DISEASE

To stem the growing tide of CKD, early detection and management are advocated. These are often initiated by simple dipstick analysis of the urine. In a simulation analysis for proteinuria dipstick testing, whole population screening was not cost-effective, except when individuals older than 60 years were screened.[11] A more realistic approach would be to screen populations at high risk, such as elderly, obese, diabetic, and hypertensive individuals; high-risk communities, such as African Americans and Native Americans in the United States and Aborigines in Australia; those

with a family history of CKD; and those with autoimmune disorders or a history of urinary tract infections.[1] Such targeted screening is supported by the observations of the American Kidney Early Evaluation Program (KEEP), wherein the prevalence of albuminuria (29%), reduced GFR (16%), and overall CKD (47%) far exceeded findings in the general population.[12]

Initial screening should consist of urinalysis (dipstick testing for albuminuria, proteinuria, and hematuria) and a blood pressure measurement. Qualitative urinalysis should be confirmed by quantitative estimation of the urine albumin-to-creatinine ratio (ACR). Ultrasonography has also been put forward by K/DOQI,[1] although this investigation is unlikely to be part of the initial screening process.

NATURAL HISTORY OF CHRONIC KIDNEY DISEASE

Most patients with CKD stages 3 to 5 progress relentlessly to ESRD. A straight-line relationship is often found between the reciprocal of serum creatinine (1/sCr) values or the estimated GFR and time (for methodologic aspects, see Chapter 69). However, a significant percentage of patients do not progress in a predictable linear fashion and have breakpoints in their progression slopes suggesting acceleration or slowing down of the rate of progression of CKD. These breakpoints could be either spontaneous or secondary to events such as infections, dehydration, changes in the adequacy of systemic blood pressure control, or exposure to nephrotoxins, in particular nonsteroidal anti-inflammatory drugs (NSAIDs) or radiocontrast agents. It is also important to appreciate that some patients with mild to moderate CKD have stable renal function for sustained periods.

The rate of progression of CKD varies according to the underlying nephropathy and among individual patients. Historically, the rate of decline in GFR of patients with diabetic nephropathy (DN) has been among the fastest, averaging about −10 ml/min/year. Control of systemic hypertension slows the rate of GFR decline to −5 ml/min/year, with further improvement (−1 to −2 ml/min/year) expected in patients whose glycemia and hypertension are optimally controlled. In nondiabetic nephropathy, the rate of progression of CKD was 2.5 times faster in patients with chronic glomerulonephritis than in those with chronic interstitial nephritis and 1.5 times faster than in those with hypertensive nephrosclerosis. The association between proteinuria and faster progression of CKD has been highlighted in a number of studies (reviewed in refs. 13, 14). Patients with polycystic kidney disease (PKD) and impaired renal function may also have a faster rate of progression compared with those with other nephropathies (Fig. 68.3).

FACTORS AFFECTING INITIATION AND PROGRESSION OF CHRONIC KIDNEY DISEASE

Susceptibility Markers and Factors
The susceptibility, initiation, and progression of CKD are all associated with risk markers and factors; markers highlight an association, whereas factors imply causality. The latter are often difficult to substantiate.

Genetic Predisposition
CKD often clusters within families. Genetic studies have suggested possible links between CKD and a variety of alterations or polymorphisms of candidate genes coding for putative mediators, including the renin angiotensin system (RAS), nitric oxide synthase, kallikrein, cytokines (such as interleukin-1 and tumor

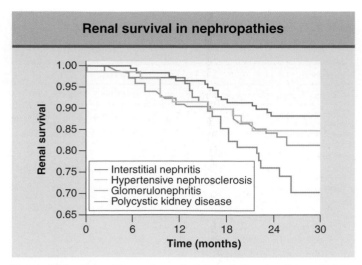

Figure 68.3 Actuarial renal survival in relation to the underlying nephropathy. (Adapted from Locatelli F, Marcelli D, Comelli M, and the Northern Italian Cooperative Study Group: Proteinuria and blood pressure as causal components of progression to end-stage renal failure. Nephrol Dial Transplant 1996;11:461–467.)

necrosis factor-α), growth factors (including platelet-derived growth factor [PDGF] and transforming growth factor-β1 [TGF-β1]), plasminogen activator inhibitor-1 (PAI-1), complement factors, and immunoglobulins.

Racial Factors

Racial factors play a role in the susceptibility to CKD as reflected by the high prevalence of hypertension- and diabetes-related CKD among African Americans and Native Americans in the United States[15] (see Fig. 68.2) and among Afro-Caribbeans and Indo-Asians in the United Kingdom. Racial predisposition has been attributed to a number of factors, including the susceptibility to diabetes mellitus and hypertension and possibly a genetic predisposition to CKD. Socioeconomic factors, such as social deprivation or low socioeconomic status, have also been linked to a higher prevalence of CKD in the developed world. Finally, exposure to high lead levels as well as raised serum uric acid levels may contribute to the increased risk for CKD in African Americans.[15]

Maternal-Fetal Factors

Maternal undernutrition during pregnancy and the ensuing fetal malnutrition may contribute to the development of hypertension, the metabolic syndrome, diabetes mellitus, and CKD in adult life. Low birth weight and the rapid catch-up growth that follows have been implicated in the pathogenesis of hypertension through a reduction in nephron numbers at birth (oligonephronia) and their inability to handle increased solute and salt load.[16] Reduced nephron numbers and the associated glomerular hypertrophy (oligomeganephronia) may also lead to glomerulosclerosis and CKD.

Other Factors

Males and the elderly may also be more susceptible to CKD and are more prevalent in RRT programs.

Initiation Markers and Factors

Hypertension, diabetes, hyperlipidemia, obesity, and smoking are risk markers or factors in the general population for the development of proteinuria and CKD.

Hypertension

The Multiple Risk Factor Intervention Trial (MRFIT) in the United States and the Japanese Okinawa survey noted an association between elevated blood pressure and the risk for ESRD in both men and women.

Dyslipidemia

The Atherosclerosis Risk in Communities (ARIC) study and the Physicians Health Study (PHS) showed an association between dyslipidemia and the risk for CKD. In contrast, in the Okinawa survey, hypertriglyceridemia but not hypercholesterolemia increased the risk for developing proteinuria, and neither was a predictor of ESRD in the general population.

Obesity, Smoking, and Other Factors

The Okinawa survey showed that obesity and smoking are associated with increased risk for proteinuria in men and that proteinuria, anemia, and hyperuricemia are risk markers of ESRD in the general population.

Common risk factors such as albuminuria appear to predispose to both renal (CKD) and cardiovascular disease (CVD) morbidity and mortality in developed countries (see Chapter 71).

Progression Markers and Factors

The progression of established CKD is variable and associated with a number of risk markers and factors.

Nonmodifiable Risk Factors

Age The rate of progression of CKD is influenced by age, with elderly patients affected by glomerulonephritis having a faster rate of GFR decline. One notable exception is type 1 diabetic nephropathy, in which young age at diagnosis is associated with a faster rate of GFR decline.

Gender In univariate analyses, male gender was often associated with more rapid GFR decline, but this was not always confirmed in multivariate analyses.

Race The incidence and prevalence of diabetic and hypertensive CKD are higher in African Americans and Hispanic Americans compared with Caucasians[15] (see Fig. 68.2). Their rate of CKD progression also seems faster, although few studies confirmed this by multivariate analysis.

In the United Kingdom, Indo-Asian patients with DN may have a faster rate of decline of GFR than Caucasians, even at comparable levels of blood pressure and with use of angiotensin-converting enzyme (ACE) inhibitors.

Genetics Diabetic and nondiabetic nephropathies cluster in families, in particular in African Americans. In diabetes mellitus, a family history of CVD or hypertension is associated, respectively, with a twofold or fourfold increase in the risk for diabetic nephropathy. Parental hypertension is also thought to be a risk factor for the progression of diabetic and IgA nephropathy (reviewed in ref. 13).

Associations have been described between certain major histocompatibility complexes (MHCs) and the rate of CKD progression. Patients with PKD carrying the genotype *PKD1* are thought to have a worse prognosis than others. Progression of CKD may also be influenced by polymorphisms of genes coding for putative mediators of renal scarring. To date, the *ACE* gene has received the most attention, with some studies linking susceptibility and progression in CKD as well as responses to antihypertensive treatment to an insertion (I)/deletion (D) polymorphism in the

ACE gene (reviewed in ref. 17). Other candidate genes include those coding for angiotensinogen, angiotensin II receptor, nitric oxide synthase, kallikrein, some cytokines, chemokines and their receptors (in particular CCR5), and growth factors. The human homologue of the rat renal failure *(Rf)* gene has been localized on the long arm of chromosome 10. In African Americans with ESRD due a variety of nephropathies, an association between two markers (D10S1435 and D10S249) spanning 21 polymorphic regions of chromosome 10 approached significance in nondiabetic patients.

Loss of Renal Mass The threshold for natural progression attributed to GFR loss appears to be crossed when reductions in nephron function exceed 50%. In contrast to unilateral nephrectomy (e.g., in living kidney donors), a further reduction in nephron function (e.g., partial nephrectomy of a solitary kidney) does lead to natural progression. A normal solitary kidney can also be vulnerable to natural progression if it is congenital or is acquired early in life.

The threshold to natural progression after nephron loss might also be lowered by the presence of hypertension, obesity, hyperlipidemia, hyperglycemia, or black race, or if the nephron loss is the result of glomerulonephritis (GN). Observations such as the latter suggest that GFR loss that results in segmental but diffuse glomerular damage (e.g., a resolved severe GN) may carry a higher risk for natural progression than an equivalent degree of GFR loss in which the surviving nephrons are normal (e.g., after unilateral nephrectomy).

Modifiable Risk Markers and Factors
Modifiable risk markers and factors include systemic hypertension, proteinuria, and metabolic factors. In addition, recent interest has focused on the contribution of cigarette smoking, alcohol consumption, and recreational drug use to the risk for ESRD (see Chapter 69).

Hypertension Strong evidence links the progression of CKD to systemic hypertension in diabetic and nondiabetic nephropathies (Fig. 68.4; reviewed in ref. 1). It is believed that the transmission of systemic hypertension into the glomerular capillary beds and the resulting glomerular hypertension contribute to the initiation of glomerulosclerosis (Figs. 68.5 and 68.6).

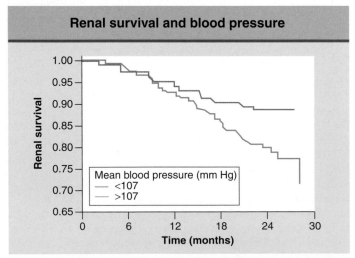

Figure 68.4 Actuarial renal survival in relation to blood pressure. (Adapted from Locatelli F, Marcelli D, Comelli M, and the Northern Italian Cooperative Study Group: Proteinuria and blood pressure as causal components of progression to end-stage renal failure. Nephrol Dial Transplant 1996;11:461–467.)

Hypotheses for the pathogenesis of glomerulosclerosis	
Hypothesis	Author(s)
Glomerular hyperfiltration/hyperperfusion	Hostetter & Brenner, 1981
Glomerular hypertension	Anderson & Brenner, 1985
Nephrotoxicity of lipids	Moorhead & El Nahas, 1982
Similarities with atherosclerosis	El Nahas, 1988 Diamond & Kamovsky, 1988
Glomerular hypertrophy	Fogo & Ichikawa, 1991
Nephrotoxicity of proteinuria	Remuzzi & Bertani, 1990
Growth factors 　Platelet-derived growth factor 　Transforming growth factor-β	Johnson et al., 1994 Border et al., 1993
Mesangial myofibroblast differentiation	Johnson et al., 1994
Low birth weight, oligomeganephronia	Brenner, 1994
Podocyte injury	Kriz, 1996

Figure 68.5 Hypotheses for the pathogenesis of glomerulosclerosis. (Adapted from El Nahas AM: Mechanisms of experimental and clinical renal scarring. In Davison AM, Cameron JS, Grunfeld J-P, et al [eds]: Oxford Textbook of Clinical Nephrology, 3rd ed. London, Oxford University Press, 2005, pp 1647–1686.)

Proteinuria A large number of studies in patients with diabetic and nondiabetic glomerular disease and nonglomerular disease confirmed, by multivariate analysis, that heavy proteinuria was associated with a faster rate of progression[1,14,18] (Fig. 68.7). Furthermore, reduction of proteinuria by diet, ACE inhibition, or angiotensin receptor blocker (ARB) predicts a better outcome.[14,19] The extent of reduction in proteinuria is often proportional to the benefit accrued by such intervention on CKD progression. Experimental data suggest that proteinuria may contribute directly to the progression of CKD (see later discussion).

The threshold for natural progression attributed to proteinuria appears to be crossed when proteinuria exceeds 500 mg/day. Nonselective proteinuria is mainly responsible for the natural progression attributed to proteinuria. Indeed, highly selective proteinuria (in which the urine protein is almost entirely albumin) can persist in the nephrotic range for more than 10 years without causing structural damage to the kidney.

Albuminuria, Chronic Kidney Disease, and Cardiovascular Disease
Urinary ACR is independently associated with the presence and severity of cardiovascular disease in the nondiabetic general population.[20] Even low-grade albuminuria (below the current microalbuminuria threshold [ACR <30 μg/mg]) in middle-aged nondiabetic and nonhypertensive individuals is associated with increased CVD risk. The risk associated with albuminuria in the general population matches, and sometimes exceeds, that attributed to better known risk factors of CVD such as hypertension and hyperlipidemia. Reduction of albuminuria not only reduces the risk for progressive CKD but also may affect the associated CVD. Diffuse endothelial dysfunction may be the common pathway linking albuminuria to the manifestations and prognosis of CKD and CVD (see Chapter 71). CKD is now defined as a CVD risk equivalent, and patients with all stages of CKD are considered in the highest-risk group for CVD.[1,21] Patients with CVD are also at a higher risk for CKD, possibly

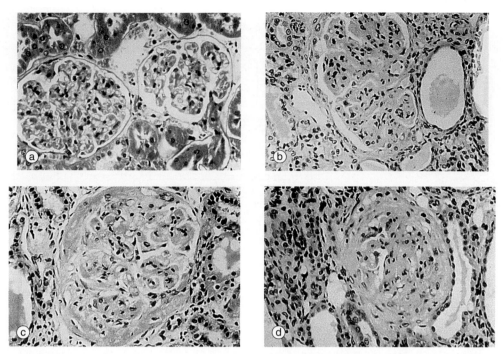

Figure 68.6 Histologic development of glomerulosclerosis. *a*, Normal glomerulus. *b*, Mesangial hypercellularity. *c* and *d*, Glomerulosclerosis of increasing severity. Note the tubular atrophy and dilatation in *b–d*, indicating the parallel development of tubulointerstitial scarring.

because of their shared risk profile, which includes hypertension, diabetes, obesity, dyslipidemia, and smoking.

Metabolic Markers and Factors

Glycemia

The evidence for a role for hyperglycemia in the progression of diabetic nephropathy is conflicting.[1]

Lipids

Dyslipidemia may contribute to glomerulosclerosis and tubulointerstitial fibrosis (Figs. 68.8 and 68.9). A number of studies of diabetic and nondiabetic nephropathies have confirmed by multivariate analysis that dyslipidemia is a risk factor for a faster rate of CKD progression.[1]

Obesity

Excessive body weight and a raised body mass index have been linked to a faster rate of progression of CKD in patients with IgA nephropathy. Anecdotal reports suggest that weight reduction lessens obesity-related renal hemodynamic changes as well as CKD-associated proteinuria.

Uric Acid

Hyperuricemia has been associated with systemic hypertension, CVD, and renal diseases[22] (see Chapter 32). Hyperuricemia may

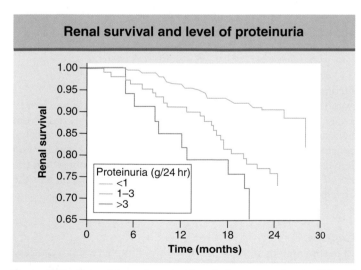

Renal survival and level of proteinuria

Renal survival (y-axis: 0.65 to 1.00) vs Time (months) (x-axis: 0 to 30)

Proteinuria (g/24 hr)
— <1
— 1–3
— >3

Figure 68.7 Actuarial renal survival in relation to proteinuria. (Adapted from Locatelli F, Marcelli D, Comelli M, and the Northern Italian Cooperative Study Group: Proteinuria and blood pressure as causal components of progression to end-stage renal failure. Nephrol Dial Transplant 1996;11:461–467.)

Hypotheses for the pathogenesis of tubulointerstitial fibrosis	
Hypothesis	Author(s)
Adaptive tubular hypermetabolism	Harris & Schrier, 1988
Adaptive tubular ammoniagenesis	Nath & Hostetter, 1985
Nephrotoxicity of lipids	Moorhead et al., 1982
Nephrotoxicity of proteinuria	Remuzzi & Bertani, 1990
Nephrotoxicity of calcium and phosphate	Alfrey, 1988
Nephrotoxicity of iron	Harris & Alfrey, 1994
Nephrotoxicity of oxygen free radicals	Nath et al., 1994
Tubular cell induction of fibrosis	Kuncio & Neilson, 1991
Tubular transdifferentiation	Okada, Strutz, & Neilson, 1994
Ischemia and hypoxia	Norman & Fine, 1998

Figure 68.8 Hypotheses for the pathogenesis of tubulointerstitial fibrosis. (Adapted from El Nahas AM: Mechanisms of experimental and clinical renal scarring. In Davison AM, Cameron JS, Grunfeld J-P, et al [eds]: Oxford Textbook of Clinical Nephrology, 3rd ed. London, Oxford University Press, 2005, pp 1647–1686.)

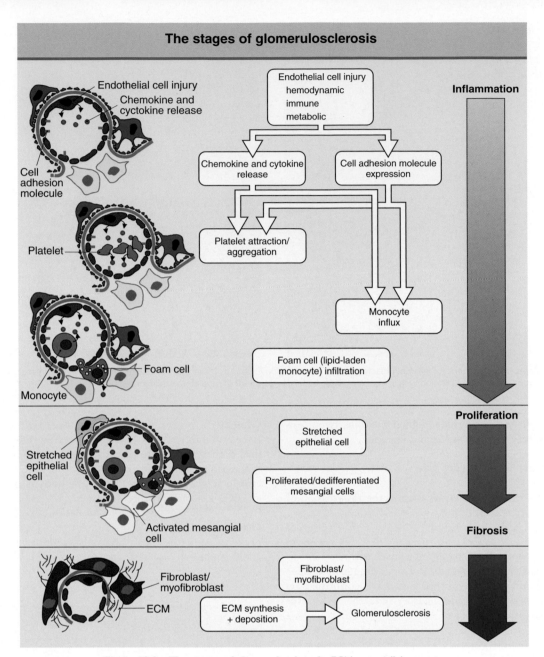

Figure 68.9 The stages of glomerulosclerosis. ECM, extracellular matrix.

cause hypertension and renal injury through crystal-independent pathways, notably a stimulation of the RAS. In a Japanese study, hyperuricemic patients with IgA nephropathy had a worse prognosis than those with normal serum uric acid levels, and a serum uric acid ≥6.0 mg/dl (359 μmol/l) was an independent predictor of ESRD in women.

Miscellaneous Factors
Smoking
Cigarette smoking increases systemic blood pressure and affects renal hemodynamics. In diabetic and nondiabetic patients, smoking is associated with a faster rate of decline of CKD. In one study of men with CKD, smoking increased the risk for ESRD threefold in patients treated with ACE inhibitors, with the odds ratio increasing to 10 in those taking other antihypertensive agents.[23]

Alcohol and Recreational Drugs
Some evidence links alcohol consumption exceeding two drinks a day to progressive renal insufficiency, perhaps through the hypertensive effect of alcohol. The association between alcohol consumption and hypertension is stronger in males than females. One analysis has suggested an association between the use of recreational drugs, and more specifically opiates, and the development of ESRD in the United States.

Caffeine
Experimental data have suggested a link between excessive exposure to caffeine and the progression of renal scarring. There are no clinical data to substantiate such risk; however, a study of a U.S. cohort of Caucasian males showed that chronic coffee drinking was associated with increased blood pressure levels.

Analgesics and Nonsteroidal Anti-Inflammatory Agents

Most studies showing an increased risk for ESRD with phenacetin, paracetamol, aspirin, and NSAIDs are confounded by the inadequacy of controls and the fact that a combination of analgesics was often used and what time the agent was ordered. Also, the interpretation of the studies was often confounded by indication.

Lead Exposure

Chronic lead intoxication has been linked in some parts of the world to the development of ESRD. Chronic low-level lead exposure has been implicated in the development of hypertension, gout, and CKD and has been associated with the pathogenesis of arteriolosclerosis.

MECHANISMS OF PROGRESSION OF CHRONIC KIDNEY DISEASE

Glomerulosclerosis

The progression of CKD is associated with the progressive sclerosis of glomeruli regardless of the nature of the underlying nephropathy. Numerous hypotheses have been put forward to explain the progressive sclerosis and fibrosis of the glomeruli (reviewed in ref. 17; see Figs. 68.5 and 68.9). Both intraglomerular and extraglomerular cells contribute to the initiation and progression of glomerulosclerosis.

Intrinsic Glomerular Cells

Glomerulosclerosis can be initiated by injury or damage to any one of the three glomerular cell lines; glomerulosclerosis may evolve in stages triggered by endothelial, mesangial, or epithelial cell injury.

Role of the Endothelium

Glomerular endothelial cells play an important role in preserving the integrity of vascular beds including the glomeruli. Within glomerular capillaries, endothelial cells are the first to be exposed to damage induced by hemodynamic (shear stress), immunologic, or metabolic insults. Glomerular endothelial injury is associated with reduction or loss of their physiologic anticoagulant and anti-inflammatory properties and the acquisition of procoagulant and inflammatory characteristics. This leads to the attraction and activation of platelets and microthrombus formation in glomerular capillaries. It is also associated with the initiation of glomerular microinflammation, with the attraction, adhesion, and infiltration of glomerular tufts by inflammatory cells (mainly monocytes). Platelets and monocytes interact with mesangial cells, stimulating their activation and proliferation and the production of extracellular matrix (ECM; see Figs. 68.5, 68.6, and 68.9). Strong similarities exist between the evolution of glomerulosclerosis and that of atherosclerosis.

Role of the Mesangium

Primary or secondary mesangial injury or activation can initiate glomerulosclerosis. For instance, after endothelial injury and the ensuing microinflammatory response, infiltrating monocytes interact with mesangial cells and stimulate their proliferation, either through direct cell-to-cell interactions or through the release of mitogens (such as PDGF). The transcription factor nuclear factor kappa B (NF-κB), as well as a variety of kinases (MAP kinases, p4/42 MAP kinase, and Jun N-terminal kinase or stress-activated protein kinase), are centrally involved in the regulation of the mesangial cell proliferative response. Mesangial hypercellularity often precedes the development of mesangial sclerosis. The turnover of mesangial cells *in vivo* appears to be regulated by complex interactions between kinases and their inhibitors. Resolution of glomerular proliferation and hypercellularity may depend on apoptosis (programmed cell death) of infiltrating and proliferating glomerular cells. However, uncontrolled apoptosis may lead to glomerular cell depletion and glomerular obsolescence.

Under the control of fibrogenic growth factors such as TGF-β1, proliferating and activated mesangial cells have the capacity to revert to a mesenchymal phenotype (myofibroblasts) expressing markers such as α-smooth muscle actin (α-SMA) and synthesizing a range of ECM components including interstitial type III collagen, not normally a component of glomerular ECM. Resolution of mesangial and glomerular sclerosis will depend on the balance between the increased ECM synthesis and its breakdown by glomerular collagenases or metalloproteinases.

Role of the Glomerular Epithelium

The relative inability of podocytes to replicate in response to injury may lead to their stretching along the GBM, exposing areas of denuded GBM that would attract and interact with parietal epithelial cells leading to the formation of capsular adhesions and subsequent segmental glomerulosclerosis.[24] This may lead to misdirected filtration with the accumulation of amorphous material in the paraglomerular space and the subsequent disruption of glomerular–tubular junction resulting in atubular glomeruli. Misdirected filtration may also contribute to tubular atrophy and interstitial fibrosis. Tuft-to-capsule adhesions may allow the influx of periglomerular fibroblasts into the glomerular tuft, thus contributing to glomerulosclerosis.

Extrinsic Cells
Platelets and Coagulation

Platelets and their release products have been detected within glomeruli in experimental and clinical nephropathies. The stimulation of the coagulation cascade is likely to activate mesangial cells and induce sclerosis. Thrombin stimulates glomerular TGF-β1 production leading to mesangial ECM production as well as that of inhibitors of metalloproteinases. Also, the upregulation within damaged glomeruli of PAI-1 is likely to affect outcome because its inhibition of the proteolytic enzyme plasmin may lead to ECM accumulation and glomerulosclerosis. Glomerulosclerosis may depend on the balance between thrombotic-antiproteolytic and anticoagulant-proteolytic activities, with a key role played by the plasminogen regulatory system.

Lymphocytes and Monocyte-Macrophages

Lymphocytes, including helper and cytotoxic T cells, as well as monocytes and macrophages, are often identified within damaged glomeruli. It has been postulated that the balance between proinflammatory Th1 and anti-inflammatory Th2 lymphocytes may be a key factor in the resolution or progression of glomerulosclerosis.

The relevance of monocyte-macrophages to the initiation and progression of glomerulosclerosis has been supported by experiments in which depletion of these cells had a protective effect. The release by these cells of cytokines, growth factors, and procoagulant factors is likely to contribute to the pathogenesis of glomerulosclerosis. However, these cells may also contribute to the termination and resolution of the glomerular inflammatory response. Phenotypic and functional macrophage changes may determine the outcome of glomerular inflammation and sclerosis.

Bone Marrow–derived Cells

Glomerular remodeling (repair and healing or scarring) may depend on the influx of hematopoietic stem cells (HSCs) with the potential for repair or scarring (reviewed in ref. 17). The detection of cells displaying embryonic mesenchymal characteristics in glomeruli has led to the hypothesis that HSCs may be involved in normal glomerular cell turnover as well as in the response of glomeruli to injury. Experiments based on bone marrow transplantation have demonstrated the potential involvement of bone marrow–derived cells in normal mesangial turnover and in glomerular repair and repopulation following experimental mesangial injury.

Tubulointerstitial Scarring

The pathogenesis of tubulointerstitial fibrosis (TIF) has also received increasing attention over recent years (see Fig. 68.8). Severity of tubulointerstitial changes correlates better with renal function than glomerulosclerosis. However, it has been argued that this is due to a sampling error because more than 90% of the renal cortex is tubulointerstitium, and detection of interstitial fibrosis is therefore much more reliable than detection of focal segmental glomerulosclerosis. TIF is likely to evolve in stages including inflammation, proliferation of interstitial fibroblasts, and excessive deposition of interstitial ECM (reviewed in ref. 17; Figs. 68.10 and 68.11). Renal tubular cells play a central role in the pathogenesis of TIF. Injured tubular cells have the capacity to act as antigen-presenting cells, to express cell adhesion molecules, and to release inflammatory mediators and autacoids as well as chemokines, cytokines, and growth factors (see Fig. 68.11). Finally, tubular cells can respond to a range of stimuli by increased synthesis of ECM.

Experimental evidence suggests that tubular cells respond to proteinuria by releasing many of the mediators mentioned earlier

as well as by the synthesis of ECM. In particular, proteins of the complement system, which are lost from the circulation in glomerular proteinuria, have been implicated in damaging tubular cells. This may establish a link between glomerular injury, proteinuria, and TIF. Tubular cells might also be stimulated by the spillover of hormones such as angiotensin II, growth factors, and cytokines from the injured glomeruli. Activation of tubular cells and their release of chemotactic factors can attract inflammatory cells, including monocytes, to the tubules and the renal interstitium, with consequent activation of renal fibroblasts. Activated renal fibroblasts acquire myofibroblast characteristics (e.g., express α-SMA and synthesize interstitial type I and III collagen), proliferate, and invade the periglomerular and peritubular spaces. The resolution of deposited ECM depends on two proteolytic pathways, the first relying on the activation of matrix metalloproteinases and the second on the activation of the proteolytic enzyme plasmin by plasminogen activators. Experimental data suggest that renal scarring is associated with the inhibition of these two collagenolytic pathways, thus disturbing the balance between ECM synthesis and breakdown to favor ECM accumulation and irreversible fibrosis.

In addition, it has been postulated that tubular cells contribute to fibrogenesis through their transformation into a myofibroblastic phenotype. Such epithelial mesenchymal transformation (EMT) is a form of reverse embryogenesis in response to injury because proximal tubules are derived ontogenetically from the metanephric mesenchyme. Experimental studies suggest that a significant percentage of renal fibroblasts may be derived from tubular cells undergoing EMT (reviewed in ref. 25).

Vascular Sclerosis

Vascular sclerosis is an integral feature of the renal scarring process. Renal arteriolar hyalinosis is present in CKD at an early

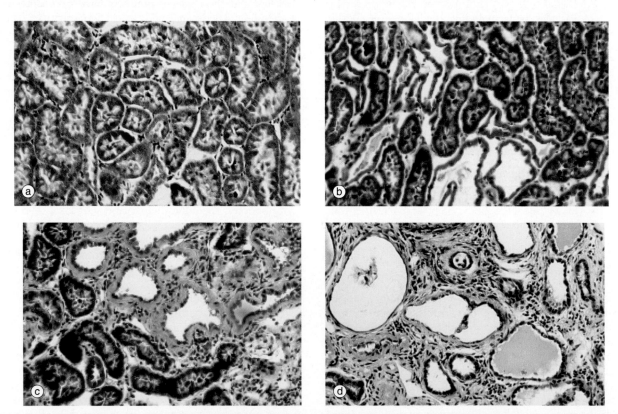

Figure 68.10 Histologic development of tubulointerstitial fibrosis. *a,* Normal tubulointerstitium. *b,* Mild tubulointerstitial scarring with tubular atrophy and interstitial edema. *c,* Segmental interstitial fibrosis. *d,* Diffuse interstitial fibrosis with tubular atrophy and dilation.

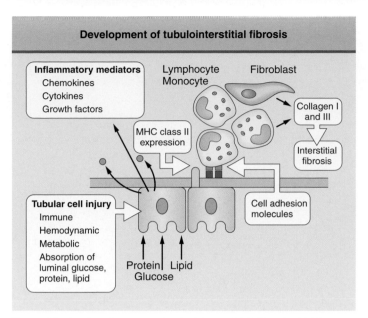

Figure 68.11 Development of tubulointerstitial fibrosis. MHC, major histocompatibility complex.

stage, even in the absence of severe hypertension. Furthermore, these vascular changes are often out of proportion to the severity of systemic hypertension. Vascular sclerosis is associated with progressive kidney failure in glomerulonephritis. Hyalinosis of afferent arterioles has been implicated in the pathogenesis of diabetic glomerulosclerosis. Changes in postglomerular arterioles and damage to peritubular capillaries may further exacerbate interstitial ischemia and fibrosis. Ischemia and the ensuing hypoxia are fibrogenic influences that stimulate tubular cells and kidney fibroblasts to produce ECM components and reduce their collagenolytic activity.[26]

Loss of peritubular capillaries has been linked in experimental models of renal scarring to a fall in the renal expression of the proangiogenic vascular endothelial growth factor (VEGF). Together with an overexpression by scarred kidneys of thrombospondin, an antiangiogenic factor, this would perpetuate microvascular deletion and ischemia.[27] The administration of VEGF preserves peritubular capillaries and improves scarring and functional outcome. Finally, the vascular adventitia may be a source of interstitial myofibroblasts, contributing to the development of interstitial renal fibrosis.

REFERENCES

1. National Kidney Foundation: K/DOQI kidney disease outcome quality initiative. Am J Kidney Dis 2002;39:(Suppl 1):S1–S266.
2. Levey AS, Eckardt KU, Tsukamoto Y, et al: Definition and classification of chronic kidney disease: A position statement from Kidney Disease: Improving Global Outcome (KDIGO). Kidney Int 2005;67:2089–2100.
3. Coresh J, Wei GL, McQuillan G, et al: Prevalence of high blood pressure and elevated serum creatinine level in the United States: Findings from the third National Health in the United States Survey, 1988–1994. Arch Intern Med 2001;161:1207–1216.
4. Iseki K, Iseki C, Ikemiya Y, et al: Risk of developing end-stage renal disease in a cohort of mass screening. Kidney Int 1996;49:800–805.
5. Hillege HL, Janssen WM, Bak AA, et al, for the PREVEND Study Group: Microalbuminuria is common, also in a nondiabetic, nonhypertensive population, and an independent indicator of cardiovascular risk factors and cardiovascular morbidity. J Intern Med 2001;249:519–526.
6. Chadban SJ, Briganti EM, Kerr PG, et al: Prevalence of kidney damage in Australian adults: The AusDiab Kidney Study. J Am Soc Nephrol 2003;14:S131–S138.
7. http://www.renalreg.com/2004.pdf.
8. U.S. Renal Data System (USRDS): 2004 Annual Data Report: Atlas of End Stage Renal Disease in the United States. Bethesda, Md, National Institutes of Health, National Institutes of Diabetes and Digestive and Kidney Diseases, 2004. Available at www.usrds.org.
9. Lysaght MJ: Maintenance dialysis population dynamics: Current trends and long-term implications. J Am Soc Nephrol 2002;13(Suppl 1):S37–40.
10. Lacson E, Kuhlmann MK, Shah K, et al: Outcomes and economics of ESRF. In El Nahas AM (ed): Kidney Disease in Developing Countries and Ethnic Minorities. New York, Taylor & Francis, 2005, pp 15–38.
11. Boulware LE, Jaar BG, Tarver-Carr ME, et al: Screening for proteinuria in US adults: A cost-effectiveness analysis. JAMA 2003;17:3101–3114.
12. National Kidney Foundation: Kidney Early Evaluation Program. Am J Kidney Dis 2005;45(2 Suppl 2):S1–135.
13. Locatelli F, Del Vecchio L: Natural history and factors affecting the progression of chronic renal failure. In El Nahas AM, Anderson S, Harris KPG (eds): Mechanisms and Management of Progressive Renal Failure. London, Oxford University Press, 2000, pp 20–79.
14. Chiurchiu C, Remuzzi G, Ruggenenti P: Angiotensin-converting enzyme inhibition and renal protection in nondiabetic patients: The data of the meta-analyses. J Am Soc Nephrol 2005;16(Suppl 1):S58–63.
15. Traver-Carr ME, Powe NR, Eberhardt MS, et al: Excess risk of chronic kidney disease among African-American versus white subjects in the United States: A population-based study of potential explanatory factors. J Am Soc Nephrol 2002;13:2363–2370.
16. Zandi-Nejad K, Luyckx VA, Brenner BM: Adult hypertension and kidney disease: The role of fetal programming. Hypertension 2006;47:502–508.
17. El Nahas AM: Mechanisms of experimental and clinical renal scarring. In Davison AM, Cameron JS, Grunfeld J-P, et al (eds): Oxford Textbook of Clinical Nephrology, 3rd ed. London, Oxford University Press, 2005, pp 1647–1686.
18. Jafar TH, Stark PC, Schmid CH, et al: Proteinuria as a modifiable risk factor for the progression of non-diabetic renal disease. Kidney Int 2001;60:1131–1140.
19. Jafar TH, Stark PC, Schmid CH, et al: Progression of chronic kidney disease: The role of blood pressure control, proteinuria, and angiotensin-converting enzyme inhibition. A patient-level meta-analysis. Ann Intern Med 2003;139:244–252.
20. Arnlov J, Evans JC, Meigs JB, et al: Low-grade albuminuria and incidence of cardiovascular disease events in nonhypertensive and nondiabetic individuals: The Framingham Heart Study. Circulation 2005;112:969–975.
21. Menon V, Sarnak MJ: The epidemiology of chronic kidney disease stages 1 to 4 and cardiovascular disease: A high-risk combination. Am J Kidney Dis 2005;45:223–232.
22. Johnson RJ, Kivlighn SD, Kim YG, et al: Reappraisal of the pathogenesis and consequence of hyperuricemia in hypertension, cardiovascular disease and renal disease. Am J Kidney Dis 1999;33:225–234.
23. Orth SR, Stockmann A, Conradt C, et al: Smoking as a risk factor for end-stage renal failure in men with primary renal disease. Kidney Int 1998;54:926–931.
24. Endlich K, Kriz W, Witzgall R: Update in podocyte biology. Curr Opin Nephrol Hypertens 2001;10:331–340.
25. El Nahas AM: Plasticity of kidney cells: Role in kidney remodeling and scarring. Kidney Int 2003;64:1553–1563.
26. Fine LG, Orphanides C, Norman JT: Progressive renal disease: The chronic hypoxia hypothesis. Kidney Int 1998;53(Suppl 65):S74–78.
27. Kang DH, Kanellis J, Hugo C, et al: Role of the microvascular endothelium in progressive renal disease. J Am Soc Nephrol 2002;13:806–816.

Retarding Progression of Kidney Disease

Nabil Haddad, Christopher Brown, and Lee A. Hebert

INTRODUCTION

A kidney disease that progresses to end-stage renal disease (ERSD) usually does so by two mechanisms: those of the primary kidney disease and those of natural progression (Fig. 69.1). Natural progression is discussed in Chapter 68. This chapter focuses on therapies to retard natural progression.[1,2] These should be used along with the therapies to treat the primary kidney disease. The goal is nephron preservation so that the vicious cycles of natural progression can be avoided.

MONITORING KIDNEY DISEASE PROGRESSION

Progression is irreversible structural kidney damage. Monitoring the structural damage itself usually is not feasible.[3] Instead, surrogate measures of structural damage, that is, changes in proteinuria and glomerular filtration rate (GFR), are used to monitor progression. For most chronic kidney disease (CKD) patients, the first evidence of natural progression is proteinuria increasing from low to heavy levels. Only later does decreasing GFR appear. However, for certain diseases such as polycystic kidney disease, a decrease in GFR or the presence of hypertension may be the heralding features.

Monitoring Proteinuria Trends

Proteinuria magnitude generally is the strongest single predictor of GFR decline (Fig. 69.2). Furthermore, therapy-induced proteinuria reduction slows GFR decline. The likely reason for these associations is that proteinuria is nephrotoxic, probably through multiple mechanisms[1] (see also Chapter 68). The most detailed analyses of proteinuria and progression are from the Modification in Diet in Renal Disease (MDRD) and Ramipril

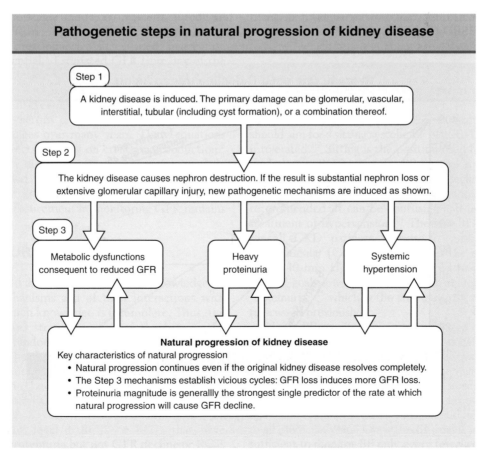

Pathogenetic steps in natural progression of kidney disease

Step 1
A kidney disease is induced. The primary damage can be glomerular, vascular, interstitial, tubular (including cyst formation), or a combination thereof.

Step 2
The kidney disease causes nephron destruction. If the result is substantial nephron loss or extensive glomerular capillary injury, new pathogenetic mechanisms are induced as shown.

Step 3
Metabolic dysfunctions consequent to reduced GFR

Heavy proteinuria

Systemic hypertension

Natural progression of kidney disease
Key characteristics of natural progression
• Natural progression continues even if the original kidney disease resolves completely.
• The Step 3 mechanisms establish vicious cycles: GFR loss induces more GFR loss.
• Proteinuria magnitude is generallly the strongest single predictor of the rate at which natural progression will cause GFR decline.

Figure 69.1   Pathogenetic steps in natural progression of kidney disease. The mechanisms of natural progression are arbitrarily categorized as those induced by decreased glomerular filtration rate (GFR), proteinuria, and systemic hypertension.

hydralazine).[1] Treating nocturnal hypertension, assessed by ambulatory BP monitoring, may also provide benefit[17] (refer to Chapter 31). A therapeutic algorithm to achieve the low BP goal in CKD[1,2] is shown in Figure 69.5.

Angiotensin-Converting Enzyme Inhibitors

Although both angiotensin-converting enzyme (ACE) inhibitors and angiotensin receptor blockers (ARBs) are kidney protective[1]; an ACE inhibitor is the first choice because it is not clear whether ARBs are cardioprotective to the level of ACE inhibitors.[1,18] ACE inhibitors should be used even if the patient is not hypertensive and regardless of the level of proteinuria.[1,8] ACE inhibitors slow progression even in those with a low grade of proteinuria, although the greatest benefit is in those with heavy proteinuria.[1,8] Measures that may increase ACE inhibitor kidney protection include a low-salt, reduced-protein diet,[1] diuretic therapy,[1,19] the low BP goal,[1,2] and statin therapy.[1] ACE inhibitors are antiproteinuric, even in inflammatory glomerulonephritis.[1] ACE inhibitors should be continued even if GFR declines to stage 4 CKD (15 to 29 ml/min/1.73 m^2).[20] To prevent hyperkalemia, dietary potassium restriction, and the concomitant use of a loop diuretic and sodium bicarbonate may be needed.[21] Long-acting ACE inhibitors are preferred.[18,21] Advancing the ACE inhibitor dose to tolerance may increase its antiproteinuric effect[1] and decrease the likelihood of aldosterone escape (increasing plasma aldosterone levels during

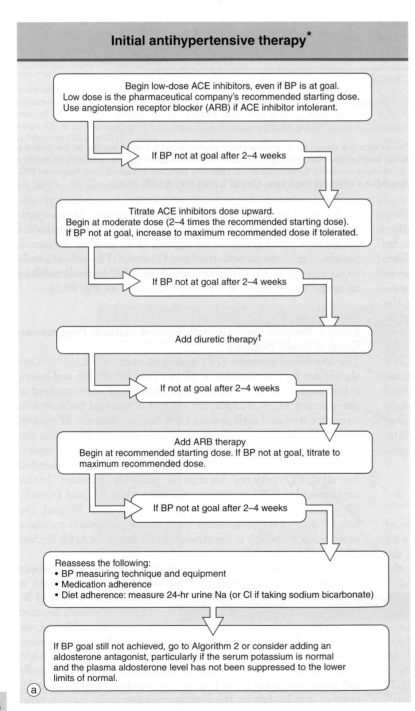

Initial antihypertensive therapy*

Begin low-dose ACE inhibitors, even if BP is at goal.
Low dose is the pharmaceutical company's recommended starting dose.
Use angiotension receptor blocker (ARB) if ACE inhibitor intolerant.

If BP not at goal after 2–4 weeks

Titrate ACE inhibitors dose upward.
Begin at moderate dose (2–4 times the recommended starting dose).
If BP not at goal, increase to maximum recommended dose if tolerated.

If BP not at goal after 2–4 weeks

Add diuretic therapy†

If not at goal after 2–4 weeks

Add ARB therapy
Begin at recommended starting dose. If BP not at goal, titrate to maximum recommended dose.

If BP not at goal after 2–4 weeks

Reassess the following:
• BP measuring technique and equipment
• Medication adherence
• Diet adherence: measure 24-hr urine Na (or Cl if taking sodium bicarbonate)

If BP goal still not achieved, go to Algorithm 2 or consider adding an aldosterone antagonist, particularly if the serum potassium is normal and the plasma aldosterone level has not been suppressed to the lower limits of normal.

(a)

Figure 69.5 Antihypertensive regimens in chronic kidney disease (CKD). *a,* Algorithm 1: initial antihypertensive therapy. *Assumes nonpharmacologic therapy to control blood pressure (BP) is in place (see text) and that the patient does not have renovascular hypertension, congestive heart failure, ischemic heart disease, or hypertensive urgency. This approach focuses on BP control in proteinuric nephropathies, but is also appropriate for hypertensive nephrosclerosis, polycystic kidney disease, and interstitial nephropathies. †The suggestion to add a diuretic before an angiotensin receptor blocker (ARB) is arbitrary but can be justified by the evidence that a diuretic increases the antihypertensive effect of an angiotensin-converting enzyme (ACE) inhibitor, is often needed in chronic kidney disease to control fluid retention, is inexpensive, and may increase the renoprotective effects of the ACE inhibitor, ARB, or the combination.[23] Emphasize salt restriction in autosomal dominant polycystic kidney disease rather than diuretic therapy, which may promote cyst growth.[2] Details of diuretic therapy were discussed previously.

stable ACE inhibitor therapy), which may diminish the ACE inhibitor renoprotection.[22]

Angiotensin Receptor Blocker Therapy

ARBs are renoprotective in the nephropathy of type 2 diabetes and likely in other nephropathies.[1,23] ARBs are recommended as initial therapy if patients are ACE inhibitor intolerant (cough, angioedema, or allergy). ARBs may increase serum potassium less than ACE inhibitors,[1] perhaps because in usual doses, ARBs do not suppress aldosterone as well as ACE inhibitors.[24] The highest tolerated ARB dose is recommended because, compared to usual ARB doses, it is more antiproteinuric[25,26] and more likely to regress left ventricular hypertrophy.[27]

Combination Angiotensin-Converting Enzyme Inhibitor and Angiotensin Receptor Blocker

The combination is more antiproteinuric[28] and appears to halt progression better than either drug alone.[23] The combination of an ACE inhibitor and an ARB is recommended if the patient fails to achieve the BP and proteinuria goals after 4 months of

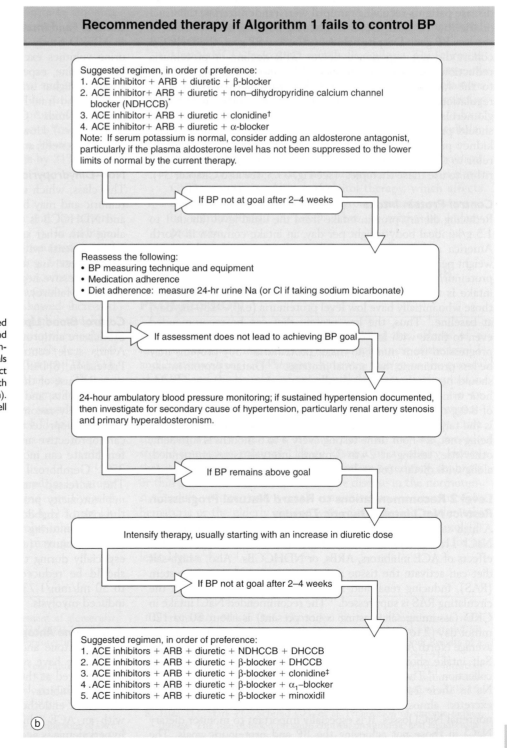

Recommended therapy if Algorithm 1 fails to control BP

Suggested regimen, in order of preference:
1. ACE inhibitor + ARB + diuretic + β-blocker
2. ACE inhibitor+ ARB + diuretic + non–dihydropyridine calcium channel blocker (NDHCCB)*
3. ACE inhibitor+ ARB + diuretic + clonidine†
4. ACE inhibitor+ ARB + diuretic + α-blocker
Note: If serum potassium is normal, consider adding an aldosterone antagonist, particularly if the plasma aldosterone level has not been suppressed to the lower limits of normal by the current therapy.

If BP not at goal after 2–4 weeks

Reassess the following:
• BP measuring technique and equipment
• Medication adherence
• Diet adherence: measure 24-hr urine Na (or Cl if taking sodium bicarbonate)

If assessment does not lead to achieving BP goal

24-hour ambulatory blood pressure monitoring; if sustained hypertension documented, then investigate for secondary cause of hypertension, particularly renal artery stenosis and primary hyperaldosteronism.

If BP remains above goal

Intensify therapy, usually starting with an increase in diuretic dose

If BP not at goal after 2–4 weeks

Suggested regimen, in order of preference:
1. ACE inhibitors + ARB + diuretic + NDHCCB + DHCCB
2. ACE inhibitors + ARB + diuretic + β-blocker + DHCCB
3. ACE inhibitors + ARB + diuretic + β-blocker + clonidine‡
4. ACE inhibitors + ARB + diuretic + β-blocker + α₁–blocker
5. ACE inhibitors + ARB + diuretic + β-blocker + minoxidil

Figure 69.5, cont'd *b*, Algorithm 2: Recommended therapy if algorithm 1 fails to control BP. *Diltiazem and verapamil sustained-release preparations are recommended. †Clonidine recommended for individuals receiving insulin because it does not greatly affect glucoregulation and for those who have difficulty with a β-blocker (e.g., bronchospasm, cardiac conduction). ‡The β-blocker/clonidine combination is usually well tolerated, but may cause bradycardia.

(b)

9. Clase CM, Garg AX, Kiberd BA: Prevalence of low glomerular filtration rate in nondiabetic Americans: Third National Health and Nutrition Examination Survey (NHANES III). J Am Soc Nephrol 2002;13: 1338–1349.

10. Levey AS, Mulrow CD: An editorial update: What level of blood pressure control in chronic kidney disease? Ann Intern Med 2005;143:79–81.

11. Sarnak MJ, Greene T, Wang X, et al: The effect of a lower target blood pressure on the progression of kidney disease: Long-term follow-up of the modification of diet in renal disease study. Ann Intern Med 2005; 142:342–351.

12. Pohl MA, Blumenthal S, Cordonnier DJ, et al: Independent and additive impact of blood pressure control and angiotensin II receptor blockade on renal outcomes in the irbesartan diabetic nephropathy trial: Clinical implications and limitations. J Am Soc Nephrol 2005;16:3027–3037.

13. Ruggenenti P, Perna A, Loriga G, et al: Blood-pressure control for renoprotection in patients with non-diabetic chronic renal disease (REIN-2): Multicentre, randomised controlled trial. Lancet 2005;365:939–946.

14. Hebert CJ, Shidham G, Hebert LA: Should the target for blood pressure control specify both a systolic and a diastolic component? Curr Hypertens Rep 2005;7:360–362.

15. Peterson JC, Adler S, Burkart JM, et al: Blood pressure control, proteinuria, and the progression of renal disease. The Modification of Diet in Renal Disease Study. Ann Intern Med 1995;123:754–762.

16. Verberk WJ, Kroon AA, Kessels AG, de Leeuw PW: Home blood pressure measurement: A systematic review. J Am Coll Cardiol 2005; 46:743–751.

17. Hermida RC, Calvo C, Ayala DE, et al: Treatment of non-dipper hypertension with bedtime administration of valsartan. J Hypertens 2005;23: 1913–1922.

18. Hebert LA, Rovin BH, Hebert CJ: Response to Dr. Brenner's comments. J Am Soc Nephrol 2004;15:1356–1357.

19. Esnault VL, Ekhlas A, Delcroix C, et al: Diuretic and enhanced sodium restriction results in improved antiproteinuric response to RAS blocking agents. J Am Soc Nephrol 2005;16:474–481.

20. Hou FF, Zhang X, Zang GH, et al: Efficacy and safety of benazepril in advanced chronic renal insufficiency. N Engl J Med 2006;354:131–140.

21. Hebert LA: Optimizing ACE inhibitor therapy for CKD. N Engl J Med 2006;354:189–191.

22. Schjoedt KJ, Rossing K, Juhl TR, et al: Beneficial impact of spironolactone in diabetic nephropathy. Kidney Int 2005;68:2829–2836.

23. Nakao N, Yoshimura A, Morita H, et al: Combination treatment of angiotensin-II receptor blocker and angiotensin-converting-enzyme inhibitor in non-diabetic renal disease (COOPERATE): A randomised controlled trial. Lancet 2003;361:117–124.

24. Haddad N, Rajan J, Agarwal A, Hebert LA: In chronic kidney disease ACE inhibition therapy suppresses plasma aldosterone levels better than angiotensin receptor blocker. J Am Soc Nephrol 2005;10:616A.

25. Rossing K, Schjoedt KJ, Jensen BR, et al: Enhanced renoprotective effects of ultrahigh doses of irbesartan in patients with type 2 diabetes and microalbuminuria. Kidney Int 2005;68:1190–1198.

26. Schmieder RE, Klingbeil AU, Fleischmann EH, et al: Additional antiproteinuric effect of ultrahigh dose candesartan: A double-blind, randomized, prospective study. J Am Soc Nephrol 2005;16:3038–3045.

27. Malmqvist K, Kahan T, Edner M, et al: Regression of left ventricular hypertrophy in human hypertension with irbesartan. J Hypertens 2001; 19:1167–1176.

28. Wolf G, Ritz E: Combination therapy with ACE inhibitors and angiotensin II receptor blockers to halt progression of chronic renal disease: pathophysiology and indications. Kidney Int 2005;67:799–812.

29. Griffin KA, Picken MM, Bidani AK: Deleterious effects of calcium channel blockade on pressure transmission and glomerular injury in rat remnant kidneys. J Clin Invest 1995;96:793–800.

30. Teixeira SR, Tappenden KA, Carson L, et al: Isolated soy protein consumption reduces urinary albumin excretion and improves the serum lipid profile in men with type 2 diabetes mellitus and nephropathy. J Nutr 2004;134:1874–1880.

31. Bayorh MA, Ganafa AA, Emmett N, et al: Alterations in aldosterone and angiotensin II levels in salt-induced hypertension. Clin Exp Hypertens 2005;27:355–367.

32. Messerli FH, Grossman E, Leonetti G: Antihypertensive therapy and new onset diabetes. J Hypertens 2004;22:1845–1847.

33. Hebert LA, Greene T, Levey AS, et al: High urine volume and low urine osmolality are risk factors for faster progression of renal disease. Am J Kidney Dis 2003;41:962–971.

34. Wenzel UO, Hebert LA, Stahl RAK, Krenz I: My doctor said I should drink a lot! Recommendations for fluid intake in patients with chronic renal disease. Clin J Am Soc Nephrol (In press).

35. LaRosa JC, Grundy SM, Waters DD, et al: Intensive lipid lowering with atorvastatin in patients with stable coronary disease. N Engl J Med 2005;352:1425–1435.

36. Tonelli M, Collins D, Robins S, et al: Gemfibrozil for secondary prevention of cardiovascular events in mild to moderate chronic renal insufficiency. Kidney Int 2004;66:1123–1130.

37. Ansquer JC, Foucher C, Rattier S, et al: Fenofibrate reduces progression to microalbuminuria over 3 years in a placebo-controlled study in type 2 diabetes: Results from the Diabetes Atherosclerosis Intervention Study (DAIS). Am J Kidney Dis 2005;45:485–493.

38. Mohanram A, Zhang Z, Shahinfar S, et al: Anemia and end-stage renal disease in patients with type 2 diabetes and nephropathy. Kidney Int 2004;66:1131-1138.

39. Gouva C, Nikolopoulos P, Ioannidis JP, Siamopoulos KC: Treating anemia early in renal failure patients slows the decline of renal function: A randomized controlled trial. Kidney Int 2004;66:753–760.

40. Siu YP, Leung KT, Tong MK, Kwan TH: Use of allopurinol in slowing the progression of renal disease through its ability to lower serum uric acid level. Am J Kidney Dis 2006;47:51–59.

41. Johnson RJ, Segal MS, Srinivas T, et al: Essential hypertension, progressive renal disease, and uric acid: a pathogenetic link? J Am Soc Nephrol 2005;16:1909–1919.

42. Curhan GC, Knight EL, Rosner B, et al: Lifetime nonnarcotic analgesic use and decline in renal function in women. Arch Intern Med 2004; 164:1519–1524.

43. Fored CM, Nyren O: Acetaminophen, aspirin, and renal failure [(letter to the editor]. N Engl J Med 2002;346:1588–1589.

44. Isnard Bagnis C, Deray G, Baumelou A, et al: Herbs and the kidney. Am J Kidney Dis 2004;44:1–11.

45. Rangan GK, Pippin JW, Coombes JD, Couser WG: C5b-9 does not mediate chronic tubulointerstitial disease in the absence of proteinuria. Kidney Int 2005;67:492–503.

46. He C, Imai M, Song H, et al: Complement inhibitors targeted to the proximal tubule prevent injury in experimental nephrotic syndrome and demonstrate a key role for C5b-9. J Immunol 2005;174:5750–5757.

47. Agarwal R, Acharya M, Tian J, et al: Antiproteinuric effect of oral paricalcitol in chronic kidney disease. Kidney Int 2005;68:2823–2828.

Clinical Evaluation and Management of Chronic Kidney Disease

David C. Wheeler and Christopher G. Winearls

INTRODUCTION

Most patients with chronic kidney disease (CKD) do not progress to end-stage renal disease (ESRD), but rather die prematurely of other causes, particularly cardiovascular events.[1] Early diagnosis of CKD is therefore becoming increasingly important because it provides opportunities not only to delay progression of kidney failure (see Chapter 69) but also to prevent complications, particularly those that may increase cardiovascular risk (see Chapter 71). Evaluation and management of such patients is likely to assume increasing global significance in coming years, not only in regions of the world with well-funded health care systems, but also in poorer countries that lack renal replacement therapy programs. Nephrologists recognize that they could be overwhelmed by this workload and will need to collaborate with their colleagues in primary care and with other specialists to develop management protocols.

DEFINITIONS

In 2002, the U.S. National Kidney Foundation published the first in a series of Kidney Disease Outcomes Quality Initiative (K/DOQI) guidelines,[2] which attempted to provide a framework for the evaluation of CKD. These guidelines, which promoted the use of the term *kidney* rather than *renal* to increase public awareness, provided a robust definition of CKD (Fig. 70.1) and outlined a five-stage classification system (see Chapter 68, Fig. 68.1). This system, which is based on disease severity rather than cause, has been widely accepted and was recently endorsed in modified format by Kidney Disease: Improving Global Outcomes (KDIGO),[3] an international organization that aims to promote

---

Criteria for definition of chronic kidney disease

Kidney damage for ≥3 months, as defined by structural or functional abnormalities of the kidney, with or without decreased GFR, that can lead to decreased GFR, manifest by either:
- Pathologic abnormalities
- Markers of kidney damage, including abnormalities in the composition of blood or urine, or abnormalities in imaging tests
- GFR <60 ml/min/1.73 m² for ≥3 months, with or without kidney damage

Figure 70.1 Criteria for definition of chronic kidney disease. GFR, glomerular filtration rate. (Adapted from National Kidney Foundation: K/DOQI clinical practice guidelines for chronic kidney disease: Evaluation, classification and stratification. Am J Kidney Dis 2002;39[Suppl 2]:S1–S266.)

---

care and improve outcomes for CKD patients worldwide. Because of the impracticalities of using radioisotopes and 24-hour urine collections, the K/DOQI classification system recommends that kidney function should be assessed by calculating the glomerular filtration rate (GFR) using an appropriate equation. Although there is continuing debate as to which is the ideal method, two formulas are in common use, one developed by Cockcroft and Gault, the other derived from the Modification of Diet in Renal Disease (MDRD) study (see Chapter 3).[4] Although the problem of standardization of creatinine assays still needs to be resolved, the K/DOQI staging system provides a useful framework for the management of CKD and is rapidly becoming accepted worldwide.

CLINICAL PRESENTATION

Many patients with CKD are already known to health care professionals because they are receiving treatment for hypertension, cardiovascular disease, or diabetes. They may be picked up because an elevated blood creatinine level or urinary abnormality is detected, become unwell due to an acute decline of kidney function (acute-on-chronic kidney failure), or remain relatively symptom free until they reach "end stage," when they present as a uremic emergency.

When to Refer to the Nephrologist

Although management of patients with early nonprogressive CKD may eventually become the responsibility of the general internist or primary care physician, nephrologists need to assess those individuals likely to progress to ESRD and require renal replacement therapy (RRT). Referral should ideally occur when such patients reach CKD stage 3. Unfortunately, because CKD is not associated with symptoms in the early stages, a substantial proportion of such patients are referred late, often at the point that they need to be started on dialysis. The problem of late referral is often avoidable,[5] particularly among patients already known to have CKD and may be explained in part by the failure of health care professionals to recognize the nonlinear relation between serum creatinine and GFR (see Chapter 3). Many patients referred late have had the progression of their kidney disease and even the development of complications well documented over sequential consultations. In other cases, late referral is unavoidable because the patient may have had a truly silent illness, or an acute presentation of a disease that causes a rapid decline in kidney function.

As a consequence of late presentation, the opportunity to prepare patients optimally for dialysis is missed, and patient choice is compromised because there is limited time to assess an individual's suitability for peritoneal dialysis, or to list for kidney transplantation before starting dialysis. Furthermore, because an arteriovenous fistula typically takes 8 to 12 weeks to mature, patients presenting late are required to start hemodialysis using central venous catheters. These are prone to infectious complications and inevitably damage central veins, leading to thromboses and stenoses, which may manifest at a later stage when venous return from one or other arm is increased by the subsequent construction of arteriovenous fistulas[6] (see Chapter 81). Late presentation of CKD prevents treatment of uremic complications such as hypertension and anemia,[7] both of which contribute to cardiovascular damage, which may ultimately limit life span.[8] These factors compound to cause psychological stress, making it more difficult for the patient to come to terms with the illness in the longer term. Importantly, late presentation is associated with a worse prognosis,[9] and the cost of initiating dialysis in ESRD patients presenting late is much higher than for those in whom an elective start is made.[10]

CLINICAL MANIFESTATIONS OF CHRONIC KIDNEY FAILURE

A more substantial discussion of the complications of CKD is provided in Chapters 71 to 79. With the exception of hypertension, there are usually few clinical manifestations during CKD stages 1 and 2 (GFR >60 ml/min), the presence of proteinuria or hematuria being dependant on the underlying cause of kidney disease. Other complications (discussed in the following sections) tend to develop progressively as GFR declines below 30 ml/min (i.e., during stages 4 to 5 CKD).

Hypertension

Between 50% and 75% of individuals with CKD stages 3 to 5 have hypertension (defined as a systolic blood pressure ≥140 mm Hg or diastolic blood pressure ≥70 mm Hg).[11] Blood pressure can be determined by random measurement (according to appropriate local guidelines), but ambulatory monitoring may be required in certain situations, for example, when it is suspected that readings taken in the hospital are not representative. In patients with atherosclerotic vascular disease and CKD, the presence of renal artery stenosis should be considered, and when appropriate, such patients are referred for specialist assessment.

Successful control of blood pressure may both slow the rate of decline of renal function (see Chapter 69) and minimize damage to both the heart and arteries, reducing the risk for cardiovascular complications. All classes of antihypertensive agent can be used in CKD patients, although multidrug regimens are usually necessary, and the underlying cause of kidney disease may influence the choice of agents[11] (see Chapter 34). Lifestyle modifications, including weight loss (where appropriate) and dietary sodium restriction to <2.4 g (100 mmol) per day, should be encouraged. Fluid retention occurs in CKD stages 3 to 5, and a diuretic should be included in the antihypertensive regimen. In general, thiazides are recommended in patients with CKD stages 1 to 3 and loop diuretics in those with more severely impaired kidney function.[11] Potassium-sparing diuretics should be avoided in CKD stages 4 to 5 and used with caution, particularly in combination with angiotensin-converting enzyme (ACE) inhibitors and angiotensin receptor blockers (ARB), in those with better preserved kidney function. The available evidence supports a target blood pressure <130/80 mm Hg for most CKD patients, but <125/75 mm Hg for those with a urinary protein excretion >1 g/24 hours.[11]

Dyslipidemia

Patients with CKD stage 3 develop a disturbance of lipoprotein metabolism characterized by the accumulation of partially metabolized very-low-density lipoprotein (VLDL) particles and a disturbance in the maturation of high-density lipoprotein (HDL).[12] Blood tests typically show hypertriglyceridemia with low HDL cholesterol concentrations. Total and low-density lipoprotein (LDL)-cholesterol levels are generally normal but may be low in patients with concomitant inflammation and malnutrition.[13] Like hypertension, treatment of dyslipidemia may have the dual benefits of both slowing the progression of CKD and reducing the likelihood of cardiovascular complications. *Post hoc* analysis of large trials of statin treatment suggests that patients with vascular disease and concomitant CKD stage 3 are likely to benefit from treatment.[14] However, to date there is no robust evidence to suggest that these drugs benefit CKD patients without overt vascular disease or those with more advanced stages of CKD. Current guidelines for the treatment of dyslipidemia in CKD patients recommend extrapolating treatment thresholds and targets from non-CKD populations.[12] The risks associated with the use of fibrates and statins, particularly muscle damage, are increased. Fibrate doses should be reduced in any patient with CKD stages 3 to 4, and these agents are best avoided in those with stage 5 disease. Statins appear to have a reasonably good safety profile, although low starting doses are recommended because of drug accumulation.[12]

Anemia

Anemia is associated with CKD stages 3 to 5[15] and is caused by a relative deficiency of erythropoietin, although reduced availability of iron and chronic inflammation are frequent contributory factors. Anemia may contribute to cardiac dysfunction by increasing cardiac output and may thereby exacerbate left ventricular hypertrophy. Although reversal of anemia with erythropoietin has been associated with regression of left ventricular hypertrophy,[16] there is currently no evidence that treatment is associated with an improved longer-term cardiac prognosis, although it can be readily justified on the basis of the associated improvements in quality of life.[17] There is ongoing debate as to the optimal target range of hemoglobin concentrations, with most guidelines recommending a level of 11 to 13 g/dl (see Chapter 72).[18] Partial correction of anemia does not accelerate the decline of renal function but may necessitate increases in antihypertensive therapy.[19] The management of anemia with erythropoietin and newer analogues with longer half-lives is covered in detail in Chapter 72.

Bone and Mineral Metabolism

Hyperphosphatemia, together with a deficiency of the 1,25-dihydroxyvitamin D_3 contributes to secondary hyperparathyroidism and ultimately to the development of renal bone disease. These biochemical and endocrine abnormalities may be evident in patients with CKD stage 3 and are well established in those who reach ESRD, even though they rarely lead to symptomatic bone disease until patients have been on dialysis for several years (see Chapter 74). Prevention of secondary hyperparathyroidism requires dietary phosphate restriction as early as possible and administration of phosphate binders.[20] Patients are also prescribed biologically active vitamin D (e.g., calcitriol) or vitamin D prohormones that are converted to active dihydroxylated compounds in the liver (e.g., 1α-hydroxyvitamin D_3).[21] Many patients with CKD stages 3 to 4 are also deficient in 25-hydroxyvitamin D_3,[22] and oral replacement with parent vitamin D_2 (ergocalciferol) may increase plasma levels of the 1,25-dihydroxy derivative.[23] As with the management of anemia, the optimal time to initiate these therapies has not been established.

Metabolic Acidosis

The metabolic acidosis associated with chronic kidney disease is caused by failure of hydrogen ion excretion and may be compounded by bicarbonate loss, particularly in interstitial kidney diseases. The clinical consequences are rarely evident until patients reach CKD stage 5, when dyspnea may occur, even on minor exertion. Similar symptoms may be attributable to anemia and pulmonary edema, emphasizing the need for careful evaluation. The development of acidosis aggravates hyperkalemia, inhibits protein anabolism, and accelerates calcium loss from bone where the hydrogen ions are buffered.[24] The presence of a severe metabolic acidosis (e.g., serum bicarbonate <20 mmol/l) associated with symptoms in a patient with CKD stage 5 is an indication to start dialysis. If dialysis is not immediately available, oral sodium bicarbonate in a dose up to 1.2 g four times daily may be considered, but sodium loading may aggravate hypertension.

Malnutrition

Malnutrition is common among patients on dialysis but may occur in those with CKD stages 4 to 5 (see Chapter 77) and is associated with an increased risk for death.[13] Its causes are multifactorial and include anorexia, acidosis, insulin resistance, inflammation, and urinary protein loss. Biochemical indicators include a fall in serum albumin, transferrin, and cholesterol. Weight should be carefully monitored in patients who progress to CKD stages 4 to 5. Serum creatinine concentrations, which in part reflect muscle mass, may stop rising despite a progressive loss of kidney function because of compromised nutritional status. If patients do not readily respond to dietary supplementation, initiation of dialysis should be considered.

Sodium and Water Retention

Sodium handling by the kidney is altered in CKD (see Chapter 7), although plasma sodium concentrations are generally within the normal range. As GFR falls, sodium homeostasis is initially maintained because a greater proportion of sodium and water filtered by the glomerulus is excreted. To produce such a change in the excretion of sodium and water requires a magnification of the normal tubular response. One of the earliest effects of CKD is to limit the ability of the kidney to compensate for large changes in sodium and water intake. Although in healthy individuals, water excretion can be varied from about 20 to 1500 ml/hour depending on hydration status, in CKD patients, this range becomes restricted. In such individuals, excessive oral water intake may lead to dilutional hyponatremia. As kidney function declines, most patients develop sodium retention and extracellular volume expansion. They may complain of ankle swelling or shortness of breath as a result of pulmonary edema. Restriction of dietary sodium intake to 2.4 g (100 mmol) per day may help to alleviate such symptoms and control the associated increase in blood pressure. Salt substitutes containing potassium should be avoided because of the risk for hyperkalemia.

Potassium

Hyperkalemia may develop in CKD stages 4 to 5 and can be managed by restricting dietary potassium to less than 60 mmol potassium daily. Unlike patients with acute kidney failure, those with CKD may tolerate high plasma potassium concentrations without electrocardiographic changes or arrhythmias. However, dialysis may be required if the serum potassium concentration is consistently above 6.5 mmol/l and no correctable exacerbating factors are identified. Ion-exchange resins are unpleasant to take, may cause severe constipation, and should not be used except in emergencies.

Endocrine Abnormalities

In addition to abnormalities in the hydroxylation of vitamin D (see Chapter 74) and the synthesis of erythropoietin (see Chapter 72), the production, protein binding, catabolism, and tissue effects of other hormones may be modified in CKD.

Thyroid Hormones

Total plasma thyroxine (T_4) levels may be low, with an associated increase in reverse triiodothyronine (T_3) as a result of impaired conversion of T_3 to T_4. Loss of thyroid-binding globulin may further lower total circulating T_4 concentrations.[25] However, patients do not become clinically hypothyroid, and measurement of thyroid-stimulating hormone remains a reliable diagnostic test for hypothyroidism in CKD.

Growth Hormone

Plasma growth hormone levels may be elevated in patients with CKD stage 5 because of delayed clearance and alterations in hypothalamic-pituitary control.[26] In children, growth retardation may result and can be corrected by treatment with exogenous recombinant growth hormone given in supraphysiologic doses.

Insulin

Decreased clearance of insulin is balanced by increased peripheral resistance to the effects of the hormone. As a result, there are usually no clinical manifestations, and patients are not particularly prone to hypoglycemia. However, in diabetic patients, these effects may lead to a falling requirement for insulin as kidney function declines, a trend that may be reversed by the initiation of dialysis.[27]

Sex Hormones

Males Prolactin levels are elevated in CKD stage 5 and may contribute to gynecomastia and sexual dysfunction. Testosterone levels are often low-normal, and gonadotropins may be raised, implying testicular failure.[28] This is accompanied by poor spermatogenesis, leading to low sperm counts and reduced fertility. It is appropriate to prescribe androgen replacement treatment if testosterone is unequivocally low, not least because this may help to prevent osteoporosis.[29] Perhaps the most important and sexual problem in males is erectile dysfunction, although this is more likely to result from neurologic, psychological, and vascular abnormalities than endocrine disturbances and may respond to phosphodiesterase type 5 inhibitors such as sildenafil citrate.

Females The pituitary-ovary axis may be disturbed CKD stages 4 to 5.[30] Although luteinizing hormone levels are raised, the normal pulsatile release and the preovulation surge are absent. Cycles are therefore often anovulatory and may be irregular, or there may be amenorrhea. Raised prolactin levels may also contribute to infertility. Rarely, women receiving dialysis conceive and very rarely carry to term (see Chapter 42).

Immunity

Infections are the second most common cause of death, after cardiovascular disease, in patients with CKD stage 5 receiving dialysis. This is explained in part by the invasive procedures required for the delivery of RRT but also reflects the fact that CKD is a state of chronic immunosuppression[31] with defects of both cellular and humoral immunity (see Chapter 73).

T cell responses to antigen are deficient, partly because of impaired antigen presentation by monocytes. Neutrophil activation is defective, and although serum immunoglobulin levels are normal, antibody responses to immunization are poor. This is a particular problem when immunizing the CKD patient against hepatitis B. Whereas more than 90% of a healthy population will respond to a standard vaccination protocol, this proportion drops to 50% to 60% of CKD patients and is directly related to the severity of kidney failure. Poor responses are also encountered when immunizing with other T cell–dependent antigens, such as *Pneumococcus* species and *Haemophilus influenzae* type b, and do not appear to be corrected by initiation of dialysis.

The clinical manifestations of these immune defects include increased susceptibility to bacterial infection (particularly staphylococcal), increased risk for reactivation of tuberculosis (typically with a negative tuberculin skin test), and failure to eliminate hepatitis B and C virus following infections. CKD patients should be immunized against hepatitis B as early as is feasible in an effort to maximize the chances of seroconversion.[32] Immunization is still worthwhile in patients presenting with CKD stage 5, but an intensified regimen is recommended (e.g., 40 μg of vaccine administered intramuscularly at 0, 1, and 6 months). Some 40% to 80% of such patients will respond to this regimen.

Psychological Manifestations

The psychological problems associated with CKD include anxiety and depression and are largely the predictable consequences of loss of health and the inevitable requirement for lifestyle changes. Most patients manage well if given sufficient information and appropriate support, whereas others may benefit from more intensive counseling. Short-term antidepressant therapy may help, and some patients benefit from night sedation, particularly during hospital admissions.

Other Complications of Chronic Kidney Disease

CKD patients, particularly those with stage 5 disease, may develop a bleeding diathesis (see Chapter 73), neurologic problems including uremic encephalopathy (see Chapter 76), and dermatologic manifestations (see Chapter 78). Uremic pericarditis may occur in CKD stage 5 and can usually be detected clinically by the presence of a pericardial rub. Administration of anticoagulants to such patients may lead to hemorrhage into the pericardial cavity, causing life-threatening tamponade.

MANAGEMENT OF CHRONIC KIDNEY DISEASE STAGES 4 TO 5

The general approach to the management of a CKD patient can be tailored according to the stage of disease, as shown in Figure 70.2. For those presenting at stage 5 who have symptoms consistent with advanced uremia, dialysis treatment may need to be initiated as an emergency. As mentioned previously, earlier presentation to a specialist increases opportunities to treat complications and to prepare patients for RRT. In an effort to optimize the management of such individuals, many centers follow patients with CKD stages 4 to 5 in dedicated "low-clearance" clinics. This allows the most productive interaction between the patient and members of the multidisciplinary team, including the nephrologist, surgeon, nurse, social worker, dietitian, and psychologist (see Chapters 80 and 81).

Treating the Uremic Emergency

For patients presenting with symptomatic uremia, the priority is to deal with life-threatening complications such as hyperkalemia, pulmonary edema, metabolic acidosis, encephalopathy, and pericarditis. This so-called uremic emergency can be the initial presentation of either acute renal failure or ESRD resulting from CKD. Whichever is the case, the immediate management is the

Management plan for chronic kidney disease patients, according to stage					
K/DOQI Class	GFR (ml/min)	Typical Serum Creatinine in a 65-kg Subject	Consequences	Action
3	30–59	2 mg/dl (170 μmol/l)	Hypertension, secondary hyperparathyroidism	Treat hypertension Start phosphate restriction and phosphate binders Start vitamin D analogue Immunize against hepatitis B
4	15–29	4 mg/dl (354 μmol/l)	+ Anemia	Restrict dietary potassium to 60 mmol/day Advise moderate protein restriction Plan renal replacement therapy, including vascular access
5	<15	8 mg/dl (707 μmol/l)	+ Sodium and water retention, anorexia, vomiting, reduced higher mental function	Plan elective start of dialysis or pre-emptive renal transplantation
5 (uremic emergency)	<5	17 mg/dl (1503 μmol/l)	+ Pulmonary edema coma, fits, metabolic acidosis, hyperkalemia, death	Start dialysis or provide palliative care

Figure 70.2 Management plan for patients with chronic kidney disease (CKD), according to stage. The table gives a rough guide to the level of blood creatinine corresponding to each stage of CKD in a typical 65-kg subject and shows the approximate timing of the anticipated clinical problems and interventions required as CKD progresses. At each stage, the action plan for the previous CKD stage should be followed if not already initiated.

same and is discussed further in Chapter 65. Patients presenting with uremic emergencies may need to be managed in an intensive care unit or in a high-dependency area. In this setting, the contribution of the nephrologist includes determination of treatment priorities, optimization of timing of dialysis, monitoring for complications, and initiation or discontinuation of medications as appropriate.

Acute Renal Failure versus Chronic Kidney Disease

After the crisis has been resolved, the next task is to distinguish between acute and chronic kidney disease, after which the diagnostic and management paths will diverge. There may be hints of a past history of kidney problems (e.g., hypertension, proteinuria, microscopic hematuria) or symptoms suggestive of prostatic disease. The physical examination is not usually helpful, although skin pigmentation (Fig. 70.3), scratch marks, left ventricular hypertrophy, and hypertensive fundal changes would favor a chronic rather than acute presentation. Of the various investigations, the renal ultrasound may be one of the most useful. Small kidneys with reduced cortical thickness, showing increased echogenicity, scarring, or multiple cysts, suggest a chronic process. Blood tests are less helpful unless they indicate evidence of an acute illness that may be the cause of kidney failure, such as systemic vasculitis or multiple myeloma. The presence of a normochromic normocytic anemia is usual in CKD, as described previously, but may also be a feature of systemic illnesses that cause acute renal failure and is not generally helpful in determining the type of presentation. The findings of low serum calcium and raised phosphate levels have little or no discriminatory value, but normal levels of parathyroid hormone are more in keeping with acute renal failure. Patients with grossly abnormal biochemical values (e.g., blood urea nitrogen [BUN] >140 mg/dl, or creatinine >1200 μmol/l [13.5 mg/dl], blood urea >50 mmol/l [>300 mg/dl]), who appear relatively well and are still passing normal volumes of urine are more likely to have chronic than acute kidney disease.

If the blood urea is disproportionately high when compared with the blood creatinine level, evidence of dehydration, gastrointestinal blood loss, infection, and other causes of hypercatabolism should be sought. In moderate to severe kidney failure the blood urea (mmol)–to–creatinine (μmol) ratio is typically about 60:1; that is, urea of 20 mmol/l coincides with creatinine of 300 μmol/l. The corresponding BUN (mg)-to-creatinine (mg) ratio is 15:1.

Establishing the Cause of Chronic Kidney Disease

Establishing the cause of CKD may be helpful for a number of reasons. First, the underlying disease may be treatable, and doing so may slow or prevent further deterioration or even lead to recovery of kidney function. Second, patients with certain genetic diseases, such as adult polycystic kidney disease, may require appropriate counseling. Third, some kidney diseases (e.g., focal segmental glomerulosclerosis) may recur after transplantation and may therefore influence the decision to place the patient on the waiting list. Although the cause may be apparent from the clinical assessment, problems may arise in patients with little or no past medical history and small kidneys on ultrasound with minimal or no abnormalities of urinalysis. Investigation should not be pursued relentlessly because the implications for treatment are often minimal. Attempting to obtain biopsy material from small kidneys is risky and may not reveal a definitive diagnosis.

Minimizing Progression of Chronic Kidney Disease

Delaying or preventing progression of kidney failure is a priority in the management of any CKD patient (see Chapter 69). The first consideration is whether the underlying cause can be modified or arrested. Whichever the case, factors that may compromise kidney function should be identified. Progression may be retarded by improving control of hypertension. The underlying nature of kidney disease influences the risk and rate of progression. For example, adult polycystic kidney disease usually leads to an inexorable decline in kidney function over time, whereas relieving obstruction of the renal tract and treated accelerated phase hypertension may stabilize kidney function.

Unexpected Deterioration of Kidney Function

CKD patients may require reassessment if kidney function suddenly declines faster than predicted during follow-up (Fig. 70.4). The possible causes for acute-on-chronic kidney failure are listed in Figure 70.5. Whatever the underlying cause of the chronic kidney disease, compromised renal perfusion may reduce the GFR sufficiently to cause a rise in blood creatinine levels over and above that predicted for the observed rate of progression, particularly in elderly patients. This may result from dehydration due to the prescription of diuretics, hot weather, diarrhea, or vomiting and is exacerbated in CKD stages 4 to 5 by the impaired concentrating ability of the kidneys. Dehydration substantial enough to cause a rise in blood creatinine may not cause symptoms, although there may be a fall in body weight of at least 3 kg and a postural drop in blood pressure. Kidney perfusion can also be compromised by heart failure, myocardial infarction, and tachyarrhythmias and may be affected by drugs, including nonsteroidal anti-inflammatory drugs (NSAIDs), ACE inhibitors, and ARB.

Drugs may also cause a sudden decline in kidney function due to direct nephrotoxicity, and a review of prescribed medications is essential in such patients. For example, a variety of different therapeutic agents may cause interstitial nephritis (e.g., antibiotics, NSAIDs, and allopurinol; see Chapter 57). A renal biopsy may help to substantiate this diagnosis, which might also be suggested by other evidence of allergy, such as skin rash, eosinophilia, or eosinophiluria. In addition to discontinuing the suspected drug, many nephrologists prescribe steroids (prednisolone, 30 mg/day

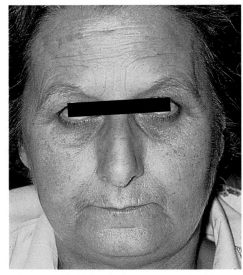

Figure 70.3 Uremic pigmentation. Diffuse brown pigmentation as seen here suggests chronic kidney disease, rather than acute kidney failure.

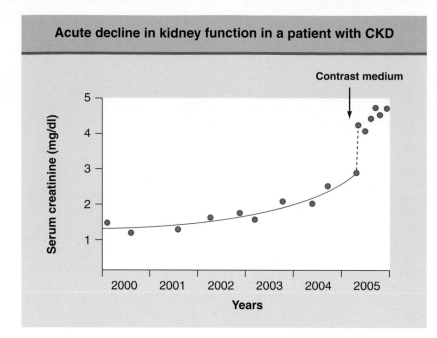

Figure 70.4 Acute decline in kidney function in a patient with chronic kidney disease. Serum creatinine plot for a 58-year-old man with CKD secondary to diabetic nephropathy. An exponential increase over time is seen between 2000 and 2004. However, an abrupt rise occurs in April 2005 when the patient receives contrast medium for coronary angiography without prior hydration. The patient's kidney function never recovered to the previous baseline, and he began hemodialysis in December 2005.

for 2 weeks), although there is no good evidence of benefit. The problem of iatrogenic drug nephrotoxicity is discussed further in Chapters 100 and 101.

Other causes of an acute decline in kidney function that should be considered in a CKD patient include renal tract obstruction, which is usually detected on ultrasound; hypercalcemia, which may be caused by the coadministration of high doses of vitamin D compounds and calcium-containing phosphate binders; accelerated-phase hypertension; and renal vein thrombosis. The clinician should also be alert to the possibility of relapse of a treated underlying disease.

Assessing Stage of Chronic Kidney Disease and Preparation for Renal Replacement Therapy

Despite all attempts to optimize the management of CKD, many patients will progress to ESRD. The KDOQI staging system (see Chapter 68, Fig. 68.1) helps to set out the management priorities according to level of kidney function (see Fig. 70.2). When GFR has fallen below 60 ml/min (CKD stage 3), prophylaxis against secondary hyperparathyroidism should be started by restricting

dietary phosphate, and if this fails to control phosphate levels (see Chapter 74), prescription of oral phosphate binders is appropriate. Patients should be checked for deficiency of 25-hydroxyvitamin D_3 and appropriate supplementation commenced if necessary. If these measures fail to prevent a rise in parathyroid hormone, 1α-hydroxyvitamin D_3 or 1,25-dihydroxyvitamin D should be commenced. Immunization against hepatitis B should also be arranged. Anemia and iron status should be evaluated, and treated or corrected if necessary (see Chapter 72).

At a GFR of 15 to 20 ml/min (late stage 4 or stage 5), patients should receive education and counseling to aid their selection of the most appropriate renal replacement modality. If hemodialysis is the preferred option, an arteriovenous fistula should be constructed, remembering that it may take 8 to 12 weeks for veins to become adequately arterialized before needling can be attempted (see Chapter 81). Because early kidney transplantation improves long-term outcome,[33] patients should be assessed for their suitability and, when feasible, activated on the waiting list before dialysis is commenced. This maximizes the chances of the potential recipient remaining in reasonably good health. The availability of a live donor should be explored to increase the chances of (pre-emptive) transplantation before the patient begins dialysis.

The decision to start dialysis is generally considered in any patient with CKD stage 5 who develops uremic symptoms, shows evidence of malnutrition, or develops life-threatening complications of CKD, such as pericarditis, hyperkalemia, acidosis, or fluid overload (see Chapter 80). The case for starting dialysis earlier than stage 5 is not strong,[34] but all patients with CKD stages 4 and 5 are best monitored regularly by a specialist team (e.g., in a low-clearance clinic). A plan for assessment of such patients in provided in Figure 70.6.

CONSERVATIVE MANAGEMENT OF TERMINAL UREMIA

There will be patients for whom dialysis is considered inappropriate and others who decide to discontinue treatment. The decision against dialysis should be made, if possible, in consultation with the patient and family long before the need arises, preferably in the context of a multidisciplinary low-clearance clinic (see

Causes of acute-on-chronic kidney failure
Dehydration
Drugs
Disease relapse
Disease acceleration
Infection
Obstruction
Hypercalcemia
Hypertension
Heart failure
Interstitial nephritis

Figure 70.5 Causes of acute-on-chronic kidney failure.

Continuing assessment of the chronic kidney disease patient
Kidney Function
Has kidney function declined?
Has kidney function declined at the predicted rate?
If not, are there exacerbating factors?
Should dialysis be started?

Are there life-threatening complications?
  Pericarditis
  Fluid overload
  Resistant hypertension
  Hyperkalemia
  Uncompensated metabolic acidosis

Should access be created or transplantation planned?
Supportive Treatment
Can salt, potassium, and fluid balance be improved by diet or diuretics?
Is the phosphate controlled?
Is the dose of vitamin D compound appropriate?
Should erythropoietin be prescribed?
Are nutritional supplements needed?
Does the patient need counseling?

Figure 70.6 Continuing assessment of the patient with chronic kidney disease (CKD). Questions to be posed when reviewing the patient.

Chapter 80). The patient will need to know the limits of what dialysis can achieve and at what cost in terms of inpatient stays, travel time, lifestyle restrictions, and complications. One compelling argument not to offer dialysis to elderly patients with high levels of associated comorbidity is that such individuals are unlikely to benefit in terms of life expectancy.[35] It may also be inappropriate to offer dialysis to patients with other concurrent conditions that lead to major limitations or limit life span, such as malignant disease.

In the context of a uremic emergency, when the background history may not be readily available and the patient's premorbid state is unknown, it is much harder not to initiate dialysis treatment, particularly when dialysis may provide symptomatic relief. However, subsequently withdrawing dialysis or dying while on dialysis treatment is traumatic for both the patient's family and staff. The ethical and legal issues are complex and require that the patient makes the decision not to receive or to discontinue dialysis when fully informed and able to do so.

Properly managed, death from uremia should be relatively free of suffering. It is important to ensure that the patient is comfortable with the decision and that family members are understanding and supportive. Symptoms such as dyspnea from pulmonary edema and acidosis are best controlled with a morphine infusion and nausea with regular chlorpromazine or ondansetron. The mouth can become dry and crusted from mouth breathing, and regular mouth washes and gum care should be offered. Pruritus can be managed by cooling the skin and by application of emollients. Myoclonic jerks are distressing and may be reduced by prescription of benzodiazepines.

REFERENCES

1. Keith DS, Nichols GA, Gullion CM, et al: Longitudinal follow-up and outcomes among a population with chronic kidney disease in a managed care organization. Arch Intern Med 2004;164:659–663.
2. National Kidney Foundation: KDOQI clinical practice guidelines for chronic kidney disease: Evaluation, classification and stratification. Am J Kidney Dis 2002;39(Suppl 2):S1–S266.
3. Levey AS, Eckardt KU, Tsukamoto Y, et al: Definition and classification of chronic kidney disease: A position statement from Kidney Disease: Improving Global Outcomes (KDIGO). Kidney Int 2005;67:2089–2100.
4. Froissart M, Rossert J, Jacquot C, et al: Predictive performance of the modification of diet in renal disease and Cockcroft-Gault equations for estimating renal function. J Am Soc Nephrol 2005;16:763–773.
5. Roderick P, Jones C, Drey N, et al: Late referral for end-stage renal disease: A region-wide survey in the south west of England. Nephrol Dial Transplant 2002;17:1252–1259.
6. Roy-Chaudhury P, Kelly BS, Melhem M, et al: Vascular access in hemodialysis: Issues, management, and emerging concepts. Cardiol Clin 2005;23:249–273.
7. Landray MJ, Thambyrajah J, McGlynn FJ, et al: Epidemiological evaluation of known and suspected cardiovascular risk factors in chronic renal impairment. Am J Kidney Dis 2001;38:537–546.
8. Go AS, Chertow GM, Fan D, et al: Chronic kidney disease and risk of death, cardiovascular events, and hospitalization. N Engl J Med 2004;351:1296–1305.
9. Winkelmayer WC, Owen WF, Levin R, Avorn J: A propensity analysis of late versus early nephrologist referral and mortality on dialysis. J Am Soc Nephrol 2003;14:486–492.
10. Lameire N, Wauters JP, Teruel JL, et al: An update on the referral pattern of patients with end-stage renal disease. Kidney Int Suppl 2002;80:27–34.
11. Kidney Disease Outcomes Quality Initiative (K/DOQI): K/DOQI clinical practice guidelines on hypertension and antihypertensive agents in chronic kidney disease. Am J Kidney Dis 2004;43(Suppl 1):S1–S290.
12. National Kidney Foundation: KDOQI clinical practice guidelines for managing dyslipidemias in chronic kidney disease. Am J Kidney Dis 2003;41(Suppl 3):S1–S92.
13. Kalantar-Zadeh K: Recent advances in understanding the malnutrition-inflammation-cachexia syndrome in chronic kidney disease patients: What is next? Semin Dial 2005;18;365–369.
14. Tonelli M, Isles C, Curhan GC, et al: Effect of pravastatin on cardiovascular events in people with chronic kidney disease. Circulation 2004;110:1557–1663.
15. Oberador GT, Pereira BJ: Anaemia of chronic kidney disease: An under-recognized and under-treated problem. Nephrol Dial Transplant 2002;17(Suppl 11):44–46.
16. Locatelli F, Pozzoni P, Del Vecchio L: Anemia and heart failure in chronic kidney disease. Semin Nephrol. 2005;25:392–396.
17. Whittington R, Barradell LB, Benfield P: Epoetin: A pharmacoeconomic review of its use in chronic renal failure and its effects on quality of life. Pharmacoeconomics 1993;3:45–82.
18. Locatelli F, Aljama P, Barany P, et al, for the European Best Practice Guidelines Working Group: Revised European best practice guidelines for the management of anaemia in patients with chronic renal failure. Nephrol Dial Transplant 2004;19(Suppl 2):1–47.
19. Jungers P, Choukroun G, Oualim Z, et al: Beneficial influence of recombinant human erythropoietin therapy on the rate of progression of chronic renal failure in predialysis patients. Nephrol Dial Transplant 2001;16:307–312.
20. Locatelli F, Cannata-Andia JB, Drueke TB, et al: Management of disturbances of calcium and phosphate metabolism in chronic renal insufficiency, with emphasis on the control of hyperphosphataemia. Nephrol Dial Transplant 2002;17:723–731.
21. Martin KJ, Gonzalez EA: Vitamin D analogues for the management of secondary hyperparathyroidism. Am J Kidney Dis 2001;38(Suppl 5):S34–S40.
22. St John A, Thomas MB, Davies CP, et al: Determinants of intact parathyroid hormone and free 1,25-dihydroxyvitamin D levels in mild and moderate renal failure. Nephron 1992;61:422–427.
23. National Kidney Foundation: K/DOQI clinical practice guidelines for bone metabolism and disease in chronic kidney disease. Am J Kidney Dis 2003;42(Suppl 3):S1–S201.
24. Alpern RJ, Sakhaee K: The clinical spectrum of chronic metabolic acidosis: Homeostatic mechanisms produce significant morbidity. Am J Kidney Dis 1997;29:291–302.
25. Lim VS: Thyroid function in patients with chronic renal failure. Am J Kidney Dis 2001;38(Suppl 1)S80–S84.
26. Johannasson G, Ahlmen J: End-stage renal disease: Endocrine aspects of treatment. Growth Horm IGF Res 2003;(Suppl A):S94–S101.

27. Snyder RW, Berns JS: Use of insulin and oral hypoglycaemic medications in patients with diabetes mellitus and advanced kidney disease. Semin Dial 2004;17:365–370.

28. Schmidt A, Luger A, Horl WH: Sexual hormone abnormalities in male patients with renal failure. Nephrol Dial Transplant 2002;17:368–371.

29. Johansen KL: Treatment of hypogonadism in men with chronic kidney disease. Adv Chronic Kidney Dis 2004;11:348–356.

30. Holley JL: The hypothalamic-pituitary axis in men and women with chronic kidney disease. Adv Chronic Kidney Dis 2004;11:337–341.

31. Descamps-Latscha B, Herbelin A, Nguyen AT, et al: Immune system dysregulation in uraemia. Semin Nephrol 1994;14:253–260.

32. Da Roza G, Loewen A, Djurdjev O, et al: Stage of chronic kidney disease predicts seroconversion after hepatitis B immunization: Earlier is better. Am J Kidney Dis 2003;42:1184–1192.

33. Wolfe RA, Ashby VB, Milford EL, et al: Comparison of mortality in all patients on dialysis, patients on dialysis awaiting transplantation, and recipients of a first cadaveric transplant. N Engl J Med 1999;341:1725–1730.

34. Korevaar JC, Jansen MA, Dekker FW, et al, for the Co-operative Study on the Adequacy of Dialysis Study Group. When to initiate dialysis: Effect of proposed US guidelines on survival. Lancet 2001;358:1046–1050.

35. Smith C, Da Silva-Gane M, Chandna S, et al: Choosing not to dialyse: Evaluation of planned non-dialytic management in a cohort of patients with end-stage renal failure. Nephron Clin Pract 2003;95:40–46.

Cardiovascular Disease in Chronic Kidney Disease

Peter Stenvinkel, Kerstin Amann, and Markus Ketteler

INTRODUCTION

The life span of chronic kidney disease (CKD) patients is reduced, and cardiovascular disease (CVD), including stroke, acute myocardial infarction (AMI), and congestive heart failure (CHF), accounts for premature death in about 50% of dialysis patients,[1] resulting in 5-year survival often worse than that of patients with cancer. Even subtle kidney dysfunction should be considered a medical condition predisposing to increased cardiovascular risk.[2] Patients on renal replacement therapy (RRT) appear to be at extraordinary risk for premature death due to cardiovascular complications. Although accelerated atherosclerosis may be one important cause of the high cardiovascular mortality in this patient group, the CVD pattern is atypical in that volume overload and left ventricular hypertrophy (LVH) are very common. In addition, the incidence of sudden cardiac death, arrhythmias, hypertension, coronary artery disease (CAD), peripheral vascular disease (PVD), and pericarditis is markedly increased, and cardiac arrest or arrhythmia is the major cause of cardiovascular death in this patient population (Fig. 71.1). The increased relative risk for cardiovascular death is greatest in young CKD patients and approaches that of elderly nonrenal patients in their 70s and 80s (Fig. 71.2). CKD patients should therefore be considered at high risk for CVD.

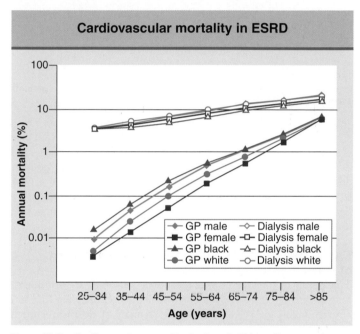

Figure 71.2 Cardiovascular mortality in chronic kidney disease end stage renal disease (ESRD). Cardiovascular mortality defined by death due to arrhythmias, cardiomyopathy, cardiac arrest, myocardial infarction, atherosclerotic heart disease, and pulmonary edema in the general population (GP) compared with those with ESRD treated by dialysis. Data stratified by age, race, and gender. (Adapted from Foley RN, Parfrey PS, Sarnak MJ: Clinical epidemiology of cardiovascular disease in chronic renal failure. Am J Kidney Dis 1998;32[Suppl 5]:S112–S119.)

EPIDEMIOLOGY

Prevalence of Cardiovascular Complications in Chronic Kidney Disease

One problem with the interpretation of epidemiologic studies on the frequency of CVD in the CKD patient is the difficulty of defining the cause of death. Clinical definitions of CVD tend to underestimate the true prevalence and incidence of atherosclerosis, autopsies are infrequently performed, the accuracy of death certificates is inherently problematic, and it is often difficult to ascribe death to a single cause in CKD patients. With falling glomerular filtration rate (GFR), the prevalence of hypertension increases progressively and is present in 75% to 85% of dialysis patients[3] (Fig. 71.3). As a consequence of hypertension (and other factors, e.g., anemia, vascular noncompliance, and volume overload), the prevalence of LVH is extremely high in CKD. About 30% of incident end-stage renal disease (ESRD) patients

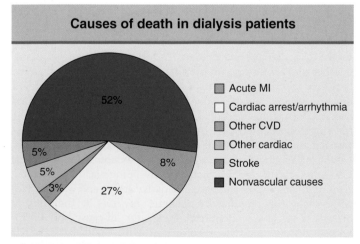

Figure 71.1 Causes of death in dialysis patients. CVD, cardiovascular disease; MI, myocardial infarction. (Data from USRDS, 2005.)

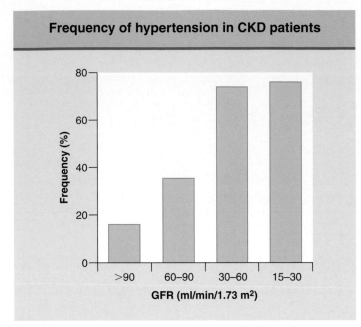

Figure 71.3 Frequency of hypertension in chronic kidney disease patients according to glomerular filtration rate (GFR). (Data from NHANES III.)

are hospitalized because of CHF within the first year of RRT (see www.usrds.org). Although occlusive CAD is commonly observed in CKD patients, AMI accounts for <10% of cardiovascular death, and rather "sudden cardiac death" is responsible for 60% to 70% of cardiac deaths in the dialysis patient population (see Fig. 71.1). Arrhythmias, electrolyte disturbances, and autonomic dysfunction may contribute to sudden deaths.

Cardiovascular Disease Is Present Before the Start of Renal Replacement Therapy

Thickening of the arterial wall and aortic stiffening are prominent long before the start of RRT. Also, patients commencing RRT are already highly preselected because chances of death are much higher than reaching dialysis in all stages of CKD. Nondialysis related factors therefore appear to be the major cause of vascular disease in dialysis patients, and interventions need to start at an early stage of CKD. Although no studies have yet shown that dialysis treatment *per se* accelerates the atherosclerotic process, several aspects of the hemodialysis procedure, such as membrane incompatibility (i.e., procoagulant and proinflammatory properties), impure dialysate, and vascular access infections might, in theory, have proatherogenic properties.

In elderly patients with CKD stage 2 or 3, traditional risk factors seem to be the major contributors to cardiovascular mortality. On the other hand, whereas the Atherosclerosis Risk in Communities (ARIC) data suggest that both traditional and nontraditional risk factors are of relevance in CKD stage 4,[4] studies in dialysis patients suggest that novel (i.e., nontraditional) risk factors are far more prevalent in this population than in the general population (Fig. 71.4). The relative importance of novel versus traditional risk factors is largely unknown and difficult to separate.

International Differences in Prevalence of Cardiovascular Disease

The differences in cardiovascular mortality in dialysis patients are striking when comparing patients from the United States, Japan, and Europe, even after adjustment for standard risk factors and dose of dialysis. Because Asian dialysis patients

treated in the United States also have a markedly lower adjusted relative risk than Caucasians, it appears that factors other than dialysis treatment characteristics (e.g., diet and genetic factors) play a role. Indeed, wide differences in mortality exist within the United States, where Hispanic, Asian, and African American dialysis patients, in general, have a better survival than Caucasians (www.usrds.org).

Reverse Epidemiology

Reverse epidemiology is the seemingly paradoxical observation in CKD patients that the well-known association between hypercholesterolemia, hypertension, obesity, and poor outcome, including cardiovascular death, in the general population does not exist or may even appear to be reversed.[5] The phenomenon of reverse epidemiology is observed not only in ESRD but also in geriatric populations and in patients with CHF. Evidence suggests that at the time of initiation of CKD, the risk factor profile is similar to the one found in the general population, but as kidney failure progresses and cardiac failure, wasting, and inflammation become more prevalent, the risk factor profile reverses. Thus, in dialysis patients, neither increased serum total cholesterol nor increased systolic blood pressure is associated with poor outcome (see later discussion).

ETIOLOGY AND RISK FACTORS

Traditional (Framingham) Risk Factors
Age, Gender, and Smoking

Most patients receiving RRT are already in an age range in which CVD is common. In the United States, the average age of patients who start dialysis is older than 60 years; the risk for death increases by 3% per year of age. In dialysis patients who were hospitalized for the first coronary revascularization procedure occurring after initiation of RRT, older age was a powerful predictor of cardiac death. The incidence of AMI is nearly 2.5 times higher in male than in female CKD patients in all age groups. However, older female patients are also at increased risk because about 70% of women on hemodialysis (HD) are menopausal before or after starting RRT, and the incidence of AMI was three to five times higher in female CKD patients than in the general female population at all age groups. Smoking is associated with CVD in CKD patients. In the Hemodialysis (HEMO) study, 52% of 936 patients either smoked cigarettes at study entry or had a previous history of smoking. Thus, cessation of smoking should be recommended to renal patients, a recommendation commonly given but less frequently followed.

Diabetes Mellitus

In the U.S. Renal Data System (USRDS) registry, the annual number of diabetic patients admitted to RRT more than doubled between 1995 and 2000 to a plateau of 45% of the incident dialysis patients and started to decrease slightly between 2002 and 2003 (www.usrds.org). Diabetes mellitus has thus become the single most important cause of ESRD, even though cardiovascular complications result in particularly poor survival of these patients. Diabetic patients starting RRT exhibit a multifactorial CVD risk factor profile, including dyslipidemia, hypertension, signs of inflammation, increased oxidative stress, and wasting. Not surprisingly, the presence of diabetes mellitus at the start of dialysis is an independent risk factor for all-cause and CVD-related deaths, and when compared with nondiabetic ESRD patients, the risk for diabetic patients increases 65% for having CAD, 36% for PVD, and 34% for dying after AMI (Fig. 71.5).

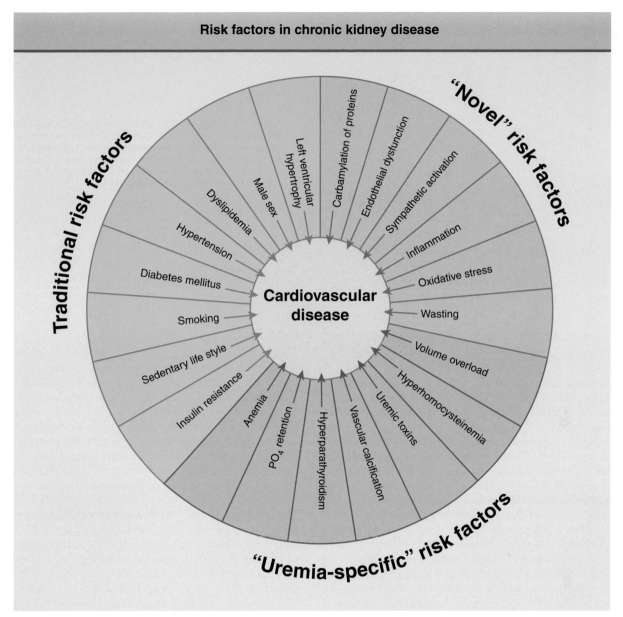

Figure 71.4 Risk factors for cardiovascular disease. Schematic overview of traditional (i.e., Framingham) risk factors *(green)*, "novel" risk factors *(orange)*, and more or less "uremia-specific" risk factors *(blue)*.

Hypertension

Low blood pressure correlated with mortality in various cohorts of dialysis patients (see Reverse Epidemiology). However, as in the general population, the presence of hypertension predicts mortality in patients before or at dialysis initiation. To explain these apparently conflicting findings, one must distinguish among the roles of systolic pressure, diastolic pressure, mean arterial pressure (MAP), and pulse pressure. Isolated systolic hypertension with increased pulse pressure is by far the most prevalent blood pressure anomaly in dialysis patients, owing to medial sclerosis of arteries with secondary arterial stiffening. Stiff vessels cause increased pulse wave velocity, resulting in an increased systolic peak pressure by a prematurely reflected pulse wave. The consequence is progressive left ventricular (LV) dysfunction and finally CHF. This may subsequently result in decreased MAP and diastolic pressure and an increased risk for cardiovascular death. Taken together, these findings suggest a U-shaped relationship between blood pressure and mortality: isolated systolic

hypertension and increased pulse pressure probably indicate a high long-term risk in dialysis patients, whereas low mean and diastolic blood pressures predict early mortality. The "invisible" hypertension danger relates to the fact that numerous CKD patients are "nondippers" (see Chapter 31) owing to autonomic dysfunction. Furthermore, sleep apnea is frequent in CKD patients and associated with nondipping, sympathetic nervous system activation, and cardiovascular risk.

Dyslipidemia

In the CKD population, the relationship among hypercholesterolemia, CVD, and mortality is weak because some of the major cardiovascular abnormalities in these patients, such as cardiomyopathy and arteriosclerosis, may be less dependent on dyslipidemia than on other factors. Paradoxically, low rather than high serum cholesterol is associated with poor survival in HD patients.[5] This "reverse epidemiology" relates to malnutrition or

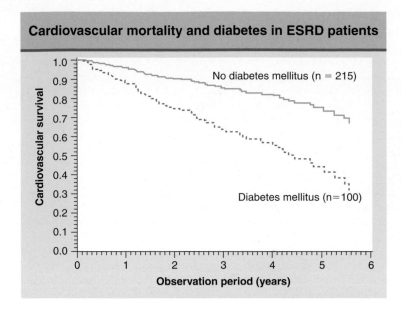

Figure 71.5 Adjusted cardiovascular mortality and diabetes in 315 incident end-stage renal disease (ESRD) patients starting renal replacement therapy in Stockholm, Sweden, divided according to the presence or absence of diabetes mellitus. Survival (likelihood ratio 46.5; $p < 0.0001$) adjusted for age, gender, inflammation (CRP >10 mg/l), and malnutrition (subjective global assessment >1).

inflammation because after adjustment for CRP levels, high cholesterol predicted risk in the noninflamed, "relatively healthy" ESRD patients.[6]

Progressive loss of renal function leads to changes in plasma composition of blood lipids that are associated with vascular disease. Renal dyslipidemia is characterized by an abnormal apolipoprotein profile, including decreased levels of apolipoprotein (apo) A–containing lipoproteins and increased levels of apoB-containing lipoproteins (Fig. 71.6). Plasma triglyceride levels are increased in most ESRD patients, whereas total serum cholesterol levels may be elevated, normal, or low, depending on nutritional status and presence of inflammation. High-density lipoprotein (HDL) cholesterol is typically reduced, and low-density lipoprotein (LDL), intermediate-density lipoprotein (IDL), and very-low-density lipoprotein (VLDL) cholesterol, as well as lipoprotein(a) [Lp(a)], levels tend to be increased. As compared with long-term HD patients, those on peritoneal dialysis (PD) more often exhibit both hypercholesterolemia and hypertriglyceridemia. Both groups are characterized by low HDL and elevated oxidized LDL cholesterol levels. Elevated Lp(a) levels are associated with increased CVD mortality both in HD and PD patients.

Insulin Resistance

Data from the National Health and Nutrition Examination Survey (NHANES) suggest that the metabolic syndrome is associated with inflammation in patients with varying levels of kidney function.[7] Although some studies have documented insulin resistance in patients with early CKD, the temporal onset of insulin resistance remains controversial. The quantitative role of insulin resistance in the composite outcome of CKD patients is currently unclear. Although correction of both acidosis and hyperparathyroidism may improve insulin sensitivity in CKD, neither has been demonstrated to improve cardiovascular outcome.

Nontraditional and Uremia-specific Risk Factors

Several large prospective population studies (e.g., Heart Outcomes Prevention Evaluation [HOPE], Artherosclerosis Risk in Communities [ARIC], Hypertension Optimal Treatment [HOT]) have shown that even mild CKD (i.e., stages 2 and 3) is an independent risk factor for CVD (Fig. 71.7). This is important new knowledge because about 10% of low-risk CVD populations and 30% of high-risk populations have mild CKD. Thus, mild renal insufficiency *per se* is now being regarded as an independent

Lipid abnormalities in renal disease

| Stage of Renal Disease | Cholesterol Levels | | | Triglycerides |
	Total	High-Density Lipoproteins	Low-Density Lipoproteins	
Nephrotic syndrome	↑↑↑	↓	↑↑	↑
Chronic renal failure	→	↓	→*	↑↑
Hemodialysis	→	↓	→*	↑↑
Peritoneal dialysis	↑	↓	↑	↑
Transplantation	↑↑	→	↑	↑

Figure 71.6 Lipid abnormalities in renal disease. Common patterns of hyperlipidemia in different stages of renal disease. *Composition altered.

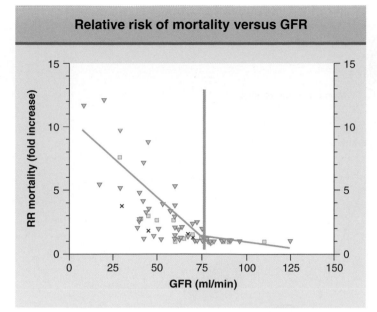

Relative risk of mortality versus GFR

Figure 71.7 Relative risk (RR) for mortality versus glomerular filtration rate (GFR). Twenty-four studies were included in this analysis. Most studies used the Cockcroft and Gault formula to estimate clearance *(green triangles)*. Studies that use the Modification of Diet in Renal Disease study formula are indicated by the *yellow squares* and unadjusted studies by the *red crosses*. The two linear regression slopes show the RR associated with nearly normal renal function *(right slope)* and decreased renal function *(left slope)*. The *thick vertical line* indicates the threshold of a GFR of 75 ml/min, below which there is a clear mortality risk. (Adapted from Vanholder R, Massy Z, Argiles A, et al: Chronic kidney disease as cause of cardiovascular morbidity and mortality. Nephrol Dial Transpl 2005; 20:1048–1056.)

cardiovascular risk factor of a similar magnitude as traditional risk factors, such as diabetes and hypertension. Moreover, data from NHANES III show that all subjects with CKD stage 4 or 5 have two or more established cardiovascular risk factors.[8] Although the exact mechanisms by which renal failure may accelerate the atherogenic process are not well established, the prevalence and magnitude of a number of nontraditional risk factors, such as oxidative stress, inflammation, vascular calcification, and advanced glycation end products (AGEs), increase as renal function deteriorates (see Fig. 71.4). In addition, several other uremic retention solutes, such as the inhibitor of NO-synthesis asymmetric dimethylarginine (ADMA), homocysteine, guanidine, indoxyl sulfate, and p-cresol, may have proatherogenic properties.[2] Finally, healthy kidneys produce substances that inhibit CVD and atherogenesis, such as renalase, a soluble monoamine oxidase that regulates cardiac function and blood pressure. In ESRD, very low plasma concentrations of this putative inhibitor of the sympathetic nervous system may contribute to sympathetic overactivity.[9]

Oxidative Stress

Clinical evidence both from nonrenal and renal patient cohorts demonstrates that increased oxidative stress, that is, an unbalanced surplus of free radicals, may be associated with accelerated atherogenesis and increased risk for atherosclerotic cardiovascular events and other complications of ESRD, such as wasting and anemia.[10] Increased production of reactive oxygen species (ROS) in the vascular wall is a characteristic feature of atherosclerosis.[10] Uremic patients are subjected to enhanced oxidative stress, as a result of reduced antioxidant systems (vitamin C and selenium deficiency), reduced intracellular levels of vitamin E, reduced activity of the glutathione system, and increased pro-oxidant

activity associated with advanced age, high frequency of diabetes, chronic inflammatory states, the uremic syndrome *per se*, and "bioincompatibility" of dialysis membranes and solutions.[10]

The most important enzymes involved in ROS production are the superoxide producer NADPH-oxidase, the hydrogen peroxide producer superoxide dismutase, the NO-producer nitric oxide synthase (NOS), and the hypochlorous acid producer myeloperoxidase (MPO). These enzymes are capable of oxidizing LDL *in vitro* and are all expressed in atherosclerotic lesions. Also, production of AGEs, including *N*-carboxymethyl-lysine (CML) and pentosidine, is accelerated under oxidative stress in ESRD patients (their potential role in cardiovascular complications is discussed later). In addition to increased generation of prooxidants, CKD patients may also be subjected to increased loss or decreased intake of antioxidants because of poor appetite. It has been demonstrated that patients with signs of malnutrition and a low serum albumin concentration have a significantly diminished plasma antioxidant capacity.[10] Inflammation and hypoalbuminemia can synergize because inflammation results in increased production of oxidants by leukocytes and hypoalbuminemia in reduced scavenging capacity for these oxidants.[10]

Inflammation

Most dialysis patients are in a state of chronic inflammation.[11] Several studies have demonstrated that various inflammatory biomarkers, such as CRP, interleukin-6 (IL-6), fibrinogen, and white blood cell count, are robust and independent predictors of mortality in CKD patients.[11] Another strong outcome predictor in CKD is hypoalbuminemia, a biochemical factor strongly associated with inflammatory biomarkers. Although both dialysis-related (e.g., bioincompatibility of the dialysis system) and dialysis-unrelated (e.g., infections, comorbidity, genetic factors, diet, and renal function loss) factors may contribute to a state of chronic inflammation in CKD, the primary causes of inflammation are not always evident. As in the general population, it is unclear in CKD patients whether the acute-phase response only reflects established atherosclerotic disease, endothelial dysfunction, vascular calcification, insulin resistance, and increased oxidative stress or if it is actually involved in the initiation or progression of atherosclerosis. However, evidence suggests that the prototypic inflammatory marker CRP, as well as other biomarkers such as IL-6 and TNF-α, may have proatherogenic properties, such as promotion of vascular calcification, oxidative stress, and endothelial dysfunction (Fig. 71.8).

Endothelial Dysfunction

Endothelial dysfunction (as evidenced by impaired endothelium-dependent vasodilation) is a prominent feature of CKD. The reasons for endothelial dysfunction in CKD include inflammation, retention of ADMA, oxidative stress, hyperhomocysteinemia, dyslipidemia, hyperglycemia, and hypertension. The importance of endothelial dysfunction in uremic vascular health is underscored by the fact that surrogate markers of endothelial dysfunction, such as ADMA and adhesion molecules, independently predict death. Recent evidence suggests that detached circulating endothelial cells (CECs) serve as a potential marker of endothelial damage in both nonrenal and renal patients, and the prognostic value of an increased number of CECs in HD patients was recently demonstrated.[12] Normally, in response to ischemic insults and cytokine stimulation, endothelial progenitor cells (EPCs) are mobilized from the bone marrow to act as repair cells in response to the endothelial injury. Because uremic patients appear to have reduced numbers of or a functional impairment of EPCs due to inflammation or uremic toxins, there appears to be an imbalance between

Effect of altered cytokine production in uremia on various target organs

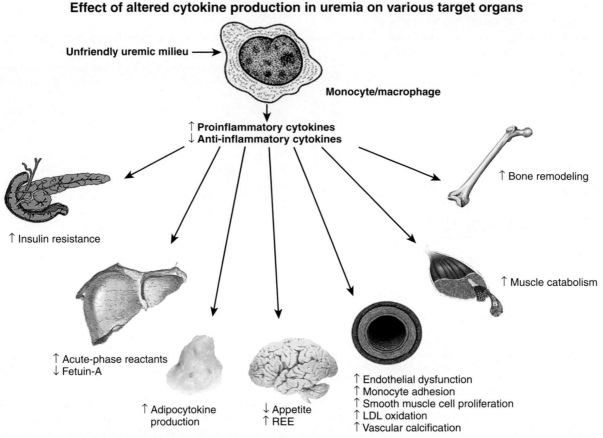

Figure 71.8 Effect of altered cytokine production in uremia on various target organs. Potential mechanisms by which altered circulating levels of proinflammatory and anti-inflammatory cytokines may promote accelerated atherosclerosis, other uremic complications, and wasting. LDL, low-density lipoprotein; REE, resting energy expenditure. (Adapted from Stenvinkel P, Ketteler M, Johnson RJ, et al: Interleukin-10, IL-6 and TNF-α: Important factors in the altered cytokine network of end-stage renal disease—the good, the bad and the ugly. Kidney Int 2005;67:1216–1233.)

CECs and EPCs, which may predispose this patient group to endothelial damage and dysfunction.

Anemia

Anemia is a major cause of LVH and LV dilation in ESRD. Partial correction of anemia with erythropoietin may result in regression of LVH, although it is currently unclear whether this intervention also has an impact on cardiovascular outcomes.

Secondary Hyperparathyroidism and Mineral Metabolism

Disturbances of calcium and phosphate metabolism start as early as CKD stage 3 and are potent triggers of accelerated calcifying atherosclerosis and arteriosclerosis. In various epidemiologic studies, hyperphosphatemia and an elevated calcium × phosphate product were strong independent mortality risk predictors, whereas hypercalcemia carries an intermediate risk and increased serum immunoreactive parathyroid hormone (iPTH) a weak, but still significant, risk.[13] The overall mortality risk prediction attributable to disorders of mineral metabolism is about 17% in HD patients.[13] Elevated serum phosphate levels are also associated with increased risk for valvular calcification and cardiac death, especially death resulting from CAD and sudden death.

Cardiovascular Calcification

Cardiovascular calcification may affect the arterial media, atherosclerotic plaques, myocardium, and heart valves (Figs. 71.9 and 71.10). Medial calcification causes arterial stiffness and consequently increased pulse pressure. The pathophysiologic role of plaque calcification is less clear because it is mostly soft plaques

that rupture and cause AMI, but it is now evident that the atherosclerotic calcification burden is a potent risk marker of cardiovascular events, at least in the normal population.[14] Valvular calcification mostly affects the aortic but also affects the mitral valves in dialysis patients and contributes to progressive stenosis and associated morbidity. Calciphylaxis (calcific uremic arteriolopathy), characterized by severe calcifications of cutaneous arterioles and exulcerating tissue necrosis, is discussed in Chapter 78. In ESRD patients, extensive vascular, in particular coronary artery, calcification can be observed in young age groups. This process frequently starts before the initiation of dialysis treatment and progresses rapidly thereafter (Fig. 71.11). The prevalence and extent of cardiovascular calcifications are strong predictors of CVD and all-cause mortality in HD and PD patients.[15] Disturbances in calcium and phosphate metabolism are an important factor in the development of cardiovascular calcification in ESRD. However, vascular calcification is not just derived from passive calcium and phosphate precipitation. Rather, it is a highly regulated active process involving differentiation of vascular smooth muscle cells toward osteoblasts induced by phosphate, calcium, and various other factors, such as calcitriol and proinflammatory mediators (Fig. 71.12). One way by which chronic inflammation promotes vascular calcification may involve downregulation of fetuin-A, the most potent circulating inhibitor of extraosseous calcification. In cross-sectional studies, dialysis patients with low serum fetuin-A levels showed a significantly poorer survival than those with normal values.[16] Apart from fetuin-A, various other inhibitors probably counteract unwanted calcification (see Fig. 71.12). Among those, leptin, matrix-gla protein (MGP),

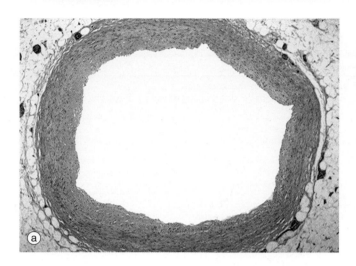

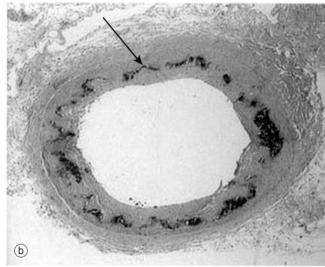

Figure 71.9 **Peripheral artery of a patient with chronic kidney disease.** *a,* The normal anatomy of a peripheral artery. *b,* Marked, nearly circumferential media calcification (*arrow*). (Hematoxylin and eosin stain.)

pyrophosphates, bone morphogenic proteins (e.g., BMP-2 and -7), and osteoprotegerin (OPG) may be related to accelerated vascular calcification in ESRD.

Advanced Glycation End Products

Pentosidine, CML, and other AGEs accumulate in CKD and may contribute to accelerated atherosclerosis and dialysis-related amyloidosis (see Chapter 75). However, neither elevated plasma pentosidine nor CML levels predict mortality in CKD patients, and the role of AGEs in renal patients therefore remains speculative.

Hyperhomocysteinemia

The prevalence of hyperhomocysteinemia in CKD stage 5 patients exceeds 90%. However, the relationship between high homocysteine (Hcy) serum levels and CVD in CKD patients has been reported variably. Some studies even noted paradoxically lower Hcy levels in uremic CVD patients.[17] The latter may

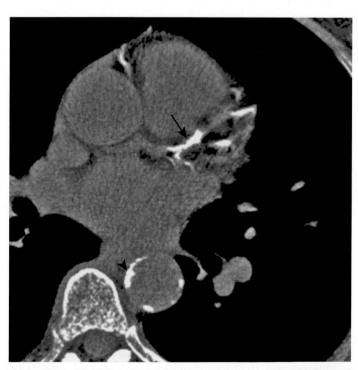

Lumen

Figure 71.10 **Coronary plaque of a patient with chronic kidney disease with heavy calcification.** (black reaction product; van Kossa stain)

Figure 71.11 **Multislice spiral computed tomography scan of the heart of a 49-year-old male Caucasian hemodialysis patient with severe coronary** (*arrow*) **and aortic** (*arrowhead*) **calcifications.**

845

Regulation and inhibition of extraosseous calcification: Experimental and clinical data with relation to CKD	
Calcium-Regulatory Factors	Potential Relation to Uremic Cardiovascular Calcification
Fetuin-A	*Experimental findings:* diffuse spontaneous calcification in knockout mice *Clinical findings:* low fetuin-A levels predict mortality risk in dialysis patients and correlate with the degree of coronary and valvular calcification
Matrix Gla protein (MGP)	*Experimental findings:* severe aortic media calcification in knockout mice *Clinical findings:* association between warfarin treatment and calciphylaxis episodes suspected
Pyrophosphates	*Experimental findings:* knockout mice of pyrophosphate transporter (ANK; periarticular manifestations) or the rate-limiting enzyme (NPP1; ligaments, tendons) cause distinct calcification phenotypes in mice *Clinical findings:* low pyrophosphate levels in hemodialysis patients; removal by hemodialysis?
Osteoprotegerin (OPG)	*Experimental findings:* aortic and renal artery calcifications in knockout mice *Clinical findings:* unexpected positive correlation of OPG with vascular calcifications in uremia
Bone morphogenic protein-7 (BMP-7)	*Experimental findings:* administration reduces vascular calcification in low-density lipoprotein receptor knockout mice with renal failure *Clinical findings:* none
Leptin	*Experimental findings:* induction of vascular smooth muscle cell calcification *in vitro* *Clinical findings:* high leptin levels in association with inflammation and cardiovascular risk

Figure 71.12 **Regulation and inhibition of extraosseous calcification.** Experimental and clinical data with relation to CKD. (Data from references 36–39.)

be another example of reverse epidemiology (discussed earlier), given the strong association between low Hcy levels and hypoalbuminemia, wasting, and inflammation.

Dialysis Modality

Reports from various U.S. dialysis registries are inconsistent, with some studies showing more favorable outcomes for patients on HD, but with others showing little or no difference and still others better outcomes for patients on PD.[18] However, valid mortality comparisons between HD and PD would require patient stratification according to the underlying cause of ESRD, age, and level of baseline comorbidity.[18] Such data are currently not available.

CLINICAL MANIFESTATIONS AND NATURAL HISTORY

Chest Pain, Coronary Artery Disease, and Acute Myocardial Infarction

Chest pain in CKD patients must be considered as seriously as in the normal population. However, it may occasionally point to uremic pericarditis, and ischemia-related complaints may not always be typical. AMI appears underrepresented as a cause of fatal outcomes in dialysis patients when compared with sudden death and arrhythmias (see Fig. 71.1). It has been suggested that there may be both undertreatment and underrecognition because of atypical clinical presentation of AMI in ESRD,[19] for example, due to autonomic neuropathy, "silent" AMI, or the frequent occurrence of pulmonary congestion associated with fluid overload. If present, poor survival characterizes the course of AMI in CKD patients, which may be also related to suboptimal diagnosis and treatment in this patient group.

Peripheral Vascular Disease

The highest risk for PVD in dialysis patients occurs in patients with diabetes and those with pre-existing atherosclerosis. In HD patients, PVD is also associated with time on dialysis, hypoalbuminemia, low PTH levels, and low predialysis diastolic blood pressure. Vascular medial calcification of large peripheral arteries may not necessarily indicate the presence of occlusive disease,

and peripheral gangrene is often caused by small-vessel disease or, rarely, calcific uremic arteriolopathy (see Chapter 78), or by multifactorial diabetic foot ulcers.

Cerebrovascular Disease

Stroke accounts for about 5% to 10% of deaths among patients on RRT (see Fig. 71.1). Strokes are related to diastolic hypertension, but atrial fibrillation is also frequent, especially in the HD population. The incidence of carotid plaques and intimal media thickness is increased in CKD patients, mostly due to an excess of hard calcified plaques and medial sclerosis. Intracerebral bleeding is more frequent in HD patients than in the normal population and is associated with a higher mortality rate.

Left Ventricular Remodeling and Hypertrophy

LVH is a potent predictor of premature mortality in patients on RRT.[3,20] Increased left ventricular mass index (LVMI) is another independent predictor of cardiac survival in dialysis patients, with a 5-year mortality rate twofold higher in those with an LVMI >125 g/mm^2 as compared with an LVMI <125 g/mm.^{2} LVH occurs early in the course of progressive CKD, probably because of the high prevalence of hypertension, including frequent nocturnal hypertension. Pressure overload, caused by hypertension and arterial stiffness, results in concentric hypertrophy. Volume overload manifests as "eccentric" hypertrophy. Asymmetric hypertrophy with predominant thickening of the septum but not of the free LV wall may be caused by sympathetic overactivity (Fig. 71.13). LV dilation is a potent predictor of poor outcome. LV dilation may simply be an end result of severe LVH, whereas diffuse ischemic damage, recurrent volume overload, or high-output arteriovenous fistula may also contribute. Diastolic dysfunction is strongly associated with LVH and with an increased risk for intradialytic hypotension because relatively small reductions in left atrial filling have significant effects on cardiac output.

Extracellular Volume Overload

Extracellular volume overload is the major cause of hypertension in dialysis patients. It is related to the progressive loss of the sodium excretory capacity. However, whether prevention of recurrent hypervolemia will reduce cardiovascular morbidity

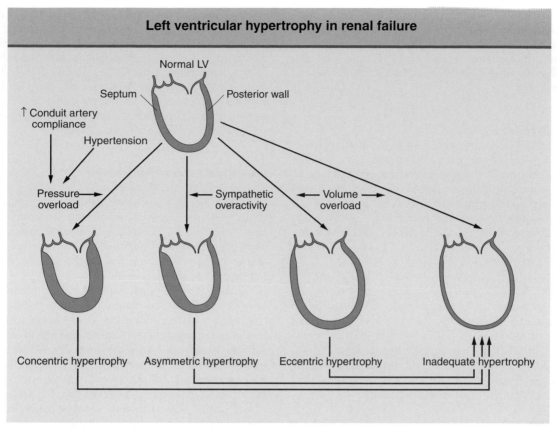

Figure 71.13 Causes of left ventricular (LV) hypertrophy in renal failure. Caution is necessary in the assessment of LV mass because echocardiographic formulas include LV diameter, which may change rapidly owing to changes in fluid balance.

and mortality remains unproved. The relationship between interdialytic weight gain and mortality is U shaped, possibly as a result of low weight gains among patients with comorbidity and advanced age. Recurrent hypervolemia may result in LVH and LV dilation, peripheral or pulmonary edema, raised jugular vein pulse, or a third heart sound, but it may also be largely asymptomatic. The tolerance of large volumes of ultrafiltration may indicate that the individual dry-weight target (see Chapter 83) has not been reached. Reaching an optimal dry weight, however, does not necessarily lead to immediate blood pressure correction because a lag phase of some weeks can precede improvements of hypertension control. Hypovolemia and dialysis-related hypotension, as well as measures to prevent them, are discussed in Chapter 84.

Pericarditis

Two types of pericarditis may occur in uremia (Fig. 71.14): uremic pericarditis has become rare and occurs in the terminal phases of untreated uremia, whereas dialysis-associated pericarditis is common and is associated with considerable mortality (up to 10%). The latter form occurs in underdialyzed patients and may be related to intercurrent illnesses, fistula recirculation, or to underlying diseases such as systemic lupus erythematosus, but the exact pathogenesis remains obscure. Fever with pericardial pain or a rub on heart auscultation should prompt echocardiography.

Autonomic Dysfunction

There is decreased baroreflex sensitivity in ESRD, which is thought to be caused by volume overload, hypertension, and aging, whereas the existence of a true uremic neuropathy has not been proven. A direct relationship between altered autonomic function

and cardiovascular mortality has not been demonstrated in CKD or ESRD. Increased sympathetic nerve discharge is common alteration in patients with ESRD. Bilateral nephrectomy eliminates sympathetic overactivity, suggesting involvement of afferent signals from the diseased kidneys. In addition, downregulation of pressor responsiveness to sympathetic stimulation may contribute to hypotension during ultrafiltration.

Valvular Disease

Disturbances of mineral metabolism, time on dialysis, hypoalbuminemia, inflammation, and advanced age are risk factors for valvular disease and calcification. Valvular calcification is associated with regurgitation or hemodynamically significant

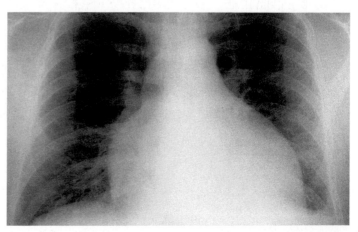

Figure 71.14 Pericardial effusion. Chest radiograph showing large pericardial effusion.

stenosis (particularly of the aortic valve) and the development of conduction disturbances, including complete heart block, due to involvement of the bundle of His. Correction of volume overload by ultrafiltration may resolve regurgitation, and this may be the only way of distinguishing between functional and structural defects.

Infective Endocarditis

Infective endocarditis has an incidence of 2% to 4% in patients with ESRD and is often related to HD treatment. Vascular access, including temporary and semipermanent catheters, is the most important source of infection. Dental infections and dental treatment are less commonly implicated. The aortic valve is infected more frequently than the mitral valve. Right-sided lesions are uncommon. Whether the degree of calcification is a risk factor is unclear.

Arrhythmias

Arrhythmias are a common clinical problem in ESRD and occur particularly frequently during HD. Sudden death, the most important cause of mortality in ESRD patients, mostly results from ventricular fibrillation, but asystolic events (about 20%) represent another significant proportion. Hyperkalemia is the most important metabolic abnormality in ESRD associated with arrhythmias and a common cause of sudden death.

PATHOLOGY

Left Ventricular Hypertrophy

LVH is the most prominent structural cardiovascular alteration in CKD patients. It starts in early CKD, is present in 75% of patients entering dialysis, and is progressive thereafter. It is therefore more appropriately also called *cardiomyopathy in CKD*. Rodent models of CKD confirmed that as early as 2 to 3 weeks after induction of renal failure, LV weight increased, numbers of cardiomyocytes decreased because of apoptosis and remaining cardiomyocytes hypertrophied[21] (Fig. 71.15), and LV

ejection fraction decreased by about 40%. LVH could not be fully explained by increased blood pressure, hypervolemia, increased activity of the sympathetic nervous system, or anemia. Additional pathogenic events may include the increased activity of the local renin angiotensin system in CKD as well as a markedly reduced elasticity module, that is, an increase in vascular stiffness of the aorta in patients with CKD leading to an increase in blood pressure amplitude and an increase in systolic peak pressure without affecting MAP.[22]

Interstitial Myocardial Fibrosis

Myocardial fibrosis develops early in CKD and is more pronounced than that observed in patients with primary hypertension or diabetes (see Fig. 71.15). In multivariate analyses, ESRD has been identified as an independent determinant of interstitial myocardial fibrosis.[23] Interstitial fibrosis in early CKD is primarily due to primary activation and proliferation of matrix-producing interstitial fibroblasts, possibly mediated by PTH and angiotensin II,[24] rather than loss of cardiomyocytes and fibrotic repair. Alterations of the three-dimensional or spatial distribution and in the composition of the connective tissue fibers (collagen isoforms) may be as important as the total net increase in interstitial volume. Myocardial fibrosis can experimentally be prevented by early treatment with angiotensin-converting enzyme (ACE) inhibitors and endothelin-1 (ET-1) receptor antagonists independent of blood pressure–lowering effects. The functional consequences of myocardial fibrosis include changes in the stress–strain relationship during systolic contraction, impairment of LV compliance during diastolic filling, and increased arrhythmogenicity.

Alterations of the Arterial and Myocardial Vasculature

The finding that CKD patients often present with cardiac ischemia despite patent coronary arteries on angiography may relate to alterations of the postcoronary intramyocardial vascular bed, in particular a significantly lower length density of intramyocardial capillaries when compared with nonrenal patients.[21] This implies that myocardial capillary angiogenesis in response to an increase in myocardial mass in LVH is impaired, leading to an increased

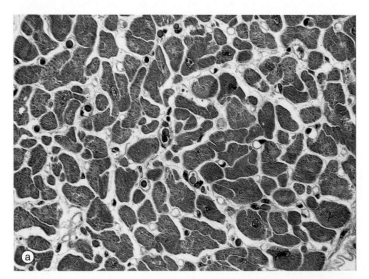
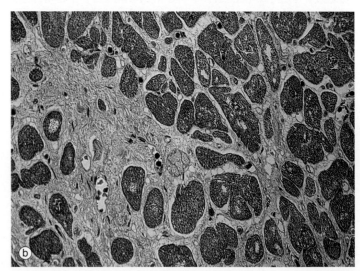

Figure 71.15 **Human myocardium.** *a,* Normal morphology of the human myocardium. *b,* Representative morphology of the myocardium of a patient with chronic kidney disease (CKD). In CKD, the typical morphology, that is, hypertrophy of cardiomyocytes, increases in interstitial tissue *(blue)*, and reduction of capillary supply can be seen.

mean intercapillary diffusion distance and significantly impaired ischemia tolerance of the heart.[21] Experimentally, improvement of myocardial vascularization can be achieved by ACE inhibitors, ET-1 receptor blockers, and sympatholytic agents.

Similar to nonrenal patients with so-called syndrome X (i.e., angina pectoris and reduced coronary reserve despite patent coronary arteries), patients with CKD also exhibit wall thickening of intramyocardial arteries. Intima and media thickness of coronary arteries in ESRD was higher in comparison to age- and sex-matched nonrenal patients, whereas plaque size was not different. In addition, more advanced stages of atherosclerotic plaques and in particular calcified plaques (see Fig. 71.10) were found in the coronary arteries of patients with ESRD.

DIAGNOSIS AND DIFFERENTIAL DIAGNOSIS

Key issues in the diagnosis of CVD are underrecognition of symptoms, underutilization of appropriate diagnostic investigations, and interpretation of those investigations.

Blood Pressure Measurements

In daily routine, outcome prediction by ambulatory blood pressure monitoring (ABPM) is not necessarily better than office blood pressure measurements, but ABPM is useful to identify the high-risk populations of nondippers and inverted dippers, with the consequence of treatment adjustments in those individuals.[20]

Electrocardiography and Echocardiography

Electrocardiography (ECG) changes in ESRD patients often result from dialysis- or diet-associated shifts in electrolytes, but signs of hypertrophy, ischemia, and infarction can be appropriately diagnosed. Holter ECG monitoring is of prognostic value in screening for cardiovascular high-risk patients suffering from QT dispersion, ventricular arrhythmias, and autonomic dysfunction (decreased heart rate variability).

Echocardiography is most valuable for the diagnosis and supervision of pericardial effusions, regional defects, and valvular disease and to judge LVMI, LVH, and LV dysfunction. It is generally recommended that all ESRD patients be evaluated for LV systolic function after a steady-state is reached following dialysis initiation, anemia correction, adequate therapy of hypertension, and revascularization procedures. The appropriate interpretation of ejection fraction may be hampered by the presence of fluid overload, and it should not be measured within 24 hours after a dialysis session or if the dry weight has not been reached. In cases of suspected high-output failure, the contribution of the fistulas, in particular if brachial or femoral, should be considered. A blood flow exceeding 1500 ml/min, measured either directly or by the alteration in cardiac output during temporary occlusion, in a patient with cardiac failure and pre-existing heart disease may require fistula banding or even ligation.

Stress Tests

CKD patients with suspected CAD, in particular those on a transplant waiting list or awaiting major surgery, should be subjected to stress testing. Positive results should always be followed by angiography. Nonetheless, stress testing is problematic in CKD patients because of its relatively low sensitivity and specificity. Exercise-limiting physical conditions (e.g., peripheral vascular disease) and ECG abnormalities caused by LVH are frequently present, rendering treadmill exercise and ECG interpretation difficult. Data on pharmacologic stress nuclear imaging are not conclusive: reported sensitivities range from 29% to 92% and specificities from 70% to 89% for detecting or excluding a coronary stenosis of >70%.[19] Except for its investigator dependency, dobutamine stress echocardiography is probably the most suitable method to detect subclinical inducible heart ischemia in ESRD patients.[19]

Coronary Angiography

Coronary angiography should be performed in ESRD patients for any reversible defect in stress testing and for significant reductions of LV ejection fraction (<40%) if the patient does not appear overhydrated. In general, recommendations are similar to conventional indications, and coronary angiography remains the gold standard in the evaluation of CAD in CKD. An algorithm for decision making in ESRD patients is shown in Figure 71.16. In CKD patients and in ESRD patients with residual renal function, fear of contrast nephropathy may play a role in a limited utilization of coronary angiography (see Chapter 64 for preventive measures). Contrast media exposure not infrequently may also precipitate an acute hyperosmolar state in ESRD patients, which may lead to hypertensive crises and pulmonary edema requiring an acute dialysis. Before any coronary angiography, ventricular function and the valvular status should be assessed by echocardiography to prevent unexpected technical difficulties and unnecessary ventriculograms.

Imaging of Vascular Calcification

Vascular calcification can be visualized by conventional x-ray techniques and multislice spiral computed tomography (CT) or electron-beam CT (see Fig. 71.11). By ultrasound techniques, valvular and large artery calcification can be visualized, and pulse wave velocity measurements provide an estimate of the severity of media sclerosis. Newly developed magnetic resonance imaging techniques also allow noninvasive evaluation of plaque size, calcification, and morphology. The value of routine imaging of vascular calcifications in CKD patients is currently not defined.

Biomarkers

Plasma brain natriuretic peptide (BNP) and the cardiac troponins (TnT, TnI) are relevant prognostic risk markers in the evaluation of heart disease in CKD and ESRD patients. BNP reflects cardiac filling pressure, whereas troponins indicate myocardial ischemia, and especially elevated TnT levels potently predict subsequent mortality. Falsely positive moderate elevations of troponins are frequently seen in patients with impaired renal function. However, fluctuations of levels (i.e., any increases even from an elevated baseline, especially when associated with clinical symptoms) must be interpreted as seriously as in acute coronary syndromes in nonrenal patients. ADMA, an endogenous NO inhibitor, is linked to hypertension and represents another important independent risk marker of progression to ESRD and of cardiovascular mortality in dialysis patients, respectively, but easy-to-perform immunoassays are only starting to become available for routine use. Currently, the predictive power of these factors appears to be relatively well established; however, how to use them in diagnostic or therapeutic decision making remains to be determined.

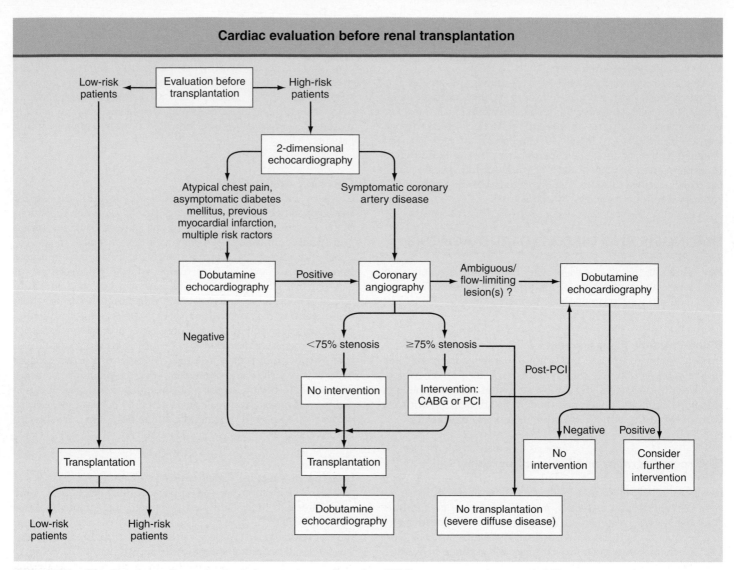

Figure 71.16 Algorithm for cardiac evaluation before renal transplantation. CABG, coronary artery bypass graft; PCI, percutaneous coronary intervention. (Redrawn from Herzog CA: How to manage the renal patient with coronary heart disease: The agony and the ecstasy of opinion-based medicine. J Am Soc Nephrol 2003;14:2556–2572.)

TREATMENT AND PREVENTION OF CARDIOVASCULAR DISEASE

Risk Factor Reduction
Smoking
It is clearly imperative to continuously encourage smoking cessation at any stage of CKD.

Weight and Diet
Lifestyle changes including balanced diets with regard to saturated fat and carbohydrates (in diabetic patients) are probably protective of cardiovascular morbidity. However, in all stages of CKD, malnutrition must be avoided, and especially in ESRD patients, an increased body mass index is associated with improved outcomes. The latter observation probably means that maintenance of appropriate energy and protein nutrition translates into a survival advantage in late CKD stages, and not that overweight should be encouraged. Low-salt diet and phosphate restriction are discussed in Chapter 77.

Hypertension and Coronary Artery Disease
Arterial hypertension is undertreated in many CKD and ESRD patients, and despite the presence of controversial data about the risk prediction by diastolic and systolic blood pressure in dialysis patients, antihypertensive treatment is associated with improved survival.[3,20] Blood pressure targets for patients with CKD and in particular those with diabetes or proteinuria exceeding 1 g/day are discussed in Chapter 69. Hallmarks of therapy are volume control, that is, finding the optimal dry weight of the patient (see Chapter 83) and preventing salt overload. Long or more frequent HD sessions may be very beneficial to control hypertension. Because of their parallel cardioprotective effects, ACE inhibitors, angiotensin receptor blockers (ARBs), and ß-blockers are the first-line drugs to treat CKD- and ESRD-related hypertension, but calcium channel blockers, as well as most other antihypertensive drugs, including centrally acting sympathetic inhibitors, are useful when administered in a complementary fashion. Pure vasodilators must be used with caution because these drugs may cause worsening of volume overload, pericardial effusions, and myocardial fibrosis (e.g., minoxidil).

CAD and CAD-related events should be treated with the same medications and with active interventions as indicated in the nonrenal population. Medical treatment includes the use of antiplatelet agents, ACE inhibitors, ARB, β-blockers, nitroglycerine, and statins. There is no rationale to be less aggressive in the therapeutic approach toward CKD and ESRD patients when compared with the normal population.

Diabetes Mellitus

Guidelines from the American Heart Association and the American Diabetes Association recommend optimal glycemic control, reaching blood pressure target levels and lipid monitoring (with subsequent dyslipidemia treatment) in diabetic CKD patients. CAD and other CVDs must be treated aggressively in this high-risk group.

Dyslipidemia

ESRD patients can be regarded as cardiovascular high-risk individuals, which would justify statin treatment of the whole population to achieve LDL cholesterol target levels of 100 mg/dl (2.6 mmol/l) or below. Alternatively, only those individuals could be treated who have an indication based on the guidelines valid for the normal population. Statin use was found to be associated with a reduction in all-cause and cardiovascular mortality in the USRDS Dialysis Morbidity and Mortality Wave 2 study. In contrast, the prospective 4D study failed to demonstrate cardiovascular outcome benefits of atorvastatin treatment in diabetic HD patients.[25] The ongoing AURORA (A study to evaluate the Use of Rosuvastatin in subjects On Regular haemodialysis: an Assessment of survival and cardiovascular events) and SHARP (Study of Heart and Renal Protection) studies may shed some more light on this issue. Until then, Kidney Disease Outcomes Quality Initiative (K/DOQI) guidelines recommend statin treatment in any CKD individual older than 20 years with LDL cholesterol levels >130 mg/dl (3.4 mmol/l) or >100 mg/dl in secondary prevention.

Volume

In the predialysis stage, sodium restriction and diuretics are important to counteract fluid retention. In ESRD, long and possibly more frequent HD sessions allow safe and mostly asymptomatic fluid removal. In the HD center in Tassin, France, 8 hours of dialysis three times per week led to >90% normotensive patients without taking antihypertensive drugs. Episodes of dialysis-related hypotension should prompt re-evaluation of the patient's dry weight, antihypertensive treatment, and the exclusion of pericardial effusions. Preliminary evidence suggests that midodrine, a short-acting α-agonist, can be used if dialysis-related hypotension persists despite these measures.

Anemia

Because anemia is contributing to the development of LVH in ESRD and partial correction of severe anemia with epoetin results in regression of LVH, epoetin treatment is advocated. Treatment of severe anemia is also associated with less ischemic symptoms in patients with CAD. However, although life quality improves after anemia correction, the evidence that epoetin therapy reduces cardiovascular mortality in ESRD is based on data from observational studies only. Randomized prospective studies on anemia treatment in both dialysis and pre-ESRD patients failed to show clear-cut outcome benefits.[26,27] The only randomized study with a primary mortality end point[26] compared partial anemia correction (hematocrit, 32%) with full correction (hematocrit, 42%) in HD patients with CVD. It was stopped prematurely because of a trend toward worse outcome in the high hematocrit group.

Similarly, the Cardiovascular risk Reduction by Early Anemia Treatment with Epoetin beta (CREATE) study testing early versus late anemia correction in CKD patients to prevent LVH failed to demonstrate a benefit of early correction.[27] Moreover, a Canadian double-blind study showed that normalization of hemoglobin in incident HD patients did not have a beneficial effect on cardiac structure, compared with partial correction.[28] Thus, a target hemoglobin interval of 11 to 12 g/dl is recommended in dialysis patients with CVD.[29]

Inflammation

Anti-inflammatory treatment strategies, such as statins and aspirin, have beneficial effects on cardiovascular mortality in the general population. In CKD and ESRD patients, such data are lacking, and until they are available, careful search for infectious processes, correction of volume status, and the use of biocompatible dialysis membranes, PD fluids, and ultrapure dialysate water appear prudent.

Oxidative Stress

An important role of oxidative stress in mediating CVD in ESRD is supported by two recent placebo-controlled interventional studies showing that vitamin E and acetylcysteine decreased the number of cardiovascular events in HD patients. Unfortunately, both studies were rather small. Because the interaction between dialysis membranes and blood neutrophils can trigger oxidative stress, specific dialysis techniques (such as vitamin E–modified cellulose membranes) have been introduced in an attempt to reduce oxidative stress. Their effect on CVD is currently unknown.

Vascular Calcification

In the prospective Treat-to-Goal Study, 200 HD patients were randomized to receive either calcium-containing phosphate binders or sevelamer.[30] The former group showed progression of coronary and aortic calcification within 1 year, whereas progression was halted in the sevelamer-treated patients. In the subsequent Dialysis Clinical Outcomes Revisited (DCOR) trial, sevelamer-based versus calcium-based phosphate binder therapy reduced mortality in patients older than 65 years and receiving sevelamer treatment for >2 years.[31] K/DOQI targets for PTH, calcium, and phosphate are discussed in Chapter 74.

Hyperhomocysteinemia

The role of homocysteine in promoting vascular injury in CKD patients is presently unclear, and folic acid or multivitamin supplementation is, in our opinion, not strongly supported by published data. Prospective randomized trials in renal cohorts (Folic Acid for Vascular Outcome In Transplantation [FAVORIT] and Homocysteine Study [HOST]) are ongoing.

Management of Pericardial Effusion and Pericarditis

Uremic patients with pericardial effusions or pericarditis should be hospitalized because of the risk for tamponade. Aggressive anticoagulation should be avoided because of an increased risk for intrapericardial hemorrhage. Spontaneous resolution is not uncommon, but nevertheless intensified dialysis should be the mainstay of therapy, avoiding episodes of cardiac underfilling. Pericardial puncture is rarely necessary.

Revascularization

Coronary intervention is superior to conservative treatment.[19] The best method of coronary revascularization is controversial, however, because percutaneous interventions show good short-term results but also high reintervention rates and a higher long-term mortality when compared with coronary artery bypass grafting (CABG). Based on USRDS data, the superiority of CABG may in part depend on procedures that include use of internal mammary grafts.[19] This observation could mean that patients who need targeted revascularization of the left anterior descending artery and who possess appropriate target vessels (and not severe diffuse coronary disease) will have a better prognosis. A recent large study reported that both interventions were equally effective concerning long-term survival in ESRD patients, but CABG was superior to percutaneous intervention in predialysis CKD patients.[32] Therefore, the choice of the optimal interventional technique depends on the local availability, and probably also the stage of CKD. The role of coated stents in CKD patients has not been established.

REFERENCES

1. Foley RN, Parfrey PS, Sarnak MJ: Clinical epidemiology of cardiovascular disease in chronic renal failure. Am J Kidney Dis 1998;32(Suppl 5):S112–S119.
2. Vanholder R, Massy Z, Argiles A, et al: Chronic kidney disease as cause of cardiovascular morbidity and mortality. Nephrol Dial Transpl 2005; 20:1048–1056.
3. Agarwal R: Hypertension and survival in chronic hemodialysis patients: Past lessons and future opportunities. Kidney Int 2005;67:1–13.
4. Muntner PHJ, Astor BC, Folsom AR, Coresh J: Traditional and nontraditional risk factors predict coronary heart disease in chronic kidney disease: Results from the atherosclerosis risk in communities study. J Am Soc Nephrol 2005;16:529–538.
5. Kalantar-Zadeh K, Block G, Humphreys MH, Kopple JD: Reverse epidemiology of cardiovascular risk factors in maintenance dialysis patients. Kidney Int 2003;63:793–808.
6. Liu Y, Coresh J, Eustace JA, et al: Association between cholesterol level and mortality in dialysis patients. Role of inflammation and malnutrition. JAMA 2004;291:451–459.
7. Beddhu S, Kimmel PL, Ramkumar N, Cheung AK: Associations of metabolic syndrome with inflammation in CKD: Results from the Third National Health and Nutrition Examination Survey (NHANES). Am J Kidney Dis 2005;46:577–586.
8. Foley RN, Wang C, Collins AJ: Cardiovascular risk factor profiles and kidney function stage in the US general population: The NHANES III study. Mayo Clin Proc 2005;80:1270–1277.
9. Xu J, Li G, Wang P, et al: Renalase is a novel, soluble monoamine oxidase that regulates cardiac function and blood pressure. J Clin Invest 2005;115:1275–1280.
10. Himmelfarb J, Stenvinkel P, Ikizler TA, Hakim RM: The elephant of uremia: Oxidative stress as a unifying concept of cardiovascular disease in uremia. Kidney Int 2002;62:1524–1538.
11. Stenvinkel P, Ketteler M, Johnson RJ, et al: Interleukin-10, IL-6 and TNF-α: Important factors in the altered cytokine network of end-stage renal disease—the good, the bad and the ugly. Kidney Int 2005;67: 1216–1233.
12. Koc M, Richards HB, Bihorac A, et al: Circulating endothelial cells are associated with future vascular events in hemodialysis patients. Kidney Int 2005;67:1079–1083.
13. Block GA, Hulbert-Shearon TE, Levin NW, Port FK: Association of serum phosphorus and calcium x phosphate product with mortality risk in chronic hemodialysis patients: A national study. Am J Kidney Dis 1998;31:607–617.
14. Vliegenthart R, Hollander M, Breteler MM, et al: Stroke associated with coronary calcification as detected by electron-bean CT: The Rotterdam Coronary Calcification Study. Stroke 2002;33:462–465.
15. Blacher J, Guerin AP, Pannier B, et al: Arterial calcifications, arterial stiffness, and cardiovascular risk in end-stage renal disease. Hypertension 2001;38:938–942.
16. Ketteler M, Bongartz P, Westenfeld R, et al: Association of low fetuin-A (AHSG) concentrations in serum with cardiovascular mortality in patients on dialysis: A cross-sectional study. Lancet 2003;361:827–833.
17. Suliman M, Barany P, Kalanthar-Zadeh K, et al: Homocysteine in uremia: A puzzling and conflicting story. Nephrol Dial Transpl 2005;20:16–21.
18. Vonesh EF, Snyder JJ, Foley RN, Collins AJ: The differential impact of risk factors on mortality in hemodialysis and peritoneal dialysis. Kidney Int 2004;66:2389–2401.
19. Herzog CA: How to manage the renal patient with coronary heart disease: The agony and the ecstasy of opinion-based medicine. J Am Soc Nephrol 2003;14:2556–2572.
20. Locatelli F, Covic A, Chazot C, et al: Hypertension and cardiovascular risk assessment in dialysis patients. Nephrol Dial Transpl 2004;19: 1058–1068.
21. Amann K, Wiest G, Zimmer G, et al: Reduced capillary density in the myocardium of uremic rats—a stereological study. Kidney Int 1992;42: 1079–1085.
22. Ritz E, Rambausek M, Mall G, et al: Cardiac changes in uraemia and their possible relationship to cardiovascular instability on dialysis. Nephrol Dial Transplant 1990;5(Suppl 1):93–97.
23. Mall G, Huther W, Schneider J, et al: Diffuse intermyocardiocytic fibrosis in uraemic patients. Nephrol Dial Transplant 1990;5:39–44.
24. Amann K, Ritz E, Wiest G, et al: A role of parathyroid hormone for the activation of cardiac fibroblasts in uremia. J Am Soc Nephrol 1994;4: 1814–1819.
25. Wanner C, Krane V, Marz W, et al: Atorvastatin in patients with type 2 diabetes mellitus undergoing hemodialysis. N Engl J Med 2005;353: 238–248.
26. Besarab A, Bolton WK, Browne JK, et al: The effects of normal as compared with low hematocrit values in patients with cardiac disease who are receiving hemodialysis and epoetin. N Engl J Med 1998;339: 584–590.
27. Macdougall IC, Steering Committee of the CREATE trial; CREATE Study Group: CREATE: New strategies for early anaemia management in renal insufficiency. Nephrol Dial Transpl 2003;18(Suppl 2):ii13–16.
28. Parfrey P, Foley RN, Wittreich BH, et al: Double-blind comparison of full and partial anemia correction in incident hemodialysis patients without symptomatic heart disease. J Am Soc Nephrol 2005;16: 2180–2189.
29. Locatelli F, Aljama P, Barany P, et al: Revised European best practice guidelines for the management of anaemia in patients with chronic renal failure. Nephrol Dial Transplant 2004;19(Suppl 2):ii1–47.
30. Chertow GM, Burke SK, Raggi P: Sevelamer attenuates the progression of coronary and aortic calcification in hemodialysis patients. Kidney Int 2002;62:245–252.
31. Suki W, Zabaneh R, Cangiano J, et al: The DCOR trial—A prospective, randomized trial assessing the impact on outcomes of sevelamer in dialysis patients (abstract). J Am Soc Nephrol 2005;16:TH–PO745.
32. Hemmelgarn BR, Southern D, Culleton BF, et al: Survival after coronary revascularization among patients with kidney disease. Circulation 2004; 110:1890–1895.

Anemia in Chronic Kidney Disease

Iain C. Macdougall and Kai-Uwe Eckardt

INTRODUCTION

Anemia is an almost universal complication of chronic kidney disease (CKD). It contributes considerably to reduced quality of life of patients with CKD and has been increasingly recognized as an adverse risk factor. Before the availability of recombinant human erythropoietin (rHuEPO, or epoetin), patients on dialysis frequently required blood transfusions and were exposed to the risks of iron overload, transmission of viral hepatitis, and sensitization, which reduced the chances of successful transplantation. The advent of rHuEPO in the late 1980s changed this situation completely. The ability to correct anemia has shown that its consequences go beyond general fatigue and reduced physical capacity to affect a broad spectrum of physiologic functions. Thus, there is a strong rationale to diagnose anemia in CKD patients, and yet the optimal treatment strategies are still incompletely defined. Apart from therapy with erythropoiesis-stimulating agents (ESAs), iron replacement is essential for anemia management. Importantly, CKD patients require different target thresholds of iron parameters than normal individuals to ensure optimal rates of red-cell production. The costs of anemia management are considerable; therefore, a rational and careful consideration of the risks and benefits are mandatory.

PATHOGENESIS

Renal anemia is typically an isolated normochromic, normocytic anemia with no leukopenia or thrombocytopenia. Both red-cell life span and the rate of red-cell production are reduced, but the latter is more important. The normal bone marrow has considerable capacity to increase the rate of erythropoiesis, and the reduction in erythrocyte life observed in association with CKD would normally be easily compensated. However, this EPO-induced compensatory increase in erythrocyte production is impaired in CKD. Serum EPO levels remain within the normal range and fail to show the inverse exponential relationship with blood oxygen content characteristic of other types of anemia. EPO is normally produced by interstitial fibroblasts in the renal cortex, located in close proximity to tubular epithelial cells and peritubular capillaries.[1,2] In addition, hepatocytes and perisinusoidal Ito cells in the liver can produce EPO (Fig. 72.1). Hepatic EPO production dominates during fetal and early postnatal life, but cannot compensate for the loss of renal production in adult organisms. Subtle changes in blood oxygen content induced by anemia, reduced environmental oxygen concentrations, or high altitude stimulate the secretion of EPO through a widespread system of oxygen-dependent gene expression.[2-4] Central to this

process is a family of hypoxia-inducible transcription factors (HIFs). The two most important members of this family, HIF-1 and HIF-2, are composed of an oxygen-regulated α-subunit (HIF-1α or HIF-2α) and a constitutive β-subunit. The production of HIF-1α and HIF-2α is largely independent of oxygen, but their degradation is related to cellular oxygen concentrations. Hydroxylation of specific prolyl and asparagyl residues of HIFα, for which molecular oxygen is required as a substrate, determines HIF proteasomal destruction and inhibits its transcriptional activity. Apart from EPO, more than 100 HIF target genes have been identified. HIF-2, rather than HIF-1, is the transcription factor primarily responsible for the regulation of EPO production.[5,6]

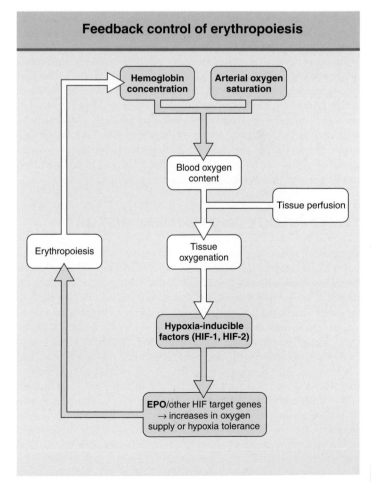

Figure 72.1   Feedback control of erythropoiesis.

The role of renal EPO production in the pathogenesis of renal anemia is supported by the observation that anemia is particularly severe in anephric individuals. However, the mechanisms impairing renal EPO production in diseased kidneys remain poorly understood. The production capacity for EPO remains significant, even in end-stage renal disease. Thus, patients with anemia and CKD can respond with a significant increase in EPO production in response to an additional hypoxic stimulus.[1] The main problem, therefore, appears to be a failure of EPO production to respond to chronically reduced hemoglobin concentrations. In line with this view, endogenous EPO production can be induced in CKD patients by pharmacologic inhibition of HIF degradation (see later discussion).

EPO is a glycoprotein hormone, consisting of a 165–amino acid protein backbone and four complex, heavily sialylated carbohydrate chains.[1,2] The latter are essential for the biologic activity of EPO *in vivo* because partially or completely deglycosylated EPO is rapidly cleared from the circulation. This is also why rHuEPO has to be manufactured in mammalian cell lines because bacteria lack the capacity to glycosylate recombinant proteins.

EPO stimulates red-cell production through binding to homodimeric EPO receptors, which are primarily located on early erythroid progenitor cells, the burst-forming units erythroid (BFU-e) and the colony-forming units erythroid (CFU-e). Binding of EPO to its receptors salvages these progenitor cells and the subsequent earliest erythroblast generation from apoptosis, thereby permitting cell division and maturation into red blood cells.[7] Inhibition of red-cell production by uremic inhibitors of erythropoiesis may also contribute to the pathogenesis of renal anemia, although they have so far not been identified. Nevertheless, dialysis *per se* can improve renal anemia and the efficacy of ESAs. Moreover, the interindividual dose requirements for ESAs vary significantly among CKD patients, and the average weekly dose is much higher than estimated production rates of endogenous EPO in healthy individuals. An alternative view to inhibitors of erythropoiesis accumulating in CKD is that in many patient there is overlap between renal anemia and the anemia of chronic disease, which is characterized by inhibition of EPO production and EPO efficacy as well as reduced iron availability, mediated through the effects of inflammatory cytokines.[8] Recently, hepcidin was discovered as a key mediator of iron metabolism. Its hepatic release is upregulated in states of inflammation; it simultaneously blocks iron absorption in the gut and promotes iron sequestration in macrophages.[9]

EPIDEMIOLOGY AND NATURAL HISTORY

In general, there is a progressive increase in the incidence and severity of anemia with declining renal function. The reported prevalence of anemia by CKD stage varies significantly and depends to a large extent on the definition of anemia and on whether study participants are selected from the general population, are at high risk for CKD, are diabetic, or are already under the care of a physician. Data from the National Health and Nutrition Examination Survey (NHANES) showed that the distribution of hemoglobin (Hb) levels starts to fall at an estimated GFR (eGFR) of less than 75 ml/min/1.73 m² in men and 45 ml/min/1.73 m² in women[10] (Fig. 72.2). The prevalence of Hb values below 13 g/dl increases below a threshold eGFR of 60 ml/min/1.73 m² in males and 45 ml/min/1.73 m² in females in the general population. Among patients under regular care and known to have CKD, the prevalence of anemia was found to be much greater, with mean Hb levels of 12.8 ± 1.5 (CKD stages 1

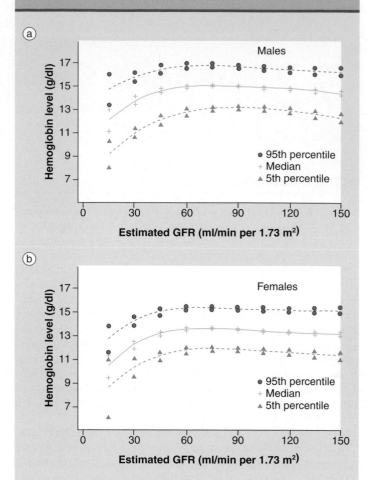

Relationship between Hb and estimated GFR

Figure 72.2 Relationship between hemoglobin (Hb) and estimated glomerular filtration rate (GFR). Data are from a cross-sectional survey of individuals randomly selected from the general U.S. population (NHANES III). Results and 95% confidence interval are shown for males (*a*) and females (*b*) at each estimated GFR interval. (From McClellan W, Aronoff SL, Bolton WK, et al: The prevalence of anemia in patients with chronic kidney disease. Curr Med Res Opin 2004;20:501–510.)

and 2), 12.4 ± 1.6 (CKD stage 3), 12.0 ± 1.6 (CKD stage 4), and 10.9 ± 1.6 (CKD stage 5).[11] Although anemia develops largely independent of the etiology of kidney disease, there are two important exceptions. Diabetic patients develop anemia more frequently, at earlier stages of CKD, and more severely at a given level of renal impairment.[12,13] Conversely, in patients with polycystic kidney disease, Hb is on average higher than in other patients with similar degrees of renal failure, and occasionally polycythemia may develop.[1]

Many patients not yet on dialysis still receive no specific treatment for their anemia. In patients on dialysis, in contrast, average Hb values have steadily increased during the past 15 years, following the advent of EPO and the development of clinical practice guidelines.[12,13] The average Hb value, however, varies considerably between countries, reflecting considerable variability in practice patterns[14] (Fig. 72.3). Moreover, a large proportion of patients continues to have Hb values below recommended target levels (see later discussion).

Hemoglobin levels in patients on dialysis						
	Among Patients on Dialysis >180 Days			Among Patients New to ESRD, at Start of Dialysis		
Country	n	Mean Hb (g/dl)	Hb <11 g/dl (% of patients)	n	Mean Hb (g/dl)	Hb <11 g/dl (% of patients)
Sweden	466	12.0	23	168	10.7	55
United States	1690	11.7	27	458	10.4	65
Spain	513	11.7	31	170	10.6	61
Belgium	442	11.6	29	213	10.3	66
Canada	479	11.6	29	150	10.1	70
Australia and New Zealand	423	11.5	36	108	10.1	70
Germany	459	11.4	35	142	10.5	61
Italy	447	11.3	38	167	10.2	68
United Kingdom	436	11.2	40	93	10.2	67
France	341	11.1	45	86	10.1	65
Japan	1210	10.1	77	131	8.3	95

Figure 72.3 Mean hemoglobin (Hb) levels and percentage of patients with Hb levels <11 g/dl who have been on dialysis therapy for more than 180 days and at the time of starting dialysis, by country. Data are from the Dialysis Outcomes and Practice Patterns Study, phase II (DOPPS II) and are derived from 308 randomly selected, representative dialysis facilities. Note that there are marked differences between countries, but at least one fourth and up to three fourths of dialysis patients and, in most countries, more than two thirds of patients starting chronic dialysis have Hb values below the recommended lower target of 11 g/dl. ESRD, end-stage renal disease. (Adapted from Pisoni RL, Bragg-Gresham JL, Young EW, et al: Anemia management and outcomes from 12 countries in the Dialysis Outcomes and Practice Patterns Study [DOPPS]. Am J Kidney Dis 2004;44:94–111.)

DIAGNOSIS AND DIFFERENTIAL DIAGNOSIS

The diagnosis of anemia and the assessment of its severity is best made by measuring the Hb concentration rather than the hematocrit (Hct). Hb is a stable analyte that is measured directly in a standardized fashion, whereas the Hct is relatively unstable, indirectly derived by automatic analyzers, and lacking in standardization. Within-run and between-run coefficients of variation in automated analyzer measurements of Hb are one-half and one-third those for Hct, respectively.[12]

There is considerable variability in the Hb threshold used to define anemia. According to the most recent definition in Kidney Disease Outcomes Quality Initiative (K/DOQI) guidelines, anemia should be diagnosed at Hb concentrations of less than 13.5 g/dl in adult males and less than 12.0 g/dl in adult females.[12] These values represent the mean Hb of the lowest 5th percentile of the sex-specific general adult population. In children, age-dependent differences in the normal values have to be taken into account. Normal Hb values are increased in high-altitude residents.[12] Adjustment is not recommended for age in adults.

In addition to the Hb value, the evaluation of anemia in CKD patients should include a complete blood count with red blood cell indices (mean corpuscular Hb concentration [MCHC]; mean corpuscular volume [MCV]), white blood cell count (including differential), and platelet count. Although renal anemia is typically normochromic and normocytic, deficiency of vitamin B_{12} or folate may lead to macrocytosis, whereas iron deficiency or inherited disorders of Hb formation (such as thalassemia) may produce microcytosis. Macrocytosis with leukopenia or thrombocytopenia suggests a generalized disorder of hematopoiesis caused by toxins, nutritional deficit, or myelodysplasia. Hypochromia likely reflects iron-deficient erythropoiesis. An absolute reticulocyte count, which normally ranges between 40,000 and 50,000 cells/μl of blood, is a useful marker of erythropoietic activity.

Iron status tests should be performed to assess the level of iron in tissue stores or the adequacy of iron supply for erythropoiesis. Although serum ferritin is so far the only available marker of storage iron, several tests reflect the adequacy of iron for erythropoiesis, including transferrin saturation (TSAT), MCV, and MCHC; the percentage of hypochromic red blood cells (PHRC); and the content of Hb in reticulocytes (CHr). Storage time of the blood sample may elevate PHRC, and MCV and MCHC are below the normal range only after long-standing iron deficiency.

It is important to identify anemia in CKD patients because it may signify the presence of nutritional deficits, systemic illness, or other conditions that warrant attention, and even at modest degrees, anemia reflects an independent risk factor for hospitalizations, cardiovascular disease, and mortality.[12] The diagnosis of renal anemia, that is, an anemia caused by CKD, requires careful judgment of the degree of anemia in relation to the degree of renal impairment and exclusion of other or additional causes. Causes of anemia other than EPO deficiency should be considered when (1) the severity of anemia is disproportionate to the deficit in renal function, (2) there is evidence of iron deficiency, or (3) there is evidence of leukopenia or thrombocytopenia. Concomitant conditions such as sickle cell disease may exacerbate the anemia, as can drug therapy. For example, inhibitors of the renin angiotensin system may reduce Hb levels by (1) direct effects of angiotensin II on erythroid progenitor cells[15]; (2) accumulation of N-acetyl-seryl-lysyl-proline (AcSDKP), an

2000 IU) 2 or 3 times weekly, either by IV or SC administration. Within 3 to 4 days, an increase in the reticulocyte count is seen, and within 1 to 2 weeks, there is a significant rise in the Hb concentration, usually on the order of 0.25 to 0.5 g/dl/week. Thus, over the course of 1 month, a significant increase of 1 to 2 g/dl in the Hb is usually achieved. If a patient fails to respond satisfactorily to ESAs, the dose is increased in stepwise upward titrations of 25% to 50%, and if there is still an inadequate response, then causes of resistance to EPO therapy should be investigated (see later discussion). The optimal target range of hemoglobin for CKD patients is 11 to 13 g/dl[12] (see earlier discussion), and iron supplementation should be administered to maximize the response to ESA therapy (see later discussion).

Hyporesponsiveness to Erythropoiesis-stimulating Agents

There is no absolute definition of hyporesponsiveness to ESA therapy, but it is usually indentified when the Hb remains below 11 g/dl despite increasing doses of ESA. The causes of resistance to ESA therapy are listed in Figure 72.7, and it is important to correct them when possible. The major causes include iron deficiency (see later discussion), infection or inflammation,[29] and underdialysis.[30] If the patient is self-administering (e.g., for peritoneal dialysis patients), poor adherence or compliance to therapy must be excluded. If there is any doubt about the possibility of iron deficiency, a trial of IV iron may be useful. Vitamin B_{12}, folate, and thyroxine deficiency may be excluded easily by requesting the appropriate laboratory tests, as may severe hyperparathyroidism. Aluminum toxicity is no longer a significant cause of ESA resistance. Depending on the ethnic origin of the patient, hemoglobinopathy should be excluded by performing Hb electrophoresis. Some patients taking ACE inhibitors may require higher doses of ESA therapy, although it is rarely necessary or indeed advisable to stop these drugs. Primary bone marrow disorders, such as myelodysplastic syndrome, should be investigated by a bone marrow examination (aspirate and trephine) if all other causes have been excluded. A bone marrow test may also be necessary in diagnosing antibody-mediated

PRCA, although measurement of the reticulocyte count and antierythropoietin antibodies may provide an earlier clue.[23] If a patient on ESA therapy has a high reticulocyte count, the bone marrow is generating more than adequate quantities of new red cells, and bleeding or hemolysis should be investigated by means of an upper gastrointestinal endoscopy, colonoscopy, or hemolysis screen (Coombs' test, bilirubin measurement, lactate dehydrogenase levels, haptoglobin levels). There is no defined upper dose limit of ESA because these agents are not regarded as being toxic in high doses, and doses of 60,000 IU per week of EPO are not uncommon in the United States. Nevertheless, dose escalation of the ESA occurs more readily in countries where the costs are reimbursed, but may be limited in countries where there are economic restraints.

Iron Management

Iron is an essential ingredient for heme synthesis, and adequate amounts of this mineral are required for the manufacture of new red cells. Thus, under enhanced erythropoietic stimulation, greater amounts of iron are utilized, and many CKD patients (particularly those on hemodialysis) have inadequate amounts of available iron to satisfy the increased demands of the bone marrow.[31] Even before the introduction of ESA therapy, many CKD patients were in negative iron balance owing to poor dietary intake, poor appetite, and increased iron losses due to occult and overt blood losses (see Chapter 73). Losses in hemodialysis patients are up to 5 or 6 mg a day, as compared with 1 mg in healthy individuals, and this may exceed the absorption capacity of the gastrointestinal tract, particularly when there is any underlying inflammation. Iron absorption capacity in patients with CKD is considerably lower than in nonuremic individuals, particularly in the presence of systemic inflammatory activity, and this is probably mediated by hepcidin (see earlier discussion).[9] For this reason also, oral iron is ineffective in many CKD patients, and parenteral iron administration is required, particularly in those receiving hemodialysis.[31]

Inadequate supply of iron to the bone marrow may be due to an *absolute* or a *functional* iron deficiency.[31] Absolute iron deficiency occurs when there are low whole body iron stores, as indicated by a serum ferritin level less than 30 μg/l. Functional iron deficiency occurs when there is ample or even increased storage iron but the iron stores fail to release iron rapidly enough to satisfy the demands of the bone marrow. Several markers of iron status are available, but none of them is ideal (Fig. 72.8). The serum *ferritin* is a marker of storage iron but is spuriously raised in inflammatory conditions and liver disease. The *transferrin saturation* is a function of the circulating plasma iron in relation to the total iron-binding capacity (TIBC) and is a better measure of available iron. The percentage of *hypochromic red cells* and the *CHr* are red-cell and reticulocyte parameters, respectively, which are indirect measures of how much iron is being incorporated into the newly developing or mature red cell.[31] No one measure of iron status is usually adequate to exclude iron deficiency, and the recommended levels for these measures are based on limited scientific evidence. Functional iron deficiency is usually diagnosed when there is a normal or increased ferritin level, and a reduced transferrin saturation (<20%) or increased hypochromic red cells (>10%). The U.S.[12] and European[13] guidelines on renal anemia management suggest that the ferritin level should be maintained in the range of 200 to 500 μg/l, with an upper limit of 800 μg/l (see Fig. 72.8). Levels of ferritin above this threshold usually do not confer any

Causes of a poor response to ESA therapy	
Major (Frequent)	**Minor (Less Common)**
Iron deficiency	Poor compliance, poor adherence to ESA therapy
Infection, inflammation	Blood loss
Underdialysis	Hyperparathyroidism
	Aluminum toxicity (rare nowadays)
	Vitamin B_{12} or folate deficiency
	Hemolysis
	Primary bone marrow disorders (e.g., myelodysplastic syndrome)
	Hemoglobinopathies (e.g., sickle cell disease)
	ACE inhibitors
	Carnitine deficiency
	Anti-EPO antibodies causing PRCA

Figure 72.7 Causes of a poor response to erythropoiesis-stimulating agent (ESA) therapy. ACE, angiotensin-converting enzyme; EPO, erythropoietin; PRCA, pure red-cell aplasia.

Markers of iron status in CKD patients

Test	Minimum/Maximum Value	Recommended Range
Serum ferritin	>100 μg/l <800 μg/l	200–500 μg/l
Transferrin saturation	> 20%	20%–40%
Hypochromic red cells	<10%	<6%
Reticulocyte hemoglobin content (CHr)	>29 pg/cell	29 pg/cell
Serum transferrin receptor	Not established	Not established
Erythrocyte zinc protoporphyrin	Not established	Not established

Figure 72.8 Markers of iron status and the recommended target ranges in chronic kidney disease (CKD).

clinical advantage and may exacerbate iron toxicity. The optimal transferrin saturation is above 20% to 30%, to ensure a readily available supply of iron to the bone marrow. Several studies support the maintenance of the percentage of hypochromic red cells at levels of less than 6%, and the CHr at levels greater than 29 pg/cell. Other measures of iron status, such as *serum transferrin receptor* levels and *erythrocyte zinc protoporphyrin* levels, are mainly research investigations.

Iron supplementation is often required in CKD patients. Oral iron is poorly absorbed in uremic individuals, and there is a high incidence of gastrointestinal side effects. Intramuscular iron is not recommended in CKD, given the enhanced bleeding tendency, the pain of the injection, and the potential for brownish discoloration of the skin. Thus, intravenous iron administration has become the standard of care for many CKD patients, particularly those receiving hemodialysis.[31] There are several IV iron preparations available worldwide, including iron dextran, iron sucrose, and iron gluconate. All of these preparations contain elemental iron surrounded by a carbohydrate shell, which allows them to be injected intravenously. The lability of iron release from these preparations varies, with iron dextran being the most stable, followed by iron sucrose, and finally iron gluconate. Iron is released from these compounds to plasma transferrin and other iron-binding proteins and is eventually taken up by the reticuloendothelial system.

In hemodialysis patients, it is easy and practical to give low doses of intravenous iron (e.g., 10–20 mg every dialysis session), or alternatively 100 mg weekly. In peritoneal dialysis and non-dialysis CKD patients, however, such low-dose regimens are impractical, and larger doses may be administered. The more stable the iron preparation, the larger the dose administration rate that can be used. For example, 1 g of iron dextran may be given by IV infusion, whereas the maximum recommended dose of iron sucrose at any one time is 500 mg. For iron gluconate, doses in excess of 125 to 250 mg are best avoided. All IV iron preparations carry a risk for immediate reactions, which may be characterized by hypotension, dizziness, and nausea. These reactions are usually short lived and caused by too large a dose given over too short a period of time. Iron dextran also carries the risk for acute anaphylactic reactions due to preformed dextran antibodies, and although this risk may be less with the lower-molecular-weight iron dextrans, the potential for anaphylaxis still remains. Other, more long-term concerns about IV iron administration include the potential for increased susceptibility to infections and oxidative stress. Much of the scientific evidence for this has been generated in *in vitro* experiments, the clinical significance of which is unclear.

There is emerging evidence that intravenous iron may also improve the anemia of chronic kidney disease in up to 30% of patients not receiving ESA therapy who have a low ferritin level.[32] In such patients, a response to IV iron alone may occur within 2 to 3 weeks of iron administration. In those already receiving ESAs, there is considerable evidence that concomitant IV iron may enhance the response to the ESAs and result in lower dose requirements.[13,14,31]

REFERENCES

1. Eckardt KU: Erythropoietin: Oxygen-dependent control of erythropoiesis and its failure in renal disease. Nephron 1994;67:7–23.
2. Jelkmann W: Molecular biology of erythropoietin. Inter Med 2004;43:649–659.
3. Schofield CJ, Ratcliffe PJ: Oxygen sensing by HIF hydroxylases. Nat Rev Mol Cell Biol 2004;5:43–54.
4. Maxwell P: HIF-1: An oxygen response system with special relevance to the kidney. J Am Soc Nephrol 2003;14:712–722.
5. Warnecke C, Zaborowska Z, Kurreck J, et al: Differentiating the functional role of hypoxia-inducible factor (HIF)-1alpha and HIF-2alpha (EPAS-1) by the use of RNA interference: Erythropoietin is a HIF-2alpha target gene in Hep3B and Kelly cells. FASEB J 2004;18:462–464.
6. Scortegagna M, Morris MA, Oktay Y, et al: The HIF family member EPAS1/HIF-2alpha is required for normal hematopoiesis in mice. Blood 2003;102:634–640.
7. Chen C, Sytkowski AJ: The erythropoietin receptor and its signalling cascade. In Jelkmann WFP (ed): Erythropoietin: Molecular Biology and Clinical Use. Johnson City, TN, Graham Publishing, 2003, pp 165–194.
8. Weiss G, Goodnough LT: Anemia of chronic disease. N Engl J Med 2005;352:11–23.
9. Verga Falzacappa MV, Muckenthaler MU: Hepcidin: Iron-hormone and anti-microbial peptide. Gene 2005;364:37–44.
10. Astor BC, Muntner P, Levin A, et al: Association of kidney function with anemia: The Third National Health and Nutrition Examination Survey, 1988–1994. Arch Intern Med 2002;162:1401–1408.
11. McClellan W, Aronoff SL, Bolton WK, et al: The prevalence of anemia in patients with chronic kidney disease. Curr Med Res Opin 2004;20:501–510.
12. K/DOQI: Anemia Guidelines in CKD patients. Am J Kidney Dis 2006;47(suppl 3):S1–S146.
13. European Best Practice Guidelines Working Group: Revised European best practice guidelines for the management of anaemia in patients with chronic renal failure. Nephrol Dial Transplant 2004;19(Suppl 2):1–47.
14. Pisoni RL, Bragg-Gresham JL, Young EW, et al: Anemia management and outcomes from 12 countries in the Dialysis Outcomes and Practice Patterns Study (DOPPS). Am J Kidney Dis 2004;44:94–111.
15. Cole J, Ertoy D, Lin H, et al: Lack of angiotensin II-facilitated erythropoiesis causes anemia in angiotensin-converting enzyme-deficient mice. J Clin Invest 2000;106:391–398.
16. Le Meur Y, Lorgeot V, Comte L, et al: Plasma levels and metabolism of AcSDKP in patients with chronic renal failure: Relationship with erythropoietin requirements. Am J Kidney Dis 2001;38:10–17.

17. Winkelmayer WC, Kewalramani R, Rutstein M, et al: Pharmacoepidemiology of anemia in kidney transplant recipients. J Am Soc Nephrol 2004;15:347–352.

18. Macdougall IC, Lewis NP, Saunders MJ, et al: Long-term cardiorespiratory effects of amelioration of renal anaemia by erythropoietin. Lancet 1990;335:489–493.

19. Parfrey PS, Foley RN, Wittreich BH, et al: Double-blind comparison of full and partial anemia correction in incident hemodialysis patients without symptomatic heart disease. J Am Soc Nephrol 2005;16:2180–2189.

20. Besarab A, Bolton WK, Browne JK, et al: The effects of normal as compared with low hematocrit values in patients with cardiac disease who are receiving hemodialysis and epoetin. N Engl J Med 1998;339:584–590.

21. Drueke TB, Locelli F, Clyne N, et al: Normalization of hemoglobin level in patients with chronic kidney disease and anemia. N Engl J Med 2006;355:2071–2084.

22. Singh AK, Szzczech L, Tang KL, et al: Correction of anemia with epoetin alfa in chronic kidney disease. N Engl J Med 2006;355:2085–2098.

23. Rossert J, Casadevall N, Eckardt KU: Anti-erythropoietin antibodies and pure red cell aplasia. J Am Soc Nephrol 2004;15:398–406.

24. Boven K, Stryker S, Knight J, et al: The increased incidence of pure red cell aplasia with an Eprex formulation in uncoated rubber stopper syringes. Kidney Int 2005;67:346–353.

25. Macdougall IC, Padhi D, Jang G: Pharmacology of erythropoiesis-stimulating agents. Nephrol Dial Transplant 2007 (in press).

26. Kaufman JS, Reda DJ, Fye CL, et al: Subcutaneous compared with intravenous epoetin in patients receiving hemodialysis. Department of Veterans Affairs Cooperative Study Group on Erythropoietin in Hemodialysis Patients. N Engl J Med 1998;339:578–583.

27. Vanrenterghem Y, Barany P, Mann JF, et al, for the European/Australian NESP 970200 Study Group: Randomized trial of darbepoetin alfa for treatment of renal anemia at a reduced dose frequency compared with rHuEPO in dialysis patients. Kidney Int 2002;62:2167–2175.

28. Macdougall IC, Eckardt KU: Novel strategies for stimulating erythropoiesis and potential new treatments for anaemia. Lancet 2006;368:947–953.

29. Macdougall IC, Cooper AC: Hyporesponsiveness to erythropoietic therapy due to chronic inflammation. Eur J Clin Invest 2005;35(Suppl 3):32–35.

30. Locatelli F, Del Vecchio L: Dialysis adequacy and response to erythropoietic agents: What is the evidence base? Nephrol Dial Transplant 2003;18(Suppl 8):29–35.

31. Macdougall IC: Monitoring of iron status and iron supplementation in patients treated with erythropoietin. Curr Opin Nephrol Hypertens 1994;3:620–625.

32. Mircescu G, Garneata L, Capusa C, Ursea N: Intravenous iron supplementation for the treatment of anaemia in pre-dialyzed chronic renal failure patients. Nephrol Dial Transplant 2006;1:120–124.

Other Blood and Immune Disorders in Chronic Kidney Disease

Walter Hörl

INTRODUCTION

Besides anemia (see Chapter 72), a variety of other changes occur in patients with advanced chronic kidney disease (CKD). These include altered platelet function, which, together with abnormal coagulation, may result in a uremic bleeding tendency but can also result in a prothrombogenic state. In addition, leukocyte function is altered, resulting in increased susceptibility to infections and abnormal immune responses, such as following vaccinations.

PLATELET DYSFUNCTION AND COAGULATION DEFECTS

Normal hemostasis (Figs. 73.1 and 73.2) begins with platelet adhesion to vascular endothelium and requires a relatively vasoconstricted vessel wall, integrity of platelet glycoproteins (GPs), and a normal quantity of large-molecular-weight, multimeric von Willebrand factor (vWF). Main platelet GPs are GPIb, the platelet receptor for vWF, involved in platelet adhesion, and GPIIb/IIIa, the platelet receptor for fibrinogen, involved in platelet aggregation. Under static conditions, GPIb and vWF have no affinity for each other. However, these molecules develop a specific affinity for one another at high shear stress, resulting in arterial platelet adhesion. Aggregated fibrinogen–platelet meshes act as a trap for binding and activation of other plasma clotting factors. The exposure of preceding clotting factors to tissue factor present on damaged endothelial cells, activated monocyte-macrophages, or other cells of the vascular wall catalyzes the conversion of prothrombin to thrombin, which converts fibrinogen to fibrin. Subsequent cross-linking of insoluble fibrin results in a stable hemostatic plug.

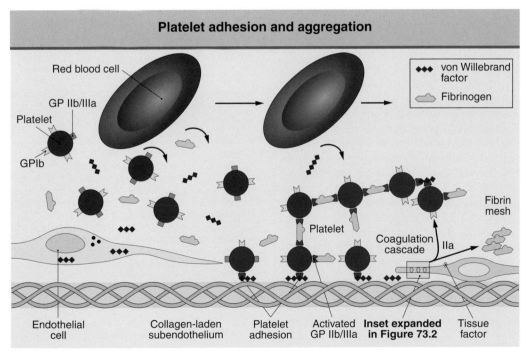

Figure 73.1   Platelet adhesion and aggregation. Platelets are pushed peripherally toward the vascular wall by red blood cells traversing centrally through the bloodstream. Damage to the vessel wall results in a rent in the nonthrombogenic endothelial cell lining and exposure of subendothelial structures. While collagen supports initial platelet adhesion (and subsequent aggregation), von Willebrand factor (vWF) deposition on the subendothelium serves as the main anchor for platelet adhesion via platelet GPIb receptor. Postadhesion conformational change in platelet GP IIb/IIIa receptor (fibrinogen/vWF receptor) results in interlinking platelet aggregation.

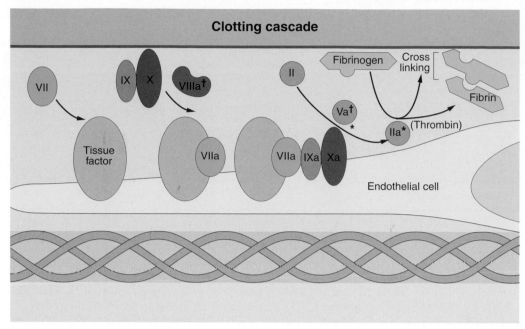

Figure 73.2   Clotting cascade. Expansion of the inset in Figure 73.1 shows the clotting cascade that takes place at the damaged vessel wall. Exposure of subendothelial tissue factor, present on pericytes and fibroblasts, allows for eventual activation of prothrombin (factor II) to thrombin. Thrombin converts fibrinogen to fibrin, activates fibrin cross-linking, stimulates further platelet aggregation, and activates anticoagulant protein C. Naturally occurring anticoagulants antithrombin III, protein C, and protein S help maintain control and counterbalance on coagulation. *Site of anticoagulant effect for antithrombin III. †Site of anticoagulant effect for protein C–protein S complex.

BLEEDING DIATHESIS IN UREMIA

Uremic bleeding caused by acquired platelet dysfunction is a major cause of morbidity and mortality in end-stage renal disease (ESRD) patients. The bleeding problems are characterized by abnormal prolongation of bleeding time and hemorrhagic symptoms, manifesting usually as ecchymoses or petechiae in the skin, epistaxis, gastrointestinal or gingival oozing, or prolonged hemorrhage from needle puncture or postoperative sites. Complications in ESRD patients may also manifest as hemorrhagic pericarditis or hemorrhagic pleural effusion, as well as intracranial, retroperitoneal, ocular, or uterine bleeding. The pathogenesis of platelet dysfunction in uremia is multifactorial (Fig. 73.3) and includes diminished adherence of platelets to vascular endothelium as well as reduced total platelet GPIb content. However, GPIb expression increases adequately after platelet stimulation. The total content of GPIIb and GPIIIa is normal, but GPIIb/IIIa expression is reduced after stimulation, indicating hyporesponsiveness of the uremic platelets under stimulatory conditions.[1] A conformational change in the GPIIb/IIIa receptor in uremia results in reduced fibrinogen binding[2]; this can be improved by hemodialysis (HD), indicating a potential role of uremic toxins.[3] Plasma vWF level is normal or elevated in uremia. However, administration of agents that increase plasma vWF or the factor VIII–vWF complex improves the bleeding tendency in uremia, suggesting abnormalities in vWF metabolism, structure, or function. Mean platelet vWF antigen is reduced in uremia. Some ESRD patients display a decrease in all components, especially those with high molecular weight, in their platelet vWF multimer pattern.

A variety of circulating plasma proteases, such as plasmin, cleave the α chain of platelet GPIb. The resulting proteolytic degradation product glycocalicin contains binding sites for thrombin and vWF. Elevated plasma glycocalicin levels in uremic patients may contribute to diminished binding of uremic platelets

to subendothelium, owing to the vWF binding site of glycocalicin. Furthermore, glycocalicin also contains the thrombin binding site of GPIb, which may also contribute to diminished platelet function in uremia.[4]

HD and peritoneal dialysis (PD) correct platelet abnormalities and prolonged bleeding time only partly, with PD being more effective than HD, possibly because of better clearance of uremic middle molecules. In addition, heparin administration is not required in PD patients. Further, platelet contact with "bioincompatible" HD membranes causes defects in platelet membrane receptors for vWF and fibrinogen (e.g., GPIb

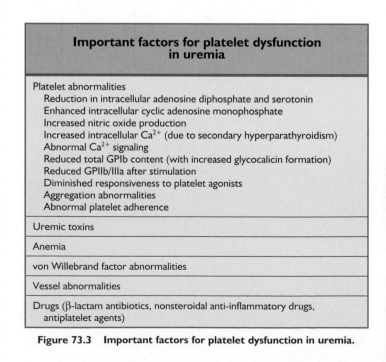

Important factors for platelet dysfunction in uremia

Platelet abnormalities
   Reduction in intracellular adenosine diphosphate and serotonin
   Enhanced intracellular cyclic adenosine monophosphate
   Increased nitric oxide production
   Increased intracellular Ca^{2+} (due to secondary hyperparathyroidism)
   Abnormal Ca^{2+} signaling
   Reduced total GPIb content (with increased glycocalicin formation)
   Reduced GPIIb/IIIa after stimulation
   Diminished responsiveness to platelet agonists
   Aggregation abnormalities
   Abnormal platelet adherence

Uremic toxins

Anemia

von Willebrand factor abnormalities

Vessel abnormalities

Drugs (β-lactam antibiotics, nonsteroidal anti-inflammatory drugs, antiplatelet agents)

Figure 73.3   Important factors for platelet dysfunction in uremia.

internalization),[5] thus preventing normal platelet–vessel wall and platelet–platelet interactions.

Nitric oxide (NO) inhibits platelet function, modulates vascular tone, and affects platelet–vessel wall and platelet–platelet interactions. Uremic platelets generate more NO than platelets obtained from healthy subjects.[6] Uremic plasma induces NO synthesis in endothelial cells. Bleeding tendency in uremic patients is related to the increased platelet nitric oxide synthase (NOS) activity. Inhibition of NOS by N(G)-monomethyl-L-arginine (L-NMMA) restores the increased bleeding time in experimental uremia to normal.[7] Influx of the NOS substrate L-arginine into uremic platelets is sustained and may contribute to platelet dysfunction even in the L-arginine–deprived uremic milieu, which is characterized by low NO levels due to accumulation of the NO inhibitor asymmetric dimethylarginine (ADMA).

Renal anemia is another determinant of the prolonged bleeding time in ESRD patients. Within the normal circulation, red blood cells increase platelet–vessel wall contact by displacing platelets away from the axial flow and toward the vessel wall. This close proximity allows the platelets to adhere to the endothelium when there is endothelial injury.[8]

The hemorrhage risk in ESRD patients can be evaluated by the determination of the bleeding time. Bleeding times of greater than 10 to 15 minutes have been associated with high risk for hemorrhage. However, the bleeding time is poorly reproducible and requires experienced operators to judge the subjective end point of the test. A multicenter study of 3242 patients before general surgery showed that routine preoperative hemostatic screening tests (prothrombin time, activated partial thromboplastin time [APTT], platelet count, and bleeding time) should not be performed routinely, but only in patients with abnormal clinical data, such as the presence of purpura, hematoma, jaundice, and signs of liver cirrhosis.[9] There is no prolongation of the prothrombin time and APTT in uremia unless there is a coexisting coagulopathy.

PLATELET NUMBER IN UREMIA

Thrombocytopenia affects 16% to 55% of ESRD patients. The platelet count is rarely less than $80 \times 10^9/l$, a number generally considered adequate for normal hemostasis.[8] During HD, acute thrombocytopenia occurs but only if complement-activating, bioincompatible dialyzer membranes are used. Heparin may also cause thrombocytopenia in ESRD patients as a result of developing antiplatelet factor 4/heparin (PF4/H) antibodies (see later discussion).

PD and HD patients exhibit 7% to 8% circulating reticulated platelets, compared with a normal of 3%, suggesting shortened platelet survival and increased turnover. Shortened platelet survival in uremia may be the result of increased exposure of negatively charged phosphatidylserine at the platelet surface in ESRD patients. This signal is recognized by macrophages and promotes phagocytosis.[10]

CORRECTION OF UREMIC BLEEDING

Correction of Anemia
Increased intraoperative complications have been reported in ESRD patients with low preoperative hematocrit levels (Fig. 73.4). If the surgery is elective, recombinant human erythropoietin (rHuEPO) or darbepoetin alfa may be administered to raise the hemoglobin to >10 g/dl (hematocrit >30%; see Chapter 72). Correction of anemia results in enhanced platelet–vessel wall interaction by the formation of a skimming layer of platelets at the

Therapeutic approaches to correct uremic bleeding tendency, ranked in order of clinical usage	
Measure	Comments
Correct anemia	Increase hemoglobin to >10 g/dl with rHuEpo or darbepoetin alfa. Use packed red blood cells in emergencies (with monitoring of serum potassium).
Adequate dialysis	Increase Kt/V >1.2 in hemodialysis and Kt/V >1.7 in peritoneal dialysis patients.
Avoid or monitor heparin usage	Note persistent anticoagulation after hemodialysis; monitor anti-Xa levels if LMWH is used at a GFR <30 ml/min; in high-risk patients on hemodialysis, reduce, eliminate, or replace heparin with citrate; administer protamine sulfate, 1 mg per 100 U of heparin infused over 10 min, in emergencies to antagonize heparin.
Withdraw antiplatelet agents	Stop dipyridamole or clopidogrel at least 72 hours before surgery; stop acetylsalicylic acid 7–10 days before surgery.
Administer DDAVP	One hour before surgery, administer DDAVP intravenously (0.3–0.4 µg/kg in 50 ml normal saline over 20–30 min), subcutaneously (0.3 µg/kg), or intranasally (2–3 µg/kg).
Administer cryoprecipitate	One hour before surgery, administer cryoprecipitate (infusion of about 10 units).
Administer estrogens	Administer conjugated estrogen, 0.6 mg/kg per day intravenously or 25–50 mg/kg per day orally, or estradiol, 50–100 µg twice weekly transdermally.

Figure 73.4 Therapeutic approaches to correct uremic bleeding tendency, ranked in order of clinical use. DDAVP, desmopressin acetate; GFR, glomerular filtration rate; LMWH, low-molecular-weight heparin; rHuEPO, recombinant human erythropoietin.

endothelial surface. It also shortens bleeding time and improves hemostasis. Red blood cells improve platelet function by releasing adenosine diphosphate, which stimulates platelet aggregation, and by inactivating vasodilatory prostacyclin, which decreases peripheral dispersion of platelets and their contact with the vessel wall. Platelet aggregation in uremia improves with rHuEPO therapy even at doses that do not influence hemoglobin by the release of young platelets to the blood. Treatment with rHuEPO increases platelet number and volume (large platelets aggregate better than small ones), improves platelet calcium signaling, reduces enhanced platelet cyclic adenosine monophosphate content, and increases platelet serotonin as well as ß-thromboglobulin. Through an increase in blood viscosity, rHuEPO enhances the risk for thrombotic events.[8]

Adequacy of Dialysis and Effects of Heparins
Adequate dialysis (see Chapters 83 and 85) improves bleeding time in ESRD patients and reduces hemorrhagic complications. Hemorrhagic problems are fewer with PD than HD, possibly because of better clearance of uremic middle molecules and no requirement of heparin. Deep-tissue biopsies or invasive surgical procedures that require improved hemostasis should ideally be scheduled 12 to 24 hours after HD. After HD, anticoagulant effects of unfractionated heparin persist as long as 2.5 to 4 hours, or even longer with the use of low-molecular-weight heparin (LMWH). LMWH-induced bleeding complications increase in renal failure because of impaired LMWH elimination, although the latter varies with different preparations. Although there is no precise glomerular filtration rate (GFR) cutoff value below

and hospitalization in HD patients. A higher lymphocyte count is associated with higher serum albumin and reduced mortality risk, whereas high neutrophil counts (which strongly correlate to WBC counts) are associated with lower serum albumin. C-reactive protein, a strong outcome predictor, correlates inversely with the lymphocyte count. Inflammation in uremia is associated with overproduction of proinflammatory cytokines due to the following:

- Elevated number of circulating monocytes, particularly the $CD14^+CD16^+$ subpopulation
- Enhanced cytokine production per cell
- Activation of mononuclear cells through complement activation during the HD procedure[19]

Lymphocyte and Immune Dysfunction

Overproduction of proinflammatory cytokines is associated with immune dysfunction in uremia. This is exemplified by hepatitis B virus (HBV) nonresponders showing the strongest overproduction in inflammatory cytokines. Production of proinflammatory cytokines is controlled by the regulatory cytokine interleukin-10 (IL-10). An association between an IL-10 genotype and the probability of a dialysis patient responding to HBV vaccination has been noted. In addition to altered cytokine production, another explanation for the low antibody titers and the short duration of protection or even nonresponsiveness to standard vaccination protocols is the defective expression of the costimulatory B7-2

molecule on monocytes of HD patients, resulting in reduced T cell function. Finally, there is an imbalance in Th1 and Th2, and sometimes the development of anergy.

Responses to Vaccinations

The immune response to vaccines, most notably *Pneumococcus* species and HBV, is often impaired in patients with advanced CKD or ESRD. Older age of ESRD patients is associated with an impaired response to HBV vaccination.[20,21] Previous studies suggested an improved immune status in PD as compared with HD patients, possibly related to better removal of middle molecules. However, in a head-to-head comparison of short-term and 2-year responses to HBV vaccination, seroconversion rates were 79% of HD patients and 77% of PD patients after injecting 40 μg of recombinant HBV vaccine into the deltoid muscle at 0, 1, 2, and 6 months.[21] Weight, albumin level, male sex, presence of diabetes, and serologic positivity for hepatitis C virus further predict the response to HBV vaccine.

Because of the apparent suboptimal response to vaccination, a four-dose schedule is recommended for uremic patients (Fig. 73.5). The intradermal vaccination is more effective than the intramuscular administration but of shorter durability of immunity. After successful vaccination and initial seroconversion, a booster dose of vaccine is generally recommended for ESRD

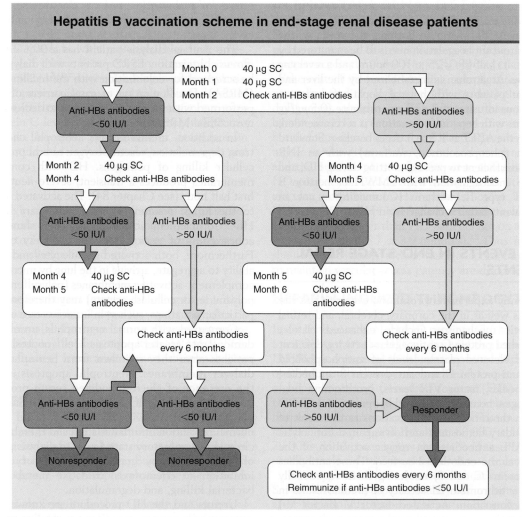

Figure 73.5 Hepatitis B vaccination scheme in end-stage renal disease patients. All patients receive 3 doses of hepatitis B vaccine 40 μg SC. An additional dose is given if anti-HBs antibody response is <50 IU/l.

patients (see Fig. 73.5) because of their immunosuppressed status, poor responses to vaccination, and environmental risks for cross-infection. Early vaccination, such as in CKD stage 3 patients, remains the best way to secure immunologic protection against HBV infection.

After *Pneumococcus* species vaccination, ESRD patients achieve lower postvaccination antibody titers with a rapid decline in antibody level. A protective response to pneumococcal vaccination 4 weeks after immunization was observed in 83% of CKD patients, but only 68% of patients retained protective antibody levels at 6 months, and only 48% at 1 year. Revaccination at 1 year produced a significant response in 50% of these patients.[22]

The typical take up rate for influenza vaccination for dialysis patients is <50% for each season. Influenza vaccination results in a significantly decreased risk for death and hospitalization in this patient population and should be performed in each ESRD patient in early October.[22]

Only 55% of CKD patients and 69% of HD patients show normal seroconversion rates after tetanus toxoid vaccination. Diphtheria vaccination results in a seroconversion rate of only 37%, and 33% of patients retain protective levels after booster administration.[22] Almost all dialysis patients may develop protective antibodies after hepatitis A vaccination is administered either intramuscularly or subcutaneously. Eighty-five percent of ESRD patients develop antibodies after administration of varicella vaccine within the first 6 months, and 76% have protective antibody titer at 1 year. However, well-designed further vaccination studies in ESRD patients are urgently needed.[22]

REFERENCES

1. Moal V, Brunet P, Dou L, et al: Impaired expression of glycoproteins on resting and stimulated platelets in uraemic patients. Nephrol Dial Transplant 2003;18:1834–1841.
2. Gawaz MP, Dobos G, Spath M, et al: Impaired function of platelet membrane glycoprotein IIb-IIIa in end-stage renal disease. J Am Soc Nephrol 1994;5:36–46.
3. Sohal AS, Gangji AS, Crowther MA, Treleaven D: Uremic bleeding: Pathophysiology and clinical risk factors. Thromb Res 2006;118:417–422.
4. Himmelfarb J, Nelson S, McMonagle E, et al. Elevated plasma glycocalicin levels and decreased ristocetin-induced platelet agglutination in hemodialysis patients. Am J Kidney Dis 1998;32:132–138.
5. Sloand JA, Sloand EM: Studies on platelet membrane glycoproteins and platelet function during hemodialysis. J Am Soc Nephrol 1997;8:799–803.
6. Noris M, Benigni A, Boccardo P, et al: Enhanced nitric oxide synthesis in uremia: Implications for platelet dysfunction and dialysis hypotension. Kidney Int 1993;44:445–450.
7. Remuzzi G, Perico N, Zoja C, et al: Role of endothelium-derived nitric oxide in the bleeding tendency of uremia. J Clin Invest 1990;86:1768–1771.
8. Boccardo P, Remuzzi G, Galbusera M: Platelet dysfunction in renal failure. Semin Thromb Hemost 2004;30:579–589.
9. Houry S, Georgeac C, Hay JM, et al: A prospective multicenter evaluation of preoperative hemostatic screening tests. The French Associations for Surgical Research. Am J Surg 1995;170:19–23.
10. Bonomini M, Sirolli V, Reale M, et al: Involvement of phosphatidylserine exposure in the recognition and phagocytosis of uremic erythrocytes. Am J Kidney Dis 2001;37:807–814.
11. Hirsh J, Raschke R: Heparin and low-molecular-weight heparin: The Seventh ACCP Conference on Antithrombotic and Thrombolytic Therapy. Chest 2004;126(Suppl 3):188S–203S.
12. Weigert AL, Schafer AI: Uremic bleeding: Pathogenesis and therapy. Am J Med Sci 1998;316:94–104.
13. Ando M, Iwata A, Ozeki Y, et al: Circulating platelet-derived microparticles with procoagulant activity may be a potential cause of thrombosis in uremic patients. Kidney Int 2002;62:1757–1763.
14. Kaufman JS, O'Connor TZ, Zhang JH, et al: Randomized controlled trial of clopidogrel plus aspirin to prevent hemodialysis access graft thrombosis. J Am Soc Nephrol 2003;14:2313–2321.
15. Goicoechea M, Caramelo C, Ochando A, et al: Antiplatelet therapy alters iron requirements in hemodialysis patients. Am J Kidney Dis 2000;36:80–87.
16. Reilly RF: The pathophysiology of immune-mediated heparin-induced thrombocytopenia. Semin Dial 2003;16:54–60.
17. Ziai F, Benesch T, Kodras K, et al: The effect of oral anticoagulation on clotting during hemodialysis. Kidney Int 2005;68:862–866.
18. Molino D, De Lucia D, Marotta R, et al: In uremia, plasma levels of anti-protein C and anti-protein S antibodies are associated with thrombosis. Kidney Int 2005;68:1223–1229.
19. Sester U, Sester M, Heine G, et al: Strong depletion of (CD14+ D16+) monocytes during haemodialysis treatment. Nephrol Dial Transplant 2001;16:1402–1408.
20. Fabrizi F, Martin P, Dixit V, et al: Meta-analysis: Effect of hepatitis C virus infection on mortality in dialysis. Aliment Pharmacol Ther 2004;20:1271–1277.
21. Liu YL, Kao MT, Huang CC: A comparison of responsiveness to hepatitis B vaccination in patients on hemodialysis and peritoneal dialysis. Vaccine 2005;23:3957–3960.
22. Dinits-Pensy M, Forrest GN, Cross AS, et al: The use of vaccines in adult patients with renal disease. Am J Kidney Dis 2005;46:997–1011.

Bone and Mineral Metabolism in Chronic Kidney Disease

Esther A. González and Kevin J. Martin

DEFINITION

Disturbances of mineral metabolism are common if not ubiquitous during the course of chronic kidney disease (CKD) and lead to serious and debilitating complications unless these abnormalities are addressed and treated. The spectrum of disorders includes abnormal concentrations of serum calcium, phosphate, and magnesium and disorders of parathyroid hormone (PTH) and vitamin D metabolism. These abnormalities, as well as other factors related to the uremic state, affect the skeleton and result in the complex disorders of bone known as *renal osteodystrophy* (ROD); it is now recommended that this term be used exclusively to define the bone pathology associated with CKD. The clinical, biochemical, and imaging abnormalities heretofore identified as correlates of renal osteodystrophy should be defined more broadly as a clinical entity or syndrome called *chronic kidney disease–mineral and bone disorder* (CKD-MBD). The spectrum of skeletal abnormalities seen in renal osteodystrophy (Fig. 74.1) includes the following:

- Osteitis fibrosa, a manifestation of hyperparathyroidism characterized by increased osteoclast and osteoblast activity and peritrabecular fibrosis
- Osteomalacia, a manifestation of defective mineralization of newly formed osteoid most often caused by aluminum deposition

- Adynamic bone disease, a condition characterized by abnormally low bone turnover
- Osteopenia or osteoporosis
- Combinations of these abnormalities termed *mixed renal osteodystrophy*
- Other abnormalities with skeletal manifestations, for example, chronic acidosis and β_2-microglobulin (β_2M) amyloidosis (see Chapter 75)

EPIDEMIOLOGY

The prevalence of the various types of renal bone disease in patients with end-stage renal disease (ESRD) is illustrated in Figure 74.2.[1] In patients on hemodialysis (HD), osteitis fibrosa and adynamic bone disease occur with almost equal frequency. In contrast, in patients on peritoneal dialysis (PD), the adynamic bone lesion predominates. Osteomalacia represents only a small fraction of cases in either group but is more common in certain ethnic groups, particularly Indo-Asians. This distribution of bony abnormalities represents considerable change from that

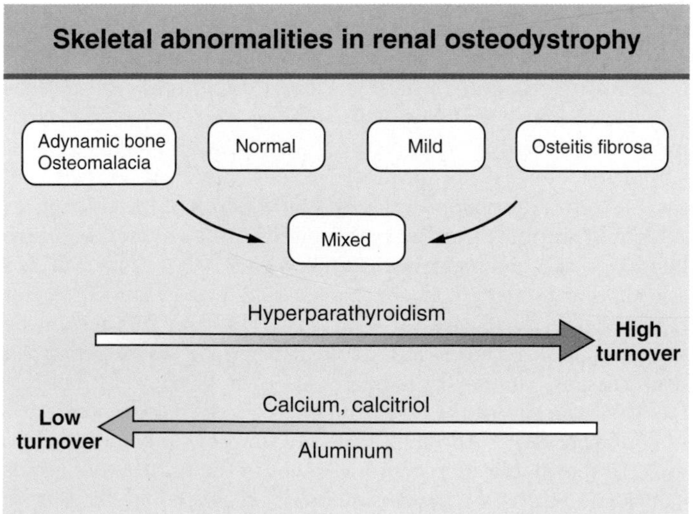

Skeletal abnormalities in renal osteodystrophy

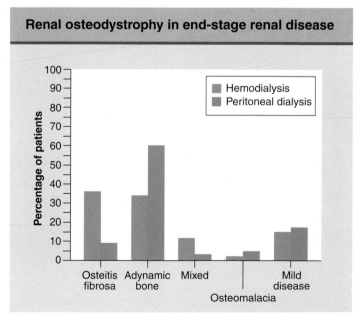

Figure 74.1 The spectrum of renal osteodystrophy. The range of skeletal abnormalities in renal bone disease encompasses syndromes with both high and low bone turnover.

Renal osteodystrophy in end-stage renal disease

Figure 74.2 Prevalence of renal osteodystrophy in patients with end-stage renal disease. The pattern of renal osteodystrophy varied with the dialysis modality in a group of patients on hemodialysis (n = 117) or peritoneal dialysis (n = 142).

identified in the late 1970s, reflecting our increased knowledge of their pathogenesis and changes in therapeutic approaches. It is important to emphasize that the abnormalities of the skeleton are not restricted to patients with ESRD, and abnormal bone histology with both increased or decreased bone turnover occurs in patients with CKD relatively early in the course of renal insufficiency.

PATHOGENESIS

Several biochemical and hormonal abnormalities that are encountered during the course of CKD contribute to renal bone disease and can be affected by prevention and therapy. The major factors that are operative in early CKD may vary as renal disease progresses. Similarly, the predominance of one particular pathogenetic mechanism over another may contribute to the heterogeneity of bone disorders.

Osteitis Fibrosa: Hyperparathyroidism

Elevated levels of PTH in blood and hyperplasia of the parathyroid glands are seen early in the course of CKD. Whereas normally the level of free (i.e., non–protein bound) calcium in blood is the principal determinant of PTH secretion, during the course of CKD, several metabolic disturbances contribute to alter the regulation of the secretion of PTH.

Abnormalities of Calcium Metabolism

There are three main body pools of calcium: the bony skeleton (mineral component), the intracellular pool (mostly protein bound), and the extracellular pool (see Chapter 10). The calcium in the extracellular pool is in continuous exchange with that of bone and cells and is altered by diet and excretion. Calcium metabolism depends on the close interaction of two hormonal systems: PTH and vitamin D. Perturbations of both of these systems occur during the course of CKD, with adverse consequences on the skeleton. Total serum calcium tends to decrease during the course of CKD, but the levels of free calcium remain within the normal range in most patients[2] (Fig. 74.3) as a result of compensatory hyperparathyroidism. A number of factors lead to hypocalcemia, including phosphate retention and decreased production of 1,25-dihydroxyvitamin D (calcitriol) from the kidney, resulting in decreased intestinal calcium absorption and skeletal resistance to the calcemic action of PTH. Because calcium is a major regulator of PTH secretion, persistent hypocalcemia is a powerful stimulus for the development of hyperparathyroidism. Persistently low levels of calcium may also contribute to parathyroid growth.

Abnormalities of Phosphate Metabolism

With progressive CKD, phosphate is retained by the kidney. However, hyperphosphatemia does not become evident until the glomerular filtration rate (GFR) has decreased to <30% of normal. Until that late stage in the course of CKD, compensatory hyperparathyroidism results in increased phosphaturia, maintaining serum phosphate levels in the normal range.

It was originally proposed that the renal retention of phosphate led to a decrease in serum free calcium, which in turn stimulated the secretion of PTH. Thus, a new steady state was achieved in which serum phosphate was restored to normal at the expense of a sustained high level of PTH. This cycle was repeated as renal function declined until sustained and severe hyperparathyroidism was present. It now appears that this is but one mechanism by which phosphate retention may lead to hyperparathyroidism (Fig. 74.4). Phosphate retention also leads to decreased production

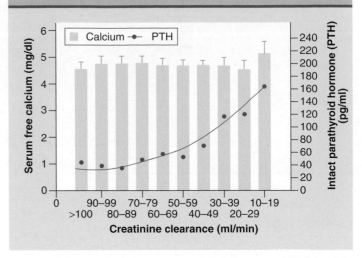

Parathyroid hormone and serum calcium levels

Figure 74.3 Ionized calcium and parathyroid hormone (PTH) levels in chronic renal failure. Levels of ionized calcium are maintained in advancing renal failure by progressive increases in PTH.

of calcitriol by the kidney, which in turn decreases intestinal calcium absorption leading to hypocalcemia, thus stimulating PTH secretion. In addition, hyperphosphatemia is associated with resistance to the actions of calcitriol in the parathyroid glands, which also favors the development of hyperparathyroidism, and also induces resistance to the actions of PTH in bone. Phosphate *per se* appears to affect PTH secretion independent of changes in serum calcium or serum calcitriol.[3,4] Phosphate may also have an effect on parathyroid growth independent of serum calcium.[5,6] Regardless of the mechanism by which phosphate retention causes hyperparathyroidism, restricting dietary phosphate in proportion to the decrease in GFR can prevent the development of hyperparathyroidism.

Abnormalities of Vitamin D Metabolism

The conversion of 25-hydroxyvitamin D to its active metabolite 1,25-dihydroxyvitamin D occurs in the kidney by the enzyme 1α-hydroxylase. The kidney is the major site of calcitriol production, and as functional renal mass decreases during the course of CKD, calcitriol production falls. Calcitriol production is also compromised in the setting of CKD by the frequently observed reductions in 25-hydroxyvitamin D levels.[7] Plasma calcitriol concentrations may be normal in patients with mild to moderate CKD; however, PTH levels are often elevated and, because PTH is a major stimulator of calcitriol production, normal levels of calcitriol may therefore be inappropriately low. Decreased production of calcitriol contributes to the pathogenesis of hyperparathyroidism by direct and indirect mechanisms (Fig. 74.5). Calcitriol has several direct effects on the parathyroid gland. Low levels of calcitriol directly release the gene for PTH from suppression by the vitamin D receptor and allow increased PTH secretion. In many tissues, vitamin D regulates its own receptor by positive feedback; the vitamin D receptor content is decreased in parathyroid tissue in CKD. Administration of calcitriol has been shown to increase the vitamin D receptor content in the parathyroid glands coincident with the suppression of PTH secretion. Studies *in vitro* have shown that calcitriol is a negative growth regulator of parathyroid cells; therefore, calcitriol deficiency in CKD may facilitate parathyroid cell proliferation. Other direct consequences

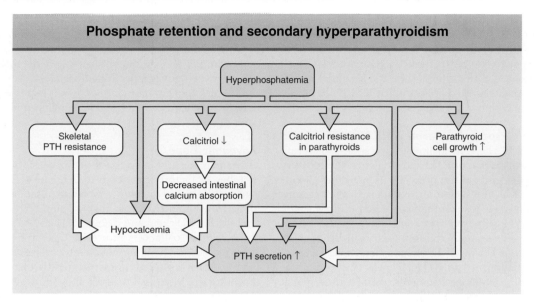

Figure 74.4 Role of phosphate retention in the pathogenesis of secondary hyperparathyroidism. Hyperphosphatemia stimulates parathyroid hormone (PTH) secretion indirectly by inducing hypocalcemia, skeletal resistance to PTH, low levels of calcitriol, and calcitriol resistance. Hyperphosphatemia also has direct effects on the parathyroid gland to increase PTH secretion and parathyroid cell growth.

of low levels of calcitriol that contribute to the pathogenesis of secondary hyperparathyroidism include increasing the parathyroid set-point for calcium-regulated PTH secretion and, possibly, decreasing levels of calcium receptors.

Low levels of calcitriol may also promote the development of hyperparathyroidism indirectly. First, decreased calcitriol production as renal function decreases can lead to progressive reductions in intestinal absorption of calcium, leading to hypocalcemia and stimulation of PTH release. Second, low levels of calcitriol have

been implicated in skeletal resistance to the calcemic actions of PTH, which may also contribute to the development of hyperparathyroidism.

Abnormalities of Parathyroid Gland Function

There are intrinsic abnormalities in parathyroid gland function in the course of CKD in addition to those caused by hypocalcemia, low levels of calcitriol, and skeletal resistance to the actions of PTH (Fig. 74.6).

Parathyroid hyperplasia is an early finding in CKD. In experimental models, hyperplasia begins within a few days following the induction of CKD. The factors responsible are unclear, but parathyroid gland hyperplasia can be prevented by dietary phosphate restriction or by the use of calcimimetic agents.[6,8] Resected parathyroids from patients with severe hyperparathyroidism have nodular areas throughout the gland, which have been shown to represent monoclonal expansions of parathyroid cells.[9] The factors involved in the genesis of these monoclonal nodules are unclear. Within these nodules, there is decreased expression of vitamin D receptors as well as calcium receptors.[10,11] In the absence of receptors for vitamin D or for calcium, efforts to regulate the secretion of these enlarged hyperplastic glands may be difficult.

The parathyroid calcium receptor is centrally involved in the regulation of PTH secretion by calcium.[12] Its expression and synthesis are decreased in parathyroid glands from hyperparathyroid subjects,[10] leading to altered calcium-regulated PTH secretion. Increased concentrations of calcium are required *in vitro* to

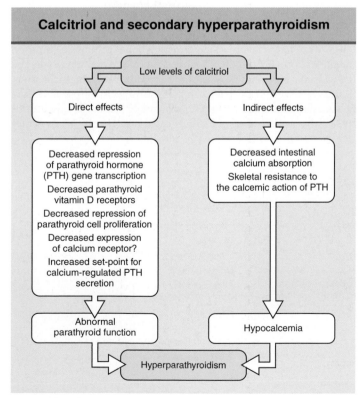

Figure 74.5 Role of low levels of calcitriol in the pathogenesis of secondary hyperparathyroidism.

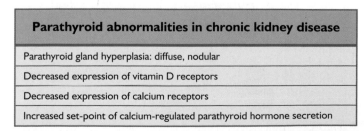

Parathyroid abnormalities in chronic kidney disease
Parathyroid gland hyperplasia: diffuse, nodular
Decreased expression of vitamin D receptors
Decreased expression of calcium receptors
Increased set-point of calcium-regulated parathyroid hormone secretion

Figure 74.6 Parathyroid abnormalities in chronic kidney disease.

suppress PTH release from the parathyroid cells of uremic patients compared with those of normal controls. Thus, the set-point for the concentration of calcium required to decrease PTH release by 50% appears to be increased. Decreased levels of calcitriol may play a role in this alteration of the set-point in that administration of calcitriol to patients with ESRD has been shown to change the set-point for PTH secretion toward normal.

Abnormal Skeletal Response to Parathyroid Hormone

In patients with CKD there is an impaired response of serum calcium to the administration of PTH and a delay in the recovery from induced hypocalcemia in the presence of larger increments in PTH levels. In CKD, the skeleton is resistant to the calcemic actions of PTH, and the resultant decrease in serum calcium levels stimulates PTH secretion and contributes to the pathogenesis of secondary hyperparathyroidism. Factors involved in the skeletal resistance to PTH in CKD include decreased levels of calcitriol, downregulation of the PTH receptor, and phosphate retention. In addition, circulating fragments of PTH, truncated at the N-terminus, which still react in the older, second-generation two-site PTH assays, may serve to oppose the calcemic actions of PTH, likely acting at a receptor for the C-terminal region of parathyroid hormone.[13]

Osteomalacia and Other Disorders of Low Bone Turnover

Because decreased levels of calcitriol are uniformly present in patients with advanced CKD, and yet osteomalacia is a relatively infrequent finding, defective mineralization of bone cannot be attributed solely to calcitriol deficiency.

Aluminum

Severe osteomalacia in patients with CKD has often been attributed to the accumulation of aluminum, which occurs mainly through the use of aluminum-containing phosphate binders. In recent years, the use of these binders has decreased markedly, and concomitantly, osteomalacia is now seen much less frequently. In addition to impairing mineralization, aluminum toxicity can decrease osteoblast proliferation as well as collagen production. Aluminum bone disease may also manifest as adynamic bone without overt osteomalacia. Although the use of aluminum-containing phosphate binders has decreased, constant vigilance is required for other sources of aluminum such as water supplies,

over-the-counter medications such as sucralfate, and other self-prescribed antacids and aluminum cookware.

In addition to osteomalacia, aluminum toxicity also induces hypochromic and microcytic anemia and causes a dementia in which myoclonus is a prominent sign.

The risk for aluminum intoxication is increased in children with CKD, in diabetic patients, and in patients co-ingesting citrate (see later discussion).

Adynamic Bone

Adynamic bone has a complex pathogenesis and likely includes a number of factors that serve to decrease PTH levels in serum, such as the use of calcium-containing phosphate binders, the use of active vitamin D sterols, high calcium dialysate for continuous ambulatory PD fluid, and diabetes[14] (Fig. 74.7). In addition, there are a number of factors in uremia that probably act directly on bone to decrease bone formation rate, such as diabetes, circulating uremic toxins, altered levels of growth factors and cytokines, malnutrition, vitamin D metabolites, downregulation of PTH-1 receptor, and possibly direct effects of C-terminal PTH fragments on bone acting at the C-terminal PTH receptor.

Clinically adynamic bone disease is associated with increased fracture risk and increased mortality. In addition, Figure 74.8 indicates a hypothetical scheme showing that when bone turn-over is abnormally low, calcium and phosphate cannot be deposited in bone. This may facilitate deposition in extraskeletal sites and contribute to vascular calcification. In support of this hypothesis, low bone turnover is associated with high arterial calcification scores in HD patients.[15]

CLINICAL MANIFESTATIONS OF RENAL OSTEODYSTROPHY

Musculoskeletal Symptoms

Clinical manifestations of hyperparathyroidism and other forms of bone disease are usually nonspecific and are often preceded by biochemical or imaging abnormalities. In patients with advanced CKD who have severe bone disease, bone pain is a common manifestation. This is often nonspecific in nature; occurs in the lower back, hips, and legs; and is aggravated by weight bearing. Acute, localized bone pain can also become manifest and may be suggestive of acute arthritis. Pain around joints may be caused by acute periarthritis, which is associated with periarticular

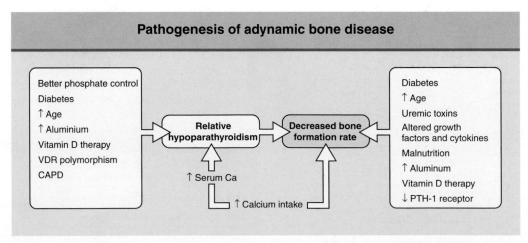

Figure 74.7 Pathogenesis of adynamic bone disease. CAPD, continuous ambulatory peritoneal dialysis; PTH, parathyroid hormone; VDR, vitamn D receptor. (Adapted from Couttenye MM, D'Haese PC, Verschoren WJ, et al: Low bone turnover in patients with renal failure. Kidney Int 1999; 56:S70–S76.)

Extraskeletal calcification in adynamic bone disease

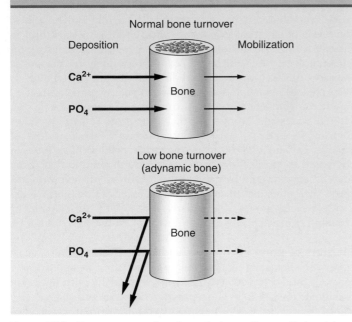

Figure 74.8 Bone turnover in adynamic bone disease. Reduced bone turnover leads to increased extraskeletal calcification.

deposition of calcium phosphate crystals, especially in patients who suffer from marked hyperphosphatemia. The symptoms may be confused clinically with gout or pseudogout and often respond to nonsteroidal anti-inflammatory drugs (NSAIDs). The gradual onset of muscle weakness is also common in patients with ESRD. Many factors are probably involved in its pathogenesis, including hyperparathyroidism and abnormalities of vitamin D. A differential diagnosis is the arthropathy associated with $\beta_2 M$ amyloidosis (see Chapter 75).

Bone deformities are common in patients with severe hyperparathyroidism, particularly in children. In adults, deformities arise as a consequence of fractures, with the axial skeleton being most commonly affected. This can lead to kyphoscoliosis or chest wall deformities. Slipped epiphysis may occur in children, and occasionally frank rachitic features are evident. Growth retardation is also common in children and, although some improvement has been shown with calcitriol, this has not been

the universal finding. The use of growth hormone may have a role in maintaining normal growth in children.

Pruritus

Another troublesome symptom in patients with advanced CKD is pruritus. As discussed in detail in Chapter 78, hyperparathyroidism can be one cause of pruritus, but parathyroidectomy should never be undertaken for pruritus alone, and only if there is also firm evidence of severe secondary hyperparathyroidism.

Metastatic Calcification and Calciphylaxis

Extraskeletal calcifications are frequently encountered in patients with advanced CKD and are aggravated by persistent elevation of the calcium-phosphate product. Most commonly, vascular calcifications are seen, but calcifications may also occur in other sites, such as the lung, myocardium, and periarticular areas (Fig. 74.9).

Calciphylaxis, or calcific uremic arteriolopathy, is discussed in detail in Chapter 78. It is a severe but uncommon form of vascular calcification, characterized by the development of painful nodules in the lower extremities, trunk, buttocks, or other areas that then become mottled or violaceous and indurated and ultimately ulcerate (see Figs. 78.6 and 78.7), leading to a high mortality rate. Calciphylaxis most commonly occurs in dialysis patients but has also been described in CKD patients who have not yet begun dialysis. Although the true prevalence is unknown, it is thought to be increasing.[16] The pathogenesis is not precisely understood, but a high calcium-phosphate product is a risk factor. The association of calciphylaxis with warfarin therapy supports the idea that an altered coagulation mechanism is present in these patients. Decreased levels of the calcification inhibitor, fetuin-A, might also be involved.[17] The principles of therapy are intense dialysis, the avoidance of calcium-containing phosphate binders, the use of low calcium dialysate, and parathyroidectomy if PTH levels are high. Newer approaches include hyperbaric oxygen, calcimimetics, and sodium thiosulfate (see Chapter 78).

DIAGNOSIS AND DIFFERENTIAL DIAGNOSIS

In addition to the clinical manifestations of renal osteodystrophy, a variety of biochemical and radiographic techniques are helpful not only to establish the specific diagnosis but also to serve as a guide for the initiation and adjustment of therapeutic

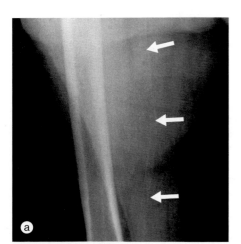
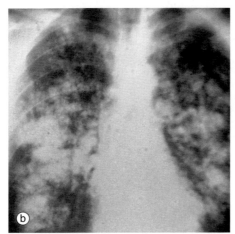
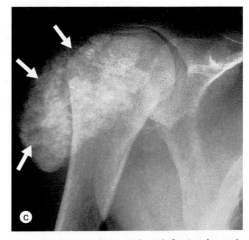

Figure 74.9 Extraskeletal calcification in chronic renal failure. *a,* Arterial calcification *(arrows). b,* Pulmonary calcification. *c,* Periarticular calcification *(arrows).*

interventions. Although bone biopsy is not widely used in clinical practice, it remains the gold standard for the diagnosis of renal osteodystrophy.

Serum Biochemistry

The levels of free calcium and phosphate in serum are usually normal in patients with mild to moderate CKD. With advanced CKD, the levels of serum calcium tend to fall; likewise, hyperphosphatemia does not become manifest until renal function has declined to <30% of normal. Hypercalcemia may occur as a result of the administration of large doses of calcium-containing antacids or the administration of vitamin D metabolites. In addition, patients with severe hyperparathyroid bone disease, as well as those with low bone turnover syndromes, have a tendency to develop hypercalcemia. It is important to differentiate between the different causes of hypercalcemia in the setting of CKD because the management will vary greatly depending on the cause. Also, the levels of serum calcium and phosphate, when used alone, are not very useful in predicting the specific type of bone disease.

Metabolic acidosis is commonly associated with CKD and contributes to osteopenia because hydrogen ions are buffered by bone carbonate, resulting in demineralization of bone.

Parathyroid Hormone

Measurements of PTH are important for diagnostic purposes and for therapeutic guidance in the management of renal osteodystrophy. With renal insufficiency, there is accumulation of circulating PTH fragments, which complicates the interpretation of PTH assays based on assessment of the midregion or the C-terminal portions of the molecule. Consequently, the preferred methods for measuring PTH have been the two-site immunoradiometric assay and immunochemiluminescence assay, which measure intact PTH (iPTH). The levels of iPTH in serum have been shown to correlate with the predominant histologic abnormality present in bone, such that elevated iPTH levels are characteristic of patients with osteitis fibrosa, whereas low levels are found in patients with low bone turnover syndromes. It is well accepted that there is an element of skeletal resistance to PTH in patients with CKD; therefore, supranormal levels of PTH are required to maintain normal bone turnover. iPTH levels two to three times normal may be appropriate for patients with advanced CKD. Serial measurements of PTH are useful in the initial evaluation of patients with renal bone disease and are essential during the management of these disorders in order to assess response to therapy and to avoid overtreatment and undertreatment because either can have detrimental effects on bone histology.

Recent refinements in PTH assays have led to the realization that these assays also measure some large fragments of PTH, which are truncated at the N-terminus and may have important biologic activity. More specific assays have been developed that exclude these fragments from measurement, which hopefully will lead to improved standardization between different PTH assays from various laboratories and various manufacturers of assay reagents,[18] and work is in progress to define the clinical utility of such more specific assays.[19,20]

Vitamin D Metabolites

Calcitriol levels remain within the normal range in patients with mild to moderate CKD because of the stimulation of 1α-hydroxylase by the high levels of PTH. With progressive decreases in renal mass and frequent decreases in the levels of 25-hydroxyvitamin D, there is impaired production of calcitriol by the failing kidney, and calcitriol levels in serum fall despite the presence of hyperparathyroidism. Although low levels of calcitriol play a very important role in the pathogenesis of secondary hyperparathyroidism, and the adynamic bone lesion has been partially attributed to overtreatment with vitamin D metabolites, the levels of calcitriol in patients with CKD are not helpful in differentiating the histologic lesions of renal osteodystrophy. Measurements of calcitriol are not used routinely for diagnostic purposes unless extrarenal production of this metabolite is suspected, as in granulomatous disorders such as sarcoidosis.

Vitamin D deficiency rarely results in osteomalacia in the United States and Europe but may contribute to hyperparathyroidism. In patients with heavy proteinuria, there is loss of vitamin D binding protein in the urine, which may result in decreased levels of 25-hydroxyvitamin D. Vitamin D deficiency may be encountered in patients with limited sun exposure, in those with intestinal malabsorption or malnutrition, and in susceptible racial groups, particularly Indo-Asians. Assessment of vitamin D nutrition is by measurement of 25-hydroxyvitamin D.

Markers of Bone Formation and Bone Resorption

Levels of circulating alkaline phosphatase offer an approximate index of osteoblast activity in patients with CKD. High levels are commonly present in hyperparathyroid bone disease, whereas low values are usually present in patients with low turnover osteodystrophy. The discriminatory power of alkaline phosphatase measurements is low. Although measurement of bone alkaline phosphatase isoenzyme is superior to that of total alkaline phosphatase, the discrimination between normal and abnormally low bone turnover remains problematic. Serial measurements of alkaline phosphatase may be useful in assessing the progression of bone disease. Osteocalcin is another marker of osteoblastic activity, but it is not superior to alkaline phosphatase for the evaluation of renal osteodystrophy. Tartrate-resistant acid phosphatase and collagen degradation products are both markers of osteoclastic activity but are not widely used in the evaluation of renal bone disease and are considered investigational at present.

Aluminum

Bone histology is the gold standard for the diagnosis of aluminum-related bone disease, demonstrating with specific stains the presence of aluminum at the mineralization front of bone. Serum aluminum levels are also useful: random serum aluminum >100 ng/ml usually indicates severe aluminum overload. However, serum aluminum levels usually reflect recent exposure, and iron status should be considered in their interpretation; in circumstances in which aluminum therapy has recently been withdrawn or iron overload is present, serum aluminum may be low despite significant tissue accumulation of aluminum. In these circumstances, liberation of aluminum from body stores by the chelator deferoxamine (desferrioxamine, DFO) may be useful. Many protocols and schedules have been described, but current recommendations state that an increase in serum aluminum of 50 mg/l (50 ng/ml) 48 hours after the administration of DFO 5 mg/kg, together with intact PTH <150 pg/ml, provides high sensitivity and specificity for aluminum overload.

Radiology of the Skeleton

Routine x-ray examination of the skeleton is relatively insensitive for the diagnosis of renal osteodystrophy, and radiographs can appear virtually normal in patients with severe histologic evidence of renal bone disease. However, subperiosteal erosions are often present in severe secondary hyperparathyroidism,

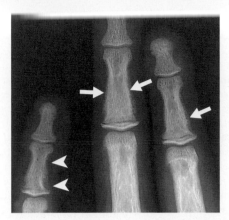

Figure 74.10 Subperiosteal erosions in hyperparathyroidism. Severe subperiosteal erosions as a manifestation of hyperparathyroidism *(arrows)*. The extensive scalloped appearance of the middle phalanx on the left *(arrowheads)* represents a small brown tumor.

detected in the hands (Fig. 74.10), clavicles, and pelvis. Skull radiographs may show focal radiolucencies and a ground-glass appearance, known as "pepper pot" skull. Osteosclerosis of the vertebrae is responsible for the "rugger-jersey" appearance of the spine (Fig. 74.11). *Brown tumors* are focal collections of giant cells that are typical of severe hyperparathyroidism and are usually seen as well-demarcated radiolucent zones in long bones, clavicles, and digits (see Fig. 74.10) and may be confused with osteolytic metastases. Looser zones or pseudofractures are characteristic of osteomalacia. The presence of β_2M amyloidosis is suggested by the presence of bone cysts and spondyloarthropathy (see Chapter 75, Fig. 75.4). Routine skeletal x-rays are not recommended.

Measurements of Bone Density

Dual-energy x-ray absorptiometry is widely used to assess bone density. However, the utility of this technique in the assessment of renal bone disease is unclear, perhaps because of the heterogeneous and complex nature of the bone histology. Other variables that may contribute to the erratic correlations of bone density measurements and bone histology in renal bone diseases

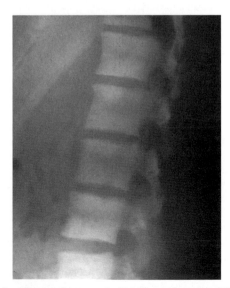

Figure 74.11 "Rugger-jersey spine" in hyperparathyroidism. Vertebral bodies show the increased density of the ground plates and central radiolucency, which gives the appearance of a rugger jersey.

include vascular and soft-tissue calcifications, age, prior therapy with corticosteroids, and limited activity secondary to chronic illness.

Bone Biopsy

Biopsy of bone and the microscopic analysis of undercalcified sections following double tetracycline labeling provide definitive and quantitative diagnosis of renal bone disease.[21] Tetracycline is administered on two occasions separated by a defined interval; the quantitation of bone mineralization rate is achieved by measuring the distance between the two fluorescent tetracycline bands. Bone biopsy is not routinely performed in clinical practice because of the invasive nature of the procedure. Biopsy is recommended for suspected osteomalacia and in patients with nondiagnostic biochemistries. At the present time, all noninvasive tests are poor at discriminating low from normal bone turnover. Although noninvasive testing is better at distinguishing normal from high bone turnover, there is considerable overlap, and therefore biopsy might be required for definitive diagnosis when biochemistries are not concordant (e.g., PTH in recommended range but bone alkaline phosphatase elevated).

Osteitis fibrosa (hyperparathyroid bone disease) is characterized by increased bone turnover, increased number and activity of osteoblasts and osteoclasts, and variable amounts of peritrabecular fibrosis (Fig. 74.12a). Osteoid may be increased but usually has a woven pattern distinct from the normal lamellar appearance. Osteomalacia is characterized by the presence of increased osteoid seam width, increase in the trabecular surface covered with osteoid, and decreased bone mineralization as assessed by tetracycline labeling (see Fig. 74.12b). The presence of aluminum can be detected on the mineralization front by specific staining (see Fig. 74.12c). Aluminum-related bone disease is defined by aluminum staining exceeding 15% of the trabecular surface and a bone formation rate <220 mm^2 per day. The adynamic bone lesion is characterized by normal or decreased osteoid volume and a reduced bone formation rate. Features of osteitis fibrosa may occur together with features of osteomalacia; the combination is termed *mixed renal osteodystrophy*.

TREATMENT

Prevention is the primary goal in the management of renal osteodystrophy. Therapy should be initiated early in the course of CKD (GFR, 50–80 ml/min) so that parathyroid gland hyperplasia can be prevented. Because renal osteodystrophy is usually asymptomatic early in the course of CKD, attention is often not paid to secondary hyperparathyroidism. By the time CKD is advanced, patients may have already developed significant skeletal abnormalities or nodular parathyroid hyperplasia, and more aggressive therapy is required to prevent the long-term consequences of renal bone disease.

Hyperparathyroid Bone Disease

Based on the multiplicity of factors involved in the pathogenesis of secondary hyperparathyroidism in CKD, the successful approach to the prevention and management of this disorder involves the integration of a variety of measures directed toward the suppression of PTH secretion and the prevention of parathyroid hyperplasia.

Prevention of Hypocalcemia

Hypocalcemia, if present, should be corrected because it is a potent stimulus for PTH secretion. In patients with hypoalbuminemia, free calcium should be measured. The initial approach

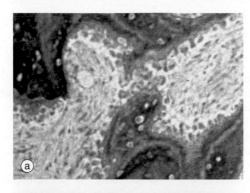

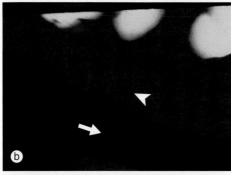

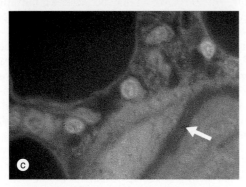

Figure 74.12   Bone histology in renal osteodystrophy. *a,* Osteitis fibrosa: characteristic manifestations of severe hyperparathyroidism with increased osteoclast and osteoblast activity and peritrabecular fibrosis. *b,* Osteomalacia: marked excess of unmineralized osteoid stained red *(arrowhead)* surrounding the mineralized bone stained black *(arrow).* *c,* Aluminum bone disease: specific red staining shows the deposition of aluminum at the mineralization front *(arrow).*

to the therapy of hypocalcemia in mild to moderate CKD is the administration of calcium supplements such as calcium carbonate, taken between meals with increasing doses as required. Assessment of vitamin D status should be undertaken by measurement of 25-hydroxyvitamin D, and this should be corrected if <30 ng/ml. Assessment of efficacy of therapy is by follow-up determinations of serum calcium and PTH. Adjunctive therapy with active vitamin D sterols should also be considered if hyperparathyroidism or hypocalcemia persists. In patients with ESRD, active vitamin D sterols are often required. The goal is to achieve levels of intact PTH of 150 to 300 pg/ml in patients on dialysis.

Control of Phosphate

Control of phosphate is the cornerstone of effective management of secondary hyperparathyroidism. In mild to moderate CKD, a normal serum phosphate does not necessarily indicate normal parathyroid status, and except for the late stages of CKD, normophosphatemia may be maintained at the expense of elevated serum PTH. Therefore, efforts to control phosphate,

including dietary phosphate restriction and the use of phosphate binders, should not be delayed until frank hyperphosphatemia develops.

Dietary Phosphate Restriction   The first step in the prevention and management of hyperparathyroidism is the restriction of dietary phosphate intake at CKD stage 2 or 3. In experimental animals with mild CKD, dietary phosphate restriction can prevent excessive PTH synthesis and secretion, as well as parathyroid cell proliferation, independent of changes in serum calcium and calcitriol concentrations. The input of a dietitian is essential for counseling and education regarding the phosphate content of various foods. Protein restriction and avoidance of dairy products are the mainstays of the regimen. In addition to reducing the rate of progression of CKD, phosphate-protein restriction has been shown to increase the serum levels of calcitriol in patients with mild to moderate CKD. Restriction of phosphate by severe dietary protein restriction should be avoided because it may lead to protein-calorie malnutrition. Restriction of the daily dietary protein intake to 0.8 g/kg should be sufficient to provide phosphate restriction without the risk for malnutrition.

Phosphate Binders   Restriction of dietary phosphate may be sufficient to prevent the development of hyperparathyroidism in early CKD. As renal function deteriorates, the control of phosphate by dietary means alone becomes difficult, and it is necessary to use agents that bind ingested phosphate in the intestinal lumen in order to limit its absorption. A variety of compounds have been used for this purpose, including aluminum hydroxide, calcium-containing antacids, magnesium salts, and in recent years, non–calcium-containing, non–aluminum-containing phosphate binders.

Aluminum-containing antacids are very effective phosphate binders, but in patients with CKD, their use can no longer be recommended because of the risk for aluminum toxicity. There are certain circumstances that limit the use of calcium-containing phosphate binders, such as hypercalcemia. In such cases, aluminum-containing antacids may be used for a short period, but the dose should be restricted to no more than 40 to 45 mg/kg per day, and frequent reassessments should be made in order to institute alternative therapy as soon as possible. Co-ingestion of aluminum-containing antacids, together with foods containing citric acid (such as fruit juices or foods with sodium, calcium, or potassium citrate) may significantly increase aluminum absorption and, therefore, should be avoided.

Calcium salts taken with meals effectively bind phosphates, limit their absorption, and have become the preferred agents for this purpose. Calcium carbonate and calcium acetate have been shown to be effective phosphate binders in 60% to 70% of patients on HD. The doses required to prevent hyperphosphatemia may vary according to the patient's compliance with dietary phosphate restriction as well as the degree of renal insufficiency, and generally range from 3 to 12 g (calcium carbonate) or 1.5 to 9 g (calcium acetate) daily. Hypercalcemia is the major potentially serious side effect related to the use of calcium carbonate. Calcium citrate potentiates aluminum uptake and should be avoided in CKD.

Magnesium salts are also effective phosphate binders for patients who become hypercalcemic on calcium-containing phosphate binders, but they should be administered with caution in patients with renal dysfunction before dialysis because hypermagnesemia may have serious adverse effects. In patients with ESRD on dialysis, magnesium carbonate (200–500 mg elemental magnesium per day) has been used successfully, with prevention of hypermagnesemia through a reduction in dialysate magnesium concentration. The use of magnesium carbonate also allows reduction of the dose of calcium carbonate required by about half, but its use is frequently complicated by diarrhea.

Because of the risks for hypercalcemia and the high calcium load of calcium-containing phosphate binders, alternative therapeutic approaches based on the use of nonabsorbable polymers have been introduced. Sevelamer hydrochloride in a dose range of 2.4 to 4.8 g daily provides effective phosphate control without hypercalcemia[22] and also produces a significant reduction in total and low-density lipoprotein cholesterol. Agents such as sevelamer may offer great advantage over calcium-containing phosphate binders, although they are significantly more expensive. At present, sevelamer should be used in patients who become hypercalcemic on calcium-containing phosphate binders and in those in whom it is desirable to limit the calcium load, until further evidence from clinical studies is available. Studies have suggested that the use of sevelamer is associated with decreased progression of vascular calcification. Sevelamer may be combined with both calcium- and magnesium-containing phosphate binders if necessary. The newer drug lanthanum carbonate is an effective phosphate binder.[23] No significant toxicity has been observed, although lanthanum appears to accumulate in bone and liver.

Use of Vitamin D Metabolites

Calcitriol and other 1α-hydroxylated vitamin D sterols, such as 1α-hydroxyvitamin D_3, 1α-hydroxyvitamin D_2, and 19-nor-1,25-dihydroxyvitamin D_2 (paricalcitol), are effective in the control of secondary hyperparathyroidism. Calcitriol lowers PTH levels and improves bone histology. In patients with very high levels of PTH and very enlarged glands that may have severe nodular hyperplasia, the effectiveness of vitamin D metabolites may be limited because the levels of vitamin D receptor are low in such tissue. Accordingly, it would appear rational to initiate treatment of secondary hyperparathyroidism with vitamin D metabolites early in the course of the disease process when the parathyroid glands are more sensitive to such therapy, and thereby prevent the progression to a refractory stage. A beneficial effect of vitamin D metabolite therapy in the treatment of secondary hyperparathyroidism in patients with mild to moderate CKD has been shown, but the concern with initiation of vitamin D therapy at this stage of CKD is acceleration of the progression of renal disease should hypercalcemia occur. Because of the effect of calcitriol to increase intestinal phosphate absorption, hyperphosphatemia and elevations in calcium phosphate product may predispose patients to the development of metastatic calcification; however, it appears that doses of 1α-hydroxyvitamin D_3 or calcitriol up to 0.5 μg/day are not commonly associated with hypercalcemia, hyperphosphatemia, or worsening renal insufficiency. Another concern with the use of vitamin D metabolites before dialysis is that oversuppression of hyperparathyroidism may increase the risk for adynamic bone. Accordingly, vitamin D therapy should be monitored carefully and should not be instituted without documentation of hyperparathyroidism, correction of 25-hydroxyvitamin D deficiency, and prior control of serum phosphate.

In patients with ESRD, indications for therapy with vitamin D metabolites are better defined; however, hypercalcemia and aggravation of hyperphosphatemia are frequent complications of therapy. Vitamin D metabolites are increasingly used as oral or intravenous pulses given intermittently (e.g., three times weekly), rather than as continuous oral therapy. There is a growing view that pulse therapy is superior to continuous therapy in the suppression of established hyperparathyroidism, although the evidence is not conclusive.

In recent years, there has been considerable interest in the development of analogues of calcitriol that have less calcemic activity than the parent compound and yet retain the ability to suppress PTH release *in vivo*. Such analogues of vitamin D studied in patients with ESRD are 22-oxacalcitriol (OCT), 1α-hydroxyvitamin D_2, and 19-nor-1α,25-dihydroxyvitamin D_2 (paricalcitol).[24-26] This last compound has been shown to decrease the levels of PTH in patients with ESRD without aggravating hypercalcemia or hyperphosphatemia. The other analogues also appear to be effective, but direct comparisons between these compounds are not available at the present time. Paricalcitol is now widely used in the United States in HD patients. It is likely that a wider therapeutic window may be offered by these analogues, which will make them the preferred treatment for hyperparathyroidism in CKD. In addition, retrospective analysis has suggested that there may be a survival advantage associated with paricalcitol compared with calcitriol.[27,28]

Role of Calcimimetic Agents

A recently introduced approach to the treatment of refractory hyperparathyroidism is use of calcimimetics, which target the calcium-sensing receptor and increase its sensitivity to calcium. The first compound in clinical use, cinacalcet, results in a significant fall in PTH levels and when administered daily can facilitate the control of hyperparathyroidism. As illustrated in Figure 74.13, the addition of cinacalcet to standard therapy in patients with iPTH serum levels exceeding 300 pg/ml while receiving standard therapy allowed significantly more dialysis patients to achieve Kidney Disease Outcomes Quality Initiative (K/DOQI) practice guideline targets for calcium, phosphate, Ca × P product, and iPTH.[29] Cinacalcet is especially useful in patients with marginal or frank hypercalcemia and can be used in conjunction with other therapies.

Role of Parathyroidectomy

Although the strategies discussed previously are effective for the control of hyperparathyroidism in many patients, there are occasions when these steps fail or are contraindicated and surgical removal of the parathyroids should be considered (Fig. 74.14). Parathyroidectomy is indicated for patients with severe hyperparathyroidism who are noncompliant with diet and phosphate binders. The presence of severe hyperphosphatemia in these patients precludes the use of vitamin D metabolites because of the risk for metastatic calcification. Some control of iPTH levels may be obtained with calcimimetics, possibly in combination with elevated dialysate calcium, once serum calcium levels decrease, but it is currently unknown whether this approach is superior to surgery, in particular in noncompliant patients. Parathyroidectomy is also indicated in advanced hyperparathyroidism that is no longer responsive to medical therapy. Some patients with severe hyperparathyroidism may become hypercalcemic in the absence of calcitriol therapy; consequently, calcitriol and calcium-containing phosphate binders cannot be administered. In this circumstance, short-term therapy with aluminum-based phosphate binders may allow vitamin D analogues to be initiated. It is important to be certain that hypercalcemia represents severe hyperparathyroidism and is not caused by adynamic bone or osteomalacia. For hypercalcemia to occur because of hyperparathyroidism in CKD, the levels of iPTH generally exceed 1000 pg/ml. Surgical parathyroidectomy might also be considered in patients with very severe

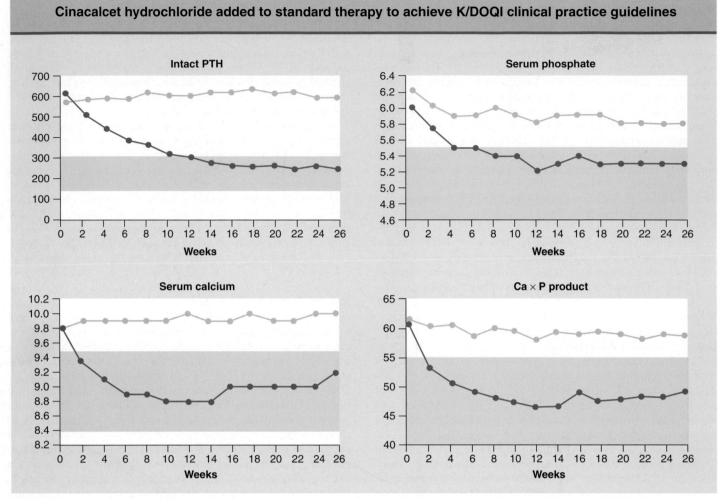

Figure 74.13 **Cinacalcet hydrochloride** *(dark blue line)* **added to standard therapy** *(light blue line)* **facilitates the achievement of the Kidney Disease Outcomes Quality Initiative (K/DOQI) clinical practice guidelines.** K/DOQI target ranges are indicated by the *shaded green* areas. PTH, parathyroid hormone. (Adapted from Moe SM, Chertow GM, Coburn JW, et al: Achieving NKF-K/DOQI bone metabolism and disease treatment goals with cinacalcet HCl. Kidney Int 2005;67:760–771.)

hyperparathyroidism who can receive a renal transplantation in the near future, particularly if they are female and have significant osteopenia. Parathyroidectomy in these cases can help to avoid post-transplantation hypercalcemia and hypophosphatemia (owing to PTH-induced phosphaturia), as well as osteopenia, and may lead to improved graft function, and possibly to less intragraft calcification. Firm guidelines have not been established for this clinical situation. Parathyroidectomy might also be considered in patients with severe hyperparathyroidism who have evidence of metastatic calcification. The development of calciphylaxis is an urgent indication for parathyroidectomy if PTH levels are elevated (see Chapter 78). Before parathyroidectomy, consideration should also be given to the possibility of coexisting aluminum accumulation, using DFO testing and bone biopsy if necessary, because this might predispose to osteomalacia after parathyroidectomy.

The choice of surgical procedure for parathyroidectomy has been controversial. The most commonly used procedures are subtotal removal of the parathyroids or total removal of the parathyroids with reimplantation of parathyroid tissue in the forearm. Recurrence of hyperparathyroidism occurs in about 10% of patients. Total parathyroidectomy alone is less commonly performed; although this is an appropriate procedure for patients remaining on dialysis, there is concern that hypoparathyroidism

after a renal transplantation may be a disadvantage of this approach. Unregulated tumor-like growth of parathyroid tissue implants has been described and may be related to the monoclonal nature of the nodular hyperplasia of severe hyperparathyroidism. Our preference is for total parathyroidectomy with forearm implant.

Recurrence of hyperparathyroidism may respond to further medical therapy, but further surgery to remove the forearm implant or further neck exploration is often necessary.

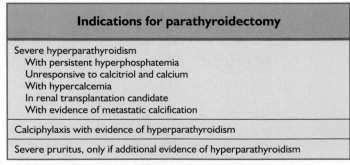

Indications for parathyroidectomy

Severe hyperparathyroidism
   With persistent hyperphosphatemia
   Unresponsive to calcitriol and calcium
   With hypercalcemia
   In renal transplantation candidate
   With evidence of metastatic calcification

Calciphylaxis with evidence of hyperparathyroidism

Severe pruritus, only if additional evidence of hyperparathyroidism

Figure 74.14 **Indications for parathyroidectomy.**

Adynamic Bone

Because therapy with vitamin D metabolites has been identified as a risk factor for adynamic bone, consideration should be given to the possibility that it represents a physiologic decrease in bone turnover as a consequence of oversuppression of PTH secretion. Aluminum should be avoided in these patients, and efforts should be made to decrease dialysate calcium in order to avoid oversuppression of PTH secretion. The use of calcium-containing phosphate binders is often problematic because of the increased frequency of hypercalcemia as a result of the altered calcium kinetics in these patients.[30] The novel phosphate binders that do not contain calcium discussed previously may potentially be beneficial in patients with the adynamic bone lesion.

Synthesis of Therapeutic Strategies

The general recommendations for the prevention and therapy of renal osteodystrophy are summarized in Figure 74.15, in which therapeutic maneuvers are stratified according to the degree of CKD.

Therapy should be initiated if possible in stage 2 or 3 CKD (GFR, 30–90 ml/min), and dietary phosphate intake should be restricted once patients enter CKD stage 3. Levels of intact PTH should be measured, and if elevated above the normal range, the levels of 25-hydroxyvitamin D should be measured and if <30 ng/ml should be corrected. If hyperparathyroidism persists, calcium-based phosphate binders, 1 to 3 g/day administered with meals, should be initiated and the dose adjusted as required to achieve control of hyperparathyroidism.

As CKD progresses to stage 3, dietary phosphate restriction should be continued or intensified, and the doses of calcium-containing phosphate binders should be adjusted based on serial measurements of iPTH, with careful attention to avoid hypercalcemia. Acidosis, if present, should be treated with oral sodium bicarbonate because persistent acidosis has deleterious effects on the skeleton. The additional sodium load may require further salt restriction or increases in diuretics. Aluminum-based phosphate binders should be avoided. If hyperparathyroidism (iPTH 100 pg/ml) persists despite these measures, consideration should be given to the addition of calcitriol (0.25–0.5 μg/day), vitamin D analogues, or vitamin D prohormones to the regimen. Such therapy should be monitored carefully to avoid hypercalcemia and acceleration of progression of renal failure.

In CKD stages 4 and 5, the preceding therapies may need to be intensified, and larger amounts of phosphate binders may be required to avoid hyperphosphatemia. The use of aluminum-containing phosphate binders is particularly undesirable at this stage in view of the increased risk for aluminum accumulation with worsening renal function. In patients on dialysis, calcitriol therapy can be intensified, with attention to the serum levels of calcium and phosphate and monitoring of iPTH levels. In CKD stage 5, iPTH levels should be maintained between 150 and 300 pg/ml to maintain normal bone turnover. Calcitriol may be administered orally either daily or intermittently (pulse therapy) or administered intravenously to patients on HD. During therapy with calcitriol, it is imperative to ensure that serum phosphate remains controlled and that elevations of serum calcium do not occur such that the calcium phosphate product is elevated to a range at which metastatic calcification is likely. The introduction of vitamin D analogues into clinical practice, which are less calcemic and phosphatemic than calcitriol and yet retain the ability to suppress the levels of PTH, may be a significant advance in our therapeutic armamentarium. The calcimimetic cinacalcet provides additional effective control of hyperparathyroidism and may be used alone or in combination with the other strategies if iPTH levels do not fall below 300 pg/ml. Parathyroidectomy needs to be considered in selected circumstances. Bone biopsy may be indicated in selected patients, particularly if aluminum

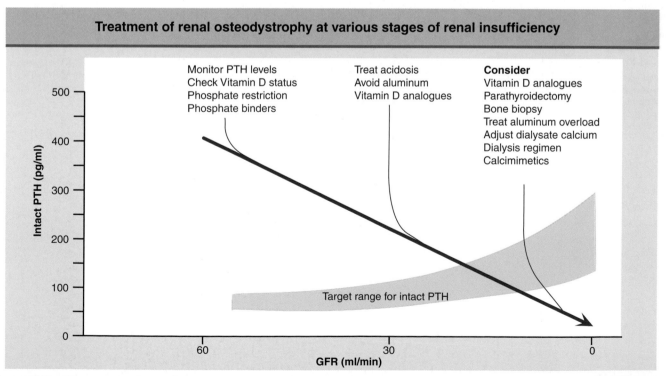

Figure 74.15 Treatment of renal osteodystrophy at various stages of renal insufficiency. GFR, glomerular filtration rate; PTH, parathyroid hormone.

overload is suspected. Aluminum overload may require chelation therapy with DFO in selected circumstances, especially if symptomatic, but in most cases, the prevention of further aluminum exposure is sufficient to allow a gradual reduction in the serum levels of aluminum. During therapy with potent vitamin D metabolites, attention should be given to the dialysate calcium concentrations because high concentrations may aggravate hypercalcemia. However, the increasingly frequent use of lower dialysate calcium levels requires careful patient monitoring to ensure compliance with calcium-containing phosphate binders and vitamin D metabolites to avoid progressive negative calcium balance. Dialysate calcium should not be taken outside the range of 1.25 to 1.75 mmol/l and, when possible, should be individually prescribed.

REFERENCES

1. Sherrard DJ, Hercz G, Pei Y, et al: The spectrum of bone disease in end-stage renal failure: An evolving disorder. Kidney Int 1993;43:436–442.
2. Martinez I, Saracho R, Montenegro J, Llach F: The importance of dietary calcium and phosphorus in the secondary hyperparathyroidism of patients with early renal failure. Am J Kidney Dis 1997;29:496–502.
3. Slatopolsky E, Finch J, Denda M, et al: Phosphorus restriction prevents parathyroid gland growth: High phosphorus directly stimulates PTH secretion in vitro. J Clin Invest 1996;97:2534–2540.
4. Almaden Y, Canalejo A, Hernandez A, et al: Direct effect of phosphorus on PTH secretion from whole rat parathyroid glands in vitro. J Bone Miner Res 1996;11:970–976.
5. Denda M, Finch J, Slatopolsky E: Phosphorus accelerates the development of parathyroid hyperplasia and secondary hyperparathyroidism in rats with renal failure. Am J Kidney Dis 1996;28:596–602.
6. Naveh-Many T, Rahamimov R, Livni N, Silver J: Parathyroid cell proliferation in normal and CKD rats: The effects of calcium, phosphate, and vitamin D. J Clin Invest 1995;96:1786–1793.
7. Gonzalez EA, Sachdeva A, Oliver DA, Martin KJ: Vitamin D insufficiency and deficiency in chronic kidney disease: A single center observational study. Am J Nephrol 2004;24:503–510.
8. Wada M, Furuya Y, Sakiyama J, et al: The calcimimetic compound NPS R-568 suppresses parathyroid cell proliferation in rats with renal insufficiency: Control of parathyroid cell growth via a calcium receptor. J Clin Invest 1997;100:2977–2983.
9. Arnold A, Brown MF, Urena P, et al: Monoclonality of parathyroid tumors in CKD and in primary parathyroid hyperplasia. J Clin Invest 1995;95:2047–2053.
10. Gogusev J, Duchambon P, Hory B, et al: Depressed expression of calcium receptor in parathyroid gland tissue of patients with hyperparathyroidism. Kidney Int 1997;51:328–336.
11. Fukuda N, Tanaka H, Tominaga Y, et al: Decreased 1,25-dihydroxyvitamin D_3 receptor density is associated with a more severe form of parathyroid hyperplasia in chronic uremic patients. J Clin Invest 1993; 92:1436–1443.
12. Brown EM, Gamba G, Riccardi D, et al: Cloning and characterization of an extracellular (Ca^{2+} sensing) receptor from bovine parathyroid. Nature 1993;366:575–580.
13. Slatopolsky E, Finch J, Clay P, et al: A novel mechanism for skeletal resistance in uremia. Kidney Int 2000;58:753–761.
14. Couttenye MM, D'Haese PC, Verschoren WJ, et al: Low bone turnover in patients with renal failure. Kidney Int 1999;56:S70–S76.
15. London GM, Marty C, Marchais SJ, et al: Arterial calcifications and bone histomorphometry in end-stage renal disease. J Am Soc Nephrol 2004;15:1943–1951.
16. Mazhar AR, Johnson RJ, Gillen D, et al: Risk factors and mortality associated with calciphylaxis in end-stage renal disease. Kidney Int 2001;60:324–332.
17. Ketteler M: Fetuin-A and extraosseous calcification in uremia. Curr Opin Nephrol Hypertens 2005;14:337–342.
18. Martin KJ, Akhtar I, Gonzalez EA: Parathyroid hormone: New assays, new receptors. Semin Nephrol 2004;24:3–9.
19. Monier-Faugere MC, Geng Z, Mawad H, et al: Improved assessment of bone turnover by the PTH-(1-84)/large C-PTH fragments ratio in ESRD patients. Kidney Int 2001;60:1460–1468.
20. Coen G, Bonucci E, Ballanti P, et al: PTH 1–84 and PTH "7–84" in the noninvasive diagnosis of renal bone disease. Am J Kidney Dis 2002;40: 348–354.
21. Malluche H, Monier-Faugere M: The role of bone biopsy in the management of patients with renal osteodystrophy. J Am Soc Nephrol 1994;4: 1631–1642.
22. Chertow GM, Burke SK, Lazarus JM, et al: Poly(allylamine hydrochloride) (RenaGel): A noncalcemic phosphate binder for the treatment of hyperphosphatemia in CKD. Am J Kidney Dis 1997;29:66–71.
23. Hutchison AJ: Calcitriol, lanthanum carbonate, and other new phosphate binders in the management of renal osteodystrophy. Perit Dial Int 1999;19(Suppl 2):S408–412.
24. Martin K, González E, Gellens M, et al: 19-Nor-1a-25-dihydroxyvitamin D_2 (paricalcitol) safely and effectively reduces the levels of intact PTH in patients on hemodialysis. J Am Soc Nephrol 1998;9:1427–1432.
25. Tan AU Jr, Levine BS, Mazess RB, et al: Effective suppression of parathyroid hormone by 1 alpha-hydroxy-vitamin D_2 in hemodialysis patients with moderate to severe secondary hyperparathyroidism. Kidney Int 1997;51:317–23.
26. Kurokawa K, Akizawa T, Suzuki M, et al: Effect of 22-oxacalcitriol on hyperparathyroidism of dialysis patients: Results of a preliminary study. Nephrol Dial Transplant 1996;11:121–124.
27. Teng M, Wolf M, Lowrie E, et al: Survival of patients undergoing hemodialysis with paricalcitol or calcitriol therapy. N Engl J Med 2003; 349:446–456.
28. Teng M, Wolf M, Ofsthun MN, et al: Activated injectable vitamin D and hemodialysis survival: A historical cohort study. J Am Soc Nephrol 2005;16:1115–1122.
29. Moe SM, Chertow GM, Coburn JW, et al: Achieving NKF-K/DOQI bone metabolism and disease treatment goals with cinacalcet HCl. Kidney Int 2005;67:760–771.
30. Kurz P, Monier-Faugere MC, Bognar B, et al: Evidence for abnormal calcium homeostasis in patients with adynamic bone disease. Kidney Int 1994;46:855–861.

75 β₂-Microglobulin–derived Amyloid

Jürgen Floege

INTRODUCTION AND DEFINITIONS

By identifying β$_2$-microglobulin (β$_2$M) as the specific amyloid precursor protein in 1985, a novel type of amyloidosis was described in patients undergoing hemodialysis.[1] It is exclusively seen in patients with chronic uremia. It can develop in patients on any type of renal replacement therapy (patients with functioning renal transplants are exceptions) and even in uremic, predialysis patients. Therefore, the amyloidosis should be referred to as β$_2$M-derived amyloid or Aβ$_2$M-amyloid rather than "dialysis amyloid" or "dialysis-associated amyloidosis." It is a systemic type of amyloidosis, but its clinical manifestations are largely confined to the musculoskeletal system. In recent years, the disease has become notably infrequent.

PATHOGENESIS

The Constituents of Aβ₂M-Amyloid Fibrils

Fibrils of Aβ$_2$M-amyloid are derived to a large extent from the circulating precursor protein β$_2$M. Other molecules that are associated with the Aβ$_2$M-amyloid fibrils include amyloid-P component, proteoglycans, antiproteases (α$_2$-macroglobulin, α$_1$-proteinase inhibitor, α$_1$-antichymotrypsin, antithrombin III, and tissue inhibitors of metalloproteinase) as well as immunoglobulin light chains.[2]

β$_2$M, an 11.8-kd protein, forms the nonvariable light chain of the human leukocyte antigen (HLA) class I complex on the surface of nearly all nucleated cells. The molecule exhibits stretches of β-pleated tertiary conformation, a prerequisite for amyloidogenesis. A 7-residue segment is of particular importance to convert β$_2$M to the amyloid state.[3]

Amyloid-P component, derived from serum amyloid-P component (SAP), is a ubiquitous constituent of nearly all types of amyloid, and may render the amyloid fibrils resistant to proteolytic degradation *in vivo*.

Pathogenetic Events in Aβ₂M-Amyloidosis

The pathogenesis of Aβ$_2$M-amyloidosis appears to involve three crucial events: (1) an increased body burden of β$_2$M, largely due to renal retention, because the amyloidosis is never observed in nonuremic subjects; (2) modifications of the β$_2$M molecule that render it more amyloidogenic; and (3) local factors that contribute to and determine the particular spatial localization of the amyloidosis.

Increased Body Burden of β₂-Microglobulin

The daily β$_2$M synthesis rate in healthy and uremic individuals ranges from 2 to 4 mg/kg. Whereas normal plasma concentrations vary between 1 and 3 mg/ml, retention occurs in renal failure, and plasma levels can be elevated as much as 60-fold in dialysis patients owing to the prolonged plasma half-life of the protein.[2] However, in dialysis patients, β$_2$M serum levels do not correlate with extent of clinical amyloid deposits, and local β$_2$M concentrations (e.g., in synovial fluid) are not increased above the serum concentration. This argues strongly against a pure "precipitation" underlying amyloid formation. Also, whereas amyloid fibrils can be generated from purified β$_2$M *in vitro*, in most studies, nonphysiologic conditions were necessary for this.[2] However, others have shown that even though first fibril stages are unstable and require stabilizing factors to remain at neutral pH, they can adapt to a neutral pH with repeated self-seeding of β$_2$M to slowly form stable fibrils.[4] Copper, derived from dialysate or dialysis membranes such as cuprophane, may promote fiber formation at physiologic conditions.[5]

Modifications of β₂-Microglobulin

Modifications of the β$_2$M molecule might facilitate its deposition in amyloid fibrils. For example, conformational intermediates with partial folding of β$_2$M can be detected.[6] More importantly, some investigators have detected a partial breakdown of native β$_2$M.[2,7] Such limited proteolysis contributes to the pathogenesis of other types of amyloid as well. Finally, different sugar-protein cross-links have been detected within Aβ$_2$M-amyloid fibrils and presumably result from oxidative or carbonyl stress in chronic dialysis patients.[8,9] Possibly, advanced glycation end product (AGE) modifications render β$_2$M more amyloidogenic or enhance the persistence of established fibrils in tissue. An unexplained finding is that radiologic signs of Aβ$_2$M-amyloid occur with similar frequency in both diabetic and nondiabetic dialysis patients, although diabetic patients have markedly higher circulating AGE levels.[2]

Local Factors

Additional local factors, perhaps proteoglycans, may facilitate amyloid formation at specific sites. Hyaluran, heparan sulfate, and chondroitin sulfate proteoglycans have been detected in or around Aβ$_2$M-amyloid fibrils. The presence of such matrix compounds, in particular heparan sulfate proteoglycans, may be related to the onset of amyloidosis.[10] Local inflammatory reactions, for example, within synovial tissue, appear to be the consequence of Aβ$_2$M-amyloid deposition. For example, *in vitro*, AGE-modified β$_2$M may initiate inflammatory reactions by activating monocytes and delaying their apoptosis.[8,9] Such inflammatory responses likely contribute to the clinical manifestation of the amyloidosis.[2,11,12]

EPIDEMIOLOGY

In rare cases, Aβ$_2$M-amyloid deposits may be detected histologically in predialysis patients.[2,8] Deposition precedes clinical manifestations by several years. Most amyloid deposits never appear to cause clinical problems, which suggests that clinical assessment markedly underestimates the prevalence of Aβ₂M-amyloidosis.[13] In histologic studies from the 1990s, the prevalence of the amyloid was already high after 2 years of chronic hemodialysis and increased to 100% in patients treated for more than 13 years.[13] Sternoclavicular joints and hips showed the highest proportion of positive samples.[2]

Both clinically and radiologically, Aβ₂M-amyloid–related symptoms rarely occur until therapy has continued for 5 years. After this time, there is an almost linear increase in the incidence, which in past evaluations reached nearly 100% after 15 years of treatment.[2,8,14] However, as described at the end of this chapter, Aβ₂M-amyloid–related symptoms have become notably rare in today's chronic dialysis populations.

Risk Factors

Main risk factors for Aβ₂M-amyloid deposition are age at onset of renal replacement therapy and the duration of (nontransplant) renal replacement therapy.[13-15] No cases of Aβ₂M-amyloidosis have yet been described in the pediatric dialysis population. Other described risk factors such as hyperparathyroidism and extraosseous calcifications, as well as iron overload, are uncertain and may be independent events also related to the duration of renal replacement therapy.

CLINICAL MANIFESTATIONS AND DIAGNOSIS

Clinical manifestations of Aβ₂M-amyloid deposition are largely confined to osteoarticular sites, in particular synovial membranes, whereas visceral manifestations are rare.[2,8] Some suggestive findings but no pathognomonic clinical or radiologic findings exist in Aβ₂M-amyloidosis.[2,11]

Carpal Tunnel Syndrome

Carpal tunnel syndrome is a characteristic, although not pathognomonic, clinical sign of Aβ₂M-amyloidosis. The pain typically worsens at night and during hemodialysis. Especially when it manifests within the first 5 years of dialysis, other reasons for the carpal tunnel syndrome, such as diabetes, heart disease, or multiple myeloma, should be considered.

Carpal tunnel syndrome induced by Aβ₂M-amyloid is often bilateral. Despite temporary relief by local measures (e.g., steroid injection) or nonsteroidal anti-inflammatory drugs (NSAIDs), it is usually progressive and requires surgical release of the transverse ligament, synovectomy of the tendon sheaths, or both. Postoperative recurrence of the carpal tunnel syndrome may be observed.

Osteoarthropathy of Peripheral Joints

Osteoarthropathy of peripheral joints is another frequent manifestation of Aβ₂M-amyloidosis and results from local amyloid deposition in periarticular bone and the synovial capsule (Fig. 75.1). It is characterized by recurrent or persistent arthralgias, stiffness of large and medium-sized joints, and swelling of capsules and adjacent tendons. Further symptoms include recurrent joint effusions and synovitis, often in the shoulders and knees, but also in the hips, wrists, elbows, acromioclavicular joints, and feet. The clinical presentation may vary from frank, acute arthritis to slow, progressive destruction of the affected joints.

In the differential diagnosis, it should be remembered that as many as 95% of patients receiving long-term hemodialysis complain of shoulder pain. Apart from Aβ₂M-amyloid deposits, this may be caused by nonamyloid-induced bursitis or tendinitis,

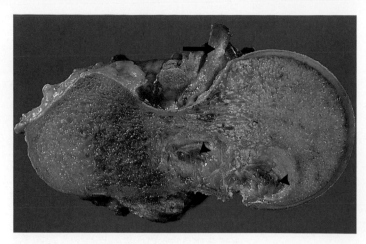

Figure 75.1   Aβ₂M-amyloid deposition in the femoral head. Postmortem specimen from a long-term hemodialysis patient. Two large lesions (*arrowheads*), partly filled with grayish amyloid and partly cystic, are noted in the femoral head. Also note the marked thickening of the synovial capsule due to amyloid deposition (*arrow*).

hydroxyapatite crystal deposition, tears in the rotator cuff, cervical radiculopathy, or septic arthritis.

Spondylarthropathy and Other Vertebral Column Involvement

Several forms of destructive spondylarthropathy are associated with long-term hemodialysis.[16] In one form, cystic bone radiolucencies dominate the picture. A second form is more destructive, with bone fragmentation and soft-tissue involvement. A third form may present with erosions and destructive changes of the intervertebral disk (Fig. 75.2). Destructive spondylarthropathy has also been noted in uremic patients before the onset of hemodialysis as well as in patients treated with peritoneal dialysis.

Destructive spondylarthropathy in patients on long-term hemodialysis was originally attributed to the deposition of hydroxyapatite crystals but is also associated with hyperparathyroidism or Aβ₂M-amyloid deposition. Deposits have been demonstrated in intervertebral disks, apophysial joints, and ligaments.

Clinical symptoms related to vertebral column involvement in the course of Aβ₂M-amyloidosis may range from asymptomatic deposits to radiculopathy, stiffness, "mechanical ache," and, finally, medullary compression with resulting paraplegia or cauda equina syndrome.[2,8] Cauda equina syndrome may result in low back pain, unilateral or usually bilateral sciatica, saddle sensory disturbances, bladder and bowel dysfunction, and variable lower extremity motor and sensory loss. Surgical decompression is controversial, as is its timing, with immediate, early, and late surgical decompression showing varying results.

Other Musculoskeletal Symptoms

In addition to carpal tunnel syndrome, various other manifestations of Aβ₂M-amyloidosis may affect the hands of patients on long-term dialysis, causing severe functional deficiencies. Camptodactyly (a flexion deformity resulting in bent fingers that cannot completely extend or straighten) can be caused by Aβ₂M-amyloid deposits along the flexor tendons of the hands and may result in prominence of the tendons upon extension ("guitar-string sign"; Fig. 75.3). Patients undergoing dialysis can also have subcutaneous tumorous deposits of Aβ₂M-amyloid; however, diffuse infiltration of the subcutaneous fat or skin has not been observed.

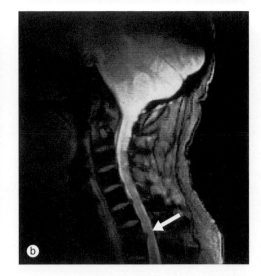

Figure 75.2 Aβ₂M-amyloidosis–associated spondylarthropathy. *a,* Destruction of an intervertebral disk *(arrow)* in the neck vertebrae of a long-term hemodialysis patient. *b,* Magnetic resonance image of the same patient as in *a.* Note destruction of the intervertebral space and protrusion of material into the spinal canal *(arrow).*

Systemic Organ Manifestations of Aβ₂M-Amyloidosis

Clinically relevant involvement of other organs with Aβ₂M-amyloidosis is rare, with most organ deposits of Aβ₂M-amyloid only showing asymptomatic microscopic foci. In cases with systemic involvement, the amyloid has been found in the walls of small blood vessels of the gastrointestinal tract, lung, heart, liver, tongue, endocrine organs, brain, and testes, as well as in the parathyroid glands.[2,8] Case reports of clinically relevant organ manifestations are almost exclusively confined to patients treated with hemodialysis for more than 15 years and have described heart failure, odynophagia, intestinal perforation of both small and large bowel, gastrointestinal bleeding and pseudo-obstruction, gastric dilation, paralytic ileus, persistent diarrhea, macroglossia or functional tongue disturbances (abnormal taste, mobility, articulation), ureteral stenosis, and renal calculi.[2,8]

Pathology

Aβ₂M-amyloidosis exhibits the typical pathology of all amyloidoses, with Congo red staining showing green dichroism under

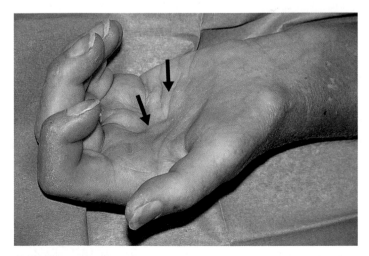

75.3 Hand involvement in Aβ₂M-amyloidosis. Hand of a long-term hemodialysis patient showing maximal extension. Note the prominence of shrunken flexor tendons *(arrows).* This is also known as the "guitar string sign."

polarized light. By immunohistochemistry, β₂M can be demonstrated within deposits, and electron microscopy reveals typical 8- to 10-nm wide fibrils.

Diagnosis

Plasma levels of β₂M are always elevated in uremia (see earlier discussion) and do not distinguish between patients with the amyloidosis and those without.

Ultrasonography is a noninvasive albeit nonspecific means of detecting synovial Aβ₂M-amyloid deposits. Thickening of the joint capsules of the hip and knee, biceps tendons, and rotator cuffs, as well as the presence of echogenic structures between muscle groups and joint effusions, have been observed in patients on long-term hemodialysis.[8]

Radiologically, affected joints may present with single or multiple juxta-articular, cystic bone radiolucencies, which are located preferentially at the insertion sites of capsules and tendons. These cystic bone radiolucencies arise from amyloid deposition in bone and are not cysts in the true sense of the word (Figs. 75.4; see also Fig. 75.1). Bone defects of this kind are prone to pathologic fractures, in particular if located in areas such as the femoral neck. However, cystic bone radiolucencies in patients undergoing chronic dialysis are not diagnostic of Aβ₂M-amyloid deposition because single, small bone cysts may be observed in 30% of nonuremic patients. Another important differential diagnosis in uremic patients is the brown tumor of secondary hyperparathyroidism. Diagnostic criteria have been developed for Aβ₂M-amyloid–induced cystic bone radiolucencies[15] (Fig. 75.5).

Computed tomography (CT) and magnetic resonance imaging (MRI) also have been used to search for evidence of Aβ₂M-amyloidosis. However, unless very strict diagnostic criteria are fulfilled, these methods are nonspecific, as is conventional scintigraphic bone scanning.[2]

Two scintigraphic methods, employing either radiolabeled SAP[2] or β₂M,[14] offer more specific detection of amyloid deposits. In long-term hemodialysis patients, intravenous injection of radiolabeled ^{123}I SAP can lead to accumulation of tracer in the wrists, knees, and shoulders. Local deposition of tracer in the hip region is rare. Splenic tracer uptake in 30% of patients was interpreted as indicating splenic amyloidosis, a conclusion not

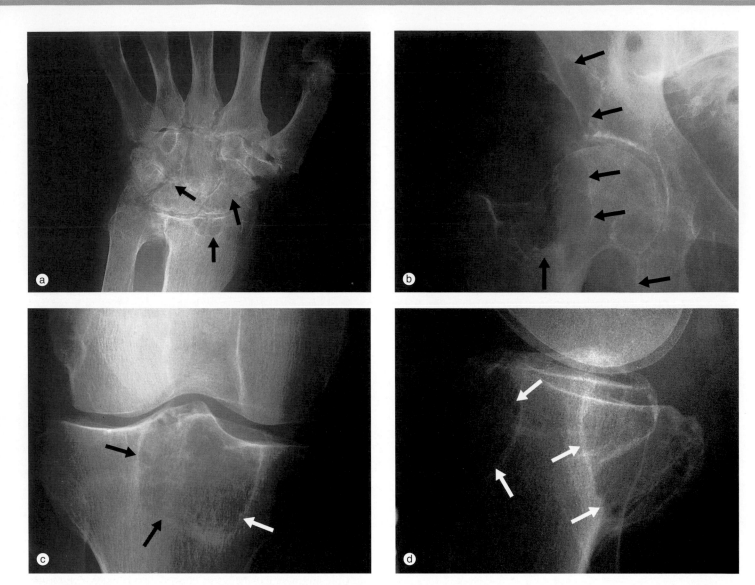

Figure 75.4   Peripheral bone "cystic" radiolucencies in Aβ₂M-amyloidosis. Radiographic findings in a long-term hemodialysis patient. *a*, Multiple cystic lesions *(arrows)* are present in the hand bones. *b*, Large cysts *(arrows)* in the neck of the femur and adjacent pelvic bones. *c* and *d*, Anterior and lateral view of the head of the tibia with two very large cystic lesions *(arrows)* resulting in posterior bulging of the tibial plateau.

Radiologic diagnostic criteria for Aβ2M-amyloidosis–associated cystic bone lesions
Diameter of lesions >5 mm in wrists and >10 mm in shoulders and hips
Normal joint space adjacent to the bone defect
Exclusion of small subchondral cysts located in the immediate weight-bearing area of the joint
Exclusion of defects of the synovial inclusion type
Increase of defect diameter >30% per year
Presence of defects in at least two joints

Figure 75.5   Radiologic diagnostic criteria for Aβ₂M-amyloidosis–associated cystic bone lesions. (From van Ypersele de Strihou C, Jadoul M, et al: Effect of dialysis membrane and patient's age on signs of dialysis-related amyloidosis. The Working Party on Dialysis Amyloidosis. Kidney Int 1991;39: 1012–1019.)

substantiated by histologic findings.[17] Therefore, although there is evidence that ^{123}I SAP can accumulate in Aβ₂M-amyloid deposits, there are, at present, uncertainties about both the specificity and sensitivity of this scan in hemodialysis patients.

Alternatively, scintigraphy with ^{131}I-labeled, or better, ^{111}In-labeled human recombinant β₂M has been used.[17] Local tracer accumulations in patients on hemodialysis correlate well with clinical, radiologic, and histologic findings. The scan has a good specificity, and its sensitivity exceeds markedly that of combined clinical and radiologic examination. However, in view of the present infrequency of Aβ₂M-amyloidosis, this scan has not been exploited commercially so far.

From a practical point of view, clinical symptoms plus ultrasound or conventional radiologic features can usually allow a tentative diagnosis of Aβ₂M-amyloidosis, and neither CT, MRI, nor conventional scintigraphy is routinely required. Unless specific amyloid scans (see earlier discussion) are available, a definitive diagnosis of Aβ₂M-amyloidosis has to rely on histology. Fat aspiration and rectal biopsy are not helpful in Aβ₂M-amyloidosis, and diagnostic material usually has to be obtained from synovial membranes or bone lesions.[2] Detritus in synovial fluid may also be used for diagnosis. In joints, amyloid deposits can be detected in articular cartilage, tendons, synovial membrane, and subchondral bone.[11]

NATURAL HISTORY

So long as patients are maintained on dialysis and have not yet received a renal transplant, the natural history of clinically manifest Aβ₂M-amyloidosis is usually one of slow but relentless progression. The prevalence after 15 years of chronic hemodialysis was almost 100% in past studies. No spontaneous remissions of clinical or radiologic findings have been described, and at best, the inflammation accompanying, for example, synovial amyloid deposits may vary in intensity.

TREATMENT AND PREVENTION

Recommendations for prevention and treatment of Aβ₂M-amyloidosis are summarized in Fig. 75.6.

Treatment
Therapy of established Aβ₂M-amyloidosis is symptomatic. NSAIDs, physical and surgical measures such as carpal tunnel decompression, endoscopic coraco-acromial ligament release, and bone stabilization in areas of cystic destruction are all used.[2,18] Preliminary data suggest that prednisone (0.1 mg/kg daily) is efficient in relieving symptoms of Aβ₂M-amyloid–associated arthropathy in uremic patients who have not undergone renal transplantation.[19] However, no follow-up data have been reported so far. Whether treating a systemic inflammatory response (e.g., with anti–tumor necrosis factor-α treatment) or subclinical infection affects the amyloidosis is unknown.

Although some dialysis modalities allow for significant β₂M removal, there is at present no convincing evidence that such a change is of therapeutic value in an established Aβ₂M-amyloidosis. However, a hemoperfusion column that absorbed β₂M relieved joint pain and stiffness, allowed for increased daily activities, and arrested progression of osteoarticular lesions.[20]

Renal transplantation is the preferred treatment because it halts further progress of the disease, but it is controversial whether this can actually lead to regression of established Aβ₂M-amyloid deposits. Renal transplantation also leads to rapid symptomatic improvement, which is probably related to the use of steroids and immunosuppressive drugs.

Prevention
A number of strategies exist for preventing the clinical manifestations of Aβ₂M-amyloidosis.[2,8,21]

Increase of β₂M Removal
Given that Aβ₂M-amyloidosis is limited to patients with severe renal insufficiency, the crucial question is whether it is possible to counteract the renal retention of β₂M in patients undergoing dialysis by an appropriate choice of renal replacement therapy. Some of the findings on nontransplantation treatment modes are summarized as follows[2]:

- Low-flux hemodialyzers with regenerated cellulosic membranes are impermeable to β₂M.
- High-flux membranes allow substantial removal of β₂M during hemodialysis through convective mass transport and adsorption. However, mass transfer is significantly lower for glycated β₂M.[22]
- Removal can be enhanced by hemodiafiltration and hemofiltration. However, currently available (nontransplantation) treatment options, even six nocturnal hemodialysis treatments per week, will not achieve normal β₂M plasma levels.[23]
- Adsorbent columns in the hemodialysis circuit have been used to increase β₂M removal. Concerns about the relative nonspecificity of β₂M adsorption, and particularly cost, have so far prevented wider use of these columns.
- Plasma levels in patients undergoing continuous ambulatory peritoneal dialysis are about 20% to 30% lower than those of patients on cuprophane hemodialysis, but there is no difference in the prevalence of Aβ₂M-amyloidosis in these two groups.[24]

Choice of Dialyzer Membranes
Available data on the clinical signs of Aβ₂M-amyloid in patients treated with cuprophane dialyzers versus high-flux hemodialyzers are inconsistent.[2] Nevertheless, three large studies suggest that high-flux dialysis or diafiltration may exert a beneficial effect on the signs of Aβ₂M-amyloidosis; there is a positive effect of long-term treatment with acrylonitrile hemodialyzers on some (bone cystic lesions) though not all (carpal tunnel syndrome)[15] Aβ₂M-amyloidosis–associated symptoms. In registry data, the risk for carpal tunnel syndrome was reduced by 40% to 50% in patients treated with high-flux hemodiafiltration[25,26] and was minimal in patients receiving on-line hemodiafiltration.[26]

Dialysate-related Factors
Three studies suggest that dialysate factors may play a central role in the clinical manifestation of Aβ₂M-amyloidosis. A dramatic reduction in the prevalence of carpal tunnel syndrome occurred in patients dialyzed with ultrapure dialysate,[27] perhaps suggesting that endotoxin or other bacterial products accelerate the clinical manifestation of the amyloidosis. In another study, an 80%

Recommendations for the prevention and management of Aβ₂M-amyloidosis
Recommendations for Prevention
Ignore the issue of Aβ₂M-amyloidosis in all patients whose life expectancy on dialysis is <5 years (i.e., the time when clinical manifestations first appear).
In all other patients, attempt renal transplantation whenever possible.
On hemodialysis, use bicarbonate-buffered dialysate and minimize microbiologic dialysate contamination.
Use high-flux hemodialysis or hemodiafiltration in those at high risk for Aβ₂M-amyloidosis (i.e., the elderly and all patients, independent of age, who have little chance of receiving a renal transplant).
Recommendations for Treatment of Symptomatic Aβ₂M-Amyloidosis
Initiate symptomatic, usually orthopedic, measures depending on musculoskeletal site and symptoms of amyloid deposits.
Attempt renal transplantation as soon as possible.
If renal transplantation is not a short-term option, consider change to hemodialysis, or preferably hemodiafiltration, using high-flux synthetic membranes and microbiologically clean dialysate (addition of adsorbent columns may also be considered, although their efficacy is less well established) to at least retard further progress.
If severe, disabling symptoms persist despite the above measures, initiate prednisone therapy at 0.1 mg/kg body weight per day.

Figure 75.6   Recommendations for the prevention and management of Aβ₂M-amyloidosis.

reduction of amyloid signs in a chronic hemodialysis population appeared to relate to dialysate factors such as microbiologic purity or the use of bicarbonate buffer.[28] Finally, in hemodialysis patients treated with a tank dialysis system, which uses essentially pyrogen-free dialysate, the prevalence of carpal tunnel syndrome compared favorably with that in various other reports.[29]

Renal Transplantation

Restoration of renal function by successful renal transplantation is the preventive measure of choice because the amyloidosis does not occur in the presence of good renal function and a successful kidney transplantation leads within days to normalization of β₂M plasma levels.

REFERENCES

1. Gejyo F, Yamada T, Odani S, et al: A new form of amyloid protein associated with chronic hemodialysis was identified as beta 2-microglobulin. Biochem Biophys Res Commun 1985;129:701–706.
2. Floege J, Ketteler M: beta2-Microglobulin-derived amyloidosis: An update. Kidney Int Suppl 2001;78:S164–171.
3. Ivanova MI, Sawaya MR, Gingery M, et al: An amyloid-forming segment of beta2-microglobulin suggests a molecular model for the fibril. Proc Natl Acad Sci USA 2004;101:10584–10589.
4. Kihara M, Chatani E, Sakai M, et al: Seeding-dependent maturation of beta2-microglobulin amyloid fibrils at neutral pH. J Biol Chem 2005;280:12012–12018.
5. Morgan CJ, Gelfand M, Atreya C, Miranker AD: Kidney dialysis-associated amyloidosis: A molecular role for copper in fiber formation. J Mol Biol 2001;309:339–345.
6. Chiti F, De Lorenzi E, Grossi S, et al: A partially structured species of beta 2-microglobulin is significantly populated under physiological conditions and involved in fibrillogenesis. J Biol Chem 2001;276:46714–46721.
7. Heegaard NH, Jorgensen TJ, Rozlosnik N, et al: Unfolding, aggregation, and seeded amyloid formation of lysine-58-cleaved beta 2-microglobulin. Biochemistry 2005;44:4397–4407.
8. Miyata T, Jadoul M, Kurokawa K, et al: Beta-2 microglobulin in renal disease. J Am Soc Nephrol 1998;9:1723–1735.
9. Nangaku M, Miyata T, Kurokawa K: Pathogenesis and management of dialysis-related amyloid bone disease. Am J Med Sci 1999;317:410–415.
10. Yamamoto S, Yamaguchi I, Hasegawa K, et al: Glycosaminoglycans enhance the trifluoroethanol-induced extension of beta 2-microglobulin-related amyloid fibrils at a neutral pH. J Am Soc Nephrol 2004;15:126–133.
11. Jadoul M, Garbar C, van Ypersele de Strihou C: Pathological aspects of (beta2microglobulin) amyloidosis. Semin Dial 2001;14:86–89.
12. Garcia-Garcia M, Argiles A, Gouin-Charnet A, et al: Impaired lysosomal processing of beta2-microglobulin by infiltrating macrophages in dialysis amyloidosis. Kidney Int 1999;55:899–906.
13. Jadoul M, Garbar C, Noel H, et al: Histological prevalence of beta 2-microglobulin amyloidosis in hemodialysis: A prospective post-mortem study. Kidney Int 1997;51:1928–1932.
14. Floege J, Burchert W, Brandis A, et al: Imaging of dialysis-related amyloid (AB-amyloid) deposits with 131I- beta 2-microglobulin. Kidney Int 1990;38:1169–1176.
15. van Ypersele de Strihou C, Jadoul M, et al: Effect of dialysis membrane and patient's age on signs of dialysis-related amyloidosis. The Working Party on Dialysis Amyloidosis. Kidney Int 1991;39:1012–1019.
16. Bindi P, Chanard J: Destructive spondyloarthropathy in dialysis patients: An overview. Nephron 1990;55:104–109.
17. Ketteler M, Koch KM, Floege J: Imaging techniques in the diagnosis of dialysis-related amyloidosis. Semin Dial 2001;14:90–93.
18. Nagoshi M, Hashizume H, Konishiike T, et al: Hemodialysis-related subacromial lesion: Diagnostic imaging and minimally invasive treatment. Clin Nephrol 2000;54:112–120.
19. Bardin T: Low-dose prednisone in dialysis-related amyloid arthropathy. Rev Rhum (Engl) 1994;61:97S–100S.
20. Kazama JJ, Maruyama H, Gejyo F: Reduction of circulating beta2-microglobulin level for the treatment of dialysis-related amyloidosis. Nephrol Dial Transplant 2001;16(Suppl 4):31–35.
21. Zingraff J, Drueke T: Can the nephrologist prevent dialysis-related amyloidosis? Am J Kidney Dis 1991;18:1–11.
22. Randoux C, Gillery P, Georges N, et al: Filtration of native and glycated beta2-microglobulin by charged and neutral dialysis membranes. Kidney Int 2001;60:1571–1577.
23. Raj DS, Ouwendyk M, Francoeur R, Pierratos A: (beta2Microglobulin) kinetics in nocturnal haemodialysis. Nephrol Dial Transplant 2000;15:58–64.
24. Tan SY, Baillod R, Brown E, et al: Clinical, radiological and serum amyloid P component scintigraphic features of beta2-microglobulin amyloidosis associated with continuous ambulatory peritoneal dialysis. Nephrol Dial Transplant 1999;14:1467–1471.
25. Locatelli F, Marcelli D, Conte F, et al: Comparison of mortality in ESRD patients on convective and diffusive extracorporeal treatments. The Registro Lombardo Dialisi E Trapianto. Kidney Int 1999;55:286–293.
26. Nakai S, Iseki K, Tabei K, et al: Outcomes of hemodiafiltration based on Japanese dialysis patient registry. Am J Kidney Dis 2001;38:S212–216.
27. Baz M, Durand C, Ragon A, et al: Using ultrapure water in hemodialysis delays carpal tunnel syndrome. Int J Artif Organs 1991;14:681–685.
28. Schwalbe S, Holzhauer M, Schaeffer J, et al: Beta 2-microglobulin associated amyloidosis: A vanishing complication of long-term hemodialysis? Kidney Int 1997;52:1077–1083.
29. Kleophas W, Haastert B, Backus G, et al: Long-term experience with an ultrapure individual dialysis fluid with a batch type machine. Nephrol Dial Transplant 1998;13:3118–3125.

INTRODUCTION

Disorders of the nervous system are associated with renal disease in patients with systemic disorders (e.g., hypertensive encephalopathy, thrombotic microangiopathies, atheroembolic and atherosclerotic disease, vasculitides), fluid and electrolyte abnormalities, multisystem disease in the intensive care unit setting, and those with chronic kidney disease (CKD). Furthermore, patients with CKD are at increased risk of toxin- and pharmacologic agent–induced neurotoxicity. This chapter focuses on the direct neurologic consequences of CKD.

UREMIC ENCEPHALOPATHY

The syndrome of uremic encephalopathy (UE) involves a spectrum of brain abnormalities that may clinically range from nearly imperceptible changes to coma and ultimately death.

Pathogenesis

The brain in CKD has decreased metabolic activity and oxygen consumption.[1,2] As long as the underlying renal disease has not affected cerebral hemodynamics and responsiveness to carbon dioxide, these functions appear intact, but subtle disturbances have been detected following dialysis.

Many theories support the role of uremic toxins that accumulate in CKD. The balance of excitatory and inhibitory neuronal pathways may be disrupted by organic substances,[3] in particular guanidino compounds, which are increased in the cerebrospinal fluid.[4,5] These compounds antagonize γ-aminobutyric acid (GABA$_A$) receptors and at the same time have agonistic effects on N-methyl-D-aspartate receptors, leading to enhanced cortical excitability. Asymmetrical dimethyl arginine,[6] which is increased in CKD, inhibits endothelial nitric oxide synthase and levels correlate with cerebrovascular complications in uremia. Disturbances in monoamine metabolism include a depletion of norepinephrine; suppression of central dopamine has been linked to the impairment of motor activity in uremic rats. Myoinositol, carnitine, indoxyl sulfate, polyamines, and decreased transport functions and increased permeability of the central nervous system have also been implicated in the neuronal dysfunction of uremia. Metabolites of drugs such as cimetidine and acyclovir may be increased in uremia due to inhibition of the OAT-3 transporter and neurotoxic syndromes may result.[7]

Secondary hyperparathyroidism may also play a role in UE[8,9] since brain calcium is increased in CKD and calcium transporters within neurons are parathyroid hormone sensitive. Increased cellular calcium may play a role in neuroexcitation.

Appetite regulation is abnormal in uremia (see Chapter 77). A high rate of tryptophan entry across the blood-brain barrier may increase the synthesis of serotonin, a major appetite inhibitor.[10] High levels of cholecystokinin, a powerful anorexigen, and low levels of neuropeptide Y, an orexigen, have been observed. Cachexia may result from anorexia, acidosis, and inflammation. Inflammatory cytokines such as leptin, tumor necrosis factor α, and interleukin-1 may signal anorexigenic neuropeptides such as pro-opiomelanocortin and α-melanocyte–stimulating hormone in the arcuate nucleus of the hypothalamus.

Clinical Manifestations

Whereas 20% of patients with acute renal failure in an intensive care unit setting developed neurologic impairment,[11] in CKD, the syndrome is more subtle, not correlating closely to the level of azotemia.[1] Cross-sectional studies in hemodialysis (HD) patients found cognitive impairment in 30% with about 10% exhibiting severe impairment. Neurocognitive deficits may have special implications for CKD in early childhood, adversely affecting development of the brain.[12]

UE can manifest as complex mental changes and/or motor disturbances (Fig. 76.1). The full-blown syndrome is a risk factor for morbidity and mortality.[1,2] Mental changes include emotional changes, depression, disturbing and disabling cognitive and memory

Clinical manifestations of uremic ecephalopathy	
Early UE	Late UE
Mental Changes	
Mood swings	Altered cognition and perception
Impaired concentration, loss of recent memory	Illusions, visual hallucinations, agitation, delirium
Insomnia, fatigue, apathy	Stupor, coma
Motor Changes	
Hyper-reflexia	Myoclonus, tetany
Tremor, asterixis	Hemiparesis
Dysarthria, altered gait, clumsiness, unsteadiness	Convulsions

Figure 76.1   Clinical manifestations of uremic encephalopathy (UE).

77 Gastroenterology and Nutrition in Chronic Kidney Disease

Gemma Bircher and Ciaran C. Doherty

GASTROINTESTINAL PROBLEMS IN CHRONIC KIDNEY DISEASE

Gastrointestinal (GI) disorders are common in chronic kidney disease (CKD), even in the absence of a primary GI disorder, and may be caused by uremia, prescribing harm, the dialysis treatment itself, or the specific disorder causing the renal failure. Some primary GI tract conditions occur with increased prevalence in chronic renal failure patients and a number of multisystem disorders can cause concurrent gut and kidney disease.

PRIMARY GASTROINTESTINAL TRACT DISORDERS WITH INCREASED PREVALENCE IN CHRONIC KIDNEY DISEASE

Gastroesophageal Reflux Disease

Upper GI symptoms are commonly reported by patients on continuous ambulatory peritoneal dialysis (CAPD) and also those with polycystic kidney disease as a result of hernia formation and gastroesophageal reflux. One study of 13 CAPD patients has suggested that gastroesophageal reflux disease (GERD) is very common among CAPD patients when 24-hour gastric pH monitoring is used to make the diagnosis.[1]

Gastroparesis

Gastroparesis is common in predialysis uremic patients and usually resolves after commencement of regular dialysis. Diabetic gastroparesis is the most severe form and is not improved by dialysis. Common symptoms are bloating, episodic vomiting, or early satiety. Delayed gastric emptying may adversely affect glycemic control as well as slowing absorption of orally administered drugs. Management can be particularly difficult in patients with a coexisting eating disorder. Treatment involves a low-fat and low-fiber diet with frequent small meals. Side effects limit the use of prokinetic drugs such as metoclopramide and domperidone, and only erythromycin is used for long-term administration. Intravenous erythromycin 250 mg every 8 hours may have a role in acute exacerbations of diabetic gastroparesis.[2] Implantation of gastric neurostimulator devices has been advocated for severe refractory cases. Enteral nutrition via a jejunostomy tube may be required.

Peptic Ulcer Disease

Uremic patients do not have an increased prevalence of peptic ulcer disease. Treatment of peptic ulcer disease in CKD patients requires avoidance of aluminum- or magnesium-containing antacids and bismuth salts, and the dose of H_2 receptor antagonists needs to be adjusted for the GFR level.[3] Proton pump inhibitors may be superior to H_2 receptor antagonists for treatment of GERD and peptic ulcer disease and do not require dose adjustment.

Acute Pancreatitis

Some evidence exists of an increased incidence of acute pancreatitis in chronic renal failure.[4] Diagnosis may be difficult since serum amylase and lipase levels increase up to fivefold in chronic renal failure due to renal retention of these two low-molecular-weight proteins. The clinical presentation of pancreatitis and peritonitis may be similar in patients on peritoneal dialysis (PD). If peritonitis fails to resolve after 2 weeks of adequate therapy, pancreatitis should be considered. An increased effluent dialysate amylase concentration (>100 U/l) favors a diagnosis of pancreatitis, and radiographic imaging may also prove helpful.

Gastritis and Duodenitis

Upper GI endoscopy in one large series of end-stage renal disease (ESRD) patients identified gastritis and duodenitis in 22% and 60%, respectively.[5] The mechanism underlying this increased mucosal inflammation is unclear, and there is poor correlation between mucosal changes and GI symptoms.

Spontaneous Colonic Perforation

Spontaneous colonic perforation in patients without renal failure is associated with diverticular disease or obstruction. In ESRD patients it may also occur in association with barium enema examination, dialysis-related amyloidosis, fecal impaction, and aluminum-containing antacids. The condition has a high mortality in uremic patients and should be considered in any ESRD patient presenting with acute abdominal pain.

Colonic Necrosis Induced by Cation Exchange Resins

Cation exchange resins used to treat hyperkalemia in patients with renal failure may cause colonic necrosis. Prevention of this complication requires that lactulose is coprescribed when polystyrene sulfonate resins (calcium resonium) or kayexalate are used orally and that sorbitol is avoided when kayexalate is given in enema form.

Fecal Impaction

Fecal impaction may occur as a complication of phosphate binders, analgesics, and iron supplements, in association with underlying motility disorders and sedentary lifestyle. Associated features may include mucosal ulceration, bleeding, perforation, and/or chronic diarrhea. Sodium docusate 100 mg once or twice per day, lactulose 15 to 30 ml/day, or bisacodyl, two 5-mg tablets once daily may help prevent this complication. Magnesium-containing salts and phosphate-containing enemas should be avoided. Manual disimpaction or surgery may be required in severe cases.

Nonocclusive Mesenteric Ischemia/Infarction

Nonocclusive mesenteric ischemia/infarction (NOMI) may cause fever, vomiting, and abdominal pain in elderly dialysis patients.[6] In this form of ischemic bowel disease, a significant proportion of patients have no arterial or venous occlusion. Predisposing factors include congestive cardiac failure, hypoxic states, or intradialytic hypotension due to excessive ultrafiltration. Mesenteric angiography in NOMI will not show critical stenosis in the major vessels but instead poor or no flow in the small submucosal resistance vessels.

Gastrointestinal Bleeding

Angiodysplasia (Fig. 77.1) and ulcerative esophagitis appear more common in patients with renal failure than in the normal population,[7,8] while peptic ulcer disease remains the most common overall cause of upper GI bleeding. In long-term dialysis patients, β_2-microglobulin amyloidosis may affect the gut and cause melena,[9] while nonsteroidal anti-inflammatory drug (NSAID)-induced enteropathy may cause mucosal damage more often in the small intestine than in the stomach.[10] Stercoral ulcers may occur in patients with constipation induced by ion exchange resins or aluminium hydroxide phosphate binders.

Diagnosis of the lesion causing GI tract bleeding in uremic patients can be difficult.[11] Small bowel enteroscopy may be necessary for diagnosis of small bowel angiodysplasia, NSAID erosions, and other lesions. Colonoscopy may be rendered impossible because of luminal blood. Angiography and radioisotope-labeled red-cell scans are of limited value.

General treatment measures for GI bleeding in the dialysis patient are removal of culpable drugs (e.g., aspirin, warfarin, NSAID, clopidogrel) and correction of uremic coagulopathy (see Chapter 73). Other general treatment measures include switching to heparin-free hemodialysis, and anecdotal reports support the use of antifibrinolytic agents such as tranexamic acid 500 mg twice daily for recurrent bleeding. The underlying causative lesion defines the specific treatment approach. Randomized trials have given conflicting results regarding the efficacy of hormone therapy for GI bleeding due to angiodysplasia. Most patients with angiodysplasia are elderly and present a poor surgical risk.

Diabetic Enteropathy

This complication affects between 8% and 22% of diabetic patients and typically produces watery and painless diarrhea that occurs at night and may be associated with fecal incontinence. The diarrhea is often episodic with intermittent normal bowel habit and bouts of constipation. Pathogenetic factors include autonomic neuropathy with disordered motility of the small bowel and colon, associated bacterial overgrowth resulting in bile acid and fat malabsorption, and concurrent celiac disease (the incidence of which is increased in diabetes). Steatorrhea due to pancreatic exocrine insufficiency in a diabetic patient suggests a diagnosis of chronic pancreatitis, often due to alcoholism. Systematic investigation to define the underlying mechanisms in an individual patient may allow treatment to be directed at the identified main cause. Appropriate investigations are stool examination for *Clostridium difficile*, bacterial pathogens, ova and parasites; barium x-rays looking for gastric retention, malabsorption pattern, and intestinal wall thickness; upper GI endoscopy with duodenal biopsy; and anorectal manometry and sensory testing if fecal incontinence is present. Small bowel enteroscopy with biopsy may be necessary in selected patients. To treat rapid intestinal transit, loperamide 2 mg qid may be tried. Some patients may respond to clonidine[12] or the somato-statin analogue octreotide.[13]

GASTROINTESTINAL-RENAL SYNDROME

Disturbed GI function may result from the specific disorder causing the renal failure, or, conversely, some primary GI tract disorders, their investigation, or treatment may cause renal failure. Concurrent gut and kidney disease may also be observed in a diverse group of multisystem disorders (Fig. 77.2).

Polycystic Kidney Disease

Abdominal wall hernia and diverticular disease prevalences are increased in patients with polycystic kidney disease (see also Chapter 43); they may occur at a younger age and may be more

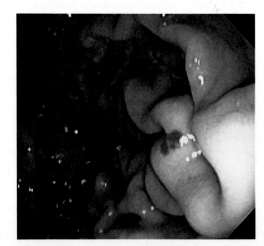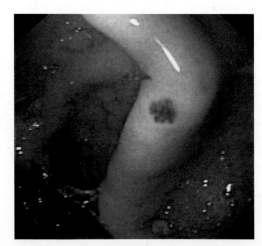

Figure 77.1 Two examples of gastric angiodysplasia in a dialysis patient. (Courtesy of Drs. R. Winograd and C. Trautwein, Aachen, Germany.)

Gastrointestinal-renal syndromes: disorders that may cause gut and kidney disease			
Disorder	Kidney	Gut	Symptoms
Polycystic kidney disease	Chronic renal failure, intracyst infection, and hemorrhage	Hepatic cystic change, gastric compression, ascites, splenomegaly, portal hypertension, hernias	Abdominal pain, distention, early satiety
Amyloidosis	Chronic renal failure, nephrotic syndrome	Malabsorption, splenic rupture	Diarrhea, weight loss, melena, acute abdomen
Systemic vasculitis	Proliferative glomerulonephritis	Mesenteric ischemia/infarction, strictures, intussusception	Abdominal pain, diarrhea, GI bleeding, peritonitis
Fabry's disease	Proteinuria, microhematuria, chronic renal failure	Autonomic dysfunction, skin angiokeratomas in bathing trunk area	Recurrent abdominal pain, episodic diarrhea and constipation
Scleroderma	Acute renal failure, chronic renal failure	Distended loops of bowel, small bowel bacterial overgrowth	Dysphagia constipation, abdominal distention, steatorrhea
Diabetes	Chronic renal failure, nephrotic syndrome	Autonomic gastropathy and enteropathy, increased incidence of celiac disease	Episodic vomiting, painless nocturnal watery diarrhea, weight loss
Ulcerative colitis	Chronic renal failure due to AA amyloidosis or sulfasalazine (Salazopyrin)-induced tubulointerstitial nephritis	Colitis, sclerosing cholangitis	Abdominal pain, diarrhea, melena jaundice
Chronic pancreatitis, small bowel disorders	Renal failure due to oxalate-induced nephrolithiasis and tubulointerstitial nephritis	Increased intestinal oxalate absorption	Upper abdominal pain radiating to the back, steatorrhea
Anorexia nervosa, bulimia, laxative or diuretic abuse	Hypokalemic nephropathy, chronic renal failure	Scaphoid abdomen, dental erosions, melanosis coli	Muscle weakness, recurrent vomiting, malnutrition
TRAPS	Nephrotic syndrome, CKD	Serositis	Recurrent abdominal pain, skin rash
Familial Mediterranean fever	Nephrotic syndrome, CKD	Serositis	Recurrent abdominal pain, skin rash
Chronic alcoholism	Secondary IgA nephropathy, hepatorenal syndrome	Esophageal varices, pancreatitis, cirrhosis, ascites	GI hemorrhage, abdominal distention
Nutcracker syndrome	Dilated left renal vain	Acute aortomesenteric angle, left-sided varicocele	Hematuria, proteinuria
Antiphospholipid syndrome	Chronic GN	Adrenal infarction and hemorrhage	Acute abdominal pain, hypotension

Figure 77.2 Gastrointestinal-renal syndromes: disorders that may cause gut and kidney disease. CKD, chronic kidney disease; GI, gastrointestinal; GN, glomerulonephritis; TRAPS, tumor necrosis factor receptor-1–associated fever syndrome.

severe.[14] Massive hepatic cysts may cause gastric compression symptoms, acute or chronic upper abdominal pain, portal hypertension, splenomegaly with hepatic insufficiency, and recurrent ascites.

Vasculitis

Systemic vasculitis involving the GI tract may cause acute mesenteric infarction or chronic mesenteric ischaemia with intestinal angina, weight loss, nausea, vomiting, and diarrhea. These patients can also present acutely with small bowel obstruction secondary to intussusception, or strictures resembling Crohn's disease. Massive GI bleeding secondary to aneurysm formation, bowel infarction, perforation, and peritonitis is a rare complication. In addition to mesenteric ischemia, systemic vasculitis can also cause ischemic hepatitis, pancreatitis, and cholecystitis. The GI tract is affected in up to 50% of patients with Henoch-Schönlein vasculitis. GI symptoms include colicky abdominal pain, nausea, vomiting, diarrhea, constipation, and GI bleeding. The course can wax and wane over several weeks and often resolves spontaneously.

In patients with systemic lupus erythematosus with abdominal pain, the causative pathology may be mesenteric vasculitis or polyserositis without evidence of vasculitis. The latter pathology is more likely to be responsive to immunosuppression.

Chronic Pancreatitis and Small Bowel Disorders

Chronic pancreatitis and small bowel disorders may cause increased intestinal oxalate absorption and oxalate-induced renal failure. Patients with alcohol-induced chronic pancreatic insufficiency who do not receive adequate enzyme supplements may develop renal failure due to this mechanism. Renal biopsy in these patients may show oxalate crystal deposition with severe tubulointerstitial scarring but only mild background diabetic nephropathy. Patients with diabetes due to chronic pancreatitis may therefore develop renal failure due to causes other than diabetic nephropathy and should be considered for renal biopsy. Treatment with adequate enzyme supplements may prevent this complication of chronic pancreatic insufficiency.

Ulcerative Colitis

Long-standing ulcerative colitis may be complicated by chronic renal failure due either to development of AA amyloidosis, secondary IgA nephropathy, or drug-induced tubulointerstitial nephritis.

Acute Phosphate Nephropathy

Acute phosphate nephropathy following an oral sodium phosphate bowel purgative may be an unrecognized cause of acute and chronic renal failure. Diffuse tubular injury and nephrocalcinosis are the causative renal lesions, and potential etiologic factors include dehydration, increased patient age, hypertension, and concurrent use of an angiotensin-converting enzyme inhibitor or angiotensin receptor blocker.[15]

Fabry's Disease

Autonomic dysfunction in Fabry's disease (see Chapter 59) contributes to the GI symptoms that may resemble irritable bowel syndrome with recurrent abdominal pain, vomiting, abdominal distention, and episodic diarrhea and constipation.

Tumor Necrosis Factor Receptor-1–Associated Fever Syndrome and Familial Mediterranean Fever

Both heredofamilial amyloidoses are associated with AA amyloid deposition, and the clinical picture is characterized by episodic abdominal pain due to serositis and fever (see Chapter 26).

Antiphospholipid Antibody Syndrome

Thrombotic events involving the mesenteric and adrenal circulation may cause acute abdominal pain, hypotension, and laboratory features suggesting adrenal insufficiency.

DRUG-INDUCED GASTROINTESTINAL DISORDERS IN CHRONIC KIDNEY DISEASE PATIENTS

Figure 77.3 lists the common drug induced gastrointestinal disorders found in patients with chronic kidney disease.

Nausea and Vomiting

Nausea and vomiting are ubiquitous drug side effects but are particularly common with codeine-containing compound analgesics, opiates, antibiotics, digoxin, azathioprine, and mycophenolate mofetil.

Intestinal Pseudo-obstruction

Intestinal pseudo-obstruction should be considered when the clinical picture suggests mechanical bowel obstruction (Fig. 77.4), but no anatomic lesion obstructing bowel transit is demonstrated. While there may be an underlying causative disorder such as amyloidosis, scleroderma, or diabetes, adverse effects of drugs such as anticholinergic antidepressants, opiates, ion-exchange resins, and calcium channel blockers often contribute to the problem. Plain radiographs of the abdomen may show distended loops of small

bowel and/or air-fluid levels. The presence of associated steatorrhea, vitamin B_{12} malabsorption, or folate excess suggests small bowel bacterial overgrowth and should prompt bacteriologic culture of a small bowel aspirate to confirm the diagnosis. Treatment may involve temporary parenteral nutrition, prokinetic agents such as erythromycin, and antibiotics for confirmed small bowel bacterial overgrowth.

Diarrhea

Diarrhea may be a side effect of many drugs (see Fig. 77.3).

DIALYSIS-INDUCED GASTROINTESTINAL DISORDERS

Figure 77.5 lists the clinical settings for dialysis-induced gastrointestinal disorders.

Idiopathic (Nephrogenic) Ascites

Idiopathic (nephrogenic) ascites is now rare due to improved nutritional therapy and refined prescribing and delivery of hemodialysis. It is necessary to exclude underdialysis and specific disorders such as constrictive pericarditis, cirrhosis, hepatic vein compression in polycystic kidney disease, occult tuberculosis, neoplastic or granulomatous peritoneal disease, and encapsulating peritoneal sclerosis. If by this process of exclusion, idiopathic dialysis ascites is diagnosed, ascitic fluid usually has a high protein content (3 to 6 g/dl).

Dialysis-Related Amyloidosis

Dialysis-related amyloidosis in very long-term dialysis patients can lead to a wide variety of GI manifestations (see Chapter 75).

Peritoneal Dialysate Inflow/Outflow Pain

This type of abdominal pain may be due to catheter malposition or the acidic pH of conventional lactate dialysate (see Chapter 86).

Hemoperitoneum

Minor blood staining of peritoneal dialysate may occur as a result of retrograde menstruation, endometriosis, or a bleeding tendency. Severe bleeding, especially if associated with pain and fever, usually indicates additional pathology such as a renal tumor, cyst rupture in polycystic kidney disease, ovarian cyst rupture, or sclerosing peritonitis. A hematocrit of >2% in a centrifuged dialysate specimen suggests the need to consider laparotomy. Peritoneal fluid white cell count, amylase, and culture should be sent in all cases as

Common drug-induced gastrointestinal disorders in chronic kidney disease	
Gastrointestinal Disorder	Commonly Implicated Drugs
Anorexia, nausea, vomiting, abdominal pain	Azathioprine, mycophenolate mofetil, sirolimus, digoxin, iron supplements, antibiotics
Intestinal pseudo-obstruction	Calcium blockers, anticholinergic antidepressants, opiate analgesics
Constipation	Iron supplements, phosphate binders, opioid analgesics
Diarrhea	Broad-spectrum antibiotics, angiotensin-converting enzyme inhibitors
Colonic necrosis	Kayexalate enema, high-dose corticosteroid
Hepatocellular jaundice	Fusidic acid
Gastrointestinal hemorrhage	Aspirin, warfarin, heparin, clopidogrel, nonsteroidal anti-inflammatory drugs, corticosteroids

Figure 77.3 Common drug-induced gastrointestinal disorders in chronic kidney disease.

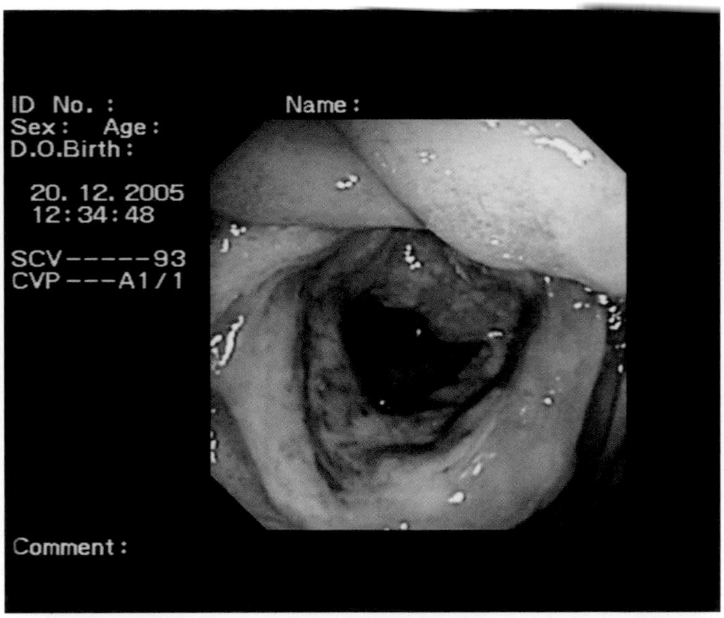

Figure 77.4 Nonsteroidal anti-inflammatory drug enteropathy in a 38-year-old hemodialysis patient taking sulindac for chronic arthritis. This concentric stricture in the ascending colon caused recurrent abdominal pain. (Courtesy of Dr. Jack Lee, Belfast, UK.)

well as coagulation studies if bleeding is heavy or recurrent. Treatment of mild cases may include withdrawing aspirin or anticoagulants, frequent exchanges, or addition of heparin (500 U/l) to the dialysate to prevent PD catheter clotting.

Culture-Negative Peritonitis

A mild form of aseptic peritonitis has been reported with the use of icodextrin solutions as a result of peptidoglycan contamination (see Chapter 86).

Encapsulating Peritoneal Sclerosis (Sclerosing Peritonitis)

Encapsulating peritoneal sclerosis is a rare but serious complication of PD (see Chapter 86). The condition may present in an indolent fashion with progressive ultrafiltration failure or as a florid febrile illness with abdominal pain and life-threatening malnutrition.

GASTROINTESTINAL TRACT DISORDERS FOLLOWING RENAL TRANSPLANTATION

Also see Chapter 94 for a discussion of the medical management of a kidney transplant recipient.

Oral Ulceration

Oral ulceration is most common during treatment of rejection. It may be nonspecific or due to herpes simplex virus or candidiasis infection. Alternately, it may be seen as a side effect of sirolimus or mycophenolate mofetil (MMF) therapy.

Esophagitis

Esophagitis (Fig. 77.6) may be caused by exacerbation of GERD, candidiasis, or diphosphonates prescribed for post-transplantation osteoporosis prophylaxis.

Dialysis-induced gastrointestinal disorders	
Disorder	Clinical Setting
Nonocclusive mesenteric infarction	Excessive ultrafiltration with intradialytic hypotension in elderly patients
β_2-microglobulin amyloidosis with visceral involvement	Long-term dialysis patients; may cause decreased motility, gastric dilatation, colonic necrosis, melena
Idiopathic (nephrogenic) ascites	Diagnosis of exclusion, rare with modern dialysis
Gastrointestinal hemorrhage	Predominantly elderly hemodialysis patients
Pseudoperitonitis	Icodextrin in peritoneal dialysis patients
Encapsulating peritoneal sclerosis	Long-term peritoneal dialysis, although 30% of cases follow bacterial peritonitis
Hemoperitoneum	Peritoneal dialysis, endometriosis
Dialysate infusion pain	Acidic dialysate, catheter malposition
Scrotal/labial swelling	Peritoneal dialysis patient with patent processus vaginalis or dissection through peritoneal membrane
Infectious peritonitis	Peritoneal dialysis

Figure 77.5 Dialysis-induced gastrointestinal disorders.

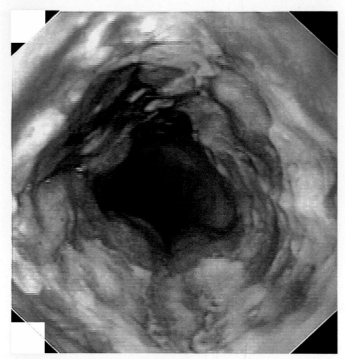

Figure 77.6 Ulcerative esophagitis in a renal transplant patient. (Courtesy of Drs. R. Winograd and C. Trautwein, Aachen, Germany.)

Upper Abdominal Pain

Upper abdominal pain following renal transplantation can result from corticosteroid-induced exacerbation of pre-existing GERD or peptic ulcer disease, cholelithiasis, acute pancreatitis, adverse drug effects, and cytomegalovirus infection. Acute pancreatitis may affect 1% to 2% of renal transplant patients, and mortality is high. Common precipitating factors are alcohol, hypercalcemia, immunosuppression, cytomegalovirus infection, and cholelithiasis.

Lower Abdominal Pain

In addition to diverticular disease and disorders causing intestinal obstruction and pseudo-obstruction, the differential diagnosis includes disorders affecting the transplanted kidney such as graft pyelonephritis, urolithiasis, segmental infarction, and lymphocele. Acute intestinal pseudo-obstruction following renal transplantation may be contributed to by retroperitoneal hematoma and opioid analgesics.

Chronic Diarrhea

Chronic diarrhea has an infectious origin in most patients (e.g., microsporidia, *Strongyloides stercoralis*, *Shigella*). In patients treated with mycophenolate mofetil, as many as 40% may show a Crohn's disease–like enterocolitis.[16] GI malignancy including lymphoma, Kaposi's sarcoma, and post-transplantation lymphoproliferative disorder may cause chronic afebrile diarrhea or may present later in the disease process with obstruction, perforation, or GI bleeding.

NUTRITION IN CHRONIC RENAL FAILURE

Nutrition plays an important role during all stages of CKD. Hypertension, obesity, hyperlipidemia, and poor diabetic control all affect CKD progress. As the glomerular filtration rate (GFR) deteriorates, retention of nitrogenous metabolites, a decreased ability to regulate levels of electrolytes and water, and certain vitamin deficiencies can be affected by dietary changes. In addition, protein-energy malnutrition predicts a poor outcome.

Malnutrition

The prevalence of malnutrition in dialysis patients ranges from 10% to 70%, depending on the choice of nutritional marker and the population studied.[17,18] There is also evidence to suggest that diminished nutritional status exists before initiation of dialysis and strongly predicts mortality on dialysis. Paradoxically, several investigators have found a significant inverse relationship between mortality risk and body size in hemodialysis populations, a phenomenon termed *reverse epidemiology* (see Chapter 71).

Several factors related to the uremic state may contribute to the high incidence of protein-energy malnutrition:

- Inadequate protein and calorie intakes of patients with CKD is probably one of the most important causes. Nutrient intake starts to decrease in the predialysis period and correlates inversely with GFR.[19] An important factor in the reduction of intake is CKD-associated anorexia. This may exist for a number of reasons, such as impaired taste acuity and diminished olfactory function, medications, autonomic gastroparesis, psychological and socioeconomic factors, and inadequate dialysis. Elevated serum leptin, a long-term regulator of appetite, has also been linked to the anorexia seen in CKD.[20]
- Nutritional losses occur during treatment: 8 to 12 g of amino acids is lost per hemodialysis treatment and 5 to 10 g of protein is lost daily during PD, related to the peritoneal membrane transport type. This may be significantly higher during episodes of PD peritonitis.
- Metabolic acidosis, periods of acute or chronic illnesses, and the use of so-called bioincompatible dialysis membranes may induce protein catabolism. This is mediated in large part through the ubiquitin-proteasome pathway of protein degradation.[21] Large doses of corticosteroids used early in the post-transplantation period, together with the stresses of surgery as well as a potentially delayed graft function, may also lead to protein loss that can further compromise patients.
- Accumulating evidence suggests that the hypoalbuminemia of kidney failure in part may be a consequence of activation of the acute-phase response (see also Chapter 71).[22]
- Endocrine disorders such as insulin resistance, increased parathyroid hormone concentrations (which may promote amino acid catabolism and gluconeogenesis), and vitamin D deficiency (which may contribute to proximal myopathy) may have an adverse effect on nutritional status.

Assessment of Nutritional Status

The measurement of nutritional status does not lend itself to one simple test, and an optimal panel of measures for screening nutritional status is still required. Figure 77.7 summarizes some of the methods used for assessing nutritional status.

Estimation of Intake

Diet history, recall, or food diaries are a mainstay for estimating dietary intake. In addition, a gradual decrease in blood urea nitrogen (BUN) and reduced phosphate and potassium levels may indicate a decrease in protein intake in dialysis-dependent patients and low serum cholesterol may indicate a poor calorie intake.

The excretion of the protein end product urea is easily measured and is often used to estimate adequacy of dialysis. The protein equivalent of total nitrogen appearance (PNA) can be

Assessment of nutritional status

Area	Assessments
Physical examination	
Assessment of dietary intake	Diet history/food diaries
Anthropometric measurements	Body weight/height/body mass index
	Percentage of weight change
	Skinfold thickness
	Midarm muscle circumference
Body composition	Neutron activation
	Ultrasonography
	Bioelectrical impedance
	Dual-energy x-ray absorptiometry
Biochemical	Serum electrolytes
determinations	Serum proteins
	PNA/PCR
	Serum cholesterol
	Creatinine index
Subjective global assessment	
Immunologic assays	Blood lymphocytes
	Delayed cutaneous hypersensitivity tests
Functional tests	Grip strength

Figure 77.7 Assessment of nutritional status. Common methods used to assess nutritional status are shown. PNA, protein equivalent of total nitrogen appearance; PCR, protein catabolic rate.

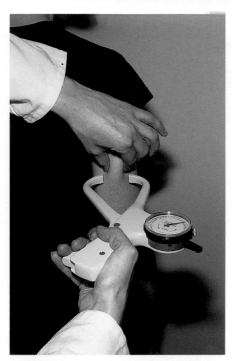

Figure 77.8 Routine measurement of skinfold thickness. The dominant arm that does not have the fistula and graft is used in patients with renal failure.

estimated from interdialytic changes in urea nitrogen concentration in serum and the urea nitrogen content of urine and dialysate. Based on the assumption that, in steady state, nitrogen excretion equals nitrogen intake, the PNA (or protein catabolic rate) has been used to approximate dietary protein intake in the short term. Results, however, need to be interpreted with caution (urea kinetic modeling and adequacy of dialysis are further discussed in Chapters 83 and 85). Equations used to estimate PNA can be found in Kidney Disease Outcomes Quality Initiative (KDOQI).[23]

Body Composition

Skinfold thickness can be used to assess body fat, and muscle mass can be assessed by measurement of mid-upper-arm muscle circumference (MAMC; Fig. 77.8). The midpoint of the upper dominant arm is used, as this is the arm less likely to have an arteriovenous fistula.

$$\text{MAMC (cm)} = \text{midarm circumference (cm)} - [3.14 \times \text{triceps skinfold (cm)}]$$

The measurement is taken after dialysis for patients on hemodialysis. Although inexpensive and relatively easy to learn and quick to carry out, these anthropometric measurements are limited by inter- and intravariability. Nevertheless, serial measures over time can be useful to track changes in the same patient when used in conjunction with other nutritional indices.

A technique known as subjective global assessment (SGA), originally used to assess surgical patients, has been shown to be a reliable nutritional assessment tool for patients on dialysis.[24] A series of questions regarding recent changes in nutrient intake are used with simple observations of the patient's body weight and muscle mass to determine subjectively the nutritional status of the individual: patients are classified as well nourished, mildly malnourished/suspected malnutrition, or severely malnourished. Figures 77.9 and 77.10 show muscle wasting in a patient on

hemodialysis classified by SGA as severely malnourished. SGA is by definition subjective and has been criticized for not being sensitive enough to show the degree of malnutrition. Other scoring systems using components of the conventional SGA are presently being evaluated.

Visceral Protein

Serum albumin is an important index of nutritional status, but its limitations must be appreciated. Fluid status, impaired liver function, age, and acute inflammatory conditions can all affect albumin levels. However, despite its relatively long half-life (20 days), albumin still remains an important measure of nutritional status and health of the patient. Clinically, it may be possible to observe the growth of white nails when there has been a transient period of hypoalbuminemia (Fig. 77.11). Other serum protein markers of malnutrition are all difficult to interpret because of the influence of factors other than nutrition: Serum transferrin is linked to body iron stores and may be altered with changes in iron status. Prealbumin levels are affected by decreased renal function because the normal kidney excretes it; levels of prealbumin also decline rapidly during episodes of acute inflammation.

With the low specificity and sensitivity of many of the anthropometric and biochemical markers of malnutrition, it becomes clear that no single factor properly reflects nutritional status. Malnutrition can be described only by integrating biochemical markers and anthropometric measurements with evaluation of the subjective well-being of the patient (Fig. 77.12).

Nutritional Guidelines

Guidelines are useful, but it is important that dietary restrictions are not unnecessarily imposed and that advice is tailored to the individual and altered as circumstances dictate. Figure 77.13 summarizes the nutritional recommendations for CKD.

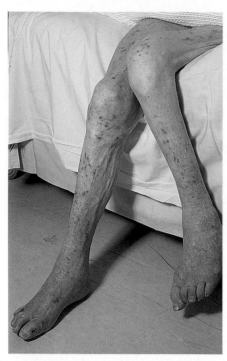

Figure 77.9 A severely malnourished hemodialysis patient. There is marked wasting of the quadriceps and calf muscles.

Hyperlipidemia

Although disturbances of lipid metabolism are commonly seen in CKD, there is a paucity of data on the effect of diet therapy in this group. A diet low in fat, particularly saturated fat, and an increased intake in soluble fiber and oily fish twice per week is recommended, but it must be remembered that a balance needs to be struck between healthy eating concepts and nutritional adequacy. Additional fiber, within the confines of the diet, has the benefit of helping to regulate bowel function. This latter point is particularly important in PD patients.

Bone Disease

KDOQI has written clinical practice guidelines for the treatment of bone metabolism and disease in CKD, which include

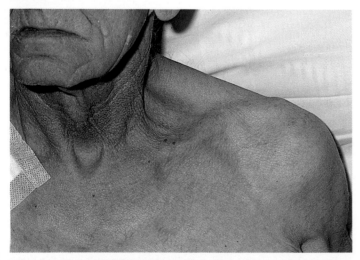

Figure 77.10 A severely malnourished hemodialysis patient. Muscle wasting around clavicle and shoulder.

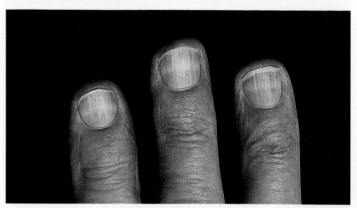

Figure 77.11 White nails in hypoalbuminemia. The white band grew during a transient period of hypoalbuminemia caused by nephrotic syndrome.

recommendations for phosphorus and calcium intake as well as vitamin D type and dose (see also Chapter 74).

Vitamins and Minerals

Vitamin and mineral abnormalities can occur with CKD. Proposed explanations include dietary restriction, dialysate losses, and/or the necessity of an intact kidney for normal metabolism of certain vitamins. However, the dietary requirements for patients with CKD are not clear cut.

Protein and/or potassium restrictions can lead to inadequate intakes of pyroxine, vitamin B_{12}, folic acid, vitamin C, iron, and zinc. The use of recombinant human erythropoietin may increase the requirement for iron and folic acid (see Chapter 72).

Increased serum homocysteine is a known risk factor for cardiovascular morbidity in CKD, and there is evidence that folic acid, B_{12}, and pyridoxine supplements may lower serum homocysteine (see also Chapter 71). It is still not established whether lowering homocysteine will lead to a reduction in cardiovascular disease, but current opinion suggests that it may be prudent to supplement maintenance dialysis patients with a daily water-

Indices of malnutrition	
Assessment	Indices
Biochemical parameters (check locally for normal biochemical ranges as they can vary)	Serum albumin below the normal range (dependent on methodology) Serum prealbumin <300 mg/l (30 mg/dl)[11] Serum cholesterol <150 mg/dl (3.8 mmol/l)[11] Low serum creatinine/phosphate/potassium/urea in patients on dialysis Low creatinine index Low PNA/PCR
Anthropometric parameters	Continuous decline in weight, skinfold thickness, midarm muscle circumference Body mass index <20 Body weight <90% of ideal Abnormal muscle strength

Figure 77.12 Indices of malnutrition. PNA, protein equivalent of total nitrogen appearance; PCR, protein catabolic rate.

Nutritional recommendations in chronic kidney disease			
Daily Intake	Predialysis CKD	Hemodialysis	Peritoneal Dialysis
Protein (g/kg body weight) (See KDOQI[11] for estimation of adjusted edema-free body weight)	0.6–1.0 (level of restriction depends on the view of the clinician) 1.0 for nephrotic syndrome	1.2[23]	1.0–1.3[23,30]
Energy (kcal/kg body weight) (See KDOQI[11] for estimation of adjusted edema-free body weight)	35[23](<60 yr) 30–35[23](>60 yr)	35[23](<60 yr) 30–35[23](>60 yr)	35,[23,30] including dialysate calories (<60 yr) 30–35,[23,30] including dialysate calories (>60 yr)
Sodium (mmol)	<100 (more if salt wasting)	<100	<100
Potassium	Reduce if hyperkalemic (>5.5 mmol/l)	Reduce if hyperkalemic (>5.5 mmol/l)	Reduce if hyperkalemic; potassium restriction is generally not required
	If hyperkalemic advice will take the form of decreasing certain fruits and vegetables, milk, and some miscellaneous foods and giving information about cooking methods		
Phosphorus	Reduce, level dependent on protein intake		
	Advice will take the form of reducing dairy products, offal, certain shellfish, and some miscellaneous foods and giving information about the timing of binders with high-phosphorus meals and snacks		
Calcium	In CKD stages 3–5 total intake of elemental calcium (including dietary calcium) should not exceed 2000 mg/day	Total intake of elemental calcium (including dietary calcium) should not exceed 2000 mg/day	Total intake of elemental calcium (including dietary calcium) should not exceed 2000 mg/day

Figure 77.13 Nutritional recommendations in chronic kidney disease (CKD). Recommendations are for typical patients, but should always be individualized based on clinical, biochemical, and anthropometric indices. KDOQI, Kidney Disease Outcomes Quality Initiative.

soluble vitamin supplement that provides the recommended vitamin profile for dialysis patients[25] (vitamin C 60 mg, biotin 300 μg, calcium pantothenate 10 mg, cyanocobalamin 6 μg, folic acid 800 μg, niacinamide 20 mg, pyridoxine 10 mg, riboflavin 1.7 mg, and thiamine 1.5 mg). Specialized multivitamins for dialysis patients are available. High-dose vitamin C supplements, as frequently taken in the nonuremic population, should not be taken as they may lead to oxalosis, and extensive soft-tissue calcification including blood vessels, heart, and retina. Supplementation with fat-soluble vitamins is generally not recommended since diets do not tend to be deficient, dialysis losses are minimal, and accumulation can occur.

Monitoring and Treatment

Monitoring of patients with CKD involves a combination of nutritional assessment, noting relevant biochemistry (potassium, phosphate, lipids), and observing fluid status. The challenge comes in giving advice that carefully balances control of electrolytes while not compromising nutritional status. Strategies to treat anorexia should be considered and nutrient intake maximized by using one or more of the methods discussed in the following sections.

Enteral Supplementation

If food fortification advice is insufficient, supplements, in the form of high-protein, high-calorie drinks, powders, and puddings, should be administered. Enteral tube feeding is also an option if nutrient intake cannot be increased sufficiently by using oral supplements, and renal-specific tube feeds and supplements are available that have lower fluid and electrolyte contents. A recent systematic review suggested that enteral multinutrient support

could significantly increase serum albumin concentration and improve total dietary intake in CKD patients receiving maintenance dialysis.[26]

Supplementation of Dialysate Fluids

Intradialytic parenteral nutrition (IDPN) can be used to provide intensive parenteral nutrient therapy with use of concentrated hypertonic solutions three times weekly during hemodialysis treatments without the need for establishing a central venous line. The nutrients, usually a mixture of amino acids, glucose, and lipid, are infused into the venous bloodline, and only about 10% of infused amino acids are lost into the dialysate. The use of IDPN in hemodialysis patients seems to be associated with decreased mortality,[27] but there is a lack of controlled studies addressing the effect of IDPN on patient outcome.

Intraperitoneal amino acid (IPAA) is sometimes used in PD. The amino acids (in a 1.1% amino acid solution) are substituted for glucose and about 80% of the amino acids are absorbed in a 4-hour period.[28] The long-term effects of IPAA on nutritional status and clinical outcomes are not known.

K/DOQI has suggested that PD and hemodialysis patients who have evidence of protein or energy malnutrition and inadequate protein or energy intake or are unable to tolerate adequate oral supplements or tube feeding may benefit from IPAA or IDPN, respectively.[23]

Appetite Stimulants and Growth Factors

The appetite stimulant of most interest is megestrol acetate: a progesterone derivative that has been shown to increase the appetite and nonfluid weight of cancer patients and, more recently, patients with acquired immunodeficiency syndrome. Pilot studies using the drug in hemodialysis patients showed an improvement in some of the nutritional parameters over a short period of time.[29]

Metabolic Acidosis

Although some trials have shown no detrimental effect of mild metabolic acidosis, many others have reported that normalizing the predialysis or stabilized serum bicarbonate concentration is beneficial for protein, nutritional status, and bone metabolism. Current guidelines recommend the correction of acidosis in CKD patients.[23,30]

REFERENCES

1. Kim MJ, Kwon KH, Lee SW: Gastroesophageal reflux in CAPD patients. Adv Perit Dial 1998;14:98–101.
2. Janssens J, Peeters TL, Vantrappen G, et al: Improvement of gastric emptying in diabetic gastroparesis by erythromycin. N Engl J Med 1990; 322:1028–1031.
3. Manlucu J, Tonelli M, Ray JG, et al: Dose-reducing H2 receptor antagonists in the presence of low glomerular filtration rate: A systematic review of the evidence. Nephrol Dial Transplant 2005;20:376–384.
4. Pitchumoni CS, Arguello P, Agarwal N, Yoo J: Acute pancreatitis in chronic renal failure. Am J Gastroenterol 1996;91:2477–2482.
5. Margolis DM, Saylor JL, Geisse G, et al: Upper gastrointestinal disease in chronic renal failure: A prospective evaluation. Arch Intern Med. 1978; 138:1214–1217.
6. Zeier M, Weisel M, Ritz E: Non-occlusive mesenteric infarction (NOMI) in dialysis patients: Risk factors, diagnosis, intervention and outcome. Int J Artif Organs 1992;15:387–389.
7. Dave PB, Romeu J, Antonelli A, Eiser AR: Gastrointestinal telangiectasias: A source of bleeding in patients receiving dialysis. Arch Intern Med 1984;144:1781–1783.
8. Zuckerman GR, Cornette GL, Clouse RE, et al: Upper gastrointestinal bleeding in patients with chronic renal failure. Ann Intern Med 1985; 102:588–592.
9. Campistol JM, Cases A, Torras A, et al: Visceral involvement of dialysis amyloidosis. Am J Nephrol 1987;7:390–393.
10. Bjarnason I, MacPherson A: The changing gastrointestinal side-effect profile of nonsteroidal anti-inflammatory drugs. A new approach for the prevention of a new problem. Scand J Gastroenterol 1989;24(Suppl 163):56–64.
11. Doherty CC: Gastrointestinal bleeding in dialysis patients. Nephron 1993;63:132–139.
12. Fedorak RN, Field M, Chang EB: Treatment of diabetic diarrhoea with clonidine. Ann Intern Med 1985;102:97–99.
13. Walker JJ, Kaplan BS: Efficacy of the somatostatin analogue octreotide in the treatment of two patients with diabetic diarrhea. Am J Gastroenterol 1993;88:765–767.
14. Morris-Stiff G, Coles G, Moore R, et al: Abdominal wall hernia in autosomal dominant polycystic kidney disease. Br J Surg 1997;84:615.
15. Markowitz GS, Stokes MB, Radhakrishnan J, D'Agati VD: Acute phosphate nephropathy following oral sodium phosphate bowel purgative: An unrecognized cause of chronic renal failure. J Am Soc Nephrol 2005;16: 389–396.
16. Maes BD, Dalle I, Geboes K, et al: Erosive enterocolitis in mycophenolate mofetil–treated renal transplant recipients with persistent afebrile diarrhea. Transplantation 2003;75:665–672.
17. Bergstom J: Nutrition and mortality in hemodialysis. J Am Soc Nephrol 1995;6:1329–1341.
18. Churchill DN, Taylor DW, Keshaviah PR: The CANUSA Peritoneal Dialysis Study Group: Adequacy of dialysis and nutrition in continuous peritoneal dialysis: Association with clinical outcomes. J Am Soc Nephrol 1996;7:198–207.
19. Kopple JD, Greene T, Chumlea W: Relationship between nutritional status and the glomerular filtration rate: Results from the MDRD Study. Int Soc Nephrol 2000;57:1688–1703.
20. Cheung W, Yu P, Little B, et al: Role of leptin and melanocortin signaling in uremia-associated cachexia. J Clin Invest 2005;115:1659–1665.
21. Mitch W: Mechanisms causing loss of lean body mass in kidney disease. Am J Clin Nutr 1998;67:359–366.
22. Stenvinkel P, Heimburger O, Paultre F, et al: Strong association between malnutrition, inflammation and atherosclerosis in chronic renal failure. Kidney Int 1999;55:1899–1911.
23. K/DOQI Clinical Practice Guidelines for Nutrition in Chronic Renal Failure. National Kidney Foundation. Am J Kidney Dis 2000;35(Suppl 2): S1–S140.
24. Enia G, Sicuso C, Alati G, Zoccali C: Subjective global assessment of nutrition in dialysis patients. Nephrol Dial Transplant 1993;8:1094–1098.
25. Makoff R: Vitamin replacement therapy in renal failure patients. Miner Electrolyte Metab 1999;25:349–351.
26. Stratton RJ, Bircher G, Foque D, et al: Multinutrient oral supplements and tube feeding in maintenance dialysis: A systematic review and meta-analysis. Am J Kidney Dis 2005;46:87–405.
27. Foulks CJ: An evidence-based evaluation of intradialytic parenteral nutrition. Am J Kidney Dis 1999;33:186–192.
28. Bruno M, Gabella P, Ramello A: Use of amino acids in peritoneal dialysis solutions. Perit Dial Int 2000;20(Suppl 2):s166–s171.
29. Rammohan M, Kalantar-Zadeh K, Liang A, Ghossein C: Megestrol acetate in a moderate dose for the treatment of malnutrition-inflammation complex in maintenance dialysis patients. J Renal Nutr 2005;15:345–355.
30. Dombros N, Dratwa M, Feriani M, et al: European best practice guidelines for peritoneal dialysis. 8. Nutrition in peritoneal dialysis. Nephrol Dial Transplant 2005; 20(Suppl 9):ix28–ix33.

Dermatologic Manifestations of Chronic Kidney Disease

Pieter Evenepoel and Dirk R. Kuypers

INTRODUCTION

Cutaneous disorders are common in patients with end-stage renal disease (ESRD), with the most prevalent disorder being hyperpigmentation. Many of these cutaneous disorders are due to the underlying renal disease, whereas others relate to the severity and duration of uremia.

Skin lesions associated with cutaneous aging have a high incidence in ESRD patients, including wrinkling, senile purpura, actinic keratoses, and diffuse hair loss. The prevalence of skin cancers does not appear to be increased, unless the patient had received or is receiving immunosuppression.

Improved treatments in dialysis patients have resulted in changes in the frequency and types of skin disorders observed in conjunction with ESRD. Dermatologic conditions such as uremic frost, erythema papulatum uremicum, uremic roseola, and uremic erysipeloid now rarely occur. Pigmentary alterations, xerosis, ichthyosis, half-and-half nails, acquired perforating dermatosis (Fig. 78.1), bullous dermatoses, pruritus, and calcific uremic arteriolopathy are prevalent, whereas the recently reported nephrogenic fibrosing dermopathy remains a rare entity.[1] The latter four skin disorders are the focus of this chapter since they are associated with significant morbidity and/or mortality and represent an ongoing diagnostic and/or therapeutic challenge.

UREMIC PRURITUS

Clinical Manifestations

Uremic pruritus (UP) is a frequent symptom of chronic renal failure with a reported prevalence ranging from 22% to 48%. Although its incidence in adult dialysis patients has declined due to improved dialysis efficacy and the introduction of biocompatible dialysis membranes, pruritus remains a frustrating problem for patients, causing serious discomfort and skin damage, often in association with disturbance of day and night rhythm, sleeping disorders, depression, anxiety, and diminished quality of life.[2] The intensity and spatial distribution of UP vary significantly between patients and over time throughout the course of renal disease. Excoriations, induced by uncontrollable scratching with or without superimposed infection, are frequently encountered in severely affected patients and rarely lead to prurigo nodularis, that is, a treatment-resistant lichenified or excoriated papulonodular chronic skin eruption (Fig. 78.2). The most frequently involved body areas are the back, limbs, chest, and face, while 20% to 50% of patients complain of generalized pruritus.[3]

Pathogenesis

Many uremic factors are thought to contribute to UP. Parathyroid hormone (PTH) and divalent ions (calcium, phosphate, and magnesium) have been implicated as itching is a frequent symptom accompanying severe secondary hyperparathyroidism and elevated calcium-phosphate product. However, the lack of consistent correlations between serum and skin levels of PTH, calcium, phosphorus, and magnesium with the severity of UP, indicates that other factors contribute to its development. Histamine released by mast cells has been implicated in UP. The number of dermal mast cells is increased in uremic patients, and higher tryptase and histamine plasma concentrations are reported in severe cases. Histamine release is triggered by substance P, a neurotransmitter involved in itch sensation. The role of elevated serotonin (5-hydroxytryptamine [5-HT3]) levels in dialysis patients with UP is debated as clinical trials using a selective inhibitor of 5-HT3 have yielded conflicting results (see later discussion). Xerosis is a very common skin problem (60% to 90%) in dialysis patients. Skin dryness is caused by primary dermal changes associated with uremia such as atrophy of sweat glands with impaired sweat secretion, disturbed stratum corneum hydration, sebaceous gland atrophy, and abnormal arborization of free cutaneous nerve fiber endings.

There are two major hypotheses of the mechanisms of UP. The opioid hypothesis proposes UP is caused by overexpression of opioid μ-receptors in dermal cells and lymphocytes. Consistent with this hypothesis, activation of the κ-opioid system using a κ-receptor agonist was efficient in reducing pruritus in a mouse model. In contrast, the immune hypothesis considers UP an inflammatory systemic disease rather than a local skin disorder. Studies examining the beneficial effects of ultraviolet B (UVB) exposure on pruritus showed that UVB attenuates the development of Th1 type lymphocytes in favor of the Th2 type. Indeed, the number of CXCR3-expressing and interferon-γ secreting CD4[+] cells (indicating Th1 differentiation) is significantly increased in the circulation of dialysis patients with pruritus compared to those without. Serum markers of inflammation such as C-reactive protein and interleukin-6 were also higher in subjects with UP.

Treatment

The treatment approach to UP is shown in Figure 78.3.

Optimizing Dialysis Therapy

Improving both dialysis efficacy and the nutritional status of the dialysis patient will result in a reduced prevalence and severity

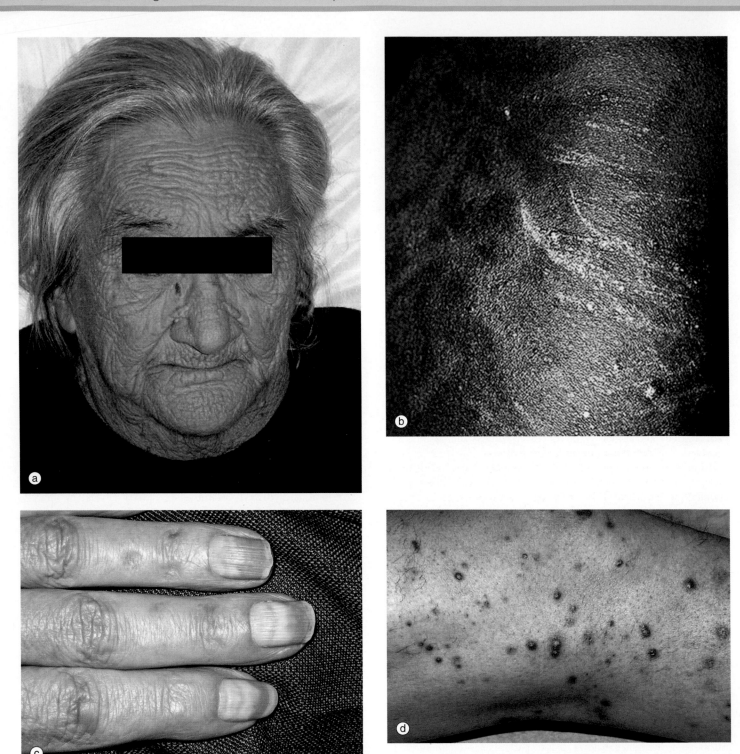

Figure 78.1   Cutaneous disorders in patients with end stage renal disease. *a*, A spectrum of pigmentary alterations occurs in dialysis patients, brownish hyperpigmentation in sun-exposed areas being the most prevalent. *b*, Xerosis, a dry or roughened skin texture, is seen in up to 75% of dialysis patients. *c*, Half-and-half nails (also termed red and white nails) occur in as many as 40% of patients on dialysis. The nails exhibit a whitish or normal proximal portion and an abnormal brown distal portion. *d*, Acquired perforating dermatosis affects approximately 10% of the dialysis population. The lesion is usually asymptomatic and consists of grouped dome-shaped papules and nodules, 1 to 10 mm in diameter. The trunk and the extremities are most commonly involved.

of UP. The use of so-called biocompatible hemodialysis (HD) membranes also has a beneficial effect. Adequate control of calcium and phosphorus plasma concentrations by using short-term low calcium and magnesium concentration dialysate ameliorated pruritus symptoms in only a few small studies and may lead to worsening of renal osteodystrophy in cases of prolonged use.

Parathyroidectomy is not advocated for relief of UP because no consistent beneficial effects have been demonstrated.

Skin Emollients

The application of emollients is probably still the primary therapeutic action undertaken by many nephrologists despite

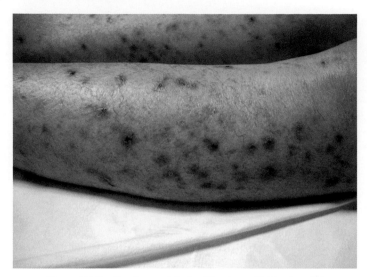

Figure 78.2   Prurigo nodularis. (Courtesy of I. Macdougall.)

contradictory results in the literature. The use of simple emollients without perfumes or other additives are preferred. Continuous bath oil therapy containing polidocanol, a mixture of monoether compounds of lauryl alcohol and macrogol, seems to be of value for some patients.

Antihistaminic Drugs
Classic antihistamines have limited efficacy and do not differ in efficacy compared to emollients; newer, second-generation antihistamines might have some effect but have not been formally tested in UP. Ketotifen (2 to 4 mg/day), a putative mast-cell stabilizer, was beneficial in a small patient group.

Phototherapy
UV light, especially UVB (wavelength 280 to 315 nm) is effective as treatment of UP and is well tolerated except for occasional sunburn. The duration of the antipruritic effect of thrice weekly

total body UVB therapy (total eight to 10 sessions) is variable but may last for several months. Potential carcinogenic effects of UV radiation require serious consideration, and its prolonged use is contraindicated in patients with a fair complexion (skin phototypes I to II).

5-Hydroxytryptamine Antagonist
Ondansetron, a selective 5-HT3 antagonist, was been used successfully in a small study in peritoneal dialysis patients. However, a subsequent larger randomized, placebo-controlled study failed to show superiority over placebo in HD patients.

Opioid Receptor Antagonists and Agonists
The oral μ-opiate receptor antagonist naltrexone seemed effective for the treatment of UP in a small randomized, crossover trial in 15 dialysis patients. In a subsequent larger trial, a significant difference in efficacy could not be demonstrated between 4 weeks of treatment with naltrexone (50 mg/day) or placebo. More recently a κ-receptor agonist, nalfurafine, given intravenously after HD, was tested in two randomized, double-blind, placebo-controlled trials comprising 144 patients. Itching intensity, excoriations, and sleep disturbances were significantly reduced in patients receiving the active compound without an excess of drug-related side effects compared to placebo.[4] In some patients, symptom relief between dialysis sessions was incomplete and central nervous system side effects such as drowsiness, dizziness, and somnolence occurred.

Gabapentin
Gabapentin, an anticonvulsant drug, was effective in reducing pruritus when administered after dialysis (300 mg). Careful dosing is advocated because of its neurotoxic side effects and narrow therapeutic window.[5]

Immunomodulators and Immunosuppressive Agents
A 7-day course of thalidomide reduced the intensity of UP by up to 80% in a placebo-controlled crossover study in 29 HD patients. Because of its strong teratogenic properties, thalidomide should probably be reserved for therapy-resistant severe UP in individuals outside the reproductive age category. Adverse effects of thalidomide such as peripheral neuropathy and cardiovascular side effects limit its continuous longer use. A prospective, single-center study of 25 chronic dialysis patients with UP demonstrated that 6 weeks of treatment with tacrolimus ointment (0.1%) significantly reduced the severity of UP. Tacrolimus was well tolerated in this trial and caused no detectable systemic exposure or side effects.[6] However, a subsequent smaller vehicle-controlled trial showed equal relief of UP with vehicle and tacrolimus. The risks of long-term topical use of these agents are currently unknown, and their prolonged use is not recommended until more data are available.

Long-Chain Essential Fatty Acids
Oral administration of γ-linoleic acid (GLA)–rich primrose oil resulted in significant improvement of UP in chronic dialysis patients. Supplementation of GLA-rich primrose oil is thought to augment synthesis of anti-inflammatory eicosanoids. Similar effects could be obtained by using fish oil, olive oil, and safflower oil.

Capsaicin
Capsaicin (trans-8-methyl-N-vanillyl-6-nonenamide) is a natural alkaloid found in the pepper plant that depletes the cutaneous type C sensory nerve endings of substance P. Two clinical studies

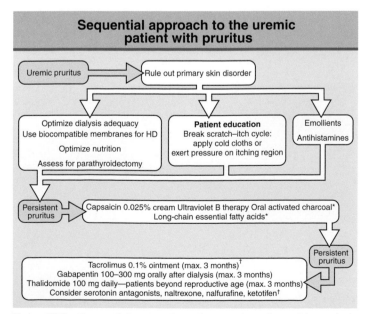

Figure 78.3   Sequential approach to the uremic patient with pruritus. *See text for details. †Therapeutic benefit in studies has been described variably; see text for details.

showed that application of a 0.025% capsaicin cream significantly alleviated UP in dialysis patients while exhibiting no side effects.

Oral Activated Charcoal

Pruritus symptoms completely disappeared or were significantly reduced in chronic dialysis patients treated with activated charcoal (6 g/day) for 8 weeks. In two different clinical studies, comparable results were obtained with this inexpensive and well-tolerated compound, rendering it a valuable alternative for patients with UP.

Miscellaneous

Various other types of therapies have been examined in the treatment of pruritus but are, despite the effectiveness of some, not considered as first choice in chronic hemodialysis patients because of undesirable side effects, cumbersome use, or incompatibility with renal replacement therapy (sauna, cholestyramine, nicergoline). Others have not been shown to effectively reduce UP in a controlled setting and are therefore not advocated (acupuncture, low-protein diet, intravenous lidocaine and mexiletine).

BULLOUS DERMATOSES

Bullous dermatoses are reported in up to 16% of patients on maintenance dialysis. They can be subdivided into true porphyrias (e.g., porphyria cutanea tarda [PCT] and variegate porphyria), pseudoporphyrias (e.g., secondary to nonporphyrinogenic drugs and chemicals and dialysis-porphyria), and other photodermatoses.[7] They are clinically and histologically similar and are characterized by a blistering photosensitive skin rash. The dorsal hands and the face are the most affected areas (Fig. 78.4).

PCT is caused by abnormalities in the porphyrin-heme biosynthetic pathway leading to an accumulation of highly carboxylated uroporphyrins in the plasma and skin. Phenotypic expression of the disease also requires one or more of a number of external contributory factors, including alcohol, estrogens, iron, and infection with hepatitis B and C. It is important to distinguish PCT from other porphyrias in which patients are at risk of developing potentially fatal neurologic attacks if exposed to porphyrinogenic drugs and other precipitants. Therapeutic options include avoidance of environmental triggers, HD with high-flux membranes, repeated small-volume phlebotomies, and iron chelators.

The term pseudoporphyria was originally used for patients with normal plasma porphyrins who exhibited PCT-like skin lesions secondary to drugs and chemicals. However, some dialysis patients also develop similar skin lesions that spontaneously heal and leave a hypopigmented area; a proportion of these have raised plasma porphyrins but without the disturbances in porphyrin metabolism classically found in the porphyrias. In rare patients, an offending medication can be identified. However, in most dialysis patients, protection from sun exposure appears to be the only preventive measure.

CALCIFIC UREMIC ARTERIOLOPATHY (CALCIPHYLAXIS)

Definition

Calcific uremic arteriolopathy (CUA), or calciphylaxis, is a devastating and life-threatening ischemic vasculopathy confined primarily to patients with renal failure. The ischemia may be so severe that frank infarction of downstream tissue develops. The most common and most noticeable damage is located in the skin and subcutaneous tissues.[8] CUA should be distinguished from benign nodular calcification (calcinosis cutis; Fig. 78.5), which can develop in patients with very high serum calcium-phosphate product.

Pathogenesis

The pathogenesis of CUA involves abnormalities in mineral metabolism in uremia that predispose to vascular and soft-tissue calcification, but no single abnormality is sufficient to predict the development of this disorder. Elevated levels of PTH and therapy with vitamin D analogues have been associated with an increased risk of CUA, although the evidence is not always striking. A perturbation of the calcium and phosphate homeostasis most probably underlies the positive association. Insufficient activation or expression of inhibitors of calcification should also be considered in the pathogenesis. Inhibitors of vascular calcification include matrix GLA protein (MGP), osteoprotegerin, and fetuin-A. MGP requires γ-carboxylation for its functional activity. As a consequence, warfarin and vitamin K deficiency may antagonize MGP function and stimulate vascular calcification. Levels of both osteoprotegerin and fetuin-A decline with inflammation. Finally, several lines of evidence indicate that a hypercoagulable state secondary to an absolute or functional protein C and/or protein S deficiency may be involved in the pathogenesis of CUA.[8]

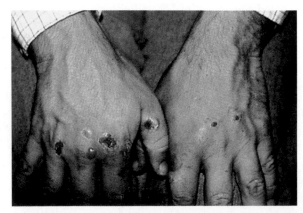

Figure 78.4 Porphyria cutanea tarda. Tense bullae, erosions, and crusts of the dorsal hands. (From Robinson-Bostom L, DiGiovanna JJ: Cutaneous manifestations of end-stage renal disease. J Am Acad Dermatol 2000;43:975–986.)

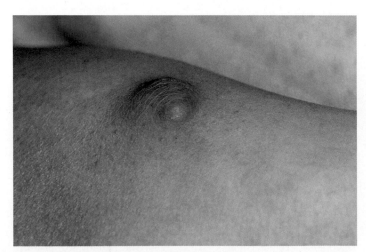

Figure 78.5 Benign nodular calcification (calcinosis cutis). Firm subcutaneous nodule adjacent to the elbow.

Epidemiology and Risk Factors

Although hard epidemiologic data are lacking, the incidence of CUA may be increasing. This might be due in part to increased physician awareness and possibly the practice of treating severe hyperparathyroidism with calcium-based phosphate binders plus vitamin D analogues. The estimated incidence rate ranges between 1 and 4 per 100 patient years.

Female gender, Caucasian race, obesity, diabetes, and dialysis vintage are established risk factors. Probable risk factors include the administration of warfarin, low serum concentrations of albumin, the use of calcium salts and vitamin D analogues, and exposure to high doses of iron salts. There is no correlation between the severity of any of these factors and the development of CUA.[8]

Clinical Manifestations

CUA is frequently precipitated by a specific event, such as local skin trauma or a hypotensive episode. CUA is typically characterized by areas of ischemic necrosis of the dermis, subcutaneous fat, and, less often, muscle. These ischemic changes lead to livedo reticularis and/or violaceous, painful, plaquelike subcutaneous nodules on the trunk, buttocks, or proximal extremity, that is, in areas of greatest adiposity (proximal CUA; Fig. 78.6a). The early purpuric plaques and nodules progress to ischemic/necrotic ulcers with eschars that often become superinfected. CUA can also affect the hands, fingers, and lower extremities, thereby mimicking atherosclerotic peripheral vascular disease (distal CUA; see Fig. 78.6b). Peripheral pulses are preserved distal to the area of necrosis. Myopathy, hypotension, fever, dementia, and infarction of the

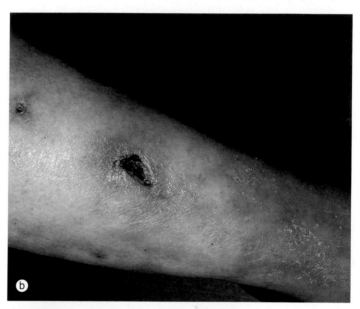

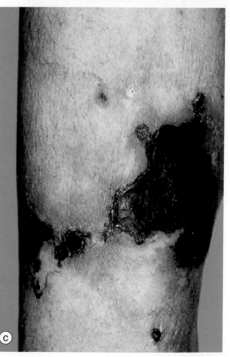

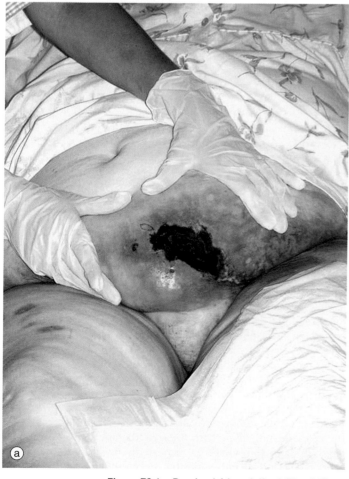

Figure 78.6 Proximal (*a*) and distal (*b*) calcific uremic arteriolopathy; (*c*), calcific uremic arteriolopathy.

central nervous system, bowel, or myocardium have been described in association with cutaneous necrosis. This condition is termed systemic CUA.[8,9]

Pathology

The histologic features of CUA are suggestive but not pathognomonic. Specimens from incisional biopsies of early lesions show subtle histologic changes. Late lesions characteristically show epidermal ulceration, dermal necrosis, and mural calcification with intimal hyperplasia of small and medium-sized blood vessels in the dermis and subcutaneous tissue (Fig. 78.7).

Diagnosis and Differential Diagnosis

Many clinicians base the diagnosis of CUA on physical examination findings only. Although ulceration is an obvious presentation of CUA, increasing awareness of the condition should allow diagnosis at an earlier, nonulcerative stage.[9] Biopsies are discouraged due to potential ulceration in the region of the incision and the risk of sample error. Other potentially useful diagnostic procedures include measurements of transcutaneous oxygen saturation, bone scintigraphy (Fig. 78.8), and xeroradiography.[9]

The following conditions should be considered in the differential diagnosis: systemic vasculitis, peripheral vascular disease, pyoderma gangrenosum, atheroemboli, cryoglobulinemia, warfarin-induced skin necrosis, and systemic oxalosis. Considering these risks, a skin biopsy should only be performed when clinical circumstances do not suggest CUA or when detailed clinical and

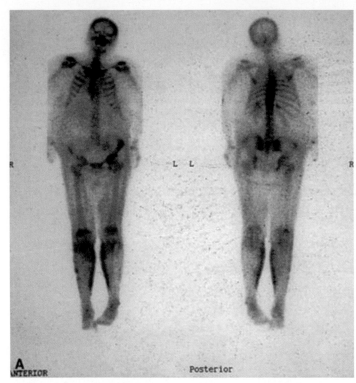

Figure 78.8 Bone scintigraphic abnormalities in calcific uremic arteriolopathy. Calf calcification in a patient with gross ulcerations in both legs from the popliteal fossae to the ankles. (From Fine A, Zacharias J: Calciphylaxis is usually non-ulcerating: Risk factors, outcome and therapy. Kidney Int 2002; 61:2210–2217.)

technical examinations, including the assessment of coagulation and immunologic parameters, point to an alternative diagnosis.

Natural History

Despite intensive combined treatments, the prognosis of CUA remains poor: the overall 1-year survival is 45% and the 5-year survival is 35%, with a relative risk of death of 8.5 compared with other dialysis patients. Patients with ulcerative and/or proximal CUA have the worst prognosis. Infection accounts for up to 60% of the mortality.[9]

Prevention and Treatment

Preventive approaches include attention to calcium, phosphorus, PTH homeostasis, and nutritional state. Specific therapeutic regimens have been limited to uncontrolled case series. A reasonable plan of intervention should include an aggressive program of wound care and prevention of superinfection, adequate pain control, and correction of underlying abnormalities in plasma calcium and phosphorus concentrations. This includes cessation of vitamin D supplementation, intensification of the dialysis treatment, and the use of a low-calcium dialysate and noncalcium-containing phosphate binders (e.g., sevelamer, lanthanum carbonate). Furthermore, local tissue trauma, including subcutaneous injections should be avoided. Parathyroidectomy has been found to be useful in the control of CUA in some series but not in others and should be reserved for patients with severe hyperparathyroidism.[8] In the latter patients, calcimimetic agents may represent a valid noninvasive alternative. Novel and experimental therapies include hyperbaric oxygen therapy and bisphosphonates. Sodium thiosulfate has repeatedly been used to enhance the solubility of calcium deposits[10] since exchange of calcium for sodium results in extremely soluble calcium thiosulfate. Besides

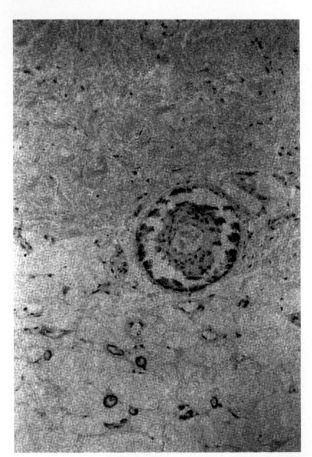

Figure 78.7 Histopathologic features of calcific uremic arteriolopathy. Medial calcification and intimal hyperplasia of an arteriole at the dermal-subcutaneous junction. Note calcification of interlobular capillaries in the subcutaneous tissue. (From Robinson-Bostom L, DiGiovanna JJ: Cutaneous manifestations of end-stage renal disease. J Am Acad Dermatol 2000;43:975–986.)

being a chelator of calcium, sodium thiosulfate is also a potent antioxidant. Sodium thiosulfate is given intravenously at the end of every HD (12.5 to 25 g over 30 to 60 minutes). Apart from nausea and vomiting, the therapy is well tolerated. The optimal duration of treatment is unknown.

NEPHROGENIC FIBROSING DERMOPATHY

Definition
Nephrogenic fibrosing dermopathy (NFD) is a recently described acquired, scleroderma-like, fibrosing disorder that develops in the setting of renal failure. The fibrotic process affects the dermis, subcutaneous tissues, fascia, and other organs, including striated muscles, heart, and lungs.[11]

Pathogenesis
The recent emergence and clustering of cases at major medical centers and renal transplantation centers suggest the possible involvement of an infectious agent or toxic contaminant. Very recently, gadolinium has been suggested to play a triggering role. Evidence points toward aberrant activation of circulating fibrocytes as a central event in the genesis of NFD. Other investigators have suspected that the strongly profibrotic mediator, transforming growth factor-β may be involved in the pathogenesis of NFD.

Epidemiology
NFD is a rare disorder. Since the identification of the first cases of NFD in 1997, the NFD registry has confirmed more than 170 cases from medical centers worldwide. NFD equally affects males and females. Besides kidney disease, conditions that may be associated with NFD include coagulation abnormalities and deep venous thrombosis, recent surgery (particularly vascular surgery), recent failure of a transplanted kidney, and sudden-onset kidney disease with severe edema of the extremities.

Clinical Manifestations and Natural History
The lesions of NFD are typically symmetrical and develop on limbs and trunk. A common location is between the ankles and midthighs and between the wrists and mid-upper arms bilaterally. Occasionally, swelling of the hands and feet, sometimes associated with bullae, is noted. The primary lesions are skin-colored to erythematous papules that coalesce into erythematous to brawny plaques with a *peau d'orange* appearance (Fig. 78.9a). These plaques have been described as having an ameboid advancing edge. Nodules are sometimes also described. Involved skin becomes markedly thickened and woody in texture. Joint contractures may develop very rapidly, with patients becoming wheelchair dependent within days to weeks of onset (see Fig. 78.9b). Patients often complain of pruritus, causalgia, and sharp pains in the affected areas.[11] In almost all cases of NFD, the disease course parallels the course of the underlying renal dysfunction. Although NFD has not been reported as a cause of death, the impairment of mobility seen in this disorder has led to fractures that ultimately resulted in a protracted hospital course and death.

Pathology
The histopathologic changes in affected skin include marked proliferation of spindle cells, the presence of numerous dendritic

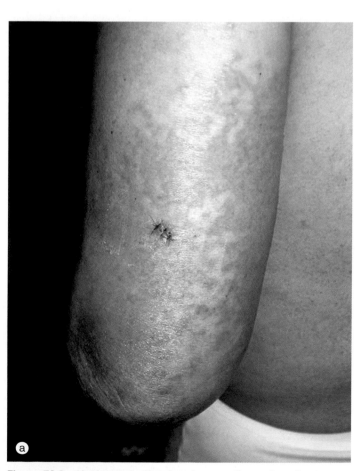
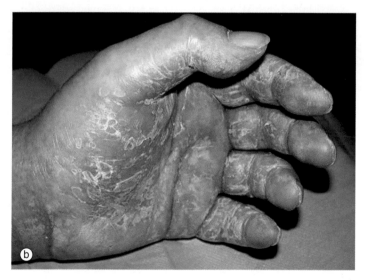

Figure 78.9 Nephrogenic fibrosing dermopathy. *a*, *Peau d'orange* appearance. *b*, Swelling of the hands, accompanied by palmar erythema, blisters, and contracture of the fingers.

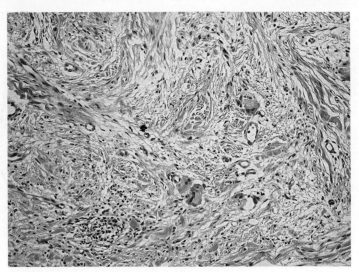

Figure 78.10 Histopathologic features of nephrogenic fibrosing dermopathy. Haphazardly arranged dermal collagen bundles with surrounding clefts and a strikingly increased number of similarly arranged spindled and plump fibroblast-like cells.

cells, and accumulation of mucinous material and thick collagen bundles (Fig. 78.10). Most dermal spindle cells in NFD have the immunophenotype of a circulating fibrocyte, a recently characterized circulating cell that expresses markers of both connective tissue cells and circulating leukocytes. Metastatic calcification and NFD may be found in the same lesion.

Diagnosis/Differential Diagnosis

The gold standard of diagnosis is histopathologic examination of skin biopsy specimens from an involved site. Skin lesions can also be visualized by [^{18}F]-fluorodeoxyglucose whole-body positron emission tomography. NFD resembles other fibrosing skin disorders including scleromyxedema, scleroderma, eosinophilic fasciitis, eosinophilia-myalgia syndrome, and Spanish toxic oil syndrome. The specific distribution of cutaneous involvement, the occurrence in the setting of renal failure, and the unique histopathologic features distinguish NFD from the other fibrotic disorders.

Treatment

At present, there is no consistently effective therapy for NFD. There is variable evidence for the efficacy of plasma exchange. Other therapeutic modalities that have been used (or are under investigation) include oral and topical steroids, selective histamine blockade, calcipotriene ointment, cyclophosphamide, cyclosporine, thalidomide, interferon-α, photophoresis, and PUVA (psoralen ultraviolet A) therapy. Intense physiotherapy is advised in every patient to prevent or reverse limb disability related to contractures of the joints.[11]

REFERENCES

1. Abdelbaqi-Salhab M, Shalhub S, Morgan MB: A current review of the cutaneous manifestations of renal disease. J Cutan Pathol 2003;30: 527–538.
2. Zucker I, Yosipovitch G, David M, et al: Prevalence and characterization of uremic pruritus in patients undergoing hemodialysis: Uremic pruritus is still a major problem for patients with end-stage renal disease. J Am Acad Dermatol 2003;49:842–846.
3. Mettang T, Pauli-Magnus C, Alscher DM: Uremic pruritus—new perspectives and insights from recent trials. Nephrol Dial Transplant 2002;17:1558–1563.
4. Wikstrom B, Gellert R, Soren D, et al: Kappa opioid system in uremic pruritus: Multicenter, randomized, double-blind, placebo-controlled clinical studies. J Am Soc Nephrol 2005;16:3742–3747.
5. Gunal AI, Ozalp G, Kurtulus Yoldas T, et al: Gabapentin therapy for pruritus in hemodialysis patients: A randomized, placebo-controlled, double-blind trial. Nephrol Dial Transplant 2004;19:3137–3139.
6. Kuypers DK, Claes K, Evenepoel P, et al: A prospective proof of concept study of the efficacy of tacrolimus ointment on uremic pruritus (UP) in patients on chronic dialysis therapy. Nephrol Dial Transplant 2004;19: 1895–1901.
7. Robinson-Bostom L, DiGiovanna JJ: Cutaneous manifestations of end-stage renal disease. J Am Acad Dermatol 2000;43:975–986.
8. Wilmer WA, Magro CM: Calciphylaxis: Emerging concepts in prevention, diagnosis, and treatment. Semin Dial 2002;15:172–186.
9. Fine A, Zacharias J: Calciphylaxis is usually non-ulcerating: Risk factors, outcome and therapy. Kidney Int 2002;61:2210–2217.
10. Guerra G, Shah RC, Ross EA: Rapid resolution of calciphylaxis with intravenous sodium thiosulfate and continuous venovenous hemofiltration using low calcium replacement fluid: Case report. Nephrol Dial Transplant 2005;20:1260–1262.
11. Cowper SE: Nephrogenic fibrosing dermopathy: The first 6 years. Curr Opin Rheumatol 2003;15:785–790.

Acquired Cystic Kidney Disease and Malignancies in Chronic Kidney Disease

Jürgen Floege and Frank Eitner

INTRODUCTION AND DEFINITION

Acquired cystic kidney disease (ACKD) was first recognized in 1847 by John Simon in patients with chronic Bright's disease. He described the development of cystic renal changes with cysts ranging from "mustard seed to as large as cocoa nuts" and also noted that they "run a slow and insidious progress during life, and often leave in the dead body no such obvious traces as would strike the superficial observer." ACKD was rediscovered by Dunnill and colleagues[1] in 1977 in kidneys of dialysis patients.

ACKD is a disease of chronic renal failure of any etiology and has to be differentiated from other types of cystic kidney disease (see Chapters 43 and 44). It is usually defined as more than three to five macroscopic cysts in each kidney of a patient who does not have a hereditary cause of cystic disease. ACKD is associated with renal neoplasms with such high frequency that some authors consider ACKD preneoplastic.[2]

PATHOGENESIS

Most cysts are lined by a single layer of epithelium composed of flat nondescript cells, cells with abundant cytoplasm and hyaline droplets, or small cuboidal cells resembling those from distal tubules or collecting ducts.[2] Others have argued that the presence of a brush border on the luminal membrane suggests that the cysts arise primarily from proliferation of proximal tubular epithelial cells. Although the mechanisms of tubule transformation into cysts are not entirely clear, tubular epithelial cell hyperplasia is currently viewed as a central early event in ACKD pathogenesis (Fig. 79.1).[3] Various factors have been implicated to explain the development of tubular hyperplasia, including plasticizer, ischemia, and uremic metabolites. However, the most important factor appears to be slow, progressive parenchymal loss, which could explain why the development or progression of ACKD does not appear to be influenced by the type of underlying renal disease or the choice of dialysis modality. The loss of intact nephrons is a strong stimulus for compensatory growth of the remaining, still intact nephrons, which is achieved by initial hypertrophy and later by hyperplasia. In these hyperplastic tubules, a cyst will develop if transepithelial fluid secretion continues and, owing to anatomic distortion or obstruction, the distal outflow is impaired.

With the continuing presence of mitogenic stimuli, the epithelial layer of the cyst becomes multilayered and atypical cells form intracystic papillary structures or mural adenomas. Activation of proto-oncogenes, chromosomal abnormalities plus additional factors such as genetic background, environmental chemicals, or sex hormones, thereafter probably account for the transition of the proliferative process into malignant growth (see Fig. 79.1).[3]

EPIDEMIOLOGY

Among patients entering dialysis treatment, the prevalence of ACKD ranging from 5% to 20% has been described. In both chronic hemodialysis and peritoneal dialysis patients, prevalence then increases at a similar rate and reaches 80% to 100% after 10 years of treatment (Fig. 79.2).[3-5] Children are also prone to develop ACKD. Several, but not all, studies have reported an increased frequency and/or faster progression in males than in females. The rate of progression appears to slow after 10 to 15 years of dialysis.

The frequency of ACKD as well as renal tumors in dialysis patients may be underestimated based on imaging methods alone. Renal cysts are detectable by ultrasonography with a minimum size of 0.5 cm. Recent data obtained in 260 native nephrectomy specimens at the time of transplantation with a median dialysis duration of 1 year only identified ACKD in 33%, renal adenomas in 14%, and renal cell carcinomas (RCCs) in 4% of the cases.[6]

Following renal transplantation, the course of ACKD is variable. There may be retardation of the progressive course of the disease or regression of the cysts, in particular if good long-term graft function is maintained. However, especially in grafts with impaired or failing renal function, there may be further progression in the native kidneys as well as the development of *de novo* ACKD in the graft.

CLINICAL MANIFESTATIONS

ACKD can manifest as unilateral or bilateral cysts, which are mostly cortical and variable in size and number. Rarely, severe ACKD can become macroscopically indistinguishable from adult polycystic kidney disease. In contrast to hereditary cystic diseases, the cysts of ACKD are strictly confined to the kidneys. The disease is usually asymptomatic and discovered accidentally during abdominal imaging procedures. Alternatively, it may manifest by potential complications or consequences of ACKD:

- Cystic hemorrhage with or without hematuria; bleeding may occur with cyst rupture with subsequent perinephric hemorrhage or retroperitoneal hemorrhage, which may in rare cases be severe enough to lead to hypovolemic shock

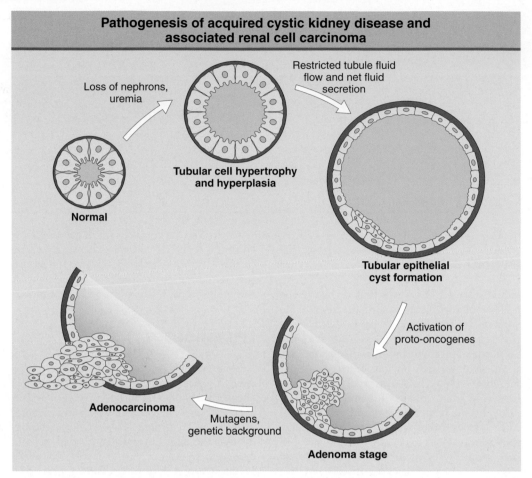

Pathogenesis of acquired cystic kidney disease and associated renal cell carcinoma

Loss of nephrons, uremia

Restricted tubule fluid flow and net fluid secretion

Tubular cell hypertrophy and hyperplasia

Normal

Tubular epithelial cyst formation

Activation of proto-oncogenes

Adenocarcinoma

Mutagens, genetic background

Adenoma stage

Figure 79.1 **Pathogenesis of acquired cystic kidney disease (ACKD) and associated renal cell carcinoma.** Diagram of events leading to the development of ACKD and subsequent malignant transformation. (Adapted from Grantham J: Acquired cystic kidney disease. Kidney Int 1991;40:143–152.)

- Calcifications in or around cysts and in rare cases stone formation (calcium-containing stones or β_2-microglobulin stones)
- Cyst infection, abscess formation, or sepsis
- Erythrocytosis in advanced cases, similar to erythrocytosis observed in polycystic kidney disease
- Malignant transformation[7]

Acquired Cystic Kidney Disease–Associated Renal Cell Carcinoma

Malignant transformation, the most feared complication of ACKD, accounts for about 80% of the renal cell neoplasms observed in uremic patients. In unselected series of chronic dialysis or transplant patients, the cumulative incidence of RCC complicating ACKD is probably <1%, although rates up to 7% have been reported in some small studies. These data indicate as much as a 40-fold increased risk of RCC in ACKD patients compared with RCC in the general population. Risk factors include male gender (male-to-female ratio, 7:1), African American ethnicity, long duration of dialysis, and severe ACKD with marked organ enlargement. It is unknown whether the risk of malignant transformation differs between hemodialysis and peritoneal dialysis patients. However, cases of malignant transformation in patients treated exclusively with peritoneal dialysis have been described.

About 85% of ACKD-associated RCCs are asymptomatic. The remaining cases mostly manifest with bleeding, usually gross hematuria, from the tumor. In cases in which nephrectomy had

to be performed in dialysis patients for intractable hematuria, RCCs, not visualized before surgery, were diagnosed in about one third of the patients. Compared with sporadic RCC, ACKD-associated RCC is characterized by younger patient age, male predominance, more frequent multicentric and bilateral manifestation, and less aggressive behavior.[2]

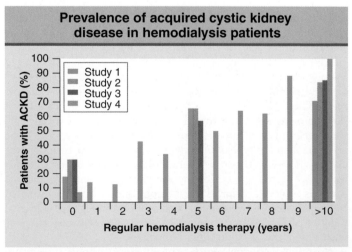

Prevalence of acquired cystic kidney disease in hemodialysis patients

Study 1
Study 2
Study 3
Study 4

Patients with ACKD (%)

Regular hemodialysis therapy (years)

Figure 79.2 **Prevalence of acquired cystic kidney disease (ACKD) in hemodialysis patients.** Summary of reported ACKD prevalences in chronic hemodialysis patients in relation to the length of hemodialysis treatment. Four separate studies are shown.

PATHOLOGY

Cystic changes in ACKD are typically bilateral but may vary between kidneys. Most ACKD kidneys are smaller than normal. An increase in size above normal can be observed in cases of cyst hematoma formation or malignant transformation. The cysts are usually restricted to the renal cortex. The size of the cysts ranges from microscopic to about 2 cm with about 60% of the cysts being <0.2 cm.[2] Preneoplastic changes can be detected in ACKD kidneys, including atypical cyst-lining cells forming multiple cell layers and intracystic nodular formations.

As many as 25% of kidneys with ACKD harbor tumors, about one third of which are carcinomas. RCCs arising from ACKD are multicentric in about 50% of cases, bilateral in about 10%, and predominantly of the papillary subtype. Transitional cell carcinoma (TCC) has been reported in ACKD, occasionally in addition to the presence of RCC. However, ACKD does not seem to increase the risk of TCC. Rather its development may be related to analgesic nephropathy as the underlying renal disease, although this notion remains speculative so far.

DIAGNOSIS AND DIFFERENTIAL DIAGNOSIS

The diagnostic approach to ACKD usually involves ultrasonography (Fig. 79.3), which is a sensitive means of detecting ACKD or large RCCs.[4,8] However, the differentiation between simple cysts and renal carcinomas can be difficult given the echogenicity of end-stage kidney parenchyma and the complexity of cysts in ACKD. Computed tomography (CT) scanning, in particular when used with early contrast enhancement, is superior to ultrasonography in detecting small malignant lesions (see Fig. 79.3).[4,8,9] Gadolinium-enhanced magnetic resonance imaging may also be useful when radiographic contrast agents cannot be administered, but its diagnostic power for detecting small carcinomas is probably no better than CT scanning.[8] Fine-needle aspiration may be necessary to clarify equivocal findings.[10] However, even with all these imaging

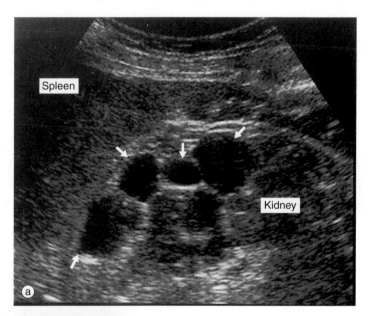

Figure 79.3 Imaging studies in acquired cystic kidney disease (ACKD). *a*, Ultrasound image of the left native kidney of a patient after 16 years of hemodialysis. Multiple cysts (*arrows*) are present in the renal cortex. *b*, Computed tomography image of a patient after 5 years of hemodialysis demonstrating multiple cysts within the right kidney (*white dashed circle*). This patient underwent a tumor nephrectomy of the left kidney 9 years prior to developing end-stage renal disease. *c*, Contrast-enhanced computed tomography image of a renal transplant recipient who developed a renal cell carcinoma originating in the left native kidney with ACKD (*white dashed circle*).

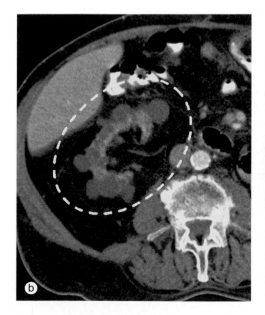

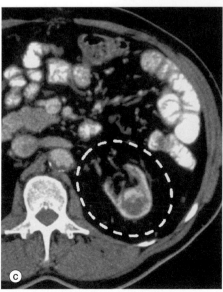

techniques, RCCs (≤8 cm) have been missed in severely distorted kidneys. Criteria that would favor the diagnosis of an RCC as opposed to a simple cyst include thickened and irregular walls, the presence of septae or renal tissue within the lesions, contrast enhancement, multilocularity, and large size (>4 cm).

Because of the risk of malignant transformation, screening for ACKD on a regular basis, as well as regular follow-up imaging in cases of established ACKD, has been advocated after 3 years of renal failure. One recent proposal, modified from Truong and associates,[7] is outlined in Figure 79.4. However, there is at present no consensus on screening strategies. This is because of the cost of screening as well as the risk-to-benefit ratio of nephrectomy in dialysis patients. A decision analysis[5] concluded that screening for ACKD (using either ultrasound or CT scanning) in young patients with a life expectancy of 25 years offers them as much as a 1.6-year gain in life expectancy. This is similar to the gain obtained in young healthy people who stop smoking. In contrast, in ACKD patients older than 60 years of age, no significant gain in life expectancy is achieved by regular screening.[5] In a different analysis of 797 dialysis patients who had developed RCCs (90% identified by screening, 10% by clinical symptoms), screening provided a mean survival benefit of 3.3 years after adjustment for age and dialysis vintage.[11] Screening during transplant evaluation by ultrasonography followed by CT in case of suspicious lesions is recommended based on recent data showing a prevalence of renal cancer in up to 4% of the patients and concerns about the role of immunosuppression in accelerating tumor growth.[12]

NATURAL HISTORY

Microscopically, cystic dilatations of renal tubules develop once the creatinine clearance decreases to <70 ml/min.[13] Macroscopic cysts start to develop when serum creatinine increases to >3 mg/dl (264 µmol/l). As discussed previously, ACKD thereafter progresses and reaches a prevalence of nearly 100% after >10 years of dialysis (sec Fig. 79.2). In malignant transformation, tumor growth rates are highly variable. The incidence of metastases at diagnosis (15%

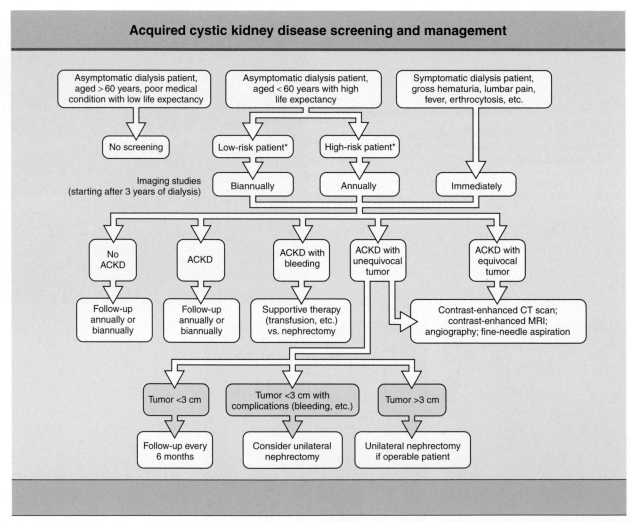

Figure 79.4 Proposed approach to ACKD screening and management of suspected renal cell carcinoma. ACKD, acquired cystic kidney disease; CT, computed tomography; MRI, magnetic resonance imaging. *Risk factors for malignant transformation in ACKD include long duration of dialysis, male gender, marked enlargement of native kidneys resulting from ACKD. (Adapted from Truong LD, Krishnan B, Cao JT, et al: Renal neoplasm in acquired cystic kidney disease. Am J Kidney Dis 1995;26:1–12; and modified according to Sarasin FP, Wong JB, Levey AS, Meyer KB: Screening for acquired cystic kidney disease: A decision analytic perspective. Kidney Int 1995;48:207–219.)

to 30% of cases) and 5-year survival rates (35%) are comparable to those observed in RCC in the general population. Death is usually associated with widespread metastases and accounts for about 2% of the deaths in renal transplant patients. It is not established whether renal transplantation affects the natural history of RCC complicating ACKD, although immunosuppression, in particular by cyclosporine, has been suggested as a risk factor for RCC in transplant patients with ACKD.[7]

TREATMENT

Treatment of ACKD is only warranted when complications such as hemorrhage, cyst infection, or malignant transformation develop. While the first two complications may be handled conservatively and only rarely require surgery, malignant transformation should raise the question of nephrectomy. Given the perioperative morbidity and mortality of nephrectomy, in particular in multimorbid dialysis or transplant patients, it is not surprising that the threshold for surgical intervention in cases of RCC is still controversial.

Most authors agree that tumors >3 cm in diameter justify nephrectomy because above this size, RCCs in the general population frequently metastasize (see Fig. 79.4).[7] However, first, it must be stressed that this strategy is based on an extrapolation from otherwise healthy persons; second, that tumor size in ACKD is often difficult to establish by imaging studies (especially given its frequent multilocular development); and, last, that metastases have been described even in ACKD where renal tumors were not detected by imaging studies.

In the case of tumors <3 cm in diameter with no complications, the slow tumor growth may justify observation with repeated imaging studies (see Fig. 79.4). Tumor enlargement should be used as an indication for nephrectomy if permitted by the patient's status. Where complications such as back pain or persistent hematuria are present, nephrectomy has been recommended by some, but not all authors.[7]

A prophylactic contralateral nephrectomy, in the case of unilateral tumors, is not routinely recommended by most investigators because of the morbidity associated with the procedure, the worsening of anemia, and the loss of residual renal function. Bilateral nephrectomy should, however, be considered in those patients likely to receive a transplant or who already received a transplant if there are concerns that immunosuppression may favor neoplastic growth.[7]

MALIGNANCIES IN DIALYSIS PATIENTS

Even if the risk of malignant transformation of ACKD is disregarded, dialysis patients have a slightly higher cancer risk as compared to the general population. Analysis of >800,000 dialysis patients in three registries from the United States, Europe, and Australia/New Zealand revealed that most of the increased risk was due to cancers of the kidney, bladder, and endocrine organs (Fig. 79.5).[14] Besides the specific risk associated with malignant transformation of ACKD, some of the increased risk is directly related to the underlying renal disease or to the immunosuppression that may have been administered in patients with immune-

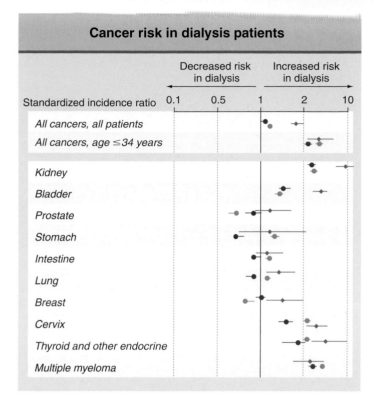

Figure 79.5 Cancer risk in dialysis patients. Relative risk of cancer (plus 95% confidence interval) compared to the general populations in 831,804 dialysis patients from Australia/New Zealand (*blue diamonds*), Europe (*red circles*), and the United States (*green circles*). (Adapted from Maisonneuve P, Agodoa L, Gellert R, et al: Cancer in patients on dialysis for end-stage renal disease: An international collaborative study. Lancet 1999;354:93–99.)

mediated renal disease. Cyclophosphamide therapy, for example, may predispose to bladder cancer that presents after patients have been started on dialysis. Renal disease or immunosuppressive therapy may underlie the apparent risk of dialysis patients to develop multiple myeloma (see Fig. 79.5). In addition, patients with analgesic nephropathy or Chinese herb nephropathy are at high risk of developing TCC of the urinary tract.[15] Especially after renal transplantation, these tumors tend to be less differentiated and in an advanced stage and the patients have a relatively poor outcome. Patients with analgesic nephropathy should therefore be screened for the presence of TCC before transplantation and annually after transplantation. It has been advocated that screening should include cystoscopy, retrograde ureteral catheterization with washings and brushings, and sonographic imaging.[16]

Other malignancies that have been observed at increased frequencies in dialysis patients include carcinoma of the cervix, thyroid, and other endocrine neoplasias (see Fig. 79.5) and, at least in the United States Renal Data System database, a 1.5- to twofold increase in risk for non-Hodgkin's lymphoma, Hodgkin's disease, and other leukemias.[14] This suggests that female dialysis patients, like the general population, should undergo at least annual gynecologic screening including cervical smear. An annual thyroid ultrasound scan is probably also justified, although no formal decision analysis is available to support this recommendation; lymphoma and leukemia screening will be difficult to impose, and instead clinical vigilance is advocated.

REFERENCES

1. Dunnill MS, Millard PR, Oliver D: Acquired cystic disease of the kidneys: A hazard of long-term intermittent maintenance haemodialysis. J Clin Pathol 1977;30:868–877.
2. Truong LD, Choi YJ, Shen SS, et al: Renal cystic neoplasms and renal neoplasms associated with cystic renal diseases: Pathogenetic and molecular links. Adv Anat Pathol 2003;10:135–159.
3. Grantham JJ: Acquired cystic kidney disease. Kidney Int 1991;40:143–152.
4. Levine E: Acquired cystic kidney disease. Radiol Clin North Am 1996;34:947–964.
5. Sarasin FP, Wong JB, Levey AS, Meyer KB: Screening for acquired cystic kidney disease: A decision analytic perspective. Kidney Int 1995;48:207–219.
6. Denton MD, Magee CC, Ovuworie C, et al: Prevalence of renal cell carcinoma in patients with ESRD pre-transplantation: A pathologic analysis. Kidney Int 2002;61:2201–2209.
7. Truong LD, Krishnan B, Cao JT, et al: Renal neoplasm in acquired cystic kidney disease. Am J Kidney Dis 1995;26:1–12.
8. Choyke PL: Acquired cystic kidney disease. Eur Radiol 2000;10:1716–1721.
9. Takebayashi S, Hidai H, Chiba T, et al: Using helical CT to evaluate renal cell carcinoma in patients undergoing hemodialysis: Value of early enhanced images. AJR Am J Roentgenol 1999;172:429–433.
10. Todd TD, Dhurandhar B, Mody D, et al: Fine-needle aspiration of cystic lesions of the kidney. Morphologic spectrum and diagnostic problems in 41 cases. Am J Clin Pathol 1999;111:317–328.
11. Ishikawa I, Honda R, Yamada Y, Kakuma T: Renal cell carcinoma detected by screening shows better patient survival than that detected following symptoms in dialysis patients. Ther Apher Dial 2004;8:468–473.
12. Gulanikar AC, Daily PP, Kilambi NK, et al: Prospective pretransplant ultrasound screening in 206 patients for acquired renal cysts and renal cell carcinoma. Transplantation 1998;66:1669–1672.
13. Liu JS, Ishikawa I, Horiguchi T: Incidence of acquired renal cysts in biopsy specimens. Nephron 2000;84:142–147.
14. Maisonneuve P, Agodoa L, Gellert R, et al: Cancer in patients on dialysis for end-stage renal disease: An international collaborative study. Lancet 1999;354:93–99.
15. Stewart JH, Buccianti G, Agodoa L, et al: Cancers of the kidney and urinary tract in patients on dialysis for end-stage renal disease: Analysis of data from the United States, Europe, and Australia and New Zealand. J Am Soc Nephrol 2003;14:197–207.
16. Swindle P, Falk M, Rigby R, et al: Transitional cell carcinoma in renal transplant recipients: The influence of compound analgesics. Br J Urol 1998;81:229–233.

CHAPTER

80 Approach to Renal Replacement Therapy

Hugh C. Rayner

MAKING DECISIONS ABOUT STARTING DIALYSIS

If every patient who developed end-stage renal disease (ESRD) was started on dialysis, the incidence rates of new dialysis patients in different countries would reflect the epidemiology of progressive renal disease. Incidence rates of treated ESRD patients are summarized in the annual report of the United States Renal Data System (USRDS). Data from 2003 show a wide variation across the world, much larger than could be explained by disease incidence alone (Fig. 80.1). This suggests that there are marked differences between countries in the way decisions are made about starting dialysis.

FACTORS INFLUENCING THESE DECISIONS

Availability of Dialysis Facilities

Renal replacement therapy (RRT) is unavailable to the majority of the world's population with renal failure.[1] There is a strong relationship between the number of patients on RRT per million population and a country's per capita income: 644 patients per million in the 15 European Union countries (average gross per capita income >US$22,000) compared with 166 in Central and Eastern European countries (average income US$4480) and 52 in Bangladesh (average income US$370). Even in affluent European and North American countries (e.g., France, the UK, and the US), lack of hemodialysis (HD) resources is given as a reason for delaying dialysis.[2,3]

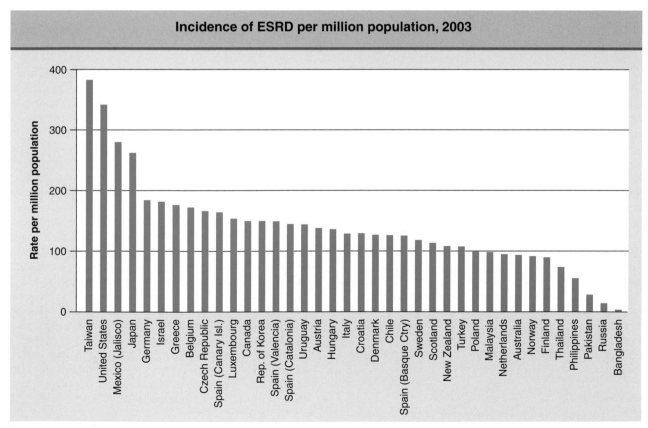

Figure 80.1 Incidence of end-stage renal disease (ESRD) per million population in 2003. Data presented only for those countries from which relevant information was available. All rates are unadjusted. Data from Israel, Jalisco (Mexico), Japan, Luxembourg, the Philippines, and Taiwan represent dialysis only. (Data supplied by the United States Renal Data System. The interpretation and reporting of these data are the responsibility of the author and in no way should be seen as an official policy or interpretation of the U.S. government.)

Patient Selection by Physicians and Nephrologists

The practice of starting dialysis in patients who are very elderly or dependent on others for their care or who have multiple comorbid conditions varies significantly among countries and among nephrologists within those countries.[2,3] For example, the percentage of patients who were living in a nursing home or who were unable to eat independently within 90 days of starting dialysis is much higher in the United States (11.6%) than in France (1.3%), Germany (6.4%), Italy (4.7%), Spain (2.0%), and the United Kingdom (1.5%).[2] That nephrologists' decisions affect the population of patients starting dialysis is confirmed by the finding that the odds of new patients being older than the age of 80 are significantly lower in units whose medical directors agree that they do not start dialysis in the very elderly.[2]

Severe intellectual impairment in a patient would much more strongly influence a nephrologist in the United Kingdom not to start dialysis than in the United States.[2,3] Furthermore, nephrologists in the United States were much more likely than those in the United Kingdom and Canada to start dialysis in patients with dementia or in a persistent vegetative state, if pressured to do so by family members. Fear of litigation was particularly influential in persuading U.S. and Canadian nephrologists to offer treatment.[3]

The Renal Physicians Association/American Society of Nephrology (RPA/ASN) guidelines for the initiation of dialysis in the United States provide a systematic approach to conflict resolution if there is disagreement regarding the benefits of dialysis (Fig. 80.2).[4]

ARE THERE OBJECTIVE CRITERIA FOR THE RATIONING OF DIALYSIS TREATMENT?

On the grounds that the greatest good should be derived from the limited resources available, it has been argued that patients who are expected to survive for only a few months should not be offered dialysis. This is supported by the view that it is preferable to avoid suffering by not starting dialysis than to withdraw treatment when the patient's condition becomes distressing.[5] Withdrawing dialysis seems more like actively causing death than withholding dialysis, where death is allowed to occur naturally.

This utilitarian approach to the allocation of resources is contrary to the instincts of most doctors to act in the patient's best interest and may be unacceptable to many physicians. Furthermore, it does not take into account the value of even a short extension of life that allows the patient and his or her family to prepare for death. It also makes only a small contribution to minimizing the use of resources as the costs of an HD program are in proportion to the length of time that the patient continues to receive treatment.

Age Criterion

Against this ethical background, are there any objective criteria that can be applied to identify patients who are unsuitable for dialysis? One criterion to be dismissed is age. Although advanced age was used as a simple exclusion criterion in the early days of dialysis, the elderly are now the most rapidly growing section of the dialysis population. Their quality of life can be good; indeed, their expressed satisfaction with life may be greater than that of younger dialysis patients.[6]

Predictive Factors

Two studies have attempted to identify other predictive factors. In a prospective Canadian study of patients starting dialysis,[7] a comorbidity scoring system was used to quantify factors likely to predict early death and the predictive value of this scoring system was compared with the value of an estimate made by the patient's nephrologist of the probability that the patient would die within 6 months. It was not possible to predict early death accurately using either the comorbidity scoring system or the clinician's opinion. Indeed, it was impossible even to identify the small proportion of patients with a very poor prognosis. Clinicians were more accurate than the scoring system in identifying patients with a <50% risk of death by 6 months, but they tended to overestimate the risk of death in the worst prognostic groups. For example, 30% of the patients whose predicted probability of death was considered to be 80% survived for >6 months.

In a UK study,[8] a high-risk group of 26 patients was identified using factors associated with poor survival in a statistical model that included poor functional status at presentation, comorbidity, and underlying disease. Although these patients had a 1-year survival rate of only 19.2%, four patients survived at least 2 years. Furthermore, the cost incurred by this high-risk group was only 3.2% of the total cost of the chronic dialysis program. These important studies should strengthen the resolve of clinicians to resist any imposition of rationing criteria on dialysis provision.

ADVISING A PATIENT ABOUT PROGNOSIS ON DIALYSIS

Despite these uncertainties, an individual patient should be given an estimate of his or her likely future on dialysis. Factors associated with a poorer prognosis in a large number of studies include advanced age, male gender, decreased serum albumin, malnutrition, impaired functional status, diabetes mellitus, and coronary heart disease. Quality of life is strongly predictive of mortality, even after statistical correction for these comorbid factors.[9]

For patients whose prognosis is particularly uncertain or where there is disagreement between the views of the patient and the dialysis team, a time-limited trial of dialysis may be offered.[4] This trial will give the patient and his or her family a better understanding of what life on dialysis entails and allow time for further discussion between all parties. The duration of the trial should be judged for each individual, and clinical and biochemical parameters reviewed regularly. In our experience of 31 patients older than the age of 79 on HD, 10 patients who were hypoalbuminemic at the start of dialysis and whose serum albumin had decreased by >3 g/l to <30 g/l after 4 weeks on dialysis had all died by 6 months. The median survival of the other 21 patients was 1.3 years (unpublished observations).

Most people would agree that patients who are certain to have an unacceptable quality of life should not be subjected to the discomfort of dialysis. In patients with multiple comorbidities, improving quality of life is more relevant than quantity. Many of the symptoms and complications of ESRD, for example, anemia, acidosis, pruritus, insomnia, depression, fluid overload, and hypertension, can be treated with medication and so a decision not to start dialysis is not the same as a decision to withhold active treatment. Such conservative therapy is best delivered by the specialist multidisciplinary team that delivers care to all patients with ESRD not yet on dialysis and should include social worker and psychologist support. The team should have close links with palliative care specialists so that there is a smooth transition from active medical therapy to terminal care.

IF THE PATIENT DOES NOT WANT DIALYSIS

Nephrologists may be presented with the dilemma of a mentally competent patient whom they would normally treat, but who does

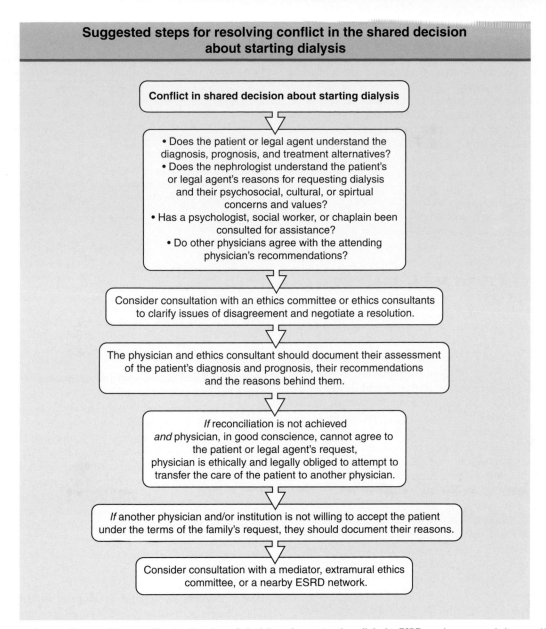

Suggested steps for resolving conflict in the shared decision about starting dialysis

Conflict in shared decision about starting dialysis

- Does the patient or legal agent understand the diagnosis, prognosis, and treatment alternatives?
- Does the nephrologist understand the patient's or legal agent's reasons for requesting dialysis and their psychosocial, cultural, or spirtual concerns and values?
- Has a psychologist, social worker, or chaplain been consulted for assistance?
- Do other physicians agree with the attending physician's recommendations?

Consider consultation with an ethics committee or ethics consultants to clarify issues of disagreement and negotiate a resolution.

The physician and ethics consultant should document their assessment of the patient's diagnosis and prognosis, their recommendations and the reasons behind them.

If reconciliation is not achieved *and* physician, in good conscience, cannot agree to the patient or legal agent's request, physician is ethically and legally obliged to attempt to transfer the care of the patient to another physician.

If another physician and/or institution is not willing to accept the patient under the terms of the family's request, they should document their reasons.

Consider consultation with a mediator, extramural ethics committee, or a nearby ESRD network.

Figure 80.2 Suggested steps for resolving conflict in the shared decision about starting dialysis. ESRD, end-stage renal disease. (Adapted from Renal Physicians Association and American Society of Nephrology: Shared Decision-Making in the Appropriate Initiation of and Withdrawal from Dialysis. Clinical Practice Guideline, Number 2. Washington, DC: Renal Physicians Association, 2000.)

not wish to have dialysis.[4] From an ethical viewpoint, decisions not to start dialysis and to withdraw dialysis are justified on the principle of individual autonomy. Similarly, in the United Kingdom, they are legally based on the individual's common-law right to self-determination and in the United States, the constitutional right of liberty. Where the patient is able to express a clear wish, the physician is obliged to respect this because to treat a patient against his or her will would constitute an assault. The physician must nonetheless ensure that all reversible factors have been addressed, such as unfounded fears about what dialysis will entail or a depressive illness affecting the patient's judgment and ideally request a psychiatric evaluation. It is not uncommon for patients to express a strong desire not to have dialysis, particularly if they are relatively asymptomatic, only to change their mind when they become more symptomatic. At this late stage, the basic will to survive comes to the fore. An advance directive written by the patient should never be held as a reason against a change of mind.

DISAGREEMENT ABOUT A DECISION TO DIALYSE A PATIENT

There will inevitably be differences of opinion about the benefits of dialysis for individual patients. Dialysis nurses may disagree with the nephrologist's decision to treat a patient. If the dialysis nurses and doctors are functioning well as a team, they should feel able to express these reservations and have the issue adequately discussed. It is very demoralizing for individual staff and the team as a whole if they feel pressured into giving treatment that they believe is inappropriate.

The nephrologist may remain unwilling to offer dialysis despite the insistence of the patient or, more often, the patient's care providers, the legal agent, or another doctor (see Fig. 80.2). Dialysis must never be given at the insistence of others if it is against the patient's clearly expressed wishes. However, if the patient insists on treatment against the nephrologist's advice, dialysis should usually be given while a resolution is reached. Extensive discussions and explanations of the treatment options and prognosis may be needed to gain a better understanding of the reasons behind the differing views. Helpful advice may be obtained from another physician, particularly the patient's family doctor who will have a broader understanding of the patient's circumstances. It may be appropriate to involve a psychologist, social worker, or religious counselor. If the conflict persists, it may be necessary to refer the case to a formal ethics committee, if one exists locally, to clarify the issues of disagreement and enable a resolution. A physician cannot be compelled to offer treatment against his or her considered professional judgment, but the physician is ethically and legally obliged to attempt to transfer the care of the patient to another physician. Only as a last resort, if no alternative dialysis unit can be found and after adequate advance notice has been given, should dialysis be withdrawn.[4]

CHOICE BETWEEN PERITONEAL DIALYSIS AND HEMODIALYSIS

The majority of patients with ESRD are suitable for treatment with either peritoneal dialysis (PD) or HD. It is difficult to envisage an ethically acceptable trial where patients are allocated randomly to PD or HD and the various possible modifications within each modality make a simple comparative trial impractical. Retrospective comparative studies have failed to indicate a consistent survival advantage for either modality.[10,11] A recent prospective cohort study from 81 U.S. dialysis clinics attempted to overcome the limitations of these studies, although it was still not a randomized study.[12] No significant difference in outcomes was found between HD and PD during the first year of treatment, but in the second year, the risk of death was significantly greater in those on PD. The increased risk was mainly in patients with cardiovascular comorbidity and is consistent with two other U.S. studies that showed patients with coronary artery disease and congestive heart failure have a shorter survival on PD than HD. This contradicts a commonly expressed opinion that PD is more gentle for such patients as it avoids rapid fluid shifts and causes less stress on the heart.[13,14]

When making their choice, patients should be aware that the chances of a change in treatment modality may be up to fivefold greater for PD (to HD) than for HD (to PD) and that change in treatment from PD to HD is associated with an increased risk of hospitalization and mortality.[15] A planned change from PD to HD may not be associated with this increased risk, although this has not been studied systematically in a large population.

Contraindications to Peritoneal Dialysis

There are a few situations where there is a consensus that PD is contraindicated (Fig. 80.3). These situations have been agreed on by the consensus panel of the National Kidney Foundation Dialysis Outcomes Quality Initiative (NKF-DOQI).[16] Relative contraindications to PD are discussed in the following sections.

Fresh Intra-abdominal Foreign Body

Patients with prosthetic aortic grafts have been successfully treated with PD. HD is usually used initially for up to 16 weeks to allow the graft to be covered with epithelium and so avoid the risk of graft infection via peritoneal dialysate. However, this risk must be balanced against that of bacterial seeding from the patient's HD access.

Contraindications to dialysis modalities	
Absolute	**Relative**
Peritoneal dialysis	
Loss of peritoneal function producing inadequate clearance	Recent abdominal aortic graft
Adhesions blocking dialysate flow	Large polycystic kidneys
Surgically uncorrectable abdominal hernia	Ventriculoperitoneal shunt
	Intolerance of intra-abdominal fluid
Abdominal wall stoma	Large muscle mass
Diaphragmatic fluid leak	Morbid obesity
Inability to perform exchanges in absence of suitable assistant	Severe malnutrition
	Skin infection
	Bowel disease
	Carriage of *S. aureus*
Hemodialysis	
No vascular access possible	Difficult vascular access
	Needle phobia
	Cardiac failure
	Coagulopathy

Figure 80.3 Contraindications to dialysis modalities. Absolute and relative contraindications to hemodialysis and peritoneal dialysis. (Adapted from NKF-DOQI: NKF-DOQI Clinical Practice Guidelines for Peritoneal Dialysis Adequacy, 2000. Am J Kidney Dis 2001;37(Suppl I):S65–S136.)

Body Size Limitations and Intolerance of Intra-Abdominal Fluid Volume

Body size can be a problem at both ends of the spectrum. Small patients may be intolerant of the volume of dialysate needed to achieve adequate dialysis, particularly if they have negligible residual renal function. Alternative methods of fluid exchange such as nocturnal automated PD can be used to overcome this limitation. It may also be difficult to achieve adequate clearances in patients with a body mass index >35 kg/m^2. Discomfort due to increased intra-abdominal volume can be significant in patients with chronic respiratory disease, low-back pain, or large polycystic kidneys. In general, it is hard to predict a patient's tolerance of intra-abdominal fluid and so these limitations usually appear after a patient has started PD.

Bowel Disease and Other Sources of Infection

The presence of ischemic bowel disease, inflammatory bowel disease, or diverticulitis is likely to increase the incidence of peritonitis due to organisms passing through the bowel wall into the peritoneum. Abdominal wall infection may lead to peritonitis via the exit site and catheter tunnel.

Nasal carriage of *Staphylococcus aureus* increases the risk of subsequent staphylococcal exit site infection and peritonitis. Clearance of nasal *S. aureus* with topical mupirocin cream has been shown to reduce significantly the risk of staphylococcal infection at the exit site.[17] Unfortunately, the reduction in staphylococcal peritonitis is compensated for by an increase in peritonitis due to gram-negative organisms.

Severe Malnutrition or Morbid Obesity

Patients should ideally commence PD in an adequate nutritional state. Severe malnutrition may lead to poor wound healing and to leakage from the catheter tunnel. In addition, peritoneal protein losses during dialysis may exacerbate hypoalbuminemia and be particularly severe with continuous ambulatory peritoneal dialysis (CAPD) peritonitis. At the other end of the spectrum, it may prove difficult to satisfactorily place a peritoneal catheter through the abdominal wall in patients with morbid obesity. Thereafter, absorption of glucose from the dialysate, which may average as much as 800 calories per day, may contribute to further weight gain.

Contraindications to Hemodialysis

Contraindications to HD are few (see Fig. 80.3). As discussed in Chapter 81, access to the circulation can usually be obtained, even in patients with extensive vascular disease or previous surgery. An aversion to needle puncture of the arteriovenous fistula is common in the early stages, but can usually be overcome by careful use of local anesthetic and nursing encouragement. Severe coagulopathy may make management of anticoagulation for the extracorporeal circuit difficult.

HOME HEMODIALYSIS

HD patients should ideally be given the option of dialyzing at home. In the past two decades, the popularity of home HD has declined. For example, in the United Kingdom, the percentage of the dialysis population on home HD decreased from 35% in 1984 to 2% in 2003. Australia and New Zealand are the only countries with a significant proportion of patients on home HD (Fig. 80.4). This situation has occurred for a variety of reasons. First, HD requires the presence of an assistant throughout the period of dialysis in case the patient becomes hypotensive and/or unconscious. As an increasing proportion of new dialysis patients are elderly, there may be no one available who is able or willing to take on this considerable responsibility. Second, there is the added cost of installing a dialysis machine and its associated water treatment, which is not required for PD. However, the subsequent running costs are less for home than in-center HD.

Home HD can provide significant benefits for appropriate patients. It removes the inconvenience of traveling to and from the dialysis facility and gives patients the freedom to dialyze at a time to suit themselves. As a result, they are able to perform more hours of treatment per week with less disruption to their lives. Although there is no randomized, controlled trial comparing hospital and home HD, comparative studies, where correction has been made for differences in comorbidity, do suggest that patients on home HD have a better outcome in terms of morbidity and mortality.[18] Selected patients are able to dialyze every night at home. This gives much greater clearance than is possible with thrice weekly dialysis, and major improvements in anemia, blood pressure, and phosphate control have been demonstrated. The inconvenience of nightly treatment is balanced by the removal of dietary restrictions and antihypertensive medications, and an improved quality of life.[19] With improvements in technology, this form of treatment may become much more widespread.

PATIENT PREFERENCE FOR HEMODIALYSIS OR PERITONEAL DIALYSIS

A number of recent studies have quantified the choices that patients would make if they were offered a free choice between HD and PD. In our facility in Birmingham (United Kingdom) all patients entering the ESRD program are given modality-neutral counseling and allowed to select their preferred mode of treatment.[20] Between 1992 and 1998, patient choice was restricted for medical reasons by the physician in 54 of 333 patients (16%), PD being contraindicated in 51. Of the remainder, 55% chose HD and 45% PD. These relative proportions are the same as those

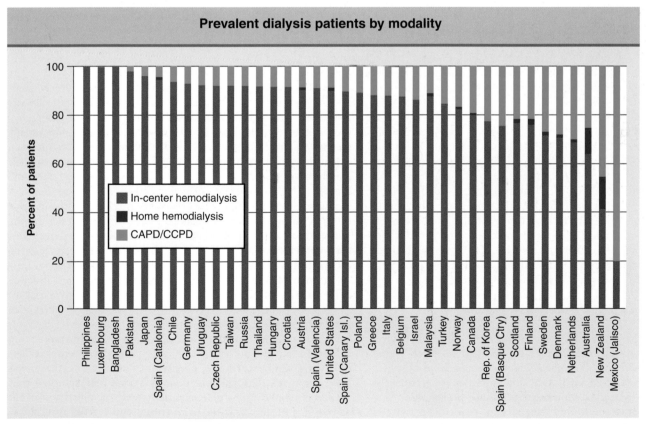

Figure 80.4 Prevalent dialysis patients by modality. Percentage of prevalent dialysis patients on each dialysis modality by country in 2003. CAPD/CCPD, continuous ambulatory peritoneal dialysis/continuous cycling peritoneal dialysis. (Data supplied by the United States Renal Data System. The interpretation and reporting of these data are the responsibility of the author and in no way should be seen as an official policy or interpretation of the U.S. government.)

found in a study of 5466 U.S. patients who received a program of predialysis education.[21] Independent predictors for choosing HD in our study were increasing age and male sex. Independent predictors for choosing CAPD in the United Kingdom and United States include being married, being counseled before the start of dialysis, and increasing distance from the base unit.[22] This last factor is a major influence in sparsely populated regions. For example, in New Zealand in 2003, 45% of patients received PD (see Fig. 80.4).

PATIENT CHOICE OF A DIALYSIS MODALITY

Of those able to choose, almost all patients can be started on their preferred modality of dialysis.[20] However, in the United States, while 45% of patients chose PD, only 33% actually started dialysis on this modality.[21] Furthermore, the major differences in dialysis modality among countries (see Fig. 80.4) suggest that the type of dialysis is more often decided by physicians rather than patients. Possible factors affecting these decisions are discussed.[23,24]

Arrangements for the Reimbursement of Physicians and Funding of Dialysis Facilities

The arrangements by which doctors and dialysis facilities are reimbursed for the cost of providing treatment vary widely around the world. There are also large differences between the levels of payment for HD and PD in many countries. For example, in French clinics, the facility is not reimbursed for PD and the physicians receive no fee. In countries such as the United Kingdom and Canada, where facilities are publicly funded from taxation, the use of more expensive types of HD, for example, high-flux hemodiafiltration, is limited. Conversely, in places such as Hong Kong, where dialysis is only available in the private sector, more patients are treated by PD than by HD, as the former is less expensive. In HD facilities, an arrangement whereby payment depends on the number of patients treated creates pressure to increase patient numbers. If the patient's nephrologist has a financial interest in the HD facility, this may also directly influence the decision on which modality of treatment to recommend.

Physician Preference

There is a strong preference for HD among some influential nephrologists on both sides of the Atlantic. In a USRDS survey reported in 1997, only 25% of HD patients remembered having PD discussed with them. In contrast, 68% of patients on PD reported discussions about HD. Interestingly, a much greater proportion of patients on HD felt that the choice had been made by the medical team rather than by either themselves or by joint decision. Since 1995, there has been a marked decline in the proportion of patients treated by CAPD in the United States (14% in 1995 to 8% in 2003) and Canada (36% in 1995 to 19% in 2003). The reasons for this are unclear.[25]

IMPORTANCE OF DIALYSIS ACCESS

In an ideal world, every patient would make an informed choice between peritoneal and HD after a period of in-depth counseling and preparation, and dialysis access would be established in advance of starting dialysis. Sadly, dialysis is frequently started in less than ideal circumstances. Late presentation is a worldwide phenomenon, indicating that no health care system has overcome the problems of identifying patients with chronic renal failure and bringing them to the attention of nephrologists in time (Fig. 80.5).[26,27]

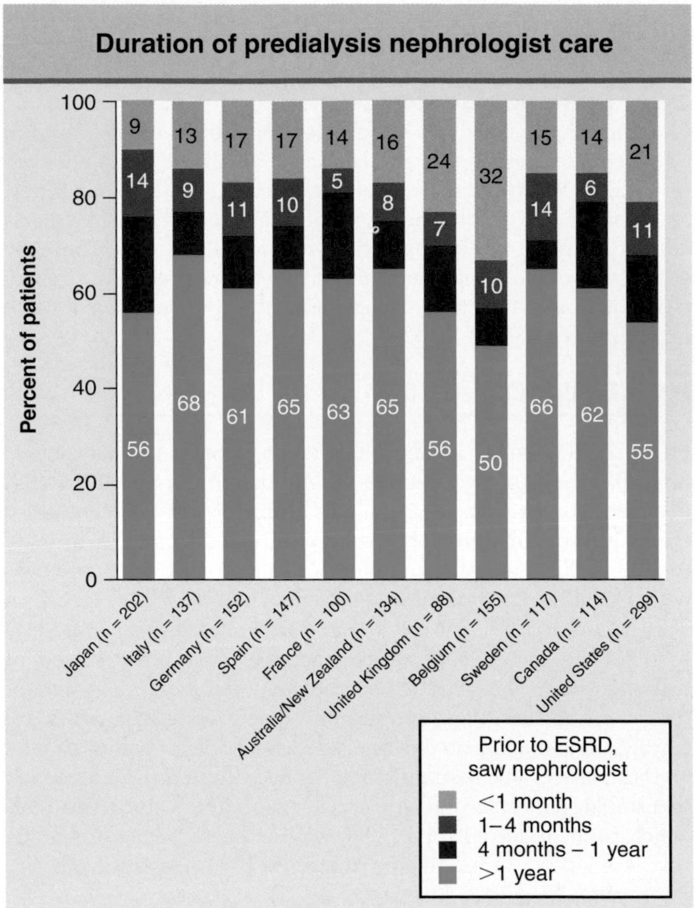

Figure 80.5 Duration of predialysis nephrologist care. Incident patients entering the DOPPS II Study (2002/2003) within 90 days of first dialysis treatment, based on patient responses. (Data from the Dialysis Outcomes and Practice Patterns Study [DOPPS], www.dopps.org.)

Reports from both Europe and the United States clearly document the excess morbidity and mortality associated with patients presenting late in ESRD and requiring dialysis as an emergency procedure.[27] Patients starting dialysis as an emergency usually receive HD via a catheter and tend to remain on HD rather than converting to PD. Compared with nonemergency patients, their length of hospital stay is significantly greater, and during this time there is a higher incidence of major complications and death. A significant part of the increased mortality is related to the use of a catheter rather than a permanent arteriovenous fistula. In the United States, many incident patients receive an arteriovenous graft rather than a fistula as it is believed that grafts can be cannulated more easily and earlier than fistulas[28] (Fig. 80.6).

International data from the Dialysis Outcomes and Practice Patterns Study showed a 37% increase in the relative risk of death in patients dialyzing via a catheter and a 19% increase in patients using a graft compared with a native arteriovenous fistula, after adjustment for a wider range of demographic and comorbid factors (both $P < 0.0001$).[29] The detrimental effects of central venous catheters persist even after the catheter has been removed. The survival rate of subsequent arteriovenous fistulas is significantly worse in patients who have had a previous catheter in place compared with those who started directly on a fistula, even after correcting for case mix and comorbidity, possibly due to central venous stenosis developing after the catheter was removed.[26] Details of vascular access surgery are

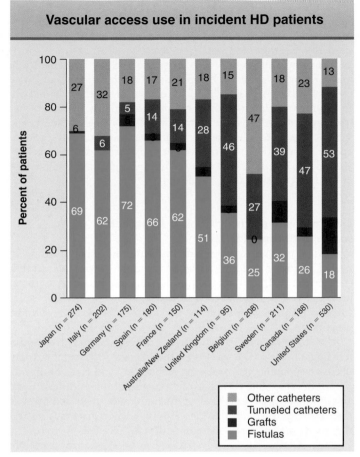

Figure 80.6 Vascular access use in incident HD patients. Entered the DOPPS II Study (2002–2004) within 5 days of starting dialysis. (Data from the Dialysis Outcomes and Practice Patterns Study [DOPPS], www.dopps.org.)

discussed in Chapter 81, and PD catheter placement is discussed in Chapter 85.

MULTIDISCIPLINARY PREDIALYSIS CARE

Predialysis care focuses on preserving residual renal function, preventing or treating complications of chronic renal failure, ensuring that the patient has sufficient understanding of their condition to decide whether they wish to have dialysis, to choose between PD and HD, and to arrange for appropriate access and, in appropriate patients, to prepare for kidney transplantation.

In addition to the nephrologist giving advice, further benefit may be gained if patients are offered education by a multidisciplinary predialysis team.[30,31] Such teams commonly include a dietitian, nurse educator, pharmacist, social worker, and sometimes a trained peer-support volunteer. Patients receiving this additional care have better biochemical results are more likely to start dialysis in a planned way with less hospitalization and may even have improved survival rates once they have started dialysis. As well as being good practice, these programs make good financial sense as the savings in inpatient costs from such programs outweigh those required to run the clinics.

Transfer to Multidisciplinary Predialysis Care

One aim of a predialysis program is to ensure that the patient and his or her family know as much as they wish to know about renal failure and its treatment before dialysis needs to be started. To achieve this aim, sufficient time is needed to allow the large amount of information to be absorbed and its implications for that individual to be understood. This may take months rather than days in patients who have difficulty accepting information about their illness and who may gain particular benefit from the program.[32] It is our practice to transfer patients to the team at least 12 months before the predicted start date of dialysis.

Predicting the start of dialysis is made easier if renal function is routinely measured by an estimated glomerular filtration rate (eGFR), such as that derived by the Modification of Diet in Renal Disease (MDRD) formula rather than serum creatinine alone (see Chapter 3). It is very easy to underestimate the severity of renal impairment from the serum creatinine alone, especially in elderly patients. Using eGFR allows thresholds to be used to generate regular reports from a computer database, identifying those patients with stage 4 chronic kidney disease (eGFR <30 ml/min per 1.73 m^2) who require careful observation for further decline in eGFR. If graphs of eGFR against time are drawn, it is easy to identify those patients whose renal function is deteriorating at a rate that predicts they will require dialysis in the next 1 to 2 years and should be referred to the multidisciplinary team (Fig. 80.7).

Designing a Predialysis Education Program

An effective program should follow the principles of adult learning, which also underlie a successful doctor-patient consultation. The three key elements are to assess the patient's existing level of knowledge and understanding, to build on this knowledge by the delivery of appropriate information in an appropriate form, and to establish that the patient has understood and accepted the information given.

Education can be delivered individually or in groups.[33] The educational value of the individual patient consultation can be increased by the physician writing a letter to the patient summarizing the patient's medical details and the discussion about his or her treatment. This can be in addition to, or replace, the conventional letter to the patient's general practitioner. In a group

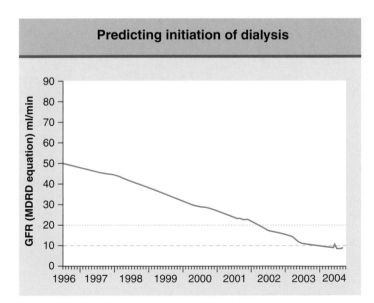

Figure 80.7 Predicting initiation of dialysis. Use of graph of glomerular filtration rate (GFR), estimated by the Modification of Diet in Renal Disease (MDRD) equation, against time to schedule preparation for dialysis. Symptoms of renal failure increase as GFR decreases to <20 ml/min per 1.73 m^2 and usually become sufficiently severe to justify dialysis at <10 ml/min per 1.73 m^2. Patient is referred to predialysis multidisciplinary clinic when GFR decreases to <20 ml/min per 1.73 m^2 or at least 12 months before the predicted need for dialysis.

session, the wide range of patients' pre-existing understanding may make it difficult for the organizer to achieve the right level of detail and complexity. On the other hand, patients probably learn as much from fellow patients within a support group as they do from the group's facilitator. Furthermore, a group will help patients and their relatives appreciate that they are not alone in facing the demands of ESRD.

The predialysis program should be delivered by representatives of all members of the multidisciplinary team, both medical and nonmedical. For example, a controlled trial from California has studied the value of social worker input to the predialysis program in reducing unemployment.[34] In the intervention group, patients and their relatives met regularly with a licensed social worker both before and after starting dialysis to explore strategies for continuing the patient's current employment. The aim of the education and counseling was to change the perception among patients, relative, and employers that dialysis patients are unable to continue working. Blue-collar workers in the intervention group were 2.8 times more likely to continue working. Patients in work had a better quality of life, greater self-esteem, and a more positive attitude to work. As it is difficult for dialysis patients to regain jobs once they are lost, this result is particularly valuable for the long-term rehabilitation of patients.

In addition to formal sessions, patients should be made aware of the wide range of educational material available. A number of books have been written specifically for dialysis patients. Many national organizations provide information on the Internet and produce patient information leaflets and audiovisual material, for example, the National Kidney Foundation (www.kidney.org).

Education about Transplantation

The possibility of kidney transplantation should be considered for each new patient with ESRD. For those who are suitable, transplantation offers the prospect of improved survival and quality of life. In a U.S. study, although the risk of death was 2.8 times higher in the first 2 weeks after transplantation compared with remaining on dialysis, the long-term mortality rate was 48% to 82% lower among transplant recipients than patients remaining on the waiting list, with relatively larger benefits among patients who were 20 to 39 years old, Caucasian, and younger with diabetes.[35]

The options of deceased donor and live donor transplants should be discussed, as well as combined kidney and pancreas transplants for diabetic patients. While outcome data from the local transplanting centers should be made available, published data can be used to inform patients.

The ideal time for the transplantation to be performed is before dialysis is ever begun, so-called pre-emptive transplantation. A U.S. study showed that pre-emptive transplantation was associated with a 52% reduction in the risk of allograft failure during the first year after transplantation, an 82% reduction during the second year, and an 86% reduction during subsequent years, compared with transplantation after dialysis. Increasing duration of dialysis was associated with increasing odds of rejection within 6 months of transplantation, possibly due to immunologic stimulation during long-term dialysis.[36]

STARTING DIALYSIS

In those patients under regular follow-up, where there is ready access to a dialysis program, it is usually recommended that dialysis should be started when subjective symptoms of uremia develop or when laboratory measurements indicate that ESRD

has been reached. The serum levels of urea and creatinine will vary according to the patient's protein intake and muscle mass, respectively, and there is no single value of either that can be used as a threshold for starting dialysis.

The mean estimated GFR at the start of dialysis is 7 to 8 ml/min per 1.73 m^2 in most HD populations. A higher threshold may used in diabetics, as they tend to tolerate uremia poorly and are frequently troubled by sodium retention and fluid overload. Other measurements to be taken into consideration include increasing serum phosphate, decreasing serum bicarbonate, and protein-energy malnutrition, which develops and persists despite vigorous attempts to optimize intake. A fall in serum albumin is a late sign of reduced protein intake and debility.

Limitations of a Purely Clinical Approach to the Initiation of Dialysis

Waiting for patients to develop uremic symptoms, such as anorexia, nausea, vomiting, and loss of lean body weight, carries the risk that the patient will start dialysis in a malnourished state with an increased risk of mortality. Renal failure itself is a catabolic state, and it is commonly difficult for patients on dialysis to regain lost weight.

Given the chronic nature of renal disease, patients frequently remain unaware of the severity of their illness. Protein intake may decrease spontaneously with the result that symptoms of uremia do not develop, but this is at the expense of a loss of lean body mass. Similarly, patients may gradually reduce their activities as their exercise tolerance declines. It is only when dialysis is started that many patients appreciate how ill they have become.

Lack of awareness is a trap that can be avoided by carefully questioning the patient for insidious symptoms of uremia. For example, the patient should be asked to compare his or her current eating habits and lifestyle with those 6 to 12 months previously. Close friends and relatives provide a useful third-party view of the patient's well-being.

Kinetic Approach to the Initiation of Dialysis

The current NKF-K/DOQI guidelines[16] recommend that residual renal function and protein intake should be measured formally and a decision to start dialysis made when these values fall below the minimum recommended for patients already on dialysis. These recommendations are based on the rationale that, just as patients on dialysis require a minimum urea and creatinine clearance and protein intake to remain healthy, patients with deteriorating native renal function should not be left for prolonged periods with inadequate renal clearance or protein intake. In other words, patients should have a healthy start to dialysis. Detailed guidelines are shown in Figure 80.8.

Arbitrary guidelines have been established to gain Medicare approval for dialysis reimbursement in the United States. These include an estimated GFR (MDRD formula[37]) of <15 ml/min/1.73 m^2 for patients older than 18 years and <20 ml/min/1.73 m^2 (Schwartz formula) for those younger than 18 years. Alternatively, adults should have a serum creatinine of >8 mg/dl (700 μmol/l) (>6 mg/dl [530 μmol/l] in diabetes) or a creatinine clearance (Cockcroft-Gault formula) of <10 ml/min (<15 ml/min in diabetics), which can be factored for body surface area (1.73 m^2). Patients may also qualify for Medicare if they do not meet the preceding criteria but have uremic symptoms (nausea, vomiting, pericardial pain, acidosis, or hyperkalemia) or pulmonary edema refractory to diuretics.

When to initiate dialysis

Unless certain conditions are met, patients should be advised to initiate some form of dialysis when the weekly renal $Kt/V_{urea}(K_rt/V_{urea})$ decreases to <2

Conditions that may indicate dialysis is not yet necessary even though the weekly K_rt/V_{urea} is <2 are as follows:
1. Stable or increased edema-free body weight; supportive objective parameters for adequate nutrition include a lean body mass of 63%, subjective global assessment score indicative of adequate nutrition, a serum albumin concentration in excess of the lower limit for the laboratory and is stable or increasing
2. Normalized protein nitrogen appearance 0.8 g/kg/day
3. Complete absence of clinical signs or symptoms attributable to uremia

A weekly K_rt/V_{urea} of 2 approximates to a renal urea clearance of 7 ml/min and a renal creatinine clearance that varies between 9 and 14 ml/min/1.73 m² . Urea clearance should be normalized to total body water (V) and creatinine clearance should be expressed per 1.73 m² of body surface area. The glomerular filtration rate, which is estimated by the arithmetic mean of the urea and creatinine clearances, will be approximately 10.5 ml/min/1.73 m² when K_rt/V_{urea} is about 2.

Figure 80.8 When to initiate dialysis. National Kidney Foundation Kidney Dialysis Outcomes Quality Initiative Clinical Practice Guidelines for initiation of dialysis. (Adapted from NKF-DOQI: NKF-DOQI Clinical Practice Guidelines for Peritoneal Dialysis Adequacy, 2000. Am J Kidney Dis 2001;37 (Suppl 1): S65–S136.) For further discussion of calculation and interpretation of K_rt/V_{urea}, see Chapters 83 and 85.

Limitations of a Purely Kinetic Approach in the Initiation of Dialysis

Routine early initiation of dialysis would need to confer significant benefits to justify the added inconvenience to the patient, the additional risk of dialysis-related complications, and the additional cost. As dialysis treatment has a finite life, either from loss of peritoneal function or failure of HD access, starting treatment earlier will bring forward the time when further procedures or a change of modality are necessary.

Another concern about a kinetic approach is the accuracy of measurements of residual renal function. These depend on timed collections of urine, which are notoriously inaccurate in clinical practice. This may lead to erroneously low values for urea and creatinine clearance and hence an unnecessarily early start for dialysis. Moreover, there is likely to be resistance from many patients to the suggestion that they should start dialysis when they have no symptoms of uremia. The nephrologist would need complete confidence in the laboratory values, as well as in the evidence supporting early commencement of dialysis, in order to persuade a reluctant, asymptomatic patient.

Starting dialysis is the first step in a lifelong commitment to RRT. Patients will be asked to comply with a wide variety of inconvenient and sometimes unpleasant treatments. A high level of compliance is required for a successful outcome, and, particularly in the United States, there is concern about the level of noncompliance associated with increased mortality.[38] It seems reasonable to presume that the commitment to dialysis is likely to be greater if the patient feels better after it has started.

In a prospective study in The Netherlands,[39] patients who started dialysis with less residual renal function (5 ml/min/1.73 m² versus 7 ml/min/1.73 m²) had a poorer quality of life in the early period after starting dialysis. However, this difference was no longer present by the end of the first 12 months of treatment. The study was too small to demonstrate a difference in mortality.

Starting dialysis earlier will lead to an apparent increase in survival if survival is measured from the time dialysis begins, so-called lead-time bias. A UK study eliminated this effect by following all patients with a creatinine clearance of <20 ml/min.[40] No association was found between creatinine clearance at the start of dialysis and survival (median creatinine clearance, 8.3 ml/min), suggesting that waiting for symptoms to develop does not jeopardize long-term outcomes.

MANAGING DISRUPTIVE PATIENTS

Most nephrologists have had experience of treating a small number of patients who, for one reason or another, will not comply with the discipline required for maintenance dialysis and who become disruptive to the staff and other patients. This behavior can range from noncompliance with treatment, which harms the patient but is merely inconvenient to the staff, to verbal or even physical aggression toward the staff and other patients in the unit. The impact of this small number of patients can be very great.

The strategy for dealing with such patients must be tailored to the individual. However, useful suggestions for resolving conflict have been provided in the RPA/ASN Clinical Practice Guideline[4] (Fig. 80.9) and are also available at www.esrdnetworks.org/networks/net6/policies/po-recom.html. They emphasize the importance of understanding, information, patience, and persistence. However, the bottom line for patients who are aggressive toward staff while on dialysis must be that they are taken off treatment and sent home (www.nhs.uk/zerotolerance/intro.htm).

Suggested steps for dealing with disruptive patients

Identify and document problem behaviors and discuss them with the patient.

Seek to understand the patient's perspective.

Identify the patient's goals for treatment.

Share control and responsibility for treatment with the patient:
Educate the patient so that he or she can make informed decisions.
Involve the patient in the treatment as much as possible.
Negotiate a behavioral contract with the patient.

Consult a psychiatrist, psychologist, or social worker for assistance in patient management or determination of decision-making capacity.

Be patient and persistent; try not to be adversarial.

Allow the patient to air concerns but do not tolerate verbal abuse or threats to staff or patients (see www.nhs.uk/zerotolerance/intro.htm).

Contact law enforcement officials if physical abuse is threatened or occurs.

If satisfactory resolution has not occured with the above strategies, contact the local end-stage renal disease network to discuss the situation and ensure due process.

Consider transferring the patient to another facility or discharging the patient.

Consult with legal counsel before proceeding with plans for discharge and do not discharge without advance notice and a full explanation of future treatment options.

Figure 80.9 Suggested steps for dealing with disruptive patients. (Adapted from Renal Physicians Association and American Society of Nephrology: Shared Decision-Making in the Appropriate Initiation of and Withdrawal from Dialysis. Clinical Practice Guideline, Number 2. Washington, DC: Renal Physicians Association, 2000.)

RESUSCITATION AND WITHDRAWAL OF DIALYSIS

Cardiopulmonary Resuscitation

If patients are to be fully involved in decision making about their treatment, two sensitive issues need to be discussed: cardiopulmonary resuscitation (CPR) and the possibility of withdrawal of dialysis. The two are not necessarily linked; patients may wish to continue with dialysis but express a desire for resuscitation not to be attempted should they suffer a cardiac arrest. Such a decision would be supported by evidence on the outcome of CPR in dialysis patients: only six of 74 dialysis patients who received CPR survived to hospital discharge and at 6 months after CPR, only two were still alive. This compares with 23 of 247 control patients not on dialysis still alive at 6 months, and this difference was not explained by age or comorbid conditions.[41] Successful CPR often resulted in a poor-quality death, with 20 of the 27 successfully resuscitated dialysis patients dying a few days later on mechanical ventilation in an intensive care unit.

A decision not to attempt CPR must be carefully documented in the patient's medical and nursing records, and all nursing staff must be made aware of it. It is important to be clear what is meant by cardiac arrest and for there to be agreement on how the nursing staff should respond should the patient suffer a hypotensive crash while on dialysis. These notes may form part of a complete advance directive, as discussed in the following section.

Withdrawal of Dialysis

As discussed earlier, it is not possible to predict accurately which patients will gain prolonged benefit from dialysis. Many nephrologists, therefore, operate a liberal policy of offering dialysis to all patients with ESRD who wish to have it. This policy ensures that no patients are denied dialysis but has the inevitable consequence that a number of patients will be started on dialysis who subsequently do not enjoy an acceptable quality of life. The possibility of withdrawing dialysis needs to be addressed if these patients are not to suffer unreasonably.

Rates of withdrawal vary widely among countries and cultures. Withdrawal rates in Italy and France are much lower than in the United Kingdom and United States.[2] In the United States, African Americans have about one third the withdrawal rate of Caucasians. Rates of withdrawal vary between dialysis units and are significantly associated with the medical director's opinion about whether withdrawal is allowed or facilitated in that unit.[2] This suggests that patients' wishes are not always fully included in these decisions. Patients may be very reticent to express a wish to withdraw from dialysis. Many see it as their duty as a patient to go along with the treatment recommended by their physician and do not wish to appear ungrateful for the efforts that are being made to keep them alive. Their physician may be the last member of the team to learn about the patient's views, and it is very important that good communication exists within the multidisciplinary team so that any clues that the patient gives are passed on and acted on.

Staff should adopt a proactive approach and raise the issue of withdrawal of dialysis with patients who are chronically not

Principles underlying withdrawal of dialysis
The ultimate responsibility for the decision rests with the physician, not the relative.
The patient's interests and dignity should be protected at all times.
The process should not be rushed. If there is any doubt about the correctness of the decision, treatment should continue.
There should be an open discussion among the multidisciplinary team to avoid any damaging disagreements.
The psychological needs of the health care team should not be overlooked.
Palliative care must be given in the most appropriate environment, e.g., a hospice or, ideally, the patient's own home.

Figure 80.10   Key principles underlying the process of withdrawal of dialysis.

thriving. There is good evidence that early discussion of these issues can lead to a more satisfactory outcome for patients, relatives, and staff when the patient eventually dies.[42] In the United States, formal advance directives play an important part in these discussions, while in the United Kingdom, there has been less enthusiasm for formalizing this process. Evidence from randomized trials suggests that implementing advance directives does not improve the quality of the end of patients' lives.[43] Advance directives are currently completed by only a minority of patients, and even if one is in place, it does not obviate the need for staff to continue to communicate closely with the patient and his or her family in case the decision changes as death comes closer.

Where a patient is no longer competent to make a decision, an advance directive can provide a clear legal basis for the decision to stop dialysis. Indeed, in the absence of clear and convincing written evidence, some states in the United States (e.g., Missouri and New York) insist that dialysis must be continued. In other states in the United States and in the United Kingdom, the physician is given the task of deciding on the patient's behalf. Helpful advice for dialysis staff and patients wishing to complete an advance directive is available in the RPA/ASN Clinical Practice Guideline[4] and at the website www.ageingwithdignity.org.

Once a patient has expressed a wish for dialysis to be withdrawn or the issue has been raised by his or her relatives, the first priority must be to identify any reversible factors that may improve the patient's health sufficiently for the decision to be reversed. In particular, any depression must be identified and treated.[44] Once all these factors have been ruled out, the process of withdrawing dialysis should be managed according to some key principles (Fig. 80.10).

Withdrawing dialysis should not be seen as an admission of failure but as a final stage in the process of RRT. This terminal phase can be uniquely rewarding, particularly if it allows a patient and his or her family and caregivers to prepare themselves for the patient's death. The opportunity for patients to complete unfinished emotional and financial business can make the subsequent bereavement period much less traumatic.

REFERENCES

1. Schieppati A, Remuzzi G: Chronic renal diseases as a public health problem: Epidemiology, social, and economic implications. Kidney Int Suppl 2005;98:S7–S10.
2. Lambie M, Rayner H, Bragg-Gresham J, et al: Starting and withdrawing hemodialysis: Associations between nephrologists' opinions and practice patterns (data from the DOPPS). Nephrol Dial Transplant 2006; 21:2814–2820.
3. McKenzie JK, Moss AH, Feest TG, et al: Dialysis decision making in Canada, the United Kingdom, and the United States. Am J Kidney Dis 1998;31:12–18.
4. Renal Physicians Association and American Society of Nephrology: Shared Decision-Making in the Appropriate Initiation of and Withdrawal from Dialysis. Clinical Practice Guideline, Number 2. Washington, DC: Renal Physicians Association, 2000.

5. Singer PA: Nephrologists' experience with and attitudes towards decisions to forego dialysis. J Am Soc Nephrol 1992;2:1235–1240.
6. Moss AH: Dialysis decisions and the elderly. Clin Geriatr Med 1994;10:463–473.
7. Barrett BJ, Parfrey PS, Morgan J, et al: Prediction of early death in end-stage renal disease patients starting dialysis. Am J Kidney Dis 1997;29:214–222.
8. Chadna SM, Schulz J, Lawrence C, et al: Is there a rationale for rationing chronic dialysis? A hospital based cohort study of factors affecting survival and morbidity. BMJ 1999;318:217–222.
9. Mapes DL, Lopes AA, Satayathum S, et al: Health-related quality of life as a predictor of mortality and hospitalization: The Dialysis Outcomes and Practice Patterns Study (DOPPS). Kidney Int 2003;64:339–349.
10. Fenton SS, Schaubel DE, Desmeules M, et al: Hemodialysis versus peritoneal dialysis: A comparison of adjusted mortality rates. Am J Kidney Dis 1997;30:334–342.
11. Held PJ, Port FK, Turenne MN, et al: Continuous ambulatory peritoneal dialysis and hemodialysis: Comparison of patient mortality with adjustment for comorbid conditions. Kidney Int 1994;45:1163–1169.
12. Jaar BG, Coresh J, Plantinga LC, et al: Comparing the risk for death with peritoneal dialysis and hemodialysis in a national cohort of patients with chronic kidney disease. Ann Intern Med 2005;143:374–383.
13. Ganesh SK, Hulbert-Shearon T, Port FK, et al: Mortality differences by dialysis modality among incident ESRD patients with and without coronary artery disease. J Am Soc Nephrol 2003;14:415–424.
14. Stack AG, Molony DA, Rahman NS, et al: Impact of dialysis modality on survival of new ESRD patients with congestive heart failure in the United States. Kidney Int 2003;64:1071–1079.
15. Rayner HC, Pisoni RL, Bommer J, et al: Mortality and hospitalization in hemodialysis patients in five European countries: Results from the Dialysis Outcomes and Practice Patterns Study (DOPPS). Nephrol Dial Transplant 2004;19:108–120.
16. NKF-DOQI: NKF-DOQI Clinical Practice Guidelines for Peritoneal Dialysis Adequacy 2000. Am J Kidney Dis 2001;37(Suppl 1):S65–S136 (www.kidney.org/professionals/doqi/index.cfm).
17. Mupirocin Study Group: Nasal mupirocin prevents *Staphylococcus aureus* exit site infection during peritoneal dialysis. J Am Soc Nephrol 1996;7:2403–2408.
18. Woods JD, Port FK, Stannard D, et al: Comparison of mortality with home hemodialysis and center hemodialysis: A national study. Kidney Int 1996;49:1464–1470.
19. Pierratos A: Daily nocturnal home hemodialysis. Kidney Int 2004;65:5975–5986.
20. Little J, Irwin A, Marshall T, et al: Predicting a patient's choice of dialysis modality: Experience in a United Kingdom renal department. Am J Kidney Dis 2001;37:981–986.
21. Golper TA, Vonesh EF, Wolfson M, et al: The impact of pre-ESRD education on dialysis modality selection. J Am Soc Nephrol 2000;11:231A.
22. Stack AG: Determinants of Modality Selection among incident U.S. dialysis patients: Results from a national study. J Am Soc Nephrol 2002;13:1279–1287.
23. Nissenson AR, Prichard SS, Cheng IKP, et al: Non-medical factors that impact on ESRD modality selection. Kidney Int 1993;43(suppl 40):S120–S127.
24. Mendelssohn DC, Mullaney SR, Jung B, et al: What do American nephrologists think about dialysis modality selection? Am J Kidney Dis 2001;37:22–29.
25. Blake PG, Finkelstein FO: Why is the proportion of patients doing peritoneal dialysis declining in North America? Perit Dial Int 2001;21:107–114.
26. Rayner HC, Pisoni RL, Young EW, et al: Creation, cannulation and survival of arteriovenous fistulae—data from the DOPPS. Kidney Int 2003;63:323–330.
27. Jungers P: Late referral: Loss of chance for the patient, loss of money for society. Nephrol Dial Transplant 2002;17:371–375.
28. Dhingra RK, Young EW, Hulbert-Shearon TE, et al: Type of vascular access and mortality in U.S. hemodialysis patients. Kidney Int 2001;60:1443–1451.
29. Pisoni RL, Albert JM, Elder SE, Ethier J, et al: Lower mortality risk associated with native arteriovenous fistula (AVF) vs graft (AVG) use in patient and facility-level analyses: Results from the DOPPS. J Am Soc Nephrol 2005;16:259A.
30. Curtis BM, Ravani P, Malberti F, et al: The short- and long-term impact of multi-disciplinary clinics in addition to standard nephrology care on patient outcomes. Nephrol Dial Transplant 2005;20:147–154.
31. Goldstein M, Yassa T, Dacouris N, McFarlane P: Multidisciplinary predialysis care and morbidity and mortality of patients on dialysis. Am J Kidney Dis 2004;44:706–714.
32. Devins GM, Mendelssohn DC, Barré PE, Binik YM: Predialysis psychoeducational intervention and coping styles influence time to dialysis in chronic kidney disease. Am J Kidney Dis 2003;42:693–703.
33. Trento M, Passera P, Borgo E, et al: A 5-year randomized controlled study of learning, problem solving ability and quality of life modifications in people with type 2 diabetes managed by group care. Diabetes Care 2004;27:670–675.
34. Razgone S, Schwankovsky L, James-Rogers A, et al: An intervention for employment maintenance among blue-collar workers with end stage renal disease. Am J Kidney Dis 1993;22:403–412.
35. Wolfe RA, Ashby VB, Milford EL, et al: Comparison of mortality in all patients on dialysis, patients on dialysis awaiting transplantation, and recipients of a first cadaveric transplant. N Engl J Med 1999;341:1725–1730.
36. Mange KC, Joffe MM, Feldman HI: Effect of the use or nonuse of long-term dialysis on the subsequent survival of renal transplants from living donors. N Engl J Med 2001;344:726–731.
37. Froissart M, Rossert J, Jacquot C, et al: Predictive performance of the Modification of Diet in Renal Disease and Cockcroft-Gault equations for estimating renal function. J Am Soc Nephrol 2005;16:763–773.
38. Saran R, Bragg-Gresham JL, Rayner HC, et al: Nonadherence in hemodialysis: Associations with mortality, hospitalization, and practice patterns in the DOPPS. Kidney Int 2003;64:154–162.
39. Korevaar JC, Jansen MA, Dekker FW, et al: Evaluation of DOQI guidelines: Early start of dialysis treatment is not associated with better health-related quality of life. National Kidney Foundation-Dialysis Outcomes Quality Initiative. Am J Kidney Dis 2002;39:108–115.
40. Traynor JP, Simpson K, Geddes CC, et al: Early initiation of dialysis fails to prolong survival in patients with end-stage renal failure J Am Soc Nephrol 2002;13:2125–2132.
41. Moss AH, Holley JL, Upton MB: Outcomes of cardiopulmonary resuscitation in dialysis patients. J Am Soc Nephrol 1992;3:1238–1243.
42. Swartz RD, Penny E: Advance directives are associated with good deaths in chronic dialysis patients. J Am Soc Nephrol 1993;3:1623–1630.
43. Anderson JP, Kaplan RM, Schneiderman LJ: Effects of offering advance directives on quality adjusted life expectancy and psychological well being among ill adults. J Clin Epidemiol 1994;47:761–772.
44. Lopes AA, Albert JM, Young EW, et al: Screening for depression in hemodialysis patients: Associations with diagnosis, treatment, and outcomes in the DOPPS. Kidney Int 2004;66:5047–5053 [Erratum in Kidney Int 2004;66:6486].

81 Vascular Access for Hemodialysis

Klaus Konner and Michael Gersch

INTRODUCTION

The maintenance of adequate, durable vascular access for hemodialysis (HD) is essential for the well-being of the patient with end-stage renal disease (ESRD). The provision of HD requires repeated vascular access that can achieve a blood flow in excess of 350 ml/min.

In the 1960s, vascular access for maintenance HD therapy was often initiated by nephrologists, the pioneers being Scribner, Brescia, Cimino, and Shaldon. However, soon, almost all vascular access creation became the domain of surgeons. The challenge to achieve successful vascular access grows as the dialysis patient population has an increasing proportion of elderly, diabetic, and hypertensive patients, many with serious cardiovascular comorbidities. Vascular access remains the Achilles heel of HD.[1]

OPTIONS IN VASCULAR ACCESS

The three main options in vascular access for HD are the arteriovenous (AV) fistula, the AV bridge graft, and tunneled and nontunneled central venous catheters. Some complex procedures that are not routinely used are also discussed.

The major contraindication to creation of any AV access is advanced calcifying arteriosclerosis. Cardiac failure, New York Heart Association grade III or IV, may also limit immediate placement of an AV fistula, although this can often be achieved after a few months of adequate HD using a venous catheter to control initial fluid overload, hypertension, and renal anemia.[2] There is no doubt that AV fistulas using native vessels have by far the best long-term function and lowest complication rates of any vascular access. Nevertheless, during the past 40 years, the United States developed different strategies for creating vascular access from those in Europe and Japan, with extensive use of AV grafts[3] (Fig. 81.1). Substantial efforts are now under way, particularly in the United States, to create more initial AV fistulas.

Many patients present as uremic emergencies requiring immediate dialysis and do not have the benefit of pre-emptive establishment of definitive vascular access. Although AV grafts offer the apparent attraction that they can be used earlier after surgery than AV fistulas, it may be preferable to accept an additional period of several weeks of dialysis using a central venous catheter while allowing an AV fistula to become usable rather than place an AV graft.

EVALUATION OF THE PATIENT FOR VASCULAR ACCESS

The earlier a patient with chronic kidney disease is referred to a nephrologist and a vascular access surgeon, the better the chances are for the patient to have a timely created and well-functioning

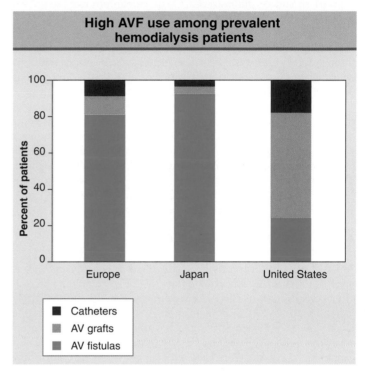

Figure 81.1 Variations in vascular access for hemodialysis. High use of arteriovenous fistulas (AVF) in prevalent hemodialysis patients in Europe and Japan compared to the United States. (Adapted from Pisoni RL, Young EW, Mapes DL, et al: Vascular access use and outcomes in the U.S., Europe, and Japan: Results from the Dialysis Outcomes and Practice Patterns Study [DOPPS]. Nephrol News Issues 2003; 17:38–47.)

access at the initiation of HD.[4] An early decision on the type, side, and site of the first vascular access, will be based on

- *Medical history* with special regard to vascular problems: peripheral ischemia, stroke, amputation or additional vascular surgery, smoking, former catheterizations of central veins, and pacemaker insertion.
- *Physical examination* with careful palpation of arterial pulses and venous vasculature, paying particular attention to the venous filling capacity using a blood pressure cuff and variable pressures and to the presence of venous collaterals and swelling; the dominant arm is not necessarily the preferred side and the decision should be based on the quality of the vessels.
- *Blood pressure* measurement in both arms.
- *Vascular mapping*, preferably using the noninvasive Doppler ultrasound technique.[5,6]

Doppler ultrasound is preferred because it provides information about the venous vasculature, particularly in obese patients, in the upper arm and the diameter of the brachial, radial, and ulnar arteries; detects vascular calcifications; and reveals the blood flow volume in the brachial artery, thus superseding clinical evaluation of arterial patency. The resistance index, a measure of arterial compliance, can be calculated from the differences between the high-resistance triphasic Doppler signal with clenched fist and the low-resistance biphasic waveform after releasing the fist. A preoperative resistance index of 0.7 in the feeding artery indicates insufficient arterial compliance so that the chance of successful creation of an AV fistula is reduced. Additional angiography is needed only in very difficult cases. The use of contrast should be minimized; CO_2 or gadolinium may be used if available.

As well as resistance index, arterial and venous diameters and the quality of the vessel wall are strong determinants for a successful first access operation. Advanced arterial calcifications with loss of elasticity, distensibility, and compliance and narrowed venous segments with wall thickening are predictive of early failure.

Based on these data the decision can be made on the side, site, and type of the first vascular access. Preservation of veins during the earlier stages of CKD is crucial for the success of vascular access and should be practiced in both arms, reducing blood sampling to the dorsum of the hand whenever possible. The best partner in venous preservation is the well-informed patient. The dominant arm is not necessarily the preferred side, and the decision should be based on the quality of the vessels.

ARTERIOVENOUS FISTULA

An AV fistula has correctly been described as not physiologic.[7] A juvenile radial artery has a blood flow rate of 20 to 30 ml/min, and after construction of the AV anastomosis, the flow immediately increases up to 200 to 300 ml/min. A well-maturing AV fistula has a flow of between 600 and 1200 ml/min a few weeks after creation. Venous dilatation, the prerequisite for safe repeated cannulation, can develop only with an excellent arterial inflow with a low venous pressure.[8] The mechanisms that initiate, regulate, and limit arterial and venous dilatation are poorly understood; remodeling of the vessels is largely an unexplored field, which lacks an *in vitro* model.

Choice of Site for an Arteriovenous Fistula

Dependent on the preoperative clinical and ultrasound findings, a first AV fistula preferably should be created peripherally at the wrist; if this is not possible, any segment of the radial or even the ulnar artery along the forearm can be used (Fig. 81.2). If there is advanced calcification of the forearm arteries and/or exhaustion of the venous vasculature, the AV anastomosis can be created in the proximal forearm using the radial, ulnar, or even the brachial artery. Failing that, the elbow region can be used with the brachial artery and a suitable vein, usually cephalic or basilic, or even one of the deep brachial veins, can be used (Fig. 81.3). There should be only a few patients in whom creation of an autologous AV fistula is not possible.

Type of Arteriovenous Anastomosis

The first AV fistulas in clinical practice used a subcutaneous artery-side-to-vein-side anastomosis at the wrist that allowed repeated cannulation. To avoid peripheral venous hypertension, ligation of the distal venous limb is helpful. An *end-to-end anastomosis* should not be used since the risk of distal ischemia is too high if an artery is cut to construct an AV anastomosis. The *artery-side-to-vein-end anastomosis* is now the preferred technique (see Fig. 81.2b). Torsion and kinking should be avoided when the venous end is transposed to the artery. In patients with calcification of the peripheral arteries, it may be necessary to consider a proximal forearm fistula using an anastomosis between the brachial artery and the perforating vein, the communicating vein between the superficial and deep vein in the proximal forearm and/or elbow[9] (Fig. 81.4). Sometimes the proximal radial or ulnar artery can be used rather than the brachial, which reduces length of the anastomosis, thereby reducing the frequency of a steal syndrome.

The aim of all vascular access surgery is to establish a high blood flow that leads to a dilated vein that can be cannulated easily and repeatedly. Where a well-filled vein cannot be cannulated because it is too deep, the vein must be brought to a subcutaneous level. This is regularly necessary with the basilic vein along the medial aspect of the upper arm, and may also be necessary in obese patients with the cephalic vein in the forearm or upper arm.

Where the anatomy only allows an anastomosis between the brachial artery and one of the brachial veins, a second procedure is always required 4 to 6 weeks after the first operation, when

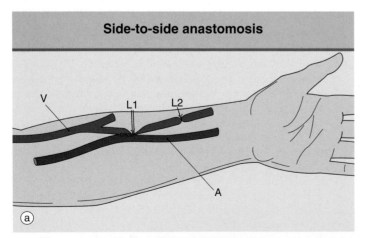

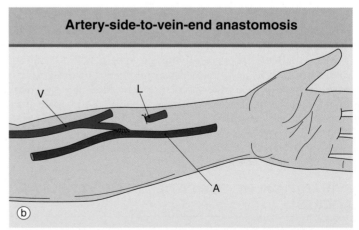

Figure 81.2 Primary radiocephalic arteriovenous fistula. *a*, A side-to-side anastomosis becomes a functional artery side-to-venous-end anastomosis by ligation of the distal venous limb close to the AV anastomosis (L1) or more distally (L2). *b*, Artery-side-to-venous-end anastomosis with ligation of the distal vein (L). A, radial artery; V, cephalic antebrachial vein.

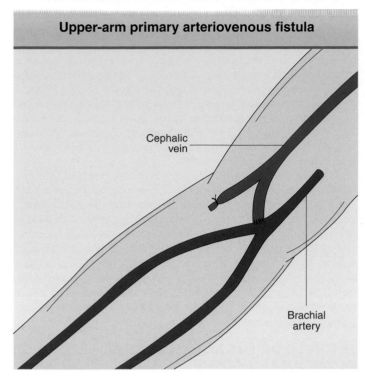

Figure 81.3 Upper arm primary arteriovenous fistula. Cephalic vein anastomosed to brachial artery. Alternatively, the basilic vein is used, but may need to be superficialized to facilitate cannulation.

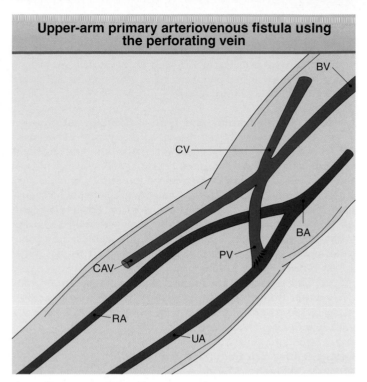

Figure 81.4 Anastomosis of the perforating vein in the proximal forearm to the ulnar artery in the proximal forearm. BA, brachial artery; BV, basilic vein; CAV, cephalic antebrachial vein; CV, cephalic vein; PV, perforating vein; RA, radial artery; UA, ulnar artery.

there has been arterial and venous dilatation. The vein can be brought subcutaneously, although this may be technically difficult to achieve. Alternatively, a forearm polytetrafluoroethylene (ePTFE) loop graft is inserted between the dilated artery and vein (Fig. 81.5).

Maturation, First Cannulation, and Early Failure of AV Fistulas

Any minor surgical error is multiplied many times and can lead to early AV fistula failure, usually early thrombosis, or delayed or absent maturation. Dissection and torsion of the vessels should be minimized, and the choice of an unsuitable calcified artery that provides an adequate arterial inflow will also lead to a high risk of failure. The primary failure rate for AV fistulas should not exceed 10%.

Although a high blood flow rate will be established 2 or 3 weeks after surgery, remodeling of the venous wall with increased mechanical stability takes a few months. Cannulation may be appropriate in the first postoperative week if the venous limb of the fistula is easily palpable, and care is taken to minimize perivascular hematoma formation, which carries a high risk of fistula failure due to mechanical narrowing. Congestion for the first cannulations with a blood pressure cuff should not exceed 40 mm Hg, with careful manual compression after decannulation.

ARTERIOVENOUS GRAFTS

ePTFE has become the most accepted synthetic graft material. While grafts generally work well in the field of vascular surgery, they often fail when used as vascular access, mainly because of repeated trauma; and there is an increased risk of infection from repeated cannulation in the context of the impaired immunity of uremia.

Indications for Arteriovenous Grafts

An AV graft is a second-line access procedure when an AV fistula cannot be successfully constructed and maintained. The use of AV grafts as initial vascular access should be a very rare event. Nevertheless, AV grafts have some advantages, including an

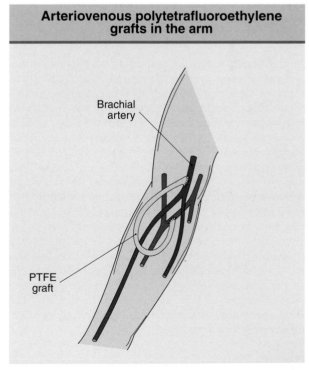

Figure 81.5 Arteriovenous polytetrafluoroethylene (PTFE) graft in the forearm.

931

initial high blood flow rate, first cannulation within 2 to 3 weeks, and, with special graft materials even a few days after insertion, easy surgical replacement, which may be segmental or total.

Indications for use of an ePTFE graft for vascular access include hypoplastic or exhausted peripheral veins, gross obesity, and severe peripheral arterial occlusive disease.

Location, Configuration, and Type of Graft Anastomoses

Theoretically, AV grafts can be placed at any site between an artery and a vein, but excellent arterial inflow and excellent venous outflow are prerequisites. A primary AV graft should use the large-bore arteries and veins in the forearm to provide good blood flow and adequate outflow, and the graft should be configured as a loop in the forearm (see Fig. 81.5). Straight forearm AV grafts may work well when there is a well-predilated radial artery following a failed AV fistula that has been used for some time, but a straight forearm radiocephalic graft as the initial access procedure is at a high risk of failure due to poor arterial inflow. The graft-vein anastomosis is the cause of most graft dysfunction due to neointimal hyperplasia within the anastomosis or stenosis of the downstream autologous vein. Early AV graft failure rates should not exceed 10%.

Postoperative Care and First Cannulation of an Arteriovenous Graft

Postoperatively, any graft can seem infected. Redness, heat, and diffuse swelling around the graft are normal findings that may persist for up to 2 weeks; this requires no specific treatment other than immobility and elevation. With decreasing swelling, the graft will become palpable. With any suspicion of a perigraft hematoma, seroma, or infectious infiltration, an ultrasound evaluation will be helpful. With normal healing, the first cannulation can be attempted after 2 or 3 weeks. In the future, new graft materials, for example, silicone-coated grafts, may allow reliable and less risky early cannulation.

MONITORING AND SURVEILLANCE OF VASCULAR ACCESS

Monitoring

Monitoring requires regular evaluation of vascular access by physical examination prior to cannulation The access should be inspected for signs of infection, hematoma, swelling, and venous collaterals. Palpation can even detect differences in intravascular pressure, suggesting early stenosis. If there is stenosis, auscultation will reveal additional high-frequency noises and a shortening of the diastolic period. The diagnosis of a hemodynamically significant stenosis can be confirmed by elevating the arm to bring the anastomosis above the level of the heart: the prestenotic venous segment will be filled to full size with palpable high intravenous pressure, whereas the poststenotic vein will collapse. Prolonged bleeding time after decannulation is also symptomatic of downstream stenosis. Documenting arterial and venous pressure during each dialysis with the cannulae at well-defined sites and an identical prescribed blood flow rate is also informative; increasing venous pressure and decreasing arterial pressure point to access dysfunction. In the authors' experience, 60% to 80% of access problems can be diagnosed on clinical assessment, using additional duplex scanning in selected cases.

Surveillance

Surveillance is the periodic evaluation of vascular access using specifically designed equipment. Intra-access flow measurement

is now accepted as the best method using ultrasound dilution, conductance dilution, thermal dilution, glucose dilution, or Doppler flow measurement. It seems likely that the simple glucose dilution technique will gain widespread acceptance, particularly in lower-income countries. A constant glucose infusion is made by a syringe pump into the arterial needle. Blood is sampled from the venous needle before the glucose infusion and then shortly after the infusion starts. Flow is easily calculated from the two glucose values.[10] Measurement of intravascular pressure or of recirculation is less useful for surveillance of vascular access than flow measurements.[11]

Criteria indicating impaired access function are blood flow rate <600 ml/min or a decrease in blood flow rate >20% per month in AV grafts and blood flow rate <300 ml/min in AV fistulas.[12] These findings should prompt pre-emptive intervention to prevent thrombosis. Monthly flow measurements for grafts and measurements every 3 months for AV fistulas are sometimes recommended and can lead to a reduced rate of thrombotic events, particularly in AV grafts but also in AV fistulas.[13] However, the authors recommend that flow measurements be reserved for patients in whom routine monitoring has detected a clinical problem to allow prompt diagnosis and intervention.

THE ROLE OF THE DIALYSIS NURSE IN VASCULAR ACCESS

Most nephrologists are not skilled in monitoring and cannulation of vascular access. Nurses and other dedicated health workers in dialysis units play a crucial role in the care and preservation of vascular access. Careful choice of cannulation sites can prolong the life of an AV fistula by minimizing the risk of stenosis (Fig. 81.6).

COMPLICATIONS OF ARTERIOVENOUS FISTULAS AND ARTERIOVENOUS GRAFTS

Complications of vascular access follow disequilibrium of the anatomic and functional status of the AV access including changes in flow volume, changes in luminal continuity such as stenoses and aneurysms, changes in shear stress, and changes from laminar to turbulent flow.

Thrombosis and Stenosis in Arteriovenous Fistulas

Thrombosis is the most frequent complication of any type of vascular access, occurring more frequently with AV grafts than AV fistulas, and is usually the result of a stenosis.

Diagnosis and Treatment of Arteriovenous Fistula Stenosis

Stenosis in the feeding artery is rare, although a centrally located arterial stenosis, for example, in the subclavian artery has a substantial impact on fistula function. Routine preoperative blood pressure checks in *both* arms can point to the problem, and angiography is needed to confirm the diagnosis. Arterial stenoses close to the anastomosis are mostly due to surgical error.

Most stenoses in AV fistulas are venous, usually found close to the AV anastomosis, and probably caused by devascularization of the venous wall during surgical dissection. Previous venous cannulation of forearm veins often results in venous segments that cannot dilate and therefore should not be used because dilatation is a prerequisite for high blood flow and cannulation. Stenoses located more cephalad develop in patients where area cannulation is the preferred type of cannulation technique[14] (see Fig. 81.6). Repeated cannulation within a limited area of the vein will result in aneurysms, narrowings, and finally in stenoses. In most patients,

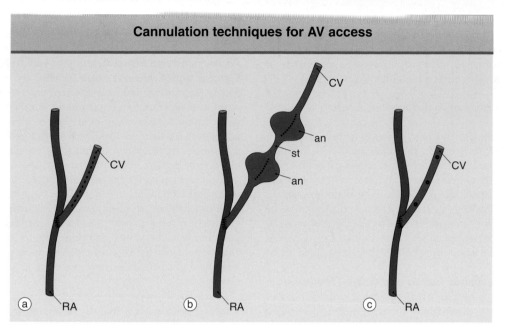

Figure 81.6 Cannulation techniques for arteriovenous access. *a*, Rope ladder technique results in moderate, but equal dilatation. *b*, Area technique results in aneurysms, often combined with interaneurysmatic narrowing or stenosis. *c*, Button-hole technique using the identical hole without cannulation-related pathology of the vein. an, aneurysm; CV, cephalic vein; RA, radial artery; st, stenosis.

physical examination can reveal the location and character of venous stenosis along the forearm and the region of the cephalic vein in the upper arm. Central venous stenoses are commonly caused by previous use of catheters. They should be confirmed by venography, preferably followed immediately by percutaneous transluminal angioplasty as the preferred therapeutic intervention.

The main objectives of intervention are to preserve the venous system as much as possible and to produce a long-term functioning access. There are two main interventions: surgery and radiologic interventional techniques. Local preferences and experience may influence selection of the procedure used. Arterial stenoses are best treated by angioplasty. Perianastomotic venous stenoses do better with creation of a new proximal AV anastomosis. Other stenoses found in the forearm and upper arm can undergo revision with various surgical techniques or with angioplasty. Restenosis is much more frequent following angioplasty, and surgery gives more stable results with less access-related morbidity. Interventional procedures for fistula stenosis are discussed in Chapter 82.

Diagnosis and Treatment of Arteriovenous Fistula Thrombosis

Thrombosis will occur when a stenosis remains undetected and any thrombotic event is an emergency. The diagnosis of thrombosis is generally clinical, confirmed by palpation and auscultation, but where palpation is difficult an ultrasound scan can give information on the length of the thrombus. Treatment consists of two stages: thrombectomy and correction of the underlying stenosis.

Surgical revision within 24 hours increases the chance of success. It minimizes the time for the thrombus to progress cephalad along the vein and avoids adherence of thrombotic material to the venous wall, which increases the risk of rethrombosis. Surgical thrombectomy involves clot removal and repair of the underlying stenosis by angioplasty or surgical revision. For interventional thrombectomy in AV fistulas, a number of mechanical and pharmacomechanical techniques have been described.[15] As with surgery, thrombectomy should be followed by correction of

the stenosis by angioplasty. Interventional techniques for the management of AV fistula thrombosis are discussed further in Chapter 82.

Thrombosis and Stenosis in Arteriovenous Grafts

The clinical appearance of thrombosis and stenosis in AV grafts is more uniform than in AV fistulas.

Sites of Arteriovenous Graft Stenosis

Arterial stenoses are rare and do not differ from those in AV fistulas. Stenoses at the arterial anastomosis are usually the result of surgical error. Midgraft stenoses due to cannulation are quite common particularly when area cannulation is used (see Fig 81.6).[14] By far the most frequent stenosis site is at the graft-vein anastomosis, due to neointimal hyperplasia. The autologous vein beyond the anastomosis may also be involved. Recurrent stenoses with subsequent thrombosis may occur and are an important comorbid risk for the patients and a major economic burden.

Diagnosis and Treatment of Arteriovenous Graft Stenosis

In the United States, where most patients have been using AV grafts, many efforts have been made to predict and prevent graft dysfunction. Measurement of blood flow is the most reliable parameter. Duplex ultrasonography gives information on anatomic and functional (e.g., flow) parameters, but for flow measurement is less reliable than transonic techniques.[16] Blood flow rate <600 ml/min and a decrease in blood flow rate >20% per month indicate graft stenosis.[11,12] Flow measurements should be made in response to clinically detected problems rather than as a routine.

Stenoses along the feeding artery are best treated by angioplasty. The best treatment for stenoses at the arterial anastomosis is uncertain and may depend on local expertise. Midgraft stenoses can be dilated by angioplasty or should be treated surgically by segmental replacement if the stenosis reduces the lumen of the graft by >50%. Graft-vein stenosis is treated similarly, and again 50% narrowing is an indication for intervention. In our experience, graft extension is the preferred intervention since patching or insertion of a jump graft does not provide a continuously identical lumen; an extension graft should be as short as possible in order to preserve the downstream vein. This is preferred to angioplasty of the graft-vein stenosis, which has a high rate of restenosis.

Diagnosis and Treatment of Arteriovenous Graft Thrombosis

As in AV fistula thrombosis, this is a clinical diagnosis, and treatment remains incomplete if only a thrombectomy is performed. Diagnosis and treatment of the underlying stenosis are vital. There is no clear preference between surgery and interventional procedures; again, local expertise should decide. The main objective is to help the patient at a time when emergency dialysis may be needed, and the use of a bridging venous catheter should be avoided if at all possible. Interventional procedures for treatment of thrombosis in AV grafts are discussed further in Chapter 82.

Prevention of Arteriovenous Fistula and Graft Thrombosis

Although there are case reports of successful use of antiplatelet agents to prevent graft thrombosis, in randomized, controlled trials both low-dose Coumadin (warfarin) therapy[17] and aspirin combined with clopidogrel[18] showed a significant increase in bleeding episodes without a reduction in graft thrombosis. Fish oil has been reported to significantly decrease graft thrombosis; however, patient compliance with fish oil supplementation is generally poor.[19] The vast majority of graft thrombosis is related to mechanical problems such as stenosis[20] rather then problems with increased coagulation. Mechanical problems should be directly addressed rather than attempting to prevent thrombosis with medications.

If a patient has two or more episodes of thrombosis in the absence of any identifiable mechanical problem, evaluation should be undertaken for inherited or acquired hypercoagulable states. If a high-risk hypercoagulable state such as antiphospholipid antibody syndrome is identified, then the patient should be anticoagulated with Coumadin. In patients with a lower-risk mutation such as the factor V Leiden mutation, the risk-benefit analysis is less clear. There has been no randomized, controlled trial examining the treatment of thrombosis of vascular access in patients with thrombophilias; however, there is a nonrandomized report that warfarin treatment did decrease vascular access thrombosis in these patients.[21]

Aneurysms and False Aneurysms in Arteriovenous Fistulas and Arteriovenous Grafts

Aneurysms are defined as local enlargements of the lumen, mostly a result of destruction of the venous wall by area cannulation and replacement by scar tissue with loss of elasticity[14] (Fig. 81.7). In autologous AV fistulas, a thinned layer of skin instead of thickened scar tissue can be observed with aneurysms that are at high risk of bleeding or rupture, particularly in the case of infection; an elective surgical revision with complete or partial resection of the aneurysm is the best treatment.

A downstream stenosis develops in many patients with an AV fistula and a venous aneurysm. Increasing prestenotic intravascular pressure can contribute substantially to increasing aneurysmal enlargement. Partial resection of the aneurysm is recommended, and the resected tissue may be used as a patch to widen the stenosis.

Occasionally, in patients with a long history of maintenance HD, a special phenomenon may be observed: calcification of aneurysmally enlarged cannulation areas (Fig. 81.8). Reconstruction can be impossible and replacement using graft material is necessary.

In AV grafts, especially ePTFE synthetic grafts, the problem is pseudoaneurysm formation caused by area cannulation. The ePTFE wall is completely destroyed and replaced by scar tissue; the enlargement is caused by high intragraft pressure and intensified if there is a graft-vein outflow stenosis. False aneurysms in ePTFE grafts can be replaced easily by a new ePTFE segment; removal of the pseudoaneurysm reduces the risk of infection.

Steal Phenomenon and Steal Syndrome in Arteriovenous Fistulas and Grafts

Steal phenomena are physiologic with AV fistulas at the wrist. Retrograde arterial inflow from the ulnar artery, palmar arch, and the peripheral limb of the radial artery contribute up to 30% of the total blood flow volume. The steal phenomenon changes to a steal syndrome when clinical symptoms appear and the syndrome has graded severity[22]:

- Grade I: pale/blue and/or cold hand without pain
- Grade II: pain during exercise and/or HD

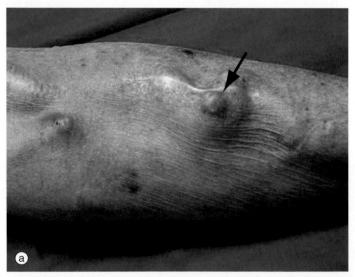
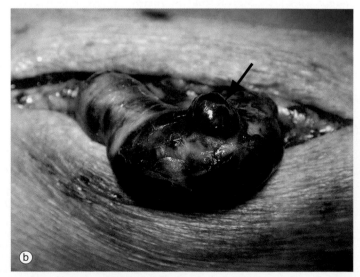

Figure 81.7   Aneurysm on an arteriovenous fistula. *a*, A thin-walled aneurysm at high risk of rupture requiring surgical revision. *b*, The same aneurysm before surgical revision.

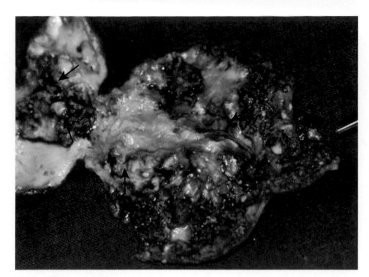

Figure 81.8 Calcification of aneurysmal cannulation area. Note extensive calcification (*arrows*) on inside of surgically resected aneurysm.

- Grade III: ischemic pain at rest
- Grade IV: ulceration, necrosis, and gangrene

Grades I and II can be managed conservatively, but grade III or IV steal syndrome requires surgery or another interventional procedure. Steal syndrome is observed more frequently with elbow/upper arm AV fistulas and AV grafts because of the higher blood flow rates, but older, diabetic, and hypertensive patients can suffer from grade III or IV steal syndrome even with blood flow as low as 300 ml/min.

Diagnosis

Physical examination with palpation of peripheral arteries and skin temperature and inspection for nonhealing wounds, necrosis, and/or gangrene helps to make the diagnosis, but it is essential to measure access blood flow to differentiate between low-flow and high-flow steal syndromes.

Treatment

High-flow AV fistulas may undergo banding procedures, although the results are not always reliable. The venous lumen should be surgically reduced to 20%, and there is only a small margin of error before iatrogenic thrombosis may occur.

Steal syndromes with normal blood flow rates can be treated by the DRIL procedure (distal revascularization and interval ligation). In brachial AV fistulas and in AV grafts, the artery is ligated close downstream from the AV anastomosis and an arterioarterial bypass, saphenous vein, or an ePTFE graft is used to bridge the ligated brachial artery (Fig. 81.9). A useful alternative with low-flow steal syndromes is the PAVA technique (proximal arteriovenous anastomosis), in which the AV anastomosis in the arm is closed and a graft is placed that is anastomosed to the axillary or other proximal artery and to the vein at the level of the closed first AV anastomosis.

Closure of the access is mandatory in AV fistulas and grafts with severe steal syndromes and blood flow rates of ≥300 ml/min. Attempts to create a new AV access in the contralateral arm usually fail because the extent of arteriosclerosis and calcification is the same in both arms, and steal again occurs.

There is a very rare but dangerous phenomenon: ischemic monomelic neuropathy. The leading symptoms are paresthesia and numbness in the dermatomal distribution of the three forearm nerves combined with paralysis of the forearm and

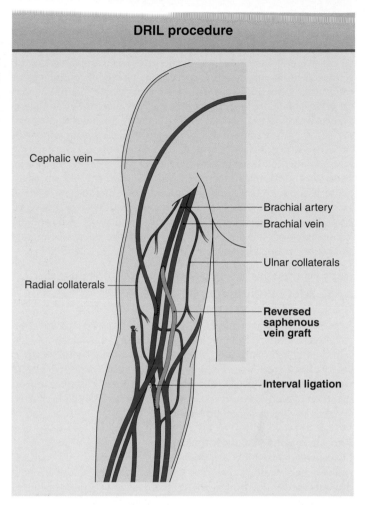

DRIL procedure

Cephalic vein

Brachial artery
Brachial vein
Ulnar collaterals

Radial collaterals

Reversed saphenous vein graft

Interval ligation

Figure 81.9 Distal revascularization and interval ligation (DRIL) procedure. This arterial bypass procedure, using a reversed saphenous vein graft from above to below the fistula corrects the steal phenomenon and allows preservation of the access.

hand muscles occurring immediately after creation of the AV anastomosis. Electromyelography reveals acute, predominantly distal denervation of all upper limb nerves. Immediate closure of the AV access is mandatory to prevent severe and irreversible neurologic injury.[23]

Cardiac Overload in Arteriovenous Fistulas and Arteriovenous Grafts

At least 50% percent of all patients starting dialysis suffer from left ventricular hypertrophy, ischemic heart disease, and some degree of cardiac failure. Nevertheless, cardiac decompensation caused by an AV fistula or graft is uncommon except in patients with advanced cardiac disease. An access blood flow exceeding 1000 to 1500 ml/min, as well as a flow/cardiac output ratio exceeding 20% should lead to concern that high flow is contributing to cardiac decompensation. Treatment initially should aim at achieving dry weight together with control of hypertension and renal anemia. In selected cases, echocardiography with acute compression of the AV fistula may allow an experienced cardiologist to assess changes in cardiac contractility. Surgery, if indicated, aims to reduce blood flow by banding procedures or interposition of narrow graft segment as well as reducing the length of the anastomosis, but results are unpredictable. Pre- and postoperative flow measurements are essential.

Edema Following Arteriovenous Access Formation—Central Venous Stenosis

If significant arm edema develops following formation of AV access, there should be an immediate evaluation for central venous stenosis, particularly if there is any history of central venous catheter placement. Use of the subclavian vein for central venous catheters should be forbidden given the very high risk of producing significant stenoses. Central venous stenosis includes stenosis of the subclavian, brachiocephalic veins, as well as the superior vena cava. If not previously identified, the most common presentation is arm edema following insertion of an AV fistula or AV graft in the upper limb. Prompt intervention will minimize the risk of inadequate HD due to recirculation, skin infection due to poor healing, and the risk of irreversible tissue damage. Contrast angiography of central veins is mandatory for proper evaluation, followed by angioplasty and stenting, which may allow the edema to regress and render the access usable.

INFECTION IN ARTERIOVENOUS FISTULAS AND ARTERIOVENOUS GRAFTS

Access infections are associated with a risk of life-threatening complications including septicemia, endocarditis, spondyloarthritis, and septic embolism. Attention should be paid to risk factors such as personal hygiene, recurrent infectious episodes, nasal carriage of pathogens, iron overload, chronic skin erosions, immunosuppressive therapy, and malnutrition. Antibiotic therapy should be started at the first clinical sign of infection.

Arteriovenous Fistula Infection

Diagnosis of infection is based on clinical evidence of warmth, redness, and swelling. The first step is to immobilize the arm and discontinue cannulation in the infected region. If pus appears in the region of the anastomosis or at cannulation sites, surgical intervention is absolutely indicated, ranging from simple drainage to removal of the anastomosis. Otherwise, appropriate antibiotic therapy and careful observation may be appropriate. Microbiologic analysis is mandatory to ensure use of the appropriate antibiotic even though most vascular access infections are caused by staphylococci and gram-negative bacilli. Antibiotic therapy must be continued for at least 2 weeks.

Arteriovenous Graft Infection

Infection of an AV graft is much more common and must be treated as an emergency. If the anastomotic area is involved, removal of all graft material is mandatory. Midgraft infections can be treated conservatively at first. Otherwise, segmental graft bypassing may be attempted, although this has a high risk of failure. In the presence of fever and/or bacteremia, the appropriate antibiotics should be given intravenously for 2 weeks and continued orally for another 4 weeks. Grafts no longer in use should be removed.[24]

CENTRAL VENOUS DIALYSIS CATHETERS

Dialysis catheters are a necessary evil, allowing dialysis in patients who do not have permanent AV access. However, they expose patients to a greater risk of complications compared to an AV fistula, including a five- to sevenfold increased risk of infection and in some studies an increase in mortality.[25,26] They are appropriately used in hospitals in patients presenting with acute renal failure; unfortunately, they are too frequently employed in chronic care of patients who have not received adequate care

prior to reaching ESRD. Use of catheters varies around the world (see Fig. 81.1), but in the United States, between 35% and 60% of patients still start dialysis using a catheter and this increased 15% between 1998 and 2002.[27]

Temporary Untunneled Catheters

Temporary dialysis catheters can be inserted at the bedside using the modified Seldinger technique with only local anesthesia. For years physicians inserted these catheters using only landmarks, but ultrasound guidance should now be used routinely if available to decrease the complication rate of the procedure. Femoral vein catheters should ideally be 24 cm in length to prevent recirculation. In the internal jugular veins, a shorter catheter should be used and the tip of the catheter is positioned just above the right atrium on a radiograph. Dialysis catheters should never be placed in the subclavian vein, as there is a significant risk of subsequent venous stenosis preventing the successful creation of a permanent vascular access. Temporary dialysis catheters should not be left in place for more than 5 to 7 days when placed in the femoral vein and not more than 3 weeks in the jugular vein. It is recommended that patients with femoral dialysis catheters remain in bed.[28] Patients should not be sent home with temporary dialysis catheters.[28]

Tunneled Cuffed Catheters

Tunneled cuffed catheters are inserted under fluoroscopic guidance, and the cuff, often made of Dacron, is positioned inside the skin tunnel allowing for fibroblast ingrowth and subsequently decreasing the risk of infection. This type of catheter is most commonly inserted in the right internal jugular vein and tunneled under the skin to the below the clavicle; however, they can be placed in any large vein if clinically indicated due to limited vascular access sites. This type of catheter is appropriate for patients who are anticipated to require dialysis for more than 3 weeks, even if they have acute renal failure.[29] The technique for tunneled catheter insertion is shown in Chapter 82.

Catheter Malfunction

Catheters can malfunction due to kinking or thrombosis. Kinking often occurs after a difficult line placement or after placement of line in very obese patients. Dialysis nurses frequently deal with these problems by positioning the patients or by subtle adjustments to the catheter. More severe problems may require repositioning or replacement of the catheter over a guidewire. In order to prevent catheter thrombosis, dialysis catheters are generally locked with heparin 5000 U/ml. A 30% trisodium citrate solution can also be used as a catheter-locking solution and may offer advantages over heparin as citrate by preventing biofilm formation and reducing the incidence of catheter associated infections.[30] Use of citrate is not yet widespread, perhaps because of concerns about accidental administration of citrate into the circulation; however, no major complications from citrate use have been reported in the clinical trials.[30]

Thrombosis in the catheter is another common cause of poor flow in both temporary and tunneled dialysis catheters. Intraluminal thrombolysis, with tissue plasminogen activator 1 mg/ml or urokinase 5000 IU/ml, to fill catheter volume are both effective treatments to restore catheter patency.

Catheter Infection

The most common complication of dialysis catheters is infection. On average, there are three episodes of infection per 1000 tunneled catheter days, and infection rates are higher with

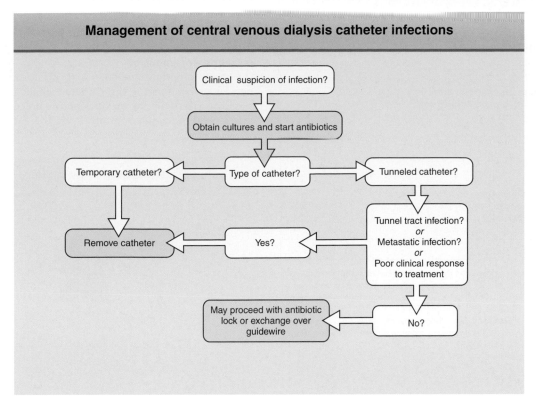

Management of central venous dialysis catheter infections

Clinical suspicion of infection?

Obtain cultures and start antibiotics

Type of catheter?

Temporary catheter?

Tunneled catheter?

Remove catheter

Yes?

Tunnel tract infection?
or
Metastatic infection?
or
Poor clinical response
to treatment

May proceed with antibiotic
lock or exchange over
guidewire

No?

Figure 81.10 Algorithm for the management of central venous dialysis catheter infections. (Adapted from NKF-K/DOQI: Clinical Practice Guidelines for Vascular Access: Update 2000. Am J Kidney Dis 2001;37:S137–S181.)

nontunneled catheters.[31] These localized infections can progress to metastatic complications of osteomyelitis, septic arthritis, epidural abscess, and endocarditis. Various societies have issued recommendations for the management of catheter infections.[29,32] The authors recommend the treatment algorithm shown in Figure 81.10.[32]

Infections Involving Temporary Catheters
When a temporary dialysis catheter becomes infected, it should always be removed. There is no role for trying to salvage temporary catheters.[29]

Exit Site versus Tunnel Tract Infections
It is critically important to distinguish exit site infections from tunnel tract infections because the treatments are quite different. An exit site infection is a localized cellulitis confined to the 1 to 2 cm where the catheter exits the skin. The majority of these cases respond well to systemic antibiotics and meticulous exit site care, and the removal of the catheter is generally not required.[29] However, exit site infections should receive prompt attention because untreated they can progress to tunnel tract infections.

By contrast, a tunnel tract infection involves the potential space surrounding the catheter and is >2 cm from the exit site (Fig. 81.11). Patients with a tunnel tract infection sometimes, but not always, have an associated exit site infection; untreated, they can rapidly develop bacteremia. Patients with a tunnel tract infection frequently present with fever as well as pain, swelling, fluctuance, and erythema along the tract of the catheter. Since tunnel tract infections involve a potential space in an area with limited vascular supply and an implanted synthetic material, they respond poorly to antibiotics alone and require catheter removal.[29]

Catheter-Associated Bacteremia
When a patient with a dialysis catheter has a fever, catheter infection must always be considered. If the patient does not have a clear and convincing alternative explanation for the fever, blood cultures should be obtained peripherally as well as through the catheter, and the patient should be started on antibiotic therapy, which is subsequently adjusted based on culture results.[29] The most common organism is *Staphylococcus*, although a wide range of gram-positive and gram-negative organisms have been reported (Fig. 81.12).[33] The percentage of patients with methicillin-resistant *Staphylococcus aureus* (MRSA) varies greatly among centers with

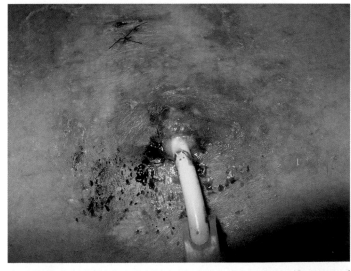

Figure 81.11 Dialysis catheter tunnel tract infection. (Courtesy of Dr. I. M. Leidig.)

Causative organisms in dialysis catheter infections

Polytmicrobial		16%
Gram positive		89%
	Staphylococcus aureus	30%
	Staphylococcus epidermidis	37%
	Enterococcus	17%
	Corynebacterium	49%
Gram negative		33%
	Enterobacter	11%
	Pseudomonas	7%
	Acinetobacter	4%
	Citrobacter	4%
	Serratia	2%
	Klebsiella	3%
	Other Gram negative	3%
Mycobacteria		2%

Figure 81.12 Causative organisms in dialysis catheter infections. Organisms isolated from a series of 123 episodes of catheter-associated bacteremia. Numbers do not add up to 100% because 16% of infections were polymicrobial. (Adapted from Weijmer MC, van den Dorpel MA, Van de Ven PJ, et al: CITRATE Study Group: Randomized, clinical trial comparison of trisodium citrate 30% and heparin as catheter-locking solution in hemodialysis patients. J Am Soc Nephrol 2005;16:2769–2777.)

higher rates associated with greater antibiotic use. In one recent outbreak of MRSA, 50% of the cases of catheter-associated bacteremia were due to MRSA[34]; therefore, empirical coverage with vancomycin for MRSA is mandatory. An aminoglycoside or a cephalosporin is a good choice for gram-negative coverage; however, local microbiologic epidemiology must be taken into consideration, especially concerning antibiotic resistance.

Catheter Removal

The decision to remove a tunneled cuffed dialysis catheter for an episode of catheter-associated bacteremia depends on the clinical condition of the patient and response to initial therapy, the presence of metastatic complications, the infecting organism, and the availability of other vascular access sites (see Fig. 81.10).

The conventional approach was formerly to remove the catheter with interval replacement at a different site after the infection resolved. This approach has drawbacks including the requirement for multiple procedures, the potential loss of the old vascular access site, and the need for an additional temporary catheter if dialysis is needed before the catheter can be replaced. Attempts to salvage an infected catheter with systemic antibiotic therapy are unsatisfactory; resolution of the infection is reported in only 25% to 37% of patients.[31] One treatment option in conjunction with systemic antibiotics is the use of antibiotic lock solutions. Many different cocktails of antibiotics mixed with either heparin or citrate have been tested; a popular regimen is vancomycin 2.5 mg/ml, gentamicin 1 mg/ml, and heparin 2500 U/ml.[29] Infection clearance rates of between 50% and 70% are reported with antibiotic locking. If catheter salvage is to be attempted, we recommend the use of an antibiotic lock solution.[32]

Several studies have reported that exchanging the catheter over a guidewire 48 hours after initial antibiotic treatment is more effective than treatment with antibiotics alone and is as effective as removal of the catheter and delayed replacement with the advantages of only one invasive procedure and preservation of the venous access site. Clinical trials of antibiotic

locking and catheter exchange over a guidewire are not yet available.

Prevention of Infection

The most important measure to prevent catheter infection is meticulous handling of the catheter at all times. The catheter should be inserted using maximal sterile precautions. The dialysis nurses need procedures for accessing the catheters under strict

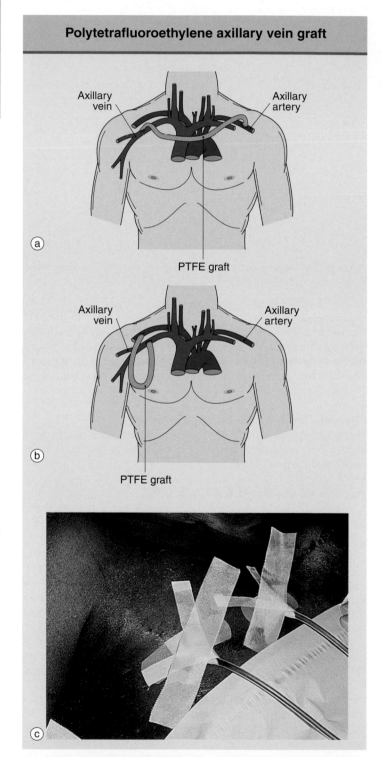

Polytetrafluoroethylene axillary vein graft

Figure 81.13 Polytetrafluoroethylene (PTFE) vein graft. *a*, Ipsilateral axillary artery to contralateral axillary vein PTFE graft. *b*, Ipsilateral axillary artery to axillary vein PTFE graft. *c*, Axilloaxillary vein PTFE graft in use.

sterile conditions, and it is of the utmost importance that these catheters are never accessed by untrained personnel. Several small trials suggest that antibiotic lock solutions significantly reduce the incidence of infection[35,36]; however, large randomized trials demonstrating both safety and efficacy are needed before these practices can be adopted.

Nasal colonization with *Staphylococcus* significantly increases the risk of infection in HD patients.[37,38] Treatment with nasal mupirocin ointment reduces the rate of colonization acutely, but recolonization is common. One small randomized study reported a significant reduction in the rates of infection in chronic dialysis patients being actively treated with nasal mupirocin.[38] Larger randomized trials and studies on the cost-effectiveness of this approach are needed. Finally, topical application of mupirocin ointment to tunneled exit sites has been reported to reduce the incidence of catheter-associated bacteremia.[39]

STRATEGIES FOR THE DIFFICULT VASCULAR ACCESS PATIENT

In general, the principle when planning vascular access should be as distal as possible for as long as possible. Once sites in both lower and then upper arms have been exhausted for AV fistulas and AV grafts, there are a variety of more difficult options.

One approach is a graft from the axillary artery to either the contralateral or ipsilateral axillary vein (Fig. 81.13). Disadvantages of this approach include difficulty in securing needles on the chest wall, problems with hemostasis after removal of the dialysis needles, and an unwanted cosmetic result (see Fig. 81.13c).

The groin is clearly not a preferred site for AV grafts because of increased infection risk as well as patient discomfort and inconvenience. However, in extreme cases of upper extremity vascular or infectious complications, a loop thigh AV graft may be constructed using ePTFE or saphenous vein (Fig. 81.14) or, rarely, an axillofemoral graft. Prior to the creation of such lower extremity

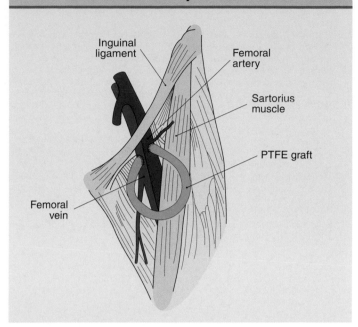

Polytetrafluoroethylene loop graft from femoral artery to femoral vein

Inguinal ligament

Femoral artery

Sartorius muscle

PTFE graft

Femoral vein

Figure 81.14 **Polytetrafluoroethylene (PTFE) loop graft from femoral artery to femoral vein.**

vascular access grafts, it is critically important to ensure that there is no overt vascular disease present that will place the limb in jeopardy with the shunting of blood through a graft. If all these procedures are exhausted, the option of conversion to peritoneal dialysis must always be seriously considered if technically feasible. Other approaches such as translumbar catheter placement into the inferior vena cava have been reported in extreme cases.

REFERENCES

1. Kjellstrand CM: The Achilles' heel of the hemodialysis patient. Arch Intern Med 1978;138:1063–1064.
2. Konner K, Hulbert-Shearon TE, Roys EC, Port FK: Tailoring the initial vascular for dialysis patients. Kidney Int 2002;62:329–338.
3. Pisoni RL, Young EW, Mapes DL, et al: Vascular access use and outcomes in the U.S., Europe, and Japan: Results from the Dialysis Outcomes and Practice Patterns Study (DOPPS). Nephrol News Issues 2003;17:38–47.
4. Avorn J, Winkelmayer WC, Bohn RL, et al: Delayed nephrologist referral and inadequate vascular access in patients with advanced chronic kidney failure. J Clin Epidemiol 2002;55:711–716.
5. Malovrh M: Native arteriovenous fistula: Preoperative evaluation. Am J Kidney Dis 2002;39:1218–25.
6. Wiese P, Nonnast-Daniel B: Colour Doppler ultrasound in dialysis access. Nephrol Dial Transplant 2004;19:1956–1963.
7. Beathard GA: Improving dialysis vascular access. Dial Transplant 2002; 31:210–219.
8. Corpataux J-M, Haesler E, Silacci P, et al: Low-pressure environment and remodelling of the forearm vein in Brescia-Cimino haemodialysis access. Nephrol Dial Transplant 2002;17:1057–1062.
9. Gracz KC, Ing TS, Soung L-S, et al: Proximal forearm fistula for maintenance hemodialysis. Kidney Int 1977;11:71–74.
10. Magnasco A, Alloatti S, Martinoli C, Solari P: Glucose pump test: A new method for blood flow measurements. Nephrol Dial Transplant 2002;17:1–5.
11. Spergel LM, Holland JE, Fadem SZ, et al: Static intra-pressure ratio does not correlate with access blood flow. Kidney Int 2004;66: 1512–1516.
12. Tessitore N, Mansueto G, Bedogna V, et al: A prospective controlled trial on effect of percutaneous transluminal angioplasty on functioning arteriovenous fistulae survival. J Am Soc Nephrol 2003;14:1623–1627.
13. Smits JHM, van der Linden J, Hagen EC, et al: Graft surveillance: Venous pressure, access flow or the combination? Kidney Int 2001;59: 1551–1558.
14. Krönung G: Plastic deformation of Cimino fistula by repeated puncture. Dial Transplant 1984;13:635–638.
15. Turmel-Rodrigues L, Pengloan J, Bourquelot P: Interventional radiology in hemodialysis fistulae and grafts: A multidisciplinary approach. Cardiovasc Intervent Radiol 2002;25:3–16.
16. Tonelli M, Klarenbach S, Jindal K, et al: Access flow in arteriovenous accesses by optodilutional and ultrasound dilution methods. Am J Kidney Dis 2005;46:933–937.
17. Crowther MA, Clase CM, Margetts PJ, et al: Low-intensity warfarin is ineffective for the prevention of PTFE graft failure in patients on hemodialysis: A randomized controlled trial. J Am Soc Nephrol 2002; 13:2331–2337.
18. Kaufman JS, O'Connor TZ, Zhang JH, et al: Veterans Affairs Cooperative Study Group on Hemodialysis Access Graft Thrombosis. Randomized controlled trial of clopidogrel plus aspirin to prevent hemodialysis access graft thrombosis. J Am Soc Nephrol 2003;14:2313–2321.
19. Schmitz PG, McCloud LK, Reikes ST, et al: Prophylaxis of hemodialysis graft thrombosis with fish oil: double-blind, randomized, prospective trial. J Am Soc Nephrol 2002;13:184–190.
20. Fan PY, Schwab SJ: Vascular access. Concepts for the 1990s. J Am Soc Nephrol 1992;3:1–11.
21. LeSar CJ, Merrick HW, Smith MR: Thrombotic complications resulting from hypercoagulable states in chronic hemodialysis access. J Am Coll Surg 1999;189:73–81.
22. Tordoir JHM, Dammers R, van der Sande FM: Upper extremity ischemia and hemodialysis vascular access. Eur J Vasc Endovasc Surg 2004;27:1–5.

23. Miles AM: Vascular steal syndrome and ischaemic monomelic neuropathy: Two variants of upper limb ischemia after hemodialysis access surgery. Nephrol Dial Transplant 1999;14:297–300.

24. Nassar GM, Ayus JC: Clotted arteriovenous grafts: A silent source of infection. Semin Dial 2000;13:1–3.

25. Combe C, Pisoni RL, Port FK, et al: Dialysis Outcomes and Practice Pattern Study: Data on the use of central venous catheters in chronic haemodialysis. Nephrologie 2001;22:379–384.

26. Dhingra RK, Young EW, Hulbert-Shearon TE, et al: Type of vascular access and mortality in U.S. hemodialysis patients. Kidney Int 2001;60:1443–1451.

27. U.S. Renal Data System: USRDS 2005 Annual Data Report: Atlas of End-Stage Renal Disease in the United States. Bethesda, MD: National Institutes of Health, National Institute of Diabetes and Digestive and Kidney Diseases, 2005.

28. Oliver MJ: Acute dialysis catheters. Semin Dial 2001;14:432–435.

29. NKF-K/DOQI: Clinical Practice Guidelines for Vascular Access: Update 2000. Am J Kidney Dis 2001;37:S137–S181.

30. Weijmer MC, van den Dorpel MA, Van de Ven PJ, et al, CITRATE Study Group: Randomized, clinical trial comparison of trisodium citrate 30% and heparin as catheter-locking solution in hemodialysis patients. J Am Soc Nephrol 2005;16:2769–2777.

31. Saad TF: Bacteremia associated with tunneled, cuffed hemodialysis. Am J Kidney Dis 1999;34: 1114–1124.

32. Gersch MS: Treatment of dialysis catheter infections in 2004. J Vasc Access 2004;5:99–108.

33. Beathard GA: Management of bacteremia associated with tunneled-cuffed hemodialysis catheters. J Am Soc Nephrol 1999;10:1045–1049.

34. Lee SC, Chen KS, Tsai CJ, et al: An outbreak of methicillin-resistant *Staphylococcus aureus* infections related to central venous catheters for hemodialysis. Infect Control Hosp Epidemiol 2004;25:678–684.

35. Saxena AK, Panhortra BR: The impact of catheter-restricted filling with cefotaxime and heparin on the lifespan of temporary hemodialysis catheters: A case controlled study. J Nephrol 2005;18:755–763.

36. Kim SH, Song KI, Chang JW, et al: Prevention of uncuffed hemodialysis catheter-related bacteremia using an antibiotic lock technique: A prospective, randomized clinical trial. Kidney Int 2006;69:161–164.

37. Kluytmans JA, Wertheim HF: Nasal carriage of *Staphylococcus aureus* and prevention of nosocomial infections. Infection 2005;33:3–8.

38. Boelaert JR, De Smedt RA, De Baere YA, et al: The influence of calcium mupirocin nasal ointment on the incidence of *Staphylococcus aureus* infections in hemodialysis patients. Nephrol Dial Transplant 1989;4: 278–281.

39. Johnson DW, MacGinley R, Kay TD, et al: A randomized controlled trial of topical exit site mupirocin application in patients with tunnelled, cuffed hemodialysis catheters. Nephrol Dial Transplant 2002;17: 1802–1807.

Diagnostic and Interventional Nephrology

W. Charles O'Neill, Haimanot Wasse, Arif Asif, and Stephen R. Ash

INTRODUCTION

A variety of procedures are essential to the care of nephrology patients and include ultrasonography, renal biopsy, insertion of hemodialysis and peritoneal dialysis (PD) catheters, creation of arteriovenous (AV) fistulas, and diagnostic and interventional procedures on hemodialysis accesses. Although some nephrologists perform certain of these procedures, they have traditionally been performed by other specialists, and this may lead to fragmented care. The desire to provide more continuity of care has led an increasing number of nephrologists to perform these procedures, a field that has recently been termed interventional nephrology. Since some of the procedures are diagnostic, we prefer diagnostic and interventional nephrology. The procedures taken on by nephrologists and the organization of interventional nephrology vary in different parts of the world. It is perhaps most developed in the United States where the American Society of Diagnostic and Interventional Nephrology (ASDIN; www.asdin.org) has established training standards and certification procedures. Certain aspects of this field are covered elsewhere in this book, and this chapter covers ultrasonography, insertion of dialysis catheters, and interventions on vascular access, focusing on their applications and their performance by nephrologists. Renal biopsy is covered in Chapter 6; placement of AV fistulas and AV grafts in Chapter 81.

ULTRASONOGRAPHY

Ultrasonography has wide utility in nephrology since it is a simple, safe, and inexpensive procedure without contraindications. An important reason for nephrologists to be involved in this procedure is that many of the findings on ultrasonography are not specific and require clinical correlation. The role and interpretation of ultrasonography are further covered in Chapter 5.

Applications and Limitations of Ultrasonography

Ultrasonography is an excellent tool for examining the kidneys and urinary tract. Under optimal conditions, both kidneys, the renal artery and vein, the proximal and distal ureter (when enlarged), and the bladder can be visualized. The ureter is usually apparent only when dilated. The middle portion of the ureter is usually obscured by overlying bowel but still may be visible when very dilated. In transplants, the entire ureter can be visualized, even when not markedly dilated, because of the proximity to the probe and the lack of overlying bowel. In very ill patients who cannot be optimally positioned or cannot control their breathing or have abdominal wounds or distention, views of the kidneys may be limited, but it is still possible in most of these patients to determine whether hydronephrosis is present.

Chronic Kidney Disease

Ultrasonography is indicated in any patient presenting with chronic renal insufficiency to establish renal size and rule out polycystic kidney disease or urinary tract obstruction. Small, echogenic kidneys indicate severe irreversible disease, eliminating the need for a biopsy.[1]

Acute Renal Failure

Although the diagnostic yield is very low in patients in whom acute tubular necrosis or prerenal azotemia is the likely cause of renal failure,[2] ultrasonography is still indicated in certain patients to rule out obstruction and to identify pre-existing chronic renal disease.

Renal Transplant

Ultrasonography is indicated in acute failure in transplant patients because urinary obstruction is common in this setting.[3] In the immediate post-transplant period, Doppler evaluation of renal blood flow should also be performed to rule out thrombosis. Additional indications in transplant patients are pain, swelling, ipsilateral leg edema, and infection. Another important indication in both native and transplanted kidneys is guidance for percutaneous biopsy, nephrostomy, or drainage of fluid collections.

Renal Biopsy

Ultrasonography is the method of choice for guiding percutaneous renal biopsy,[4] which is discussed further in Chapter 6. Except in rare cases, computed tomography offers no advantages over ultrasonography[5] and results in unnecessary radiation.

Urinary Bladder

Ultrasonography is the procedure of choice for measuring postvoid residual volume because it is painless and sufficiently accurate[6] and, when a scanner is readily available, a simple task. Additional indications include checking the location and patency of Foley catheters and examination of the distal ureters. Placement of the catheter in the proximal urethra is uncommon but not rare, and obstruction of catheters is frequent, so examination of the bladder should always be considered when urine output decreases. Prostatic hypertrophy, prostatitis, bladder carcinoma, mucosal edema, blood clots, stones, stents, and other foreign bodies can all be recognized by ultrasonography, but transabdominal ultrasonography is not the appropriate test for bladder or prostatic cancer.

Hemodialysis Access

Ultrasonography is essential in the management of vascular access, including guidance of catheter insertion, evaluation of fistula dysfunction, preoperative vein mapping, and monitoring of access flow. Of these, the first two can be readily performed by nephrologists. Guidance of catheterization is best performed with a dedicated scanner but can be done with any scanner that has a vascular probe and does not require Doppler imaging. Examination of dysfunctional fistulas is also straightforward and does not necessarily require Doppler analysis. Vein mapping and monitoring of access flow are both best performed by an experienced vascular technician.

Renovascular Ultrasonography
Doppler ultrasonography of renal arteries and veins is a difficult study requiring an experienced operator and is not usually practical for nephrologists.

Equipment
Important considerations in the choice of equipment are image quality, probe type and frequency, cost, size, portability, and output. Image quality is difficult to quantitate and is related to the number of elements (crystals) in the probe and the number of channels that can be processed. Probes should be electronic and in the frequency range of 2.0 to 5.0 MHz. (up to 7.5 MHz for pediatric use) for abdominal imaging. Preferably these should be variable frequency, curvilinear probes. Probes for vascular imaging are usually linear probes with a frequency between 7.5 and 12 MHz. For gray-scale renal ultrasonography, very portable, light-weight scanners with good image quality are available; Doppler capability can add to the cost but is increasingly being offered as a standard feature. Larger and more expensive scanners are difficult to maneuver and have additional features that are of little use to the nephrologist. Numerous controls on the scanner allow adjustment of scanning depth, focal length, time-gain compensation, sound intensity, and the gray scale. While this seems a daunting number of variables, adjustment is usually straightforward and mostly empirical. Images can be printed directly or digitally stored.

Procedure
Description of the scanning procedures cannot be a substitute for actual hands-on training since scanning is an acquired skill that requires practice. Ideally the patient should be fasting for abdominal scanning to minimize interference from intestinal gas, but this is not essential for examination of kidneys and of no consequence for examination of the bladder or transplanted kidneys. There must be an airtight connection between the probe and the skin, which is accomplished by placing gel on the probe or skin and applying firm pressure against the skin. However, to avoid compression of the vessels, minimal pressure should be applied for vascular examinations, with the use of more gel. Gel specifically designed for ultrasonography should be used since other gels, such as lubricating gel, give poorer image quality. Ambient light should be dimmed to optimize viewing of the monitor.

The patient should be flat in the supine or lateral decubitus position with imaging through the abdomen for examination of native kidneys. Initial attempts should be made in the former position before resorting to the latter. Imaging through the back is not recommended for diagnostic imaging because of sound attenuation by muscle and fascia and limitations on angling of the probe. Placement of the ipsilateral arm over the head, removal of pillows from under the head, and deep inspiration aid in moving overlying ribs superiorly. Transplanted kidneys and the urinary bladder are examined in the supine position, but the patient need not be completely flat.

Initially, longitudinal images should be obtained to determine maximal kidney length. On the right side, this view should be obtained through the liver if possible (Fig. 82.1a). The probe should be oriented so that the upper pole is toward the left hand side of the image. The probe should then be rotated 90 degrees to obtain transverse views (see Fig. 82.1b) and the kidney is scanned from pole to pole to ensure visualization of the entire kidney. Examination of each kidney should include longitudinal images with adjacent liver or spleen if possible, as well as transverse images through the midkidney and each pole.[7] Measurements other than length are of no clinical utility, and sonographic measurements of kidney volume are very inaccurate and no better than length in judging kidney size.[8] Sagittal and transverse views of the urinary bladder are obtained with the probe just superior to the symphysis pubis and angled inferiorly (see Fig. 82.1c and d). Volume is obtained by multiplying the two transverse dimensions and the sagittal length by 0.523.[6] The technique for renal biopsy is discussed in Chapter 6.

Training and Certification
There are no data on what constitutes adequate training for renal ultrasonography and few data for abdominal ultrasonography in general. Training is required for both performance and interpretation and should include didactic, formal hands-on, and supervised components. The last can vary considerably depending on case volume and particularly type since any quantity of studies will be inadequate if they are all normal. Thus, the number of studies required for competence is inversely related to the frequency of pathology. Minimal qualifications for physician-sonographers have been established by the American Institute for Ultrasound in Medicine[9] and the American College of Radiology,[10] but neither organization has developed guidelines for limited abdominal ultrasonography. ASDIN (www.asdin.org) has established training standards for ultrasonography limited to kidneys and bladder[11] that specify 50 hours of training and 125 studies (at least 80 being supervised and the remaining having confirmatory follow-up). Since renal ultrasonography is not an established component of training in nephrology, a course for nephrologists has been established in the United States[12] (www.medicine.emory.edu/renal/ultrasound). Training and certification are available in vascular ultrasonography but are not limited to applications specific to nephrology. Such training is important for vascular studies of kidneys but not necessary for examination of dysfunctional AV fistulas and grafts (unless flow is measured) since this does not require Doppler analysis. There are currently no guidelines or training established for vascular ultrasonography related to nephrology.

PERITONEAL DIALYSIS CATHETERS

Successful PD is dependent on proper catheter insertion and management. The feasibility, safety, and success of these procedures when performed by nephrologists have been well documented,[13–16] and this leads to greater use of PD.[13,17] Chronic PD catheters are constructed of silicone rubber or polyurethane with a 5-mm external diameter and internal diameters of 2.6 to 3.5 mm. Some commonly used designs of PD catheters are shown in Fig. 82.2 and also Fig. 85.6. The intraperitoneal portion can be straight, straight with perpendicular silicone disks, or curled with side holes, or T shaped with linear grooves or slots rather than side holes. These designs are all created to diminish outflow obstruction. The subcutaneous portion is either straight or bent and has one or two extraperitoneal Dacron cuffs that prevent fluid leaks and bacterial migration around the catheter. The subcutaneous catheter shapes

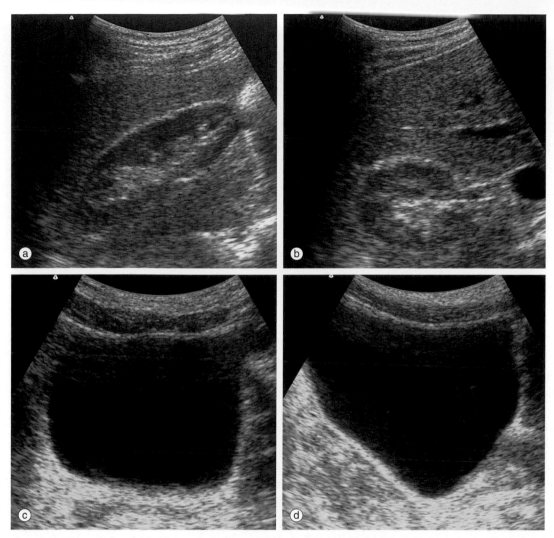

Figure 82.1 Imaging planes for renal and bladder sonography. *a*, Longitudinal image of right kidney. Upper pole should be on left side of the image. *b*, Transverse image of right kidney through the renal hilum. *c*, Transverse image of urinary bladder. Anteroposterior and mediolateral dimensions are obtained in this plane. *d*, Sagittal image of the urinary bladder. Superior portion of the bladder is to the left. Superoinferior dimension is obtained in this plane.

all provide a lateral or downward direction of the exit site. An upward directed exit site collects debris and fluid, increasing the risk of exit site infection. Currently, the method of placement of the catheter has more effect on the outcome than catheter choice.

Catheter Insertion

The three techniques for PD catheter insertion are dissective or surgical, the blind or modified Seldinger, and peritoneoscopic.[18] Only the last two are feasible for nephrologists. Peritoneoscopic insertion uses a small (2.2-mm diameter) optical peritoneoscope for direct inspection of the peritoneal cavity and identification of a suitable site for the intraperitoneal portion of the catheter[18] and is therefore the only technique allowing direct visualization of the intraperitoneal structures. The preference of one technique over another must take into account the incidence of complications (pericatheter leakage, exit site, and tunnel infection) and long-term catheter survival associated with each technique, costs, ease and timely insertion of the catheter, and factors contributing to mortality risk (general anesthesia). Both randomized and nonrandomized studies have documented the superiority of the peritoneoscopic technique with fewer catheter complications (infection, outflow failure, pericatheter leak) and improved catheter survival.[15,16,19–21] The superior results with peritoneoscopic placement may relate to

direct visualization of the abdominal cavity, less tissue dissection, and avoidance of general anesthesia. Since it also avoids the need for an operating room and attendant staff and anesthesiologist, catheter placement can often be expedited.[13] Since tissue dissection is minimal with the peritoneoscopic technique, the postoperative course is brief and the catheter can be used immediately (after 36 hours) for intermittent dialysis, although a 2- to 3-week postoperative period for complete wound healing is recommended before implementing continuous ambulatory PD.[13] During this period, the goal is to avoid ambulation with a filled abdomen. A patient can use manual or automated PD exchanges during the evening and overnight while in bed and drain in the morning. These therapies are generally adequate to avoid uremia and hemodialysis until the catheter is well healed in place.

For peritoneoscopic insertion (Fig. 82.3), a small skin incision (2 to 3 cm) is made and dissection is carried down only to the subcutaneous tissue. The anterior rectus sheath is identified but not incised. A preassembled cannula with trocar and a spiral sheath is then inserted into the abdominal cavity through the rectus muscle (Figs. 82.3a and 82.4). The trocar is then removed and replaced by the peritoneoscope to confirm the intra-abdominal position of the cannula (Figs. 82.3b and 82.5). Six hundred to 1000 ml of air is then infused to separate visceral

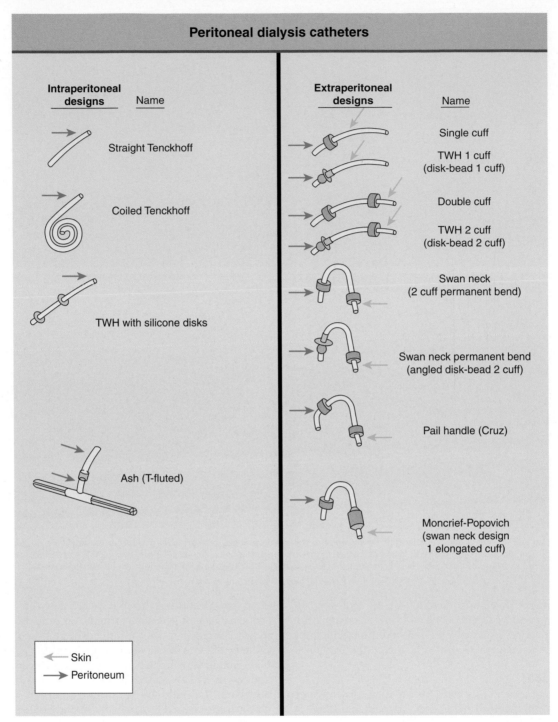

Figure 82.2 Peritoneal dialysis catheters. Various combinations of these intraperitoneal and extraperitoneal designs are available. (Redrawn from Gokal R, Alexander S, Ash S, et al: Peritoneal catheters and exit site practices: Toward optimum peritoneal access, 1998 update. Perit Dial Int 1998;18:11–33.)

and parietal peritoneal surfaces. Bowel loops, the dome of the bladder, and any intraabdominal adhesions are identified. The cannula and spiral sheath are advanced into the pelvis (see Fig. 82.3c). The cannula and the peritoneoscope are then removed, the spiral sheath is dilated to 6 mm diameter (see Fig. 82.3d), and the catheter is inserted through the sheath using an internal stylette (see Fig. 82.3e). The deep cuff is implanted into the rectus muscle using an Implanter Tool without dissection of the anterior rectus sheath or the muscle (see Fig. 82.3f). A tunnel and an exit site are created (Fig. 82.6), and the superficial cuff is implanted into the subcutaneous tissue. The subcutaneous tissue is sutured using absorbable material while the skin is

closed with nylon. No sutures are placed on the external rectus sheath or at the skin exit site. If the catheter will not be used immediately, it can be buried under the skin for weeks to months before it is tunneled to the outside and used.[22] The catheter is tied off with silk suture or plugged, and then coiled into a subcutaneous pouch. This allows ingrowth of tissue into the cuffs of the catheter without an opportunity for bacterial colonization and eliminates early pericatheter infections.[22–24] Catheters buried in this fashion have been successfully used up to 1 year after insertion.[25] We recommend burial when use of the catheter is not anticipated for at least a month after insertion.

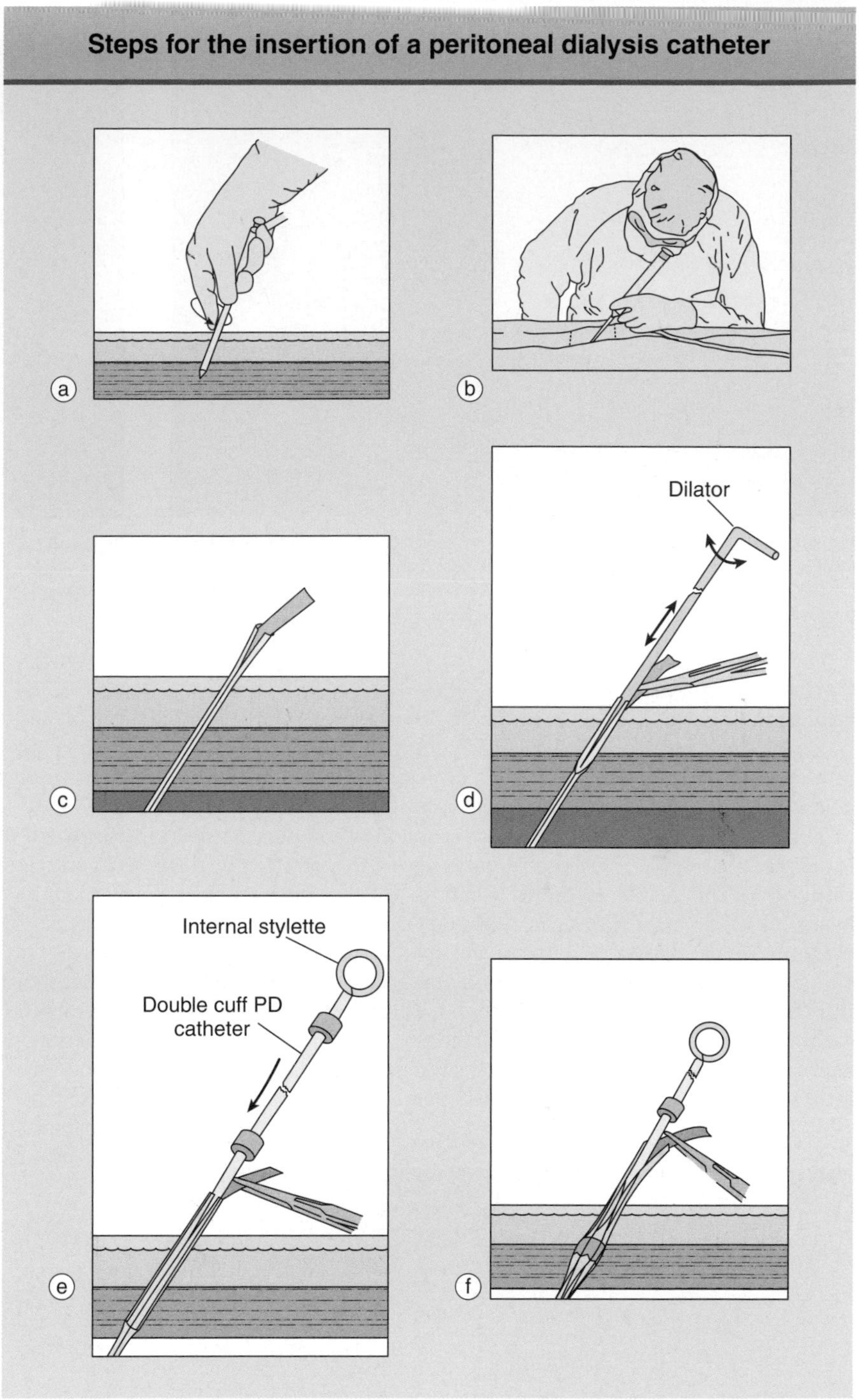

Steps for the insertion of a peritoneal dialysis catheter

Figure 82.3 **Steps for the insertion of a peritoneal dialysis (PD) catheter.** *a*, A trocar and cannula with a sheath are inserted into the abdominal cavity. *b*, The trocar and cannula are removed and a peritoneoscope passed through the sheath. *c*, The sheath has been advanced into the abdominal cavity and the peritoneoscope removed. *d*, The sheath is secured with a forceps while it is being dilated. *e*, A PD catheter (with double cuff) is passed through the dilated sheath using an internal stylette. *f*, The deep cuff is implanted into the rectus muscle. (Redrawn from Y-Tec Instructions: Laparascopic and Peritoneoscopic Placement of Peritoneal Dialysis Catheters. Medigroup Inc. [division of Janin Group, Inc], Oswego, IL, 2004, pp1–5.)

Complications of Peritoneal Dialysis Catheter Insertion

Bowel perforation is the most feared complication of catheter insertion. The incidence is 1% to 1.4% with surgical insertion[26,27] but 0% to 0.8% with the peritoneoscopic insertion.[14,15,28,29] The diagnosis is established by direct peritoneoscopic visualization of bowel mucosa, bowel contents or hard stool, return of fecal material, or emanation of foul-smelling gas through the cannula in a majority of the cases. Whereas some investigators suggest that this complication should be treated with surgical intervention,[30] successful conservative management of bowel perforation using bowel rest and intravenous antibiotics has also been reported.[28,31,32]

To minimize the risk of perforation, a needle (such as a Veress needle) that is smaller and has a blunt, self-retracting end can be used instead of a trocar to gain access to the abdominal cavity.[33] Previous abdominal surgery is mentioned as a relative contraindication to PD due to intraperitoneal adhesions,[34,35] but catheter insertion can be successfully accomplished in this situation.[13,16,28] With the use of peritoneoscopy, which can identify intraperitoneal adhesions, assess their extent, and locate a suitable site for catheter placement, the incidence of bowel perforation is no higher than in patients without prior abdominal surgery, and the success rate exceeds 95%.[16,28]

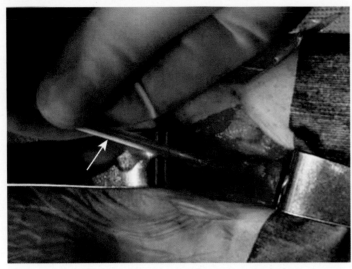

Figure 82.4 Peritonescopic insertion of a peritoneal dialysis catheter. During peritoneoscopic insertion of a peritoneal dialysis catheter a Quill Guide trocar and cannula (*arrow*), with its wrapped spiral sheath, is being inserted through the rectus muscle under local anesthesia.

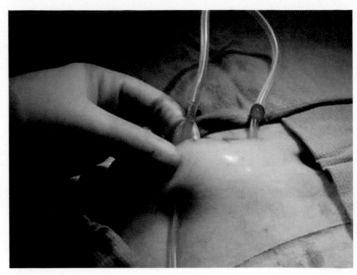

Figure 82.6 Peritonescopic insertion of a peritoneal dialysis catheter. Using a disposable tool, a subcutaneous tunnel is created for the catheter. The superficial cuff shown will be implanted in the subcutaneous tunnel.

Catheter Repositioning

Migration of the PD catheter to the upper abdomen is a frequent cause of outflow problems and catheter failure.[36–40] A variety of techniques have been used to combat migration, including guidewire or stylet insertion, Fogarty catheters, and laparoscopy, and are feasible for nephrologists, but the long-term success rate is only 27% to 48%,[36,38–40] probably because the migration of the catheter is the result of encasement by the omentum. Thus, insertion of a new catheter is required in many cases. Fogarty catheter manipulation is perhaps the most cost-effective, safe, and simple intervention to reposition a migrated PD catheter. In this technique, a Fogarty catheter is advanced into the PD catheter to a premarked point at which the end of the Fogarty is near the end of the PD catheter. Sterile saline (0.5 ml) is injected into the catheter to inflate its balloon. Manipulation is then performed by tugging movements to reposition the catheter into the pelvic area. Infusion and drainage of dialysate as well as radiography are performed to determine patency and position of PD catheter, respectively.

Removal of Peritoneal Dialysis Catheters

A peritoneoscopically inserted PD catheter can be safely removed without need for an operating room or general anesthesia.[13,26] Local anesthetic is infiltrated at the site of the primary incision, and dissection is carried down to the subcutaneous portion of the catheter using longitudinal incisions with scissors while holding the catheter with toothed forceps. The catheter is clamped with a hemostat, a nylon suture is placed in the catheter beyond the hemostat as a tag, and the catheter is cut between the two. Dissection is continued toward the deep cuff (Fig. 82.7), and additional anesthetic is infiltrated around the deep cuff. For catheters that have been in place for less than a month, blunt dissection is usually sufficient to free the deep cuff. Older catheters require

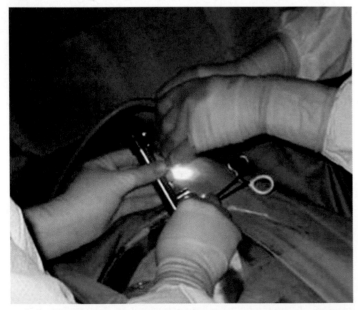

Figure 82.5 Peritonescopic insertion of a peritoneal dialysis catheter. A peritoneoscope has been introduced into the abdominal cavity through the cannula and the fibro-optic light source is being connected to the scope.

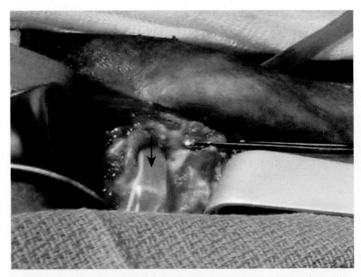

Figure 82.7 Peritoneal dialysis catheter removal. The catheter (*arrow*) has been exposed by dissection of the subcutaneous tunnel.

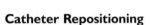

sharp dissection. Exposure of the deep cuff and the anterior rectus sheath is required. Once the deep cuff is separated from the surrounding tissue, the intraperitoneal portion of the catheter is gently withdrawn from the peritoneal cavity. The defect in the rectus sheath is closed with an absorbable pursestring suture using an absorbable material. The nylon tag is then pulled to expose the remaining subcutaneous portion of catheter segment, and dissection is performed in the direction of the superficial cuff. Once the superficial cuff is free, this portion of the catheter is removed through the primary incision site or the exit site. Absorbable suture material such as Vicryl is used to close the subcutaneous tissue while nylon is used to close the skin. The exit site is not sutured.

Training and Certification

The ASDIN has established training guidelines and criteria for certification of physicians in the insertion of PD catheters[41] (www.asdin.org). In addition to appropriate didactic training, there should be two practice insertions (into models, animals, or human cadavers), observation of two insertions into patients, and then six successful insertions into patients as primary operator.

TUNNELED HEMODIALYSIS CATHETERS

Central venous catheters are used as a temporary hemodialysis access, as a bridge to AV fistula or graft use, and when all others permanent access sites have been exhausted. Nontunneled catheters are used when a limited number of dialysis sessions are anticipated or there are contraindications to tunneled catheters (systemic infection, risk of bleeding) and are only appropriate for use in the inpatient setting. Tunneled catheters can be placed in both inpatient and outpatient settings, can be inserted at multiple vein locations, are relatively low in cost, and provide immediate access. However, there are significant disadvantages, including morbidity due to infection and thrombosis, and risk of central vein stenosis or occlusion.[42,43] The role of tunneled dialysis catheters in the provision of vascular access for HD is discussed further in Chapter 81. The right internal jugular vein is the preferred catheter location compared with the left internal jugular or subclavian vein sites and provides a straight route to the right atrium, thereby reducing the risk of central vein stenosis.[44] Catheters may also be placed in the femoral veins. The vein should be cannulated under ultrasound guidance in order to detect anatomic variation or venous thrombosis.

Catheter Insertion

Catheter insertion is performed in a sterile setting, ideally in an operating room environment with fluoroscopy available or, at a minimum, in a dedicated procedure room with cardiac monitoring. Prior to cannulation, the vein should be located by ultrasonography. The patient's neck is then prepared and draped in sterile fashion, and under ultrasound guidance, the vein is cannulated with a micropuncture needle (18 to 22 gauge), and a micropuncture guidewire is inserted and positioned in the superior vena cava. The needle is then removed, and a micropuncture dilator is inserted over the guidewire so that it can be replaced with a standard guidewire. The use of the smaller needle, rather than the standard 15-gauge needle, minimizes trauma to the vein. A small subcutaneous incision is made adjacent to the dilator or guidewire, additional dilation is performed, and the catheter is placed over the guidewire with care being taken to hold the guidewire in place. If a tunneled catheter is to be placed, a catheter exit site is selected inferior to the clavicle and sufficiently lateral to the venotomy to avoid a kink in the catheter. A 1-cm superficial incision is made at this point, and a subcutaneous track adjacent to the venotomy is infiltrated with lidocaine. A double-lumen catheter, generally 28 or 32 cm in length, is attached to a tunneling device, inserted into the exit site, and forced through the subcutaneous tissue in a curved path to the venotomy. A guidewire is passed through the dilator and into the inferior vena cava. The venotomy site is then serially dilated over the guidewire. The catheter can then be inserted over the guidewire through the venous port. When using a split-tip catheter, the guidewire is passed in and out of two venous ports and through the arterial port or through a hollow intracatheter stiffener. Alternatively, a peel-away sheath is placed over the guidewire, and the catheter inserted through the sheath after the removal of the guidewire; however, this method has greater potential for blood loss and air embolism. Fluoroscopy is used to confirm tip placement at the level of the right atrium, with the arterial port facing away from the atrial wall, and to ensure that there are no kinks in the catheter (Fig. 82.8). Each port of the catheter is then flushed with saline and locked with the appropriate amount of heparin, based on catheter length and designated priming volume, followed by placement of the catheter hub caps.

Catheter Dysfunction

Catheter dysfunction is defined as the failure to reach and maintain a blood flow sufficient to perform hemodialysis without significantly extending treatment time and generally reflects a blood flow <300 ml/min.[44] Causes of immediate dysfunction include a kink in the catheter, incorrect position or orientation (arterial port against the vessel wall), and errant venous cannulation. These problems should be ascertained and corrected at the time of catheter placement. Catheter thrombosis is the most common cause of late dysfunction. Extrinsic thrombosis is less common than intrinsic thrombosis and is caused by central vein, mural, or right atrial thrombosis. Intrinsic obstruction results from thrombus within the catheter lumen or tip or most

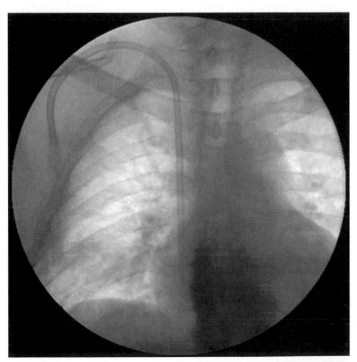

Figure 82.8 Insertion of a venous catheter for hemodialysis. Chest radiograph confirming that the tip of the catheter is at the junction of the superior vena cava and the right atrium.

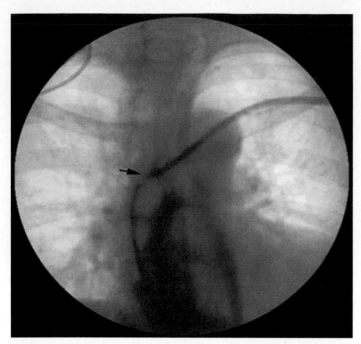

Figure 82.9 Fibrin sheath on a tunneled venous catheter. Contrast has been injected into a tunneled catheter after the tip (*arrow*) has been pulled back into the innominate vein. The contrast fills a sheath that extends from the catheter tip.

commonly from a fibrin sheath. Fibrin sheaths typically develop weeks to months after catheter insertion, initially forming at the venotomy site, and then extending to encase the catheter tip, creating a flap-valve (Fig. 82.9). If flow becomes insufficient, instillation of a fibrinolytic enzyme is used. Tissue plasminogen activator (tPA) is commonly used and may be more effective in restoring patency and adequate flow than urokinase.[45,46] Typically, 2 mg tPA is instilled into the occluded catheter lumen and allowed to dwell 30 minutes.[47] If this fails, the catheter should be exchanged. Strategies to minimize dialysis catheter thrombosis are discussed in Chapter 81.

Catheter Exchange and Fibrin Sheath Removal
Catheter exchange over a guidewire is useful in the setting of catheter thrombosis or bacteremia and allows for the preservation of the venotomy, tunnel, and exit sites. The tunnel and exit sites must appear free of infection if the same sites are to be used. Under sterile conditions, the exit site is anesthetized and the cuff is freed. Once the catheter is pulled back 8 to 10 cm, radiographic contrast is injected through the catheter under fluoroscopy to check for a fibrin sheath (see Fig. 82.9). To obliterate a sheath, a guidewire is passed down the venous port of the catheter and into the inferior vena cava. The catheter is then removed, and a balloon catheter is inserted over the guidewire to the sheath location and inflated to disrupt the sheath. The guidewire is then wiped with Betadine, and a new catheter is inserted over the guidewire. When the catheter tip is beyond the venotomy site, near the superior vena cava, contrast can be injected again to check for sheath removal, before proceeding with catheter insertion.

Training and Certification
The ASDIN guidelines for Hemodialysis Vascular Access Procedure Certification specify formal didactic training in central venous anatomy, sonographic examination of central veins, fluoroscopy, and catheter design and complications. In addition,

practical training for certification includes satisfactory insertion of 25 tunneled long-term catheters.[48] More information may be obtained at www.asdin.org.

PROCEDURES ON ARTERIOVENOUS FISTULAS AND GRAFTS

The most common indications for intervention are inadequate flow during dialysis, thrombosis, and failure of AV fistulas to mature. Specific interventions include angiography, thrombectomy, angioplasty, and stenting. All these procedures require a dedicated facility, either inpatient or outpatient, with fluoroscopy, monitoring equipment, and staff to assist with the procedures and deliver conscious sedation. There are many different approaches to and methods of performing AV access procedures, and few data to indicate superiority of one method over the other, so the choice is generally one of personal preference and cost. However, the first step should always include a careful physical and ultrasound examination of the access. An examination will generally identify the problem and allow for detection of access infection, an absolute contraindication to intervention. Appropriate intervention can then be planned. Monitoring and management of vascular access to minimize stenosis, thrombosis and failure are discussed further in Chapter 81.

Percutaneous Balloon Angioplasty
Stenosis in AV grafts and fistulas is routinely managed by percutaneous balloon angioplasty, which can be safely performed on an outpatient basis, causes minimal discomfort and allows for immediate use of the access. Not all stenotic lesions are responsive, however, and some require repeated treatment. In fistulas, the stenosis is most commonly located adjacent to the anastomosis at the swing point, the portion of the native vein mobilized during creation of the AV anastomosis (Fig. 82.10), while in grafts, the venous anastomosis is the most common site of stenosis.[49-53] Angioplasty is indicated if the stenosis is >50% and is associated with clinical or physiologic abnormalities.[3] Treatment of stenosis increases access blood flow and longevity, reduces access thrombosis, and reduces vascular access-related hospitalization.[51,54,55] A relative contraindication to angioplasty is a newly created access (<4 to 6 weeks old).

The access is cannulated with an introducer needle, a sheath is inserted, and an initial angiogram is obtained. This should include views of the access, draining veins (peripheral and central), and arterial anastomosis, and is used to confirm the location and degree of stenosis (Fig. 82.11a). Angioplasty is recommended for stenoses >50% of the lumen diameter and associated with a clinical or physiologic abnormality.[44] Unless contraindicated, sedation and analgesia are then given with short-acting agents once a lesion has been identified on the initial angiogram, as angioplasty is painful.

A guidewire is passed through the sheath and across the stenosis. An angioplasty balloon catheter is passed over the guidewire, positioned at the stenotic site, and inflated with a syringe to 18 to 20 atm. A variety of sheaths, guidewires, balloon sizes, and maximum pressures are available. The guidewire is left in place, and a repeat angiogram is obtained to identify residual stenosis or any complications (see Fig. 82.11b). Angioplasty is repeated for residual stenosis or when multiple lesions are present and may require a second cannulation of the access in the opposite direction for inflow stenoses. Following removal of all devices, hemostasis at the cannulation site is achieved by manual pressure or suture placement. According to Kidney Disease Outcomes Quality Initiative guidelines, a successful angioplasty is achieved when there

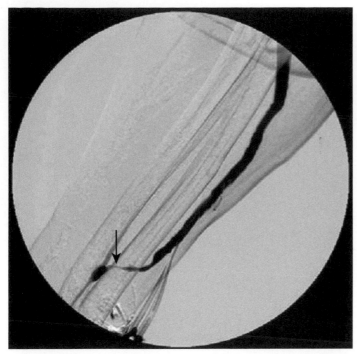

Figure 82.10 Juxta-anastomotic stenosis in a radiocephalic arteriovenous fistula. Contrast was injected at the arterial anastomosis (*bottom left of image*) and demonstrates a narrowing in the initial portion of the fistula (*arrow*).

is no more than 30% residual stenosis and physical indicator(s) of stenosis have resolved.[44]

Percutaneous Thrombectomy

There are a variety of techniques for thrombus removal, and in selecting a procedure effectiveness, efficiency, safety, and economy must be considered. Currently, thromboaspiration is the least costly of all the techniques and is equally as effective and efficient as mechanical and pharmacomechanical thrombolysis, in which low-dose tPA is instilled into the thrombosed access, the clot is manually macerated, flow returns, and angioplasty is used to dilate access stenoses.[56] Thrombectomy by thromboaspiration combines angiography with balloon angioplasty and thrombectomy by clot aspiration, and the sequence varies by operator. Absolute contraindications to thromboaspiration include access infection and known right to left cardiac shunt, while relative contraindications include a large clot burden and long-standing access occlusion.

The access is cannulated in an antegrade direction, and a guidewire is passed to the level of the central veins. A straight catheter is inserted over the wire to the central veins and an angiogram is performed to confirm central venous patency. Anticoagulation and short-acting sedative and analgesic medications are administered in the central circulation. An angiogram is then obtained as the catheter is pulled back to identify the location of stenosis. The guidewire is then inserted beyond the stenotic lesion, followed by an angioplasty balloon catheter. The balloon catheter is insufflated by hand using a syringe, and the stenotic lesion is dilated. The access is then cannulated in the retrograde direction, a sheath is inserted, and a Fogarty catheter is passed across the arterial anastomosis, inflated and pulled back through the entire length of the access, while clot fragments are aspirated. Upon return of flow through the access, an angiogram is obtained to evaluate the inflow and the arterial anastomosis, and angioplasty is repeated if necessary. Hemostasis is achieved via manual pressure or a suture at the cannulation sites.

Stents

The precise role of the endovascular stent in AV fistulas and grafts has not been fully defined. Stents are expensive and have often been used in situations where their use will not extend the life of the access. Appropriate indications include certain situations,[57,58] such as failed balloon angioplasty (an elastic lesion) in central or peripheral veins, when there are few remaining access sites and when an outflow vein ruptures following balloon angioplasty[57,58] (Figs. 82.12 and 82.13). Finally, a stent may be useful in the setting of an expanding pseudoaneurysm.[59]

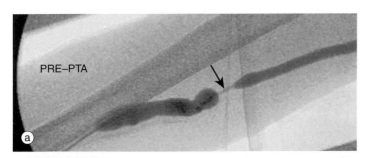

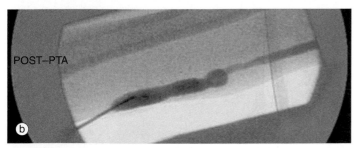

Figure 82.11 Arteriovenous (AV) graft stenosis. *a,* Stenosis in the outflow vein of an upper arm AV graft (*arrow*). *b,* Angiogram performed immediately after percutaneous angioplasty.

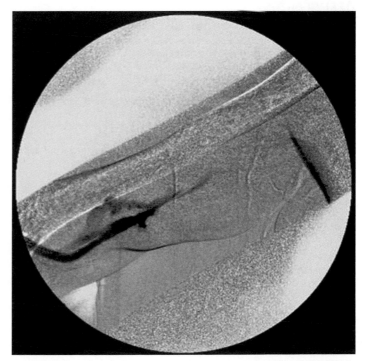

Figure 82.12 Vein rupture. A postangioplasty angiogram of an arteriovenous fistula showing extravasation of dye indicative of a vein rupture. (Image courtesy of Dr. G. Beathard.)

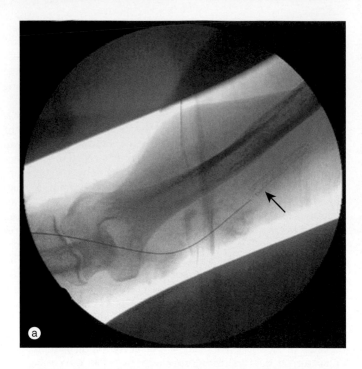

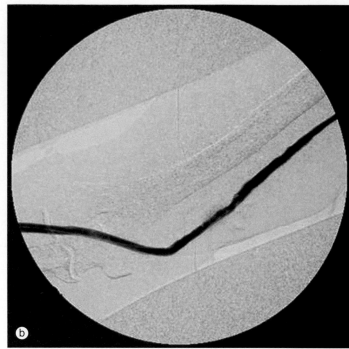

Figure 82.13   Treatment of vein rupture with an intraluminal stent. *a*, Placement of the stent (*arrow*). *b*, An angiogram obtained after stent placement showing that venous outflow has been re-established. (Courtesy of Dr. G. Beathard.)

Training and Certification

The ASDIN guidelines for Hemodialysis Vascular Access Procedure Certification[48] specify didactic training in venous anatomy, fluoroscopy, procedural equipment, sedation, and analgesia. Requirements for practical training include 25 cases in both fistulas and grafts of each of the following: angiography, angioplasty, and thrombectomy as primary operator (please refer to www.asdin.org for more information). In general, several times that number of cases as secondary operator is required to become a primary operator.

REFERENCES

1. Moghazi S, Jones E, Schroepple J, et al: Correlation of renal histopathology with sonographic findings. Kidney Int 2005;67:1515–1520.
2. Gottlieb RH, Weinberg EP, Rubens DJ, et al: Renal sonography: Can it be used more selectively in the setting of an elevated serum creatinine level? Am J Kidney Dis 1997;29:362–367.
3. O'Neill WC, Baumgarten DA: Ultrasonography in renal transplantation. Am J Kidney Dis 2002;39:663–678.
4. Korbet SM: Percutaneous renal biopsy. Semin Nephrol 2002;22:254–267.
5. Nass K, O'Neill WC: Bedside renal biopsy: Ultrasound guidance by the nephrologist. Am J Kidney Dis 1999;34:955–959.
6. Riccabona M, Nelson TR, Pretorius DH, Davidson TE: In vivo three-dimensional sonographic measurement of organ volume: Validation in the urinary bladder. J Ultrasound Med 1996;15:627–632.
7. American Institute of Ultrasound in Medicine: AIUM guidelines. J Ultrasound Med 1995;14:979–981.
8. Emamian SA, Nielsen MB, Pedersen JF: Intraobserver and interobserver variations in sonographic measurements of kidney size in adult volunteers. Acta Radiol 1995;36:399–401.
9. American Institute of Ultrasound in Medicine: Training guidelines for physicians who evaluate and interpret diagnostic ultrasound examinations. Laurel, MD: American Institute of Ultrasound in Medicine, 1997.
10. American College of Radiology: ACR Standard for Performing and Interpreting Diagnostic Ultrasound Examinations. Reston, VA: American College of Radiology, 1996.
11. American Society of Diagnostic and Interventional Nephrology: Guidelines for training, certification, and accreditation in renal sonography. Semin Dialysis 2002;15:442–445.
12. O'Neill WC: Renal ultrasonography: A procedure for nephrologists. Am J Kidney Dis 1997;30:579–585.
13. Asif A, Byers P, Gadalean F, Roth D: Peritoneal dialysis underutilization: The impact of an interventional nephrology peritoneal dialysis access program. Semin Dial 2003;16:266–271.
14. Ash SR, Handt AE, Bloch R: Peritoneoscopic placement of the Tenckhoff catheter: Further clinical experience. Perit Dial Bull 1983;3:8–12.
15. Pastan S, Gassensmith C, Manatunga AK, et al: Prospective comparison of peritoneoscopic and surgical implantation of CAPD catheters. Trans Am Soc Artif Organ 1991;37:M154–M156.
16. Gadallah MF, Pervez A, EI-Shahawy MA, et al: Peritoneoscopic versus surgical placement of peritoneal dialysis catheters: A prospective randomized study on outcome. Am J Kidney Dis 1999;33:118–122.
17. Gadallah MF, Ramdeen G, Torres-Rivera C, et al: Changing the trend: A prospective study on factors contributing to the growth rate of peritoneal dialysis programs. Adv Perit Dial 2001;17:122–126.
18. Ash SR: Chronic peritoneal dialysis catheters: Procedures for placement, maintenance and removal. Semin Nephrol 2002;22:221–236.
19. Scalamonga A, De Vecchi A, Castelnovo C, Ponticelli C: Peritoneal catheter outcome effect of mode of placement. Perit Dial Int 1994;14(Suppl 1):S81.
20. Handt AD, Ash SR: Longevity of Tenckhoff catheters placed by the y-tec® Peritoneoscopic technique. Perspect Perit Dial 1984;2:30–33.
21. Chadha I, Mulgaonkar S, Jacobs M, et al: Outcome of laparoscopic Tenckhoff catheter insertion (LTCI) versus surgical Tenckhoff catheter insertion (STCI): A prospective randomized comparison. Perit Dial Int 1994;14(Suppl 1):S89.
22. Moncrief JW, Popovich RP, Simmons EE, et al: The Moncrief-Popovich catheter: A new peritoneal access technique for patients on peritoneal dialysis. Trans Am Soc Artif Intern Organs 1994;39:62–65.
23. Moncrief JW, Popovich RP, Simmons EE, et al: Peritoneal access technology. Perit Dial Int 1993;13:S112–S123.

24. Prischl F, Wallner M, Kalchmair H, et al: Initial subcutaneous embedding of the peritoneal dialysis catheter—a critical appraisal of this new implantation technique. Nephrol Dial Transplant 1997;12:1661–1667.

25. Ash SR: Chronic peritoneal dialysis catheters: Overview of design, placement, and removal procedures. Semin Dial 2003;16:323–334.

26. Ash SR: Who should place peritoneal catheters? A nephrologist's view. Nephrol News Issues 1993;7:33–34.

27. Thibodeaux LC: Bowel perforation associated with continuous ambulatory peritoneal dialysis. Nephron 1995;70:265.

28. Asif A, Byers P, Vieira CF, et al: Peritoneoscopic placement of peritoneal dialysis catheter and bowel perforation: Experience of an interventional nephrology program. Am J Kidney Dis 2003;42:1270–1274.

29. Ash SR: Bedside peritoneoscopic peritoneal catheter placement of Tenckhoff and newer peritoneal catheters. Adv Peritoneal Dial 1998;14:75–79.

30. Simkin EP, Wright FK: Perforating injuries of the bowel complicating peritoneal catheter insertion. Lancet 1968;1:64–66.

31. Kahn SI, Garella S, Chazan JA: Nonsurgical treatment of intestinal perforation due to peritoneal dialysis. Surg Gynecol Obstet 1973;136:40–42.

32. Rubin J, Oreopoulos DG, Lio TT, et al: Management of peritonitis and bowel perforation during chronic peritoneal dialysis. Nephron 1976;16:220–225.

33. Asif A, Tawakol J, Khan T, et al: Modification of the peritoneoscopic technique of peritoneal dialysis catheter insertion: Experience of an interventional nephrology program. Semin Dial 2004;17:171–173.

34. Nkere Nkere UU: Postoperative adhesion formation and the use of adhesion preventing techniques in cardiac and general surgery. ASAIO J 2000;46:654–656.

35. Brandt CP, Franceschi D: Laparoscopic placement of peritoneal dialysis catheters in patients who have undergone prior abdominal operations. J Am Coll Surg 1994;178:515–516.

36. Gadallah MF, Aurora N, Arumugam R, Moles K: Role of Fogarty catheter manipulation in management of migrated, nonfunctional peritoneal dialysis catheters. Am J Kidney Dis 2000;35:301–305.

37. Gadallah MF, Mignon J, Torres C, et al: The role of peritoneal dialysis catheter configuration in preventing catheter tip migration. Adv Perit Dial 2000;16:47–50.

38. Siegel RL, Nosher JL, Gesner LR: Peritoneal dialysis catheters: Repositioning with new fluoroscopic technique. Radiology 1994;190:899–901.

39. Kappel JE, Ferguson GM, Kudel RM, et al: Stiff wire manipulation of peritoneal dialysis catheters. Adv Perit Dial 1995;11:202–207.

40. Simons ME, Pron G, Voros M, et al: Fluoroscopically-guided manipulation of malfunctioning peritoneal dialysis catheters. Perit Dial Int 1999;19:544–549.

41. The American Society of Diagnostic and Interventional Nephrology: Guidelines for training, certification, and accreditation in placement of permanent tunneled and cuffed peritoneal dialysis catheters. Semin Dial 2002;15:440–442.

42. Schwab SJ, Beathard G: The hemodialysis catheter conundrum. Hate living with them, but can't live without them. Kidney Int 1999;56:1–17.

43. Vanherweghem JL, Yassine T, Goldman M, et al: Subclavian vein thrombosis: A frequent complication of subclavian vein cannulation for hemodialysis. Clin Nephrol 1986;26:235–238.

44. National Kidney Foundation: K/DOQI clinical practice guidelines for vascular access, 2000. Am J Kidney Dis 2001;37(Suppl 1):S137–S181.

45. Haire WD, Atkinson JB, Stephens LC, Kotulak GD: Urokinase versus recombinant tissue plasminogen activator in thrombosed central venous catheters: A double-blinded, randomized trial. Thromb Haemost 1994;72:543–547.

46. Zacharias JM, Weatherston CP, Spewak CR, Vercaigne LM: Alteplase versus urokinase for occluded hemodialysis catheters. Ann Pharmacother 2003;37:27–33.

47. Beathard GA: Catheter thrombosis. Semin Dial 2001;14:441–445.

48. The American Society of Diagnostic and Interventional Nephrology Application for Certification in Interventional Nephrology: Hemodialysis Vascular Access Procedures, 2004.

49. Falk A, Teodorescu V, Lou WY, et al: Treatment of "swing point stenoses" in hemodialysis arteriovenous fistulae. Clin Nephrol 2003;60:35–41.

50. Beathard GA, Arnold P, Jackson J, Litchfield T: Aggressive treatment of early fistula failure. Kidney Int 2003;64:1487–1494.

51. Beathard GA: Angioplasty for arteriovenous grafts and fistulae. Semin Nephrol 2002;22:202–210.

52. Maya ID, Oser R, Saddekni S, et al: Vascular access stenosis: Comparison of arteriovenous grafts and fistulas. Am J Kidney Dis 2004;44:859–865.

53. Sivanesan S, How TV, Bakran A: Sites of stenosis in AV fistulae for hemodialysis access. Nephrol Dial Transplant 1999;14:118–120.

54. Schwab SJ, Oliver MJ, Suhocki P, McCann R: Hemodialysis arteriovenous access: Detection of stenosis and response to treatment by vascular access blood flow. Kidney Int 2001;59:358–362.

55. Schwab SJ, Harrington JT, Singh A, et al: Vascular access for hemodialysis. Kidney Int 1999;55:2078–2090.

56. Schon D, Mishler R: Pharmacomechanical thrombolysis of natural vein fistulas: Reduced dose of TPA and long-term follow-up. Semin Dial 2003;16:272–275.

57. Vesely TM, Hovsepian DM, Pilgram TK, et al: Upper extremity central venous obstruction in hemodialysis patients: Treatment with wallstents. Radiology 1997;204:343–348.

58. Funaki B, Szymski GX, Leef JA, et al: Wallstent deployment to salvage dialysis graft thrombolysis complicated by venous rupture: Early and intermediate results. AJR Am J Roentgenol 1997;169:1435–1437.

59. Vesely TM: Use of stent grafts to repair hemodialysis graft-related pseudoaneurysms. J Vasc Interv Radiol 2005;16:1301–1307.

83 Hemodialysis: Technology, Adequacy, and Outcomes

Peter Kotanko, Martin K. Kuhlmann, and Nathan W. Levin

INTRODUCTION

Despite the widespread use of peritoneal dialysis and renal transplantation, hemodialysis (HD) remains the main renal replacement therapy in most countries worldwide. Currently more than 1.4 million patients worldwide are on HD with an estimated growth to 2.0 millions in 2010. Despite significant advances in our understanding of the biology of chronic kidney disease and the risk factors for poor outcome on HD, and improved dialysis technology, the annual mortality in HD patients remains as high as 15% to 25% internationally depending on demographic factors.

DIALYSIS SYSTEM

The aim of the HD system is to deliver blood in a fail-safe manner from the patient to the dialyzer, enable an efficient removal of uremic toxins and fluid, and to pass the cleared blood back to the patient.[1] The main components of the dialysis system are the extracorporeal blood circuit, the dialyzer, the dialysis machine, and the water purification system.[2] The dialysis machine delivers dialysis fluid with the intended flow rate, temperature, and chemical composition. The dialysis machine has monitoring and safety systems, blood and dialysate pumps, a heating system, a dialysate mixing and degassing unit, and an ultrafiltrate balancing system. The role of the water purification system is to produce water for dialysis that complies with set standards.

DIALYZER DESIGNS

The dialyzer provides controllable transfer of solutes and water across the semipermeable membrane. The flows of dialysate and blood are separated and countercurrent. The dialyzer (Fig. 83.1) has four ports, one inlet and one outlet port for each for blood and dialysate, respectively. The semipermeable dialysis membrane separates the blood compartment and the dialysate compartment. The transport processes across the membrane are diffusion (dialysis) and convection (ultrafiltration). The removal of small solutes occurs primarily by diffusion, while larger components such as β_2-microglobulin are more effectively removed by convection. The hollow fiber dialyzer represents currently the most effective design (see Fig. 83.1); it delivers high dialysis efficiency with low resistance to flow.

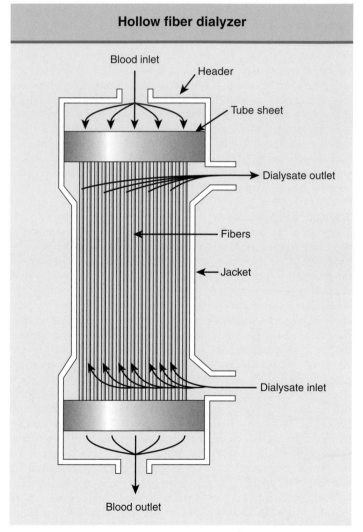

Hollow fiber dialyzer

Blood inlet · Header · Tube sheet · Dialysate outlet · Fibers · Jacket · Dialysate inlet · Blood outlet

Figure 83.1   Design of a modern hollow-fiber dialyzer.

DIALYSIS MEMBRANE

Membranes vary with respect to chemical structure, biophysical properties such as transport characteristics, and biocompatibility (Fig. 83.2).[1]

Dialysis membrane properties			
Membrane	Membrane Name (example)	High or Low Flux	Biocompatibility
Cellulose semisynthetic cellulose			
Cellulose diacetate	Cellulose acetate	High and low	Intermediate
Cellulose triacetate	Cellulose triacetate	High	Good
Diethylaminoethyl-substituted cellulose	Hemophane	High	Intermediate
Synthetic polymers			
Polymethylmethacrylate	PMMA	High	Good
Polyacrylonitrile methacrylate copolymer	PAN	High	Good
Polyacrylonitrile methallyl sulfonate copolymer	PAN/AN-69	High	Good
Polyamide	Polyflux	High	Good
Polycarbonate/Polyether	Gambrane	High	Good
Polyethylene/Vinyl alcohol	EVAL	High	Good
Polysulfone	Polysulfone	High	Good

Figure 83.2 Dialysis membrane properties.

Materials

The basic membrane material has been cellulose, which is made up of repetitive polysaccharide units containing hydroxyl groups. Cellulose acetate is a modification, in which 80% of the hydroxyl groups are replaced by acetate radicals; despite this alteration, biocompatibility is still low. To increase it, synthetic tertiary amino compounds are added during cellulose membrane synthesis (cellulosynthetic membranes). More recent membranes are not cellulose based but instead are built of entirely synthetic materials, such as polyacrylonitrite, polysulfone, polycarbonate, polyamide, and polymethylmethacrylate. These synthetic membranes provide superior biocompatibility.

Transport Properties

Transport of molecules across the dialysis membrane is due to (1) the concentration gradient (diffusive transport) and (2) the pressure across the membrane (convective transport) and is dependent on membrane pore size. Dialyzer efficiency in terms of urea removal depends on the surface area (usually 0.8 to 2.1 m^2). High-efficiency dialyzers have a high surface area irrespective of pore size and possess a superior clearance for small molecules but may have small pores and thus a low ability to remove large molecules such as β_2-microglobulin. The dialyzer mass transfer area coefficient for urea (KoA) is a measure of the theoretically maximal possible urea clearance (ml/min) at infinite blood and dialysate flow rates. Dialyzer efficiency can be categorized according to KoA as low (<500 ml/min), moderate (500 to 700 ml/min), and high (>700 ml/min). High-flux dialyzers have pores large enough to allow the passage of larger molecules such as β_2-microglobulin (molecular weight 11800 d). Water permeability is described by the ultrafiltration coefficient (Kuf) in ml transmembrane ultrafiltration/hr/mm Hg transmembrane pressure. Kuf is high in high-flux dialyzers, with ultrafiltration coefficients up to 80 ml/hr/mm Hg. During high-flux HD, backfiltration may result in a transfer of 5 to 10 liters of dialysate into the blood. Therefore, water quality is of paramount importance when using high-flux dialyzers.

SAFETY MONITORS

Safety monitors are important integral parts of the dialysis machine. Pressure monitors are in most machines integrated to monitor the system pressure in critical positions (Fig. 83.3)[2]:

- Between the arterial side and the blood pump (arterial pressure) to assess the suction pressure; overly negative values may signal reduced arterial inflow and access problems
- Between the blood pump and the dialyzer inlet (dialyzer inflow pressure) to assess the dialyzer inflow pressure; a high pressure may signal dialyzer clotting
- Between the dialyzer outlet and the air trap (venous pressure) to control the return pressure; a high pressure may point toward an obstruction in the venous limb; it is important to consider that in the event of venous needle displacement, the venous pressure will remain positive because of the needles' flow resistance

A venous air detector and air trap are located downstream of the venous pressure monitor. The air trap prevents air from passing into the patient; a positive signal at the air detector automatically clamps the venous line and stops the blood pump. A blood leak detector is placed in the dialysate outflow line. Dialysate temperature is constantly monitored. Dialysate is produced by a proportioning system that mixes acid and bicarbonate concentrates with water. The osmolarity of the dialysate translates into conductivity, which is measured by the dialysis conductivity monitor. The ultrafiltration rate has to be controlled precisely, nowadays in most machines by a volumetric control system. This issue is of great importance especially with the use of high-flux dialyzers.

ANTICOAGULATION

Usually unfractioned or, in some countries, low molecular weight (LMW) heparin is used to prevent blood clotting in the extracorporal circuit. Constant infusion of heparin, repeated-bolus of heparin, or single bolus of LMW heparin is used.

A typical routine prescription of constant infusion heparin is to administer an initial bolus of 2000 IU followed by a heparin infusion (800 to 1200 IU/hr) until 30 to 60 minutes before the end of the session. Applying the repeated-bolus method, an initial heparin bolus of, for example, 4000 IU is followed by, for example, 1000 to 2000 IU after 2 hours. Initially, measurement of whole-blood partial thromboplastin time may be necessary to avoid bleeding complications, but routine monitoring of whole-blood partial thromboplastin time or activated clotting time is usually not necessary. LMW heparin is given as a bolus at the beginning of the session. Antifactor Xa activity measurement to monitor LMW heparin treatment is usually not necessary. In some institutions, regional citrate anticoagulation is used routinely, but we recommend limiting its use to patients with recent surgery, coagulopathies, thrombocytopenia, active bleeding, intracerebral

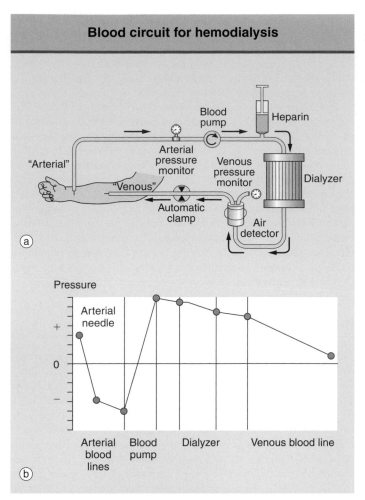

Figure 83.3   Blood circuit for hemodialysis. *a*, The blood circuit. *b*, The pressure profile in the blood circuit with an arteriovenous fistula as the vascular access.

hemorrhage, pericarditis, and heparin-associated side effects (such as immune-mediated heparin-induced thrombocytopenia (type 2), pruritus, rapidly progressive osteoporosis, alopecia). Heparin-free dialysis may be an alternative in some circumstances. In the event of heparin-induced thrombocytopenia type 2, regional citrate anticoagulation, danaparoid, recombinant hirudin (lepirudin), or argatroban can be used instead (see Chapter 73).

DIALYSATE FLUID

Water and Water Treatment
A standard 4-hour HD session, with a dialysate flow of 500 ml/min, exposes the patient to 120 liters of water. Therefore, water quality is of paramount importance to the patients' well-being. Water for the dialysate may be subjected to filtration, softening, and deionization, but it is ultimately purified in most centers by reverse osmosis. Reverse osmosis entails forcing water through a semipermeable membrane at very high pressure to remove microbiologic contaminants and > 90% of dissolved ions.

Standards for clinical quality of water are widely accepted, but there is less consensus as to acceptable levels of bacterial and endotoxin contamination. Municipal water supplies may contain a variety of contaminants that are toxic to HD patients. Substances added to the water such as aluminum and chloramines cause

significant morbidity. The clinical sequelae of water contents are listed in Figure 83.4. Current AAMI water standards are available at www.betterwater.com/documents/manuals/PBManB.pdf.

Aluminum may result in a severe neurologic disorder (speech abnormalities, muscle spasms, seizures, and dementia), bone disease, and erythropoietin-resistant anemia. Plasma aluminum concentration should be monitored regularly, levels should be <1 µmol/l levels >2 µmol/l should prompt the search for excessive exposure (aluminum-based phosphate binders may be an important source). Chloramines have been associated with hemolysis, and methemoglobinemia. Copper and zinc may leach from plumbing components and may cause hemolysis. Lead has been associated with abdominal pain and muscle weakness. Nitrate and nitrite may cause nausea and seizures. High concentrations of calcium may cause the hard water syndrome, characterized by an acute hypercalcemia and hypomagnesemia, hemodynamic instability, nausea, vomiting, muscle weakness, and somnolence.

Gram-negative bacteria produce endotoxins (pyrogenic lipopolysaccharides from the outer bacterial cell wall) and fragments of these endotoxins may well be responsible for some dialysis-related symptoms. Endotoxin fragments of 3 to 4 kd are able to cross even cellulose-based membranes and are capable of inducing cytokines such as interleukin-1 and tumor necrosis factor. Exposure to bacteria and endotoxin is associated with rigors, hypotension, and fever; even low levels of microbiologic contaminants may contribute to chronic inflammation in HD patients. Bacteria may proliferate in the biofilm, a coating on surfaces consisting of microcolonies of bacteria embedded in an extracellular matrix secreted by the cells, protecting the bacteria from antibiotics and disinfectants. The microbiologic standards for HD water vary between countries (Fig. 83.5).

The harm done by endotoxin passing through the dialysis membrane by backfiltration includes stimulation of inflammation, decreased response to erythropoiesis stimulating agents, and possible aggravation of atherosclerosis. Use of a polysulfone or polyamide filter in the dialyzer may be adequate to remove endotoxins, but smaller molecules including bacterial DNA fragments may pass through the dialyzer. In the absence of routine hot water disinfection of the machine and the connections to the water loop, the only way that endotoxin concentration can be kept low is by frequent measurement and use of disinfection when concentration exceeds accepted standards.

Clinical sequelae of water contamination in hemodialysis	
Water Contamination	Clinical Sequelae
Al, chloramine, nitrate, Pb, Cu, Zn, Si	Anemia
Al, fluoride, Si	Bone disease
Bacteria, endotoxins	Fever
Ca, Mg, Na	Hypertension
Bacteria, endotoxins, nitrates	Hypotension
Low pH, sulfate	Acidosis
Ca, Mg	Muscle weakness
Bacteria, endotoxins, chloramine, low pH, nitrate, sulfate, Ca, Mg, Cu, Zn	Nausea/vomiting
Al, Pb, Ca, Mg	Neurologic distubances

Figure 83.4   Clinical sequelae of water contamination in hemodialysis.

Recommendations for water quality for hemodialysis

Fluid/Organization	Bacteria (cfu/ml)	Endotoxin (EU/ml)
Water for Hemodialysis		
AAMI	<200	<2
AAMI action level	50	1
UK Renal Association	<100	<0.25
European Best Practice Guidelines	<100	<0.25
European Pharmacopeia	<100	<0.25
Japan Society for Dialysis Therapy	<100	<0.25
Ultrapure water	<0.1	<0.03
Sterile water	<0.000001	<0.03

Figure 83.5 Recommendations for water quality for hemodialysis. Acceptable bacterial and endotoxin levels. AAMI, Association for the Advancement of Medical Instrumentation; cfu, colony-forming units; EU, endotoxin units.

Ultrapure water is defined as bacterial count <0.1 colony-forming units/ml and endotoxin <0.03 endotoxin units/ml and is recommended by both European and American guidelines for use with high-flux dialyzers. Ultrapure water represents a basic prerequisite for dialysis modalities using online production of substitution fluid (online hemofiltration [HF] or hemodiafiltration [HDF]).

Liquid bicarbonate dialysis fluid concentrate may be a source of bacterial growth; bacterial growth is not seen in acetate concentrate and bicarbonate powder.

Short bacterial DNA fragments, oligodeoxynucleotides (ODNs) of six to 20 nucleotides (five nucleotides ~1250 d) are stimulatory to immune cells. Bacterial ODNs are able to diffuse through regular high-flux dialyzer membranes; the clinical consequences of ODNs are under investigation.[3]

Dialysis Solution

Dialysis fluid can be considered as a drug to be adjusted to the individual patients' needs. In modern machines, dialysate is made by mixing two concentrate components, which may be provided as liquid or dry (powder) concentrates. The bicarbonate component contains sodium bicarbonate and sodium chloride, the acid component contains chloride salts of Na^+, K^+ (if needed), Ca^{2+}, Mg^{2+},

Composition of dialysates for bicarbonate dialysis

Component	Concentration	
	Range	Typical
Electrolytes		
Sodium (mmol/l)	135–145	140
Potassium (mmol/l)	0–4.0	2.0
Calcium (mmol/l)	0–2.0	1.25
Magnesium (mmol/l)	0.5–1.0	0.75
Chloride (mmol/l)	87–124	105
Buffers		
Acetate (mmol/l)	2–4	3
Bicarbonate (mmol/l)	20–40	35
pH	7.1–7.3	7.2
Pco_2 (mm Hg)	40–100	
Glucose (mg/dl)	0–200	100

Figure 83.6 Composition of dialysates for bicarbonate dialysis.

acetate (or citrate), and glucose (optional). These two components are mixed simultaneously with purified water to make the dialysate. Dialysate proportioning pumps ensures proper mixing. The relative amounts of water, bicarbonate and acid component define the final dialysate composition (Fig. 83.6). Bicarbonate has replaced acetate as the dialysate buffer in most countries.

Commercially available dialysates can be further modified by changing the mixing fraction and by adding salt solutions. Modern machines allow an alteration of the bicarbonate concentration by changing the mixing ratio of water to bicarbonate. A variable sodium option allows the adaptation of the dialysate sodium concentration to the patients' needs. A dialysate sodium concentration below the plasma concentration leads to a net Na^+ loss and may promote muscle cramps and hemodynamic instability. A dialysate Na^+ concentration in excess of the plasma concentration causes increased thirst, high intradialytic weight gain, and high blood pressure. Potassium may be changed by adding potassium to the acid concentrate. Glucose is usually added to prevent intradialytic hypoglycemia. The advantages and disadvantages of dialysate modifications are shown in Figure 83.7.

BIOCOMPATIBILITY

The contact of blood with lines and membranes triggers an inflammatory response akin to that seen in infection. Biocompatibility indicates a membrane is biologically compatible by not producing a toxic, injurious, or immunologic response on contact with blood. Although many components of the dialysis procedure contribute to the degree of biocompatibility, it is the membrane itself that is most important. Biocompatibility is of particular importance with the use of cellulose membranes, whereas synthetic membranes and reused membranes activate complement to a lesser extent (see Fig. 83.2). Blood contact with the dialysis membrane activates the complement cascade, the coagulation cascade, and cellular mechanisms (Fig. 83.8). Activation of complement peaks at 15 minutes after the start of dialysis and lasts up to 90 minutes.

HEMOFILTRATION

HF differs markedly from HD by the mechanisms by which the composition of the blood is modified. In the simplest form of HF, blood under pressure passes down one side of a highly permeable membrane allowing both water and substances up to a molecular weight of about 20 kd to pass across the membrane by convective flow. During HF, the filtrate is discarded and the patient receives a substitution fluid either before (predilution) or after (postdilution) the dialyzer (Fig. 83.9). The substitution fluid contains the major crystalloid components of the plasma at physiologic levels. Both bicarbonate and lactate are used as buffers. The rate of fluid removal and substitution fluid infusion can be adapted to the patient's need. In patients with fluid overload, a negative fluid balance can be obtained by replacing less fluid through infusion that is removed. HF is particularly useful as a continuous renal replacement therapy in an intensive care setting.[4] The hemodynamic stability characteristic of convective therapies is confirmed also in comparison with modern HD.

HEMODIAFILTRATION

HDF combines the benefits of HD (high transport rate of low molecular weight solutes by diffusion) and HF (high convective transport of substances; Fig. 83.10). HDF is used both as a

Advantages and disadvantages of modifications in the dialysate composition

Component	Advantage	Disadvantage
Sodium		
Increased	Hemodynamic stability	Thirst, intradialytic weight gain, high blood pressure
Decreased	Reduced osmotic stress in the presence of predialytic hyponatremia	Intradialytic hemodynamic instability
Potassium		
Increased	Fewer arrhythmias with digoxin intoxication and hypokalemia; may improve hemodynamic stability	Hyperkalemia
Decreased	Increased dietary potassium intake	Arrhythmias; risk of sudden death
Calcium		
Increased	Suppresses PTH, increased hemodynamic stability	Hypercalcemia, vascular calcification, adynamic bone disease due to PTH suppression
Decreased	Permits more liberal use of calcium-containing phosphate binders	Stimulation of PTH, reduced hemodynamic stability
Bicarbonate		
Increased	Acidosis control improved	Postdialytic alkalosis
Decreased	No postdialytic alkalosis	Promotes acidosis
Magnesium		
Increased	Hemodynamic stability, fewer arrhythmias, suppresses PTH	Altered nerve conduction, pruritus, renal bone disease
Decreased	Permits use of magnesium-containing phosphate binders, improved bone mineralization, less bone pain	Arrhythmias, muscle weakness and cramps, elevated PTH

Figure 83.7   Advantages and disadvantages of modifications in the dialysate composition. PTH, parathyroid hormone.

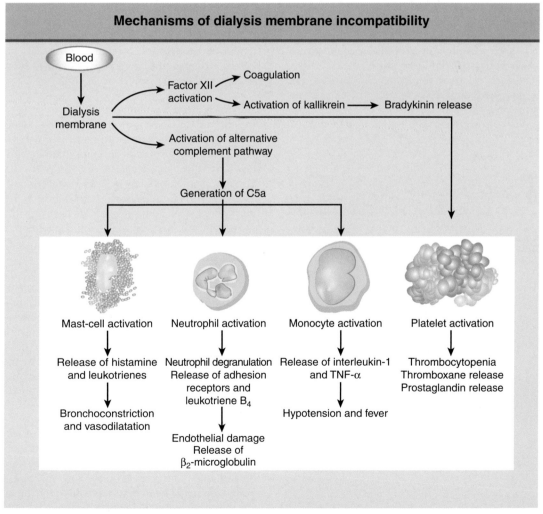

Figure 83.8   Mechanisms of dialysis membrane incompatibility. TNF, tumor necrosis factor.

Circuit for hemofiltration

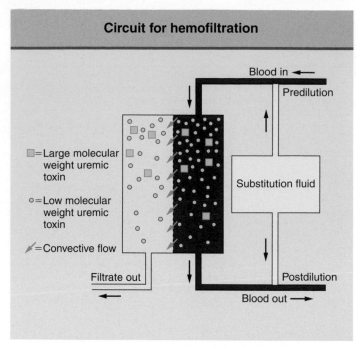

Figure 83.9 Circuit for hemofiltration.

continuous and an intermittent renal replacement therapy. HDF offers a potential benefit regarding anemia correction, inflammation, oxidative stress, lipid profiles, and calcium-phosphate product[5] and possibly the prevention of long-term complications such as dialysis amyloidosis, a disease exacerbated by the low clearance of β_2-microglobulin with conventional HD techniques. Higher costs and, in some countries, the decisions of regulatory boards prevent the widespread use of HDF, despite its likely benefits over conventional HD.

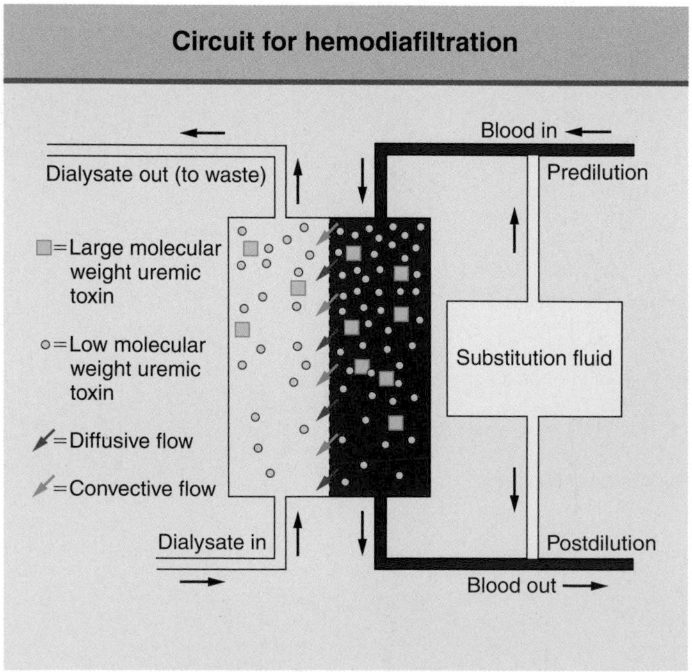

Circuit for hemodiafiltration

Figure 83.10 Circuit for hemodiafiltration.

ADDITIONAL DEVICES AND TECHNOLOGIES

Blood Volume Monitor

A decrease in blood volume due to ultrafiltration is one of the main causes of intradialytic hypotension. Blood volume monitors provide continuous noninvasive monitoring of changes in blood volume by continuous measurement of plasma protein concentration by ultrasonography or hematocrit by optical scattering (Fig. 83.11). Too rapid changes in blood volume from baseline indicate decreased plasma refilling rates and may precede intradialytic hypotension. Blood volume monitoring can be used for monitoring is particularly useful for hemodynamically unstable dialysis patients.

Ultrafiltration Profiling

The ultrafiltration rate is usually kept constant, but can be changed during the dialysis session in a preprogrammed manner. It may be advantageous to remove a large proportion of the ultrafiltration volume in the first half of the HD session. Because of a high initial plasma refilling rate, severely overhydrated patients may tolerate a higher ultrafiltration rate in the early stages and dry weight may be reached more easily. In some machines, predefined ultrafiltration profiles are incorporated. The clinical benefits of ultrafiltration profiling are under debate

Sodium Modeling

Normally, the dialysate sodium concentration is kept constant throughout the dialysis treatment. The variable sodium option allows dynamic changes of the dialysate sodium concentration during the treatment. Patients with hemodynamic instability or significant interdialytic weight gains may benefit from this option, although the general applicability of sodium modeling has not yet been accepted.

Dialysate Urea Sensor

The dialysate urea sensor measures the concentration of urea in the spent dialysate at multiple time points during the dialysis therapy. This information in combination with data on dialysis flow and ultrafiltration rate can be used to compute online the amount of urea removed and consequently the Kt/V (see "Adequacy of Hemodialysis"); the whole body water distribution volume (V) is approximated applying formulas based on anthropometric data derived from urea kinetic modeling.

Online Clearance Monitor

Sodium and urea clearances are identical for practical purposes. Since the conductivity of the dialysate is largely a function of the dialysate sodium concentration, online clearance monitors can use this feature to compute the urea clearance (K) of a dialyzer. Changes in inflow dialysate sodium concentration are related to the respective changes of conductivity in the dialysate outflow. The conductivity clearance is equivalent to urea clearance and Kt is easily calculated. Together with measures of total body water, Kt/V can be determined with each treatment.

Blood Temperature Monitor

During standard HD, the core temperature usually increases. Since the thermoregulatory response to rising core temperature (dilation of thermoregulatory vessels) may offset the vascular response to hypovolemia (vasoconstriction), this increase in internal heat production might be in part responsible for the intradialytic hemodynamic instability. Reducing dialysate temperature has been shown to improve vascular stability during dialysis. The core

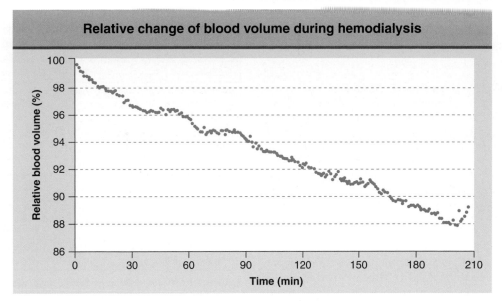

Figure 83.11   Relative change of blood volume during hemodialysis as recorded by a blood volume monitor.

temperature can be controlled by the blood temperature monitor, which adapts the dialysate temperature according to the desired core temperature. This intervention results in fewer hypotensive episodes.[6]

ADEQUACY OF HEMODIALYSIS

Hemodialysis, as well as peritoneal dialysis, needs to be prescribed and dosed according to the patient's individual needs. The term adequacy of dialysis was originally used exclusively to describe dialysis dosing but now includes broader aspects of the management of complications and comorbidities of chronic kidney disease that affect outcome. From a clinical perspective, probably the best marker of adequacy is a physically active, well-nourished, nonanemic, normotensive patient with no complaints. Adequacy purely in terms of dialysis dose refers to delivery of a treatment dose that is considered high enough to promote an optimal long-term outcome.

Assessment of Dialysis Dose
Urea serves as surrogate marker for water soluble small molecular weight toxins, and in clinical practice, dialysis dose is expressed by urea reduction ratio or by the treatment index Kt/V. Simply following predialysis BUN (blood urea nitrogen) (or serum urea) levels is insufficient to assess dialysis dose because a low BUN may much more reflect inadequate protein intake as a consequence of malnutrition rather than sufficient dialytic urea removal.

Urea Kinetics
Dialyzers are highly efficient in removing urea from the blood, reducing the urea concentration during one passage by 80% to 90%. During dialysis, the urea concentration in the blood compartment is always lower than in the tissue compartments. The urea rebound after dialysis is the period of equilibration between blood and tissue compartments and takes about 30 to 60 minutes.

Urea kinetics were originally described by single compartment (pool) models, assuming that full equilibration between blood and tissue compartments occurs immediately and without time delay. In such models, the change in BUN follows first-order kinetics with a linear decline in BUN and no urea rebound

(Fig. 83.12, dashed line). The *in vivo* situation is more accurately described by double-pool models that take into account delayed intercompartmental urea redistribution and urea rebound (see Fig. 83.12, solid line). The timing of the post-HD blood sample is critical for analysis of urea kinetics. In daily practice, blood samples for post-HD BUN are collected right after termination of dialysis. Most methods for assessment of dialysis dose are based on the pre-/post-HD difference in BUN.

Urea Reduction Ratio
Urea reduction ratio is a simple but rather imprecise way to quantify dialysis dose.

$$URR(\%) = \left(1 - \frac{C_t}{C_0}\right) \times 100\%,$$

where C_t = postdialysis and C_0 = predialysis BUN concentration.

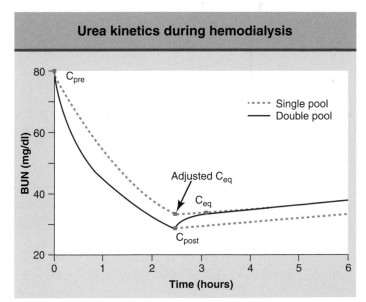

Figure 83.12   Urea kinetics during hemodialysis. BUN, blood urea, nitrogen; C_{eq}, equilibrated BUN concentration postdialysis; C_{post}, BUN concentration postdialysis; C_{pre}, BUN concentration predialysis.

URR correlates well with dialysis outcome, and despite its limitations, it is an accepted method for assessment of dialysis adequacy (www.kidney.org/professionals/).

Single-Pool Kt/V(spKt/V): Urea Kinetic Modeling

The treatment index Kt/V is the most widely used parameter to assess dialysis dose. Kt/V may be applied to any substance but in clinical practice is almost exclusively used for urea, where K is defined as the whole-body clearance rate of urea, t as the effective treatment time, and V as the body's urea distribution volume (which equates closely to total body water). The dimensionless treatment index Kt/V relates the total volume cleared from urea during a dialysis session (K × t) to the patient urea distribution volume (V):

$$K \times t/V = \ln (C_0/C_t)$$

This equation has been the basis for the further development of formal urea kinetic modeling (UKM), which is used to model spKt/V from information on dialyzer characteristics (KoA), blood and dialysate flow rates, and treatment time, as well as anthropometric patient data. The modeled spKt/V is then compared to delivered spKt/V assessed from pre-/post-BUN concentrations. Additional benefits of formal UKM in addition to Kt/V include estimation of normalized protein catabolic rate and V. Because of its mathematical complexity, UKM requires computer support. UKM is the currently most rigorous method for prescribing and evaluating dialysis dose.

Single-Pool Kt/V: Daugirdas' Formula

spKt/V can be approximated by the second-generation formula developed by Daugirdas,[7] which is widely used due to its simplicity:

$$spKt/V = -\ln[R - 0.008 \times t] + [4 - 3.5 \times R] \times UF/W$$

where ln is the natural logarithm, R is the postdialysis/predialysis BUN ratio, t is the effective treatment time (hours), UF is ultrafiltration volume (liters), and W is the patient's postdialysis weight (kilograms). This equation has been validated by UKM for a Kt/V range between 0.8 and 2.0.

Equilibrated Kt/V (eKt/V)

Using nonequilibrated BUN (or serum urea) overestimates urea reduction. Dialysis dose is more accurately estimated using equilibrated post-HD BUN; the resulting measure is called equilibrated Kt/V (eKt/V) and is derived using the equilibrated BUN. Equilibrated BUN can be measured either 30 to 60 minutes after HD or estimated (without additional blood sampling) from nonequilibrated BUN and the rate of the intradialytic urea decline (Kt/V per time unit = K/V):

$$eKt/V = spKt/V - (0.6 \times spK/V) + 0.03$$

This equation is valid when the vascular access is an arteriovenous fistula or graft. When a central venous catheter is used a different equation has to be applied:

$$eKt/V = spKt/V - (0.47 \times spK/V) + 0.02$$

In patients on short high-flux HD, dialysis dose is overestimated by spKt/V. Typical results on spKt/V and eKt/V for identical treatment characteristics are shown in Figure 83.13.

spKt/V or (better) eKt/V should be assessed monthly. Formal UKM should be used in patients not achieving adequacy targets.

Computation of dialysis dose: results derived from different model equations		
Formula	Result	Comment
URR = $(1 - C_t/C_0) \times 100\%$	67%	Urea rebound, urea generation, and ultrafiltration not taken into account
Kt/V = $\ln (C_0/C_t)$	1.10	Urea rebound, urea generation, and ultrafiltration not taken into account
spKt/V = $-\ln (R - 0.008 \times t) +$ $(4 - 3.5 \ R) \times UF/W$	1.33	Single pool model; urea rebound not taken into account
eKt/V = spKt/V $- 0.6 \times$ spKt/V/t $+ 0.03$	1.16	Equilibrated double pool model for arteriovenous access
eKt/V = spKt/V $- 0.47 \times$ spKt/V/t $+0.02$	1.20	Equilibrated double pool model for central venous access

Figure 83.13 Computation of dialysis dose: results derived from different model equations. Calculations based on dialysis duration (t) = 4 hours; prehemodialysis (HD) BUN (C_0) = 90 mg/dl; nonequilibrated post-HD BUN (C_t) = 30 mg/dl; ultrafiltration volume (UF) = 3 liters; post-HD body weight (W) = 72 kg; R = C_t/C_0. Kt/V, URR, urea reduction ratio.

Prescribing Dialysis

Delivered dialysis dose depends on blood flow rate, dialyzer efficiency (K), session length (t), and the patient's body water volume (V). A standard dialysis prescription includes a minimum treatment time of 4 hours, a blood flow rate between 250 and 300 ml/min, and a dialysate flow rate of 500 ml/min. In a new dialysis patient, V is unknown and has to be estimated (e.g., using the Watson formula) or as percentage of body weight (e.g., 58% for males). Once V is obtained, K and t are computed to meet the 1.2-fold of V.

Example

Male, body weight: 76 kg; V = 58% of body weight = 44 liter
Target blood flow rate: 300 ml/min; dialyzer efficiency: 80%; effective dialyzer urea clearance (K_d) = 240 ml/min; target Kt/V = 1.2
Required treatment time (min): 1.2 × V(ml)/K_d(ml/min) = 220 min

Once delivered and Kt/V has been measured, the prescription is adjusted to meet the Kt/V target. In case of severe and long-standing uremia, the target dose is approached slowly over the course of several sessions to avoid disequilibrium syndrome.

Factors Affecting Delivered Kt/V

The effective clearance K depends on blood and dialysate flow rate, dialyzer KoA, effective surface area, hematocrit, anticoagulation, and recirculation. Treatment time t is important for reaching the Kt/V target. Effective treatment time can be substantially shorter than prescribed treatment time due to intermittent pump stops or patient demand. V does not substantially change during a single HD but may change over time. Dialysis dose needs to be adjusted for an increase in V. On the contrary, if there is a loss in body mass, which is associated with a decrease in V, Kt/V should not be reduced but rather adjusted to the higher, ideal patient V.

Confronted with an inadequate delivered Kt/V, it is sensible to check whether the studied session was representative of an

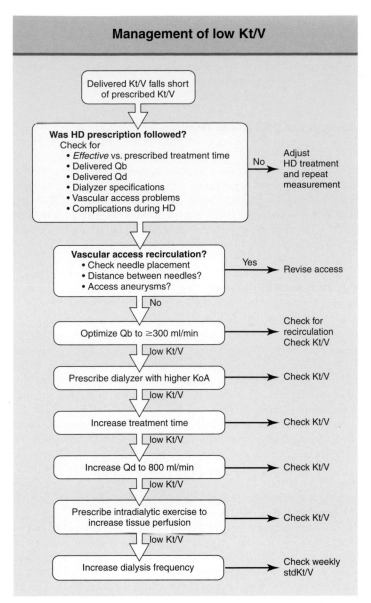

Figure 83.14 Management of low Kt/V. HD, hemodialysis; KoA, the dialyzer mass transfer area coefficient for urea.

Comparing Different Dialysis Frequencies: Weekly Dialysis Dose

In patients not receiving a standard thrice-weekly HD schedule, assessment of just one representative Kt/V value is insufficient since target Kt/V values for these variations have not been defined. Expressing dialysis efficiency as a weekly dose allows comparison between different dialysis frequencies, but weekly dialysis dose is not equivalent to the product of Kt/V times the number of treatments per week. The urea mass removed per time unit decreases with increasing dialysis time and dose (Fig. 83.15). About 63% of total body urea fraction is removed with Kt/V of 1.0 and doubling of Kt/V to 2.0 increases the removed urea fraction only by an additional 24%.

Weekly dialysis dose can be expressed as standard Kt/V (stdKt/V), which combines treatment dose with treatment frequency and allows for intermittent therapies of any frequency to be compared to continuous therapy.[8] stdKt/V is derived by plotting eKt/V for a representative dialysis session onto the respective frequency curve (Fig. 83.16). A maximum stdKt/V of 3.0 can be achieved with thrice-weekly dialysis; higher stdKt/V can be reached with more frequent dialysis. Residual renal function (RRF) expressed as weekly urea Kt/V can simply be added to dialysis stdKt/V. stdKt/V allows direct comparison of dialysis doses delivered by PD and HD.

Recommendations for Dialysis Dose Adequacy

Current recommendations in the United States are as follows:
- A minimum spKt/V of at least 1.2 for both adult and pediatric HD patients. When using URR, the delivered dose should be equivalent to a Kt/V of 1.2, that is, an average URR of 65%.

average session since unusual problems may have occurred (e.g., shortened time, single-needle HD). A frequent cause of low Kt/V is access recirculation. Blood sampling errors should be considered since delayed post-HD sampling will reduce Kt/V. Blood sampling procedures should be standardized in each center (for recommendations, see www.kidney.org/professionals/kdoqi/guidelines).

If, despite these checks, a low Kt/V remains unexplained, treatment time should be increased to 4.5 or 5 hours. Prescribing a more efficient dialyzer and higher blood and dialysate flow rates should also be considered (Fig. 83.14). Muscle exercise during dialysis can increase Kt/V. Delivered Kt/V should be checked whenever the dialysis prescription has been modified substantially. Online clearance monitoring allows for assessment of Kt/V during each single session without blood sampling.

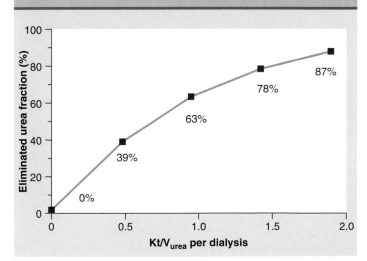

Total body urea fraction removed in relation to Kt/V

Figure 83.15 Total body urea fraction removed in relation to Kt/V. In this example, 63% of total body urea fraction is removed with Kt/V of 1, and doubling of Kt/V to 2 increases the removed urea fraction only by an additional 24%.

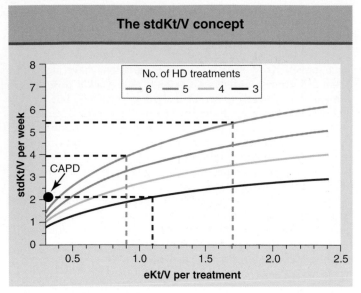

Figure 83.16 The stdKt/V concept. stdKt/V for any hemodialysis (HD) frequency is derived by plotting eKt/V of a representative dialysis session onto the respective frequency curve.

- To prevent the delivered dose of HD from falling below the recommended minimum dose, the prescribed dose of HD should be spKt/V 1.3, which corresponds to an average URR of 70%.
- The delivered dose of HD should be measured at least once per month in all adult and pediatric HD patients.

Details on these recommendations can be found at www.kidney.org/professionals/. A comparison with recommendations from other countries (Australia, Canada, Europe, United Kingdom) can be found at www.kdigo.org.

Adequacy of Dietary Protein and Calorie Intake

HD patients are at risk of malnutrition due to increased catabolism, decreased appetite, infection and other intercurrent illnesses, hospital admissions, and skipped meals after dialysis. The recommended daily intake of 1.0 to 1.2 g protein/kg ideal body weight and 35 kcal/kg ideal body weight is often not met. The nutritional status of HD patients should be assessed regularly by clinical and biochemical means (see Chapter 77).

Significance of Residual Renal Function for Dialysis Adequacy

Patients starting dialysis may still have considerable RRF. The majority of HD patients have lost RRF by the end of the first year, but 10% to 20% of patients still have RRF after more than 3 years. A RRF of 2 to 3 ml/min urea clearance contributes significantly to the elimination of uremic toxins. RRF translates into lower β_2-microglobulin levels; better hemoglobin, phosphate, potassium, and urate levels; enhanced nutritional status; better quality of life (QoL) scores; and a reduced need for dietary and fluid restrictions. Loss of RRF is associated with left ventricular hypertrophy.[9] The quantitative contribution of RRF to total delivered dialysis dose is assessed by weekly stdKt/V. For a patient with an estimated total body water of 40 liters, a residual urea clearance of 2 to 3 ml/min is equivalent to a weekly stdKt/V of 0.5 to 0.75.

Risk factors for loss of RRF include activation of the immune system (bioincompatible membranes, water impurities), intradialytic hypotension, use of nephrotoxic agents (e.g., nonsteroidal anti-inflammatory drugs and angiotensin-converting enzyme inhibitors), and hypercalcemia.

Adequacy of Phosphate Removal by Hemodialysis

Hyperphosphatemia is one of the major problems in HD[10] (see Chapters 71 and 74). Hyperphosphatemia management is based on phosphate removal by dialysis, dietary phosphate restriction, and intestinal phosphate binding. Phosphate is removed less efficiently by dialysis, but it can be increased by HDF. More frequent dialysis, such as short daily or daily nocturnal home HD further increase phosphate elimination. Long frequent dialysis schedules may result in hypophosphatemia.

OUTCOMES IN HEMODIALYSIS

The outcomes of dialysis patients expressed in terms of mortality, hospitalization, and QoL measurement are comparable to those observed in patients with solid organ cancer.[1]

Some major factors influencing outcome are common to all patients with end-stage renal disease and include cardiovascular disease (Chapter 71), anemia (Chapter 72), and control of mineral metabolism (Chapter 74).

Acute complications of HD are discussed in Chapter 84. Here we focus on the factors influencing outcome that are specific to patients receiving maintenance HD (Fig. 83.17).

Unfortunately, randomized, controlled trials are few in HD, and lower grades of evidence have often been resorted to in issuing authoritative dialysis clinical practice guidelines, which are listed in Figure 83.18.

The life expectancy of the average patient on HD in the United States is 4 years at 59 years of age with an annual mortality of approximately 20% (www.usrds.org). In patients in South East Asia, in some Mediterranean countries, in South America and Mexico, and in the United States in Hispanics and African American patients, mortality rates are lower. The Dialysis Outcomes and Practice Pattern Study suggests that variations in practice patterns account for some of these differences.

Uremic Toxins

The catalog of retained (or noncatabolized) uremic toxins is long but few compounds have been specifically associated with outcomes. A continuously updated list of uremic toxins is provided at http://eutoxdb.ukbf.fu-berlin.de/eutoxdb/index.php. Mortality is associated with the clearance of urea (acting presumably as a marker for other protein-derived small molecules).

Current dialysis and dialysis-related treatments do not remove any significant quantity of substances of molecular weight >10 to 15 kd. Sorbents may be necessary to remove the higher molecular weight toxins or of lower molecular weight substances bound to proteins. Of commonly measured protein-derived substances, only the concentrations of β_2-microglobulin correlate with mortality.[11]

Influences of Dialysis Treatment on Chronic Outcomes

The major dialysis-related factors that may influence patient outcome are shown in Figure 83.19.

Factors related to dialysis outcomes

Factor	Effects of Dialysis	Effect on Dialysis	Effect on Outcome
Hemoglobin	May increase sharply during dialysis ultrafiltration	High hemoglobin in hollow fiber may limit phosphate removal	Anemia associated with left ventricular mass ↑
EPO resistance	Appropriate dose of dialysis could improve	Suggests change from catheter to fistula	Association with poor survival
EPO variability	—	—	Possibly associated with poor outcomes
Vitamin D deficiency	—	Hypocalcemia, hemodynamic instability	Associated with osteomalacia
Vitamin D supplementation	—	—	Vitamin D use associated with increased survival
PTH	Moderately decreased by increased dialysate calcium	Hypocalcemia → vascular instability	↑ PTH possible relation to morbidity outcomes.
IV iron	—	—	↓ Iron → EPO resistance ↑ Iron → hemosiderosis
Diabetes mellitus	Worse metabolic control; falsely lower HbA,C	Autonomic dysfunction → ↑ interdialytic weight gain	Profound effect on increasing mortality due to CVD; increased risk of calciphylaxis
Age	—	Hemodynamic instability	Profound increase in CVD
Race/ethnicity	—	—	Definite effects on cardiac outcomes, especially atherosclerosis, which may be dependent on background population risk
Body size	—	Requires longer treatment time	Worse outcomes in small people
↑ Blood pressure	Increase or decrease	Very low BP → ↑ dialysis time	Both low and high BP associated with increased mortality
Cardiomyopathy	May be worsened	Makes ultrafiltration difficult	Is associated with poorer survival
Depression; anxiety	Possibly	Missed treatments	Increased morbidity; QoL
Inflammation	Increased by LPS or other mechanisms?	Choice of access	Increased morbidity and mortality: EPO resistance
Malnutrition Including ↓ albumin ↓ cholesterol	May be benefited by high flux treatment	Volume control poorer	Increased morbidity and mortality
Hyperphosphatemia	Conventional, no; Long nocturnal, yes	—	Increased morbidity and mortality
Low albumin concentration	Indirectly by dialysate endotoxin	May limit refilling of plasma volume	Profound effect of hypoalbuminemia
Overhydration	To variable degree	Easier dialysis due to rapid plasma refilling	Increased morbidity and mortality
Calcium	Dependent on dialysate calcium	Increased cardiac output and BP with high dialysate calcium and vice versa	May be associated with increased mortality
β_2 microglobulin	Reduced with high-flux dialyzers	—	↑ plasma concentration associated with increased mortality
Hyperlipidemia	Possible reduction in triglycerides and and LDL with high flux		Associated with ↑ morbidity
Use of permanent catheters	—	Reduced dose due to thrombosis and infection	Associaited with increased mortality, EPO resistance, inflammation

Figure 83.17 Factors related to dialysis outcomes. BP, blood pressure; CVD, cardiovascular disease; EPO, erythropoietin; HDF, hemodiafiltration; LDL, low-density lipoprotein; LPS, lipopolysaccharide; PTH, parathyroid hormone; QoL, quality of life.

Web-based resources for hemodialysis
Guidelines
NKF-KDOQI (National Kidney Foundation–Kidney Disease Outcomes Quality Initiative); www.kidney.org/professionals/kdoqi/guidelines.cfm
European Best Practice Guidelines for Haemodialysis (Part 1)–European Renal Association–European Dialysis and Transplant Association ndt.oupjournals.org/content/vol17/suppl7/index.shtml
CARI (Caring for Australians with Renal Impairment)–Australian and New Zealand Society of Nephrology (ANZSN) and Kidney Health Australia (KHA) www.cari.org.au/guidelines.php
The Renal Association (United Kingdom) Treatment of Adults and Children with Renal Failure Standards and Audit Measures; www.renal.org/standards/standards.html
Canadian Society of Nephrology Clinical Practice Guidelines, 1999; csnscn.ca/local/files/guidelines/CNS-Guidelines-1999.pdf
National Guideline Clearinghouse lists an index of clinical practice guidelines of various organizations; www.guideline.gov/browse/guideline_index.aspx
Foundations, Associations and Initiatives
USRDS (United States Renal Data System); comprehensive analyses of renal disease epidemiology in United States; www.usrds.org
NKF (National Kidney Foundation); committed to education of health care professionals and public, research support, expanding health care resources, and shaping health policies in the field of nephrology; www.kidney.org
KDIGO (Kidney Disease Improving Global Outcomes); international cooperation in the development and implementation of clinical practice guidelines in nephrology; www.kdigo.org
Kidney and Urology Foundation of America; promoting renal research and accessibility of new therapies to renal disease patients; www.kidneyurology.org/
HDCN (Hypertension, Dialysis and Clinical Nephrology); an official educational program of Renal Physicians Association and American Society of Nephrology; www.hdcn.com

Figure 83.18   Web-based resources for hemodialysis.

Dialysis Dose

The HEMO study showed no primary benefit on outcome of different dialysis dose, expressed as eKt/V, and different degrees of membrane flux (low and high, based on clearance of β_2-microglobulin). However, analysis of secondary outcomes has shown that women benefit from higher dialysis dose[12] and that cardiac deaths were decreased with use of high- flux dialyzers, as was overall mortality with high flux dialyzers in patients who had been on dialysis for >3.7 years. There was also a correlation of serum β_2-microglobulin concentration with mortality.[11]

Effect of Fluid Removal

The process of ultrafiltration of excess extracellular fluid causes no symptoms until plasma water refilling rate does not keep the blood volume at a level at which blood pressure and tissue perfusion can still be maintained by compensatory increases in cardiac output and peripheral resistance. This depends on adequate cardiac and autonomic nervous system function. In patients without significant cardiac disease, blood volume may decrease to 80% to 85% without hypotension occurring. However, when the left ventricular wall is stiff and compensation for reduced blood volume by increased contractility or increased pulse rate is inadequate, even a small further reduction in the blood volume will result in a blood pressure decrease.

Diabetes is the most important cause of autonomic dysfunction that manifests as both inadequate arterial and venous constriction during fluid removal. Increased interdialytic weight gain aggravates the problem of adequate fluid removal. A positive intradialytic sodium balance may occur when dialysate sodium is higher than the patient's own plasma sodium concentration. In hemodynamically unstable patients, only lower rates of ultrafiltration and therefore longer dialysis treatments can accomplish the goal of adequate fluid removal.

Dry Weight

There are no accurate clinical techniques for identifying a patient as having a normal extracellular fluid volume, the so-called dry weight. Methods such as inferior vena cava diameter measurement, measurement of circulating natriuretic peptide levels, relative blood volume change, and clinical symptoms of hypovolemia (including intradialytic hypotension and cramps) are all impractical or unreliable, especially in patients with plasma refilling problems or cardiac disease (as discussed previously). New bioimpedance techniques may be helpful in indicating dry weight, but further clinical evaluation is required.[13]

Dialysis treatment factors in relationship to outcomes	
Dialysis Treatment Factor	**Outcomes**
Inadequate dose	Mortality and hospitalizations increased Quality of life decreased
Short dialysis time	Inability to remove fluid → cardiac disease
Hypotension	Decreased cerebral perfusion, CNS damage Decreased coronary artery and peripheral vascular perfusion
Acidosis	Bone disease; ↑ sympathetic overactivity
Alkalosis	Reduced cerebral perfusion
Membrane incompatibility (predominantly cellulose)	Complement activation, leukocyte sequestration; β_2 microglobin ↑
Membrane flux (high)	Removal of β_2 microglobin ↑ Survival ↑ EPO requirements ↓
Lipopolysaccharide transfer from dialysate to plasma	Inflammation and its consequences
Sodium overload	Thirst ↑ Interdialytic weight gain ↑ Hypertension Cardiac failure
Dialyzer reuse	If performed correctly fewer negative effects

Figure 83.19   Dialysis treatment factors in relationship to outcomes. EPO, erythropoietin.

Dialysis Prescription and Delivered Dose

The HEMO study did not show an overall improvement in mortality with eKt/V between 1.3 and 1.7, although women did benefit by the higher dose. Lower eKt/V, for example, <1.0, in observational studies, is associated with increased mortality.

In many dialysis facilities, and especially when kinetic modeling or other quantities measurement is not used, no definite information about the dose actually delivered is available. The increasing use of devices measuring conductive clearance (equivalent to urea clearance) makes it more likely that underdialysis would be recognized. Reasons for not delivering the prescribed dose include reductions in treatment time, access recirculation, high negative arterial and positive venous pressures with misleadingly high blood flow rates, and refusal to be dialyzed for the time prescribed. The result of constant underdialysis is increased cardiovascular morbidity and even missing one treatment per month results in a measurable increase in mortality.

Vascular Access in Relationship to Inflammation and EPO Resistance

Central venous catheters are associated with markers of inflammation, such as low serum albumin and elevated neutrophil count, and an impaired response to erythropoietin. Every attempt should be made to avoid catheters and to use arteriovenous fistulas or grafts instead (see Chapter 81).

Physician Attendance

Physician attendance during dialysis is a treatment variable that occasions controversy and is significantly influenced by health care organization in different countries. Objective evidence of its importance is rare,[14] but recent studies suggest better improved hemoglobin control and dialysis adequacy with more frequent physician visits. There are no available data on the impact of the attendance of other health professionals.

Role of the Patient

The range of activities requiring patient compliance is broad and all have measurable consequences. They include not missing treatments or reducing treatment times, adhering to dietary advice (phosphate, potassium, and sodium intake) and taking all prescribed drugs.[15] Another practical compliance issue is walking unaided after dialysis with consequent risk of falls.

Quality Control in the Dialysis Unit

Factors that may be of value in assessing quality in the dialysis unit include serum levels of phosphate, bio-intact parathyroid hormone, albumin, and hemoglobin; eKdrt/V and normalized protein catabolic rate; and percentage use of native arteriovenous fistulas for vascular access.

It is important to ensure that the basic elements of dialysis therapy are met; that is, dose of dialysis, safe water and dialysate, appropriate maintenance of dry weight, appropriate vascular access. Psychosocial assistance may be required. Other factors requiring attention include adequate nutrition and treatment of obesity; eradication of infection; treatment of anemia; management of phosphate excess, calcium, and PTH; smoking cessation programs; and control of diabetes.

Assessments of QoL by SF-36, of performance by the Karnofsky Performance Status Scale, and of depression by the Beck Depression Inventory are useful in assessing treatment efficacy. Identification of patients for whom dialysis appears to be an unacceptable burden should stimulate an intensive search for reversible adverse factors. Failure to find these can prompt conversation and discussion of a decision to cease therapy in a small minority of patients.

Quality of Life

A combination of physical and psychological disturbances accompanied by lifestyle changes are commonly reported in patients on dialysis and represent an important outcome. Health-related QoL measures may be among the most sensitive indicators of the effect of dialysis therapies.[16] QoL is influenced by patient travel time, waiting time before being placed on dialysis, availability of desirable dialysis times, interference with employment or family responsibilities, lost educational or recreational opportunities, sexual problems, and sleep disturbances. Patients will often express feelings of guilt for the unintended neglect of their families resulting from the many hours involved in the treatment. Every effort must be made to accommodate those issues that are within the scope of the dialysis unit's operations.

Among psychosocial problems, depression appears to be the most prominent. Depression correlates with measures of anxiety and of inflammation.[17] Chronic pain may be a significant factor in causing depression and insomnia and may cause patients to consider withdrawal for dialysis.[18] Patients with increased C-reactive protein and hypoalbuminemia should be evaluated for depression after somatic causes have been managed.[19]

Comparison of outcomes between dialysis facilities and in different geographic areas is made difficult by varying case mix. Nonspecific inflammatory and nutritional markers cannot replace the use of comorbid indicators for patient care.[20] QoL indices such as the Index of Coexistent Disease have been proposed as valid predictors of mortality.[21]

Changing Future Outcomes
Increased Frequency of Dialysis

In the United States, a randomized trial is comparing six times weekly versus three times weekly dialysis with primary endpoints of changes in left ventricular mass index as measured by magnetic resonance imaging scanning, and QoL including cognitive measures. The outcome of this study may have major implications for the management of dialysis patients and might promote a resurgence of home hemodialysis.

Hemodiafiltration

High-volume HDF (removing and replacing 15 to 50 liters per treatment) is in common use in parts of Europe and Asia. The beneficial effects are controversial, but a recent study suggests favorable short-term outcomes.[5] A large randomized, controlled trial is in preparation.[22]

Sorbents

Use of sorbents to absorb molecules that are nondialysable due to size or other reasons will test the relevance as uremic toxins of the many protein-derived substances that accumulate in the plasma of uremic patients. The relevance of glycation of proteins, as affected by sorbent absorption, may also be addressed by this approach.

REFERENCES

1. Pastan S, Bailey J: Dialysis therapy. N Engl J Med 1998;338:1428–1437.
2. Misra M: The basics of hemodialysis equipment. Hemodial Int 2005;9: 30–96.
3. Schindler R, Beck W, Deppisch R, et al: Short bacterial DNA fragments: Detection in dialysate and induction of cytokines. J Am Soc Nephrol 2004;15:3207–214.
4. Forni LG, Hilton PJ: Continuous hemofiltration in the treatment of acute renal failure. N Engl J Med 1997;336:1303–1309.
5. Vaslaki L, Major L, Berta K, et al: On-line haemodiafiltration versus haemodialysis: Stable haematocrit with less erythropoietin and improvement of other relevant blood parameters. Blood Purif 2005;24:163–173.
6. van der Sande FM, Kooman JP, Burema JH, et al: Effect of dialysate temperature on energy balance during hemodialysis: Quantification of extracorporeal energy transfer. Am J Kidney Dis 1999;33:1115–1121.
7. Daugirdas JT: Second generation logarithmic estimates of single-pool variable volume Kt/V: An analysis of error. J Am Soc Nephrol 1993; 4:1205–1213.
8. Gotch FA: The current place of urea kinetic modelling with respect to different dialysis modalities. Nephrol Dial Transplant 1998;13(Suppl 6):10–14.
9. Bargman JM, Golper TA: The importance of residual renal function for patients on dialysis. Nephrol Dial Transplant 2005;20:671–673.
10. Levin NW, Gotch FA, Kuhlmann MK: Factors for increased morbidity and mortality in uremia: Hyperphosphatemia. Semin Nephrol 2004;24: 396–400.
11. Cheung AK, Rocco MV, Yan G, et al: Serum beta-2 microglobulin levels predict mortality in dialysis patients: Results of the HEMO Study. J Am Soc Nephrol 2006;17:546–555.
12. Eknoyan G, Beck GJ, Cheung AK, et al: Effect of dialysis dose and membrane flux in maintenance hemodialysis. N Engl J Med 2002;347: 2010–2019.
13. Kuhlmann MK, Zhu F, Seibert E, Levin NW: Bioimpedance, dry weight and blood pressure control: New methods and consequences. Curr Opin Nephrol Hypertens 2005;14:543–549.
14. Plantinga LC, Jaar BG, Fink NE, et al: Frequency of patient-physician contact in chronic kidney disease care and achievement of clinical performance targets. Int J Qual Health Care 2005;17:115–121.
15. Bander SJ, Walters BA: Hemodialysis morbidity and mortality: Links to patient non-compliance. Curr Opin Nephrol Hypertens 1998;7: 649–653.
16. Unruh ML, Weisbord SD, Kimmel PL: Health-related quality of life in nephrology research and clinical practice. Semin Dial 2005;18:82–90.
17. Dogan E, Erkoc R, Eryonucu B, et al: Relation between depression, some laboratory parameters, and quality of life in hemodialysis patients. Ren Fail 2005;27:695–699.
18. Davison SN, Jhangri GS: The impact of chronic pain on depression, sleep, and the desire to withdraw from dialysis in hemodialysis patients. J Pain Symptom Manage 2005;30:465–473.
19. Kalender B, Corapcioglu Ozdemir A, Koroglu G: Association of depression with markers of nutrition and inflammation in chronic kidney disease and end-stage renal disease. Nephron Clin Pract 2005;102: c115–c121.
20. Miskulin D: Characterizing comorbidity in dialysis patients: Principles of measurement and applications in risk adjustment and patient care. Perit Dial Int 2005;25:320–332.
21. Miskulin DC, Athienites NV, Yan G, et al: Comorbidity assessment using the Index of Coexistent Diseases in a multicenter clinical trial. Kidney Int 2001;60:1498–1510.
22. Penne EL, Blankestijn PJ, Bots ML, et al: Effect of increased convective clearance by on-line hemodiafiltration on all cause and cardiovascular mortality in chronic hemodialysis patients—the Dutch CONvective TRAnsport STudy (CONTRAST): Rationale and design of a randomised controlled trial [ISRCTN38365125]. Curr Control Trials Cardiovasc Med 2005;6:8.

DIALYSIS REACTIONS

During hemodialysis (HD), blood is exposed to surface components of the extracorporeal circuit including the dialyzer, tubing, sterilization processes, and other foreign substances related to the manufacturing and reprocessing procedures. This interaction between the patient's blood and the extracorporeal system can lead to various adverse reactions (Fig. 84.1).[1]

Anaphylactic and Anaphylactoid Reactions
Clinical Presentation

Anaphylaxis is the result of an IgE-mediated acute allergic reaction in a sensitized patient, whereas anaphylactoid reactions result from the direct release of mediators by host cells. The onset of symptoms usually occurs within the first 5 minutes of initiating dialysis, although a delay of up to 20 minutes is possible. Symptoms vary from subtle to quite severe and include burning/

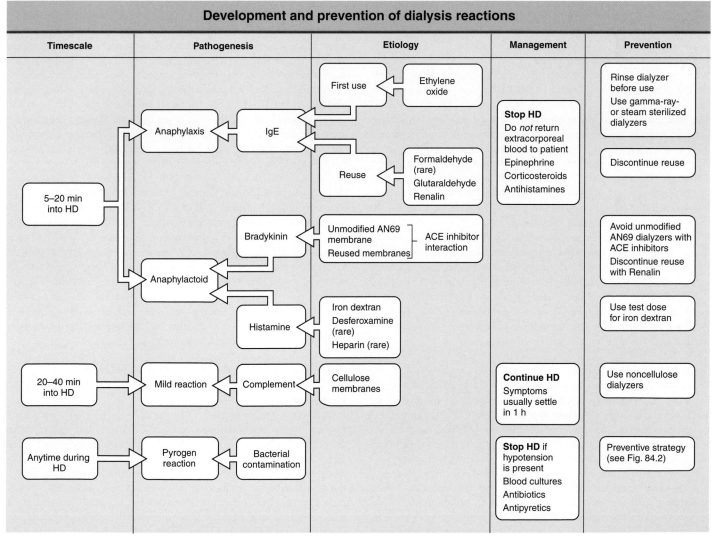

Figure 84.1   Development and prevention of dialysis reaction. ACE, angiotensin-converting enzyme; HD, hemodialysis.

heat throughout the body or at the access site; dyspnea, chest tightness, angioedema/laryngeal edema; paresthesias involving the fingers, toes, lips, or tongue; rhinorrhea; lacrimation; sneezing or coughing; skin flushing; pruritus; nausea/vomiting, abdominal cramps; and diarrhea. Predisposing factors include a history of atopy, elevated total serum IgE, eosinophilia, and the use of angiotensin-converting enzyme (ACE) inhibitors. The etiology of dialysis reactions is diverse and requires a thorough investigation.

First Use Reactions

The majority of these reactions are ascribed to the manufacturer's dialyzer sterilant ethylene oxide (ETO). The potting compound that anchors the hollow fibers in the dialyzer housing acts as a reservoir for ETO and may impede its washout from the dialyzer, leading to sensitization. When conjugated to human serum albumin (HSA), ETO acts as an allergen. Using a radioallergosorbent test (RAST), specific IgE antibodies against ETO-HSA are detected in two thirds of patients with such reactions. However, 10% of patients with no history of dialysis reactions have a positive RAST result.

Reuse Reactions

As most residual ETO is washed out of the dialyzer during first use, reuse reactions are likely to be due to the disinfectants used for dialyzer reprocessing. These agents include formaldehyde, glutaraldehyde, and peracetic acid/hydrogen peroxide (renalin), and, in allergic patients, specific IgE antibodies against formaldehyde are occasionally detectable.

Bradykinin-Mediated Reactions

In the early 1990s, anaphylactoid reactions appeared in Europe among patients dialyzed with AN69 dialyzers who were also taking ACE inhibitors. Investigation of these incidents revealed that binding of factor XII to this sulfonate-containing, negatively charged membrane resulted in the formation of kallikrein and release of bradykinin, which, in turn, led to the production of prostaglandin and histamine, with subsequent vasodilatation and increased vascular permeability. ACE inactivates bradykinin, and, therefore, ACE inhibitors can prolong the biologic activities of bradykinin.[2] These membranes have since been chemically modified, thereby reducing this risk.

Anaphylactoid reactions have also been observed in patients on ACE inhibitors who were dialyzed with membranes that had been reprocessed. Renalin was the sterilant used, and the reactions abated once reprocessing was discontinued, despite continued use of ACE inhibitors. It has been speculated that Renalin may oxidize cysteine-containing proteins that are adsorbed on the dialyzer membrane, leading to the formation of cysteine sulfonate and contact activation of factor XII.

Drug-Induced Reactions

Anaphylactoid reactions to parenteral iron dextran occur in 0.6% to 1% of HD patients. Significantly higher rates of anaphylactoid reactions have been observed among users of higher molecular weight compared with lower molecular weight iron dextran.[3] In vitro, dextran produces a dose-dependent basophil histamine release. At a clinical dose >250 mg, iron dextran is associated with hypotension, and a serum sickness–like syndrome may ensue. It is therefore recommended to initiate iron dextran as a 25-mg test dose, with staff available to respond to reactions, followed by a course of 100 mg/dialysis session for 10 doses.[4] Intravenous iron gluconate and sucrose are alternative preparations that have rapidly replaced iron dextran for patients requiring intravenous

iron supplementation because of rare anaphylactoid reactions associated with high-molecular-weight dextran. Finally, patients who rarely exhibit hypersensitivity to heparin formulations usually respond by substituting beef with pork heparin or vice versa.

Treatment and Prevention

Treatment of anaphylactic/anaphylactoid reaction requires the immediate cessation of HD without returning the extracorporeal blood to the patient. Epinephrine, antihistamines, corticosteroids, and respiratory support should be provided, if needed. Specific preventive measures include rinsing the dialyzer immediately before first use, substituting ETO- with gamma ray– or steam-sterilized dialyzers, avoiding unmodified AN69 membranes in patients on ACE inhibitors, and discontinuing reprocessing procedures in selected cases.

Mild Reactions

Mild reactions occur 20 to 40 minutes after initiating dialysis with unsubstituted cellulose dialyzers and consist of chest/back pain. Dialysis can be continued as symptoms usually abate after the first hour, suggesting a relation to the degree of complement activation. Indeed, these reactions decrease with the use of substituted and reprocessed unsubstituted cellulose membranes. Oxygen therapy and analgesics are usually sufficient. Preventive measures include automated cleansing of new dialyzers or using noncellulose dialyzers.

Microbial Contamination

Several factors that are operative during dialysis place patients at risk of exposure to bacterial products, including contaminated water/bicarbonate dialysate, improperly sterilized dialyzers, use of central venous dialysis catheter, and cannulation of infected grafts or fistulas.[1] Soluble bacterial products can diffuse across the dialyzer into the blood, resulting in cytokine production and, consequently, pyrogen reactions. When bacterial contamination becomes excessive, pyrogen reactions with or without bacteremia can result.

Pyrogen reaction is a diagnosis of exclusion, as bacteremia should first be ruled out. Careful examination of the dialysis access is warranted, and blood cultures should be obtained. Treatment includes antipyretics, broad-spectrum antibiotics, cessation of ultrafiltration whenever hypotension is present, and selective hospitalization. An outbreak of bacteremia among several patients involving a similar organism should prompt a thorough search for bacterial contaminants in the dialysis equipment.[1] Attention should also be paid to single-use vials that are punctured several times, such as erythropoietin, which has been linked to an outbreak of bloodstream infection.[5] Strategies for the prevention of pyrogen reactions are summarized in Figure 84.2.

CARDIOVASCULAR COMPLICATIONS

Hypotension

Intradialytic hypotension occurs in 10% to 30% of treatments, ranging from asymptomatic episodes to marked compromise of organ perfusion resulting in myocardial ischemia, cardiac arrhythmias, vascular thrombosis, loss of consciousness, seizures, or death. Further, in patients with acute renal failure, intradialytic hypotension may induce further renal ischemia and retard recovery of renal function. Intradialytic hypotension and postdialysis orthostatic hypotension have been shown to be independent risk factors for mortality.[6] The pathogenesis of intradialytic hypotension is complex[7] and is summarized in Figure 84.3.

Strategies to prevent bacterial contamination

Strict adherence to the AAMI standards

Type of Fluid	Microbial Count	Endotoxin
Water products	<200 cfu/ml	<2 EU
Dialysate	<2000 cfu/ml	No standard
Reprocessed dialyzers	No growth	—

Use appropriate germicide
  4% formaldehyde[*]
  1% formaldehyde heated to 40°C[*†]
  Glutaraldehyde[†]
  Hydrogen peroxide/peracetic acid mixture (Renalin)[*†]
  Heat sterilization (105°C for 20 hours) for reprocessing of polysulfone
    membranes.[†]

Wash and rinse the vascular access arm with soap and water

Prior to cannulation, inspect vascular access for local signs of inflammation

Scrub the skin with povidone iodine or chlorhexidine and allow to dry for
  5 minutes prior to cannulation

Record temperature before and after dialysis

When central delivery system is used
  Clean and disinfect connecting pipes regularly
  Remove residual bacteria or endotoxin by additional filtration

When single-patient proportioning dialysis machine is used
  Freshly prepare bicarbonate dialysate on a daily basis
  Discard unused solutions at the end of each day
  Rinse and disinfect containers with fluids that meet AAMI standards
  Air-dry containers prior to dialysate preparation

Follow manufacturer's guidelines for use of preservative-free medications

Figure 84.2 Strategies to prevent bacterial contamination. *A minimum of 11- or 24-hour exposure to peracetic acid or formaldehyde is required, respectively. †These germicides are all equivalent or superior to 4% formaldehyde. AAMI, Association for the Advancement of Medical Instrumentation; cfu, colony-forming units; EU, endotoxin units.

The immediate treatment is to restore the circulating blood volume by placing the patient in the Trendelenburg position, reducing or stopping ultrafiltration, and infusing isotonic normal saline. With the advent of newer dialysis engineering principles, better preventive strategies have emerged. These include the use of bicarbonate dialysate, volumetric control of ultrafiltration, sodium modeling, and better assessment of patient's dry weight. Midodrine—an oral selective α_1-agonist, and cool dialysate—a measure that increases the release of catecholamines and therefore induces vasoconstriction, are also two useful preventive therapies.[8] Salt poor albumin offers no advantage over normal saline and costs more. Other preventive strategies include correction of anemia and hypoalbuminemia, withdrawal of antihypertensive drugs before dialysis, avoidance of food before and during dialysis, counseling patients about weight gain, and treatment of congestive heart failure or arrhythmias. Online blood volume monitoring and biofeedback techniques have also been used to improve intradialytic cardiovascular stability.[9] Short daily HD plays a role in preventing intradialytic hypotension as well.[10] Finally, a new device with thermal sensors able to measure blood temperature at the arterial and venous sides of the extracorporeal circuit and accordingly modify the dialysate temperature has been developed. This technique allows isothermic dialysis and has been shown to reduce symptomatic intradialytic hypotension.[11]

Hypertension

Hypertension during or immediately after dialysis constitutes an important risk factor for cardiovascular mortality. Its mechanism is primarily volume dependent. However, in a number of patients, blood pressure remains elevated despite fluid removal, a syndrome called dialysis-refractory hypertension. These patients are usually young with pre-existing hypertension and have excessive interdialytic weight gain and a hyperactive renin angiotensin system in response to fluid removal.[12]

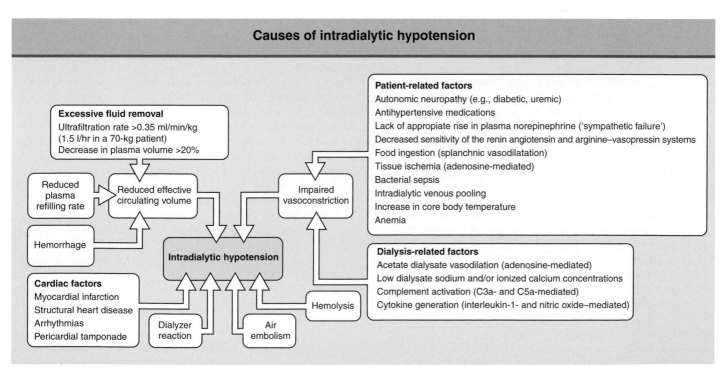

Figure 84.3 Pathogenesis and causes of intradialytic hypotension.

Erythropoietin and other erythropoeisis-stimulating agents have been associated with a 20% to 30% incidence of new-onset or exacerbation of hypertension. Further, among patients receiving intravenous (not subcutaneous) erythropoietin, elevated levels of endothelin-1 (a potent vasoconstrictor) have been shown to correlate with increased blood pressure. Intradialytic hypertension can be precipitated by the use of hypernatric dialysate, which is intended to mitigate the intradialytic decrease in serum osmolality that occurs with the diffusive removal of urea and sodium.[13] Although this approach stabilizes blood pressure during dialysis, hypernatric dialysate results in a positive intradialytic sodium balance and is associated with increased postdialysis thirst, resulting in significant weight gain in the interdialytic period. To circumvent these problems, sodium modeling has been adopted as an approach that uses variable sodium concentrations in the dialysate, generally with sodium reduced in a continuous or stepwise manner from an initial level of 150 to 154 mmol/l to 138 to 142 mmol/l. Finally, clinicians should also be aware of possible dialytic removal of certain antihypertensive drugs such as ACE inhibitors and β-blockers.

Treatment requires an accurate determination of the patient's dry weight. It is reasonable to avoid the use of hypernatric dialysate but adopt instead sodium modeling targeting serum sodium concentrations of 138 to 142 mmol/l at the end of dialysis, reduce the dry weight in 0.5-kg increments, observe the clinical response, and reevaluate periodically. Once dry weight is achieved, optimization of antihypertensive drug therapy is warranted, including withholding antihypertensive medication before dialysis.

Cardiac Arrhythmias

Intradialytic arrhythmias are common and are often multifactorial in origin.[14,15] Left ventricular hypertrophy, congestive cardiomyopathy, uremic pericarditis, silent myocardial ischemia, and conduction system calcification are frequently encountered in adult dialysis patients. In addition, polypharmacy coupled with the constant alterations in fluid, electrolyte, and acid-base homeostasis may precipitate intradialytic arrhythmias. Hypocalcemia and hypomagnesemia have additive effects to hypokalemia, whereas hypercalcemia and hypokalemia can precipitate arrhythmias in patients on digoxin. Further, myocardial ischemia due to a decrease in myocardial oxygen delivery (e.g., intradialytic hypotension) or an increase in myocardial oxygen consumption (e.g., volume overload) can trigger arrhythmias in patients with underlying coronary artery disease. The range of electrocardiographic abnormalities that may be encountered in renal failure are shown in Figure 84.4. QTc dispersion, the difference between maximum and minimum QTc interval on a standard 12-lead electrocardiogram, is prolonged prolonged following HD and has been proposed as a prognostic indicator of cardiac complications in dialysis patients.[16]

Preventive measures include the use of bicarbonate dialysate and careful attention to dialysate potassium and calcium levels. Use of zero potassium dialysate should be discouraged due to its arrhythmogenic potential, particularly in patients on digoxin, should serum potassium decrease to <3.5 mmol/L. Serum digoxin levels should be regularly monitored and the need for the drug regularly reassessed. Finally, maintenance of an adequate hemoglobin level, treatment of hypertension or congestive heart failure, and antianginal prophylaxis offer additional precautions against arrhythmias.

Sudden Death

Cardiac arrest occurs at a rate of 7 per 100,000 HD sessions and is more common in the elderly, patients with diabetes, and patients using central venous catheters.[17] Some 80% of sudden deaths

Electrocardiographic abnormalities in renal failure	
Function	**Abnormality Seen in Renal Failure**
P-R interval	Usually normal; prolongation in long-term hemodialysis
	Calcification of mitral valve annulus may involve His bundle, giving complete heart block
QRS interval	
Amplitude	Increases during ultrafiltration (correlates with reduction in left ventricular [LV] dimensions)
	LV hypertrophy (LVH) on voltage criteria found in up to 50%
Duration	Prolonged (within normal range) by hemodialysis
	Late potentials increased only in patients with pre-existing ischemic heart disease
	Prolonged in hyperkalemia
ST segment	Depression during hemodialysis does not predict coronary artery disease
	Depression or elevation may occur in hyperkalemia
	Depression during ambulatory monitoring poorly predictive of coronary artery disease
Q-T$_c$ interval	Increases during hemodialysis (correlates with reduction in [K$^+$] and [Mg^{2+}])
	Increased Q-T dispersion reported in patients on dialysis
T wave	Peaking or inversion may occur in hyperkalemia
	Inversion in anterolateral leads in LVH with strain pattern
Rhythm	High incidence of atrial and ventricular arrhythmias during hemodialysis

Figure 84.4 Electrocardiographic abnormalities in renal failure. Risk factors include LV dysfunction, wall motion abnormalities, known coronary artery disease, positive thallium redistribution tests (even without coronary artery disease), use of cardiac glycosides, and low dialysate K$^+$.

during dialysis are due to ventricular fibrillation and are more frequently observed after the long interdialytic interval on thrice-weekly dialysis.[18,19] Although ischemic heart disease increases the risk of sudden death, other catastrophic intradialytic events need to be ruled out. The prompt recognition and treatment of life-threatening hyperkalemia, often encountered in young, noncompliant patients, is imperative. Profound generalized muscle weakness may be a warning sign of imminent life-threatening hyperkalemia. When cardiopulmonary arrest occurs during dialysis, an immediate decision must be made as to whether the collapse is due to an intrinsic disease or technical errors such as air embolism, unsafe dialysate composition, overheated dialysate, line disconnection, or sterilant in the dialyzer have occurred. Air in the dialysate, grossly hemolyzed blood, and hemorrhage due to line disconnection can be easily detected. However, if no obvious cause is identifiable, blood should not be returned to the patient, particularly if the arrest occurred immediately on initiation of dialysis. A patient exposed to formaldehyde may have complained earlier of burning at the access site. If the possibility of a problem with dialysate composition is remote, blood may be returned to the patient. However, blood and dialysate samples should be immediately sent for electrolyte analysis, the dialyzer and bloodlines saved for later analysis, and the dialysis machine replaced until all its safety features have been thoroughly evaluated for possible malfunction. It should be a standard practice to have defibrillators in dialysis units. While the management of cardiopulmonary arrest during dialysis should follow the standard principles of cardiopulmonary resuscitation, the diagnosis and management of technical errors are discussed later.

Dialysis-Associated Steal Syndrome

The construction of an arteriovenous fistula or graft frequently results in reduction of blood flow to the hand. Although clinically significant ischemia does not usually result, symptoms are by no means rare, particularly in diabetics or elderly patients with peripheral vascular disease. Dialysis-associated steal syndrome has been reported in 6.4% and 1% of patients with radiocephalic fistulas and grafts, respectively. The clinical presentation, differential diagnosis, and evaluation of dialysis-associated steal syndrome are summarized in Figure 84.5 and are discussed further in Chapter 81.[20,21]

Treatment depends on the clinical severity of ischemia and vascular access anatomy.[21] Severe ischemia can cause irreparable injury to nerves within hours and must be considered a surgical emergency. Mild ischemia, manifested by subjective coldness and paresthesias and objective reduction in skin temperature but with no loss of sensation or motion, is common and generally improves with time.[22] Patients with mild ischemia should undergo symptom-specific therapy (e.g., wearing a glove) and frequent physical examination, with special attention to subtle neurologic changes and muscle wasting.[23] Failure to improve may require surgical intervention with banding or access correction or ligation. The simplest way to improve distal perfusion is ligation of the venous outflow of the fistula/graft. This procedure provides immediate improvement in perfusion but results in the elimination of a site for vascular access and the immediate need to construct another one. Other techniques that do not sacrifice the access and yet improve distal perfusion include ligation of the artery distal to the origin of the fistula/graft with or without establishing an arterial bypass (see Chapter 81) or narrowing of the fistula/graft to reduce flow, thereby improving distal perfusion. Percutaneous luminal angioplasty or laser recanalization is reserved for patients with inflow or outflow arterial disease. A modified brachiocephalic fistula extension technique, in which the median vein is anastomosed to the radial or ulnar artery just below the brachial bifurcation, is thought to preserve part of the blood supply to the hand and prevent the arterial steal syndrome.[24] Persistence of symptoms after an apparently successful correction of the vascular access flow should alert the clinician to other unrelated causes.

NEUROMUSCULAR COMPLICATIONS

Muscle Cramps

Muscle cramps occur in 5% to 20% of patients late during dialysis and frequently involve the legs. They account for 15% of premature discontinuations of dialysis.[25] Electromyography shows increased tonic muscle electrical activity throughout dialysis, and serum creatinine kinase may be elevated.

Although the pathogenesis is unknown, dialysis-induced volume contraction and hypo-osmolality are common predisposing factors. However, hypomagnesemia and carnitine deficiency may also play a role.

The acute management is directed at increasing plasma osmolality. Parenteral infusion of 23.5% hypertonic saline (15 to 20 ml), 25% mannitol (50 to 100 ml), or 50% dextrose in water (25 to 50 ml) are equally effective. However, hypertonic saline may result in postdialytic thirst, and both hypertonic saline and mannitol cause transient warmth/flushing during the infusion. Furthermore, large and repetitive infusions of mannitol may lead to increased thirst, interdialytic weight gain, and fluid overload. Overall, dextrose in water is preferred, particularly in nondiabetics.

Preventive measures include dietary counseling about excessive interdialytic weight gain. In patients without clinical signs of fluid overload, it is reasonable to increase the dry weight by 0.5 kg and observe the clinical response. Quinine sulfate (260 to 325 mg) or oxazepam (5 to 10 mg) given 2 hours prior to dialysis may also be effective. Although in the United States, the U.S. Food and Drug Administration regards quinine sulfate as both unsafe and ineffective for the prevention of cramps, this drug works very well in some patients, and in most parts of the world, it is used freely. The use of sodium gradient during dialysis is effective as well. Proposed strategies include starting with a dialysate sodium concentration of 145 to 155 mmol/l and a linear decrease to 135- to 140 mmol/l by the completion of the treatment. A comparison of sodium modeling using an exponential, linear, or step program has yielded similar results.[26] In anecdotal reports, 5 mg enalapril twice weekly may be effective, presumably by inhibiting angiotensin II–mediated thirst. Finally, stretching exercises, creatine monohydrate,[27] and L-carnitine supplementation (20 mg/kg per dialysis session) may also be beneficial.[28] An intradialytic blood volume biofeedback control system has been shown to effectively reduce the incidence of muscle cramps.[29]

Restless Legs Syndrome

Restless legs syndrome occurs in a significant portion of chronically dialyzed patients. Patients complain of crawling sensations in their legs that occur exclusively during sleep or inactive seated or recumbent wakefulness, particularly during dialysis. Although the tendency to move can be momentarily suppressed, it is ultimately irresistible to move the legs, which yields prompt relief. Some patients also complain of pain at the same site. As a consequence, most patients have insomnia, and some suffer from anxiety or mild depression and have a poor quality of life. The results of neurologic and electromyographic examinations are generally unremarkable.

Iron deficiency anemia, vascular insufficiency, chronic lung disease, caffeine abuse, hyperphosphatemia, and psychological factors have all been implicated in the pathogenesis of restless

---

Dialysis-associated vascular steal syndrome

Clinical presentations (symptoms often aggravated on dialysis)
  Hand numbness, pain, or weakness
  Coolness of distal arm
  Diminished pulses
  Acrocyanosis, gangrene

Differential diagnosis
  Dialysis-associated cramp
  Polyneuropathy—diabetes, uremia
  Entrapment neuropathy—Aβ_2M-amyloid
  Reflex sympathetic dystrophy
  Calciphylaxis

Evaluation of steal severity
  Pulse oximetry
  Plethysmography
  Doppler flow
  Angiography

Treatment options (depending on severity)
  Symptomatic (e.g., gloves)
  Surgical, with preservation of vascular access: banding to reduce flow,
    DRIL procedure (see Fig. 81.9)
  With loss of vascular access; ligation

Figure 84.5 Dialysis-associated vascular steal syndrome. DRIL, distal revascularization and interval ligation.

legs.[30] The use of tricyclic antidepressants, selective serotonin reuptake inhibitors, lithium, and dopamine antagonists might exacerbate this condition. The differential diagnosis is peripheral neuropathy, in which paresthesias are constant and unrelieved by activity. When symptoms develop in a stable dialysis patient, anxiety, peripheral vascular disease, and inadequate dialysis need to be considered.

Whereas temazepam (a short-acting benzodiazepine) is temporarily effective when administered at bedtime, opiates are remarkably efficient but have the potential for abuse and development of tolerance. Carbamazepine and levodopa have also been advocated, but tolerance may develop rapidly. Hence, a reasonable approach is to alternate chemically unrelated agents on a weekly/biweekly basis. More recently, gabapentin has been found to be superior to levodopa and can also improve sleep disturbances.[31] These agents should be given early enough before dialysis to allow for absorption. Transcutaneous electric nerve stimulation and methadone use[32] should be reserved for refractory cases. More recently, ropinirole, a dopamine receptor agonist, has shown promising outcomes in dialysis patients.[33]

Dialysis Disequilibrium Syndrome

Despite a decline in its incidence, dialysis disequilibrium syndrome (DDS) is still observed sporadically in patients who are initiated on HD with large surface area and high-flux dialyzers and shorter dialysis time. Risk factors include young age, severe azotemia, low dialysate sodium concentration, and pre-existing neurologic disorders (see also Chapter 76).

DDS commonly presents with restlessness, headache, nausea, vomiting, blurred vision, muscle twitching, disorientation, tremor, and hypertension. More severe manifestations include obtundation, seizures, and coma. DDS usually develops toward the end of dialysis but may be delayed for up to 24 hours. Although cerebral edema is a consistent finding on computed tomographic scanning, DDS remains a clinical diagnosis since laboratory tests, including electroencephalography, are nonspecific. It is usually self-limiting, but full recovery may take several days.

The pathogenesis of DDS is still a subject of debate. The reverse urea effect theory, which proposes that a transient osmotic disequilibrium occurs during dialysis as a result of a more rapid removal of urea from blood than from cerebrospinal fluid (CSF), has been disputed.[34] In animals undergoing rapid dialysis, despite the correction of systemic acidosis, a paradoxical CSF acidosis develops that is aborted by slower dialysis. Additional mechanisms include the intracerebral accumulation of idiogenic osmoles such as inositol, glutamine, and glutamate.

In high-risk patients, preventive measures include the use of volumetric-controlled machines, bicarbonate dialysate, sodium modeling, earlier recognition of uremic states, and earlier initiation of dialysis. In addition, short and more frequent dialysis treatments are recommended using small-surface area dialyzers and reduced blood flow rates. The target reduction in plasma urea should initially be limited to 30%. The prophylactic use of mannitol or anticonvulsants is not recommended.

Seizures

Intradialytic seizures occur in <10% of patients and tend to be generalized but easily controlled. However, focal or refractory seizures warrant evaluation for focal neurologic disease, particularly intracranial hemorrhage. Causes of seizures are summarized in Figure 84.6 and are discussed further in Chapter 76.

Treatment of established seizures requires cessation of dialysis, maintenance of airway patency, and investigation for metabolic abnormalities. Intravenous diazepam, alprazolam or clonazepam, and phenytoin may be required. Intravenous 50% dextrose in water should be administered promptly if hypoglycemia is suspected.

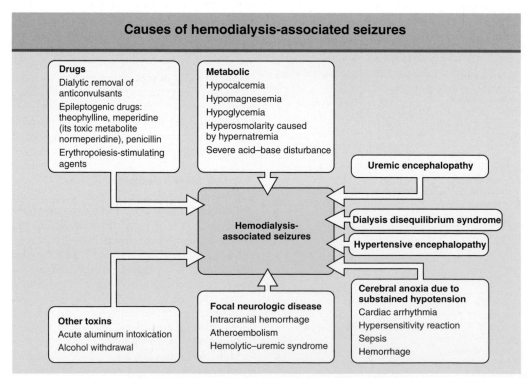

Figure 84.6 Causes of hemodialysis-associated seizures.

Headache

Dialysis headache is common and consists of a bifrontal discomfort that develops during dialysis and may become intense and throbbing, accompanied by nausea and vomiting. It is usually aggravated by the supine position, but there are no visual disturbances.

Although its etiology has not been elucidated, dialysis headache may be a subtle manifestation of DDS or may be related to the use of acetate dialysate. Furthermore, it may be a manifestation of caffeine withdrawal due to dialytic removal of caffeine.

Management consists of oral analgesics (e.g., acetaminophen [paracetamol]), and preventive measures include slow dialysis with reduced blood flow rates, change to bicarbonate dialysate, sodium and ultrafiltration modeling, coffee ingestion during dialysis, and use of reprocessed dialyzers.

HEMATOLOGIC COMPLICATIONS

Complement Activation and Dialysis-Associated Neutropenia

During dialysis with unsubstituted cellulose dialyzers, the free hydroxyl groups present on the membrane cause activation of the alternative pathway of complement.[35] This results in activation and increased adherence of circulating neutrophils to the endothelial capillary pulmonary vasculature, leading to transient neutropenia that reaches a nadir after 15 minutes of dialysis, followed by a rebound leukocytosis 1 hour later. Neutropenia has also been detected with other more widely used dialyzer membranes including cellulose acetate and polysulfone, but to a lesser degree. Although the long-term clinical relevance of this phenomenon remains speculative, its contribution to acute intradialytic morbidity is discussed later.

Intradialytic Hemolysis

Acute hemolysis can be due to faulty dialysis equipment, chemicals, drugs, toxins, or patient-related factors[36] (Fig. 84.7). With the advent of better dialysis equipment and the widespread use of deionization systems, traumatic red blood cell fragmentation caused by poorly designed blood pumps and methemoglobinemia caused by water contamination with chloramine or copper are never seen today. However, nitrate/nitrite intoxication causing methemoglobinemia still occurs sporadically in patients on home HD who use well water that is contaminated with urine from domesticated animals. Further, during dialyzer reprocessing, formaldehyde retention can result in hemolysis by inducing formation of cold agglutinins or inhibiting red cell metabolism.

The diagnosis of acute hemolysis is self-evident when grossly translucent hemolyzed blood is observed in the tubing. Patients with methemoglobinemia have nausea, vomiting, hypotension, and cyanosis, and oxygen therapy does not improve the black-colored blood present in the extracorporeal circuit. Copper contamination should be suspected in the presence of skin flushing and abdominal pain or diarrhea.

Evaluation should include reticulocyte count, haptoglobin, lactate dehydrogenase, blood smear, Coombs' test, and measurement of methemoglobin.[51]Cr-RBC survival and bone marrow examination may occasionally be indicated if there is recurrent hemolysis. More importantly, analysis of tap water for chloramines and metal contaminants and thorough analysis of the dialysis equipment for clues of increased blood turbulence are recommended.

Hemorrhage

Bleeding complications are commonly related to the use of intradialytic anticoagulation, which further confounds the uremic bleeding diathesis[37] (see Chapter 73). In addition, dialysis patients are prone to spontaneous bleeding at specific sites, such as gastrointestinal arteriovenous malformations; subdural, pericardial, pleural, retroperitoneal, and hepatic subcapsular spaces; and the ocular anterior chamber. Despite its limitations, the bleeding time remains the best indicator of hemorrhagic tendency. In addition to specific measures directed to the site of hemorrhage, reversal of

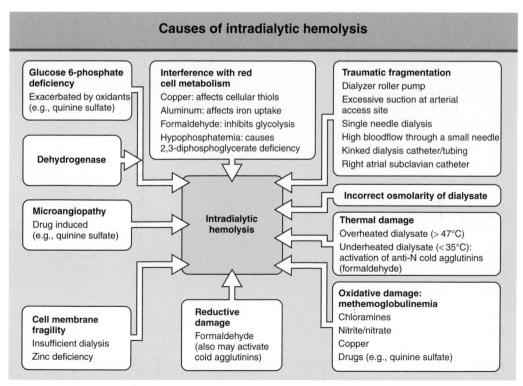

Figure 84.7 Causes of intradialytic hemolysis.

uremic platelet dysfunction is imperative. Strategies include the use of erythropoiesis-stimulating agents or RBC transfusions to achieve a hematocrit >30% in order to improve rheologic platelets–vessel wall interactions, intravenous conjugated estrogens at 0.6 mg/kg/day for 5 consecutive days, intravenous/subcutaneous 1-deamino-8-D-arginine vasopressin (DDAVP) at 0.3 μg/kg over 15 to 30 minutes, and/or intravenous infusion of cryoprecipitate (see Fig. 73.4). For patients experiencing severe bleeding, it is advisable to consider heparin-free dialysis, using normal saline flushes every 15 to 30 minutes with ultrafiltration adjustments, regional heparin or citrate anticoagulation, low-molecular-weight heparin, heparin modeling, or prostacyclin. More recently, the use of heparin-bound hemophan dialyzers has been advocated in patients at risk of bleeding.[38] In patients scheduled for elective surgery or invasive procedures, aspirin should be stopped a week earlier, the dose of anticoagulant reduced to minimum, and the hematocrit maintained at >30%. In some cases, DDAVP and/or estrogens may also be required. Tranexamic acid, a potent fibrinolytic inhibitor, has recently been used as an adjuvant treatment for controlling hemorrhage in dialysis patients.[39]

PULMONARY COMPLICATIONS

Dialysis-Associated Hypoxemia

In most patients, the arterial PaO_2 decreases by 5 to 20 mm Hg (0.6 to 4.0 kPa) during dialysis, reaching a nadir at 30 to 60 minutes, and resolves within 60 to 120 minutes following discontinuation of dialysis. This decrease is usually of no clinical significance to patients unless there is pre-existing chronic cardiopulmonary disease.

Hypoventilation is the main implicated factor and is primarily central in origin due to a decrease in carbon dioxide production following acetate metabolism (specific to acetate dialysate), loss of carbon dioxide in the dialyzer (with both acetate and bicarbonate dialysate), and rapid alkalinization of body fluids (specific to bicarbonate dialysate, particularly with large surface-area dialyzers).[40] In addition, acetate-induced respiratory muscle fatigue can lead to hypoventilation, especially in acutely ill patients. Further, a commonly observed ventilation-perfusion mismatch may be due to pulmonary leukoagglutination (due to complement activation) and/or impaired cardiac output (due to acetate-induced myocardial depression).

In high-risk patients with fluid overload, preventive measures consist of using intradialytic oxygen supplementation, conventional bicarbonate dialysate, and biocompatible membranes. Optimizing hematocrit values and performing sequential ultrafiltration followed by HD may further reduce the likelihood of hypoxemia.

TECHNICAL MALFUNCTIONS

Air Embolism

The most vulnerable source of air entry into the extracorporeal circuit is the prepump tubing segment, where significant subatmospheric pressures prevail. However, other sources need to be considered including intravenous infusion circuits especially with glass bottles, air bubbles from the dialysate, and dialysis catheters. High blood flow rates may allow rapid entry of large volumes of air despite small leaks.

Clinical manifestations depend on the volume of air introduced, the site of introduction, patient's position, and the speed at which air is introduced.[41] In the sitting position, air entry through a peripheral vein bypasses the heart and causes venous emboli in the cerebral circulation. The acute onset of seizures and coma in the absence of precedent symptoms such as chest pain or dyspnea is highly suggestive of air embolism. In the supine position, air introduced through a central venous line will be trapped in the right ventricle where it forms foam, interferes with cardiac output, and, if large enough, leads to obstructive shock. Dissemination of microemboli to the pulmonary vasculature results in dyspnea, dry cough, chest tightness, or respiratory arrest. Further, passage of air across the pulmonary capillary bed can lead to cerebral or coronary artery embolism. In the left Trendelenburg position, air emboli migrate to the lower extremity venous circulation, resulting in ischemia, due to increased outflow resistance. Foam may be visible in the extracorporeal tubing and cardiac auscultation may reveal a peculiar churning sound.

The immediate management of clinically suspected air embolism is summarized in Figure 84.8. Prevention depends primarily on dialysis machines that are equipped with venous air bubble traps and foam detectors located just distal to the dialyzer and a venous pressure monitor at the venous end. The detector is attached to a relay switch that simultaneously activates an alarm, shuts off the blood pump, and clamps the venous bloodline if air is detected. Therefore, dialysis should never be performed in the presence of an inoperative air detection alarm system. Glass bottles should be avoided since they create vacuum effects that can permit air entry into the extracorporeal system. Dialysis catheters should be aspirated and flushed with saline prior to connection. Dialyzer rinsing, prior to use, should expand all compartments to remove residual air bubbles.

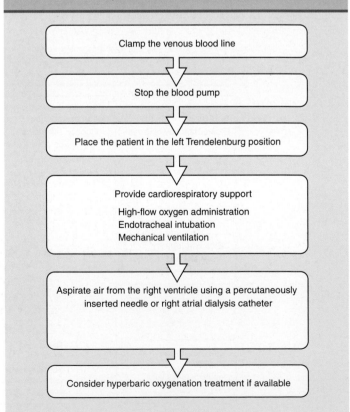

Figure 84.8   Management of clinically suspected air embolism.

Incorrect Dialysate Composition

Incorrect dialysate composition occurs as a result of technical or human errors. Since the primary solutes constituting the dialysate are electrolytes, the dialysate concentration will be reflected by its electrical conductivity (see Chapter 83). Therefore, proper proportioning of concentrate to water can be achieved by the use of a meter that continuously measures the conductivity of the dialysate solution as it is being fed to the dialyzer. Life-threatening electrolyte and acid-base abnormalities are avoidable if the conductivity alarm is functioning properly and the alarm limits are set correctly. However, in dialysis machines that are equipped with conductivity-controlled mixing systems, the system automatically changes the mixing ratio of the concentrates until the dialysate solution conductivity falls within the set limits. This may inadvertently lead to dialysate without any bicarbonate, with apparently acceptable conductivity. Therefore, if conductivity-controlled systems are used, it is safer to also check the dialysate pH prior to dialysis. Conductivity monitors can fail or can be improperly adjusted due to human error. Therefore, it is important to add human monitoring of dialysate composition before every treatment, whenever a machine has been sterilized or moved about, or whenever a new concentrate is used. Furthermore, many nonstandardized solutions are available, some of which may be used with an inappropriate proportioning system. Therefore, it is also essential that the supplies match the machine-proportioning ratio for which they were prepared to obtain the appropriate final dialysate composition.

Hypernatremia

Hypernatremia occurs when concentrate or the ratio of concentrate to water is incorrect, and the conductivity monitors or the alarms are not functioning properly. Hyperosmolality results in intracellular water depletion. Clinical manifestations include thirst, headache, nausea, vomiting, seizures, coma, and death. Aggressive treatment is mandatory and includes cessation of dialysis, hospitalization, and infusion of 5% dextrose in water. Dialysis should be resumed using a different machine, and the dialysate sodium level should be 2 mmol/l lower than the plasma level and isotonic saline should be concurrently infused. Dialysis against a sodium level 3 to 5 mmol/l lower than the plasma level may increase the risk of disequilibrium. Ultrafiltration with equal volume replacement with normal saline is another option.

Hyponatremia

Failure to add concentrate, inadequate concentrate to water ratio, or conductivity monitor or alarm malfunction can cause hyponatremia. Hyponatremia can also occur during the course of dialysis with a proportioning system, if the concentrate container runs dry and the conductivity set limits are inappropriate. Acute hypoosmolality causes hemolysis with hyperkalemia and hemodilution of all plasma constituents. Symptoms include restlessness, anxiety, pain in the vein injected with the hypotonic hemolyzed blood, chest pain, headache, nausea, and occasional severe abdominal/lumbar cramps. Pallor, vomiting, and seizures may be observed. Treatment consists of clamping the bloodlines and discarding the hemolyzed blood in the extracorporeal circuit. High-flow oxygen and cardiac monitoring is imperative because of hyperkalemia and potential myocardial injury. Dialysis should be restarted with a new dialysate batch containing low potassium, and high transmembrane pressure should be applied to remove excess water. Correction of plasma sodium concentration should be achieved by no more than 1 to 2 mmol/l/hr. Anticonvulsants are indicated for seizures and blood transfusions for severe anemia. Successful correction of severe hyponatremia has been reported using a single 3-hour hemodialysis session using a dialysate sodium concentration of 135 mmol/l without sustaining any adverse neurologic consequences despite a serum sodium correction rate of 3 mmol/l/hr.[42] This suggests elevated blood urea levels might protect uremic patients from the development of demyelinating syndromes when hyponatremia is rapidly corrected.

Metabolic Acidosis

Although acute intradialytic metabolic acidosis can be a manifestation of improper mixing of concentrates or failure of pH monitors, other causes need to be ruled out including diabetic or alcoholic ketoacidosis, lactic acidosis, toxic ingestions, or dilutional acidosis.[43] The diagnosis is usually suggested by the acute onset of hyperventilation during HD and confirmed by laboratory evaluation. In most circumstances, correcting the underlying cause and using bicarbonate dialysate at the appropriate concentration (35 mmol/l) are adequate measures.

Metabolic Alkalosis

Severe intradialytic metabolic alkalosis is rare and may be due to error in dialysate concentrates, reversed connection of bicarbonate and acid concentrate containers to the entry ports of the dialysis machine, pH monitor malfunction, or the use of regional citrate anticoagulation. The most common cause, however, is hydrochloric acid loss as a result of vomiting or nasogastric suction. Attention should also be directed at identifying sources of added alkali.[44] Further, the combination of sodium polystyrene sulfonate and aluminum hydroxide can lead to absorption of alkali that is normally neutralized in the small intestine.

Acute treatment is rarely necessary unless a technical error has occurred. Usually, removal of the alkali source is sufficient, and H2-antagonists or proton pump inhibitors may be successful if there is gastric acid loss. The administration of sodium chloride to anephric patients with chloride-sensitive alkalosis will not repair the alkalosis. If a more rapid reduction in plasma bicarbonate is desired, modifying the dialysate bath by replacing alkali with chloride, substituting bicarbonate with acetate dialysate, using acid dialysate, or infusing hydrochloric acid are effective, but cumbersome, measures. The use of conventional or low bicarbonate (25 to 30 mmol/l) dialysate is probably as effective.

Temperature Monitor Malfunction

Malfunction of the thermostat in the dialysis machine can result in the production of excessively cool or hot dialysate. Whereas cool dialysate is not dangerous and may have beneficial hemodynamic effects, overheated dialysate can cause immediate hemolysis and life-threatening hyperkalemia, particularly if the dialysate temperature increases to >51°C. In such an event, dialysis must be stopped immediately and blood in the system be discarded. The patient should be monitored for hemolysis and hyperkalemia. Dialysis should be resumed to cool the patient by using a dialysate temperature of 34°C to treat hyperkalemia and to allow blood transfusions if necessary. Visual and audible alarms are mandatory to prevent this complication.

Blood Loss

Intradialytic blood loss can result from arterial or venous needle disengagement from the access, separation of the venous or arterial line connections, femoral or central line dialysis catheter perforation or dislodgment, or rupture of a dialysis membrane with or without malfunction of the blood leak detector. Clinical findings include hypotension, loss of consciousness, or cardiac arrest. In addition, following traumatic insertion of a dialysis catheter, blood loss can result in pain/mass from a rapidly expanding hematoma; chest, shoulder, or neck pain from intrapericardial blood loss; back, flank, groin, or lower abdominal pain/distention from retroperitoneal bleeding; or hemoptysis from pulmonary bleeding. Acute management includes the discontinuation of HD, pressure application for local hemostasis, hemodynamic support, oxygen administration, and surgical intervention if needed.

MISCELLANEOUS COMPLICATIONS

Postdialysis Syndrome

An ill-defined washed-out feeling or malaise during or after HD is a common nonspecific symptom that is observed in about one third of patients[45] and has multifactorial origins. Reduced cardiac output, peripheral vascular disease, depression, poor conditioning, postdialysis hypotension, hypokalemia or hypoglycemia, mild uremic encephalopathy, myopathy due to carnitine deficiency, and membrane bioincompatibility through cytokine production have all been incriminated. The use of glucose/bicarbonate dialysate and L-carnitine supplementation (20 mg/kg/day) has been shown to improve postdialysis well-being. A recent trial of thrice-weekly L-carnitine at 20 mg/kg for 6 months resulted in a marked decrease in C-reactive protein level, which was paralleled by an increase in body mass index.[46] Although there are insufficient data to support the use of L-carnitine to improve quality of life in unselected dialysis patients, the most promising of the proposed applications is for the treatment of erythropoietin-resistant anemia.[47]

Pruritus

Pruritus is common, and the etiology is often multifactorial including xerosis, hyperparathyroidism, neuropathy, derangements in the immune system, and inadequate dialysis. In many cases, pruritus is more severe during or after dialysis and may be an allergic manifestation to heparin, ETO, formaldehyde, or acetate. In this subgroup of patients, use of gamma ray–sterilized dialyzers, discontinuation of formaldehyde use, switching to bicarbonate dialysate, and use of low dialysate calcium and magnesium might result in cessation of itching. Eczematous reactions to antiseptic solutions, rubber glove or puncture needle components, puncture needles, or collophane used to secure dialysis needles should also be considered.[48]

Therapies include the use of emollients and antihistamines, activated charcoal, ultraviolet therapy, sunbathing, ketotifen (a mast cell stabilizer), erythropoietin therapy, topical capsaicin, or topical tacrolimus ointment. Finally, dialysis adequacy should always be assessed. The management of uremic pruritus is discussed further in Chapter 78 (see Fig. 78.3).

Priapism

Priapism occurs in <0.5% of male HD patients. It is not related to sexual activity and occurs while on dialysis. The patient is usually awakened from sleep by a painful erection. Although the majority of cases are idiopathic, secondary causes include heparin-induced hyperviscosity; high hematocrit due to androgen or epoetin therapy; dialysis-induced hypoxemia and hypovolemia due to excessive ultrafiltration, particularly in African American males with sickle cell disease; and the use of α-blockers, such as prazosin, or an antidepressant such as trazodone.

Urologic referral is mandatory. Acute treatment consists of corporal aspiration and irrigation. Although surgical bypass provides venous egress from the corpora cavernosa, secondary impotence commonly develops but may be effectively treated by a penile prosthesis.

Hearing and Visual Loss

Intradialytic hearing loss may be due to bleeding in the inner ear as a consequence of anticoagulation or cochlear hair cell injury from edema.

Intradialytic visual loss is rare, but can be caused by central retinal vein occlusion, precipitation of acute glaucoma, ischemic optic neuropathy secondary to hypotension, or Purtscher's-like retinopathy secondary to leukoembolization.

Finally, concomitant ocular and hearing impairment can occur following the use of outdated cellulose acetate dialyzer membranes.[49]

REFERENCES

1. Jaber BL, Pereira BJG: Dialysis reactions. Semin Dial 1997;10:158–165.
2. Coppo R, Amore A, Cirina P, et al: Bradykinin and nitric oxide generation by dialysis membranes can be blunted by alkaline rinsing solutions. Kidney Int 2000;58:881–888.
3. Chertow GM, Mason PD, Vaage-Nilsen O, Ahlmen J: On the relative safety of parenteral iron formulations. Nephrol Dial Transplant 2004;19:1571–1575.
4. National Kidney Foundation–Dialysis Outcome Quality Initiative: NKF-DOQI clinical practice guidelines for the treatment of anemia of chronic renal failure. Am J Kidney Dis 1997;30:192S–240S.
5. Grohskopf LA, Roth VR, Feikin DR, et al: Serratia liquefaciens bloodstream infections from contamination of epoetin alfa at a hemodialysis center. N Engl J Med 2001;344:1491–1497.
6. Shoji T, Tsubakihara Y, Fujii M, Imai E: Hemodialysis-associated hypotension as an independent risk factor for two-year mortality in hemodialysis patients. Kidney Int 2004;66:1212–1220.
7. Daugirdas JT: Dialysis hypotension: a hemodynamic analysis. Kidney Int 1991;39:233–246.
8. Cruz DN, Mahnensmith RL, Brickel HM, Perazella MA: Midodrine and cool dialysate are effective therapies for symptomatic intradialytic hypotension. Am J Kidney Dis 1999;33:920–926.
9. Locatelli F, Buoncristiani U, Canaud B, et al: Haemodialysis with on-line monitoring equipment: Tools or toys? Nephrol Dial Transplant 2005;20:22–33.
10. Okada K, Abe M, Hagi C, et al: Prolonged protective effect of short daily hemodialysis against dialysis-induced hypotension. Kidney Blood Press Res 2005;28:68–76.
11. Cogliati P: Thermal sensor and on-line hemodialfiltration. G Ital Nefrol 2005;22(Suppl 31):S111–S116.
12. Rahman M, Dixit A, Donley V, et al: Factors associated with inadequate blood pressure control in hypertensive hemodialysis patients. Am J Kidney Dis 1999;33:498–506.
13. Sang GL, Kovithavongs C, Ulan R, Kjellstrand CM: Sodium ramping in hemodialysis: A study of beneficial and adverse effects. Am J Kidney Dis 1997;29:669–677.
14. Bailey RA, Kaplan AA: Intradialytic cardiac arrhythmias: I. Semin Dial 1994;7:57–58.
15. Kant KS: Intradialytic cardiac arrhythmias: II. Semin Dial 1994;7:58–60.
16. Nakamura S, Ogata C, Aihara N, et al: QTc dispersion in haemodialysis patients with cardiac complications. Nephrology (Carlton) 2005;10:113–118.
17. Karnik JA, Young BS, Lew NL, et al: Cardiac arrest and sudden death in dialysis units. Kidney Int 2001;60:350–357.
18. Chazan J: Sudden deaths in patients with chronic renal failure on hemodialysis. Dial Transplant 1987;16:447–448.
19. Bleyer AJ, Russell GB, Satko SG: Sudden and cardiac death rates in hemodialysis patients. Kidney Int 1999;55:1553–1559.
20. Kwun KB, Schanzer H, Finkler BA, et al: Hemodynamic evaluation of angioaccess procedures for hemodialysis. Vasc Surg 1979;13:170–177.
21. Schanzer H, Skladany M, Haimov M: Treatment of angioaccess-induced ischemia by revascularization. J Vasc Surg 1992;16:861–866.
22. NKF-K/DOQI: Clinical practice guidelines for vascular access: Update 2000. Am J Kidney Dis 2001;37:137S–181S.

23. Mattson WJ: Recognition and treatment of vascular steal secondary to hemodialysis prostheses. Am J Surg 1987;154:198–201.

24. Ehsan O, Bhattacharya D, Darwish A, Al-khaffaf H: "Extension technique": A modified technique for brachio-cephalic fistula to prevent dialysis access-associated steal syndrome. Eur J Vasc Endovasc Surg 2005;29:324–327.

25. Canzanello VJ, Burkart JM: Hemodialysis-associated muscle cramps. Semin Dial 1992;5:299–304.

26. Sadowski RH, Allred EN, Jabs K: Sodium modeling ameliorates intradialytic and interdialytic symptoms in young hemodialysis patients. J Am Soc Nephrol 1993;4:1192–1198.

27. Chang CT, Wu CH, Yang CW, et al: Creatine monohydrate treatment alleviates muscle cramps associated with haemodialysis. Nephrol Dial Transplant 2002;17:1978–1981.

28. Eknoyan G, Latos DL, Lindberg J; National Kidney Foundation Carnitine Consensus Conference: Practice recommendations for the use of L-carnitine in dialysis-related carnitine disorder. National Kidney Foundation Carnitine Consensus Conference. Am J Kidney Dis 2003;41:868–876.

29. Basile C, Giordano R, Vernaglione L, et al: Efficacy and safety of haemodialysis treatment with the Hemocontrol biofeedback system: A prospective medium-term study. Nephrol Dial Transplant 2001;16:328–334.

30. Krueger BR: Restless legs syndrome and periodic movements of sleep. Mayo Clin Proc 1990;65:999–1006.

31. Micozkadioglu H, Ozdemir FN, Kut A, et al: Gabapentin versus levodopa for the treatment of restless legs syndrome in hemodialysis patients: An open-label study. Ren Fail 2004;26:393–397.

32. Ondo WG: Methadone for refractory restless legs syndrome. Mov Disord 2005;20:345–348.

33. Pellecchia MT, Vitale C, Sabatini M, et al: Ropinirole as a treatment of restless legs syndrome in patients on chronic hemodialysis: An open randomized crossover trial versus levodopa sustained release. Clin Neuropharmacol 2004;27:178–181.

34. Arieff AI: Dialysis disequilibrium syndrome: Current concepts on pathogenesis and prevention. Kidney Int 1994;45:629–635.

35. Cheung AK: Biocompatibility of hemodialysis membranes. J Am Soc Nephrol 1990;1:150–161.

36. Eaton JW, Leida MN: Hemolysis in chronic renal failure. Semin Nephrol 1985;5:133–139.

37. Remuzzi G: Bleeding in renal failure. Lancet 1988;1:1205–1208.

38. Lee KB, Kim B, Lee YH, et al: Hemodialysis using heparin-bound Hemophan in patients at risk of bleeding. Nephron Clin Pract 2004;97:c5–c10.

39. Sabovic M, Lavre J, Vujkovac B: Tranexamic acid is beneficial as adjunctive therapy in treating major upper gastrointestinal bleeding in dialysis patients. Nephrol Dial Transplant 2003;18:1388–1391.

40. Cardoso M, Vinay P, Vinet B, et al: Hypoxemia during hemodialysis: A critical review of the facts. Am J Kidney Dis 1988;11:281–297.

41. O'Quin RJ, Lakshminarayan S: Venous air embolism. Arch Intern Med 1982;142:2173–2176.

42. Oo TN, Smith CL, Swan SK: Does uremia protect against the demyelination associated with correction of hyponatremia during hemodialysis? A case report and literature review. Semin Dial 2003;16:68–71.

43. Gennari FJ: Acid-base balance in dialysis patients. Semin Dial 2000;13:235–240.

44. Gennari HJ, Rimmer JM: Acid-base disorders in end-stage renal disease: Part II. Semin Dial 1990;3:161–165.

45. Parfrey PS, Vavasour HM, Henry S, et al: Clinical features and severity of nonspecific symptoms in dialysis patients. Nephron 1988;50:121–128.

46. Savica V, Santoro D, Mazzaglia G, et al: L-carnitine infusions may suppress serum C-reactive protein and improve nutritional status in maintenance hemodialysis patients. J Ren Nutr 2005;15:225–230.

47. NKF-K/DOQI: Clinical practice guidelines for nutrition in chronic renal failure. Am J Kidney Dis 2000;35:S54–S55.

48. Weber M, Schmutz JL: Hemodialysis and the skin. Contr Nephrol 1988;62:75–85.

49. Hutter JC, Kuehnert MJ, Wallis RR, et al: Acute onset of decreased vision and hearing traced to hemodialysis treatment with aged dialyzers. JAMA 2000;283:2128–2134.

Peritoneal Dialysis: Principles, Techniques, and Adequacy

Bengt Rippe

INTRODUCTION

Peritoneal dialysis (PD) is a treatment for end-stage renal disease (ESRD), currently used by ~120,000 patients worldwide, representing approximately 8% to 9% of the total dialysis population. In PD, the peritoneal cavity, which is the largest serosal space in the body, is used as a container for 2.0 to 2.5 liters of sterile, usually glucose-containing, dialysis fluid, which is exchanged four to five times daily via a permanently indwelling catheter. The dialysis fluid is provided in plastic bags. The peritoneal membrane via the peritoneal capillaries acts as an endogenous dialyzing membrane. Across this membrane waste products diffuse to the dialysate, while excess body fluid is removed by osmosis induced by the glucose or another osmotic agent in the dialysis fluid, usually denoted ultrafiltration (UF). PD is usually provided 24 hours per day and 7 days per week in the form of continuous ambulatory peritoneal dialysis (CAPD). Approximately one third of the patients in most centers are on automated peritoneal dialysis (APD), in which nightly exchanges are delivered via an automatic PD cycler, by which rather large dialysate volumes (10 to 20 liters) can be exchanged during a limited period of time. Patients in APD usually have one or two manual exchanges when they are off the machine (a so-called wet day).

Advantages and Limitations of Peritoneal Dialysis

Assuming the patients or their caregiver are competent to undertake PD, the only absolute contraindications are large diaphragmatic defects, excessive peritoneal adhesions, surgically uncorrectable abdominal hernias, or acute ischemic or infectious bowel disease. These and other relative contraindications are discussed further in Chapter 80. PD is best used for patients with some residual renal function (RRF), although anuric patients may also do very well. Most patients who start PD will eventually, after several years, transfer to other modalities of renal replacement therapy, such as hemodialysis (HD), if adequacy cannot be maintained, or due to other complications, such as recurrent peritonitis or exit site or catheter problems. Only rarely do HD patients transfer to PD.

PD offers a number of advantages over HD, at least during the first 2 or 3 years of treatment. First, PD represents a slow, continuous, physiologic mode of removal of small solutes and of excess body water, associated with a seemingly stable blood chemistry and body hydration status. Second, there is no need for vascular access. The absence of vascular access and the absence of the blood-membrane contact of HD make catabolic stimuli less prominent in PD than in HD. This and the continuous nature of PD may be the

major reason why the small-solute clearance needed to yield an adequate dialysis is only ~50% of that in HD. Thus, for the same protein intake in PD, compared to HD, the need for clearance of uremic waste products is reduced. Furthermore, RRF is better preserved in PD patients compared to HD patients.

PD is a home-based therapy, and most patients are trained to do the bag exchanges themselves. Generally, home dialysis patients have a better quality of life than those on other types of dialysis. The number of hospital visits is reduced, while the ability to travel is increased. According to some studies, PD patients are more likely to be employed than those on HD.[1] There is also some evidence that PD patients may be better candidates for transplantation than HD patients; several studies have shown a lower incidence and severity of delayed graft function in PD patients after transplantation.[2] In children, PD (usually APD) is usually the preferred dialysis modality since it is noninvasive and socially acceptable, reducing hospital visits and allowing the child to attend school. Advocates of PD often recommend that renal replacement therapy should ideally begin with PD according to the patient's choice and then proceed, as required when RRF declines, to HD or transplantation. PD should thus be regarded as part of an integrated renal replacement therapy together with HD and transplantation.[3] Factors influencing the choice of dialysis modality between PD and hemodialysis as well as global variations in the use of PD are discussed further in Chapter 80.

PRINCIPLES OF PERITONEAL DIALYSIS

Three-Pore Model

The major principles governing solute and fluid transport across the peritoneal membrane are diffusion, driven by concentration gradients, and convection (filtration or ultrafiltration), driven by osmotic or hydrostatic pressure gradients. The barrier separating the plasma in the peritoneal capillaries from the fluid in the peritoneal cavity is represented by the capillary wall and the interstitium, which can be regarded as a barrier coupled in series with that of the capillary wall, while the mesothelium lining the peritoneal cavity is of much less significance as a transport hindrance. For the transport of fluid (UF) and of large solutes, the capillary wall is by far the dominating transport barrier. However, for small-solute diffusion the interstitium accounts for approximately one third of the transport (diffusion) resistance. The permeability of the capillary wall can be described by a three-pore model of membrane transport[4,5] (Fig 85.1). In the capillary wall, the major route for small-solute and fluid exchange between the plasma and the peritoneal cavity is the space between individual endothelial cells, the

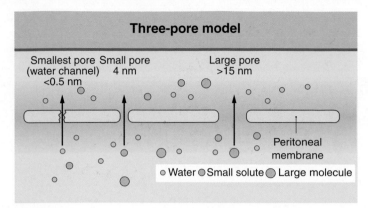

Figure 85.1 Three-pore model. The small pores represent the major pathway across the peritoneum through which small solutes move by diffusion and water by convection driven by hydrostatic, colloid osmotic, and crystalloid osmotic pressure differences. Across large pores (*to the right*) macromolecules move out slowly by convection from plasma to the peritoneal cavity. The smallest pores (*to the left*) are represented by aquaporins permeable to water, but impermeable to solutes. Water moves here exclusively by crystalloid osmotic pressure.

so-called interendothelial clefts. The functional radius of the permeable pathways in these clefts, denoted small pores, is 40 to 50 Å, which is slightly larger than the radius of albumin (36 Å). The size of these pores markedly impedes the transit of albumin and completely prevents the passage of larger molecules (e.g., immunoglobulins and α_2-macroglobulin). However, larger proteins can transit via very rare large pores (radius ~250 Å) in capillaries and in postcapillary venules. The large pores constitute only 0.01% of the total number of capillary pores, and the transport across them occurs by hydrostatic pressure-driven unidirectional filtration from the plasma to the peritoneal cavity. In addition, the capillary wall has a high permeability to osmotic water transport via the presence of water-only pores of radius ~2 Å, present in the endothelial cell membranes. These pores have been identified as aquaporin-1 (AQP-1) channels[6] (Fig. 85.2).

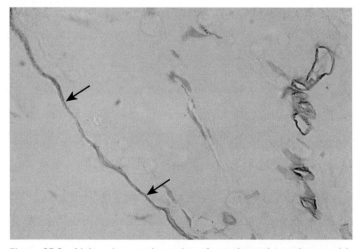

Figure 85.2 Light microscopic section of a peritoneal membrane with capillaries and venules (*to the right*) in an amorphous interstitium. The peritoneum is lined by a thin layer of mesothelium (*arrows*). Capillaries and venules, as well as the mesothelium, are immunocytochemically stained brown for aquaporin-1. (From Carlsson O, Nielsen S, Zakaria el R, Rippe B: In vivo inhibition of transcellular water channels [aquaporin-1] during acute peritoneal dialysis in rats. Am J Physiol 1996;271:H2254–H2262.)

Fluid Kinetics

Under normal conditions, most transport occurs via the small pores; only 2% of the peritoneal water transport occurs via AQP-1. In PD, fluid removal is markedly enhanced by infusing a hyperosmolar dialysate into the peritoneal cavity. The type of osmotic agent used affects the mechanism of osmosis. Very small osmotic agents (such as glycerol) will exert a rather low osmotic effect on the small pores and thereby work primarily on AQP-1 channels. By contrast, glucose will induce fluid flow through both AQP-1 (~40%) and small pores (~60%), while large molecules, such as polyglucose (icodextrin) will remove fluids mainly via small pores (~90%). Thus, glycerol will result in a more rapid dilution of the peritoneal dialysate than, for example, glucose, as reflected by a decrease in sodium concentration (sodium sieving) during the first 2 hours of the dialysate dwell due to relatively greater transport via the water-only AQP-1 channel; this tends to correct later as diffusion across the small pores eventually increases the sodium concentration to that present in the plasma.

Glucose, the commonly used osmotic agent, is usually available at three concentrations: 1.36%, 2.27%, or 3.86%. Figure 85.3a demonstrates the intraperitoneal fluid kinetics over 12 hours of dwell time for 1.36% and 3.86% glucose in the PD fluid together with that of isotonic saline. Glucose is an intermediate-sized osmolyte with a low osmotic efficiency (osmotic reflection coefficient [σ] = 0.03) across small pores, whereas glucose is 100% efficient as an osmotic agent across AQP-1 (σ = 1). For that reason, glucose will markedly (30-fold) boost the transport of fluid through AQPs and thus redistribute fluid transport away from the small pores toward AQP-1, resulting in significant sodium sieving. For example, for 3.86% glucose in the PD solution, the dialysate Na^+ concentration will decrease from 132 to 123 mmol/l in 60 to 100 minutes, and later increases toward plasma Na^+ concentration (see Fig. 85.3b). In addition to the size of the osmotic agent, the degree of sodium sieving is dependent on the presence and quantity of AQP-1 as well as on the total rate of net UF (the glucose concentration) and the diffusion capacity of Na^+.

A high rate of small-solute transport, and thereby of sodium diffusion, occurs in so-called high transporters, who have rapid equilibration of small solutes (creatinine and glucose) in the peritoneal equilibration test (PET; see later discussion). This will also reduce sodium sieving. If glucose is replaced by glycerol as an osmotic agent, the degree of sodium sieving will increase for equivalent rates of UF. This is because glycerol is a smaller solute than glucose, and glycerol is thus even less efficient than glucose as an osmolyte across small pores. It will therefore repartition the fluid flow away from the small pores toward AQP-1 in a more pronounced manner than does glucose. On the other hand, polyglucose (icodextrin) with an average molecular weight (MW) of 17 kd, has a high osmotic efficiency (σ ~0.5) *vis-à-vis* the small pores, and, in relative terms, is rather inefficient across aquaporins. Hence, during icodextrin-induced osmosis, only a very minor fraction of the UF will occur through AQP-1, producing insignificant sodium sieving.

In the absence of an osmotic agent in the PD fluid, the dialysate would be reabsorbed to the plasma within a few hours (see Fig. 85.3a), mainly driven by the difference in colloid osmotic pressure between plasma and the peritoneum. This absorption will to a major extent occur via small pores, whereas ~30% of the peritoneal fluid would be absorbed by lymphatic absorption. The partial fluid flows in the peritoneal membrane modeled across different fluid conductive pathways in the three-pore model (for 3.86% glucose) are shown in Figure 85.4. It is the presence of relatively high concentrations of glucose in the peritoneal fluid that

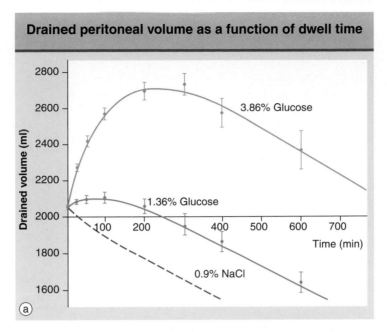

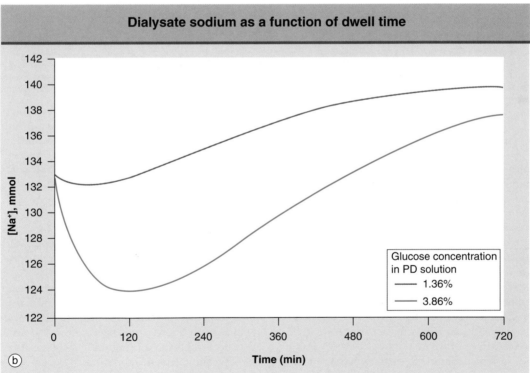

Figure 85.3 **Effects of dwell time on fluid volumes in PD.** *a*, Drained peritoneal volume as a function of dwell time for 3.86% and 1.36% glucose together with that for isotonic saline (NaCl), computer simulated using the three-pore model of peritoneal transport. *b*, Dialysate sodium as a function of dwell time for 3.86% and 1.36% glucose computer simulated according to the three-pore model. (*a*, From Rippe B, Stelin G, Haraldsson B: Fluid exchange across the peritoneal membrane during CAPD. Computer simulations using modified two-pore model. In Ota K, Maher JF, Winchester, JF, et al [eds]: Current Concepts in Peritoneal Dialysis. Amsterdam: Elsevier Science, 1992, pp 42–48.)

prevents the reabsorption of fluid to the plasma during the first few hours of the dwell.

Patients who have a high rate of sodium diffusion (high transporters) will have more difficulty in achieving effective fluid removal as opposed to low transporters. This is because in high transporters, the dissipation of the glucose osmotic gradient occurs rapidly (via the small pores), and therefore fluid reabsorption occurs earlier. The maximum UF volume is reduced, and the peak of the UF versus time curve occurs earlier than in normal patients. To the extent that water permeability (L_pS) of the peritoneum is

increased, there is also a more rapid reabsorption of fluid in the late phase of the dwell. The issue of fluid loss from the peritoneum is, however, very controversial since some authors claim that the peritoneal fluid loss occurring in the late phase of the PD dwell is dominated by lymphatic absorption.[7]

Effective Peritoneal (Vascular) Surface Area
The functional surface area of the peritoneum reflects the effective surface area of the peritoneal capillaries.[8] The transport of small solutes, such as urea, creatinine, and glucose, is partly limited

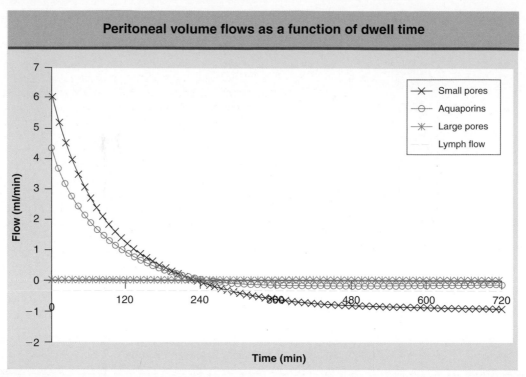

Figure 85.4 Peritoneal volume flows as a function of dwell time. Peritoneal volume flows as a function of dwell time for 3.86% glucose partitioned among aquaporins, small pores, large pores, and lymphatic absorption. The small pore volume flow is initially approximately 60% of total volume flow and becomes negative after peak time (220 minutes). The aquaporin-mediated water flow becomes slightly negative after approximately 250 minutes. The large-pore volume flow is negligible and remains constant throughout the dwell, as does lymphatic absorption (0.3 ml/min). (From Venturoli D, Rippe B: Validation by computer simulation of two indirect methods for quantification of free water transport in peritoneal dialysis. Perit Dial Int 2005;25:77–84.)

by the degree of perfusion of these capillaries, the effective peritoneal membrane blood flow. Furthermore, as mentioned previously, some of the diffusion resistance for the smallest solutes (urea and creatinine) is located in the interstitium. Vasodilatation of arterioles results in an increase in the number of effectively perfused capillaries, whereas vasoconstriction results in a reduction. These alterations often occur without large changes in the fluid permeability (hydraulic conductance, L_pS) of the peritoneum. Thus, during vasodilatation or vasoconstriction, there is usually a dissociation between changes in the permeability–surface area product (PS) for small solutes and in the hydraulic conductance (L_pS) of the membrane. Vasodilatation, with recruitment of capillary surface area, occurs early in the dwell when glucose is used as the osmotic agent, causing early, transient increases in PS.[9]

Peritonitis is also associated with marked vasodilatation, again leading to increases in small solute PS, in the absence of large changes in L_pS, during the first 60 to 100 minutes of the dwell. However, in some subjects with peritonitis, an increase in L_pS will result in relative increased fluid transport across the small pores. Furthermore, there is usually an opening of large pores in the capillaries (and postcapillary venules) resulting in enhanced leakage of macromolecules (e.g., albumin and immunoglobulins) from plasma to peritoneum. Peritonitis may thus result in relative difficulty with removing fluid (due to rapid dissipation of intraperitoneal glucose), reduced sodium sieving (due to the reduced UF and increased Na^+ diffusion), and increased protein losses (via enhanced transport across the large pores).

The contact area between the dialysate and the peritoneal tissue varies due to posture and fill volume. Adult subjects usually tolerate 2.0 to 2.5 liters of instilled volume. An intraperitoneal hydrostatic pressure (IPP) <18 cm H_2O (supine position) is usually tolerated.[10] At higher pressures (>18 cm H_2O), the patient usually feels some discomfort. At intraperitoneal volumes <2 liters, there is a reduction in small-solute PS, whereas PS is only moderately increased at high fill volumes. Overall, an increased fill volume implies a more efficient exchange both with regard to small-solute exchange and UF, with the latter being much more pronounced for hypertonic solutions.[11] For a long time, it was thought that increased fill volumes would directly affect peritoneal fluid reabsorption by the hydrostatic pressure effect (increases in IPP). However, since ~80% of the increase in IPP is transmitted via venous compression back to the capillaries, the actual changes in the transcapillary hydrostatic pressure gradient, which governs UF, will be rather small.[12] On the other hand, to the extent that an elevated IPP will cause peritoneal tissue edema and subsequently a lower tissue oncotic pressure, an elevated IPP may actually (moderately) increase fluid reabsorption across the peritoneal capillaries.

PERITONEAL ACCESS

The key to successful chronic PD is a safe and permanent access to the peritoneal cavity (Fig. 85.5). Despite improvements in catheter survival over the past few years, catheter-related complications still occur, causing significant morbidity, sometimes forcing the removal of the catheter. Catheter-related problems are a cause of permanent transfer to HD in up to 20% of patients. Most catheters nowadays are derived from the one originally devised by Tenckhoff and Schechter.[13] The Tenckhoff catheter is a silastic tube with side holes along its intraperitoneal portion. There are usually one or two Dacron cuffs, allowing tissue ingrowth, which secure the catheter in place and prevent pericatheter leakage and infection. The Tenckhoff catheter is straight, having one cuff lying

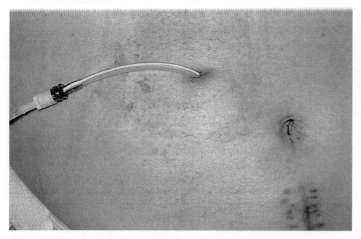

Figure 85.5   A recently implanted peritoneal dialysis catheter *in situ*.

on the peritoneum, with the catheter tip pointing in the caudal direction, and the outer cuff is close to the skin exit. Several centimeters of the catheter is thus located transcutaneously. There have been a variety of catheter designs based on the original Tenckhoff catheter. Intraperitoneal and transcutaneous catheter modifications continue to appear, indicating that no single design is perfect (Fig. 85.6). A number of studies comparing the arcuate swan-neck catheter to straight catheters report less frequent catheter drainage failures using the swan-neck design. The latter design appears superior to a straight catheter when the latter is *not* tunneled through an arcuate pathway with a downwardly directed exit site. A cranially directed exit site may result in an increased risk of exit site infection. It should be kept in mind, however, that previous catheter studies have not taken into account confounding factors such as nasal carriage of *Staphylococcus aureus* and comorbid conditions such as diabetes mellitus, both known as risk factors for exit site infection, which may put these results into doubt. Thus, there is no hard evidence that any of the modified

catheters on the market are actually superior to the original (one- or two-cuff) Tenckhoff catheter.[14]

Ideally, catheter insertion should be undertaken by an experienced operator under operating room sterile conditions. In different centers, that operator may be a surgeon or a nephrologist trained in interventional nephrology techniques. Presurgical assessment of the patient is essential, especially concerning the presence of herniation or any weakness of the abdominal wall. If present, it may be possible to correct these at the time of catheter insertion. Eradication of nasal carriage *S. aureus* with locally applied antibacterials (such as mupirocin) prior to the operation has shown significant reduction in exit site infection rates. It is also recommended that a single dose of first- or second-generation cephalosporin be given intravenously prior to the operation. To avoid development of vancomycin-resistant *Enterococcus* infection, vancomycin should not be used as a prophylactic agent. Several placement techniques have been described and practiced: surgical minilaparotomy and dissection, blind placement using the Tenckhoff trocar, blind placement using a guidewire (Seldinger technique), minitrocar peritoneoscopy placement, and laparoscopy. These techniques are discussed further in Chapter 82.

TECHNIQUES OF PERITONEAL DIALYSIS

In CAPD, 2.0 to 2.5 liters of dialysis fluid is exchanged with the peritoneal cavity four or five times daily. In 4 to 5 hours, there is nearly full (95%) equilibration of urea and approximately 65% equilibration of creatinine, while the glucose gradient has dissipated to approximately 40% of the initial value. For glucose as an osmotic agent, 4 to 5 hours is a suitable dwell time, although for night dwell exchanges, longer dwell times can be accepted (8 to 10 hours). Furthermore, there is room for individual exchange schedules that can be adjusted to suit individual patient convenience. Dwell times shorter than 4 to 5 hours can be performed using a machine (cycler) and can be used when the patient needs to reduce intraperitoneal volume, for example, to minimize leakage. This is often the case in conjunction with catheter insertion, hernia repair, or abdominal operations. Rapid exchanges may also be required during treatment for peritonitis or in patients with fluid overload when the patient's hydration status needs to be rapidly corrected.

Nowadays, double-bag systems (so-called Y systems) are in general use according to the "flush before fill" principle. The double-bag system contains the unused dialysis fluid connected to an empty sterile drain bag via a Y-set tubing system. After the patient has connected the system and flushed the connection (for 2 to 3 seconds) a frangible (breakable) pin to the drain bag is opened, and the peritoneal cavity drained during 10 to 15 minutes to fill the drain bag. Then, this bag is clamped, and the fresh bag opened to fill the peritoneal cavity during another 10 to 15 minutes. The time for exchange (instillation and drainage), if the catheter is in good order, should not exceed a total of 30 minutes. Usually the first 1.6 to 1.8 liters will drain rapidly (at ≥200 ml/min), whereas the last 200 to 300 ml will drain much more slowly. The breakpoint between the rapid and the slow phase may vary markedly from individual to individual.

APD refers to PD that is assisted by a cycler. APD is often performed overnight (8 to 10 hours), during which large volumes (10 to 20 liters) can be exchanged. During daytime, the APD patient has usually a so-called wet day, that is, a long dwell, usually with polyglucose as the osmotic agent in the dialysis fluid. Some patients with nightly APD perform one daily exchange so that there are two long (6 to 8 hours) daily dwells. Most cyclers can be

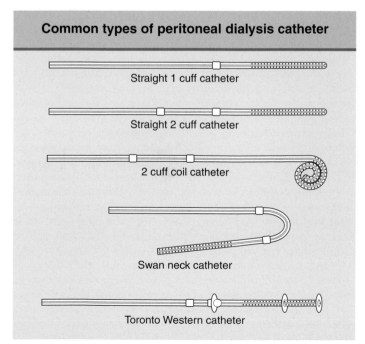

Common types of peritoneal dialysis catheter

Straight 1 cuff catheter

Straight 2 cuff catheter

2 cuff coil catheter

Swan neck catheter

Toronto Western catheter

Figure 85.6   Common types of peritoneal dialysis catheter.

programmed to vary inflow volume, inflow time, dwell time, and drain time. Cyclers usually warm the fluid prior to inflow and also monitor outflow volume and the excess drainage (= UF volume). Current APD machines have alarms for inflow failure, overheating, and poor drainage. Some cyclers interrupt drainage at the breakpoint between the fast and slow phases to make the exchange more efficient. Another way to accelerate exchanges is to allow a considerable sump volume in the peritoneal cavity by not letting all the fluid drain. Subsequent inflow volumes are proportionally reduced, and after a number of cycles, complete drainage occurs. This technique is called tidal peritoneal dialysis.

The exchange volume should be adjusted according to the patient's size. Adult patients weighing <60 kg should start with 1.5-liter bags. The average patient (60 to 80 kg) should receive 2-liter exchanges, and if >80 kg, then 2.5 liters should be used. If pressure monitoring systems are available, the intraperitoneal hydrostatic pressure (IPP) may yield a clue as to which volumes should be used. In the supine position, most patients have an IPP of 12 cm H_2O. If the IPP is >18 cm H_2O, the patient usually feels some discomfort.

PERITONEAL DIALYSIS FLUIDS

The majority of PD fluids used today have the composition of a lactate-buffered, balanced salt solution devoid of potassium, with glucose (1.36%, 2.27%, and 3.86%) as the osmotic agent. Lactate is used as a buffer instead of bicarbonate because bicarbonate and Ca^{2+} may precipitate (to form calcium carbonate) during storage. However, with the advent of newer multichambered PD delivery systems, it is nowadays possible to replace lactate with bicarbonate and to make a number of other solution modifications, which previously were not feasible. However, the high cost of a number of the newer, more physiologic fluid formulations should be borne in mind.

Electrolyte Concentration

In current PD fluids, the concentrations of Na^+, Cl^-, Ca^{2+}, and Mg^{2+} are selected to be close to the plasma (equilibrium) concentration. The removal of these ions across the peritoneum is therefore due to the low diffusion gradient, more or less completely dependent on convection. For every deciliter of fluid removed in a 4-hour dwell, there is approximately 10 mmol/l of Na^+ and 0.1 mmol/l of Ca^{2+} removed, provided that plasma Na^+ and Ca^{2+} are within the normal concentration ranges.[12,15]

The frequent use of calcium-containing phosphate binders emphasizes the necessity to understand Ca^{2+} kinetics for various types of dialysis fluids to avoid hypercalcemia. The calcium concentration of current PD solutions is usually 1.25 to 1.75 mmol/l. However, since Ca^{2+}, like Na^+ and Mg^{2+}, has a UF-dominated transport, 1.25 mmol/l may be considered appropriate only for 1.36% glucose to achieve a zero (neutral) peritoneal calcium removal. To reach the same objective for 3.86% glucose, then the dialysis fluid Ca^{2+} should be increased to 2.3 mmol/l in order to prevent (UF-driven) Ca^{2+} loss during a 4-hour dwell. Using a three-compartment system for the PD bags, it is actually possible to adapt the dialysis fluid Ca^{2+} concentration to either obtain net zero peritoneal Ca^{2+} transport across the peritoneum or to reach a preset calcium removal target for each PD fluid glucose concentration (1.36%, 2.27%, and 3.86%) used.[16] Since in currently available PD solutions, Ca^{2+} concentration is not variable as a function of glucose concentration, using 1.25 mmol/l Ca^{2+} is recommended when patients use calcium-containing phosphate binders. However, net peritoneal calcium removal with this dialysis fluid Ca^{2+}

level can only be achieved by PD fluids containing 2.27% or 3.86% glucose.

The Mg^{2+} concentration commonly used in current PD solutions is 0.25 to 0.75 mmol/l. For 1.36% glucose, 0.25 mmol/l would be appropriate for zero Mg^{2+} transport during the dwell, whereas for higher dialysis fluid glucose concentrations, there will be net Mg^{2+} loss with this concentration. The K^+ concentration in current PD fluids is zero to aid control of potassium balance.

Osmotic Agents

Glucose is the principal osmotic agent used for fluid removal (UF) in PD. Alternative osmotic agents are glycerol, amino acids, and icodextrin, of which only amino acids and icodextrin are commercially available. Icodextrin is a polydisperse glucose polymer with a (weight average) MW of 17 kd.[17] However, due to the polydispersity of icodextrin, ~70% of the molecules have a MW ≤3 kd.[11] Icodextrin is available as a 7.5% solution with essentially the same electrolyte composition as glucose-based dialysates. The osmolality of the glucose polymer solution, unlike that of 1.36% glucose (osmolality = 350 mOsmol/kg) dialysis fluid, is within the same range, or actually slightly lower, than that of normal plasma. The presence of larger molecules in the icodextrin solution compared to those in glucose-based solutions improves the osmotic efficiency markedly across the small pores ($\sigma = 0.5$) and also reduces the dissipation of the osmotic gradient over time. This yields a sustained UF over 8 to 12 hours (Fig. 85.7). Therefore, polyglucose is preferred for long-dwell exchanges, for example, overnight, and particularly for patients who tend to absorb glucose rapidly (high transporters, see later discussion).

A second alternative osmotic agent, which is commercially available, is a 1.1% amino acid mixture having the same osmolality as 1.36% glucose.[18] According to some studies, regular use of this dialysate may increase certain nutritional indices, although there is some evidence that amino acid solutions have a tendency to increase acidosis and increase plasma urea. Both icodextrin-based and amino acid–based solutions may be used to reduce the glucose exposure of the peritoneal membrane and the total glucose load to the patient. However, there are no data yet demonstrating a clear-cut clinical benefit of replacing two of the daily glucose exchanges with icodextrin or amino acids.

Until recently, conventional PD solutions have had a low pH and a high concentration of glucose degradation products (GDPs). GDPs are reactive carbonyl compounds that form during heat sterilization and/or storage of glucose-based solutions. GDPs are toxic to a variety of cells *in vitro* and also potentially toxic *in vivo*.[19] By the use of multicompartment systems, it has been possible to compose new solutions with much lower concentrations of GDPs and a neutral pH and also to use bicarbonate or bicarbonate/lactate mixtures as buffer.[20-22] Solutions using bicarbonate or bicarbonate/lactate mixtures result in significantly less infusion pain and are as effective as lactate in correcting acidosis when used at the same total buffer ion concentration.[23] Prospective, randomized studies of such fluids have been associated with the improvement in dialysate effluent markers of peritoneal membrane integrity, particularly elevation of cancer antigen 125 (CA-125), a measure of peritoneal mesothelial cell mass.[20-22] There are also some indications of an improved RRF in patients with PD solutions low in GDP.[22] The long-term effect on peritoneal membrane function, however, remains to be determined.

Glycerol, an even smaller osmolyte than glucose with a lower reflection coefficient across small pores ($\sigma \sim 0.02$), has not entered clinical practice because of the risk of accumulation of glycerol in plasma. Pyruvate is an alternative buffer to lactate (or

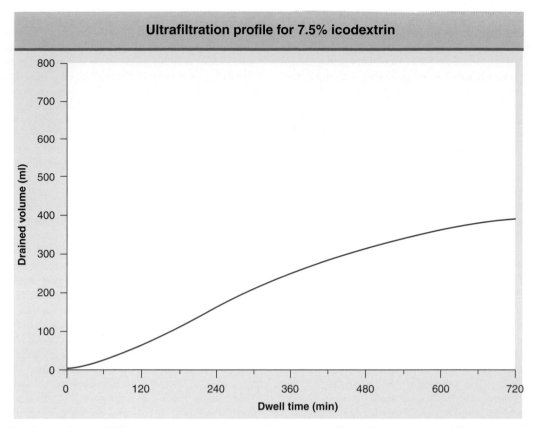

Figure 85.7   Ultrafiltration profile for 7.5% icodextrin. Profile is computer simulated according to the three-pore model in an average patient who is *not* naïve to icodextrin.[11]

bicarbonate) but is not yet clinically available. Finally, certain additives may help to preserve the peritoneal membrane, such as N-acetylglucosamine (NAG), hyaluronic acid (HA), and low MW heparin (LMWH). LMWH, 4500 IU in every morning bag daily for 3 months, increased UF due to reduced glucose reabsorption during the dwell. This perhaps occurred by reducing the initial vasodilatation that regularly occurs on intraperitoneal instillation of glucose-based PD solutions.[24] HA seems to reduce the reabsorption of fluid that occurs in the late phase of the dwell, possibly by producing a filter cake at the peritoneal surface.[25] While LMWH has been shown clinically to increase UF,[24] the advantage of using HA to improve UF has only been shown in animal models. None of these additives (NAG, HA, or LMWH) or buffers (pyruvate) can yet be recommended in clinical practice, and further evidence is awaited.

ASSESSMENTS OF PERITONEAL SOLUTE TRANSPORT AND ULTRAFILTRATION

Small Solute Removal

The net removal of solutes and fluid during PD, in excess of urinary excretion, can be measured in a relatively straightforward way by evaluating the dialysate drained. For this purpose, the concentrations of urea and creatinine are measured in dialysate and plasma. The dialysate-to-plasma concentration (D/P) ratios of either of these solutes multiplied by the daily drain volume gives the 24-hour clearance. Weekly creatinine and urea clearance is obtained by multiplying these figures by 7. For comparison between patients, creatinine clearance is conventionally related to body standard surface area (1.73 m^2), while urea clearance (mostly for comparison with HD) is expressed as Kt/V (in which

Kt is the weekly clearance and V the volume of distribution of urea). The latter parameter cannot be routinely assessed unambiguously in PD, in contrast to the situation in HD, in which V can be mathematically derived directly from urea kinetics. Preferably, V should be determined by direct techniques, such as from the dilution of isotopic water (total body water). In practice, however, V is usually approximated from standard tables using body weight and height together with gender.[26] The Kt/V concept in conjunction with PD is open to criticism, mostly due to the uncertainty of determining a correct value for V.

Large Solute Removal

To gain more insight into peritoneal transport, the clearance of larger solutes such as β$_2$-microglobulin, as well as markers for transport across the large pores, such as albumin, immunoglobulins, and α$_2$-macroglobulin, can be measured. While many centers assess the daily peritoneal removal of total protein and/or albumin, measurements of most other solutes are not made in routine clinical practice.

Ultrafiltration

UF can be assessed with a 24-hour collection. Even if done accurately, there is a considerable dwell-to-dwell and day-to-day variability in UF depending on drainage conditions, varying levels of residual (sump) intraperitoneal volume, posture, and so forth. Reasonably accurate estimations of daily UF volume can be obtained by averaging collections of all fluid during a period of several days. In clinical practice, the patient's own daily dialysis records should also be examined with respect to dwell-to-dwell UF volumes and the number of hypertonic bags used per day.

UF volume can also be determined by the peritoneal equilibration test (PET), as described later. For a 3.86% glucose dwell, a UF volume <400 ml will indicate insufficient UF, that is, UF failure. For the ordinary 2.27% glucose, PET (see later discussion), <200 ml of UF in 4 hours signals UF failure. More accurate determination of intraperitoneal volume can be achieved as a function of time using an intraperitoneal volume marker, such as ^{125}I-human serum albumin (radioactive iodinated serum albumin [RISA]) or dextran 70 (while correcting for marker clearance from the peritoneal fluid). With such marker techniques, rather precise UF volume estimations can be done, which is a prerequisite for accurate estimations of true membrane parameters in terms of PS for small solutes or clearance (Cl) for macromolecules. Detailed UF volume estimations with RISA and dextran 70 are not yet recommended in routine clinical practice.

Peritoneal Membrane Function
Peritoneal Equilibration Test
The PET yields approximate estimations of the rate of peritoneal transport of small solutes and of UF capacity.[27] The rate of small-solute transport is dependent on the effective peritoneal surface area, which is essentially dependent on the number of effectively perfused capillaries available for exchange (and the blood flow). The volume ultrafiltrated in 4 hours is a function of the osmotic conductance to glucose (the peritoneal UF coefficient × the reflection coefficient for glucose) as well as the rate of dissipation of the glucose osmotic gradient (= rate of small-solute transport). Generally, when the rate of glucose disappearance is high (for high transporters, see later discussion), UF volume is low. The PET procedure is summarized in Figure 85.8. After an overnight dwell (8 to 12 hours), the dialysate fluid is drained, and a 2-liter 2.27% glucose bag is infused for 10 minutes with the patient in supine position (rolling from side to side every 2 minutes). At 10 minutes (after start), at the completion of the infusion, 200 ml is drained into the drainage bag, mixed, and a zero-time dialysate sample taken. At the end of the 4-hour dwell period, dialysate is drained and measured. The net volume is noted. Concentrations of glucose and creatinine in the outflow and plasma are measured, as well as the concentration of glucose in the zero-time sample. The results

are expressed at the ratio of dialysate to plasma (D/P) solute concentration ratio and as the glucose at 4 hours–to–dialysate glucose at time zero (D/D_0) concentration ratio. The higher D/P ratio is for creatinine, the faster the rate of transport is for small solutes. According to D/P ratios for creatinine or D/D_0 for glucose, patients can be divided into low, low average, high average, or high transporters (Fig. 85.9). It should, however, be emphasized that D/P measurements only give an approximate estimation of small-solute transport rate. An increased D/P-creatinine is usually accompanied by a lower UF volume, but it should be noted that a lower UF volume will *per se* (due to less dilution) tend to increase the D/P.

Standard Permeability Analysis and the Fast-Fast Peritoneal Equilibration Test
In the standard permeability analysis (SPA), a 3.86% glucose bag is instilled, but the test is otherwise performed as the PET.[28] After a dwell time of 1 hour, a dialysate sample is taken and the sodium concentration is compared to that of the time-zero value. This is done to assess the degree of sodium sieving and hence to get a measure of AQP-mediated water flow.[29] In SPA, a UF volume <400 ml (4 hours) suggests the presence of UF failure. A variant of SPA advocates complete drainage of a 3.86% glucose bag at 1 hour and assessment of the total drained volume.[30] By such a technique, it is theoretically possible to assess the fraction of "free" water transport (across AQP-1) in the early phase of the dwell when Na^+ diffusion is negligible from the (1 hour) drained volume. First, the peritoneal clearance of sodium in 1 hour, that is, the mass of sodium drained minus that instilled divided by the average Na^+ concentration in plasma, is calculated. The peritoneal clearance of sodium approximately equals the peritoneal small-solute clearance of fluid (water) during the first hour of the dwell. This value is then subtracted from total UF volume. Thereby, a surprisingly accurate estimate of the free (AQP-mediated) water transport during the first 60 minutes is obtained. This estimation becomes even more accurate after the application of a correction algorithm.[31]

If a fast-fast (1 hour) 3.86% PET is combined with a fast-fast (1 hour) 1.36% PET it is possible to calculate UF volumes after 1 hour for the two glucose strengths. From the measured difference in UF volume at 1 hour (between 3.86% and 1.36% glucose), it is possible to calculate a value of the osmotic conductance to glucose ($L_pS \cdot \sigma_g$), independently of the transport rate (D/D_0) of glucose.[12] This parameter may decline in long-term patients with UF failure, often combined with increases in D/P creatinine and a decline in D/D_0 glucose. During the first 1 to 2 years of PD treatment, there is usually an increase in D/P creatinine without any changes in 4-hour UF in a standard PET.[32] When UF failure occurs, often after several years of PD, the osmotic conductance to glucose is usually affected (reduced). Then, the UF volume is usually ≤400 ml (in 4 hours) for 3.86% glucose. In patients with UF failure, an SPA can thus give additional information compared to the conventional PET. Furthermore, the combination of 3.86% and 1.36% glucose fast-fast PET is recommended in UF failure to assess the presence of a reduced peritoneal osmotic conductance.

Residual Renal Function
In PD, the presence of RRF is of considerable importance for patient and technique survival. RRF is better preserved over treatment time in PD than in HD.[33] Residual renal function can be assessed by collecting all urine during a day and by assessing

Peritoneal equilibration test
1. The night bag (8–12 hours) must be 1.36% or 2.27% glucose, drained for 20 minutes with patient sitting.
2. 2 liters (warm) 2.27% fluid instilled for 10 minutes with the patient supine and rolling from side to side every 2 minutes.
3. Exactly at 10 minutes after start of the infusion, 20 ml is drained into the bag. Draw 5 ml (discard); 5 ml taken for creatinine and glucose determination.
4. After 2 hours, new samples collected as under 3.
5. After 4 hours (exactly) drainage during 20 minutes. Note total bag weight. Subtract empty bag weight. Take samples (after mixing) for creatinine and glucose.
6. The glucose at 4 hours to dialysate glucose at time zero for glucose and dialysate to plasma ratio for creatinine are D/D_0 plotted versus time in a graph demonstrated in Figure 85–9a. The drained volume is noted (D/P-creatine)

Figure 85.8 Peritoneal equilibration test.

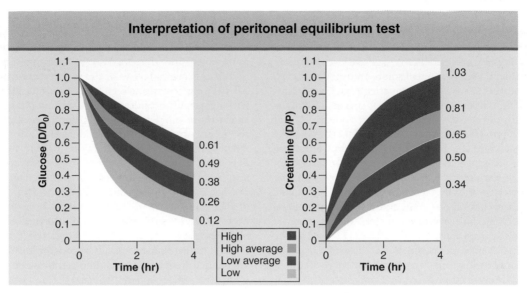

Figure 85.9 **Interpretation of the peritoneal equilibration test.** Changes in solute concentration during a peritoneal equilibration test (PET) allow classification into different transport types. (From Twardowski ZJ, Nolph DK, Khanna R, et al: Peritoneal equilibration test. Perit Dial Bull 1987;7:138–147.)

the urine concentrations of urea and creatinine and total urine volume. Since renal creatinine clearance, due to tubular secretion, yields an overestimate of the glomerular filtration rate (GFR; by 1 to 2 ml/min), when GFR is ≤10 ml/min, and renal urea clearance yields an underestimate of GFR (by 1 to 2 ml/min) in the same interval of (reduced) GFR, a good estimate of actual GFR can be calculated as the average of renal creatinine clearance *and* urea clearance. However, if the daily urine volume is <200 ml, then the RRF will be too small to be measured accurately.

ADEQUACY

An important measure of dialysis adequacy is the general clinical state of the patient, as manifested by a good nutritional status (maintained muscle mass), the absence of anemia, edema, hypertension, electrolyte and acid-based disturbances, neurologic symptoms, pruritus, and insomnia. Management of uremic anemia and renal osteodystrophy are discussed in Chapters 72 and 74, respectively. Some criteria for PD adequacy are given in Figure 85.10.

Small Solute Clearance

There are few prospective, randomized studies to set the target for adequate PD. From a clinical point of view, it was previously suggested that a weekly Kt/V >1.7 and a weekly creatinine clearance >50 l/1.73 m^2 would be (minimally) adequate for patients on CAPD. This represents only approximately 50% to 60% of the urea and creatinine clearance considered adequate in HD patients. In a large prospective study in the United States and Canada, the CANUSA study, the outcome for a cohort of 680 patients starting CAPD was studied with an average follow-up of 2 years.[34] In the CANUSA study, patients who maintained a high Kt/V or creatinine clearance over time did better than those who

did not. An increase of 0.1 unit of Kt/V (peritoneal + renal) per week was associated with a 5% decrease in relative risk of death, and an increase of 5 l/1.73 m^2 of creatinine clearance per week (peritoneal + renal) was associated with a 7% decrease in the relative risk of death. Further analysis of the CANUSA study indicated that the survival advantage of patients with higher total small-solute clearance was entirely attributed to the RRF. For each increase of 250 ml of urine output per day, there was a 36% decrease in the relative risk of death. In the ADEMEX study,[35] a large, randomized, controlled clinical trial designed to test the value of increasing peritoneal small-solute clearance in a Mexican PD cohort, there was no obvious survival advantage of increasing

Criteria for peritoneal dialysis adequacy	
Clinical	The patient feels well and has a stable lean body mass. No symptoms of anorexia, asthenia, nausea, emesis, insomnia Stable nerve conductance velocity
Small solute clearance	Weekly Kt/V urea >1.7 (renal + peritoneal) Weekly creatinine clearance >50 l/1.73 m^2
Large solute clearance	Albumin clearance <0.15 ml/min
Fluid balance	No edema No hypertension No postural hypotension
Electrolyte balance	Serum potassium <5 mmol/l
Acid-base balance	Serum bicarbonate >24 mmol/l
Nutrition	Daily protein intake ≥1.2 g/kg Caloric intake >35 kcal/kg/day Serum albumin >3.5 g/l Body mass index 20–30 Stable midarm muscle circumference

Figure 85.10 **Criteria for peritoneal dialysis adequacy.**

the peritoneal clearance to obtain a total creatinine clearance >60 l/1.73 m² compared to <50 l/1.73 m².

From these studies, it seems that renal clearance and peritoneal clearance are not mutually comparable. A high RRF is of greater survival advantage than a high peritoneal solute transport capacity. The mere fact that the survival of PD patients is equal to or supersedes that of HD patients during the first 2 years of dialysis (see later discussion), despite the fact that PD provides ~50% of the total Kt/V of HD, indicates that the benefit of PD goes beyond the clearance of small solutes. In the European APD Outcome Study, small solute clearance did not correlate with survival in anuric patients.[36] On the contrary, total volume removal and the patients' hydration were important factors. Still, there is reasonably good evidence that a weekly Kt/V >1.7 and a weekly creatinine clearance >50 l/1.73 m² are adequacy targets that should be reached and maintained in a majority of patients. Hence, as the RRF declines one should attempt to increase the dose of dialysis by increasing the exchange volumes or by prescribing more frequent exchanges. It should be again emphasized that the concept of Kt/V, a kinetic parameter obtained from the HD practice, is somewhat questionable in PD. Theoretically, body surface area would be superior to urea distribution volume to normalize urea clearance. Furthermore, the long-term PD patient is often overhydrated and/or has an increased fat mass, which makes the estimation of V very cumbersome.[37] A patient with a high solute transport will achieve peritoneal creatinine clearance targets rather easily, while obese individuals may have difficulties in reaching an adequate Kt/V urea.

There are at least three computer programs commercially available that can predict urea and creatinine clearance and peritoneal UF performance together with suggestions of treatment options, based on drained volumes and plasma and dialysate creatinine and urea values. These parameters are often obtained by a PET or standardized schedules for specified dwell exchanges. Some of the programs yield an estimate of peritoneal albumin clearance, which to a great extent is dependent on the filtration occurring across large pores, being increased in inflammation. Recommended dialysis schedules based on the categorization of the PET are given in Figure 85.11.

Fluid Balance

As in all types of renal replacement therapy, long-term maintenance of an adequate fluid and electrolyte balance is of crucial importance for the survival of patients on PD. As already mentioned, the outcome of PD is directly related to the presence of RRF, particularly a high urine output. Furthermore, patients with high transport in the PET (a more rapid absorption of glucose and a more rapid loss of the osmotic gradient) have a reduced technique survival. It seems evident that after 2 or 3 years of PD, when RRF is low, most patients on PD are fluid overloaded. It is likely that volume overload not only aggravates hypertension but also leads to progression of left ventricular hypertrophy, often present already at the start of PD. However, during the first year of PD, there is often a decrease in blood pressure and a reduced need for antihypertensive agents. Unfortunately, with time on PD, blood pressure usually increases and the number of antihypertensive drugs needed usually again increases.[38] Therefore, it is advisable to regularly assess fluid removal over time, at least every 6 months, either separately (using, e.g., SPA) or in conjunction with PET measurements.

Management of Fluid Overload

As total urinary water (and sodium) excretion and peritoneal UF volume decline, it is advisable to instruct the patients to restrict salt and water intake. There is one study reporting increased thirst in PD patients compared either to normal subjects or HD patients, further emphasizing the need for dietary salt restriction.[39] In view of the difficulty in compliance with respect to restricted salt intake, however, the use of PD solutions with lowered sodium concentration has been advocated. Preliminary studies of low sodium PD solutions have been very promising, reducing the need for blood pressure–lowering drugs to control hypertension.[40] At present, however, low sodium solutions are not commercially available. Loop diuretics (furosemide), 250 to 500 mg/day, can be used to maintain urine volumes but do not maintain renal clearance. In the next step, UF can be enhanced by increasing the dialysis glucose concentration to 2.27% or 3.36%. Patients with alterations in peritoneal membrane function, appearing over the first few years of PD, usually have an

Typical PD regimens required to achieve adequate solute clearances				
Patient Body Surface Area (m²)	Peritoneal Solute Transport Characteristics—D/P Creatinine at 4 Hours			
	Low (<0.5)	Low Average (0.5 to <0.65)	High Average (0.65–0.82)	High (>0.83)
<1.7	CAPD/APD	CAPD/APD+	APD+*	APD*
	10–12.5 liters	10–12.5 liters	10–12.5 liters	10–12.5 liters
1.7–2.0	CAPD+/APD	APD+	APD+*	APD+*
	12.5–15 liters	12.5–15 liters	12.5–15 liters	12.5–15 liters
>2.0	CAPD+, HD	APD+	APD+*	APD+*
		15–20 liters	15–20 liters	15–20 liters

Figure 85.11 Peritoneal dialysis (PD) regimens. Typical peritoneal dialysis regimens required to achieve adequate solute clearance according to patient size and membrane characteristics in anuric patients. The total volume of dialysate fluid required increases with body size, using 2.5- or even 3.0-liter exchanges. As solute transport increases, the use of automated peritoneal dialysis (APD) using shorter overnight exchanges is favored over continuous ambulatory peritoneal dialysis (CAPD). Both CAPD and APD may have to be augmented by the use of an additional exchange (denoted by +); this is given by way of an additional afternoon exchange in CAPD patients or by employing an exchange device that delivers a single additional exchange at night. HD, hemodialysis. *The use of glucose polymer (icodextrin) solution for the long exchange will enhance both solute clearance and ultrafiltration.

increased small solute transport combined with a moderately increased UF capacity of the peritoneum.[32] In these patients, there is an increased reabsorption of fluid in the late phase of the dwell. These patients can benefit from switching to APD and to the use of polyglucose dialysis fluid (icodextrin) for one of the day time exchanges. Randomized, controlled trials using icodextrin for the long daytime dwell in APD have demonstrated an improved UF and a reduced extracellular fluid volume with this regimen.[41] Patients who have been on PD for several years may have a reduced UF capacity (reduced osmotic conductance to glucose).[32] These patients would theoretically benefit much less from switching to icodextrin because of the reduced UF capacity.

Nutrition

During their first year of treatment, CAPD patients typically have evidence of net anabolism; the average weight gain may exceed 5 kg without any clinical signs of fluid overload. Contributing to this weight gain is the peritoneal glucose reabsorption (on average being 100 to 150 g/day), which adds 400 to 600 kcal of energy intake daily. As RRF declines, the nutritional and metabolic abnormalities in CAPD become increasingly manifest, implying reductions in lean body mass. The main cause of protein-energy malnutrition and wasting are, except for poor food intake, the impaired metabolism of protein and energy in uremia. Despite glucose absorption, many patients on long-term CAPD have signs of energy malnutrition, a major component of the uremic wasting syndrome. Contributing factors are (low-grade) inflammation associated with carbonyl and oxidative stress and with accelerated atherosclerosis, the so-called malnutrition inflammation atherosclerosis syndrome.[42] It is important that CAPD patients are prescribed an adequate amount of protein (1.2 to 1.3 g protein/kg/day) and energy (total energy intake >35 kcal/kg/day) and a sufficient dose of dialysis, enabling the patient to ingest this diet. Daily loss of protein to the dialysate is approximately 7 to 8 g/day, of which ~4 to 5 g is albumin, thus comparable to the losses in nephrotic range proteinuria. The nutritional management of PD patients should include frequent assessments of their nutritional status, which is discussed further in Chapter 77.

OUTCOME OF PERITONEAL DIALYSIS

Several sets of registry data[43] have indicated a lower risk of death in patients treated with PD during the first 2 years of treatment compared to those treated with HD. Overall, the mortality in PD versus HD is not significantly different, however. Survival differences seem to vary substantially according to the underlying cause of ESRD, age, and level of baseline comorbidity. In a recent study based on U.S. Medicare registry data,[44] HD was associated with a higher risk of death among diabetic patients with *no* comorbidity and among younger patients (age 18 to 44), while PD implied a higher risk of death among older patients (age 45 to 64). In patients with baseline comorbidity, adjusted mortality rates were not different between HD and PD among nondiabetic patients and among younger diabetic patients (age 18 to 44), but higher in PD in older diabetic patients with baseline comorbidity.

REFERENCES

1. van Manen JG, Korevaar JC, Dekker FW, et al: Changes in employment status in end-stage renal disease patients during their first year of dialysis. Perit Dial Int 2001;21:595–601.
2. Bleyer AJ, Burkart JM, Russell GB, Adams PL: Dialysis modality and delayed graft function after cadaveric renal transplantation. J Am Soc Nephrol 1999;10:154–159.
3. Coles GA, Williams JD: What is the place of peritoneal dialysis in the integrated treatment of renal failure? Kidney Int 1998;54:2234–2240.
4. Rippe B, Stelin G: Simulations of peritoneal solute transport during continuous ambulatory peritoneal dialysis (CAPD). Application of two-pore formalism. Kidney Int 1989;35:1234–1244.
5. Rippe B, Stelin G, Haraldsson B: Computer simulations of peritoneal fluid transport in CAPD. Kidney Int 1991;40:315–325.
6. Carlsson O, Nielsen S, Zakaria el R, Rippe B: In vivo inhibition of transcellular water channels (aquaporin-1) during acute peritoneal dialysis in rats. Am J Physiol 1996;271:H2254–H2262.
7. Krediet RT: The effective lymphatic absorption rate is an accurate and useful concept in the physiology of peritoneal dialysis. Perit Dial Int 2004;24:309–317.
8. Flessner MF: Peritoneal transport physiology: Insights from basic research. J Am Soc Nephrol 1991;2:122–135.
9. Waniewski J, Heimbürger O, Werynski A, Lindholm B: Diffusive mass transport coefficients are not constant during a single exchange in continuous ambulatory peritoneal dialysis. ASAIO J 1996;42:M518–M523.
10. Fischbach M, Dheu C: Hydrostatic intraperitoneal pressure: An objective tool for analyzing individual tolerance of intraperitoneal volume. Perit Dial Int 2005;25:338–339.
11. Rippe B, Levin L: Computer simulations of ultrafiltration profiles for an icodextrin-based peritoneal fluid in CAPD. Kidney Int 2000;57:2546–2556.
12. Rippe B, Venturoli D, Simonsen O, de Arteaga J: Fluid and electrolyte transport across the peritoneal membrane during CAPD. Perit Dial Int 2005;1:10–27.
13. Tenckhoff H, Schechter H: A bacteriologically safe peritoneal access device. Trans Am Soc Artif Intern Organs 1973;10:363–370.
14. Flanigan M, Gokal R: Peritoneal catheters and exit-site practices toward optimum peritoneal access: A review of current developments. Perit Dial Int 2005;25:132–139.
15. Heimbürger O, Waniewski J, Werynski A, Lindholm B: A quantitative description of solute and fluid transport during peritoneal dialysis. Kidney Int 1992;41:1320–1332.
16. Simonsen O, Wieslander A, Venturoli D, et al: Mass transfer of calcium across the peritoneum at three different peritoneal dialysis fluid Ca and glucose concentrations. Kidney Int 2003;64:208–215.
17. Mistry CD, Gokal R, Peers E: A randomized multicenter clinical trial comparing isosmolar icodextrin with hyperosmolar glucose solutions in CAPD. MIDAS Study Group. Multicenter Investigation of icodextrin in Ambulatory Peritoneal Dialysis. Kidney Int 1994;46:496–503.
18. Kopple JD, Bernard D, Messana J, et al: Treatment of malnourished CAPD patients with an amino acid based dialysate. Kidney Int 1995;47:1148–1157.
19. Wieslander AP, Nordin MK, Kjellstrand PT, Boberg UC: Toxicity of peritoneal dialysis fluids on cultured fibroblasts, L-929. Kidney Int 1991;40: 77–79.
20. Rippe B, Simonsen O, Heimbürger O, et al: Long-term clinical effects of a peritoneal dialysis fluid with less glucose degradation products. Kidney Int 2001;59:348–357.
21. Jones S, Holmes CJ, Krediet RT, et al: Bicarbonate/lactate-based peritoneal dialysis solution increases cancer antigen 125 and decreases hyaluronic acid levels. Kidney Int 2001;59:1529–1538.
22. Williams JD, Topley N, Craig KJ, et al: The Euro-Balance Trial: The effect of a new biocompatible peritoneal dialysis fluid (balance) on the peritoneal membrane. Kidney Int 2004;66:408–418.

23. Mactier RA, Sprosen TS, Gokal R: Bicarbonate and bicarbonate/lactate peritoneal dialysis solutions for the treatment of infusion pain. Kidney Int 1996;53:1061–1067.

24. Sjøland JA, Smith Pedersen R, Jespersen J, Gram J: Intraperitoneal heparin reduces peritoneal permeability and increases ultrafiltration in peritoneal dialysis patients. Nephrol Dial Transplant 2004;19:1264–1268.

25. Rosengren B-I, Carlsson O, Rippe B: Hyaluronan and peritoneal ultrafiltration: A test of the "filter-cake" hypothesis. Am J Kidney Dis 2001;37:1277–1285.

26. Watson PE, Watson ID, Batt RD: Total body water volumes for adult males and females estimated from simple anthropometric measurements. Am J Clin Nutr 1980;33:27–39.

27. Twardowski ZJ, Nolph DK, Khanna R, et al: Peritoneal equilibration test. Perit Dial Bull 1987;7:138–147.

28. Pannekeet MM, Imholz AL, Struijk DG, et al: The standard peritoneal permeability analysis: A tool for the assessment of peritoneal permeability characteristics in CAPD patients. Kidney Int 1995;48:866–875.

29. Smit W, Struijk DG, Ho-Dac-Pannekeet MM, Krediet RT: Quantification of free water transport in peritoneal dialysis. Kidney Int 2004;66:849–854.

30. La Milia V, Di Filippo S, Crepaldi M, et al: Mini-peritoneal equilibration test: A simple and fast method to assess free water and small solute transport across the peritoneal membrane. Kidney Int 2005;68:840–846.

31. Venturoli D, Rippe B: Validation by computer simulation of two indirect methods for quantification of free water transport in peritoneal dialysis. Perit Dial Int 2005;25:77–84.

32. Davies SJ: Longitudinal relationship between solute transport and ultrafiltration capacity in peritoneal dialysis patients. Kidney Int 2004;66:2437–2445.

33. Rottembourg J, Issad B, Gallego JL, et al: Evolution of residual renal function in patients undergoing maintenance haemodialysis or continuous ambulatory peritoneal dialysis. Proc Eur Dial Transplant Assoc 1983;19:397–403.

34. Adequacy of dialysis and nutrition in continuous peritoneal dialysis: Association with clinical outcomes. Canada-USA (CANUSA) Peritoneal Dialysis Study Group. J Am Soc Nephrol 1996;7:198–207.

35. Paniagua R, Amato D, Vonesh E, et al: Effects of increased peritoneal clearances on mortality rates in peritoneal dialysis: ADEMEX, a prospective, randomized, controlled trial. J Am Soc Nephrol 2002;13:1307–1320.

36. Brown EA, Davies SJ, Rutherford P, et al: Survival of functionally anuric patients on automated peritoneal dialysis: The European APD Outcome Study. J Am Soc Nephrol 2003;14:2948–2957.

37. Johansson AC, Samuelsson O, Attman PO, et al: Limitations in anthropometric calculations of total body water in patients on peritoneal dialysis. J Am Soc Nephrol 2001;12:568–573.

38. Faller B, Lameire N: Evolution of clinical parameters and peritoneal function in a cohort of CAPD patients followed over 7 years. Nephrol Dial Transplant 1994;9:280–286.

39. Wright M, Woodrow G, O'Brien S, et al: Polydipsia: A feature of peritoneal dialysis. Nephrol Dial Transplant 2004;19:1581–1586.

40. Nakayama M, Kawaguchi Y, Yokoyama K, et al: Anti-hypertensive effect of low Na connection (120 mEq/l) solution for CAPD patients. Clin Nephrol 1994;41:357–363.

41. Davies SJ, Woodrow G, Donovan K, et al: Icodextrin improves the fluid status of peritoneal dialysis patients: Results of a double-blind randomized controlled trial. J Am Soc Nephrol 2003;14:2338–2344.

42. Stenvinkel P, Heimburger O, Paultre F, et al: Strong association between malnutrition, inflammation, and atherosclerosis in chronic renal failure. Kidney Int 1999;55:1899–1911.

43. USRDS: United States Renal Data System. Am J Kidney Dis 2005;45(Suppl 1):S1–S270.

44. Vonesh EF, Snyder JJ, Foley RN, Collins AJ: The differential impact of risk factors on mortality in hemodialysis and peritoneal dialysis. Kidney Int 2004;66:2389–2401.

Complications of Peritoneal Dialysis

Simon J. Davies and John D. Williams

CHANGES IN PERITONEAL STRUCTURE AND FUNCTION ON PERITONEAL DIALYSIS

Loss of peritoneal function is a major factor leading to late treatment failure in peritoneal dialysis (PD). Although the precise biologic mechanisms responsible for these changes have not been defined, it is widely assumed that alterations in peritoneal function are related to structural changes in the peritoneal membrane. There is accumulating, albeit indirect, evidence that continuous exposure to bioincompatible dialysis solution components, as well as repeated episodes of bacterial peritonitis (Fig. 86.1), plays a major role in the long-term changes seen in peritoneal function (ultrafiltration loss and increased solute clearance). While the relationship between structure and function has not been fully defined, increased solute transport is likely to reflect a greater vascular surface area, which in turn causes reduced ultrafiltration due to early loss of the osmotic gradient and enhanced fluid reabsorption (type 1 ultrafiltration failure). There is also evidence of an additional mechanism by which membranes exhibit a reduced ultrafiltration capacity for a given osmotic gradient (type 2 failure) that might be explained by progressive fibrosis.[1] Although a number of studies have identified various mesothelial, vascular, and interstitial changes in peritoneal morphology during PD, neither the factors responsible for these changes nor the time scale over which they develop have been identified. The changes observed include loss or degeneration of mesothelium, submesothelial thickening (variously described as fibrosis or sclerosis),

changes in the structure and number of blood vessels, and vascular basement membrane reduplication.

Recent studies have quantified the changes within the submesothelial collagenous zone and demonstrated a progressive increase in thickness with time on PD (Fig. 86.2). Changes within the peritoneal vascular bed have also been identified. These include progressive changes to the structure of small venules ranging from subtle thickening of the subendothelial matrix through to complete obliteration of vessels (Fig. 86.3).[2] In one study, the extent of these changes in a small group of patients correlated with the loss of ultrafiltration.[3] There is thus accumulating evidence that changes occur in both the interstitial and vascular compartments of the dialyzed peritoneal membrane. While it is likely that these changes are related to time on dialysis, peritonitis, and perhaps dialysis solution components, the exact relationships are poorly understood as is the possible contribution of uremia. In response to these concerns, new more biocompatible dialysis solutions have been developed that are characterized by low concentrations of glucose degradation products (GDPs), normal pH, and, in some cases, the use of bicarbonate as a buffer. Early studies would suggest that these solutions improve markers of membrane damage and reduce circulating GDPs.[4-6] Whether these will translate into improved clinical outcomes remains to be determined.

Encapsulating Peritoneal Sclerosis

In a small proportion of patients, there is extensive thickening and fibrosis of the peritoneal membrane (Fig. 86.4). It was originally described following exposure to acetate in the dialysate, the use of chlorhexidine as an antiseptic, and the administration of the β-blocker practolol. This can occur after severe or recurrent peritonitis, although it is also recognized as a complication of long-term PD, even when there is no recorded history of peritonitis. Clinically, it usually presents with poor ultrafiltration and reduced peritoneal transport.

Some patients develop an encapsulating, sclerotic reaction, in which the bowel is enveloped in a thick cocoon of fibrous tissue, causing obstruction (Fig. 86.5). Such individuals present with anorexia, nausea, malnutrition, and partial or complete intestinal obstruction. Whether this is a variant of extensive peritoneal fibrosis or a separate entity is unknown. The treatment of encapsulating sclerosing peritonitis remains controversial. Most agree that PD should be stopped to avoid continued exposure to nonphysiologic dialysis solutions, although continued irrigation with physiologic Hartman's solution is undertaken by some. Surgical debridement has been pioneered in Japan, although this practice requires prolonged surgery and considerable experience.[7] Several reports have suggested the use of tamoxifen as an antifibrotic agent, although the results are by no means uniform.[8]

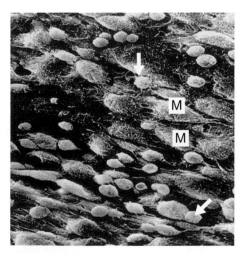

Figure 86.1 Peritonitis. Scanning electron micrograph of the peritoneum from a patient receiving peritoneal dialysis who has peritonitis. The small round cells (*arrows*) are phagocytes, which are widely distributed among the mesothelial cells (M) (×1800).

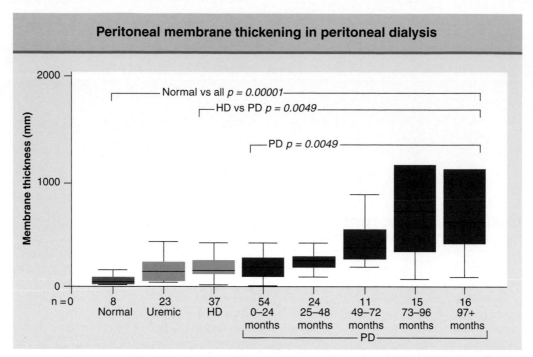

Figure 86.2 shows a box plot titled "Peritoneal membrane thickening in peritoneal dialysis" with y-axis "Membrane thickness (mm)" ranging 0 to 2000, and x-axis categories with n values: n=0, 8 Normal, 23 Uremic, 37 HD, 54 0–24 months, 24 25–48 months, 11 49–72 months, 15 73–96 months, 16 97+ months (PD). Significance brackets: Normal vs all p = 0.00001; HD vs PD p = 0.0049; PD p = 0.0049.

Figure 86.2 Peritoneal membrane thickening in peritoneal dialysis (PD). The thickness of the submesothelial collagenous zone of the peritoneal membrane in normal individuals, in undialyzed uremics, in hemodialysis (HD), and in those who have received PD for different periods of time. Membrane thickness is significantly increased in all uremic and dialysis patients compared to normal. Membrane thickness increases significantly with duration of PD and is increased in PD patients as a group compared to HD.

INFECTIOUS COMPLICATIONS

Peritonitis

While the introduction of disconnect delivery systems has reduced the incidence of peritonitis, it remains one of the most important complications of long-term PD and is a major cause of treatment failure. Guidelines for the diagnosis and management of PD peritonitis are published by the International Society of Peritoneal Dialysis (ISPD; www.ispd.org).[9]

Diagnosis of Peritonitis

The diagnosis of peritonitis should be suspected in any patient who develops a cloudy bag and/or abdominal pain. Fever may also be present but is not a universal feature of peritonitis. Patients should be advised to contact their dialysis unit immediately if they observe a cloudy bag or develop persistent abdominal pain. Samples of the dialysate should be taken for cell count and microbiologic examination. The diagnosis of peritonitis is confirmed by finding >100 white blood cells/mm³ (1×10^7 cells/l). A Gram stain of the spun deposit should also be performed to help to identify the type of causative organism, although initial treatment will often have to be empirical pending culture and sensitivity results. Various culture techniques have been proposed, but white cell lysis is often helpful in increasing the yield of a positive growth.

The dialysate leukocyte count will be affected by dwell length, and this needs taking into account in automated PD (APD)

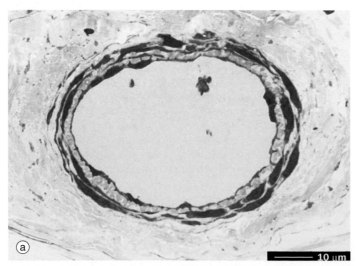

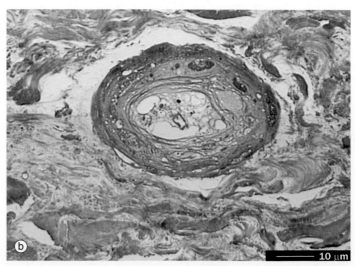

Figure 86.3 Blood vessels in the parietal peritoneum: transverse sections of peritoneal arterioles. *a*, Normal. *b*, Vasculopathy in a patient on peritoneal dialysis; the vascular lumen is occluded by connective tissue containing fine calcific stippling.

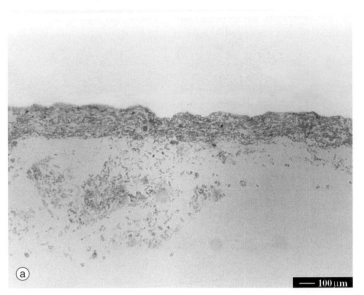

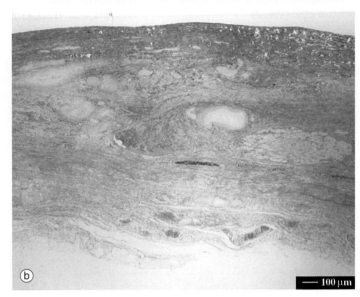

Figure 86.4 Morphologic changes in the parietal peritoneal membrane. *a*, Normal. *b*, A patient who has been on peritoneal dialysis for 10 years. Note the marked thickening of the submesothelial compact zone (toluidine blue).

patients. In short dwells, the count will be lower, and under these circumstances, if the proportion of cells that are neutrophils exceeds 50%, then empirical treatment for peritonitis should be commenced. Conversely, if the patient has had a dry abdomen during the day, the initial drain on connection may be cloudy. This will, however, clear within one or two cycles, and the majority of the cells found will be mononuclear leukocytes.

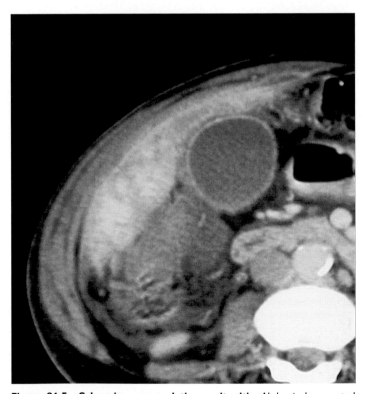

Figure 86.5 Sclerosing encapsulating peritonitis. Abdominal computed tomography scan of a patient with sclerosing encapsulating peritonitis, showing extensive peritoneal thickening.

Treatment of Peritonitis

The empirical treatment of peritonitis will vary according to center and should be developed in close collaboration with the local microbiologic service. Initial regimens must cover both gram-positive and gram-negative organisms and in the latest ISPD guidelines examples of appropriate antibiotics include vancomycin, cephalosporins, and aminoglycosides.[9] Dosing regimens will depend on whether the patient is on continuous ambulatory PD (CAPD) or APD. For CAPD, the antibiotic is administered as a loading dose in the first bag and then as a maintenance dose in subsequent bags. Although it was customary to transfer APD patients to CAPD for the purpose of treating peritonitis, this is no longer necessary. APD patients are now given large loading doses into dialysis fluid with a minimum 6-hour dwell (e.g., vancomycin 30 mg/kg) and then are given further doses every 3 to 5 days according to checked blood levels. Once the culture result is available, the regimen should be modified accordingly (Fig. 86.6). If the organism is methicillin-resistant *Staphylococcus aureus* (MRSA), vancomycin will continue as part of the regimen.

If the culture is negative, then empirical therapy should be continued for 2 weeks, assuming there is a clinical response. If a gram-negative organism is identified, the subsequent management will depend on the sensitivity (Fig. 86.7). The isolation of multiple organisms including anaerobes strongly suggests major bowel pathology. Metronidazole should be added to the regimen and consideration given to surgical intervention.

A wide variety of antibiotics other than those cited have been used with success. In particular, a commonly used strategy is to include an oral quinolone, such as ciprofloxacin, instead of an aminoglycoside since ototoxicity and loss of residual renal function may occur with aminoglycosides. Current recommendations are that for gram-positive organisms, therapy should be for 14 days except in the case of *S. aureus*, for which 21 days is suggested. For culture-negative episodes, 14 days of therapy should suffice. The same is true in the case of single organism gram-negative peritonitis. For *Pseudomonas, Xanthomonas* species, or multiple organisms, 21 days is recommended.

Many patients can be treated successfully as outpatients. It is extremely important, however, that they are followed up either

Antibiotic regimens for PD peritonitis	
Culture	Antibiotic
Enterococci (including vancomycin-resistant enterococci)	Ampicillin
*Staphylococcus aureus** Methicillin-resistant*	Cephalosporin/floxacillin (flucloxacilin) Vancomycin
Other gram-positive organism[†]	Cephalosporin/floxacillin
Gram-negative organisms (including *Pseudomonas* species)*	Cefazolin, quinolone, or aminoglycoside, [†]depending on sensitivities and residual renal function
Multiple/anaerobic organisms*	Metronidazole ± laparotomy
Culture negative[‡]	Continue empirical treatment

Figure 86.6 Antibiotic regimens for bacterial peritoneal dialysis (PD) peritonitis. Suggested antibiotic regimens when dialysate fluid culture is available. Except for culture-negative episodes, empirical treatment is stopped once the sensitivities are known. All antibiotic regimens should be developed in consultation with local microbiology practices. *Three-week treatment. [†]Two-week treatment. [‡]Avoid unnecessary use if residual function is present.

in the clinic or by telephone. In most cases, clinical resolution, as judged by the clearing of the bags, starts within 48 hours. If there is no improvement within 96 hours, despite using the correct antibiotic, as judged by sensitivity tests, the fluid must be retested by cell count, Gram stain, and culture. In the case of a persistent *S. aureus* infection, an underlying tunnel infection should be excluded. In all other situations where there is a failure to improve, serious consideration should be given to removing the catheter. In addition, the possibility of intra-abdominal or gynecologic pathology or the presence of unusual organisms such as mycobacteria should be considered. Under these circumstances, a mini-laparotomy should be performed to exclude intra-abdominal pathology, and if mycobacterial infection is suspected, a peritoneal biopsy specimen should be obtained for culture.

Fungal Peritonitis

If peritonitis is caused by yeasts or fungi, then the peritoneal catheter should always be removed. There is limited experience with drug treatment. The recommendation for adults is daily fluconazole at an oral or intraperitoneal dose of 200 mg and flucytosine at a loading dose of 2 g orally with a maintenance dose of 1 g/day. Amphotericin is no longer recommended. Unfortunately, oral flucytosine is not universally available. Oral treatment should be continued for at least 10 days after catheter removal.[9]

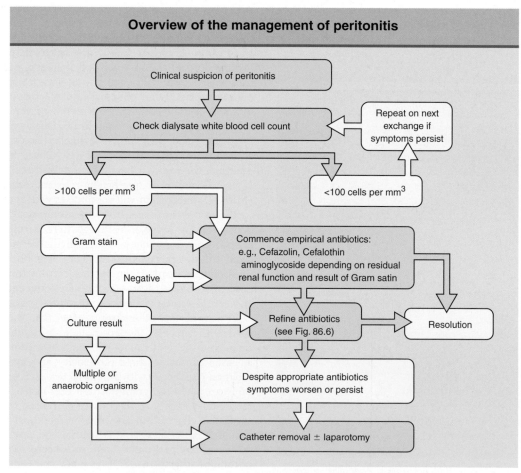

Figure 86.7 Overview of the management of peritonitis.

Relapsing Peritonitis

Relapsing or recurrent peritonitis is defined as a separate infective episode caused by the same organism within 4 weeks of completing an appropriate course of antibiotics. In the case of a relapsing gram-positive infection, a 4-week course of intra-peritoneal cephalosporin together with oral rifampin (rifampicin) should be tried. Recurrence of *S. aureus* infection should trigger the search for pericatheter infection. Relapsing MRSA peritonitis will require a prolonged course (4 weeks) of intraperitoneal vancomycin or clindamycin. If enterococci or gram-negative organisms are the cause of a relapse, then the possibility of intra-abdominal pathology or an abscess should be considered (although these organisms are frequently water borne). If a patient has other gastrointestinal symptoms, such as change in bowel habit, then colonoscopy should be performed, but this is only essential if multiple organisms have been isolated. Again, a repeat course of antibiotics chosen by sensitivity testing should last 4 weeks. Removal of the catheter should be considered if there is no improvement within 4 days of commencing treatment, or earlier if clinically indicated. Current practice in most units is to allow a period of up to 3 weeks before a new catheter is inserted. Some centers, however, have practiced simultaneous removal and replacement of the catheter, under antibiotic cover, with success.[10]

Prevention of Peritonitis

The latest ISPD guidelines place increased emphasis on prevention of peritonitis. Antibiotic cover at the time of catheter insertion is recommended to prevent subsequent exit-site infection and peritonitis.[9] No particular catheter design has been shown to reduce infection rates, but a downward pointing exit-site of the catheter assists in catheter care. Enhanced training schedules and improved exit-site care have been shown in a randomized study to reduce infection rates.[11] Flush-before-fill dialysate delivery systems have been shown to reduce infections associated with touch contamination and should now be standard.[12]

S. aureus nasal carriage is associated with an increased chance of peritonitis caused by this organism. Regular use of mupirocin either intranasally or applied to the catheter exit site reduces the rate of *S. aureus* peritonitis; occasional resistance has been reported but to date this has not been a significant problem. A recent randomized trial has shown a reduction in *Pseudomonas* peritonitis associated with topical gentamicin applied to the exit site (see later discussion).[13]

Eosinophilic Peritonitis

Eosinophilic peritonitis is diagnosed when a patient presents with a cloudy bag of effluent containing eosinophils rather than neutrophils. The fluid is also culture negative. It is an uncommon event, but tends to occur within the first few weeks of starting PD. The cause is unknown, but assumed to be some form of reaction to the cannula or the dialysate. The condition is usually self-limiting, and no treatment is required.

Exit Site Infection

Exit site infection is an important complication of long-term PD, occurring on average at a rate of 0.48 episodes per patient-year. The diagnosis is suspected on clinical grounds, usually by the presence of marked erythema and/or discharge from the exit site (Fig. 86.8). A scoring system for exit sites has been developed to determine the likelihood of infection and to grade its severity, with 1 to 2 points awarded for crusting, swelling, pain, and discharge

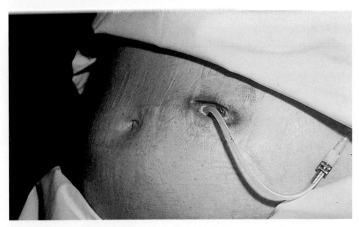

Figure 86.8 Exit site infection. A severe exit site infection that has exposed the outer cuff of the cannula.

according to severity (score >4 indicating infection), although if the discharge is purulent, this mandates treatment.[9] Extension of the infection into the tunnel may be assessed either clinically or by ultrasonography, enabling measurement of any abscess formation. The most common infecting organism is *S. aureus*. Regular use of topical mupirocin can reduce the frequency of infection episodes substantially with the additional benefit of reducing the risk of peritonitis due to this organism. Otherwise, the most common pathogen is *Pseudomonas*, and a recent randomized trial comparing mupirocin and gentamicin cream at the exit site found that both staphylococcal and pseudomonal infections (exit site and peritonitis) were less common in those using gentamicin. While regular application of gentamicin to exit sites infected at any stage with gram-negative organisms is currently advised, the routine application of gentamicin cream for all patients raises concerns over bacterial resistance, although this has not yet been reported.[13]

Initial treatment should be with an antibiotic effective against *S. aureus* unless there is prior evidence that the patient carries MRSA or *Pseudomonas*, for example, flucloxacillin (500 mg 4 times a day), or a cephalosporin if the patient is allergic to penicillin. In most patients, the drug can be given orally, but if the individual is systemically ill, the antibiotics should be administered intravenously until clinical improvement occurs. Hospitalization, parenteral antibiotics, and often urgent catheter removal are required if there is evidence of spread into the tunnel. If the infection is MRSA, eradication therapy should be attempted using systemic vancomycin, as for peritonitis. Should the culture grow a gram-negative organism, ciprofloxacin 500 mg bid orally will be effective empirical treatment in most patients.

Treatment is recommended for a minimum of 2 weeks. In gram-positive infections, if there is no improvement within 7 days, rifampin 600 mg/day can be added. If complete healing does not take place after 4 weeks of therapy, further measures should be considered, such as exteriorizing and shaving the outer cuff. Should this cuff be visible or even close to the exit site, it is likely to be involved in the infection. There is often temporary resolution of infection following this procedure. If despite this step the infection persists or relapses, catheter removal must be considered since there is a high risk of the exit site infection leading to peritonitis. It is important that the new exit site is formed in a different part of the anterior abdominal wall. If the infection is controlled and there is no evidence of sepsis along the tunnel, it is possible to insert a new catheter under antibiotic cover at the same time that the old one is removed.

NONINFECTIOUS COMPLICATIONS

Reduced Ultrafiltration and Ultrafiltration Failure

There is increasing evidence that reduced ultrafiltration is associated with poor survival in PD.[14-16] The cause and effect in this relationship are not clear since the studies are observational, but in the only study with a preset ultrafiltration target (>750 ml/day), mortality was significantly worse in those patients who were identified as having reduced peritoneal ultrafiltration capacity, resulting in daily ultrafiltration consistently below this level.[15] Ultrafiltration failure, often defined as <400 ml at 4 hours following a 3.86% exchange, is also associated with technique failure. This occurs in up to 31% of patients by 6 years of treatment.[13] Problems with ultrafiltration should be suspected if patients have signs of fluid overload, are using excessive numbers of hypertonic exchanges, or when the total fluid removal per day (urine plus dialysate) is <1 liter. It is important to check the actual drainage volumes by asking the patient to bring their bags to the unit and to remember to include the overfill flush volume in the calculation of net ultrafiltration. In these circumstances, peritoneal membrane function tests should be performed to establish the solute transport and ultrafiltration capacity of the membrane (see Figs. 85.8 and 85.9). If membrane function is normal and ultrafiltration adequate, it is likely that fluid intake is excessive, and educational measures must be undertaken to correct this. Diabetics may require improved blood glucose control, which will be helped by reducing the glucose prescription and using icodextrin and amino acid solutions.[17] If the ultrafiltration capacity is <200 ml using a routine peritoneal equilibration test (PET) with 2.27% glucose or <400 ml using a modified standard permeability analysis (SPA) with 3.86% glucose, then treatment strategy is determined by transport status.

Management of High Solute Transport Ultrafiltration Failure (Dialysate-to-Plasma Creatinine Ratio >0.64)

In observational studies, increased solute transport is consistently associated with increased mortality and technique failure, independent of age, gender, and comorbidity. In patients with high transport, there is a more rapid absorption of glucose from the peritoneal cavity, which results in the early loss of the osmotic gradient. Short dwell periods reduce the degree of fluid reabsorption, and a change to APD using several (typically four) short overnight cycles may improve the situation. If there is a significant urine output, a loop diuretic in high dose (e.g., furosemide 250 mg/day) should be tried. This has been shown in a randomized study to maintain urine volume and sodium excretion without affecting clearances.[18]

For the long dwells, icodextrin, a glucose polymer that is iso-osmotic with plasma and can generate prolonged ultrafiltration due to a sustained oncotic pressure gradient, should be used. A number of randomized trials have shown that this prevents fluid reabsorption in the long dwell, resulting in a significant benefit when compared to glucose 2.27% in high transporters.[19] It also improves the fluid status of these patients by reducing the extracellular fluid volume, usually by ~15%.[20,21] Care needs to be taken when commencing patients on icodextrin that a rapid change in fluid status is avoided, typically seen in individuals in whom excessive fluid reabsorption was occurring, as this might result in a loss of residual renal function. When icodextrin has been used in long-term studies (e.g., in anuric patients using APD), high peritoneal transport is no longer a risk factor for mortality and technique failure, and there is stable membrane function.

Management of Low Transport Ultrafiltration Failure (Dialysate-to-Plasma Creatinine Ratio <0.64)

Although less common, the management of low transport ultrafiltration failure is more difficult. It is essential to exclude any form of mechanical failure, such as an occult peritoneal cuff leak or an inguinal hernia, using contrast-enhanced computed tomography (CT) scanning. Once mechanical problems have been excluded, it is possible to determine whether the poor ultrafiltration is due to a failure of ultrafiltration or of excessive fluid reabsorption by determining whether sodium sieving is present. Typically, low transport patients will have a sustained glucose gradient and will therefore exhibit sodium sieving (a decrease in the dialysate sodium concentration) during the first 60 minutes of a 3.86% dwell. This occurs because of the convective transport of water through water exclusive pathways, now known to be capillary aquaporins. Lack of sieving indicates failure of the membrane to generate an ultrafiltrate. Patients with loss of sodium sieving will require regular hypertonic exchanges as well as strategies to preserve urine volume, such as using diuretics[18] or angiotensin-converting enzyme inhibitors.[22] For many of these patients, a planned transfer to hemodialysis is the only practical outcome.

Catheter Malfunction

Inflow Failure

A 2-liter bag of dialysate should take ≤15 minutes to run into the peritoneal cavity. If inflow is significantly slowed or even stopped completely, mechanical causes should first be eliminated. After checking that the tubing and catheter are not kinked, that all clamps or rollers are open to the inflow position, and that any frangible seal is fully broken, the catheter should be flushed vigorously with 20 ml heparinized saline. If the catheter is cleared, then heparin should be added (500 U/l) to the next few cycles since the cause of the blockage is often a fibrin plug. Should the catheter remain blocked, a plain abdominal radiograph is required. If this shows that the catheter is in a satisfactory position in the pelvis, an attempt to restore patency should be made using urokinase. Urokinase (25,000 U in 2 ml of saline) is infused into the lumen of the catheter and left *in situ* for 2 to 4 hours. The catheter is then flushed. If inflow is restored, heparin should be added to the dialysate for the next few cycles. Should this procedure not be successful, but fibrin is still thought to be the cause, an endoscopy brush may sometimes prove successful in unblocking the catheter.

If the radiograph shows the catheter to be malpositioned (Fig. 86.9), an attempt should be made to reposition the catheter tip into the pelvis. This can be done using a sterile semirigid rod, shaped into a curve and slid down the lumen of the catheter under radiographic screening control. The rod is then rotated. Sometimes the catheter will move easily and slide back into the pelvis. (For further discussion see Chapter 82.) This technique is not practical when the cannula has a swan-neck configuration. Alternatively, the cannula can be repositioned at laparotomy or peritoneoscopy. Often the cannula will be found to be wrapped in omentum, and the only solution will be to carry out an omentectomy or an omental hitch, a surgical procedure in which the omentum is temporarily held away from the cannula by a dissolvable suture.

Outflow Failure

The most common reason for outflow failure is constipation, although causes of inflow failure discussed previously should also be considered. Loading of the bowel with fecal material is often

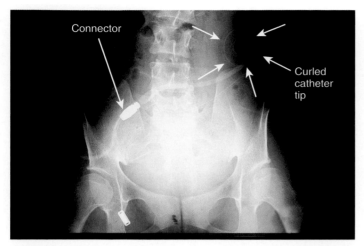

Figure 86.9 Catheter malposition. Plain radiograph of the abdomen with curled catheter (*arrows*) misplaced in the upper left abdomen.

obvious on a plain radiograph, but treatment for constipation should be initiated without recourse to this investigation as it is so common. Constipation should be treated with oral laxatives or an enema. Subsequently, bowel action should be kept regular by increasing the fiber in the diet and, if necessary, the addition of a mild laxative such as lactulose or senna. Slow outflow can be a problem in APD patients resulting in excessive machine alarms. This is best dealt with by switching to tidal APD and using a relatively large residual volume (>50% of the fill volume).

Fibrin in the Dialysate

During peritonitis, fibrin in the dialysate is common. If fibrin causes restriction to dialysate flow, heparin (500 U/l) should be added to each bag. A small number of patients have fibrin formation in the absence of peritonitis. Immediately on drainage, the bag may appear cloudy, but on standing, the fibrin will aggregate. The first time this happens, a sample must be sent to the microbiology laboratory to exclude infection. If this proves negative, the patient can be reassured. If catheter plugging occurs subsequently, regular use of heparin is recommended.

Fluid Leaks

External Leaks

On occasion, fluid may leak from the exit site or even the incision used to insert the cannula into the peritoneal cavity. This is usually a problem that occurs early, particularly if dialysis is started soon after cannula insertion. Whenever possible, elective insertion of the catheter should be performed at least 10 days before dialysis is required. In addition, the use of the paramedian approach for the peritoneal entry site is thought to minimize the chances of this complication. If a leak occurs, PD should be withheld for as long as possible. If dialysis is necessary, APD can be used overnight with a dry day for at least 10 days.

Internal Leaks

Isolated edema of the abdominal wall suggests an internal leak from the peritoneal cavity, either spontaneously or in association with a surgical hernia. In contrast, genital edema suggests an inguinal hernia or patent processus vaginalis. Occasionally both can be present. The site of the leak can be visualized by CT scanning following intraperitoneal instillation of contrast. It may be necessary for the patient to stand or perform other maneuvers to

increase intra-abdominal pressure before the leak is demonstrated (Fig. 86.10a). An alternative diagnostic test is to perform scintigraphy after injecting a compound such as technetium-99m-diethylenetriamine pentaacetic acid ($^{Tc-99m}$DTPA; see Fig. 86.10b). A surgical repair will be required if a major leak is visualized and

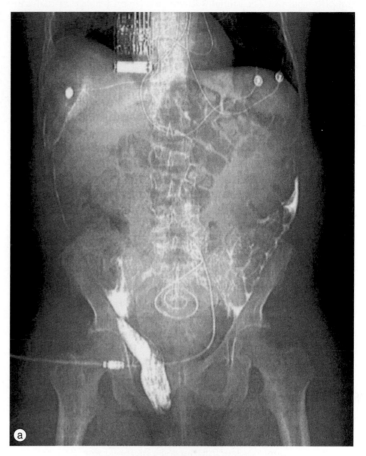

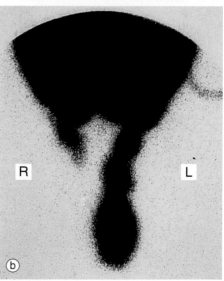

Figure 86.10 Inguinal hernia during peritoneal dialysis. *a*, Computed tomography scan following intraperitoneal injection of contrast in a male patient showing dialysate flowing into a right inguinal hernia. *b*, Peritoneal scintigram of a male patient on peritoneal dialysis, showing bilateral inguinal hernias. The left hernia extends into the scrotum; the right hernia is less extensive. (*a*, From Tintillier M, Coche E, Malaise J, Goffin E: Peritoneal dialysis and an inguinal hernia. Lancet 2003;362:1893.)

should always be considered if in association with a hernia. Most leaks, however, will heal following resting or the use of APD, using dry days or temporary HD.

Hydrothorax

A pleural effusion can occur with generalized fluid overload or local lung disease, but occasionally it is caused by a leakage of dialysate through the diaphragm (Fig. 86.11). This more commonly occurs on the right side. A leak is most simply confirmed by aspirating a sample of the effusion and finding that its glucose concentration is higher than the patient's blood glucose. Initially, conservative measures should be tried. These include stopping PD, aspirating the effusion to dryness, and leaving the abdomen dry for 2 weeks (using hemodialysis, if necessary). This regimen is effective in a number of patients. If the condition recurs, then pleurodesis can be tried; various agents have been advocated, including tetracycline, talc, autologous blood, and fibrin glue, but there are no comparative studies to indicate the best regimen.

Pain

Inflow Pain

Soon after starting PD, patients may experience pain during fluid inflow. This is particularly likely to occur if dialysis begins immediately or within a few days of catheter insertion. It is either related to blunt trauma of the peritoneum or the low dialysate pH. This problem usually disappears with time but may temporarily require simple analgesics. Slowing the rate of fluid inflow will often reduce the symptoms. Peritonitis should be excluded and treated. A small number of individuals get persistent inflow pain. A randomized, controlled trial has demonstrated that bicarbonate dialysis fluid at physiologic pH is associated with a dramatic improvement in infusion pain in such individuals.[23]

Backache

Backache occurs in a minority of PD patients; the presence of a large volume of fluid in the abdomen distorts the normal posture, exacerbating any tendency to lordosis of the spine. Patients with pre-existing back problems are most likely to have an exacerbation of their backache, though not all will be affected. It is important to

investigate the symptom to exclude treatable or serious disease. Adjusting the dialysis regimen to reduce the daytime volume or leaving the abdomen empty of fluid during the day can help symptoms, provided treatment is not compromised.

Outflow Pain

Some patients have discomfort or even pain when the fluid runs out. This emptying sensation is abolished when the next cycle runs in. This commonly occurs during peritonitis but may be experienced in the absence of infection during the first few weeks of treatment. Switching to tidal APD will often solve this problem. Tidal therapy enables a prescribed amount of fluid to remain in the peritoneal cavity throughout treatment. If this is set to between 50% and 80% of the inflow volume, pain and drainage alarms are often prevented.

Bleeding
Exit Site

The exit site can be a source of blood loss at any time while a peritoneal catheter is in place. A common cause is the removal of a crust before natural separation has occurred. The bleeding almost invariably stops with local pressure but a new raw area that is liable to become infected remains. Regular cleansing of the exit site with povidone-iodine will reduce the chances of this complication. Patients must be instructed not to pull off the crust but await its natural separation. Severe infection of the exit site may, on occasion, be accompanied by secondary hemorrhage. This will usually respond to firm pressure. The subsequent management is the same as for any exit site infection.

Blood-Stained Dialysate

Blood-stained dialysate is uncommon. It is rarely serious but causes considerable alarm to the patient. There is sometimes a clear history of trauma to the abdomen or of unexpected strain. A few female patients relate the episode to their menstrual cycle at the time of ovulation or menstruation. The treatment is to flush the abdomen with a few cycles of dialysate containing heparin (500 U/l) to minimize the chances of clotting in the cannula. The problem usually resolves spontaneously and often is only visible in one outflow. It is unusual for the blood-stained dialysate to be associated with infection, although it is wise to have the fluid cultured. Routine use of antibiotics is not necessary.

Nutritional Problems
Malnutrition

Cross-sectional surveys of patients receiving PD show that about 40% have malnutrition and 8% having severe protein-calorie depletion. Malnutrition is an adverse risk factor for morbidity and mortality of patients on PD; this poor nutrition is multifactorial. The assessment and management of malnutrition are discussed further in Chapter 77. It has been suggested that ideally patients should consume daily at least 1.2 to 1.3 g protein/kg body weight. In practice, many subjects take only 0.8 g/kg/day and seem to be nutritionally stable. It is likely that they have achieved a steady state but with a lower total body nitrogen or lean body mass.

Patients on CAPD have abnormal eating behavior with smaller meals, slow eating, and impaired gastric emptying compared with normal subjects. The full peritoneal cavity may produce easy satiety, and some patients complain of feeling bloated. However, studies have shown that there is no actual difference in food consumption with or without dialysate in the abdomen.

One obvious contributing factor is protein loss via the peritoneum, which averages 8 g/day but can be as high as 20 g/day. It

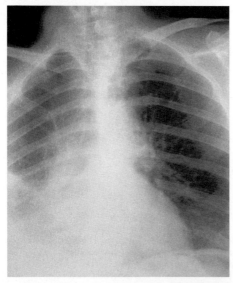

Figure 86.11 Hydrothorax in peritoneal dialysis. Chest radiograph showing a right-sided pleural effusion caused by a diaphragmatic leak.

increases considerably during peritonitis. Patients with high solute transport also have high peritoneal protein losses, in particular albumin. In both cases, the protein loss is a reflection of a larger effective peritoneal surface area. The ensuing hypoalbuminemia complicates poor ultrafiltration and exacerbates the extracellular fluid expansion in these patients.

Acid-Base Status

Another important influence on nutrition is the acid-base status of the patient. Correction of acidosis reduces protein catabolism. One study compared the use of 35 mmol/l lactate dialysate with fluid containing 40 mmol/l lactate.[24] After 1 year, the group receiving the higher lactate concentration had increased serum bicarbonate levels and, more importantly, had gained more weight with a greater increase in midarm muscle circumference. This implies that protein anabolism had taken place as the result of better acid-base correction. Correction of malnutrition is not easy. Clearly patients should be encouraged to increase protein and calorie intake. Food supplements are of particular value during intercurrent illness. One report suggested that the regular use of a calorie supplement was associated with increased total body nitrogen after several months, but this remains to be confirmed. Correction of acidosis is best achieved by using dialysate with higher levels of potential buffer,[25] but if necessary oral bicarbonate may be added.

Amino acid–based dialysate improves nitrogen balance in malnourished patients, but the long-term benefits are still unclear.[26] Usually one bag per day is recommended during the daytime when calories are being consumed in order to promote anabolism and avoid the risk of the absorbed amino acids being used for energy production. Earlier reports noted a tendency to

acidosis with this type of dialysate, which would negate any beneficial effect. Close observation of the plasma bicarbonate is necessary, with supplementation as required.

Lipids and Obesity

The use of glucose-based hyperosmolar solutions for PD results in a significant increase in the glucose load experienced by the patient. A number of reports have measured the daily glucose absorption, which is estimated to be 100 and 200 g/day, producing 400 to 800 kcal. The resultant metabolic effect is a persistent tendency for patients on CAPD to develop obesity, hyperglycemia, and hyperinsulinemia; they may even develop frank diabetes. Serum triglycerides and cholesterol increase during the first year on CAPD, with increases in very-low-density and low-density lipoproteins. The greater the degree of hyperlipidemia at the start of therapy, the worse will be the changes with time on CAPD. In addition, there is some evidence that lipoprotein (a) levels may increase with time on CAPD (although this has not been consistently confirmed). Proatherogenic lipid levels are more common in patients on CAPD than on hemodialysis. A number of studies have demonstrated the effectiveness of cholesterol-lowering agents in patients on CAPD. Statins are of proven efficacy in reducing total cholesterol and low-density lipoprotein cholesterol while increasing high-density lipoprotein cholesterol. However, the long-term effects of such intervention on cardiovascular morbidity and mortality in CAPD patients have yet to be established.

There is no evidence to suggest that PD should be avoided in obese patients despite these concerns. The survival advantage seen in hemodialysis associated with a higher body mass index is not seen.[27]

REFERENCES

1. Davies SJ: Longitudinal relationship between solute transport and ultra-filtration capacity in peritoneal dialysis patients. Kidney Int 2004;66:2437–2445.
2. Williams JD, Craig KJ, Topley N, et al: Morphologic changes in the peritoneal membrane of patients with renal disease. J Am Soc Nephrol 2002;13:470–469.
3. Honda K, Nitta K, Horita S, et al: Morphological changes in the peritoneal vasculature of patients on CAPD with ultrafiltration failure. Nephron 1996;72:171–176.
4. Jones S, Holmes CJ, Krediet RT, et al: Bicarbonate/lactate-based peritoneal dialysis solution increases cancer antigen 125 and decreases hyaluronic acid levels. Kidney Int 2001;59:1529–1538.
5. Rippe B, Wieslander A, Musi B: Long-term results with low glucose degra-dation product content in peritoneal dialysis fluids. Contrib Nephrol 2003:140:47–55.
6. Williams JD, Topley N, Craig KJ, et al: The Euro-Balance Trial: The effect of a new biocompatible peritoneal dialysis fluid (balance) on the peritoneal membrane. Kidney Int 2004;66:408–418.
7. Yamamoto R, Otsuka Y, Nakayama M, et al: Risk factors for encapsu-lating peritoneal sclerosis in patients who have experienced peritoneal dialysis treatment. Clin Exp Nephrol 2005;9:148–152.
8. Summers AM, Clancy MJ, Syed F, et al: Single-center experience of encapsulating peritoneal sclerosis in patients on peritoneal dialysis for end-stage renal failure. Kidney Int 2005;68:2381–2388.
9. Piraino B, Bailie GR, Bernardini J, et al: Peritoneal dialysis-related infections recommendations: 2005 update. Perit Dial Int 2005;25:107–131.
10. Paterson AD, Bishop MC, Morgan AG, Burden RP: Removal and replacement of Tenckhoff catheter at a single operation: Successful treatment of resistant peritonitis in continuous ambulatory peritoneal dialysis. Lancet 1986;2:1245–1247.

11. Hall G, Bogan A, Dreis S, et al: New directions in peritoneal dialysis patient training. Nephrol Nurs J 2004;31:149–154, 159–163.
12. MacLeod A, Grant A, Donaldson C, et al: Effectiveness and efficiency of methods of dialysis therapy for end-stage renal disease: Systematic reviews. Health Technol Assess 1998;2:1–166.
13. Bernardini J, Bender F, Florio T, et al: Randomized, double-blind trial of antibiotic exit site cream for prevention of exit site infection in peritoneal dialysis patients. J Am Soc Nephrol 2005;16:539–545.
14. Jansen MA, Termorshuizen F, Korevaar JC, et al: Predictors of survival in anuric peritoneal dialysis patients. Kidney Int 2005;68:1199–1205.
15. Brown EA, Davies SJ, Rutherford P, et al: Survival of functionally anuric patients on automated peritoneal dialysis: The European APD Outcome Study. J Am Soc Nephrol 2003;14:2948–2957.
16. Ates K, Nergizoglu G, Keven K, et al: Effect of fluid and sodium removal on mortality in peritoneal dialysis patients. Kidney Int 2001;60:767–776.
17. Marshall J, Jennings P, Scott A, et al: Glycemic control in diabetic CAPD patients assessed by continuous glucose monitoring system (CGMS). Kidney Int 2003;64:1480–1486.
18. Medcalf JF, Harris KP, Walls J: Role of diuretics in the preservation of residual renal function in patients on continuous ambulatory peritoneal dialysis. Kidney Int 2001;59:128–133.
19. Wolfson M, Piraino B, Hamburger RJ, Morton AR: A randomized con-trolled trial to evaluate the efficacy and safety of icodextrin in peritoneal dialysis. Am J Kidney Dis 2002;40:1055–1065.
20. Konings CJ, Kooman JP, Schonck M, et al: Effect of icodextrin on volume status, blood pressure and echocardiographic parameters: A randomized study. Kidney Int 2003;63:1556–1563.
21. Davies SJ, Woodrow G, Donovan K, et al: Icodextrin improves the fluid status of peritoneal dialysis patients: Results of a double-blind random-ized controlled trial. J Am Soc Nephrol 2003;14:2338–2344.

22. Li PK, Chow KM, Wong TY, et al: Effects of an angiotensin-converting enzyme inhibitor on residual renal function in patients receiving peritoneal dialysis. A randomized, controlled study. Ann Intern Med 2003;139: 105–112.
23. Mactier RA, Sprosen TS, Gokal R, et al: Bicarbonate and bicarbonate/lactate peritoneal dialysis solutions for the treatment of infusion pain. Kidney Int 1998;53:1061–1067.
24. Stein A, Moorhouse J, Iles-Smith H, et al: Role of an improvement in acid-base status and nutrition in CAPD patients. Kidney Int 1997;52: 1089–1095.
25. Mujais S: Acid base profile in patients on PD. Kidney Int 2003(Suppl): 88:S26–S36.
26. Li FK, Chan LY, Woo JC, et al: A 3-year, prospective, randomized, controlled study on amino acid dialysate in patients on CAPD. Am J Kidney Dis 2003;42:173–183.
27. Abbott KC, Glanton CW, Trespalacios FC, et al: Body mass index, dialysis modality, and survival: Analysis of the United States Renal Data System Dialysis Morbidity and Mortality Wave II Study. Kidney Int 2004;65:597–605.

Acute Renal Replacement Therapy in the Intensive Care Unit

Emil P. Paganini and Mark R. Marshall

INTRODUCTION

Acute renal replacement therapy (ARRT) for critically ill patients with acute renal failure (ARF) has been a clinical reality for >50 years. Over this period, technologic progress has made ARRT safer and easier, but mortality in this population remains high, although outcomes may be gradually improving despite a higher degree of prevalent illness severity. Mortality attributable to ARF is due to nonresolving infection; hemorrhage; or nonresolving shock, despite optimal care. Such conditions may therefore comprise an acute uremic syndrome that is specific to ARF and the target for modulation with ARRT, as opposed to the traditional uremic syndrome of end-stage renal disease (ESRD).

Therapeutic goals for ARRT are not well defined. The usual minimum recommendation is to correct acidosis or hyperkalemia, refractory hypervolemia, and traditional uremic features such as pericarditis or coma. Serum electrolyte and bicarbonate concentrations should be maintained in the normal range. Targets for uremic solute control are discussed later in this chapter. Importantly, the process of ARRT itself should not jeopardize the patient by exacerbating hemodynamic instability, increasing end-organ damage, or delaying renal recovery.

Increasingly, efforts are being made to facilitate clearance of unconventional uremic markers and mediators such as proinflammatory cytokines, which might contribute to the purported acute uremic syndrome due to their cardiodepressant, vasodilatory, and immunomodulatory properties. Since ARRT will remove both pro- and anti-inflammatory cytokines, there is the potential to inadvertently exacerbate the inflammatory milieu.[1] Presently, there are insufficient data on the therapeutic benefit of clearing such mediators to justify a change in ARRT practice patterns.

The four main modalities of ARRT are acute intermittent hemodialysis (IHD), continuous renal replacement therapy (CRRT), sustained low-efficiency dialysis/dialfiltration (SLED), and acute peritoneal dialysis (PD). Globally, CRRT is the most popular modality, although practice patterns vary regionally due to cost, availability of technology, and reimbursement policies. SLED is becoming more popular, and for reasons of cost and convenience may become the dominant ARRT in the future. Acute PD is now only rarely used in adults and is not considered further in this chapter.

MECHANISMS OF SOLUTE REMOVAL IN ACUTE RENAL REPLACEMENT THERAPY

Diffusive blood purification occurs during hemodialysis (HD) by solute transfer through a semipermeable membrane down its concentration gradient. Diffusion favors removal of small uremic solutes <300 d and is enhanced by increased blood and dialysate flows (Qb, Qd) in the hemodialyzer. Convective solute removal occurs during hemofiltration (HF) when solutes are dragged though the membrane with ultrafiltered plasma water when transmembrane hydrostatic pressure is applied. Blood purification occurs when replacement fluid is returned to the patient, thereby diluting the concentration of retained solutes. Convection favors the removal of both small and medium-sized uremic solutes (<12 kd) and is enhanced by increased ultrafiltration rate (UFR). Figure 87.1 demonstrates the contrast between these mechanisms.[2]

Mass transfer across the membrane may not be the main mechanism for the extracorporeal removal of some uremic solutes, which, despite being water soluble, have a sieving coefficient (proportionality constant between the rate of solute movement and fluid movement across the membrane) <1, and their removal is not significantly different between diffusive and convective ARRT using conventional operating parameters. Studies have confirmed an adsorptive mechanism resulting in up to 10-fold higher removal of such mediators in comparison to convective removal alone.[1] In these studies, mediators only appeared in filtrate after complete saturation of the membrane. Adsorption is critically dependent on membrane composition and structure: for example, an open pore structure and hydrophobic (e.g., synthetic) membrane is necessary for binding to the hydrophobic amino acids in the polypeptide structure of cytokines.

ACUTE INTERMITTENT HEMODIALYSIS

Acute IHD is still a widely used modality for the management of ARF when the patient has sufficient hemodynamic stability. HD techniques and adequacy are discussed in the context of maintenance treatment for ESRD in Chapter 83.

Techniques for Acute Intermittent Hemodialysis

Acute IHD is categorized according to hemodialyzer membrane and mechanism of solute removal. High-flux membranes allow greater convective removal of middle and larger solutes, but there are only limited clinical data on high-flux dialysis in the critically ill with ARF, and these do not show obvious advantages.[3] Biocompatibility defines a membrane with a low capacity for activating complement and leukocytes during HD. Following complement activation, there is stasis of leukocytes in the lungs, renal parenchyma, and other organs and the release of products of leukocyte activation. By minimizing these processes, use of biocompatible membranes should in principle favorably affect

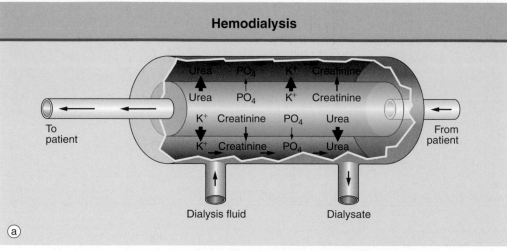

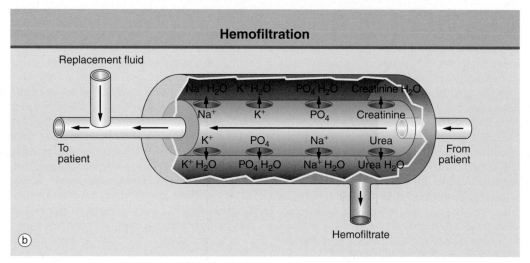

Figure 87.1 Comparison of hemodialysis and hemofiltration fluid and solute movements across the membrane. Demonstrates this movement in hemodialysis (*a*) and in hemofiltration (*b*). The arrows that cross the membrane indicate the predominant direction of movement of each solute through the membrane; the relative size of the arrows indicates the net amounts of the solute transferred. Other arrows indicate the direction of flow. (From Forni LG, Hilton PJ: Continuous hemofiltration in the treatment of acute renal failure. N Engl J Med 1997;336:1303–1309.)

mortality and recovery of renal function in critically ill ARF patients. Unfortunately, studies to resolve this issue have often been confounded by poor design, and recent meta-analyses have not clarified this issue. Although more studies are needed, a reasonable recommendation can be made against the use of bioincompatible unsubstituted cuprophane membranes in the critically ill.

Hemodialfiltration (HDF) is usually performed in the intensive care unit (ICU) as a continuous modality. However, acute intermittent HDF can be performed in this setting with standard machinery, using sterile online replacement fluid generated from ultrapure dialysate, which is then diverted by a separate pump to be infused directly into the extracorporeal blood circuit. As with high-flux dialysis, limited clinical data do not show obvious advantages.

Dialysate for the single-pass machines is generated online with a proportionating system from concentrate using reverse osmosis–treated tap water. There is concern about the possibility of back-filtration of bacterial contaminants, specifically endotoxin, from the dialysate compartment into the patient, which could perpetuate microcirculatory insult and cytokine-mediated injury. As a minimum, dialysate for IHD should be of the same purity as that accepted for routine maintenance HD. Online replacement fluid

for intermittent HDF is produced by cold sterilization using ultrafilters in the dialysate pathway fluid and does not differ from commercial HF solutions and depyrogenated saline in terms of microbial counts, endotoxin concentration, and cytokine-inducing activity. Dialysate cold sterilization is also suggested by some for IHD, but there are insufficient data to support a strong recommendation and further studies are warranted.

Hemodynamic stability of critically ill patients during IHD is facilitated by accurate fluid removal, and computerized volumetric ultrafiltration control is therefore preferred. The capability for sodium profiling, ultrafiltration profiling, and blood temperature monitoring may be desirable (see later discussion).

Strategies to Reduce Intradialytic Hemodynamic Instability

Hypotension is detrimental for end-organ function and recovery in critically ill patients. Fresh ischemic lesions in kidney biopsy specimens can be found in patients with ARF of >3 weeks duration. The relatively high UFR with IHD often leads to intradialytic hypotension, which reduces residual renal function. A frequent schedule of IHD and prolonged treatment time will minimize ultrafiltration goals and rates and is the most effective measure to minimize hypotension.

Bicarbonate-buffered dialysate should be used routinely in critically ill ARF patients. It is associated with less hypotension than acetate dialysate, which has a peripheral vasodilating and myocardial depressant effect.

The rapid reduction in serum osmolality with IHD promotes water movement into cells, thus reducing effective circulating volume. Sodium profiling mitigates this process by promoting water flux into the vascular compartment, although the simpler approach of a high sodium dialysate without profiling also may achieve this and needs to be tested in the ICU setting. A randomized study showed that patients receiving IHD with sodium profiling (160 mmol/l initially reducing to 140 mmol/l) combined with ultrafiltration profiling (50% of ultrafiltration volume removed in first third of treatment) improved hemodynamic stability despite a larger ultrafiltration volume.[4] Profiling therefore seems to be safe and effective, although it should be used judiciously in the treatment of dysnatremias where a dialysate sodium should be chosen that allows for the slow correction of the serum sodium. Serum sodium should not be corrected faster than in the nondialysis population to minimize the risk of neurologic complications (see Chapter 8).

Blood volume monitoring with a biofeedback system automatically adjusts UFR and dialysate sodium content in response to a decrease in circulating blood volume, usually assessed by real-time hematocrit or plasma protein monitoring. Although effective for ESRD patients, a prospective observational study has suggested no benefit for critically ill ARF patients.[5]

High dialysate calcium (1.75 mmol/l) may increase cardiac output and peripheral vascular resistance and improve hemodynamic stability during IHD in ESRD patients with cardiomyopathy. This technique is limited by the development of hypercalcemia, however, and has not been studied in the critically ill ARF population.

Vasoconstriction due to lower body temperatures has been used to increase vascular resistance and improve hemodynamic stability during IHD in ESRD. Hypothermia, however, may be undesirable in critically ill patients due to an adverse effect on myocardial function, end-organ perfusion, blood clotting, and probably renal recovery. With blood temperature monitoring, the patients' blood temperature is maintained precisely at target value by a series of feedback loops controlling thermal transfer to and from the dialysate and is effective in ameliorating hemodynamic instability for ESRD patients. Blood temperature monitoring might conceivably allow for controlled cooling in critically ill ARF patients without the risk of hypothermic damage, but it has not been evaluated in this setting.

A number of observational studies in ESRD have suggested superior hemodynamic stability during intermittent HDF in comparison to conventional IHD. This could theoretically be related to heat loss in the circuit, lower sodium removal, higher calcium flux, and enhanced removal of endogenous vasoactive substances leading to increased peripheral vasoconstriction. Two prospective, controlled studies of HDF involving ESRD patients are contradictory with respect to hemodynamic stability,[6,7] and both have methodologic inadequacies.

Measures to reduce hemodynamic instability during IHD are summarized in Figure 87.2.[8] Should these measures fail, modality change to SLED or CRRT is recommended.

Dosing of Acute Intermittent Hemodialysis

Two recent studies support a relationship between acute IHD dose and mortality. A retrospective observational study showed

Measures to improve hemodynamic stability during intermittent HD

Minimize ultrafiltration rate requirements by
  Increased frequency of treatments (up to daily)
  Increased duration of treatments (up to 6 hours) then consider SLED or
  CRRT

Bicarbonate-buffered dialysate
Sodium/ultrafiltration profiling
? Increase dialysate [Ca^{2+}]
? Change modality from hemodialysis to hemodiafiltration
? Blood temperature monitoring

Figure 87.2 Measures to improve hemodynamic stability during intermittent hemodialysis (HD). CRRT, continuous renal replacement therapy; SLED, sustained low-efficiency dialysis. (Modified from Marshall M, Golper T: Intermittent hemodialysis. In Murray P, Brady H, Hall J [eds]: Intensive Care in Nephrology. Oxon, UK: Taylor & Francis, 2006, pp 181–198.)

that a delivered single-pool Kt/V (fractional clearance of body water for urea) >1.0 per treatment significantly improved outcome in patients with intermediate illness severity.[9] This study did not attempt to relate outcomes to the frequency of IHD. Most recently, a prospective, controlled trial demonstrated substantially improved outcomes with a cumulative single pool Kt/V of 6.0 versus 3.0 per week (by simple addition), and daily versus alternate-day treatments.[10] In this study, the time-averaged blood urea nitrogen (BUN) in the lower dose group (104 mg/dl) indicates underdialysis by contemporary standards, possibly exaggerating the result in the higher dose group. A further study is under way to confirm these findings.[11]

It is a reasonable recommendation to deliver a Kt/V >1.0 on at least 6 days per week. The required Kt/V for less frequent treatments can be established from the nomogram shown in Figure 87.3 that expresses combinations of IHD dose and treatment frequency as a continuous small-solute clearance.[12] These recommendations do not constitute consensus guidelines and do not account for any effect of IHD on the control of larger solutes.

Delivered IHD dose tends to be low in critically ill ARF patients. Measures to increase dialysis dose are summarized in Figure 87.4.[8]

CONTINUOUS RENAL REPLACEMENT THERAPY

CRRT involves the application of lower solute clearances and UFR for substantial periods every day. Solute removal is achieved using diffusion, convection, or a combination. CRRT was originally promoted for ultrafiltration of anuric patients, and it has now been shown effective as renal replacement therapy in patients hemodynamically intolerant to a regimen of conventional bicarbonate IHD.

CRRT is used to complement or supplant IHD in critically ill ARF patients. CRRT provides comparatively better hemodynamic stability and steady-state control of uremia, especially for severely catabolic patients. Consistent solute control avoids the water shifts during IHD that increase brain edema. However, interruptions to CRRT because of circuit clotting or out-of-unit procedures lead to a reduction in dose from down time as well as expense related to blood circuitry changes. Mean operating time for CRRT has been reported at 21.9 hr/day.[13]

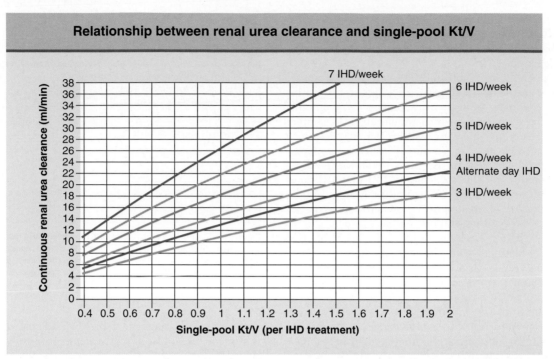

Figure 87.3   Relationship between corrected continuous renal urea clearance and single-pool Kt/V (fractional clearance of body water for urea) per treatment for a frequency of three to seven treatments per week. IHD, intermittent hemodialysis. (From Casino F, Lopez T: The equivalent renal urea clearance: A new parameter to assess dialysis. Nephrol Dial Transplant 1996;11:1574–1581.)

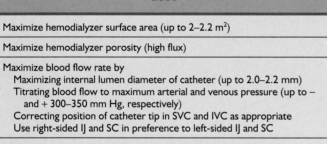

Measures to increase intermittent hemodialysis dose
Maximize hemodialyzer surface area (up to 2–2.2 m²)
Maximize hemodialyzer porosity (high flux)

Maximize blood flow rate by
  Maximizing internal lumen diameter of catheter (up to 2.0–2.2 mm)
  Titrating blood flow to maximum arterial and venous pressure (up to −
  and + 300–350 mm Hg, respectively)
  Correcting position of catheter tip in SVC and IVC as appropriate
  Use right-sided IJ and SC in preference to left-sided IJ and SC

Minimize access recirculation by correcting position of catheter tip in
  superior or inferior vena cava as appropriate using internal jugular and
  subclavian, rather than femoral, catheters

Maximize dialysate flow (up to 800–1000 ml/min)
Add postdilution HDF
Optimize anticoagulation to reduce hemodilyzer fiber bundle clotting
Optimize circulation to reduce compartmental urea sequestration
Increased treatment frequency (up to daily)
Increased treatment duration (up to 6–8 hours, then consider SLED or   CRRT)

Figure 87.4   Measures to increase intermittent hemodialysis dose. CRRT, continuous renal replacement therapy; HDF, hemodialfiltration; SLED, sustained low-efficiency dialysis. (Modified from Marshall M, Golper T: Intermittent hemodialysis. In Murray P, Brady H, Hall J [eds]: Intensive Care in Nephrology. Oxon, UK: Taylor & Francis, 2006, pp 181–198.)

Techniques of Continuous Renal Replacement Therapy

The Acute Dialysis Quality Initiative group (www.adqi.net) has proposed standardized classification, with nomenclature based on the type of vascular access and the method of solute removal.

Arteriovenous (AV) denotes an extracorporeal blood circuit in which an arterial catheter allows blood to circulate by systemic blood pressure. A venous catheter is placed for return. AV circuits are simple, but involve arterial puncture, which can lead to distal embolization, hemorrhage, and vessel damage. Qb 90 to 150 ml/min is typical in patients with mean arterial pressure >80 mm Hg, although flow can be erratic predisposing to clotting. Venovenous (VV) denotes a single- or dual-lumen catheter placed in a central vein, achieving more reliable and rapid Qb ~250 ml/min by a mechanical pump. Pumped VV circuits have the disadvantage of a possible inadvertent disconnection of the lines, resulting in hemorrhage or air embolism with continued pump operation; this risk is minimized but not eliminated by monitors and alarms.

Mechanisms of Solute Removal
Hemodialysis

Continuous HD provides diffusive small-solute transport that can be quantified according to the degree to which dialysate is saturated with urea (expressed as the ratio of dialysate to blood urea nitrogen or DUN/BUN). Qb and Qd during CRRT are usually relatively low (100 to 200 ml/min and 1 to 2 l/hr, respectively). Under these conditions, DUN/BUN is 1.0, indicating complete saturation. Urea clearance therefore equals Qd and is unaffected by Qb until it decreases to <50 ml/min.

With increasing Qd, there are proportionally decreasing gains in small-solute clearance as the DUN/BUN progressively decreases. Figure 87.5 illustrates this principle.[14] The flattening of the curves describes the conditions where increasing Qb does not enhance clearance. At Qb of 200 ml/min, urea clearance will correspond to Qd at a rate of 2 l/hr (or less) and will not increase with increased Qb. If Qd is increased to 4 l/hr, this will correspond to a

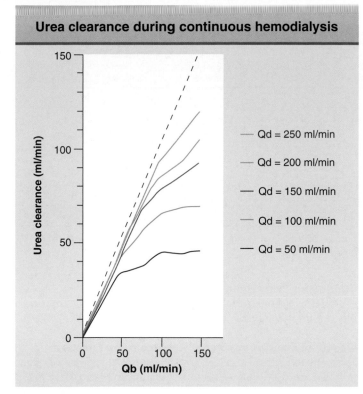

Figure 87.5 Determinants of urea clearance during continuous hemodialysis. Relationship among urea clearance, Qb (blood flow), and Qd (dialysate flow) during continuous hemodialysis. The flattening of the urea clearance curves describes the conditions in which increases in Qb do not enhance clearance. (From Kudoh Y, Iimura O: Slow continuous hemodialysis—new therapy for acute renal failure in critically ill patients—Part 1. Theoretical considerations and new technique. Jpn Circ J 1988;52:1171–1182.)

urea clearance of ~3 l/hr that will progressively increase with increased Qb.

Hemofiltration

Continuous HF provides convective small- and medium-sized–solute transport that can also be quantified by filtrate saturation with urea nitrogen (FUN/BUN). An important determinant of clearance is the site of fluid replacement, which can be infused either into the arterial blood line leading to the hemofilter (predilution) or into the venous blood line leaving the hemofilter (postdilution). The standard method is postdilution. However, higher UFR can lead to hemoconcentration in the hemofilter, increased resistance in the blood flow pathway, reductions in Qb, and ultimately hemofilter clotting. In practice, UFR should not exceed 30% of the plasma water flow rate (i.e., filtration fraction should be <0.30). The problem can be resolved by increasing Qb to 200 to 250 ml/min or more or by diluting the blood and clotting factors with replacement fluid before it reaches the hemofilter (predilution), thereby improving filter patency and decreasing anticoagulant requirements.

The disadvantage of predilution is that ultrafiltrate is generated from blood diluted with replacement fluid and therefore contains a lower concentration of uremic solutes. Lower small-solute clearances of about 15% are noted at low UFR, although this figure increases to about 40% with a higher UFR.[15,16] The clearance on any given solute during postdilution continuous HF is

$$K = UFR \times S,$$

where K is clearance (ml/min) and S is the sieving coefficient of the solute.

The clearance in predilution is

$$K = UFR \times S \times [Qbw/(Qbw + Qr)],$$

where Qbw is blood water flow rate and Qr is the replacement fluid rate.

Modern CRRT practice involves the generation of large ultrafiltrate volumes to achieve dose targets, resulting in higher filtration fractions and more hemofilter clotting. Predilution may therefore be preferable to improve filter life. The prime disadvantage of the predilution mode is the cost of increased fluid replacement.

Hemodialfiltration

Continuous HDF refers to a combination of the preceding techniques. With large enough membranes, the small solute clearances obtained approach the sum of the individual techniques.[15]

Specific Techniques

CRRT techniques are shown in Figures 87.6 and 87.7. The choice of technique is dependent on equipment availability, clinician expertise, prospects for vascular access, and whether the primary need is for fluid and/or solute removal. This last factor is often the most important since each technique provides different rates of solute and fluid removal. The substantially enhanced clearance capabilities of continuous AV (CAV)-HD/CAV-HDF or continuous VV (CVV)-HD/CVV-HDF allow these techniques to be applied to hypercatabolic or intoxicated patients. Most clinicians prefer pumped VV circuits because of reliable Qb and therefore higher solute clearance, as well as lower vascular complications rates, by avoiding arterial puncture. The potential complications of the techniques are listed in Figure 87.8.[17]

Slow Continuous Ultrafiltration

Slow continuous ultrafiltration (SCUF) is a dehydrating procedure providing slow fluid removal by filtration. Convective solute clearance is equal to the UFR (generally 4 to 5 ml/min). When solute control is important, such as for uremic or hypercatabolic patients, SCUF must be supplemented with either IHD or continuous HD.

Continuous Arteriovenous Hemofiltration

CAV-HF is similar to SCUF except that UFR is greater than that required for the restoration of euvolemia, and replacement fluid is administered to prevent hypovolemia. UFR and hence convective solute clearance tend to be lower in CAV-HF than pumped CRRT techniques as a result of erratic and lower Qb.

Continuous Venovenous Hemofiltration

CVV-HF is similar to CAV-H except that the VV access and pumped circuit allows for a higher UFR and convective solute clearance. CVV-HF is therefore preferable to CAV-HF when solute control is important.

Continuous Arteriovenous Hemodialysis

CAV-HD differs from CAV-HF in that solute removal is diffusive and dependent on Qb and Qd. Unlike CAV-HF, UFR is not maximized, but set as required to restore euvolemia.

Continuous Venovenous Hemodialysis

CVV-HD is similar to CAV-HD except that the VV access and pumped circuit allow for higher Qb and diffusive solute clearance. A prospective study comparing CVV-HD with CAV-HD did not show a survival difference (52% versus 43%) when urea clearances were not different (37 l/day versus 33 l/day).[18]

Comparison of continuous renal replacement modalities

Modality	Blood Pump	Dialysate (D) Replacement Fluid (RF)	Urea Clearance (l/day)	Urea Clearance (ml/min)	Middle Molecular Clearance	Complexity
Slow continuous ultrafiltration	Yes/no	No	1–4	1–3	+	+
Continuous arteriovenous hemofiltration	No	RF	10–15	7–10	++	+
Continuous venovenous hemofiltration	Yes	RF	22–24	15–17	+++	++
Continuous arteriovenous hemodialysis	No	D	24–30	17–21	–	+
Continuous venovenous hemodialysis	Yes	D	24–30	17–21	–	++
Continuous arteriovenous hemodiafiltration	No	RF+D	36–38	25–26	+++	+++
Continuous venovenous hemodiafiltration	Yes	RF+D	36–38	25–26	+++	+++

Figure 87.6 **Comparison of different continuous renal replacement modalities.** +, simplest; +++, most complex. (Modified from Manns M, Sigler MH, Teehan BP: Continuous renal replacement therapies: An update. Am J Kidney Dis 1998;32:185–207.)

Continuous Arteriovenous Hemodialfiltration

CAV-HDF is similar to CAV-HD, except that UFR is greater than that required for the restoration of euvolemia, and replacement fluid is required to prevent hypovolemia. CAV-HDF combines diffusion, which favors small-solute removal, with convection, which removes both small and medium-sized solutes.

Continuous Venovenous Hemodialfiltration

CVV-HDF is similar to CAV-HDF except that VV access and a blood pump are used.

Dosing of Continuous Renal Replacement Therapy

A recent large, prospective, randomized trial comparing three doses of postdilution continuous HF determined that UFR of

Continuous renal replacement therapies

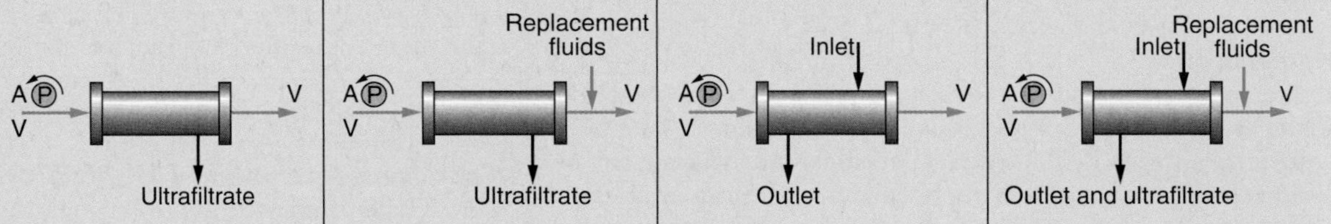

	Slow continuous ultrafiltration	Continuous hemofiltration	Continuous hemodialysis	Continuous hemodiafiltration
Arteriovenous (AV) or venovenous (VV)	AV or VV	AV or VV	AV or VV	AV or VV
Blood flow (ml/min)	50–100	50–200	50–200	50–200
Dialysate flow (ml/min)	–	–	10–20	10–20
Clearance (l/24 hr)	–	12–36	14–36	20–40
Ultrafiltration rate (ml/min)	2–5	8–25	2–4	8–12
Blood filter	Highly permeable filter	Highly permeable filter	Low-permeability dialyzer with countercurrent flow through the dialyzer compartment	High permeability dialyzer with countercurrent flow through the dialyzer compartment
Ultrafiltrate	Corresponds exactly to the patient's weight loss	Replaced in part or completely to achieve purification and volume control	Corresponds to patient's weight loss; solute clearance by diffusion	In excess of patient's weight loss; solute clearance by both diffusion and convection
Replacement fluid	None	Yes	None	Yes, to achieve fluid balance
Efficiency	Used only for fluid control in overhydrated states	Clearance for all solutes equals ultrafiltration	Limited to small molecules	Extends from small to large molecules

Figure 87.7 **Continuous renal replacement therapy modalities.** The pump (P) is used only in venovenous modes. (Modified from Ronco C: Continuous renal replacement therapies for the treatment for acute renal failure in intensive care patients. Clin Nephrol 1993;40:187–198.)

Complications of continuous renal replacement therapy	
Technical	Clinical
Vascular access malfunction	Hemorrhage
Circuit clotting	Hematomas
Catheter and circuit kinking	Thrombosis
Line disconnections	Hypothermia
Insufficient blood flow	Allergic reactions
Air embolism	Nutrient losses
Fluid balance errors	Insufficient clearance
Loss of efficiency	Hypotension
	Arrhythmias

Figure 87.8 Complications of continuous renal replacement therapy. (Reproduced from Ronco C, Bellomo R: Complications with renal replacement therapy. Am J Kidney Dis 1996;28[Suppl 3]:S100–S104.)

>35 ml/hr/kg (based on premorbid or pre-ICU weight) was associated with highest survival. The broad relevance of the study may be limited by the small patient size (average patient weight 68 kg) and the predominantly postsurgical causes of ARF (sepsis comprised only 12% of the cases, trauma 12%, medical causes 13%). Two further studies are under way to determine whether these findings can be extrapolated to continuous HDF,[11,19] although a reasonable interim recommendation can be made for all CRRT to deliver a minimum small-solute clearance of 35 ml/hr/kg. In predilution continuous HF, the UFR required to achieve small-solute clearance targets can be calculated[20]:

$$ UFR = \frac{Qbw \times K_{target} \times (Wt/60)}{(Qbw - K_{target} \times (Wt/60))} \times 60/Wt $$

where Wt is body weight, where K_{target} is the small-solute clearance target (here being 35 ml/hr/kg). For example, a UFR of 42.4 ml/hr/kg should be prescribed to deliver this K_{target} to an 80kg person using predilution continuous HF with Qb of 267 ml/min in a patient with a hematocrit of 0.25. These recommendations do not constitute consensus standards and do not account for the effect of CRRT on the control of larger solutes. Optimal patient outcomes with continuous HF therefore appear to require ultrafiltrate volumes of approximately 60 l/day.

High-volume HR (UFR >100 ml/hr/kg) has been used recently to facilitate removal of proinflammatory cytokines in septic shock. Preliminary data suggest improved hemodynamic stability, but need corroboration in controlled studies.

Technical Aspects of Continuous Renal Replacement Therapy
Equipment
VV CRRT requires a blood pump, a hemofilter or hemodialyzer, arterial and venous pressure monitors, an air detection system, a method for removing air bubbles, and a system to balance dialysate inflow/replacement fluid with dialysate outflow/filtrate. Integrated machinery dedicated to CRRT are commercially available with computerized volumetric balancing allowing accurate and reliable treatment delivery.

Hemofilters
Specific artificial kidneys for CRRT are usually referred to as hemofilters. However, conventional inexpensive hemodialyzers can serve as hemofilters by occluding one of the dialysate ports and connecting the other to a drainage system. To achieve adequate UFR, the surface area must be large ($\sim$2 m^2) for low-flux or, alternatively, more modest ($\sim$0.5 m^2) for high-flux hemodialyzers. Some CRRT machines, however, require the use of a specific hemofilter because of a unique cartridge system (e.g., Prisma-Gambro/Hospal). Sieving coefficients of small solutes are usually preserved throughout the life of all such hemofilters.

A promising innovation has been the recent use of super-flux hemofilters with molecular weight cutoff of 100 to 150 kd. When used with CRRT and IHD *ex vivo* or in healthy volunteers, significant convective removal of proinflammatory cytokines can be achieved, and studies are under way in the critically ill ARF population.

Replacement Fluids and Dialysate
CRRT requires sterile replacement fluid or dialysate for blood purification, with composition that is determined by the clinical requirements for acid-base control and electrolyte management. Fluids can be prepared aseptically in hospital pharmacies or are available commercially, although this adds greatly to cost. A commonly used regimen consists of a blended mixture of 1 liter of each of four different solutions, which are kept separately until allowed to mix via a multiprong adapter just before entering the blood pathway:
1. Isotonic saline (0.9% NaCl) plus 7.5 ml 10% calcium chloride (5.2 mmol calcium)
2. Isotonic saline plus 1.6 ml 50% magnesium sulfate (3.2 mmol magnesium)
3. Half-isotonic saline
4. Half-isotonic saline plus 150 mmol sodium bicarbonate

Options for replacement fluids are summarized in Figure 87.9.

Buffer choice is between bicarbonate and lactate, which metabolizes in the liver to bicarbonate in a 1:1 ratio. Although many patients tolerate lactate solutions, bicarbonate solutions are superior in terms of acid-base control, hemodynamic stability, urea generation, cerebral dysfunction, and possibly survival in patients with a history of cardiovascular disease. Overall, bicarbonate has become the buffer of choice and is preferred in patients with lactic acidosis and/or liver failure. If lactate-buffered fluids are used, the development of lactate intolerance (>5 mmol/l increase in serum lactate during CRRT) may require a switch to bicarbonate-based fluid. Bicarbonate concentrations in fluid are typically 25 to 35 mmol/l: concentrations in the lower part of this range are indicated during high-dose or prolonged CRRT and during regional citrate anticoagulation therapy to prevent metabolic alkalosis.

Glucose concentrations in fluids range from 0.1% in commercially prepared fluids to 1.5% to 4.25% in PD fluids adapted for use with CRRT. Up to 3600 kcal/day may be derived from these latter solutions, although hyperglycemia may supervene to the detriment of patient outcomes. It is recommended that glucose intake is <5 g/kg/day and that glucose concentration in fluid is $\sim$100 to 180 mg/dl ($\sim$5.5 to 10 mmol/l) to maintain zero glucose balance.

Intravenous phosphate supplementation is often required during CRRT and is usually administered separately due to the potential for precipitation with calcium and magnesium in dialysate or replacement fluid. This concern may have been overstated in the past, and phosphate has been safely supplemented by injecting phosphate into these solutions.

Replacement fluids for CRRT							
Component (mmol/l)	Dialysis Machine Generated*	Peritoneal Dialysis Fluid†	Lactated Ringer's Solution	Accusol† (2.5-liter bag)	Primasate‡ (5-liter bag)	Nxstage§ (5-liter bag)	Normocarb‖
Sodium	140	132	130	140	140	140	140
Potassium	Variable	—	4	0 or 2 or 4	0 or 2 or 4	0 or 2 or 4	0
Chloride	Variable	96	109	109.5 to 116.3	108 to 120.5	109 to 113	106
Bicarbonate	Variable	—	—	30 or 35	22 or 32	35	35
Calcium	Variable	3.5	2.7	2.8 or 3.5	0 or 2.5 or 3.5	3	0
Magnesium	1.5	0.5	—	1 or 1.5	1.0 or 1.5	1	1.5
Lactate	2	40	28	0	3	0	0
Glucose (mg/dl)	100	1360	—	0 or 110	0 or 110	100	—
Preparation method	6-liter bag via membrane filtration	Premix	Premix	Two-compartment bag	Two-compartment bag or Premix	Two-compartment bag or Premix	Vial mix added to 3-liter sterile water bag
Sterility	No	Yes	Yes	Yes	Yes	Yes	Yes

Figure 87.9 Replacement fluids for continuous renal replacement therapy (CRRT). Examples of replacement fluids that are suitable for CRRT. Dialysis machine generated ultrapure dialysate and peritoneal dialysis fluid are used for continuous hemodialysis (HD) only. Lactated Ringer's solution and commercial hemodialfiltration (HDF) fluids are used for continuous HD, HF (hemofiltration), and HDF. *Leblanc et al.[30] †Dianeal 1.5%, Baxter Healthcare Corp. ‡Gambro Renal Products. §Nxstage Medical Inc. ‖B. Braun Medical Inc.

A novel method of preparing bicarbonate buffered fluid is by ultrafiltering dialysate using a standard HD machine and storing the solution in 6-liter drainage bags used for automated PD. Fluid prepared in this manner is usually used promptly, although it is reported to remain sterile for up to a month, with endotoxin levels below the limit of detection. Such solutions are used for dialysate rather than replacement fluid and are combined with ultrafiltration to prevent backfiltration through the hemodialyzer. Pioneered by the Cleveland Clinic Foundation, there have been no reported adverse events in the 10-year experience of this technique.

SUSTAINED LOW-EFFICIENCY DIALYSIS

Experience is increasing with so-called hybrid therapies that use standard IHD equipment and accessories, but with lower solute clearances and UFR maintained for prolonged periods of time.[21] The systems are fully monitored and have computerized volumetric ultrafiltration control. Qd and urea clearances are higher than in conventional CVV-HD, which allows for scheduled down time without compromise in dialysis dose.

SLED provides a high dose of dialysis with minimal urea disequilibrium, online bicarbonate dialysate, excellent control of electrolytes, and good tolerance to ultrafiltration. Clearance is predominantly diffusive, although there is increasing experience combined diffusive and convective clearance via HDF using online replacement fluid. Hemodialyzer clotting is a common complication; monitoring the degree to which dialysate is saturated with urea may enable elective blood circuit changes and optimization of anticoagulation prior to complete clotting. Survival in the reported observational series has not differed from that predicted by a variety of illness severity scores. ARRT that is easiest to administer will be the most popular if all such outcomes are equivalent, and SLED may become the therapy of choice in this setting, as it is safe, convenient, inexpensive, and effective in achieving goals for solute and fluid removal.

VASCULAR ACCESS

A prerequisite for all ARRT modalities is reliable vascular access. This is usually via uncuffed single- or double-lumen polyurethane or silicone catheters in the internal jugular (IJ), subclavian (SC), or femoral (FE) veins. SC catheters are associated with a higher incidence of procedural complications, venous stenosis, and thrombosis.

For CRRT, Qb <250 ml/min is usually sufficient. For IHD, higher Qb is required to provide sufficient solute clearance and can be safely increased until venous and arterial pressures are plus and minus 350 mm Hg, respectively, after which hemolysis can occur. Left-sided IJ and SC catheters provide flows that are more erratic and up to 100 ml/min lower than elsewhere because their tips abut the vein walls. FE and right-sided IJ or SC catheters provide the best Qb.[22] Catheters with larger bore lines are preferred.

Using ultrasound dilution, access recirculation for all sites is approximately 10% at Qb 250 to 350 ml/min and may increase to as much as 35% at Qb >500 ml/min. Recirculation depends on the site of the catheter; it is negligible in IJ catheters and highest in FE catheter <20 cm. Up to half of acute IHD treatments will require catheters to be used in reversed configuration, such that the original venous line is used as for blood inflow (relative to dialyzer), and the original arterial line for outflow. Access recirculation in this situation doubles to ~20% at 250 to 350 ml/min.[22] Access recirculation also affects dialysis dose; in one study, the urea reduction ratio was significantly higher with SC (62.5%) versus FE (54.5%) catheters despite identical IHD operating parameters.[23]

Infection of temporary catheters is common. Bacteremia, exit site infection, and distant infection occurred in one series at 6.2, 3.6, and 1.1 episodes per 1000 catheter days.[22] The risk of bacteremia is highest with FE catheters and lowest with SC catheters. Although there are generally fewer data than for tunneled catheters, both povidone and mupirocin ointments with dry gauze exit site dressings have been shown to reduce the risk of bacteremia in temporary catheters.

The Centers for Disease Control and Prevention recommend that temporary catheters in the ICU setting should be changed when clinically indicated rather than routinely since the risks of the catheterization outweigh the supposed benefit of reduced infection risk.[24] K-DOQI (Kidney Disease Outcomes Quality Initiative)[25] recommends that SC and IJ catheters should be changed after 3 weeks and FE catheters after 5 days in the non-ICU setting due to increased infection risk.

ANTICOAGULATION IN ACUTE RENAL REPLACEMENT THERAPY

Anticoagulation during ARRT ideally should prevent clotting in the extracorporeal circuit without producing significant systemic anticoagulation. Most commonly, unfractionated heparin is infused into the most proximal part of the extracorporeal circuit keeping the activated partial thromboplastin time (APTT) in the venous blood line 1.5 to two times the control value and the systemic APTT <50 seconds. This typically requires an initial bolus dose of ~2000 U and maintenance infusion of ~500 U/hr. Low-molecular-weight heparin is theoretically advantageous because of increased antithrombotic activity and decreased hemorrhagic risk. However, disadvantages include a prolonged half-life (approximately doubled in renal failure), incomplete reversal with protamine, and limited availability of appropriate monitoring by serial anti–factor Xa determinations. Most experience is with dalteparin, and the optimal dose appears to be an initial bolus of ~20 to 30 U/kg (IHD and CRRT), followed by an infusion of ~10 U/kg/hr (CRRT). Other systemic anticoagulants include lepirudin (recombinant hirudin) and argatroban, which are direct thrombin inhibitors, and fondaparinux, which is a synthetic pentasaccharide that inhibits factor Xa by binding to antithrombin. Experience with these anticoagulants is limited, although they are the anticoagulants of choice in patients with heparin-induced thrombocytopenia who also require ARRT.

For those receiving systemic anticoagulation with heparin, the incidence of significant bleeding complications is between 25% and 30%, and 4% of such patients die as a result of hemorrhage. Most patients can successfully avoid any anticoagulation during IHD, but only a minority during CRRT. Alternatives to systemic anticoagulation include regional citrate anticoagulation (RCA), regional heparin anticoagulation, and prostacyclin (epoprostenol), which is a potent inhibitor of platelet aggregation that essentially acts as a regional anticoagulant. The lowest rates of hemorrhage and greatest prolongation of filter life are associated with RCA, and it is the preferred regional technique.

RCA involves calcium chelation in the extracorporeal blood circuit with calcium reversal. For IHD, this most commonly involves an infusion of 4% trisodium citrate (TSC) into the proximal circuit, with an infusion of calcium chloride into the venous blood line. A simpler approach has been described in which the TSC infusion is combined with normal calcium dialysate and no calcium infusion. The positive calcium flux through the hemodialyzer maintains calcium balance without the need for a separate infusion and provides partial chelation of the undialyzed citrate.

For CRRT, RCA may be performed using 4% TSC or with ACD-A solution (anticoagulant citrate dextrose A) containing 3% combined TSC (2.2 g/100 ml), citric acid (0.73 g/100 ml),

and dextrose (2.45 g/100 ml). ACD-A is preferred over TSC as it is less hypertonic and commercially widely available, potentially reducing complications from overinfusion and mixing errors. For continuous HD, a prefilter infusion of 3% to 7% of Qb with a postfilter infusion of calcium chloride is used. This requires dialysate that is hyponatremic and devoid of alkali because citrate metabolizes to bicarbonate in the liver in a 1:3 ratio. For continuous HF, a prefilter infusion of substitution fluid can be used that contains no calcium but citrate as buffer (Fig. 87.10). Frequent monitoring and titration of citrate dose are needed to keep the ionized calcium within a therapeutic range. The major complications of RCA are systemic hypocalcemia and metabolic alkalosis from citrate toxicity, particularly in patients with liver dysfunction.

Regional heparin anticoagulation involves neutralization of heparin by infusion of protamine into the venous blood line. It may be complicated by rebound bleeding, occurring when neutralization with protamine wears out faster than the anticoagulation from heparin. Furthermore, protamine may cause sudden hypotension, bradycardia, or anaphylactoid reactions.

Prostacyclin is an effective alternative anticoagulant. However, it is a vasodilator, causing a variable but occasionally marked decrease in blood pressure.

OUTCOMES AND MODALITY CHOICE IN ACUTE RENAL REPLACEMENT THERAPY

The prime advantage of CRRT appears to be the increased hemodynamic stability it affords in the critically ill. Observational reports have previously suggested improved survival with CRRT, but numerous confounding variables have made definitive comparison with IHD difficult. A recent randomized, controlled study did not demonstrate any differences in mortality, length of hospital stay, and recovery of renal function between groups treated with CRRT and IHD.[26] Although this study is difficult to interpret because of irregularities in the randomization process, a report in which patients were well matched after randomization and received equivalent dialysis dose also showed no difference in survival or duration of ARF.[27] To resolve this question will require large studies with rigorous standardization of patient care between groups.

The relationship between modality choice and outcomes is currently under study in specific clinical situations such as acute lung injury, sepsis, and acute cardiac decompensation. Such studies may yet yield definitive data, but in the interim, modality choice depends on the patient's condition and the clinical objectives. IHD can provide safe and effective renal replacement therapy in most cases, with recourse to other therapies as the individual situation dictates. For example, CRRT will be more appropriate for a patient unable to achieve ultrafiltration goals using IHD because of hemodynamic instability, and intermittent high-efficiency postdilution HDF may be more appropriate than IHD for a highly catabolic patient.

The skill and experience of the staff providing renal replacement therapy probably influence patient outcomes as much as the choice of modality.[28] In many parts of the world, all modalities of ARRT are now delivered by ICU staff; in other countries, support from nephrology staff is still sought. As machinery platforms are becoming universal for CRRT and IHD, it is likely that ICU expertise in all modalities of RRT will grow, provided in-service education and support are sufficient to develop and maintain the medical and nursing skill base.

	Modality	Blood Flow (ml/min)	Replacement Fluid Composition (mmol/l)	Dialysis Fluid Composition (mmol/l)	Citrate Source
Comparison of regional citrate anticoagulation protocols					
Mehta et al.[31] (1990)	CAV-HD	52–125	Normal saline	Na 117, Cl 122.5, Mg 0.75, K 4, dextrose 2.5%	4% Trisodium citrate
Palsson and Niles[32] (1999)	CVV-HD	180	Citrate 13.3, Na 140, Cl 101.5, Mg 0.75, dextrose 0.2%	—	Customized citrate solution
Tolwani et al.[33] (2001)	CVV-HD	125–150	—	Normal saline + MgSO$_4$ 1.0, KCl 3	4% Trisodium citrate
Hofmann et al.[34] (2002)	CVV-HD	125	Prefilter: normal saline + KC14, alternate with 0.45% saline + KC14 Postfilter: 0.45% saline +MgSO$_4$+ CaCl$_2$	—	4% Trisodium citrate
Tobe et al.[35] (2003)	CVV-HDF	100	Normal saline	Normocarb	ACD-A
Mitchell et al.[36] (2003)	CVV-HD	75	—	Variable Ca 1.75–1.78	ACD-A
Swartz et al.[37] (2004)	CVV-HD	200	—	Na 135, HCO$_3$ 28, Cl 105, MgSO$_4$ 1.3, glucose 1g/l	ACD-A
Gupta et al.[38] (2004)	CVV-HDF	150	Normal saline ±MgSO$_4$ and KCl	PD fluid: Na 132, Ca 1.25, Cl 95, Mg 0.5, lactate 360 mg/dl, 1.5% dextrose	ACD-A

Figure 87.10 Comparison of regional citrate anticoagulation protocols. ACD-A, anticoagulant citrate dextrose form A; CAV-HD, continuous arteriovenous hemodialysis; CVV-HD, continuous venovenous hemodialysis; CVV-HDF, continuous venovenous hemodialfiltration.

COST OF ACUTE RENAL REPLACEMENT THERAPY

Extracorporeal circuits and artificial kidneys for CRRT are more expensive than those for IHD. In the United States, the reimbursement structure inflates the cost of replacement fluid that is prepared in hospital pharmacies. CRRT is therefore more expensive than IHD in the United States, but this is not necessarily so elsewhere. For example, a comparison at Guys Hospital, London, in the late 1990s showed no substantial difference between the estimated cost of CVV-HD (US$1190 [£750] weekly) and intermittent HD (US$1152 [£700] weekly).[29]

DRUG DOSING IN ACUTE RENAL REPLACEMENT THERAPY

For patients undergoing CRRT, 20 liters of daily filtrate correspond to a glomerular filtration rate (GFR) of ~14 ml/min, and the dose of drugs should be calculated as for a patient with a GFR of 14 ml/min. Although losses of dopamine, epinephrine, and norepinephrine do occur, these agents are usually dosed by titration. Any drug with a low therapeutic index that can be readily measured should be measured frequently early in the course of ARRT, until a stable pattern appears. One day of CRRT is in general comparable to one IHD treatment with regard to drug removal.

REFERENCES

1. De Vriese AS, Colardyn FA, Philippe JJ, et al: Cytokine removal during continuous hemofiltration in septic patients. J Am Soc Nephrol 1999; 10:846–853.
2. Forni LG, Hilton PJ: Continuous hemofiltration in the treatment of acute renal failure. N Engl J Med 1997;336:1303–1309.
3. Ponikvar J, Rus R, Kenda R, et al: Low-flux versus high-flux synthetic dialysis membranes in acute renal failure: Prospective randomized study. Artif Organs 2001;25:946–950.
4. Paganini E, Sandy D, Moreno L, et al: The effect of sodium and ultrafiltration modeling on plasma volume and haemodynamic stability in intensive care patients receiving haemodialysis for acute renal failure: A prospective, stratified, randomized, cross-over study. Nephrol Dial Transplant 1996; 11(Suppl):32–37.
5. Tonelli M, Astephen P, Andreou P, et al: Blood volume monitoring in intermittent hemodialysis for acute renal failure. Kidney Int 2002;62: 1075–1080.
6. Locatelli F, Mastrangelo F, Redaelli B, et al: Effects of different membranes and dialysis technologies on patient treatment tolerance and nutritional parameters. Kidney Int 1996;50:1293–1302.
7. Movilli E, Camerini C, Zein H, et al: A prospective comparison of bicarbonate dialysis, hemodiafiltration, and acetate-free biofiltration in the elderly. Am J Kidney Dis 1996;27:541–547.
8. Marshall M, Golper T: Intermittent hemodialysis. In Murray P, Brady H, Hall J (eds): Intensive Care in Nephrology. Oxon, UK: Taylor & Francis, 2006, pp 181–198.
9. Paganini EP, Tapolyai M, Goormastic M, et al: Establishing a dialysis therapy/patient outcome link in intensive care unit acute dialysis for patients with acute renal failure. Am J Kidney Dis 1996;28(Suppl): S81–S89.
10. Schiffl H, Lang S, Fischer R: Daily hemodialysis and the outcomes of acute renal failure. N Engl J Med 2002;346:305–310.
11. Palevsky P, O'Conner T, Zhang J, et al: Design of the VA/NIH Acute Renal Failure Trial Network (ATN) Study: Intensive versus conventional renal support in acute renal failure. Clin Trials 2005;2:423–435.
12. Casino F, Lopez T: The equivalent renal urea clearance: A new parameter to assess dialysis. Nephrol Dial Transplant 1996;11:1574–1581.
13. Frankenfield D, Reynolds H, Wiles C, et al: Urea removal during continuous hemodiafiltration. Crit Care Med 1993;22:407–412.

14. Kudoh Y, Iimura O: Slow continuous hemodialysis—new therapy for acute renal failure in critically ill patients—Part 1. Theoretical considerations and new technique. Jpn Circ J 1988;52:1171–1182.

15. Brunet S, Leblanc M, Geadah D, et al: Diffusive and convective solute clearances during continuous renal replacement therapy at various dialysate and ultrafiltration flow rates. Am J Kidney Dis 1999;34:486–492.

16. Troyanov S, Cardinal J, Geadah D, et al: Solute clearances during continuous venovenous hemofiltration at various ultrafiltration flow rates using Multiflow-100 and HF1000 filters. Nephrol Dial Transplant 2003;18:961–966.

17. Ronco C, Bellomo R: Complications with renal replacement therapy. Am J Kidney Dis 1996;28(Suppl 3):S100–S104.

18. Bellomo R, Parkin G, Love J, et al: A prospective comparative study of continuous arteriovenous hemodiafiltration and continuous venovenous hemodiafiltration in critically ill patients. Am J Kidney Dis 1993;21:400–404.

19. http://www.clinicaltrials.gov/ct/show/NCT00221013

20. Marshall M: The current status of dosing and quantification of acute renal replacement therapy. Nephrology 2006;11:181–191.

21. Marshall MR, Golper TA, Shaver MJ, et al: Sustained low-efficiency dialysis for critically ill patients requiring renal replacement therapy. Kidney Int 2001;60:777–785.

22. Oliver M: Acute dialysis catheters. Semin Dial 2001;14:432–435.

23. Leblanc M, Fedak S, Mokris G, et al: Blood recirculation in temporary central catheters for acute hemodialysis. Clin Nephrol 1996;45:315–319.

24. Centers for Disease Control and Prevention: Guidelines for the prevention of intravascular catheter-related infections. MMWR 2002;51(RR-10).

25. National Kidney Foundation: K/DOQI clinical practice guidelines for vascular access, 2000. Am J Kidney Dis 2001;37(Suppl 1):S137–S181.

26. Mehta RL, McDonald B, Gabbai FB, et al: A randomized clinical trial of continuous versus intermittent dialysis for acute renal failure. Kidney Int 2001;60:1154–1163.

27. Augustine JJ, Sandy D, Seifert TH, et al: A randomized controlled trial comparing intermittent with continuous dialysis in patients with ARF. Am J Kidney Dis 2004;44:1000–1007.

28. Lameire N, Van Beisen W, Vanholder R: Dialysing the patient with acute renal failure in the ICU: The emperor's clothes? Nephrol Dial Transplant 1999;14:2570–2573.

29. Silvester W: Outcome studies of continuous renal replacement therapy in the intensive care unit. Kidney Int 1998;53(Suppl 66):S138–S141.

30. Leblanc M, Moreno L, Robinson OP, et al: Bicarbonate dialysate for continuous renal replacement therapy in intensive care unit patients with acute renal failure. Am J Kidney Dis 1995;26:910–917.

31. Mehta RL, McDonald BR, Aguilar MM, et al: Regional citrate anticoagulation for continuous arteriovenous hemodialysis in critically ill patients. Kidney Int 1990;38:976–981.

32. Palsson R, Niles JL: Regional citrate anticoagulation in continuous venovenous hemofiltration in critically ill patients with a high risk of bleeding. Kidney Int 1999;55:1991–1997.

33. Hofmann RM, Maloney C, Ward DM, et al: A novel method for regional citrate anticoagulation in continuous venovenous hemofiltration (CVVHF). Ren Fail 2002;24:325–335.

34. Tolwani AJ, Campbell RC, Schenk MB, et al: Simplified citrate anticoagulation for continuous renal replacement therapy. Kidney Int 2001;60:370–374.

35. Tobe SW, Aujla P, Walele AA, et al: A novel regional citrate anticoagulation protocol for CRRT using only commercially available solutions. J Crit Care 2003;18:121–129.

36. Mitchell A, Daul AE, Beiderlinden M, et al: A new system for regional citrate anticoagulation in continuous venovenous hemodialysis (CVVHD). Clin Nephrol 2003;59:106–114.

37. Swartz R, Pasko D, O'Toole J, et al: Improving the delivery of continuous renal replacement therapy using regional citrate anticoagulation. Clin Nephrol 2004;61:134–143.

38. Gupta M, Wadhwa NK, Bukovsky R: Regional citrate anticoagulation for continuous venovenous hemodiafiltration using calcium-containing dialysate. Am J Kidney Dis 2004;43:67–73.

88 Plasma Exchange

Jeremy Levy and Charles D. Pusey

INTRODUCTION

The place of plasma exchange (plasmapheresis) in the management of renal disease remains controversial, largely because of the paucity of controlled studies comparing plasma exchange with other treatments. The techniques for separating plasma from cells were initially developed during the 1940s and 1950s, but only put into widespread clinical use after early reports of the beneficial effects in Goodpasture's disease in the mid-1970s. More recently, plasma exchange has been used to remove many large-molecular-weight substances from plasma, including pathogenic antibodies, cryoglobulins, and lipoproteins. Newer techniques have also been developed to allow more selective removal of plasma components, such as double filtration plasmapheresis, cryofiltration, and immunoadsorption.

TECHNIQUES

Therapeutic plasma exchange can be carried out either by centrifugal cell separators or, more commonly in renal units, with hollow-fiber plasma filters and standard hemodialysis equipment (Figs 88.1 and 88.2). Centrifugal devices allow withdrawal of plasma from a bowl with either synchronous or intermittent return of blood cells to the patient. There is no upper limit to the molecular weight of proteins removed by this method. The bowls and circuits are single use and disposable, and blood flow rates generally relatively low (90 to 150 ml/min). Platelet loss is a particular problem with centrifugal devices, and platelet counts can decrease by as much as 50%. Membrane plasma filtration uses highly permeable hollow fibers with membrane pores 0.2 to 0.5 μm. Plasma readily passes through the membrane, while the cells are simultaneously returned to the patient. All immunoglobulins will cross the membrane (IgG more efficiently than IgM); however, some large immune complexes and cryoglobulins may not be adequately cleared, although many membranes allow for clearance of molecules up to 3 million daltons. There is no loss of platelets, but hemolysis can occur if transmembrane pressures are too high (a rare complication). Blood flow rates are generally between 90 and 200 ml/min, and there is no increase in rate of plasma filtration at higher blood flows, but an increased risk of hemolysis. Membranes used in plasma filters are generally synthetic and may be polysulfone, polypropylene, cellulose diacetate, polymethylmethacrylate, or polyacrylonitrile. It has been suggested that the adsorptive properties of the membrane for cytokines and other biomolecules may account for some of the beneficial effects of plasma filtration. There have been occasional reports of mild adverse reactions in patients taking angiotensin-converting enzyme inhibitors when plasma is filtered using ethylene vinyl alcohol or acrylic copolymer membranes. Reuse of plasma filters is not advised, but performance data does not indicate a major loss of function during routine plasma exchange.

All methods of plasma exchange require vascular access. Generally, this is achieved using standard central venous catheters, but if a patient already has an arteriovenous fistula, then of course this can be used. However, it is also possible to perform plasma exchange using peripheral access through large-bore, short, intravenous cannulas, placed in the antecubital fossa, since the blood flow rates required are low. Single-needle access is also relatively easy to accommodate, especially for centrifugal plasma exchange, in which the blood removal and return can be asynchronous, but also for membrane filtration. Anticoagulation is almost always needed and must be carefully managed in patients with a bleeding risk, for example, those with hemolytic uremic syndrome (HUS), recent or ongoing pulmonary hemorrhage, or a recent renal biopsy. Generally, citrate is used for centrifugal plasma exchange, and heparin for membrane plasma filtration; however, citrate has particular advantages in patients at higher bleeding risk in view of its lack of systemic anticoagulant actions. Where heparin is used, higher doses may be needed than in hemodialysis as a result of increased losses during the procedure (heparin is protein bound). Bolus doses of unfractionated heparin 2000 to 5000 U are given initially, and then 500 to 2000 U/hr. Anticoagulant is administered prefilter. Citrate toxicity (by inducing hypocalcemia) can occur even if citrate is not used for anticoagulation since fresh-frozen plasma (FFP) contains a high concentration of citrate (up to 14% by volume) and manifests initially as perioral tingling and paresthesias.

Both methods of plasma exchange require large volumes of colloid replacement. A single plasma volume exchange will lower plasma macromolecule levels by approximately 60%, and five exchanges over 5 to 10 days will clear 90% of the total body immunoglobulin (Fig. 88.3).[1] For most patients, this is achieved by removing 50 ml/kg plasma at each procedure (~4 liters for a 75-kg person). Daily plasma exchange is likely to be most effective in rapidly depleting total body load in view of redistribution of immunoglobulins from the extravascular compartments, but there is no good evidence that intensity of exchanges has a major effect on outcomes except in patients with HUS with poor prognostic markers (see later discussion). Indeed, alternate-day exchanges are of proven efficacy in antineutrophil cytoplasmic antibody (ANCA)–associated diseases. Replacement with crystalloid is untenable because of the need to maintain colloid oncotic pressure. Synthetic gelatin–based plasma expanders can be used as part of a replacement regimen but have a shorter half-life than human albumin. As a result, human albumin remains the mainstay of fluid replacement. The major disadvantage of albumin solutions is the lack of clotting factors, with the potential development of depletion coagulopathy after plasma exchange. FFP is also used as replacement colloid, usually in addition to

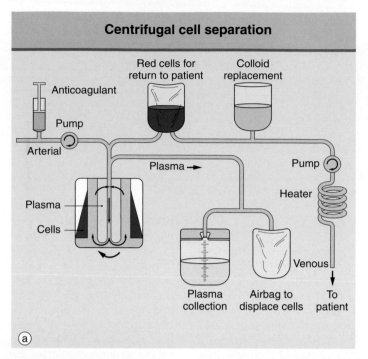

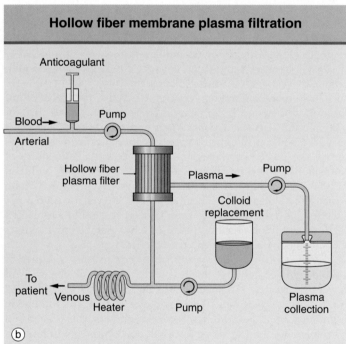

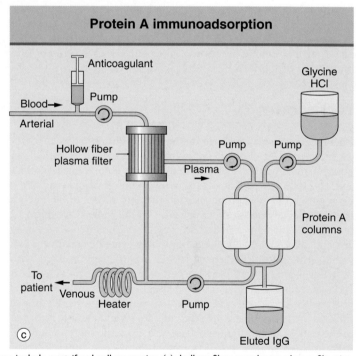

Figure 88.1 **Plasma exchange and immunoadsorption techniques.** Techniques include centrifugal cell separation (*a*), hollow-fiber membrane plasma filtration (*b*), and protein A immunoadsorption (*c*).

human albumin solution, in patients at particular risk of bleeding. However, almost all the serious complications of plasma exchange (hypotension, anaphylaxis, citrate-induced paresthesia, urticaria) have been reported in patients receiving FFP rather than albumin (see later discussion).[2] Both human products carry a tiny risk of transmission of infectious diseases, especially viral. Standard regimens for plasma exchange are summarized in Figure 88.4. Human albumin solution should be used for all exchanges except in HUS/thrombotic thrombocytopenia purpura (TTP; where plasma should provide the total exchange), and FFP should form part of the exchange where bleeding risk is high (ongoing pulmonary hemorrhage or within 48 hours of biopsy or surgery). If

fibrinogen levels decrease to <1.25 to 1.5 g/l or prothrombin time is increased 2 to 3 seconds above normal, then FFP should also be administered.

Double filtration plasmapheresis (or cascade filtration) uses membrane filtration to separate cells from plasma, and then a secondary plasma filtration (pore size 0.01 to 0.03 μm) to remove plasma solutes based on molecular size. Most albumin is therefore returned to the patient, together with lower molecular weight proteins, reducing the need for replacement fluids. Cryofiltration uses a similar principle but exposes the filtrate to 4°C during the procedure, with the aim of precipitating cryoproteins. These techniques are not widely available.

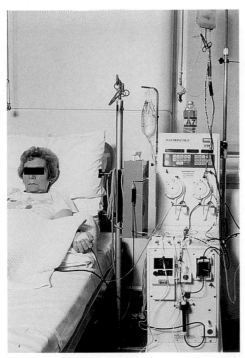

Figure 88.2 A centrifugal cell separator used for plasma exchange.

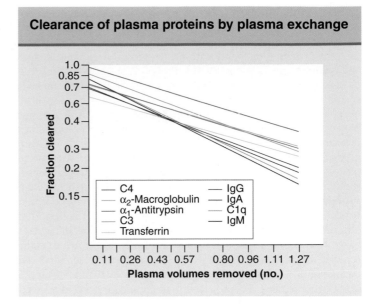

Figure 88.3 Clearance of plasma proteins by plasma exchange. Clearance from the intravascular compartment varies with the plasma volume exchanged and between individual proteins. (Adapted from Derksen RH, Schuurman HJ, Meyling FH, et al: The efficacy of plasma exchange in the removal of plasma components. J Lab Clin Med 1984;104:346–354.)

Regimens for plasma exchange in renal disease

Indication	Antiglomerular Basement Membrane Antibody (anti-GBM) Disease	Small Vessel Vasculitis	Cryoglobulinemia	Recurrent FSGS After Transplantation	HUS/TTP
Duration of treatment	Daily, at least 14 days until anti-GBM antibodies 20%	Daily, 7–10 days depending on clinical response	At least 7–10 days or until clinical response	Daily, at least 10 days initially, then continuing less frequently, often for months	Daily for 7–10 days or until platelet count 80–100 × 10⁹/l (sometimes needed twice daily)
Exchange volume	50 ml/kg each treatment	As for anti-GBM disease	As for anti-GBM disease	As for anti-GBM disease	As for anti-GBM disease
Replacement fluid	Human albumin 5% (unless bleeding risk)	As for anti-GBM disease	As for anti-GBM disease	As for anti-GBM disease	Fresh-frozen plasma (FFP) or cryo-poor FFP
Additions to replacement fluid	20 ml 10% calcium gluconate (occasionally more), 3 ml 15% KCl if not dialysis dependent, heparin 5000–10,000 U (unless citrate anticoagulation)	As for anti-GBM disease	As for anti-GBM disease	As for anti-GBM disease	As for anti-GBM disease (may need more calcium because of increased volume of FFP-containing citrate)
Immunosuppression	Prednisolone and cyclophosphamide	As for anti-GBM disease	Prednisolone and cyclophosphamide in type II (caution if HCV positive)	None	None
Variations	FFP 5–8 ml/kg as part of exchange volume if hemorrhage risk (renal biopsy in last 48 hr, lung hemorrhage, platelets <40 ×10⁹/l, fibrinogen <1.5 g/l); immunoadsorption may be as effective	As for anti-GBM disease Immunoadsorption may be as effective	As for anti-GBM disease	As for anti-GBM disease; may need to include replacement immunoglobulins if continuing long term; immunoadsorption may be as effective	

Figure 88.4 Practical regimens for plasma exchange in renal disease. FSGS, focal segmental glomerulosclerosis; HCV, hepatitis C virus; HUS/TTP, hemolytic uremic syndrome/thrombotic thrombocytopenic purpura.

Selective and specific immunoadsorption techniques are increasingly available. Protein A immunoadsorption has been used to remove immunoglobulin alone from plasma, without the need for replacement fluids and without depletion of clotting factors and complement (see Fig. 88.1c). Protein A selectively binds the Fc domains of immunoglobulin molecules, and the immunoadsorption columns can be repeatedly regenerated. Columns have been used for 1 year for a single patient on up to 30 occasions; however, the repeated acid stripping during regeneration does reduce the efficacy of antibody binding. This technique has been used to treat conditions in which autoantibodies are thought to play a key pathogenic role and usually in place of plasma exchange, such as in Goodpasture's disease, rheumatoid arthritis, and systemic lupus, vasculitis, and to remove anti-HLA antibodies in highly sensitized transplant recipients. In general, the reported efficacy has been equal to that of plasma exchange. Specific ligands have also been immobilized onto columns for more specific removal of potentially pathogenic serum factors; ligands used include anti-human IgG, C1q, phenylalanine, hydrophobic amino acids, acetylcholine receptor, and β-adrenoreceptor peptides, and blood group–related oligosaccharides.

COMPLICATIONS

Plasma exchange is expensive (mostly the cost of replacement fluids) and time consuming and requires trained staff and large-bore vascular access. However, the complication rate is not great. The Swedish registry reported no fatalities during 20,485 procedures, and an overall adverse incidence rate of only 4.3% of all exchanges (0.9% for severe adverse events) of which 27% were paresthesias, 19% transient hypotension, 13% urticaria, and 8% nausea.[3] The Canadian apheresis registry has collected data on 144,432 apheresis procedures since 1981 and reported adverse events occurring in 12% of procedures (mostly minor), and overall in 40% of patients. Severe events only occurred in 0.4% of procedures. Three deaths were probably related directly to the procedure: one from a transfusion-related acute lung injury and two from complications from central venous catheters.[4] An overall complication rate of 1.4% has been reported in more than 15,000 treatments in patients receiving albumin, and 20% in patients receiving FFP.[2,3]

Other complications directly attributable to plasma exchange include citrate-induced hypocalcemia and citrate-induced metabolic alkalosis. Citrate is usually present in the FFP or is administered in the extracorporeal circuit as an anticoagulant; it binds free calcium in plasma. Some patients experience symptomatic hypocalcemia, which can be averted by infusing 10 to 20 ml 10% calcium gluconate during each plasma exchange. Alkalosis is rare and is caused by metabolism of citrate to bicarbonate and failure to excrete the latter in patients with renal impairment.

Plasma exchange predictably increases the risk of bleeding as a result of depletion of coagulation factors in patients receiving albumin as sole replacement colloid. Prothrombin time is increased by 30%, and partial thromboplastin times by 100% after a single plasma volume exchange. Patients at risk of bleeding (alveolar hemorrhage, postbiopsy, postoperative) should receive FFP (300 to 600 ml) with replacement fluids. Dilutional hypokalemia is avoided by adding potassium to the replacement albumin. An increased incidence of infection secondary to hypogammaglobulinemia has not been confirmed in recent series.[4] Sepsis related to intravenous access is the most common infectious complication of plasma exchange. Cascade filtration can lead to hemolysis (in up to 20% patients), but rarely necessitates transfusion.

MECHANISM OF ACTION

Plasma exchange removes large molecular weight substances from the plasma, including antibodies, complement components, immune complexes, endotoxin, lipoproteins, and von Willebrand factor (vWF) multimers. The pathogenicity of autoantibodies in antiglomerular basement membrane (anti-GBM) disease provided the impetus for developing plasma exchange therapy, but it is now clear that antibodies, although necessary, are not alone sufficient to cause the necrotizing glomerulonephritis in Goodpasture's disease. Therefore, plasma exchange may well have benefits in addition to simply clearance of autoantibodies. Plasma exchange has been successfully used in a number of other diseases characterized by autoantibodies, including myasthenia gravis, hemolytic anemia, Eaton-Lambert syndrome, and ANCA-associated systemic vasculitis and in patients with cytotoxic anti-HLA antibodies. The clearance of antibodies from patients is variable and depends on a number of factors, including the rate of equilibration of macromolecules between the intra- and extravascular compartments. IgM antibodies are cleared more effectively by centrifugal plasma exchange than other classes of immunoglobulin as they are retained in the vascular compartment almost wholly. Rebound increase in antibody production will occur unless there is concomitant immunosuppression to prevent resynthesis.

Plasma exchange has also been shown to remove immune complexes, which may have clinical significance in cryoglobulinemia and systemic lupus and fibrinogen and complement components. Plasma exchange improves reticuloendothelial clearance of senescent red blood cells. There is no good evidence that removal of cytokines has any clinical significance. Plasma exchange reduces plasma viscosity, with consequent improved blood flow in the microvasculature.

INDICATIONS FOR PLASMA EXCHANGE

Evidence to support specific indications for plasma exchange is variable in quality. Randomized, controlled trials are few and often involve regimens with considerable variations in dose and frequency of plasma exchange and in immunosuppressive and other adjunctive therapy, making direct comparisons between trials unsatisfactory. Here, evidence from available randomized trials is discussed alongside observational data. The indications are summarized in Figure 88.5.

Antiglomerular Basement Membrane Antibody Disease

Plasma exchange removes anti-GBM antibodies very effectively. Most patients can be depleted of pathogenic antibodies after 7 to 10 plasma volume exchanges if further antibody synthesis is inhibited by the concurrent use of cyclophosphamide and corticosteroids. Prior to the introduction of this therapy, the mortality from Goodpasture's disease was >90%, and only 11% of patients who were not dialysis dependent at presentation survived with preserved renal function. The use of plasma exchange improved the outcome considerably: 70% to 90% of patients now survive. However, only 50% of survivors retain independent renal function overall, and 10% (at best) of those who are dialysis dependent at presentation (Fig. 88.6). There has only been one small controlled trial of plasma exchange in the treatment of Goodpasture's disease

Renal conditions for which plasma exchange has an established role or may be useful			
Conditions for which Plasma Exchange Has an Established Role		**Conditions for which Plasma Exchange May Be Useful**	
Condition	Comment	Condition	Comment
Antiglomerular basement membrane antibody disease	Especially nonoliguric renal failure predialysis and for pulmonary hemorrhage	Nephrotic proteinuria post-transplantation caused by recurrent focal segmental glomerulosclerosis (FSGS)	Transient reduction in proteinuria in most patients; 50% achieve long-term remission
Antineutrophil cytoplasmic antibody–associated vasculitis	Only for patients with dialysis-dependent renal failure and/or pulmonary hemorrhage	Acute vascular allograft rejection	May help in patients with resistant rejection
Hemolytic uremic syndrome (HUS) in adults or nondiarrheal HUS in children	Plasma exchange or infusion may both be beneficial, although exchange allows greater volume of plasma to be infused; full exchange for plasma rather than albumin	Highly sensitized transplant recipients	May help remove anti-HLA antibodies and allow successful transplantation
Thrombotic thrombocytopenic pupura	Plasma exchange or infusion both beneficial, although exchange allows greater volume of plasma to be infused; full exchange for plasma rather than albumin	Systemic lupus	May be of use in the most severe disease, cerebral lupus, or catastrophic antiphospholipid syndrome; no clear benefit in moderately severe renal involvement
Types I and II cryoglobulinemia	Patients improve symptomatically, vasculitic syndrome improves, variable effect on renal function No controlled trials	Crescentic IgA nephropathy	Possible short-term benefit
ABO incompatible transplantation	Plasma exchange allows successful transplantation	Primary FSGS	Up to 40% remission rate of nephrotic syndrome in steroid–resistant patients

Figure 88.5 Renal conditions for which plasma exchange has an established role or may be useful.

that used a low intensity of plasma exchange.[5] A total of 17 patients were randomized to receive steroids and cyclophosphamide, with or without plasma exchange. Only two of the eight receiving plasma exchange developed end-stage renal disease compared with six of the nine receiving drugs alone.

Long-term data from 71 patients with Goodpasture's disease confirmed the benefit of a treatment regimen including plasma exchange since most patients with mild to moderate renal failure retained independent renal function over 10 to 25 years,[6] and renal recovery was possible even in some of those with the most severe renal disease. Combining all the available published data for patients with Goodpasture's disease, 76% of patients presenting with serum creatinine <5.7 to 6.6 mg/dl (500 to 600 μmol/l) will retain renal function, in contrast to 8% of those presenting dependent on dialysis (see Fig. 88.6).

Plasma exchange in Goodpasture's disease		
	SCr <6.6 mg/dl at Presentation	SCr >6.6 mg/dl at Presentation
Independent renal function at 1 yr	109/162 (67%)	18/241 (7.5%)
Number receiving plasma exchange	122	126

Figure 88.6 Plasma exchange in Goodpasture's (anti-GBM) disease. Summation of available patient outcome in observational and randomized, controlled trials. SCr, serum creatinine.

Recommendation

All patients presenting predialysis should receive intensive plasma exchange with daily 4-liter exchanges initially for 14 days, using 4.5% albumin solution (supplemented with calcium) as replacement fluid. Fresh plasma (300 to 600 ml) is added for patients actively bleeding or those who have had recent surgery or biopsy. We reserve plasma exchange with immunosuppression for dialysis-dependent patients with biopsy or clinical evidence of recent-onset disease. Pulmonary hemorrhage is an independent indication for plasma exchange. Treatment of Goodpasture's disease is discussed further in Chapter 22.

Small Vessel Vasculitis

The majority of patients with rapidly progressive glomerulonephritis (RPGN), other than anti-GBM disease, have small-vessel vasculitis with ANCA detectable in their serum, and there is now good evidence that these autoantibodies are pathogenic (see Chapter 23). Plasma exchange was initially introduced in such patients because of the similarity of the histologic changes to those seen in Goodpasture's disease, and the supposition that immune complexes may be instrumental in disease pathogenesis. Seven trials of plasma exchange in non–anti-GBM RPGN have been reported (Fig. 88.7).[7–13] Most of the early trials[7–12] included patients with a variety of diseases, used a low intensity of plasma exchange, and often excluded those with oligoanuria. These trials showed no overall benefit of plasma exchange in addition to conventional immunosuppression; however, those patients with the most severe disease did seem to benefit. Combining the results of the controlled trials, 31 of 42 (74%) dialysis-dependent patients

Plasma exchange in non–anti GBM rapidly progressive glomerulonephritis		
	Successfully Treated with Plasma Exchange	Successfully Treated with Oral or Intravenous Drugs Alone
6 reports, 1991–2002[7–12]		
Nonrandomized studies	79/108 (73%)	79/132 (60%)
Randomized, controlled trials	73/103 (71%)	38/88 (43%)
Dialysis-dependent patients in randomized studies	31/42 (74%)	8/25 (32%)
MEPEX trial 2006[13]		
SCr >5.5 mg/dl (500 μmol/l) at presentation	50/70 (71%)	33/67 (49%)

Figure 88.7   Plasma exchange in non–antiglomerular basement membrane (GBM) rapidly progressive glomerulonephritis. Summation of available patient outcome data in observational and randomized, controlled trials. SCr, serum creatinine.

treated with plasma exchange recovered renal function compared with only 8 of 25 (32%) treated with drugs alone. The most recent randomized, controlled trial (MEPEX) randomized 137 patients with ANCA-associated systemic vasculitis and serum creatinine >5.5 mg/dl (500 μmol/l) to plasma exchange or intravenous methylprednisolone in addition to oral steroids and cyclophosphamide.[13] Seventy-one percent of patients recovered renal function when treated with plasma exchange compared with 49% of those receiving intravenous methylprednisolone. Patients with both ANCA and anti-GBM antibodies (so-called double-positive patients) and RPGN do not seem to respond so well to plasma exchange and rarely, if ever, recover renal function.[14]

Recommendation

We perform plasma exchange in patients with small-vessel vasculitis who present with dialysis-dependent renal failure or pulmonary hemorrhage. Exchanges are performed with albumin replacement unless there is a bleeding risk (as in anti-GBM disease).

Other Crescentic Glomerulonephritis

Crescent formation is a common histologic finding in a number of other patterns of glomerulonephritis (GN), including postinfectious GN, GN associated with infective endocarditis, IgA nephropathy, membranoproliferative glomerulonephritis (MPGN), and membranous nephropathy. Plasma exchange has been used in the treatment of a number of these conditions, despite the lack of substantive evidence that the renal injury is caused by circulating antibodies or immune complexes. There are no controlled trials. In crescentic IgA nephropathy, there are anecdotal reports of short-term benefit in patients with severe renal impairment but longer-term follow-up has proved disappointing.

Recommendation

We reserve plasma exchange in IgA nephropathy and other GN for patients with rapidly deteriorating renal function and extensive fresh crescents in the biopsy.

Focal Segmental Glomerulosclerosis

Plasma exchange and protein A immunoadsorption have been used to treat patients with primary FSGS. The results have been less good than in patients with recurrent disease after transplantation, and in general <40% of patients achieve either partial or complete remission,[15] and we do not recommend plasma exchange in this setting.

Hemolytic Uremic Syndrome/Thrombotic Thrombocytopenic Purpura

In both HUS and TTP, endothelial activation leads to thrombotic microangiopathy, but through independent mechanisms (see Chapter 28).

Diarrhea-Associated Hemolytic Uremic Syndrome

Childhood diarrhea-associated HUS (D+ HUS) is usually caused by bacterial verotoxins and has a good prognosis. Most children will recover fully with supportive care and management of fluid and electrolyte imbalance and hypertension. Two controlled trials of plasma infusion (at least 10 ml/kg daily) in childhood HUS complicated by dialysis-dependent renal failure could not demonstrate any clinical benefit (as determined by hypertension, renal dysfunction, and proteinuria) in either short- or medium-term follow-up.[16] There has been no study of plasma exchange in childhood D+ HUS. Plasma exchange and infusion have not been subjected to any controlled trials in adult D+ HUS, but uncontrolled observations suggest benefit.[17]

Thrombotic Thrombocytopenic Purpura

Patients with TTP have a defective vWF cleaving protease (ADAMTS13), an enzyme that normally degrades large vWF multimers, either due to inherited deficiency or to autoantibodies directed against the protease. Accumulation of VWF multimers leads to systemic platelet activation under conditions of high shear stress (the microcirculation) and thrombosis. The rationale for plasma infusion and plasma exchange in TTP is therefore to replenish vWF cleaving protease, to remove antibodies against it, and to remove the large vWF multimers from circulation.

A prospective, controlled trial compared plasma infusion with plasma exchange (1 to 1.5 plasma volumes at least 7 times in the first 9 days).[18] All patients received aspirin and dipyridamole. Of patients receiving plasma exchange, 47% had a platelet count >150 × 10^9 cells/l and no new neurologic features, compared with only 25% of those receiving plasma infusion over the first 2 weeks. At 6 months, survival was substantially better in the plasma exchange group (50% versus 78%). More recent series using plasma exchange have reported mortality rates as low as 15%,[17] and there may be an association of reduced early mortality with more intensive plasma exchange. Renal impairment is not an independent predictor of poor outcome in TTP and does not in itself warrant more intensive therapy. Fever, age older than 40 years, and hemoglobin <9 g/dl have been associated with a worse outcome.[19] Whether FFP or its cryosupernatant fraction is better as replacement fluid remains unclear.

D- Hemolytic Uremic Syndrome

The cause of adult HUS remains unclear in most cases in which there is no clear diarrheal prodrome (D-HUS). Some patients have defective regulation of the complement pathway (e.g., factor H deficiency) leading to uninhibited activation of complement, while in others, infections or drugs cause platelet or leukocyte activation and complement activation and consumption. Direct activation of endothelial cells may also be a cause. Plasma exchange and infusion has not been subjected to any controlled trials in adult D-HUS, but uncontrolled series suggest benefit.[17] HUS/TTP occurring after renal transplantation has also responded to plasma exchange.

Recommendation

We use plasma exchange in all adults with HUS/TTP and perform all exchanges against FFP or cryo-poor FFP.

Systemic Lupus

Plasma exchange has been used extensively in patients with lupus. Most studies have included patients with diverse patterns of disease and often only mild renal involvement. A randomized, prospective trial could show no benefit of plasma exchange over conventional immunosuppression for renal, serologic, or clinical outcomes, both in the short and long term.[20] However, patients with crescentic lupus nephritis and those with the most severe renal dysfunction (dialysis dependency) were excluded. Anecdotal evidence suggests that plasma exchange may benefit patients with crescentic nephritis, pulmonary hemorrhage, cerebral lupus, catastrophic antiphospholipid syndrome, lupus-associated TTP, or severe lupus unresponsive to conventional drugs or in patients for whom cytotoxic therapy has been withdrawn because of bone marrow suppression or other toxicity. Immunoadsorption may be more successful in the severe forms of lupus nephritis. A variety of techniques have been used including standard protein A and anti-Ig absorption, and also phenylalanine, tryptophan, and dextran sulfate ligands, all of which bind immunoglobulin, rheumatoid factors, and immune complexes to varying degrees and all of which have been reported to induce remission in patients with severe disease after failure of conventional therapy.[21]

Recommendation

We reserve plasma exchange for lupus patients with rapidly progressive renal failure and class IV renal histology, often with neurologic involvement and hemolysis, for those likely to suffer bone marrow suppression from cyclophosphamide, and for those with catastrophic antiphospholipid syndrome. The treatment of lupus is further discussed in Chapter 24.

Cryoglobulinemia

In type I cryoglobulinemia, usually associated with myeloma or lymphoma, a monoclonal immunoglobulin causes hyperviscosity and cryoprecipitation. Such antibodies are easily removed by plasma exchange, often with immediate benefit for the patient. Cytotoxic agents are used simultaneously to inhibit further paraprotein production. There are no controlled trials of the use of plasma exchange, but symptoms are closely related to the presence of the cryoimmunoglobulin, and hence treatment with plasma exchange appears effective.

Patients with type II (mixed essential) cryoglobulinemia develop a monoclonal antibody (usually IgM) with specificity for a second, usually polyclonal, immunoglobulin. Type II cryoglobulins occur most commonly in association with lymphoma and hepatitis C virus infection. The resulting immune complexes can be deposited in the microcirculation and are particularly associated with MPGN (see Chapter 20). Plasma exchange is effective at clearing the immune complexes, although in long-term follow-up, the cryoglobulins often recur, and sustained benefit has not been clearly demonstrated. Despite these reservations, many of the acute features of cryoglobulinemia do resolve with plasma exchange, particularly arthralgia, skin lesions, and digital necrosis, and patients with RPGN can recover renal function. Concomitant immunosuppression with cytotoxic agents or rituximab may prevent resynthesis of the cryoproteins, although some patients require long-term intermittent plasma exchange to control symptoms. Immunosuppressive treatment should be used with caution in patients with hepatitis C virus–associated cryoglobulinemia who may respond to antiviral therapies such as interferon or ribavirin. Cryofiltration apheresis (in which the separated plasma is cooled to precipitate the cryoglobulin) selectively removes cryoglobulins, avoids large volumes of replacement fluids, and avoids deficiency of clotting factors, but needs to be combined with immunosuppression to prevent synthesis of further cryoglobulin. Few centers currently perform this technique.

Myeloma

Plasma exchange has been reported to be of benefit in patients with myeloma and either cast nephropathy or light-chain renal toxicity. Two small controlled trials performed over 15 years ago provided conflicting results.[22,23] Recently, a large prospective, controlled trial was reported in which 97 patients with myeloma and progressive acute renal failure (creatinine >200 μmol/l [2.3 mg/dl] with an increase >50 μmol/l over the previous 2 weeks despite conventional management) were randomized to receive plasma exchange (five to seven sessions of 50 ml/kg over 10 days) in addition to chemotherapy (VAD or melphalan and prednisolone).[24] This study showed no benefit of plasma exchange on mortality or recovery of renal function.

Recommendation

The most recent trial suggests that plasma exchange should not be routinely used for myeloma patients with acute renal failure, but that aggressive hydration, correction of other reversible causes (such as hypercalcemia and sepsis), and early initiation of chemotherapy are more important factors in recovery of renal function.

Transplantation
Vascular Rejection

Vascular rejection is associated with both anti-HLA and antiendothelial antibodies. Studies in the 1980s suggested that combining plasma exchange with cyclophosphamide could deplete circulating antibodies and improve renal function. Subsequent controlled studies have been performed in heterogeneous patient populations, with conflicting results. A review of 157 patients included in five trials could not demonstrate any significant difference in the outcome of acute vascular rejection in patients treated with or without plasma exchange.[25] Another study documented reversal of acute (but not chronic) rejection in 75% of 62 patients treated with plasma exchange.[26] A number of reports indicate that plasma exchange is effective at reversing up to 50% of episodes of acute vascular rejection resistant to corticosteroids, but there are no studies comparing plasma exchange with antibody therapy in resistant rejection. There is no convincing evidence that plasma exchange has any role in the treatment of chronic rejection.

Anti-HLA Antibodies

Highly sensitized patients with preformed anti-HLA antibodies have been treated both pre- and post-transplantation with plasma exchange or immunoadsorption to reduce cytotoxic antibody levels.[27] Patients usually received intensive immunoadsorption or plasma exchange before transplantation to ensure a current negative cross-match immediately prior to transplantation; some received longer-term immunoadsorption/plasma exchange in combination with steroids and cyclophosphamide in the months preceding transplantation. Treatment of 100 patients with high-titer cytotoxic antibodies with plasma exchange or immunoadsorption in addition to cyclophosphamide and prednisolone[27] led to graft survival rates at 1 and 4 years of 77% and 64%, respectively, in living donor recipients, and 70% and 57%, respectively, in first cadaveric graft recipients.

ABO Incompatible Renal Transplantation

Plasma exchange is widely used to remove natural anti-A or anti-B blood group antibodies from the recipient prior to living related transplantation from an ABO incompatible donor. Various protocols are in use, but all rely on depleting specific antibody over 4 to 6 days prior to transplantation by exchanging a single plasma volume for human albumin solution (in addition to routine immunosuppression, sometimes including rituximab and intravenous immunoglobulin). Plasma exchange is sometimes continued for one or two sessions after transplantation or if antibody-mediated rejection occurs.[28] One-year graft survival rates of up to 85% have been reported with such protocols, although rejection episodes are more common than in ABO compatible transplants. More recently, immunoadsorption using synthetic A- or B-oligosaccharide epitopes linked to Sepharose has been developed.

Such columns specifically remove anti-A or anti-B antibodies, but whether this will in fact be an advantage is yet to be determined.

Recurrent Focal Segmental Glomerulosclerosis

Plasma exchange, double-filtration plasmapheresis, and protein A immunoadsorption have all been used to treat recurrence of nephrotic syndrome after transplantation in patients with recurrent focal segmental glomerulosclerosis.[29,30] An undefined factor causing increased permeability of glomerular capillaries can be found in most patients with recurrent disease (see Chapter 96). There are no controlled trials of plasma treatments in recurrent FSGS, and most series are small. One study demonstrated an 82% reduction in urinary protein excretion in eight patients with recurrent nephrosis during plasma protein adsorption; however, the effect was transient and persisted for <2 months in seven of the eight patients.[30] Other investigators have obtained remissions in approximately 50% patients, and a significant reduction in graft loss due to recurrent disease compared with historic controls. More intensive treatment regimens have led to more persistent remissions. All three apheresis modalities have also been used prophylactically in patients deemed to be at high risk of recurrence with variable success.[31]

REFERENCES

1. Derksen RH, Schuurman HJ, Meyling FH, et al: The efficacy of plasma exchange in the removal of plasma components. J Lab Clin Med 1984; 104:346–354.
2. Reutter JC, Sanders KF, Brecher ME, et al: Incidence of allergic reactions to FFP or cryo-supernatant in the treatment of thrombotic thrombocytopenic purpura. J Clin Apheresis 2001;16:134–138.
3. Norda R, Stegmayr B: Therapeutic apheresis in Sweden. Transfus Apheresis Sci 2003;9:159–166.
4. Rock G, Clark B, Sutton D, et al: The Canadian apheresis registry. Transfus Apheresis Science 2003;29:167–177.
5. Johnson JP, Whitman W, Briggs WA, Wilson CB: Plasmapheresis and immunosuppressive agents in antibasement membrane antibody-induced Goodpasture's syndrome. Am J Med 1978;64:354–359.
6. Levy JB, Turner AN, Rees AJ, Pusey CD: Long term outcome of anti-glomerular basement membrane antibody disease treated with plasma exchange and immunosuppression. Ann Intern Med 2001;134:1033–1042.
7. Glockner WM, Sieberth HG, Wichmann HE, et al: Plasma exchange and immunosuppression in rapidly progressive glomerulonephritis: A controlled multi-center study. Clin Nephrol 1988;29:1–8.
8. Pusey CD, Rees AJ, Evans DJ, et al: Plasma exchange in focal necrotizing glomerulonephritis without anti-GBM antibodies. Kidney Int 1991;40:757–763.
9. Cole E, Cattran D, Magil A, et al: A prospective randomized trial of plasma exchange as additive therapy in idiopathic crescentic glomerulonephritis. Canadian Apheresis Study Group. Am J Kidney Dis 1992; 20:261–269.
10. Guillevin L, Fain O, Lhote F, et al: Lack of superiority of steroids plus plasma exchange to steroids alone in the treatment of polyarteritis nodosa and Churg Strauss syndrome. A prospective randomised trial in 78 patients. Arthritis Rheum 1992;35:208–215.
11. Guillevin L, Lhote F, Cohen P, et al: Lack of superiority of corticosteroids plus pulse cyclophosphamide and plasma exchanges to corticosteroids plus pulse cyclophosphamide alone in the treatment of polyarteritis nodosa and Churg Strauss syndrome patients with poor prognostic factors. A prospective randomised trial in 62 patients. Arthritis Rheum 1995;38: 1638–1645.
12. Zauner I, Bach D, Kramer BK, et al: Predictive value of initial histology and effect of plasmapheresis on long term prognosis of rapidly progressive glomerulonephritis. Am J Kidney Dis 2002;39:28–35.
13. Rasmussen N, Jayne DRW, Abramowicz D, et al: European therapeutic trials in ANCA associated systemic vasculitis: Disease scoring, consensus regimens and proposed clinical trials. Clin Exp Immunol 1995; 101(Suppl 1):29–34.
14. Levy JB, Hammad T, Coulthart A, et al: Clinical features and outcome of patients with both ANCA and anti-GBM antibodies. Kidney Int 2004;66:1535–1540.
15. Bosch T, Wendler T: Extracorporeal plasma exchange in primary and recurrent focal segmental glomerulosclerosis. A review. Ther Apheresis 2001;5:155–160.
16. Rizzoni G, Claris-Appiani A, Edefonti A, et al: Plasma infusion for hemolytic uremic syndrome in children. J Pediatr 1988;112:284–290.
17. Nguyen TC, Stegmayr B, Busund R, et al: Plasma therapies in thrombotic syndromes. Int J Art Organs 2005;28:459–465.
18. Rock GA, Shumak KH, Buskard NA, et al: Comparison of plasma exchange with plasma infusion in the treatment of thrombotic thrombocytopenic purpura. Canadian Apheresis Study Group. N Engl J Med 1991;325:393–397.
19. Wyllie BF, Garg AX, Macnab J, et al: TTP/HUS: A new index predicting response to plasma exchange. Br J Haematol 2005;132:204–209.
20. Korbet SM, Lewis EJ, Schwartz MM, et al: Factors predictive of outcome in severe lupus nephritis. Lupus Nephritis Collaboration Group. Am J Kidney Dis 2000;35:904–914.
21. Gaubitz M, Seidel M, Kummer S, et al: Prospective randomized trial of two different immunoadsorbers in severe SLE. J Autoimmun 1998;11: 495–501.
22. Zucchelli P, Pasquali S, Cagnoli L, Ferrari G: Controlled plasma exchange trial in acute renal failure due to multiple myeloma. Kidney Int 1988; 33: 1175–1180.
23. Johnson WJ, Kyle RA, Pineda AA, et al: Treatment of renal failure associated with multiple myeloma. Arch Intern Med 1990;150:863–869.
24. Clark WF, Stewart AK, Rock GA, et al: Plasma exchange when myeloma presents as acute renal failure. Ann Intern Med 2005;143:777–784.
25. Gurland HJ, Blumenstein M, Lysaght MJ, et al: Plasmapheresis in renal transplantation. Kidney Int 1983;23(Suppl 14):82–84.
26. Frasca GM, Martella D, Vangelista A, Bonomini V: Ten years experience with plasma exchange in renal transplantation. Int J Artif Organs 1991; 14:51–55.
27. Reisaeter AV, Leivestad T, Albrechtsen D, et al: Pretransplant plasma exchange or immunoadsorption facilitates renal transplantation in immunized patients. Transplantation 1995;60:242–248.
28. Winters JL, Gloor JM, Pineda AA, et al: Plasma exchange conditioning for ABO-incompatible renal transplantation. J Clin Apheresis 2004;19: 79–85.
29. Otsubo S, Tanabe K, Shinmura H, et al: Effect of post transplant DFPP on recurrent FSGS in renal transplant recipients. Ther Apher Dial 2004;8:299–304.
30. Dantal J, Bigot E, Bogers W, et al: Effect of plasma protein adsorption on protein excretion in kidney-transplant recipients with recurrent nephrotic syndrome. N Engl J Med 1994;330:7–14.
31. Gohh RY, Yango AF, Morrissey PE, et al: Pre-emptive plasmapheresis and recurrence of FSGS in high-risk renal transplant recipients. Am J Transplant 2005;5:2907–2912.

CHAPTER
89 Immunologic Principles of Kidney Transplantation

Luis G. Hidalgo, Gunilla Einecke, and Philip F. Halloran

INTRODUCTION

Kidney transplantation between nongenetically identical humans leads to the activation of a large number of alloreactive T lymphocytes that can exert effector functions leading to the destruction of the transplant. The massive response is invoked due to the large number of T cells capable of recognizing allogeneic major histocompatibility complex (MHC). Unlike most responses to intrinsic (cognate) antigens where approximately $1/10^6$ of the T cell population may respond, up to 5% of the T cell population may respond to an allogeneic stimulus. Many arms of the immune system are activated during rejection including the generation of T cell effector mechanisms (cytotoxic T lymphocytes [CTLs], delayed-type hypersensitivity [DTH] responses), and formation of alloantibodies. The relationship between tissues of individuals is called syngeneic for identical twins, allogeneic for nonidentical members of the same species, and xenogeneic for members of different species. The prefixes allo- and xeno- designate components of the respective immune response, for example, alloantibody. This chapter is devoted to allotransplantation but alludes briefly to xenotransplantation. The mechanism of action, pharmacokinetics, administration, and side effects of immunosuppressives are discussed in detail in Chapter 90.

Initiation of the Alloimmune Response

Alloimmune responses are initiated by activation of antigen-presenting cells (APCs) through innate immune recognition systems. In the graft and surrounding tissues, dendritic cells of donor and host origin become activated and move to T cell areas of secondary lymphoid organs (SLOs). Naive T cells are triggered by the encounter of donor antigen, which is presented by dendritic cells in SLO.[1,2] Antigen experienced memory cells may be activated by other cell types, such as graft endothelium.[3] These memory cells may have been activated previously by alloantigenic stimuli or much more commonly by viral antigens that cross-react with alloantigens.[4] B cells are activated when antigen engages their antigen receptors, usually in lymphoid follicles or in extrafollicular sites, such as red pulp of spleen,[5] or possibly in the transplant,[6] leading to the production of alloantibody against donor HLA antigens.

The presentation of donor antigen on the surface of dendritic cells triggers T cells through cognate T cell receptors (TCRs). Dendritic cells provide costimulation, leading to the activation of three signal transduction pathways: the calcium-calcineurin pathway, the renin angiotensin system mitogen-activated protein kinase pathway, and the nuclear factor-κB (NF-κB) pathway.[7]

These pathways activate transcription factors that trigger the expression of many additional molecules, including interleukin (IL)-2, CD154, and the IL-2 receptor α-subunit (CD25) that provide the trigger for cell proliferation. Proliferation and differentiation lead to a large number of effector T cells. Thus, within days, the immune response generates the effector mechanisms—effector T cells and alloantibody—that can damage the organ and mediate allograft rejection.

EFFECTORS OF REJECTION

Rejection is defined as tissue injury produced by the effector mechanisms of the adaptive alloimmune response, leading to deterioration in renal function. There are two types of rejection: T cell–mediated rejection (TCMR) and antibody-mediated rejection (ABMR). The cellular infiltrate observed in rejection is composed of mononuclear cells including T cells, macrophages, B cells, and plasma cells. T cells serve as the main effectors and regulators of the alloimmune response. Macrophages are possible effectors and aid in the removal of apoptotic cells. Theoretically, B cells and plasma cells could contribute to the production of alloantibodies within the graft but are not part of the criteria for ABMR; in fact, infiltration by B cells and plasma cells into the graft is seen more often in TCMR as part of the cellular infiltrate. In ABMR, the high-affinity damaging IgG antibodies are probably made in SLO or in the marrow.

Alloresponses involve two groups of immune cells: lymphocytes and APCs. T and B lymphocytes mediate adaptive immune responses through their antigen-specific receptors, which permit them to display specificity, adaptation and tolerance, memory, and self-/nonself-recognition. NK cells are not antigen specific, but express receptors for MHC class I and may have roles in transplantation, especially bone marrow transplantation. However, their role in allotransplantation remains unclear. APCs are cells required for the activation of T cells, engulfing and destruction of microorganisms, and the generation of successful immune responses. The most effective APCs are dendritic cells (DCs), which are specialized cells in peripheral tissues and lymphoid tissues belonging mainly to the monocyte lineage. Macrophages may serve as APCs at the inflamed site and can also exert effector functions.

T Cells

T cells arise in the thymus from bone marrow–derived precursors, somatically rearranging the genes for their antigen-specific T cell receptors (TCRs). Each T cell expresses a unique TCR that is expressed by all its daughter cells, forming a T cell clone. As

T cells mature in the thymus, they undergo positive and negative selection. Positive selection identifies useful clones recognizing foreign antigens in the context of self MHC. Negative selection prevents potentially destructive autoreactive clones from maturing. Mature T cells expressing their clone-specific TCRs then leave the thymus. T cells are divided into two subpopulations: CD4 T cells (also called helper cells) and CD8 T cells. CD4 T cells direct many aspects of the antigen-specific immune responses, while CD8 T cells are precursors of potent CTLs, which are major effectors against intracellular pathogens. The TCRs of CD4 T cells are selected to interact with class II MHC molecules, and the TCRs of CD8 T cells with class I MHC molecules.

B Cells

B cells arise and mature in the bone marrow. B cells express immunoglobulin (Ig) as their B cell receptors (BCRs). The precursors somatically rearrange their BCR (Ig) genes to express clone-specific Ig receptors. They are also selected negatively, deleting strong autoreactivity. When they leave the bone marrow, they express BCRs on their surface. When a BCR is stimulated by antigen, the B cell secretes Ig (antibodies) of the same specificity as their BCRs. The antibodies interacting with antigen activate the effector systems such as complement, natural killer (NK) cells, phagocytes, and mast cells. B cells can differentiate into plasma cells that are very efficient in secreting antibody. Antibody-mediated responses are called humoral and play an important role in some types of kidney allograft rejection.

Antigen-Presenting Cells

APCs are specialized cells capable of activating T cells. Antigen is endocytosed by APCs and then displayed on MHC molecules on their surface. T cells recognize and interact with antigen MHC to become activated. Additional costimulatory molecules are expressed by APCs that allow for the optimal activation of T cells. DCs, macrophages, and B cells are considered APCs with DCs being the most effective APCs. Immature DCs live in the interstitial areas of the kidney and are activated by stimuli (innate immunity, endotoxin, possibly tissue injury) to mature and move to the T cell areas of SLOs. Resident macrophages are also present in kidney interstitium and although activated by the same stimuli as DCs, they do not migrate to lymphoid tissues.

T CELL ACTIVATION

The activation of T cells is a crucial step in the generation of immune responses to specific antigens (Fig. 89.1). It begins with naive T cells, which have not yet encountered their cognate antigen, that is, the MHC peptide complex whose shape engages their TCRs with sufficient affinity to trigger activation. The trafficking pattern of naive T cells is restricted to SLOs such as the lymph nodes and spleen. They cannot enter organs such as the kidney. They traverse from blood to lymphoid organs, where they pass through the T cell areas, enter lymph vessels, and return to the blood.

Within SLOs, naive T cells interact with DCs that have migrated from the periphery in response to infection or injury. DCs are the sentinels of the immune system. Immature DCs pick up material for surveillance and sense environmental disturbances in the peripheral tissues. They respond to disturbances such as endotoxin by maturing into potent APCs and migrating to SLOs.[8] DCs are highly intelligent cells, interpreting the environment and determining whether the environment suggests that antigen

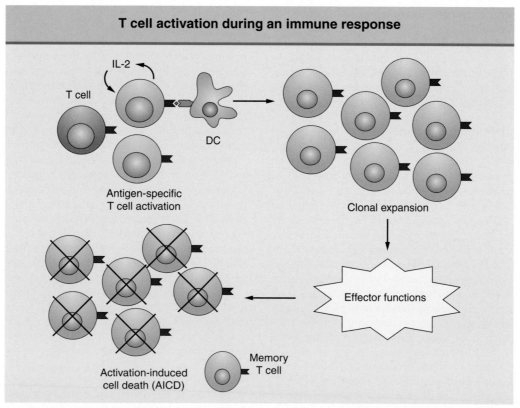

T cell activation during an immune response

IL-2

T cell

DC

Antigen-specific
T cell activation

Clonal expansion

Effector functions

Activation-induced
cell death (AICD)

Memory
T cell

Figure 89.1 T cell activation during an immune response. Only those naive T cells specific for the antigen being presented by a dendritic cell (DC) are activated and begin to produce interleukin (IL)-2. IL-2 drives the clonal expansion of the activated clones, which go on to become effector cells. The majority of the activated clones undergo apoptosis by activation-induced cell death; others become memory T cells.

should lead to an immune response, no response (ignorance), or deletion of responsiveness (tolerance).

Thus, the movement of DCs and the movement of naive T cells are coordinated to bring them into contact in the T cell areas of SLOs. If naive T cells encounter their cognate antigen presented on mature DCs, they become activated. Following activation, CD4 T cells move to the B cell region of SLOs to provide help to B cells, permitting them to class switch from IgM to IgG and to become antibody-producing plasma cells. Activated T cells also leave SLOs and are now able to enter peripheral tissues, particularly into sites of inflammation to apply their effector functions.[9]

CD4 T cells can become effector cells but also are important regulatory cells in both the development and prevention of autoimmunity. They exert their effects mainly through the production of cytokines and by direct contact between their surface molecules and other cells. CD4 T cells are required to provide help for the generation of plasma cells and CTLs. One important type of CD4 T cell is the $CD4^+CD25^+$ regulatory T cell population (discussed later).

As the host defense challenge subsides, the majority of T cells generated in an immune response will be deleted through cell death, either activation-induced cell death (AICD) triggered by antigen, or cell death secondary to antigen withdrawal, which acts by stopping growth factor production. Programmed cell death spares only antigen-specific memory cells that maintain the capacity to produce an efficient, rapid secondary response on reexposure to the same antigen.

Antigen Presentation

Allografts (tissue transplants between members of the same species) induce alloimmune responses due to the recognition of nonself antigens from the graft by recipient T cells. Recipient T cells may encounter alloantigen through either direct or indirect pathways.[10]

Indirect antigen presentation is the way antigen is normally presented in immune responses. Antigen is taken up by APCs, processed intracellularly, and then presented as peptides on MHC molecules. In alloimmune responses, graft-derived cells or released antigens can be taken up by recipient APCs. Recipient APCs process donor antigens, present donor MHC-derived peptides on recipient MHC molecules to T cells, and initiate the alloimmune response (Fig. 89.2a).

Direct antigen presentation involves the recognition of intact donor MHC on the surface of donor cells. Donor APCs may migrate from the graft to recipient lymphoid organs and activate alloreactive T cells to begin the alloimmune response (see Fig. 89.2b). Direct antigen presentation also occurs when recipient T cells encounter the allograft and recognize nonself antigens within the allograft. B cells also recognize intact donor MHC antigen by their B cell receptors, leading to alloantibody production. The best evidence of direct recognition is the strong *in vitro* responses generated by cultured T cells with allogeneic APCs (mixed lymphocyte reaction [MLR]).

Major Histocompatibility Complex

MHC genes (in humans, HLA) encode molecules crucial to the initiation and propagation of immune responses. The HLA locus maps to a 3.5-million base-pair region on chromosome 6 and is divided into three regions: the class II region, the class III region, and the class I region. Only the class I and class II regions encode proteins involved in antigen presentation. The key MHC genes are the class I genes (namely, HLA-A, -B, and -C) and the class II genes (including HLA-DP, -DQ, and -DR).

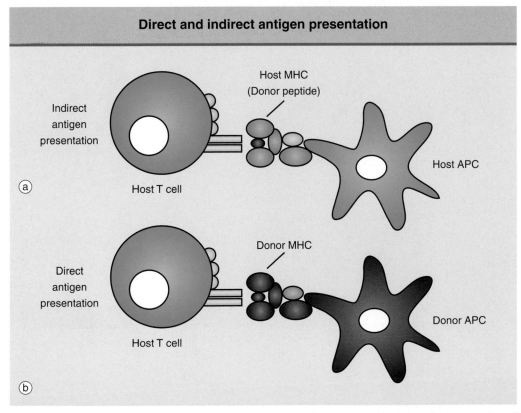

Direct and indirect antigen presentation

Figure 89.2   Direct and indirect antigen presentation. *a,* Indirect antigen presentation. Donor antigen (shown in red) is presented to a T cell by a host dendritic cell. *b,* Direct antigen presentation. A donor antigen-presenting cell (APC) interacts directly with a host T cell. MHC, major histocompatibility complex.

The class I and II proteins share overall structural homology but are functionally different.[11] MHC class I molecules are single polypeptide chains of 45-kd noncovalently associated with a smaller 12-kd protein, β_2-microglobulin. The class I heavy chain consists of three α domains (α1, α2, and α3) and a short cytoplasmic tail (Fig. 89.3a). The membrane proximal α3 domain and β_2-microglobulin are Ig domains, while the α1 and α2 domains are sheet-and-helix domains, each constructed to form a long α helix and an antiparallel β sheet. The two sheet and helix domains assemble face to face to form a long β sheet bounded by two α helices, making up the peptide-binding groove. The membrane-proximal Ig domain binds to β_2-microglobulin, which is like a single Ig domain. Thus, the structural elements of class I are two α helices, a β-pleated sheet, and two membrane-proximal Ig domains, with a membrane anchor.

Class II proteins are heterodimers of an α and a β chain each crossing the membrane. The α2 and β2 domains are adjacent to the cell membrane and are Ig domains, while the peptide-binding groove is composed of the α1 and β1 domains (see Fig. 89.3b). The structural elements of class II are two α helices, a β pleated sheet, and two membrane-proximal Ig domains, with two membrane anchors.

Class I molecules present peptide (usually derived from endogenously synthesized proteins) to CD8 T cells. Class II proteins present peptides (usually derived from endocytosed proteins synthesized outside the cell) to CD4 T cells. Each molecule contains a groove that can hold peptides of 8 to 10 amino acids for class I or 8 to 25 amino acids for class II.

MHC class I and class II genes are highly polymorphic in the regions that encode the peptide-binding groove. The polymorphism helps to ensure survival of a population by increasing the variety of peptides that can be presented to T cells. MHC polymorphism decreases the chance of encountering pathogens that may induce poor immune responses within a population leading to the demise of the population due to disease. However, the polymorphism also predisposes to allograft rejection as the antigen-presenting structures of one person are seen as foreign by another person.

The primary HLA products that contribute to rejection are the most polymorphic including HLA-A, -B, and -DR. HLA-A and

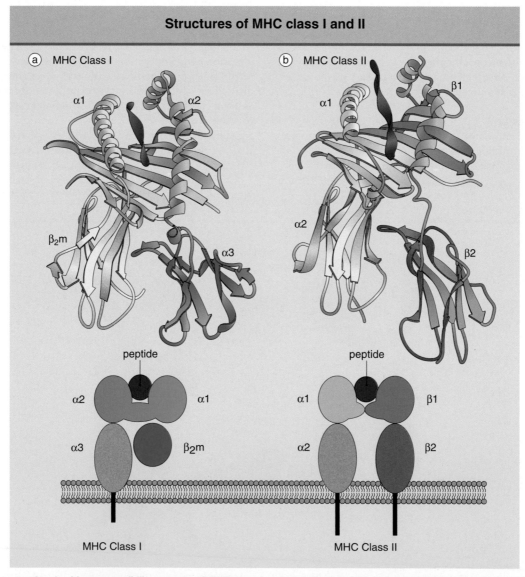

Figure 89.3   Structures of major histocompatibility complex (MHC) class I and class II. MHC class I is composed of a heavy chain divided into α1, α2, and α3 domains, noncovalently associated with β_2-microglobulin (β_2-m). The α1 and α2 domains make up the floor and the walls of the peptide-binding groove. MHC class II is a dimer composed of an α and a β chain. Each chain is divided into two domains, with α1 and β1 making up the floor and walls of the peptide-binding groove.

HLA-B products are expressed on most somatic cells, but the amount expressed varies. DR antigens also are widely expressed or inducible and serve as important transplantation antigens. Efforts are made to match HLA-A and -B and DR genes and proteins in kidney transplantation. Although class II expression is mainly restricted to marrow-derived APCs including DCs, B cells, macrophages, and Langerhans cells, humans also express class II products on some endothelial cells and epithelial cells. Moreover, both class I and class II antigens can be induced on many cells by interferon (IFN)-γ, in synergy with other cytokines. In the absence of IFN-γ, little MHC can be induced in the kidney, even during strong inflammatory stimuli such as allograft rejection.[12,13]

Function of Major Histocompatibility Complex

Class I and class II systems are designed for the presentation of antigen from different sources and for different purposes. The class I system is designed to sample cytosolic proteins and detect foreign proteins that would indicate an intracellular pathogen such as a virus or intracellular bacteria. Class I proteins are recognized by CD8 T cells and thus provide a surveillance mechanism to target infected cells for destruction. The class II system is designed to sample extracellular proteins by specialized APCs, which are very efficient in taking up material by phagocytosis or endocytosis. Class II proteins are recognized by CD4 T helper cells and allow for the generation of immune responses to invading pathogens that are phagocytosed by APCs early on in the infection.

MHC products also play important roles in the regulation of T cell function, including the positive and negative selection of developing T cells, stimulation of naive T cells that is necessary for their survival, the induction of T cell tolerance and anergy, and interaction with NK and other inhibitory and activating receptors.

HLA Matching and Transplantation

The class I and class II HLA genes are the most polymorphic in the human genome. Originally polymorphisms were defined by HLA serologic typing using sera from multiparous women or persons who had received multiple blood transfusions. Approximately 30 serotypes have been identified for HLA-A, 70 for HLA-B, and 10 for HLA-C. The development of molecular biology techniques (polymerase chain reaction [PCR], sequencing) has made possible the analyses of the HLA allelic sequence diversity at the DNA level. By DNA typing, many more polymorphisms have been identified: >230 for HLA-A, >470 for HLA-B, nearly 120 for HLA-C, and >380 for HLA-DR. The most currently updated source for HLA alleles can be found at the website www.anthonynolan.com/HIG/index.html. Currently, PCR methods allow for rapid DNA sequence-based typing of human populations, although serologic methods (antibodies) are still sometimes used for identifying HLA antigens.

HLA Profiles

HLA genes are codominantly expressed, meaning that both copies of each HLA gene will be expressed as antigens. Tissue typing identifies the two alleles encoded at each of the three loci (A, B, DR). One allele for each of HLA-A, -B, and -DR (i.e., one haplotype) will have been inherited from the mother, and a second haplotype will have been inherited from the father. Using mendelian genetics, it could be predicted that siblings from the same set of parents will have a 25% chance of having zero mismatches, 50% chance of having one mismatch, and a 25% chance of two mismatches. HLA typing identifies the specific alleles carried by a person. The term *HLA matching* means assigning a donor kidney to a recipient, after typing both, with as few mismatches as possible.

The degree of HLA matching at the HLA-A, B, and DR loci affects the survival of kidney allografts, as demonstrated by data from the United Network for Organ Sharing database (UNOS).[14] This is reflected in the 3-year graft survival rates: 93% and 85% for HLA-matched and mismatched living related donors, respectively. The same trend is observed in cadaveric donor grafts with 82% and 76% survival rates for HLA-matched and mismatched living related donors, respectively. Differences in survival rates and graft half-life are observed despite the improved immunosuppression in use today. However, most of the benefit of HLA matching is in those who receive zero mismatches: the number of mismatches seems less important once there are HLA mismatches. One important benefit of HLA matching is the protection from antibody-mediated rejection since the great majority of alloantibody-mediated rejection is due to anti-HLA.

Another useful test is the cross-matching test: the serum of a potential recipient is incubated with cells from the possible donor to see whether the recipient has antidonor antibodies, usually against the HLA antigens of the donor. If they do, there is a strong likelihood that the recipient would destroy the transplant by antibody-mediated rejection. Cross-matching donors and recipients helps to determine whether a kidney transplantation should occur (see Chapter 91).

Anti-HLA antibodies in the serum of a person can be assessed as panel-reactive antibodies (PRAs). This is determined by testing the serum of the patient against a panel of cells or antigens prepared from many different donors using cytotoxicity or flow cytometry. The results are expressed as the percentage of positive donors. PRAs can also be identified in enzyme-linked immunosorbent assay–based methods, using purified HLA antigens instead of cells from each donor. Alloreactive antibodies can be generated by prior sensitization through blood transfusions, previous transplantations, or by pregnancy.

Cross-matching prevents a transplant from being given to a recipient who has preexisting antibodies to the transplant. PRA measurement determines how many anti-HLA antibodies a person has, which predicts whether he or she will have difficulty getting a transplant.

GENERATION OF T CELL EFFECTOR FUNCTIONS

Alloreactive T cells can be found in the naive and memory T cell populations, but both require recognition of nonself-MHC molecules to become activated. Naive T cells may be triggered by donor or recipient APCs to proliferate and develop effector functions in SLOs. Memory cells may be activated in the same manner or may also become activated by recognizing cells in the allograft directly. The difference is that naive cells are restricted to trafficking only within SLOs, while memory cells can enter peripheral tissues. Reactions mediated by naive T cells take longer to develop than those mediated by memory T cells, which can be generated more quickly and with higher numbers of cells (secondary response). During allograft rejection, both populations are activated simultaneously.

Antigen-induced T cell activation and proliferation occur in SLOs and are driven by T cell growth factors such as IL-2. Proliferation of alloreactive clones generates a considerable number of responding T cells including CD4 and CD8 T cells and B cells. These can injure the allograft through the generation of alloantibody by B cells, the generation of CTLs, and by mediating DTH responses. Each CD4+ T helper cell can activate several B cells to produce antibody or recruit and activate a large number of macrophages for a DTH response. CTLs can destroy the cells of the allograft directly. Although CTLs can only kill one target at a time, a single CTL can kill multiple targets over a short period of time.

T Cell Receptor

T cells express TCRs that recognize peptide-MHC complexes on the surface of other cells. TCRs are heterodimers composed of α and β chains, or γ and δ chains. Expression of αβ and γδ TCRs are mutually exclusive. The majority of T cells (approximately 95%) have αβ TCRs and account for all T cell functions in kidney transplantation. A minority (approximately 5%) express γδ TCRs but are generally restricted to epithelial tissues, and their role in alloimmunity is not known.

Each α chain and β chain contains a constant domain and a variable domain. These domains are similar to the C and V domains of Ig and are in the Ig superfamily. The diversity in the TCR repertoire is encoded in the V domains of the α and β chains. These V domains have three hypervariable loops or complementary determining regions (CDRs) that form the antigen-binding site at the end of the TCR, interacting with the sheet and helix domains of the MHC and the presented peptide. Of these CDRs, CDR3 is most variable. Much of the peptide contact is made by the CDR3 loop. This interaction enhances the specificity of antigen recognition by T cells since the most variable region of the TCR interacts with the diverse peptides that are presented in MHC molecules.[15]

Normally an individual's TCRs recognize a universe of MHC peptide shapes that form the surface of MHC peptide molecules that are viewed as self and do not lead to T cell activation. This is the concept of central tolerance in which each T cell expressing individual self-reactive TCRs are deleted in the thymus by negative selection. MHC peptide shapes that are later encountered are identified as nonself or potentially infected self, such as a peptides from a virus that create a new MHC peptide shape, and this triggers an immune response. The shapes of one person's MHC peptide universe differ from those of another because of peptides they contain or because of polymorphisms in the amino acids of the peptide-binding regions of the MHC itself. Thus, the predisposition to alloreactivity is often a cross-reactivity of T cells specific for pathogenic peptides in the context of self-MHC that can also be activated by allogeneic peptides presented on self- or donor MHC.

CD4 and CD8 Coreceptors

TCR-MHC interaction alone is not enough to invoke T cell activation. Specific coreceptor molecules are also found on the T cell surface that enhance the affinity of TCR interaction with a peptide-MHC complex and help recruit signaling molecules to engaged TCRs. CD4 and CD8 bind to conserved regions of MHC molecules. CD4 is monomeric membrane glycoprotein containing four Ig-like domains. CD8 can be an αβ heterodimer or an αα homodimer, each chain consisting of a single Ig-like domain. Both CD4 and CD8 have a cytoplasmic tail that can associate with signaling proteins important in T cell activation.

Expression of CD4 and CD8 divides mature T cells into two distinct subsets due to their mutually exclusive expression. T helper cells that recognize MHC class II molecules on APCs express CD4, while CTLs that recognize MHC class I molecules on target cells express CD8. Both coreceptors interact with the nonpolymorphic regions of their respective MHC molecules; CD4 binds the membrane proximal β2 domain of class II and CD8 interacts mostly with the α3 and the α2 domains of class I.

T Cell Signaling: The Three-Signal Model

T cell activation by antigen on APCs requires signal 1 (antigen) and signal 2 (costimulation). Proliferation and emergence of effector function require cytokine signaling (signal 3).

T Cell Receptor Engagement of Antigen: Signal 1

The antigen-specific receptor of T cells (TCR) does not have signaling properties directly associated with it, having only short cytoplasmic tails that are unable to transduce signals. The signaling complex noncovalently associated with TCRs is known as the CD3 complex and is composed of three different chains: CD3γ, CD3δ, and CD3ε (Fig. 89.4). A homodimer of ξ chains completes the signaling complex.

Engagement of the TCR by MHC, along with the other required receptor engagements, initiates the signaling process from the CD3 complex.[16] The first event to occur following TCR engagement is the activation of the protein tyrosine kinase *lck* associated with CD4 or CD8 molecules. Activated *lck* phosphorylates tyrosine residues on the CD3 molecules that then serve as anchoring sites for the protein tyrosine kinase ZAP-70. ZAP-70 phosphorylates several downstream substrates including adaptor and linker molecules that lead to the activation of phospholipase C (PLC-γ1).

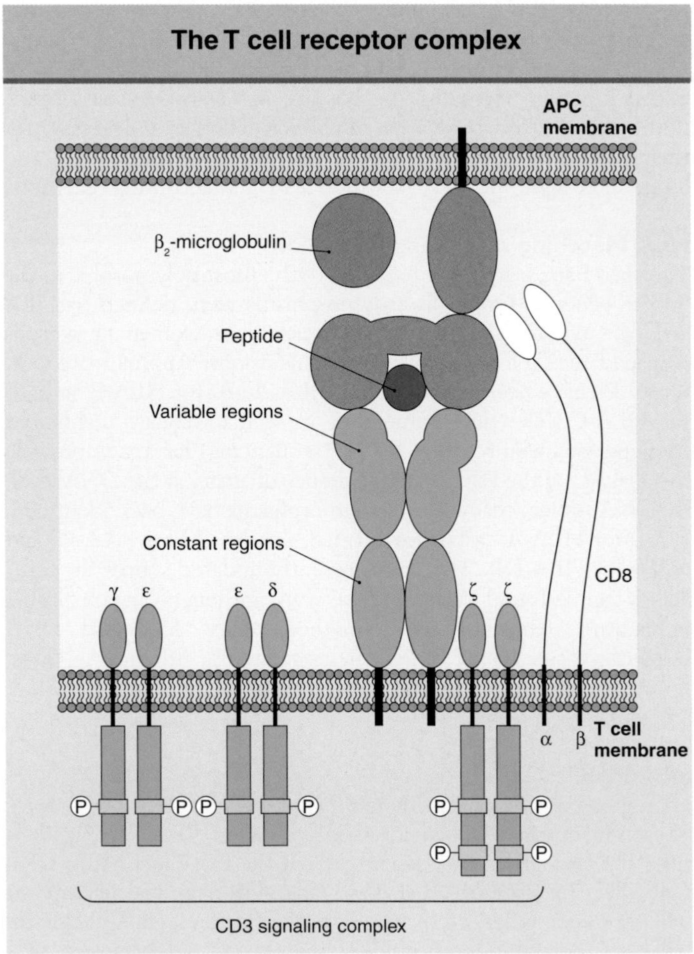

The T cell receptor complex

Figure 89.4 The T cell receptor (TCR) complex. Antigenic peptides are presented in the groove of an HLA molecule and are recognized by the variable regions of the TCR. Binding of CD8 (or CD4) to the HLA molecules increases the affinity of the TCR–major histocompatibility complex interaction. Triggering of the TCR by antigen initiates a signaling cascade started by the signaling complex made up of CD3 γ, ε, and δ chains as well as the ξ chain homodimer. APC, antigen-presenting cell.

PLC-γ1 hydrolyzes phosphatidylinositol-4,5-bisphosphate to the potent second messengers inositol triphosphate (IP_3) and diacylglycerol (DAG). DAG activates protein kinase C leading to the activation of the NF-κB pathway, while IP_3 acts on the endoplasmic reticulum to induce the release of intracellular Ca^{2+}.

The release of intracellular Ca^{2+} from the endoplasmic reticulum opens calcium channels that are linked to depletion of endoplasmic reticulum calcium stores, the so-called calcium release–activated calcium (CRAC) channels. These channels generate a calcium current (I_{CRAC}). The I_{CRAC} then activates the protein serine phosphatase calcineurin. Calcineurin dephosphorylates the transcription factor NF-AT (nuclear factor of activated T cells) allowing it to translocate into the nucleus. Translocation of NF-AT and NF-κB, along with other transcription factors, allows for the transcription of the genes for IL-2 and other cytokines, as well as the genes for the high-affinity subunit of the IL-2 receptor (CD25), and thus enhances clonal expansion. Cyclosporine and tacrolimus are immunosuppressive due to their ability to inhibit calcineurin and prevent translocation of NF-AT (see Chapter 90).

Immune Synapse The molecular interaction between a T cell and an APC results in a structure known as the immune synapse.[17] The mature immune synapse is characterized by the bull's-eye arrangement of supramolecular activation clusters (SMACs) that form during T cell–APC contact. The center of the SMAC contains the TCR and important cytoplasmic signaling molecules on the T cell and MHC peptide complexes on the APC. The peripheral SMAC contains the integrin LFA-1 on the T cell and its ligand intercellular adhesion molecule (ICAM)-1 on the APC. Immune synapse stabilization correlates with T cell activation and is dependent on TCR signaling.

Costimulation: Signal 2

Costimulation is the second signal required for the activation of T helper cells. Signal 1 is provided by the recognition of peptide MHC by the TCR, but signal 2 is necessary for optimal IL-2 production, IL-2 receptor expression, and cell-cycle progression according to the two-signal model of T cell activation. The TCR dictates the specificity of the response, while costimulation amplifies and prolongs the response and allows for the generation of effector function. Costimulation is probably a checkpoint developed by the immune system to prevent the generation of autoimmune cells. The activation of a naive T helper cell in the absence of signal 2 leads to anergy, through an incompletely understood mechanism. Thus, costimulation removes this inhibition and determines whether a T cell will proceed with clonal expansion and development of effector function or become anergic (Fig. 89.5).

CD28 was the first costimulatory molecule identified on T cells and binds to B7 molecules on the APCs. CD28 costimulation is mostly required by T helper cells but does not appear to be as important in the activation of CTLs.[18] Blockade of this costimulation can be mediated by the administration of CTLA-4Ig, a fusion protein with high-affinity for B7 molecules (see Fig. 89.5).

The CD40-CD40L system plays an ancillary role as an amplifier of costimulation. CD40L (a member of the tumor necrosis factor [TNF] superfamily) is expressed on activated T cells and binds to CD40 expressed on B cells, DCs, macrophages, and endothelial cells. When CD40L engages CD40, a differentiation signal is sent that allows the APCs to perform more specialized tasks. CD40 ligation on B cells induces class switching, allowing for the production and secretion of specialized, higher affinity antibodies. DCs must also have CD40 engaged by T helper cells to allow for proper

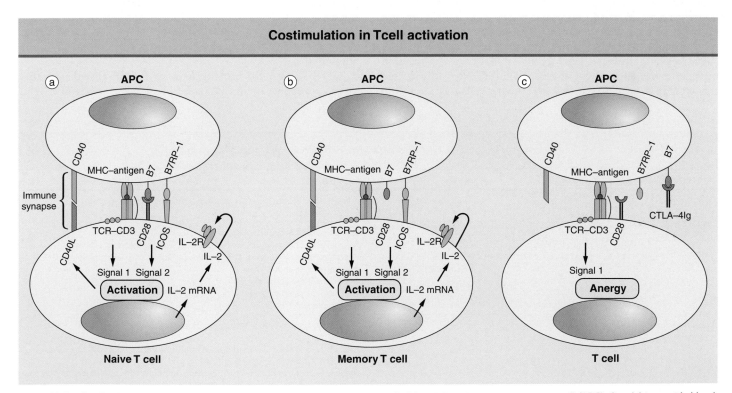

Figure 89.5 Costimulation in T cell activation. *a*, Naive T cells require ligation of CD28 by B7 on the antigen-presenting cell (APC). Signal 1 is provided by the recognition of antigen by the T cell receptor (TCR) while signal 2 is provided by ligation of CD28 and inducible costimulator (ICOS) by their respective ligands. Signals 1 and 2 lead to activation of the T cell and expression of interleukin (IL)-2, IL-2R, and CD40L. *b*, Memory T cells do not require costimulation through CD28 to become activated. Costimulation through ICOS is sufficient for memory T cell activation. *c*, Absence of B7 or blocking of B7 with CTLA-4 Ig leads to anergy of the T cell. APC, antigen-presenting cell; MHC, major histocompatibility complex. B7RP–1, B7-related protein-1.

priming of precursor CTLs. The roles of CD40-CD40L in modulating costimulation and class switching in the immune system make it a potential target for immunosuppression. However, clinical trials using anti-CD40L antibody have proved disappointing.

The B7 superfamily and their receptors are also involved in costimulation. Of these, B7-related protein-1 (B7RP-1) and its T cell counterpart, inducible costimulator (ICOS), are important. ICOS is a member of the CD28 family that is induced on activated T cells within 24 to 48 hours of activation. Engagement of ICOS increases production of IFN-γ, IL-4, IL-10, and IL-2 independent of CD28. Antibody production requires ICOS-B7RP-1 interactions, highlighting its role in T cell–dependent B cell activation. Unlike CD28 or CD40L, ICOS is expressed on memory T cells, suggesting an important role for ICOS in the regulation of effector and memory T cells.[19] Lack of signaling through CD28 leads to termination of the T cell response (see later discussion).

Trigger for T Cell Proliferation (Clonal Expansion) and Differentiation: Signal 3

CD4 and CD8 T cells are both produced in the thymus from which they leave to enter the circulation as naive T cells. Naive T cells are restricted to recirculating between SLOs and blood until they encounter antigen. DCs enter lymph nodes and migrate into the T cell region in the paracortex. On encountering a DC-expressing antigenic MHC and costimulatory receptors, T cells are induced to undergo gene transcription and differentiate into effector T cells.

Signals 1 and 2 activate three signal transduction pathways: the calcium-calcineurin pathway, the renin angiotensin system–mitogen-activated protein kinase pathway, and the NF-κB pathway.[7] These pathways activate transcription factors that trigger the expression of many new molecules, including IL-2, CD154, and CD25. IL-2 and other cytokines (e.g., IL-15) activate the target of rapamycin pathway to provide signal 3, the trigger for cell proliferation. One of the first cytokines produced is IL-2, which helps to drive T cell division during clonal expansion through the mamalian target of rapamycin (mTOR) pathway (see Chapter 90). A subset of activated T helper cells migrate to the

B cell region of the lymph node located in the cortex and provide help to differentiating B cells. The remainder of the effector T cells leaves the lymph node and proceeds to the inflamed site.

As T cells leave the lymph node, they have undergone multiple rounds of division and express their respective effector molecules between 3 and 5 days following activation. After activation, T cells change their chemokine receptor expression to permit them to enter the peripheral tissues. Those that enter the graft promote inflammation. The activated T cells become responsive to inflammatory chemokines and home to inflamed sites (Fig. 89.6). The activated T cells rapidly accumulate in the interstitium of the allograft as the response mounts in the first few days.

Effector Functions of T Cells

CD4 and CD8 T cells have different roles during immune responses. CD4 T cells may be both effectors and regulators. CD4 T cells are cytokine-secreting cells that express IL-2 and later a wide variety of cytokines. After prolonged stimulation, CD4 T cells sometimes tend to express groups of several cytokines, probably depending on the local environment, the nature of the antigen, and the APCs. The T helper 1 (Th1) pattern of cytokines includes IL-2, IFN-γ, and lymphotoxin, while the Th2 pattern includes IL-4, IL-5, IL-10, and IL-13. However, these cytokine patterns are never observed as unique patterns in transplantation. Thus, rejecting grafts typically have high levels of IFN-γ, TNF-α, and IL-10 mRNA and cannot be called a pure Th1 response.

CD4 T helper cells may release numerous cytokines (Fig. 89.7) that affect the alloimmune response. For example, they may promote a DTH response that involves stimulating production of nitric oxide, reactive oxygen species, and TNF-α in macrophages (Fig. 89.8). They may also become cytolytic T cells, similar to CD8 CTLs. One mechanism is by expression of the apoptosis-triggering molecule Fas ligand (FasL). However, whether this is important in killing graft cells is unknown. FasL is important in killing lymphocytes in normal immune homeostasis, and disruptions in the FasL-Fas system manifest lymphoproliferation and autoimmunity.

CD4 T cells also provide help to B cells to enhance their antibody production in the SLOs. In addition, regulatory T cells

Proteins involved in the recruitment of leukocytes into allografts

Protein Type	Name	Ligand	Function
Selectins	L-selectin	Sialated glycoproteins	Present on activated EC mediates initial rolling of leukocytes on endothelium
Chemokines	MCP-1/CCL2	CCR2	Recruitment of monocytes, immature DC, T cells, and NK cells
	MIP-1α/CCL3	CCR1	Recruitment of monocytes, immature DC, T cells, and neutrophils
	RANTES/CCL5	CCR1, CCR4, CCR5	Recruitment of monocytes, DC, T cells, NK cells, and neutrophils
	IL-8/CXCL8	CXCR1, CXCR2	Recruitment of neutrophils
	MIG/CXCL9	CXCR3	Recruitment of activated/memory T cells
	IP-10/CXCL10	CXCR3	Recruitment of activated/memory T cells
	Lymphotactin/XCL1	XCR1	Recruitment of T cells
Immunoglobulin superfamily	ICAM-1	LFA-1	Present on activated EC, mediates tight adhesion of leukocytes to endothelium
	ICAM-2, -3	LFA-1	Present on activated EC, mediates tight adhesion of leukocytes to endothelium (not as strong as ICAM-1)
	VCAM-1	VLA-4	Present on activated EC, mediates rolling and tight adhesion of leukocytes to endothelium
	CD31	CD31	Present at intercellular junctions on EC, mediates extravasation of leukocytes across endothelium

Figure 89.6 Proteins involved in the recruitment of leukocytes into allografts. DC, dendritic cells; EC, endothelial cells; ICAM, intercellular adhesion molecule; MHC, major histocompatibility complex; NK, natural killer; VCAM, vascular cell adhesion molecule.

Cytokines involved in allograft rejection

Cytokine	Source	Biologic Activity
IL-1	Macrophages, EC, NK cells	Proinflammatory, costimulates T cell and macrophage activation, enhances NK-cell activity
IL-2	Activated T cells	Promotes T cell proliferation, induces NK-cell activity, responsible for AICD of activated T cells
IL-4	Activated T cells	B and T cell growth factor, promotes allergic responses, increases MHC expression on B cells
IL-5	Activated T cells	Eosinophil growth factor and chemoattractant
IL-6	Macrophages, EC, T cells	Lymphocyte differentiation, stimulates production of acute-phase proteins
IL-10	T cells, macrophages	Anti-inflammatory, suppresses cytokine production and MHC expression on APC
IL-12	Macrophages, DC, B cells	Proinflammatory, stimulates interferon-γ production by T and NK cells, enhances NK cell activity
IL-15	Epithelial cells, stroma cells, macrophages	T cell growth factor, supports NK-cell development, required for memory T cell survival
Interferon-γ	Antigen-engaged T and NK cells	Increases MHC expression, increases cytotoxic activity of macrophages, promotes recruitment of activated T cells by EC
Transforming growth factor-β	T and B cells, macrophages, platelets	Anti-inflammatory, promotes wound healing
Tumor necrosis factor-α	Macrophages and NK, T, and B cells	Proinflammatory, cytotoxic, activates ECs and fibroblasts

Figure 89.7   Cytokines involved in allograft rejection. AICD, activation-induced cell death; APC, antigen-presenting cells; DC, dendritic cells; EC, endothelial cells; IL, interleukin; MCH, major histocompatibity complex; NK, natural killer.

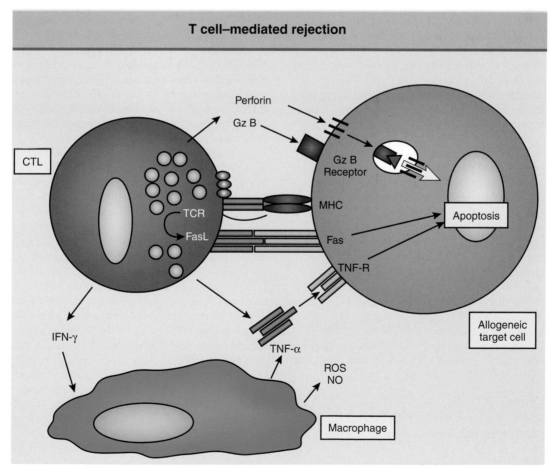

Figure 89.8   T cell–mediated rejection. T cell receptor (TCR) of alloreactive cytotoxic lymphocytes (CTL) recognize allogeneic major histocompatibility complex (MHC) on target cells. CTL mobilize cytotoxic granules containing perforin and granzyme B (Gz B) toward the target cell releasing the cytotoxic molecules into the intercellular space. Perforin inserts into the target cell membrane and Gz B binds to its receptor and both are internalized to induce apoptosis. TCR stimulation increases expression of Fas ligand (FasL) on the CTL surface and binds the Fas receptor, triggering the apoptotic cascade. CTL can produce the cytotoxic cytokine tumor necrosis factor α (TNF-α), which binds the TNF-R on the target cell leading to apoptosis. CTL can also release interferon (IFN)-γ, which will activate the macrophage to release proinflammatory substances. NO, nitric oxide; ROS, reactive oxygen species.

may have important roles in suppressing immune responses and maintaining tolerance.

Many cells in the graft express and present class II MHC to alloreactive CD4 T cells. IFN-γ is released by both CD4 and CD8 cells during rejection and induces MHC class II expression on endothelium and increases class I expression on vascular endothelial cells, epithelial cells, and parenchymal cells in the graft. Ischemic injury to the graft also induces class II expression. A mild increase in MHC expression caused by ischemic injury can serve as the alloantigen for infiltrating alloreactive CD4 and CD8 T cells to induce secretion of IFN-γ and other effector cytokines that further amplify MHC expression and inflammation. The precise role of class II expression by donor cells in the graft remains controversial because mouse kidney grafts lacking all class II are rejected more vigorously.[20] Thus, MHC is an antigen and an antigen-presenting structure, but IFN-γ probably has other signaling roles that actually help to stabilize the graft.

Alloantibody responses are generated simultaneously with T cell responses against foreign MHC antigens, particularly the class I antigens. T helper cell–dependent B cell activation is an important component of the effector functions of graft rejection. Naive or memory B cells become activated by the cross-linking of the BCR by intact antigen (donor MHC). They also express donor peptides in their class II molecules to permit them to be recognized and helped by peptide-specific primed T cells. T helper cells stimulate B cells to become antibody-producing plasma cells through CD40L, which engages CD40 on B cells. Alloantibody produced during rejection is mainly IgG and primarily participates in the destruction of the vascular endothelium of the graft (e.g., peritubular capillaries).

CD8 T cells express many effector functions, including cytokine production (e.g., IFN-γ) and cytotoxicity. They participate in rejection through DTH or through cytotoxicity. The role of CD8 effector functions is discussed in more detail (see "T Cell–Mediated Rejection").

Termination of the T Cell Response

T cell activation is terminated through a number of events, one of which is the membrane expression of the inhibitor of costimulation CTLA-4. CTLA-4 is similar to CD28 in that it also interacts with B7 but, unlike CD28, it sends an inhibitory signal and is not expressed on resting T cells. TCR engagement causes CTLA-4 expression but only following 24 hours of stimulation, thus providing an effective regulatory feedback mechanism. Although CTLA-4 surface levels are not as high as CD28, its higher affinity for B7 molecules allows it to outcompete CD28 for B7 binding. Thus, CTLA-4 has two effects: it removes B7 from CD28, eliminating the CD28 signal, and it delivers a poorly understood negative signal to terminate T cell activation. The higher affinity of CTLA-4 for B7 is the reason behind the immunosuppressive effects of the soluble fusion protein CTLA-4 Ig that efficiently blocks B7 expressed on APCs.

GRAFT REJECTION

Recruitment of Cells into the Interstitium of Kidney Allografts

Rejection is defined as tissue injury produced by the effector mechanisms of the adaptive alloimmune response, leading to deterioration in renal function. There are two types of rejection: T cell–mediated rejection and antibody-mediated rejection. Both types of rejection can be early or late, fulminant and rapid, or relatively indolent and slow. The leukocytic infiltrate observed in rejection is composed of mononuclear cells including T cells, macrophages, B cells, and plasma cells. T cells serve as the main effectors and regulators of the alloimmune response. Macrophages serve as possible effectors and aid in the removal of apoptotic cells, while B cells and plasma cells serve in the production of alloantibodies. The recruitment of these cells into the graft is a result of the combination of chemokine expression and adhesion molecule expression by the endothelium of the graft (see Fig. 89.6). The endothelium of postcapillary venules in the graft serves as the entry point of recipient leukocytes from the bloodstream into the allograft. Graft endothelial cells are activated by proinflammatory cytokines and injury to express adhesion molecules and chemokines necessary for transendothelial migration. The general model for leukocyte movement across the endothelium of the microcirculation is that they roll on selectins; receive chemokines signals, which activate the leukocyte integrins; and then flatten due to integrin engagement of their ligands and diapedese through endothelial cell junctions.

The recruitment of leukocytes is initiated by the release of chemokines by tubular cells, interstitial cells, endothelial cells, and infiltrating recipient cells within the allograft. Thus, effector T cells expressing the respective chemokine receptors extravasate through the endothelium and are guided by a chemokine gradient. In the interstitium, they engage alloantigen and mediate DTH.

Binding of chemokines to chemokine receptors induces a conformational change on integrins, which are normally present on circulating leukocytes in an inactive state. Tight adhesion occurs when activated integrins bind their Ig superfamily ligands such as ICAM and vascular cell adhesion molecule (VCAM). The most common integrins present on lymphocytes are LFA-1, which binds ICAM-1 and -2, and VLA-4, which that binds with VCAM-1. ICAM-1, VCAM-1, and E-cadherin are expressed on the tubular epithelium of rejecting grafts where they play a role in the development of tubulitis. Unfortunately, blocking of adhesion has not been that successful for treating rejection, likely due to redundancy among the multiple adhesion molecules and ligands that mediate leukocyte adhesion.

As a result of cytokines from infiltrating T cells, the graft changes its pattern of gene expression. For example, IFN-γ from T cells induces a massive increase in MHC expression in the epithelium and endothelium of the graft. Expression of other genes, such as those for adhesion molecules, is also induced.

T Cell–Mediated Rejection

Most rejection in clinical kidney transplantation is mediated by T cells (see Fig. 89.8) and may most closely correspond to a DTH response, even though many cells with CTL capabilities (i.e., granzyme B, perforin) are present. Activated CD4 or CD8 effector T cells secrete cytokines that induce the influx of nonspecific inflammatory cells—macrophages—and activate them to organize a DTH response. DTH responses can induce tissue injury through direct effects of soluble products on the epithelium, alterations in the interstitial matrix, and stimulation of macrophages to release reactive oxygen species, proteolytic enzymes, eicosanoids, and other products.

Deterioration of renal function in T cell–mediated rejection correlates with invasive lesions involving the tubules (tubulitis; Fig. 89.9) and arterial arteritis, which is much less common (endothelialitis; Fig. 89.10). At a certain point, the effector T cells move toward the tubules of the graft where they cross the basement membrane and engage the basolateral membrane of the epithelial cells in a process known as tubulitis. Some studies suggest that tubulitis may involve a specific subset of CTLs expressing the integrin CD103, which binds to its ligand E-cadherin on epithelial

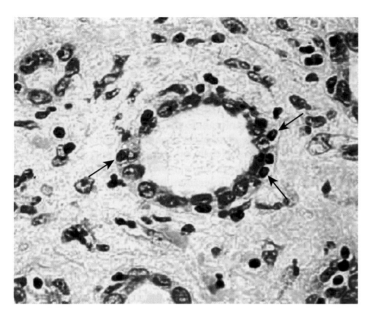

Figure 89.9 Tubulitis. Infiltration of tubular epithelium by T lymphocytes (*arrows*) that have crossed the basement membrane.

cells.[21,22] However, a special role for CD103-E-cadherin interactions in creating tubulitis lesions may not be necessary. Another view is that the inflammatory changes in the interstitium cause changes in the epithelium that lead to loss of the ability of the epithelium to exclude inflammatory cells. Thus, tubulitis may not be the cause of tubular cell deterioration, but a sign that the tubule cells have already deteriorated. Either way, it is a useful marker for T cell–mediated rejection when other criteria support that diagnosis.

While cytotoxicity is an attractive mechanism for explaining epithelial deterioration, the data that it is necessary for kidney injury are poor. Although CTLs are present in large numbers in renal allograft rejection, mice lacking cytotoxic molecules still reject grafts relatively briskly. T cell cytotoxicity *in vitro* results from two principal mechanisms. First, activated CTLs may kill

their targets by releasing the cytotoxic molecules perforin and granzyme B from stored granules that initiate a cascade of events that leads to apoptosis (see Fig. 89.8). Second, activated CTLs and T helper cells also use the Ca^{2+}-independent Fas/FasL pathway. Engagement of Fas on target cells by FasL from CTLs results in apoptotic death of the target cell.

Alloantibody-Mediated Rejection

Alloantibody-mediated rejection is classically associated with the triad of decreased renal function, the presence of antidonor antibody in recipient serum, and a renal biopsy specimen showing neutrophils in peritubular capillaries with endothelial damage.[23] Alloantibodies are cytotoxic through their ability to activate complement as well as by recruiting leukocytes with receptors for immunoglobulins (FcR) or complement (C3b). The demonstration of C4d deposition in the peritubular capillaries is now the basis for the diagnosis of antibody-mediated rejection (see Chapter 93).[24]

If recipients have been sensitized by previous transfusions, pregnancies, or transplants bearing donor MHC molecules, they may have preformed alloantibody against the donor. This can lead to disastrous hyperacute rejection, even on the operating table.[25] The entire endothelium of the graft is injured, and the large vessels usually fail (Fig. 89.11). This is prevented by cross-matching. For the same reason, recipients must be compatible with the donor at the ABO blood group locus. Hyperacute rejection is now very rare due to cross-matching practices.

Late Deterioration of Kidney Transplants

Approximately 40% of late graft loss is due to nonspecific deterioration in the absence of other specific diseases, often described as chronic rejection. Chronic rejection of kidney transplants is commonly defined as an alloimmune response causing the slow deterioration of renal function accompanied with pathology showing tubular atrophy, interstitial fibrosis (Fig. 89.12), and fibrous intimal thickening of arteries (Fig. 89.13). Unfortunately, the term *chronic rejection* is ambiguous as it fails to differentiate between the presence of an active alloimmune response causing tissue damage (rejection) and the state of the transplanted tissue (e.g., fibrosis and atrophy).[23] Whereas some cases of late slow graft deterioration are due to immune mechanisms, other cases may represent the consequences of hypertension, chronic calcineurin toxicity, or other diseases.

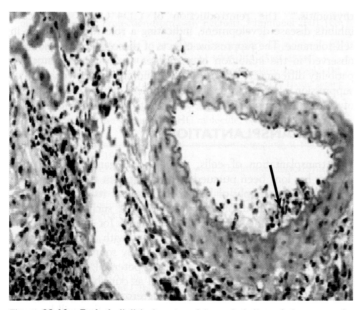

Figure 89.10 Endothelialitis. Invasion of the endothelium of a large artery by graft-infiltrating lymphocytes (*arrow*).

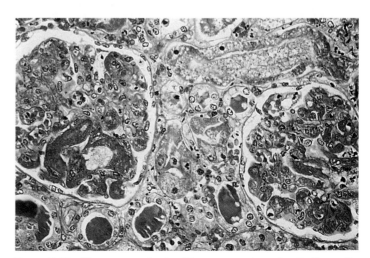

Figure 89.11 Hyperacute rejection. Hyperacute rejection showing glomerular and peritubular capillary infiltration and thrombosis with tubular injury and cast formation.

42. Larsen CP, Elwood ET, Alexander DZ, et al: Long-term acceptance of skin and cardiac allografts after blocking CD40 and CD28 pathways. Nature 1996;381:434–438.

43. Wells AD, Li XC, Li Y, et al: Requirement for T cell apoptosis in the induction of peripheral transplantation tolerance. Nat Med 1999;5:1303–1307.

44. Coates PT, Thomson AW: Dendritic cells, tolerance induction and transplant outcome. Am J Transplant 2002;2:299–307.

45. Takahashi T, Tagami T, Yamazaki S, et al: Immunologic self-tolerance maintained by CD25(+) CD4(+) regulatory T cells constitutively expressing cytotoxic T lymphocyte-associated antigen 4. J Exp Med 2000;192:303–310.

46. Sakaguchi S, Sakaguchi N, Shimizu J, et al: Immunologic tolerance maintained by CD25+ CD4+ regulatory T cells: Their common role in controlling autoimmunity, tumor immunity, and transplantation tolerance. Immunol Rev 2001;182:18–32.

47. Taylor PA, Noelle RJ, Blazar BR: CD4(+)CD25(+) immune regulatory cells are required for induction of tolerance to alloantigen via costimulatory blockade. J Exp Med 2001;193:1311–1318.

48. Lai L, Kolber-Simonds D, Park KW, et al: Production of alpha-1,3-galactosyltransferase knockout pigs by nuclear transfer cloning. Science 2002;295:1089–1092.

90

Immunosuppressive Agents Used in Transplantation

Gunilla Einecke, Anette Melk, and Philip F. Halloran

INTRODUCTION

Suppression of allograft rejection remains the central issue for successful organ transplantation. Current regimens of immunosuppression yield excellent 1-year rates of patient and graft survival; however, 5-year survival rates are only 66% and 79% for recipients of kidneys from cadaveric and living related donors, respectively. Paradoxically, some commonly used drugs, while effective for immunosuppression, may contribute to late allograft loss and death by virtue of their side effects; they are nephrotoxic or have adverse effects on blood pressure, lipid levels, and glucose homeostasis and thus promote cardiovascular disease and chronic allograft nephropathy. The current goal is to use immunosuppressive agents that are potent, selective, and reversible, with reliable delivery and long-term safety. These therapies suppress immune-response mechanisms but are not immunologically specific, and a careful balance is required between prevention of rejection (the therapeutic effect) and toxic effects: complications of immunodeficiency (development of infection and certain types of cancer) and nonimmune toxicities such as nephrotoxicity or hyperlipidemia. The variety of therapeutic options for transplant immunosuppression continues to broaden and become more complex, as do the possibilities for potential drug combinations and protocols. The present chapter focuses on immunosuppressive agents that are either approved or in phase II or phase III clinical trials in kidney transplantation.

IMMUNE RESPONSE

We briefly review a model of the alloimmune response to illustrate how immunosuppressive medications act. For a more extensive discussion of the principles of antigen recognition and the alloimmune response, see Chapter 89. Alloimmune responses are initiated by activation of APCs through innate immune-recognition systems. Once activated, dendritic cells of donor and host origin move to secondary lymphoid organs such as lymph nodes and spleen where they present donor antigen to naive T cells.[1,2] Previously stimulated or "antigen-experienced" memory cells may be activated by other cell types, such as graft endothelium.[3] B cells are activated when antigen engages their antigen receptors, usually in lymphoid follicles or in extrafollicular sites, such as red pulp of spleen[4] and possibly in the transplant,[5] producing alloantibody against donor HLA antigens.

The activation of the T cell requires three events (Fig. 90.1). Presentation of donor antigen on the surface of dendritic cells via the T cell receptor (TCR) constitutes signal 1 and is transduced

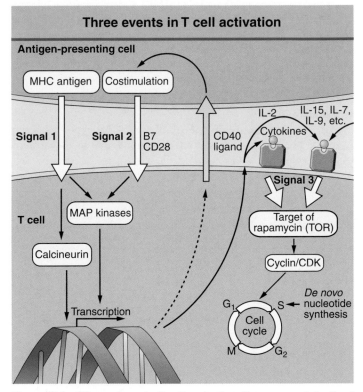

Figure 90.1 Three events in T cell activation. Engagement of the T cell receptor with the antigenic peptide in the context of self major histocompatibility complex (MHC) class II molecule leads to the activation of the calcineurin pathway and results in the induction of cytokine genes (e.g., interleukin [IL]-2) (signal 1). Signal 2, the costimulatory signal, involves the engagement of CD28 with members of the B7 family. This synergizes with signal 1 to induce cytokine production. Interaction between cytokine production and its corresponding receptor leads to induction of cell division, probably through the target of rapamycin pathway. This constitutes signal 3. MAP, mitogen-activated protein.

through the CD3 complex. Dendritic cells provide costimulation, or signal 2, delivered when B7.1 (CD80) and B7.2 (CD86) on the surface of dendritic cells engage CD28 on T cells. Signals 1 and 2 activate three signal transduction pathways: the calcium-calcineurin pathway, the renin angiotensin system–mitogen-activated protein (MAP) kinase pathway, and the nuclear factor-κB pathway.[6] These pathways activate transcription factors that trigger the expression of many new molecules, including interleukin (IL)-2, CD154, and CD25. IL-2 and other cytokines (e.g., IL-15) activate the target of rapamycin pathway to provide signal 3, the trigger for cell proliferation. Proliferation and differentiation lead to a large number of effector T cells. Thus, within days, the immune response generates the effector mechanisms—effector T cells and alloantibody—that can damage the organ and mediate allograft rejection. The two major types of rejection are T cell–mediated rejection and antibody-mediated rejection (see Chapter 89). Suppression of established antibody responses is a particularly challenging problem requiring immunosuppressive therapy.

IMMUNOSUPPRESSIVE AGENTS

Immunosuppression can be achieved by depleting lymphocytes, diverting lymphocyte traffic, or blocking lymphocyte response pathways. In transplantation, immunosuppressive agents are used for induction, maintenance, and treatment and reversal of established rejection.[7] The common immunosuppressive agents used in transplantation include small-molecule drugs (corticosteroids, azathioprine, mycophenolate mofetil [MMF], the calcineurin inhibitors cyclosporine and tacrolimus, inhibitors of the target of rapamycin), and protein drugs (polyclonal and monoclonal antibodies to cell surface antigens on lymphocytes, fusion proteins, and intravenous immunoglobulins; Fig. 90.2). Summaries of the effects of immunosuppressive drugs are presented in Figures 90.3 through 90.5.

Corticosteroids
Corticosteroids represent one of the principal types of agent used for both maintenance immunosuppression and treatment of acute rejection[8] (Fig. 90.6).

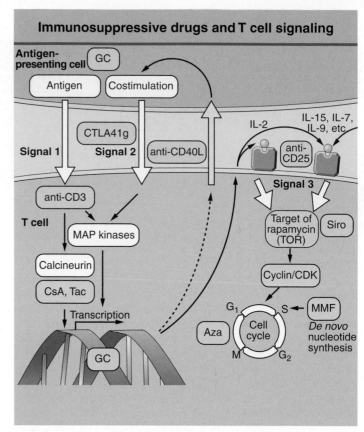

Figure 90.3 Immunosuppressive drugs and T cell signaling. Aza, azathioprine; CD25, interleukin 2–receptor α chain; CsA, cyclosporine; CTLA4Ig, fusion protein; Tac, tacrolimus; GC, glucocorticoids; MMF, mycophenolate mofetil; Siro, sirolimus.

Classification of immunosuppressive therapies

Pharmaceutical Therapies	Examples
Small molecule drugs	
Glucocorticoids	
Antimetabolites	Azathioprine
Immunophilin-binding drugs	Calcineurin inhibitors: cyclosporine, tacrolimus
	Target of rapamycin inhibitors: sirolimus, everolimus
Inhibitors of nucleotide synthesis	Purine synthesis (IMPDH inhibitors): mycophenolate mofetil (mizoribine, only in Japan)
	Pyrimidine synthesis (DHODH) inhibitors: leflunomide FK778
Sphingosine-1-phosphate-receptor antagonists	FTY720
Protein drugs	
Depleting antibodies	Polyclonal antibody: horse or rabbit antithymocyte globulin
	Murine monoclonal anti-CD3 antibody (muronomab-CD3)
	Humanized monoclonal anti-CD52 antibody (alemtuzumab)
	B cell depleting monoclonal anti-CD20 antibody (rituximab)
Nondepleting antibodies and fusion proteins	Humanized or chimeric monoclonal anti-CD25 antibody (daclizumab, basiliximab)
	Anti-CD40L
	Fusion protein with natural binding properties: CTLA4-Ig (LEA29Y)
Intravenous immunoglobulin	

Figure 90.2 Classification of immunosuppressive therapies. DHODH, dihydro-orotate dehydrogenase inhibitors IMPDH, inosine monophosphate dehydrogenase.

Pharmacokinetics and Absorption
The major corticosteroids used are prednisone or prednisolone (given orally with comparable efficacy) and methylprednisolone (given intravenously with 25% more potency). These agents are rapidly absorbed and have short plasma half-lives (60 to 180 minutes) but long biologic half-lives (18 to 36 hours). The effect of prednisone (dose/weight) is greater in the setting of renal failure or hypoalbuminemia in women and in the elderly, whereas less prednisone effect is observed in children. Prednisone should be dosed on body weight independent of obesity, whereas methylprednisolone should be administered based on ideal weight. In practice, methylprednisolone is given in standard doses. Certain drugs can decrease steroid efficacy by increasing metabolism: rifampin, phenytoin, phenobarbital, and carbamazepine. In contrast, increased corticosteroid effects may be observed in patients receiving oral contraceptives, estrogens, ketoconazole, and erythromycin.

Mechanism of Action
Corticosteroids have both anti-inflammatory and immunosuppressive effects. Lymphopenia and monocytopenia occur, with inhibition of lymphocyte proliferation, survival, activation, homing, and effector functions. Corticosteroids suppress production of numerous cytokines and vasoactive substances, including IL-1, tumor necrosis factor α (TNF-α), IL-2, major histocompatibility complex (MHC) class II, chemokines, prostaglandins (via inhibition of phospholipase A_2), and proteases. Corticosteroids also cause neutrophilia (often with a left shift), but neutrophil chemotaxis and adhesion are inhibited. They also affect nonhematopoietic cells.

Comparison of small-molecule immunosuppressive drugs

Agent	Action	Toxicity	Uses in Renal Transplantation
Corticosteroids (prednisone, prednisolone, methylprednisolone)	Binds to steroid receptor; complex enters the nucleus and binds to DNA and/or interacts with transcription factors and activators to alter transcription; acts particularly through regulation of factors AP-1 and NF-κB	Cushingoid features, skin thinning, osteoporosis, diabetes	Prophylaxis against rejection; reversal of rejection; used in short-term high doses or long-term maintenance doses
Azathioprine	Prodrug that releases 6-mercaptopurine; incorporated as a purine into DNA; interferes with DNA synthesis; other effects on purine metabolism	Leukopenia, anemia, thrombocytopenia, megaloblastoid changes	Commonly used with cyclosporine or tacrolimus, plus steroids in maintenance therapy
Cyclosporine	11-Amino-acid cyclic peptide from *Tolypocladium inflatum*; binds to cyclophilin; complex inhibits calcineurin phsophatase and T cell activation	Nephrotoxicity, hyperlipidemia, hypertension, gum hyperplasia, skin changes; less neurotoxicity and diabetes than tacrolimus	Long-term oral maintenance therapy against rejection, usually with steroids
Tacrolimus	Macrolide antibiotic from *Streptomyces tsukubaensis*; binds to FKBP12 complex inhibits calcineurin phosphatase and T cell activation	Nephrotoxicity, more neurotoxicity and diabetes but less hypertension, gum hyperplasia, skin changes than cyclosporine	Long-term maintenance therapy against rejection; rescue of patients with severe or refractory rejection, usually with steroids
Sirolimus/everolimus	Triene macrolide antibiotic from *Streptomyees hygroscopius*; binds to FKBP12, complex inhibits target of rapamycin (TOR) and IL-2–driven T cell proliferation (everolimus is a derivative of sirolimus)	Hyperlipidemia, thrombocytopenia II, leukopenia, impaired wound healing	Long-term maintenance therapy; often used in calcineurin-sparing protocols usually used with steroids
Mycophenolate mofetil	Prodrug that releases mycophenolic acid, a fermentation product from *Penicillium* species; blocks *de novo* purine synthesis by inhibiting IMPHDH; prevents proliferation of T and B cells	Gastrointestinal symptoms (mainly diarrhea), neutropenia, occasional mild anemia	Usually used with cyclosporine or tacrolimus in maintenance therapy
FK778	Modification of A77 1726 (active derivative of leflunomide); inhibitor of pyrimidine synthesis, blocks proliferation of T and B cells	Anemia; other effects not known	In phase II trials
FTY720	Sphingosine-like derivative of myriocin from ascomycete fungus; functional antagonist of sphingosin-1-phosphate receptors on lymphocytes; enhances homing to lymphoid tissues; reduces number of circulating lymphocytes	Reversible first-dose bradycardia; increased liver enzyme levels	On hold
CP-609, 550	Synthetic molecule; binds to cytoplasmic tyrosine kinase JAK3, inhibits cytokine-induced signaling	Anemia	In phase II trials

Figure 90.4 **Comparison of small-molecule immunosuppressive agents.** FKBP12, FK binding protein 12; NF-κB, nuclear factor-κB.

Corticosteroids act as agonists of glucocorticoid receptors, but at higher doses, they have receptor-independent effects. Corticosteroid receptors (CRs) belong to a family of ligand-regulated transcription factors called nuclear receptors. CRs are normally present in the cytoplasm in an inactive complex with heat shock proteins (HSP90, HSP70, and HSP56). The binding of corticosteroids to the CRs dissociates HSP from the CR and forms the active corticosteroid-CR complex, which migrates to the nucleus and dimerizes on palindromic DNA sequences in many genes, called the corticosteroid response element. The binding of CR in the promoter region of the target genes can lead to either induction or suppression of gene transcription (e.g., of cytokines). CR also exert effects by interacting directly with other transcription factors independent of DNA binding. Two of the key ways corticosteroids regulate immune responses is by regulating the transcription factors AP-1 and nuclear factor-κB (NF-κB). Normally, NF-κB is in

Protein immunosuppressive drugs			
Agent	Action	Toxicity	Uses in Renal Therapy
Depleting antibodies			
Polyclonal horse or rabbit antilymphocyte or antithymocyte globulin (ALG, ATG)	Contains many antibodies against proteins on lymphocytes that alter traffic, trigger, kill, and sequester the T and B lymphocytes	First-dose cytokine-release syndrome; thrombocytopenia, leukopenia	Prophylaxis against rejection; reversal of severe rejection
Mouse monoclonal anti-CD3 (OKT3)	Binds to CD3 complex associated with T cell receptor (TCR), triggers, and then blocks the TCR and inactivates or kills the T cell; short half-life and eventually neutralized by antibody response	First-dose cytokine-release syndrome (fever, chills, flulike symptoms) plus occasional acute pulmonary edema, acute renal failure, encephalopathy	Prophylaxis against rejection; reversal of severe rejection; daily IV dose for 7–14 days
Humanized monoclonal anti-CD52 antibody (alemtuzumab)	Depletion of peripheral and central lymphoid cells	First-dose reactions, neutropenia, anemia, and (rarely) pancytopenia and autoimmunity; risks of immunodeficiency complications (infections and cancer) are unknown	Alemtuzumab is used off-label for induction in some centers, but controlled trials are needed to establish dosing, safety, and efficacy
B cell depleting monoclonal anti-CD20 antibody (rituximab)	Targets CD20 and directly inhibits B cell proliferation by antibody-dependent, cell-mediated, cytotoxicity with depletion of circulating and tissue-based B cells; decreases the production of activated B cells and limits antibody production as well as antigen presentation	Virtually none	Treatment of steroid-resistant acute rejection; treatment of post-transplantation lymphoproliferative disease; may be an effective agent to reduce high-titer anti-HLA antibodies in hyperimmunized patients
Nondepleting antibodies			
Humanized or chimeric monoclonal anti-CD25 (basiliximab and daclizumab)	Binds to CD25 in IL-2 receptor complex; rendering all T cells resistant to IL-2; long half-life (same as human IgG, 21 days) once CD25 is saturated	Virtually none	Prophylaxis against rejection; interval dosing to saturate the CD25 for 4–16 weeks; usually used with cyclosporine plus steroid
Anti-CD40L	Costimulatory blockade	Thromboembolic events	Currently not in clinical use; a chimeric monoclonal is in development to minimize side effects
Belatacept (LEA29Y)	Fusion protein consisting of the extracellular domain of CTLA-4 the Fc domain of an IgG molecule; saturates CD80/86 and delivers a negative signal, resulting in costimulatory blockade of the CD28 pathway		Long-term maintenance immunosuppression; may allow calcineurin and steroid-sparing protocols

Figure 90.5 Protein immunosuppressive agents. ALG, antilymphocyteglobulin; ATG, antithymocyte globulin; IL, interleukin.

an inactive complex with inhibitor of nuclear factor κB (IκB) but can be released by IκB kinase (Fig. 90.7a) Corticosteroids stimulate IκB, which then compete with the IκB–NF-κB complex for degradation by the IκB kinase (see Fig. 90.7b).[9] Corticosteroids also stimulate lipocortin, which inhibits phospholipase A$_2$, thereby inhibiting the production of leukotrienes and prostaglandins. The total immunosuppressive effect of corticosteroids is complex, reflecting effects on cytokines, adhesion molecules, apoptosis, and activation of inflammatory cells.

Administration

In many transplantation centers, high-dose intravenous corticosteroids (e.g., methylprednisolone 250 mg to 1g, depending on the local protocol) are administered in the perioperative period as induction therapy, although the need for such high steroid pulses has not been established. This is followed by oral corticosteroids, usually in the form of prednisone (e.g., 30 mg/day) followed by a gradual taper to a maintenance dose of 2.5 to 5 mg/day or on

alternate days. Complete steroid withdrawal or induction regimens that are completely corticosteroid sparing are now used in many centers, despite being associated with higher rates of rejection (see Chapter 93). For many clinicians, the benefits in terms of reduced toxicity seem to offset slight increases in rejection rates. Variations include complete avoidance, use in the first few days only, early tapering and withdrawal, later tapering and withdrawal, and alternate-day dosing. One concern about these protocols is the long-term prevention of late rejection, which needs to be established. The first-line treatment of acute rejection is usually intravenous methylprednisolone at 250 to 500 mg/day for 3 days. This regimen reverses about 75% of acute rejection episodes.

Side Effects

Side effects of corticosteroid therapy are common and associated with significant morbidity, particularly cataracts, osteoporosis, and avascular necrosis of the femoral heads. Other side effects include hypertension, hyperglycemia, dyslipidemia, cushingoid

Corticosteroid structures

Hydrocortisone (cortisol)

Cortisone

Prednisolone (Δ_1 cortisol)

Prednisone (Δ_1 cortisone)

6α-methylprednisolone

Figure 90.6   Structural formulas of the corticosteroids cortisol, cortisone, prednisolone, prednisone, and 6α-methylprednisone.

facies, psychiatric disturbances, sleep disorders, peptic ulcer disease, pancreatitis, colonic perforation, and increased appetite and weight gain. Infection risk is also increased and is excessive if high-dose pulse therapy is prolonged (>3 days). Corticosteroid dose should, therefore, be decreased gradually during rejection treatment even if serum creatinine fails to improve. Interestingly, corticosteroids are not associated with increased risk of malignancy. Corticosteroids are generally safe in pregnancy due to efficient metabolism by the placenta with protection of the fetus; however, cases of fetal adrenal suppression have been reported. Strategies to

minimize the numerous side effects of steroids include reduction in the daily administered dose of steroids, use of alternate-day dosing regimens, steroid withdrawal post-transplantation, and complete steroid avoidance (see Chapter 93).

Calcineurin Inhibitors

Cyclosporine, a lipophilic cyclic peptide of 11-amino-acid residues, and tacrolimus, a macrolide antibiotic, are drugs with similar mechanisms of action and have become major maintenance immunosuppressive agents used in transplantation. The use of the more potent

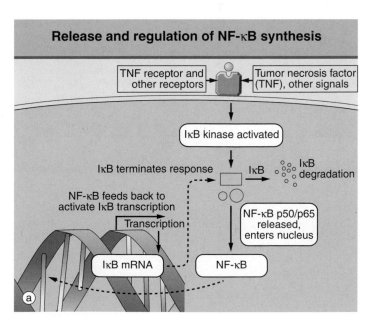

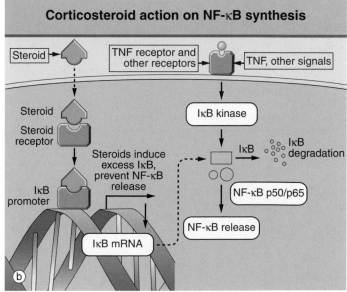

Figure 90.7   Corticosteroids and regulation of transcription factors. *a*, The mechanism of nuclear factor-κB (NF-κB) and its regulation by induction of synthesis of its inhibitor IκB. Activation of IκB kinase leads to IκB degradation; released NF-κB enters the nucleus and activates IκB transcription. Synthesis of IκB feeds back to terminate the cycle. *b*, The mechanism of corticosteroid immunosuppression by inhibition of NF-κB. The corticosteroid-corticosteroid receptor complex migrates to the nucleus and interacts with the promoter of the IκB gene to induce the synthesis of excess IκB, the natural inhibitor of NF-κB. IκB in excess prevents the release of NF-κB to the nucleus upon stimulation by cytokines such as tumor necrosis factor.

tacrolimus has increased steadily, and it is now the dominant calcineurin inhibitor. However, most transplantation programs exploit the strengths of both tacrolimus and cyclosporine, depending on the risks in individual patients. Tacrolimus is often considered for patients at greater risk of rejection, for those in which lower doses of corticosteroids are desired (such as the growing child), and for those with cardiovascular disease due to the fact that tacrolimus is associated with less hypertension and hyperlipidemia than cyclosporine (see "Side Effects"). Switching from cyclosporine to tacrolimus has also been reported as an effective rescue therapy for subjects with recurrent rejection. In contrast, cyclosporine seems to be more beneficial in those who experience or are at risk of the side effects of tacrolimus, such as the development of diabetes. Tacrolimus has been suspected of inducing more BK-virus nephropathy, especially when used with mycophenolate mofetil, but renal function may be better with tacrolimus. Due to the ability of both drugs to cause chronic nephrotoxicity, some centers are electively withdrawing calcineurin inhibitors late following transplantation, whereas others are attempting calcineurin inhibitor–sparing protocols. However, in many of these protocols, the rate of rejection and long-term safety of this practice remain to be established (see Chapter 93).

Pharmacokinetics and Drug Interactions

Cyclosporine and tacrolimus are both variably absorbed and are metabolized extensively by the cytochrome P-450 system in the liver. Cyclosporine is excreted primarily by the biliary system. The absorption of some cyclosporine preparations may be bile dependent and, therefore, may be reduced in the presence of cholestatic liver disease. The absorption of the microemulsion formulation of cyclosporine or of tacrolimus is bile independent. Neither cyclosporine nor tacrolimus is affected by alterations in renal function. Both cyclosporine and tacrolimus bind to cells and to plasma components (primarily lipoproteins for cyclosporine and albumin for tacrolimus) in the blood; consequently, they must be assayed in whole blood. Many drugs and agents can affect cyclosporine and tacrolimus levels through effects on their absorption or metabolism (Fig. 90.8).

Cyclosporine is usually administered initially as 8 to 10 mg/kg/day in divided doses (or intravenously using one third the oral dose over a 24-hour period) during the induction phase, with target trough blood levels of 150 to 300 μg/l for the first 6 months. (Some investigators recommend monitoring the level 2 hours after the dose [C2 monitoring], but the clinical benefits of this approach have not been established.). Doses are reduced after 6 months (typically 4 to 6 mg/kg/day); long-term target blood levels of 75 to 125 μg/l appear to provide comparable patient and graft survival as higher blood levels but with less risk of malignancy. The microemulsion formulation of cyclosporine gives more reliable and slightly higher absorption. Generic forms of cyclosporine are available and a chemically modified cyclosporine, ISA(TX)247, is under development.[10] However, oral formulations of cyclosporine may not be equivalent and readily interchangeable, and knowledge of the characteristics of the oral formulations is necessary before switching between them.

The more widely used calcineurin inhibitor is tacrolimus, which has 20- to 30-fold higher potency than cyclosporine on a molecular weight basis and is therefore administered at a 20-fold lower dose. Initial dosing is usually 0.2 mg/kg/day in divided doses orally (or 0.05 to 0.1 mg/kg intravenously over 24 hours) and target trough levels are 5 to 20 μg/l. New developments include a preparation of modified-release tacrolimus to permit once-daily dosing.

Drug interactions with cyclosporine and tacrolimus		
Increased Cyclosporine or Tacrolimus Blood Levels	Decreased Cyclosporine or Tacrolimus Blood Levels	Increased Cyclosporine or Tacrolimus Nephrotoxicity
Ketoconazole Fluconazole Erythromycin Diltiazem Verapamil Nicardipine Metoclopramide Methylprednisolone Sirolimus (increases cyclosporine levels)	Anticonvulsants: phenytoin, phenobarbital, carbamazepine, others Antibiotics: rifampin, rifabutin Nonsteroidal anti-inflammatory drugs Grapefruit juice	Amphotericin B Aminoglycosides Cisplatin

Figure 90.8   Drug interactions with cyclosporine and tacrolimus.

Cyclosporine and tacrolimus can be used in pregnancy and result in fetal blood levels approximately half of that observed in the mother with some immunosuppressive effects. However, they have not been associated with teratogenicity to date.

Mechanism of Action

Cyclosporine and tacrolimus act by inhibiting the calcium-dependent serine phosphatase calcineurin, which normally is rate limiting in T cell activation (Fig. 90.9). Cyclosporine is a prodrug that engages cyclophilin, an intracellular protein of the immunophilin family, forming a complex that engages the calcium-dependent serine phosphatase calcineurin and blocks interactions with its key substrates. Similarly, tacrolimus engages another immunophilin, FK-binding protein 12 (FKBP12), to create an active complex that blocks calcineurin with greater molar potency than does cyclosporine.

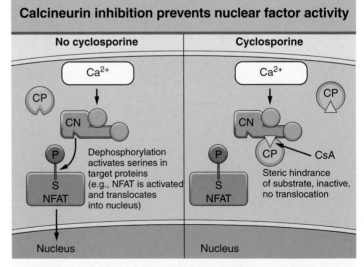

Calcineurin inhibition prevents nuclear factor activity

Figure 90.9   Calcineurin inhibition prevents nuclear factor (NFAT) dephosphorylation, activation, and translocation. In the absence of cyclosporine, calcium activates calcineurin by exposing its phosphatase site, which, in turn, activates its target protein, for example, the transcription factor NFAT. Cyclosporine forms a complex with cyclophilin (CP), which binds to calcineurin (CN) and sterically hinders the phosphatase site. P, phosphorylation (*triangle*) site; S, serine.

Calcineurin is usually activated by the engagement of the TCR via activation of tyrosine kinases and phospholipase Cγ, release of inositol triphosphate, release of calcium stored in the endoplasmic reticulum, and opening of membrane calcium channels. A high cytoplasmic calcium concentration activates calcineurin, which then dephosphorylates regulatory sites in key transcription factors, the nuclear factors of activated T lymphocytes (NFAT$_p$ and NFAT$_c$). This causes the NFAT proteins to translocate (with calcineurin) into the nucleus and bind to their DNA target sequences in the promoters of cytokine genes. Calcineurin has been implicated in the dephosphorylation of transcription factor Elk-1 and indirectly in the activation of Jun/AP-1 and NF-κB. Calcineurin provides an essential step for transducing signal 1 to permit cytokine and CD40L transcription and is normally rate limiting in T cell activation (see Figs. 90.3 and 90.9). The inactivity of calcineurin bound to cyclosporine-cyclophilin or tacrolimus-FKBP12 is the key to the immunosuppressive effect and some of the toxic effects of these drugs.

Cyclosporine and tacrolimus partially inhibit the calcineurin pathway at therapeutic blood levels (e.g., trough levels of 50–200 μg/l cyclosporine or 5 to 20 μg/l tacrolimus).[11] However, even partial inhibition of calcineurin reduces the transcription of many genes associated with T cell activation (e.g., IL-2, interferon [IFN]-γ, granulocyte-macrophage colony-stimulating factor, TNF-α, IL-4, CD40L). The functional consequence of partial calcineurin inhibition is probably a quantitative limitation in cytokine production, CD40L expression, and lymphocyte proliferation. The effect of cyclosporine and tacrolimus on calcineurin *in vivo* is rapidly reversible, emphasizing the importance of patient compliance, drug monitoring, and reliable formulations for delivery.

Side Effects

Cyclosporine and tacrolimus have similarities and differences in their toxicity profiles (see Fig. 90.4). Both can cause nephrotoxicity, hyperkalemia, hyperuricemia (with occasional gouty attacks), hypomagnesemia (secondary to urinary loss), hypertension, diabetes, and neurotoxicity (especially tremor). Certain side effects, such as gingival hyperplasia, hirsutism, hypertension, hyperuricemia, and hyperlipidemia, are more commonly observed with cyclosporine,

whereas tremor and glucose intolerance are more common with tacrolimus. Cyclosporine may also be associated with coarsening of facial features, especially in children. Bone pain that is responsive to calcium channel blockers may also occur with cyclosporine use and sometimes may require changing to tacrolimus. In contrast, tacrolimus is more commonly associated with post-transplant diabetes. Tacrolimus has also been suspected of inducing more BK-related polyomavirus nephropathy.

The most common serious problem with the calcineurin inhibitors is nephrotoxicity, with both a reversible hemodynamic component and an irreversible (structural) component. Both cyclosporine and tacrolimus, but especially cyclosporine, can cause acute elevations in serum creatinine that is reversible with dose reduction and is mediated by acute renal vasoconstriction. The vasoconstriction is caused by direct vascular effects of the calcineurin inhibitors but also due to activation of the renin angiotensin system, endothelin, thromboxane, and the sympathetic nervous system. Over time, chronic renal injury occurs, which is characterized by a characteristic lesion of afferent arteriolar hyalinosis and tubulointerstitial fibrosis (Fig. 90.10). This lesion appears to result from long-standing renal vasoconstriction with ischemia. Experimentally, chronic cyclosporine nephropathy is exacerbated in the presence of sodium restriction/volume depletion (which stimulates the renin angiotensin system) and can be ameliorated by angiotensin-converting enzyme (ACE) inhibitors or angiotensin receptor blockers (ARBs) and to a lesser extent by other vasodilators. As a consequence, ACE inhibitors are increasingly being used in transplant recipients following the initial stabilization of renal function after transplantation. There are also provocative experimental data suggesting that lowering uric acid with xanthine oxidase inhibitors might provide protection.

The importance of chronic calcineurin inhibitor nephrotoxicity is apparent from studies in cardiac and liver transplant recipients, in which the larger doses of cyclosporine or tacrolimus that are used are associated with progression to end-stage renal disease (ESRD) in many patients.

Finally, calcineurin inhibitors can cause hemolytic uremic syndrome, probably by directly causing endothelial injury and dysfunction. This complication, which is usually associated with markedly elevated (>300 μg/l and >25 μg/l trough levels

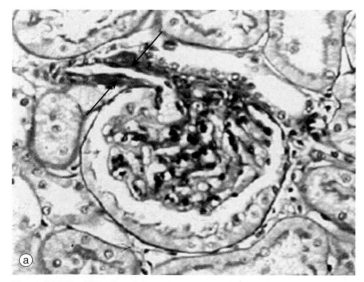
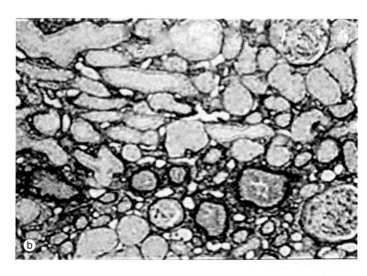

Figure 90.10 Chronic calcineurin nephrotoxicity. Biopsy specimen of a rat with chronic cyclosporine nephrotoxicity showing characteristic arteriolar hyalinosis (*a*) (*arrows*), and tubulointerstitial fibrosis, noted by type IV collagen staining (*black*) (*b*). (Courtesy of Dr. Richard J. Johnson.)

of cyclosporine and tacrolimus, respectively) drug levels, may respond to withdrawal of cyclosporine or tacrolimus, empirical plasma exchange, and switching to another class of immunosuppressive drug (see Chapter 93).

Azathioprine

Azathioprine, an antimetabolite that is a purine analogue, is still used with prednisolone and a calcineurin inhibitor in maintenance immunosuppressive regimens (see Chapter 93). It has a good safety profile and has been one of the more commonly used immunosuppressives in renal transplantation for over three decades. When calcineurin inhibitors emerged, azathioprine became a second-line drug in combined regimens. With the emergence and superiority of MMF, azathioprine was displaced from these combinations, although it is still used (see Chapter 93).

Pharmacokinetics

Azathioprine is administered orally at 2 to 3 mg/kg/day but is often used at lower doses when it is supplementing cyclosporine or tacrolimus. It is metabolized in the liver to 6-mercaptopurine and further converted to the active metabolite thio-inosinic acid by hypoxanthine-guanine phosphoribosyltransferase. Because allopurinol (a xanthine oxidase inhibitor) will increase the levels of thio-inosinic acid, doses of azathioprine must be reduced by two thirds in subjects taking allopurinol. Azathioprine is generally considered safe in pregnancy, although some fetal immunosuppression may occur.

Mechanism of Action

Azathioprine suppresses the proliferation of activated B and T cells and reduces the number of circulating monocytes by arresting the cell cycle of promyelocytes in the bone marrow. This antiproliferative effect is mediated by the metabolites of azathioprine, which include 6-mercaptopurine, 6-thiouric acid, 6-methyl-mercaptopurine, and 6-thioguanine. These compounds are incorporated into replicating DNA and halt replication. They also block the *de novo* pathway of purine synthesis by formation of thio-inosinic acid. This latter effect confers specificity of action on lymphocytes that lack a salvage pathway for purine synthesis. Other possible mechanisms include converting the costimulatory signal of CD28 into an apoptotic signal, thereby deleting activated lymphocytes.

Side Effects

The major side effect of azathioprine is bone marrow suppression, leading to leukopenia, thrombocytopenia, and anemia. The mean cell volume is commonly increased in patients on full-dose azathioprine, and red cell aplasia can eventually result in occasional cases. The hematologic side effects are dose related and can occur late in the course of therapy. They are usually reversible on dose reduction or temporary discontinuation of the drug. Other important side effects include increased susceptibility to infection, increased risk of malignancy (especially skin cancers), hepatotoxicity, and hair loss. Interactions between azathioprine and ACE inhibitors have been reported, causing anemia and leukopenia.

Mycophenolate Mofetil

MMF has now become one of the current standard immunosuppressives in renal transplantation and is commonly used as a replacement for azathioprine. Several studies demonstrate that its use is associated with better short- and long-term graft survival (see Chapter 97).

Pharmacokinetics and Drug Interactions

MMF is a prodrug and an ethyl ester of mycophenolic acid (MPA). MMF is rapidly and completely absorbed and hydrolyzed by esterases to yield the active drug MPA. The usual dose varies from 250 mg to 1.5 g orally twice daily with higher doses reserved for subjects at high risk of rejection (such as the African American). Doses are usually tapered gradually following transplantation. MPA levels are usually not measured in most centers. Enteric-coated MPA has also been introduced as an alternative to MMF.[12]

MPA has an extensive enterohepatic circulation. Ultimately, MPA is metabolized in the liver by β-glucuronidase enzymes to the glucuronide (MPAG), and the excretion of MPAG into the gut may explain many of its gastrointestinal side effects (see later discussion). MPAG levels are also high in patients on MMF, particularly in patients in renal failure, but the MPAG is itself probably inactive.

MMF is not absorbed well in the setting of antacids or cholestyramine use. There is also an important drug-drug interaction with cyclosporine, in that cyclosporine lowers MPA levels. MMF does not appear to interact with tacrolimus.

MMF should not be used in pregnant transplant recipients since it is teratogenic in experimental animal models, and one clinical case of major fetal malformations has been described.[13]

Mechanism of Action

MPA acts by blocking *de novo* purine synthesis in lymphocytes. Purines can be generated either by *de novo* synthesis or by recycling (salvage pathway), and lymphocytes preferentially use *de novo* purine synthesis, whereas other tissues such as brain use the salvage pathway. MPA noncompetitively inhibits inosine monophosphate dehydrogenase (IMPDH), which is the rate-limiting enzyme in the *de novo* synthesis of guanosine monophosphate (GMP; Fig. 90.11). Inhibition of IMPDH creates a relative deficiency of GMP and

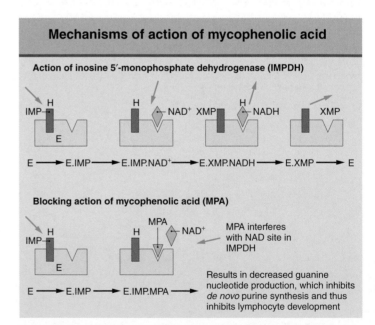

Mechanisms of action of mycophenolic acid

Action of inosine 5′-monophosphate dehydrogenase (IMPDH)

$E \longrightarrow E.IMP \longrightarrow E.IMP.NAD^+ \longrightarrow E.XMP.NADH \longrightarrow E.XMP \longrightarrow E$

Blocking action of mycophenolic acid (MPA)

MPA interferes with NAD site in IMPDH

$E \longrightarrow E.IMP \longrightarrow E.IMP.MPA \longrightarrow$

Results in decreased guanine nucleotide production, which inhibits *de novo* purine synthesis and thus inhibits lymphocyte development

Figure 90.11 Mechanism of action of mycophenolic acid (MPA). Inosine 5′-monophosphate (IMP) dehydrogenase (IMPDH) catalyzes the oxidized nicotinamide adenine dinucleotide (NAD⁺)–dependent oxidation of IMP to xanthosine 5′-monophosphate (XMP) (*top*). MPA, a noncompetitive inhibitor of IMPDH, binds to IMPDH after the release of reduced nicotinamide adenine dinucleotide (NADH) but before the production of XMP; it interferes with the NAD⁺ site by mimicking the nicotinamide portion of the NAD⁺ cofactor and a catalytic water molecule (*bottom*). E, enzyme; H, hydrogen molecule.

a relative excess of adenosine monophosphate (AMP). GMP and AMP levels act as a control on *de novo* purine biosynthesis; therefore, MPA, by inhibiting IMPDH, creates a block in *de novo* purine synthesis that selectively interferes with proliferative responses of T and B cells, inhibiting clonal expansion and thus inhibiting antibody production, the generation of cytotoxic T cells, and the development of delayed-type hypersensitivity.

The drug mizoribine also inhibits IMPDH but differs from MMF in being a purine and a competitive inhibitor. Mizoribine is used for transplant immunosuppression in Japan.

Side Effects

The major side effects of MMF are gastrointestinal and include oral ulcerations, nausea and vomiting, diarrhea, and colonic ulcers. Diarrhea and/or nausea are often major symptoms that require dose adjustment (using either lower doses or dividing the dose into three or four smaller daily doses). Bone marrow suppression with leukopenia or anemia may also occur. MMF also increases the risk of certain infections, particularly cytomegalovirus (CMV). In contrast, MPA has been associated with protection from *Pneumocystis carinii* pneumonia (PCP) and may actually have some anti-PCP activity because *P. carinii* has IMPDH activity.

Target of Rapamycin Inhibitors

Sirolimus is a macrolide product of a soil organism found in Easter Island (Rapa Nui). It inhibits signal 3 by preventing cytokine receptors from activating the cell cycle. Like tacrolimus, sirolimus is a prodrug that engages FKBP12, but unlike tacrolimus-FKBP12, the sirolimus-FKBP12 complex cannot inhibit calcineurin (Fig. 90.12). Everolimus (RAD) is an analogue of sirolimus that is in clinical trial with effectiveness and side effect profile similar to those of sirolimus.

Sirolimus is currently used in transplantation in a variety of regimens often with the intent of sparing calcineurin inhibitor use (see Chapter 93). Sirolimus, however, has been associated with its own set of toxicities that have prevented its widespread use (see later discussion).

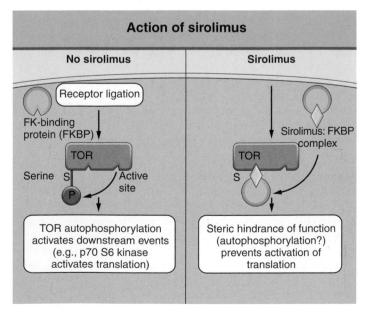

Action of sirolimus

No sirolimus	Sirolimus
Receptor ligation	
FK-binding protein (FKBP)	Sirolimus: FKBP complex
TOR	TOR
Serine S — Active site	S
P	
TOR autophosphorylation activates downstream events (e.g., p70 S6 kinase activates translation)	Steric hindrance of function (autophosphorylation?) prevents activation of translation

Figure 90.12 Action of sirolimus. In the absence of sirolimus, receptor ligation causes activation of a kinase enzyme called target of rapamycin (TOR). Sirolimus prevents the activation of TOR by binding to FK-binding proteins and preventing autophosphorylation of TOR through steric hindrance.

Pharmacokinetics and Drug Interactions

Sirolimus is available as tablet or oral solution and is usually administered as a once-daily dose of 2 or 5 mg. Maximal concentrations are reached after 1 hour with excellent penetration into most tissues, including blood cells. Trough levels of 5 μg/l are considered therapeutic. The drug is metabolized by the cytochrome P-450 system, similar to tacrolimus and cyclosporine. The drug is primarily (90%) excreted by the biliary system. Hepatic impairment may result in markedly elevated levels.

Sirolimus has numerous drug and food interactions. High-fat meals increase sirolimus levels. Drugs that induce the cytochrome P-450 system also increase sirolimus levels, including diltiazem and ketoconazole; in contrast, rifampin and anticonvulsants decreased sirolimus levels. Importantly, sirolimus increases the blood levels of several immunosuppressive agents, including cyclosporine (usually twofold) and tacrolimus. The simultaneous use of sirolimus and cyclosporine increases cyclosporine toxicity, for example, nephrotoxicity, and hypertension. Sirolimus in combination with tacrolimus probably has similar effects. Sirolimus blood levels are also increased by the use of cyclosporine (especially the microemulsion form).

Mechanism of Action

Sirolimus binds to FKBP but does not inhibit calcineurin or the calcium-dependent activation of cytokine genes (see Figs. 90.3 and 90.12). Instead, sirolimus inhibits signal 3 and thus cell division driven by certain cytokine receptors (e.g., IL-2). Unlike cyclosporine or tacrolimus, sirolimus blocks IL-2–mediated signal transduction and cell proliferation and blocks lymphocyte responses to IL-4, IL-7, IL-15, and other cytokines and growth factors. Sirolimus-FKBP12 engages a kinase enzyme called target of rapamycin or TOR.[14] TOR is critical in transducing a signal from these cytokine receptors to the mechanisms controlling cell division. TOR acts to inhibit an inhibitor, 4E-BP1, and activates a ribosomal enzyme, p70 S6 kinase. Both of these proteins are important for the translation of the mRNAs for certain proteins needed for progression from the G_1 phase to the S phase of DNA synthesis. Therefore, cytokines must activate these steps to trigger G_1-to-S progression and act via TOR and its effects on 4E-BP1 and p70 S6 kinase. Unlike cyclosporine or tacrolimus, sirolimus blocks IL-2–mediated signal transduction and cell proliferation and blocks lymphocyte responses to IL-4, IL-7, IL-15, and other cytokines and growth factors.[14]

Side Effects

Sirolimus and everolimus have a wide variety of toxicities. These include hematologic complications such as thrombocytopenia and leukopenia. Impaired wound healing is common and may predispose to wound dehiscence. Hyperlipidemia is common, especially hypertriglyceridemia. Cases with aphthous mouth ulcers have been described. Increased risk of infection, especially *P. carinii*, has been reported in some studies.[15] However, no significant differences were observed with relation to CMV or Epstein-Barr virus infection. There have also been reports of cases of hemolytic uremic syndrome, and there is concern that at higher doses sirolimus may inhibit endothelial cell growth. Nephrotoxicity, however, when observed, is often due to the ability of sirolimus to potentiate blood levels of cyclosporine and tacrolimus. Sirolimus prolongs delayed graft function in kidney transplants and aggravates proteinuria.

Sirolimus and everolimus may also have antineoplastic effects due to their ability to inhibit cell growth. Indeed, some clinicians regard sirolimus as the preferred immunosuppressive agent in transplant patients who develop malignancies, but more evidence is needed on this point. Furthermore, sirolimus-impregnated stents are used to prevent restenosis in coronary arteries after angioplasty, perhaps because of its ability to reduce healing.

PROTEIN IMMUNOSUPPRESSIVES

Protein immunosuppressives, particularly antibodies directed to lymphocyte populations or receptors, have often been used in transplantation, particularly during induction or in the treatment of rejection. While many antibodies are polyclonal and are derived from horses or rabbits, others are as murine monoclonal antibodies. However, because foreign proteins can often elicit their own immune response, there has been an attempt to replace murine monoclonal products with humanized or chimeric monoclonal antibodies (Fig. 90.13). To humanize a mouse monoclonal, the sequences encoding the antigen-combining sites are transferred into human immunoglobulin genes, which are transfected into mouse hybridomas to secrete the new product with the specificity of the original mouse monoclonal antibody in a human immunoglobulin framework. Chimeric antibodies use the same strategy but for the entire V region. Humanized mouse monoclonal antibodies have been introduced, and other monoclonal or fusion proteins, such as CTLA4Ig (belatacept), are being evaluated. Figure 90.5 gives an overview of protein- or peptide-based biologic immunosuppressives.

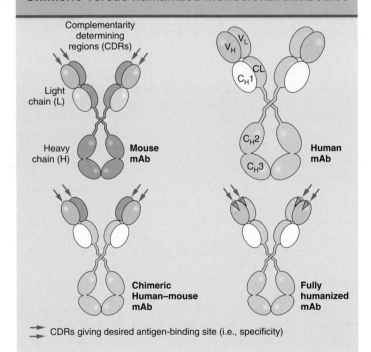

Chimeric versus humanized monoclonal antibodies

Complementarity determining regions (CDRs)

Light chain (L)

Heavy chain (H) **Mouse mAb**

V_L
V_H
CL
C_H1
C_H2
C_H3 **Human mAb**

Chimeric Human–mouse mAb

Fully humanized mAb

CDRs giving desired antigen-binding site (i.e., specificity)

Figure 90.13   Chimeric versus humanized monoclonal antibodies. Chimeric monoclonal antibodies consist of human constant (C) regions and mouse heavy and light chain variable (V) regions. A chimeric antibody therefore retains the binding specificity of the original mouse antibody but contains fewer amino acid sequences foreign to the human immune system. Humanized monoclonal antibodies retain only minimum necessary parts of the mouse antibody. These complementary-determining regions are built into a human antibody, that is, only the antigen-binding site is combined with human V region framework and human C region sequences. These monoclonal antibodies retain the ability to recognize the target sequence. mAb, monoclonal antibody.

Polyclonal Antibodies

Polyclonal antithymocyte globulin (ATG) is currently a favored method for induction therapy and is produced by immunizing rabbits (or horses) with human thymus-derived lymphoid cells. Currently ATG is the most commonly used pan-T cell–targeted antibody, but historically horse antilymphocyte globulin was also used.

Current regimens consist of daily intravenous doses of ATG for 3 to 7 days used either for induction or treatment of steroid-resistant rejection. ATG is an extremely potent immunosuppressive and will cause systemic lymphocyte depletion that may persist for a week following administration. The lack of specificity coupled with marked immunosuppression increases the risk of infection and malignancies, and repeated courses are generally not recommended. The initial lysis and activation of T cells associated with administration of ATG may also generate significant first-dose effects, with release of TNF-α, IFN-γ, and other cytokines, causing a first-dose reaction (flulike symptoms, fever, and chills; see later discussion).

Mouse Monoclonal Anti-CD3 Antibody (OKT3)

Although rarely used today, the first monoclonal antibody for routine antirejection therapy in renal transplantation was murine monoclonal anti-CD3 (OKT3). The CD3 complex is the transducer associated with the TCR and is essential for T cell triggering. OKT3 binds to the ε-chain of this complex and paralyzes T cell recognition, but at the expense of triggering the T cells to release TNF-α and other cytokines, which produce fever and other flulike first-dose symptoms. OKT3 is highly effective in reducing CD3 counts and creates potent suppression of T cells for several days, during which there is virtually no T cell function. As such, it was found to be both effective as an agent used in induction phase following transplantation as well as for the treatment of steroid-resistant rejection (see Chapter 93).

However, numerous toxicities complicate its use. First, the use of OKT3 was associated with severe first-dose effects or cytokine release syndrome with fever and capillary leak syndrome and, rarely, pulmonary edema, acute renal failure, or even cerebral edema or cortical blindness. Prolonged or repeated courses of OKT3 were also found to increase the risk of post-transplantation lymphoproliferative disease.[16] Finally, being a mouse protein, the monoclonal antibody evokes a host antibody response that not uncommonly resulted in the development of antimurine antibodies that decreased the efficacy of OKT3 and potentially necessitated higher doses. With the introduction of newer small-molecule immunosuppressive drugs, the use of OKT3 has declined. Several humanized anti-CD3 monoclonal antibodies (huOKT3g1, HuM291) have been generated, but their future use remains in question.[17]

Monoclonal Anti-CD25 Antibody (Daclizumab, Basiliximab)

The α-subunit of the IL-2 receptor (CD25) is expressed on activated T cells and engagement by IL-2 triggers the activated T cell to undergo rapid proliferation. Blockade of CD25 therefore selectively prevents the IL-2–induced T cell activation. Because expression of CD25 requires T cell activation, anti-CD25 antibody causes little depletion of T cells, preventing increased risk of infection and malignancy commonly seen with other immunosuppressants.

IL-2 receptor functions are partially redundant because of overlapping functions of other cytokine receptors, for example, IL-15 receptors. Saturating IL-2 receptors thus produces stable but relatively mild immunosuppression and is only effective in combination with other immunosuppressives (e.g., cyclosporine, corticosteroids). As such, anti-CD25 antibody is primarily used in conjunction with cyclosporine and corticosteroids during induction therapy, where it has been reported to reduce rejection by about one third with minimal toxic effects.[18-21] They have also been used in subjects with increased risk of delayed graft function to avoid use of calcineurin inhibitors in the immediate post-transplantation period. They are not used for treatment of established acute rejection and may not be optimal for preventing rejection in highly sensitized recipients (for details, see Chapter 93).

There are two types of anti-CD25 monoclonal antibodies: one humanized (daclizumab) and one chimeric (basiliximab). The studies on the two monoclonal antibodies produced similar results,[18,20,22] and both antibodies are approved for clinical use. The use of anti-CD25 antibodies did not result in increased infections, malignancies, or post-transplantation lymphoproliferative disorders.

B Cell–Depleting Monoclonal Anti-CD20 Antibody (Rituximab)

Rituximab is a high-affinity monoclonal antibody directed against the CD20 antigen on B lymphocytes that is currently used off-label to treat some forms of antibody-mediated transplant rejection, particularly those associated with anti-HLA antibodies. Treatment is often combined with plasma exchange and intravenous immunoglobulin. Rituximab is also used to treat some post-transplantation lymphoproliferative diseases in organ transplant recipients in whom remission was achieved with minimized immunosuppression, rituximab, and sirolimus or radiotherapy.[23,24] More experience with rituximab has been achieved outside transplantation where it is used to treat non-Hodgkin's lymphoma as well as a variety of humorally mediated autoimmune diseases.

Rituximab directly inhibits B cell proliferation by antibody-dependent, cell-mediated, and complement-mediated cytotoxicity.[25] A rapid and sustained depletion of circulating and tissue-based B cells follows its intravenous administration. B cell recovery begins approximately 6 months after completion of treatment. Although plasma cells are usually CD20 negative, many are short-lived and require replacement from CD20-positive precursors. In addition, CD20-positive B cells can act as secondary APCs, thereby enhancing T cell responses. By targeting CD20 on precursor B cells, rituximab decreases the production of activated B cells and limits antibody production as well as antigen presentation.

In addition to reversing established rejection episodes, rituximab may be an effective agent to reduce high-titer anti-HLA antibodies in hyperimmunized patients awaiting kidney transplantation. A phase I study in nine dialysis patients with >50% panel-reactive antibodies obtained favorable results with a significant reduction in the anti-HLA antibody titer in two patients and loss of specificity of these antibodies in five other patients.[26] Controlled trials are needed to confirm the efficacy and safety of rituximab in large patient cohorts.

Intravenous Immunoglobulin

There is a considerable potential for intravenous immunoglobulin (IVIG) in control of antibody responses and possibly other responses in transplantation. It is used in studies together with plasma exchange, tacrolimus, and MMF to desensitize highly immunized patients before transplantation and as a therapeutic approach for humoral rejection after transplantation. IVIG reduces high levels of preformed anti-HLA antibody and produces long-term suppression or elimination of anti-HLA reactive T cells.

The mode of action of IVIG is not understood. The most important effect appears to be a reduction of alloantibodies through inhibition of antibody production and increased catabolism of circulating antibodies. Additional potential mechanisms include inhibition of complement-mediated injury, inhibition of inflammatory cytokine generation, and neutralization of circulating antibodies by anti-idiotypes.[27]

Side effects related to IVIG administration occur in 12% to 23% of patients and include minor self-limited reactions, such as flushing, chills, headache, myalgia, and arthralgia. Rarely, anaphylactic reactions may occur. Delayed reactions include severe headache and aseptic meningitis, which respond to analgesics. More recently, serious thrombotic events have been linked to the administration of IVIG products. Of particular importance to transplant recipients is the development of acute renal failure following IVIG administration, which is due to osmotic injury to the proximal tubular epithelium mediated by carbohydrate (sucrose) additives contained in the IVIG preparation. Patients with impaired baseline renal function may suffer further transient deterioration of function that may necessitate dialysis. The tubular injury is self-limiting and typically resolves within several days.

IVIG appears to offer significant benefits in the desensitization of highly HLA-sensitized and ABO incompatible patients as well as in the treatment of antibody-mediated rejection. However, its high cost and limited supply are serious barriers to its frequent use. Further studies are necessary to define which patients would benefit most from this therapy.

IMMUNOSUPPRESSIVE AGENTS IN CLINICAL TRIALS

Humanized Monoclonal Anti-CD52 Antibody

CD52 is a membrane glycoprotein found on B cells and T cells, monocytes, macrophages, natural killer (NK) cells, and granulocytes. Alemtuzumab (Campath-1H) is a humanized monoclonal antibody against CD52, which was first used in the treatment of B cell chronic lymphocytic leukemia resistant to alkylating agents and fludarabine. Alemtuzumab induces severe and long-lasting depletion, recovering slowly over months or years. More recently, alemtuzumab has been used during induction therapy in which it is administered once daily for 2 days. Treatment results in a rapid and effective depletion of peripheral and central lymphoid cells that may take months to return to pretransplantation levels. Although promising, the clinical efficacy and safety profile of alemtuzumab for prophylaxis in renal transplantation have not been established in phase III trials. Side effects of alemtuzumab include first-dose reactions, neutropenia, anemia, and (rarely) pancytopenia and autoimmunity (e.g., hemolytic anemia, thrombocytopenia, and hyperthyroidism).[28] The risks of immunodeficiency complications (infections and cancer) with alemtuzumab are also unclear. Further controlled trials are needed to establish dosing, safety, and efficacy.

Dihydro-orotate Dehydrogenase Inhibitors (FK778)

FK778 is a synthetic malononitrilamide, derived from leflunomide, with immunosuppressive as well as antiproliferative effects. FK778 inhibits T cell and B cell function by blocking dihydro-orotate dehydrogenase, which is a key enzyme in pyrimidine synthesis. In multiple experimental transplant models, FK778 has been shown to prevent or reverse acute allograft rejection.[29–31] In addition, FK778 suppresses neointimal formation in vascular smooth muscle cells and exerts moderate antiviral activity against polyomavirus and CMV.[32,33] In a double-blind, randomized multicenter phase II study of 149 patients, both active treatment arms showed efficacy of FK778 to reduce acute graft rejection. Anemia was the most commonly reported adverse event and was dose related, while mean total cholesterol and low-density lipoprotein cholesterol levels were reduced.[34] Currently, FK778 is undergoing additional clinical trials in liver and renal transplantation.

Janus Kinase 3 (JAK3) Inhibitors

JAK3 is a tyrosine kinase expressed at high levels in NK cells and thymocytes and is inducible in T cells, B cells, and myeloid cells but not expressed in resting T cells. It is important in the immune cell response to a variety of cytokines (including IL-2 and IL-15). Blockade of JAK3 with the JAK3 inhibitor CP-690,550 has resulted in strong immunosuppression and significant improvement in allograft survival in experimental models.[35–37] CP-690,550 is currently undergoing phase II clinical trials.

Sphingosine-1-Phosphate-Receptor Antagonists

FTY720 is a novel immunosuppressive agent that acts as a high-affinity agonist at the sphingosine 1-phosphate receptor-1. FTY720 causes alterations in the chemokine pathways that govern lymphocyte homing and result in the sequestration of T cells to secondary lymphoid organs such as the spleen without affecting their function or properties.[38] This reduces migration of effector cells to inflammatory tissues and graft sites. Both phase I and II clinical trials suggest that the drug in combination with cyclosporine is well tolerated, causing transient lymphocytopenia and reducing rejection.[38,39] The toxicities have included bradycardia during the first doses and macular edema, both of which raised safety concerns. The clinical development of FTY720 for renal transplantation is delayed by concerns about safety and efficacy in the phase III trials. Analogues directly against this unique mechanism are also being developed.

Monoclonal Anti-CD154 (Antibody)

CD40 is constitutively expressed on APCs, such as B cells, macrophages, and dendritic cells, but can also be induced on endothelial cells and fibroblasts. It interacts with its ligand CD154 (CD40L) on activated CD4 T cells, as well as on a subset of CD8 on T cells, NK cells, and eosinophils. The CD40-CD154 interaction serves primarily to provide a costimulatory signal to the APCs rather than to the T cells, thereby significantly augmenting the ability of the APCs to present antigen and to deliver positive costimulatory signals. These in turn indirectly promote T cell activation.

Although it emerged as a promising immunosuppressive strategy for clinical use in transplantation, an initial clinical trial failed to protect patients from acute rejection episodes, and phase I studies also were associated with a high incidence of thromboembolic events. This complication may reflect enhanced platelet aggregation mediated by platelet surface expression of CD154.

Future studies using anti-CD40L or chimerized anti-CD40L are likely to be limited.

CTLA-4-IgG

Activated T cells upregulate CTLA-4, a molecule that is structurally similar to CD28 but binds to CD80/86 with higher affinity. This molecule provides a negative signal for T cell activation, resulting in the termination of T cell responses. Initial immunosuppressive drug development in this area focused on a recombinant fusion protein CTLA-4-Ig, consisting of the extracellular domain of CTLA-4 and the Fc domain of an IgG molecule (Fig. 90.14). CTLA-4-Ig saturates CD80/86 and thereby blocks the CD28 costimulatory pathway.

A second-generation and more potent CTLA-4-Ig, LEA29Y (belatacept), was developed that does provide effective rejection prophylaxis in nonhuman primates. Its mechanism of action, acting extracellularly on a specific target, may limit toxicity compared to conventional immunosuppressants. Belatacept is being developed for use as chronic maintenance immunosuppression. A recent phase II study suggested that the belatacept-based regimen was as effective as standard therapy with cyclosporine in preventing acute rejection at 12 months and with less renal toxicity, hypertension, or dyslipidemia.[40] Phase III studies are in progress to determine whether belatacept, used in protocols with mycophenolate and steroids and anti-CD25 induction, can provide equivalent immunosuppression to calcineurin inhibitors without their associated toxicities. This would open the possibility of long-term administration of protein immunosuppressive drugs to reduce the burden of nonimmune toxicity from the calcineurin inhibitors.

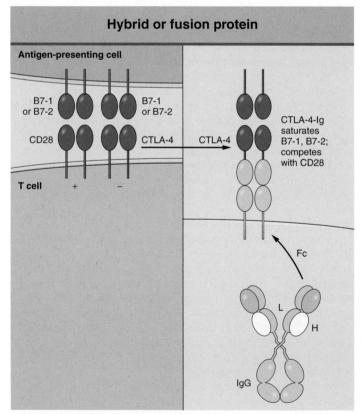

Figure 90.14 Hybrid or fusion protein. A ligand is combined with the Fc portion of the IgG H chain, e.g., CTLA-4-Ig. In theory, this fusion should prevent the costimulatory signal required for activation of T lymphocytes (see text). +, activates costimulation; –, blocks costimulation.

REFERENCES

1. Lakkis FG, Arakelov A, Konieczny BT, Inoue Y: Immunologic "ignorance" of vascularized organ transplants in the absence of secondary lymphoid tissue. Nat Med 2000;6:686–688.
2. Zhou P, Hwang KW, Palucki D, et al: Secondary lymphoid organs are important but not absolutely required for allograft responses. Am J Transplant 2003;3:259–266.
3. Biedermann BC, Pober JS: Human endothelial cells induce and regulate cytolytic T cell differentiation. J Immunol 1998;161:4679–4687.
4. MacLennan IC, Toellner KM, Cunningham AF, et al: Extrafollicular antibody responses. Immunol Rev 2003;94:8–18.
5. Sarwal M, Chua MS, Kambham N, et al: Molecular heterogeneity in acute renal allograft rejection identified by DNA microarray profiling. N Engl J Med 2003;349:125–138.
6. Wang D, Matsumoto R, You Y, et al: CD3/CD28 Costimulation-induced NF-kappaB activation is mediated by recruitment of protein kinase C-theta, Bcl10, and IkappaB kinase beta to the immunological synapse through CARMA1. Mol Cell Biol 2004;24:164–171.
7. Halloran PF: Immunosuppressive drugs for kidney transplantation. N Engl J Med 2004;351:2715–2729.
8. Rhen T, Cidlowski JA: Antiinflammatory action of glucocorticoids—new mechanisms for old drugs. N Engl J Med 2005;353:1711–1723.
9. Karin M: New twists in gene regulation by glucocorticoid receptor: Is DNA binding dispensable? Cell 1998;93:487–490.
10. Stalder M, Birsan T, Hubble RW, et al: In vivo evaluation of the novel calcineurin inhibitor ISATX247 in non-human primates. J Heart Lung Transplant 2003;22:1343–1352.
11. Batiuk TD, Kung L, Halloran PF: Evidence that calcineurin is rate-limiting for primary human lymphocyte activation. J Clin Invest 1997;100:1894–1901.
12. Gabardi S, Tran JL, Clarkson MR: Enteric-coated mycophenolate sodium. Ann Pharmacother 2003;37:1685–1693.
13. Le Ray C, Coulomb A, Elefant E, et al: Mycophenolate mofetil in pregnancy after renal transplantation: A case of major fetal malformations. Obstet Gynecol 2004;103:1091–1094.
14. Sehgal SN: Immunosuppressive profile of rapamycin. Ann NY Acad Sci 1993;696:1–8.
15. Murgia MG, Jordan S, Kahan BD: The side effect profile of sirolimus: A phase I study in quiescent cyclosporine-prednisone-treated renal transplant patients. Kidney Int 1996;49:209–216.
16. Swinnen LJ, Costanzo-Nordin MR, Fisher SG, et al: Increased incidence of lymphoproliferative disorder after immunosuppression with the monoclonal antibody OKT3 in cardiac-transplant recipients. N Engl J Med 1990;323:1723–1728.
17. Norman DJ, Vincenti F, de Mattos AM, et al: Phase I trial of HuM291, a humanized anti-CD3 antibody, in patients receiving renal allografts from living donors. Transplant 2000;70:1707–1712.
18. Vincenti F, Kirkman R, Light S, et al: Interleukin-2-receptor blockade with daclizumab to prevent acute rejection in renal transplantation. Daclizumab Triple Therapy Study Group. N Engl J Med 1998;338:161–165.
19. Nashan B, Light S, Hardie IR, et al: Reduction of acute renal allograft rejection by daclizumab. Daclizumab Double Therapy Study Group. Transplantation 1999;67:110–115.
20. Nashan B, Moore R, Amlot P, Schmidt AG, et al: Randomised trial of basiliximab versus placebo for control of acute cellular rejection in renal allograft recipients. CHIB 201 International Study Group. Lancet 1997;350:1193–1198.
21. Kahan BD, Rajagopalan PR, Hall M: Reduction of the occurrence of acute cellular rejection among renal allograft recipients treated with basiliximab, a chimeric anti-interleukin-2-receptor monoclonal antibody. United States Simulect Renal Study Group. Transplantation 1999;67:276–284.
22. Bumgardner GL, Hardie I, Johnson RW, et al: Results of 3-year phase III clinical trials with daclizumab prophylaxis for prevention of acute rejection after renal transplantation. Transplantation 2001;72:839–845.
23. Garcia VD, Bonamigo Filho JL, Neumann J, et al: Rituximab in association with rapamycin for post-transplant lymphoproliferative disease treatment. Transpl Int 2003;16:202–206.
24. Molnar I, Keung YK: Treatment of post-transplant lymphoproliferative disorder with rituximab and radiation in a patient with second renal allograft. Nephrol Dial Transplant 2001;16:2114–2115.
25. Grillo-Lopez AJ: Rituximab: An insider's historical perspective. Semin Oncol 2000;27(Suppl 12):9–16.
26. Vieira CA, Agarwal A, Book BK, et al: Rituximab for reduction of anti-HLA antibodies in patients awaiting renal transplantation: 1. Safety, pharmacodynamics, and pharmacokinetics. Transplantation 2004;77:542–548.
27. Jordan S, Cunningham-Rundles C, McEwan R: Utility of intravenous immune globulin in kidney transplantation: Efficacy, safety, and cost implications. Am J Transplant 2003;3:653–664.
28. Coles AJ, Wing M, Smith S, et al: Pulsed monoclonal antibody treatment and autoimmune thyroid disease in multiple sclerosis. Lancet 1999;354:1691–1695.
29. Jin MB, Nakayama M, Ogata T, et al: A novel leflunomide derivative, FK778, for immunosuppression after kidney transplantation in dogs. Surgery 2002;132:72–79.
30. Bilolo KK, Ouyang J, Wang X, et al: Synergistic effects of malononitrilamides (FK778, FK779) with tacrolimus (FK506) in prevention of acute heart and kidney allograft rejection and reversal of ongoing heart allograft rejection in the rat. Transplantation 2003;75:1881–1887.
31. Qi S, Zhu S, Xu D, et al: Significant prolongation of renal allograft survival by delayed combination therapy of FK778 with tacrolimus in nonhuman primates. Transplantation 2003;75:1124–1128.
32. Zeng H, Waldman WJ, Yin DP, et al: Mechanistic study of malononitrileamide FK778 in cardiac transplantation and CMV infection in rats. Transplantation 2005;79:17–22.
33. Chong AS, Zeng H, Knight DA, et al: Concurrent antiviral and immunosuppressive activities of leflunomide in vivo. Am J Transplant 2006;6:69–75.
34. Vanrenterghem Y, van Hooff JP, Klinger M, et al: The effects of FK778 in combination with tacrolimus and steroids: A phase II multicenter study in renal transplant patients. Transplantation 2004;78:9–14.
35. Changelian PS, Flanagan ME, Ball DJ, et al: Prevention of organ allograft rejection by a specific Janus kinase 3 inhibitor. Science 2003;302:875–878.
36. Borie DC, Larson MJ, Flores MG, et al: Combined use of the JAK3 inhibitor CP-690,550 with mycophenolate mofetil to prevent kidney allograft rejection in nonhuman primates. Transplantation 2005;80:1756–1764.
37. Borie DC, Changelian PS, Larson MJ, et al: Immunosuppression by the JAK3 inhibitor CP-690,550 delays rejection and significantly prolongs kidney allograft survival in nonhuman primates. Transplantation 2005;79:791–801.
38. Brinkmann V, Cyster JG, Hla T: FTY720: sphingosine 1-phosphate receptor-1 in the control of lymphocyte egress and endothelial barrier function. Am J Transplant 2004;4:1019–1025.
39. Tedesco-Silva H, Mourad G, Kahan BD, et al: FTY720, a novel immunomodulator: Efficacy and safety results from the first phase 2A study in de novo renal transplantation. Transplantation 2005;79:1553–1560.
40. Vincenti F, Larsen C, Durrbach A, et al: Costimulation blockade with belatacept in renal transplantation. N Engl J Med 2005;353:770–781.

INTRODUCTION

Successful renal transplantation improves the life span and quality of life of the recipient.[1] The greatest benefit occurs when the patient receives a transplant either before or shortly after initiating dialysis (Fig. 91.1).[2] For a full discussion of the outcomes of renal transplantation, see Chapter 97.

Unfortunately, the number of patients who would be predicted to benefit from renal transplantation vastly outstrips the supply of donor organs. As such, there is a need to maximize the potential for organ donation from both deceased and live donors, to identify ways to allocate a scarce deceased donor organ to a single individual from a large recipient pool, and to exclude those recipients who would be predicted to experience an early unacceptable survival risk.

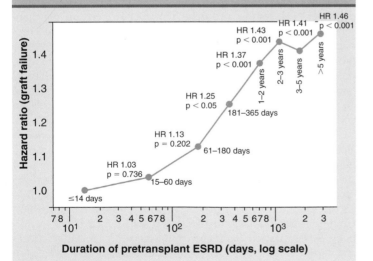

Graft survival increases with less time on dialysis

Duration of pretransplant ESRD (days, log scale)

Figure 91.1   Graft survival increases with less time on dialysis. Hazard ratio (HR) of the graft failure in different categories of the pretransplantation end-stage renal disease (ESRD) duration. Compared with the reference (ESRD duration 14 days), the hazard ratio of graft failure became significant only after 180 days of pretransplantation ESRD. The hazard ratio increased from this point in a linear fashion, until the ESRD duration reached 3 years, when there was no further increase in the risk of graft failure. (From Goldfarb-Rumyantzev A, Hurdle JF, Scandling J, et al: Duration of end-stage renal disease and kidney transplant outcome. Nephrol Dial Transplant 2005;20:167–175.)

RECIPIENT EVALUATION

In this section, extensive use has been made of guidelines published by the American Society of Transplantation and the American Society of Transplant Surgeons in 2001[3] as well as the European Best Practice Guidelines for Renal Transplantation published on behalf of the European Renal Association–European Dialysis and Transplant Association in 2000.[4] A key goal in the workup is to rapidly identify patients for whom transplantation is not an appropriate option, in part to avoid costly investigation and also to carefully evaluate those who would benefit even if they possess comorbidities that need special assessment. A summary of the overview of the routine evaluation is shown in Figure 91.2.

HISTOCOMPATIBILITY

Histocompatibility testing is performed to help identify recipient and donor combinations that would be expected to result in poor graft survival. ABO typing is critical as an incompatible match can result in hyperacute rejection; the only exception is the transplantation of an A2 kidney into an O- or B-positive recipient in whom low titer anti-A antibodies are present.

Both donors and recipients should also undergo HLA typing in which the HLA-A, HLA-B, and HLA-DR antigens of the major histocompatibility complex (MHC) are determined. For cadaveric donors, a complete six-antigen match is associated with a 5% to 10% increased survival over 3 to 10 years, compared to mismatched kidneys, and hence such "full-house" donor kidneys are often given preference in donor-recipient selection. In contrast, it is harder to show differences in graft survival in the presence of one or more mismatches. For living related kidneys, a complete match is also associated with improved patient and graft survival compared to haploidentical or zero-antigen matched kidneys.

HLA Antibodies and Cross-matching

It is imperative that all subjects undergoing transplantation be tested for the presence of antibodies to HLA antigens from the donor. Antibodies may occur from previous transplantation of (mismatched) organs, after pregnancies (due to exposure to paternal antigens carried by the fetus), after blood transfusions, and rarely without known risk factors.

The principle of screening is shown in Figure 91.3. IgG antibodies against class I (HLA-A and HLA-B) antigens (positive crossmatch) are highly associated with acute rejection and are a contraindication to transplantation. IgM antibodies against HLA antigens may also predict rejection if they are present in current

Recipient evaluation

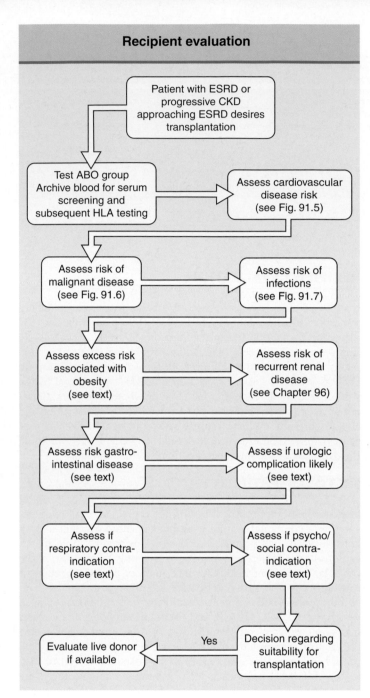

Figure 91.2 Recipient evaluation. CKD, chronic kidney disease; ESRD, end-stage renal disease.

Principle of screening for anti-HLA antibodies

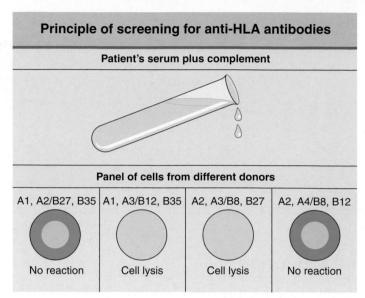

Figure 91.3 Principle of screening for anti-HLA antibodies. The patient's serum is tested with a panel of cells of known HLA types. The most common HLA antigens are represented in such panels. In this example, the A3 antigen is the only antigen present in the two lysed cell populations and absent from the nonlysed samples. Therefore, the patient's serum contains anti-HLA A3 antibodies.

Minimizing the degree of HLA mismatch between donor and recipient also reduces the risk of HLA sensitization should the graft fail. Current recommendations for detection and characterization of clinically relevant antibodies in solid organ transplantation have been summarized by the British Society of Histocompatibility and British Transplantation Society and are available at www.bts.org.uk.

Another issue is the presence of antibodies to class II (HLA-DR) antigens in the absence of antibody to class I antigens. While hyperacute rejection does not occur in these subjects, there is concern that antibody-mediated graft damage may occur, and in general transplantation is not recommended.

While conventional crossmatching involves complement-dependent cell lysis assays, many centers also perform the more sensitive flow cytometric crossmatching. Several multicenter studies have confirmed a benefit of performing flow crossmatch as it can better predict graft outcome.[5,6] As with all crossmatch tests, it is the specificity of the antibody that is crucial, and each unit will have a protocol agreed on between laboratory and clinical staff to allow decisions to be made as to the course of action to be taken consequent to the pattern of the results.

While the presence of ABO incompatibility or the presence of a positive crossmatch is used to exclude the possibility of donation, in recent years several groups have published case reports of successful transplantations in this situation using combinations of intravenous immunoglobulin and plasma exchange as well as antibody conditioning, particularly with anti-CD20 antibodies. Comprehensive reviews of the largest experience of HLA antibody desensitization have been published in the United States and Japan, particularly related to ABO-incompatible live donor renal transplantation. Summary guidelines relating to antibody incompatible transplants are available at www.bts.org.

CARDIOVASCULAR DISEASE

Cardiovascular disease is a major contributor to the increased premature mortality rate seen in renal transplant recipients. An algorithm for the work-up overview is shown in Figure 91.5.

but not past sera; however, they may also be false positive. Prior treatment of sera with dithiothreitol can remove IgM antibodies and aid in the interpretation of the test (Fig. 91.4). Autoantibodies (such as may occur in lupus) may also give false-positive results and can be determined by prior absorption with autologous lymphocytes.

Some patients may have antibodies that react with an antigen ("public epitope") present on numerous class I HLA antigens. In such subjects with a high panel of reactive antibodies (defined as antibodies present to >85% of the HLA class I antigens), it may be difficult if not impossible to find a compatible donor. To reduce the risk of this, exposure to blood transfusions should be avoided if possible for waitlisted patients and, if performed, should use leukocyte-depleted blood to reduce the risk of sensitization.

Interpretation of the crossmatch test					
	Crossmatch (normal procedure)		**Crossmatch (dithiothreitol)**		**Antibody-Mediated Graft**
Antibody to MHC Class	T Cells	B Cells	T Cells	B Cells	Damage
IgG against class I	+	+	+	+	Yes
IgM against class I	+	+	–	–	Yes, IgM class I antibodies may be harmless if present in old sera only but not in the current serum
IgG against class II	–	+	–	+	Yes
IgM against class II	–	+	–	–	Unknown
IgM autoantibodies	+	+	–	–	No

Figure 91.4 Interpretation of the crossmatch test.

Ischemic Heart Disease

We recommend that asymptomatic patients undergo further assessment if they are older than 50 years, are diabetic, have smoked cigarettes in the past 5 years, or have a resting electrocardiogram that shows a rhythm disturbance or ST segment abnormalities. We recommend beginning with a noninvasive test of occult cardiac ischemia, but it is not possible to justify any one particular test. Exercise tests probably have the most discriminating power but may not be practical, making pharmacologically driven cardiac stress testing more popular. Combined dipyridamole and exercise thallium imaging or dobutamine stress echocardiography are the most commonly used tests (see also Chapter 71). The discovery of significant reversible ischemia requires coronary imaging with management subsequently directed by conventional protocols. If left ventricular function is adequate and symptoms are controlled, then transplant listing is recommended.

Cerebrovascular Disease

There is no evidence to support screening asymptomatic potential renal transplant recipients for cerebrovascular disease.[7] Patients with a completed stroke or a transient ischemic attack within the past 6 months should be referred for neurologic assessment and transplantation reconsidered after medical and surgical management has been optimized and the patient is free of recurrent transient ischemic attacks for 6 months. Screening in the presence of an asymptomatic carotid bruit is prudent, but further investigations rarely alter the clinical decision.

Peripheral Vascular Disease

If patients are asymptomatic with good femoral pulses, then only plain radiographs are recommended to rule out extensive vascular calcification.[8] In contrast, patients with claudication or lack of palpable femoral pulses require vascular imaging and a surgical assessment of whether it is technically possible to implant the graft and whether the transplant would be predicted to lead to steal and critical ischemia in the distal leg.

CANCER

Cancer rates are increased in patients with end-stage renal disease (ESRD) on dialysis.[9] For a potential recipient who has been previously treated for cancer, the question is whether a delay before transplantation will reduce the risk of relapse of occult metastatic disease, perhaps accelerated by immunosuppression. Transplant registries have demonstrated that recurrence rates of cancer are less the longer the waiting time is, with 53% recurring within 2 years, 34% between years 2 and 5, and the last 13% recurring after 5 years.[10] Given the survival advantages of transplantation over dialysis, a reasonable compromise is to wait 2 years after successful treatment for most cancers prior to transplant listing. Exceptions in which there is no recommended delay include asymptomatic incidentally discovered renal cell carcinoma confined to the kidney, *in situ* cancer of the bladder or cervix, and basal cell and squamous cell carcinomas of the skin. In contrast, cancers with a high risk of recurrence, such as colorectal cancer, malignant melanoma, and cancer of the body of the uterus, should have a 5-year delay. It is difficult to know how best to advise patients with treated breast cancer because the majority of relapses occur after 3 years; breast cancer is also twice as common in renal transplant recipients compared to the general population.[11] For patients treated for breast cancer, we recommend an interval of 2 years after curative treatment. As breast (and many other cancers) are heterogeneous conditions with a variable prognosis depending on staging, an individualized approach is recommended in consultation with an oncologist. Current guidelines are summarized in Figure 91.6.

The issue of screening for cancer in both potential renal transplant recipients and patients post-transplantation is contentious. The numbers needed to screen to save one life varied from 338 to >5000 for colorectal, breast, and prostate cancers.[12] We therefore do not recommend routine screening but rather use an individualized approach with cancer screening based on symptoms, signs, or in the presence of conditions known to predispose to cancer such as von Hippel–Lindau disease or analgesic nephropathy.

INFECTIOUS COMPLICATIONS

The primary tests required for screening are shown in Figure 91.7.[13] Geographic location determines screening requirements for some occult infections. In regions of the world where human herpesvirus 8 infection is common, it may be helpful to know the serology of individuals prior to grafting, given the strong association of the virus with Kaposi's sarcoma. Recipients who have negative Epstein-Barr virus (EBV) titers who receive EBV-positive renal transplants have a sevenfold increased risk of developing post-transplantation lymphoproliferative disorder. The knowledge of recipient serologies may therefore influence post-transplantation immunosuppressive strategies. In particular, the cytomegalovirus serology at the time of grafting helps guide antiviral prophylactic strategies.[14]

While human immunodeficiency virus (HIV) infection was originally viewed as an absolute exclusion for transplantation, the

Workup algorithm for cardiovascular disease

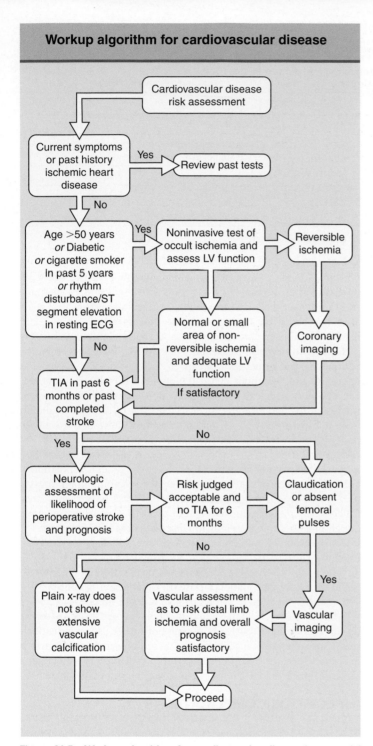

Figure 91.5 **Workup algorithm for cardiovascular disease in potential transplant recipient.** ECG, electrocardiogram; LV, left ventricular; TIA, transient ischemic attack.

Guidelines for transplantation in patients with previous malignancies

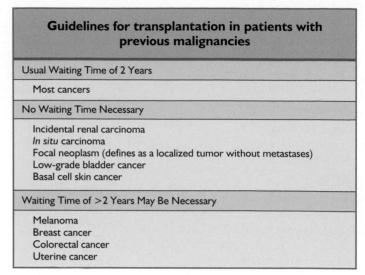

Figure 91.6 **Guidelines for transplantation in patients with previous malignancies.** (From Penn I: The effect of immunosuppression on pre-existing cancers. Transplantation 1993;55:742–747.)

Carriers of hepatitis B surface antigen may receive renal transplantation provided there is no evidence of active viral replication (hepatitis B virus [HBV] DNA or hepatitis B early [HBe] antigen positive) or evidence of chronic active hepatitis or cirrhosis. Patients with active viral infection are recommended to undergo liver biopsy to stage the disease and to receive antiviral treatment (lamivudine or interferon-α) before transplantation. Patients with cirrhosis and active viral replication have a poor prognosis, and immunosuppressive therapy in these subjects can lead to an increase in viral replication with worsening of the liver disease. In addition, patients should be monitored for the increased risk of hepatocellular carcinoma with yearly serum α-fetoprotein estimations and/or liver ultrasonography. The indications for liver or combined liver/ kidney transplantation are discussed in Chapter 99.

Candidates who have antibodies to hepatitis C virus (HCV) should be tested for HCV RNA (by polymerase chain reaction) and also undergo liver biopsy since there is only a weak relationship between viral RNA load, derangement of conventional liver function tests and liver histology. Subjects with mild liver disease and active infection should be treated with pegylated interferon while

use of concomitant retroviral therapy in subjects with low viral load and without features of the acquired immunodeficiency syndrome have allowed kidney transplantation with some reports of graft and patient survival that are comparable to non–HIV-infected recipients.[15] The workup is complex and is likely to change in the near future. Guidelines have been produced by the British HIV Association and are available via the British Transplantation Society website at www.bts.org.uk/ and information about HIV and transplantation in the United States is available at www.clinicaltrials.gov/.

Screening tests for occult infection

Routine Serology	Where Indicated, Tests for	Other Routine Investigations
Hepatitis B virus	Human herpesvirus 8	Urine culture
Hepatitis C virus	HTLV	Chest radiograph
HIV	*Strongyloides stercoralis*	
Cytomegalovirus	Malaria	
Epstein-Barr virus	*Trypanosoma cruzi*	
	Schistosomiasis	

Figure 91.7 **Screening tests for occult infection.** Routine screening tests for occult infection. HIV, human immunodeficiency virus; the replacement lymphotropic virus.

still on dialysis. In the event that infection is not cleared, subjects may undergo renal transplantation, for even though viremia may increase with the immunosuppression, the survival of HCV-positive transplant recipients is improved compared to those remaining on dialysis.[16] In contrast, in subjects found to have advanced liver disease on biopsy, a liver-kidney transplant may be entertained.

Tuberculosis may reactivate following transplantation. As such, all patients should undergo chest radiography to look for inactive disease and have a tuberculin skin (purified protein derivative [PPD]) test. While a positive PPD correlates with past infection, false-negative skin tests in the uremic patient are common. In one study, the PPD test result was positive in only 20% to 25% of patients pretransplantation who developed active tuberculosis post-transplantation.[17] Patients identified as at high risk (history of tuberculosis, positive chest radiograph, positive PPD test result, or living in an endemic area) and who have not received isoniazid in the past in many centers should receive daily isoniazid post-transplantation for 9 months.

OBESITY

Obese subjects carry increased risk during surgery, including increased risk of wound infections and perioperative complications. According to the United States Renal Data System database, an advantage for transplantation for obese subjects could be shown for live donors, whereas for deceased donors, the survival benefit was only shown in the recipient who had a body mass index (BMI) <40 kg/m^2.[18] We therefore do not recommend transplantation of deceased donor kidneys for recipients with BMI >40 kg/m^2. Obese subjects also need assessment for potential comorbidities (such as hypertension or diabetes) during the workup.

RECURRENT DISEASE

Graft loss attributed to recurrent disease has increased in recent years but is still only thought to be responsible for about 5% of graft loss.[19] The risks and management of recurrent disease are discussed in Chapter 96.

GASTROINTESTINAL

The rate of colonic perforation after renal transplantation is approximately 1% and is most commonly associated with diverticular disease. Screening of asymptomatic patients is not justified as a study found none of the patients with significant diverticular disease had symptomatic disease post-transplantation.[20] Patients with symptomatic disease should undergo imaging and consideration given to resection of extensive disease. Screening of asymptomatic individuals for peptic ulcer disease is not recommended because of the low morbidity rate even in patients with past peptic ulcer disease.[21] The issue of how best to manage incidentally noted cholelithiasis is not straightforward. The strategy adopted in any one unit will in part be determined by access to laparoscopic cholecystectomy and whether cholecystectomy will significantly delay listing, which may more seriously disadvantage the patient compared to the risk of subsequent biliary sepsis post-transplantation. In a recent decision analysis, expectant management was recommended as the preferred strategy for kidney transplant recipients with asymptomatic cholelithiasis, and this is our advice.[22]

GENITOURINARY

Routine screening of potential transplant candidates is unnecessary. Appropriate urologic investigations should be carried out in the pediatric population when congenital obstructive uropathy is suspected or in adult practice where bladder outlet obstruction or a neurogenic bladder resulting in high intravesical pressures is suggested by clinical history and examination. Whether urinary diversion, bladder augmentation, or intermittent self-catheterization is the best option will depend on the result of specialist evaluation.

Native nephrectomy is rarely indicated prior to transplant waitlisting. Removal of both kidneys may be indicated for persistent sepsis, especially in the presence of nephrolithiasis and/or pronounced reflux. Uninephrectomy of a large polycystic kidney is occasionally required to make space for the allograft or if it is harboring infection; there is no compelling evidence favoring whether the surgery should be pre-emptive or at the time of transplantation. Similarly, the removal of a failed allograft may be required prior to waitlisting if it is the source of sepsis or causing systemic inflammation from rejection or to allow space for a new allograft. Whether surgical removal of a failed graft minimizes the degree of HLA sensitization is not clear. In practice, grafts that fail within 6 months are usually removed. The decision to remove a failed graft after 6 months will need to balance surgical morbidity against the resistance to erythropoietin that is seen with a failed graft *in situ*, the advantage of rapid tapering of immunosuppression, and whether any urine output contributes meaningfully to fluid balance. Slow tapering of immunosuppression mostly to avoid hypoadrenalism is usually safe if the graft is not removed.

PULMONARY

Pulmonary function tests are generally performed in the preparation for surgery if the clinical history or examination suggests chronic lung disease.[23] All patients who smoke cigarettes should be advised to quit since active smokers have a 5.5-times increased risk of perioperative pulmonary complications compared to those who do not smoke. Patients with bronchiectasis require careful assessment as they carry significant risk of serious septic complications post-transplantation.

PSYCHOSOCIAL

A number of psychosocial variables can affect transplantation evaluation. If an adult has impaired capacity for consent, proxy arrangements consistent with the local jurisdiction need to be put in place, as some of these individuals, despite irreversible cognitive impairment, may be judged as likely to benefit from transplantation. This appears particularly true under conditions in which medication compliance is supervised.

Another concern relates to issues associated with treatment adherence and compliance. Successful postoperative transplant care inevitably requires frequent hospital attendance and adherence to a complex drug regimen. Some individuals can be identified prior to listing for whom additional support post-procedure can minimize the risk of premature graft failure due to inability to comply with management. Other individuals may be deemed to have demonstrated such poor adherence to medical management advice that withholding the offer of transplantation waitlisting is appropriate. It is usual in these circumstances to collate views from several of the health professionals involved in the patient's care as well as from the patient and immediate family members.

RE-EVALUATION OF PATIENTS ON THE WAITING LIST

Following placement on the waiting list, a number of patients wait years before receiving the offer of a transplant. It is logical that a re-evaluation of suitability is undertaken at intervals, but there are no data to help decide how often this should be. Guidelines have been proposed but are significantly more rigorous than those recommended for initial evaluation in this chapter and would, if followed, have very significant resource implications and logistic demands.[24] Regular assessment of hepatitis and HIV viral status will occur as a part of routine dialysis care. However, re-evaluation for progression of asymptomatic ischemic heart disease and atherosclerotic disease is the area most expected to be of medical benefit. In one observational study, no benefit of cardiac surveillance after listing could be shown.[25] Nevertheless, we recommend that, in the absence of symptoms, cardiac reevaluation be performed every 4 years on nondiabetics and every 2 years on diabetic transplant waitlisted candidates using similar workups as in the initial evaluation.

DECEASED DONORS

Deceased donors can be categorized as heart-beating donors with brainstem death (standard donor) or donors after cardiac death, also known as non–heart-beating donors. Donations following cardiac death constitute 2% of the deceased donors in the United States and a rapidly increasing proportion in Europe. Extended criteria donors are heart-beating donors older than 60 years of age or 50 to 59 years old with two or three of the following: a history of hypertension, serum creatinine >1.5 mg/dl (130 μmol/l) at donation, and/or dying of a cerebrovascular accident. On average, the survival of extended criteria and kidneys retrieved from some categories of non–heart-beating donors are inferior to that seen from standard criteria donors. Most matching schemes attempt to allocate these grafts to recipients who are predicted to have a lower than average overall survival.

Potential deceased donors are screened by coordinators who evaluate current clinical records and primary physician notes and conduct relative interviews. The review focuses on health history, social history, and laboratory evidence of renal impairment, cancer, and infectious disease (Fig. 91.8). Patients with sepsis, acute hepatitis, HIV infection, West Nile virus, or a history of malignancy are excluded from donation. Donors carrying HBV or HCV are accepted only for those positive for HBV or HCV antibody, respectively. The risk of an unknown donor malignancy is about 1.3%, and the risk of transmitting a donor malignancy is about 0.2%.[26] The possibility of permanent renal disease is determined by history, urinalysis, serum creatinine, and biopsy, if indicated. Serum creatinine at admission should be in the near normal range (estimated creatinine clearance >60 ml/min), but a temporary decline in renal function with subsequent signs of improvement is acceptable. The presence of proteinuria (>0.5 g/24 hr) indicates structural renal damage and is a valid reason for nonacceptance. However, the use of gelatin-based plasma expanders can interfere with several urinary protein assays, leading to apparently high protein concentrations while the dipstick reaction remains negative.

Deceased donor evaluation checklist
Medical History
Hypertension Diabetes Infections (TB, hepatitis, HIV) Malignancy Transfusions Trauma Surgical Hospitalizations Reason for hospitalization Recent infections
Social History
Intravenous drug abuse Alcohol Sexual behavior Acupunture Tattoo Travel Incarceration TB exposure
Examination
Blood pressure Cardiac Vascular Lymphadenopathy Abdominal
Laboratory/Technical
Creatinine Urinalysis Urine culture Transaminase Coagulation profile Complete blood count Blood culture Virology: antibodies to CMV, EBV, HSV-1 and -2, HHV-6, -7, -8, HCV, HBV (include HBsAg, anti-HBc IgG, and IgM), HIV, West Nile, rabies, HTLV-I Parasites depending on geographic region: malaria, babesiosis, toxoplasmosis, Chagas, syphilis Fungi in appropriate regions: coccidiodes, histoplasmosis Tuberculosis (depending on geographic region) Chest radiograph Electrocardiogram Biopsy if there is concern for chronic renal disease
Operating Room Evaluation
Intra-abdominal examinate to detect occult malignancy
Contraindications for Deceased Donation
Sepsis Acute hepatitis HIV (unless recipient positive) Infection with West Nile virus or rabies High-risk behavior for HIV unless testing negative and life-saving transplantation History of malignancy (unless nonmetastatic skin tumor or noninvasive brain tumor) Chronic renal insufficiency Advanced age with poor estimated renal function, but potentially could be used for older recipients

Figure 91.8 Deceased donor evaluation checklist. CMV, cytomegalovirus; EBV, Epstein-Barr virus; HBc, hepatitis B core antigen; HBsAg, hepatitis B surface antigen; HBV, hepatitis B virus; HCV, hepatitis C virus; HHV, human herpesvirus; HIV, human immunodeficiency virus; HTLV-I, human T-lymphocyte virus type I; TB, tuberculosis.

Kidneys from very small donors typically younger than 6 years of age are generally regarded as being at high risk of failure, especially from vascular thrombosis; on occasions, two kidneys are transplanted *en bloc* using the aorta and inferior vena cava as conduits.

In the brain-dead donor, maintenance of an adequate stable blood pressure and oxygenation and a continuous diuresis to avoid warm ischemic injury is important. The use of pressor agents, volume resuscitation, and other conditioning strategies is complex and has been the subject of several guideline documents (see www.ics.ac.uk). In this category of donor, the kidneys are not subject to significant warm ischemia at the time of organ retrieval.

Donation after cardiac death can occur via several mechanisms.[27] One scenario is that an individual dies soon after the elective withdrawal of ventilatory support in the intensive care unit, followed by a rapid surgical exposure of the great vessels and cooling of the organs followed by prompt retrieval. Donation after cardiac death may also occur following failed cardiopulmonary resuscitation after unanticipated cardiac arrest in which the kidneys are cooled *in situ* by inserting perfusion catheters via the femoral vessels. Surgical retrieval then takes place after a delay to allow family counseling and donor assessment. Donation after cardiac death is inevitably associated with a warm ischemic injury to the kidneys. This is responsible for the higher rate of delayed graft function that is seen in this group. The need for dialysis support post-transplantation is on average 50% but varies from 30% to 90%, depending on the category of donor.[27]

The time to assess a potential deceased donor is always limited, and it is obvious that cadaveric kidneys cannot be "quality assured." A few recipients of renal transplants experience primary nonfunction and often require removal of the graft. These individuals are certainly disadvantaged by renal transplant surgery. However, there is a serious shortage of donor organs, so it is important to retrieve from all donors where there is a good chance of using the kidneys to provide good-quality rehabilitation and a survival advantage to the recipient.

LIVING DONORS

Living donors may be related, unrelated, altruistic, or part of a donor exchange or list-exchange program. Live donation results in the best recipient renal function and survival. Since 2001 in the United States, more than half of all transplantations use living donors. In Japan, Brazil, and the Middle East, >80% of donors are living donors. More than 30% of the live kidney donors in the United States are from living unrelated donors, that is, genetically unrelated to their recipient. The superior success of live donors compared to deceased donor transplants independent of the donor-recipient match has supported the development of live donor paired exchange and live donor-deceased donor exchange. In the first instance, live donors who are incompatible with their intended recipients are exchanged between recipients. In the other instance, the donor donates to the waitlist in exchange for their intended recipient receiving priority on the list. In some countries, either a state-organized or free-market system results in the purchase of live donor kidneys; this is a highly controversial area and under active international policy development.[28]

Death following Living Donation
The underlying premise of living kidney donation is that the removal of one kidney does not impair survival or long-term kidney function. Nevertheless, the donor profile has changed over time to include those with isolated medical abnormalities such as essential hypertension, an increased BMI, isolated hematuria, dyslipidemia,

and previous stone disease. While donation appears to be safe in the short term for these subjects, in many cases, follow-up has not been long enough to be confident that various comorbid conditions will not adversely influence long-term survival.

Donor death is not only related to acute surgical complications. Common medical conditions may develop such as cancer or vascular disease, but of special concern is the contribution of donation to the psychological state of the donor and the impact on accident-, homicide-, and suicide-related deaths. In particular, younger donors need to be evaluated for thought processes that might put them at increased risk of self-destructive behavior following donation as there is evidence that the rate of accidental death, homicide, and suicide are at rates slightly above the average.[29]

Perioperative Complications
Reports of relatively homogeneous Northern European populations after nephrectomy for trauma and for kidney donation suggest that uninephrectomy is safe.[30] This is illustrated by Figure 91.9, which shows the improved life expectancy of live donors relative to the general population in Sweden.[31] The perioperative mortality risk of open surgery is estimated at 1 in 3000. Laparoscopic surgical techniques have been credited for the recent increase in living kidney donation achieving shorter hospital stay, less incisional discomfort, and an earlier return to work. A comparison of complications between procedures is shown in Figure 91.10.[32] Laparoscopic donor nephrectomy is associated with open conversion in 2%, more frequent readmission for gastrointestinal complications, and rarely the development of chylous ascites.

End-Stage Renal Disease following Living Donation
In a large program in Norway, of 1800 (0.4%) living donors had developed ESRD.[33] More recent published data suggest that between 0.4% and 0.7% of donors of Northern European descent have developed ESRD.[34] In a preliminary evaluation of the Scientific Registry of Transplant Recipients and Centers for Medicare and Medicaid Services ESRD databases, the overall incidence of ESRD in Caucasian donors was estimated as a maximum to be 0.10% and 0.52% in Black donors.[35] Supporting the concern over

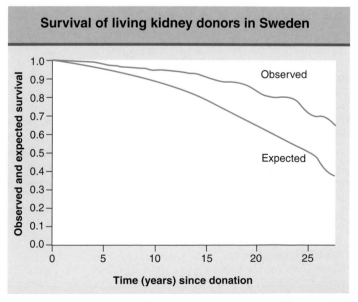

Figure 91.9 Survival of living kidney donors in Sweden. The survival of living related donors is superior to the expected survival derived from the general population. (Adapted from Fehrman-Ekholm I, Elinder CG, Stenbeck M, et al: Kidney donors live longer. Transplantation 1997;64:976–978.)

Complications of donor nephrectomy

	Open Procedure	Hand-Assised Laproscopic Nephrectomy	Nonhand-Assisted Laproscopic Nephrectomy
Number of procedures	5660	2239	2929
Reoperation	0.4%	1.0%	0.9%
Readmission	0.6%	1.6%	1.6%
Nonoperative complications	0.3%	1.0%	0.8%
DVT/PE	0.02%	0.09%	0.1%
Bleeding	0.1%	0.45%	0.2%
Rhabdomyolysis	0	0.09%	0.13%
Mortality	0	0.04%	0.07%

Figure 91.10 Complications of donor nephrectomy. Complications noted after different types of donor nephrectomy. DVT/PE, deep venous thrombosis/pulmonary embolus; Open, open nephrectomy. (Adapted from Matas AJ, Bartlett ST, Leichtman AB, Delmonico FL: Morbidity and mortality after living kidney donation, 1999–2001: Survey of United States transplant centers. Am J Transplant 2003;3:830–834.)

Renal function pre- and postdonor nephrectomy in Blacks and Caucasians

Variable	Black	Caucasian	P Value
Precreatinine (mg/dl)	1 ± 0.1	0.8 ± 0.2	NS
Postcreatinine (mg/dl)	1.5 ± 0.3	1.2 ± 0.2	NS
ΔScr >50%	75%	25%	<0.05

Figure 91.11 Renal function pre- and postdonor nephrectomy in Blacks and Caucasians. Black donors show a greater increase in serum creatinine compared to Caucasian living kidney donors. HTN, hypertension; SCr, serum creatinine. (Adapted from Ahmed J, Shah V, Malinzak L, et al: Comparison of the increase in serum creatinine post kidney donation between African American and Caucasian donors. Am J Transplant 2005;5:A416.)

increased risk of ESRD in African American donors were data showing that, although the serum creatinine was not different at donation between donors of different ethnicities, the number of donors with a serum creatinine that increased >50% was higher in African American donors (Fig. 91.11).[36] The renal evaluation for African American donors needs to be undertaken with special care.

Medical Evaluation of the Live Donor

Medical evaluation of the living donor has been standardized by two large conferences with broad representation from the transplant community.[37,38] An outline of the usual donor evaluation is shown in Figure 91.12 and includes blood and urine screening tests, chest radiography, electrocardiography, an age- and family history–appropriate cardiac stress test, and radiographic assessment of the kidneys and vessels. An assessment of the anatomy may be achieved by renal arteriography, computed tomography angiography, or magnetic resonance angiography.

Renal Function and Live Kidney Donation

The threshold of acceptable donor renal function has declined with time. Ideally, living donors should have a glomerular filtration rate (GFR) at the average of the age-specific GFR. Furthermore, as GFR declines with age, a donor's projected GFR at age 80 should be ≥40 to 50 ml/min per 1.73 m.[2] The majority of centers have chosen a GFR of 80 ml/min per 1.73 m² to be the lower limit for donation.[37,38] An age-related threshold has been adopted in the revised British Transplantation Society/Renal Association UK guidelines for living donor kidney transplantation (available at www.bts.org.uk/). This is shown in Figure 91.13.

Donor Hypertension

The evaluation for hypertension should include blood pressure measurements on three separate occasions; verification of elevated levels should be undertaken with ambulatory blood pressure monitoring. If elevated blood pressure is detected and the prospective donor is still under consideration, then chest radiography, electrocardiography, echocardiography, and ophthalmologic evaluation

Live donor evaluation checklist

History (look for/ask about)

Hypertension
Diabetes
Nonsteroidal anti-inflammatory inhibitors/medications/herbs
Family history
Intravenus drug abuse
Infections
Vascular
Vocation/avocation
Willingness to donate

Physical Exam (evaluate/look for)

Blood pressure
Weight/height
Arthritis
Autoimmunity
Cancer
  Prostate
  Breast
  Colorectal
  Lymph node
  Skin
Cardiovascular disease

Laboratory

Urinalysis
Electrolytes, liver panel
Fasting blood glucose and lipid profile
Complete blood count with platelets, coagulation screen
24-hour urine, creatinine clearance, protein excretion or glomerular
    filtration rate measurement (iothalamate clearance), and protein
    determination
Antiviral screening: HCV, HBV, HIV, EBV, CMV, HSV
Purified protein derivative test (PPD; controversial in nonendemic areas),
    rapid plasmin reagin tests
Electrocardiogram, chest radiograph
PAP smear, prostate examination
Age/family history determined
    Exercise tolerance test, echocardiography
    Colonoscopy, ultrasonography
    Mammography/prostate-specific antigen

Anatomic Evaluation per the Local Expertise

Computed tomography angiography
Magnetic resonance imaging angiography
Arteriography

Figure 91.12 Live donor evaluation checklist. CMV, cytomegalovirus; HBV, hepatitis B virus; HCV, hepatitis C virus; HIV, human immunodeficiency virus; HSV, herpes simples virus.

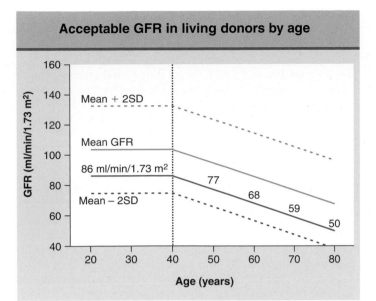

Figure 91.13 Acceptable glomerular filtration rate (GFR) in living donors by age. Diagram explaining the minimum acceptable age-associated GFR in living donor candidates. *Solid orange line* shows the variation with age of mean GFR. The *outer dashed lines* show the plus and minus two population standard deviation limits. GFR is constant up to the age of 40 years and then declines at the rate of 9 ml/min per 1.73 m² per decade. The reference plot is based on an analysis of data for 428 live renal transplant donors who had ^{51}Cr-ETDA GFR measurements. The *solid blue line* shows the safety limit of 86 ml/min per 1.73 m² for young adults declining to 50 ml/min per 1.73 m² at age 80. For transplant donors with preoperative GFR values above the *solid blue line*, the GFR of the remaining kidney will still be >37.5 ml/min per 1.73 m² at age 80. (Adapted from with permission from the revised British Transplantation Society/Renal Association UK guidelines for living donor kidney transplantation available at www.bts.org.uk/.)

should be performed looking for secondary consequences of hypertension. Donation may be acceptable for hypertensive individuals if blood pressure is controlled, GFR is as expected for donation and age, and there has been no increase in protein or albumin excretion.[39] However, more detailed information about these donors and their long-term outcomes is needed before generally accepting hypertensive individuals as donors.

Donor Obesity or Family History of Diabetes

One importance of obesity for the living donor is its impact on perioperative complications, future renal function, and cardiovascular health. Obesity is a risk factor for the development of nephrolithiasis, renal cell cancer, and ESRD. For ESRD, the relative risk is 3 for a BMI between 30 and 34.9 kg/m² and 4.7 for a BMI of 35 to 39.9 kg/m².[40] Obese individuals may be more prone to develop renal disease following donation. In one study, obese (BMI >30) subjects had an increased rate of proteinuria and renal impairment 10 to 20 years after nephrectomy.[41] Despite these concerns, many programs accept obese living donors.

Obesity greatly increases the future risk of diabetes, and, as a consequence, all obese prospective donors or those nonobese subjects with a first-degree relative with diabetes or with a history of gestational diabetes should be evaluated with an oral glucose tolerance test. An abnormal glucose tolerance is a contraindication to donation.

Nephrolithiasis

Those with a history of bilateral or recurrent stones and those with systemic conditions associated with recurrent stone disease should not donate. An asymptomatic potential donor with a current single stone is suitable if the donor does not have a high risk of recurrence, the stone is <1.5 cm in size, and especially if it is potentially removable during transplantation.[42] The evaluation of an asymptomatic donor with a single prior episode of nephrolithiasis should include evaluation of serum calcium, creatinine, albumin, and parathyroid hormone levels; spot urine for cystine; a urinalysis; and urine culture; a spiral computed tomography scan; chemical analysis of the stone if available; and 24-hour urine for oxalate, urate, and creatinine.

History of Malignancy and Infectious Disease

A history of the following malignancies excludes live kidney donation: melanoma, testicular cancer, renal cell cancer, choriocarcinoma, hematologic malignancy, bronchial cancer, breast cancer, and monoclonal gammopathy.[37] A history of malignancy may be acceptable for donation if prior treatment of the malignancy does not decrease renal reserve or place the donor at increased risk of ESRD and prior treatment of malignancy does not increase the operative risk of nephrectomy. A history of malignancy may be acceptable if the specific cancer is curable and transmission of the cancer can reasonably be excluded; consultation with an oncologist may be required. Consent to receive a renal transplant must include a discussion with the donor and the recipient that risk of transmission of malignant disease cannot be completely excluded.

Active Infections

A living donor should not be accepted if there is a history of active infection that requires nephrotoxic treatments or that would put the donor at risk of developing renal disease. These include HIV, HCV, HBV, recurrent urinary tract infections, endocarditis, and malaria.[37]

Venous Thromboembolism

Unless the history suggests a medical condition that would necessitate a comprehensive coagulation profile, these tests are not likely to yield useful information. A previous thromboembolism is a relative contraindication to live donation and will require an evaluation of the likelihood of recurrence. Oral contraceptives and hormone replacement therapy are commonly used and present an increased risk of postoperative venous thrombosis and thus should be withheld for at least 1 month prior to elective surgery.

Renovascular Disease

Fibromuscular dysplasia is found on average in 2% to 4% of prospective donors. Donors with severe and diffuse disease should not be selected for donation. The age of the prospective donor should also be considered, with the outcome in donors older than 50 seemingly more predictable and benign than in younger donors.[43]

Atherosclerotic renal vascular disease (ARVD) is a relative contraindication for living donation. If ARVD is present, the donor should be normotensive, have normal renal function, and have only unilateral disease.[44] Careful evaluation for coronary disease and peripheral vascular disease should be undertaken given the significant association of renovascular disease with atherosclerosis elsewhere.

Isolated Hematuria

Isolated hematuria in a prospective donor necessitates consideration of thin basement membrane nephropathy and IgA nephropathy as well as urinary tract infection, malignancy, and nephrolithiasis. This is a relatively common problem; a mass screening study in Japan found a single test point prevalence of 4% of adult men and 10% of adult women.[45]

Some investigators have reported the development of ESRD in individuals with thin basement membrane nephropathy. Currently, one approach to prospective donors with hematuria and thin basement membrane nephropathy would be to limit selection to those older than age 50 who have the least risk[46] and those with predictable family histories of disease and normal functional studies.

IgA nephropathy is a contraindication to live donation. The implications of isolated mesangial IgA without other manifestations of nephropathy require further study, and donation should be decided on in the context of family history, absolute renal function, the presence of interstitial disease, and age.[47] If during live donor evaluation, persistent isolated asymptomatic hematuria is detected, a workup should include a renal biopsy because, in that setting, the biopsy is often abnormal and aids the decision-making process.[48]

Autosomal-Dominant Polycystic Kidney Disease

Familial studies have shown the sensitivity of ultrasonography to be 100% in individuals at risk of autosomal-dominant polycystic kidney disease (ADPKD) who are age 30 or older. Wherever possible, linkage analysis should be performed in prospective donors at risk who are younger than age 30 as well as ultrasound imaging. If genetic testing is not possible, computed tomography and/or magnetic resonance imaging may provide better sensitivity than ultrasonography.

Cardiopulmonary Disease

Cardiac evaluations need to be performed based on family history, personal history, physical examination, electrocardiogram, and chest radiograph. If the history, examination, and test results suggest ischemia or valvular disease, then an exercise or pharmacologic stress test and/or echocardiography should be performed. An individual with myocardial dysfunction or coronary ischemia should not donate. Absolute contraindications to donation are symptomatic valvular disease, severe valvular disease even if asymptomatic, and valvular disease with abnormal cardiac function and/or ischemia. The possibility of valvular abnormalities should be particularly considered in family members of those with ADPKD. Relative contraindications are the presence of a prosthetic valve and moderate regurgitant valvular disease with otherwise normal echocardiographic findings. Finally, the donor with valvular disease should be informed of the risk of perioperative endocarditis even with antimicrobial prophylaxis, bleeding in those treated with anticoagulants, and thromboembolism during changes in anticoagulation.

Pulmonary contraindications to donation include chronic lung diseases that significantly increase the anesthetic risk. If indicated by history and examination, pulmonary function testing, echocardiography, and/or sleep studies should be performed. In all cases, donors should cease smoking for at least 4 to 8 weeks before surgery to minimize the risk of pneumonia. Optimally, donors should stop smoking permanently due to the increased risk of vascular disease, renal arteriosclerosis, and cancer.

Quality of Life following Living Donation

Physical and psychological function in living donors is higher than the community norm. Physical issues reported by donors following donation frequently include a decrease from baseline in energy, while some note a longer time to full recovery (up to 4 months) than they had anticipated and incision pain that lasts longer than they expected. Psychological factors usually include an improved relationship with the recipient, an improved self-image, and frequently a positive effect on the donor's life. Even though most donors have a very positive experience, a small number do regret the decision to donate (0% to 5%).[49]

DAY OF TRANSPLANTATION MANAGEMENT

The potential recipient will undergo a clinical evaluation with particular attention paid to changes in symptoms that may indicate the development of significant disease that contraindicates transplantation. As well as biochemistry and hematology blood tests, chest radiography and electrocardiography are routinely performed but no other special investigations.

All subjects undergo crossmatch using the patient's serum and donor peripheral white cells and lymphoid tissue in a way similar to that performed in serum screening (see Fig. 91.3). Conventionally, both current and archived recipient serum taken in the past as part of the serum screening program is tested. Often a "historical" serum sample from the recipient with the highest reactivity to a panel of HLA antigens is selected (a peak positive specimen). Interpretation may be difficult when a historical serum has a positive crossmatch with the donor cells while current sera are negative. Successful transplantation in the presence of current negative peak (or past) positive is commonly performed in many transplant programs, but it is the specificity of the antibodies that is crucial and the potential to alter the subsequent immunosuppressive protocol that is often necessary to ensure an acceptable outcome.

With the advent of genomic HLA typing of donor and recipient, as well as the improved ability to characterize circulating antibodies in stored blood specimens, the rate of day of transplantation-positive (unacceptable) crossmatch due to donor relevant HLA sensitization has become low. Many units are therefore using the most recent specimens to perform the crossmatch where it is known that there are no sensitizing events since the last blood sample or performing the crossmatch retrospectively post-transplantation. Both of these strategies have the potential to reduce cold ischemic time in cadaveric transplantation by several hours but can only be undertaken where careful characterization of the patient's risk of sensitization can be established and where there are serial blood samples to document any such sensitization.

Preoperative hemodialysis may be necessary if the patient is significantly hyperkalemic or fluid overloaded. Most clinicians prefer to avoid presurgery hemodialysis if possible. There is anxiety that both intravascular dehydration and the generation of cytokines during hemodialysis may contribute to delayed graft function. At the least, it may contribute to a delay and increase the risk of bleeding because of systemic heparinization.

REFERENCES

1. Simmons RG, Abress L: Quality-of-life issues for end-stage renal disease patients. Am J Kidney Dis 1990;15:201–208.
2. Goldfarb-Rumyantzev A, Hurdle JF, Scandling J, et al: Duration of end-stage renal disease and kidney transplant outcome. Nephrol Dial Transplant 2005;20:167–175.
3. Kasiske BL, Cangro CB, Hariharan S, et al: The evaluation of renal transplant candidates: Clinical practice guidelines. Am J Transpl 2001; 1(Suppl 2):3–95.
4. Berthoux F, Abramowicz D, Bradley B, et al: European best practice guidelines for renal transplantation (part 1). Nephrol Dial Transpl 2000; 15(Suppl 7):1–85.

5. Ogura K, Terasaki PI, Johnson C, et al: The significance of a positive flow cytometry crossmatch test in primary kidney transplantation. Transplantation 1993;56:294–298.

6. Cho YW, Cecka JM: Crossmatch tests—an analysis of UNOS data from 1991–2000. In Cecka M, Terasake PI (eds): Clinical Transplants 2001. Los Angeles: UCLA Press, 2002, pp 237–246.

7. Massy ZA, Mamzer-Bruneel MF, Chevalier A, et al: Carotid atherosclerosis in renal transplant recipients. Nephrol Dial Transplant 1998;13:1797–1798.

8. Brekke IB, Lien B, Sodal G, et al: Aortoiliac reconstruction in preparation for renal transplantation. Transpl Int 1993;6:161–163.

9. Maisonneuve P, Agodoa L, Gellert R, et al: Cancer in patients on dialysis for end-stage renal disease: An international collaborative study. Lancet 1999;354:93–99.

10. Penn I: The effect of immunosuppression on pre-existing cancers. Transplantation 1993;55:742–747.

11. Kasiske BL, Snyder JJ, Gilbertson DT, Wang C: Cancer after kidney transplantation in the United States. Transpl Int 2005;18:779–784.

12. Kiberd BA, Keough-Ryan T, Clase CM: Screening for prostate, breast and colorectal cancer in renal transplant recipients. Am J Transplant 2003;3:619–625.

13. Kasiske BL, Cangro CB, Hariharan S, et al: The evaluation of renal transplant candidates: Clinical practice guidelines. Am J Transplant 2001; 1(Suppl 2):3–95.

14. Newstead C, Griffiths PD, O'Grady JG, Parameshwar JK: Guidelines for the Prevention and Management of Cytomegalovirus Disease after Solid Organ Transplantation, 2nd ed. British Transplantation Society, 2004.

15. Abbott KC, Swanson SJ, Agodoa LY, Kimmel PL: Human immunodeficiency virus infection and kidney transplantation in the era of highly active antiretroviral therapy and modern immunosuppression. J Am Soc Nephrol 2004;15:1633–1639.

16. Pereira BJ, Natov SN, Bouthot BA, et al: Effects of hepatitis C infection and renal transplantation on survival in end-stage renal disease. The New England Organ Bank Hepatitis C Study Group. Kidney Int 1998;53:1374–1381.

17. Abbott KC, Klote MM: Update on guidelines for prevention and management of mycobacterium tuberculosis infections after transplant. Am J Transplant 2005;5:1163.

18. Glanton CW, Kao TC, Cruess D, et al: Impact of renal transplantation on survival in end-stage renal disease patients with elevated body mass index. Kidney Int 2003;63:647–653.

19. Chadban S: Glomerulonephritis recurrence in the renal graft. J Am Soc Nephrol 2001;12:394–402.

20. McCune TR, Nylander WA, van Buren DH, et al: Colonic screening prior to renal transplantation and its impact on post-transplant colonic complications. Clin Transpl 1992;6:91–96.

21. Troppman C, Papalois BE, Chiou A, et al: Incidence, complications, treatment, and outcome of ulcers of the upper gastrointestinal tract after renal transplantation during the cyclosporine era. J Am Coll Surg 1995;180:433–443.

22. Kao LS, Flowers C, Flum DR: Prophylactic cholecystectomy in transplant patients: A decision analysis. J Gastrointest Surg 2005;9:965–972.

23. Zibrak JD, O'Donnell CR: Indications for preoperative pulmonary function testing. Clin Chest Med 1993;14:227–236.

24. Matas AJ, Kasiske B, Miller L: Proposed guidelines for re-evaluation of patients on the waiting list for renal cadaver transplantation. Transplantation 2002;73:811–812.

25. Gill JA, Ma I, Landsberg D, et al: Cardiovascular events and investigation in patients who are awaiting cadaveric kidney transplantation. J Am Soc Nephrol 2005;16:808–816.

26. Morath C, Schwenger V, Schmidt J, Zeier M: Transmission of malignancy with solid organ transplants. Transplantation 2005;80:S164–S166.

27. Bernat JL, D'Alessandro AM, Port FK, et al: Report of a National Conference on Donation after cardiac death. Am J Transplant 2006;6:281–291.

28. Friedman EA, Friedman AL: Payment for donor kidneys: Pros and cons. Kidney Int 2006;69:960–962.

29. Jordan JC, Sann U, Janton A, et al: Living kidney donors' long-term psychological status and health behavior after nephrectomy—a retrospective study. J Nephrol 2004;17:728–735.

30. Ramcharan T, Matas AJ: Long-term (20–37 years) follow-up of living kidney donors. Am J Transplant 2002;2:959–964.

31. Fehrman-Ekholm I, Elinder CG, Stenbeck M, et al: Kidney donors live longer. Transplantation 1997;64:976–978.

32. Matas AJ, Bartlett ST, Leichtman AB, Delmonico FL: Morbidity and mortality after living kidney donation, 1999–2001: Survey of United States transplant centers. Am J Transplant 2003;3:830–834.

33. Hartmann A, Fauchald P, Westlie L, et al: The risk of living kidney donation. Nephrol Dial Transplant 2003;18:871–873.

34. Fehrman-Ekholm I, Thiel GT: Long-term Risks after Kidney Donation. London and New York: Taylor & Francis, 2005.

35. Davis C, Ojo AO: Living donor risks. American Transplant Congress, 2005.

36. Ahmed J, Shah V, Malinzak L, et al: Comparison of the increase in serum creatinine post kidney donation between African American and Caucasian donors. Am J Transplant 2005;5:A416.

37. Delmonico FL: A report of the Amsterdam forum on the care of the live kidney donor: Data and medical guidelines. Transplantation 2005;79:S53–S66.

38. Bia MJ, Ramos EL, Danovitch GM, et al: Evaluation of living renal donors. The current practice of US transplant centers. Transplantation 1995;60:322–327.

39. Textor SC, Taler SJ, Driscoll N, et al: Blood pressure and renal function after kidney donation from hypertensive living donors. Transplantation 2004;78:276–282.

40. Hsu C, McCulloch CE, Iribarren C, et al: Increased body mass index is an independent risk factor for end-stage renal disease: The Kaiser Multiphasic Health Checkup Cohort Study. J Am Soc Nephrol 2004;15:43A.

41. Praga M, Hernandez E, Herrero JC, et al: Influence of obesity on the appearance of proteinuria and renal insufficiency after unilateral nephrectomy. Kidney Int 2000;58:2111–2118.

42. Delmonico FL: The consensus statement of the Amsterdam Forum on the care of the live kidney donor. Transplantation 2004;78:491–492.

43. Indudhara R, Kenney, Bueschen AJ, Burns JR: Live donor nephrectomy in patients with fibromuscular dysplasia of the renal arteries. J Urol 1999;162:678–681.

44. Zierler RE, Bergelin RO, Davidson RC, et al: A prospective study of disease progression in patients with atherosclerotic renal artery stenosis. Am J Hypertens 1996;9:1055–1061.

45. Iseki K, Ikemiya Y, Iseki C, Takishita S: Proteinuria and the risk of developing end-stage renal disease. Kidney Int 2003;63:1468–1474.

46. Nieuwhof CM, de Heer F, de Leeuw P, van Breda Vriesman PJ: Thin GBM nephropathy: Premature glomerular obsolescence is associated with hypertension and late onset renal failure. Kidney Int 1997;51:1596–1601.

47. Lai KN, Chan LY, Leung JC: Mechanisms of tubulointerstitial injury in IgA nephropathy. Kidney Int Suppl 2005;94:S110–S115.

48. Koushik R, Garvey C, Manivel JC, et al: Persistent, asymptomatic, microscopic hematuria in prospective kidney donors. Transplantation 2005;80:1425–1429.

49. Johnson EM, Anderson JK, Jacobs C, et al: Long-term follow-up of living kidney donors: Quality of life after donation. Transplantation 1999;67:717–721.

Kidney Transplantation Surgery

Nicholas R. Brook and Michael L. Nicholson

KIDNEY DONORS

The usual and most frequent source of kidney for transplantation has been the heart-beating cadaveric donor, defined dead by brainstem death criteria.[1] The increasing worldwide discrepancy between the availability of and need for renal allografts[2] has led to the increasing use of alternative source of organs, from non–heart-beating cadaveric donors and living donors. The evaluation and selection of donors are discussed in Chapter 91. Here we discuss surgical aspects of retrieval and transplantation of kidneys.

HEART-BEATING CADAVERIC KIDNEY DONORS

The potential heart-beating cadaveric donor is maintained by artificial ventilation in a critical care setting until death has been diagnosed by brainstem death criteria, the consent of the next of kin for donation has been given, and the necessary legal and institutional approvals have been obtained.

The donor is then moved to the operating room, ventilation is discontinued, and surgery begins. The priorities of the organ retrieval team are influenced by the range of organs being donated. Heart, lung, and liver retrieval take priority over kidney retrieval, which may significantly lengthen the warm ischemic time. The kidneys are removed *en bloc*, and typically the artery is retrieved with a cuff of aorta (Carrel patch), with the maximum achievable length of renal vein, and 10 to 15 cm of ureter. Care is taken to avoid damage to polar and other accessory arteries, especially the lower pole artery, which may supply the ureter; stripping of adventitial tissue from the ureter must also be avoided, which may also compromise its blood supply.

The kidneys are flushed with ice cold preservation fluid until the effluent is clear and then are stored for transport in crushed ice or on a perfusion machine (see "Renal Preservation").

NON–HEART-BEATING KIDNEY DONORS

Prior to consensus on the definition of brainstem death, non–heart-beating donors (NHBDs) were the main source of transplant organs. These donors were intensive care unit based and had suffered head injuries or cerebrovascular accidents deemed irrecoverable, but organ retrieval could proceed only after cardiorespiratory death. This changed with the introduction of brainstem death legislation, but the use of NHBDs has recently increased again in response to the shortage of suitable organs for transplantation.

An international consensus has defined categories of NHBDs[3] (Fig. 92.1) to facilitate legal and ethical discussion and to highlight possible differences in organ viability. NHBD kidneys suffer a period of warm ischemia (the period between cardiac death and the time that *in situ* cold perfusion is started). The duration

Categories of non–heart-beating donor	
Uncontrolled	
I	Dead on arrival
II	Failed resuscitation
Controlled	
III	Awaiting cardiac arrest
IV	Cardiac arrest after brain stem death*
V	Unexpected cardiac arrest in intensive care unit*

Figure 92.1 Categories of non–heart-beating donor. Maastricht classification. *Less controlled.

of ischemia correlates with rates of primary nonfunction, delayed graft function (DGF), acute rejection, allograft, and patient survival. The main requirement of organ procurement from NHBDs is therefore to achieve rapid *in situ* perfusion of the kidneys to limit warm ischemia. This requires an emergency response team of surgeons and transplant coordinators, with considerable on-call and logistic commitments.

NHBDs may be either uncontrolled (Maastricht categories I and II) or controlled (Maastricht categories III through V). In controlled donors, cardiac arrest is expected and it is therefore possible to reduce the warm ischemia time to only a few minutes, as the transplantation team will be on standby. Uncontrolled donor cardiac arrest occurs suddenly, and this may result in prolonged warm ischemia times. The duration of reversible warm ischemia time that the human kidney can sustain is unknown, but NHBD kidneys should probably not be used for transplantation if warm ischemia exceeds 60 minutes.

Non–Heart-Beating Donor Protocol

Centers involved with NHB donation should adhere to the Maastricht protocol,[4] which includes the following principles:

- Approval by the local medical ethics committee
- Diagnosis of death by doctors who are independent of the transplantation team
- 10-minute rule (after declaration of cardiac death, the body is left untouched for a period of 10 minutes prior to intervention)
- Rapid *in situ* cooling using a catheter inserted into the aorta
- Organ retrieval using standard surgical techniques

Uncontrolled Non–Heart-Beating Donors

After a period of unsuccessful resuscitation and confirmation of cardiac death and observation of the 10-minute rule, cardiac

In situ perfusion of non–heart-beating donor kidneys

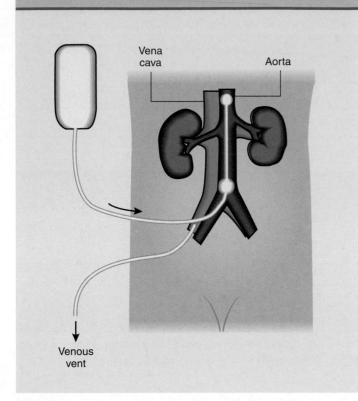

Figure 92.2 **Technique for *in situ* perfusion of non–heart-beating donor kidneys.** A double-lumen, double-balloon arterial catheter is introduced through the femoral artery and the lower balloon inflated at the aortic bifurcation and the upper balloon above the renal arteries. Ice-cold perfusion fluid is introduced and vented through the femoral vein until the effluent becomes clear.

massage and ventilation with 100% oxygen are recommended in an attempt to deliver oxygenated blood to the kidneys. A mechanical resuscitation device may be used. *In situ* renal cooling is effected by placing a double-balloon, triple-lumen perfusion catheter into the aorta via a femoral artery cut-down (Fig. 92.2), with instillation of preservation solution. Alternatively, the donor can be moved to an operating room as soon as death has occurred, and the aortic perfusion catheter is placed directly at laparotomy rather than via a femoral artery cut-down.

Controlled Non–Heart-Beating Donors

Here the transplantation team awaits cardiac arrest; after confirmation of death, the 10-minute rule is observed, and then the perfusion catheter is inserted via the femoral artery. Alternatively, the patient can be taken to the operating room before cardiac death if the next of kin gives consent.

LIVING KIDNEY DONORS

While cadaveric transplant rates remain more or less static, living donor transplantation has increased threefold in the United States over the past decade, where it now accounts for 49% of renal transplant activity.[5] In the United Kingdom, 27% of all renal transplants were from live donors in 2005.[6] Superior recipient post-transplantation outcome compared to cadaveric kidneys,[7] the

potential for pre-emptive transplantation before dialysis, and the ability to plan the procedure (allowing optimization of recipient condition) are major advantages and justify this growth in live donation.

Preoperative Imaging

Preoperative imaging of live donors confirms the presence of two functioning kidneys, indicates pathology that would preclude donation, and provides anatomic information necessary for planning the procedure. Imaging assumes paramount importance before minimal access donor nephrectomy because of the reduced operative exposure and particular difficulties in the identification of complex renal vein tributaries. The location, size, and number of renal veins and tributaries needs to be accurately described preoperatively. Angiography combined with excretion urography is now obsolete. For preoperative description of the main renal artery and vein anatomy, magnetic resonance angiography and computed tomography angiography are comparable,[8] but computed tomography angiography is more sensitive and specific for complex vascular anatomy and provides excellent correlation between imaging and surgical findings[9] (Fig. 92.3).

Minimal Access Donor Nephrectomy

The live donor nephrectomy operation has traditionally been performed through an open incision, necessitating a prolonged period of recovery. This and the cosmetic implications of a large flank wound may discourage potential donors (Fig. 92.4). To reduce such disincentives, there has been a move toward minimally invasive donor nephrectomy, first performed as a transperitoneal laparoscopic procedure (laparoscopic donor nephrectomy [LapDN]).[10] LapDN is associated with decreased severity and duration of postoperative pain, shorter in-patient stay, quicker return to work and normal activities, and improved cosmetic result when compared to open donor nephrectomy[11] (Fig. 92.5). Furthermore, the overall societal cost of LapDN is lower and recipient quality-of-life scores are higher.[12] The procedure is, however, technically demanding, and there is potential for damage to the renal parenchyma, vessels, and ureter during dissection. It takes longer than open nephrectomy and exposes the allograft to a short period of warm ischemia. There is also the potential for reduced graft perfusion before extraction in the presence of a pneumoperitoneum.

Nevertheless, retrospective data suggest that minimal access donor nephrectomy not only offers postoperative advantages to the donor, but also increases the number of transplants performed by reducing donor disincentives: estimates range from a 25% to a 100%[13] increase in transplantation activity. In the United States in 2005, 80% of live kidney donor procedures were performed laparoscopically. The United Kingdom is demonstrating year-on-year increases in live donor transplant activity,[6] and with accumulating evidence that laparoscopically procured kidneys yield high-quality grafts, more centers are adopting minimally invasive donor surgery.[14]

Three approaches have been described: transperitoneal, extraperitoneal, and hand-assisted live donor nephrectomy. Each approach is discussed in the following sections.

Transperitoneal Laparoscopic Donor Nephrectomy

Pneumoperitoneum is established and four laparoscopic ports are usually required (Fig. 92.6). After laparoscopic dissection, control, and division of the artery, vein, and ureter, a Pfannenstiel incision is made through which the kidney is brought out within an endoscopy retrieval bag.

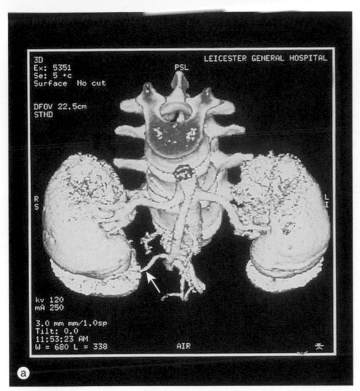

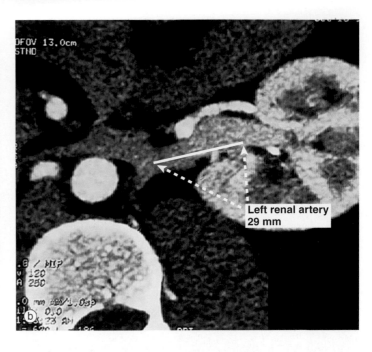

Figure 92.3 Living donor preoperative computed tomography angiography. *a*, Three-dimensional reconstruction of arterial supply. Note the lower pole artery to the right kidney (*arrow*), which may supply the ureter as well as the lower pole parenchyma. *b*, Measurement of renal vessels to give precise preoperative guidance to the surgeon.

Hand-Assisted Laparoscopic Donor Nephrectomy

The hand-assisted technique allows tactile sense to facilitate dissection, retraction, and exposure. It is said to be easier to learn and can be safely and efficiently performed by surgeons with less laparoscopic experience. The hand-assist device allows the operator's nondominant hand to enter the abdomen through an airtight system.

Retroperitoneoscopic Operative Technique

The retroperitoneal approach avoids breaching the peritoneum, displays the renal anatomy in a very different manner, and may be easier to harvest the full length of the vessels, especially on the right side. The disadvantage is that a more limited operating space is available than with the transperitoneal or hand-assisted laparoscopic techniques.

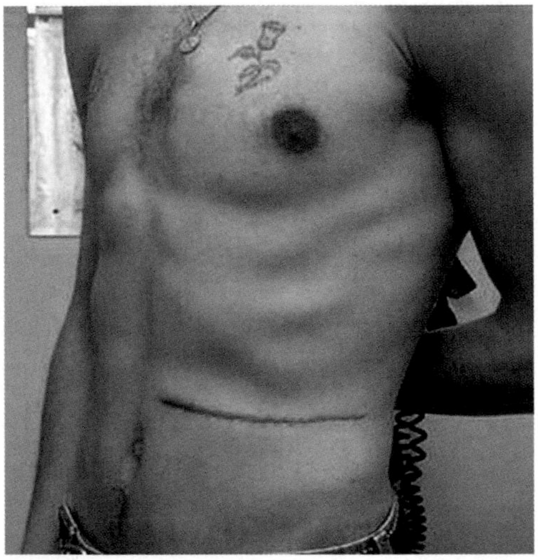

Contraindications to Minimal Access Donor Nephrectomy

There are no absolute contraindications other than those applying to the open operation. The relative contraindications are dictated by donor factors and the experience of the surgeon. The donor must be fit for anesthesia, including the physiologic stress of pneumoperitoneum. Obesity is a relative contraindication for both open and laparoscopic surgery, and the hand-assisted approach may be better suited in such patients. Previous abdominal surgery is a further relative contraindication because of the potential for adhesions. Multiplicity of renal vessels should not hinder LapDN.

Effect of Pneumoperitoneum

Transient intraoperative oliguria secondary to decreased renal blood flow is a frequent occurrence during laparoscopic procedures.

Figure 92.4 Flank wound from open nephrectomy.

Donor benefits of minimally invasive donor nephrectomy
Shorter incisions
Less pain
Shorter hospital stay
Shorter recovery
Better cosmetic appearance

Figure 92.5 Donor benefits of minimally invasive donor nephrectomy.

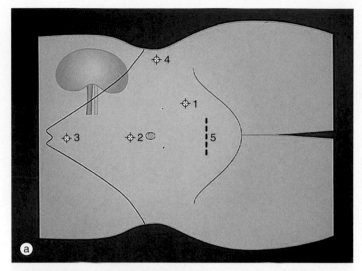

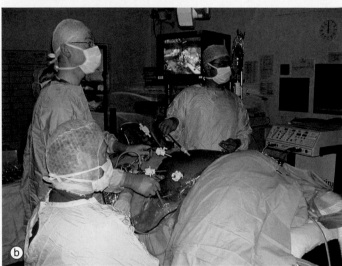

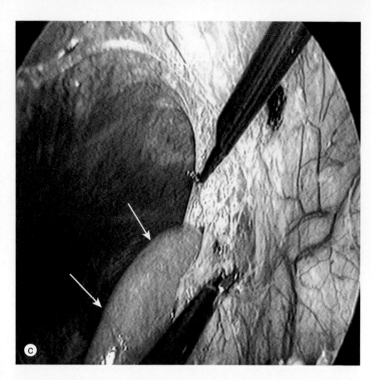

Figure 92.6 Technique for laparoscopic donor nephrectomy. *a*, Positions for four laparoscopic ports (1 to 4) and Pfannenstiel incision (5) through which the kidney is removed. *b*, Operative approach. *c*, Intraoperative view showing connective tissue being dissected away from the kidney (*arrows*).

Proposed mechanisms include decreased cardiac output, renal vein compression, ureteral obstruction, renal parenchymal compression, and systemic hormonal effects. Intracranial pressure increases during pneumoperitoneum, with release of vasoconstrictor agents that decrease renal blood flow. Use of a lower pressure reduces the adverse effects of pneumoperitoneum on renal perfusion. In donor nephrectomy, impaired renal blood flow may compromise early allograft function and compound the damaging effects of warm and cold ischemia and operative manipulation of the kidney. Laparo-scopically derived donor kidneys have higher serum creatinine up to 1 month post-transplantation compared to open surgery,[13] but thereafter graft function is equivalent.[13] The pioneers of LapDN report using high volumes of crystalloid pre- and intraoperatively to maintain renal perfusion in the presence of pneumoperitoneum. The authors have seen two episodes of unilateral pulmonary edema in the dependent lung, and we now recommend volume loading the donor with 2 liters of crystalloid the night before surgery and using replacement fluid only during surgery. This protocol has led to no apparent detriment to renal function.

Graft Function and Acute Rejection

There is no consistent evidence that graft function differs between kidneys retrieved by open, laparoscopic, or hand-assisted donor nephrectomy. The exception is that rates of DGF and acute rejection may be higher in pediatric recipients, especially the 0- to 5-year age group.

Pretransplantation ischemia could, in theory, render the donor kidney more immunogenic by inducing major histocompatibility complex (MHC) class II expression. However, despite the longer warm ischemia time, acute rejection rates and severity of rejection are not higher in laparoscopic than in open live donor kidneys.

Technical Issues

Ureteral ischemia was more common in early experience of LapDN, but can be avoided if care is taken to ensure that suffi-cient periureteral tissue is taken and that the dissection does not occur too close to the renal pelvis.

Multiple arteries need not be a barrier to successful use of grafts from laparoscopic donors. In open donor nephrectomy, the right kidney is retrieved in 20% to 30% of cases, whereas LapDN uses the right kidney in <10%,[14] reflecting concern over the operative safety of the right-sided laparoscopic operation, principally the difficulties involved in obtaining an adequate length of renal vein. It has been argued that this practice has led to compromise of the principle that the better kidney should remain with the donor. With newer laparoscopic techniques, however, there is no difference between right and left nephrec-tomy in operative complication rates.[15]

Postoperative Recovery

After uneventful open nephrectomy, the donor can expect to be discharged from the hospital in 5 to 6 days and return to work in 8 to 12 weeks. After LapDN the donor usually leaves hospital in 2 to 4 days and can return to work in 4 to 6 weeks.

Choice of Donor Operative Technique

The choice of operative procedure depends on the local expertise of the surgeons. There is accumulating evidence that the laparoscopic operation removes some of the disincentives to donation, and this approach is likely to be adopted widely in the future.

RENAL PRESERVATION

Preservation of cadaveric organs is crucial to allow time for matching, sharing of organs, and preparation of the recipient. Damage from hypothermia and reperfusion must be minimized. There is little standardization of the type of preservation solution used. Marshall's hyperosmolar citrate solution and histidine-tryptophan-ketoglutarate are popular choices in Europe but University of Wisconsin (UW) solution is more commonly used in the United States as extended preservation times are more common there.

Organs can be preserved by cold storage (kept in crushed ice after flushing with preservation solution) or by machine-driven pulsatile perfusion. The proposed benefits of machine perfusion come from allowing aerobic function through provision of oxygen and substrate and removal of metabolic end products. Although machine perfusion has been used for many years, there is still no consensus about its superiority to cold storage nor about the best perfusion parameters.

Decisions on the use of a kidney from a marginal donor can be supported by data from machine perfusion; high perfusion pressures are associated with primary nonfunction and DGF.

RENAL TRANSPLANTATION PROCEDURE

The transplanted kidney is placed heterotopically in one or other iliac fossa. The inferior epigastric vessels are ligated, as is the round ligament of the uterus in female patients. In males, the spermatic cord is mobilized and preserved. The peritoneum should not be breached, but instead swept superiorly to reveal the extraperitoneal bed into which the transplanted kidney will be placed. The iliac blood vessels are then mobilized, taking care meticulously to ligate all the associated lymphatic channels to reduce the risk of post-transplantation lymphatic leak.

Vascular Anastomosis

The renal vein is anastomosed end to side to the external iliac vein. The arterial anastomosis can be performed either end to side to the external iliac artery or end to end to the divided internal iliac artery (Fig. 92.7). The end-to-side anastomosis is technically easier and is the usual method employed in cadaveric transplantation, where it is possible to include a Carrel aortic patch with the renal artery.

With live donor kidneys, it is not possible to include a Carrel patch, and it is preferable to anastomose the renal artery end to end to the divided internal iliac artery. If there is no Carrel patch and the internal iliac artery is not available for anastomosis because of severe atheroma, it is possible to anastomose the renal artery directly to the external iliac artery without a patch. However, the

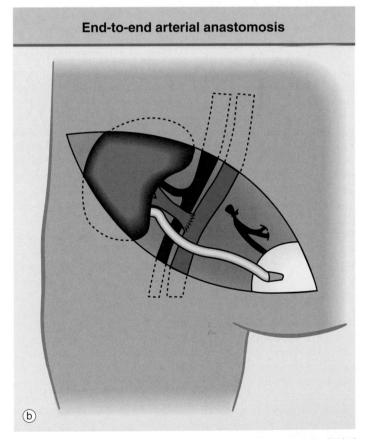

End-to-side arterial anastomosis	End-to-end arterial anastomosis
(a)	(b)

Figure 92.7 Vascular anastomosis techniques for renal transplantation. *a*, End-to-side anastomosis to the external iliac artery. *b*, End-to-end to the divided internal iliac artery, suitable for live donor transplantation in which no aortic patch is available.

external iliac artery has a much thicker wall than the renal vessel, increasing the likelihood of technical errors, in particular, narrowing of the anastomosis.

After completion of the vascular anastomoses, the kidney must sit in such a position that the renal vessels are not kinked. The transplanted kidney can be placed laterally in the iliac fossa or may be placed in a subrectus pouch fashioned specifically for the purpose.[16] In the latter case, the renal vessels run laterally from the kidney, and this needs to be noted when performing a post-transplantation biopsy. An operative diagram of the position of the kidney and vessels is therefore a vital component of the clinical notes.

If there are multiple renal vessels, the number of anastomoses should be minimized. This can usually be achieved by careful bench surgery before implantation. If there are two or more renal arteries, their aortic patches are joined in such a way that a single arterial anastomosis is required. If necessary, recipient iliac artery or saphenous vein is used to facilitate reconstruction. Occasionally, small polar arteries will only be recognized after a kidney has been retrieved, and it is particularly important to reanastomose lower polar arteries accurately as these may provide all the ureteral blood supply. In the case of double renal veins, the most common course of action is simply to ligate the smaller vein; the larger one is usually sufficient to drain the whole kidney. If there are two equally sized veins, both may need to be anastomosed separately to the external iliac vein.

Urinary Drainage

The traditional method of ureteral anastomosis is the Politano-Leadbetter technique, involving a transvesical ureteroneocystostomy with creation of a submucosal antireflux tunnel. The end of the transplanted ureter is drawn through a submucosal tunnel from outside to inside and sutured to the bladder mucosa. Many surgeons now prefer the technically simpler extravesical ureteroneocystostomy onlay in which the spatulated end of the ureter is anastomosed to the cystostomy and the divided muscle layer is then resutured over the ureter to create a short antireflux muscle tunnel. The onlay method has the advantage of being possible with only a short length of ureter. The shorter the ureter, the less likely it is that there will be an inadequate blood supply to the distal end, thereby reducing the risks of ischemic ureteral leaks or stenosis. A temporary double-J ureteral stent is usually placed. Stents reduce the impact of small technical errors while the ureter is leaking, and reduce major urological complications to an incidence of 1.5%.[17] However, they are a potential source of urinary infection, can become encrusted or blocked by debris, and can migrate or fragment. A further danger is the forgotten stent that has not been removed, which should always be considered in patients with unexplained and persistent lower urinary tract symptoms after transplantation. Stents are usually removed 4 to 6 weeks post-transplantation, and this can be performed without general anesthesia using a flexible cystoscope.

Alternative Techniques of Urinary Reconstruction

Renal transplantation is quite commonly performed in patients who have abnormal bladders. In many cases, it is possible to anastomose the transplanted ureter to the bladder in the hope that the bladder can be rehabilitated, if necessary, using post-transplantation intermittent self-catheterization. Nonetheless, some patients require urinary diversion using an ileal conduit. The conduit should be fashioned at least 6 weeks before transplantation, but it may have been present for many years. If so, a contrast study (a conduitogram) should be performed before transplantation to exclude the development of conduit stenosis, although this condition is rare. The transplanted kidney is best placed in the ipsilateral iliac fossa to avoid tension in the ureter, and it may be preferable to deliberately place the transplanted kidney upside down so that the ureter runs cranially and has a more direct route to the conduit. After revascularization, the peritoneum is opened and the ureter is anastomosed to the conduit over a double-J stent. Excellent long-term results have been achieved using this technique.[18]

Drainage and Wound Closure

Both the transplant bed and the subcutaneous tissues are drained using a closed suction drainage system to prevent the accumulation of serosanguinous fluid or lymph around the transplanted kidney. The skin is best closed with a subcuticular absorbable suture and then dressed with a clear adhesive dressing so that ultrasound scanning can be performed early without disturbing the wound. For this reason, metal clips are never used for the skin.

Postoperative Course

The recipient is nursed in a general ward with standard precautions and no need for reverse barrier nursing. If recovery is straightforward, the bladder catheter and wound drains are usually removed by day 5, and the recipient is fit for discharge after 7 to 10 days to be kept under close outpatient monitoring.

SURGICAL COMPLICATIONS OF RENAL TRANSPLANTATION

There is a small but significant incidence of technical complications, which can be minimized by avoiding damage to the kidneys at the time of the retrieval. Nonetheless, the presence of multiple renal vessels and donor atherosclerotic disease do increase the likelihood of technical problems in the recipient, as do recipient obesity, atherosclerosis, and previous transplantation.

Vascular Complications

Transplant vascular thrombosis is a feared complication that may cause early and irreversible graft failure. Although there are also significant hemorrhagic risks, routine perioperative prophylaxis should be given with subcutaneous heparin and some units prescribe aspirin for the first few postoperative months.

Bleeding from Vessels in the Renal Hilum

Careful postoperative observations, with regular hemoglobin and hematocrit measurements are crucial for the early detection of bleeding. Output from the transplant drains may give an early indication of heavy blood loss. Unsecured small vessels in the renal hilum may not be obvious during surgery, but they may start bleeding postoperatively. This form of blood loss can be slow, persistent, and serious. If the patient's condition allows, urgent imaging may be performed to secure a diagnosis, but the best course of action is usually emergency exploration of the transplant under general anesthesia.

Anastomosis Hemorrhage

This is a rare occurrence, usually due to a technical surgical error, and is more common with multiple arteries.[19] Early after transplantation, the patient may complain of pain over the graft. This symptom should always be taken seriously. There may also be pain in the back or the rectum caused by a tension hematoma in the retroperitoneum or pelvis. Significant hemorrhage will be attended by circulatory collapse, with tachycardia and hypotension. There will be a decrease in the hemoglobin and hematocrit, sometimes to alarmingly low levels. The patient must be returned to the operating theater immediately and the transplant re-explored.

Hemorrhage can also occur some weeks after transplantation due to the development of a mycotic aneurysm of the renal artery. In the rare case of a ruptured mycotic aneurysm, an immediate graft nephrectomy is required, but the mortality is high.

Renal Artery Thrombosis

This is a rare event, occurring in <1% of transplants. The usual outcome is loss of the kidney. Acute arterial thrombosis may occur intraoperatively or during the first days or weeks post-transplantation. Potential causes including hyperacute rejection or a procoagulant state, but most cases are due to a technical error during the anastomosis of small or atheromatous vessels.[20] Successful vascular anastomosis requires that the vessels are not under tension and that there is a smooth transition between the two intimal surfaces; sutures must be placed through all layers of the vessel walls so that an intimal flap is avoided. Vascular adventitia is thrombogenic and must be excluded from the lumen of the anastomosis.

Renal arterial thrombosis presents with sudden anuria, the differential diagnoses being a blocked urinary catheter, dehydration, acute tubular necrosis, or a urologic complication. A high index of suspicion is required to make this diagnosis, particularly in the immediate postoperative period. The only worthwhile investigation is an urgent duplex ultrasound scan, but if the diagnosis is seriously entertained, then the only hope of saving the transplant is to re-explore it immediately in the hope that a correctable cause can be found. The reality is that, unless the acute arterial thrombosis occurs on-table, there is little chance of saving the transplanted kidney. Acutely thrombosed grafts must nevertheless be explored and removed to avoid the development of sepsis in a necrotic graft, a potentially fatal complication.

Renal Vein Thrombosis

Renal vein thrombosis is more common than arterial thrombosis and occurs in 1% to 6% of renal transplants.[21] While it may result from a technical error at the time of surgery, its cause is usually less certain. The renal vein can certainly be twisted or kinked if it is not correctly placed after completion of the vascular and ureteral anastomoses. The peak incidence of renal vein thrombosis is 3 to 9 days post-transplantation[22]; a transplant with good initial graft function will have a sudden loss of urine output associated with severe pain arising from swelling and (very rarely) rupture of the allograft. The ipsilateral leg may also swell if there is involvement of the iliac venous system. Renal vein thrombosis may also be occult and is one differential diagnosis of DGF. Color Doppler duplex ultrasound scanning is the best investigation. In an established renal vein, thrombosis this may show an obviously swollen allograft with surrounding hematoma and an absence of renal perfusion. Lesser degrees of thrombosis, or indeed incipient thrombosis, may be highlighted by an absence of arterial flow in diastole. An even later development is a reversal of flow in diastole. Isotope renography is an alternative test that will show a nonperfused graft but ultrasonography is usually more rapidly available.

As with arterial thrombosis, if this diagnosis is entertained, then the best course of action is to re-explore the transplant as an emergency. The renal vein anastomosis can be opened to allow clot to be extracted, and the venotomy is then closed and the kidney observed for improvement. A more radical alternative is to immediately explant the kidney by taking down the arterial, venous, and ureteral anastomoses. The kidney can then be reflushed with cold perfusion fluid on the backtable and held in preservation fluid at 4°C. This allows much more time to assess the cause of the venous thrombosis, and if the kidney remains viable, the transplant operation can then be repeated. If the transplant is already infarcted or cannot be adequately flushed with preservation fluid, then the organ will need to be discarded anyway and nothing is lost by immediate explantation. Successful emergency surgical exploration with subsequent long-term function is rare. Interventional radiographic techniques offer an alternative to surgery. The renal vein can be selectively catheterized via the ipsilateral femoral vein, and graft thrombolysis may then be attempted.

Transplant Renal Artery Stenosis

Transplant renal artery stenosis is a later complication occurring from 3 to 48 months after transplantation. Not all stenoses are of functional or clinical significance, as shown by studies in which all functioning transplants have undergone angiography.[23] Causal factors include donor and recipient atherosclerosis, factors associated with surgical technique, and severe acute rejection.[24] The presentation and management of transplanted renal artery stenosis are discussed in Chapter 61.

Lymphocele

Small, clinically insignificant lymphatic collections can be demonstrated by ultrasound scan in up to 50% of renal transplants.[25] Larger lymphoceles that cause complications or require treatment occur in 2% to 10% of cases.[26] The source of peritransplant lymph leaks is the lymphatic channels around the iliac arterial system rather than the lymphatics of the transplanted kidney itself.[27] Therefore, during the dissection of the iliac arterial system, all the surrounding lymphatic channels must be meticulously secured with nonabsorbable ligatures or metals clips. Wound suction drains should not be removed postoperatively until <30 ml of fluid is produced on 2 consecutive days. It is safe to leave drains in place for several weeks post-transplantation to allow a low-volume lymphatic leak to seal by gradual fibrosis. Despite the theoretical risk of infection, this does not seem to be a problem in practice. If necessary, the patient can be discharged from hospital with the drain *in situ*.

Compression of the transplanted ureter leading to renal dysfunction is only produced by very large lymphoceles (volume >300 ml). The peak incidence is at 6 weeks, but a lymphatic collection may present between 2 weeks and 6 months post-transplantation.[25] Most lymphatic collections are found anterior to the iliac vessels and lying between the transplant and the bladder (Fig. 92.8). Presenting features may include wound or ipsilateral thigh swelling in association with suprapubic discomfort and urinary frequency due to bladder compression. Other presentations include pain over the transplanted kidney sometimes associated with fever, ureteral obstruction with graft dysfunction, and ipsilateral thrombophlebitis. However, the vast majority are asymptomatic and present as an incidental finding during an ultrasound scan being performed for another reason. It is important to aspirate all peritransplant fluid collections under ultrasound control in order to aid diagnosis. Macroscopic findings are usually sufficient to differentiate infected from noninfected lymph, and biochemical analysis of the fluid allows a urine leak to be excluded. Computed tomography or magnetic resonance imaging is an essential investigation if surgery is being contemplated, particularly if a laparoscopic procedure is planned. This allows accurate definition of the relationship between the lymphocele

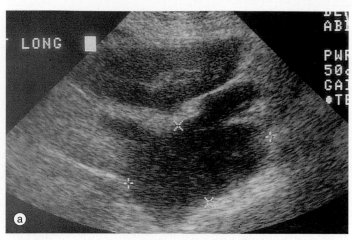 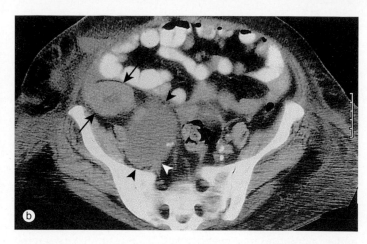

Figure 92.8 Post-transplantation lymphocele. *a*, Ultrasound appearance. A large echolucent lymphocele can be seen inferior to the transplanted kidney. *b*, Computed tomography appearance. A 5 × 5-cm lymphocele (*arrowheads*) is present under the transplanted kidney (*arrows*).

and the transplanted ureter. If the ureter is bow-strung across the superior surface of the lymphocele, then it could be damaged during a laparoscopic fenestration procedure.

Many small lymphoceles are asymptomatic and will resolve spontaneously given enough time. If action is deemed necessary, first-line treatment is aspiration under ultrasound control. If there is a recurrence, further aspirations can be performed or an external drain can be placed with ultrasound guidance. If these simple measures fail, then open or laparoscopic surgical drainage may be required. A 5-cm diameter disk of the lymphocele wall is removed to create a large opening into the peritoneal cavity, allowing reabsorption of the lymph through the abdominal lymphatic drainage system. These peritoneal fenestrations have a tendency to heal before the lymphocele is completely reabsorbed, leading to early recurrence; a metal plug may avoid this.

Urologic Complications

Urinary tract complications are relatively common after renal transplantation, with an incidence of between 5% and 14%.[28] While they can be difficult to manage, they only rarely cause graft loss or mortality. The relatively high incidence of urologic problems is a consequence of the tenuous blood supply of the transplanted ureter. After kidney retrieval, the only ureteral blood supply that is preserved is derived from the renal artery near the hilum of the kidney, and this can be easily damaged during retrieval.

Urinary Leaks

These most commonly occur because of ischemic necrosis in any part of the transplanted urinary collecting system. The distal ureter has the poorest blood supply and is therefore the most common site. Less commonly, leaks occur from the renal pelvis or the mid-portion of the ureter, which may be due to unrecognized direct damage to the ureter during organ retrieval. Urinary leaks tend to occur in the first few days after transplantation but can present much later. The usual presentation is with straw-colored fluid leaking directly from the transplant wound or accumulating in the drains in association with oliguria. Alternatively, extravasating urine may accumulate as a peritransplant fluid collection. This presents as a painful swelling of the wound, and the patient may have a fever. In either case, the extravasated fluid must be differentiated from lymph by biochemical analysis of the fluid and a simultaneous serum sample. Urine will have markedly elevated urea and

creatinine levels compared to the patient's serum, whereas lymph will have a similar biochemical profile.

The presence of a urinary fistula should be confirmed by antegrade or retrograde pyelography. Both of these techniques present challenges. Antegrade puncture of a nondilated pelvical-iceal system is technically difficult but usually possible. Retrograde cannulation of the transplanted ureteral orifice can be attempted using a flexible cystoscope. This is also a difficult maneuver

Ureteral reconstruction using native ureter

Proximal native ureter

Renal transplant

Stenosed transplant ureter

Native ureter

Figure 92.9 Ureteral reconstruction using native ureter.

because the transplanted ureter is implanted into the dome of the bladder rather than at its base. If the urine leak is contained as a urinoma, ultrasonography will demonstrate a fluid collection between the transplanted kidney and the bladder, which can be sampled by needling or drained by the placement of a suitable percutaneous catheter.

The management of urinary leaks has changed significantly in recent years. The former practice of early re-exploration and surgical reconstruction[29] is no longer always necessary. Interventional radiographic techniques offer an alternative, at least for initial treatment. The aim is to place a double-J ureteral stent across the region of damage via an antegrade nephrostomy; this may allow time for the urinary fistula to heal.[30] This technique, however, is unlikely to be successful if there is significant ischemic necrosis of the ureter, in which case, surgery still has a role. Re-exploration of kidney transplants is straightforward in the early postoperative period but may be a considerable challenge later on because of the development of an intense peritransplant fibrotic reaction. The choice of operative procedure for a necrotic distal ureter depends on the length of remaining viable ureter. If there is sufficient length after excision of the necrotic distal portion, the transplanted ureter may be simply reimplanted into the bladder. If this is not possible, the urinary tract should be reconstructed using the patient's native ureter. Depending on length of viable transplanted ureter, there is a choice between anastomosing the native ureter

to the transplanted ureter proximal to the ischemic segment (uretero-ureterostomy) or to the transplanted renal pelvis (ureteropyelostomy; Fig. 92.9). Whichever technique is chosen, the anastomosis should be protected with a double-J stent. Although these techniques require the native ureter to be ligated proximally, there is usually no need to perform an ipsilateral nephrectomy.[31] Postoperatively, the antegrade nephrostomy can be left *in situ* so that a contrast study can be performed after 7 to 10 days to confirm healing of the new anastomosis. If the transplanted recipient has undergone an ipsilateral nephrectomy in the past or the native ureter is too diseased to be used for reconstruction, a Boari bladder flap can be used to reconstruct the urinary tract.

Ureteral Obstruction

Obstruction of the transplanted ureter may occur at anytime after transplantation. It should always be considered in the differential diagnosis of acute transplant dysfunction and excluded by ultrasound examination. The management of transplant ureteral obstruction is summarized in Figure 92.10. Early obstruction is uncommon and suggestive of a technical error, such as creating a submucosal bladder tunnel that is too tight, kinking of a redundant length of ureter, and incorrect suture placement during anastomosis. Early obstruction may also be caused by blood clot in the ureter, bladder, or catheter. Bleeding may occur from the

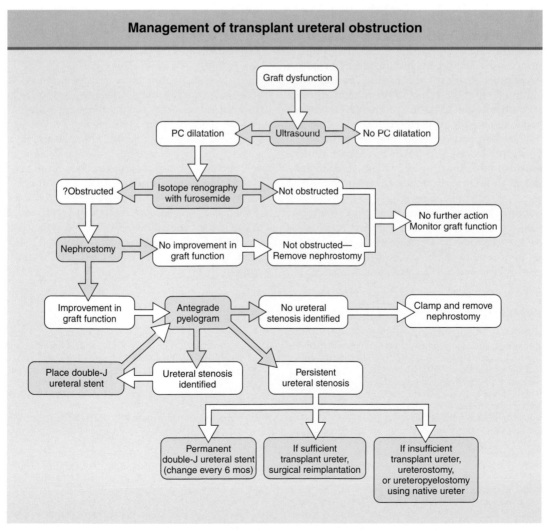

Figure 92.10 Management of transplant ureteral obstruction. PC, pelvicaliceal.

ureterovesical anastomosis or cystostomy or after a transplant biopsy. It is common practice to drain the urinary bladder using a three-way irrigating catheter as small-diameter two-way Foley catheters are easily blocked by blood clot.

Late ureteral obstruction may occur at the vesico-ureteral or pelviureteral junctions. Ischemia that is not severe enough to cause necrosis is presumed to be the cause of most vesico-ureteral obstructions. Renal transplants invariably excite a pronounced perigraft fibrotic response, and this is more likely to be the cause of an obstruction at the level of the pelviureteral junction. It is also possible that acute rejection episodes contribute to subsequent fibrosis.[32]

An ultrasound scan will demonstrate a dilated pelvicaliceal system. However, long-standing kidney transplants may have quite marked pelvicaliceal dilatation without being obstructed. This most commonly causes uncertainty when assessing whether obstruction may be contributing to chronic allograft dysfunction in a patient with biopsy-proven chronic allograft nephropathy. Further investigation is needed to confirm or refute the presence of obstruction and to define its anatomy. Retrograde pyelography has a low success rate because of the difficulty of catheterizing the transplanted ureteral orifice at cystoscopy. Isotope renography can be used to confirm obstruction; in equivocal cases, the study is more discriminating if a diuresis is stimulated by the administration of furosemide (see Chapter 49, Fig. 49.21). Isotope renography does not provide good anatomic localization of the obstruction; therefore, percutaneous nephrostomy followed by antegrade pyelography is the investigation of choice in suspected transplant ureteral obstruction. The nephrostomy is performed under antibiotic cover using ultrasound control, and the nephrostomy tube should be left in place for a few days. If serum creatinine decreases during this period, then obstruction is confirmed. If there is no improvement in renal function, significant obstruction can be confidently excluded. This simple observation avoids the need for an antegrade pressure study (Whittaker test), which may be difficult to interpret in transplanted kidneys. Following external decompression of the transplanted kidney for a few days, an antegrade pyelogram is obtained to accurately define the anatomy of the obstructing lesion.

Nonoperative approaches for the treatment of transplant ureteral stricture are often preferred.[33] The simplest approach is to place a double-J stent across the stricture via a percutaneous nephrostomy. This may require initial balloon dilatation.[34] The stent can be removed after 6 weeks, but the restenosis rate is high.

An alternative is long-term stenting, changing the stent every 6 months. The disadvantage of this method is a high incidence of urinary tract infection, with potential severe consequences for immunosuppressed patients, and long-term antibiotic prophylaxis is a sensible precaution. Open surgical management still has a place in the management of ureteral obstruction. The operation performed depends on the site of obstruction and the remaining length of healthy transplanted ureter proximal to the obstruction (see "Urinary Leaks"). Not all cases of obstruction require intervention. Where there is a mild degree of obstruction not associated with urinary tract infection and in a long-standing kidney that is affected by chronic allograft nephropathy, then it may be better to simply monitor transplant function, reserving intervention for a later date should it become necessary.

Complications in the Transplant Bed

A number of nerves may be encountered in the retroperitoneal dissection required for kidney transplantation. These include the lateral femoral cutaneous nerve and the femoral, obturator, and sacral nerves. Each of these may be damaged by a traction injury, particularly when modern fixed wound retraction systems are used as these can exert a great deal of pressure on the surrounding tissues. Such neurapraxias should recover completely, but this may take some months, and they can be very disabling.

In male transplant recipients, the spermatic cord must be mobilized during the dissection to gain access to the retroperitoneal space. Damage to the testicular artery in the cord can result in testicular atrophy.

TRANSPLANT NEPHRECTOMY

An early graft nephrectomy may be required for arterial thrombosis, capsular rupture (due to severe rejection or venous thrombosis), or other technical reasons. Graft nephrectomy may also be required after graft failure for persisting pain, malaise, fever, and thrombocytopenia; although usually a nonfunctioning graft left *in situ* will usually shrink and become fibrotic. Early graft nephrectomy is straightforward, but after the first few weeks, kidney transplants usually develop quite intense perigraft fibrosis, and this can make late allograft nephrectomy a difficult technical challenge. A subcapsular dissection is preferred, and after removal of the kidney, the hilum is sutured, leaving a cuff of donor vessels in place. Careful hemostasis is required, and the whole raw capsular bed should be cauterized. The wound is usually closed without drains.

REFERENCES

1. Criteria for the diagnosis of brain stem death. Review by a working group convened by the Royal College of Physicians and endorsed by the Conference of Medical Royal Colleges and their Faculties in the United Kingdom. J R Coll Physicians Lond 1995;29:381–382.
2. Koffman G, Gambaro G: Renal transplantation from non-heart-beating donors: A review of the European experience. J Nephrol 2003;16:334–341.
3. Kootstra G, Daemen JH, Oomen AP: Categories of non-heart-beating donors. Transplant Proc 1995;27:2893–2894.
4. Daemen JW, Kootstra G, Wijnen RM, et al: Nonheart-beating donors: The Maastricht experience. Clin Transpl 1994:303–16.
5. The Organ Procurement and Transplantation Network. Donors Recovered in the U.S. by Donor Type, 2005. Available at: www.optn.org/latestData/rptData.asp.
6. Statistics and Audit Directorate: United Kingdom Transplant More transplants—New lives. Transplant Activity in the UK 2004–2005. Available at: www.uktransplant.org.uk/ukt/statistics/transplant_activity_report/current_activity_reports.jsp/ukt/tx_activity_report_2005_uk_complete-v2.pdf.
7. Ratner LE, Montgomery RA, Kavoussi LR: Laparoscopic live donor nephrectomy: The four year Johns Hopkins University experience. Nephrol Dial Transplant 1999;14:2090–2093.
8. Rankin SC, Jan W, Koffman CG: Noninvasive imaging of living related kidney donors: Evaluation with CT angiography and gadolinium-enhanced MR angiography. AJR Am J Roentgenol 2001;177:349–355.
9. Namasivayam S, Small WC, Kalra MK, et al: Multidetector-row CT angiography for preoperative evaluation of potential laparoscopic renal donors: How accurate are we? Clin Imaging 2006;30:120–126.
10. Ratner LE, Ciseck LJ, Moore RG, et al: Laparoscopic live donor nephrectomy. Transplantation 1995;60:1047–1049.
11. Brown SL, Biehl TR, Rawlins MC, Hefty TR: Laparoscopic live donor nephrectomy: A comparison with the conventional open approach. J Urol 2001;165:766–769.
12. Pace KT, Dyer SJ, Phan V, et al: Laparoscopic v open donor nephrectomy: A cost-utility analysis of the initial experience at a tertiary-care center. J Endourol 2002;16:495–508.

13. Ratner LE, Buell JF, Kuo PC: Laparoscopic donor nephrectomy: Pro Transplantation 2000;70:1544–1546.
14. Brook NR, Nicholson ML: An audit over 2 years' practice of open and laparoscopic live-donor nephrectomy at renal transplant centres in the UK and Ireland. BJU Int 2004;93:1027–1031.
15. Montgomery RA, Kavoussi LR, Su L, et al: Improved recipient results after 5 years of performing laparoscopic donor nephrectomy. Transplant Proc 2001;33:1108–1110.
16. Wheatley TJ, Doughman TM, Veitch PS, Nicholson ML: Subrectus pouch for renal transplantation. Br J Surg 1996;83:419.
17. Wilson CH, Bhatti AA, Rix DA, Manas DM: Routine intraoperative ureteric stenting for kidney transplant recipients. Cochrane Database Syst Rev 2005;4:CD004925.
18. Abusin K, Rix D, Mohammed M, et al: Long-term adult renal graft outcome after ureteric drainage into an augmented bladder or ileal conduit. Transpl Int 1998;11(Suppl 1):S147–S149.
19. Osman Y, Shokeir A, Ali-el-Dein B, et al: Vascular complications after live donor renal transplantation: Study of risk factors and effects on graft and patient survival. J Urol 2003;169:859–862.
20. Nerstrom B, Ladefoged J, Lund F: Vascular complications in 155 consecutive kidney transplantations. Scand J Urol Nephrol 1972;6(Suppl 15):65–74.
21. Reuther G, Wanjura D, Bauer H: Acute renal vein thrombosis in renal allografts: Detection with duplex Doppler US. Radiology 1989;170:557–558.
22. Beyga ZT, Kahan BD: Surgical complications of kidney transplantation. J Nephrol 1998;11:137–145.
23. Lacombe M: Arterial stenosis complicating renal allotransplantation in man: A study of 38 cases. Ann Surg 1975;181:283–288.
24. Bruno S, Remuzzi G, Ruggenenti P: Transplant renal artery stenosis. J Am Soc Nephrol 2004;15:134–141.
25. Pollak R, Veremis SA, Maddux MS, Mozes MF: The natural history of and therapy for perirenal fluid collections following renal transplantation. J Urol 1988;140:716–720.
26. Zincke H, Woods JE, Leary FJ, et al: Experience with lymphoceles after renal transplantation. Surgery 1975;77:444–450.
27. Ward K, Klingensmith WC 3rd, Sterioff S, Wagner HN Jr: The origin of lymphoceles following renal transplantation. Transplantation 1978;25:346–347.
28. Mundy AR, Podesta ML, Bewick M, et al: The urological complications of 1000 renal transplants. Br J Urol 1981;53:397–402.
29. Palmer JM, Chatterjee SN: Urologic complications in renal transplantation. Surg Clin North Am 1978;58:305–319.
30. Nicholson ML, Veitch PS, Donnelly PK, Bell PR: Urological complications of renal transplantation: The impact of double J ureteric stents. Ann R Coll Surg Engl 1991;73:316–321.
31. Lord RH, Pepera T, Williams G: Ureteroureterostomy and pyeloureterostomy without native nephrectomy in renal transplantation. Br J Urol 1991;67:349–351.
32. Brook NR, Waller JR, Pattenden CJ, Nicholson ML: Ureteric stenosis after renal transplantation: No effect of acute rejection or immunosuppression. Transplant Proc 2002;34:3007–3008.
33. Goldstein I, Cho SI, Olsson CA: Nephrostomy drainage for renal transplant complications. J Urol 1981;126:159–163.
34. Streem SB, Novick AC, Steinmuller DR, et al: Long-term efficacy of ureteral dilation for transplant ureteral stenosis. J Urol 1988;140:32–35.

Prophylaxis and Treatment of Kidney Transplant Rejection

Karl L. Womer and Bruce Kaplan

INTRODUCTION

The era of clinical organ transplantation began in 1962 with the discovery that azathioprine in conjunction with corticosteroids was clinically useful as an immunosuppressive regimen. In the ensuing decades, improvements in both immunosuppression and surgical technique resulted in an incremental increase in both short- and long-term renal allograft graft survival.[1] In 1984, the introduction of cyclosporine heralded a new era in immunosuppressive therapy with markedly decreased acute rejection episodes and allowed for the widespread use of transplantation as a therapy for end-stage organ disease. In the 1990s, the introduction of more potent immunosuppressive agents led to an even further decrease in the incidence of acute rejection.[2] Acute rejection remains one of the strongest risk factors for the development of chronic allograft nephropathy (CAN) and ultimately long-term graft loss.[3] The risk is highest in those acute rejection episodes that are late,[4] recurrent,[5] exhibiting a vascular component,[6] and, importantly, result in impaired renal function at the time of diagnosis[7] and following treatment.[8] Despite the dramatic reduction of acute rejection rates, long-term graft survival rates in the current era do not appear to be improving,[9] suggesting that a point of diminishing return may have been reached with regard to immunosuppressive therapy. Current strategies are aimed at minimizing immuno-suppression, with the goal of avoiding their myriad untoward side effects, while maintaining a low incidence of acute rejection.

ETIOLOGY/PATHOGENESIS

The principal targets of the immune response to allografts are the major histocompatibility complex (MHC) molecules present on donor cells. After implantation, donor and/or recipient antigen-presenting cells (APCs) leave the graft and migrate to secondary lymphoid tissues where T cell recognition of alloantigen presented by cell surface MHC molecules occurs. Such allorecognition occurs directly (via donor APCs) or indirectly (via recipient APCs) and depends on the necessary costimulatory molecules present on these "professional" APCs (see Chapter 89). It has been proposed that early rejection episodes are mediated through the direct pathway since newly engrafted tissue typically contains a high density of passenger leukocytes, mostly dendritic cells, that are capable of presenting antigen by this pathway. The corollary hypothesis is that direct allorecognition becomes less important as passenger leukocytes are depleted with time post-transplantation. Once activated, T cells initiate the cascade of immunologic events responsible for destruction of the allograft, including the cytokine production and cell contact required for cytotoxic T cell, monocyte/macrophage, and B cell/antibody responses.

Memory T cells do not require professional APCs for activation and can recognize alloantigen presented by MHC molecules on inflamed endothelial cells. As a result, memory T cells can enter the graft and mediate damage without circulating to the draining lymph node. Memory T cells can be generated after a sensitizing event, such as pregnancy, transfusion, and previous transplantation. In addition, there is evidence that memory T cells generated by other immunizing events can cross-react with alloantigen. Memory CD8[+] T cells in peripheral tissue can lyse target cells without undergoing clonal expansion and differentiation. Furthermore, activated memory T cells acquire a heightened ability to recruit additional inflammatory cells into the graft. Hence, early rejection may reflect memory T cell involvement.[10]

Antibody-mediated rejection involves the binding of antibody to MHC molecules on the allograft vascular endothelium. This antibody response, including isotype switching from IgM to IgG, is dependent on T helper–cell function. Antibodies are cytotoxic through their ability to activate complement as well as by recruiting leukocytes with receptors for attached antibody (FcR) or complement. In addition to alloantibody responses, rejection following ABO incompatible transplantation is characterized by antibody binding to carbohydrate blood group antigens on endothelial cells. These antibody responses are not dependent on T helper–cell function.

EPIDEMIOLOGY

In 2003, 13% of kidney transplant recipients in the United States experienced an acute rejection episode in the first year after transplantation.[11] This number represents a decline from 15% in 2002 and 17% in 2001, confirming the continuing trend toward improvement in the prevention of acute rejection (Fig. 93.1). The availability of newer, more efficacious immunosuppressive agents has been instrumental in this trend for decreased acute rejection and also has helped narrow the gap between traditional high-risk and low-risk groups. The presence of delayed graft function (DGF) following transplantation is a strong risk factor for the development of acute rejection.[12] The risk of DGF is associated with powerful factors also known to influence acute rejection rates, including donor age, recipient race, and sensitization, making dissection of the effects of DGF from the effects of these other factors extremely difficult. Numerous reports have confirmed historically higher rates of acute rejection in the African American population compared to other races,[13] although with immunosuppression dosing tailored to race, these differences have

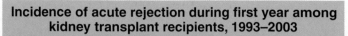

Incidence of acute rejection during first year among kidney transplant recipients, 1993–2003

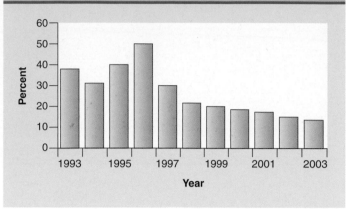

Figure 93.1 Incidence of acute rejection during the first year among kidney transplant recipients, 1993–2003. (Adapted from U.S. Transplant–Scientific Registry of Transplant Recipients: 2005 OPTN/SRTR Annual Report. Ann Arbor, MI: University Renal Research and Education Association with the University of Michigan, 2005.)

Risk factors for acute rejection
High Risk
African American recipient

Sensitization (high panel reactive antibody percentage)
    Previous transplantation
    Pregnancy
    Transfusion

Delayed graft function
    Deceased donor source
    Increased donor age
    Prolonged ischemic time
    Donor brain death
    Donor acute renal dysfunction

HLA mismatching
Positive pretransplantation B-cell crossmatch
ABO incompatibility
Corticosteroid minimization

Infection
    Pyelonephritis
    Cytomegalovirus

Adolescent recipient
Previous rejection episode
Low Risk
Zero HLA mismatch
Elderly recipient of young donor kidney
Pre-emptive transplantation
Living donor source
First transplant

Figure 93.2 Risk factors for acute rejection.

begun to narrow. Interestingly, acute rejection rates were found to be similar between patients of Caucasian or African origin in France, including sub-Saharan African and Caribbean patients.[14] Since African Europeans and African Americans share the same genetic background, it would appear that factors other than race are operative. Initial reports indicated lower acute rejection rates in the elderly population, likely due to a relatively incompetent immune system compared to their younger counterparts.[15] However, more careful analysis reveals that the reduction in risk only holds for elderly recipients of younger donor kidneys.[16] The remaining high-risk group includes those patients with sensitization to alloantigen (high panel reactive antibody), either through previous transplantation, blood transfusion, or pregnancy. A special population at particular high risk of rejection includes recipients of ABO blood group–incompatible renal transplants (Fig. 93.2). This section reviews the current induction and maintenance immunosuppressive agents as they relate to the risk of acute rejection.

Induction

Induction therapy refers to the temporary use of high doses of immunosuppressive medications in the early post-transplantation period, when the risk of acute rejection is highest (see Chapter 90). Recipients treated with induction immunosuppression typically receive a brief course of antibody therapy that is intended to reduce or modify early immune system activity against the transplanted organ. Traditionally, induction therapy has been reserved for those recipients at higher risk of acute rejection. However, recent data demonstrating superior acute rejection prophylaxis with rabbit antithymocyte globulin (ATG) and the emerging trend toward more corticosteroid avoidance protocols have prompted more centers to use this agent routinely. In the United States, the trend for increasing use of induction therapy in the perioperative period continues, from 25% in 1994 to 72% in 2004. Rabbit ATG was the most commonly used agent, and its use increased from 26% in 2002 to 37% in 2004. In 2004, the two interleukin (IL)-2 receptor antagonist (IL-2RA) preparations basiliximab and daclizumab accounted for 19% and 11% of induction therapy, respectively. Administration of equine ATG and monoclonal anti-T cell–receptor antibody (OKT3) for induc-

tion therapy continued to decline to only 1.8% and 0.3% of kidney transplant recipients, respectively.[11] Use of the humanized monoclonal anti-CD52 antibody alemtuzumab nearly doubled from 4% of all patients in 2003, the first year the agent was reported, to 7% in 2004. Although historically the use of induction therapy has been lower in Europe, a trend toward more frequent use of ATG, similar to that in the United States, is emerging.

Compared to no induction, patients receiving polyclonal antibody induction experience fewer acute rejection episodes, including a reduction in steroid-resistant cases and less frequent recurrent rejection.[17,18] Furthermore, these agents provide adequate rejection prophylaxis for patients in whom calcineurin inhibitor therapy is delayed until allograft recovery occurs.[19] Compared to equine ATG, the rabbit preparation is superior at preventing acute rejection when used as an induction agent.[20] Recent reports show that a 3-day course of rabbit ATG induction is as effective as a 7-day course in reducing acute rejection. OKT3 is also effective in preventing acute rejection as an induction agent. However, since the development of blocking antibodies limits its efficacy on repeated exposure, this powerful immunosuppressant is more often reserved for serious rejection episodes. The ability of IL-2RAs to reduce acute rejection episodes when used as an induction agent is well established.[21,22] However, these agents are ineffective in forestalling acute rejection alone and should be used in combination with a three-drug regimen.[23] Although IL-2RA administration appears to be without major side effects, polyclonal antibody induction therapy is associated with increased relative risk of early infectious death and long-term malignancy-related death.[24] This risk, however, should be taken in context with the potential benefits of this therapy.

The anti-CD20 humanized monoclonal antibody rituximab, along with plasma exchange and immunoglobulin, has been used successfully in lieu of splenectomy to suppress antibody formation following ABO-incompatible renal transplantation.[25]

Maintenance

Corticosteroids remain a cornerstone of modern immunosuppression, although the numerous untoward side effects have prompted the development of various protocols in which these medications are weaned and eventually withdrawn from the maintenance regimen. After an initial intravenous bolus of pulse corticosteroids, particularly during induction therapy, oral corticosteroid doses are tapered rapidly to 20 to 30 mg/day at the time of discharge. Over the ensuing weeks, this medication is reduced further to 5 to 10 mg/day for maintenance, depending on the center (Fig. 93.3). Early experience with corticosteroid withdrawal during the azathioprine era led to higher rates of acute rejection. More recent attempts with steroid avoidance in the mycophenolate mofetil (MMF) era have yielded similar results, particularly in African American recipients, as well as those patients with elevated serum creatinine and a history of rejection.[26,27] More recent protocols have addressed complete corticosteroid avoidance. A large nonrandomized study using a 10-day course of cyclosporine, and MMF with complete corticosteroid avoidance has yielded excellent results, but unfortunately lacked a control group.[28] A recent trial found no increased acute rejection in African Americans compared to non–African Americans following complete corticosteroid avoidance.[29] Despite the associated risk of increased acute rejection, many centers continue to use corticosteroid avoidance protocols.

Compared to only 3% in 1999, 20% of kidney transplant recipients in the United States were discharged on a corticosteroid-free protocol in 2004.[11]

There has been a substantial improvement in both short- and long-term graft and patient survival rates after kidney transplantation since the introduction of cyclosporine in the early 1980s.[30] With two commercially available calcineurin inhibitors, cyclosporine and tacrolimus, the transplantation community has committed many resources in an effort to identify the superior agent. Several studies have concluded that tacrolimus results in lower acute rejection rates.[31] However, conclusions drawn from these studies are difficult to interpret because the conventional form of cyclosporine (Sandimmune) was used for the comparison. The older formulation of cyclosporine has less predictable absorption and elimination, which diminishes the efficacy compared to the newer microemulsion formulation (Neoral). In a recent multicenter randomized European trial, the rates of biopsy-confirmed acute rejection and steroid-resistant rejection were lower in patients assigned to tacrolimus versus the microemulsion formulation of cyclosporine. However, in this study, azathioprine was used as the antimetabolite, raising the question of whether tacrolimus offers a true benefit over cyclosporine in the MMF era. In fact, a recent trial comparing tacrolimus and cyclosporine in a quadruple immunosuppressive regimen consisting of rabbit ATG induction and MMF with corticosteroids found no significant difference in acute rejection rates.[32] Despite the lack of solid evidence favoring one agent over the other, the use of tacrolimus continues to increase in the United States (from 67% in 2003 to 72% in 2004), while the number of recipients treated with cyclosporine preparations declined over the same period, from 26% to 21%.[11] Given the well-documented nephrotoxic effects of calcineurin inhibitors,[33] these agents are often withheld for a few days during the early post-transplantation period, particularly during DGF. However, such an approach does result in significantly more acute rejection episodes. For standard target levels of these two calcineurin inhibitors, see Figure 93.3.

Three large multicenter trials have confirmed that MMF significantly reduces acute rejection episodes compared to its antimetabolite counterpart azathioprine in patients receiving the older formulation of cyclosporine.[34–36] In a *post hoc* subgroup analysis, it was determined that acute rejection episodes in the African American population were equivalent to those in other populations with 1.5 g twice daily dosing compared to the typical dose of 1 g twice daily.[37] More recent reports have questioned whether there is a benefit of MMF over azathioprine in patients receiving the microemulsion formulation of cyclosporine.[38] MMF is often poorly tolerated, requiring dose reduction or complete discontinuation because of side effects (gastrointestinal, bone marrow suppression). Dose reductions are not without risk, however, as there is a 4% increase in acute rejection episodes for every week that the patient is kept on suboptimal doses of MMF.[39] Cyclosporine blocks the enterohepatic recirculation of mycophenolic acid (MPA), the active metabolite of MMF, in the terminal ileum, resulting in lower MPA levels. This interaction does not occur with tacrolimus and may explain many of the reported differences in acute rejection rates between the two calcineurin inhibitors when equivalent doses are delivered. In fact, most centers reduce the dose of MMF for patients receiving tacrolimus within the first month to 1000 mg twice daily in African Americans and 750 mg twice daily in other patient groups (see Fig. 93.3). Given its apparent superior ability to reduce acute rejection episodes, MMF was used in >83% of renal transplant recipients at discharge in the United States, in

Maintenance immunosuppressive medication dose ranges		
1 Month Post-transplantation		
	C_0 (trough)	C_2 (2 hr peak)
Cyclosporine	200–400 ng/ml	1200–1600 ng/ml
Tacrolimus	8–12 ng/ml	
Mycophenolate mofetil	Daily dose 3.0 g AA/2.0 g others (cyclosporine) 2.5 g AA/2.0 g others (tacrolimus)	
Prednisone	0–30 mg	
1 Year Post-transplantation		
	C_0 (trough)	C_2 (2 hr peak)
Cyclosporine	100–200 ng/ml	400–800 ng/ml
Tacrolimus	3–8 ng/ml	
Mycophenolate mofetil	Daily dose 3.0 g AA/2.0 g others (cyclosporine) 2.0 g AA/1.5 g others (tacrolimus)	
Prednisone	0–10 mg	

Figure 93.3 Maintenance immunosuppressive medication dose ranges. Standard immunosuppressive medication doses and blood levels for kidney transplant recipients at q month and q year post-transplantation. AA, African American; C_0, 12-hour trough level; C_2, 2-hour level.

2004, while azathioprine was given to <2% of patients.[11]

Sirolimus has yet to find its ideal place in current immunosuppressive protocols. After a rapid increase in the use of sirolimus from 3% in 1998 to 17% in 2000, the number of kidney transplant recipients on this drug has decreased to 12% in 2004.[11] The medication is clearly not as effective as cyclosporine in preventing acute rejection since attempts to wean cyclosporine from a sirolimus-corticosteroid regimen result in a higher acute rejection rate at 1 year.[40] Although ultimate graft survival was improved in the cyclosporine withdrawal group, this report lacked a conventional cyclosporine-based but sirolimus-free treatment group for comparison.[41] It is now clear from several studies that sirolimus and the related compound everolimus both enhance cyclosporine toxicity.[42-44] Multicenter trials are currently under way using sirolimus-MMF-corticosteroid combinations or substitution of cyclosporine with sirolimus after the early post-transplantation period.

CLINICAL PRESENTATION

Most often experienced by patients who are noncompliant with their medications or office visits, acute rejection episodes may befall even the most ideal of patients. Approximately 75% of acute rejection episodes occur in the first 3 months post-transplantation. Early recognition and prompt treatment are essential in preventing premature allograft loss, as acute rejection episodes successfully treated within 60 days of transplantation do not appear to affect adversely the long-term survival of the allograft.[4] Elevation of serum creatinine is generally the precipitating event alerting the clinician to the possibility of acute rejection. The classic triad of fever, oliguria, and graft tenderness, however, is uncommon in the current era of heightened immunosuppression. Likewise, the clinical signs of acute antibody-mediated rejection are also nonspecific, varying from mild dysfunction to complete cessation of graft function with oligoanuria. Furthermore, the differential diagnosis for reduced graft function in a transplant recipient is broad and depends on the time frame after transplantation (Fig. 93.4). Therefore, any significant increase in serum creatinine should prompt a comprehensive review of the patient's overall clinical status, including physical examination, medication review, interval medical history, measurement of immunosuppressive medication levels, urinalysis, complete blood count, and virologic analysis (focusing on cytomegalovirus [CMV] and BK virus). Based on this assessment, therapeutic measures to correct obvious causes of renal dysfunction, including volume depletion, urinary tract or other infection, bladder outlet obstruction, congestive heart failure, and hypotension should be initiated. Nephrotoxic medications, including nonsteroidal anti-inflammatory drugs, aminoglycosides, and amphotericin, and other drugs that affect renal function and/or serum creatinine levels such as trimethoprim-sulfamethoxazole, angiotensin-converting enzyme inhibitors, angiotensin receptor blockers, and diuretics should be discontinued when appropriate. Sudden anemia, thrombocytopenia, increased serum lactate dehydrogenase, and abnormally low haptoglobin levels should raise suspicion of thrombotic microangiopathy (recurrent, *de novo*, or calcineurin inhibitor induced). Consideration of recurrent glomerular disease, particularly focal segmental glomerulosclerosis, should be made if there is new-onset heavy proteinuria. The absence of plasma or whole blood BK virus DNA by quantitative polymerase chain reaction essentially rules out the diagnosis of BK virus nephropathy.

Differential diagnosis of renal allograft dysfunction
Week 1 Post-transplantation
Acute tubular necrosis
Hyperacute/accelerated rejection

Urologic
    Obstruction
    Urine leak

Vascular thrombosis
    Renal artery
    Renal vein

<12 Weeks Post-transplantation
Acute rejection
Calcineurin inhibitor toxicity
Volume contraction
Urologic   Obstruction

Infection
    Pyelonephritis
    Viral infections

Interstitial nephritis
Recurrent disease
>12 Weeks Post-transplantation
Acute rejection
Volume contraction
Calcineurin inhibitor toxicity
Urologic   Obstruction

Infection
    Pyelonephritis
    Viral infections

Chronic allograft nephropathy
Recurrent disease
Renal artery stenosis
Post-transplantation lymphoproliferative disorder

Figure 93.4   Differential diagnosis of renal allograft dysfunction.

DIAGNOSIS

Renal transplant imaging by ultrasonography is mandatory, although the morphologic alterations seen in acute rejection are nonspecific. Duplex ultrasound measures the resistive index, which is nonspecific as it is elevated in acute rejection, acute tubular necrosis, acute pyelonephritis, and cyclosporine toxicity. Ultrasound imaging is important, however, to rule out obstruction. In addition, ultrasonography can identify fluid collections, which may indicate a urine leak or formation of a hematoma or lymphocele obstructing urine or blood flow. Radionuclide imaging may also be of value in the diagnosis of urinary extravasation and, along with Doppler ultrasonography, can confirm adequate arterial flow to the allograft. Finally, ultrasonography is required to confirm an adequate window for allograft biopsy, which remains the gold standard for confirming the diagnosis of acute rejection.

Adequacy of renal transplant biopsy	
Adequacy of Sample	
Unsatisfactory	<7 glomeruli and no arteries
Marginal	7 glomeruli with one artery
Adequate	≥ 10 glomeruli with at least two arteries
Pathologic Analysis (minimum sampling)	
7 slides	3 H&E, 3 PAS or silver stains, and 1 trichrome, section thickness 3–4 μm

Figure 93.5 Adequacy of renal transplant biopsy. H&E, hematoxylin and eosin; PAS, periodic acid–Schiff. (Adapted from Racusen LC, Solez K, Colvin RB, et al: The Banff 97 working classification of renal allograft pathology. Kidney Int 1999;55:713–723.)

If the patient has normal clotting parameters, informed consent is obtained and a transplant ultrasound scan is performed to determine the optimal site at which to perform a biopsy. Local anesthetic is delivered followed by a slow advancement of the biopsy needle to the capsule of the kidney. An 18- or 16-gauge needle as part of a spring-loaded biopsy gun is thrown between 0.5 and 1.5 cm into the parenchyma of the kidney. In some centers, a pathologist is present to confirm the origin of the tissue and the adequacy of the sample. The Banff 97 classification (discussed later)[45] defines an adequate specimen as a biopsy with ≥10 glomeruli and at least two arteries, while the threshold for a minimal sample is seven glomeruli and one artery (Fig. 93.5). Two separate cores containing cortex should be obtained since histologic evidence of rejection may be focal (Fig. 93.6) and

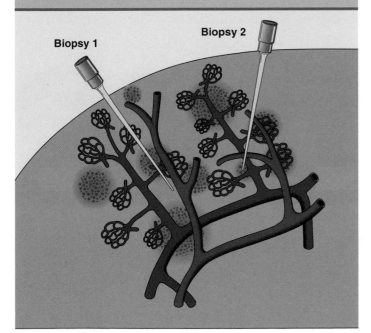

Effect of sample site on the diagnosis of rejection

Figure 93.6 Effect of sample site on the diagnosis of rejection. Acute rejection begins as patchy, focal infiltrates and only becomes homogeneous in advanced stages. The intensity of mononuclear infiltrate seen on biopsy would differ between core 1 and core 2. Routinely taking two core biopsy samples can help decrease the sampling errors, which can affect the histologic interpretation of rejection.

individual histopathologic stains may require differential fixation techniques.

PATHOLOGY

The renal allograft biopsy should ideally provide answers to at least three important clinical questions:
- The cause of graft dysfunction
- The current activity of the process
- The degree of irreversible damage that has already occurred, which has significant implications for therapy

Standardization of renal allograft biopsy interpretation is necessary to guide therapy and to establish an objective endpoint for clinical trials in renal transplantation, which frequently involve multiple centers. The Banff Working Classification of Renal Allograft Pathology is an international schema published originally in 1993 to meet this need. The Banff meeting has been held every 2 years to review and update the criteria for rejection. This series of meetings culminated in what is referred to as the Banff 97 scoring criteria.[45] The initial Banff criteria focused on cell-mediated injury. However, in 2001, the criteria were updated to include antibody-mediated rejection[46] (Fig. 93.7).

The following areas of the parenchyma are examined on biopsy specimens: the interstitium, glomeruli, tubules, and vessels. A score of 0 to 3 is given to each of these areas to indicate the degree of inflammation (ranging from none to severe). The Banff schema focuses on inflammatory infiltration of tubules (tubulitis) and/or

Banff 97 Classification of renal allograft biopsies
1. Normal
2. Antibody-mediated rejection Rejection due, at least in part, to documented antidonor antibody (suspicious for if antibody not demonstrated); may coincide with categories 3 and 4 Type (grade) I. ATN-like C4d+, minimal inflammation II. Capillary margination and/or thromboses, C4d+ III. Arterial, severe vascular arteritis, C4d+
3. Borderline changes: Suspicious for acute cellular rejection This category is used when no intimal arteritis is present, but there are foci of mild tubulitis (one to four mononuclear cells/tubular cross section) and at least 10%–25% interstitium affected; may coincide with category 2
4. Acute/active cellular rejection T cell–mediated rejection; may coincide with category 2 Type (grade) Histopathologic findings IA: Cases with significant interstitial infiltrate (>25% of parenchyma affected) and foci of moderate tubulitis (more than four mononuclear cells/tubular cross section or group of 10 tubular cells) IB: Cases with significant interstitial infiltrate and foci of severe tubulitis (>10 mononuclear cells/tubular cross section or group of 10 tubular cells) IIA: Cases with mild to moderate intimal arteritis IIB: Cases with severe intimal arteritis comprising >25% of the luminal area III: Cases with transmural arteritis and/or fibrinoid change and necrosis of medial smooth muscle cells with accompanying lymphocytic inflammation

Figure 93.7 Banff 97 classification of renal allograft biopsies. (Adapted from Racusen LC, Colvin RB, Solez K, et al: Antibody-mediated rejection criteria—an addition to the Banff 97 classification of renal allograft rejection. Am J Transplant 2003;3:708–714.)

vessel walls (arteritis) to establish the diagnosis and to grade the severity of rejection. Interstitial infiltrates are a constant feature in renal allograft rejection and are required to make the diagnosis. However, these infiltrates are not specific for rejection and have been demonstrated in protocol biopsies of well-functioning grafts. Furthermore, there is no correlation between the degree of interstitial inflammation and response to antirejection therapy.

The tubule is the main target of cellular rejection. Tubulitis involves mononuclear cell infiltration across the tubular basement membrane, with cells generally below or between the tubular epithelial cells. Periodic acid–Schiff and silver stains, which highlight the basement membrane, are the best for localization of inflammatory cells. One to four cells per affected tubule may be seen in acute tubular necrosis and in areas of scarring and therefore are nonspecific findings. When associated with at least 10% to 25% involvement of the interstitium, these findings are deemed suspicious for acute rejection and are present in approximately 30% of biopsy specimens in the first 3 months post-transplantation. Whether these changes represent an early acute rejection remains an unanswered question, and thus these findings should be interpreted in the appropriate clinical context. A recent retrospective analysis of borderline infiltrates found that an increase in serum creatinine, persistently elevated creatinine after the initial kidney biopsy, and histologic findings of glomerulitis were statistically associated with progression of these infiltrates into acute rejection in the short term.[47] However, only more severe tubulitis (more than four cells per tubular cross section) is specific for rejection, which is supported by the observation that treatment of this degree of tubulitis after protocol biopsies resulted in better allograft function after 2 years of follow-up.[48] According to the Banff schema, type I is defined as cases with tubulointerstitial rejection without vascular involvement (Fig. 93.8) and is further subdivided into type IA with moderate tubulitis and type IB with severe tubulitis. It is often difficult to make the diagnosis of acute rejection during active BK virus nephropathy, which is characterized histopathologically by an interstitial infiltration of mononuclear cells and may contain tubulitis.

Intimal arteritis (type II), which is mononuclear cell infiltration beneath the endothelium, is the pathognomonic feature of acute vascular rejection (Fig. 93.9). This grade is further subcategorized into type IIA or IIB, depending on the degree of involvement.

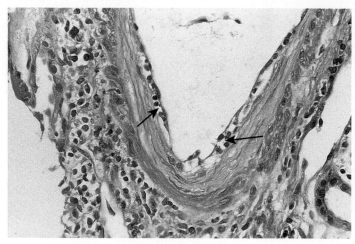

Figure 93.9 Type II acute cellular rejection. Type II rejection, called acute vascular rejection, is manifested by endothelialitis with mononuclear cell infiltration beneath the arterial endothelium (periodic acid–Schiff stain, ×200). (Courtesy of Dr. Agnes Fogo.)

These findings are differentiated from arteritis (type III), which has inflammation in the media and/or fibrinoid necrosis of the vessel wall (Fig. 93.10). As with scoring for tubulitis, the vessel with the most severe lesions should be graded. Data from single-center reports and larger multicenter trials confirm that the presence of vasculitis portends a poor prognosis.

Antibody-mediated rejection can occur alone or in combination with cell-mediated rejection. Traditionally, there has been difficulty documenting the presence of antibody-mediated injury on renal biopsy because staining for complement and immunoglobulin was typically absent. In landmark observations from the early 1990s, Halloran and colleagues[49] were the first to identify acute rejection of kidney transplants associated with the development of *de novo* anti-HLA donor-specific antibody production as a definite clinicopathologic entity carrying a

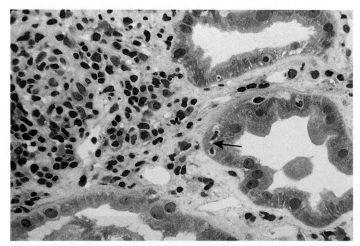

Figure 93.8 Type I acute cellular rejection. Type I acute rejection is manifested by interstitial mononuclear cell infiltration (*arrow*) with invasion of the tubules (periodic acid–Schiff, ×200).

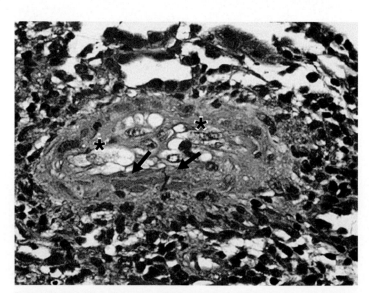

Figure 93.10 Type III acute cellular rejection. Severe small-vessel vasculitis with transmural mononuclear cell infiltration, fibrinoid necrosis (*arrows*), and very swollen endothelial cells (*asterisks*) (periodic acid–Schiff, ×400). (From Racusen LC, Colvin RB, Solez K, et al: Antibody-mediated rejection criteria—an addition to the Banff 97 classification of renal allograft rejection. Am J Transplant 2003; 3:708–714.)

poor prognosis. The Banff criteria can be used to identify pathologic features of acute rejection associated with donor-specific antibody.[50] The most consistent finding was neutrophils in the capillaries. Also seen are severe vasculitis, glomerulitis, and fibrinoid necrosis, whereas typical features of cell-mediated rejection, such as tubulitis, were absent. The complement-split product C4d was present in renal biopsies from individuals with early graft loss,[51,52] and subsequent studies have shown a strong association between peritubular capillary C4d staining and antidonor antibodies.[53] Staining for C4d has now become a routine practice at many centers and identifies grafts that are at higher risk of early graft loss[54] (Fig. 93.11). Rejection with severe vessel involvement and fibrinoid changes, thrombosis, glomerulitis, and focal interstitial hemorrhage strongly suggests antibody-mediated rejection and warrants a repeat crossmatch. The updated Banff schema includes three types of antibody-mediated rejection, graded according to severity, which may coincide with the other categories (see Fig. 93.7). Type III antibody-mediated rejection includes immediate (hyperacute) rejection, which occurs in the setting of preformed antibodies and is characterized by a cyanotic and flaccid graft immediately after vascular anastomosis is complete (Fig. 93.12). Histopathologic findings include polymorphonuclear leukocyte accumulation in the glomerular and peritubular capillaries, endothelial damage, and diffuse microcirculatory thrombosis. Also included in this type is accelerated rejection, which typically occurs between 3 and 14 days post-transplantation and often presents as an abrupt decline in urine output in a previously functioning graft. Graft loss following ABO-incompatible transplantation typically results from antibody-mediated rejection.

Glomerular lesions (glomerulitis) are graded depending on the number of glomeruli involved. Glomerulitis is defined as mononuclear cells in the glomerular capillaries and enlargement of the glomerular endothelial cells (Fig. 93.13). Glomerulitis, however, is not specific for rejection, although there is some evidence that a monocyte/macrophage infiltrate in glomeruli and peritubular capillaries is specific for antibody-mediated acute rejection and portends a worse prognosis.[55,56] If polymorphonuclear leukocytes are present, antibody-mediated rejection or early thrombotic microangiopathy should be considered.

TREATMENT

The choice of treatment for acute rejection depends largely on the histologic severity of the rejection process as determined by biopsy and, to a lesser degree, by the clinical context in which the episode occurs. Unfortunately, very few recent multicenter trials have specifically addressed the treatment of acute rejection, focusing instead on the prevention of acute rejection with newer immunosuppressive agents and with differing combinations of existing medications. The treatment options include high-dose oral/intravenous corticosteroids, polyclonal antilymphocyte antibodies (rabbit, equine), monoclonal anti–T cell–receptor antibody (OKT3) and, more recently, the humanized monoclonal antibodies against CD52 (alemtuzumab) and CD20 (rituximab). According to U.S. Renal Transplant Registry data, in 2003, only 13% of kidney transplant recipients required treatment of acute rejection within 1 year of transplantation.[11] Corticosteroids are still the mainstay of treatment, used alone or in combination with antibodies in 78% to 80% of cases since 1998. The use of antilymphocyte antibodies has also remained relatively stable at

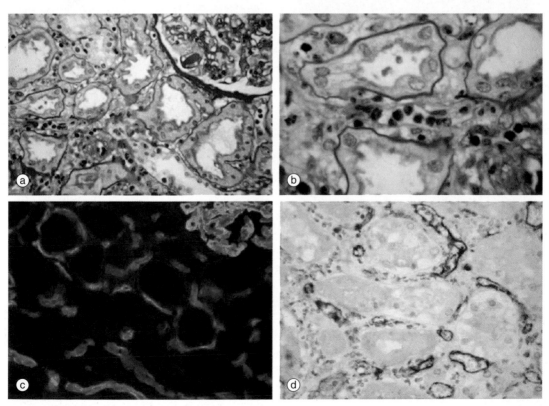

Figure 93.11   Acute antibody-mediated rejection. *a*, Peritubular and glomerular capillaries contain numerous polymorphonuclear leukocytes and mononuclear cells. *b*, Numerous polymorphonuclear leukocytes are observed in a peritubular capillary. Interstitial edema is noted (periodic acid–Schiff, ×200). *c*, Immunofluorescence staining of peritubular capillaries with C4d (fresh-frozen tissue sample, ×250). *d*, Immunohistochemistry demonstrating peritubular capillary staining of C4d (paraffin-embedded tissue, ×480). (From Moll S, Pascual M: Humoral rejection of organ allografts. Am J Transplant 2005;5:2611–2618.)

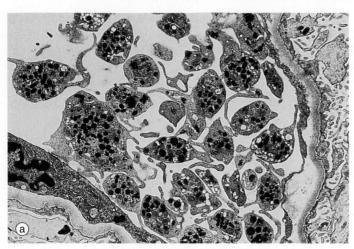
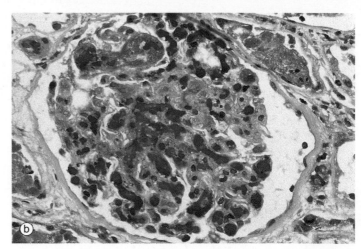

Figure 93.12 Hyperacute rejection. Hyperacute rejection refers to immediate rejection of the kidney due to preformed antibodies to alloantigens of the endothelium. *a,* Hyperacute rejection is associated with massive platelet accumulation within a glomerular capillary (by electron microscopy). *b,* This is followed by further endothelial damage, resulting in capillaries filled with sludged red blood cells and fibrin (hematoxylin and eosin). (*a,* Courtesy of Dr. Charles Alpers; *b,* Courtesy of Dr. Agnes Fogo.)

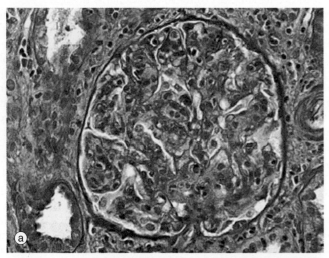

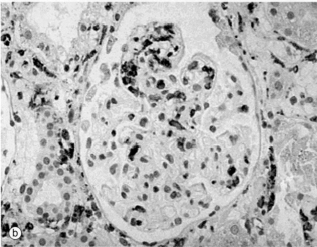

Figure 93.13 Glomerulitis. *a,* Infiltrating mononuclear cells and swollen endothelial cells (periodic acid–Schiff, ×400). *b,* Immunoperoxidase staining for monocyte/macrophages (KP-1) demonstrating numerous positive cells in glomerular capillaries and peritubular capillaries (×400). (From Racusen LC, Colvin RB, Solez K, et al: Antibody-mediated rejection criteria—an addition to the Banff 97 classification of renal allograft rejection. Am J Transplant 2003; 3:708–714.)

36% to 39% since 1998. Rabbit ATG has largely replaced OKT3 as the principal antibody given as antirejection treatment.

Acute Cellular Rejection

Initial treatment for mild acute rejection (Banff types IA and IB) is usually pulse intravenous methylprednisolone 250 to 500 mg/day for 3 to 5 days. If there has been no decrease in serum creatinine by that time, in the absence of any other factors contributing to allograft dysfunction, steroid therapy should be judged ineffective, and an alternative therapy and/or repeat renal biopsy should strongly be considered. The determination of successful treatment is generally based on a decrease in serum creatinine. Follow-up biopsies after clinically successful antirejection therapy have revealed the continued presence of lymphocytic infiltrates.[57,58] The significance of this finding is unclear, as this may represent residual/resolving rejection, the presence of regulatory T cells, or ongoing graft infiltration due to inadequate therapy. Unfortunately, there are no reliable markers to distinguish among these possibilities, and the clinical context becomes of paramount importance in determining the need for further therapy.

An initial diagnosis of acute vascular rejection (Banff type IIA or higher) or the failure of high-dose corticosteroid therapy to reverse milder rejections should prompt treatment with an antilymphocyte antibody preparation. Combined clinical data confirm the superiority of antilymphocyte regimens over corticosteroid therapy. However, studies comparing monoclonal to polyclonal antilymphocyte antibody preparations have generally been inconclusive, although rabbit ATG appears superior to the equine preparation in reversing acute rejection and preventing recurrent rejection.[59] Side effects commonly seen with the first dose of OKT3, the so-called cytokine release syndrome, have limited its use as a first-line agent. Treatment of recurrent rejection episodes with repeated doses of monoclonal or polyclonal antilymphocyte agents is often problematic, as patients may develop neutralizing antibodies. These findings are best documented with OKT3, but can also occur with polyclonal preparations. Monitoring of lymphocyte cell counts during therapy is useful to determine efficacy as well as duration of therapy. Multiple doses of antibody therapy in close succession or as a prolonged course greatly increase the risk of serious infections and lymphoproliferative disease and should be undertaken with great caution.

Another important consideration in the overall approach to the treatment of acute rejection includes modification of the existing immunosuppressive regimen following successful treatment of the rejection episode. Options generally include increased dose of the same medications, addition of another immunosuppressant, and substitution of a different immunosuppressant. Common substitutions include MMF for azathioprine and tacrolimus for cyclosporine. Reinstitution of corticosteroids may be indicated for those patients experiencing a rejection episode following steroid discontinuation or avoidance.

Acute Antibody-Mediated Rejection

Antibody-mediated acute rejections are highly unlikely to respond to high-dose corticosteroid therapy, and graft loss at 1 year is dramatically higher compared to cellular rejection alone.[60] The overall goal in treatment of antibody-mediated rejection is removal of antidonor antibody and inhibition of further antibody synthesis. This feat has been accomplished using a variety of approaches, including high-dose tacrolimus and MMF, immunoadsorption, plasma exchange, intravenous immunoglobulin, and antilymphocyte therapy. Although the titer of serum antidonor antibody, if present, is often monitored during therapy for antibody-mediated rejection, the correlation with immunologic events in the allograft is variable and should not be relied on solely to determine therapy. Rituximab may play a role as its anti-B cell effects have been shown to reduce antidonor antibody production.

No therapy has been found to be effective for hyperacute rejection, and immediate graft nephrectomy is generally indicated. Donor-specific antibody may be detected in a repeat crossmatch at the time of graft dysfunction or later. However, the inability to detect antibody does not preclude the diagnosis of hyperacute rejection since antibodies may be adsorbed in the graft and not reappear until weeks later. A poorly understood entity called delayed hyperacute rejection, characterized by sudden severe graft dysfunction or thrombosis 24 to 48 hours after implantation, may result from the same mechanism of preformed antibody along with a component of cellular rejection and on occasion is reversible. Accelerated rejection requires aggressive therapy with antilymphocyte antibodies and usually plasma exchange or immunoadsorption. Unfortunately, only 30% of these cases can be expected to recover to baseline function following treatment.

ANTIMICROBIAL PROPHYLAXIS

A major concern during treatment of acute rejection, particularly with the use of antilymphocyte antibodies, is CMV reactivation. Those patients at highest risk of reactivation during treatment early after transplantation are CMV-seronegative recipients who receive a kidney from a seropositive donor. Initial reports used low-dose intravenous ganciclovir for the prevention of CMV in high-risk patients receiving antilymphocyte therapy.[61] Later studies compared pre-emptive therapy, which involved treatment based on positive polymerase chain reaction results for CMV, and deferred therapy, in which treatment was withheld unless clinical symptoms were present.[62] Deferred therapy was not significantly different in its control of CMV morbidity and mortality, but was more cost effective. Although intravenous ganciclovir is still routinely used in many centers, oral valganciclovir has a bioavailability of nearly 70% (compared to 7% for oral ganciclovir) and at doses of 900 mg produces ganciclovir levels that are similar to intravenous administration of ganciclovir at 2.5 to 5 mg/kg.[63] Based on these reports, many centers have begun the exclusive use of oral valganciclovir. As both agents are renally excreted, dosing is based on the level of renal function. The major side effect during therapy is leukopenia, particularly in those patients also receiving MMF and/or sirolimus.

Prophylactic regimens shown to be effective against *Pneumocystis carinii* in kidney transplant recipients include trimethoprim-sulfamethoxazole (usually given as one single-strength tablet daily or one double-strength tablet three times weekly). This agent is also useful for the prevention of urinary tract infections, other bacterial infections, toxoplasmosis, and *Nocardia* infection. Alternative therapy in those patients allergic to sulfa includes aerosolized pentamidine, dapsone, and atovaquone. In centers that do not continue *P. carinii* prophylaxis indefinitely after initial transplantation, prophylaxis is generally reinstituted in patients who receive therapy for acute rejection. During treatment of acute rejection, oral nonabsorbable antifungal agents, such as clotrimazole or nystatin, are typically administered to prevent mucocutaneous *Candida* infection. These agents are ineffective in preventing systemic fungal infections, and prophylaxis with a systemic antifungal agent may be indicated during prolonged treatment, particularly with persistent candiduria.

REFERENCES

1. Sayegh MH, Carpenter CB: Transplantation 50 years later—progress, challenges, and promises. N Engl J Med 2004;351:2761–2766.
2. Denton MD, Magee CC, Sayegh MH: Immunosuppressive strategies in transplantation. Lancet 1999;353:1083–1091.
3. Womer KL, Vella JP, Sayegh MH: Chronic allograft dysfunction: Mechanisms and new approaches to therapy. Semin Nephrol 2000;20:126–147.
4. Basadonna G, Matas A, Gillingham K, et al: Early versus late acute renal allograft rejection: Impact on chronic rejection. Transplantation 1993;55:993–995.
5. Matas AJ, Gillingham KJ, Payne WD, Najarian JS: The impact of an acute rejection episode on long-term renal allograft survival (t1/2). Transplantation 1994;57:857–859.
6. Kuypers DR, Chapman JR, O'Connell PJ, et al: Predictors of renal transplant histology at three months. Transplantation 1999;67:1222–1230.
7. Heaf JG, Ladefoged J: The effect of acute rejection on long-term renal graft survival is mainly related to initial renal damage. Transpl Int 1998;11(Suppl 1):S26–S31.
8. Hariharan S, McBride MA, Cherikh WS, et al: Post-transplant renal function in the first year predicts long-term kidney transplant survival. Kidney Int 2002;62:311–318.
9. Meier-Kriesche HU, Schold JD, Srinivas TR, Kaplan B: Lack of improvement in renal allograft survival despite a marked decrease in acute rejection rates over the most recent era. Am J Transplant 2004;4:378–383.
10. Valujskikh A, Lakkis FG: In remembrance of things past: Memory T cells and transplant rejection. Immunol Rev 2003;196:65–74.
11. U.S. Transplant–Scientific Registry of Transplant Recipients: 2005 OPTN/SRTR Annual Report. Ann Arbor, MI: University Renal Research and Education Association with the University of Michigan, 2005.
12. Ojo AO, Wolfe RA, Held PJ, et al: Delayed graft function: Risk factors and implications for renal allograft survival. Transplantation 1997;63:968–974.
13. Young CJ, Gaston RS: Renal transplantation in black Americans. N Engl J Med 2000;343:1545–1552.

14. Pallet N, Thervet E, Alberti C, et al: Kidney transplant in black recipients: Are African Europeans different from African Americans? Am J Transplant 2005;5:2682–2687.

15. Doyle SE, Matas AJ, Gillingham K, Rosenberg ME: Predicting clinical outcome in the elderly renal transplant recipient. Kidney Int 2000;57:2144–2150.

16. de Fijter JW, Mallat MJ, Doxiadis II, et al: Increased immunogenicity and cause of graft loss of old donor kidneys. J Am Soc Nephrol 2001;12:1538–1546.

17. Hardinger KL, Schnitzler MA, Miller B, et al: Five-year follow up of thymoglobulin versus ATGAM induction in adult renal transplantation. Transplantation 2004;78:136–141.

18. Lange H, Muller TF, Ebel H, et al: Immediate and long-term results of ATG induction therapy for delayed graft function compared to conventional therapy for immediate graft function. Transpl Int 1999;12:2–9.

19. Stratta RJ, D'Alessandro AM, Armbrust MJ, et al: Sequential antilymphocyte globulin/cyclosporine immunosuppression in cadaveric renal transplantation. Effect of duration of ALG therapy. Transplantation 1989;47:96–102.

20. Brennan DC, Flavin K, Lowell JA, et al: A randomized, double-blinded comparison of thymoglobulin versus Atgam for induction immunosuppressive therapy in adult renal transplant recipients. Transplantation 1999;67:1011–1018.

21. Nashan B, Moore R, Amlot P, et al: Randomised trial of basiliximab versus placebo for control of acute cellular rejection in renal allograft recipients. CHIB 201 International Study Group. Lancet 1997;350:1193–1198.

22. Vincenti F, Kirkman R, Light S, et al: Interleukin-2-receptor blockade with daclizumab to prevent acute rejection in renal transplantation. Daclizumab Triple Therapy Study Group. N Engl J Med 1998;338:161–165.

23. Hong JC, Kahan BD: A calcineurin antagonist-free induction strategy for immunosuppression in cadaveric kidney transplant recipients at risk for delayed graft function. Transplantation 2001;71:1320–1328.

24. Meier-Kriesche HU, Arndorfer JA, Kaplan B, Division of Nephrology: Association of antibody induction with short- and long-term cause-specific mortality in renal transplant recipients. J Am Soc Nephrol 2002;13:769–772.

25. Sonnenday CJ, Warren DS, Cooper M, et al: Plasmapheresis, CMV hyperimmune globulin, and anti-CD20 allow ABO-incompatible renal transplantation without splenectomy. Am J Transplant 2004;4:1315–1322.

26. Ahsan N, Hricik D, Matas A, et al: Prednisone withdrawal in kidney transplant recipients on cyclosporine and mycophenolate mofetil—a prospective randomized study. Steroid Withdrawal Study Group. Transplantation 1999;68:1865–1874.

27. Vanrenterghem Y, Lebranchu Y, Hene R, et al: Double-blind comparison of two corticosteroid regimens plus mycophenolate mofetil and cyclosporine for prevention of acute renal allograft rejection. Transplantation 2000;70:1352–1359.

28. Birkeland SA: Steroid-free immunosuppression in renal transplantation: A long-term follow-up of 100 consecutive patients. Transplantation 2001;71:1089–1090.

29. Anil Kumar MS, Moritz MJ, Saaed MI, et al: Avoidance of chronic steroid therapy in African American kidney transplant recipients monitored by surveillance biopsy: 1-year results. Am J Transplant 2005;5:1976–1985.

30. Hariharan S, Johnson CP, Bresnahan BA, et al: Improved graft survival after renal transplantation in the United States, 1988 to 1996. N Engl J Med 2000;342:605–612.

31. Knoll GA, Bell RC: Tacrolimus versus cyclosporin for immunosuppression in renal transplantation: Meta-analysis of randomised trials. BMJ 1999;318:1104–1107.

32. Hardinger KL, Bohl DL, Schnitzler MA, et al: A randomized, prospective, pharmacoeconomic trial of tacrolimus versus cyclosporine in combination with thymoglobulin in renal transplant recipients. Transplantation 2005;80:41–46.

33. Nankivell BJ, Borrows RJ, Fung CL, et al: The natural history of chronic allograft nephropathy. N Engl J Med 2003;349:2326–2333.

34. Placebo-controlled study of mycophenolate mofetil combined with cyclosporin and corticosteroids for prevention of acute rejection. European Mycophenolate Mofetil Cooperative Study Group. Lancet 1995;345:1321–1325.

35. A blinded, randomized clinical trial of mycophenolate mofetil for the prevention of acute rejection in cadaveric renal transplantation. The Tricontinental Mycophenolate Mofetil Renal Transplantation Study Group. Transplantation 1996;61:1029–1037.

36. Sollinger HW: Mycophenolate mofetil for the prevention of acute rejection in primary cadaveric renal allograft recipients. U.S. Renal Transplant Mycophenolate Mofetil Study Group. Transplantation 1995;60:225–232.

37. Neylan JF: Immunosuppressive therapy in high-risk transplant patients: Dose-dependent efficacy of mycophenolate mofetil in African-American renal allograft recipients. U.S. Renal Transplant Mycophenolate Mofetil Study Group. Transplantation 1997;64:1277–1282.

38. Remuzzi G, Lesti M, Gotti E, et al: Mycophenolate mofetil versus azathioprine for prevention of acute rejection in renal transplantation (MYSS): A randomised trial. Lancet 2004;364:503–512.

39. Knoll GA, MacDonald I, Khan A, Van Walraven C: Mycophenolate mofetil dose reduction and the risk of acute rejection after renal transplantation. J Am Soc Nephrol 2003;14:2381–2386.

40. Johnson RW, Kreis H, Oberbauer R, et al: Sirolimus allows early cyclosporine withdrawal in renal transplantation resulting in improved renal function and lower blood pressure. Transplantation 2001;72:777–786.

41. Oberbauer R, Segoloni G, Campistol JM, et al: Early cyclosporine withdrawal from a sirolimus-based regimen results in better renal allograft survival and renal function at 48 months after transplantation. Transpl Int 2005;18:22–28.

42. Kahan BD: Efficacy of sirolimus compared with azathioprine for reduction of acute renal allograft rejection: A randomised multicentre study. The Rapamune US Study Group. Lancet 2000;356:194–202.

43. MacDonald AS: A worldwide, phase III, randomized, controlled, safety and efficacy study of a sirolimus/cyclosporine regimen for prevention of acute rejection in recipients of primary mismatched renal allografts. Transplantation 2001;71:271–280.

44. Nashan B, Curtis J, Ponticelli C, et al: Everolimus and reduced-exposure cyclosporine in de novo renal-transplant recipients: A three-year phase II, randomized, multicenter, open-label study. Transplantation 2004;78:1332–1340.

45. Racusen LC, Solez K, Colvin RB, et al: The Banff 97 working classification of renal allograft pathology. Kidney Int 1999;55:713–723.

46. Racusen LC, Colvin RB, Solez K, et al: Antibody-mediated rejection criteria—an addition to the Banff 97 classification of renal allograft rejection. Am J Transplant 2003;3:708–714.

47. Meehan SM, Siegel CT, Aronson AJ, et al: The relationship of untreated borderline infiltrates by the Banff criteria to acute rejection in renal allograft biopsies. J Am Soc Nephrol 1999;10:1806–1814.

48. Rush D, Nickerson P, Gough J, et al: Beneficial effects of treatment of early subclinical rejection: A randomized study. J Am Soc Nephrol 1998;9:2129–2134.

49. Halloran PF, Schlaut J, Solez K, Srinivasa NS: The significance of the anti-class I response. II. Clinical and pathologic features of renal transplants with anti-class I-like antibody. Transplantation 1992;53:550–555.

50. Trpkov K, Campbell P, Pazderka F, et al: Pathologic features of acute renal allograft rejection associated with donor-specific antibody, analysis using the Banff grading schema. Transplantation 1996;61:1586–1592.

51. Feucht HE, Felber E, Gokel MJ, et al: Vascular deposition of complement-split products in kidney allografts with cell-mediated rejection. Clin Exp Immunol 1991;86:464–470.

52. Feucht HE, Schneeberger H, Hillebrand G, et al: Capillary deposition of C4d complement fragment and early renal graft loss. Kidney Int 1993;43:1333–1338.

53. Collins AB, Schneeberger EE, Pascual MA, et al: Complement activation in acute humoral renal allograft rejection: Diagnostic significance of C4d deposits in peritubular capillaries. J Am Soc Nephrol 1999;10:2208–2214.

54. Herzenberg AM, Gill JS, Djurdjev O, Magil AB: C4d deposition in acute rejection: An independent long-term prognostic factor. J Am Soc Nephrol 2002;13:234–241.

55. Magil AB: Infiltrating cell types in transplant glomerulitis: Relationship to peritubular capillary C4d deposition. Am J Kidney Dis 2005;45:1084–1089.

56. Magil AB, Tinckam K: Monocytes and peritubular capillary C4d deposition in acute renal allograft rejection. Kidney Int 2003;63:1888–1893.

57. Gaber LW, Moore LW, Gaber AO, et al: Correlation of histology to clinical rejection reversal: A thymoglobulin multicenter trial report. Kidney Int 1999;55:2415–2422.

58. Mazzucchi E, Lucon AM, Nahas WC, et al: Histological outcome of acute cellular rejection in kidney transplantation after treatment with methylprednisolone. Transplantation 1999;67:430–434.

59. Gaber AO, First MR, Tesi RJ, et al: Results of the double-blind, randomized, multicenter, phase III clinical trial of thymoglobulin versus

Atgam in the treatment of acute graft rejection episodes after renal transplantation. Transplantation 1998;66:29–37.

60. Schroeder TJ, Moore LW: Efficacy Endpoints Conference on Acute Rejection in Kidney Transplantation: Summary report of the database. Am J Kidney Dis 1998;31(6 Suppl 1):S31–S39.

61. Hibberd PL, Tolkoff-Rubin NE, Conti D, et al: Preemptive ganciclovir therapy to prevent cytomegalovirus disease in cytomegalovirus antibody-positive renal transplant recipients. A randomized controlled trial. Ann Intern Med 1995;123:18–26.

62. Brennan DC, Garlock KA, Singer GG, et al: Prophylactic oral ganciclovir compared with deferred therapy for control of cytomegalovirus in renal transplant recipients. Transplantation 1997;64:1843–1846.

63. Wiltshire H, Hirankarn S, Farrell C, et al: Pharmacokinetic profile of ganciclovir after its oral administration and from its prodrug, valganciclovir, in solid organ transplant recipients. Clin Pharmacokinet 2005; 44:495–507.

94

Medical Management of the Kidney Transplant Recipient

Phuong-Thu T. Pham, Gabriel M. Danovitch, and Phuong-Chi T. Pham

While renal transplantation improves both patient survival and quality of life compared to dialysis, there are numerous medical issues that arise in the transplant recipient. Cardiovascular disease, hypertension, dyslipidemia, diabetes mellitus, and malignancies are some of the most important factors associated with increased morbidity and mortality after renal transplantation. This chapter provides an approach to the medical management of these patients. A discussion of the use of immunosuppressive medications and the management of acute and chronic rejection is provided elsewhere (see Chapter 93).

CARDIOVASCULAR DISEASE

Death with a functioning graft is one of the major causes of late graft loss, with cardiovascular disease (CVD) being the most frequent cause. When compared to the general population, cardiovascular mortality in transplant recipients is increased by nearly 10-fold among patients within the age range of 35 and 44 and at least doubled among those between the ages of 55 and 64.[1] While renal transplantation ameliorates many CVD risk factors by restoring renal function, it introduces new cardiovascular risks derived in part from immunosuppressive medications such as calcineurin inhibitors or corticosteroids; these include impaired glucose tolerance or diabetes mellitus, hypertension, and dyslipidemia. Management of CVD risk factors begins in the early post-transplantation period and should remain an integral part of long-term care in renal transplant recipients. Although the determinants of enhanced CVD risks in renal transplant recipients have not been well defined, both traditional and nontraditional risk factors have been suggested to be contributory (see Chapter 71).

Hypertension

Hypertension is an independent risk factor for allograft failure and mortality and is present in 50% to 90% of renal transplant recipients. Systolic blood pressure (BP) is highest immediately after transplantation and declines during the first year. In the Collaborative Transplant Study (CTS) registry analysis involving 24,723 recipients of deceased donor transplants, only 8% had systolic BP <120 mm Hg at 1 year, 33% had BP in the prehypertension range, 39% had stage 1 hypertension, and 20% had stage 2 hypertension despite antihypertensive therapy.[2] Preexisting hypertension, tacrolimus, and, to a greater degree, cyclosporine, corticosteroids, chronic allograft nephropathy, excess weight gain, acute rejection, recurrent or de novo glomerulonephritis, and transplant renal artery stenosis have all been implicated in post-transplantation hypertension. Excess

renin output from the native kidneys may contribute to post-transplantation hypertension in rare cases.

The results of the CTS Registry suggest that BP control after transplantation is suboptimal. Management of post-transplantation hypertension should include attempts to identify and treat the underlying etiology, lifestyle modifications, and treatment of associated cardiovascular risk factors. Lifestyle modifications should be similar to those used in the nontransplant population (see Chapter 33). Potassium-based salt substitutes must be used with caution or should be avoided due to the high incidence of hyperkalemia among patients receiving cyclosporine or tacrolimus immunosuppression.

Controlled clinical trials to determine the superiority of one class of hypertensive agent over the other in the transplant setting are lacking. In general, there are no absolute contraindications to the use of any antihypertensive agent in renal transplant recipients. Nondihydropyridine calcium channel blockers and diuretics are frequently used in the early post-transplantation period, the former due to their beneficial effect on renal hemodynamics and the latter due to their ability to eliminate salt and water in these subjects who are frequently volume expanded. In a single-center retrospective study to identify coronary artery disease (CAD) risk after renal transplantation, Kasiske and colleagues[3] unexpectedly found an association between the use of dihydropyridine calcium channel antagonists and an increased CAD risk. Although the mechanism(s) for the potential adverse effects of dihydropyridine calcium channel blockers on the cardiovascular risk profile is unclear, the use of amlodipine has been reported to be associated with increased catecholamine levels.[4] While further recommendations await results of large, ongoing, randomized, controlled trials in the general population, dihydropyridine calcium channel antagonists should be used with caution.

The use of angiotensin-converting enzyme (ACE) inhibitors and/or angiotensin receptor blockers (ARBs) has gained increasing popularity due to their safety, efficacy, and well-established renoprotective, antiproteinuric, and cardioprotective effects. Nonetheless, an increase in serum creatinine (i.e., >30% above baseline) associated with their use should alert the clinician of possible transplant renal artery stenosis. Caution should be exercised when used with diuretics as ACE inhibitors and/or ARBs may potentiate volume depletion–induced renal hypoperfusion. In patients with slow or delayed graft function, ACE inhibitors and/or ARBs are generally not recommended until recovery of allograft function. Mild to moderate renal allograft dysfunction, however, does not exclude their use if serum potassium and creatinine can be closely monitored. β-Blockers should be considered in patients with known CAD or other atherosclerotic vascular disease, whereas α_2-blockers may be beneficial in patients with benign prostatic hypertrophy and neurogenic bladder. Although aggressive blood pressure control is vital in reducing cardiovascular morbidities and mortalities as well as improving graft survival, this is not recommended in the early perioperative period due to the risk of precipitating acute tubular necrosis and/or graft thrombosis.

Post-transplantation Diabetes Mellitus

Post-transplantation diabetes mellitus (PTDM) is a well-known complication following solid organ transplantation and has been reported to occur in 4% to 25% of renal transplant recipients. Potential risk factors for PTDM include African American, Indo-Asian, and Hispanic ethnicity, obesity, age older than 40 years, male gender, family history of diabetes among first-degree relatives, impaired glucose tolerance before transplantation, recipients of deceased donor kidneys, hypertriglyceridemia, hypertension, hepatitis C virus (HCV) and cytomegalovirus (CMV) infection, and immunosuppressive therapy including corticosteroids, tacrolimus, and, to a lesser extent, cyclosporine. The presence of certain HLA antigens such as A30, B27, and B42, increasing HLA mismatches, acute rejection history, and male donor may also be associated with an increased risk of PTDM. Azathioprine and mycophenolate mofetil (MMF) do not appear to be diabetogenic. In contrast, the use of azathioprine and MMF has been associated with a lower risk of PTDM and the diabetogenic effect of tacrolimus may be mitigated by concomitant use of MMF. (See p. 1101.)

The management of PTDM should follow the conventional approach for patients with type 2 diabetes mellitus such as recommended on the International Federation Global Guideline website (www.d4pro.com/diabetesguidelines/index.htm). Additional intervention may include adjustment or modification in immunosuppressive medications and pharmacologic therapy to achieve a target hemoglobin A1C level of <6.5%. Corticosteroid dose reduction may significantly improve glucose tolerance during the first year after transplantation.[5] Steroid-sparing regimens or steroid-avoidance protocols should be tailored to each individual patient. Tacrolimus to cyclosporine conversion therapy may be considered in patients who fail to achieve target glycemic control or in those with difficult-to-control diabetes. Alternative management has included calcineurin inhibitor withdrawal in a regimen that consists of sirolimus and/or MMF. Nevertheless, manipulation of immunosuppressive therapy to alleviate adverse effects must be balanced against the risk of allograft rejection and graft loss. Clinicians must be familiar with the patients' immune history such as history of acute rejection, highly sensitized recipients, or recipients of a re-allograft transplant prior to manipulating their immunosuppressive regimen.

Insulin therapy may be necessary in up to 40% of patients,[6] particularly in the early post-transplantation period. Of the oral hypoglycemic agents, metformin is preferred for overweight patients but should be avoided in patients with impaired allograft function due to the increased risk of metformin-induced lactic acidosis. Sulfonylurea derivatives must also be prescribed carefully for patients with impaired allograft function or elderly patients due to the increased risk of hypoglycemia. In general, it is best to start with a low dose and titrate upward every 1 to 2 weeks. The nonsulfonylureas meglitinides are insulin secretagogues with a mechanism of action similar to that of the sulfonylureas. They have a more rapid onset and shorter duration of action, and the risk of hypoglycemia and the amount of weight gain appear to be less than those seen with the sulfonylureas. These agents are best suited for patients whose food intake is erratic, elderly patients, and patients

with impaired graft function. They are best taken before meals, and the dose may be omitted if a meal is skipped.

The thiazolidinedione derivatives are insulin sensitizers, and their use may allow a reduction in the insulin requirement. However, potential adverse effects of these agents include weight gain, peripheral edema, anemia, pulmonary edema, and congestive heart failure. Peripheral edema is common when thiazolidinedione derivatives are used in combination therapy with insulin. Drug-drug interactions must also be considered. The meglitinide derivatives repaglinide and, to a lesser extent, nateglinide are metabolized by cytochrome P-450 isozyme CYP 3A4. Combination of repaglinide with a strong CYP 3A4 inhibitor (e.g., cyclosporine, gemfibrozil, the azole antifungals) may result in an increased risk of hypoglycemia, whereas the coadministration of an inducer of CYP 3A4 (such as rifampin, carbamazepine, and phenytoin) may result in higher glucose levels.

Monitoring of patients with PTDM should include measuring hemoglobin A1C levels every 3 months and screening for diabetic complications including microalbuminuria, regular ophthalmologic examinations, and regular foot care. Figure 94.1 shows the suggested guidelines for the management of PTDM.

Management of post-transplantation diabetes mellitus
Dietary Modification
Dietitian referral For diabetic dyslipidemia: a diet low in saturated fats and cholesterol and high in complex carbohydrates and fiber is recommended
Lifestyle Modification
Exercise Weight reduction or avoidance of excessive weight gain Smoking cessation
Adjustment or Modification in Immunosuppressive Medications*
Rapid steroid taper, steroid-sparing or steroid-avoidance protocols Tacrolimus cyclosporine conversion therapy Calcineurin inhibitor withdrawal†
Pharmacologic Therapy
Acute, marked hyperglycemia (may require in-patient management) Intensive insulin therapy (consider insulin infusion when glucose ≥400 mg/dl [22 mmol/l])
Chronic Hyperglycemia: Treat to Target Hemoglobin A$_{1c}$<6.5%
Oral glucose-lowering agent monotherapy or combination therapy‡ and/or insulin therapy Consider diabetologist referral if hemoglobin A1C remains ≥9.0%
Monitoring of Patients with PTDM
Hemoglobin A1C every 3 months Screening microalbuminuria Regular ophthalmologic examination Regular foot care Annual fasting lipid profile Aggressive treatment of dyslipidemia and hypertension

Figure 94.1 **Management of post-transplantation diabetes mellitus (PTDM).** *Clinicians must be familiar with the patients' immune history prior to manipulating their immunosuppressive therapy (see text). †Calcineurin inhibitor withdrawal may be considered to a regimen that consists of sirolimus and/or mycophenolate mofetil, although the diabetogenic effects of such regimens have not been well studied. ‡The choice of a particular agent should be based on the characteristics of each individual patient (see text).

Post-transplantation Dyslipidemia

Dyslipidemia is common following transplantation. Many immunosuppressive agents, including corticosteroids, cyclosporine, tacrolimus, and sirolimus adversely affect lipids. While tacrolimus-based therapy has been suggested to be associated with better lipid profiles than cyclosporine-based therapy, sirolimus has been shown to be associated with a significantly greater incidence and severity of dyslipidemia than cyclosporine-based therapy, including higher total cholesterol and triglyceride (TG) levels. Other factors contributing to post-transplantation dyslipidemia include age, diet, rapid weight gain, hyperinsulinemia, pre-existing hypercholesterolemia, allograft dysfunction, proteinuria, the use of β-blockers and diuretics, and probably hypomagnesemia.[6]

Although hyperlipidemia often improves within the first 6 months after transplantation as immunosuppression is reduced, total and low-density lipoprotein (LDL) cholesterol goals rarely meet guidelines (such as defined by the National Cholesterol Education Program guidelines www.nhlbi.nih.gov/about/ncep/index.htm) and lifestyle changes and pharmacotherapy are often required. Statins (3-hydroxy-3-methylglutaryl coenzyme A reductase inhibitors) are effective and safe in transplant recipients and usually are the agent of choice. However, the use of statins with calcineurin inhibitors (particularly cyclosporine) often results in severalfold increase in statin blood level and an increased risk of myopathy and rhabdomyolysis.[7] Cyclosporine increases plasma fluvastatin levels by twofold, simvastatin by threefold, atorvastatin by sixfold, pravastatin by five- to 23-fold, and lovastatin by up to 20-fold. Approximate therapeutic equivalencies are achieved by 10 mg atorvastatin, 20 mg simvastatin, 40 mg pravastatin, 40 mg lovastatin, and 80 mg fluvastatin. At these doses, LDL cholesterol decreases approximately 34% with minimal change in high-density lipoprotein (HDL) levels.[7]

Other lipid-lowering agents include fibric derivatives, nicotinic acid, bile acid sequestrants, and the newer lipid-lowering agent ezetimibe. Ezetimibe, which blocks intestinal absorption of dietary cholesterol, potentiates the effects of statins to reduce LDL cholesterol levels. Experience with ezetimibe in transplantation is currently limited, but to date no significant interaction with the calcineurin inhibitors or sirolimus has been reported.

Severe hypertriglyceridemia (TG >500 mg/dl) is more frequent since the introduction of sirolimus. Management includes sirolimus dose reduction, addition of a fibric acid derivative, or nicotinic acid. In refractory cases, a switch from sirolimus to MMF or tacrolimus may be indicated.

Careful monitoring for side effects from the lipid-lowering agents is indicated (see Ballantyne and colleagues[7] for a complete list). Of the major fibric acid medications (bezafibrate, ciprofibrate, fenofibrate, and gemfibrozil), the first three have been reported to cause increases in serum creatinine in cyclosporine-treated patients as well as higher plasma homocysteine levels. When used in combination with statins, fibrates (especially gemfibrozil) may result in elevations of creatine phosphokinase (CK), with or without overt rhabdomyolysis and myopathy. Niacin monotherapy has not been reported to cause myopathy, but its combined use with lovastatin, pravastatin, or simvastatin may be associated with rhabdomyolysis. Bile acid sequestrants must be used with caution due to their potential interference with the absorption of other medications vital to the renal transplant recipients. Suggested guidelines for pharmacologic treatment of dyslipidemia are shown in Figure 94.2.

Obesity

Obesity is common in renal transplant recipients. Patients on prednisone therapy may overeat as they often experience constant

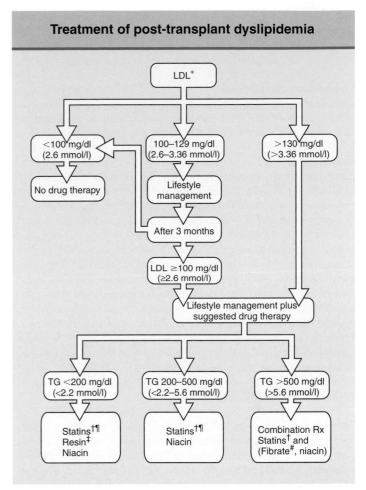

Treatment of post-transplant dyslipidemia

Figure 94.2 Suggested guidelines for the treatment of post-transplantation dyslipidemia. All transplant recipients should be regarded as coronary heart disease risk equivalent. Goals: low-density lipoprotein (LDL) <100 mg/dl (2.6 mmol/l), triglycerides <200 mg/dl, (2.2 mmol/l), high-density lipoprotein >45 mg/dl (1.16 mmol/l). *A goal of LDL <70 mg/dl has been suggested for very high risk patients (National Cholesterol Education Program and guidelines). †Statins are the most effective drugs and should be the agents of first choice. Start at a low dose in patients on cyclosporine and tacrolimus. Monitor for myosytis and transaminitis, particularly in those receiving combination therapy. ‡Bile acid sequestrants should probably not be taken at the same time as cyclosporine. #Extreme caution should be used with statin and fibrate combination therapy. ¶If LDL targets not achieved with statins, consider cholesterol absorption inhibitors.

hunger or craving for sweets. The release from pretransplantation dietary restriction and habitual physical inactivity may also result in rapid post-transplantation weight gain. In liver transplant recipients, tacrolimus immunosuppression was associated with a lower likelihood of post-transplantation weight gain compared to cyclosporine (27% versus 46%, respectively),[8] an effect that was suggested to be due to its better steroid-sparing effect compared to cyclosporine. Nonetheless, cyclosporine has not always been found to independently predict post-transplantation obesity. Other possible predictors for increased weight gain after transplantation include pretransplantation obesity, greater donor body mass index, and higher cumulative doses of prednisone.

Enrollment in a diet support group and/or exercise program can be invaluable. Steroid reduction or withdrawal must be balanced against the risk of allograft rejection and graft loss. The use of pharmacologic agents for weight reduction in the post-transplantation period is currently not recommended due to unknown potential drug-drug interactions. In morbidly obese patients, gastric bypass surgery has been shown to be a safe and effective means for achieving significant long-term weight loss and relief of comorbid conditions after transplantation.

Hyperhomocysteinemia

Hyperhomocysteinemia (see Chapter 71) occurs in two thirds of renal transplant recipients and is associated with an increased risk of cardiovascular complications of 6% for every μmol/l increase in homocysteine.[9] In a recent single-center prospective study consisting of 733 renal transplant recipients, baseline fasting plasma total homocysteine levels independently predicted the risk of death and kidney allograft loss.[10] Important determinants of total plasma homocysteine levels include folate, B_6 (pyridoxine), B_{12} (cyanocobalamin), and impaired renal function. In a small prospective, randomized, placebo-controlled study consisting of 56 stable hyperhomocysteinemic renal transplant recipients, vitamin supplementation with folic acid 5 mg/day, vitamin B_6 50 mg/day, and vitamin B_{12} 400 μg/day significantly decreased fasting homocysteine level and improved carotid intima-media thickening compared to placebo-treated patients.[11] Although definitive results from large randomized trials are needed, treatment of hyperhomocysteinemia may be beneficial. In addition, unless contraindicated, antiplatelet therapy (such as the use of low-dose aspirin) should be considered in all patients.

INFECTIOUS DISEASES

Despite the routine use of prophylactic therapy against common bacterial, viral, and opportunistic pathogens in the peri- and postoperative period, infection remains an important cause of morbidity and mortality following organ transplantation. The time to occurrence of different infections in the immunocompromised transplant recipients follows a timetable pattern[12] (Fig. 94.3).

In the first month after transplantation, infections are most frequently caused by common nosocomial bacterial microorganisms and *Candida* species. Except for herpes simplex virus (HSV), other viral infections are uncommon during this period. Similar to those following any major surgical procedure, the sources of infections after solid organ transplantation include surgical wounds, surgical drainage catheters, indwelling urethral catheters, bacteremia from vascular access devices, aspiration

pneumonia, and urinary tract infections. Potential sources of infections specific to renal transplant recipients include perinephric fluid collections due to lymphoceles, wound hematomas or urine leaks, indwelling urinary stents, and anatomic or functional genitourinary tract abnormalities such as ureteral stricture and vesicoureteric reflux, and neurogenic bladder. Although bacterial pathogens vary from center to center, urinary tract infections in renal transplant recipients are commonly caused by aerobic gram-negative bacteria (*Escherichia coli*, *Enterobacteriaceae*, and *Pseudomonas*) and aerobic gram-positive bacteria (*Enterococcus*). Preventive measures to reduce urinary tract infections include early urethral catheter removal and antibiotic prophylaxis. Trimethoprim-sulfamethoxazole or ciprofloxacin prophylaxis during the first 3 months after transplantation effectively reduces the frequency of urinary tract infections to <10% and essentially eliminates urosepsis unless urine flow is unknowingly obstructed. Although strict aseptic surgical techniques and perioperative use of first-generation cephalosporins reduce the incidence of wound infections, risk factors including diabetes mellitus and obesity at the time of transplantation remain problematic.

After the first post-transplantation month, infections with viruses including CMV, HSV, varicella-zoster virus, Epstein-Barr virus (EBV), hepatitis B virus (HBV), and HCV may occur either due to the overall state of immunosuppression, exogenous infection, or reactivation of latent disease. Repeated courses of antibiotics and corticosteroid therapy increase the risk of fungal infections, whereas infections with immunomodulating viruses may render the patients more susceptible to opportunistic infections. Causative opportunistic agents include *Pneumocystis jiroveci* (previously known as *Pneumocystis carinii*), *Aspergillus* species, *Listeria monocytogenes*, *Nocardia* species, and *Toxoplasma gondii*. Trimethoprim-sulfamethoxazole prophylaxis eliminates or reduces the incidence of pneumocystis pneumonia, *L. monocytogenes* meningitis, *Nocardia* species infection, and *T. gondii* infection.

Beyond 6 months following transplantation, patients can be arbitrarily divided into three categories in terms of infection risks.[13]

The first category consists of the majority of transplant recipients (70% to 80%) who have satisfactory or good allograft function and who have no history of chronic viral infection. These

Infections following renal transplantation		
Month 1 After Transplantation	Months 1–6	After 6 Months

Postoperative bacterial infections
  Urinary tract
  Respiratory
  Vascular access related
  Wound
Nosocomial, including *Legionella*
  species
Viral: HSV
Fungal: *Candida*
Organisms transmitted with donor organ
Untreated infection in recipient
	Opportunistic or unconventional infections
	  Viral: CMV, HHV-6, HHV-7, EBV, VZV,
	    influenza, RSV, adenovirus
	  Fungal: *Aspergillus* species, *Cryptococcus*, *Mucor*
	  Bacterial: *Nocardia*, *Listeria*,
	    Mycobacterium species, *Legionella*, tuberculosis
	  Parasitic: *Pneumocystis carinii*,
	    Toxoplasma and *Strongyloides* species,
	    leishmaniasis
	  HBV, HCV, HIV
		Late opportunistic infections
		  Cryptococcus, CMV retinitis
		  or colitis, VZV, parvovirus B-19,
		  polyomavirus (BK, JC),
		  Listeria, tuberculosis
		  Persistent infections: HBV, HCV
		Associated with malignancy
		  EBV, papillomavirus, HSV, HHV-8
		Community acquired
		Unusual sites, e.g., paravertebral abscess

Figure 94.3 Infections following renal transplantation. Geographically focused infections will need to be considered in certain cases, such as malaria, leishmaniasis, trypanosomiasis, and strongyloidiasis. CMV, cytomegalovirus; EBV, Epstein-Barr virus; HBV, hepatitis B virus; HCV, hepatitis C virus; HHV, human herpesvirus; HIV, human immunodeficiency virus; RSV, respiratory syncytial virus; VZV, varicella-zoster virus. (Adapted from Fishman JA, Rubin RH: Infection in organ transplant recipients. N Engl J Med 1998;338:1743.)

Suggested prophylactic therapy for recipients of renal transplants	
	Comments
Trimethoprim-sulfamethoxazole* (TMP/SMX)	Its routine use reduces or eliminates the incidence of *Pneumocystis carinii*, *Listeria monocytogenes*, *Nocardia asteroides*, and *Toxoplasma gondii* In renal transplant recipients, TMP/SMX reduces the incidence of urinary tract infection from 30%–80% to <5%–10%
Monthly intravenous or aerosolized pentamidine >dapsone[†]> or atovaquone[‡]	Replaces TMP/SMX for patients with sulfa allergies
Nystatin 100,000 units/ml, 4 ml after meals and before bedtime	For fungal prophylaxis
Acyclovir, valganciclovir, ganciclovir	For cytomegalovirus prophylaxis, see Figure 94.5

Figure 94.4 Suggested prophylactic therapy for recipients of renal transplants. *Prophylactic therapy the first 3 months after transplantation is generally recommended. For those patients receiving sirolimus immunosuppression, 1 year of therapy is recommended. [†]Check glucose-6-phosphate dehydrogenase deficiency before initiation of therapy. [‡]In order of efficacy. (Modified from Pham PT, Pham PC, Wilkinson AH: Medical and urological complications of pancreas and kidney/pancreas transplantation. In Hakim N, Stratta R, Gray D [eds]: Pancreas and Islet Transplantation. New York: Oxford University Press, 2002, pp 167–189.)

patients are usually maintained on a relatively low level of immunosuppression; hence, their risk of infection is similar to that of the general population, with community-acquired respiratory viruses constituting the major infective agents.[12] Opportunistic infections are unusual unless environmental exposure has occurred.

The second group of patients (approximately 10% of patients) consists of those with chronic viral infection that may include HBV, HCV, CMV, EBV, polyoma BK virus, or papillomavirus. In the setting of immunosuppression, such viral infections may result in progressive liver disease or liver cirrhosis (HBV, HCV), polyomavirus BK nephropathy, post-transplantation lymphoproliferative disease (EBV), or squamous cell carcinoma (papillomavirus).

The third group of patients (approximately 10% of patients) consists of those who experience multiple episodes of rejection requiring repeated exposure to heavy immunosuppression. These patients are the most likely candidates for chronic viral infections and superinfection with opportunistic organisms. Causative opportunistic pathogens include *P. jiroveci*, *L. monocytogenes*, *Nocardia asteroides*, *Cryptococcus neoformans*, and geographically restricted mycoses (coccidioidomycosis, histoplasmosis, blastomycosis, and paracoccidioidomycosis). In these high-risk candidates, lifelong prophylactic therapy with trimethoprim-sulfamethoxazole 80 mg/400 mg daily has been advocated. In addition, antifungal prophylaxis should be considered and environmental exposure minimized. Suggested prophylactic therapy in renal transplant recipients is shown in Figure 94.4.

Cytomegalovirus

CMV infection occurs primarily after the first month post-transplantation and continues to be a significant cause of morbidity during the first 6 months. CMV infection may occur as a primary infection in a seronegative recipient (donor seropositive, recipient

seronegative), reactivation of endogenous latent virus (donor seropositive or seronegative, recipient seropositive), or superinfection with a new virus strain in a seropositive recipient (donor seropositive, recipient seropositive). Primary CMV infection often results in more severe disease than reactivation or superinfection. The clinical manifestations of CMV infection span the spectrum of asymptomatic seroconversion, mononucleosis-like syndrome or flulike illness with fever and leukopenia, and/or thrombocytopenia to widespread tissue invasive disease. The latter may result in clinical hepatitis, esophagitis, gastroenteritis, colitis, pneumonia, and allograft dysfunction, among others. Donor and recipient seropositive status and the use of blood products from CMV-seropositive donor are well-established risk factors for CMV infection. Other factors associated with an increased risk of CMV infection include prolonged or repeated courses of antilymphocyte preparations, episodes of allograft rejection, comorbid illnesses, and neutropenia. MMF has also been variably reported to be associated with an increased incidence of CMV viremia and CMV disease. The risk is particularly increased in patients receiving MMF 3 g/day. Management of CMV infection consists of preventive (prophylactic and/or pre-emptive therapy) and therapeutic measures. Prophylactic therapy involves antiviral therapy beginning in the immediate postoperative period (Fig. 94.5), whereas pre-emptive therapy involves treatment of those who are found to seroconvert by use of laboratory assays such as CMV DNA polymerase chain reaction (PCR) or pp65 antigenemia during surveillance studies. In a recent study, Hadaya and associates[14] demonstrated that the peak viral loads were significantly higher in patients with CMV-related complications (median, 5000 DNA copies/ml) than in those without symptoms (1160 DNA copies/ml) ($P = 0.048$). Although further studies are needed, treatment is probably warranted when viral load is >5000 copies/ml. Established clinical CMV disease should be treated with intravenous ganciclovir. The usual course consists of 3 weeks (range, 2 to 4 weeks) of intravenous therapy in conjunction with

Suggested cytomegalovirus prophylaxis protocol*
For CMV-negative recipients of a CMV-negative organ Acyclovir 400 mg/day for herpes prophylaxis Check for CMV DNA every 2 weeks for 3 months
For CMV-negative recipients of a CMV-positive organ During antibody treatment, ganciclovir[†] 2.5 mg/kg /day IV Following antibody treatment, valganciclovir[†] 900 mg/day PO for 6 months If no antibody treatment, valganciclovir 900 mg/day for 6 months Check for CMV DNA every 2 weeks for 3 months
For CMV-positive recipients of a CMV-negative organ During antibody treatment, ganciclovir 2.5 mg/kg/day IV Following antibody treatment, valganciclovir[†] 900 mg/day PO for 3 months If no antibody treatment, acyclovir 400 mg/day for 3 months Check for CMV DNA every 2 weeks for 3 months
For CMV-positive recipients of a CMV-positive organ During antibody treatment, ganciclovir 2.5 mg/kg/day IV Following antibody treatment, valganciclovir 900 mg/day PO for 3 months If no antibody treatment, acyclovir 400 mg/day for 3 months Check for CMV DNA every 2 weeks for 3 months

Figure 94.5 Suggested cytomegalovirus (CMV) prophylaxis protocol. *If CMV status is unknown, give intravenous ganciclovir until CMV status is determined. [†]Dose adjustment for renal function necessary.

reduction of immunosuppression for severe CMV disease. In patients with tissue invasive disease, intravenous ganciclovir is recomended, followed by a 2-month course of oral ganciclovir or valganciclovir in seropositive individuals and for 3 to 4 months in those with primary infection.[12] In patients slow to respond to therapy, the addition of CMV hyperimmune globulin or intravenous pooled gamma globulin (IVIG) can be of therapeutic benefit. Although oral valganciclovir provides good bioavailability and may be effective in mild to moderate CMV disease,[15] its use in the treatment of CMV disease has not been well studied. In renal transplant recipients with CMV infection with or without tissue invasive disease, treatment failure to valganciclovir necessitating intravenous ganciclovir has been reported.[16] The use of cidofovir and foscarnet should be reserved for those with clinically suspected ganciclovir-resistant strains due to their associated nephrotoxicity. Suggested CMV prophylaxis protocol is shown in Figure 94.5.

Candida Infection

Candida species are the most common fungal pathogens encountered in the immunocompromised transplant recipients, with *Candida albicans* and *Candida tropicalis* accounting for 90% of the infections followed by *Candida glabrata*. Diabetes mellitus, high-dose corticosteroids, and broad-spectrum antibacterial therapy predispose patients to mucocutaneous candidal infections such as oral candidiasis, intertriginous candidal infections, esophagitis, vaginitis, and urinary tract infections. Superficial infections involving the mouth or intertriginous areas can be treated with nystatin and topical clotrimazole, whereas candidal urinary tract infections are usually treated with systemic antifungal therapy with fluconazole, or more rarely with amphotericin bladder washes, liposomal amphotericin, or caspofungin for fluconazole-resistant species (see Chapter 52). Whenever possible, foreign objects such as bladder catheter, surgical drains (such as percutaneous nephrostomy tube), and urinary stents should be promptly removed.

Polyomavirus (BK) Infection

Over the past decade, polyoma infection due to BK virus has emerged as an important cause of allograft failure following renal transplantation. BK virus is a ubiquitous human virus with a peak incidence of primary infection in children 2 to 5 years of age and a seroprevalence rate of >60% to 90% among the adult population worldwide. Following primary infection, BK virus preferentially establishes latency within the genitourinary tract and frequently reactivates in the setting of immunosuppression. In renal transplant recipients, BK virus is associated with a range of clinical syndromes including asymptomatic viruria with or without viremia, ureteral stenosis and obstruction, interstitial nephritis, or BK allograft nephropathy. In most series, 30% to 40% of renal transplant recipients develop BK viruria, 10% to 20% develop BK viremia, and 2% to 5% develop BK nephropathy (BKN).

BKN most commonly presents with an asymptomatic increase in serum creatinine between 2 to 60 months (median, 9 months) after transplantation. The diagnosis of BKN is made by allograft biopsy showing BK virus inclusions in renal tubular and glomerular epithelial cells (Fig. 94.6a). Variable degrees of interstitial inflammation (see Fig. 94.6b), degenerative changes in tubules, and focal tubulitis can be seen and may mimic acute tubular necrosis (ATN) or acute rejection. In the absence of classic histologic findings, distinguishing between BKN, acute rejection, and the presence of both processes can be a diagnostic challenge. Immunohistochemistry (see Fig. 94.6c), *in situ* hybridization or electron microscopy is often required to confirm the diagnosis of BKN. In the late stage

of BKN, few characteristic intranuclear inclusions are seen, and the histopathologic changes are indistinguishable from those of chronic allograft nephropathy including interstitial fibrosis and scarring. Urine cytology for decoy cells or quantitative determinations of viruria and of viral load in blood measured by PCR are also used as surrogate markers for the diagnosis of BKN.

There is no standard protocol for the treatment of BKN. The mainstay of treatment includes reduction or discontinuation of antimetabolites (MMF or azathioprine) with judicious reduction in calcineurin inhibitor therapy or other immunosuppressive regimen. The level of reduction in immunosuppression has not been clearly defined. Switching from tacrolimus to cyclosporine or to sirolimus has resulted in resolution of BKN and viremia/viruria in anecdotal case reports.[17] Adjunctive antiviral therapy with cidofovir or leflunomide has been used with variable response rates.[18] Low-dose cidofovir (0.25 to 0.33 mg/kg intravenously biweekly) has been proposed in refractory cases. More recently, IVIG in conjunction with reduction in immunosuppression has been reported to result in clearance of viremia and stabilization of serum creatinine.[19] Anecdotal reports suggest that IVIG may be effective in treating steroid-resistant rejection and its use may be beneficial in patients with simultaneous rejection and BKN.

Despite various treatment strategies, up to 30% to 50% of patients with established BKN developed progressive decline in renal function with graft loss. Early diagnosis and intervention may improve prognosis. Intensive monitoring of urine and serum for BK by PCR during the first year post-transplantation and pre-emptive reduction of immunosuppressive therapy are associated with resolution of viremia and absence of BKN without acute rejection or graft loss.[20] More recently, a panel of experts has suggested that all renal transplant recipients should be screened for BK virus replication in the urine: (1) every 3 months during the first 2 years post-transplantation, (2) when allograft dysfunction is noted, and (3) when allograft biopsy is performed. A positive screening result should be confirmed in <4 weeks and assessed by quantitative assays (e.g., BK virus DNA load in plasma or urine). A definitive diagnosis of BKN requires an allograft biopsy.[21] In the absence of active viral replication, patients with graft loss due to BKN can safely undergo retransplantation. Active surveillance for BK virus reactivation after transplantation is recommended. Figure 94.7 shows the currently recommended guidelines for post-transplantation screening and monitoring for polyomavirus replication.

Other Infections

Tuberculosis (TB) is an important cause of morbidity and mortality in renal transplant recipients, and its incidence varies according to the prevalence in the general population (e.g., the incidence of TB in transplant recipients has been reported to occur in 0% to 1.3% in the United States, in 0.8% to 1.6% in Spain, in 3.5% in Saudi Arabia, in 11% in South Africa, in 11.8% in India, and in 14.5% in Pakistan).[22] Although TB can be contracted by the inhalation of airborne bacilli, it more commonly emerges due to the reactivation of dormant lesions in the setting of immunosuppressive therapy. Hence, all potential renal transplantation candidates should have a purified protein derivative (PPD) skin test (tuberculin skin test) with controls placed prior to transplantation. A positive skin test or a history of tuberculosis mandates further evaluation to rule out active disease. Isoniazid (INH) prophylaxis for a total of 9 months is recommended for those who have a positive skin test. In patients with a known history of adequately treated TB infection, we have advocated the use of INH prophylaxis the first 9 months after

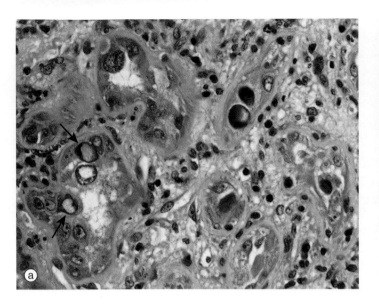

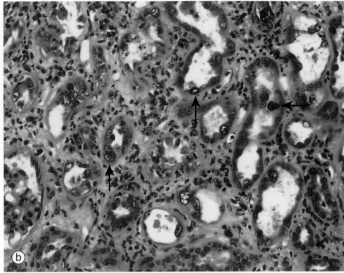

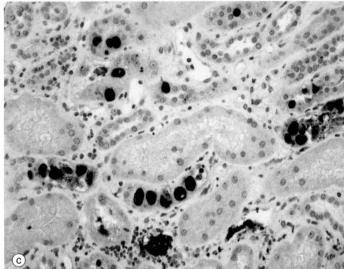

Figure 94.6 BK polyoma virus infection. *a*, Prominent intranuclear viral inclusions are present within tubular epithelial cells (*arrows*) (hematoxylin and eosin, original magnification ×400). *b*, Tubulointerstitial nephritis with diffuse intranuclear polyomavirus inclusions (*arrows*) (hematoxylin and eosin, original magnification ×200). *c*, Immunohistochemistry staining highlights intranuclear polyomavirus inclusions (SV40 immunoperoxidase stain, original magnification ×200). (Courtesy of Charles Lassman and William Dean Wallace.)

transplantation and during intensification of immunosuppression. Others, however, have suggested that INH prophylaxis is not indicated for those patients whose TB had been properly treated.[23] Clinical, radiographic, and/or culture evidence of active TB infection is a contraindication to transplantation.

A rare but important cause of infection in transplant recipients is *Strongyloides*, which is observed particularly in patients from endemic areas such as Southeast Asia. In the presence of immunosuppression, a hyperinfection syndrome may be observed with parasitic pneumonia (Fig. 94.8) and gastrointestinal (GI) involvement.

Immunizations before and after Transplantation

A history of immunization should be obtained in all potential renal transplantation candidates to ensure adequate immunizations for common infections prior to transplantation such as HBV, pneumovax, and other standard immunization appropriate for age. Up-to-date recommendations for routine adult immunizations are available through the Centers for Disease Control and Prevention website (www.cdc.gov/nip/rec/adult-schedule.pdf). Ideally all potential transplantation candidates should complete

all recommended immunizations at least 4 to 6 weeks before transplantation to achieve optimal immune response and to minimize the possibility of live vaccine–derived infection in the post-transplantation period.[15] Household members, close contacts, and health care workers should also be fully immunized.

Live virus or live organism vaccines should be avoided after transplantation. These include measles-mumps-rubella (MMR), live oral polio (which is also contraindicated for household contacts), smallpox (vaccinia), varicella, yellow fever, adenovirus, live oral typhoid (Ty21a), bacille Calmette-Guérin, and intranasal influenza vaccine. Additionally, exposure to persons who have chickenpox or herpes zoster should be avoided until the lesions have crusted over and no new lesions are appearing. Vaccinations using inactivated or killed microorganisms, component, and recombinant moieties are safe for transplant recipients. These include hepatitis A virus and HBV, intramuscular influenza A and B, pneumococcal, *Haemophilus influenzae B*, inactivated-polio vaccine, diphtheria-pertussis-tetanus, and *Neisseria meningitides*.

In general, vaccination should be avoided in the first 6 months post-transplantation. Administration of immunizations during this period may be associated with a higher chance of graft dysfunction and rejection. In addition, vaccinations within the first 6 months

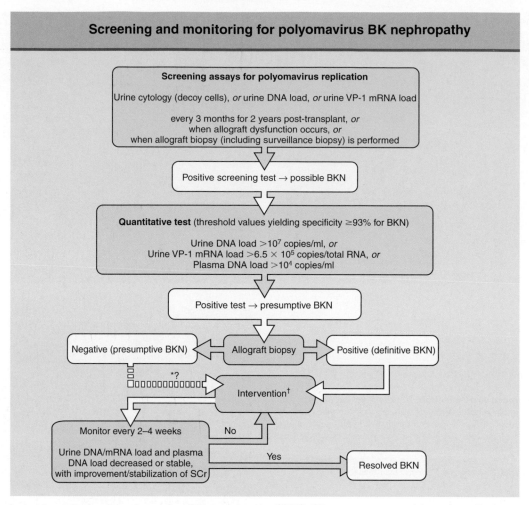

Screening and monitoring for polyomavirus BK nephropathy

Screening assays for polyomavirus replication

Urine cytology (decoy cells), *or* urine DNA load, *or* urine VP-1 mRNA load

every 3 months for 2 years post-transplant, *or*
when allograft dysfunction occurs, *or*
when allograft biopsy (including surveillance biopsy) is performed

Positive screening test → possible BKN

Quantitative test (threshold values yielding specificity ≥93% for BKN)

Urine DNA load >10^7 copies/ml, *or*
Urine VP-1 mRNA load >6.5×10^5 copies/total RNA, *or*
Plasma DNA load >10^4 copies/ml

Positive test → presumptive BKN

Negative (presumptive BKN) ← Allograft biopsy → Positive (definitive BKN)

*?

Intervention†

Monitor every 2–4 weeks — No

Urine DNA/mRNA load and plasma DNA load decreased or stable, with improvement/stabilization of SCr — Yes — Resolved BKN

Figure 94.7 Screening and monitoring for polyomavirus BK nephropathy (BKN). SCr, serum creatinine; (–), negative. *Pre-emptive immunosuppression reduction may be associated with resolution of viremia and decreased incidence of BKN. †See text.

after transplantation may result in ineffective protection due to heavy immunosuppression. For prevention of infection in adult travelers after solid organ transplantation, readers are referred to Kotton and associates.[24] Recommended vaccinations before and after transplantation are listed in Figure 94.9.

TRANSPLANT-ASSOCIATED MALIGNANCIES

Recipients of organ transplants are at an increased risk of developing neoplasms compared to the general population. Similar to post-transplantation infectious complications, the time to occurrence of

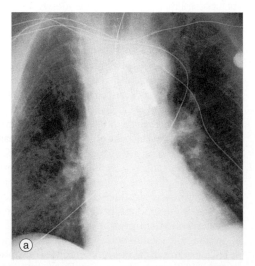
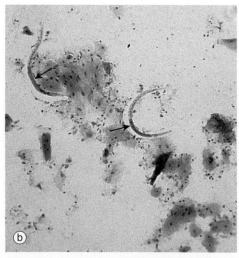

Figure 94.8 Disseminated stronglyodiasis in an immunocompromised patient. *a*, Chest radiograph showing a diffuse bilateral interstitial process. *b*, Gram stain of sputum from the same patient shows filariform lavae of *Strongyloides stercoralis (arrows).* (Courtesy of R. Johnson.)

Recommended immunizations before and after transplantation		
Vaccine	Before	After
Measles/mumps/rubella	Yes	—
Diphtheria/tetanus/pertussis	Yes	Diptheria and tetanus*
Varicella	Yes	Controversial
Poliovirus	Yes	—
Haemophilus influenzae B	Yes	Yes
Influenza	Yes	Yes[†]
Pneumococcus	Yes	Yes[‡]
Hepatitis B	Yes	Yes[§]
Hepatitis A	Yes	Yes[#]

Figure 94.9 Recommended immunizations before and after transplantation. *Booster every 10 years. [†]Annually. [‡]Every 3 to 5 years. [§]Monitor titers. [#]For travelers to endemic areas.

different types of malignancies following transplantation appears to follow a timetable pattern.[25] The Israel Penn International Transplant Tumor Registry data on the time of appearance of different neoplasms following solid organ transplantation is shown in Figure 94.10. Post-transplantation lymphoproliferative disease (PTLD) generally occurs early after transplantation, while skin cancers occur in increasing frequency with time. The intensity and duration of immunosuppression as well as the ability of these agents to promote replication of various oncogenic viruses have been suggested to be important risk factors. The association of human papillomaviruses with cervical and vulvar carcinoma, EBV, with PTLD, HBV, and HCV with hepatocellular carcinoma, and human herpesvirus 8 with Kaposi's sarcoma is well established. Interestingly, transplant recipients show no increase and even a decrease in the incidence of certain neoplasms commonly seen in the general population such as cancer of the lung, breast, prostate, colon, and invasive uterine cancer.[25] Nonetheless, adherence to standard cancer surveillance

Time of appearance of neoplasms following transplantation and initiation of immunosuppression	
Type of Cancer	Median (months)
Lymphomas	12
Kaposi's sarcoma	12.5
Carcinomas of kidney	41
Sarcomas (excluding Kaposi's)	43.5
Carcinomas of cervix	46
Hepatobiliary carcinomas	67.5
Skin cancers	69
Carcinoma of vulva/perineum	113.5
All cancers	46

Figure 94.10 Time of appearance of neoplasms following transplantation and initiation of immunosuppression. (Adapted from Pham PT, Pham PC, Wilkinson AH: Medical and urological complications of pancreas and kidney/pancreas transplantation. In Hakim N, Stratta R, Gray D [eds]: Pancreas and Islet Transplantation. New York: Oxford University Press, 2002, pp 167–189.)

appropriate for age is recommended (Fig. 94.11). In patients with a history of pre-existing malignancies, close monitoring for malignancy recurrences in the post-transplantation period is mandatory. Among the pretransplantation-treated cancers, the highest recurrence rates have been observed with multiple myeloma (67%), nonmelanoma skin cancers (53%), bladder carcinomas (29%), sarcomas (29%), symptomatic renal cell carcinomas (27%), and breast carcinomas (23%).[26] It has been suggested that immunosuppressive therapy facilitates the growth of residual cancers.

Post-transplantation Lymphoproliferative Disorder

PTLD occurs in 1% to 5% of renal and liver transplant recipients; 2% to 3% of pancreas/simultaneous pancreas kidney transplants; 2% to 10% of heart, lung, and heart-lung transplants; and 11% to 15% of recipients of bowel transplants. PTLD is the most common post-transplantation malignancy in children, whereas in adults, it is the second most common malignancy after skin cancer. The high incidence of PTLD observed in thoracic organs and bowel transplants have been largely attributable to the use of more intensive immunosuppression in these patients.

The majority of PTLD is of B cell origin, where >80% to 90% are linked to EBV infection. Based on the World Health Organization classification, PTLD can be divided into three distinct morphologic groups including (a) diffuse B cell hyperplasia, (b) polymorphic PTLD (usually monoclonal), and (c) monomorphic PTLD that includes high-grade invasive lymphoma of B or T lymphocyte centroblasts. Diffuse B cell hyperplasia is usually seen in children and young adults and commonly occurs within the first year after transplantation. Polymorphic PTLD represents the most common type of PTLD in both children and adults and may occur at any time after transplantation. In contrast, monomorphic B cell PTLD is often seen several years after transplantation and may resemble non-Hodgkin's lymphoma similar to that seen in the general population.[27] In a retrospective analysis of the Israel Penn International Transplant Tumor Registry of 402 recipients of kidney transplants, PTLD occurred at a median of 18 months (range, 1 to 310) after transplantation.[28]

PTLD may present with constitutional symptoms such as fevers, night sweats, and weight loss or with localized symptoms of the respiratory tract (such as infection, mass, tonsillitis, or even gingival involvement), GI tract (diarrhea, pain, perforation, bleeding, mass), or central nervous system (headache, seizure, confusion). PTLD involving the renal allograft occurs in 20% to 26% of patients and may mimic acute rejection clinically and histologically. In contrast to lymphomas in the general population where lymph nodes are almost always involved, lymph node involvement is absent in >80% of patients with PTLD.

Risk factors for PTLD include primary EBV infection; younger age; history of CMV disease; immunosuppression with cyclosporine, tacrolimus, or MMF; and use of antilymphocyte antibody such as ATG/ALG or OKT3. A history of pretransplantation malignancy and fewer HLA matches have also been reported to be associated with an increased risk of PTLD. Cyclosporine and tacrolimus may enhance the development of EBV-associated PTLD by directly promoting the survival of EBV-infected B cells; indeed, cyclosporine- and tacrolimus-treated EBV-transformed cells are protected from apoptosis.[25] In contrast, sirolimus has no effect on growth or viability of PTLD-derived lymphoid cell lines.

Reduction or discontinuation of immunosuppressive therapy, particularly antilymphocyte antibody, cyclosporine, tacrolimus, and MMF, is recommended as first-line treatment while prednisone is increased to 10 to 15 mg/day to prevent allograft rejection.

Preventive care recommendations for adult cancer surveillance			
Screening for	Starting at Age	Preventive Care	Screening Frequency
Colorectal cancer	Average risk: 50	Colonoscopy *or* FOBT + Flexible sigmoidoscopy	Colonoscopy: every 10 years FOBT: every year Flex sig: every 5 years
	Increased risk: 40	Colonoscopy *or* *or*	(a) Every 5 years if a parent or sibling had colorectal cancer at ≤ 60 years of age (b) At 10 years younger than the youngest family member with cancer (c) Every 10 years if the relative was 60 years (d) Consider referral to medical genetics if two or more first-degree relatives had colorectal cancer
Females			
Breast cancer	40	Breast exam and screening mammography	*Every year for 3 years*
	Before age 30 (if mother or sister had breast cancer)		
Cervical cancer	18	Pap smear and pelvic exam	*Every year for 3 years* If all three smears are normal, begin having pap smear every 3 years if patient does not have any of the following risk factors: HIV positivity Infection with certain types of HPV Cigarette smoking Multiple sex partners Prior abnormal pap smear or cervical dysplasia Chronic immunosuppression for organ transplantation Every year if patient has any of the above risk factors
Males			
Prostate cancer	50 (40*)	Digital rectal exam and PSA testing	*Every year* Discuss with your physician

Figure 94.11 Preventive care recommendations for adult cancer surveillance. *If African American, a family history of prostate cancer, or receiving long-term immunosuppression for organ transplantation. Flex sig, flexible sigmoidoscopy; FOBT, fecal occult blood testing; HIV, human immunodeficiency virus; HPV, human papillomavirus; PSA, prostate specific antigen. (Adapted from the Cleveland Clinic Foundation Cancer Surveillance Task Force, 2001.)

Sirolimus has a strong antiproliferative effect on PTLD-derived B cell lines,[29] but whether sirolimus may limit B cell lymphoma growth while simultaneously providing immunosuppression to prevent graft rejection awaits studies. Acyclovir or ganciclovir therapy and reduction in immunosuppression may be beneficial and curative in benign polyclonal B cell proliferation. The role of antiviral therapy in B cell monoclonal malignant transformation is less well defined. Fifty percent to 90% mortality has been reported despite antiviral therapy. Surgical resection, with or without adjunctive local radiation, has been suggested for localized disease. Local radiation has been advocated as the treatment of choice for PTLD involving the central nervous system.

In lesions not amenable to surgery or for more aggressive monoclonal types of PTLD, chemotherapy has been used with favorable results compared to reduction in immunosuppression alone. The most frequently used regimen includes CHOP (cyclophosphamide, Adriamycin, vincristine, and prednisone) and VAPEC-B (Adriamycin, etoposide, cyclophosphamide, methotrexate, bleomycin, and vincristine). Adverse effects of chemotherapy include high mortality rates from sepsis and treatment-related toxicities. Rituximab, a chimeric monoclonal antibody with murine variable regions targeting the CD20 antigen and human IgG1-κ constant regions, has antitumor activity against CD20-expressing B cell lymphomas. Early experience with rituximab (two to six weekly doses of 375 mg/m²) in patients with PTLD (in conjunction with reduction in immunosuppression) has shown promising results.[27] Longer-term results are needed to determine relapse rates. Remission has also been reported with cytokine-based therapy such as interferon-α and anti–interleukin-6. The routine use of either agent, however, is yet to be validated as an increased risk of allograft rejection is seen with the former and clinical experience remains limited with the latter.

Factors that adversely affect survival include multiple versus single site involvement, increasing age, B cell predominance, the use of ALG/ATG and OKT3, and early versus late onset (within 6 to 12 months versus >12 months). For patients with PTLD restricted to the renal allograft alone, transplant nephrectomy may improve survival.

Skin Cancer

Skin cancers are the most common *de novo* post-transplantation tumors in the adult transplant recipient population and may occur 20 to 30 years earlier in immunosuppressed patients compared to the general population. Furthermore, the incidence of skin cancers may be up to 20 times higher in sun-exposed areas and seven times higher in non–sun-exposed areas.[25]

Risk factors for skin cancers among immunosuppressed post-transplant recipients include light skin color, intensity of sun exposure, and duration of follow-up following transplantation. Geographic risks for the development of skin cancers appear to reflect higher sun exposure areas including residence in Australia and countries at higher altitudes such as Canada, Sweden, and Scotland. Azathioprine has been particularly associated with an increased risk of skin cancer. In addition, immunosuppression in combination with enhanced sunlight exposure may induce malignant changes in papilloma-induced warts.

The clinical presentation of skin cancers differs in transplant recipients compared to the general population.[25] First, the incidence of squamous cell carcinoma is approximately twice that of basal cell carcinoma (up to 16:1 in Australia) among transplant recipients compared to a ratio of 0.2:1.0 in the general population. Second, multiple cancerous lesions of different types may be observed (i.e., concomitant appearance of squamous cell carcinoma and basal cell carcinoma). Third, malignant melanoma is twice as common. Fourth, skin cancers in transplant recipients tend to behave more aggressively with a higher incidence of metastatic disease and mortality (5.8% versus 1% to 2%).

Interestingly, recent studies have demonstrated a lower incidence of skin cancer with sirolimus-based therapy without cyclosporine or sirolimus maintenance therapy after early cyclosporine withdrawal compared to those who remained on cyclosporine and sirolimus combination therapy.[30] It is conceivable that the protective effect of sirolimus against skin cancer is due to its inhibition of several ultraviolet ray–induced mechanisms involved in skin carcinogenesis.

COMMON LABORATORY ABNORMALITIES

Anemia

Mild anemia is common in the early post-transplantation period, but generally improves within several weeks to months. Assessment of baseline iron stores at the time of transplantation may be invaluable and, if present, should be treated with intravenous iron as tolerated. Erythropoietin therapy is generally effective in patients who have impaired allograft function and adequate iron stores. Refractory or severe anemia mandates aggressive evaluation to exclude the possibility of surgical postoperative bleeding or other possibilities including GI bleed, tertiary hyperparathyroidism, underlying inflammatory conditions, or parvovirus B19 infection. Sirolimus, MMF, azathioprine, ACE inhibitors, and ARBs may also cause or exacerbate anemia. Sirolimus inhibits erythropoiesis by interfering with intracellular signaling in erythroid cells,[31] and while it may correct with higher doses of erythropoietin, in some cases erythropoietin-resistant anemia may result.

Leukopenia and Thrombocytopenia

Leukopenia and thrombocytopenia may occur in transplant recipients and are usually due to side effects from azathioprine, MMF, antilymphocyte antibody treatment, sirolimus,[32,33] and trimethoprim-sulfamethoxazole. Withholding the offending agent or dose reduction generally corrects these hematologic abnormalities. Severe leukopenia may require treatment with granulocyte-stimulating factor. The presence of thrombocytopenia and hemolytic anemia should also raise the possibility of thrombotic microangiopathy, whereas low platelets and low leukocyte counts may be seen with CMV infection. Parvovirus B19 infection may present with refractory anemia, pancytopenia, and thrombotic microangiopathy.

Erythrocytosis

Post-transplantation erythrocytosis (PTE) occurs in 20% to 25% of transplant recipients within the first 2 years. Diagnosis is based on excluding secondary causes such as renal artery stenosis, polycystic kidney disease, renal cell carcinoma, cerebellar hemangioblastoma, or chronic hypoxia in heavy tobacco users as clinically indicated.[6]

Risk factors for PTE include the presence of native kidneys, male gender, excellent graft function and the absence of rejection episodes, smoking, hypertension, and diabetes mellitus. Suggested pathogenic mechanism(s) include defective feedback regulation of erythropoietin metabolism, direct stimulation of erythroid precursors by angiotensin II, and/or abnormalities in circulating insulin-like growth factor-I levels (IGF-I).[6] Erythropoietin levels are inconsistently elevated. Treatment is recommended for hemoglobin (Hb) levels >17 to 18 g/dl or hematocrit level >52% to 55% due to the risk of thromboembolic complications, hypertension, and headaches. Both ACE inhibitors and ARBs help correct PTE, although phlebotomy is occasionally necessary. In one study, treatment with enalapril 5 mg/day resulted in a greater reduction in Hb levels compared to therapy with losartan 50 mg. The better reduction in Hb levels in enalapril-treated patients was associated with a reduction in circulating IGF-I levels that was not observed in the losartan-treated patients.[34]

Hyperkalemia

Mild hyperkalemia is common, especially in the early post-transplantation period when relatively high-dose calcineurin inhibitors are given. It is often associated with a type IV renal tubular acidosis with mild hyperchloremic acidosis and urine with an acidic pH. Suggested mechanism(s) of calcineurin inhibitor–induced hyperkalemia include hyporeninemic hypoaldosteronism, aldosterone resistance, end-organ defect in potassium excretion, or inhibition of cortical collecting duct potassium secretory channels.[6] Cyclosporine decreases Na^+-K^+-ATPase activity in K^+ secretory cells in the cortical and outer medullary collecting tubules, thereby decreasing intracellular K^+ accumulation required for urinary secretion.

In patients receiving calcineurin inhibitors, a potassium level between 5.2 and 5.5 mmol/l is common and generally does not require treatment. However, dietary potassium restriction is recommended (2 g/day [52 mmol/day]). Higher potassium levels, especially in the presence of drugs that may exacerbate hyperkalemia such as ACE inhibitors, ARBs, or β-blockers may require treatment. Caution should be used when a potassium-containing phosphorus supplement is prescribed. Although trimethoprim can cause hyperkalemia via an amiloride-like effect, the routine use of low-dose trimethoprim-sulfamethoxazole for pneumocystis and urinary tract infection prophylaxis is rarely the cause of significant hyperkalemia in renal transplant recipients.

Most patients respond to diuretics, and this therapy is appropriate since volume expansion and hypertension are common. Potassium exchange resin (sodium polystyrene or kayexalate) is occasionally needed. In the event of life-threatening hyperkalemia, more aggressive approaches are required (see Chapter 9).

Hypokalemia

Sirolimus may be associated with hypokalemia, possibly due to renal potassium wasting. In an early trial using sirolimus, azathioprine, and corticosteroids, hypokalemia occurred in 34%, and potassium supplementation was required in 27% of patients.[32] This finding has been confirmed in a separate trial.[33]

Hypophosphatemia

Hypophosphatemia is common following successful renal transplantation and may represent persistent hyperparathyroidism (in which hypercalcemia is usually present), primary renal phosphate wasting syndrome, or even malnutrition. Early after transplantation, hypophosphatemia has been attributed to a massive initial diuresis, particularly following a living-donor renal transplant, defective renal phosphate reabsorption due to allograft injury, glycosuria, magnesium depletion, and corticosteroid use, the latter by inhibiting proximal tubular reabsorption of phosphate. A non–parathyroid hormone (PTH) circulating factor (possibly phosphatonin, also known as FGF-23, see Chapters 10 and 74) has also been suggested to cause hypophosphatemia early after a successful kidney transplantation by increasing the fractional excretion of phosphate.[35] Treatment of hypophosphatemia involves correcting the underlying conditions and phosphate replacement therapy. Mild hypophosphatemia (<0.65 mmol/l or 2 mg/dl) can be managed with a high phosphorus dietary intake, while oral or intravenous phosphate supplementation may be necessary for more severe hypophosphatemia.

Hypercalcemia

Hypercalcemia after transplantation is generally due to persistent secondary hyperparathyroidism. The concomitant presence of severe hypophosphatemia, particularly in patients with excellent graft function, may exacerbate hypercalcemia through stimulation of renal proximal tubular 1α-hydroxylase. Resolution of soft-tissue calcifications, high-dose corticosteroid therapy, and immobilization are potential contributing factors. In two thirds of cases, hypercalcemia resolves spontaneously within 6 to 12 months. However, spontaneous resolution occurs in less than half of those whose hypercalcemia existed before transplantation. Severe hypercalcemia or persistent hypercalcemia (>12 months) requires further evaluation. Initial assessment should include an intact parathyroid hormone level. Imaging studies including neck ultrasonography or parathyroid technetium 99mTc-sestamibi scan should be done at the clinician's discretion to exclude parathyroid adenoma or parathyroid gland hyperplasia and/or hyperplastic nodular formation of the parathyroid glands. Parathyroidectomy is warranted in patients with tertiary hyperparathyroidism or persistent severe hypercalcemia for >6 to 12 months, symptomatic or progressive hypercalcemia, nephrolithiasis, persistent metabolic bone disease, calcium-related renal allograft dysfunction, or progressive vascular calcification and calciphylaxis.[36]

Persistent hyperparathyroidism has generally been attributed to continued autonomous production of PTH from nodular hyperplastic glands, reduced density of calcitriol receptors, and decreased expression of the membrane calcium sensor receptors that render cells more resistant to physiologic concentrations of calcitriol and calcium. The risk of developing persistent hyperparathyroidism is increased with the duration of dialysis and the severity of pretransplantation hyperparathyroidism.

In a recent study involving 11 renal transplant recipients with persistent hyperparathyroidism (>6 months post-transplantation) and good allograft function (creatinine clearance >40 ml/min per 1.73 m²) treatment with cinacalcet (a calcium-sensing receptor antagonist) resulted in significant reduction in serum calcium and PTH levels with an increase in serum phosphate and unchanged calcium × phosphate product.[37] In a separate study, cinacalcet treatment also decreased serum calcium; however, unlike the prior study, there was a slight reduction in renal allograft function at months 2 and 3.[38] Further studies on the safety and efficacy of cinacalcet in renal transplant recipients are warranted.

Hypomagnesemia

Hypomagnesemia is a common side effect of calcineurin inhibitors and is due to urinary magnesium wasting. Sirolimus has also been shown to cause urinary magnesium wasting and hypomagnesemia.

Other contributory factors include loop diuretic therapy, postobstructive polyuria, and/or renal tubular acidosis. In addition, the propensity toward hypomagnesemia may be more pronounced among diabetics. In the first 3 months following transplantation, a magnesium level <0.62 mmol/l (1.5 mg/dl) is common. Dietary magnesium intake is usually insufficient and high-dose oral magnesium supplement (i.e., 400 to 800 mg magnesium oxide three times daily) may be required for treatment. Intravenous magnesium is administered in severe hypomagnesemia (<0.4 mmol/l or 1.0 mg/dl), particularly in patients with a history of coronary artery disease or cardiac arrhythmias and in those taking digitalis. Aggressive treatment may benefit renal transplant recipients by improving lipid profiles (decreased total cholesterol, decreased LDL, and decreased total cholesterol/HDL ratio), cyclosporine-induced neurotoxicity, and hypertension.

Abnormal Liver Function Tests

Elevated hepatic enzymes (transaminases) are common in the early post-transplantation period and usually due to drug-related toxicity. Potential culprits include acyclovir, ganciclovir, trimethoprim-sulfamethoxazole, cyclosporine, tacrolimus, sirolimus, statin therapy, and proton pump inhibitors. Cyclosporine and, less commonly, tacrolimus, may cause transient, self-limited, dose-dependent elevations of transaminase levels and mild hyperbilirubinemia secondary to defective bile secretion. Drug-related hepatotoxicity usually improves or resolves following drug discontinuation or dose reduction.

Persistent or severe elevation in hepatic liver enzymes should prompt further evaluation to exclude infectious causes including CMV, HBV, and HCV. In high-risk candidates for primary CMV infections (recipient seronegative, donor seropositive), it may occasionally be necessary to initiate CMV therapy while awaiting laboratory results, particularly, when there is a high index of clinical suspicion (fever, fatigue, malaise, gastroenteritis, leukopenia, and/or thrombocytopenia). Evidence of post-transplantation HBV reactivation should be treated with lamivudine (elevated alanine aminotransferase, histologic hepatitis, and serum DNA >10⁵ copies/ml). Some programs routinely initiate lamivudine prophylaxis in all HBsAg–positive candidates at the time of transplantation. Pretransplantation lamivudine prophylactic therapy is recommended in renal transplantation candidates who have HBV DNA >10⁵ copies/ml and active liver disease defined as alanine aminotransferase more than two times the upper limit of normal or biopsy-proven hepatic disease.[39]

There is currently no effective treatment for chronic HCV in renal transplant recipients. Although treatment with interferon-α may result in clearance of HCV RNA in 25% to 50% of cases, rapid relapse following drug withdrawal is nearly universal. More importantly, interferon-α treatment may precipitate acute allograft rejection and graft loss and is therefore not recommended. Management of HCV infection in this patient population should rely on reduction of immunosuppressive therapy. Since corticosteroid therapy and antilymphocyte antibody treatment may enhance viral replication and increase the risk of progression to cirrhosis, it is advisable to avoid antilymphocyte antibody induction therapy and minimize steroid dose in transplant recipients with chronic HCV infection. Although early reports suggested that MMF may reduce HCV replication and delay the recurrence of HCV in the transplant recipient,[40] the antiviral properties of MMF and its impact on HCV replication and HCV recurrence have not been consistently demonstrated[41] in subsequent studies. A suggested algorithm for the management of renal transplant recipients with elevated hepatic enzymes is shown in Figure 94.12.

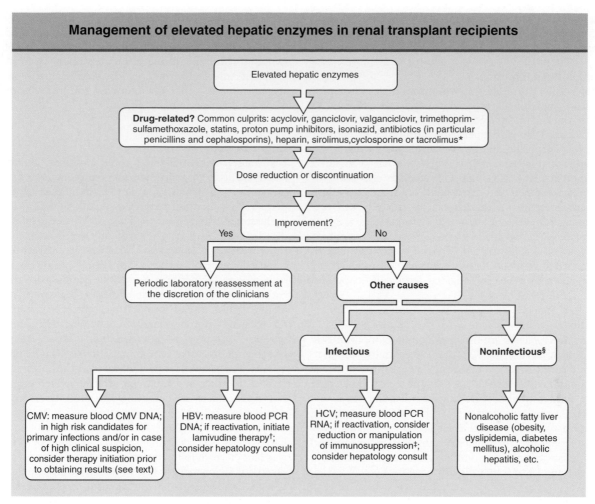

Figure 94.12 **Suggested algorithm for the management of elevated hepatic enzymes in renal transplant recipients.** *Cyclosporine and less commonly tacrolimus may cause transient, self-limited, dose-dependent elevations of aminotransferase levels and mild hyperbilirubinemia secondary to defective bile secretin. †Some programs routinely start lamivudine prophylactic therapy in all hepatitis B virus surface antigen–positive candidates at the time of transplantation. ‡There is currently no effective treatment for chronic hepatitis C in renal transplant recipients (see text). §Appropriate evaluation and management similar to nontransplantation settings. CMV, cytomegalovirus; PCR, polymerase chain reaction.

GASTROINTESTINAL DISEASE

Post-transplantation GI complications are common as they can arise from a number of etiologies involving drugs, infections, mucosal injury and ulceration, biliary tract diseases, diverticular diseases, perforations, pancreatitis, and malignancy.[42] Only selected complications are discussed; for a comprehensive review of post-transplantation GI complications, readers are referred to Helderman and Goral.[42]

Drug-related Gastrointestinal Complications

MMF commonly causes GI side effects, including nausea, vomiting, dyspepsia, anorexia, flatulence, and diarrhea. Dose reduction, transient discontinuation of the drug, or dividing the dose into three or four times daily often ameliorates or resolves the symptoms. The enteric-coated formulation of MMF, developed to improve GI tolerability, has not been shown to be better than the original formulation. Nonetheless, switching to enteric-coated MMF has resulted in symptomatic relief in a subset of patients (unpublished observations).

Sirolimus may cause oral mucocutaneous lesions and should be differentiated from those related to viral causes such as herpetic

or CMV infections. Drug-related oral ulcers usually resolve after discontinuation of the offending agent. Sirolimus, tacrolimus, and cyclosporine have all been suggested to cause diarrhea to variable extents.

Infections

Post-transplantation infections of the GI tract may be viral, fungal, or bacterial in etiology. Viral infections are most commonly caused by CMV and HSV, whereas C. *albicans* and C. *tropicalis* are common opportunistic fungal infections. Commonly encountered bacterial pathogens include *Clostridium difficile* and *Helicobacter pylori*.

Cytomegalovirus Infection

CMV can affect any segment of the GI tract and remains an important cause of morbidity and mortality in recipients of organ transplantation. Clinical signs and symptoms may include dysphagia, odynophagia, (pain on swallowing), nausea, vomiting, gastroparesis, abdominal pain, diarrhea, or GI bleeding.[42] Leukopenia and/or elevated transaminases are common. Persistent or unexplained symptoms of nausea, vomiting, or diarrhea, particularly in the early post-transplantation period or during intensification of immunosuppression, warrant further investigation with upper and/or lower endoscopies and biopsies. Risk factors and management of CMV infection are discussed in the section on infectious diseases.

Herpes Simplex Virus Infection

HSV infection results primarily from reactivation of endogenous latent virus causing clinical infection within the first 1 to 2 months after transplantation. Patients commonly present with oral mucocutaneous lesions or gingivostomatitis with or without odynophagia and dysphagia due to esophageal involvement. An increased incidence of herpes simplex esophagitis has been noted to occur in patients receiving high-dose steroids and antilymphocyte preparations for the treatment of acute rejection. Limited oral mucocutaneous lesions can be treated with oral acyclovir, whereas extensive infections may require intravenous acyclovir or ganciclovir, particularly when there is concomitant CMV or EBV infection. Untreated herpetic ulcers can lead to hemorrhage or esophageal perforation. Hence, unexplained GI symptoms should be further investigated with endoscopy and biopsy.

Fungal Infections

C. *albicans* and C. *tropicalis* are the most common opportunistic fungal organisms affecting the GI tract after transplantation. Patients may present with stomatitis or epiglottitis, with or without odynophagia or dysphagia due to esophagitis. GI bleeding or perforation with formation of tracheoesophageal fistulas has been reported. Prophylactic nystatin swish and swallow during the first post-transplantation month is recommended. In high-risk candidates, including liver or pancreas transplant recipients and those receiving antilymphocyte antibody therapy, fluconazole prophylactic therapy (3 to 6 months) is warranted.

Clostridium *Infection*

C. *difficile* infection encompasses a wide spectrum of clinical syndromes including asymptomatic carrier states, diarrhea and intestinal obstruction to fulminant pseudomembranous colitis with toxic megacolon and perforation. Rarely intra-abdominal abscesses and bacteremia may occur.[15] In recipients of solid organ transplants, C. *difficile* colitis has been reported to occur in 3.5% to 16% of patients.[43] Suggested risk factors include young recipient age (<5 years), female gender, the use of monoclonal antibodies to treat acute rejection episodes, and intra-abdominal graft placement. Among transplant recipients receiving antimicrobial therapy, C. *difficile*–associated diarrhea develops in approximately 50% of patients.[43] In mild cases, oral metronidazole is as effective as oral vancomycin and is the preferred first-line treatment. Treatment failure, however, requires treatment with oral vancomycin. In severely ill patients with GI dysmotility or ileus where oral agents may not reach the colonic mucosa, metronidazole should be administered intravenously.[15]

Helicobacter *Infection*

H. *pylori* infection may also cause gastritis and peptic ulcer disease in transplant recipients. Treatment should include a triple-drug regimen consisting of two antibiotics and an acid-suppressive agent such as an H_2-blocker or a proton pump inhibitor. In recipients of an orthotopic heart transplant, triple-drug therapy resulted in a lower eradication rate compared to the general population, suggesting that immunosuppression may hinder the clearance of H. *pylori*. Unexplained dyspeptic or reflux symptoms should be investigated further with endoscopy

and biopsy to exclude malignancy. An increased risk of gastric cancer–associated with H. *pylori* infection has been reported. More recently, cases of mucosa-associated lymphoid tissue (MALT) lymphoma have been described in renal transplant recipients infected with H. *pylori*. MALT lymphoma may be less aggressive than other lymphomas, and the disorder may be cured by eradication of H. *pylori*.[44]

Colon Disorders

Post-transplantation colonic complications may be life threatening and difficult to diagnose because symptoms may be masked by immunosuppressive therapy, particularly in the early postoperative period. The major disease entities include diverticulitis and colonic perforations. The former may be related to the high incidence of diverticulosis in end-stage renal disease patients, particularly in those with adult polycystic kidney disease. Diverticulitis complicated by perforation, abscess formation, phlegmon, or fistula has been reported to occur in 1.1% of renal transplant recipients.[42] In patients with polycystic kidney disease and symptoms suggestive of diverticular disease or in those with documented history of diverticulitis, pretransplantation screening with either a barium enema or colonoscopy is warranted. Pretransplantation surgical resection of extensive symptomatic disease should be considered.

Post-transplantation perforations of the GI tract commonly involve the colon and can be arbitrarily divided into those occurring early and those occurring late after transplantation. Early perforations have largely been attributed to heavy immunosuppression, particularly with high-dose corticosteroids, diverticulitis, CMV colitis, and intestinal ischemia, whereas perforations occurring late or years following transplantation are commonly due to diverticulosis or malignancy. Mortality from colonic perforations is high, although aggressive diagnostic evaluation and treatment may improve prognosis. Management includes prompt exterioration of the perforated colon, early and broad-spectrum antimicrobial therapy, and minimization of immunosuppressive therapy.

MUSCULOSKELETAL DISORDERS

Osteoporosis

Post-transplantation reduction in bone mineral density (BMD) is most pronounced in the first 6 to 12 months and correlates with higher corticosteroid exposure in the early post-transplantation period. The rate of bone loss varies from 3% to 10% and is most apparent in the lumbar spine or axial skeleton. This early rapid decrease in BMD is usually followed by a slower rate of bone loss and reflects cumulative steroid dose. Nonetheless, controversies exist as to whether bone loss continues to decline, stabilizes, or even reverses after the first year.[45] A decrease in BMD averaging 1.7% per year in later post-transplantation years has been reported, whereas stabilization during the second year, followed by an improvement of 1% to 2% per year thereafter, was observed by others.[46] Yet, osteopenia and osteoporosis prevalence rates range from 31% to 41%, respectively, 20 years after renal transplantation.[47]

Corticosteroids act on the skeletal system by directly inhibiting osteoblastogenesis and cause apoptosis of osteoblasts and osteocytes. Other adverse effects of corticosteroids include inhibition of intestinal calcium absorption, enhancement of renal calcium excretion, secondary hyperparathyroidism, and direct suppression of gonadal hormones. Other factors that may contribute to post-transplantation BMD loss include the duration of chronic kidney disease and dialysis, persistent metabolic acidosis, persistent hyperparathyroidism, vitamin D deficiency or resistance, phosphate depletion, diabetes mellitus, hypogonadism, and smoking. Experimental animal models suggest that cyclosporine and tacrolimus may also contribute to post-transplantation bone loss by stimulating bone resorption. The effects of calcineurin inhibitor in humans remains speculative, although increasing alkaline phosphatase and osteocalcin and increased osteoblast and osteoclast activity have been reported with cyclosporine treatment relative to azathioprine. Although Heaf and coworkers[45] have previously related low whole body and lumbar spine BMD to high cyclosporine concentrations, a number of studies have shown no or only minor toxic effect of cyclosporine on bone.

Evaluation of patients for bone loss or osteoporosis relies on the measurement of BMD using dual-energy x-ray absorptiometry (DEXA) scan. The T scores obtained by the DEXA scan are based on BMD comparisons with young adults and are used to describe a fracture threshold (>2.0 standard deviations [SDs] below the mean reference value of young adults) and osteoporosis itself (>2.5 SD below).

Preventive measures to minimize post-transplantation bone loss should be initiated early after transplantation. Adequate calcium and vitamin D supplementation is generally recommended to prevent rapid bone loss in the first post-transplantation year. In long-term, stable transplant recipients, corticosteroids should be kept at a safe minimum. Early steroid withdrawal during the first post-transplantation year has been shown to significantly reduce the incidence of osteoporosis and should be considered in low immunologic risk candidates. Patients with established osteoporosis, particularly those at risk of osteoporosis-related fracture, should receive oral bisphosphonates, calcium, and vitamin D supplements. For those who cannot tolerate oral bisphosphonates, calcitonin nasal spray may be a useful alternative. However, in the presence of adynamic bone disease, bisphosphonate therapy is not recommended due to its potential oversuppression of bone metabolism. Unless contraindicated, estrogen replacement therapy should be considered in postmenopausal transplant recipients. In patients with an intact uterus, progesterone must also be given to prevent endometrial cancer. Although testosterone deficiency has been implicated in the development of bone loss and fractures following transplantation, the role of hormonal replacement therapy in men with hypogonadism is less well defined. Smoking cessation, avoidance of excess alcohol and/or caffeine consumption, and weight-bearing exercise should be encouraged. Caution should be exercised to prevent stress fractures in diabetic patients with peripheral neuropathy.

Avascular Necrosis

Post-transplantation osteonecrosis (avascular necrosis [AVN]) occurs at an incidence of 3% to 16%[45] and most commonly affects the femoral head and neck. It usually occurs within the first few years after transplantation and may affect other joints including the knees, shoulders, and, less commonly, ankles, elbows, and wrists. Early avascular necrosis of the femoral head commonly presents with hip or groin pain and/or referral knee pain. Symptoms may be aggravated by weight bearing but may also be paradoxically worse at night. Use of crutches to avoid weight bearing on the affected side is advisable. Core decompression with or without bone grafting before the femoral head collapse may relieve pain, but approximately 60% of cases require total hip arthroplasty.[48] Drastic corticosteroid dose reduction or discontinuation has little if any effect on altering the course of established AVN and may

jeopardize renal allograft function. Magnetic resonance imaging is the most sensitive technique for early detection. Plain radiographs are of limited diagnostic value in the early stage. Predisposing factors for the development of AVN include greater exposure to intravenous corticosteroid pulse therapy, low bone mass, hyperparathyroidism, increasing dialysis duration, excessive weight gain, hyperlipidemia, and microvascular thrombosis. Recent studies have shown that renal transplant recipients maintained on steroid-free immunosuppressive regimen have had low rates of AVN at 3-year follow-up.[49] More recently, the use of cyclosporine compared to tacrolimus has been implicated as a risk factor for AVN, possibly due to lower prednisolone dose in the tacrolimus-versus cyclosporine-treated groups. Whether tacrolimus has a more favorable effect on post-transplantation bone disease compared to cyclosporine remains to be determined.

Gout

Hyperuricemia and gout are common among renal transplant recipients receiving cyclosporine-based immunosuppression with a reported prevalence of 30% to 84% and 2% to 28%, respectively.[50] Cyclosporine impairs renal excretion of uric acid secondary to decreased filtration due to the associated decrease in glomerular filtration rate (GFR) as well as increased net uric acid reabsorption by the proximal tubule. Potential contributing risk factors for the development of post-transplantation hyperuricemia and gouty arthritis include diuretic use, pretransplantation hyperuricemia, allograft impairment, and obesity. Although tacrolimus may also cause hyperuricemia, cases of gout associated with tacrolimus appear rare.

Management of the acute gouty attack includes topical ice and rest of the inflamed joint. Pharmacologic treatments include colchicine, increased corticosteroid dose, or nonsteroidal anti-inflammatory drugs (NSAIDs). The use of NSAIDs, however, should be avoided in patients with impaired allograft function (GFR <60 ml/min). Other treatment options have included intra-articular steroids and parenteral adrenocorticotropic hormone—the latter being reserved for patients with multiple medical problems such as allograft impairment, GI bleeding, or gouty arthritis refractory to conventional therapy.

Management of chronic gout is directed at lowering uric acid levels. Allopurinol, a xanthine oxidase inhibitor, should be started at a low dose (100 to 200 mg/day), particularly in the presence of impaired allograft function since renal insufficiency predisposes to severe allopurinol toxicity due to retention of the metabolite oxipurinol.[50] Allopurinol should be used cautiously in patients taking azathioprine due to the inhibition of azathioprine metabolism by allopurinol. Dose reduction of both drugs may be necessary (i.e., azathioprine dose may be quartered and allopurinol initiated at 100 mg/day with close monitoring). Complete blood count and hepatic and renal function should be monitored closely. Allopurinol dose reduction is not necessary in patients taking MMF. In allopurinol-allergic patients with preserved allograft function (GFR >50 ml/min) and no history of urolithiasis, uricosuric agents such as probenecid or losartan (an ARB that uniquely reduces serum uric acid) can be used.

Long-term prophylaxis may include reduction or discontinuation of diuretics, long-term allopurinol therapy, dietary modification, and consideration of alternative immunosuppressive therapy. Cyclosporine to tacrolimus switch has been reported to result in resolution of severe polyarticular gout refractory to conventional therapy. Small doses of colchicine at 0.5 or 0.6 mg/day may also prevent recurrent gouty attacks.

OUTPATIENT CARE

The frequency of outpatient clinic visits may vary between centers. We recommend that patients be seen two to three times weekly for the first 2 weeks after transplantation, twice weekly for the next 2 weeks, and weekly for the next month. After the first 2 months, the frequency of outpatient visits depends on the complexity of the patient's early postoperative course. Patients with stable graft function and an uneventful postoperative course can return to work or their regular daily activities 2 to 3 months post-transplantation. Laboratory assessment during the first month after transplantation should include serum creatinine, immunosuppressive drug levels, a complete blood count with platelets, urinalysis, electrolytes, and a comprehensive metabolic panel. After the first post-transplantation month, pertinent laboratory evaluation should be performed at the discretion of the clinician. After the first post-transplantation year, annual follow-up at a transplantation center is generally recommended.

REFERENCES

1. Hollar K, Butterly D: Team management of cardiovascular disease after transplantation. Graft 2005;7:62–73.
2. Opelz G, Wujciak T, Ritz E, et al: Association of chronic kidney graft failure with recipient blood pressure. Kidney Int 1998;53:217–222.
3. Kasiske BL, Chakkera HA, Roel J: Explained and unexplained ischemic heart disease risk after renal transplantation. J Am Soc Nephrol 2000;11:1735–1743.
4. de Champlain J, Karas M, Nguyen P, et al: Different effects of nifedipine and amlodipine on circulating catecholamine levels in essential hypertensive patients. J Hypertens 1998;16:1357–1369.
5. Hjelmesaeth J, Hartmann A, Kofstad J, et al: Tapering off prednisolone and cyclosporine the first year after renal transplantation: The effect on glucose tolerance. Nephrol Dial Transplant 2001;16:829–835.
6. Pham PT, Pham PC, Wilkinson AH: The early management of the renal transplant recipient. In Davidson AM, Cameron JS, Grunfeld JP, et al (eds): Oxford Textbook of Clinical Nephrology, 3rd ed. New York: Oxford University Press, 2005, pp 2087–2101.
7. Ballantyne CM, Corsini A, Davidson MH, et al: Risk for myopathy with statin therapy in high-risk patients. Arch Intern Med 2003;163:553–564.
8. Canzanello VJ, Schwartz L, Tater SJ, et al: Evolution of cardiovascular risk after liver transplantation: A comparison of cyclosporine A and tacrolimus FK(506). Liver Transpl Surg 1997;3:1–9.
9. Ducloux D, Motte G, Challier B, et al: Serum total homocysteine and cardiovascular disease occurrence in chronic, stable renal transplant recipients: A prospective study. J Am Nephrol 2000;11:134–137.
10. Winkelmayer WC, Kramar R, Curhan GC, et al: Fasting plasma total homocysteine levels and mortality and allograft loss in kidney transplant recipients: A prospective study. J Am Soc Nephrol 2005;16:255–260.
11. Marcucci R, Zanazzi M, Bertoni E, et al: Vitamin supplementation reduces the progression of atherosclerosis in hyperhomocysteinemic renal-transplant recipients. Transplantation 2003;9:1551–1555.
12. Fishman JA, Rubin RH: Infection in organ transplant recipients. N Engl J Med 1998;338:1741–1751.
13. Fishman JA, Ramos E: Infection in renal transplant recipients. In Pereira BJG, Sayegh MH, Blake P (eds): Chronic Kidney Disease, Dialysis, and Transplantation, 2nd ed. Philadelphia: Elsevier Saunders, 2005, pp 681–697.
14. Hadaya K, Wunderdi W, Deffernez C, et al: Monitoring of cytomegalovirus infection in solid-organ transplant recipients by an ultrasensitive plasma PCR. J Clin Microbiol 2003;41:3757–3764.
15. Kubak BM, Maree CL, Pegues D, et al: Infections in kidney transplantation. In Danovitch GM (ed): Handbook of Kidney Transplantation, 4th ed. Philadelphia: Lippincott Williams & Wilkins, 2005, pp 279–333.
16. Humar A, Siegal D, Moussa G, et al: A prospective assessment of valganciclovir for the treatment of cytomegalovirus infection and disease in transplant recipients. J Infect Dis 2005;192:1154–1157.
17. Wali RK, Drachenberg C, Hirsch HH, et al: BK virus-associated nephropathy in renal allograft recipients: Rescue therapy by sirolimus-based immunosuppression. Transplantation 2004;74:1069–1073.
18. Vats A, Shapiro R, Randhawa PS, et al: Quantitative viral load monitoring and cidofovir therapy for the management of BK virus-associated nephropathy in children and adults. Transplantation 2003;75:102–112.
19. Cibrik DM, O'Toole JF, Norman SP, et al: IVIG for the treatment of BK nephropathy [abstract]. Am J Transplant 2003;3(Suppl):370.
20. Brennan DC, Agha I, Bohl DL, et al: Incidence of BK with tacrolimus versus cyclosporine and impact of preemptive immunosuppression reduction. Am J Transplant 2005;3:582–594.
21. Hirsch HH, Brennan DC, Drachenberg CB, et al: Polyomavirus-associated nephropathy in renal transplantation: Interdisciplinary analyses and recommendations. Transplantation 2005;27:1277–1286.
22. Park YS, Choi JY, Cho CH, et al: Clinical outcomes of tuberculosis in renal transplant recipients. Yonsei Med J 2004;45:865–872.
23. Riska H, Gronhagen-Riska C, Ahonen J: Tuberculosis and renal transplantation. Transplant Proc 1987;19:4096–4097.
24. Kotton CN, Ryan ET, Fishman JA: Prevention of infection in adult travelers after solid organ transplantation. Am J Transplant 2005;5:8–14.
25. Pham PT, Pham PC, Wilkinson AH: Medical and urological complications of pancreas and kidney/pancreas transplantation. In Hakim N, Stratta R, Gray D (eds): Pancreas and Islet Transplantation. New York: Oxford University Press, 2002, pp 167–189.
26. Penn I: Evaluation of transplant candidates with pre-existing malignancies. Ann Transplant 1997;2:14–17.
27. Taylor AL, Marcus R, Bradley JA: Post-transplant lymphoproliferative disorders (PTLD) after solid organ transplantation. Crit Rev Oncol Hematol 2005;56:155–167.
28. Trofe J, Buell JF, Beebe TM, et al: Analysis of factors that influence survival with post-transplant lymphoproliferative disorder in renal transplant recipients: The Israel Penn International Transplant Tumor Registry Experience. Am J Transplant 2005;5:775–780.
29. Nepomuceno RR, Balatoni CE, Natkunam Y, et al: Rapamycin inhibits the interleukin 10 transduction pathway and the growth of Epstein-Barr virus B cell lymphomas. Cancer Res 2003;63:4472–4480.
30. Euvrard S, Ulrich C, Lefrancois N: Immunosuppressants and skin cancers in transplant patients: Focus on rapamycin. Dermatol Surg 2004;30:628–633.
31. Jaster R, Bittorf T, Klinken SP, et al: Inhibition of proliferation but not erythroid differentiation of j2E cells by rapamycin. Biochem Pharmacol 1996;51:1181–1185.
32. Kreis H, Cisterne JM, Land W, et al: Sirolimus in association with mycophenolate mofetil induction for the prevention of acute graft rejection in renal allograft recipients. Transplantation 2000;69:1252–1260.
33. Groth CG, Backman L, Morales JM, et al: Sirolimus (rapamycin)-based therapy in human renal transplantation. Similar efficacy and different toxicity compared with cyclosporine. Transplantation 1999;67:1036–1042.
34. Wang AY, Yu AW, Lam CW, et al: Effects of losartan or enalapril on hemoglobin, circulating erythropoietin, and insulin-like growth factor-1 in patients with and without posttransplant erythrocytosis. Am J Kidney Dis 2002;39:600–608.
35. Green J, Debby H, Lederer E, et al: Evidence of a PTH-independent humoral mechanism in posttransplant hypophosphatemia and phosphaturia. Kidney Int 2001;60:1182–1196.
36. Pham PC, Pham PT: Parathyroidectomy. In Nissenson AR, Fine RN (eds): Dialysis Therapy, 2nd ed. Philadelphia: Hanley and Belfus, 2002, pp 410–415.
37. Serra AL, Schwarz AA, Wick FH, et al: Successful treatment of hypercalcemia with cinacalcet in renal transplant recipients with persistent hyperparathyroidism. Nephrol Dial Transplant 2005;20:1315–1319.
38. Kruse AE, Eisenberger U, Frey FJ, et al: The calcimimetic cinacalcet normalizes serum calcium in renal transplant patients with persistent hyperparathyroidism. Nephrol Dial Transplant 2005;20:1311–1314.
39. Gane E, Pilmore H: Management of chronic viral hepatitis before and after renal transplantation. Transplantation 2002;74:427–437.
40. Fasola CG, Netto G, Chritsensen LL, et al: Delay of hepatitis C recurrence in liver transplant recipients treated with mycophenolate mofetil. Transpl Proc 2002;34:1561–1562.
41. Bahra M, Neumann UIF P, Jacob D, et al: MMF and calcineurin taper in recurrent hepatitis C after liver transplantation: Impact on histological course. Am J Transplant 2005;5:406–411.
42. Helderman JH, Goral S: Gastrointestinal complications of transplant immunosuppression. J Am Soc Nephrol 2002;13:277–287.

43. Ponticelli C, Passerini P: Gastrointestinal complications in renal transplant recipients. Transpl Int 2005;18:643–650.
44. Hsi ED, Singleton TP, Swinnen L, et al: Mucosa-associated lymphoid tissue-type lymphomas occurring in post-transplantation patients. Am J Surg Pathol 2000;24:100–106.
45. Heaf JG: Bone disease after renal transplantation. Transplantation 2003;75:315–325.
46. Yazawa K, Ishikawa T, Ishikawa Y, et al: Positive effect of kidney transplantation on bone mass. Transplant Proc 1998;30:3031–3033.
47. Braun WE, Yadlapalli NG: The spectrum of long-term renal transplantation: Outcomes, complications, and clinical studies. Transplant Rev 2002;16:22–50.
48. Sahadevan M, Kashiski B: Long-term posttttransplant management and complications. In Danovitch GM (ed): Handbook of Kidney Transplantation, 4th ed. Philadelphia: Lippincott Williams & Wilkins, 2005, pp 234–278.
49. Khwaja K, Asolati M, Harmon J, et al: Outcome at 3 years with a prednisone-free maintenance regimen: A single center experience with 349 kidney transplant recipients. Am J Transplant 2002;4:980–987.
50. Clive DM: Renal transplant-associated hyperuricemia and gout. J Am Soc Nephrol 2000;11:974–979.

CHAPTER ADDENDUM

Early clinical trials suggest that sirolimus is devoid of diabetogenic effect. However, subsequent studies in animal models and in recipients of renal transplants suggest that sirolimus is associated with reduced insulin sensitivity and a defect in the compensatory β-cell response. Studies in diabetic mice transplanted with islet cells suggest that sirolimus is associated with reduced islet engraftment and impaired β-cell function in transplants.

Chronic Allograft Nephropathy

Bertram L. Kasiske

INTRODUCTION AND DEFINITIONS

The first quarter century of kidney transplantation brought remarkable improvements in short-term allograft survival. In the early days of transplantation, more than half of kidneys were lost to acute rejection during the first year after transplantation. Now >90% of kidneys are still functioning at 1 year. Unfortunately, the rate of graft failure after the first year has changed very little (see Chapter 97).

Slightly more than half of kidney allograft failures are due to patients returning to dialysis or requiring retransplantation. The remainder of allograft failures are due to death with a functioning kidney, most commonly from cardiovascular disease, infection, or malignancy; poor graft function is an important risk factor for mortality. Hence, chronic allograft dysfunction directly or indirectly contributes to most kidney allograft failure.

Chronic allograft dysfunction is the term used to describe a persistent (over weeks to months) decrease in transplant GFR, with or without persistent proteinuria. There are many causes of chronic allograft dysfunction, including recurrent disease and calcineurin inhibitor (cyclosporine and tacrolimus) toxicity. However, the most common cause is chronic allograft nephropathy, which is always associated with chronic allograft dysfunction and/or proteinuria.

Chronic allograft nephropathy (CAN) is a histologic diagnosis characterized by nonspecific chronic changes, including glomerulosclerosis, fibrointimal thickening of large and medium-sized arteries, and tubulointerstitial fibrosis (Fig. 95.1). Some patients with CAN also have evidence of inflammation (e.g., inflammatory cells in blood vessels and tubules), and this subset of patients is often referred to as having chronic rejection. Previously, the term *chronic rejection* was used synonymously with CAN, but this has largely been abandoned with recognition that not all CAN is accompanied by evidence of ongoing immunologic damage or inflammation (Fig. 95.2).

EPIDEMIOLOGY

CAN is the leading cause of death-censored graft failure late after transplantation. The incidence and prevalence of CAN are difficult to determine because the onset of CAN is often insidious and difficult to define, especially when not every patient undergoes biopsy. However, in some studies, protocol biopsy specimens have been obtained in all patients at predetermined intervals after transplantation. In these studies, evidence of CAN was found in 24% of protocol biopsy specimens at 3 months[1] and in 62% to 72% of protocol biopsies at 2 years after transplantation, in recipients treated with calcineurin inhibitors.[2]

PATHOGENESIS

The pathogenesis of CAN is unknown. Most of our understanding of likely pathogenic mechanisms is not derived from direct mechanistic studies, but from identification of risk factors associated with either late allograft failure or histologic evidence of CAN[3] (Figs. 95.3 and 95.4). These risk factors can be conveniently classified as antigen dependent (immune mediated) or antigen independent (nonimmune mediated). There is no direct proof they cause CAN; the associations may be explained by other shared risk factors or mechanisms.

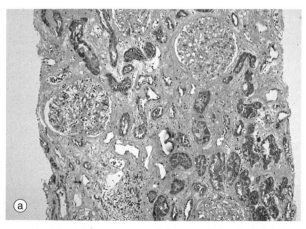
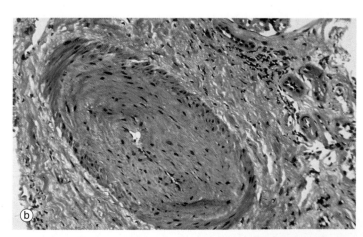

Figure 95.1 **Histologic changes typical of chronic allograft nephropathy.** *a*, Interstitial fibrosis, glomerulosclerosis, and tubular atrophy (trichrome). *b*, Fibrointimal proliferation in an intrarenal artery (hematoxylin and eosin).

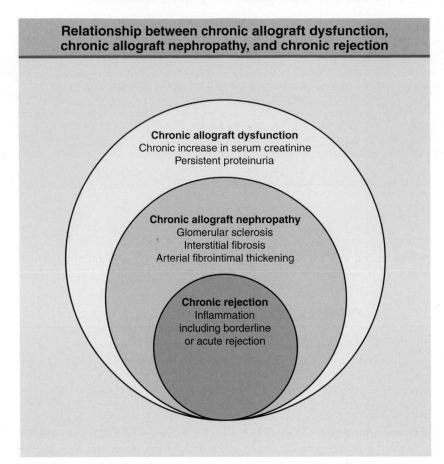

Relationship between chronic allograft dysfunction, chronic allograft nephropathy, and chronic rejection

Chronic allograft dysfunction
Chronic increase in serum creatinine
Persistent proteinuria

Chronic allograft nephropathy
Glomerular sclerosis
Interstitial fibrosis
Arterial fibrointimal thickening

Chronic rejection
Inflammation
including borderline
or acute rejection

Figure 95.2   Relationship between chronic allograft dysfunction, chronic allograft nephropathy (CAN), and chronic rejection. *Chronic allograft dysfunction* is a term usually used to describe a persistent (over weeks to months) increase in serum creatinine, with or without persistent proteinuria. There are many causes, including recurrent disease and calcineurin inhibitor toxicity, but the most common cause is CAN, which is always associated with chronic graft dysfunction and/or proteinuria. Some with patients with CAN also have inflammation, and this subset of patients is often referred to as having chronic rejection.

Risk factors for chronic allograft nephropathy
Alloantigen-Dependent (Immune) Risk Factors
Acute rejection, especially if late, multiple, and/or severe
Subclinical acute rejection
MHC antigen mismatches
Prefomed anti-HLA antibodies
Previous transplantation
Younger recipient
Deceased (versus living) donor
Delayed graft function (?)
Cytomegalovirus infection (?)
Alloantigen-Independent (Nonimmune) Risk Factors
Kidney size mismatch
Older donor age
Proteinuria
Hypertension
Dyslipidemias
Cigarette smoking

Figure 95.3   Risk factors for chronic allograft nephropathy.

Antigen-dependent Mechanisms

Increasing circumstantial evidence suggests that antigen-dependent or immune mechanisms play a major role in CAN and that part of what we call CAN is truly chronic rejection. Otherwise, it is difficult to account for the association of major histocompatibility complex (MHC) mismatches, preformed antibodies, younger recipient age, and previous transplantation with CAN.

Acute Rejection

One of the best predictors of late graft failure is acute rejection,[4,5] and acute rejection is a strong risk factor for biopsy-proven CAN.[6] However, not all acute rejection episodes lead to late graft failure and CAN. Although it is not possible to predict with certainty which acute rejection episodes herald late graft failure and CAN, some studies indicate that acute rejection episodes that are more severe, as determined by a greater decline in renal function, are more likely to be associated with graft failure, as are acute rejections occurring after the first 3 months post-transplantation, and recurrent acute rejections.[7] Acute rejection episodes that show histologic evidence of antibody or vascular involvement, including C4d deposition,[8] are also more likely to be associated with late graft failure and CAN.[7] The effect of early acute rejections on late graft failure appears to be greater in recent years, even as the incidence of early acute rejections declines.[9] This may be a result of more potent immunosuppressive agents effectively preventing mild rejections, thereby increasing the proportion of early rejections that are more severe and refractory to treatment and lead on to CAN.[9]

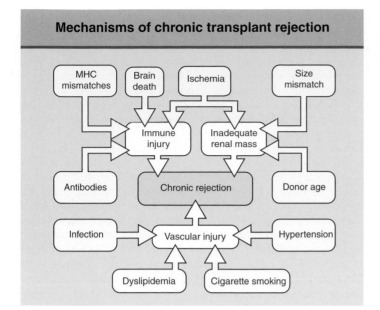

Figure 95.4 Some possible immune and nonimmune mechanisms of injury leading to chronic allograft nephropathy. Antigen-dependent and antigen-independent risk factors may be involved. MHC, major histocompatibility complex.

Subclinical Acute Rejection

Subclinical rejection, defined as histologic evidence of Banff 97 acute rejection (see Chapter 93) without acute decline of renal function, correlates with chronic interstitial fibrosis and chronic arterial fibrointimal thickening at 12 months and is also associated with increased MHC mismatch and with previous acute rejection,[1] but is not clear whether this association is mediated through the presence of previous acute rejection or MHC mismatch.[1]

MHC Antigen Mismatches

The number of MHC antigen matches has a significant effect on long-term graft survival[9] and histologic CAN.[10] A retrospective study showed histologic changes of CAN in recipients of deceased donor kidney transplants, but not in the recipients of MHC identical living related donor kidneys. However, this study could not exclude the effect of confounding factors such as less cold ischemia, less delayed graft function, and differences in calcineurin inhibitor use in the living donor recipients.[11]

Preformed Antibodies

Preformed antibodies to MHC antigens are usually the consequence of previous transplants, pregnancies, and blood transfusions; the degree of sensitization or cytotoxicity is usually measured as the percentage of panel reactive antibodies (PRAs), the percentage of lymphocytes from a random sample of individuals that react to antibodies in the recipient's serum. High PRA is an independent risk factor for graft failure, early and late after transplantation, is also a risk factor for histologic CAN.[12]

There is some evidence that patients with CAN have circulating antibodies to MHC antigens.[13] Circulating alloantibodies and peritubular capillary C4d deposition have both been linked to a higher risk of CAN and graft failure.[8]

Cytomegalovirus Infection

The role of cytomegalovirus (CMV), or other infections, in the pathogenesis of CAN is controversial. Some studies indicate an association between CMV infection and long-term graft failure, which may be a consequence of the association of CMV infection and acute rejection episodes.[14]

Previous Transplantation

Previous kidney transplantation is associated with late allograft failure[15,16] and histologic changes of CAN. This is independent of acute rejection, but may be mediated by subclinical acute rejection.

Younger Recipient Age

Younger recipients are more likely to have late allograft failure and to develop histologic findings of CAN. Younger individuals are more likely to have acute rejection and are more likely to be noncompliant with immunosuppressive medications. The association between recipient age and CAN is likely due to antigen-dependent (immune-mediated) mechanisms since most antigen-independent mechanisms are more prevalent in older individuals.

Antigen-Independent Mechanisms

It is difficult to explain many of the clinical risk factors associated with CAN solely by antigen-dependent mechanisms. Major antigen-independent mechanisms include chronic calcineurin toxicity, vascular injury, and perhaps nephron dosing.

Chronic Calcineurin Inhibitor Toxicity

Virtually all the histologic changes that characterize CAN can be caused by toxicity due to calcineurin inhibitors (cyclosporine and tacrolimus). CAN is, however, common in patients who have never been treated with calcineurin inhibitors; otherwise, it might be suspected that CAN is entirely caused by these agents. Protocol biopsy studies have shown that many of the CAN changes that develop during the first year post-transplantation are associated with inflammation, that is, acute clinical and subclinical rejection.[15] Thus, antigen-dependent mechanisms of CAN may be dominant during the first year after transplantation. However, after the first year, there is little evidence of inflammation and the presumption is that calcineurin inhibitor toxicity is a major cause of CAN changes after the first post-transplantation year. Consistent with these assumptions, elective withdrawal of calcineurin inhibitors can cause a higher incidence of acute rejection without causing a higher incidence of late graft failure.[16]

Deceased Donor Kidneys

Kidneys from living donors, regardless of their relationship with the recipients, survive longer than kidneys from deceased donors. Recipients of living donor kidneys have less late allograft failure and less histologic evidence of CAN.[17] Living donor kidneys survive longer than deceased donor kidneys because of reduced ischemia time or because of the negative influence of deceased donor brain death, which causes an upregulation of cytokines and growth factors in the kidney and other organs, perhaps related to increased catecholamine release. Experimental data suggest that the increase in tissue cytokines resulting from brain death may enhance rejection. Brain death is also associated with tissue ischemia, which is more severe in brain death related to intracerebral hemorrhage compared to head trauma. Retrospective analyses identify a cardiovascular or cerebrovascular cause of donor death as a risk factor for decreased long-term allograft survival.

Delayed Graft Function

Delayed graft function, usually defined by the need for dialysis in the first week after transplantation, is a risk factor for histologic CAN.[18] There are also independent associations between delayed graft function and late graft failure and between delayed graft function and graft failure that is mediated by acute rejection. Major risk factors for delayed graft function are prolonged cold ischemia time, donor age older than 50 years, and peak PRA >50%.[19] Ischemia and oxidative injury resulting from reperfusion of an ischemic kidney may cause an upregulation of MHC antigens and/or proinflammatory cytokines, predisposing to acute rejection.

Nephron "Dosing"

It has also been suggested that an inadequate functioning renal mass may lead to CAN, just as it contributes to progressive disease in native kidneys, possibly as a result of glomerular hyperfiltration.[20] Proteinuria from hyperfiltration could cause chronic interstitial injury. Senescence of the allograft, perhaps accelerated by injury response mechanisms, could also play a role.[21]

Factors predicted to reduce functioning nephron number are associated with worse graft survival including donor age, donor kidney size, female donors, donor race, and graft function at time of discharge after transplantation.[20] However, the effects of these factors on graft survival are already fully manifest 1 year after transplantation, when the incidence of graft failure owing to chronic allograft dysfunction is still relatively low.[20]

Donor Age

One of the strongest risk factors for late graft failure is the age of the donor.[3,4] Older donor age is a strong risk factor for late graft failure and histologic evidence of CAN.[10,11] Pretransplantation donor kidney changes may contribute.

Cardiovascular Risk Factors

The vasculopathy in CAN resembles systemic vascular disease, raising the possibility that conventional cardiovascular disease risk factors may be implicated. Hypertension occurs in >50% of transplant recipients. In a multicenter, retrospective study of 29,751 kidney transplant recipients with 7 years of follow-up, elevated systolic and diastolic blood pressures were associated with chronic graft failure in a multivariate analysis.[22] Hypertension is associated with histologic CAN. Dyslipidemias, including increased levels of total cholesterol, high-density lipoprotein cholesterol, and triglycerides, have been associated with late graft failure.[4] Cigarette smoking is associated with late graft failure,[4,23] either by a direct toxic effect on the allograft or more likely mediated by hypertension or other cardiovascular risk factors. In health systems where patients must meet the cost of their immunosuppressive medication, it is also possible that cigarette smoking may identify patients more likely to be noncompliant with immunosuppressive medications for socioeconomic reasons.

Proteinuria

Proteinuria is a major risk factor for late renal allograft failure[4,7] and is associated with histologic changes of CAN.[24] It is not possible to determine whether proteinuria is just an early marker of CAN or directly contributes to renal injury.

Uric Acid

The renal histologic appearances in gout have some similarity to those of CAN, and there is some evidence that uric acid is an independent predictor of progressive graft failure. Experimental evidence also suggests uric acid may play a role in calcineurin inhibitor toxicity.

CLINICAL MANIFESTATIONS

Chronic allograft nephropathy usually presents as a decline in glomerular filtration rate (GFR) and/or an increase in urine protein excretion. Unless advanced renal failure is present, there are no clinical features of CAN. All too often CAN is first detected when it is already far advanced because clinical methods for detecting early declines in GFR are relatively insensitive. Serum creatinine remains the routine parameter for detecting changes in GFR in kidney transplant recipients. While an acute increase in serum creatinine is a relatively sensitive, albeit nonspecific indicator of acute allograft dysfunction from any cause, chronic changes in serum creatinine are not very sensitive for detecting chronic allograft dysfunction and CAN. Furthermore, patients with CAN may have lower muscle mass, resulting in serum creatinine values lower than expected for the GFR. Estimation of GFR using the Cockcroft-Gault formula or the Modification of Diet in Renal Disease formula may be helpful to supplement information from serial serum creatinine estimations. Serum cystatin C may ultimately prove superior to serum creatinine, but is not routinely available. The value and limitations of measurement and estimation of GFR are discussed further in Chapter 3.

Proteinuria may also be the first manifestation of CAN. Few studies have prospectively evaluated proteinuria as a tool for screening to detect CAN or other causes of allograft dysfunction. CAN is found in more than half of patients who undergo allograft biopsy for proteinuria, and in 40% of those who have nephrotic-range proteinuria.[25] Transplant glomerulopathy (see later), one histologic manifestation of CAN, is almost always accompanied by proteinuria. Except for proteinuria, the urinalysis is usually unremarkable in CAN.

PATHOLOGY

CAN is a pathologic diagnosis (Fig. 95.5), and because most of the pathologic changes are nonspecific, CAN is largely a diagnosis of exclusion. The most widely used pathologic diagnostic criteria for rejection were developed by the Banff consortium.[26] The Banff 97

Histologic findings in chronic allograft nephropathy
Glomeruli
Mesangial expansion
Global sclerosis
Focal segmental sclerosis
Basement membrane reduplication
Tubulointerstitium
Tubular atrophy
Interstitial fibrosis
Arteries
Fibrointimal proliferation
Peritubular Capillaries
Reduplication of tubular basement membranes (electron microscopy)

Figure 95.5 Histologic findings in chronic allograft nephropathy.

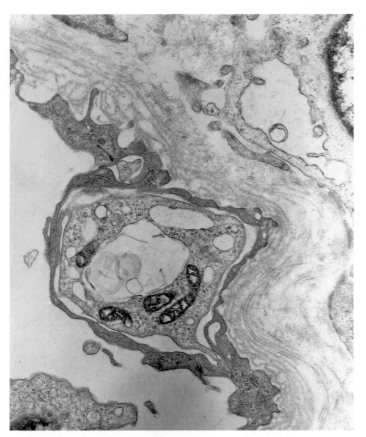

Figure 95.6 Electron microscopic appearances in chronic allograft nephropathy. Note the multiple layers of peritubular capillary basement membranes. (Courtesy of Dr. David Grange.)

schema grades CAN on the light microscopic features as grade I (mild), II (moderate), or III (severe). These changes include glomerulosclerosis, interstitial fibrosis, tubular atrophy, and fibrointimal proliferation in arteries (see Fig. 95.1). If the chronic vascular changes are accompanied by evidence of acute inflammation (e.g., disruption of the internal elastic lamina, inflammatory cells in the intima, proliferation of myofibroblasts), then the CAN grade is designated "b"; otherwise, it is "a."

One of the most consistent histologic features of CAN is peritubular capillary basement membrane reduplication on electron microscopy[27] (Fig. 95.6). The more basement membrane layers that are present, the more likely the diagnosis is CAN. Given

the association between peritubular capillary C4d deposition and CAN, the basement membrane reduplication may be the result of antibody-mediated injury, but this is unproven.

Transplant Glomerulopathy

Transplant glomerulopathy (Fig. 95.7) is the one pathogno-monic histologic pattern of CAN, and it is always associated with proteinuria. Transplant glomerulopathy is associated with circulating anti-HLA antibodies,[28] but no other pathogenic processes distinct from other patterns of CAN have yet been identified.

Light microscopic findings in transplant glomerulopathy are diffuse mesangial expansion often leading to a lobular appearance, with endothelial and mesangial cell swelling and mononuclear cell infiltration. There is also diffuse thickening and splitting of the glomerular capillary walls.[29] Immune microscopy may show deposits of IgM and to a lesser extent C3. Electron microscopy shows no glomerular electron-dense deposits but glomerular basement membrane reduplication and sometimes subendothelial deposition of electron-lucent material as well as peritubular capillary basement membrane reduplication. The light microscopic appearances are not distinguishable from those of membranoproliferative glomerulonephritis (MPGN). However, in MPGN, immune microscopy will reveal dominant capillary wall deposits of C3 and smaller deposits of IgG and IgM, whereas IgM is dominant in transplant glomerulopathy. Electron microscopy in MPGN will show subendothelial (type I) or intramembranous (type II) dense deposits (see Chapter 20).

DIAGNOSIS

The diagnosis of CAN is made by biopsy, unless contraindicated, in patients with chronic renal allograft dysfunction, with or without proteinuria. It is a diagnosis of exclusion in patients who have no evidence of acute rejection, acute calcineurin inhibitor toxicity, *de novo* glomerulonephritis, or recurrent renal disease.

DIFFERENTIAL DIAGNOSIS

Chronic renal allograft dysfunction is common and can have many causes (Fig. 95.8).

Prerenal Causes

Prerenal causes of allograft dysfunction include reversible hemodynamic alterations that may occur from dehydration or congestive

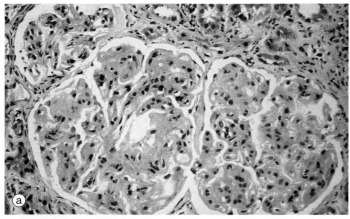

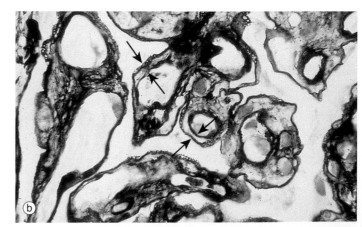

Figure 95.7 Histologic changes of transplant glomerulopathy. *a,* Transplant glomerulopathy with mesangial matrix expansion and thickening of capillary loops (hematoxylin and eosin). *b,* Transplant glomerulopathy showing membrane reduplication in capillary loops (*between arrows*) (methenamine silver).

Differential diagnosis of chronic allograft dysfunction

Prerenal, reversible hemodynamic dysfunction
  Dehydration
  Congestive heart failure
  Antihypertensive medications
  Nonsteroidsal anti-inflammatory drugs
  Graft renal artery stenosis or proximal arterial stenosis

Intrinsic renal parenchymal disease
  Acute rejection*
  Calcineurin inhibitor toxicity
  Recurrent kidney disease
  De novo glomerulonephritis
  Lymphomatous infiltration
  Allergic interstitial nephritis, drug induced*
  Viral infection: cytomegalovirus, polyomavirus*
  Bacterial pyelonephritis*

Postrenal, reversible obstruction

Figure 95.8 Differential diagnosis of chronic allograft dysfunction. *More often presents as acute allograft dysfunction, but should always be considered in the differential diagnosis of chronic allograft dysfunction.

heart failure. Graft renal artery stenosis, or stenosis of arteries proximal to the kidney allograft can cause a decline in kidney function. This is usually associated with difficult-to-control hypertension. Rarely, cholesterol emboli can present as a decrease in function late after transplantation.

Intrinsic Renal Causes

Acute rejection can occur late after transplantation and present as a gradual increase in serum creatinine with or without proteinuria. Often late acute rejection is the result of patient noncompliance with immunosuppressive medications. The diagnosis and management of acute deterioration of allograft function are discussed further in Chapter 93.

Viral infections, including cytomegalovirus and polyomaviruses, especially BK virus, can also cause acute or chronic graft dysfunction. BK virus infection is now the most common, suspected on finding BK virus in the plasma or urine and confirmed by detecting virus in kidney tissue with either antibody staining or *in situ* hybridization. Histologic changes associated with BK nephropathy can resemble acute rejection, but renal tubular cell cytopathic changes may also be seen in BK nephropathy. Acute rejection and BK nephropathy can occur together.

Allergic interstitial nephritis, often medication induced, and acute bacterial pyelonephritis are usually differentials for acute rather than chronic allograft dysfunction.

Calcineurin inhibitor toxicity may occur even when monitoring shows that drug levels are within recommended therapeutic ranges. Histologic changes include striped interstitial fibrosis and arteriolar hyalinosis, but these changes are nonspecific, and calcineurin inhibitor toxicity cannot reliably be distinguished from CAN, with which it will often coincide.

Proteinuria, with or without a decline in kidney function, may be caused by *de novo* or recurrent glomerular diseases. The most common *de novo* glomerular disease causing clinical proteinuria is membranous nephropathy. Membranous nephropathy can also recur in the allograft, but this usually occurs within the first 1 to 2 years after transplantation, whereas *de novo* membranous nephropathy is a late event. MPGN is a very important differential for the histologic features of transplant glomerulopathy (see

"Pathology"). Other recurrent diseases in the renal transplant are discussed in Chapter 96.

Postrenal Causes

Postrenal causes should also be considered. Although uncommon, ureteral obstruction can occur late after transplantation. Bladder dysfunction or prostatic hypertrophy can also cause allograft dysfunction.

PREVENTION AND TREATMENT

Since the pathogenesis of CAN is uncertain, it is not surprising that there are no specific preventive measures and treatments for CAN that have been established in randomized trials. Current recommendations are shown in Figure 95.9.

Prevention

The first goal should be to minimize the incidence and severity of acute rejection. Early detection by frequent monitoring of serum creatinine remains the first line of defense against acute rejection. Therapeutic levels of immunosuppressive medications, especially calcineurin inhibitors, should be carefully monitored. Patients who fail to come to clinic appointments designed to monitor graft function may be those more likely to be noncompliant with their immunosuppressive medications.

Although randomized trials have established that several newer immunosuppressive agents, for example, mycophenolate mofetil (MMF), tacrolimus, and sirolimus, are effective in reducing the incidence of acute rejection, there are as yet no large randomized trials showing that such immunosuppression effectively reduces the incidence of subsequent CAN.

The role of protocol biopsies in detecting subclinical acute rejection, and thereby preventing chronic rejection, remains to be firmly established. Noninvasive techniques to detect early acute rejection including imaging, and urinary excretion of cytokines and other low-molecular-weight proteins are as yet of insufficient specificity for routine clinical use.

Strategies to prevent, diagnose, and treat chronic allograft dysfunction

Minimize acute rejection
  Use adequate immunosuppression
  Monitor graft function and urine protein
  Perform biopsy for unexplained increases in serum creatinine or urine
    protein

Minimize subclinical acute rejection
  Use adequate immunosuppression
  Consider protocol biopsies (currently research tool only)

Consider elective withdrawal of calcineurin inhibitors after 1 year
Reduce proteinuria   ACE inhibitors and/or ARB
Control blood pressure   <130/80 mm Hg (proteinuria <1 g/24 hr)   <125/75 mm Hg (proteinuria >1 g/24 hr)

Treat other cardiovascular disease risk factors
  Keep low-density lipoprotein cholesterol <100 mg/dl (3.5 mmol/l)
  Encourage smoking cessation

Figure 95.9 Strategies to prevent, diagnose, and treat chronic allograft dysfunction. ACE, angiotensin-converting enzyme; ARB, angiotensin receptor blockers.

It remains controversial whether treatment of subclinical acute rejection prevents chronic rejection. A small randomized trial found subclinical acute rejection occurred in 80% of 36 patients who underwent multiple, serial protocol biopsies. Treatment of the subclinical acute rejection resulted in fewer changes of CAN at 6 months and better graft function at 2 years compared to a control group who did not have protocol biopsies.[30] However, lower serum creatinine in the treatment group might be explained by a reduction in muscle mass from the additional treatment with corticosteroids rather than an improvement in graft function. These results require confirmation before protocol biopsies become part of routine management.

Maintenance Immunosuppression

There is emerging evidence that improvements in immunosuppression may have led to a reduction in the incidence of late allograft failure, and presumably CAN, as suggested by the decreasing rate of decline in allograft function in some studies.[31,32] However, the optimum maintenance immunosuppression protocol to prevent CAN remains to be established. Calcineurin inhibitors are still the mainstay of maintenance immunosuppression because of their proven efficacy despite the problem of calcineurin inhibitor toxicity. There are a few randomized trials showing that changing immunosuppressive medications may alter the course of CAN once it has become established. A small randomized trial in patients treated with cyclosporine and prednisone showed that biopsy-proven CAN at 1 year was less in patients treated with MMF compared to those treated with azathioprine.[33] MMF may have additional beneficial effects on antigen-independent mechanisms of CAN by blocking fibroblast activation and vascular smooth muscle cell proliferation.

A number of randomized trials have examined the effects of elective withdrawal of cyclosporine during the first year after transplantation. Meta-analysis of these studies showed an increase in acute rejection, but no effect of withdrawing cyclosporine on graft failure.[34] However, two of these studies have now reported longer-term follow-up, and both showed that patients who had electively stopped cyclosporine had better kidney function and long-term graft survival than patients who continued on cyclosporine.[35,36] Thus, strategies that limit the use of calcineurin inhibitors to the first few months after transplantation may be effective in preventing nephrotoxicity and CAN.

Hypertension

Blood pressure targets recommended for progressive disease in native kidneys are also appropriate for management of CAN (see Fig. 95.9), although such targets have not been subject to formal trial evaluation in transplant recipients so have not been proven to delay progression of CAN.

Proteinuria

Reducing proteinuria by aggressively treating hypertension, including renin-angiotensin blockade using angiotensin-converting enzyme (ACE) inhibitors or angiotensin receptor blockers (ARBs) or their combination is well established for delaying progressive renal disease in native kidneys. It seems logical that the same approach would be beneficial in CAN, although this has not been explored with adequate clinical trials.[37] When ACE inhibitors or ARB are introduced, graft function should always be monitored carefully; rarely, a catastrophic decrease in GFR can follow if there is undetected transplant renal artery stenosis.

Dyslipidemia

A randomized trial of lipid reduction with fluvastatin in kidney transplant recipients showed no improvement in kidney function or graft survival.[38] Nevertheless, treatment of dyslipidemias and other risk factors in patients with CAN is justified to minimize cardiovascular disease (see Chapter 71).

REFERENCES

1. Nankivell BJ, Fenton-Lee CA, Kuypers DR, et al: Effect of histological damage on long-term kidney transplant outcome. Transplantation 2001; 71:515–523.
2. Solez K, Vincenti F, Filo RS: Histopathologic findings from 2-year protocol biopsies from a U.S. multicenter kidney transplant trial comparing tacrolimus versus cyclosporine: A report of the FK506 Kidney Transplant Study Group. Transplantation 1998;66:1736–1740.
3. Joosten SA, Sijpkens YW, van Kooten C, Paul LC: Chronic renal allograft rejection. Kidney Int 2005;68:1–13.
4. Matas AJ, Gillingham KJ, Humar A, et al: Immunologic and nonimmunologic factors: Different risks for cadaver and living donor transplantation. Transplantation 2000;69:54–58.
5. Fellstrom B, Holdaas H, Jardine AG, et al: Risk factors for reaching renal endpoints in the assessment of Lescol in renal transplantation (ALERT) trial. Transplantation 2005;79:205–212.
6. Schwarz A, Mengel M, Gwinner W, et al: Risk factors for chronic allograft nephropathy after renal transplantation: A protocol biopsy study. Kidney Int 2005;67:341–348.
7. Massy ZA, Guijarro C, Wiederkehr MR, Ma JZ, et al: Chronic renal allograft rejection: Immunologic and nonimmunologic risk factors. Kidney Int 1996;49:518–524.
8. Sijpkens YW, Joosten SA, Wong MC, et al: Immunologic risk factors and glomerular C4d deposits in chronic transplant glomerulopathy. Kidney Int 2004;65:2409–2418.
9. Meier-Kriesche HU, Ojo AO, Hanson JA, et al: Increased impact of acute rejection on chronic allograft failure in recent era. Transplantation 2000;70:1098–1100.
10. Lehtonen SR, Taskinen EI, Isoniemi HM: Histological alterations in implant and one-year protocol biopsy specimens of renal allografts. Transplantation 2001;72:1138–1144.
11. Legendre C, Thervet E, Skhiri H, et al: Histologic features of chronic allograft nephropathy revealed by protocol biopsies in kidney transplant recipients. Transplantation 1998;65:1506–1509.
12. Sijpkens YW, Doxiadis II, van Kemenade FJ, et al: Chronic rejection with or without transplant vasculopathy. Clin Transpl 2003;17:163–170.
13. Lee PC, Terasaki PI, Takemoto SK, et al: All chronic rejection failures of kidney transplants were preceded by the development of HLA antibodies. Transplantation 2002;74:1192–1194.
14. Dickenmann MJ, Cathomas G, Steiger J, et al: Cytomegalovirus infection and graft rejection in renal transplantation. Transplantation 2001; 71:764–767.
15. Nankivell BJ, Borrows RJ, Fung CL, et al: The natural history of chronic allograft nephropathy. N Engl J Med 2003;349:2326–2633.
16. Kasiske BL, Chakkera HA, Louis TA, Ma JZ: A meta-analysis of immunosuppression withdrawal trials in renal transplantation. J Am Soc Nephrol 2000;11:1910–1917.
17. Cosio FG, Grande JP, Larson TS, et al: Kidney allograft fibrosis and atrophy early after living donor transplantation. Am J Transplant 2005; 5:1130–1136.
18. Kuypers DRJ, Chapman JR, O'Connell PJ, et al: Predictors of renal transplant histology at three months. Transplantation 1999;67:1222–1230.
19. McLaren AJ, Jassem W, Gray DW, et al: Delayed graft function: Risk factors and the relative effects of early function and acute rejection on long-term survival in cadaveric renal transplantation. Clin Transpl 1999;13:266–272.
20. Terasaki PI, Koyama H, Cecka JM, Gjertson DW: The hyperfiltration hypothesis in human renal transplantation. Transplantation 1994;57:1450–1454.

21. Halloran PF, Melk A, Barth C: Rethinking chronic allograft nephropathy: The concept of accelerated senescence. J Am Soc Nephrol 1999;10: 167–181.

22. Opelz G, Wujciak T, Ritz E: Association of chronic kidney graft failure with recipient blood pressure. Collaborative Transplant Study. Kidney Int 1998;53:217–222.

23. Sung RS, Althoen M, Howell TA, et al: Excess risk of renal allograft loss associated with cigarette smoking. Transplantation 2001;71:1752–1757.

24. McLaren AJ, Fuggle SV, Welsh KI, et al: Chronic allograft failure in human renal transplantation: A multivariate risk factor analysis. Ann Surg 2000;232:98–103.

25. Yakupoglu U, Paranowska-Daca E, Rosen D, et al: Post-transplant nephrotic syndrome: A comprehensive clinicopathologic study. Kidney Int 2004;65:2360–2370.

26. Racusen LC, Solez K, Colvin RB, et al: The Banff 97 working classification of renal allograft pathology. Kidney Int 1999;55:713–723.

27. Gough J, Yilmaz A, Miskulin D, et al: Peritubular capillary basement membrane reduplication in allografts and native kidney disease: A clinicopathologic study of 278 consecutive renal specimens. Transplantation 2001;71:1390–1393.

28. Palomar R, Lopez-Hoyos M, Pstor JM: Impact of HLA antibodies on transplant glomerulopathy. Transplant Proc 2005;37:3830–3832.

29. Joosten SA, Sijpkns YWJ, an Kooten C, Paul LC: Chronic renal allograft rejection: Pathophysiologic considerations. Kidney Int 2005;68:1–13.

30. Rush D, Nickerson P, Gough J, et al: Beneficial effects of treatment of early subclinical rejection: A randomized study. J Am Soc Nephrol 1998;9:2129–2134.

31. Kasiske BL, Gaston RS, Gourishankar S, et al: Long-term deterioration of kidney allograft function. Am J Transplant 2005;5:1405–1414.

32. Gourishankar S, Hunsicker LG, Jhangri GS, et al: The stability of the glomerular filtration rate after renal transplantation is improving. J Am Soc Nephrol 2003;14:2387–2394.

33. Merville P, Berge F, Deminiere C, et al: Lower incidence of chronic allograft nephropathy at 1 year post-transplantation in patients treated with mycophenolate mofetil. Am J Transplant 2004;4:1769–1775.

34. Kasiske BL, Chakkera HA, Louis TA, Ma JZ: A meta-analysis of immunosuppression withdrawal trials in renal transplantation. J Am Soc Nephrol 2000;11:1910–1917.

35. Hilbrands LB, Hoitsma AJ, Koene RAP: Randomized, prospective trial of cyclosporine monotherapy versus azathioprine-prednisone from three months after renal transplantation. Transplantation 1996;61: 1038–1046.

36. Gallagher MP, Hall B, Craig J, et al: A randomized controlled trial of cyclosporine withdrawal in renal-transplant recipients: 15-year results. Transplantation 2004;78:1653–1660.

37. Stigant CE, Cohen J, Vivera M, Zaltzman JS: ACE inhibitors and angiotensin II antagonists in renal transplantation: An analysis of safety and efficacy. Am J Kidney Dis 2000;35:58–63.

38. Fellstrom B, Holdaas H, Jardine AG, et al: Effect of fluvastatin on renal end points in the Assessment of Lescol in Renal Transplant (ALERT) trial. Kidney Int 2004;66:1549–1555.

Recurrent Disease in Kidney Transplantation

Steven J. Chadban

INTRODUCTION

Kidney transplantation is a treatment, not a cure. While transplantation may restore kidney function to the recipient, it does not necessarily remove the cause of the recipient's original kidney disease. Glomerulonephritis (GN) and diabetes are the two leading causes of end-stage renal disease (ESRD) worldwide and are the primary diseases afflicting the majority of patients considered for kidney transplantation. Both diseases may recur despite the different antigens expressed within the new kidney and the altered state of systemic immunosuppression.

The longer that a transplant remains *in situ*, the more likely it is to be affected by recurrence. As graft survival rates have increased over the past 30 years, mostly due to more effective antirejection therapies that prevent early graft loss, the incidence of recurrence has grown.[1] Within cohorts reassessed over time, an increase in the prevalence of recurrent disease with longer follow-up is also evident. An analysis of U.S. Renal Allograft Disease Registry data demonstrated a prevalence of 2.8% at 2 years, 9.8% at 5 years, and 18.5% at 8 years follow-up after transplantation, and such patients were twice as likely to experience graft failure as compared to those without recurrence.[2]

Recurrence has a powerful impact on transplant survival and one that is increasingly apparent with time after transplantation. Analysis of data from the Australasian registry (ANZDATA) of >1500 patients with biopsy-proven GN who received a kidney transplant, biopsy-proven recurrence was found to cause graft loss in 0.5% within 1 year after transplantation, 3.7% within 5 years, and 8.4% within 10 years after transplantation[3] (Fig. 96.1). Several studies have found recurrent disease to be the third most common cause of graft failure beyond the first year after transplantation, falling behind death with function and chronic allograft nephropathy (CAN), but substantially ahead of acute rejection[3,4] (see Fig. 96.1).

This chapter reviews the pathogenesis, clinical features, diagnostic and management issues, and outcome data of relevance to clinicians and their patients in contemplating transplantation as a treatment for kidney failure caused by diseases with a propensity to recur.

De novo GN and post-transplantation diabetes may also affect the transplanted kidney. Like recurrent disease, the prevalence of both appears to increase with time after transplantation. Given the high incidence of post-transplantation diabetes, coupled with general increases in graft survival,[5] it is likely that *de novo* diabetic nephropathy in particular will be a significant clinical problem in the future. Both conditions may be difficult to distinguish

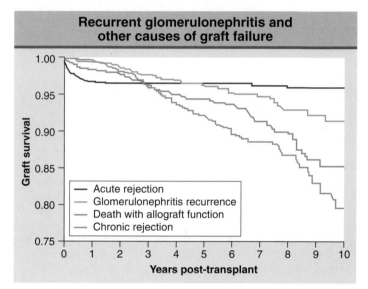

Figure 96.1 Recurrent glomerulonephritis and other causes of graft failure. Kaplan-Meier analysis of the relative contributions of acute rejection, glomerulonephritis recurrence, death, and chronic allograft nephropathy to graft loss during the first 10 years post-transplantation among patients who underwent transplantation because of end-stage renal disease caused by glomerulonephritis. (Modified from Briganti EM, Russ GR, McNeil J, et al: Risk of renal allograft loss from recurrent glomerulonephritis. N Engl J Med 2002;347:103–109.)

from recurrence and indeed from CAN and are discussed in "Differential Diagnosis."

Defining Recurrence and Interpreting the Literature

The diagnosis of recurrence almost invariably requires histologic demonstration of the same disease involving both the native and transplanted kidneys. In addition, the diagnosis of recurrence causing graft failure requires a clinical decision that recurrence was the dominant contributor to graft loss (other contributors may be present, such as CAN). A histologic diagnosis of the primary kidney disease is not obtained for all patients with ESRD, and the majority of transplant recipients do not undergo biopsy to look specifically for recurrent disease (which requires electron microscopic and immunohistologic examination of the biopsy specimen).[1] Coupled with the tendency of clinicians to make a clinical diagnosis of CAN and thereby avoid biopsy in patients with declining graft function and proteinuria, the true incidence of disease recurrence is not known and is almost certainly underestimated by existing literature.

Additional factors cloud the available evidence. Many reports of disease recurrence are retrospective, single-center studies. Recall bias and incomplete documentation, changes in practice over time, and peculiarities of local patient populations and local practices may limit relevance to other populations. The most definitive reports have come from analyses of the large registry databases of Europe, the United States, and Australasia. Registries capture data on large numbers of patients; however, unit participation rates; quantity and type of data collected; accuracy, uniformity, and consistency of reporting by units; and the reliability of data entry vary between the registries, which may introduce bias to the data. How recurrence is defined and diagnosed and which outcomes were measured is crucial. For example, IgA nephropathy (IgAN) has been demonstrated to recur in 58% of cases in one series in which all recipients underwent biopsy,[5] but in approximately 25% of cases in which biopsy was performed only when clinically indicated. When graft loss due to IgAN recurrence is the outcome measure, the risk decreases to approximately 10% at 10 years of follow-up.[3] Thus, definition of recurrence, outcome measures, study design, and source of data all need to be considered in assessing the published literature regarding recurrence.

RECURRENT GLOMERULONEPHRITIS

Virtually all recognized forms of GN may recur post-transplantation; however, the rate and consequences of recurrence vary enormously. For example, antiglomerular basement membrane (GBM) disease (Goodpasture's disease) recurs only rarely, but when it does, it is likely to cause rapid graft loss. In contrast, type II membranoproliferative GN recurs in >80% of cases; however, the disease tends to be very slowly progressive and graft survival beyond 10 years is typical. Numerically, recurrence of focal and segmental glomerulosclerosis (FSGS), IgAN, and membranous nephropathy (MN) are the most frequently encountered clinical problems (Fig. 96.2).

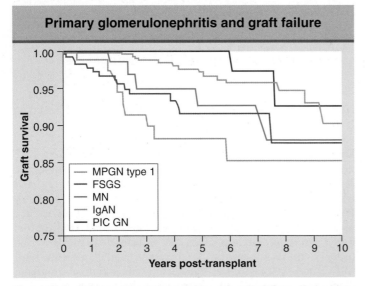

Primary glomerulonephritis and graft failure

Graft survival vs. Years post-transplant

- MPGN type 1
- FSGS
- MN
- IgAN
- PIC GN

Figure 96.2 Primary glomerulonephritis and graft failure. Kaplan-Meier analysis of freedom from graft loss caused by recurrent glomerulonephritis during the first 10 years after kidney transplantation among patients with a primary diagnosis of glomerulonephritis. FSGS, focal and segmental glomerulosclerosis; IgAN, IgA nephropathy; MN, membranous nephropathy; MPGN, membranoproliferative glomerulonephritis; PIC GN, pauci-immune crescentic glomerulonephritis. (Adapted from Briganti EM, Russ GR, McNeil J, et al: Risk of renal allograft loss from recurrent glomerulonephritis. N Engl J Med 2002;347:103–109.)

Factors in addition to the underlying type of GN may influence the risk of recurrence. Time of follow-up is clearly important and may be related to the duration of exposure of the graft to the nephritogenic factors responsible for causing GN.[1] In general, grafts that are lost early due to rejection are exposed relatively briefly and rarely develop recurrence. In contrast, those grafts that survive long term are exposed to nephritogenic factors for longer and are more likely to develop recurrent GN. Consistent with this concept, recipients of HLA-identical transplants rarely suffer rejection, enjoy prolonged graft survival, but have a high rate of recurrent GN.[6] In one report of HLA-identical recipients, recurrent GN was present in 36% to 42% of those in whom biopsy was performed and resulted in 24% of graft losses, thereby being the second most frequent cause of graft loss after death in this group.[6]

Higher rates of recurrence have also been reported in pediatric transplant recipients in whom recurrent GN has been the cause of 6% of first allograft losses and 12% of subsequent graft losses.[7] Patients suffering first allograft loss from recurrent GN are also at higher risk of recurrence in a subsequent graft, documented at up to 48%.[8]

The impact of choice of immunosuppressive agents is likely to be significant; however, data in this area is sparse. *Post hoc* analyses of corticosteroid withdrawal trials suggest that this strategy does not lead to increased rates of recurrence.[9] Many researchers have postulated that mycophenolate mofetil, an agent increasingly used in the management of proliferative GN, may have benefits in preventing or treating recurrent disease; however, clear demonstration of this is lacking. Inclusion or addition of cyclophosphamide has been effective in the management of recurrent vasculitis affecting the graft.[10] Of major interest and concern is the tendency for patients maintained on, or particularly switched to, sirolimus to develop proteinuria and renal dysfunction. This effect appears to be more common among those with a primary diagnosis of GN, suggesting that sirolimus may either facilitate recurrence or more likely accelerate its impact on the graft.[11] Effects of individual agents are likely to be disease specific, and much needs to be learned in this area.

Strategies to reduce the risk of recurrence have been reported. Bilateral native nephrectomy as a means of eliminating persistent antigenic stimulation appears unhelpful as nephrectomized patients experienced a higher incidence of recurrence compared to those with native kidneys left *in situ* in one large single-center, retrospective study.[12] Induction of disease remission prior to transplantation and prolonged time on dialysis pretransplantation, both aimed at permitting disease "burnout," do not appear to be effective except in the case of anti-GBM disease in which a delay in transplantation until the patient has been serologically negative for at least 6 months virtually eliminates the risk of recurrence.[3] Avoidance of living related donation has been debated for years and may be a relevant factor in individual disease settings (see later discussion).

Clinical Features and Differential Diagnosis of Recurrent Glomerulonephritis

As is the case with GN in native kidneys, proteinuria, hematuria, and deterioration in kidney function are the cardinal manifestations of recurrent GN. The pattern of renal and extrarenal manifestations is frequently similar to that of the native disease, except that, in the opinion of the author, the rate of progression may be slower. Extrarenal features of the primary condition may recur, such as thrombocytopenia and hemolysis in hemolytic uremic syndrome (HUS) and extrarenal vasculitis in recurrent

Wegener's granulomatosis. Serology may be helpful in some cases, such as anti-GBM antibody detection in Goodpasture's disease, but may be inconsistent in others such as recurrent lupus nephritis (LN).

The differential diagnosis of recurrent GN is clinically important as management may vary according to the diagnosis (Fig. 96.3). CAN and diabetic nephropathy, recurrent or *de novo*, may both present with progressive graft dysfunction, proteinuria, and hypertension and may therefore be clinically indistinguishable from recurrence. *De novo* GN should also be considered. Viral disease of the kidney, particularly BK nephropathy, is an important alternative to consider as a reduction in immunosuppression and specific antiviral therapy may provide benefit. The need to exclude obstructive uropathy and tumors involving the graft warrant an ultrasound scan. Finally, recurrence may coexist with CAN or calcineurin inhibitor toxicity. Indeed, every condition that can lead to chronic graft dysfunction should be considered in the differential diagnosis of recurrence (see Fig. 96.3 and Chapter 95).

Histologic evidence of recurrence is required in all cases. Biopsy can provide the diagnosis, exclude alternative diagnoses that may require different approaches to treatment, and provide important prognostic information pertinent to the affected graft and also relevant to any future consideration of retransplantation. Full evaluation of the biopsy specimen by light microscopy, immunohistology, and electron microscopy is desirable and in many cases essential to confirm recurrence.[13,14] Light microscopy and immunohistology are necessary to differentiate recurrent from *de novo* GN, rejection, and calcineurin inhibitor toxicity. The presence of tubulitis should suggest acute rejection. CAN may produce chronic interstitial inflammation and transplant glomerulopathy, which may be indistinguishable from membranoproliferative glomerulonephritis (MPGN) by light microscopy (Fig. 96.4; see also Chapter 95). The use of immunohistology to define the content of immune deposits and electron microscopy to establish the structure of basement membrane and location of deposits may clarify the diagnosis.[14] Histologic appearances are typically no different from the patterns of GN in native kidneys and are illustrated in the relevant chapters of Section 4, Glomerular Disease. The risk of recurrence in common patterns of renal disease is summarized in Figure 96.5.

IgA Nephropathy and Henoch-Schönlein Purpura

IgAN is the most common form of GN leading to ESRD, and these patients are frequently transplant recipients. Histologic recurrence is frequent and increases with time; one study in which all recipients were subjected to protocol biopsy found recurrence in 58%.[6] Recurrence is difficult to predict. Patient characteristics, pretransplantation course, serum IgA glycosylation, and angiotensin-converting enzyme genotype have been found to have no predictive value.[1,15] Immunosuppression posttransplantation, including the use of mycophenolate mofetil,[16] and post-transplantation course have no impact.[15] Living related donor transplantation has been associated with an increased risk of recurrence and graft loss in some series but not in others[3] and does not justify the avoidance of living related donor transplantation in patients with IgAN.

The clinical expression of disease is variable and time dependent. Graft loss within the first 3 years after transplantation is uncommon (see Fig. 96.2), although it can be seen, particularly when there is extensive crescentic GN retransplantation following previous graft loss due to recurrence.[15] The longer-term outlook

Differential diagnosis of recurrent glomerulonephritis					
Diagnosis	Frequency and Timing	Clinical Features	Lab Features	Biopsy Features	Management
Recurrent glomerulonephritis	Common; variable timing, days to years	Proteinuria, hematuria, renal impairment, hypertension	Similar to primary glomerulonephritis; serology may be negative	Same as primary glomerulonephritis[4,5]	Disease specific
De novo glomerulonephritis	Uncommon; variable timing but typically later than recurrence	Proteinuria, hematuria, renal impairment	Hemolysis and thrombocytopenia in HUS	Type specific[4,5,8]	Antiprogression strategies (see Chapter 69)
Chronic allograft nephropathy	Very common; increasing incidence with time	Hypertension, proteinuria, renal impairment Calcineurin inhibitor exposure		Tubulointerstitial fibrosis, arteriolar hyalinosis, transplant glomerulopathy	Minimize calcineurin inhibitor and antiprogression strategies (see Chapter 69)
Graft pyelonephritis	Uncommon Typically early after transplantation	Fever Renal impairment, pyuria	Positive blood or urine cultures	Neutrophil infiltration	Antibiotics
BK nephropathy	Uncommon; typically 1–5 yr after transplantation	Renal impairment, decoy cells in urine	Serum BK PCR positive	Tubulitis with tubular cell atypia and inclusions, normal glomeruli	Antiviral drugs and minimize immunosuppression
Acute rejection	Common; early	Renal impairment, oliguria	Nonspecific	Tubulitis ± vasculitis[15]	Increase immunosuppression
Renal tumor/PTLD	Uncommon, rare; early or late	Renal impairment, renal mass	Anemia, EBV positive	Atypical cells, mitoses, monoclonality	Minimize immunosuppression, ? chemotherapy

Figure 96.3 Differential diagnosis of recurrent glomerulonephritis. EBV, Epstein-Barr virus; PCR, polymerase chain reaction; PTLD, post-transplantation lymphoproliferative disease; HUS, hemolytic uremic syndrome.

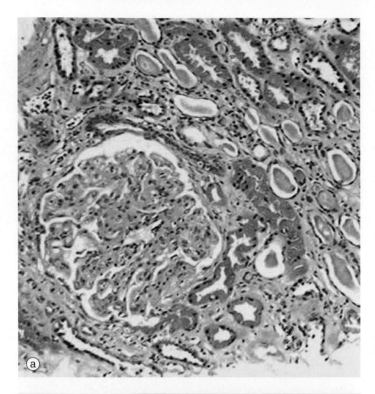

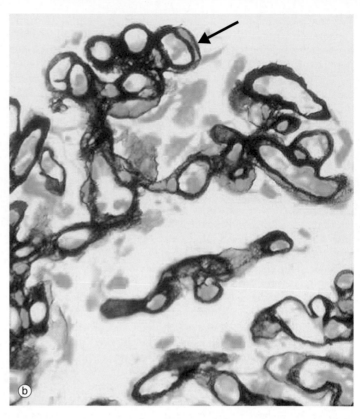

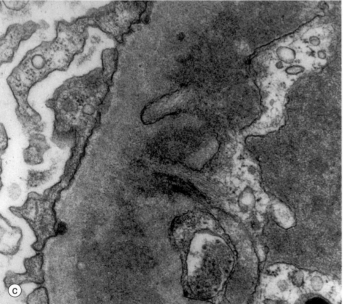

Figure 96.4 Transplant glomerulopathy and membranoproliferative glomerulonephritis (MPGN). Transplant biopsy specimen from a patient with end-stage renal disease due to biopsy-proven idiopathic MPGN type I, who received a kidney transplant and had a progressive reduction in glomerular filtration rate with proteinuria 1.5 g/day and hypertension. *a*, Light microscopy. Glomerular hypercellularity and lobulation on a background of chronic interstitial inflammation and fibrosis, with protein casts within dilated tubules (hematoxylin and eosin, ×100). *b*, Subendothelial deposits and basement membrane reduplication (*arrow*) (methenamine silver, ×400). *c*, Electron microscopy showing subendothelial electron-dense deposits (×7500). There were also prominent C3 deposits on immunofluorescence (not shown). Light microscopy was therefore suggestive of recurrent MPGN, but was also consistent with chronic allograft nephropathy (CAN) with transplant glomerulopathy associated with CAN. Immunofluorescence and electron microscopy (subendothelial deposits) confirmed recurrence of MPGN. (Compare Chapter 95, Figures 95.6 and 95.7.) (*a* and *b*, Courtesy of Dr. Paul McKenzie.)

is not benign as progressive graft loss over time has been documented by all major studies. In one registry study that included 587 subjects with biopsy-proven IgAN, the risk of graft loss due to IgA recurrence was approximately 10% within 10 years post-transplantation.[3]

Recurrence of Henoch-Schönlein purpura (HSP) nephritis is less well characterized but appears to be similar to IgAN in all respects. The largest report that pooled patients from Belgium and Japan found recurrence in 35% and graft loss in 11% at 5 years of follow-up.[18]

Treatment of recurrent IgAN and HSP has not been systematically evaluated, and specific therapies such as corticosteroids, mycophenolate mofetil, fish oil, and antiplatelet agents cannot be

recommended. The use of nonspecific measures to prolong kidney survival, such as tight blood pressure control, renin-angiotensin blockade, and avoidance of nephrotoxins, is appropriate.

Focal Segmental Glomerulosclerosis

Patients with renal failure due to FSGS incur a risk of recurrence of 20% to 30% for first transplants.[19,20] FSGS is a heterogeneous group of conditions, and those with familial or sporadic forms associated with mutation of slit-diaphragm proteins such as podocin, those with FSGS secondary to vascular disease, and those with a very slow rate of progression are at substantially lower risk, whereas patients with an aggressive initial course (heavy proteinuria and renal failure within 3 years of onset), are younger than 15 years,

Recurrent diseases in renal transplants and effects on graft survival		
Disease	Clinical Recurrence Rate (%)	Graft Loss in Recurrent Disease (%)
Primary focal segmental glomerulosclerosis	20–50 (children), 10–15 (adults)	40–50
Membranoproliferative glomerulonephritis Type I Type II	 20–30 80–100	 30–40 20
Hemolytic uremic syndrome (HUS) Classic D+HUS Atypical D–HUS Familial HUS	 0–13 30–50 57	 Uncommon 55–100 Approaching 100
IgA nephropathy	29–39 increases with longer duration of follow-up (30%–60% histologic recurrence rate)	16–33
Henoch-Schönlein purpura	Rare (despite 50% histologic recurrence rate)	Rare
Membranous nephropathy	10–29 (histologic recurrence may be more common)	≤50
Systemic vasculitis, including Wegener's granulomatosis and microscopic polyangiitis	10–20 overall (WG MPA)	20–50
Antiglomerular basement membrane antibody-mediated glomerulonephritis	<5	50
Systemic lupus erythematosus	1–30	Rare
Amyloidosis	5–25	10–20

Figure 96.5 Recurrent diseases in renal transplants and effects on graft survival.

with mesangial proliferation on biopsy, or with recurrence in a previous graft are at greatest risk.[19,20] The rate of recurrence is >75% in subsequent grafts when the first graft was lost due to recurrence.[21] Living related donor transplantation has been implicated as a risk factor for recurrence; however, a major analysis of U.S. Renal Data System (USRDS) refutes this notion.[13]

Recurrence occurs early, typically within the first month post-transplantation, and is commonly manifested by heavy proteinuria, hypertension, and graft dysfunction. Patients with recurrent disease appear more susceptible to acute rejection and acute renal failure,[22] as well as graft loss. Recurrence has been associated with early graft loss in up to 40% to 50% of cases[20]; however, the adoption of plasma exchange appears to have delayed graft loss in many cases and decreased the incidence of overall graft failure[3] (see Fig. 96.2).

A circulating 50-kd plasma protein that is bound to immunoglobulin appears to cause recurrent FSGS. The protein remains unidentified but is capable of inducing proteinuria when applied to rat kidneys.[23,24] Attempts to use the presence of the circulating "permeability factor" as a guide to the risk of recurrence have not produced a clinically useful test. Plasma exchange or immunoadsorption effectively removes the "permeability factor" because it is bound to immunoglobulin and as a result provides an effective therapy for many patients who develop recurrent FSGS.[23,24] Although not subjected to a randomized, controlled, prospective trial, several series have found disease remission in the majority of patients who receive treatment within 2 weeks of recurrence.[24,25] A minority of patients with an incomplete response or relapse following cessation of initial therapy will require repeated or long-term plasma exchange or concurrent treatment with cyclophosphamide.[25] Pretransplantation plasma exchange has not been shown to be of benefit in the prevention of recurrence in the graft. The role of concomitant immunosuppressive therapy, in addition

to that required to prevent acute rejection, is unclear. See Figure 96.6 for an approach to the management of recurrent FSGS.[26]

Minimal change disease is a far less frequent cause of ESRD. Recurrence of disease after transplantation has been reported; however, it is difficult to be sure that the underlying disease was not FSGS.

Congenital Nephrotic Syndrome

Congenital nephritic syndrome of the Finnish type has been reported to recur following transplantation and to cause graft loss; however, it is likely that the mechanism of kidney damage is quite different between primary and recurrent disease. In cases where the primary disorder is caused by a mutation of the *NPHS1* gene that results in complete absence of nephrin, transplantation causes *de novo* exposure to nephrin in the transplanted kidney. Neoantigen exposure causes antibody development and deposition that damages the slit diaphragm and produces a type of membranous nephropathy with podocyte fusion on electron microscopy and a clinical picture of heavy proteinuria and ultimately graft failure. Cyclophosphamide-based rescue therapy may be successful.[27]

Membranous Nephropathy

Data on recurrent MN is clouded by two key issues: the small number of subjects in reported series and the frequency of *de novo* MN post-transplantation. *De novo* MN has been reported in 2% to 15% of transplant recipients and tends to present more insidiously and later than recurrent MN.[28]

The largest series (pooled from centers in Belgium and France) reported a recurrence rate of 29% in 30 patients at 3 years post-transplantation[28] and graft survival of 38% at 5 years and 52% at 10 years follow-up. Recurrence is a significant clinical event causing proteinuria, nephrotic syndrome, and graft loss in 12% of recipients within 10 years after transplantation.[3] Clinical factors

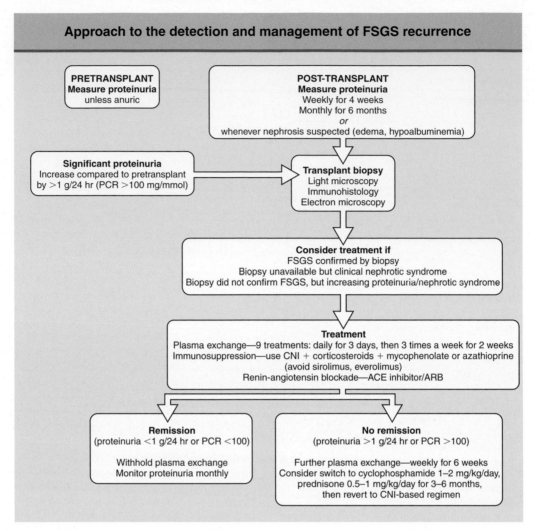

Figure 96.6 Approach to the detection and management of focal and segmental glomerulosclerosis (FSGS) recurrence. ACE, angiotensin-converting enzyme; ARB, angiotensin receptor blocker; CNI, calcineurin inhibitor; PCR, urine protein: creatinine ratio. Author's recommendation based on Davenport.[26]

including pretransplantation disease course, duration of dialysis, HLA genotype, graft source, and immunosuppression are not predictive of risk. However, those with a previous graft loss due to recurrence are at high risk if retransplanted.[29]

Management of recurrent MN is based on anecdotal reports and extrapolation of data on the management of native kidney MN. Spontaneous remissions appear to be less common. The cumulative exposure to immunosuppressive therapy should be considered as these patients may be at increased risk of lymphoma. Live donor transplantation appears warranted for first grafts but, in the opinion of the author, should probably be avoided for second grafts if the first was lost early due to recurrence.

Thrombotic Microangiopathy and Hemolytic Uremic Syndrome

The diagnosis of recurrent thrombotic microangiopathy and HUS is complicated by the fact that *de novo* HUS is seen in 1% to 5% of kidney transplant recipients, most commonly associated with the use of calcineurin inhibitors (both tacrolimus and cyclosporine carry a similar risk), sirolimus, OKT3, or acute vascular rejection. A meta-analysis, which examined 10 reports covering 159 grafts in 127 patients, reported recurrence in 28% of cases, and this was strongly associated with a poor outcome: 1-year graft survival was 33% for those with recurrence versus 77% in those free from

recurrence ($P < 0.001$).[30] Recurrence risk is clearly associated with the type of HUS. Typical childhood postdiarrheal (D+) HUS seldom recurs, whereas recurrence of atypical (D–) HUS is frequent and in hereditary forms associated with mutation of complement factor H exceeds 50%. Within these groups, recurrence is associated with an older age at onset, rapid progression of the original disease, earlier transplantation, living-related transplantation, and the use of calcineurin inhibitors.[30] Recurrence is generally within the first 6 months post-transplantation; however, late recurrences have been reported.[30] The clinical presentation may be gradual or abrupt, with thrombocytopenia, hemolysis, and progressive renal dysfunction.

While *de novo* disease may respond to withdrawal of the inciting agent, management of recurrent disease is unproven. The author recommends withdrawal of any potential causative agent such as calcineurin inhibitors, and if this is not effective after 48 hours, a trial of plasma exchange should be initiated with three half-plasma volume exchanges performed on three consecutive days using fresh-frozen plasma for replacement. As an increased incidence of acute rejection has been reported in patients with recurrence,[31] underimmunosuppression following calcineurin inhibitor withdrawal should be avoided by a temporary increase in the dose of corticosteroids. In cases of life-threatening thrombocytopenia or hemolysis, hematologic stability may be restored by transplant nephrectomy. The prognosis of recurrent disease is poor. More than 50% of grafts are lost within the first year and graft survival beyond 5 years is quite uncommon.[30] Combined liver-kidney transplantation has been reported to prevent recurrence in one case of complement factor H deficiency–associated HUS, with the liver graft facilitating restoration of a normal complement synthesis.[32] There is no evidence that calcineurin inhibitor avoidance is useful in preventing recurrence.

Antineutrophil Cytoplasmic Antibody–Associated Pauci-immune Vasculitis

A pooled analysis of all reported case series examining recurrence of antineutrophil cytoplasmic antibody (ANCA)–associated vasculitis, incorporating 127 patients, has largely clarified the behavior of this group of disorders following transplantation.[33] Disease recurrence was detected in 17% of cases after 4 to 89 months of follow-up, with renal involvement demonstrated in approximately 60% of cases and graft losses reported in a minority of these. Clinical parameters were not useful in predicting those patients likely to suffer a relapse post-transplantation. Pretransplantation disease course, duration of dialysis, ANCA titers at time of transplantation and during follow-up, cytoplasmic ANCA or peripheral ANCA specificity, disease subtype (Wegener's, microscopic polyangiitis, or renal-limited vasculitis), and donor source had no significant impact on recurrence rate.[33]

The prevention and management of relapse has not been prospectively examined. In most reports, patients did not receive a transplant until they were in clinical remission; however, successful transplantation in the face of persisting ANCA positivity is well recognized. In the absence of evidence, the author recommends that clinical remission be maintained for at least 6 months prior to transplantation to reduce the risk of recurrence and also to avoid the risks associated with transplanting a debilitated patient. Patients with renal relapses have generally been managed with cyclophosphamide-based immunosuppression, reported to be successful in inducing a remission in 11 of 16 (69%) cases.[33] The negative impact of using cyclophosphamide to treat relapse has not been reported, but would clearly include a significant increase in the risk of bladder cancer.

Kidney transplantation for ANCA-associated vasculitis is associated with a reduction in the frequency of disease relapse by approximately 50% compared to patients without transplants, and patient and graft survival post-transplantation is similar to other transplant recipients.[33]

Goodpasture's Disease

Histologic recurrence of anti-GBM disease (Goodpasture's disease) is seen in 50% of patients who receive a transplant while circulating anti-GBM antibodies persist,[34] but rarely when patients undergo transplantation 6 months or more after the disappearance of anti-GBM antibodies. With delayed transplantation, the rate of clinical recurrence is very low, and since the implementation of this practice in Australia, no grafts were lost following transplantation in 47 cases followed for up to 10 years.[3] Rare episodes of recurrence should be treated as for native kidney disease with corticosteroids, cyclophosphamide, and aggressive plasma exchange (see Chapter 22).

Recurrent anti-GBM disease is distinct from *de novo* anti-GBM disease, which is seen in up to 15% of transplant recipients with Alport's syndrome who develop anti-GBM antibodies in response to neoantigen exposure (α-chain of type IV collagen) via the transplant.[34] This is also discussed further in Chapter 22.

Membranoproliferative Glomerulonephritis

Recurrent MPGN bears major clinical and histologic similarities with the subgroup of patients with CAN who have transplant glomerulopathy, and comprehensive assessment of transplant biopsies (see Fig. 96.4 and compare Figs. 95.6 and 95.7) as well as accurate diagnosis of the native kidney disease is crucial in making this distinction (see Fig. 96.3). MPGN is suggested by the presence of crescents on light microscopy, stronger staining for C3, and weaker staining for IgM on immunohistology and by the presence of subendothelial or intramembranous dense deposits on electron microscopy.[14] This distinction has important clinical implications, particularly as a recurrence carries a higher risk of subsequent recurrence should retransplantation be considered.

Membranoproliferative Glomerulonephritis Type I

This disorder appears to be mediated by glomerular deposition of immune complexes, triggered by exposure to endogenous or exogenous (e.g., hepatitis C virus [HCV]) antigens. As the antigens are not necessarily removed by transplantation, recurrence of disease is possible and is seen in 20% to 33% of graft recipients.[35] Graft loss has been reported in up to 40% of those with recurrence, and the risk of recurrence in subsequent grafts approaches 80%.[36] Significant geographic diversity in the risk of recurrence is evident, largely linked to the prevalence of HCV, with much higher rates of graft loss due to recurrence being reported in areas where the majority of patients with MPGN are HCV positive, such as Spain,[37] as compared to low HCV prevalence areas, such as Australia.[3] Patients receiving HLA-identical grafts appear to be at increased risk of recurrence in some series[35] but not in others.[3]

No form of treatment is proven, and the underlying cause of recurrent MPGN should be considered in each case. Prevention may be effective in HCV-associated MPGN, as interferon-based therapy appears to be effective for virus elimination if undertaken while the patient is on maintenance dialysis, and this provides substantial protection from HCV viremia and MPGN recurrence after subsequent transplantation.[38] By contrast, the use of interferon post-transplantation is associated with acute rejection and should be avoided. Other forms of MPGN type I have been treated with immunosuppression or plasma exchange with success in single cases.

Membranoproliferative Glomerulonephritis Type II (Dense Deposit Disease)

This disease has been found to recur in 50% to 100% of grafts, typically presenting with proteinuria, hematuria, and slowly progressive loss of kidney function.[39] The disease course tends to be slow, and while graft loss due to recurrence is ultimately seen in 10% to 25% of cases, this generally occurs beyond the first 10 years after transplantation.[3,39] Graft loss has been associated with male gender, crescents on biopsy, and heavy proteinuria.[39] No effective therapy is known, and although plasma exchange and immunosuppression have been described, these are not warranted in the opinion of the author and control of blood pressure and proteinuria with renin-angiotensin blockade is the preferred therapy.

Membranoproliferative Glomerulonephritis Type III

Recurrence of this rare disease has been reported, resulting in graft loss in the longer term.[40]

Lupus Nephritis

The reported recurrence rate of lupus nephritis (LN) has varied from 1% to 30%.[41,42] Recurrence has been reported early (days) and late (years) after transplantation, with a mean time to recurrence of 3.1 years in the largest series reported.[43] The clinical and histologic pattern of recurrence is variable, but is typically more benign in histology and clinical expression than the patient's original disease. Whereas the majority of patients with ESRD caused by lupus have had diffuse proliferative disease (class III or IV), mesangial proliferative (class II) disease is the most commonly described lesion post-transplantation, followed by class III and membranous (class V).[44] Duration of dialysis prior to transplantation and serologic activity do not predict recurrence and antinuclear antibody titer and complement levels are unreliable markers of disease recurrence post-transplantation. There is no reliable relationship between recurrence of nephritis and activity of extrarenal lupus post-transplantation.

The long-term outcome for lupus patients following transplantation is controversial but appears similar to the general post-transplantation population.[41] While recurrence is an uncommon cause of graft loss within the first 10 years after transplantation, with no cases of graft loss reported from 86 recipients in one registry analysis,[3] late graft losses do occur. It is clear that lupus patients, particularly those with a lupus anticoagulant, are at increased risk of thrombotic events following transplantation including graft thrombosis.[41]

Management of recurrent LN has not been formally studied; however, the use of corticosteroids, cyclophosphamide, and plasma exchange has been reported, with variable results.[44] The impact of mycophenolate mofetil, which is effective in management of diffuse proliferative LN in native kidneys, remains to be proven. Anticoagulation during the perioperative and early post-transplantation phases should be considered for those with a history of thrombosis or lupus anticoagulant positivity. Successful retransplantation has been reported following graft loss due to recurrence.[43]

Scleroderma

An analysis of 86 patients reported to the United Network for Organ Sharing registry after receiving a kidney transplant for scleroderma demonstrated graft survival of 62% at 1 year and 47% at 5 years post-transplantation; 24% of recipients died during the 10-year observation period.[45] The recurrence rate could not be accurately determined; however, recurrence was responsible for graft loss in 21% of cases in which the cause was identified, which is consistent with previously accepted recurrence rates. Risk factors for recurrence were not identified and cyclosporine use did not appear to affect the recurrence rate.[45] The effect of transplantation on the extrarenal manifestations of scleroderma has not been well documented. The management of scleroderma post-transplantation is unstudied; however, the use of angiotensin-converting enzyme inhibitors post-transplantation to treat hypertension would seem appropriate. Overall, the post-transplantation course of scleroderma appears to be similar to that of LN,[45] and renal transplantation appears to be an appropriate treatment for those with ESRD.

AMYLOID, LIGHT CHAIN DISEASE, AND FIBRILLARY AND IMMUNOTACTOID GLOMERULOPATHIES

Amyloidosis

The risk and impact of recurrence for patients who underwent transplantation because of systemic amyloidosis is clearly dependent on its cause. Management of AL amyloid is primarily directed at treating the underlying plasma cell dyscrasia, most commonly

by high-dose chemotherapy and bone marrow transplantation. Recurrence after transplantation will occur if the malignancy is not fully controlled and may be susceptible to further chemotherapy.

Secondary (AA) amyloidosis is typically a more insidious disease; renal failure is a relatively frequent complication and renal transplantation is frequently effective. The risk of recurrence of AA amyloid depends on the ability to eradicate the underlying cause of chronic inflammation. Recurrence is unlikely in AA amyloid due to chronic infection if the infection can be eradicated pretransplantation, whereas conditions such as rheumatoid arthritis may persist after transplantation and lead to recurrent amyloid in the graft. Patients with AA amyloid associated with familial Mediterranean fever, which can be managed post-transplantation with colchicine, have recurrence in <5% of cases at 10 years post-transplantation.[46] A Norwegian series of 62 transplants in patients with AA amyloid, mostly secondary to rheumatic diseases, demonstrated a recurrence rate of 10% at an average of 5 years of follow-up, causing graft loss in two cases only. Overall, patient and graft survival rates were 65% and 62%, respectively, at 5 years, with most losses due to infection.[47]

Light Chain Nephropathy

Patients with light chain nephropathy have occasionally received transplants; however, recurrence is the norm, with one case series reporting recurrence in five of seven patients at a range of 2 to 45 months post-transplantation. Those with recurrence developed proteinuria, hypertension, and progressive graft dysfunction. One of seven has enjoyed long-term graft function, and one died soon after transplantation because of myeloma.[48] Kidney transplantation is therefore generally inadvisable for patients with this disease, unless performed in conjunction with bone marrow transplantation as a means of curing the underlying disease.

Fibrillary and Immunotactoid Glomerulopathies

Fibrillary and immunotactoid glomerulopathies are known to recur in approximately 50% of those undergoing transplantation for these diseases, and although early graft loss due to recurrence has been reported, decline in graft function is most commonly slow and does not appear to have an impact on 5-year graft survival rates.[49]

RECURRENCE OF METABOLIC DISEASES AFFECTING THE KIDNEY TRANSPLANT

Diabetes Mellitus

Diabetes mellitus is the most common cause of ESRD in many parts of the world; however, these patients undergo transplantation less commonly than those with GN because of a higher prevalence and severity of cardiovascular comorbidity. Recurrence of diabetic nephropathy is well recognized both histologically and clinically, affecting at least 25% of recipients at an average follow-up of 6 years with some cases diagnosed within 3 years of transplantation.[49] Histologic and clinical features are similar to those of native kidney diabetic nephropathy. The risk of graft loss due to recurrence has not been well documented, but appears to be less than with GN, probably due to the competing risk of death due to cardiovascular disease. New-onset diabetes after transplantation is also common and has been reported to cause nephropathy in the graft in a similar proportion of cases, also commonly manifesting within 5 years of transplantation. The extent to which this contributes to graft loss also awaits clarification, but is likely to be significant. As is the case in native kidney

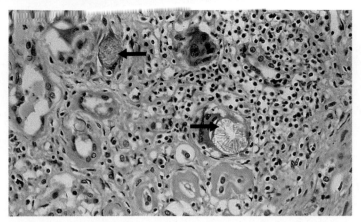

Figure 96.7 Recurrent primary hyperoxaluria. Light microscopy demonstrates oxalate crystals within the tubular lumen (*arrows*) with a secondary interstitial inflammatory infiltrate.

diabetic nephropathy, it is likely that transplant diabetic nephropathy further increases the cardiac risk of those affected.

Primary Hyperoxaluria

Primary hyperoxaluria (see Chapter 54) is a rare autosomal recessive disease caused by defective or absent hepatic production of alanine glyoxylate aminotransferase, resulting in systemic accumulation of calcium oxalate (oxalosis). Kidneys and blood vessels in particular are affected. Kidney transplantation alone is frequently complicated by hyperoxaluria and consequent recurrence in the graft and ultimately graft loss (Fig. 96.7). By contrast, combined liver-kidney transplantation corrects the underlying metabolic deficit and permits long-term kidney graft survival. In an analysis of the USRDS that included 190 adults with oxalosis who went on to renal transplantation, 134 patients who received a kidney transplant alone experienced 48% 8-year death-censored graft survival. This was inferior to 56 patients who received a liver as well (76%) and inferior to a control group with a primary diagnosis of GN (61%).[50] Aggressive removal of residual oxalate pretransplantation by dialysis and post-transplantation by pyridoxine

supplementation and maintaining high urine volumes may also decrease the risk of graft damage.

Fabry's Disease

Fabry's disease results from a defect in lysosomal α-galactosidase A enzyme, which results in tissue accumulation of trihexosylceramide eventually causing ESRD (see Chapter 45). Recurrent Fabry's disease has been documented within the graft; however, graft survival does not appear to be affected. The development of recombinant α-galactosidase A, should this become widely available, is likely to reduce the risk of ESRD and also that of recurrence.

RECURRENCE OF VIRUS-ASSOCIATED NEPHROPATHIES AND TUMORS IN THE TRANSPLANTED KIDNEY

Virus-associated kidney diseases may recur following transplantation. Hepatitis B and C virus–associated MPGN and MN are known to recur; however, the risk of this can be substantially decreased by successful antiviral therapy prior to retransplantation (see Chapter 20). Retransplantation has been reported in patients experiencing graft loss due to BK nephropathy. In the largest series, recurrence was documented in 1 of 10 transplant recipients at an average follow-up of 3 years.[51] Measures to decrease the risk of recurrence included delay in retransplantation by an average of 13 months and transplant nephroureterectomy in seven cases. Calcineurin inhibitor–based triple immunosuppressive therapy was used in all cases, and the one case of recurrence experienced stabilization of graft function following a reduction in their immunosuppression.[52] Thus, retransplantation, ideally delayed until BK virus is not detectable in serum by polymerase chain reaction, appears to be safe and effective.

Patients who develop post-transplantation lymphoproliferative disease and incur graft loss due to direct infiltration or rejection following the withdrawal of immunosuppression may safely and successfully undergo retransplantation after a period of recovery. There was no evidence of recurrence reported in one series of five cases.[52]

REFERENCES

1. Chadban SJ: Glomerulonephritis recurrence in the renal graft. J Am Soc Nephrol 2001;12:394–402.
2. Hariharan S, Adams MB, Brennan DC, Davis CL: Recurrent and de novo glomerular disease after renal transplantation: A report from Renal Allograft Disease registry (RADR). Transplantation 1999;68: 635–641.
3. Briganti EM, Russ GR, McNeil J, et al: Risk of renal allograft loss from recurrent glomerulonephritis. N Engl J Med 2002;347:103–109.
4. Ponticelli C, Villa M, Cesana B, et al: Risk factors for late kidney allograft failure. Kidney Int 2002;62:1848–1854.
5. Hariharan S, Johnson CP, Breshahan BA, et al: Improved graft survival after renal transplantation in the United States, 1988 to 1996. N Engl J Med 2000;342:605–612.
6. Andresdottir MB, Hoitsma AJ, Assmann KJ, et al: The impact of recurrent glomerulonephritis on graft survival in recipients of human histocompatibility leucocyte antigen-identical living related donor grafts. Transplantation 1999;68:623–627.
7. Baqi N, Tejani A: Recurrence of the original disease in paediatric renal transplantation. J Nephrol 1997;10:85–92.
8. Douglas Briggs J, Jones E, on behalf of the ERA-EDTA Registry: Recurrence of glomerulonephritis following renal transplantation. Nephrol Dial Transplant 1999;14:564–565.
9. Ibrahim H, Rogers T, Casingal V, et al: Graft loss from recurrent glomerulonephritis is not increased with a rapid steroid discontinuation protocol. Transplantation 2006;81:214–219.

10. Nachman PH, Segelmark M, Westman K, Hogan SL: Recurrent ANCA-associated small vessel vasculitis after transplantation: A pooled analysis. Kidney Int 1999;56:1544–1550.
11. Ruiz JC, Campistol JM, Sanchez-Fructuso A, et al: Increase of proteinuria after conversion from calcineurin inhibitor to sirolimus-based treatment in kidney transplant patients with chronic allograft dysfunction. Nephrol Dial Transplant 2006;21:3252–3257.
12. Odorico JS, Knechtle SJ, Rayhill SC, Pirsch JD: The influence of native nephrectomy on the incidence of recurrent disease following renal transplantation for primary glomerulonephritis. Transplantation 1996; 61:228–234.
13. Cibrik DM, Kaplan B, Campbell DA, Meier-Kriesche HU: Renal allograft survival in transplant recipients with focal segmental glomerulosclerosis. Am J Transplant 2003;3:64–67.
14. Andresdottir MB, Assmann KJ, Koene RA, Wetzels JF: Immunohistological and ultrastructural differences between recurrent type I membranoproliferative glomerulonephritis and chronic transplant glomerulopathy. Am J Kidney Dis 1998;32:582–588.
15. Ohmacht C, Kliem V, Burg M, Nashan B: Recurrent immunoglobulin A nephropathy after renal transplantation: A significant contributor to graft loss. Transplantation 1997;64:1493–1496.
16. Chandrakantan A, Ratanapanichkich P, Said M, et al: Recurrent IgA nephropathy after renal transplantation despite immunosuppressive regimens with mycophenolate mofetil. Nephrol Dial Transplant 2005; 20:1214–1221

17. Kowalewska J, Yuan S, Sustento-Reodica N, et al: IgA nephropathy with crescents in kidney transplant recipients. Am J Kidney Dis 2005;45: 167–175.

18. Meulders Q, Pirson Y, Cosyns JP, et al: Course of Henoch-Schonlein nephritis after renal transplantation. Report on 10 patients and review of the literature. Transplantation 1994;58:1179–1186

19. Senggutuvan P, Cameron JS, Hartley RB, et al: Recurrence of focal segmental glomerulosclerosis in transplanted kidneys: Analysis of incidence and risk factors in 59 allografts. Pediatr Nephrol 1990;4:21–28.

20. Artero M, Biava C, Amend W, et al: Recurrent focal glomerulosclerosis: Natural history and response to therapy. Am J Med 1992;92:375–383.

21. Stephanian E, Matas AJ, Mauer SM, et al: Recurrence of disease in patients retransplanted for focal segmental glomerulosclerosis. Transplantation 1992;53:755–757.

22. Kim EM, Striegel J, Kim Y, et al: Recurrence of steroid resistant nephrotic syndrome in kidney transplants is associated with increased acute renal failure and acute rejection. Kidney Int 1994;45:1440–1445.

23. Savin VJ, Sharma R, Sharma M, et al: Circulating factor associated with increased glomerular permeability to albumin in recurrent focal segmental glomerulosclerosis. N Engl J Med 1996;334:878–883.

24. Dantal J, Godfrin Y, Koll R, et al: Antihuman immunoglobulin affinity immunoadsorption strongly increases proteinuria in patients with relapsing nephrotic syndrome. J Am Soc Nephrol 1998;9:1709–1715.

25. Andresdottir MB, Ajubi N, Croockewit S, Assmann KJ. Recurrent focal glomerulosclerosis: Natural course and treatment with plasma exchange. Nephrol Dial Transplant 1999;14:2650–2656.

26. Davenport RD: Apheresis treatment of recurrent focal segmental glomerulosclerosis after kidney transplantation: Re-analysis of published case-reports and case-series. J Clin Apher 2001;16:175–178.

27. Patrakka J, Ruotsalainen V, Reponen P, et al: Recurrence of nephrotic syndrome in kidney grafts of patients with congenital nephrotic syndrome of the Finnish type: Role of nephrin. Transplantation 2002;73:394–403.

28. Schwarz A, Krause PH, Offerman G, Keller F: Impact of de novo membranous glomerulonephritis on the clinical course after kidney transplantation. Transplantation 1994;58:650–654.

29. Cosyns JP, Couchoud C, Pouteil-Noble C, Squifflet JP: Recurrence of membranous nephropathy after renal transplantation: Probability, outcome and risk factors. Clin Nephrol 1998;50:144–153.

30. Ducloux D, Rebibou JM, Semhoun-Ducloux S, Jamali M: Recurrence of hemolytic-uremic syndrome in renal transplant recipients: A meta-analysis. Transplantation 1998;65:1405–1407.

31. Artz MA, Steenbergen EJ, Hoitsma AJ, et al: Renal transplantation in patients with hemolytic uremic syndrome: High rate of recurrence and increased incidence of acute rejections. Transplantation 2003;76: 821–826.

32. Remuzzi G, Ruggenenti P, Codazzi D, et al: Combined kidney and liver transplantation for familial haemolytic uraemic syndrome. Lancet 2002; 359:1671–1672.

33. Westman KWA, Bygren PG, Olsson H, Ranstam J: Relapse rate, renal survival and cancer morbidity in patients with Wegener's granulomatosis or microscopic polyangiitis with renal involvement. J Am Soc Nephrol 1998;9:842–852.

34. Gobel J, Olbricht CJ, Offner G, et al: Kidney transplantation in Alport's syndrome: Long-term outcome and allograft anti-GBM nephritis. Clin Nephrol 1992;38:299–304.

35. Cruzado JM, Gil-Vernet S, Ercilla G, et al: Hepatitis C virus-associated membranoproliferative glomerulonephritis in renal allografts. J Am Soc Nephrol 1996;7:2469–2475.

36. Andresdottir MB, Assmann KJ, Hoitsma AJ, Koene RA: Recurrence of type 1 membranoproliferative glomerulonephritis after renal transplantation: Analysis of the incidence, risk factors, and impact on graft survival. Transplantation 1997;63:1628–1633.

37. Kamar N, Toupance O, Buchler M, et al: Evidence that clearance of hepatitis C virus RNA after alpha-interferon therapy in dialysis patients is sustained after renal transplantation. J Am Soc Nephrol 2003;14: 2092–2098.

38. Andresdottir MB, Assmann KJ, Hoitsma AJ: Renal transplantation in patients with dense deposit disease: Morphological characteristics of recurrent disease and clinical outcome. Nephrol Dial Transplant 1999; 14:1723–1731.

39. Morales JM, Martinez MA, Munoz de Bustillo E: Recurrent type III membranoproliferative glomerulonephritis after kidney transplantation. Transplantation 1997;63:1186–1188.

40. Moroni G, Tantardini F, Gallelli B, et al: The long-term prognosis of renal transplantation in patients with lupus nephritis. Am J Kidney Dis 2005; 45:903–911.

41. Goral S, Ynares C, Shappell SB, et al: Recurrent lupus nephritis in renal transplant recipients revisited: It is not rare. Transplantation 2003;75: 651–656.

42. Stone JH, Millward CL, Olson JL, Amend WJ: Frequency of recurrent lupus nephritis among ninety-seven renal transplant patients during the cyclosporine era. Arthritis Rheum 1998;41:678–686.

43. Goss JA, Cole BR, Jendrisk MD, et al: Renal transplantation for systemic lupus erythematosus and recurrent lupus nephritis: A single-centre experience and a review of the literature. Transplantation 1991;52: 805–810.

44. Chang YJ, Spiera H: Renal transplantation in scleroderma. Medicine (Baltimore) 1999;78:382–385.

45. Sherif AM, Refaie AF, Sobh MA, et al: Long-term outcome of live donor kidney transplantation for renal amyloidosis. Am J Kidney Dis 2003;42:370–375.

46. Leung N, Lager DJ, Gertz MA, et al: Long-term outcome of renal transplantation in light-chain deposition disease. Am J Kidney Dis 2004;43: 147–153.

47. Hartmann A, Holdaas H, Fauchald P, et al: Fifteen years experience with renal transplantation in systemic amyloidosis. Transpl Int 1992;5: 15–18.

48. Pronovost PH, Brady HR, Gunning ME, Espinoza O: Clinical features, predictors of disease progression and results of renal transplantation in fibrillary/immunotactoid glomerulopathy. Nephrol Dial Transplant 1996; 11:837–842.

49. Bhalla V, Nast CC, Stollenwerk N, et al: Recurrent and de novo diabetic nephropathy in renal allografts. Transplantation 2003;75:66–71.

50. Cibrik DM, Kaplan B, Arndorfer JA, Meier-Kriesche HU: Renal allograft survival in patients with oxalosis. Transplantation 2002;74:707–710.

51. Ramos E, Vincenti F, Lu WX, et al: Retransplantation in patients with graft loss caused by polyoma virus nephropathy. Transplantation 2004;77: 131–133.

52. Birkeland SA, Hamilton-Dutoit S, Bendtzen K: Long-term follow-up of kidney transplant patients with posttransplant lymphoproliferative disorder: Duration of posttransplant lymphoproliferative disorder-induced operational graft tolerance, interleukin-18 course, and results of retransplantation. Transplantation 2003;76:153–158.

Outcomes of Renal Transplantation

Colm C. Magee, Glenn M. Chertow, and Edgar L. Milford

INTRODUCTION

The most clinically useful method of assessing renal transplantation outcomes is measurement of allograft survival. Other important measures include allograft function (typically measured by serum creatinine), patient survival, number and severity of acute rejection episodes, days of hospitalization, and quality-of-life indices. Most of the data described here are derived from the U.S. Renal Database System (USRDS)[1] and the Collaborative Transplant Study (CTS).[2] The USRDS reports on almost all transplant recipients in the United States; the CTS on some, but not all, transplant recipients throughout the world.

Registry data are very useful for analyzing allograft survival, although their accuracy is dependent on complete and correct reporting of outcomes to the registries.[3] In practice, randomized, controlled trials of interventions (typically new immunosuppressive drugs) are of limited benefit in comparing effects on allograft survival, as it is difficult to demonstrate statistically significant differences within the short periods of follow-up normally used in such trials. Hence, there has been interest in developing surrogate markers of long-term outcomes.[3-5] Examples of proposed surrogates for allograft survival are creatinine clearance and other estimates of glomerular filtration rate (GFR) and renal histology.

Actual and Actuarial Allograft and Patient Survival

Allograft survival is calculated from the day of transplantation to the day of reaching a defined endpoint (i.e., return to dialysis, retransplantation, or death, whichever occurs first). In practice, survival is usually calculated by actuarial methods. These methods imply estimation or projection of survival as not all patients will have been followed for the same period of time. Also, as not all patients will have reached the defined endpoint, censoring of such patients is required. Projected survival estimates must be interpreted with caution; projected survival may ultimately not be as impressive as actual survival.[6] One-, 5-, and 10-year actuarial survival rates are frequently presented. Another actuarial measure commonly used is graft half-life (median graft survival).

Traditionally, graft survival (or its inverse, graft loss) is assessed under two distinct-time phases: early and late. Early graft loss refers to loss in the first 12 months and late loss to any time thereafter. This distinction is empirical but makes clinical sense. In the first 12 months, graft loss is relatively common because of technical complications such as graft thrombosis and severe rejection. After 12 months, the incidence of graft loss is lower but remains quite stable over time. Usually, analysis of long-term survival is restricted to those allografts that have survived to 12 months post-transplantation. The causes of late graft loss are also different and are discussed later.

Note that using this definition, patient death is equivalent to graft loss. Graft survival can also be calculated after censoring for patient death. Death with a functioning allograft is not necessarily a bad outcome (at least in adult recipients) and in fact is probably the best outcome, provided survival after transplantation is prolonged.

SURVIVAL BENEFITS OF RENAL TRANSPLANTATION

Comparison of survival between the general dialysis population and transplant recipients is greatly affected by selection bias; only relatively healthy patients are referred for transplantation. Thus, comparisons between patients on the waiting list who do or do not receive a transplant are usually performed instead (the large increase in the number of patients on the waiting list has allowed such meaningful statistical analyses). Of course, such analyses assume that the two groups (having received a transplant or still on the list) are otherwise equivalent in factors that affect outcomes, and this is not necessarily true. For example, a patient with serious medical problems might be kept on the waiting list (in the hope that these problems resolve) but would not be called in for a transplantation if a deceased donor kidney were offered to them.

One study of the USRDS database found that during the first 106 days after transplantation, the relative risk of death was greater than remaining on the waiting list (on dialysis).[7] This mainly reflected the risks associated with the transplantation procedure itself. Thereafter, however, transplantation conferred a survival benefit (Fig. 97.1). Based on 3 to 4 years of follow-up, transplantation was associated with a 68% lower risk of death. Transplantation appeared to be particularly effective among patients with diabetes, but improved survival was observed in all patient subgroups.

SHORT TERM OUTCOMES IN RENAL TRANSPLANTATION

Current adjusted 1-year survival probabilities for deceased donor allografts (first or subsequent transplant) are 89% and 95% for living donor allografts (first or subsequent transplant).[1] First transplants consistently have slightly better survival than subsequent ones. One-year graft survival has improved steadily over the past 25 years (Fig. 97.2). The principal causes of graft loss in the first post-transplantation year are acute rejection, graft vessel thrombosis, primary nonfunction, and patient death.

The current adjusted 1-year survival probability for recipients of deceased donor allografts (first or subsequent transplant) is

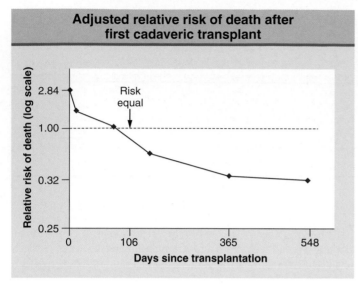

Adjusted relative risk of death after first cadaveric transplant

Risk equal

Figure 97.1 Adjusted relative risk of death among 23,275 recipients of a first cadaveric transplant. The reference group was the 467,164 patients on dialysis who were on the waiting list (relative risk, 1.0). Values were adjusted for age, sex, race, cause of end-stage renal disease, year of placement on the waiting list, geographic region, and time from first treatment for end-stage renal disease to placement on the waiting list. (Adapted from Wolfe RA, Ashby VB, Milford EL, et al: Comparison of mortality in all patients on dialysis, patients on dialysis awaiting transplantation, and recipients of a first cadaveric transplant. N Engl J Med 1999;341:1725–1730.)

91%; this has slowly but steadily improved over the past 25 years. The current adjusted 1-year survival probability for recipients of living donor allografts (first or subsequent transplant) is 95%. These outcomes have also improved over the past 25 years (Fig. 97.3). The principal causes of patient death in the first year are cardiovascular disease and infection (malignancy is a much less common cause) (Fig. 97.4).

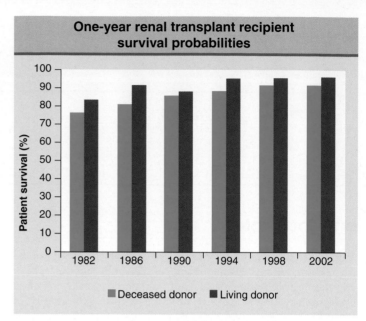

One-year renal transplant recipient survival probabilities

■ Deceased donor ■ Living donor

Figure 97.3 One-year renal transplant recipient survival probabilities (first transplants), adjusted by age, gender, race, primary survival diagnosis. (Data from U.S. Renal Data System: 2005 Annual Data Report. Available at www.usrds.org.)

LONG TERM OUTCOMES IN RENAL TRANSPLANTATION

There has also been a steady improvement in long-term allograft survival (Fig. 97.5). Recently this increase has occurred mainly in higher risk patients, such as those undergoing retransplantation (Fig. 97.5 includes a large percentage of such patients). When first deceased donor transplants alone are assessed, recent improvements are less impressive (Fig. 97.6). These findings

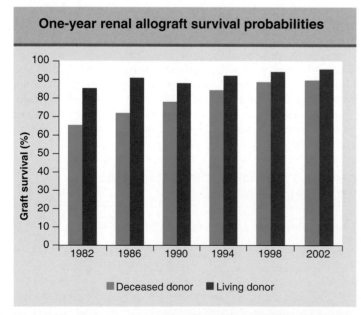

One-year renal allograft survival probabilities

■ Deceased donor ■ Living donor

Figure 97.2 One-year renal allograft survival probabilities (all transplants), adjusted by age, gender, race, primary diagnosis, transplant number. (Data from U.S. Renal Data System: 2005 Annual Data Report. Available at www.usrds.org.)

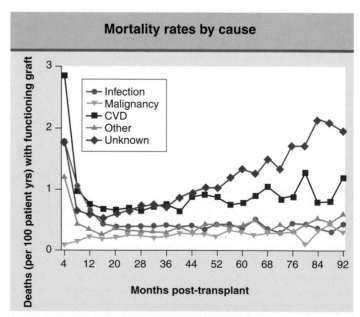

Mortality rates by cause

- Infection
- Malignancy
- CVD
- Other
- Unknown

Figure 97.4 Mortality rates by cause, as a function of time after transplantation. CVD, cardiovascular disease. (Data from U.S. Renal Data System: 2005 Annual Data Report. Available at www.usrds.org.)

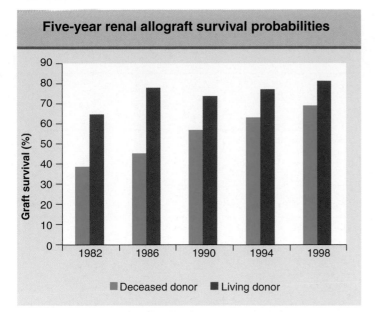

Figure 97.5 Five-year renal allograft survival probabilities (all transplants; conditional on surviving 1 year post-transplantation), adjusted by age, gender, race, primary diagnosis. (Data from U.S. Renal Data System: 2005 Annual Data Report. Available at www.usrds.org.)

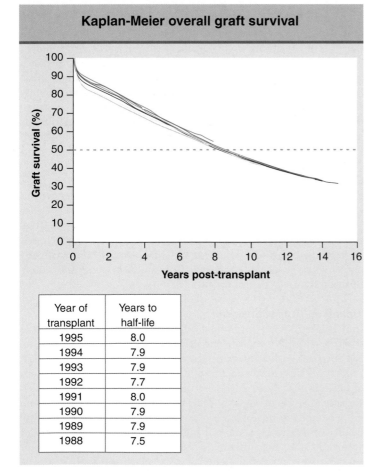

Year of transplant	Years to half-life
1995	8.0
1994	7.9
1993	7.9
1992	7.7
1991	8.0
1990	7.9
1989	7.9
1988	7.5

Figure 97.6 Kaplan-Meier overall graft survival by year of transplantation: first deceased donor transplants 1988 to 1995. The survival curves for each year from 1988 to 1995 are not significantly different. Graft half-life (*lower panel*) varies from 7.5 to 8 years over the same period. (From Meier-Kriesche HU, Schold JD, Kaplan B: Long-term renal allograft survival: Have we made significant progress or is it time to rethink our analytic and therapeutic strategies? Am J Transplant 2004;4:1289–1295.)

indicate that improving long-term allograft survival is not just a matter of preventing early acute rejection.

Beyond the first post-transplantation year, the principal causes of renal allograft loss are patient death and chronic allograft nephropathy; less common causes are late acute rejection and recurrent disease.[8] *Chronic allograft nephropathy* is a nonspecific term and in practice often encompasses chronic damage due to ischemia, rejection, and calcineurin inhibitor toxicity. Some have advocated use of more precise histopathologic definitions.[9] Chronic allograft nephropathy is discussed further in Chapter 95. The number one cause of death post-transplantation remains cardiovascular disease, followed by infection and malignancy (see Fig. 97.4). In children, however, death is a much less common cause of graft loss; conversely, in the elderly, it is more common.

FACTORS AFFECTING RENAL ALLOGRAFT SURVIVAL

Prospective studies and analyses of registry data have shown that many factors are associated with renal allograft survival. These can be considered as either donor, recipient, or donor-recipient. An alternative classification is based on factors being considered either alloantigen dependent or alloantigen independent. Many of the factors considered here contribute to the development of chronic allograft nephropathy, which is the most common cause of nondeath graft failure (see Chapter 95).

Donor-Recipient Factors
Delayed Graft Function
Delayed graft function (DGF) is considered here because both donor and recipient factors are associated with it. DGF is usually defined as failure of the renal allograft to function immediately post-transplantation, with the need for one or more dialysis sessions within a specified period, usually 1 week. DGF is associated with poorer graft survival, poorer graft function, and higher risk of patient death,[10] in part because of the association of DGF with higher rates of acute rejection. Rejection may be more common because ischemia-reperfusion injury increases the immunogenicity of the graft. Most studies have also demonstrated that, even in the absence of documented acute rejection, DGF is associated with poorer long-term graft function and survival.[11] Although the incidence of acute rejection continues to decrease (Fig. 97.7), rates of DGF have declined only slightly, to just over 20% of deceased donor grafts (Fig. 97.8).

DGF reflects a variable combination of chronic pretransplantation injury (e.g., advanced donor age) and peritransplantation injury (e.g., ischemia-reperfusion). Risk factors for DGF are shown in Figure 97.9. Warm ischemia time is probably also a risk factor, but as it is often not accurately recorded, its role is difficult to assess.

Slow graft function (SGF) defines a group of recipients with moderate early graft dysfunction; one definition is plasma creatinine >3.0 mg/dl (264 μmol/l) and no dialysis within 1 week of transplantation.[10] SGF appears also to be associated with poorer graft function and survival. Thus, measures that simply convert grafts from DGF to SGF may be of limited benefit.[10]

HLA Matching
Registry data from many countries clearly demonstrate that, even with current immunosuppression regimens, better HLA-matched deceased donor allografts still have better survival[12] (Fig. 97.10).

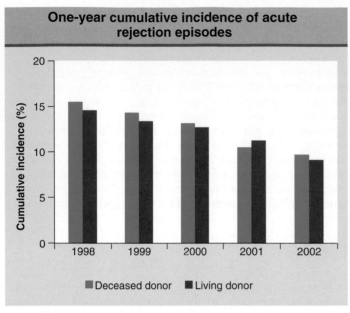

Figure 97.7 One-year cumulative incidence of acute rejection episodes. Recipients of first kidney-only transplants, 1998 to 2002 (N = 58,215). Does not include acute rejection episodes at the time of transplantation or acute rejections listed as the cause of graft failure. (Data from U.S. Renal Data System: 2005 Annual Data Report. Available at www.usrds.org.)

Risk factors for delayed graft function

Risk Factor	Odds Ratio
Donor age (10–40 yr)	
<10 yr	1.2
41–55 yr	1.7
>55 yr	2.1
Cold Ischemia time (<12 hr)	
13–12 hr	1.4
25–36 hr	2.3
>36 hr	3.5
Recipient race (non-Black)	
Black	1.6
PRA (<50%)	
>50%	1.2
HLA mismatch (>0)	
0 mismatches	0.8
Duration of dialysis	
Per year	1.1

Figure 97.9 Risk factors for delayed graft function. PRA, panel reactive antibody. (Adapted from Halloran PF, Hunsicker LG: Delayed graft function: State of the art. Am J Transplant 2001;1:115–120.)

This is why many countries operate national or international sharing systems for zero-mismatched renal allografts, even though this prolongs cold ischemia times. The hazard ratio of graft failure for recipients of a zero-mismatched allograft in the 1998 to 2003 cohort was 0.85 (0.78 to 0.92) compared to 1.24 (1.15 to 1.34) for recipients of a three-mismatched allograft.[1] The better outcomes are presumably related to fewer immunologic failures. There is some evidence, however, that the benefits of HLA matching are diminishing, probably because of more effective immunosuppression.[12]

The effect of HLA matching is much less pronounced in living donor recipients (although a large survival advantage is still seen in those with two haplotype matched grafts).[1] Possible reasons are that the transplantation surgery itself is associated with minimal ischemic injury (such injury probably increases the immunogenicity of allografts) and that living donor recipients might have better compliance with post-transplantation immunosuppression. The very limited effect of HLA mismatching on living donor transplant survival is important as this means that there is no contraindication to living unrelated transplant from a general immunologic perspective.

Cytomegalovirus Status of Donor and Recipient

Registry data show a small but definite effect of donor and recipient cytomegalovirus (CMV) serologic status on renal allograft and recipient survival.[1] Donor negative–recipient negative pairings have the best outcomes, whereas donor positive–recipient negative pairings have the worst. CMV probably affects graft outcomes via overt infection, but subclinical effects on immune function may also be important.

Timing of Transplantation

In the case of living donor renal transplantation, there is evidence that pre-emptive—before initiation of dialysis—transplantation is associated with a lower risk of allograft failure.[13] This, in part, reflects a higher risk of acute rejection in patients with a history of prolonged dialysis. Although this important study used multivariable analysis of registry data, the results may still have been influenced by unmeasured confounders such as differences in the quality of medical care and of self-care between the two patient groups. Minimizing time on dialysis before transplantation has of course many potential benefits; this strategy should thus be considered where possible.

Center Effect

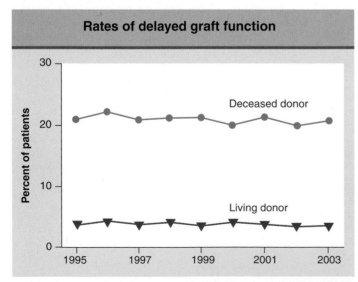

Figure 97.8 Rates of delayed graft function between 1995 and 2003, according to type of donor. Includes only patients with functioning grafts on discharge. (Data from U.S. Renal Data System: 2005 Annual Data Report. Available at www.usrds.org.)

Not surprisingly, outcomes have varied widely among transplantation centers. This reflects normal statistical variance as well as center expertise. It is important to note that outcomes

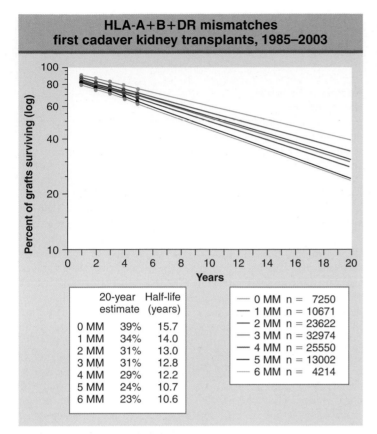

HLA-A+B+DR mismatches
first cadaver kidney transplants, 1985–2003

	20-year estimate	Half-life (years)
0 MM	39%	15.7
1 MM	34%	14.0
2 MM	31%	13.0
3 MM	31%	12.8
4 MM	29%	12.2
5 MM	24%	10.7
6 MM	23%	10.6

	n =
0 MM	7250
1 MM	10671
2 MM	23622
3 MM	32974
4 MM	25550
5 MM	13002
6 MM	4214

Figure 97.10   Effects of HLA mismatching on renal allograft survival. MM, mismatch. (Data from Collaborative Transplant Study, 2005. Available at www.ctstransplant.org.)

will be confounded by many donor and recipient factors that differ across centers. Thus, between-center comparisons are difficult. USRDS data suggest minimal difference in outcomes between small and large transplantation centers in the United States.[14]

Year of Transplant

Long-term allograft survival is slowly increasing (see Fig. 97.5). This presumably reflects multiple factors, including more effective but not significantly more toxic immunosuppressive regimens, better pre- and post-transplantation general medical care, and more effective prevention and treatment of opportunistic infections (particularly CMV).

Genetic Polymorphism

It has been hypothesized that genetic variation (with regard to the organ donor or recipient) may influence post-transplantation outcomes such as susceptibility to infections, susceptibility to acute rejection, and allograft survival. Candidate polymorphic genes would be those encoding cytokines, chemokines, adhesion molecules, and their relevant receptors. Some studies have suggested that polymorphisms of such molecules can influence outcomes. There are many caveats with regard to the current literature on this topic: studies have been retrospective and usually single center, have not incorporated multivariable analysis, and, in some cases, have yielded contradictory results. Thus, it is premature to alter immunosuppression or other facets of post-transplantation care based on the data available. It is hoped that prospective, multicenter studies will be performed to assess the clinical importance of polymorphisms of candidate molecules.

Donor Factors

The quality of the kidney immediately prior to transplantation has a major impact on long-term graft function and the risk of developing chronic allograft nephropathy.

Donor Source: Deceased versus Living Donor

The donor source is one of the most important predictors of short- and long-term graft outcomes. In general, living donor grafts are superior to deceased donor grafts. Figures 97.2 and 97.5 clearly show how the short- and long-term survival rates of living donor allografts are higher than for deceased donor grafts. The better outcomes reflect several factors: healthy living donors, the absence of brain death, the general benefits of elective as opposed to semi-emergency surgery, avoidance of ischemia-reperfusion injury, high nephron mass, and probably the effects of a shorter waiting time (see previous discussion). Better compliance by the recipient may also play a role. Excellent results are now being demonstrated with living unrelated kidney transplantation where HLA matching is not optimum.[15] This finding further emphasizes the importance of the healthy transplant kidney effect.

Donor Age

Deceased donor and living donor allografts from those aged older than 50 years, and particularly older than 65 years, have poorer outcomes.[1] These results are thought to reflect a higher incidence of DGF and of "nephron underdosing." Grafts from older donors have fewer functioning nephrons because of the aging process and donor-related conditions such as hypertension and atherosclerosis. However, because of the organ donor shortage, more elderly donors are being used.

Deceased donor age younger than 5 years is also associated with poorer outcomes, which likely reflects relatively high rates of technical complications and probably nephron underdosing (see later discussion). *En bloc* transplantations (consisting of both kidneys with a segment of aorta and inferior vena cava) from donors aged 0 to 5 years may significantly improve survival, however.[16]

Cold Ischemia Time

Prolonged cold ischemia time is associated with higher risk of DGF and poorer allograft survival.[17] Registry data suggest that >24 hours is particularly deleterious to the graft.[1] (DGF has been discussed previously.)

Donor Race

In the United States, the survival of deceased donor grafts obtained from African Americans is poorer than grafts from Caucasians. One theory is that a lower nephron number in African Americans is important.

Donor Sex

There is evidence that grafts from deceased female donors have slightly poorer survival, particularly in male recipients.[1,18] This probably reflects "nephron underdosing" (see later discussion), as females have smaller renal mass than males. However, differences in the antigenicity of female grafts may also be a factor.[18]

Donor Nephron Mass

An imbalance between the metabolic/excretory demands of the recipient and the functional transplant mass has been postulated to play a causative role in the development and progression of chronic allograft nephropathy. "Nephron underdosing," exacerbated by perioperative ischemic damage and postoperative nephrotoxic drugs, might lead to nephron overwork and eventual failure, similar to the mechanisms occurring in native kidney disease. Thus, kidneys from small donors transplanted into recipients of large body surface area or large body mass index (BMI) would be at highest risk of this problem. There is support for this hypothesis from animal studies and retrospective human studies. Prospective human trials to determine the role of inadequate nephron mass are not available, however.

Expanded Criteria Donors

As the discrepancy between the number of patients awaiting kidney transplantation and the number of available organs increases, many countries are now using expanded criteria donor (ECD) allografts.[19] By definition, ECD allografts have poorer survival than ideal deceased donor allografts; the definition of an ECD allograft involves an estimated relative risk of failure of >1.7 compared to an ideal reference group.[19] The clinical criteria used to define ECD are shown in Figure 97.11. Survival of ECD kidneys is, on average, shorter than regular deceased donor kidneys for two general reasons: first, as Figure 97.11 shows, the baseline GFR of these kidneys is likely to be lower and, second, ECD kidneys tend to be transplanted into older recipients who have higher rates of post-transplantation death. It should be emphasized that transplantation with an ECD kidney confers a significant survival advantage compared to remaining on the transplant waiting list (on dialysis).[20] Different allocation algorithms are often used for ECD allografts to minimize cold ischemia times.

Other nontraditional donors (in which there has been renewed interest) are non–heart-beating donors. The use of non–heart-beating donors has been controversial as short-term outcomes are inferior to those seen with standard deceased donor kidneys. This reflects the longer period of warm ischemia. Rates of DGF and primary nonfunction are generally higher than with standard donors. There is accumulating evidence, however, that long-term graft survival is similar to heart-beating deceased donors, although renal function may be inferior.[21] Experience in the United Kingdom has shown that more use of carefully selected non–heart-beating donors has the potential to significantly increase transplantation rates.

Recipient Factors
Recipient Age

In general, graft survival rates are poorer in those at the extremes of age: younger than 17 and older than 65 years.[1] In the young, technical causes of graft loss such as vessel thrombosis are relatively more common. Acute rejection is also a more common cause of graft loss; conversely, death with a functioning graft is relatively rare.

In most Western countries, the elderly (those older than 65 years) are forming an increasing percentage of the incident and prevalent end-stage renal disease (ESRD) population. Many of these patients have significant comorbid disease, particularly cardiovascular disease and type 2 diabetes mellitus. Nevertheless, age *per se* is not a contraindication to transplantation: among elderly patients carefully screened and deemed fit for the procedure, long-term outcomes are clearly better with transplantation than dialysis.[7] It is therefore appropriate that transplantation in elderly recipients is becoming more common. Not surprisingly, compared with younger recipients, death with a functioning graft is a more common cause of graft loss in the elderly (responsible for >50% of graft failures). Conversely, acute rejection *may* be less common. Thus, although randomized, controlled trials are not available, it seems reasonable, in general, to use less aggressive immunosuppression in the elderly (see Chapter 93).

Recipient Race

In the United States, African American recipients have poorer deceased donor graft survival compared to Caucasians.[1] There is also a trend toward poorer survival of living donor grafts in African American as opposed to non–African American recipients. This probably reflects multiple factors including higher incidence of DGF, higher incidence of acute and late acute rejection, stronger immune responsiveness, a predominantly Caucasian donor pool (with resultant poorer matching of HLA and non-HLA antigens), altered pharmacokinetics of immunosuppressive drugs, and a higher prevalence of hypertension. Socioeconomic factors associated with inability to pay for transplant medications (an issue in the United States where universal health coverage does not exist), poorer access to high-quality medical care, and noncompliance probably also play a role. There is some evidence to suggest Blacks have outcomes equivalent to those of Caucasians in Europe.[22] In the United States, Asian and Hispanic recipients have outcomes superior to those of Caucasians.

Strategies that should improve outcomes in African American recipients include increasing living and deceased donation by African American and, possibly, use of higher dose immunosuppression in African American recipients (see Chapter 93).

Recipient Gender

Registry studies of the association of recipient gender with transplantation outcomes have yielded differing results. In the CTS database, female recipients had slightly better allograft survival than male recipients of deceased donor kidneys or HLA-identical kidneys.[18] Data solely from U.S. transplantation centers have shown better graft survival in male as opposed to female recipients of living donor kidneys.[1,23] An important difference between

Defining an expanded criteria donor		
	Donor Age	
Donor Condition	50–59 Yrs	>59 Yrs
CVA + hypertension + creatinine >1.5 mg/dl (133 µmol/l)	X	X
CVA + hypertension	X	X
CVA + creatinine >1.5 mg/dl (133 µmol/l)	X	X
Hypertension + creatinine >1.5 mg/dl (133 µmol/l)	X	X
CVA		X
Hypertension		X
Creatinine >1.5 mg/dl (133 µmol/l)		X
None of the above		X

Figure 97.11 Defining an expanded criteria donor. CVA, cerebrovascular accident. (Adapted from Metzger RA, Delmonico FL, Feng S, et al: Expanded criteria donors for kidney transplantation. Am J Transplant 2003;3(Suppl 4):114–125.)

female and male transplantation candidates is the higher degree of sensitization of the former to HLA antigens and possibly non-HLA antigens. Females tend to be more sensitized because of pregnancy and possibly because of more blood transfusions related to menstruation.

Recipient Sensitization: before or after Transplantation

Patients who are broadly sensitized (e.g., panel reactive antibody [PRA] status >50%) at the time of transplantation generally have poorer early and late graft survival compared to nonsensitized recipients. This is mainly related to an increased incidence of complications in the early post-transplantation period such as DGF and acute rejection. The principal reasons for sensitization are previous transplants, pregnancy, and previous blood transfusions. Highly sensitized patients are often given more intensive immunosuppression to reduce the risk of rejection, but this also exposes them to risk.

There is accumulating evidence that the presence of donor-specific and nondonor-specific HLA antibodies are associated with inferior graft survival.[24] This evidence suggests that low-grade antibody–mediated rejection is an important cause of graft damage.

Recipient Hepatitis C Virus Antibody and Hepatitis B Virus Surface Antigen Positivity

Recipients who are hepatitis C virus (HCV) antibody positive at the time of transplantation have poorer allograft survival and poorer survival.[1,25] Higher mortality rates appear to be related to infection and worsening liver disease.[25] Nevertheless, it seems that transplantation of selected HCV-positive patients confers a survival benefit as opposed to remaining on the waiting list.[26]

The adverse effects of hepatitis B virus (HBV) surface antigen positivity on post-transplantation outcomes are much less pronounced. This may in part reflect the better anti-HBV therapies available for transplant recipients that have been introduced in recent years.

Acute Rejection

Acute rejection has been consistently associated with an increased risk of graft loss. This is due to irreversible graft injury at the time of acute rejection and probably ongoing subclinical immune-mediated injury. Such damage accentuates the effects of poor-quality donor tissue, perioperative ischemic injury, nephron underdosing, and so forth. Acute rejection refractory to steroids, acute rejection where creatinine does not return near baseline, and late acute rejection (occurring after the first 6 months) are particularly associated with poorer graft and patient outcomes.[6] More severe histologic changes (e.g., Banff grade II or III cellular rejection) or severe acute antibody-mediated rejection are also associated with poorer graft survival. Although current immunosuppressive regimens have steadily decreased rates of acute rejection, this has not necessarily translated into a major improvement in long-term graft survival.[27]

Recipient Immunosuppression

Undoubtedly, the improvements in short- and long-term allograft survival reflect, in part, the effectiveness of the newer antirejection drugs such as the calcineurin inhibitors (CNIs) and mycophenolate mofetil. As discussed earlier, the short-term improvements in allograft survival have been particularly impressive. The contribution of long-term CNI therapy, particularly with currently used maintenance doses, to chronic renal allograft dysfunction (and loss) remains controversial. The increases in short- and long-term

graft survival in the CNI era (cyclosporine became widely used in the early 1980s) suggest that these antirejection effects override the nephrotoxic effects. The debate as to whether cyclosporine is preferable to tacrolimus, or vice versa, continues. One recent meta-analysis found that tacrolimus was more effective than cyclosporine in preventing acute rejection and allograft loss but at the expense of higher rates of diabetes mellitus.[28]

There is limited evidence (registry data, not randomized trials) that mycophenolate mofetil improves long-term graft survival both by preventing overt acute rejection and possibly by other mechanisms. Short-term studies of sirolimus have shown contradictory results.[29,30] In fact, one registry study suggests that sirolimus use is associated with inferior allograft survival.[31]

Although antilymphocyte antibody preparations (e.g., antithymocyte globulin or interleukin-2 receptor blockers) are widely used, particularly in the setting of DGF, their effects on long-term graft survival have not been well studied. Recent United Network of Organ Sharing data suggest that antibody induction protocols slightly reduce early acute rejection episodes in recipients with DGF and slightly improve graft survival. It is important to note that aggressive immunosuppression could adversely affect graft survival by promoting BK (polyoma) virus nephropathy or higher rates of death from opportunistic infections.

Recipient Compliance

Poor compliance with the immunosuppressive regimen is known to increase the risk of acute rejection, particularly late acute rejection, and chronic allograft dysfunction. The magnitude of this problem is difficult to define. In one study of patients followed up to 5 years after transplantation, 22.6% were identified as being noncompliant; this was associated with a large increase in risk of late acute rejection and of higher plasma creatinine (and likely poorer allograft survival eventually).[32]

Obesity

Obesity is increasingly common in ESRD patients and is associated with more transplantation surgery–related complications, more DGF, higher mortality (related to cardiovascular complications), and poorer graft survival.[33] Similar evidence of poorer patient and graft outcomes has been reported by USDRS.[1] The poorer long-term graft survival probably reflects the effects of DGF, nephron overwork, and more difficult dosing of immunosuppressive drugs. Nevertheless, most studies of patients with BMI >30 kg/m^2 suggest transplantation provides a survival benefit over remaining on the waiting list (on dialysis), at least up to a BMI of 41 kg/m^2.

Recipient Hypertension: Renin Angiotensin System

Retrospective studies have shown that the greater the severity of post-transplantation hypertension is, the higher is the risk of graft loss.[34] Of course, hypertension could also be secondary to graft damage and not just a cause. No prospective human studies of the effect of treating hypertension on allograft outcomes are available. However, control of hypertension is associated with improved allograft survival.[35] Common sense dictates that treatment of hypertension should be the goal to prevent both its renal and nonrenal complications.

Multiple studies have confirmed the ability of angiotensin-converting enzyme (ACE) inhibitors and angiotensin receptor blockers (ARBs) to slow the progression of both diabetic and nondiabetic proteinuric native kidney disease. Some have argued that ACE inhibitors and ARBs should be similarly beneficial in transplant kidney disease and thus should be used more frequently. While several studies have shown that both classes of drugs are effective in treating post-transplantation hypertension and reducing proteinuria in the short-term, no long-term studies of their effects on progression of transplant kidney dysfunction have been published. In one randomized, controlled trial, patients randomized to nifedipine had sustained improvement in GFR up to 2 years after transplantation; no improvement was seen in the lisinopril group. This may reflect the ability of nifedipine to attenuate CNI-induced vasoconstriction of the afferent arteriole.[33]

Recipient Dyslipidemia

The prominence of the vascular lesions in CAN and the similarity of these lesions to atherosclerosis suggest that dyslipidemia plays a role in the pathogenesis of CAN and graft failure. Some studies have suggested that hypercholesterolemia and/or hypertriglyceridemia are associated with poorer graft outcomes.

Recurrence of Primary Disease

Determining the incidence and prevalence of recurrent or *de novo* renal disease is difficult. The original cause of ESRD is often unknown; most relevant studies are small and retrospective with variable follow-up periods. In one of the best performed studies of transplant recipients whose cause of ESRD was glomerulonephritis, the cumulative incidence of graft loss at 10 years was 8.4%.[36] Recurrence was the most important cause of loss, after chronic rejection and death. It is likely that as renal allograft survival continues to improve, recurrent or *de novo* disease will be increasingly diagnosed (both clinically and histologically) and will become a more important cause of late graft loss. Recurrent disease in renal transplants is discussed further in Chapter 96.

Proteinuria

The degree of proteinuria correlates with poorer renal outcome in both native and transplant kidney disease. Proteinuria may simply be a marker of renal damage, but there is speculation that proteinuria *per se* may accelerate allograft loss from CAN. The role of ACE inhibitors and ARBs in slowing the progression of proteinuric transplant renal diseases is discussed further in Chapter 95.

Measures that should improve renal allograft survival
Measure
Increased living kidney donation: both related and nonrelated
Preemptive transplantation
Increased donatin from younger, previously healthy deceased donors
Preferential matching of younger deceased donors with younger recipients
Zero mismatching of HLA antigens
Improved organ preservation
Faster matching and transplantation; reduced cold ischemia time
Nephron dosing (e.g., matching of donor-recipient sex, body mass index)
Calcineurin inhibitor–sparing immunosuppressive protocols
Angiotensin-converting enzyme inhibitors, angiotensin receptor blockers
High-quality general medical care (e.g., aggressive control of hyperlipidemia, hypertension)
Comment
Under-used in many countries
Under-used in many countries
Difficult to achieve; Spain best example of successful high donation rates
Requires more debate
Already practised in many countries
Controversial if machine perfusion improves long-term graft function
Difficult to achieve
No large randomized controlled trials; complex to administer in practice
Controversial; no long-term data from randomized controlled trials
Minimal data in transplant patients *per se* showing that renal function is better preserved; reasonable to extrapolate from native kidney disease
No randomized controlled trials showing survival benefits in transplant patients but benefits likely

Figure 97.12 Measures that should improve renal allograft survival.

IMPROVING RENAL ALLOGRAFT OUTCOMES

Measures that would likely further improve allograft survival are summarized in Figure 97.12. Probably the most important (in terms of achievable impact) is increased use of living kidney donors. In the United Kingdom, for example, the percentage of living donors is increasing, but is still only about 27% of the total compared to 40% to 50% in the United States or Australasia. Ideally, most living donor kidneys would be transplanted just before the recipient needs to start dialysis, both to improve allograft survival[13] and because this is usually patient preference. It is critical, however, that donation should only be allowed when the risk of medical and psychological complications to the donor is minimal.

The criteria used for allocation of deceased donor allografts can have an important impact on overall allograft survival. A purely utilitarian approach would imply directing organs to those who possess certain demographic and clinical characteristics (e.g., younger patients with minimal comorbidities). In practice, a balance must be struck between utility and equity (ensuring that anyone medically fit for a transplant has a reasonable chance of obtaining one). In many countries, this balance is achieved by means of a points system, points being awarded for zero-HLA mismatching, time on the waiting list, and so forth.

There is evidence that preferential allocation of organs of younger donors to younger recipients (as opposed to the current system where some organs of younger donors are transplanted into elderly patients with a limited life span) would significantly improve overall allograft survival.[37] Considerable debate is required before such a strategy can be implemented in the United States. Results from the Eurotransplant Senior Program of transplanting older kidneys to older patients are encouraging.[38]

REFERENCES

1. U.S. Renal Data System: 2005 Annual Data Report. Available at www.usrds.org.
2. Collaborative Transplant Study, 2005. Available at www.ctstransplant.org.
3. Meyers CM, Kirk AD: Workshop on late renal allograft dysfunction. Am J Transplant 2005;5:1600–1605.
4. Hariharan S, McBride MA, Cohen EP: Evolution of endpoints for renal transplant outcome. Am J Transplant 2003;3:933–941.
5. Lachenbruch PA, Rosenberg AS, Bonvini E, et al: Biomarkers and surrogate endpoints in renal transplantation: Present status and considerations for clinical trial design. Am J Transplant 2004;4:451–457.
6. Meier-Kriesche HU, Schold JD, Kaplan B: Long-term renal allograft survival: Have we made significant progress or is it time to rethink our analytic and therapeutic strategies? Am J Transplant 2004;4:1289–1295.
7. Wolfe RA, Ashby VB, Milford EL, et al: Comparison of mortality in all patients on dialysis, patients on dialysis awaiting transplantation, and recipients of a first cadaveric transplant. N Engl J Med 1999;341:1725–1730.
8. Pascual M, Theruvath T, Kawai T, et al: Strategies to improve long-term outcomes after renal transplantation. N Engl J Med 2002;346:580–590.
9. Halloran PF: Call for revolution: A new approach to describing allograft deterioration. Am J Transplant 2002;2:195–200.
10. Halloran PF, Hunsicker LG: Delayed graft function: State of the art, November 10–11, 2000. Summit meeting, Scottsdale, Arizona, USA. Am J Transplant 2001;1:115–120.
11. Shoskes DA, Cecka JM: Deleterious effects of delayed graft function in cadaveric renal transplant recipients independent of acute rejection. Transplantation 1998;66:1697–1701.
12. Su X, Zenios SA, Chakkera H, et al: Diminishing significance of HLA matching in kidney transplantation. Am J Transplant 2004;4:1501–1508.
13. Mange KC, Joffe MM, Feldman HI: Effect of the use or nonuse of long-term dialysis on the subsequent survival of renal transplants from living donors. N Engl J Med 2001;344:726–731.
14. Terasaki PI, Cecka JM: The center effect: Is bigger better? Clin Transpl 1999;317–324.
15. Gjertson DW, Cecka JM: Living unrelated donor kidney transplantation. Kidney Int 2000;58:491–499.
16. Dharnidharka VR, Stevens G, Howard RJ: En-bloc kidney transplantation in the United states: An analysis of United Network of Organ Sharing (UNOS) data from 1987 to 2003. Am J Transplant 2005;5:1513–1517.
17. Salahudeen AK, Haider N, May W: Cold ischemia and the reduced long-term survival of cadaveric renal allografts. Kidney Int 2004;65:713–718.
18. Zeier M, Dohler B, Opelz G, Ritz E: The effect of donor gender on graft survival. J Am Soc Nephrol 2002;13:2570–2576.
19. Metzger RA, Delmonico FL, Feng S, et al: Expanded criteria donors for kidney transplantation. Am J Transplant 2003;3(Suppl 4):114–125.
20. Ojo AO, Hanson JA, Meier-Kriesche H, et al: Survival in recipients of marginal cadaveric donor kidneys compared with other recipients and wait-listed transplant candidates. J Am Soc Nephrol 2001;12:589–597.
21. Cooper JT, Chin LT, Krieger NR, et al: Donation after cardiac death: The University of Wisconsin experience with renal transplantation. Am J Transplant 2004;4:1490–1494.
22. Pallet N, Thervet E, Alberti C, et al: Kidney transplant in black recipients: Are African Europeans different from African Americans? Am J Transplant 2005;5:2682–2687.
23. Kayler LK, Rasmussen CS, Dykstra DM, et al: Gender imbalance and outcomes in living donor renal transplantation in the United States. Am J Transplant 2003;3:452–458.
24. Hourmant M, Cesbron-Gautier A, Terasaki PI, et al: Frequency and clinical implications of development of donor-specific and non-donor-specific HLA antibodies after kidney transplantation. J Am Soc Nephrol 2005;16:2804–2812.
25. Fabrizi F, Martin P, Dixit V, et al: Hepatitis C virus antibody status and survival after renal transplantation: Meta-analysis of observational studies. Am J Transplant 2005;5:1452–1461.
26. Pereira BJ, Natov SN, Bouthot BA, et al: Effects of hepatitis C infection and renal transplantation on survival in end-stage renal disease. The New England Organ Bank Hepatitis C Study Group. Kidney Int 1998;53:1374–1381.
27. Meier-Kriesche HU, Schold JD, Srinivas TR, Kaplan B: Lack of improvement in renal allograft survival despite a marked decrease in acute rejection rates over the most recent era. Am J Transplant 2004;4:378–383.
28. Webster AC, Woodroffe RC, Taylor RS, et al: Tacrolimus versus ciclosporin as primary immunosuppression for kidney transplant recipients: Meta-analysis and meta-regression of randomised trial data. BMJ 2005;331:810.
29. Mendez R, Gonwa T, Yang HC, et al: A prospective, randomized trial of tacrolimus in combination with sirolimus or mycophenolate mofetil in kidney transplantation: Results at 1 year. Transplantation 2005;80:303–309.
30. Watson CJ, Firth J, Williams PF, et al: A randomized controlled trial of late conversion from CNI-based to sirolimus-based immunosuppression following renal transplantation. Am J Transplant 2005;5:2496–2503.
31. Meier-Kriesche HU, Schold JD, Srinivas TR, et al: Sirolimus in combination with tacrolimus is associated with worse renal allograft survival compared to mycophenolate mofetil combined with tacrolimus. Am J Transplant 2005;5:2273–2280.
32. Vlaminck H, Maes B, Evers G, et al: Prospective study on late consequences of subclinical non-compliance with immunosuppressive therapy in renal transplant patients. Am J Transplant 2004;4:1509–1513.
33. Midtvedt K, Hartmann A, Foss A, et al: Sustained improvement of renal graft function for two years in hypertensive renal transplant recipients treated with nifedipine as compared to lisinopril. Transplantation 2001;72:1787–1792.
34. Opelz G, Wujciak T, Ritz E: Association of chronic kidney graft failure with recipient blood pressure. Collaborative Transplant Study. Kidney Int 1998;53:217–22.
35. Opelz G, Dohler B: Improved long-term outcomes after renal transplantation associated with blood pressure control. Am J Transplant 2005;5:2725–2731.
36. Briganti EM, Russ GR, McNeil JJ, et al: Risk of renal allograft loss from recurrent glomerulonephritis. N Engl J Med 2002;347:103–109.
37. Meier-Kriesche HU, Schold JD, Gaston RS, et al: Kidneys from deceased donors: maximizing the value of a scarce resource. Am J Transplant 2005;5:1725–1730.
38. Fabrizii V, Kovarik J, Bodingbauer M, et al: Long-term patient and graft survival in the Eurotransplant Senior Program: A single-center experience. Transplantation 2005;80:582–589.

Pancreas and Islet Transplantation

Jonathan S. Fisher, Jonathan R.T. Lakey, Mohammadreza Mirbolooki, R. Paul Robertson, and Christopher L. Marsh

INTRODUCTION

Pancreas transplants are performed for the amelioration of insulin-requiring diabetes. Initially pancreas transplants were performed only in those diabetic patients with chronic kidney disease who needed kidney transplants; these patients underwent simultaneous pancreatic-kidney transplantation (SPK). Today, pancreas transplantation alone (PTA) or pancreas transplantation after living related or unrelated kidney transplantation (PAK) is increasingly common. By the end of 2004, >23,000 pancreas transplants had been performed worldwide, with >75% being done in the United States.[1] Of the 1417 pancreas transplants reported in the United States in 2002, 65% were SPKs, 26% PAKs, and 9% PTAs (Fig. 98.1).[1] More recently, there has been an increase in the number of patients receiving islet cell transplants. As the experience in islet cell transplantation grows with improved outcome, it may become the modality of choice.

PATIENT SELECTION CRITERIA FOR PANCREAS OR ISLET TRANSPLANTATION

Indications for Transplantation

Indications for pancreas or islet transplantation include (1) insulin-dependent diabetes with associated diabetic complications (nephropathy, neuropathy, and retinopathy) and (2) diabetes with episodes of hypoglycemic unawareness.

So why give one patient a pancreas transplant and another an islet transplant? Since giving sufficient islets remains a limiting factor, islet transplants are more appropriate for patients with smaller insulin requirements, typically slender women. Larger patients (with generally higher insulin requirements) are more reliably served with whole-organ pancreatic transplants. Islet transplantation is performed by a radiographic procedure and therefore is better suited for patients who cannot tolerate the increased surgical stress of whole-organ transplantation, such as older patients with severe coronary artery disease.

Pancreas or islet transplants are not routinely performed for type 2 diabetes mellitus since the defect in type 2 diabetes is insulin resistance, not insulin deficiency. There may be a role for pancreas transplantation in type 2 diabetic patients who develop pancreatic burnout after years of insulin resistance. Interestingly, similar outcomes have been observed between insulin-dependent type 1 and type 2 diabetic recipients of SPKs. The vast majority of pancreata for transplantation come from cadaveric donors. However, one approach to increasing the donor supply has involved living donor laparoscopic distal pancreatectomy with or without simultaneous laparoscopic nephrectomy.[2]

Should living kidney donor recipients be offered a pancreatic transplant? An analysis of the United Network for Organ Sharing (UNOS) database revealed no difference in survival of SPK recipients and living kidney donor recipients at up to 8 years of follow-up.[3] However, a recent European study showed an improved 10-year patient survival (83% in SPKs versus 70% in kidney transplants alone) and noted a significantly lower progression of macrovascular diseases (cerebrovascular, coronary, and peripheral vascular) in the SPK group.[4] Therefore, pancreas transplantation after a living donor kidney transplant should perhaps be offered to patients with significant vascular disease or worsening hypoglycemic unawareness.

Recently the practice of performing pancreas transplants in the setting of preserved renal function has also been questioned. An analysis of the UNOS database demonstrated worse survival for those with diabetes and preserved kidney function receiving a PTA than for those who remained on the waiting list and received conventional therapy.[5] This analysis, however, has been challenged by a subsequent review of both the UNOS database and the International Pancreas Transplant Registry, which demonstrated an improvement in 1-year pancreas graft survival rates from 1988/1989 to 2002/2003 (an increase from 55% to 78% in the case of PAKs and 45% to 77% in the case of PTAs; Fig. 98.2).[1] Further close study is warranted, keeping in mind that a prospective, randomized trial of pancreas transplantation versus conservative therapy is not practical. Once again, one must emphasize careful patient selection.

Medical Evaluation

The medical evaluation for the prospective pancreatic transplantation candidate is similar to that of the kidney-only recipient (see Chapter 91), although the cardiac workup is more extensive. The best candidates for transplantation are younger than the age of 50 and have a limited number of major complications of diabetes such as hypoglycemic unawareness or diabetic neuropathy. Additional complications such as vascular disease, orthostatic hypotension, and severe gastroparesis put patients at higher risk of post-transplant complications, but none of these factors by themselves exclude a patient from transplantation. The patient's cardiovascular status is the primary deciding factor for transplantation eligibility because the surgery, infections, risk of thrombotic complications, and, until recently, rejection are more severe in the pancreatic transplant recipient, demanding that the cardiovascular system be strong enough to withstand multiple

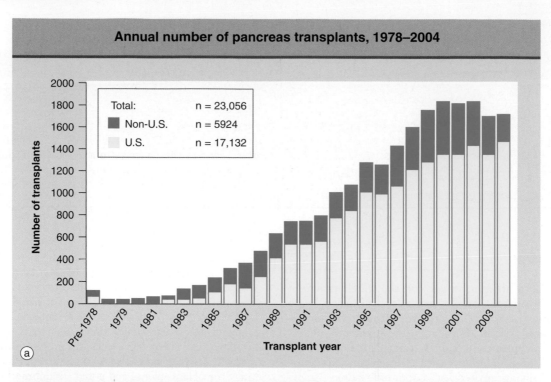

Annual number of pancreas transplants, 1978–2004

Total: n = 23,056
Non-U.S. n = 5924
U.S. n = 17,132

(a)

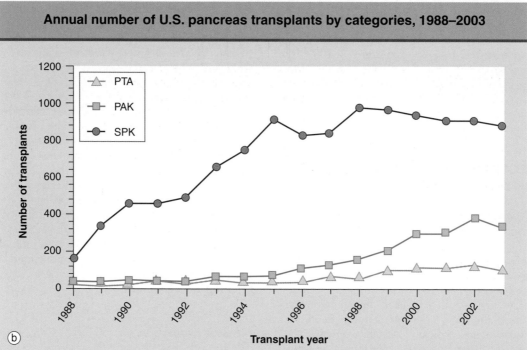

Annual number of U.S. pancreas transplants by categories, 1988–2003

PTA
PAK
SPK

(b)

Figure 98.1 Pancreas transplantation. *a*, Annual number of U.S. and non-U.S. pancreas transplantations reported to the International Pancreas Transplant Registry, 1978 to 2004. *b*, Annual number of pancreas transplants in the United States, 1988 to 2003. PAK, pancreas transplantation after living related or unrelated kidney transplantation; PTA, pancreas transplantation alone; SPK, simultaneous pancreas-kidney transplantation. (Redrawn from Gruessner AC, Sutherland DE: Pancreas transplant outcomes for United States [US] and non-US cases as reported to the United Network for Organ Sharing [UNOS] and the International Pancreas Transplant Registry [IPTR] as of June 2004. Clin Transplant 2005;19:433–455.)

prolonged hemodynamically stressful events. All patients require noninvasive cardiac stress evaluation because of the limited exercise capabilities of many patients. Cardiac catheterization is performed based on the results of noninvasive testing or performed first for high-risk patients: those older than age 45,

those with diabetes duration of >25 years, smokers of more than five pack-years, and/or those with an abnormal electrocardiogram. Peripheral vascular disease is evaluated by clinical examination and frequently by arterial duplex ultrasonography. Patients with limb-threatening ischemia are typically poor pancreas transplant

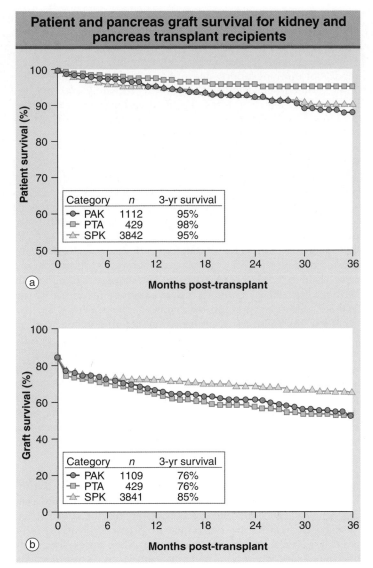

(a)

(b)

Figure 98.2 Patient and graft survival for kidney and pancreas transplant recipients. Outcomes for U.S. primary pancreas transplants by recipient category, 2000 to 2004. *a*, Patient survival rates. *b*, Pancreas graft functional survival (insulin-independence) rates. PAK, pancreas transplantation after living related or unrelated kidney transplantation; PTA, pancreas transplantation alone; SPK, simultaneous pancreas-kidney transplantation. (Redrawn from Gruessner AC, Sutherland DE: Pancreas transplant outcomes for United States [US] and non-US cases as reported to the United Network for Organ Sharing [UNOS] and the International Pancreas Transplant Registry [IPTR] as of June 2004. Clin Transplant 2005;19:433–455.)

candidates. The medical evaluation for islet transplantation is similar to that for pancreatic transplantation, but exclusion criteria are fewer due to fewer surgical and inflammatory risks.

The last criteria for transplantation are that the donor and recipient be matched for ABO blood type and the recipient sera be crossmatch negative against donor T cells using either the standard antiglobulin or flow cytometry crossmatch.

PANCREATIC TRANSPLANTATION

Patient and Graft Survival

Pancreatic allograft survival rates have increased as a result of improvement of surgical techniques (see later discussion), improvement in the composition of the preservation fluid, and

more efficiency in immunosuppressive treatments, despite an increasing proportion of high-risk patients.

The most commonly used cold storage solution is the University of Wisconsin (UW) solution, which has increased early pancreatic graft function and reduced the occurrence of preservation pancreatitis. A second cold storage solution, histidine-tryptophan-ketoglutarate (HTK), is also effective. Approaches using either a two-layer storage method with UW or an HTK solution and a second layer of highly oxygenated perfluorocarbon (PFC), or the attachment of the pancreas to a low-pressure pulsatile perfusion are currently being investigated.

The current gold standard immunosuppression for pancreas transplants is antibody induction therapy, tacrolimus, mycophenolate mofetil, and corticosteroids; this has led to a 40% decrease in incidence of rejection and an increase in 1-year graft survival to >90%.[6] UNOS registry data show that HLA matching has no effect on the outcome in SPK, while for PAK and PTA, a beneficial effect is seen by matching at the A and B loci.[7] Using these techniques and criteria, the reported 1-, 3-, and 5-year patient and graft survival rates are given in Figure 98.2.[1]

Surgical Procedure

Current practice is to transplant the whole pancreas with a cuff of duodenum, which preserves the blood supply of the head of the pancreas and provides a means to drain exocrine secretions into either the small bowel (enteric drainage) or the bladder (Figs. 98.3 and 98.4).[1] From 2000 to 2004, the majority of the pancreas transplants in the United States were enterically drained (81% of SPKs, 67% of PAKs, 56% of PTAs; Fig. 98.5a).[1] The graft may be placed in the right iliac fossa like a kidney, intraperitoneally, and vascularized from the common iliac vessels so that the insulin output enters the systemic circulation. However, an alternative is to construct the venous anastomosis to the superior mesenteric vein of the recipient, allowing more physiologic insulin output via the portal circulation. Currently 20%–30% of enterically drained transplants use portal drainage (see Fig. 98.5b).

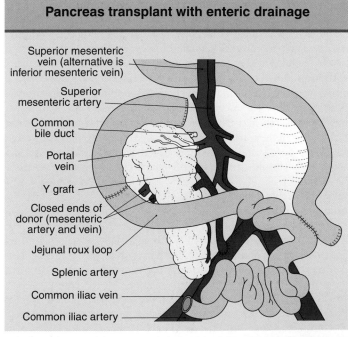

Pancreas transplant with enteric drainage

Superior mesenteric vein (alternative is inferior mesenteric vein)

Superior mesenteric artery

Common bile duct

Portal vein

Y graft

Closed ends of donor (mesenteric artery and vein)

Jejunal roux loop

Splenic artery

Common iliac vein

Common iliac artery

Figure 98.3 Pancreas transplant with enteric (portal) drainage.

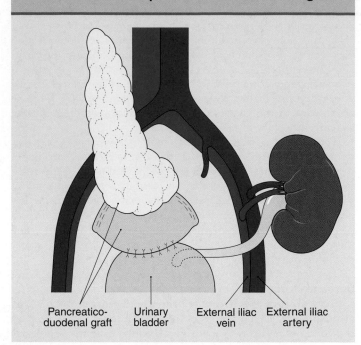

Pancreatic transplant with bladder drainage

Pancreatico-
duodenal graft | Urinary bladder | External iliac vein | External iliac artery

Figure 98.4 Pancreatic transplantation with bladder drainage. The pancreas may be placed in either the intra- or extraperitoneal position.

Bladder drainage allows monitoring for rejection by measurement of urinary amylase and also avoids enterotomy-associated risks of infection and leak. The disadvantages of bladder drainage include susceptibility to dehydration, metabolic acidosis, and frequent bladder-related complications. Primary enteric drainage avoids these complications and is more physiologic but does not allow urinary amylase monitoring. With improved surgical techniques, increased use of real-time ultrasonography, and percutaneous needle biopsy, the outcomes of portal enteric drainage now match those of bladder drainage. Bladder drainage is still appropriate in the following settings: (1) history of major abdominal surgery, (2) the presence of Crohn's or other small bowel disease, and (3) older patients with less cardiovascular reserve in whom a laparotomy may be avoided through a smaller lower quadrant retroperitoneal incision similar to that for a kidney transplant. Pancreas transplants with venous outflow to the superior mesenteric vein can be placed either anterior to the small bowel mesentery or in a retroperitoneal position behind the ascending colon, where the superior mesenteric vein is reached from the side. Surgical outcomes have not differed whether the venous drainage is systemic or portal. Although portal drainage is considered as more physiologic and avoids hyperinsulinemia, these benefits are not well characterized.

Postoperative Management
Immunosuppression
Most centers use antibody induction therapy during the first 1 to 2 weeks post-transplantation. OKT3 has largely been replaced by antithymocyte globulin (ATG).[6] Other centers use an interleukin-2 receptor antagonist (basiliximab, daclizumab) or, most recently, an anti-CD25 antibody (alemtuzumab).[8,9] Most centers employ triple-drug maintenance immunosuppression with tacrolimus (or less commonly cyclosporine), mycophenolate mofetil (or rarely azathioprine), and prednisone. There is increasing evidence of equivalent success with rapid steroid elimination or steroid-

avoidance protocols.[10,11] Some centers replace the calcineurin inhibitor or mycophenolate mofetil with sirolimus. With the more profound immunosuppressive induction produced by the newer antibodies (particularly alemtuzumab), there have been reports of immunosuppression protocols limited to a depleting antibody and a single additional agent.[9] Fortunately, cytomegalovirus (CMV) infection rates appear to be lower in steroid-free regimens,[11] although there has been some increase in CMV in those receiving depleting antibody therapies.[8]

Graft Monitoring
The causes of pancreatic allograft dysfunction and the evaluation process are shown in Figures 98.6 through 98.8.

During the immediate perioperative phase, intravenous insulin is used to decrease the stress on the transplanted pancreas by maintaining serum glucose around 100 to 120 mg/dl (5.5 to 6.6 mmol/l). Serum glucose values are not a particularly accurate marker of pancreatic dysfunction; elevations are observed only after significant parenchymal pancreatic damage has occurred. With bladder drainage, urinary amylase excretion is measured on 12-hour collections and reported as units per hour. During the first 1 to 2 weeks following transplantation, serum amylase may be elevated and urinary amylase decreased due to pancreatic preservation injury. Stable serum and urinary levels are usually attained within 2 weeks after transplantation. Thereafter, an elevated serum amylase and/or decreased urinary amylase indicate possible pancreatic allograft injury, which must be evaluated. Enterically drained transplants, as well as bladder-drained transplants, may manifest elevated serum amylase and serum lipase, which are moderately sensitive markers of pancreatic rejection. However, other conventional causes of pancreatitis can still occur.

Pancreatic transplant ultrasonography is performed frequently in the early post-transplantation period to rule out vascular thrombosis. If the pancreas cannot be well visualized by ultrasound scan, magnetic resonance imaging and angiography may be informative.

Allograft biopsies are performed by protocol, or at times of graft dysfunction, to identify rejection or other causes of pancreatic injury before irreversible tissue damage has occurred. The easiest approach is a percutaneous biopsy using ultrasound or computed tomography (CT) scan guidance; cystoscopic biopsy is used in bladder-drained transplants in situations where the percutaneous technique is not possible because of difficult visualization or an overlying bowel.[12] The most frequent complication of percutaneous biopsy is a perigraft hematoma or transient hematuria, but rarely seen are pancreatitis, arteriovenous fistula, abdominal hemorrhage, bowel perforation requiring exploration, or even graft loss.

Treatment of pancreatic rejection is similar to that used for kidney rejection and generally involves pulse intravenous steroids or antilymphocyte antibodies (see Chapter 93).

Antimicrobial Prophylaxis
The antimicrobial prophylaxis is much like that for a kidney transplant alone with trimethoprim-sulfamethoxazole for the prevention of urinary tract infections and *Pneumocystis*, oral clotrimazole or nystatin for the prevention of oral candidiasis, with some centers using fluconazole for prophylaxis of *Candida* urinary tract infections and intra-abdominal fungal or yeast infections. Oral acyclovir is given to patients with a history of herpes simplex infection and to patients who are CMV negative and receive CMV-negative donor organs. Otherwise, valacyclovir or ganciclovir is given for 3 months following transplantation to all patients who are CMV positive or who receive CMV-positive organs. Patients treated for

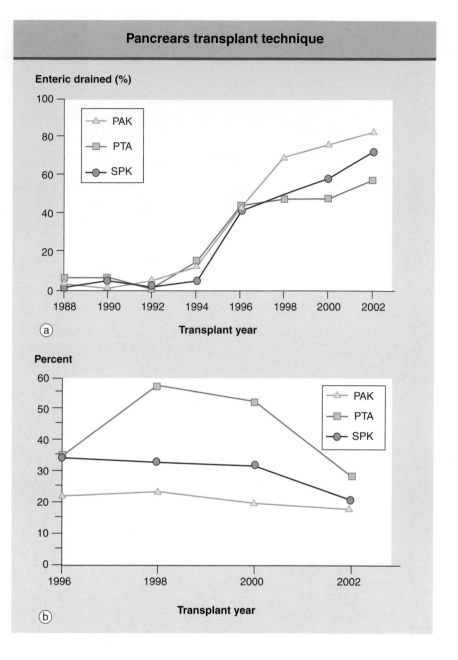

Figure 98.5 Pancreas transplant technique. *a,* Percentage of U.S. primary pancreas transplantations using enteric drainage, by recipient category and era, 1988 to 2002. There has been a shift toward enterically drained compared to bladder-drained pancreas transplantations in the past few years. *b,* Percentage of U.S. enteric drainage primary pancreas transplants done with portal drainage, by recipient category and era, 1996 to 2003. PAK, pancreas transplantation after living related or unrelated kidney transplantation; PTA, pancreas transplantation alone; SPK, simultaneous pancreas-kidney transplantation. (Redrawn from Gruessner AC, Sutherland DE: Pancreas transplant outcomes for United States [US] and non-US cases as reported to the United Network for Organ Sharing [UNOS] and the International Pancreas Transplant Registry [IPTR] as of June 2004. Clin Transplant 2005;19:433–455.)

rejection are typically returned to any discontinued anti-infectious prophylaxis for 1 to 3 months after rejection therapy.

Metabolic Monitoring

In addition to monitoring the serum and urinary amylase and the serum lipase, serum creatinine, potassium, magnesium, phosphorus, and bicarbonate must be monitored. With bladder drainage, there is high urinary loss of bicarbonate in pancreatic exocrine secretions, which may require ≥130 mmol/day of replacement. Without replacement, patients develop metabolic acidosis with nausea and vomiting, which may lead to volume depletion, hypotension (exacerbated by underlying autonomic neuropathy), and graft thrombosis. Intravenous 5% dextrose in water with 50 to 150 mmol sodium bicarbonate may be used for repletion. Oral sodium bicarbonate, typically 2 g four times daily, is needed. Fluid intake should be 2.5 to 3 l/day to accommodate pancreatic and renal fluid outputs. This volume may be difficult to consume because abdominal bloating from diabetic gastroparesis is exacerbated by large fluid intake and

the gas released from bicarbonate tablets. Patients who are unable to maintain adequate oral intake may require long-term intravenous access for fluid administration.

Surgical Complications

Surgical complications of pancreas transplantation are shown in Figure 98.9. Superficial infections and deep-seated abscesses are commonly fungal. The source of fungal contamination is thought to be the duodenal segment. Therefore, topical antibiotic and antifungal solutions are used to irrigate the organ during procurement and implantation. Patients commonly receive 24 to 48 hours of postoperative antibiotics and fluconazole.

The causes of wound drainage are seroma, lymphocele, pancreatic fistula either from the tail or the anastomosis to the bladder or bowel, wound dehiscence, and preservation pancreatitis. Preservation pancreatitis may lead to wound drainage of whitish-yellow, thick, noninfectious material formed from the enzymatic digestion of tissue leading to fat necrosis

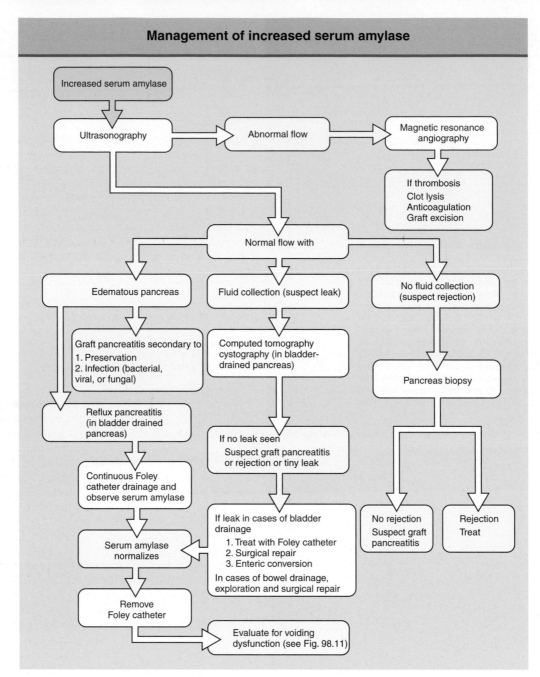

Figure 98.6   Management of increased serum amylase after pancreatic transplantation.

and saponification. Wound drainage is seen more often with the extraperitoneal placement of the pancreas and also occurs when using a pancreas from an obese donor. It is also associated with a mild increase in serum amylase, low urinary amylase excretion, and variable changes in the serum glucose.

Vascular complications occur in about 5% of patients and include arteriovenous fistulas due to surgery or biopsy, venous and arterial thrombosis, and rarely mycotic aneurysms. The pancreas is a low blood flow organ; vascular thrombosis rates were previously as high as 10%, but current rates are <5%. Means of reducing the rate of thrombosis include minimization of warm and cold ischemia, procurement procedures involving a no-touch technique using the duodenum and spleen as handles, and postoperative anticoagulation; aspirin may be sufficient or in other circumstances, heparin is indicated. Partial thrombosis may resolve with thrombolytic

therapy or anticoagulation. More extensive thrombosis requires urgent surgical intervention. Complete graft thrombosis, especially in the immediate postoperative period, mandates urgent graft removal to prevent sepsis syndrome or a more diffuse hypercoagulable state, leading to further vascular thrombotic complications such as myocardial infarction.

Nonsurgical Complications
Nausea and vomiting are common, and causes include gastroparesis, constipation, cholelithiasis, or esophageal reflux developing from motility problems and esophagitis with or without CMV disease. Antiemetics plus histamine H_2 blockers or proton pump inhibitors are usually effective therapy and are given for 2 to 3 months following transplantation. Persistent symptoms may require prokinetic agents (metoclopramide or erythromycin).

Causes of pancreas graft dysfunction
Rejection
Ductal obstruction
Vascular: arterial/venous thrombosis (partial/complete), arteriovenous fistula
Volume depletion
High calcineurin inhibitor levels
Graft pancreatitis (preservation, viral, bacterial, or fungal)

In cases of bladder drainage
    Reflux pancreatitis
    Urinary tract infection
    Anastomotic leak
    Bladder outflow obstruction

In cases of enteric drainage
    Anastomotic leak
    Bowel obstruction

Figure 98.7   Causes of pancreas graft dysfunction.

Diarrhea can be caused by immunosuppressive medications, intrinsic gut motility problems, food intolerance, or CMV or other infection. Constipation is treated with increased fluid intake, dietary modification, increased activity, and a regular low-dose schedule of stool softeners or laxatives.

Orthostatic hypotension may worsen following transplantation as a consequence of prolonged bed rest in the presence of diabetic autonomic neuropathy. Treatment may include a salt-loading diet, with a mineralocorticoid (fludrocortisone) or an α-adrenergic agonist (midodrine).[13]

Urologic Complications

Urologic complications are common after bladder drainage (Fig. 98.10).[14] Pretransplantation bladder dysfunction caused by diabetic autonomic neuropathy causes a large-capacity bladder, decreased bladder sensation, increased residual urine volume, and decreased urinary flow rates. Bladder function is worsened by the autoaugmentation of the bladder by the added duodenal segment and also because of poor muscle contraction and outlet dysfunction created by pre-existing pelvic nerve neuropathy. Preoperative urodynamics

Evalution of pancreas graft dysfunction	
Assessment	Tests
Laboratory tests	Serum amylase, blood glucose, human anodal trypsinogen, cyclosporine or tacrolimus levels, C-peptide In bladder-drained cases, urinary amylase and urine culture
Doppler ultrasonography	Pancreatic blood flow, peripancreatic fluid collection, pancreatic ductal dilatation In bladder-drained cases, evidence of bladder outlet obstruction
Computed tomography ± cystography	Looking for leak and collections; this is performed by cystography in bladder-drained cases

Figure 98.8   Evaluation of pancreas graft dysfunction.

are abnormal in up to 43% of patients but do not predict post-transplantation urologic complications such as reflux pancreatitis or infections.[15]

Urinalysis is difficult to interpret with the bladder-drained pancreas. The urine contains white cells from duodenal mucosal sloughing and may be leukocyte esterase positive without bacteriuria. Urine protein excretion is elevated to 1 to 3 g/day in most patients and comprises pancreatic enzymes, immunoglobulins, other globulins, albumin, and digested fragments of these proteins. Urinary albumin, if measurable in the presence of enzymatic degradation, may come from the transplanted or native kidneys.

Hematuria is seen in up to 28% of bladder-drained pancreatic recipients. Early hematuria is usually related to surgical trauma to the bladder or duodenal mucosa near the cystoduodenostomy site and usually clears with diuresis or bladder irrigation.[14] Continuous bladder irrigation requires caution because the cystoduodenostomy is vulnerable to rupture if the drainage catheter becomes obstructed. Late hematuria, beyond 2 to 4 weeks post-transplantation, can arise from anastomotic bleeding, duodenal mucosal sloughing or ulceration, reflux pancreatitis, cystitis, graft thrombosis, rarely arteriovenous fistulas, and pseudoaneurysms. Evaluation should include ultrasonography, urine culture, cystoscopy, and, possibly, pancreatic biopsy.

Urinary Tract Infections

Risk factors for urinary tract infection following pancreatic transplantation include large bladder capacity, incomplete bladder emptying, high bladder urine pH (due to pancreatic bicarbonate), bladder and urethral mucosal irritation from activated pancreatic enzymes with the loss of mucosal barrier, prolonged bladder catheterization, and immunosuppression.[16] Most centers administer oral antibacterial and antifungal prophylaxis for up to 6 to 12 months or indefinitely following transplantation.

Urinary reflux pancreatitis, which causes pancreatic allograft dysfunction, may be associated with periallograft abdominal pain and fever. It is often a result of poor bladder function and requires drainage with a bladder catheter for 5 to 7 days and assessment of bladder dysfunction (Fig. 98.11).

A urethritis dysuria syndrome occurs in 2% to 8% of pancreas recipients with bladder drainage and is caused by uroepithelial exposure to the activated pancreatic proenzymes trypsinogen, chymotrypsinogen, and procarboxypeptidase. Pancreatic exocrine secretions consist of bicarbonate, amylase, lipase, and proenzymes, which are activated by the enterokinase in the allograft duodenal brush border. Increased intravesical enzyme activation occurs with low-grade urinary infections and urinary stasis and patients will develop voiding pain and/or penile, glandular, meatal, or vulval ulceration. Enzyme activation may be minimized by treating low-count bacteriuria, increasing fluid intake, and frequent voiding. If emptying does not improve with α-blockers, continuous Foley catheter drainage for 7 to 10 days has been effective.

Enteric Conversion

This is an option for most of the chronic urologic complications associated with bladder-drained pancreas transplant. The indications are urethral disruption, recurrent urine leak, persistent bleeding, chronic urinary tract infection, dysuria, recurrent hypovolemia, and metabolic acidosis. The conversion rate varies from 8% to 14%. It is ideal to wait until 6 to 12 months after transplantation, when possible, to allow monitoring of urine amylase for early rejection episodes.

Surgical complications following pancreas transplantation

Type of Complication	Presentation	Diagnostic Findings and Testing	Treatment Options
Abscess	Fever, erythema of wound, wound drainage	Elevated white cell count (WBC), fluid collection on computed tomography (CT) scan, pus on aspiration	Open or percutaneous drainage
Graft pancreatitis	Pain over allograft, lower abdominal pain	Elevated serum amylase, enlarged pancreas allograft	Octreotide or somatostatin Foley catheter if bladder drained
Lymphocele	Mass on palpation, urgency if bladder compression	Fluid collection on CT scan, clear fluid on aspiration	Open or percutaneous drainage
Wound drainage	Pancreatic goo, no erythema	Culture, CT scan to rule out deep abscess	Local wound care
Dehiscence	Wound open		Wound care/surgical closure
Arteriovenous fistula	Hematuria, abdominal bleeding	Doppler ultrasonography, angiography	Embolization, surgical repair
Graft thrombosis	Elevated blood sugars Bloody urine if bladder drained	Low serum and urine amylase, sepsis-like syndrome, ultrasound or magnetic resonance imaging	If partial, thrombolytic therapy or anticoagulation (high risk of bleeding), graft pancreatectomy
Pancreatic fistula/leak (bowel drained)	Pain over allograft, sepsis, peritonitis, fever	Elevated WBC, fluid collection on CT scan	Surgical drainage and repair

Figure 98.9 Surgical complications following pancreas transplantation.

IMPACT OF PANCREAS TRANSPLANTATION ON DIABETIC COMPLICATIONS

Pancreatic transplantation is performed to eliminate the need for exogenous insulin and the risk of severe hypoglycemic episodes and to stop or reverse the consequences of hyperglycemia. Well-functioning pancreas transplants result in normal fasting blood glucose, normal glycated hemoglobin levels, and only slightly abnormal oral glucose tolerance testing.[17]

Hypoglycemia

Although severe hypoglycemia is rare, mild hypoglycemia may develop in patients with a well-functioning pancreatic allograft once low baseline immunosuppression has been reached, especially in those patients who have gained back little weight following transplantation and who are physically active. Postprandial hypoglycemic episodes are not always symptomatic. They are associated with high-carbohydrate meals, excessive intake of caffeine or alcohol, excessive exercise, and possible evidence of anti-insulin antibodies in some patients with hypoglycemia. This is not often a significant clinical problem and is usually resolved by avoiding carbohydrate-rich meals.

A major benefit of pancreatic transplantation is restoration of glucagon secretory responses to hypoglycemia. Type 1 diabetics invariably have defective glucagon responses to hypoglycemia, even though they have normal glucagon responses to intravenous arginine. The absence of functional β-cells within the islet eliminates the normal physiologic response by which intraislet insulin tonically dampens secretion of glucagon from α-cells. Consequently, diabetic subjects are usually at risk of prolonged hypoglycemia secondary to injected insulin because there is failure of the normal counterregulatory action of glucagon on the liver to increase glycogenolysis. Despite the fact that the transplanted pancreas is placed ectopically and does not develop vagal control, the transplanted organ has normal glucagon responses to insulin-induced hypoglycemia and resultant counterregulation of hypoglycemia via increased hepatic glucose production. This procedure is also associated with full return of symptoms and partial return of defective epinephrine secretion during insulin-induced hypoglycemia.

Hyperglycemia

Post-transplantation hyperglycemia may be caused by pancreatic graft dysfunction, inadequate insulin release secondary to high tacrolimus or occasionally cyclosporine levels, resistance to insulin secondary to corticosteroids, weight gain, and inadequate physical activity. Although the use of tacrolimus has reduced pancreatic allograft rejection, it also decreases insulin gene transcription. If laboratory and imaging evaluations (see Fig. 98.8) are normal, hyperglycemia is likely a result of decreased insulin production and/or peripheral insulin resistance, which can be identified by measuring glucose utilization rates and glucose/arginine-potentiated insulin secretion. Treatment of nonimmunologic post-transplantation hyperglycemia includes dietary intervention, exercise, and minimizing the tacrolimus dose or changing to cyclosporine. Insulin may be needed initially but can often be discontinued as oral hypoglycemic agents begin to take effect. Sulfonylureas are very effective therapy. Hyperglycemia secondary to rejection is a late event and indicates the irreversible graft damage.

Microvascular Complications
Retinopathy

In a prospective fundoscopic study of SPK patients over 45 months, there was a decreased need for post-transplantation laser therapy, and the diabetic retinopathy showed stabilization in 62%, improvement in 21%, and progression in 17%.[18] The incidence of cataracts of all types increased after transplantation. In the postoperative period, patients may develop neoproliferation and retinal hemorrhages if preoperative blood glucose control is very poor and blood glucose normalizes rapidly following the transplantation. Patients continue to remain at risk of retinal detachment because of scarring secondary to previous retinal damage.

Urologic complications of bladder-drained pancreas transplants				
Complication	Etiology	Presentation	Evaluation	Treatment Options
Urinary tract infection (UTI)	Diabetic bladder dysfunction (DBD)	Asymptomatic, or dysuria, fever, sepsis	Urine culture; check postvoid residual, if elevated urodynamics	Culture-specified antibiotics, prophylactic antibiotics Female: double and timed voiding, clean intermittent catheterization (CIC) Male: α-adrenoeptor blockers to aid bladder emptying, CIC, bladder neck/prostate incision. If treatment failure enteric conversion: Foley catheter drainage
Reflux pancreatitis	DBD	Asymptomatic of pain over pancreas allograft, elevated serum amylase	Check serum amylase, computed tomography (CT) cystogram to exclude leak or duct obstruction	If DBD: double and timed voiding, CIC, α-blockers to aid bladder emptying. If multiple and symptomatic episodes: bladder neck/ prostate incision or enteric diversion
Duodenal cystotomy leak	Ischemic injury to duodenal cuff, cytomegalovirus or other infection, rejection, DBD	Pain over allograft, or peritonitis, elevated serum amylase	Check serum amylase, elevated creatinine, leak on CT cystogram	Foley catheter drainage, if small If early, open surgical repair with resection and closure of layers, evaluate for DBD post recovery. If late, consider enteric conversion
Urethritis/dysuria syndrome, occasional urethral disruption	UTI or DBD causing activation of pancreatic enzymes with digestion of urethral mucosa	Dysuria, urinary retention, hematuria	Check postvoid residual, low-grade UTI; once recovered, evaluate for DBD	Foley catheter, analgesics, empirical treatment of UTI If multiple and symptomatic: enteric conversion

Figure 98.10 **Urologic complications of bladder-drained pancreas transplants.**

Neuropathy

Sensory and motor nerve conduction velocities improve rapidly following pancreas transplantation and then stabilize.[19] The largest degree of recovery is seen in nonobese, younger, shorter patients and in those not receiving renal replacement therapy. The recovery of action potential amplitudes is gradual, continuing improve up to 5 years beyond transplantation. Recovery is more complete in sensory than in motor nerves. More improvement is noted in nonobese patients, those with better initial amplitudes, and, perhaps, those who use angiotensin-converting enzyme inhibitors or angiotensin receptor blockers for the treatment of hypertension.[19]

Improvement in autonomic reactivity and stabilization or improvement in gastric emptying is noted in pancreatic/kidney recipients compared to diabetic kidney-only transplant recipients.[20] If autonomic symptoms are severe at the time of pancreatic transplantation, improvement is unlikely.

Nephropathy

Early diabetic nephropathy is characterized by increased glomerular basement membrane thickness and an increase in mesangial volume. Renal transplant biopsy specimens from diabetics with kidney/pancreas and kidney-only transplants within 2.5 years of transplantation show glomerular basement membrane thickness within the normal range.[21] After 2.5 years from transplantation, 92% of the biopsy samples from the kidney/pancreas recipients have a normal glomerular basement membrane thickness compared to only 35% of the biopsy samples from the kidney-only group, while relative mesangial volume was normal in 82% of the biopsy specimens from pancreas/kidney recipients compared with only 12% in the kidney-only recipients.[22] Thus, concurrent pancreas transplantation decreases the occurrence of the changes of diabetic nephropathy that may result in allograft loss.[21]

Vascular Disease

Successful kidney/pancreas transplantation results in a significant improvement in the control of hypertension compared to kidney transplant alone in type 1 diabetics.[23] Increase in peripheral vascular disease has been correlated to kidney/pancreas transplant recipients compared with kidney-alone transplant recipients.[24] However, another study found the same prevalence of peripheral vascular disease following pancreas transplantation, as occurred in diabetic kidney-only recipients who refused pancreas transplantation for nonmedical reasons and in nondiabetic renal transplant recipients.[25] Encouragingly, one recent study showed that after a 10-year mean observation period, the progression of macrovascular diseases (cerebrovascular, coronary, and peripheral vascular) were significantly lower in recipients with a functioning SPK compared to a kidney transplant alone.[4]

A study using intravital microscopic evaluation of nailbeds and conjunctival vasculature found improved vascularization (as assessed by a reduction in venular diameter, increased number of arterioles per unit area, and elevation of the perfusion capacity) only in the kidney/pancreas recipients.[26]

Quality of Life and Social Issues

Similar to other types of transplantation, pancreas transplantation is a very stressful event and can tax even the strongest of family relationships. Pretransplantation debilities (decreased vision, neuropathy, muscle weakness, orthostatic symptoms) can

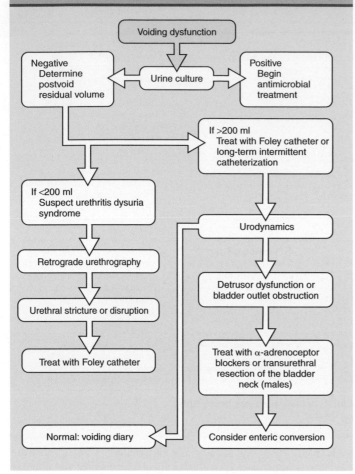

Managing voiding dysfunction in bladder-drained pancreas transplants

Figure 98.11 Management of post-transplantation voiding abnormalities. (From Kuhr CS, Bakthavatsalam R, Marsh CL: Urologic aspects of kidney-pancreas transplantation. Urol Clin North Am 2001;28:751–758.)

be exacerbated by the surgery and immunosuppressive medications. Furthermore, patients who smoke and/or drink and are without family support do not survive as long following transplantation. However, kidney/pancreatic transplant recipients with social support and well-functioning allografts report an increased global quality of life and frequently return to work, although the number returning to work is not much different from that in those receiving a kidney transplant alone.[27]

Pregnancy Following Pancreatic Transplantation

Within 1 year of transplantation, menstruation and ovulation return in most women of child-bearing age, making pregnancy possible following kidney/pancreatic transplantation. The National Transplantation Pregnancy Registry has reported 36 pregnancies in 27 patients.[28] The outcomes were 31 live births, three therapeutic and three spontaneous abortions (one twin reduction), and one ectopic twin pregnancy. The newborn outcomes were prematurity (24/31), low birth weight (20/31), newborn complications (17/31), and neonatal death (1/31). Six patients had rejections that resulted in losing the graft (four kidneys, two pancreas and kidney) and 50% of the patients required cesarean section. Optimal outcome was seen when the mother had a serum creatinine <1.5 mg/dl (132 μmol/l) at the beginning of pregnancy.

Hypertension, prematurity, preeclampsia, and growth retardation frequently complicated the pregnancies, even with good renal function. Urinary tract infections occurred in up to 73% of pregnant pancreas recipients. To prevent rejection, cyclosporine or tacrolimus levels, which often decline during pregnancy, require close monitoring. Cesarean section is not mandatory; vaginal deliveries, however, must be observed for signs of allograft duodenal rupture. The average gestational period is 35 ± 2 weeks; the average birth weight is 2150 ± 680 g. To date, most children of transplant recipients have developed normally.

The management of other medical issues does not differ from those in kidney-only transplant recipients (see Chapter 94). However, there seems to be an increased risk of post-transplantation lymphoproliferative disorder, presumably due to the enhanced immunosuppressive regimens compared to kidney-only protocols.

ISLET CELL TRANSPLANTATION

There were sporadic reports in the 1990s of insulin-independence for extended periods following islet allotransplantation.[29–32] Auto-transplantation studies then demonstrated that a critical mass of 300,000 islet equivalence could reestablish and maintain insulin independence beyond 2 years.[33] To date, the longest period of insulin independence following autotransplantation is >13 years.[34] Of the 237 well-documented allotransplants recorded in the Islet Transplant Registry from 1990 to 2000, <12% of recipients were insulin free at 1 year post-transplantation. The reasons for this failure rate may include a subtherapeutic islet implant mass, a high rate of engraftment failure, islet damage in the liver (the site of implantation) by direct local toxic effects of the immunosuppressants, ineffective immunosuppression failing to prevent rejection and recurrent autoimmune diabetes, and islet functional exhaustion. Four criteria have been associated with insulin independence: (1) the critical islet implant mass >6000 IE (islet equivalents)/kg, (2) cold ischemia (preservation) time <8 hours, (3) use of polyclonal antibodies such as antilymphocyte globulin or ATG in depleting cytotoxic T cells, and (4) the liver as the favored implantation site. Early immunosuppressive regimens were relatively ineffective in preventing allograft rejection when compared to their effect on vascularized pancreatic grafts. Most, if not all agents, were associated with impaired β-cell function and reduced graft revascularization.

Insulin-independence was reported in nonuremic type 1 diabetics transplanted with an average of approximately 800,000 islets using the Edmonton protocol, a corticosteroid-free immunosuppression regimen of daclizumab, sirolimus, and low-dose tacrolimus. Follow-up of this cohort has since confirmed long-term insulin independence with therapy that is safe and well tolerated.[30,35] There has since been an exponential increase in clinical islet transplant activity; more patients with type 1 diabetes have now received islet transplants in the past 5 years than in the entire preceding 30-year history of islet transplantation.

Technique of Islet Transplantation

The current technique of islet transplantation involves cadaveric pancreas procurement, organ preservation, enzymatic isolation of the islets, purification, and percutaneously injection of sterile islets into the liver through the portal vein by a catheter placed under radiographic guidance (Fig. 98.12). Although accessing the portal vein percutaneously is relatively invasive, the entire procedure can be performed on an outpatient basis. Effective

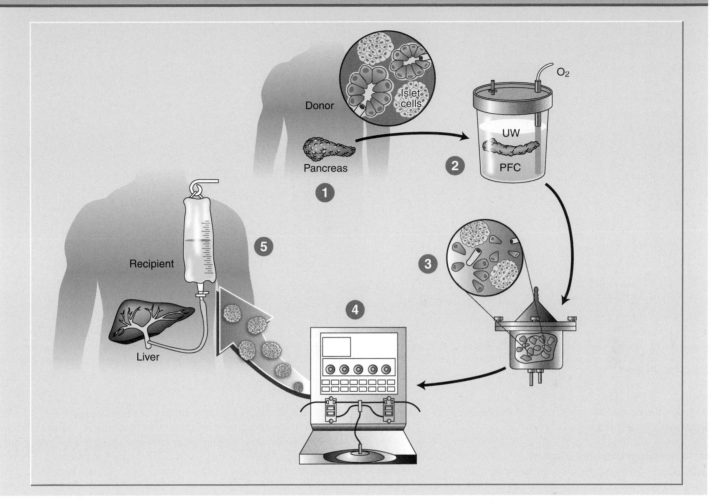

Figure 98.12 Current clinical islet cell transplantation protocol. The retrieved donor pancreas (1) is preserved (2) with a two-layer storage method using University of Wisconsin solution (UW) over a layer of highly oxygenated perfluorocarbon (PFC). The pancreas is distended with collagenase and placed in a digestion chamber (3). The disrupted exocrine and endocrine elements are purified by centrifugation (4) and the islet preparation free from exocrine elements is transplanted by intrahepatic portal vein infusion (5). (Adapted from Mirbolooki M, et al: A perspective on clinical transplantation. Curr Med Chem in press.)

mechanical and physical methods to seal the catheter tract reduce the risk of postprocedural bleeding.[36]

Bleeding related to the procedure (23%), thrombus in segmental branches of the portal vein (8%), and punctured gallbladder (3%) are the most observed acute complications after islet transplantation.[37]

Medical Complications

There are significant medical problems reported after islet transplantation.[35] Changes consistent with fatty liver are reported in 22% of subjects who had MRI post-transplantation. Mouth ulcers occur in 90% of subjects, usually responding to simple antiseptic measures or topical triamcinolone ointment together with a reduction in the dose of sirolimus. Diarrhea is frequent (60%), and acne occurred in 52%. Forty-three percent of subjects complained of edema, and in 12%, was severe enough to necessitate a change in the immunosuppressive regimen. Weight loss is common.

Glycemic Control and Insulin Independence

Successful islet transplantation establishes normal levels of hemoglobin A_{1c} (HbA_{1c}), although the fasting glucose levels tend to be slightly elevated, and there is often impaired glucose

tolerance. Another difference between successful pancreas and islet transplants is that placement of islets within the liver results in failure of the α-cell response to hypoglycemia, even though they are responsive to intravenous arginine.

In a recent combined analysis, 82% of 118 islet recipients in three North American centers were insulin free at 1 year.[37] However, a 5-year follow-up in Edmonton[35] revealed that, although the majority of subjects (82%) have C-peptide present after islet transplantation, only a minority (7.5%) maintain insulin independence (Fig. 98.13). The median duration of insulin independence was 15 months.

Technical Progress

Islet transplantation can relieve glucose instability and problems with hypoglycemia, but there is still a need for further progress in the availability of transplantable islets, improving islet engraftment, and preserving islet function. Use of the two-layer oxygenated PFC system usually allows for better pancreatic transportation. PFC-based preservation also optimizes islet recovery and post-transplantation graft function without inducing oxidative stress.[39] Islet culture for 24 to 48 hours in antioxidant-enriched medium has

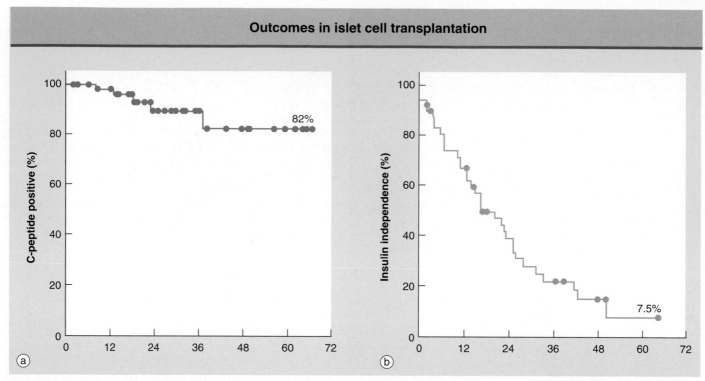

Figure 98.13 Outcomes in islet cell transplantation. *a*, Persistence of C-peptide secretion over time. The curves are dated from the time of the final transplant. *b*, Persistence of insulin independence over time. (Redrawn from Ryan EA, Paty BW, Senior PA, et al: Five-year follow-up after clinical islet transplantation. Diabetes 2005;54:2060–2069.)

improved the quality of islet preparations and facilitated the shipment of islets between centers.[40]

Immunosuppressive Regimens

Tacrolimus, cyclosporine, and corticosteroids are clearly diabetogenic through increased peripheral insulin resistance or by direct islet cell toxicity. Oral administration increases portal venous drug concentrations and the possibility of significant injury to intrahepatic islet allografts. Most programs use steroid-free and calcineurin inhibitor–sparing protocols for islet and/or kidney recipients using different combinations of mycophenolate mofetil and sirolimus. Mycophenolate mofetil has been shown to reduce early pancreatic rejection rates. Insulin independence has now been achieved with islet grafts derived from non–heart-beating donors and following sequential kidney/islet transplantations using sirolimus-based therapy. Islet engraftment can also be improved using a calcineurin inhibitor–free regimen with profound T cell depletion.[35] Anti–T cell therapy using ATG or OKT3 may be associated with a cytokine storm, which is toxic to islets, and hence the newer induction agents (anti–interleukin-2 receptor blockers) may be particularly useful to minimize cytokine release.

A number of new immunosuppressive agents that offer the potential for more islet friendly approaches are now entering clinical trials. These include combinations of biologic agents such as ATG, rituximab, and alemtuzumab; novel anti–T cell biologic agents, some of which offer the prospect of inducing tolerance based on animal studies; and also agents that produce costimulatory blockade.

Future Directions in Islet Transplantation
Single Donor Islet Transplantation

The critical shortage of donor pancreata and the inability to recover large numbers of high-quality islets from a single pancreas

are major obstacles to the widespread application of clinical islet transplantation. Some clinicians have advocated blood glucose stability rather than insulin independence as the goal of islet transplantations. Although this would benefit more patients, diabetics disabled by hypoglycemic unawareness and marked metabolic lability would be reluctant to accept the potential risks of long-term immunosuppressive therapy if they were to have only partial control of their diabetes. While multiple-donor transplants continue to be the norm, single-donor to single-recipient transplantation may soon become a reality as better methods are developed for pancreatic preservation, islet isolation and purification, and islet engraftment. An encouraging study of islet allotransplantation with a mean of 7271 IE/kg prepared from a single cadaver donor pancreas enabled eight recipients to achieve insulin independence and freedom from hypoglycemia; five remained insulin independent for longer than 1 year.

Clinical autotransplantation studies have shown that if ischemic injury and immune reactivity can be minimized, normoglycemia can be maintained with fewer islets.

Living Donor Islet Transplantation

Recent experience indicates that live donor segmental-pancreatic transplants have only a modest increase in procedure-related complications. Live donation of a segmental graft specifically for islet transplantation is an attractive option, but the risk of inducing diabetes or creating a pancreatic fistula in an otherwise healthy donor remains a major concern.

Islet Transplantation in Children

Because end-organ damage evolves over many years, the trade-off of exchanging frequent blood glucose testing, daily insulin injections, and dietary restrictions for lifelong immunosuppression cannot be justified in most children or adolescents. However, islet cell transplantation may be appropriate for children with recurrent episodes of unexplained severe hypoglycemia and its life-threatening sequelae,[41] those with progressive microvascular complications (particularly retinopathy and nephropathy) indicating a risk of severe disability and premature death in early or mid-adulthood, those requiring concurrent immunosuppressive therapy for a comorbidity (such as a kidney, heart, or liver transplant) that can be safely and effectively treated with a steroid-free regimen.

Islet Transplantation in Type 2 Diabetes

The underlying metabolic defect in type 2 diabetes is insulin resistance, but β-cell dysfunction can also coexist. Combined islet-liver allografts in patients with cirrhosis and overt type 2 diabetes (which occurs in about 20% of cirrhotic patients) have given much improvement in insulin requirements, HbA$_{1C}$ levels, and overall metabolic control than one would expect in liver transplant–alone patients. It is unclear at this time whether islet or pancreatic transplantation can override the abnormal insulin demand caused by peripheral insulin resistance without β-cell exhaustion.

Stem-Cell Technology and Xenotransplantation

Islet transplantation in its present form would benefit <0.5% of type 1 diabetics. It has been long recognized that alternative sources of insulin-producing, glucose-responsive tissue must be developed. Islet farming may be one solution. Adult and embryonic stem cells can be transformed into islet-like cells *in vitro*, but it is not yet clear whether they can maintain physiologic glucose homeostasis and will not undergo senescence, or malignant degeneration, over time.

Xenotransplantation remains a promising approach, although transplantation of porcine islet cell clusters has not yet achieved insulin independence in human diabetics. Many technologic and biologic limitations as well as ethical, political, and regulatory obstacles must be overcome before such radical approaches become realistic in clinical practice.

REFERENCES

1. Gruessner AC, Sutherland DE: Pancreas transplant outcomes for United States (US) and non-US cases as reported to the United Network for Organ Sharing (UNOS) and the International Pancreas Transplant Registry (IPTR) as of June 2004. Clin Transplant 2005; 19:433–455.
2. Tan M, Kandaswamy R, Sutherland DE, Gruessner RW: Laparoscopic donor distal pancreatectomy for living donor pancreas and pancreas-kidney transplantation. Am J Transplant 2005;5:1966–1970.
3. Reddy KS, Stabelin D, Taranto S, et al: Long-term survival following simultaneous kidney-pancreas transplantation versus kidney transplantation alone in patients with type 1 diabetes mellitus and renal failure. Am J Kidney Dis 2003;41:464–470.
4. Biesenbach G, Konigsrainer A, Gross C, Margreiter R: Progression of macrovascular diseases is reduced in type 1 diabetic patients after more than 5 years successful combined pancreas-kidney transplantation in comparison to kidney transplantation alone. Transpl Int 2005;189: 1054–1060.
5. Venstrom JM, McBride MA, Rother KI, et al: Survival after pancreas transplantation in patients with diabetes and preserved kidney function. JAMA 2003;290:2817–2823.
6. Demartines N, Schiesser M, Clavien PA: An evidence-based analysis of simultaneous pancreas-kidney and pancreas transplantation alone. Am J Transplant 2005;5:2668–2697.
7. Gruessner AC, Sutherland DE: Pancreas transplant outcomes for United States and non–United States cases as reported to the United Network for Organ Sharing (UNOS) and the International Pancreas Transplant Registry. Clin Transplant 2004;19:433–455.
8. Burke GW 3rd, Kaufman DB, Millis JM, et al: Prospective randomized trail of the effect of antibody induction in simultaneous pancreas and kidney transplantation: Three-year results. Transplantation 2004;77: 1269–1275.
9. Gruessner RW, Kandaswamy R, Humar A, et al: Calcineurin inhibitor- and steroid-free immunosuppression in pancreas-kidney and solitary pancreas transplantation. Transplantation 2005;79:1184–1189.
10. Sundberg AK, Roskopf JA, Harmann EL, et al: Pilot study of rapid steroid elimination with alemtuzumab induction therapy in kidney and pancreas transplantation. Transplant Proc 2005;37:1294–1296.
11. Axelrod D, Leventhal JR, Gallon LG, et al: Reduction of CMV disease with steroid-free immunosuppression in simultaneous pancreas-kidney transplant recipients. Am J Transplant 2005;5:1423–1429.
12. Perkins JD, Engen DE, Munn ST, et al The value of cystoscopically-directed biopsy in human pancreaticoduodenal transplantation. Clin Transpl 1989;3:306–315.
13. Hurst GC, Somerville KT, Alloway RR, et al: Preliminary experience with midodrine in kidney/pancreas transplant patients with orthostatic hypotension. Clin Transpl 2000;14:42–47.
14. Kuhr CS, Bakthavatsalam R, Marsh CL: Urologic aspects of kidney-pancreas transplantation. Urol Clin North Am 2001;28:751–758.
15. Taylor RJ, Mays SD, Grothe TJ, Stratta RJ: Correlation of preoperative urodynamic findings to postoperative complications following pancreas transplantation. J Urol 1993;150:1185–1188.
16. Smets YF, van der Pijl JW, van Dissel JT, et al: Infectious disease complications of simultaneous pancreas kidney transplantation. Nephrol Dial Transplant 1997;12:764–771.
17. Robertson RP, Sutherland DE, Kendall DM, et al: Metabolic characterization of long term successful pancreas transplants in type I diabetes. J Invest Med 1996;44:549–555.
18. Koznarova R, Saudek F, Sosna T, et al: Beneficial effect of pancreas and kidney transplantation on advanced diabetic retinopathy. Cell Transplant 2000;9:903–908.
19. Allen RD, Al Harbi IS, Morris JG, et al: Diabetic neuropathy after pancreas transplantation: Determinants of recovery. Transplantation 1997; 63:830–838.
20. Hathaway DK, Abell T, Cardoso S, et al: Improvement in autonomic and gastric function following pancreas-kidney versus kidney-alone transplantation and the correlation with quality of life. Transplantation 1994;57:816–822.
21. Fioretto P, Steffes MW, Sutherland DER, et al: Reversal of lesions of diabetic nephropathy after pancreas transplantation. N Engl J Med 1998;339:69–75.
22. Hariharan S, Smith RD, Viero R, First MR: Diabetic neuropathy after renal transplantation. Clinical and pathologic features. Transplantation 1996;62:632–635.
23. Elliot MD, Kapoor A, Parker MA, et al: Improvement in hypertension in patients with diabetes mellitus after kidney/pancreas transplantation. Circulation 2001;104:563–569.
24. Morrissey PE, Shaffer D, Monaco AP, et al: Peripheral vascular disease after kidney-pancreas transplantation in diabetic patients with end-stage renal disease. Arch Surg 1997;132:358–361.
25. Kausz A, Brunzell J, Marcovina S, et al: Lipid profile and peripheral vascular disease among diabetic patients receiving kidney-pancreas or kidney transplants. J Am Soc Nephrol 1998;9:A680.
26. Cheung AT, Chen PC, Leshchinsky TV, et al: Improvement in conjunctival microangiopathy after simultaneous pancreas-kidney transplants. Transplant Proc 1997;29:660–661.
27. Adang EM, Engel GL, van Hooff JP, Kootstra G: Comparison before and after transplantation of pancreas-kidney and pancreas-kidney with loss of pancreas: A prospective, controlled quality of life study. Transplantation 1996;62:754–758.
28. Wilson GA, Coscia LA, McGrory CH: National Transplantation Pregnancy Registry: Postpregnancy graft loss among female pancreas-kidney recipients. Transplant Proc 2001;33:1667–1669.
29. Warnock GL, Kneteman NM, Ryan E, et al: Normoglycaemia after transplantation of freshly isolated and cryopreserved pancreatic islets in type 1 (insulin-dependent) diabetes mellitus. Diabetologia 1991;34: 55–58.

30. Ryan EA, Lakey JR, Paty BW, et al: Successful islet transplantation: Continued insulin reserve provides long-term glycemic control. Diabetes 2002;51:2148–2157.

31. Shapiro AM, Ricordi C, Hering B: Edmonton's islet success has indeed been replicated elsewhere. Lancet 2003;362:1242.

32. Shapiro AM, Lakey JR, Ryan EA, et al: Islet transplantation in seven patients with type 1 diabetes mellitus using a glucocorticoid-free immunosuppressive regimen. N Engl J Med 2000;343:230–238.

33. Farney AC, Hering BJ, Nelson L, et al: No late failures of intraportal human islet autografts beyond 2 years. Transplant Proc 1998;30:420.

34. Robertson RP, Lanz KJ, Sutherland DE, Kendall DM: Prevention of diabetes for up to 13 years by autoislet transplantation after pancreatectomy for chronic pancreatitis. Diabetes 2001; 50:47–50.

35. Ryan EA, Paty BW, Senior PA, et al: Five-year follow-up after clinical islet transplantation. Diabetes 2005;54:2060–2069.

36. Owen RJ, Ryan EA, O'Kelly K, et al: Percutaneous transhepatic pancreatic islet cell transplantation in type 1 diabetes mellitus: Radiologic aspects. Radiology 2003;229:165–170.

37. Shapiro AM, Ricordi C: Unraveling the secrets of single donor success in islet transplantation. Am J Transplant 2004;4:295–298.

38. Ricordi C, Fraker C, Szust J, et al: Improved human islet isolation outcome from marginal donors following addition of oxygenated perfluorocarbon to the cold-storage solution. Transplantation 2003;75:1524–1527.

39. Gaber AO, Fraga DW, Callicutt CS, et al: Improved in vivo pancreatic islet function after prolonged in vitro islet culture. Transplantation 2001;72:1730–1736.

40. The Diabetes Control and Complications Trial Research Group: Hypoglycemia in the Diabetes Control and Complications Trial. Diabetes 1997;46:271–286.

Kidney Disease in Liver, Cardiac, Lung, Intestine, and Hematopoietic Cell Transplantation

Akinlolu O. Ojo

INTRODUCTION

Allogeneic transplantation with solid organs (heart, intestine, kidney, liver, lung, and their combinations) has become a successful and widely accepted therapy for end-stage organ failure. Recipients of these organs now survive for many decades in part because of remarkable advances in transplant immunosuppressive regimens and surgical techniques. More than 150,000 heart, liver, lung, or intestinal transplants were performed worldwide between 1980 and 2005. Chronic kidney disease (CKD) has emerged as a common complication of nonrenal solid organ transplantation with significant adverse influence on both patient and allograft survival. In the immediate perioperative period following a nonrenal organ transplantation, 50% to 60% of recipients may experience acute renal failure (ARF) and up to 30% of recipients require urgent renal replacement therapy (RRT). CKD is even more common; >75% of some nonrenal transplant recipients will eventually develop some impairment of renal function. Both ARF and CKD complicate the medical management of solid organ recipients and contribute in substantial measure to excessive mortality in the post-transplantation period.

Hematopoietic cell transplants are increasingly used treatments for hematologic malignancies and are more common than solid organ transplants: 15,000 bone marrow and stem cell transplants are performed annually worldwide. This chapter also considers the distinctive problems of renal disease following hematopoietic cell transplants.

EPIDEMIOLOGY OF RENAL DISEASE FOLLOWING NONRENAL SOLID ORGAN TRANSPLANTATION

Acute Renal Failure

A commonly used definition of ARF in transplantation medicine is an increase in serum creatinine of 0.5 mg/dl (44 μmol/l) above baseline or an acute need for RRT within 30 days of the transplant or during the initial transplantation hospital stay. Perioperative ARF is common in all types of nonrenal organ transplantation.

Figure 99.1 shows the incidence of ARF in nonrenal organ transplant recipients and the main predisposing risk factors. ARF is more common after liver and lung transplantation than cardiac transplantation, but only a proportion of each type of transplant recipient requires RRT. Although there are no large studies of ARF following intestinal transplantation, case reports suggest a high risk.

Chronic Kidney Disease

Most studies of CKD in nonrenal organ transplantation predate the adoption of the CKD classification developed from the National Kidney Foundation Disease Outcomes Quality Index initiative. The

Epidemiology of acute renal failure in cardiac, liver, and lung transplant recipients			
	Cardiac Transplantation	Liver Transplantation	Lung Transplantation
Incidence	20%–30%	46%–61%	50%–60%
Requiring RRT	10%–15%	20%–25%	8%–10%
Preoperative reduced renal function is a major risk factor in cardiac, liver, and lung transplants			
	Ischemic cardiomyopathy	MELD >21 Age Retransplant ICU stay >3 days	Mechanical ventilation >1 day Diagnosis other than COPD Amphotericin
1-year patient survival Without ARF With ARF	91% 36%	93% 48%	82% 22%

Figure 99.1 Epidemiology of acute renal failure in cardiac, liver, and lung transplant recipients. COPD, chronic obstructive pulmonary disease; ICU, intensive care unit; MELD, Mayo Endstage Liver Disease score; RRT, renal replacement therapy. (Adapted from Ojo AO, Held PJ, Port FK, et al: Chronic renal failure after transplantation of a nonrenal organ. N Engl J Med 2003;349:931–940.)

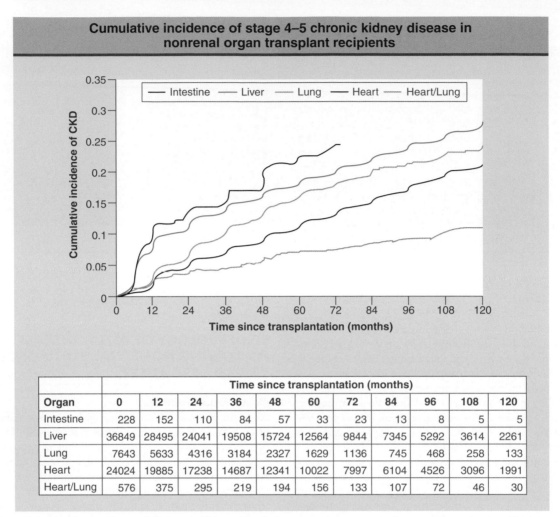

Figure 99. 2 Cumulative incidence of stage 4–5 chronic kidney disease in nonrenal organ transplant recipients. Lower table shows number of patients in each cohort at each time point. Stage 4–5 CKD = GFR <30 ml/min. (Adapted from Ojo AO, Held PJ, Port FK, et al: Chronic renal failure after transplantation of a nonrenal organ. N Engl J Med 2003;349:931–940.)

most common definitions previously in use are persistent elevation of serum creatinine >2.0 mg/dl (176 µmol/l), increase in serum creatinine of 0.5 mg/dl (44 µmol/l) above pretransplant level for ≥6 months, or end-stage renal disease (ESRD). Because of variable definitions, an accurate assessment of the incidence of post-transplantation CKD is difficult to make. In cardiac transplantation, 8% to 10% of recipients alive at 10 years post-transplantation are on RRT. The lung transplant recipient population has a 10% prevalence of ESRD 10 years after transplantation. In most series, there are prevalence rates for CKD of 25% to 35% for liver transplant recipients.

The findings in the U.S. Registry of approximately 70,000 nonrenal transplant recipients are shown in Figure 99.2. There is an ESRD incidence of 1.5% to 2% per year for each type of non-renal transplant organ among recipients who survived 6 months beyond transplantation.[1]

ETIOLOGY AND PATHOGENESIS

Common Risk Factors

Older age and preoperative renal function are two well-established risk factors for postoperative ARF in all nonrenal organ recipients. Hemodynamic instability occurring before transplantation or

intraoperatively, most commonly due to bleeding, sepsis, or myocardial ischemia, also significantly increase in risk of ARF in heart, lung, and liver transplant recipients. The necessary use of nephrotoxic agents may also contribute to acute renal injury.

There are also risk factors for CKD common to all types of nonrenal organ transplantation, including hypertension, diabetes mellitus, and advancing age. Hypertension is found in 65% to 90% of heart, lung, and liver recipients. Diabetes mellitus is present in 1% to 2% of patients before nonrenal organ transplantation, and post-transplantation diabetes mellitus develops in 10% to 30%. Dyslipidemia is a probable but unproven risk factor for CKD, which is highly prevalent in the organ transplant recipient population affecting 45% to 80% of liver and thoracic organ recipients. Another major etiologic factor is the use of calcineurin inhibitors (CNIs) (tacrolimus and cyclosporine), which remain the mainstay of post-transplantation immunosuppression (see later discussion).

The potency of these common risk factors for CKD has been well characterized in epidemiologic studies. Each 10-year increase in age after age 18 years confers a 36% greater risk of post-transplantation CKD. For reasons that have not been well elucidated, pediatric recipients are much more susceptible to post-transplantation CKD. Recipients who required intervention with RRT in the 6 months prior to transplantation are twice as likely to develop both ARF and CKD in the post-transplantation period; presumably the renal injury from the preoperative insult may not have resolved completely. It is not known whether postponing transplantation to allow for further renal recovery would have prevented further postoperative renal dysfunction, but in most cases, this is a theoretical consideration because the transplant is often a life-saving procedure with no opportunity for elective timing. Reduced pretransplantation glomerular filtration rate (GFR) increases the risk of post-transplantation CKD by 38%, 125%, and 240% for postoperative GFR of 60 to 80, 30 to 39, and <30 ml/min per 1.73 m², respectively, compared to recipients with a preoperative GFR of ≥90 ml/min per 1.73 m². Systemic hypertension and diabetes mellitus increase the risk of CKD by 18% and 42%, respectively. The presence of pretransplantation chronic hepatitis C virus (HCV) infection also confers a 15% greater risk of post-transplantation CKD in all categories of organ recipients.

Calcineurin Inhibitor Toxicity

The two widely used CNI, cyclosporine and tacrolimus, have a similar degree of acute and chronic nephrotoxicity (see also Chapters 90 and 95). Acute CNI nephrotoxicity is principally mediated by reversible intrarenal hemodynamic changes, with higher concentrations of CNI also producing tubular injury. Chronic CNI nephrotoxicity is characterized by progressive interstitial fibrosis with arterial hyalinosis and intimal hyperplasia.

Chronic CNI nephrotoxicity is estimated as the predominant etiology in 70% of CKD in cardiac, lung, and liver transplant recipients.[2] However, its perceived prevalence is mainly based on clinical evaluation with limited histologic evidence because renal biopsy is infrequently performed in solid organ recipients with renal failure. Reasons for infrequent renal biopsy include the finding of shrunken kidneys at the time of referral, a relative contraindication to a safe and informative renal biopsy, the acquired bleeding disorders related to allograft dysfunction in many liver recipients, and the volume overload, heart failure, or pulmonary disease present in many patients that makes it difficult to lie prone or cooperate with respiratory maneuvers required for the biopsy procedure.

In one of the few series where renal histology was available, the predominant histologic lesions were CNI arteriolopathy in 46%, diabetic nephropathy in 34%, and focal segmental glomerulosclerosis (FSGS) in 34%.[3] In another series with renal biopsy data following liver transplantation, predominant findings were CNI nephrotoxicity in 73%, FSGS in 7%, cystic kidney disease in 7%, and other diagnoses in 7%.[4] In a series of heart transplant recipients, lesions attributable to CNI toxicity were found in 60%, hypertensive nephrosclerosis in 30%, FSGS in 16%, and diabetic nephropathy in 6%.[2] The reasons for the high incidence of CNI toxicity in nonrenal as opposed to renal transplantation are not fully understood. It may in part be explained by the higher CNI serum levels sometimes recommended compared to renal transplantation. It has also been proposed that the denervated state of the renal transplant may afford some protection from CNI toxicity compared to the native kidney, but there is limited evidence for this. Progression of renal disease often continues even after withdrawal of CNI.

Thrombotic Microangiopathy

Thrombotic microangiopathy (TMA) is characterized by microangiopathic hemolysis, thrombocytopenia, and renal failure and may occur in recipients of any nonrenal organ transplant at any time from a few weeks to 10 years after transplantation. It is a major

Organ-specific risk factors for chronic kidney disease following liver, heart, or lung transplantation

Liver
HBV- or HCV-associated glomerulonephritis
IgA nephropathy
Hepatorenal syndrome
Oxalosis
Repeat liver transplant

Heart
Systemic atherosclerosis
Renal hypoperfusion due to congestive heart failure
Cyanotic congenital heart disease

Lung
Cystic fibrosis
Pulmonary hypertension

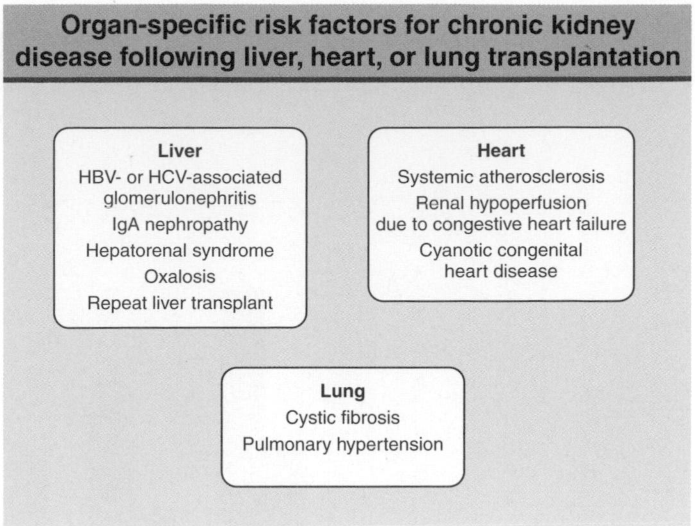

Figure 99.3 Organ-specific risk factors for chronic kidney disease following liver, heart, or lung transplantation. HBV, hepatitis B virus; HCV, hepatitis C virus.

cause of both ARF and CKD. CNI-induced endothelial injury appears to be the initiating factor in many but not all patients.

Organ-Specific Risk Factors

Figure 99.3 shows the common organ-specific risk factors for CKD after liver, cardiac, or lung transplantation, which are discussed in further detail in the context of each type of organ transplant. The general implication of these underlying predispositions is that the nephrologist providing post-transplantation care should consider the underlying cause of end-organ failure as a risk factor for post-transplantation renal dysfunction even if clinically overt renal disease was not manifest prior to transplantation.

IMPACT OF ACUTE RENAL FAILURE AND CHRONIC KIDNEY DISEASE ON CLINICAL OUTCOME

ARF and CKD complicate the care of organ transplant recipients. Drug treatment with immunosuppressants, anti-infectives, and other agents may be hampered because of contraindications or complex dosing adjustment. The relative imprecision of serum creatinine as an indicator of renal function is not always appreciated, leading to the potential for increased drug toxicity. Many studies have shown that both ARF and CKD are associated with increased frequency of hospitalization and infectious complications in nonrenal organ recipients. Because of extracellular fluid retention, the severity of pre-existing hypertension may worsen. The use of diuretics and the renal disease itself may result in electrolyte abnormalities such as hyponatremia, disordered calcium-phosphate regulation, and acid-base disturbances.

Liver and cardiac transplant recipients with CKD have a higher incidence of allograft dysfunction, although this relationship may not be causally linked. The most significant impact of post-transplantation renal disease is an increase in mortality. ARF in the early post-transplantation period is associated with a two- to threefold increase in mortality, which is even higher when RRT is required acutely (see Fig. 99.1). CKD is also associated with a two- to fourfold excess risk of mortality (Fig. 99.4). The effect of CKD on mortality is detectable even before recipients reach stage 4 or 5 CKD.

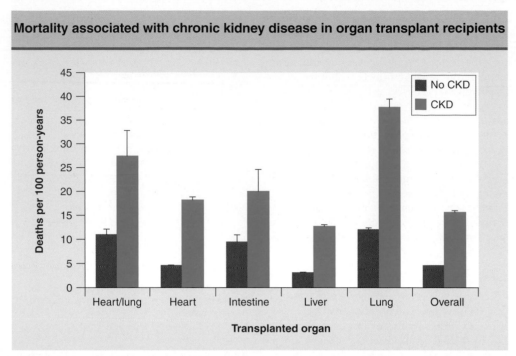

Figure 99.4 **Mortality associated with stage 4 and 5 chronic kidney disease (CKD) in organ transplant recipients.** (Data from Scientific Registry of Transplant Recipients.)

GENERAL MANAGEMENT OF KIDNEY DISEASE IN NONRENAL ORGAN RECIPIENTS

Pretransplantation Evaluation

Pretransplantation assessment of renal function is valuable even when serum creatinine values are within the reference range; malnourished patients with end-organ failure may have unusually low serum creatinine for GFR because of muscle wasting, and a more precise assessment of renal function, such as isotopic determination of GFR, should be considered and can provide the basis for calculation of medication doses to minimize drug toxicity. Pretransplantation evaluation should include urinalysis with microscopy of a freshly voided urine specimen. A renal biopsy should be performed pretransplantation if renal function is significantly depressed in the absence of a hemodynamic explanation or if serologic evaluation or urinary sediment suggests an active and potentially treatable renal disease.

Perioperative Care

In the perioperative period, the appropriate type of RRT should be initiated with minimal delay and should be performed with no systemic anticoagulation whenever feasible. Close attention must be paid to the composition and volume of all intravenous infusions. In particular, liver transplantation is almost always accompanied by massive intravenous volume expansion, and iatrogenic electrolyte abnormalities or coagulopathy may supervene quickly if intravenous fluids are not carefully calibrated.

Minimizing Calcineurin Inhibitor Treatment

The introduction of newer immunosuppressants has given the opportunity to delay the initiation of CNI or withdraw CNI at various times after transplantation. Induction therapy with basiliximab, daclizumab, or antithymocyte globulin is now used in cardiac, liver, and lung transplant recipients to delay initiation of CNI therapy for up 7 to 10 days post-transplantation. This spares the acute nephrotoxic effect of CNI, which would otherwise

be superimposed on acute ischemic renal injury resulting from perioperative hemodynamic instability. Although rational, this approach is yet to be proven in randomized clinical trials as an effective strategy to minimize postoperative ARF.

Reduction in dose or complete withdrawal of CNI several months to years after organ transplantation has become increasingly common practice in recipients with post-transplantation CKD. These renal-sparing maintenance protocols typically rely on sirolimus or everolimus in combination with mycophenolate mofetil (MMF) to prevent rejection. A number of small studies have shown modest improvement in renal function following CNI withdrawal with sirolimus or MMF substitution in cardiac and liver transplant recipients with established CKD. This improvement may represent relief from the reversible vasoconstrictive effect of CNIs, but some renal dysfunction is likely to be irreversible because histologic evidence of chronic glomerular and tubulointerstitial injury is often seen after 3 to 6 months of continuous CNI exposure. In some cases, increased risk of an acute rejection episode has been reported following CNI withdrawal. At present, there is insufficient evidence to recommend initial CNI-free regimens for heart, lung, and liver allograft recipients.

Reduction in CNI dose can produce sustained improvement in renal function. In one series, a 30% reduction in mean CNI dose in heart transplant recipients was associated with improvement in mean serum creatinine from 2.8 mg/dl (250 μmol/l) to 1.8 mg/dl (160 μmol/l). However, there are no studies showing reduction in the risk of ESRD with CNI dose modification.

Calcium channel blockers are potent vasodilators that may counteract the vasoconstrictive effect of CNI. Their benefit may be limited to the early stages of CNI toxicity when afferent arteriolar vasoconstriction has not resulted in irreversible ischemic injury. Calcium channel blockers have not been evaluated specifically in nonrenal organ transplantation.

Other treatments shown to ameliorate experimental chronic CNI-induced nephrotoxicity include antioxidant nutrients, angiotensin receptor blockers (ARBs), nitric oxide enhancement, melatonin, and pentoxifylline. None of these agents have been prospectively evaluated in the clinical setting of nonrenal organ transplantation, apart from pentoxifylline, which has not shown benefit.

Blood Pressure Control

Aggressive blood pressure control with renin-angiotensin blockade using angiotensin-converting enzyme (ACE) inhibitors and ARBs is key to the treatment of CKD in the nontransplant recipient population and would be expected to have beneficial effects in nonrenal organ transplant recipients, although substantial clinical studies to confirm this in such patients have not been reported.

Renal Replacement Therapy

Management of CKD in organ recipients does not differ substantially from that required for a CKD patient without an allograft. The patient should be assessed for dialysis or renal transplantation in stage 4 CKD or if the patient enters an accelerated phase of decline during stage 3 CKD. Cardiac, liver, and lung transplant recipients with ESRD who subsequently received a living or deceased donor transplant have a 44% to 60% reduction in long-term mortality compared to their dialysis-treated counterparts. In one series, the 6-year survival in liver recipients after the onset of ESRD was 27% if they were on maintenance dialysis compared to 71% if kidney transplantation was performed. Preemptive kidney transplantation is also beneficial in these recipients. Nonrenal organ transplant recipients with ESRD who are treated with maintenance dialysis have an annual mortality rate of 28% to 40% compared to 17% to 20% in dialysis-treated ESRD patients who did not receive a prior nonrenal organ transplant. It is a challenging issue deciding whether a potential cardiac or liver transplantation candidate with advanced renal disease should undergo multiorgan transplantation including a kidney transplantation. This decision should be based on the duration and severity of renal function along with a renal biopsy to assess chronicity of disease. If a percutaneous renal biopsy is not feasible, a transjugular approach may be considered. The decision to recommend a cardiac or liver transplantation candidate for simultaneous renal transplantation should not be based on the severity of renal dysfunction alone.

LIVER TRANSPLANTATION

Renal Disease before Liver Transplantation
Glomerular Disease

Many patients with end-stage liver disease (ESLD) have histologic glomerular abnormalities.[5] HCV infection is associated with cryoglobulinemic membranoproliferative glomerulonephritis (MPGN) (see Chapter 20) and hepatitis B infection (HBV) with membranous nephropathy. Patients with ESLD of any etiology may develop a renal lesion resembling IgA nephropathy (see Chapter 21). A characteristic lesion of ESLD is hepatic glomerulosclerosis, which histologically resembles MPGN with mesangial sclerosis and splitting of the capillary basement membranes, occasionally with IgM and IgA deposition and with subendothelial widening on electron microscopy.[5] Despite the frequency of histologic changes, microscopic hematuria and low-grade proteinuria are observed in <20% of all patients with ESLD and <40% of patients with HCV-associated ESLD.

Acute Renal Failure

Patients with ESLD awaiting orthotopic liver transplantation (OLT) often have renal insufficiency, usually the result of hepatorenal syndrome (HRS) or acute tubular necrosis (ATN). HRS

has been reported in 5% of children and 10% to 15% of adults awaiting OLT. Treatment of HRS is discussed in Chapter 67. Prolonged severe HRS may be lead to ATN or ATN may be precipitated by infection, bleeding, or administration of radiocontrast. Pretransplantation dialysis is required in 10% to 20% of patients with HRS. Hemodialysis and ultrafiltration are often poorly tolerated because of peripheral vasodilatation and shunting caused by ESLD. Intermittent dialysis may also lead to transient increases in intracranial pressure as a result of osmotic shifts and decreased perfusion pressure. This is of greatest concern in patients with fulminant hepatic failure in whom intracranial pressures are often elevated. These patients are best treated with continuous slow dialysis therapies or peritoneal dialysis. In patients with fulminant hepatic failure, intracranial pressure should be monitored, and dialysis should be discontinued if it increases to >30 to 40 mm Hg (normal <10 mm Hg).

Renal Disease after Liver Transplantation
Acute Renal Failure

ARF within 30 days of transplantation is associated with poor preoperative renal function, preoperative HRS, poor liver allograft function, induction with CNIs, use of other nephorotoxic drugs, rhabdomyolysis, sepsis, and reoperation for bleeding. Perioperative ARF is associated with prolonged hospitalization and an increased risk of infection and death. CNI avoidance is usually recommended in those with renal dysfunction or poor hepatic graft function until renal function improves. Fifteen percent of patients with ARF do not recover renal function and require maintenance RRT.[6]

Hemolysis Associated with an ABO-Incompatible Transplant

Hemolysis causing ARF may occur in an A or B blood group liver recipient of an O type (universal donor) organ due to passenger lymphoid tissue that is capable of producing anti-A or anti-B antibodies. Anti-A or anti-B antibodies are usually detected between 10 and 25 days after transplantation but then resolve spontaneously.[7] Treatment of hemolysis consists of plasma exchange, urinary alkalinization, and the use of type O blood for transfusion.

Glomerular Disease

Glomerular disease is common after liver transplantation. The greatest risk is for patients with HCV infection; proteinuria >1 g/day is seen in 5% of HCV-positive and 3% of HCV-negative patients at transplantation, increasing to a maximum of 25% in the HCV-positive and 5% in HCV-negative patients at 2 years[8] (Fig. 99.5). Renal biopsy typically shows MPGN (with or without

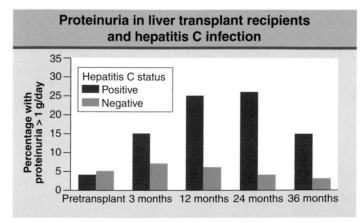

Figure 99.5 Proteinuria in liver transplant recipients and hepatitis C virus infection.

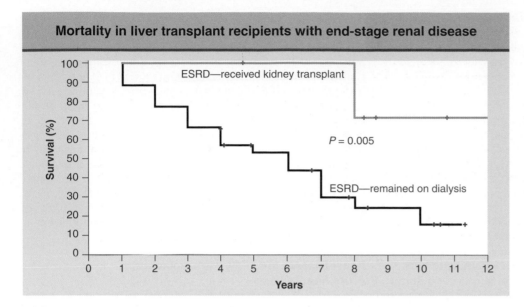

Figure 99.6 Mortality in liver transplant recipients with end-stage renal disease (ESRD). Impact of renal transplantation on mortality for 1602 liver transplant recipients with ESRD. (Adapted from Paramesh AS, Rooyaie S, Doan Y, et al: Post-liver transplant acute renal failure. Factors predicting development of end-stage renal disease. Clin Transplant 2004;18: 94–99.)

cryoglobulinemia) or mesangial proliferative glomerulonephritis. Despite these histologic findings, HCV-positive patients maintain renal function similar to that of HCV-negative recipients in the early years post-transplantation.[8] Florid cryoglobulinemic disease including glomerulonephritis, pulmonary vasculitis, purpura, and arthralgias may respond to interferon with or without ribavirin and plasma exchange. However, the long-term benefits of interferon on renal function and proteinuria are uncertain in the liver recipient, and even after a virologic response, relapse is common. HCV-infected patients are also more likely to develop diabetes post-transplantation (31% versus 7% in HCV-negative patients).[8]

Combined Liver-Kidney Transplantation

A difficult problem is determining whether a patient on dialysis for >2 months after the onset of HRS or ATN has developed permanent renal failure and, therefore, should be offered a concurrent renal transplantation. There is no definitive strategy to manage this situation, although some centers do list such patients for both transplantations and only place the kidney if an intraoperative renal biopsy shows significant glomerulosclerosis or interstitial fibrosis.

End-Stage Renal Disease after Liver Transplantation

Long-term patient survival is decreased in liver recipients developing ESRD.[4] By 13 years after transplantation, survival in those developing ESRD is 28% compared to 55% in controls without renal failure (Fig. 99.6). Mortality is most often due to dialysis access–related sepsis. In addition to sepsis, patients are often plagued with blood pressure instability and are at risk of both hemorrhagic and thrombotic complications. Six-year patient survival after developing ESRD is 27% for patients on dialysis compared to 71% for those who subsequently receive a renal transplant.[2,4] Patients with HCV liver disease do well after kidney transplantation with 71% patient and 61% kidney graft 3-year survival rates.[10]

CARDIAC TRANSPLANTATION

Renal Disease before Cardiac Transplantation

Renal insufficiency frequently accompanies cardiac failure as a result of impairment of renal perfusion and occasionally due to associated primary renal disorders. Cardiac failure causes a decrease in renal plasma flow, with a relative preservation of GFR through an increase in efferent arteriolar pressure, which increases glomerular hydraulic pressure causing an increased filtration fraction. Consequently, the kidneys are unable to augment function during a further insult such as hypotension. The increase in glomerular hydrostatic pressure may be associated with mild proteinuria (generally <500 mg/day), as well as glomerular changes, including mesangiolysis and mesangial proliferation. Progressive cardiac dysfunction eventually leads to decompensation resulting in renal functional impairment and volume overload.

Attempts to improve cardiac output with the use of ACE inhibitors and ARBs may be complicated by worsening renal function or hyperkalemia. Intra-aortic balloon pumps may improve systemic and renal perfusion, but can cause renal failure due to occlusion of the renal arteries, cholesterol embolization, cortical necrosis, excessive exit site bleeding with hypotension, or sepsis. Left ventricular assist devices increase cardiac output and are increasingly used as a bridge to cardiac transplantation; their use has improved renal function at transplantation and decreased the incidence of postoperative ARF, but is associated with increased risks of infection and coagulopathy.[11] Pretransplantation RRT may be required and is ideally accomplished by continuous rather than intermittent modalities.

The most common cause of end-stage heart failure is ischemic heart disease, and in heart transplant recipients with this condition, systemic atherosclerosis involving small and large renal vessels is almost always present before transplantation. In addition, significant, irreversible chronic renal ischemic injury (glomerular collapse) is common in heart transplantation candidates with low-output cardiac failure. Pretransplantation renal histology in cardiac transplantation candidates commonly shows advanced arteriolar hyalinosis and obsolescent glomeruli.

Chronic glomerular hypoxia associated with cyanotic congenital heart disease is associated with secondary FSGS.

Renal Disease after Cardiac Transplantation
Acute Renal Failure

The newly transplanted heart may have temporary right heart failure (because of recipient pulmonary hypertension) leading to acute left heart failure and renal hypoperfusion. ARF following cardiac transplantation is multifactorial including CNI-induced renal vasoconstriction in combination with the effects of anesthesia, pressor support, the bypass procedure, poor graft function, and blood loss (Fig. 99.7). CNI therapy is usually replaced by treatment with antilymphocyte or anti–interleukin-2 receptor antibody, and CNIs are started only after renal function improves.

Chronic Kidney Disease

As well as CNI toxicity, other possible etiologies of CKD include hemodynamic instability secondary to cardiac allograft rejection, toxicity from other medications, thrombotic microangiopathy, sepsis, and possibly renal viral infection. Urinary decoy cells and BK and JCV viral genomes can be found in the urine of long-term heart transplant recipients, although this has not been clearly associated with virus-induced renal failure.[12]

End-Stage Renal Disease after Cardiac Transplantation

Overall, the risk of death in heart transplant recipients with ESRD is double that of patients of comparable age with ESRD without a heart transplant, and the risk of death for patients treated with peritoneal dialysis (PD) is significantly higher than that of patients on hemodialysis (HD; Fig. 99.8).[13] PD in heart transplant recipients is complicated by more frequent peritonitis and PD failure following infection than in nontransplant recipients. The proportion of patients remaining on PD at 24 months after initiation of therapy may be as low as 25%. The increased mortality of PD patients compared to HD is likely related to patient selection for PD based on the presence of cardiac dysfunction.[14] Special management problems for RRT following heart transplantation include difficulty achieving adequate arteriovenous fistulas due to poor peripheral vasculature and difficulty placing renal allografts due to severe aortoiliac arteriopathy. Patients selected for renal transplantation may do well, with 1-year graft survival rates >80%. However, because of additional exposure to immunosuppression, there is increased risk of the development of post-transplantation lymphoproliferative disease and other malignancies.

Combined Heart-Kidney Transplantation

One treatment option for those with intrinsic renal disease is combined heart-kidney transplantation. The dual procedure is usually

Factors contributing to acute renal failure after cardiac transplantation
Acute cardiac allograft rejection with impaired function
Other causes of impaired cardiac allograft function
Vasopressor use
Cardiopulmonary bypass
Contrast nephrotoxicity
Drug nephrotoxicity Calcineurin inhibitors Amphotericin Angiotensin-converting enzyme inhibitors Angiotensin receptor blockers
Hemorrhage
Rhabdomyolysis
Thrombotic microangiopathy
Hemolysis

Figure 99.7 Factors contributing to acute renal failure after cardiac transplantation.

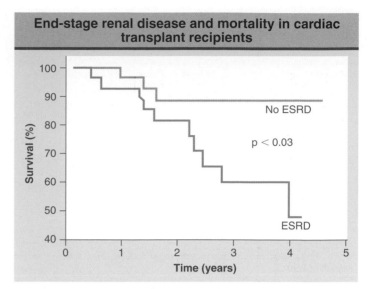

Figure 99.8 End-stage renal disease (ESRD) and mortality in cardiac transplant recipients. Mortality with and without ESRD (N = 1211). (Adapted from Sénéchal M, Dorent R, duMontcel S, et al: End-stage renal failure and cardiac mortality after heart transplantation. Clin Transpl 2004;18:1–6.)

staged and the renal transplant is placed during a second operation to allow for hemodynamic and coagulation stabilization. Renal allograft survival after combined transplantation may approach 90% 2 years after transplantation.[15] Dual transplantation should only be performed in those with fixed, irreversible renal disease and not those with hemodynamic-induced renal failure. Ideally, a renal biopsy would be performed to determine the degree of fixed renal injury prior to a decision for kidney transplantation; however, anticoagulation, which cannot be uninterrupted, often prevents biopsy.

LUNG TRANSPLANTATION

Renal Disease before Lung Transplantation

Lung transplantation candidates with cystic fibrosis are prone to systemic oxalosis, urolithiasis, and medullary nephrocalcinosis; have an increased risk of diabetes; and are at increased risk of post-transplantation renal failure.

Renal disease was once regarded as a relative contraindication to lung transplantation, but it is now recognized that renal blood flow may be markedly impaired in the setting of pulmonary failure and that this may improve after successful lung transplantation.[16]

Renal Disease after Lung Transplantation

CKD in the lung recipient is largely attributed to CNI nephrotoxicity; however, sepsis, other nephrotoxic agent use, and TMA may also contribute. Minimizing CNI toxicity in the lung transplant patient may be more difficult than other allograft recipients due to the high risk of rejection.

KIDNEY DISEASE IN HEMOPOIETIC CELL TRANSPLANT RECIPIENTS

Acute Renal Failure

Both allogeneic and autologous bone marrow transplantation (BMT) as well as stem cell transplantation are associated with increased risk of renal dysfunction. The incidence of ARF after BMT ranges from 30% to 50%. The risk of ARF within 1 month of transplantation is greater for allogeneic BMT (36%) compared to autologous BMT (10% to 12%). Forty percent to 50% of

Risk factors for acute renal failure after bone marrow transplantation
Advanced age
Pretransplantation renal function
Calcineurin inhibitor nephrotoxicity
Tumor lysis syndrome
Veno-occlusive disease
Conditioning chemoradiation
Hemolytic uremic syndrome
Nephrotoxic antibiotics
Sepsis

Figure 99.9   Risk factors for acute renal failure after bone marrow transplantation.

Causes of early onset acute renal failure after bone marrow transplantation
Volume depletion (due to nausea, vomiting, diarrhea) associated with graft-versus-host disease or chemotherapy

Acute tubular necrosis
  Nephrotoxins (including aminoglycosides, amphotericin, ifosfamide, bisphosphonates, carboplatin)
  Sepsis

Interstitial nephritis due to medication
  Penicillins
  Cephalosporins
  Allopurinol

Obstruction
  Fungus ball in collecting system
  Clot from hemorrhagic cystitis

Hepatorenal-like syndrome associated with veno-occlusive disease

Figure 99.10   Causes of early onset acute renal failure after bone marrow transplantation.

patients with ARF after BMT require RRT. The risk factors for ARF are shown in Figure 99.9. The risk of ARF is increased when the conditioning therapy includes fractionated total body irradiation; there is an inverse relationship between the prescribed radiation dose and risk of ARF. Bone marrow transplant recipients with ARF have significantly higher mortality compared to those without ARF. When RRT is required within the first 3 months after transplantation, mortality can be as high as 80%.

Immediate-Onset Renal Failure

Renal failure presenting within 5 days of transplantation is usually caused by tumor lysis syndrome (TLS) or toxicity from the infused marrow. TLS refers to the metabolic derangements that follow release of tumor-derived intracellular constituents, including uric acid, phosphate, and xanthine (which have low urinary solubilities) after cytoreductive therapy. TLS is surprisingly uncommon in bone marrow transplant recipients, in part because of routine preventive measures with allopurinol or recombinant urate oxidase and also because patients undergoing transplantation do not have *de novo* disease but rather have disease in relapse, in which the tumor burden is not as extreme.[17] If TLS does occur, the prognosis for recovery from ARF is excellent. Volume depletion is a major risk factor for the development of TLS; aggressive volume repletion can minimize tubular precipitation of uric acid, phosphate, and xanthine. Urinary alkalinization to maintain the urine pH between 6.5 and 7.5 also increases uric acid solubility.

Cryopreservation is necessary for the storage and maintenance of autologous marrow used for transplantation. Dimethyl sulfoxide (DMSO) is frequently employed as a protectant. During marrow infusion, patients are exposed to toxic products of cell lysis as well as to DMSO. Hemoglobin is noted in the urine of 75% to 100% of patients and is possibly caused by DMSO-induced disruption of red cells in the infusate. Although hemoglobinuria is common, ARF is not because volume loading and bicarbonate diuresis are routinely instituted.

Early-Onset Renal Failure

The most common period for the development of ARF is between 10 and 20 days after BMT. During this period, the complications of radiochemotherapy are most likely to manifest; these include pancytopenia, sepsis, pneumonitis, mucositis, and gastrointestinal and hepatic toxicity. Although the differential diagnosis is wide (Fig. 99.10), the large majority of patients with ARF early after

BMT develop a clinical disorder that is reminiscent of HRS, and is preceded in 90% of patients by veno-occlusive disease (VOD) of the liver. VOD is thought to result from hepatic venule endothelial cell injury, induced by radiochemotherapy, leading to thrombosis, fibrin deposition, and sinusoidal and portal hypertension.[18] Liver biopsy is seldom performed due to thrombocytopenia and coagulopathy, so the diagnosis is most often made on clinical grounds. VOD has been reported in up to 50% of bone marrow transplant recipients. The incidence is increasing, possibly as a result of more aggressive cytoreductive regimens. Approximately 25% to 30% of reported cases of VOD are severe, and mortality in these patients has been >90% despite treatment. Although hepatic endothelial injury plays a central role, a superimposed clinical event is usually necessary to trigger renal failure. Sepsis is the most frequent event, and fungemia is common. Histologic findings at autopsy have not shown structural changes to explain the ARF, lending further support to the assertion that this is a problem of renal hemodynamic disturbance. Management of VOD-associated ARF is for the most part supportive (Fig. 99.11). Prophylaxis against fungal infection is usually given with fluconazole (400 mg/day). Liposomal

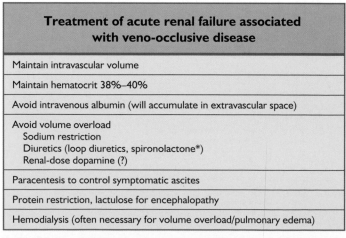

Treatment of acute renal failure associated with veno-occlusive disease
Maintain intravascular volume
Maintain hematocrit 38%–40%
Avoid intravenous albumin (will accumulate in extravascular space)

Avoid volume overload
  Sodium restriction
  Diuretics (loop diuretics, spironolactone*)
  Renal-dose dopamine (?)

Paracentesis to control symptomatic ascites
Protein restriction, lactulose for encephalopathy
Hemodialysis (often necessary for volume overload/pulmonary edema)

Figure 99. 11   Treatment of acute renal failure associated with veno-occlusive disease. *Use spironolactone with care to avoid hyperkalemia.

amphotericin is as effective as conventional amphotericin for proven antifungal therapy, but may be less nephrotoxic and has fewer infusion-related reactions.

Ursodeoxycholic acid has been shown in a controlled trial to prevent VOD in allogeneic BMT recipients, and is used routinely at some centers.[19] Low-dose heparin (100 U/kg) has also shown promise in some, but not all, studies. No therapy for established VOD has been shown to be effective in a controlled study.

Chronic Kidney Disease
Calcineurin Inhibitor Toxicity

Renal disease occurring >1 month after BMT is often the result of CNI use to prevent graft-versus-host-disease (GVHD). Cyclosporine or tacrolimus is usually used in combination with prednisone, methotrexate, or MMF to prevent GVHD, which if severe has a mortality of 50%. CKD in this setting correlates with trough serum CNI levels. In patients without GVHD, CNIs are used only for a short time and chronic CNI toxicity is not seen. As more unrelated grafts are used, it is likely that chronic GVHD will be seen more often, and chronic CNI toxicity may become more common. Rarely, patients with GVHD present with the nephrotic syndrome due to membranous nephropathy.[20]

Bone Marrow Transplant Thrombotic Microangiopathy

The syndrome of delayed chronic renal insufficiency, anemia, and hypertension not attributable to CNI use is thought to be a form of radiation nephropathy. This syndrome is observed in 10% to 25% of bone marrow transplant recipients and presents 6 to 12 months after BMT. Histologic features are suggestive of TMA[21] (Fig. 99.12). In mild cases, the hemolytic anemia and thrombocytopenia may be minimal or absent. There is a more severe acute presentation with hypertension, proteinuria, hematuria, red blood cell casts, and rapidly progressive renal failure, with microangiopathic hemolytic anemia. Central nervous system abnormalities may also occur.

Current evidence suggests that BMT TMA is primarily a consequence of total body irradiation and resultant endothelial cell damage. Although CNIs given to prevent GVHD may contribute, TMA has been described in patients who have not received these agents. The conditioning regimen for BMT usually includes 8 to 14 Gy of radiation, a dose comparable to that given to patients who develop radiation nephropathy.[21]

The histologic features and clinical presentation of BMT-associated TMA show a striking similarity to acute radiation nephropathy.[21] The histopathology reveals enlarged hypocellular glomeruli with mesangiolysis (see Fig. 99.12). There is accumulation of spongiform material along the inner aspect of the glomerular basement membrane that extends into the glomerular capillary

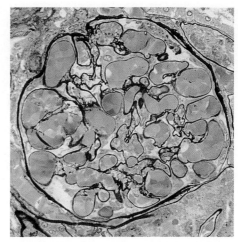

Figure 99.12 Thrombotic microangiopathy. Mesangiolysis in a patient with thrombotic microangiopathy associated with bone marrow transplantation.

loops, producing a double-contour appearance. There is marked narrowing of the arteriolar lumen caused by mucoid intimal thickening.

Once TMA is established, treatment is supportive and includes aggressive treatment of hypertension as well as RRT. ACE inhibitors have been shown in animal models of BMT nephropathy to prevent and treat the syndrome and therefore may be preferable to other agents, but definitive proof in humans is lacking. Plasma exchange is not of proven benefit. Although it is unlikely that CNI use alone is responsible for causing BMT-associated TMA, attempts at CNI dose reduction seem reasonable, but discontinuation is inappropriate given the risks of GVHD. The natural history of patients with BMT-associated TMA is variable. Symptoms may be mild and resolve on their own without specific treatment; others will progress to ESRD.

End-Stage Renal Disease

ESRD develops in up to 10% of bone marrow transplant recipients. The prognosis of ESRD after BMT is very poor. When there is concomitant GVHD, HD sessions are often attended by turbulent episodes of hemodynamic instability. PD is often ineffective because of poor peritoneal circulation associated with GVHD. One-year mortality rate as high as 75% has been reported in bone marrow transplant recipients receiving maintenance dialysis, with infection the leading cause of death. Success of renal transplantation from the bone marrow transplant donor is excellent and requiring no immunosuppression.[22] Cadaveric or non–bone marrow donor renal transplantation requires immunosuppression. Furthermore, bone marrow transplant recipients may be more sensitive to cytotoxic agents and careful monitoring is necessary.

REFERENCES

1. Ojo AO, Held PJ, Port FK, et al: Chronic renal failure after transplantation of a nonrenal organ. N Engl J Med 2003;349:931–940.
2. Coopersmith CM, Brennan DC, Miller B, et al: Renal transplantation following previous heart, liver, and lung transplantation: An 8-year single-center experience. Surgery 2001;130:457–462.
3. Pillebout E, Nochy D, Hill G, et al: Renal histopathological lesions after orthotopic liver transplantation (OLT). Am J Transplant 2005;5:1120–1129.
4. Gonwa TA, Mai ML, Melton LB, et al: End-stage renal disease (ESRD) after orthotopic liver transplantation (OLTX) using calcineurin-based immunotherapy. Risk of development and treatment. Transplantation 2001;72:1934–1939.
5. Crawford DH, Endre ZH, Axelsen RA, et al: Universal occurrence of glomerular abnormalities in patients receiving liver transplants. Am J Kidney Dis 1992;19:339–344.
6. Paramesh AS, Rooyaie S, Doan Y, et al: Post-liver transplant acute renal failure. Factors predicting development of end-stage renal disease. Clin Transpl 2004;18:94–99.
7. Triulzi DJ, Shirey RS, Ness PM, Klein AS: Immunohematologic complications of ABO-unmatched liver transplants. Transfusion 1992;32:829–833.
8. Kendrick EA, McVicar JP, Kowdley KV, et al: Renal disease in hepatitis C-positive liver transplant recipients. Transplantation 1997;63:1287–1293.

9. Fraley DS, Burr R, Bernardini J, et al: Impact of acute renal failure on mortality in end-stage liver disease with or without transplantation. Kidney Int 1998;54:518–524.

10. Molmenti EP, Jain AB, Shapiro R, et al: Kidney transplantation for end-stage renal failure in liver transplant recipients with hepatitis C viral infection. Transplantation 2001;71:267–271.

11. Bank AJ, Mir SH, Nguyen DQ, et al: Effects of left ventricular assist devices on outcomes in patients undergoing heart transplantation. Ann Thorac Surg 2000;69:1369–1375.

12. Etienne I, Francois A, Redonnet M, et al: Does polyomavirus infection induce renal failure in cardiac transplant recipients? Transplant Proc 2000;32:2794–2795.

13. Sénéchal M, Dorent R, duMontcel S, et al: End-stage renal failure and cardiac mortality after heart transplantation. Clin Transpl 2004;18:1–6.

14. Jayasena SD, Riaz A, Lewis CM, et al: Outcome in patients with end-stage renal disease following heart or heart-lung transplantation receiving peritoneal dialysis. Nephrol Dial Transplant 2001;16:1681–1685.

15. Blanche C, Kamlot A, Blanche DA, et al: Combined heart-kidney transplantation with single-donor allografts. J Thorac Cardiovasc Surg 2001;122:495–500.

16. Navis G, Broekroelofs J, Mannes GP, et al: Renal hemodynamics after lung transplantation. A prospective study. Transplantation 1996;61:1600–1605.

17. Zager RA: Acute renal failure in the setting of bone marrow transplantation. Kidney Int 1994;46:1443–1458.

18. McDonald GB, Hinds MS, Fisher LD, et al: Veno-occlusive disease of the liver and multiorgan failure after bone marrow transplantation: a cohort study of 355 patients. Ann Intern Med 1993;118:255–267.

19. Essell JH, Schroeder MT, Harman GS, et al: Ursodiol prophylaxis against hepatic complications of allogeneic bone marrow transplantation. A randomized, double-blind, placebo-controlled trial. Ann Intern Med 1998;128:975–981.

20. Lin J, Markowitz GS, Nicolaides M, et al: Membranous glomerulopathy associated with graft-versus-host disease following allogeneic stem cell transplantation. Report of 2 cases and review of the literature. Am J Nephrol 2001;21:351–356.

21. Cohen EP: Radiation nephropathy after bone marrow transplantation. Kidney Int 2000;58:903–918.

22. Butcher JA, Hariharan S, Adams MB, et al: Renal transplantation for end-stage renal disease following bone marrow transplantation: A report of six cases, with and without immunosuppression. Clin Transpl 1999;13:330–335.

CHAPTER
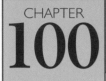
100   Poisoning and Drug Overdose

Haresh Dodeja and John Feehally

POISONING THROUGH DELIBERATE AND ACCIDENTAL SELF-HARM

Poisoning may be iatrogenic through failure to appreciate the principles and practice of prescribing described in Chapter 101. Poisoning may also be caused by deliberate self-harm (attempted suicide), accidental self-harm (most commonly in children), or deliberate harm (homicide or war). It may also be caused by environmental exposure (industrial poisons or poisonous wildlife). Usually the event is acute and the presentation to hospital early, although chronic poisoning may also occur.

The nephrologist is involved in the clinical care of poisoning for several reasons:

- Iatrogenic drug nephrotoxicity may require active management.
- Acute renal failure (ARF) is a common consequence of many poisonings.
- The metabolic consequences of poisoning may require intervention.
- Many agents are excreted via the kidney, and drug removal may occasionally require promotion at controlled urinary pH.
- Drug removal using extracorporeal techniques, usually by hemodialysis or hemoperfusion may be valuable.

Epidemiology of Poisoning

In the developed world, deliberate self-harm is a common cause for emergency admission: about 1% of all hospital admissions. Admissions for poisoning steadily increased until the 1970s; since that time, there has been a gradual decline. Deliberate self-harm has a peak incidence around 25 years of age and is more common in women; the majority of these incidents are not serious suicide intents.

In serious cases of poisoning, the individual dies before admission; this particularly includes carbon monoxide (car exhaust) poisoning, which is the most common cause of death by suicide in males age 15 to 44 years. After admission, 50% are discharged from the emergency department, and in-hospital mortality from poisoning is extremely low. Only 4% of all cases of self-poisoning require hospital admission, and among these, mortality is only 1% to 2%.

One factor in the decreasing mortality is the changing pattern of drugs involved. Until the 1970s, barbiturates and other lipid-soluble sedatives such as glutethimide and meprobamate were widely available and frequently produced severe clinical effects in overdose. They were subsequently replaced by safer hypnotic agents such as benzodiazepines.[1] Mortality from acute sedative overdose was 45% in 1945, had decreased to 1% by the mid-1960s and was no more than 0.2% by the late 1990s. Paraquat has also been taken less commonly in overdose as other safer herbicides have come into horticultural and agricultural use. Among common drug poisonings, few require extracorporeal drug removal (Fig. 100.1).

Approximately 75% of accidental self-harm occurs in children younger than 4 years of age; this is decreasing in frequency. Only 15% have symptoms of poisoning, and deaths are rare. The majority results from exposure to household commodities including alcohol and domestic cleansing agents, as well as pharmaceutical preparations.

In the developing world, patterns of poisoning are very different and include animal, plant, and chemical poisons. Of the 2000 species of snakes worldwide, about 400 are poisonous.[2] ARF occurs with 5% to 25% of all snake bites. The most common are viper bites, which cause extensive bleeding, followed by disseminated intravascular coagulation (DIC), hypotension, and ARF. Sea snake bites cause rhabdomyolysis and ARF. Early administration of antivenom (available as monovalent or polyvalent serum) is vital given as a bolus dose followed by a maintenance infusion. Whole blood clotting time can be used to monitor the response to treatment. Bee, wasp, and hornet stings can occasionally cause hemolysis and rhabdomyolysis, leading to acute tubular necrosis (ATN),[3] while spider venoms are the most potent, causing DIC and ARF. Plant poisons include mushrooms of the genera *Amanita*, *Galerina*, and *Cortinorius*, which cause gastrointestinal symptoms, followed by hypotension and ARF. The nephrotoxic constituent is amatoxin cyclopeptide, and this poisoning has a 50% mortality.[4] Djenkol beans grown in Southeast Asia are considered a delicacy and consumed raw. In large quantities, they cause nonglomerular hematuria, renal pain, and hypotension leading to ATN. Poisoning can be prevented by cooking the beans and by liberal fluid intake.[5] Ingestion of raw carp bile is known to impair visual acuity and induce hepatitis, hypotension, and ATN.[6]

Deliberate or accidental ingestion of chemicals, such as copper sulfate used in the leather industry, is known to cause hemolysis and ATN, while paraquat, widely used as a pesticide in Southeast Asia is a known nephrotoxin that causes ATN. Treatment involves forced diuresis, with occasional need for hemodialysis and hemofiltration. Glue sniffing is another form of chemical poisoning; toluene is the poison involved that causes ATN and hepatorenal syndrome and, with long-term exposure, may lead to renal tubular acidosis, proteinuria, and renal calculi.[7]

There are very large numbers of poisons for which detailed information must be readily available to influence immediate management. This information is beyond the scope of this chapter. There are published reference texts that are frequently updated.[8] Poison information centers are freely accessible by telephone or the Internet for urgent advice. For example, in the United Kingdom, there are six regional poisons information centers (www.doh.gov.uk/npis.htm); in the United States, there are state

Pattern of poisoning in accidental and deliberate self-harm		
Drug/Class	Specific Antidote Available	Extracorporeal Drug Removal May Be Indicated
Acetaminophen (paracetamol)	N-acetylcysteine	No
Benzodiazepines	Flumezanil	No
Antidepressants (most commonly amitriptyline)	No	No
Street drugs (including opioids and stimulants)	Naloxone	No
Other analgesics including opioids and NSAIDs	Naloxone	No
Aspirin	No	Yes
Anticonvulsants	No	Yes
Household compounds	No	No
Theophylline	No	Yes
Lithium	No	Yes

Figure 100.1   Pattern of poisoning in accidental and deliberate self-harm. The most common categories of drugs taken in deliberate and accidental self-harm listed in descending order of frequency. NSAIDs, nonsteroidal anti-inflammatory drugs. (Adapted from data reported by National Poisons Information Service, United Kingdom [www.doh.gov.uk/npis.htm] and the American Association of Poison Control Centers [www.aapcc.org]).

centers within the American Association of Poison Control Centers (www.aapcc.org), which publishes data annually.[9]

MANAGEMENT OF POISONING

General Management
The diagnosis of poisoning is not always straightforward since the patient may deny intoxication or may be comatose or otherwise unable to give the necessary information. Poisoning may present as unexplained coma, unexplained ARF, or a metabolic disorder. High-anion-gap metabolic acidosis is a characteristic presentation of several poisonings including ethylene glycol and methanol, while salicylate poisoning may present with a mixed acid-base disorder.

The primary aim of the management of poisoning is not to retrieve the poison but to save a life. The mainstay of treatment for most poisonings is supportive care while spontaneous excretion or metabolism of the drug occurs. It may include correction of fluid, electrolyte, and acid-base derangements, cardiovascular support, and respiratory support, including artificial ventilation.

Acute Renal Failure in Poisoning
ARF may develop in poisoning (Fig. 100.2) as a result of circulatory collapse or the hepatorenal syndrome when there is severe hepatic toxicity. Rhabdomyolysis may result from prolonged coma or seizures. In addition, a range of poisons are directly nephrotoxic. ATN may be caused by direct toxicity or myoglobinuria,

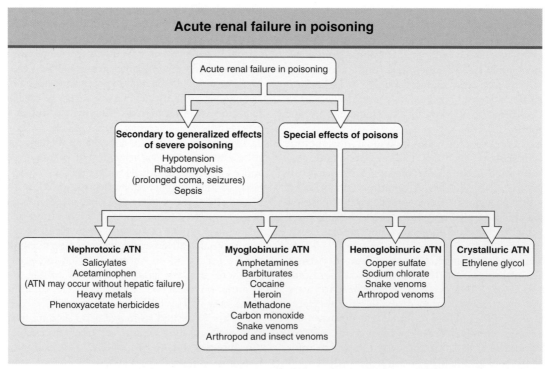

Figure 100.2   Acute renal failure in poisoning. ATN, acute tubular necrosis.

hemoglobinuria, or crystalluria.[10] Acetone, taken itself or derived from metabolism of isopropyl alcohol ingestion, interferes with colorimetric assays for creatinine and may produce false elevations of serum creatinine with normal blood urea nitrogen levels.

Specific Antidotes

In a small minority of poisonings, a specific antidote is available (Fig. 100.3) that may prevent life-threatening consequences. Antidotes are valuable when toxicity develops too rapidly and irreversibly to wait for spontaneous excretion or to introduce techniques that accelerate drug removal.[11] Most commonly this is because the poison or a metabolite fixes in tissues and does not remain in the plasma to be accessible for removal.

Prevention of Drug Absorption

Absorption is usually gastrointestinal after oral intoxication, but other routes to consider are intravenous injection, through the skin, or by inhalation.

Gastric Lavage

Gastric lavage (via an orogastric tube) is a long-established treatment to remove a drug from the stomach before it is absorbed. However, recent evidence indicates it is relatively ineffective at removing solid tablet accretions and may actually promote absorption by propelling some gastric contents into the duodenum. It no longer has a place in routine management[12] but is of value when the patient presents within 1 hour of overdosing or when the drug taken slows gastric emptying (e.g., aspirin or tricyclic antidepressants).

Emesis by syrup of ipecacuanha no longer has a role in the management of poisoning.[12] It has been shown to be no more efficient than lavage or activated charcoal, leaving significant gastric solids behind and carrying important side effects: up to 15% of those treated will have vomiting and drowsiness, which may be confused with the toxicity of the poisoning agent; aspiration pneumonitis may also occur. It may reduce the effectiveness of activated charcoal, oral antidotes, and whole bowel irrigation.

Activated Charcoal

Activated charcoal (50 g orally) is now the mainstay of immediate treatment for most poisoning in the emergency department.[12] The charcoal is activated by exposure to gas or chemicals, which increases the internal pore structure, expanding the surface area available for adsorption. It is sometimes given with a laxative (often sorbitol) to speed elimination of the poison, but this is not of proven benefit. Multiple doses of activated charcoal for up to 72 hours may continue to reduce absorption[13] since it decreases absorption of any residual drug in the gut (particularly relevant for slow-release formulations and drugs that delay gastric emptying). Activated charcoal also adsorbs drug secreted in the bile, interrupting intestinal reabsorption, and adsorbs any drug permeating from the circulation into the gut, thus blocking enteroenteric circulation. However, based on recent experimental and clinical studies, multiple-dose activated charcoal should be considered only if a patient has ingested a life-threatening amount of carbamazepine, dapsone, phenobarbitone, quinine, or theophylline.

Whole Bowel Irrigation

Whole bowel irrigation should be considered for poisons that are not absorbed by charcoal (e.g., iron, lithium), for sustained-release preparations where absorption of a poison into the circulation may be long lasting (e.g., theophylline, verapamil), or for toxins that may form pharmacobexaors (e.g., salicylates). The patient takes large volumes (15 to 25 ml/kg/hr) orally or by nasogastric tube of an iso-osmolar solution of polyethylene glycol, which is not absorbed. An antiemetic may be needed. The endpoint is to have a clear rectal effluent, which usually occurs after 4 to 5 liters of fluid (2 to 4 hours). It is contraindicated in patients with bowel obstruction, ileus, or perforation.[14]

TOXICOKINETICS

The great majority of poisonings require no specific removal strategies. Once absorption has been minimized, supportive treatment is given while spontaneous metabolism or excretion takes place.

However, it is necessary to be aware of factors affecting drug removal since these will influence the decision to employ additional drug removal techniques in the small minority of patients in which they are valuable. Normal pharmacokinetics for any drug do not necessarily apply in overdose. Toxicokinetics may differ since the poison may damage an organ that contains the major route of elimination or the usual routes of excretion and metabolism may be saturable. Alternatively, in chronic overdose, clearance may be increased by enzyme induction (e.g., carbamazepine), so extracorporeal removal will not have the same value for the drug as in acute overdose. Several toxicokinetics factors must be considered, as follows.

Time since Overdose

Accidental poisoning will usually present immediately. Deliberate poisoning (suicide or homicide) may present hours or days later, so irreversible organ damage may have occurred; although it may still be possible to remove toxin from blood and tissues, it may be futile, having no impact on outcome.

Toxic and Lethal Doses

Toxic and lethal doses are defined from previous case reports, but toxic and lethal plasma concentrations correlate better with clinical evidence of severity. The precise dose taken is often not known and will be influenced by subsequent vomiting and gastric lavage. Gastrointestinal absorption is usually rapid but may be

Antidotes of proven value in common causes of poisoning	
Poison	Antidote
Acetaminophen	N-acetylcysteine, methionine
Benzodiazepines	Flumazenil
Carbon monoxide	Oxygen
Coumadin (warfarin)	Vitamin K
Cyanide	Amyl nitrite, sodium nitrite, sodium thiosulfate, dicobalt edetate
Digoxin	Digoxin-specific Fab antibodies
Ethylene glycol	Fomepizole, ethanol
Iron salts	Desferoxamine
Methanol	Ethanol
Methemoglobinemia	Methylene blue
Opioids	Naloxone
Organophosphate insecticides	Atropine, pralidoxime

Figure 100.3   Antidotes of proven value in common causes of poisoning.

prolonged (e.g., by anticholinergics); the efficacy of drug removal depends on the availability of drug in the plasma in the period between absorption and redistribution.

Plasma Protein Binding

Protein binding limits drug removal by hemodialysis and hemofiltration, but not by hemoperfusion or plasma exchange. Protein binding is reversible, allowing distribution of drug into other compartments. Protein binding may be saturated in severe poisoning with the result that more drug than expected is available for clearance; rapid removal of unbound drug will also liberate further bound drug, making it accessible to removal.

Ionization

Nonionized (lipid-soluble) drugs redistribute easily through cell membranes; ionized drugs can only redistribute slowly through membrane pores. Ionized drugs are, therefore, more susceptible to extracorporeal removal. Many drugs are weak acids and bases, and their degree of ionization *in vivo* is predicted by the pK_a; for example, the weak acid diazepam ($pK_a = 3.3$) is mostly nonionized in the circulation; as a result, it is rapidly redistributed and is a poor candidate for extracorporeal removal.

Volume of Distribution and Redistribution

Volume of distribution (V_D) is an imaginary space for drug distribution measured in volume per body weight units (l/kg). It is not a single space: absorbed drug moves rapidly from the blood compartment (8% of total volume) to a central compartment comprising the major organs (heart, lungs, kidneys, and liver) (7%), then slowly to the peripheral compartment comprising muscle, adipose tissue, skin, and bone (75%). At equilibration, 70% of a drug will usually be in the peripheral compartment. This pattern may vary if a toxin becomes concentrated in a specific tissue, for example, carbon monoxide in hemoglobin or paraquat in the lung. Toxins may also become concentrated in a nontoxic site. For example, lead is stored in bone where it is nontoxic, but it is toxic in soft tissues.

A large V_D will reduce clearance efficacy, for example, amitriptyline, which has a volume of distribution of 20 l/kg. Extracorporeal removal will be efficient if the V_D is <0.5 l/kg (e.g., alcohols, lithium, salicylate, theophylline) and if rapid removal from central and peripheral compartments will allow redistribution into the empty plasma compartment. Extracorporeal removal may be too rapid, removing toxin faster than it can be redistributed from the peripheral space; as a result, it may be more effective to discontinue removal and restart later (e.g., for lithium). This additional deferred treatment will have no value if the initial distribution has produced irreversible target organ damage.

Saturation of Metabolic Pathways

Excretory and metabolic pathways may be saturated in overdose, which delays the proportional excretion rates.

IMPLEMENTATION OF DRUG-REMOVAL TECHNIQUES

In making a decision to use drug-removal techniques, measurements of plasma drug levels must be interpreted with the toxicokinetic factors described in the context of clinical signs and symptoms of severity.

Early Signs

Nausea and vomiting, fatigue, and grade I/II coma are not usually indications for extracorporeal treatment unless the toxin is known to have a silent period.

Late Signs

Grade III/IV coma, cardiorespiratory failure, and hyper- and hypothermia may be indications for extracorporeal treatment.

Irreversible Late Signs

Some signs and symptoms indicate irreversible damage. Extracorporeal measures are usually useless in late organ injury when tissue damage is irreversible, for example, hepatic failure caused by acetaminophen or the *Amanita phalloides* mushroom.

DRUG REMOVAL BY DIURESIS

Although the majority of drugs and poisons are renally excreted, enhanced diuresis only occasionally makes a worthwhile contribution to accelerated drug removal.

Forced Diuresis

The provocation of a large increase in urine volumes was widely used in the past. The aim was to reduce the tubular concentration of freely filtered intact drug by increasing urine flow rate, thus reducing passive reabsorption by minimizing the increasing concentration gradient that would otherwise develop in the distal tubule. Maintaining fluid balance required vigilance, and, particularly in the elderly, pulmonary edema caused by fluid overload, hypotension caused by volume depletion, and electrolyte disturbance were not uncommon. Forced diuresis now has no place in the management of poisoning.

Diuresis at Controlled pH

In some poisonings, alteration of urine pH will substantially alter the rate of excretion. Nonionized drugs are lipid soluble and will diffuse through cell membranes relatively easily, promoting passive reabsorption of filtered drug. By contrast, drug in the ionized state is very poorly reabsorbed. For weak acids and alkalis, pK_a dictates that the proportion of ionized to nonionized drug can be significantly increased within the range of urine pH.

In common practice, alkaline diuresis only applies to salicylate, phenobarbitone, and phenoxyacetate herbicides. Salicylate is a weak acid ($pK_a = 3.5$), and its urine excretion is significantly enhanced in alkaline urine (pH 8.0). Alkaline diuresis is achieved by administering isotonic sodium bicarbonate, with careful monitoring of serum potassium to avoid hypokalemia, aiming for a urine pH target of 7.5 to 8.5. Maintaining an alkaline urine will also minimize tubular toxicity induced by myoglobinuria in poisonings associated with rhabdomyolysis.

Amphetamine is a weak alkali ($pK_a = 9.8$) and its excretion is significantly enhanced in acid urine (pH 5.0). Urine can be acidified by administration of ammonium chloride, but this approach is not used regularly since amphetamine may also cause rhabdomyolysis, and maintaining a low urinary pH will increase the risk of myoglobinuric ATN.

REMOVAL OF POISONS BY EXTRACORPOREAL TREATMENT

The original description of hemodialysis by Abel and colleagues[15] in 1913 was an attempt to remove salicylate, and this was next described in the 1960s. Over the next 30 years, increasing

Indications for extracorporeal detoxification
Ingestion of a dose that will cause serious toxicity or death, for which supportive care is ineffective
Extracorporeal treatment known to eliminate significant amounts of drugs (It is generally accepted that extracorporeal elimination is worthwhile if it increases total body clearance by 30%)
Clinical evidence of severe toxicity Grade IV coma Hypotension Hypothermia Respiratory depression
Impaired clearance of the toxic compound Excretory/metabolic pathways saturated Genetic defect in metabolism Coincidental hepatic or renal dysfunction (pre-existing or acute)
Undue susceptibility because of concurrent disease states or age (very young and elderly)

Figure 100.4   Indications for extracorporeal detoxification.

numbers of drugs were reported that could be removed by extracorporeal techniques. Since many poisons have small molecular size, they are accessible to removal from the plasma by hemodialysis or hemofiltration.[16] Many can also be removed by hemoperfusion in which the poison is adsorbed to activated charcoal in an extracorporeal circuit.[16]

However, nephrologists have become less involved since the 1980s in the management of poisoning as the indications for extracorporeal drug removal have become fewer. Even for those relatively frequently encountered poisons in which it is effective, there is often no demonstrable advantage over simple supportive treatment measures combined with oral activated charcoal. Extracorporeal treatment was only used in two per 1000 of all poisonings registered by the American Association of Poisons Control Centers in the 1990s.[9] Even among those poisonings requiring admission to an intensive care unit, only 1% require extracorporeal drug removal.

No extracorporeal detoxification treatments have been the subject of prospective, randomized, controlled trials to test the hypothesis that they reduce morbidity and mortality. Retrospective studies have sometimes shown worse outcome in the treated groups, which is usually attributed to the selection of more severely poisoned patients.[17] The small number of appropriate cases means that prospective, randomized trials may never be performed.

Extracorporeal detoxification is indicated only if it will provide a significant addition to removal by biotransformation, renal excretion, or pulmonary excretion (Fig. 100.4). If extracorporeal treatment is indicated, it should be started as soon as possible, provided there is sufficient cardiovascular stability. There is no absolute contraindication to extracorporeal treatment; the usual restriction is circulatory insufficiency in the severely ill patient.

Techniques of Extracorporeal Drug Removal
Hemodialysis
Small molecules that are free in the plasma (i.e. not protein bound) will be removed using hemodialysis by diffusion down a concentration gradient from plasma into dialysate. Toxins of molecular mass up to 2000 d can pass unhindered through all dialysis membranes; the cut off for high-flux membranes is above 10,000 d. Clearance is determined by both the blood flow rate and also ultrafiltration rate.

Removal efficacy by hemodialysis depends on the volume of distribution of the drug and the rate of equilibration between peripheral tissues and the plasma once removal has been started. There is no time limit to the dialysis treatment; efficiency does not lessen since fresh dialysate is continually presented and the membrane permeability is not affected. Hemodialysis may be combined with other strategies, for example, with induction of alcohol dehydrogenase by ethanol or fomepizole for the treatment of ethylene glycol or methanol poisoning.[18] Hemodialysis is ineffective when poisons are lipid soluble or significantly protein bound.

Hemodialysis is also indicated as a supportive therapy when ARF complicates poisoning and as adjunctive therapy for the complications of poisoning, including electrolyte disturbance, acidosis, hyper- and hypothermia, pulmonary edema, and volume overload.

Peritoneal dialysis is inefficient compared with hemodialysis, achieving low mass transfer of solute relatively slowly. It should be used in poisoning only when hemodialysis is not rapidly available or is contraindicated.

Hemofiltration
Hemofiltration (see Chapter 83) generates convective transport of solute through the membrane and allows high flux up to a molecular mass of 40,000 d. Since most poisons have molecular weights of <1000 d, hemofiltration usually offers no particular advantages over hemodialysis but is occasionally needed for larger substances, for example, metal chelating complexes such as desferoxamine and sodium ethylenediamine tetraacetic acid (EDTA), and aminoglycosides.

Hemoperfusion
In hemoperfusion, blood comes into direct contact with a sorbent system by passage in the extracorporeal circuit through an adsorbent cartridge (Fig. 100.5). The first usable cartridge containing charcoal was introduced in 1954. Early use was complicated particularly by platelet depletion, which was overcome by microencapsulation of the charcoal with a polymer such as cellulose nitrate, rendering the surface biocompatible. Currently available devices use activated charcoal that adsorbs uncharged toxin molecules to carbon by van der Waals interactions. The rate-limiting step for coated carbon is diffusion through the polymer membrane. Nonionic polystyrene exchange resins are also available. Amberlite may be superior to charcoal for lipophilic molecules.

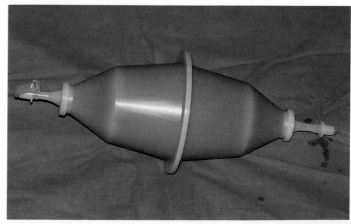

Figure 100.5   A charcoal hemoperfusion cartridge.

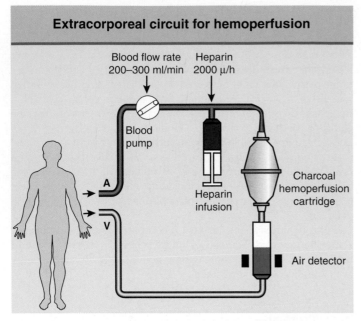

Extracorporeal circuit for hemoperfusion

Blood flow rate 200–300 ml/min

Heparin 2000 μ/h

Blood pump

A

Heparin infusion

Charcoal hemoperfusion cartridge

V

Air detector

Figure 100.6 Extracorporeal circuit for hemoperfusion.

The extracorporeal circuit for hemoperfusion is shown in Figure 100.6. Hemoperfusion requires careful monitoring for, and treatment of, potential complications. The main complications are

- Mild thrombocytopenia caused by adsorption: the platelet counts usually decrease by <30%; if the decrease is >30% or initial thrombocytopenia existed, prostacyclin treatment should be considered
- Mild leukopenia resulting from margination owing to complement activation on surface contact
- Low fibrinogen (and other coagulation factors) caused by adsorption
- Hypothermia
- Hypocalcemia
- Hypoglycemia

The crucial difference from hemodialysis is that hemoperfusion is time limited. After 4 to 8 hours, the capacity of the adsorbents is exhausted because of clotting and adherence of cellular debris and plasma proteins on the adsorbent. Heparin itself is adsorbed, and clotting of the cartridge is not uncommon. The heparin infusion rate should be at least 2000 U/hr at a blood flow rate of 200 to 300 ml/min.

At one time hemoperfusion was heralded as the universal antidote. But it does not remove ionized or protein-bound toxins, and although it removes many poisons, it does not offer superior clearance to hemodialysis in the great majority of circumstances. The use of hemoperfusion is now steadily declining. Although hemoperfusion can remove many poisons, in the majority of cases it has no advantage over hemodialysis, which in turn is used less and less as simpler measures are proving to be equally effective.

Hemodialysis-Hemoperfusion

Although expensive, the concurrent use of hemodialysis and hemoperfusion is theoretically the treatment of first choice since it offers a very effective combination of removal by adsorption and diffusion.[19] The perfusion cartridge is placed upstream of the dialyzer. This system is very efficient for toxins with a small volume of distribution, achieving total removal in 4 to 6 hours. For larger volumes of distribution (1 to 3 l/kg), it is slower and >10 hours of treatment may be needed, with further treatment later when the toxin becomes redistributed into the plasma. There have been few systematic reports of combined hemodialysis-hemoperfusion, but its effective use is described for theophylline[20,21] and *Amanita phalloides* mushroom poisoning.[22]

Exchange Transfusion

Exchange transfusion has a role for poisoning complicated by massive hemolysis, for example, sodium chlorate or arsine, since it will remove not only the poison but also red cell fragments and free hemoglobin. Exchange transfusion is also indicated when poisoning with hydrogen sulfide is complicated by methemoglobinemia and sulfhemoglobinemia.

Extracorporeal Liver Support

Newer techniques developed to maintain patients with acute hepatic failure are designed to remove both water-soluble and protein-bound toxins. They should therefore also be effective at removing most poisons that remain in the circulation. Fifty-five percent of all patients referred to specialized centers with acute hepatic failure develop renal failure due to hepatorenal syndrome or drug toxicity, of which the most common is intoxication due to acetaminophen and mushroom (*Amanita*) poisoning.

There are two available systems, both combining removal of water soluble and albumin-bound toxins. In the Molecular Adsorbents Recirculating System (Fig. 100.7a), an albumin-impermeable high-flux membrane is impregnated with human albumin and the dialysate enriched with albumin to facilitate removal of albumin-bound toxins from the blood, a process relying on dissociation of the toxins from the albumin and their diffusion through the membrane. The albumin is regenerated by passage through activated charcoal and an anion exchanger. In fractionated plasma separation (see Fig. 100.7b), the blood passes through an albumin-permeable membrane; the albumin is removed by convection and then passes through neutral and anion exchange adsorbers for regeneration.[23]

These systems have great potential for the management of poisoning associated with acute hepatic and renal failure, both by achieving extracorporeal removal of the poisons and supporting the patient's associated organ failures. However, published experience in the management of poisoning with these systems remains sparse.

Clinical Decision Making in Poisoning

The final decision to deploy an extracorporeal drug-removal technique in any individual case requires the interpretation of the known toxicokinetics for that drug in the context of the clinical severity.[24] In clinical practice, the measurement of serum levels of drugs and poisons only influences clinical decision making for a few agents, so only for these is it necessary to have round-the-clock availability of a rapid assay (Fig. 100.8). The kinetics characteristics of poisons that make them amenable to the different modalities of extracorporeal removal are shown in Figure 100.9. The lack of controlled trials means that even the best-documented indications are still being debated. The common poisonings for which extracorporeal removal are presently indicated are shown in Figure 100.10.

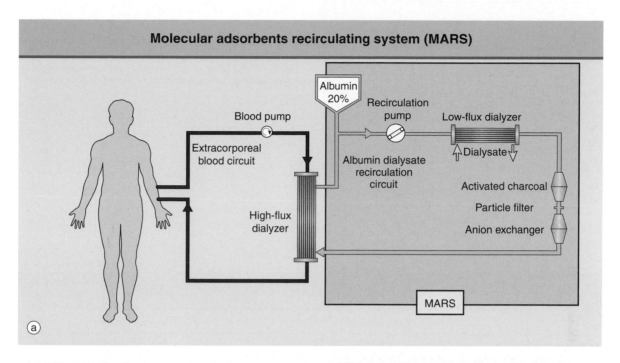

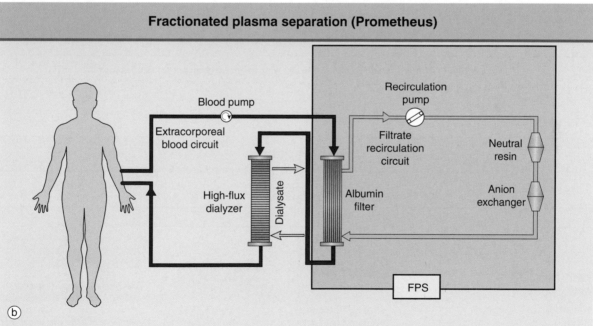

Figure 100.7 Extracorporeal liver support techniques. *a*, Molecular Adsorbents Recirculating System (MARS): an albumin-impermeable high-flux membrane is impregnated with human albumin and the dialysate enriched with albumin to facilitate removal of albumin-bound toxins from the blood. The albumin is regenerated by passage through activated charcoal and an anion exchanger. A low- flux dialyzer is in series to remove water-soluble toxins. *b*, Fractionated Plasma Separation (FPS) (Prometheus): blood passes through an albumin-permeable membrane; the albumin is removed by convection and then passes through neutral and anion exchange adsorbers to regenerate the albumin. A high-flux dialyzer is in series to remove water-soluble toxins.

Drug assays necessary for management of poisoning

Drug assays necessary for management of poisoning
Acetaminophen
Carbamazepine
Digoxin
Ethylene glycol
Ethanol
Lithium
Methemoglobin
Methanol
Phenobarbitone
Salicylate
Theophylline
Valproate

Figure 100.8   Drug assays necessary for management of poisoning. Drug assays that should be readily available around the clock for management of poisoning.

Kinetic characteristics that assist extracorporeal drug removal

Hemodialysis	Hemofiltration	Hemoperfusion
Relative molecular mass <500 d Small volume of distribution (V$_D$) (<1 l/kg) Poorly bound to plasma proteins Single-compartment kinetics Low endogenous clearance (<4 ml/min/kg)	Relative molecular mass less than cutoff of filter fibers (usually 40,000 d) Small V$_D$ (<1 l/kg) Poorly bound to plasma proteins Single-compartment kinetics Low endogenous clearance (<4 ml/min/kg)	Adsorbed by activated charcoal Small V$_D$ (<1 l/kg) Single-compartment kinetics Low endogenous clearance (<4 ml/min/kg)

Figure 100.9   Kinetic characteristics of drugs that assist extracorporeal drug removal.

Common poisonings for which extracorporeal removal may be indicated

	Drug Level or Other Criterion for Extracorporeal Treatment	Comment
Hemodialysis		
Ethanol	>5 g/l (108 mmol/l)	Combine with fomepizole 15 mg/kg IV over 30
Methanol	>50 mg/l (15 mmol/l)	min, then 10 mg/kg every 4 hours during
		hemodialysis
Ethylene glycol	>500 mg/l (8 mmol/l)	
Lithium	>4 mmol/l; >2.5 mmol/l if severe symptoms	Postdialysis rebound as intracellular lithium
		diffuses into extracellular fluid
Methanol	>500 mg/l (15 mmol/l)	
Salicylate	>800 mg/l (5.8 mmol/l)	Lower threshold if renal impairment or if fluid
		overload restricts treatment with sodium
		bicarbonate
Hemofiltration		
Aminoglycosides	Various	
Hemoperfusion		
Amanita mushroom	Clinical severity	
Barbiturates	Phenobarbitone 150 mg/l (630 mmol/l)	
Carbamazepine	Clinical severity	
Paraquat	Clinical severity	
Theophylline	Acute >100 mg/l	Chronic >40 mg/l
Valproic acid	>1 g/l	

Figure 100.10   Common poisonings for which extracorporeal removal may be indicated.

REFERENCES

1. Macnamara AF, Riyat MS, Quinton DN: The changing profile of poisoning and its management. J R Soc Med 1996;89:608–610.
2. Chugh KS, Sakhuja V: Renal failure from snake bites. Int J Artif Organs 1980;3:319–321.
3. Sert M, Tetiker T, Paydas S: Rhabdomyolysis and acute renal failure due to honeybee stings as an uncommon cause. Nephron 1993;55:146–151.
4. McClain JL, Hause DW, Clark MA: *Amanita phalloides* mushroom poisoning: A cluster of four fatalities. J Forensic Sci 1989;34:83–87.
5. Ejam-Ong S, Sitprija V: Tropical plant associated nephropathy. Nephrology 1998;4:313–314.
6. Park SK, Kim DG, Kang SK: Toxic acute renal failure and hepatitis after ingestion of raw carp bile. Nephron 1990;56:188–193.
7. Crowe AV, et al: Substance abuse and the kidney. Q J Med 2000;93:147–152.
8. Seyffart G: Poison Index: The Treatment of Acute Intoxication. Lengerich, Germany: Pabst Science, 1997.
9. Litovitz TL, Klein-Schwartz W, White S, et al: 2000 Annual report of the American Association of Poison Control Centers Toxic Exposure Surveillance System. Am J Emerg Med 2001;19:337–395.
10. Abuelo GJ: Renal failure caused by chemicals, foods, plants, animal venoms and misuse of drugs. Arch Intern Med 1990;150:505–510.
11. Lheureux P, Even-Adin D, Askenasi R: Current status of antidotal therapies in acute human intoxications. Acta Clin Belg Suppl 1990;13:29–47.
12. Vale JA: Review in medicine. Clinical toxicology. Postgrad Med J 1993;69:19–32.
13. Position statement and practical guidelines on the use of multidose activated charcoal in the treatment of acute poisoning. J Toxicol Clin Toxicol 1999;37:731–751.
14. Tenenbein M: Position statement: Whole bowel irrigation. American Academy of Clinical Toxicology; European Association of Poisons Centres and Clinical Toxicologists. J Toxicol Clin Toxicol 2000;38:689–690.
15. Abel JJ, Rowntree LG, Turner BB: On the removal of diffusible substances from the circulating blood by means of dialysis. Trans Assoc Am Phys 1913;28:51–54.
16. Winchester JF: Active methods of detoxification. In Haddad LM, Shannon MW, Winchester JF (eds): Clinical Management of Poisoning and Drug Overdose, 3rd ed. Philadelphia: WB Saunders, 1997, pp 175–186.
17. Pond SM: Extracorporeal techniques in the treatment of poisoned patients. Med J Aust 1991;154:617–622.
18. Brent J, McMartin K, Phillips S, et al: Fomepizole for the treatment of methanol poisoning. N Engl J Med 2001;344:424–429.
19. Verpooten GA, de Broe M: Combined hemoperfusion-hemodialysis in severe poisoning. Kinetics of drug extraction. Resuscitation 1984;11:275–289.
20. Higgins RM, Hearing S, Goldsmith DJA, et al: Severe theophylline poisoning: Charcoal haemoperfusion or haemodialysis? Postgrad Med J 1995;71:224–226.
21. Heath A, Knudsen K: Role of extracorporeal drug removal in acute theophylline poisoning: A review. Med Toxicol 1987;2:294–308.
22. Sabeel AI, Kurkus J, Lindholm T: Intensive haemodialysis and hemoperfusion treatment of *Amanita* mushroom poisoning. Mycopathologia 1995;131:107–114.
23. Lahdenpara A, Koivusalo A-M, et al: Value of albumin dialysis therapy in severe liver insufficiency. Transpl Int 2005;17:717–723.
24. Richlie DG, Anderson RJ: Contemporary management of salicylate poisoning: Should hemodialysis and hemoperfusion be used? Semin Dial 1996;9:257–264.

Principles of Drug Dosing and Prescribing in Renal Failure

Ali J. Olyaei and William M. Bennett

INTRODUCTION

Optimal management of patients with renal failure requires the use of pharmacotherapeutic agents for comorbid conditions. The kidney is the major organ in which drug elimination from the body occurs. Renal insufficiency and dialysis alter the pharmacokinetics and pharmacodynamics of most commonly used drugs. A recent report from the U.S. Renal Data System (USRDS) indicates that the median number of medications prescribed in renal failure is eight different classes of drugs per patient. In comparison to the general population, patients with renal insufficiency experience significantly more adverse drug reactions. Therefore, clinicians should be familiar with the pharmacokinetics behavior of each agent and the impact of renal failure on the drug elimination process. A particular area of concern is that patients with chronic kidney disease (CKD) also grow older, and this also may affect drug disposition. Approximately 80% of patients with renal failure are concomitantly prescribed a phosphate binder, antihypertensive agent, iron supplement, and antihypercholesterolemic drug in addition to other medications. Because these patients take multiple medications, they are at a greater risk of drug-drug interactions.

This chapter highlights the most common prescribing issues for the practicing nephrologist. It describes the principles of pharmacotherapy in patients with renal disease of varying severity and proposes prescribing guidelines for physicians who care for patients with renal impairment. This is particularly important since physiologic changes associated with CKD affect virtually every organ system in the body and, thus, drug disposition. Specific dosing guidelines and pharmacokinetic information are beyond the scope of this chapter. They can be obtained from a number of references or websites.[1–3]

GENERAL PRINCIPLES OF DRUG PHARMACOKINETICS

Pharmacokinetics is the study of drug behavior (absorption, distribution, metabolism, and elimination) in the body. The key elements of drug pharmacokinetics are shown in Figure 101.1. Following oral administration, only a certain proportion of the drug is absorbed and reaches the systemic circulation (bioavailability). Drugs can be highly bound to plasma proteins or unbound. Only the free or unbound concentration of the drug interacts with specific receptors at the site of pharmacologic action. The three major processes affecting drug excretion and/or elimination from the body are metabolism by the liver, metabolism by the gastrointestinal tract (cytochrome P-450 and P-glycoproteins) or elimination, and metabolism by the kidney.

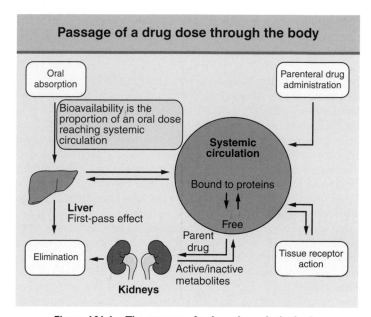

Passage of a drug dose through the body

Figure 101.1   The passage of a drug through the body.

The kidney remains the most important organ for drug elimination, both of the parent compound and of drug metabolites.[1] The liver can also metabolize drugs in the first pass as the drug is absorbed into the portal circulation or later when the drug is delivered to the liver via the systemic blood flow prior to reaching the systemic circulation. First-pass metabolism can significantly reduce the rate and extent of drug absorption. Lidocaine, for example, is metabolized extensively before it reaches the systemic circulation; renal failure may decrease its biotransformation and ultimately the first-pass metabolism. Changes in cardiac output in patients with renal failure may also reduce the rate and extent of drug metabolism of drugs with significant first-pass metabolism. For example, increased bioavailability has been reported in patients with renal failure for propranolol and dihydrocodeine, which both undergo a significant first-pass metabolism. In one report, the overall drug exposure in 24 hours and plasma drug concentration of dihydrocodeine were significantly higher in patients with renal failure.[1]

Pharmacokinetic drug interactions are a common problem among patients with CKD and after renal transplantation. Cyclosporine, tacrolimus, and sirolimus are metabolized through the cytochrome P-450 enzyme system. Many drugs routinely used following transplantation or in the treatment of hypertension or hyperlipidemia are also metabolized through this system. Drug interactions are common and require vigilance. Calcineurin inhibitor interactions frequently present practical problems. Common interactions with these drugs are shown in Figure 90.8.

Bioavailability

The percentage of a drug dose that appears in the systemic circulation following oral administration compared to the intravenous route for the same drug defines its bioavailability. In general, drugs given by the intravenous route reach the central compartment directly and usually have a more rapid onset of action. Drugs given by other routes must pass through a series of biologic membranes before entering the systemic circulation. For many drugs, only a fraction of the administered dose may reach the circulation to exert any pharmacodynamic effect. CKD may influence drug absorption and bioavailability. Edema of the gastrointestinal tract is a limiting factor in drug absorption. Drug absorption is particularly a problem when patients have diabetes mellitus as a cause of CKD. Gastrointestinal neuropathy may decrease gastric emptying time and slow the rate and extent of drug absorption. In addition, since gastrointestinal symptoms are common in advanced renal failure of any cause, nausea and vomiting often impair drug dosing and contact time between the individual drug and the mucosa of the gastrointestinal tract. In advanced CKD with uremia, there is an alkalinizing effect of salivary urea, which is converted to ammonia by urease. This effect decreases the absorption of drugs that are optimally absorbed in an acid milieu (Fig. 101.2). For example, supplemental iron requires conversion by acid from the ferrous to the ferric state for absorption. The administration of histamine H_2-receptor blockers may also contribute to an alkalinizing effect and impair the absorption of iron. In addition, other drugs used as phosphate-binding agents and even dairy products themselves may decrease drug absorption by chelating and formation of nonabsorbable complexes. Hypertensive crisis has been reported following administration of the orally active lipase inhibitor orlistat in hypertensive patients. Finally, food and phosphate binders can alter the pharmacokinetics of a number of drugs used in patients with CKD (Fig. 101.3). Grapefruit juice interacts with a number of drugs used in patients with CKD and following transplantation. Cyclosporine, tacrolimus, sirolimus, calcium channels blockers, and antihyperlipidemic and hypertensive agents are metabolized through cytochrome P-450 system, and the flavonoid component of grapefruit inhibits cytochrome P-450 3A4 isoenzymes in the intestinal wall, in hepatocytes, and potentially in the kidney, resulting in significant increases in plasma levels of these agents, increasing the risk of drug toxicity.[3]

Effect of food and phosphate binders on drug absorption	
Drugs	Effect of Food
Acetaminophen, aspirin, digoxin	Decreased/delayed drug absorption
ACE inhibitors (captopril and moexipril)	Significant decrease in serum drug levels
Fluoroquinolones and tetracycline	Avoid taking with phosphate binders, antacids and iron products; significantly decreased drug absorption
Lovastatin, spironolactone	Food, especially high-fat meals, improves drug absorption; take with food or within 2 hours of a meal
Famotidine	Decreased/delayed drug absorption
Verapamil	Decreased pharmacodynamic effects with calcium-based phosphate binders
Iron, levodopa, penicillins (most), tetracycline, erythromycin	High-carbohydrate meals decrease drug absorption

Figure 101.3   Effect of food and phosphate binders on drug absorption. ACE, angiotensin-converting enzyme.

If possible, combination of these agents with grapefruit should be avoided or plasma level monitoring with dose adjustment is highly recommended.

Hepatic first-pass metabolism may also be altered in patients with stage 4 and 5 CKD. Decreased biotransformation of drugs to inactive metabolites may lead to an increased amount of active drug reaching the systemic circulation. Some drugs have increased bioavailability in renal failure, leading to increased pharmacologic effects after a relatively small dose (e.g., zidovudine). The P-glycoprotein pump may also affect the drug delivery system. The P-glycoprotein is an efflux pump expressed in many tissues including the gastrointestinal tract, liver, and brain. Drugs that induce P-glycoproteins may decrease drug absorption or decrease active drug moiety at the pharmacologic site.[4] Because the interactions of drug absorption and hepatic metabolism are very complex, the situation in individual patients is difficult to predict from general principles. Therefore, drug bioavailability should always be considered as a factor in either increased or decreased pharmacologic effects of a given dose of drug administered to a patient with CKD.[3]

Drug Distribution
Volume of Distribution

There is a characteristic volume of distribution (V_D) for any drug, which represents the ratio of the administered dose to the resulting plasma concentration at equilibrium. This is really an apparent V_D since this mathematical construct does not correspond to a specific anatomic space but instead relates the amount of drug in the body to its plasma concentration. It is obvious that for drugs with a low plasma concentration relative to the dose, such as digoxin, this apparent V_D may exceed the total body water. Conversely, drugs that are highly protein bound and thus are restricted to the circulation have low V_D relative to the dose. The concept of V_D is useful in predicting loading doses of drugs to achieve the desired

Effect of urea on gastrointestinal absorption

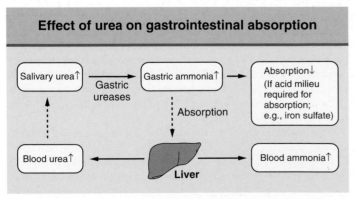

Figure 101.2   Effect of urea levels on gastrointestinal absorption.

plasma concentration relative to the dose prior to drug administration. The mathematical formula relating apparent V_D to the dose and blood concentration is V_D = dose/blood concentration. Highly protein-bound agents or drugs that are water soluble tend to be restricted to the extracellular fluid space and have a relatively small V_D, while drugs that are lipid soluble penetrate body tissues and have a large V_D.

Any factor that alters the V_D will alter plasma drug levels and hence their effects. CKD may alter the apparent drug V_D. Increases in the V_D occur in massive edema or ascites, particularly for drugs that are water soluble or are ordinarily protein bound. If the usual drug doses are given to patients with hypoalbuminemia or dehydration, low plasma drug levels may result. By comparison, muscle wasting or volume depletion may decrease the apparent V_D of water-soluble drugs. In these cases, giving the usual dose may result in unexpectedly high blood concentrations of the drug.[5]

Plasma Protein Binding

Plasma protein binding is often altered in patients with renal insufficiency, and this has an important effect on the V_D of any drug. Since the quantity of drug that is free or unbound is the pharmacologically active component, this fraction determines the amount available for pharmacologic action as well as the degree to which a particular therapeutic agent will be metabolized by the liver or excreted by the kidneys. Protein-bound drugs attach reversibly to either albumin or various glycoproteins in plasma. Organic acids usually have a single binding site on albumin, whereas organic bases tend to have multiple binding sites and their behavior in the presence of advancing CKD is less predictable. In general, acidic drugs reduce plasma protein binding in patients with renal failure. This reduction is attributable to a combination of decreased albumin concentration and a reduction in albumin affinity, which is, in turn, influenced by either structural changes in the albumin molecule or accumulation of competing endogenous inhibitors of protein binding.

Common drugs that have plasma protein binding changes in renal dysfunction are shown in Figure 101.4. This list is clearly not complete but is chosen to represent drugs of different classes. The consequences to the patient of impaired plasma protein binding are important since the unbound fraction of the drug may be substantially increased, resulting in toxicity. The best clinical example is phenytoin, which has marked decreases in plasma protein binding with concomitant increased pharmacologic effects, particularly if plasma concentrations are assumed to be in the usual therapeutic range for the nonuremic patient. If protein binding is reduced, pharmacologic effects may be seen at lower plasma levels, particularly if such levels correspond to total drug. Furthermore, decreased protein binding may increase the apparent V_D of any drug. However, predicting the clinical consequences of protein-binding abnormalities is difficult because, although more free drug may be available to the site of drug action, lower plasma

Protein binding of drugs in renal disease	
Albumin: Binding Sites for Acidic Compounds	
Protein binding reduced in nephrotic syndrome (hypoalbuminemia) and renal failure (altered albumin affinity). Increased risk of drug toxicity	
Major Effects	Minor Effects
Barbiturates	Ascorbic acid
Benzodiazepine	Bilirubin
Carbamazepine	Fatty acids
Fibrates	Nafcillin
Furosemide	Phenylbutazone
Mycophenolate mofetil	Probenecid
Penicillins	Thiopental
Phenytoin	
Sulfonamides	
Tetracyclines	
Globulins: Binding Site for Basic Compounds	
Effect of altered protein binding less predictable in renal disease	
Major Effects	Minor Effects
Digitoxin	Adenosine
Methadone	Amitriptyline
Propranolol	Chloramphenicol
Warfarin	Chlorpromazine
	Nortriptyline
	Quinine

Figure 101.4 Protein binding of drugs in renal disease.

concentrations of the drug after a given dose can also occur. When more unbound drug is available for metabolism or renal excretion, the half-life of a drug in the body may actually be decreased rather than increased by altered protein binding. Again, the clinician must be vigilant for unexpected adverse reactions and not rely on the numerical value of any plasma level but instead observe carefully.

Drug Metabolism

Progressive CKD obviously affects most body biochemical processes, and this includes drug biotransformation. In general, reduction and hydrolysis reactions are slowed, but glucuronidation, sulfation, conjugation, and microsomal oxidation reactions occur at normal rates. Since there may be significant patient variation, no prior assumptions will substitute for careful clinical evaluation. Furthermore, some drugs have pharmacologically active metabolites, which, although unimportant in patients with normal renal function, may accumulate in patients with renal insufficiency, causing adverse drug reactions. Some of these pharmacologic reactive metabolites may account for the high incidence of adverse drug reactions in patients with CKD. Some of the best-known examples of this phenomenon are the accumulation of pharmacologically active metabolites of meperidine causing seizures, nitrofurantoin causing peripheral neuropathy, and morphine sulfate causing respiratory depression.[5]

Renal Handling of Drugs

The renal excretion of drugs depends primarily on the glomerular filtration rate (GFR) and the balance between reabsorption and secretion of drugs in the renal tubules. In turn, the GFR of drugs depends on molecular size and protein binding of the agent. Therefore, for drugs that have decreased protein binding in CKD, increased amounts of drug may be secreted by the renal tubule in compensation. However, when GFR is impaired, the clearance of drugs eliminated primarily by the kidney is decreased and usually the plasma half-life of drugs is prolonged. The quantitation of drug elimination by the kidney is usually expressed as clearance, which equals the volume of blood or plasma from which the drug is cleared per unit of time. This depends on renal blood flow and the ability of the kidney to extract the drug. For the whole body, the clearance is expressed as the drug dose divided by the area under the drug concentration curve. For the kidney, this is the well-understood clearance formula (Fig. 101.5). The drug half-life describes the rate of drug removal from the body related to the V_D and the clearance (see Fig. 101.5). If the drug half-life increases, the renal clearance is usually decreased. Occasionally, there is compensation by extrarenal elimination pathways in a patient with CKD. Clinically, it is very difficult to measure tubular function, and the secretion of drugs that are eliminated by active tubular transport systems may also be affected in patients with renal disease. For practical purposes, as GFR decreases, drugs dependent on renal tubular secretion are also excreted more slowly.[5,6]

Pharmacokinetics

Pharmacokinetics is the study and mathematical expression of the time course of drugs in the body. Mathematical equations can explain the behavior of an individual drug with regard to its absorption, distribution, metabolism, and excretion (for both the parent drug and any metabolites). After the administration of a drug, there is a high initial plasma concentration of the drug, followed by a decrease in the drug level as the drug is distributed

Mathematics of drug elimination
Total body drug clearance equals drug dose over **AUC**
where AUC is the area under the concentration curve for the drug
Renal clearance equals total amount of drug in urine sample over **Plasma drug concentration**
where the total amount of the drug in the urine sample is the urine drug concentration × volume of the sample collected in a fixed time
Renal clearance rate equals clearance over **Sample collection time**
Clearance has units of volume (since the units of concentration in plasma and urine cancel out), and clearance rate has units of volume per time (e.g., ml/min)
Drug half-life ($t_{1/2}$) equals V_D × 0.693 over **Drug clearance**
V_D is volume of distribution (dose/blood concentration)

Figure 101.5   Mathematics of drug elimination.

from the plasma into an extravascular compartment. Along with this absorption and distribution, drug metabolism and elimination are beginning. At steady state, drug concentrations in plasma reach equilibrium with concentrations in body tissue. It is useful to determine the behavior of a given drug in patients at varying stages of CKD. This is usually done by comparing pharmacokinetics data from individuals with normal renal function to those from patients with CKD. This is the basis for most dose recommendations. However, individual patient factors almost always limit the utility of broad generalities when the physician is confronted with a complex, sick individual. It is here that the judgment of the physician in regard to a particular patient's ability to handle a drug or chemical substance is paramount. There is no easy substitute for knowing the pharmacology of the drug under normal circumstances, and there is no easy way to understand dosing other than to consider individual patient factors. The pharmacokinetic parameters usually used in describing drug behavior are shown in Figure 101.6.

Pharmacokinetic parameters	
Parameter (abbreviation)	Clinical Application
Bioavailability (*F*)	Determines the amount of drug reaching the systemic circulation and therefore the amount at the site of action
Volume of distribution (V_D)	Determines the size of a loading dose
Clearance (C)	Determines the maintenance dose
Half-life ($t_{1/2}$)	Determines the amount of time needed to reach steady-state serum concentrations

Figure 101.6   Pharmacokinetic parameters.

The key effects of renal dysfunction on drug handling that will affect dosing are
- Accumulation of drugs normally excreted
- Accumulation of active drug metabolites
- Changes in drug distribution: protein binding
- Decreases in renal drug metabolism

PRESCRIBING FOR THE PATIENT WITH CHRONIC KIDNEY DISEASE

The thought process that goes into prescribing drugs for patients with CKD should be systematic and careful because of the high incidence of adverse drug reactions. A stepwise approach is outlined in Figure 101.7. The goal of therapy, of course, is to maintain efficacy while avoiding drug accumulation and associated adverse reactions.

Dosing for the Renal Patient
When the GFR is reduced, the elimination of many compounds and pharmacologically active metabolites declines proportionally. The prolongation of a drug's elimination half-life is proportional to the reduction in GFR. Although drug accumulation may occur at any stage of CKD, such adverse events are relatively uncommon when the GFR remains >50 ml/min. If dose restrictions are excessive because of fears of toxicity, inadequate therapy may result. In acute renal failure,[8] the decline in GFR is virtually total, so patients should be dosed as if they have a GFR <10 mL/min until a steady state is reached.[6,7]

Dosing of Individual Drugs
Patients with renal failure are heterogeneous, and their responses to drug therapy are variable. Dose nomograms, tables, and computer-assisted dosing recommendations are helpful but are not necessarily associated with better therapeutic outcomes. Any fixed approach to dosing will probably fail because of the clinical complexity of renal failure.[8] In reference sources,[1–3] dosing recommendations are made based on various levels of renal function, but

it must be realized that these doses vary with the specific needs of each patient. It should be emphasized that physicians should use their clinical judgment to evaluate every individual situation, choose a dosage regimen based on factors present in that patient, and continually reevaluate the patient's response to therapy.

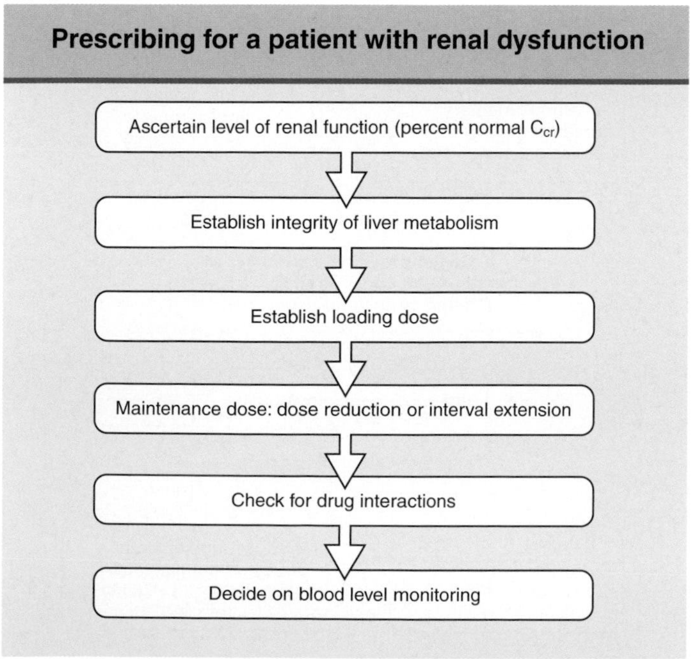

Initial Assessment
A targeted history and physical examination constitute the first step in assessing dose in patients with CKD. Previous drug toxicity or intolerance should be ascertained, if possible. The patient's current medication list (both prescription and nonprescription formulations) must be reviewed to identify potential drug interactions and nephrotoxins. Physical findings suggest the patient's volume status, provide height and weight data used in calculating ideal body mass, and determine whether extrarenal diseases such as hepatic dysfunction are present and requiring additional dose adjustment.

Estimating Renal Function for Drug Dosing
Renal function and GFR can be estimated by measuring the clearance of certain compounds (see Chapter 3). Blood urea nitrogen (BUN) and serum creatinine levels are insensitive measures of renal function. Creatinine clearance (C_{cr}) has traditionally been used to approximate GFR, calculated by the Cockcroft-Gault formula. Alternatively, the four-variable Modification of Diet in Renal Disease equation can be used to estimate GFR, which has the practical advantage that it is not necessary to know the patient's body weight. Using either method is appropriate and reliable for estimating GFR for drug dosing in CKD patients. It is important to remember that these formulas represent only an approximation of renal function (see Chapter 3). If a patient has acute renal failure, residual GFR of <10 ml/min should be assumed for purposes of drug dose adjustment.

Loading Dose
For most drugs in the setting of normal renal function, a steady-state concentration is achieved after five drug half-lives. Because CKD may prolong the drug's half-life, simply reducing drug doses would be a therapeutic error because such a strategy would delay achievement of steady-state concentrations and therapeutic drug levels. Therefore, a loading dose needs to be given for most drugs. This dose usually does not vary much from the initial dose given to patients with normal renal function. An exception to this rule is digoxin, for which 50% to 75% of the usual loading dose should be given because of its reduced V_D in renal failure. In patients with significant volume contraction superimposed on CKD, it is prudent to lower the standard loading doses of aminoglycosides by 20% to 25% to avoid toxicity.

Maintenance Dosing
Reference sources provide general dosing guidelines but patient-specific factors, risk of drug-drug interactions, and general risk of adverse events for a particular agent should always be considered prior to starting pharmacotherapy. After a loading dose has been given, a maintenance dosing regimen should be calculated.[9] The maintenance dose may be determined by one of two methods. First, the dosing interval can be lengthened by the use of the following formula:

$$\text{Dosing interval} = \frac{\text{Normal } C_{cr}}{\text{Patient's } C_{cr}} \times \text{Normal interval}$$

Alternatively, each individual dose can be reduced and given at standard intervals.

Prescribing for a patient with renal dysfunction

Ascertain level of renal function (percent normal C_{cr})

↓

Establish integrity of liver metabolism

↓

Establish loading dose

↓

Maintenance dose: dose reduction or interval extension

↓

Check for drug interactions

↓

Decide on blood level monitoring

Figure 101.7 Prescribing for a patient with renal dysfunction. C_{cr}, creatinine clearance

The first or varying interval method can potentially lead to periods of subtherapeutic drug concentrations. The latter or varying dose method allows for more constant drug levels but risks toxicity owing to higher trough levels. For these reasons, the interval method is appropriate for aminoglycosides, whereas the dosing method is more applicable to anticonvulsants and antiarrhythmics. An example of calculations for the dose of aminoglycosides is shown in Figure 101.8. Because the elimination half-life of aminoglycosides is markedly prolonged as renal function declines, maintenance dose intervals should be carefully extended in patients with CKD. Once-daily aminoglycoside dosing may be less nephrotoxic for a given total daily dose in both patients with normal renal function and those with CKD.

Drug Level Monitoring

Simply varying the dose or dosing interval is usually not sufficient when adjusting drug regimens for patients with complex disease including renal failure. Monitoring drug levels when possible may be necessary to ensure therapeutic levels while avoiding toxicity. Drug assays usually measure only total blood concentrations and may significantly underestimate plasma levels of the active or free form of the drug. Phenytoin represents a prototype. As a result of opposing pharmacokinetics changes in protein binding and distribution factors, no dose adjustment is generally needed. The therapeutic range, however, is reduced to 4 to 8 mg/l (16 to 32 mmol/l) from 10 to 20 mg/l (40 to 80 mmol/l), reflecting the increased proportion of active or free drug present. In clinical practice, drug level monitoring is necessary to assist prescribing in renal failure for only a minority of drugs, especially those with a narrow therapeutic index. The drugs for which such monitoring is recommended are shown in Figure 101.9.

Drugs in Nephrotic Syndrome

Drug handling in patients with heavy proteinuria and nephrotic syndrome is complex. In patients with low serum albumin and coexisting renal dysfunction, drug binding to plasma proteins may be altered. In this case, greater free drug is available for any total drug concentration; this may result in adverse effects or more rapid metabolism, depending on the clinical circumstances. Furthermore, when albumin is lost in the urine, bound drug may also be lost. This may be a partial explanation for the refractoriness of some nephrotic patients to diuretic therapy. Some drugs produce adverse effects more readily in nephrotic patients, for example, clofibrate, which can provoke severe muscle necrosis; all fibrates should be used with caution in patients with nephrotic syndrome (see Fig. 101.4).

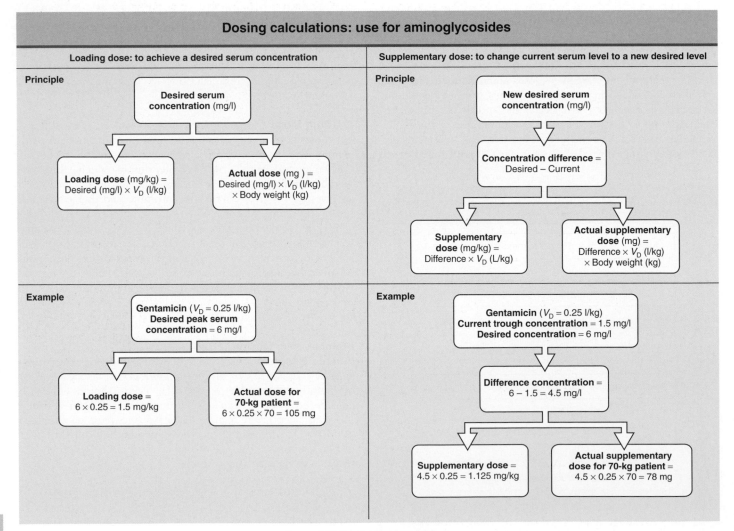

Figure 101.8 Dosing calculations.

Therapeutic drug monitoring in renal insufficiency			
Drug Name	Therapeutic Range	When to Draw Sample	How Often to Check Levels
Aminoglycosides (conventional dosing): gentamicin, tobramycin, amikacin	Gentamicin and tobramycin Trough: 0.5–2 mg/l Peak: 5–8 mg/l Amikacin Peak: 20–30 mg/l Through: <10 mg/l	Trough: immediately prior to dose Peak: 30 min after a 30-min infusion	Check peak and trough with 3rd dose. For therapy 72 hr, levels not necessary. Repeat drug levels weekly or if renal function changes
Aminoglycosides (24-hr dosing): gentamicin, tobramycin, amikacin	0.5–3 mg/l	Obtain random drug level 12 hr after dose	After initial dose. Repeat drug level in 1 wk or if renal function changes
Carbamazepine	4–12 μg/ml	Trough: immediately prior to dosing	Check 2–4 days after first dose or change in dose
Cyclosporine	50–200 μg/ml	Trough: immediately prior to dosing	Daily for first week, then weekly
Digoxin	0.8–2 μg/ml	12 hr after maintenance dose	5–7 days after first dose for patients with normal renal and hepatic function; 15–20 days in anephric patients
Lidocaine	1–5 μg/ml	8 hr after IV infusion started or changed	
Lithium	Acute: 0.8–1.2 mmol/l Chronic: 0.6–0.8 mmol/l	Trough: before AM dose at least 12 hr since last dose	
Phenobarbitone	15–40 μg/l	Trough: immediately prior to dosing	Check 2 wk after first dose or change in dose. Follow-up level in 1–2 mo
Phenytoin Free phenytoin	10–20 μg/ml 1–2 μg/ml	Trough: immediately prior to dosing	5–7 d after first dose or after change in dose
Procainamide NAPA (N-acetyl procainamide), a procainamide metabolite	4–10 μg/ml Trough: 4 μg/ml Peak: 8 μg/ml 10–30 μg/ml	Trough: immediately prior to next dose or 12–18 hr after starting or changing an infusion Draw with procainamide sample	
Quinidine	1–5 μg/ml	Trough: immediately prior to dosing	
Sirolimus	10–20 μg/dl	Trough: immediately prior to dosing	
Tacrolimus	10–15 μg/ml	Trough: immediately prior to dosing	
Theophylline PO or aminophylline IV	15–20 μg/ml	Trough: immediately prior to dosing	
Valproic acid (divalproex sodium)	40–100 μg/ml	Trough: immediately prior to dosing	Check 2–4 days after first dose or change in dose
Vancomycin	Trough: 5–15 mg/l Peak: 25–40 mg/l	Trough: immediately prior to dosing Peak: 60 min after a 60 min infusion	With 3rd dose (when initially starting therapy, or after each dose adjustment). For therapy <72 hr, levels not necessary. Repeat drug levels if renal function changes

Figure 101.9 Therapeutic drug monitoring in renal insufficiency. Drugs for which monitoring of drug levels is routinely recommended.

Extracorporeal Drug Losses
Hemodialysis
For patients receiving hemodialysis, attention must be paid to dose scheduling and the need to give supplemental doses to replace lost body stores.[10,11] Dialysis clearance of a drug depends primarily on its molecular weight and degree of protein binding. As protein binding increases, dialysis clearance decreases. Likewise, the smaller the compound is (<500 d), the more drug is removed during a dialysis treatment. In general, scheduled doses should be given after dialysis, if possible. Additionally, if a significant portion of a drug is removed, supplemental doses should be given after each dialysis session. Commonly used drugs for which supplemental postdialysis dosing may be required are shown in Figure 101.10.

Peritoneal Dialysis
Many of the same properties of drugs that affect removal by hemodialysis also apply to peritoneal dialysis, but the latter treatment is very inefficient. For significant removal to occur by peritoneal dialysis, the drug must have a very low V_D, low protein binding, and few other routes of drug elimination. Therefore, for most drugs in

Commonly used drugs that require replacement dosing following intermittent hemodialysis					
Acebutolol	Cefamandole	Ceftizoxime	Gabapentin	Metronidazole	Ticarcillin
Acetaminophen	Cefazolin	Cefuroxime	Ganciclovir	Mezlocillin	Tobramycin
Acyclovir	Cefdinir	Chloral hydrate	Gentamicin	Minoxidil	Trimethoprim
Allopurinol	Cefdroxil	Chloramphenicol	Ifosfamide	Nadolol	Valacyclovir
Amikacin	Cefepime	Cyclophosphamide	Imipenem	Ofloxacin	Vigabatrin
Amoxicillin	Cefmenoxime	Disopyramide	Iodixanol	Penicillin	Zidovudine
Ampicillin	Cefmetazole	Enalapril	Isosorbide	Piperacillin	
Aspirin	Cefotaxime	Esmolol	Lisinopril	Procainamide	
Atenolol	Cefotetan	Ethosuximide	Lithium	Pyrazinamide	
Aztreonam	Cefoxitin	Famciclovir	Loracarbef	Sotalol	
Captopril	Cefpirome	Fluconazole	Meropenem	Streptomycin	
Carboplatin	Cefradine	Flucytosine	Methotrexate	Sulfamethoxazole	
Cefaclor	Ceftazidime	5-Fluorouracil	Methylprednisolone	Sulfisoxazole	
Cefalexin	Ceftibuten	Foscarnet	Metoprolol	Theophylline	

Figure 101.10   Commonly used drugs that require replacement dosing following intermittent hemodialysis.

clinical use, there is little evidence of significant drug removal during chronic peritoneal dialysis.[11] It is also generally true that if hemodialysis does not remove a drug significantly, neither will peritoneal dialysis. As an example, one conventional hemodialysis treatment removes about two thirds of the body stores of aminoglycoside antibiotics, whereas 24 hours of continuous ambulatory peritoneal dialysis will remove only 25% to 30% of the drug.

Continuous Renal Replacement Therapy

Continuous therapies with arteriovenous hemofiltration or venovenous hemofiltration use relatively porous membranes with convective transport of solute. If dialysate is added, diffusion of solutes can also occur. Therefore, low-molecular-weight drugs are removed at a greater rate using these continuous techniques. The rate of removal is determined by the drug protein binding and the device filtration rate. A series of sieving coefficients is available that allows calculation of the amount of drug actually lost if the ultrafiltration flow rate is known.[11] It is difficult to adjust doses except by carefully timed and interpreted blood measurements.

COMMON PRESCRIBING ISSUES IN CHRONIC KIDNEY DISEASE

Even when the principles of drug dosing in CKD are followed, a substantial risk remains of drug-related adverse events. If there is still residual renal function, drugs may aggravate established CKD. Furthermore, other drugs may aggravate the metabolic problems of CKD or cause nervous system or other toxicities because of accumulation.

Nephrotoxicity

A wide range of drugs may cause nephrotoxicity with or without pre-existing renal insufficiency (Fig. 101.11). Idiosyncratic nephrotoxic effects are unpredictable and independent of dose. Acute interstitial nephritis and acute tubular necrosis are both common. Chronic effects result from interstitial nephritis or glomerulonephritis, most commonly membranous nephropathy with gold or D-penicillamine.

Predictable nephrotoxic effects are dose related. The four most common classes of drug that aggravate renal impairment are aminoglycosides, angiotensin-converting enzyme (ACE) inhibitors and angiotensin receptor blockers (ARB), nonsteroidal anti-inflammatory drugs (NSAIDs), and radiographic contrast media. Other examples include vancomycin, amphotericin, cisplatin, and the calcineurin inhibitors cyclosporine and facrolimus.

Aminoglycosides

Because of a narrow therapeutic window and GFR-dependent excretion, close attention must be paid to aminoglycoside dosing regimens, drug levels, changes in renal function, and concomitant nephrotoxic drug use. As aminoglycosides accumulate, the risk of nephrotoxicity and ototoxicity increases. Bactericidal efficacy of aminoglycosides correlates with therapeutic peak concentrations. Toxicity, however, corresponds to rising trough levels. Therefore, dose adjustment for these antimicrobial agents should primarily involve the varying interval approach (see Fig. 101.6). Individual dose reductions are also occasionally necessary. Assessment of peak and trough aminoglycoside serum levels as well as GFR is required to monitor therapy and avoid toxicity.[12] As well as aggravating pre-existing renal impairment, aminoglycoside toxicity may cause *de novo* acute renal failure. Nephrotoxicity is usually reversible, but ototoxicity may cause irreversible vestibular damage with long-term disability. If possible, concomitant use of high-dose loop diuretics (furosemide, bumetanide, and especially ethacrynic acid) should be avoided. The combination of these agents may greatly increase the risk of ototoxicity.

Angiotensin-Converting Enzyme Inhibitors and Angiotensin Receptor Blockers

Worsening of renal impairment or even acute oliguric renal failure may occur when prescribing an ACE inhibitor or ARB in patients with pre-existing renal disease. Those with atherosclerotic renal

Drug-induced kidney injury					
Drug	Risk Factor	Incidence	Pathophysiology	Prevention	Management
Antimicrobials					
Acyclovir	High dose, IV bolus dose	5%–25%	Deposition of acyclovir crystals → intratubular obstruction and foci of interstitial inflammation → ARF Crystal nephropathy Proximal tubulopathy	Avoid bolus dose, slow drug infusion over 1–2 hr Prior hydration (maintain urine output >75 ml/hr)	Discontinue hydration and loop diuretic
Adefovir dipivoxil	Dose ≥30 mg/day Duration of therapy Renal impairment Pre-existing tubular dysfunction	1% Fanconi syndrome	Depletion of mitochondrial DNA from proximal tubular cells → enlargement and dysmorphia of mitochondria of PCT → acute tubular degeneration		Discontinue
Aminoglycosides	Dose, duration, and frequency of administration Concurrent renal ischemia or administration of nephrotoxins Liver disease plasma concentration >10 mg/dl peak and >2–3 trough	5%–20%	In proximal tubule aminoglycoside bound to anionic phospholipid, delivered to megalin, endocytic uptake into the cell. Within cell, accumulates → direct toxicity → ARF	Maintain therapeutic range Give once-daily dose if necessary	Decrease dose, frequency, and duration of therapy
Amphotericin	High dose and long duration of therapy	5%–80%	Afferent vasoconstriction and direct action → ↓ GFR Distal tubular injury via creation of pores that increase membrane permeability → hypokalemia, hypomagnesemia, renal tubular acidosis, polyuria due to nephrogenic diabetes insipidus	Use liposomal formulation (does not contain deoxycholate) Sodium loading (500–1000 ml normal saline 30 min prior to administration) Regularly monitor serum Na, K, Mg	
Cidofovir		8%	Induces apoptosis in proximal tubule → tubular dysfunction, diabetes insipidus, renal failure		Probenecid (human organic anion transporter inhibitor) →reduce tubular uptake of cidofovir
Foscarnet	Duration of therapy Renal impairment Pre-existing tubular dysfunction	27%	Direct tubular toxicity → acute tubular necrosis, nephrogenic diabetes insipidus Crystals in glomerular capillary lumen and proximal tubular lumen	0.5–1 liters normal saline infusion	
Indinavir	Bolus dose	4%–14%	Crystal nephropathy, Nephrolithiasis → obstructive ARF	Hydration Establish high urine flow Avoid bolus dose	Discontinue
Sulfonamide (sulfadiazine and sulfamethoxazole)	High dose Urine pH <5.5	7%	Intrarenal precipitation → kidney stone formation	Fluid intake >3 l/day, monitor urine for crystals; if crystals seen; alkalinize urine to pH >7.1	

Figure 101.11 Drug-induced kidney injury. All drugs in this table should be dosed based on renal function. Avoid concomitant use of nephrotoxic medications and diuretics. Monitor renal function before and during treatment. Patient-related risk factors for all these drugs include age, pre-existing chronic kidney disease, volume depletion, concurrent use of nephrotoxic drugs. Adequate hydration prior to therapy and during the treatment of acute renal failure because volume depletion is one of the most important risk factors. ACE, angiotensin-converting enzyme; ARF, acute renal failure; FDA, U.S. Food and Drug Administration; GFR, glomerular filtration rate; NSAIDs, nonsteroidal anti-inflammatory drugs. *Continued*

Drug-induced kidney injury—cont'd					
Drug	Risk Factor	Incidence	Pathophysiology	Prevention	Management
Tenofovir	Dose Duration	Few case reports	Tubular cell karyomegaly, degeneration, and necrosis → interstitial nephritis, diabetes insipidus, ARF Fanconi syndrome		
Immune-modulating and Chemotherapeutic Agents					
Cyclosporine/ tacrolimus	Dose Age Postoperative ARF Diabetes Hypertension		↓ PG and ↑ 20-HETE acid production → vasoconstriction generation of H_2O_2 resulting in depleted glutathione → ↓ GFR, ischemic collapse or scarring of the glomeruli, vacuolization of the tubules, and focal areas of tubular atrophy and interstitial fibrosis	Maintain in therapeutic range Avoid drugs that raise levels (CYP 3A4 inhibitors) Calcium channel blockers	Discontinue or reduce dose
Interferon		15%–20% proteinuria	Prerenal ARF Tubulointerstitial nephritis Thrombotic microangiopathy Membranoproliferative glomerulonephritis		Discontinue
Intravenous immunoglob-ulin	Sucrose-containing product Dehydration	90% contained sucrose	Accumulation of sucrose in PCT forms vesicles, ↑ osmolarity → cell swelling, vacuolization, and tubular luminal occlusion	Infusion rate <3 mg sucrose/kg/min Avoid coadministration of radiocontrast Avoid sucrose-containing product	Hydration Discontinue sucrose-containing product
Methotrexate	Acidic urine High dose		Precipitates in the urine and induces tubular injury	Prior hydration Alkalinize urine to pH >7.0 (3 l of 5% dextrose in water + 44–66 mmol of $NaHCO_3$ per day)	Loop diuretic Leukovorin rescue with or without thymidine for systemic toxicities
Chemotherapeutic Agents					
Cisplatin	Low chloride High dose	25%–42%	Chloride in cis position replaced by H_2O → highly reactive hydroxyl radical via Cyp450 → DNA injury tubular cell death Nephrogenic diabetes insipidus Hypomagnesemia (may be persistent)	Forced diuresis: 2.5 l/hr normal saline before and several hours after administration Mannitol or furosemide Thiophosphate, thiosulfate	Discontinue Mg supplementation
Ifosfamide	Coprescription of cisplatin	Almost 100%	Direct tubular injury and mitochondrial damage → renal tubular acidosis, Fanconi-like syndrome, nephrogenic diabetes insipidus, hypokalemia	Mesna	Discontinue
Other Agents					
ACE inhibitor			Vasoconstriction → prerenal ARF	Avoid in bilateral renal artery stenosis	

Figure 101.11, cont'd

			Drug-induced kidney injury—cont'd		
Drug	Risk Factor	Incidence	Pathophysiology	Prevention	Management
Lithium	Renal impairment Dehydration Hyponatremia Diuretic use, especially thiazide	20%–54% develop urine concentration defect 12% frank diabetes insipidus (defect persists in 63% despite withdrawal of lithium)	Impairment of collecting duct concentrating ability → diabetes insipidus Chronic tubulointerstitial nephropathy (tubular atrophy and interstitial fibrosis)	Therapeutic range (0.6–1.2 mmol/l) Prevent dehydration Avoid low-sodium diet Avoid thiazide	Amiloride for nephrogenic diabetes insipidus Fluid restoration Furosemide up to 40 mg/hr Acetazolamide + $NaHCO_3$ Na, K supplement Hemodialysis (rebound can occur if stop too early) Discontinue
NSAIDs	Volume and sodium depletion Diuretic use Large dose and long therapy Severe liver disease	1%–5%	Hemodynamically induced ARF due to vasoconstriction via reduced prostaglandin production → Acute and chronic tubulointerstitial nephritis, with or without nephrotic syndrome Direct toxicity → chronic interstitial nephritis and papillary necrosis	Avoid coprescription of diuretic Avoid large dose	
Radiocontrast media	Dose and frequency Osmolarity of contrast media	<10% in patients with normal GFR 12%–25% if GFR ↓	High osmolarity, medullary vasoconstriction, ↑ active transport in thick ascending loop of Henle → ↑ O_2 demand	Hydration before and after administration Acetylcysteine unproven	

Figure 101.11, cont'd

artery stenosis are at greatest risk, but these drugs may also cause deterioration of renal function in the absence of conduit artery stenosis, particularly in dehydrated patients or where renal perfusion is compromised. Monitoring renal function is necessary 7 to 10 days after starting therapy to ensure that there has been no precipitous decline in GFR or hyperkalemia. Renal impairment caused by ACE inhibitors is usually, but not always, reversible on withdrawal of the drug.

Nonsteroidal Anti-inflammatory Drugs

By far the most common nephrotoxic effect of NSAIDs is acute deterioration in renal function due to renal vasoconstriction caused by renal prostaglandin inhibition. The consequent acute renal failure may be oliguric or nonoliguric. The newer cyclooxygenase 2 [COX-2] inhibitors (celecoxib and rofecoxib) have significantly fewer gastrointestinal complications than conventional NSAIDs. However, the COX-2 enzyme is constitutively expressed and regulates important physiologic functions in the kidney, and available evidence indicates COX-2 inhibitors are no less nephrotoxic than other NSAIDs.[13–14]

Another uncommon form of NSAID nephrotoxicity involves drug hypersensitivity, resulting in interstitial nephritis with nephrotic-range proteinuria, with histology showing glomerular podocyte changes similar to minimal change nephrotic syndrome. These changes are thought to result from the effects on glomerular permeability of cytokines released from infiltrating interstitial T cells. This form of renal failure typically has a protracted course; it is insidious in onset and slow in resolution. Long-term use of NSAIDs has also been linked to the development of renal papillary necrosis.

In patients at risk of developing acute renal failure or worsening CKD, NSAID use should be avoided. If NSAID use is necessary, particularly on a continuous basis, close monitoring of renal function, as well as urinalysis, should be performed at regular intervals.

Radiographic Contrast Media

Worsening of renal impairment by radiographic contrast media is common, particularly if large contrast volumes are used (e.g., in vascular imaging). Nonionic contrasts are safer but do not eliminate the risk. Fluid depletion aggravates the risk. The prevention and management of contrast nephrotoxicity are discussed further in Chapter 5 and Chapter 63.

Aggravation of Metabolic Effects of Renal Impairment

A number of drugs have no direct adverse influence on renal function but when used inappropriately in patients with renal impairment will aggravate the metabolic consequences of renal failure (Fig. 101.12).

Hyperkalemia

As well as potassium supplements and potassium-sparing diuretics (spironolactone, amiloride), hyperkalemia may also occur with ACE inhibitors, ARBs, NSAIDs, and potassium citrate mixture. Tetracyclines are catabolic and provoke release of intracellular potassium into the extracellular fluid; this produces significant problems in stage 4 and 5 CKD.

Uremia

Protein catabolic drugs will accelerate urea production and, therefore, aggravate uremia with no change in renal excretory function. Corticosteroids will provoke a modest increase in urea whenever they are used in the context of renal impairment. Tetracyclines are extremely catabolic and may rapidly worsen uremia and produce life-threatening hyperkalemia. They are absolutely contraindicated in stage 3 to 5 CKD. Second-generation tetracyclines such as doxycycline and minocycline are, however, safe in this regard.

Sodium and Water Retention

Most patients with renal impairment are intolerant of sodium loading, which may provoke fluid overload and hypertension. All sodium-containing medications and those that promote sodium and water retention should, therefore, be used with caution. These include sodium chloride, sodium bicarbonate, sodium-containing antacids (e.g., alginate preparations such as Gaviscon), fludrocortisone, and carbenoxolone.

Acidosis

Both acetazolamide and metformin aggravate metabolic acidosis and are contraindicated in renal failure. Although very rare, lactic acidosis is an important and potentially fatal adverse reaction of metformin (approximately 0.06 per 1000 patient-years). The predisposing factors for metformin-induced lactic acidosis include serum creatinine >1.4 mg/dl (125 µmol/l), liver disease, sepsis, and exposure to radiographic contrast media. In all patients, metformin should be discontinued at least for 48 hours before radiographic procedures (or on admission for an emergency procedure) and not restarted for 24 hours.

Coagulopathy

The platelet dysfunction of uremia may be aggravated by aspirin. Low-dose aspirin (up to 150 mg/day) is widely used, with few problems, in the management of coronary and cerebral vascular disease in CKD. Nevertheless, there may be a major clinical bleeding problem when the uremic patient on aspirin requires surgery or renal biopsy. Aspirin in a full anti-inflammatory dose is contraindicated in CKD.

Drug Accumulation in Chronic Kidney Disease

Many other drugs and their metabolites accumulate in stage 4 and 5 CKD unless adequate dose reductions are made, usually by increasing dosing intervals. Fortunately, only a small minority of drugs produce clinically important adverse effects. Some important examples are aluminum (confusion and dementia), nitrofurantoin (peripheral neuropathy), acyclovir (confusional state), morphine (obtundation and coma), digoxin (cardiotoxicity), fibrates (myopathy), and allopurinol (rash).

CKD alters the pharmacokinetic properties of morphine, meperidine, and propoxyphene. Toxicity can develop from accumulation of the parent drug or an active metabolite. Morphine is metabolized to two active morphine analogues; morphine-3-glucuronide (M3G) and morphine-6-glucuronide (M6G). These active metabolites are both renally excreted. M6G is a potent opiate with a half-life >60 hours in CKD patients and has been associated with respiratory depression in patients with CKD. M3G is not a potent opiate but may precipitate a dystonic reaction (neurotoxicity). Codeine is metabolized to morphine; therefore, it possesses the same risk of neuro- and respiratory toxicity. Meperidine is metabolized to its active metabolite normeperidine, which can accumulate in patients with CKD. Normeperidine may induce tremor, pupillary dilatation, and seizures. Fentanyl and oxycodone have no active metabolites and can be used in CKD with minimal side effects at appropriate doses. Hydromorphone is metabolized to an active hydromorphine-3-glucuronide. However, this metabolite has minor activity and does not accumulate substantially in renal failure.[16]

Aggravation by drugs of the metabolic effects of pre-existing renal impairment	
Metabolic effect	Drugs
Hyperkalemia	Potassium supplements, potassium-sparing diuretics (especially combination diuretics), nonsteroidal anti-inflammatory drugs, potassium citrate, tetracyclines, angiatensin-converting enzyme inhibitors, angiotensin II receptor antagonists
Uremia	Corticosteroids, tetracyclines
Sodium and water retention	Sodium chloride, sodium bicarbonate, sodium-containing antacids (e.g., Gaviscon), fludrocortisone, carbenoxolone
Metabolic acidosis	Acetazolamide, metformin
Coagulopathy	Aspirin

Figure 101.12   Aggravation by drugs of the metabolic effects of pre-existing renal impairment.

REFERENCES

1. Drug prescribing in renal failure. Available at www.kdp-baptist.louisville.edu/renalbook.
2. Dosing of antiretroviral drugs in adults with renal insufficiency and hemodialysis. Available atwww.globalrph.com/renaldosing2.htm.
3. Olyaei AJ, deMattos AM, Bennett WM: Drug-drug interactions and most commonly used drugs in renal transplant recipients. In Weir M (ed): Medical Management of Kidney Transplantation. Philadelphia: Lippincott Williams & Wilkins, 2005, pp 512–532.
4. Zhang Y, Benet LZ: The gut as a barrier to drug absorption: Combined role of cytochrome P450 3A and P-glycoprotein. Clin Pharmacokinet 2001; 40:159–168.
5. Aronoff GR, Brier ME: Prescribing drugs in renal disease. In Brenner BM (ed): The Kidney. Philadelphia, Saunders, 2004, pp 2849–2870.
6. Benedetti P, de Lalla F: Antibiotic therapy in acute renal failure. Contrib Nephrol 2001;132:136–145.
7. Olyaei AJ: Drug dosing in renal failure. In Bennett WM (ed): Treatment Strategies in Nephrology and Hypertension. PocketMedicine.com Inc., 2001.
8. Bennett WM: Guide to drug dosage in renal failure. In Speight TM, Holford N (eds): Avery's Drug Treatment, 4th ed. Auckland: ADIS International, 1997, pp 1725–2792.
9. Aronoff GR, Golper TA, Morrison G, et al: Drug Prescribing in Renal Failure. Philadelphia: American College of Physicians, 1999.
10. Olyaei AJ, de Mattos AM, Bennett WM: Principle of drug usage in dialysis patients. In Nissenson Ar, Fine RN (eds): Dialysis Therapy. Philadelphia: Hanley & Belfus Inc., 2001, pp 435–442.
11. Olyaei AJ, de Mattos AM, Bennett WM: Drug usage in dialysis patients. In Nissenson AR, Fine RN, Gentile DE (eds): Clinical Dialysis. Norwalk, CT: Appleton and Lange, 2001, pp 891–926.
12. Nicolau DP, Freeman CD, Belliveau PP, et al: Experience with a once-daily aminoglycoside program administered to 2184 adult patients. Antimicrob Agent Chemother 1995; 39:650–655.
13. Brater DC: Effects of nonsteroidal anti-inflammatory drugs on renal function: Focus on cyclooxygenase-2-selective inhibition. Am J Med 1999;107(Suppl):65S–70S.
14. Perazella MA, Tray K: Selective cyclooxygenase-2 inhibitors: A pattern of nephrotoxicity similar to traditional nonsteroidal anti-inflammatory drugs. Am J Med 2001;111:64–67.
15. Whelton A, Fort JG, Puma JA, et al: SUCCESS VI Study Group. Cyclooxygenase-2-specific inhibitors and cardiorenal function: A randomized, controlled trial of celecoxib and rofecoxib in older hypertensive osteoarthritis patients. Am J Ther 2001;8:85–95.
16. Reid C, Gibbins J, Hanks G: Pain is an issue in renal impairment. BMJ 2006;332:448–449.

Index

Note: Page numbers followed by f indicate figures.

A

AA-amyloidosis, 320f, 324–325, 325f
  recurrent post-transplantation, 1118
AASK (African American Study of Kidney
    Disease), 378, 414, 419, 420f, 828
AASKD (African American Study for Kidney
    Disease and Hypertension),
    469–470, 470f
Aβ₂M amyloidosis. See β₂-Microglobulin–
    derived (β₂M)-amyloidosis.
Abacavir, renal syndromes associated with,
    314f
ABCD (Appropriate Blood Pressure Control
    in Diabetes) trial, 368, 419f
Abdominal aortic aneurysm
  autosomal dominant polycystic kidney
    disease with, 511
  renal arterial disease with, 734
Abdominal compartment syndrome, acute
    renal failure due to, 767
Abdominal obesity, 405
Abdominal pain
  drug-induced, in chronic renal failure, 896f
  after kidney transplantation, 898
Abluminal membrane, 6
ABMR. See Alloantibody-mediated rejection
    (ABMR).
ABO typing, for kidney transplantation,
    1049, 1050
ABO-incompatible liver transplantation, 1149
ABO-incompatible renal transplantation,
    plasma exchange for, 1017f, 1020
Abscess(es)
  after pancreas transplantation, 1135,
    1138f
  renal, 611, 611f
    glomerulonephritis due to, 310
    imaging of, 60f
    nephritic syndrome due to, 203f
Acanthocytes, in urine sediment, 39f
ACE. See Angiotensin-convertin enzyme
    (ACE).
ACE gene, and chronic kidney disease, 815
ACE-Inhibition in Progressive Renal Disease
    study group, 414
Acetaminophen (paracetamol)
  acute renal failure due to, 763
  poisoning, 1156f, 1157f
Acetate, in dialysate fluid, 956f
Acetazolamide
  and metabolic acidosis, 1176
  volume contraction due to, 83
  for volume expansion, 89, 89f
acetoacetate, in urine, 37
Acetoacetic acid, 154
Acetone, in urine, 37
Acetylcysteine, for prevention of acute renal
    failure, 784
Acetylsalicylic acid poisoning, metabolic
    acidosis due to, 155–156
Acid, net production of, 141
Acid excretion, net, 142, 142f, 144
Acid-base balance, 141–145, 142f–144f
  in peritoneal dialysis, 987f, 999
  during pregnancy, 478

Acid-base disturbance(s), 174
  in acute renal failure, 787f, 792–793
  metabolic acidosis as. See Acidosis,
    metabolic.
  metabolic alkalosis as. See Alkalosis,
    metabolic.
  mixed, 174–179
    classification of, 174–177, 174f–177f
    clinical manifestations of, 178
    diagnosis of, 178–179, 179f
    etiology and pathogenesis of, 174
    treatment of, 179
  respiratory acidosis as. See Acidosis,
    respiratory.
  respiratory alkalosis as. See Alkalosis,
    respiratory.
  due to sickle cell nephropathy, 581–582
  triple, 177
Acidosis
  during dialysis, 964f
  metabolic
    in acute renal failure, 787f, 792–793
    aggravation by drugs of, 1176, 1176f
    in chronic kidney disease, 829, 833,
      874, 902
    due to hemodialysis, 975
    hyperchloremic, in Fanconi syndrome,
      565
    with metabolic alkalosis, 175f, 176
    mixed, 175f, 177
    after pancreas transplantation, 1135
    with respiratory acidosis, 174, 175f
    with respiratory alkalosis, 176, 178f
    secondary response to, 169f
  respiratory, 167–171
    acute, 168, 168f, 170f
    acute on chronic, 175f
    chronic, 168, 168f, 170f
    clinical manifestations of, 169
    diagnosis of, 169
    etiology and pathogenesis of, 167–168,
      167f, 168f
    with metabolic acidosis, 174, 175f
    with metabolic alkalosis, 174–176, 175f,
      177f
    secondary physiologic response to,
      168–169, 169f
    treatment of, 169–171, 170f
Acid-sterile pyuria, 617
Acquired cystic kidney disease (ACKD),
    911–915
  clinical manifestations of, 530f, 911–912
  diagnosis and differential diagnosis of,
    913–914, 913f, 914f
  epidemiology of, 911, 912f
  malignant transformation of, 912,
    912f–914f, 913, 915
  natural history of, 914–915
  pathogenesis of, 911, 912f
  pathology of, 913
  in renal failure, 532
  screening for, 914
  treatment of, 915
Acquired immunodeficiency syndrome
    (AIDS). See Human
    immunodeficiency virus (HIV).
Acquired perforating dermatosis, due to
    chronic kidney disease, 904f

ACR (albumin-creatinine ratio), and
    cardiovascular disease, 816–817
Acromegaly, 449–450
  clinical manifestations of, 449, 450f
  diagnosis of, 450, 450f
  epidemiology of, 449
  hyperphosphatemia due to, 133
  hypertension due to, 389f, 449–450
  treatment of, 450
Actin cytoskeleton, disruption of, and acute
    tubular necrosis, 759
α-Actinin-4
  in focal segmental glomerulosclerosis, 218
  in proteinuria, 187, 187f
Activated charcoal, 1157
  for uremic pruritus, 905f, 906
Activation-induced cell death (AICD),
    1022f, 1023, 1032
Active transport, 17
ACTN4 gene, 187, 339
Acute Candesartan Cilexitil Evaluation in
    Stroke Survivors trial, 462
Acute Dialysis Quality Initiative, 1004
Acute fatty liver of pregnancy, 492
Acute intermittent hemodialysis,
    1001–1003, 1003f, 1004f, 1008
Acute interstitial nephritis (AIN), 681–688
  acute renal failure due to, 755f, 756f, 766
  diagnosis of, 685–686, 686f
  drug-induced, 681–687
    clinical manifestations of, 681–684, 684f
    drugs responsible for, 683f
    natural history of, 686, 686f
    pathology of, 684–685, 685f
    treatment of, 686–687
  epidemiology of, 681
  with HIV infection, 769f
  idiopathic, 688
  due to infectious diseases, 687, 687f
  due to malignancies, 688
  due to nephrotoxic agents, 761f
  pathogenesis of, 681, 682f
  and renal allografts, 688
  due to systemic diseases, 687–688, 688f
Acute kidney injury (AKI). See Acute renal
    failure (ARF).
Acute myocardial infarction (AMI), with
    chronic kidney disease, 846
Acute on chronic kidney failure, 835–836,
    835f
Acute renal failure (ARF), 755, 771
  biopsy for, 69, 69f
  after bone marrow transplantation,
    1151–1153, 1152f
  changing spectrum of, 772–774, 773f
  vs. chronic kidney disease, 774, 835, 835f
  classic, 771
  classification of, 771–772, 771f
  clinical evaluation of, 774–781
    algorithm for, 774, 775f
    history and record review in, 774–775
    imaging in, 779–781, 780f, 781f
    laboratory tests in, 775–779, 776f–779f
    physical examination in, 775, 775f
    renal biopsy in, 781
  drugs to promote recovery from, 784
  in elderly, 750
  epidemiology of, 772–774, 772f–774f